CRITICAL CARE NURSING PROCEDURES—*Continued*

AACN
PROCEDURE MANUAL *for* CRITICAL CARE

Edited by:

Debra Lynn-McHale Wiegand, PhD, RN, CCRN, FAAN

Assistant Professor, University of Maryland School
of Nursing
Baltimore, Maryland;
Staff Nurse, Surgical Cardiac Care Unit, Thomas Jefferson
University Hospital
Philadelphia, Pennsylvania

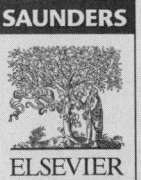

SAUNDERS

ELSEVIER

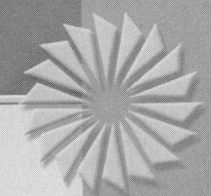

AMERICAN
ASSOCIATION
of CRITICAL-CARE
NURSES

Sixth Edition

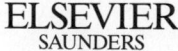

3251 Riverport Lane
St. Louis, Missouri 63043

AACN PROCEDURE MANUAL FOR CRITICAL CARE   ISBN: 978-1-4160-6218-9
Copyright © 2011 by Saunders, an imprint of Elsevier Inc.

Notice

Nursing is an ever-changing field. Standard safety precautions must be followed, but as new research and clinical experience broaden our knowledge, changes in treatment and drug therapy may become necessary or appropriate. Readers are advised to check the most current product information provided by the manufacturer of each drug to be administered to verify the recommended dose, the method, and duration of administration, and contraindications. It is the responsibility of the licensed prescriber, relying on experience and knowledge of the patient, to determine dosages and the best treatment for each individual patient. Neither the publisher nor the author assume any liability for any injury and/or damage to persons or property arising from this publication.

Library of Congress Cataloging-in-Publication Data

AACN procedure manual for critical care / edited by Debra J. Lynn-McHale Wiegand.—6th ed.
    p. ; cm.
  Other title: Procedure manual for critical care
  Rev. ed. of: AACN procedure manual for critical care / edited by Debra
J. Lynn-McHale Wiegand, Karen K. Carlson. 5th ed. c2005.
  Includes bibliographical references and index.
  ISBN 978-1-4160-6218-9 (pbk. : alk. paper)
  1. Intensive care nursing—Handbooks, manuals, etc. I. Wiegand, Debra
J. Lynn-McHale. II. American Association of Critical-Care Nurses.
 III. Title: Procedure manual for critical care.
  [DNLM: 1. Critical Care—methods—Handbooks. 2. Critical
Illness—nursing—Handbooks. WY 49 A111 2011]
  RT120.I5A17 2011
  616.02'8—dc22

                                                              2010020639

Acquisitions Editor: Maureen Iannuzzi
Senior Developmental Editors: Robin Levin Richman and Jennifer Ehlers
Publishing Services Manager: Jeff Patterson
Senior Project Manager: Anne Konopka
Designer: Kim Denando

Printed in the United States of America.

Last digit is the print number: 9 8 7 6 5 4 3 2

This edition of the *AACN Procedure Manual for Critical Care* is dedicated to the memory of my dear friend and colleague, Karen Carlson. Karen and I coedited the fourth and fifth editions of the *AACN Procedure Manual for Critical Care*, and we had every intention of coediting this edition too. However, Karen's cancer progressed, and she lost her battle with cancer in December of 2007. This edition of the *AACN Procedure Manual for Critical Care* is dedicated to Karen.

Section Editors

Michael W. Day, RN, MSN, CCRN
Trauma Care Coordinator, Providence Sacred Heart Medical
  Center and Children's Hospital
Spokane, Washington

Eleanor Fitzpatrick, MSN, RN, CCRN
Clinical Nurse Specialist, Surgical Intensive Care Unit and
  Intermediate Surgical Intensive Care Unit, Thomas Jefferson
  University Hospital
Philadelphia, Pennsylvania

Mary Beth Flynn Makic, RN, PhD, CNS, CCNS
Research Nurse Scientist, University of Colorado Hospital;
  Assistant Professor, Adjoint, University of Colorado, Denver,
  College of Nursing,
Aurora, Colorado

Teresa Preuss, MSN, RN, CCRN
Clinical Charge Nurse, Medical Coronary Care Unit, Thomas
  Jefferson University Hospital
Philadelphia, Pennsylvania

Debra Lynn-McHale Wiegand, PhD, RN, CCRN, FAAN
Assistant Professor, University of Maryland School of Nursing
  Baltimore, Maryland;
Staff Nurse, Surgical Cardiac Care Unit, Thomas Jefferson
  University Hospital
Philadelphia, Pennsylvania

Contributors

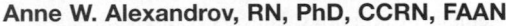

Anne W. Alexandrov, RN, PhD, CCRN, FAAN
Professor of Clinical Nursing, and NET SMART Program
  Director, University of Alabama
Birmingham, Alabama
Procedure 93: *Transcranial Doppler Monitoring*

Tracey Anderson, RN, MSN, FNP-BC
Nurse Practitioner, Neurology Intensive-Care Unit, University of
  Colorado
Aurora, Colorado
Procedure 124: *Wound Closure*
Procedure 125: *Suture and Staple Removal*

**Richard B. Arbour, MSN, RN, CCRN, CNRN, CCNS,
  FAAN**
Critical Care Clinical Nurse Specialist, Albert Einstein Healthcare
  Network
Philadelphia, Pennsylvania
Procedure 86: *Bispectral Index Monitoring*

Sonia M. Astle, RN, MS, CCRN, CCNS
Clinical Nurse Specialist, Critical Care, Inova Fairfax Hospital
Falls Church, Virginia
Procedure 112: *Continuous Renal Replacement Therapies*
Procedure 113: *Hemodialysis*
Procedure 114: *Peritoneal Dialysis*
Procedure 116: *Apheresis and Therapeutic Plasma Exchange
  (Assist)*

Robin M. Beard, RN, MS, CRNI, PCCN
Vascular Access Nurse, Kootenai Medical Center
Coeur d'Alene, Idaho
Procedure 19: *Autotransfusion*

Deborah E. Becker, RN, PhD, CRNP, APRN, BC
Assistant Professor of Nursing, Director, Acute Care Nurse
  Practitioner & Adult Health Clinical Nurse Specialist Programs,
  Biobehavioral & Health Sciences Division, School of Nursing,
  University of Pennsylvania
Philadelphia, Pennsylvania
Procedure 45: *Pericardiocentesis (Perform)*
Procedure 46: *Pericardiocentesis (Assist)*
Procedure 53: *Temporary Transvenous Pacemaker Insertion
  (Perform)*
Procedure 61: *Arterial Catheter Insertion (Perform)*

Stephanie A. Bloom, ACNP-BC
Nurse Practitioner, NeuroCritical Care, Hospital of the
  University of Pennsylvania
Philadelphia, Pennsylvania
Procedure 87: *Brain Tissue Oxygen Monitoring: Insertion
  (Assist), Care, and Troubleshooting*

Jenny Bosley, RN, MS, CEN
Clinical Nurse Specialist, Emergency Department, Thomas
  Jefferson University Hospital
Philadelphia, Pennsylvania
Procedure 109: *Peritoneal Lavage (Perform)*
Procedure 110: *Peritoneal Lavage (Assist)*

Joel M. Brown II, BS, RRT
Respiratory Staff Development Specialist, Department of Respiratory
  Care, Christiana Care Health System
Newark, Delaware
Procedure 80: *Arterial Puncture*

Linda Bucher, RN, PhD
Professor, School of Nursing, University of Delaware and
  Nursing Research Facilitator, Christiana Care Health System;
  and Per Diem Staff Nurse, Emergency Department, Virtua
  Memorial Hospital
Newark, Delaware; and Mount Holly, New Jersey
Procedure 80: *Arterial Puncture*
Procedure 85: *Peripherally Inserted Central Catheter*

Kathy Bunzli, RN, MS, CCRN-CMC
Clinical Nurse Educator, Medical Intensive Care Unit, University
  of Colorado Hospital
Aurora, Colorado
Procedure 104: *Esophagogastric Tamponade Tube*

Shelley Burcat, MSN, RN, AOCNS
Clinical Nurse Specialist, Blood and Marrow Transplant Unit,
  Thomas Jefferson University Hospital
Philadelphia, Pennsylvania
Procedure 139: *Calculating Doses and Flow Rates and
  Administering Continuous Intravenous Infusions*

Suzanne M. Burns, MSN, RN, RRT, ACNP, CCRN, FAAN
Director PNSO Clinical Research Program, School of Nursing,
  University of Virginia
Charlottesville, Virginia
Procedure 28: *Noninvasive Positive Pressure Ventilation:
  Continuous Positive Airway Pressure (CPAP) and Bilevel
  Positive Airway Pressure (BiPAP)*
Procedure 29: *Arterial-Venous Oxygen Content Difference and
  Oxygen Transport (Delivery) and Consumption Calculations*
Procedure 30: *Auto–Positive End-Expiratory Pressure (Auto-PEEP)
  Calculation*
Procedure 31: *Compliance and Resistance Measurement*
Procedure 32: *Manual Self-Inflating Resuscitation Bag-Valve Device*
Procedure 33: *Indices of Oxygenation*
Procedure 34: *Shunt Calculation*
Procedure 35: *Invasive Mechanical Ventilation (Through an
  Artificial Airway): Volume and Pressure Modes*

Procedure 36: *Standard Weaning Criteria: Negative Inspiratory Force or Pressure, Positive Expiratory Pressure, Spontaneous Tidal Volume, Vital Capacity, and Rapid Shallow Breathing Index*
Procedure 37: *Weaning Process*

Margaret L. Campbell, PhD, RN, FAAN
Director, Nursing Research, Detroit Receiving Hospital
Detroit, Michigan
Procedure 135: *Determination of Death in Adult Patients*
Procedure 137: *Donation After Cardiac Death*

Mary G. Carey, PhD, RN
Assistant Professor, University of Buffalo
Buffalo, New York
Procedure 59: *Continuous ST-Segment Monitoring*

Deborah Castellucci, RN, MPA, CCRN
Medical & Surgical Cardiac Intensive Care, Thomas Jefferson University Hospital
Philadelphia, Pennsylvania
Procedure 55: *Intraaortic Balloon Pump Management*

Susan Chioffi, RN, MSN, CCRN, ACNP-BC
Nurse Practitioner, Neuroscience ICU, Duke University Medical Center
Durham, North Carolina
Procedure 95: *Lumbar Puncture (Perform)*
Procedure 96: *Lumbar Puncture (Assist)*

Marianne Chulay, RN, PhD, FAAN
Consultant, Clinical Research and Critical Care Nursing
Gainesville, Florida
Procedure 12: *Suctioning: Endotracheal or Tracheostomy Tube*

Christine A. Cottingham, RN, MS, CCRN
Assistant Director, Clinical Education Department; Trauma Clinical Nurse Specialist, Harborview Medical Center
Seattle, Washington
Procedure 122: *Intracompartmental Pressure Monitoring*

Bonnie L. Curtis, RN, CCRN
Core Charge Nurse, Intensive Care Unit, St Cloud Hospital
St Cloud, Minnesota
Procedure 5: *Extubation/Decannulation (Perform)*
Procedure 6: *Extubation/Decannulation (Assist)*
Procedure 10: *Nasopharyngeal Airway Insertion*
Procedure 11: *Oropharyngeal Airway Insertion*
Procedure 13: *Tracheal Tube Cuff Care*
Procedure 14: *Tracheostomy Tube Care*

Janice Y. Dawson, BSN, RN
Staff Nurse, Department of Cardiology, Lankenau Hospital, Jefferson Health System
Wynnewood, Pennsylvania
Procedure 79: *Transesophageal Echocardiography (Assist)*

Jeffrey Dawson, RN, CCRN, EMP-P
Flight Nurse, Northwest Medstar
Spokane, Washington
Procedure 1: *Combitube Insertion and Removal*
Procedure 7: *Laryngeal Mask Airway*

Michael W. Day, RN, MSN, CCRN
Trauma Care Coordinator, Providence Sacred Heart Medical Center and Children's Hospital
Spokane, Washington
Procedure 84: *Intraosseous Devices*

Barbara J. Drew, PhD, RN, FAAN
Lillian & Dudley Aldous Professor of Nursing Science, Clinical Professor of Medicine, Cardiology, University of California
San Francisco, California
Procedure 58: *Extra Electrocardiographic Leads: Right Precordial and Left Posterior Leads*

Margaret M. Ecklund, MS, RN, CCRN, ACNP-BC
Clinician VI/Nurse Practitioner, Pulmonary Medicine, Rochester General Hospital
Rochester, New York
Procedure 133: *Percutaneous Endoscopic Gastrostomy (PEG), Gastrostomy, and Jejunostomy Tube Care*
Procedure 134: *Small-Bore Feeding Tube Insertion and Care*

Eileen C. Finnegan, RN, MS, CRNP, APRN-BC, CCRN
Nurse Practitioner, Hematopoietic Transplant Unit, Thomas Jefferson University Hospital
Philadelphia, Pennsylvania
Procedure 117: *Bone Marrow Biopsy and Aspiration (Perform)*
Procedure 118: *Bone Marrow Biopsy and Aspiration (Assist)*

Eleanor Fitzpatrick, MSN, RN, CCRN
Clinical Nurse Specialist, Surgical Intensive Care Unit and Intermediate Surgical Intensive Care Unit, Thomas Jefferson University Hospital
Philadelphia, Pennsylvania
Procedure 107: *Paracentesis (Perform)*
Procedure 108: *Paracentesis (Assist)*
Procedure 111: *Endoscopic Therapy*

Desiree A. Fleck, RN, MSN, CRNP
Nurse Practitioner, Philadelphia Adult Congenital Heart Center, Children's Hospital of Philadelphia and The Hospital of the University of Pennsylvania, University of Pennsylvania
Philadelphia, Pennsylvania
Procedure 56: *Ventricular Assist Devices*
Procedure 72: *Pulmonary Artery Catheter Insertion (Perform)*
Procedure 81: *Central Venous Catheter Insertion (Perform)*
Procedure 82: *Central Venous Catheter Insertion (Assist)*

Janet G. Whetstone Foster, PhD, APRN, CNS
Adult Associate Professor, Texas Woman's University College of Nursing
Houston, Texas
Procedure 38: *Peripheral Nerve Stimulators*

John J. Gallagher, MSN, RN, CCNS, CCRN, RRT
Clinical Nurse Specialist, Hospital of the University of Pennsylvania
Philadelphia, Pennsylvania
Procedure 106: *Intraabdominal Pressure Monitoring*

Karen A. Gilbert, MSN, RN, CRNP, CNSC
Nutrition Support Clinical Specialist, Thomas Jefferson University Hospital
Philadelphia, Pennsylvania

Procedure 132: *Small-Bore Feeding Tube Insertion Using an Electromagnetic Guidance System (CORTRAK®)*

Paula Gipp, RN, BSN, CWOCN
Clinical Registered Nurse, Specialty Areas, University of Colorado Hospital
Aurora, Colorado
Procedure 131: *Negative-Pressure Wound Therapy*

Karen K. Giuliano, RN, PhD, FAAN
Principal Scientist, Philips Healthcare
Andover, Massachusetts
Procedure 16: *Continuous Venous Oxygen Saturation Monitoring*

Vicki S. Good, MSN, RN, CCNS, CENP
Director of Nursing Practice Integration, Nursing Administration, Cox Health Care System
Springfield, Missouri
Procedure 15: *Continuous End-Tidal Carbon Dioxide Monitoring*

Cynthia A. Goodrich, RN, MS, CCRN
Flight Nurse, Airlift Northwest
Seattle, Washington
Procedure 2: *Endotracheal Intubation (Perform)*
Procedure 3: *Endotracheal Intubation (Assist)*
Procedure 25: *Needle Thoracostomy (Perform)*

Charlotte A. Green, RN, MN
Director of Clinical Programs, Carlson Consulting Group
Bellevue, Washington
Procedure 39: *Automated External Defibrillation*

Patricia L. Hahn, RN, MN, ARNP
Internal Medicine Hospitalist, Providence Sacred Heart Medical Center
Spokane, Washington
Procedure 8: *Surgical Cricothyrotomy (Perform)*
Procedure 9: *Surgical Cricothyrotomy (Assist)*

Cynthia Hambach, MSN, RN, CCRN
Adjunct Clinical Faculty, Drexel University College of Nursing and Health Professions; Staff Nurse, Cardiovascular Intensive Care Unit, Doylestown Hospital
Philadelphia, Pennsylvania; and Doylestown, Pennsylvania
Procedure 40: *Cardioversion*
Procedure 41: *Defibrillation (External)*

Mary Hanson, MN, RN-BC
Spine Clinical Nurse Educator, Harborview Medical Center
Seattle, Washington
Procedure 97: *Cervical Tongs or Halo Ring: Application for Use in Cervical Traction (Assist)*
Procedure 98: *Halo Ring and Vest Care*
Procedure 99: *Pin Site Care: Cervical Tongs and Halo Pins*
Procedure 100: *Cervical Traction Maintenance*

Jan M. Headley, RN, BS
Director, Strategic Alliances & Professional Education, Edwards Lifesciences
Irvine, California
Procedure 16: *Continuous Venous Oxygen Saturation Monitoring*

Julie Lynn Henderson, RN, MSN, ANP, FNP-C
Nurse Practitioner, University of Colorado Hospital
Aurora, Colorado
Procedure 127: *Débridement: Pressure Ulcers, Burns, and Wounds*

Linda M. Hoke, PhD, RN, CCNS, ACNS-BC, CCRN
Clinical Nurse Specialist, Cardiac Intermediate Care Unit, Hospital of the University of Pennsylvania
Philadelphia, Pennsylvania
Procedure 79: *Transesophageal Echocardiography (Assist)*

Shannon Johnson, RN, MS, CCNS
Clinical Nurse Specialist, University of Colorado Hospital
Aurora, Colorado
Procedure 123: *Pressure Redistribution Surfaces: Continual Lateral Rotation Therapy and RotoRest™ Lateral Rotation Surface*

Sharon R. Josephson-Keeven, RN, MS, APRN, BC
Department of Cardiology, Kaiser Permanente Mid-Atlantic States
Fairfax, Virginia
Procedure 50: *Implantable Cardioverter-Defibrillator*

Maribeth Kelly, MSN, RN, PCCN
Clinical Nurse Specialist, Medical Telemetry, Thomas Jefferson University Hospital
Philadelphia, Pennsylvania
Procedure 139: *Calculating Doses and Flow Rates and Administering Continuous Intravenous Infusions*

Mary Ellen Kern, RN, MSN, CCRN, APN-BC
Clinical Nurse Specialist, Critical Care Units and the Emergency Department, Methodist Division, Thomas Jefferson University Hospital
Philadelphia, Pennsylvania
Procedure 63: *Arterial Pressure-Based Cardiac Output Monitoring*
Procedure 78: *Pericardial Catheter Management*

Peggy Kirkwood, RN, MSN, ACNPC
Cardiovascular Nurse Practitioner, Mission Hospital
Mission Viejo, California
Procedure 22: *Chest Tube Removal (Perform)*
Procedure 23: *Chest Tube Removal (Assist)*

Deborah G. Klein, MSN, RN, CCRN, CS
Clinical Nurse Specialist, Cleveland Clinic Foundation
Cleveland, Ohio
Procedure 67: *Cardiac Output Measurement Techniques (Invasive)*

Nicole L. Kupchik, RN, MN, CCRN-CMC
Clinical Nurse Specialist, Harborview Medical Center
Seattle, Washington
Procedure 94: *External and Intravascular Warming/Cooling Devices*

Sarah-Jane Lawless, RN, BSN
Duke University School of Nursing, Nurse Anesthesia
Durham, North Carolina;
Procedure 101: *Epidural Catheters: Assisting with Insertion and Pain Management*
Procedure 103: *Peripheral Nerve Blocks: Assisting with Insertion and Pain Management*

Barbara Leeper, MN, RN, CNS M-S, CCRN
Clinical Nurse Specialist, Cardiovascular Services, Baylor University Medical Center
Dallas, Texas
Procedure 71: *Left Atrial Catheter: Care and Assisting with Removal*

Paul Luehrs, RRT, BSRT, BSE
Supervisor, Adult Critical Care, CoxHealth
Springfield, Missouri
Procedure 15: *Continuous End-Tidal Carbon Dioxide Monitoring*

Paula A. Lusardi, PhD, RN, CCRN, CCNS
Critical Care Clinical Nurse Specialist, Baystate Medical Center
Springfield, Massachusetts
Procedure 20: *Chest Tube Placement (Perform)*
Procedure 21: *Chest Tube Placement (Assist)*

Mary Beth Flynn Makic, RN, PhD, CNS, CCNS
Research Nurse Scientist, University of Colorado Hospital;
Assistant Professor, Adjoint, University of Colorado, Denver, College of Nursing
Aurora, Colorado
Procedure 91: *Lumbar Subarachnoid Catheter Insertion (Assist) for Cerebrospinal Fluid Drainage and Pressure Monitoring*
Procedure 128: *Wound Management with Excessive Drainage*
Procedure 129: *Drain Removal*
Procedure 130: *Fecal Containment Devices and Bowel Management System*

Margaret M. Mahon, PhD, CRNP, FAAN
Associate Professor, College of Health and Human Services, George Mason University
Fairfax, Virginia
Procedure 138: *Withholding and Withdrawing Life-Sustaining Therapy*

Eileen Maloney-Wilensky, MSN, RN, CRNP
Director, Clinical Research Division & Clinical Staff Practitioners, Department of Neurosurgery, Hospital of the University of Pennsylvania
Philadelphia, Pennsylvania
Procedure 87: *Brain Tissue Oxygen Monitoring: Insertion (Assist), Care, and Troubleshooting*

Maj. Elizabeth A. Mann, RN, MS, CCRN, CCNS, CNS, AN
US Army Institute of Surgical Research, Army Burn Center
San Antonio, Texas
Procedure 119: *Donor Site Care*
Procedure 120: *Burn Wound Care*

Mary G. McKinley, RN, MSN, CCRN
Critical Connections, Healthcare Consulting Partner
Wheeling, West Virginia

Procedure 57: *Electrocardiographic Leads and Cardiac Monitoring*
Procedure 60: *Twelve-Lead Electrocardiogram*

Lorie Ann Meek, MSN, RN
Alumnus CCRN, Clinical Nurse Educator, Clinical Education and Professional Development, Duke University Health System
Durham, North Carolina
Procedure 102: *Patient-Controlled Analgesia*

Anne C. Muller, RN, MSN, BC-CNS
Clinical Nurse Specialist, Hospital of the University of Pennsylvania
Philadelphia, Pennsylvania
Procedure 83: *Implantable Venous Access Device: Access, Deaccess, and Care*

Carol A. Offutt, RN, MSN, CRNP
Kaiser Permanente, Mid-Atlantic States
Silver Spring, Maryland
Procedure 50: *Implantable Cardioverter-Defibrillator*
Procedure 51: *Permanent Pacemaker (Assessing Function)*

Michele M. Pelter, RN, PhD
Assistant Professor, Orvis School of Nursing, University of Nevada
Reno, Nevada
Procedure 59: *Continuous ST-Segment Monitoring*

Joya D. Pickett, MSN, CCNS, ACNS-BC
Clinical Instructor, University of Washington, Biobehavioral Nursing and Health Sciences and Critical Care Clinical Nurse Specialist, Swedish Medical Center
Seattle, Washington
Procedure 24: *Closed Chest Drainage System*

Jan Powers, PhD, RN, CCRN, CCNS, CNRN, FCCM
Director, Clinical Nurse Specialists and Nursing Research, Critical Care Clinical Nurse Specialist, St Vincent Hospital
Indianapolis, Indiana
Procedure 18: *Pronation Therapy*

D. Nathan Preuss, MA, RN, CCRN
Clinical Charge Nurse, Neurovascular Intensive Care Unit, Thomas Jefferson University Hospital
Philadelphia, Pennsylvania
Procedure 92: *Intraventricular Catheter with External Transducer for Cerebrospinal Fluid Drainage and Intracranial Pressure Monitoring*
Procedure 115: *Use of a Massive Transfusion Device and a Pressure Infusor Bag*
Procedure 136: *Organ Donation: Identification of Potential Organ Donors, Request for Organ Donation, and Care of the Organ Donor*

Teresa Preuss, MSN, RN, CCRN
Clinical Charge Nurse, Medical Coronary Care Unit, Thomas Jefferson University Hospital
Philadelphia, Pennsylvania
Procedure 47: *Atrial Electrogram*
Procedure 65: *Blood Sampling from a Central Venous Catheter*
Procedure 66: *Blood Sampling from a Pulmonary Artery Catheter*
Procedure 68: *Central Venous Catheter Removal*

Procedure 69: *Central Venous Catheter Site Care*
Procedure 70: *Central Venous/Right Atrial Pressure Monitoring*
Procedure 73: *Pulmonary Artery Catheter Insertion (Assist) and Pressure Monitoring*
Procedure 74: *Pulmonary Artery Catheter Removal*
Procedure 75: *Pulmonary Artery Catheter and Pressure Lines, Troubleshooting*
Procedure 76: *Single-Pressure and Multiple-Pressure Transducer Systems*

Mark Puhlman, RN, MSN, ARNP
Mechanical Heart/Research Coordinator, Inland Northwest Thoracic Transplant Program, Sacred Heart Medical Center
Spokane, Washington
Procedure 56: *Ventricular Assist Devices*

Marylou V. Robinson, RN, PhD, FNP, CCRN
Assistant Professor, University of Colorado, Denver, College of Nursing
Aurora, Colorado
Procedure 126: *Cleaning, Irrigating, Culturing, and Dressing an Open Wound*

Linda V. Sanderson, RN, MSN, CRNI
Injury Prevention Educator, Christiana Care Health Services
Newark, Delaware
Procedure 85: *Peripherally Inserted Central Catheter*

Linda Schakenbach, MSN, RN, CNS, CCRN, CWCN, ACNS-BC
Clinical Nurse Specialist, Inova Fairfax Hospital/Inova Heart and Vascular Institute
Falls Church, Virginia
Procedure 42: *Defibrillation (Internal)*
Procedure 43: *Emergent Open Sternotomy (Perform)*
Procedure 44: *Emergent Open Sternotomy (Assist)*
Procedure 48: *Atrial Overdrive Pacing (Perform)*
Procedure 49: *Epicardial Pacing Wire Removal*

Sandra L. Schutz, RN, MSN
Clinical Nurse Specialist, Cardiology, Overlake Hospital and Medical Center
Bellevue, Washington
Procedure 17: *Oxygen Saturation Monitoring with Pulse Oximetry*

Finn Scott, RN, MSN, CEN
Clinical Nurse Specialist, Emergency Department, Baystate Medical Center
Springfield, Massachusetts
Procedure 20: *Chest Tube Placement (Perform)*
Procedure 21: *Chest Tube Placement (Assist)*

Robin Scott, RN, MS, CNS, CEN
Clinical Nurse Specialist/Educator, University of Colorado Hospital
Aurora, Colorado
Procedure 84: *Intraosseous Devices*

Susan S. Scott, MSN, RN, CCRN
ICU Educator, Baystate Medical Center
Springfield, Massachusetts
Procedure 20: *Chest Tube Placement (Perform)*
Procedure 21: *Chest Tube Placement (Assist)*

Dawn Lequatte Sculco, RN, MS, CCRN
Clinical Nurse Specialist, St Anthony Summit Medical Center
Frisco, Colorado
Procedure 121: *Skin Graft Care*

Maureen A. Seckel, APN, ACNS, BC, CCNS, CCRN
Clinical Nurse Specialist, Medical Pulmonary Critical Care, Christiana Care Health Services
Newark, Delaware
Procedure 12: *Suctioning: Endotracheal or Tracheostomy Tube*

Rose B. Shaffer, RN, MSN, ACNP-BC, CCRN, FAHA
Cardiology Nurse Practitioner, Thomas Jefferson University Hospital
Philadelphia, Pennsylvania
Procedure 62: *Arterial Catheter Insertion (Assist), Care, and Removal*
Procedure 64: *Blood Sampling from an Arterial Catheter*
Procedure 77: *Arterial and Venous Sheath Removal*

Kirsten N. Skillings, RN, MA, CCNS, CCRN
ICU Clinical Nurse Specialist
St Cloud Hospital
St Cloud, Minnesota
Procedure 5: *Extubation/Decannulation (Perform)*
Procedure 6: *Extubation/Decannulation (Assist)*
Procedure 10: *Nasopharyngeal Airway Insertion*
Procedure 11: *Oropharyngeal Airway Insertion*
Procedure 13: *Tracheal Tube Cuff Care*
Procedure 14: *Tracheostomy Tube Care*

Tess Slazinski, RN, MN, APRN, CCRN, CNRN
ICU Clinical Nurse Specialist, Neurological ICU/Med-Surg, Cedars-Sinai Medical Center
Los Angeles, California
Procedure 88: *Intracranial Bolt and Fiberoptic Catheter Insertion (Assist), Intracranial Pressure Monitoring, Care, Troubleshooting, and Removal*
Procedure 89: *Combination Intraventricular/Fiberoptic Catheter Insertion (Assist), Monitoring, Nursing Care, Troubleshooting, and Removal*
Procedure 90: *Jugular Venous Oxygen Saturation Monitoring: Insertion (Assist), Patient Care, Troubleshooting, and Removal*

Mary Lou Sole, PhD, RN, FAAN
Professor, School of Nursing, University of Central Florida
Orlando, Florida
Procedure 4: *Endotracheal Tube and Oral Care*

Valerie Spotts, BSN, RN
University of Michigan Hospitals and Health System
Ann Arbor, Michigan
Procedure 52: *Temporary Transcutaneous (External) Pacing*
Procedure 54: *Temporary Transvenous and Epicardial Pacing*

Michael F. Stiefel, MD, PhD
Associate Director, Neurocritical Care Director, Comprehensive Cerebrovascular and Endovascular Neurosurgery Program, Penn Comprehensive Neuroscience Center; Assistant Professor of Neurosurgery, Hospital of the University of Pennsylvania
Philadelphia, Pennsylvania
Procedure 87: *Brain Tissue Oxygen Monitoring: Insertion (Assist), Care, and Troubleshooting*

Kathleen M. Vollman, MSN, RN, CCNS, FCCM, FAAN
Clinical Nurse Specialist, Educator, Consultant, Advancing
  Nursing LLC
Northville, Michigan
Procedure 4: *Endotracheal Tube and Oral Care*
Procedure 18: *Pronation Therapy*

Debra Lynn-McHale Wiegand, PhD, RN, CCRN, FAAN
Assistant Professor, University of Maryland School of Nursing
Baltimore, Maryland;
Staff Nurse, Surgical Cardiac Care Unit, Thomas Jefferson
  University Hospital
Philadelphia, Pennsylvania
Procedure 47: Atrial Electrogram
Procedure 65: *Blood Sampling from a Central Venous Catheter*
Procedure 66: *Blood Sampling from a Pulmonary Artery Catheter*
Procedure 68: *Central Venous Catheter Removal*
Procedure 69: *Central Venous Catheter Site Care*
Procedure 70: *Central Venous/Right Atrial Pressure Monitoring*
Procedure 73: *Pulmonary Artery Catheter Insertion (Assist) and
  Pressure Monitoring*
Procedure 74: *Pulmonary Artery Catheter Removal*
Procedure 75: *Pulmonary Artery Catheter and Pressure Lines,
  Troubleshooting*
Procedure 76: *Single-Pressure and Multiple-Pressure
  Transducer Systems*
Procedure 91: *Lumbar Subarachnoid Catheter Insertion (Assist)
  for Cerebrospinal Fluid Drainage and Pressure Monitoring*
Procedure 138: *Withholding and Withdrawing Life-Sustaining
  Therapy*

Ann G. Will, MS, RN, CNS
ICU Clinical Nurse Specialist, Poudre Valley Hospital
Fort Collins, Colorado
Procedure 105: *Gastric Lavage in Hemorrhage and Overdose*

Patricia H. Worthington, MSN, RN, CNSC
Nutrition Support Clinical Specialist, Thomas Jefferson
  University Hospital
Philadelphia, Pennsylvania
Procedure 132: *Small-Bore Feeding Tube Insertion Using an
  Electromagnetic Guidance System (CORTRAK®)*

Shu-Fen Wung, PhD, MS, ACNP-BC, FAHA, FAAN
Associate Professor, College of Nursing, The University of
  Arizona
Tucson, Arizona
Procedure 58: *Extra Electrocardiographic Leads: Right
  Precordial and Left Posterior Leads*

Susan Yeager, MS, RN, CCRN, ACNP
The Ohio State University Medical Center
Columbus, Ohio
Procedure 26: *Thoracentesis (Perform)*
Procedure 27: *Thoracentesis (Assist)*

Reviewers

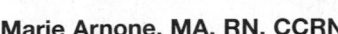

Marie Arnone, MA, RN, CCRN
Professional Development Specialist,
Cardiac Services, Swedish Medical Center
Seattle, Washington

Mary Pat Aust, MS, RN
Clinical Practice Specialist, American
Association of Critical-Care Nurses
Aliso Viejo, California

Mary Kay Bader, RN, MSN, CCNS, CCRN, CNRN, FAHA
Neuro/Critical Care CNS, Mission Hospital
Mission Viejo, California

Linda Bell, RN, MSN
Clinical Practice Specialist, American
Association of Critical-Care Nurses
Aliso Viejo, California

Maj. Kimberlie A. Biever, RN, MS, ACNP-BC, ANP-BC, CCNS, CCRN
Critical Care Clinical Nurse Specialist,
Walter Reed Army Medical Center
Washington, DC

Shelley Burcat, MSN, RN, AOCNS
Clinical Nurse Specialist, Blood and
Marrow Transplant Unit, Thomas
Jefferson University Hospital
Philadelphia, Pennsylvania

Kimberly R. Bush, RN, MSN
Nurse Educator, Intermediate Surgical
Intensive Care Unit, Thomas Jefferson
University Hospital; Adjunct Clinical
Assistant Professor, Villanova University
Philadelphia, Pennsylvania; and Villanova,
Pennsylvania

Cathleen Carlen-Lindauer, RN, MSN, CEN
Clinical Nurse Specialist, Department of
Emergency Medicine, The Johns Hopkins
Hospital
Baltimore, Maryland

Amy P. Callahan, RN, MSN, CNE, APRN-BC
Clinical Nurse Specialist, Nurse Practitioner,
Medical Intensive and Intermediate Care
Units, Thomas Jefferson University Hospital
Philadelphia, Pennsylvania

Barbara Chesnutt, RN, MSN, ACNP-BC
Critical Care Nurse Practitioner, Colorado
Pulmonary Intensivists, Inc., Littleton
Adventists Hospital
Littleton, Colorado

Barbara Cilento, RN, MEd, MSN
Critical Care Clinical Nurse Specialist,
National Naval Medical Center
Bethesda, Maryland

Doyle M. Coons, BSN, RN
Unit Coordinator, Medical ICU, University
of Kansas Hospital
Kansas City, Kansas

Damon B. Cottrell, MS, RN, CCNS, CCRN, ACNS-BC, CEN
Clinical Nurse Specialist, Washington
Hospital Center
Washington, DC

Sarah E. Courneya, RN, BSN, CCRN
Staff Nurse, 2N CICU, Providence Sacred
Heart Medical Center
Spokane, Washington

Kathleen M. Cox, MS, APRN, ACNP, CCNS
Critical Care Nurse Practitioner, Department
of Surgery, William Beaumont Army
Medical Center
El Paso, Texas

Joni Hentzen Daniels, MSN, RN, CEN
Clinical Nurse Specialist, Emergency
Care Regional Director, Clinical Services,
EmCare, Inc.
San Antonio, Texas

Susan Davis, MSN
Nurse Practitioner Cardiac Surgery, Sinai
Hospital
Baltimore, Maryland

Laura Dechant, RN, MSN, CCRN, CCNS, BC
Critical Care Staff Development Specialist,
Christiana Care Health System
Newark, Delaware

Bridget DeLeo, RN-BC, BSN
Staff Development Nurse, Transplant and
Urology Surgery 7N/NE, Thomas Jefferson
University Hospital
Philadelphia, Pennsylvania

Gail Delfin, MSN, RN, CCRN
Clinical Nurse Specialist, Cardiac Care Unit,
Hospital of the University of Pennsylvania
Philadelphia, Pennsylvania

Christina Marie Dennis, MSN, RN, CCRN, CNRN, APRN
Clinical Nurse Specialist, Neurosciences,
WakeMed Health & Hospitals
Raleigh, North Carolina

Karlene A. Dewar, RN, BSN
Facility Administrator, DaVita Dialysis
Services, Thomas Jefferson University
Hospital
Philadelphia, Pennsylvania

Joni L. Dirks, RN, MS, CCRN
Critical Care Educator, Providence Sacred
Heart Medical Center
Spokane, Washington

Phyllis Dubendorf, RN, MSN, CNRN
Clinical Nurse Specialist, University of
Pennsylvania Medical Center; Lecturer,
Clinical Nurse Specialist, University of
Pennsylvania School of Nursing
Philadelphia, Pennsylvania

Lisa Erickson, MSN, RN, ACNP-BC
Trauma Nurse Practitioner, Christiana Care
Health System
Newark, Delaware

RoseMarie Faber, MSN/ED, RN, CCRN
Clinical Practice Specialist, American
Association of Critical-Care Nurses
Aliso Viejo, California

Anna Gawlinski, RN, DNSc, FAAN
Adjunct Professor, School of Nursing/
UCLA School of Nursing, Ronald Reagan
UCLA Medical Center
Los Angeles, California

Lori E. Geisler, RN, MSN, CCRN
Clinical Nurse Specialist, Shore Health
System, University of Maryland Medical
System
Baltimore, Maryland

Paula Gipp, RN, BSN, CWOCN
Clinical Registered Nurse, Specialty Areas,
    University of Colorado Hospital
Aurora, Colorado

Vicki S. Good, MSN, RN, CCNS, CENP
Director of Nursing Practice Integration,
    Nursing Administration, Cox Health Care
    System
Springfield, Missouri

Carla P. Grant, RN, BSN
Supervisor, Clinical Education, Kootenai
    Medical Center
Coeur d'Alene, Idaho

Linda Hale, RN, CNSC
Nurse Clinician, Nutrition Support Service,
    William Beaumont Hospital
Royal Oak, Michigan

Nancy C. Edger Hall, RN, BSN, MBA
Supervisor, Blood Donor Center, Blood
    Bank, Thomas Jefferson University
    Hospital
Philadelphia, Pennsylvania

**Jillian Hamel, ACNP-BC, MS, CCNS,
CCRN**
Nurse Practitioner, Division of Cardiology,
    University of Maryland Medical Center
Baltimore, Maryland

Deborah S. Harper, MS, RN
Advanced Practice Nurse, Cardiovascular
    Critical Care, Heart Center, Sinai Hospital
    of Baltimore
Baltimore, Maryland

John P. Harper, MSN, RN-BC
Per Diem, Nursing, Crozer-Chester Medical
    Center
Upland, Pennsylvania

Jane H. Hawks, RN, DNP, CS, CPAN
Clinical Nurse Specialist, Harborview
    Medical Center
Seattle, Washington

Jan M. Headley, RN, BS
Director, Strategic Alliances & Professional
    Education, Edwards Lifesciences
Irvine, California

Elizabeth Helvig, MS, RN, CWOCN
Clinical Nurse Specialist, Rochester
    General Hospital
Rochester, New York

**Kiersten Henry, MS, ACNP-BC,
CCNC, CCRN-CMC**
Cardiac and Vascular Nurse Practitioner,
    Montgomery General Hospital
Olney, Maryland

Susan Hodges, CRNP
Hematology/BMT Nurse Practitioner,
    Greenebaum Cancer Center, University of
    Maryland Hospital
Baltimore, Maryland

**Linda M. Hoke, PhD, RN, CCNS,
ACNS-BC, CCRN**
Clinical Nurse Specialist, Cardiac
    Intermediate Care Unit, Hospital of the
    University of Pennsylvania
Philadelphia, Pennsylvania

**Reneé S. Holleran, RN, PhD, CEN,
CCRN, CFRN, CTRN, FAEN**
Staff Nurse, Emergency Department,
    Intermountain Medical Center
Salt Lake City, Utah

**Jennifer M. Joiner, MSN, RN,
CCRN-CSC**
Clinical Nurse Educator, Cardiac Surgery,
    Robert Wood Johnson University Hospital
New Brunswick, New Jersey

**Victoria A. Kark, RN, MSN, CCRN,
CCNS, CSC**
Open Heart Clinical Specialist, The NIH
    Heart Center at Suburban Hospital
Bethesda, Maryland

**Kate Kennedy, RN, MN, CNRN,
ARNP**
Neurology Nurse Practitioner, Swedish
    Neuroscience Institute
Seattle, Washington

Tamarah Kent, RN, BSN
Senior RN, Blood Donor Center, Thomas
    Jefferson University Hospital
Philadelphia, Pennsylvania

**Michael J. Kingan, RN, MSN,
CWOCN**
Clinical Specialist, Washington Hospital
    Center
Washington, DC

Peggy Kirkwood, RN, MSN, ACNPC
Cardiovascular Nurse Practitioner, Mission
    Hospital
Mission Viejo, California

Elizabeth Kozub, RN, MS, CNRN
Nurse Clinician, Neurology Critical Care
    Unit, Johns Hopkins Hospital
Baltimore, Maryland

Tracy Krimmel, AOCN, APRN-BC
Advanced Practice Nurse, Hematology/
    Oncology/BMT, The Cancer Institute of
    New Jersey
New Brunswick, New Jersey

**Sarah A. Layman, BS, BSN, MSN,
ARNP, PNP**
Teaching Associate, Department of
    Neurological Surgery, University of
    Washington School of Medicine;
    Senior Clinical Expert, Harborview
    Medical Center
Seattle, Washington

**Rosemary Koehl Lee, RN-CNS, MSN,
ACNP-BC, CCRN, CCNS**
Clinical Nurse Specialist, Critical and
    Progressive Care Units, Homestead
    Hospital
Homestead, Florida

**Barbara Leeper, MN, RN, CNS M-S,
CCRN**
Clinical Nurse Specialist, Cardiovascular
    Services, Baylor University Medical
    Center
Dallas, Texas

Jeanne R. Lowe, RN, CWCN
Research Assistant and Doctoral Student,
    Biobehavioral Nursing and Health
    Systems, University of Washington;
    Clinical Instructor, University of
    Washington School of Nursing
Seattle, Washington

**Laurence M. Lysne, MAE, CRNA,
ARNP**
Staff Nurse Anesthetist/Clinical Preceptor,
    Gonzaga University/Sacred Heart Medical
    Center, School of Anesthesia
Spokane, Washington

Jane MacIver, RN-NP, MSc, CCN(C)
Nurse Practitioner, Heart Failure/Heart
    Transplant, Toronto General Hospital
Toronto, Ontario, Canada

Karen March, RN, MN, CNRN, CCRN
Director of Clinical Development, Integra
    LifeSciences; Clinical Faculty,
    Biobehavioral Nursing, University
    of Washington School of Nursing
Seattle, Washington

**Christina Marino, RN, MSN, FNP,
AOCNS**
Clinical Nurse Specialist, UCLA Health
    System
Los Angeles, California

Norma D. McNair, RN, CCRN, CNRN
Assistant Clinical Professor, School of
Nursing, University of California Los
Angeles; Clinical Nurse Specialist,
Ronald Reagan UCLA Medical Center
Los Angeles, California

**Laura J. McNamara, RN, MSN,
CCRN**
Clinical Practice Specialist, American
Association of Critical-Care Nurses
Aliso Viejo, California

Karen A. McQuillan, RN, MS, CCRN
Clinical Nurse Specialist, R. Adams
Cowley Shock Trauma Center, University
of Maryland Medical Center
Baltimore, Maryland

**Marion E. McRae, RN, MScN,
CCRN-CSC-CMC, CCN(C),
ACNP-BC, ACNPC**
Nurse Practitioner, Cardiovascular Surgery
and the Toronto Congenital Cardiac
Centre for Adults, Peter Munk Cardiac
Centre, Toronto General Hospital,
University Health Network; Clinical
Associate, Lawrence S. Bloomberg
Faculty of Nursing, University of Toronto
Toronto, Ontario, Canada

Reba McVay, MSN, RN
Clinical Nurse Specialist, Medical ICU,
University of Maryland Medical Center
Baltimore, Maryland

Carol Metcalf, BSN, MN
Adult Nurse Practitioner, Department
of Anesthesiology and Pain Medicine,
University of Washington; Nurse
Practitioner Pain Relief Service,
Harborview Medical Center
Seattle, Washington

Bernadette E. Michel, RN, BS
Clinical Nurse Specialist, Johns Hopkins
University
Baltimore, Maryland

Mary Jo Moore, RN, MA, CCRN
Nurse Manager 2 South ICU, Providence
Sacred Heart Medical Center
Spokane, Washington

Mark R. Oherrick, MSN, CEN, RN
Acute Care Nurse Practitioner, Nationally
Registered Paramedic, Advanced Practice
Nurse, Department of Emergency
Medicine, Fulton County Medical Center
McConnellsburg, Pennsylvania

DaiWai M. Olson, PhD, RN, CCRN
Assistant Professor, Department of Medicine/
Neurology, Duke University Medical
Center; Staff Nurse Level 4, Duke
Neurocritical Care Unit
Durham, North Carolina

Cherryl Parcon, RN
Peritoneal Dialysis Nurse, DaVita Dialysis
Services, Thomas Jefferson University
Hospital
Philadelphia, Pennsylvania

**Kristine J. Peterson, MS, RN, CCRN,
CCNS**
Critical Care Clinical Nurse Specialist, Park
Nicollet Methodist Hospital
St Louis Park, Minnesota

**Joya D. Pickett, MSN, CCNS,
ACNS-BC, CCRN**
Clinical Instructor, University of Washington,
Biobehavioral Nursing and Health
Sciences; Critical Care Clinical Nurse
Specialist, Swedish Medical Center
Seattle, Washington

**Pamela Popplewell, RN, MSN,
ANP-BC, CCRN**
Nurse Practitioner, General Surgery, Director
of Nursing, Surgical and Perioperative
Care, VA Puget Sound Health Care
System
Seattle, Washington

**Jan Powers, PhD, RN, CCRN, CCNS,
CNRN, FCCM**
Director, Clinical Nurse Specialists and
Nursing Research, Critical Care Clinical
Nurse Specialist, St Vincent Hospital
Indianapolis, Indiana

**Kimberly L. Quinn, RN, BSN, MSN,
ACNP, ANP, CCRN**
Associate Professor, Department of Nursing
College of Notre Dame; Adult Nurse
Practitioner in Thoracic Surgery, Union
Memorial Hospital
Baltimore, Maryland

Ann B. Rayburn, RN, BSN, CPTC
Senior Manager of Professional Education,
Alabama Organ Center
Birmingham, Alabama

Robert E. St. John, MSN, RN, RRT
Director, US Marketing, Covidien Respira-
tory and Monitoring Solutions
Boulder, Colorado

**Maureen A. Seckel, APN, ACNS, BC,
CCNS, CCRN**
Clinical Nurse Specialist, Medical
Pulmonary Critical Care, Christiana
Care Health System
Newark, Delaware

Pamela Shellner, RN, MA
Clinical Practice Specialist, American
Association of Critical-Care Nurses
Aliso Viejo, California

Erin Shepherd, RD, LD, CNSD
Clinical Dietitian, Trauma and Critical
Care, Baylor University Medical Center
Dallas, Texas

**Sarah K. Shingleton, MS, RN, CCRN,
CCNS**
Clinical Nurse Specialist, Burn Unit and F6/6
(GYN, Plastics, ENT, Urology), University
of Wisconsin Hospital and Clinics
Madison, Wisconsin

**Deborah Sidor, NP, MSN, ACNS-BC,
CCRN**
Clinical Nurse Specialist, Providence Park
Hospital
Novi, Michigan

**Debra Siela, PhD, RN, CCNS,
ACNS-BC, CCRN, CNE, RRT**
Assistant Professor, School of Nursing,
Critical Care CNS, Ball Memorial Hospital
Muncie, Indiana

Marty Slate, RN, BSN
Clinical Nurse, ABLS National Faculty,
University of Colorado Hospital
Aurora, Colorado

Michelle D. Smeltzer, MSN, RN, CEN
Clinical Nurse Specialist for Emergency
Services, Albert Einstein Health Network
Philadelphia, Pennsylvania

**Christine L. Sommers, RN, MN,
CCRN**
Staff Nurse, Intensive Care Unit, Kadlec
Regional Medical Center; Faculty,
Washington State University
Richland, Washington

Marcus Soper RN, MS, CRNA
Nurse Anesthetist, Providence Sacred Heart
Medical Center and Children's Hospital
Spokane, Washington

**Kathleen M. Stacy, RN, CNS, CCRN,
PCCN, CCNS**
Critical Care Clinical Nurse Specialist–IMC,
Palomar Pomerado Health
Escondido, California

Andrea L. Strayer, MS, A/GNP-BC, CNRN
Neurosurgery Nurse Practitioner, Department of Neurological Surgery, Hospital and Clinics, University of Wisconsin School of Medicine and Public Health
Madison, Wisconsin

Doris Strother, MSN, RN
Advanced Nursing Coordinator, University Hospital
Birmingham, Alabama

Shilta Subhas, RN, MS
Clinical Nurse Specialist, The Johns Hopkins Hospital
Baltimore, Maryland

Erica Thibault, MS, RN, CNS, APN, CWON
Medical Surgical Clinical Nurse Specialist, St Anthony Hospital
Denver, Colorado

Tamekia L. Thomas, MSN, RN, PCCN
Critical Care Education Coordinator, Christiana Care Health System
Newark, Delaware

Paul A. Thurman, RN, MS, ACNPC, CCNS, CCRN, CNRN
Clinical Nurse Specialist, R. Adams Cowley Shock Trauma Center, University of Maryland Medical Center
Baltimore, Maryland

Michael L. Tidwell, CRNP
Hematology/Oncology Nurse Practitioner Greenebaum Cancer Center
University of Maryland Hospital
Baltimore, Maryland

Terry L. Tucker, RN, MS, CCRN, CEN
Critical Care Clinical Nurse Specialist, Nursing Education and Research Center, Veterans Affairs Maryland Health Care System
Baltimore, Maryland

Elizabeth Visco, CRNA
Chief Nurse Anesthetist, Harborview Medical Center
Seattle, Washington

Kathleen M. Vollman, MSN, RN, CCNS, FCCM
Clinical Nurse Specialist, Educator, Consultant, Advancing Nursing LLC
Northville, Michigan

Eloise Wagner, RN, MSN
Nurse Educator, Department of Surgery, The Johns Hopkins Hospital
Baltimore, Maryland

Teresa A. Wavra, RN, MSN, CNS, CCRN
Cardiovascular Clinical Nurse Specialist, Cardiac Intensive Care Unit and Cardiac Telemetry Unit, Mission Hospital
Mission Viejo, California

Christine G. Westphal, APN, MSN, ACNS-BC, AHCPN, CCRN
Director/Nurse Practitioner, Palliative and Restorative Integrated Services Model, Oakwood Healthcare System
Dearborn, Michigan

Sue Wingate, RN, PhD, CRNP
Cardiology Nurse Practitioner, Kaiser Permanente Mid-Atlantic States
Silver Spring, Maryland

Elizabeth Zink, RN, MS, CCRN, CNRN
Clinical Nurse Specialist, Neurosciences Critical Care Unit, The Johns Hopkins Hospital
Baltimore, Maryland

Preface

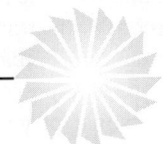

In this time of dramatic change in healthcare, it is with great pleasure that we present the sixth edition of the *AACN Procedure Manual for Critical Care*. The changes that our colleagues will find in this edition are a direct reflection of the ongoing knowledge and technology explosion that has been a part of the new century. Although every attempt was made to capture current clinical practice, we recognize that critical care clinical practice is dynamic, and therefore, any resource to support that practice must be considered a work in progress.

AACN is dedicated to the care of patients with critical illness or injury and their families. AACN's vision is of a healthcare system driven by the needs of patients and their families in which critical care nurses make their optimal contribution. Toward that vision, our hope is that this edition of the *AACN Procedure Manual for Critical Care* will be a useful resource for critical care nurses in providing quality patient care.

The sixth edition of the *AACN Procedure Manual for Critical Care* will be an asset for nurses across the spectrum of acute and critical care practice. The manual includes a comprehensive review of state-of-the-art information on acute and critical care procedures. The following procedures related to new and emerging trends have been added:

- Surgical Cricothyrotomy (Perform and Assist)
- Noninvasive Positive Pressure Ventilation: Continuous Positive Airway Pressure (CPAP) and Bilevel Positive Airway Pressure (BiPAP)
- Arterial Pressure-Based Cardiac Output Monitoring
- Fecal Containment Devices and Bowel Management System
- Small-Bore Feeding Tube Insertion Using an Electromagnetic Guidance System (CORTRAK®)
- Intraosseous Devices

All procedures have been revised to reflect changes in practice. With the increased presence of advanced practice nurses in critical care units, this edition of the *AACN Procedure Manual for Critical Care* not only contains procedures commonly performed by critical care nurses but also includes an even greater number of procedures performed by advanced practice nurses than the fifth edition. Each advanced practice procedure has an AP designation in the Table of Contents and a special AP icon and explanatory footnote on the first page of each procedure.

Because we recognize that the procedures included in this manual are only a portion of the repertoire needed by today's critical care practitioners to skillfully care for critically ill patients, we recommend it be used in conjunction with *AACN Core Curriculum for Critical Care Nursing*, *AACN Certification and Core Review for High Acuity and Critical Care*, and *AACN Advanced Critical Care Nursing*.

The *AACN Procedure Manual for Critical Care* is designed so that information within each procedure can be found quickly. To provide high-quality care to seriously ill patients, we need resources that provide us with readily available need-to-know information. This edition, like the fifth, is organized in units, with most of the units having several sections. All procedures are designed in the same style and begin with the following:

- Purpose of the procedure.
- Prerequisite Nursing Knowledge, which includes information the nurse needs before performing the procedure.
- Equipment list, which includes equipment necessary to perform the procedure. Some of the procedures identify additional equipment that may be necessary based on individual situations.
- Patient and Family Education, which identifies essential information that should be taught to patients and their families.
- Patient Assessment and Preparation, which includes specific assessment criteria that should be obtained before the procedure and describes how the patient should be prepared for the procedure.

Each step-by-step procedure includes:

- Steps, Rationales, and for some steps, Special Considerations.
- Associated research and appropriate figures and tables.
- Expected Outcomes, including the anticipated results of the procedure.
- Unexpected Outcomes, including potential complications or untoward outcomes of the procedure.
- Patient Monitoring, which includes information related to assessments and interventions that should be completed. The rationale for each item is described, and conditions that necessitate notification of an advanced practice nurse or physician are identified.
- Documentation that describes what should be documented after the procedure is performed.
- References are included, and the majority of procedures also include Additional Readings.

This edition of the *AACN Procedure Manual for Critical Care* includes several icons that are common to many of the procedures. These icons include:

AP A procedure with the *AP* icon should be performed only by physicians, advanced practice nurses, and other healthcare professionals (including critical care nurses) with additional knowledge, skills, and demonstrated competence per professional licensure or institutional standard.

HH A procedure step with the *HH* icon designates that hand hygiene should be performed. This step is essential to reduce the transmission of microorganisms and is part of Standard Precautions.

PE A procedure step with the *PE* icon designates that personal protective equipment should be applied. Personal protective equipment may include gloves, protective eyeglasses, masks, gowns, and any additional equipment needed to protect the nurse or provider performing the procedure. The application of personal protective equipment reduces the transmission of microorganisms, minimizes splash, and is part of Standard Precautions.

VP A procedure step with the *VP* icon designates that the correct patient is identified using two identifiers. It is essential that prior to performing a procedure, the nurse ensures the correct identification of the patient for the intended intervention.

CR A reference with the *CR* icon is a classic reference. A classic reference is a reference that is more than 5 years old at the time the procedure was written and meets the following criteria:

- It is widely cited in the literature and impacts practice.
- It is considered a standard work of established excellence.
- It is the foundation for practice.

In the nursing profession, the quest to have our practice driven by research has never been greater. Once again, this edition of the *AACN Procedure Manual for Critical Care* uses a research-based leveling system. As available, this research-based information is provided to indicate the research-based strength of recommendation for various interventions. Although we believe that this is a major step forward in promoting research-based practice, the paucity of research available in many procedures also speaks loudly to the need for further investigation. The research-based leveling system is the same as is used for *AACN Protocols for Practice* and includes:

- Level A: Meta-analysis of quantitative studies or metasynthesis of qualitative studies with results that consistently support a specific action, intervention, or treatment.
- Level B: Well-designed controlled studies with results that consistently support a specific action, intervention, or treatment.
- Level C: Qualitative studies, descriptive or correlational studies, integrative reviews, systematic reviews, or randomized controlled trials with inconsistent results.
- Level D: Peer-reviewed professional organizational standards with clinical studies to support recommendations.
- Level E: Multiple case reports, theory-based evidence from expert opinions, or peer-reviewed professional organizational standards without clinical studies to support recommendations.
- Level M: Manufacturer's recommendations only.

Given the nature of critical care, many of the included procedures use electrical equipment. This manual makes the assumption that all equipment is maintained by the institution's bioengineering department according to accepted national and state regulations for the individual piece of equipment.

We hope that you find this book an essential resource for clinical practice.

Debra Lynn-McHale Wiegand

Acknowledgments

This edition of the *AACN Procedure Manual for Critical Care* could not have been published without the help of numerous invaluable individuals. First, I want to thank AACN for giving me the opportunity to edit this edition. My deepest gratitude is extended to Ellen French, who was Publishing Director for AACN. Ellen believed in Karen Carlson and me when we first started coediting the *AACN Procedure Manual for Critical Care,* and she continued to support me when I was faced with the challenge of editing this text without Karen at my side. I am especially thankful for Ellen's expertise, time, advice, support, and understanding during the development of this book.

I am very grateful that I had the opportunity to work with the talented, hard-working, and dedicated editorial staff at Elsevier. I want to extend a special thank you to Maureen Iannuzzi, my editor. Maureen's leadership was an essential component to the success of the publication. Maureen provided important guidance and support throughout the entire publication process. I also want to thank Robin Levin Richman and her predecessor, Jennifer Ehlers, Senior Developmental Editors, for coordinating the day-to-day progress of the book. Jennifer and Robin were fun to work with and approached challenges with patience and kindness. I also want to thank Julia Curcio, Editorial Assistant; Anne Konopka, Senior Project Manager; Karen Moehlman, Copyeditor; Kim Denando, Designer; and Jeff Patterson, Publishing Services Manager for all of their hard work and commitment to the process of producing this book. In addition, I want to thank Suzanne Toppy, Managing Editor, Mosby Nursing Skills, for all of her work as she coordinated the review process. The Elsevier team worked very hard to produce this quality textbook.

I want to extend a huge thank you to each of the section editors: Michael Day, Eleanor Fitzpatrick, Mary Beth Makic, and Teresa Preuss. The section editors coordinated the development and revision of each of the procedures within their sections. I am very appreciative of all of their hard work and commitment to a quality product. I tremendously enjoyed working with such an expert team.

This book would not be possible without the hard work and commitment from the contributors. The contributors are the staff nurses and advanced practice nurses who revised the procedures and developed new procedures. Each contributor worked very hard to ensure that each procedure included all of the information needed so that acute and critical care nurses would have the most helpful information at their fingertips. I cannot thank each of the contributors enough for their commitment to this book.

I also want to thank the staff nurses and advanced practice nurses who reviewed each of the procedures. At least two reviewers critiqued each procedure and provided important feedback to the contributors. The reviewers' critiques improved the quality of each procedure. I am also grateful to Laura McNamara and Mary Pat Aust, Clinical Practice Specialists at the AACN National Office, who dedicated a tremendous amount of time and energy reviewing this work. Their critiques contributed to ensuring the quality of the *AACN Procedure Manual for Critical Care.*

On a personal note, I want to thank the critical care nurses who cared for my mother and my son when they were critically ill. Nurses make a difference every day in the lives of patients and families. I also want to extend the biggest thank you ever to my husband, Jim. There is not another man in the world that I would rather have by my side.

Contents

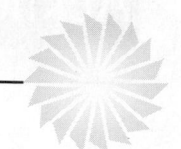

Unit I
Pulmonary
System

SECTION ONE
Airway Management

PROCEDURE
1

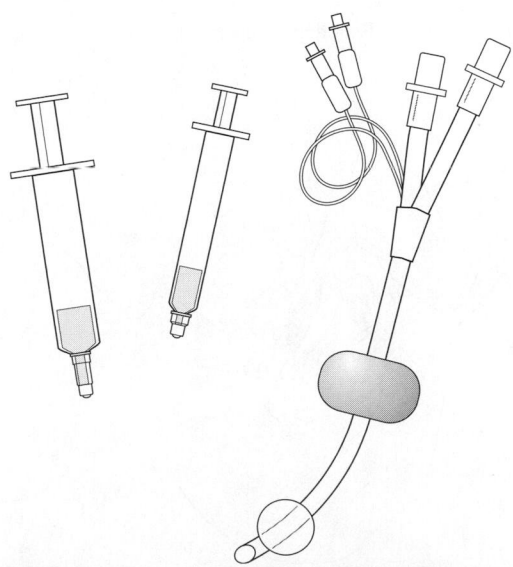 **AP** Combitube Insertion and Removal

P U R P O S E :   A Combitube may be used to provide an emergency airway during resuscitation of a profoundly unconscious patient who needs artificial ventilation when endotracheal intubation is not readily available or has failed in successfully establishing an airway.

Jeffrey Dawson

PREREQUISITE NURSING KNOWLEDGE

- Anatomy and physiology of the upper airway should be understood.
- The Combitube does not require direct visualization of the airway for insertion and is inserted in a "blind" fashion, as an adjunct when endotracheal intubation attempts fail or trauma makes visualization of the airway difficult.[1,8] The Combitube (Fig. 1-1) is available in two sizes, determined by patient height.[12]
  - ❖ The 37F size is used for patients 48 to 66 inches tall (122 to 168 cm).
  - ❖ Either size 37F or size 41F is applicable in patients 60 to 66 inches tall (152 to 168 cm).[12]
- For patients greater than or equal to 66 inches (168 cm), the 41F size should be used.
- The Combitube has a unique design that includes:
  - ❖ A double-lumen, semirigid airway
    - ○ Blue lumen opening to the perforations between the cuffs
    - ○ White lumen opening distal to the distal cuff
    - ○ Each lumen fitted with a 15-mm male adapter
  - ❖ Two cuffs for occlusion
    - ○ Proximal cuff (85 mL or 100 mL, depending on tube size) to occlude the hypopharynx
    - ○ Distal cuff (12 mL or 15 mL, depending on tube size) to occlude either the esophagus or the trachea

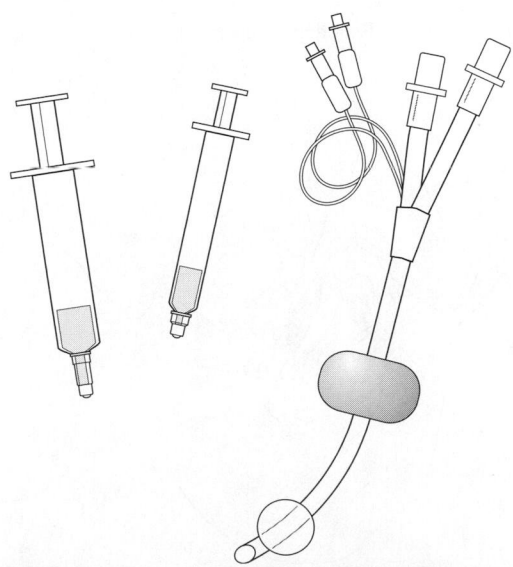

FIGURE 1-1   Components of the Combitube.

AP   This procedure should be performed only by physicians, advanced practice nurses, and other healthcare professionals (including critical care nurses) with additional knowledge, skills, and demonstrated competence per professional licensure or institutional standard.

○ Each cuff connected to a pilot balloon and valve: blue for proximal (No. 1), white for distal (No. 2)

❖ Two black lines indicate the position of the patient's teeth or gum line when the device is first inserted.

❖ Because of the large inflated cuff in the hypopharynx, the Combitube needs no stabilization or securing after placement.

• The correct placement of a Combitube in the airway is as follows:

❖ Esophageal insertion (Figs. 1-2 and 1-3), in which the distal cuff occludes the esophagus and the proximal balloon occludes the hypopharynx, allows ventilation via the blue lumen.

• Tracheal insertion (Fig. 1-4), in which the distal cuff occludes the trachea and the proximal balloon occludes the hypopharynx, allows ventilation through the white lumen.

• Before the insertion of a Combitube, adequate ventilation of an unconscious patient with a mouth-to-mask or a bag-valve-mask device is necessary.

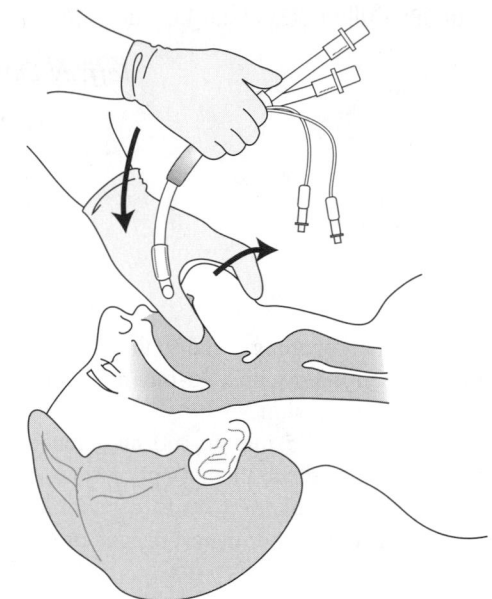

FIGURE 1-2   Esophageal insertion of a Combitube.

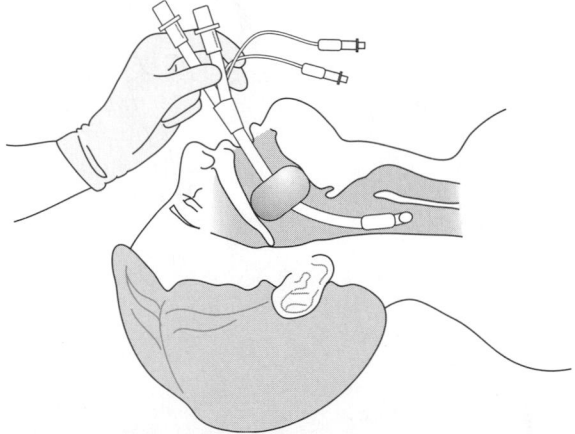

FIGURE 1-3   Combitube in esophageal position.

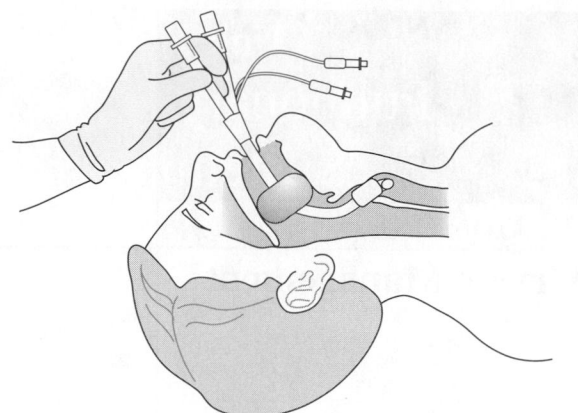

FIGURE 1-4   Combitube in tracheal position.

• Use of the Combitube is contraindicated for airway management[8,12] in the following cases:
  ❖ Patients with an intact gag reflex
  ❖ Patients with known esophageal disease
  ❖ Patients who have ingested caustic substances
  ❖ Patients with a known or suspected foreign body in the hypopharynx
  ❖ Pediatric patients

• The Combitube contains latex and may cause an allergic reaction in patients or in personnel who handle the device with a sensitivity to latex.[12]

• The Combitube is supplied either in a complete kit (with all of the necessary components for insertion), in soft or rigid packaging, or as a single individual device (without any of the necessary components for insertion). If the single individual device is used, additional components are necessary for insertion.

• Initial and ongoing training is needed to maximize insertion success and minimize complications.[7]

• Medications delivered via endotracheal tube cannot be used with a Combitube in the esophageal position. Medications may not reach the alveolar surfaces of the lung for absorption.

• The Combitube is intended for use up to 8 hours only.[13]

EQUIPMENT

• Combitube, of the appropriate size for the patient's height
• Large (100-mL) Luer-tip syringe
• Small (20-mL) Luer-tip syringe
• Water-soluble lubricant
• Mouth-to-mask or self-inflating manual resuscitation bag-valve-mask device and mask attached to a high-flow oxygen source
• Oxygen source and tubing
• Gloves, mask, gown, and eye protection
• Suction equipment (suction canister with control head, tracheal suction catheters, Yankauer suction tip)
• Fluid deflector elbow

PATIENT AND FAMILY EDUCATION

- If time allows, provide the family with information about the Combitube and the reason for insertion. ➤*Rationale:* This information assists the family in understanding why the procedure is necessary and decreases family anxiety.

PATIENT ASSESSMENT AND PREPARATION

Patient Assessment

- Assess level of consciousness and responsiveness. ➤*Rationale:* In an emergency situation, the Combitube should be inserted only into a patient who is profoundly unconscious, unresponsive, and unable to maintain adequate ventilation. Administration of neuromuscular blocking agents and sedation may be needed to ensure that the patient's gag reflex does not return while the Combitube is in place.[9,13]
- Assess history and patient information for possibility of esophageal disease or caustic substance ingestion. ➤*Rationale:* A Combitube is contraindicated in patients with these conditions.[8]

- Assess patient's height. ➤*Rationale:* This assessment allows the selection of an appropriately sized Combitube.[13]
- Assess risk for hypertensive bleeding and take precautions if increased catecholamine stress response is likely. ➤*Rationale:* Combitube insertion may cause pronounced catecholamine response.[5,10]

Patient Preparation

- Verify correct patient with two identifiers. ➤*Rationale:* Prior to performing a procedure, the nurse should ensure the correct identification of the patient for the intended intervention.
- Ensure adequate ventilation and oxygenation with either a mouth-to-mask or a self-inflating manual resuscitation bag-valve-mask device. ➤*Rationale:* The patient is nonresponsive and unable to maintain adequate ventilation without assisted ventilation before the Combitube insertion.
- Ensure that the suction equipment is assembled and in working order. ➤*Rationale:* The patient may regurgitate during insertion or while the Combitube is in place and need oropharyngeal or tracheal suctioning or both.
- Perform a pre-procedure verification and time out, if nonemergent. ➤*Rationale:* Ensures patient safety.

Procedure for Combitube Insertion

Steps	Rationale	Special Considerations
1. **HH**	Minimizes possible contamination of Combitube.	
2. **PE**	Minimizes possible contamination of Combitube.	
3. Open the package and test the integrity of both cuffs. **(Level M*)**	Ensures that the device is not defective and will work as indicated.	
A. Pull the plunger back on the large syringe to the appropriate volume for the size of the tube and attach it to the proximal (blue) valve, marked "No. 1."	Readies the syringe for inflating the cuff.	Use 85 mL volume for the 37F size and 100 mL volume for the 41F size.[12,13]
B. Inflate the proximal cuff with the appropriate volume and assess for leaks.	Ensures that the device is not defective and will work as indicated.	If a leak is found, discard the device and secure another.
C. Actively deflate the proximal cuff, leaving the syringe attached to the valve.	Provides for smoother insertion and readies the syringe for inflation after insertion.	
D. Pull the plunger back on the small syringe to the appropriate volume for the size of the tube and attach it to the distal (white) valve, marked "No. 2."	Readies the syringe for inflating the cuff.	Use 12 mL volume for the 37F size and 15 mL volume for the 41F size.[12,13]
E. Inflate the distal cuff with the appropriate volume and assess for leaks.	Ensures that the device is not defective and will work as indicated.	If a leak is found, discard the device and secure another.

*Level M: Manufacturer's recommendations only

Procedure continues on following page

Procedure   for Combitube Insertion—*Continued*

Steps	Rationale	Special Considerations
F. Actively deflate the distal cuff, leaving the syringe attached to the valve.	Provides for smoother insertion and readies the syringe for inflation after insertion.	
4. Lubricate the device with water-soluble lubricant. **(Level M*)**	Facilitates and eases insertion.	
5. Attach a fluid deflector to the clear lumen marked "No. 2." **(Level M)**	Diverts any fluid that may be regurgitated through the tube during insertion away from the person inserting the device.	A fluid deflector is included in the kits but not in the single individual devices.
6. Grasp the patient's jaw with one hand and pull up (or forward if the patient is in a sitting position), maintaining the head in a neutral position (see Fig. 1-4).[9] **(Level M)**	Pulls the tongue forward and away from the hypopharynx.	With facial trauma, assess for the presence of broken teeth (real or artificial) and remove loose fragments. Maintain cervical spine precautions with suspected or known spine trauma. Use extreme caution to avoid puncturing the balloons during insertion.[12]
7. Grasp the Combitube in the other hand so that it curves toward the patient's feet. **(Level M)**	Places the Combitube in the appropriate position for insertion.	
8. Insert the tip of the Combitube into the patient's mouth and advance it in a downward curving motion, maintaining a midline position, until the teeth or gum line is between the two black marks on the device. **(Level M)**	Allows the Combitube to follow the patient's hypopharynx until it is in the correct position.	***Do not force the Combitube.[12]*** If it does not easily advance, attempt to redirect or remove and reinsert.[12]
9. Inflate the proximal cuff with the appropriate volume, using the blue valve, marked "No. 1." **(Level M)**	Inflates and seats the proximal cuff into the posterior hypopharynx and seals it.	Use 85 mL volume for the 37F size and 100 mL volume for the 41F size.[12,13] Significant resistance is felt as the cuff is inflated. Keep the syringe plunger depressed while removing it from the valve to prevent air escaping from the cuff.[3] If an air leak develops, add 10 mL of air at a time until the leak seals. Volumes of 150 mL may be needed for some individuals.[3,12]
10. Inflate the distal cuff with the appropriate volume, using the white valve, marked "No. 2." **(Level M)**	Inflates the distal cuff and seals the esophagus (or trachea) depending on locations. Both locations allow the establishment of an effective airway.	Use 12 mL volume for the 37F size and 15 mL volume for the 41F size.[12,13]
11. Connect the self-inflating manual resuscitation bag-valve device to the 15-mm adapter on the blue lumen, marked "No. 1," and ventilate. **(Level M)**	Most of the time, the distal balloon is in the esophagus.[2,12,13] With both cuffs inflated, the only place the ventilation can go is into the trachea.	

*Level M: Manufacturer's recommendations only

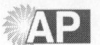

Procedure for Combitube Insertion—*Continued*

Steps	Rationale	Special Considerations
12. Assess for tube placement. **(Level M*)**	Determines placement of the tube and which lumen should be used to ventilate.	
A. Assess for gurgling over the epigastrium, chest rise and fall, and breath sounds in the lung fields with each ventilation.	If the distal cuff is in the esophagus, no gurgling is heard over the epigastrium and the ventilation expands the lungs, causing the chest to rise and fall and breath sounds to be heard over the lung fields. **Go to Step 12**. If the distal cuff is in the trachea, gurgling is heard over the epigastrium and no rise and fall of the chest is seen or breath sounds heard over the lung fields. **Go to Step 11B**. If no gurgling or breath sounds are noted with each ventilation, the Combitube may have been advanced too far into the esophagus, blocking the perforations from the blue lumen. **Go to Step 11C**.	Listening over the epigastrium initially provides rapid determination that the ventilation is going into the esophagus.[1] When assessing for the presence of breath sounds, always consider the possibility of a pneumothorax. This condition can change the breath sounds presentation and lead the inserter to believe that the Combitube is misplaced.
B. Immediately switch the self-inflating manual resuscitation bag-valve device to the clear lumen, marked "No. 2," and attempt to ventilate, assessing for gurgling over the epigastrium, chest rise and fall, and breath sounds in the lung fields with each ventilation.	If the distal cuff is in the trachea, no gurgling is heard over the epigastrium and the ventilation expands the lungs, causing the chest to rise and fall and breath sounds to be heard over the lung fields. **Go to Step 12**.	Listening over the epigastrium initially provides rapid determination that the ventilation is going into the esophagus.[1] When assessing for the presence of breath sounds, always consider the possibility of a pneumothorax. This condition can change the breath sounds presentation and lead the inserter to believe that the Combitube is misplaced.
C. Deflate the proximal cuff, using a syringe on the blue valve, marked "No. 1," withdraw the Combitube approximately 2 to 3 cm, and reinflate the "No. 1" cuff.	Allows for the repositioning of the Combitube so that the blue lumen perforations no longer are occluded by the soft tissue of esophagus. **Return to Step 11**.	If repositioning of the Combitube does not establish an effective airway, remove the device and establish an airway with alternative means.
13. Further assess device placement with an end-tidal carbon dioxide device.[2,11,13] or an esophageal detector device.[2,11] **(Level E*)**	Confirms proper placement with two additional methods.[3,4]	
14. Continue ventilation through whichever lumen provides the airway. **(Level M)**	Adequate ventilation can be achieved with the distal cuff of the Combitube in either the esophagus or the trachea.	
15. Remove personal protective equipment.		
16. **HH**		
17. Document the procedure in the patient's record.		

*Level E: Multiple case reports, theory-based evidence from expert opinions, or peer-reviewed professional organizational standards without clinical studies to support recommendations

*Level M: Manufacturer's recommendations only

Procedure continues on following page

Procedure for Combitube Removal

Steps	Rationale	Special Considerations
1. **HH**	Minimizes contamination of Combitube.	
2. **PE**	Minimizes contamination of Combitube.	
3. To remove the Combitube[12,13]: **(Level E*)**	Removal is indicated within 8 hours of insertion or when the patient's airway can be managed by skilled personnel.[13]	A fiberoptic scope may be used to replace a Combitube with an endotracheal tube. If the Combitube has been placed in the trachea, cricoid pressure should be established and maintained until the new airway is established.
A. Decompress the stomach.	Removes any contents from the stomach, which makes regurgitation less likely with removal of the device.	If the Combitube is placed in the esophagus, a small suction catheter may be inserted through the white "No. 2" lumen to decompress the stomach.
B. Attach a 100-mL syringe to the blue valve, marked "No. 1," and deflate the cuff.	Deflates the proximal cuff and allows suctioning of the hypopharynx.	
C. Suction the hypopharynx.	Removes secretions that may have accumulated in the hypopharynx.	
D. Attach a 20-mL syringe to the white valve, marked "No. 2," and deflate the cuff.	Deflates the distal cuff and allows the Combitube to be withdrawn.	
E. Withdraw the Combitube from the airway, and administer supplemental oxygen.	Allows the patient to breathe on his or her own and supplies supplemental oxygen to counter any hypoxia.	
4. Remove personal protective equipment.		
5. **HH**		
6. Document the procedure in the patient's record.		

*Level E: Multiple case reports, theory-based evidence from expert opinions, or peer-reviewed professional organizational standards without clinical studies to support recommendations

Expected Outcomes

- Establishment of an effective airway in an emergency situation
- Maintenance of adequate ventilation and oxygenation
- Recovery of spontaneous ventilation

Unexpected Outcomes

- Complications from use of the Combitube related to insertion technique or excessive cuff pressures
- Sore throat[6]
- Dysphagia[6]
- Bleeding[14]
- Pharyngeal perforation[14]
- Esophageal lacerations[14]
- Esophageal rupture[14]
- Improper placement, resulting in hypoventilation

Patient Monitoring and Care

Steps	Rationale	Reportable Conditions
		These conditions should be reported if they persist despite nursing interventions.

1. Monitor ventilation effectiveness while the Combitube is in place by monitoring:
  A. Difficulty of ventilation.
  B. Oxygen saturation (SpO_2).
  C. End-tidal carbon dioxide ($PetCO_2$).
	Determines that the Combitube is functioning correctly and providing adequate ventilation and oxygenation.	• Increased difficulty in ventilation
		• Unexplained decreases in SpO_2 or $PetCO_2$ levels

2. Monitor for return of spontaneous attempts at breathing.	May indicate need either to remove the device or use medications (sedatives or nondepolarizing neuromuscular blockade) to prevent the gag reflex.[13,6]	

Documentation

Documentation should include the following:
- Assessment findings that indicate the need to insert a Combitube
- Confirmation of adequacy of ventilation, with auscultation of gastric area and lung fields with $PetCO_2$
- Any difficulties with placement of the Combitube
- $PetCO_2$ levels
- Need for sedation or neuromuscular blockade or both
- Assessment findings on removal of the Combitube, including work of breathing, breath sounds, and SpO_2 levels

- Assessment findings after insertion of the Combitube that indicate which lumen ventilates the patient
- Secondary confirmation of adequacy of ventilation, or an esophageal detection device, in conjunction with SpO_2 levels with ventilation
- Ongoing monitoring of difficulty or ease of ventilation
- SpO_2 levels
- Assessment findings that indicate the need to remove the Combitube or replace it with an endotracheal tube

References

1. American Heart Association: *ACLS Resource Text (ACLS)*, Dallas, 2008, AHA.
2. Calkins T, et al: Success and complication rates with prehospital placement of an esophageal-tracheal Combitube as a rescue airway, *Prehosp Disaster Med* 21(2 Suppl 2):97-100, 2006.
3. Frass M: Combitube, *Internet J Anesthesiol* 5(2): 2001. Text available at www.ispub.com, retrieved June 22, 2009.
4. Frass M, et al: Evaluation of esophageal Combitube in cardiopulmonary resuscitation, *Crit Care Med* 15:609-611, 1987.
5. Kayhan D, et al: Which is responsible for hemodynamic response due to laryngoscopy and endotracheal intubation? Catecholamines, vasopression or angiotensin? *Eur J Anaesthesiol* 22(10):780-785, 2005.
6. Keller C, et al: The influence of cuff volume and anatomic location on pharyngeal, esophageal, and tracheal mucosal pressures with the esophageal tracheal Combitube, *Anesthesiology* 96:1074-1077, 2002.
7. Kory P, et al: Initial airway management skills of senior residents: Simulation training compared with traditional training, *Chest* 132(6):1927-1931, 2007.
8. Lavery G, McCloskey B, et al: The difficult airway in adult critical care, *Crit Care Med* 39(7):2163-2173, 2008.
9. Mace SE: Challenges and advantages in intubation: Rapid sequence intubation, *Emerg Med Clin North Am* (26)4:1043-1068, 2008.
10. Oczenski W, et al: Hemodynamic and catecholamine stress responses to insertion of the Combitube, laryngeal mask airway, and tracheal intubation, *Anesth Analg* 88(6):1389-1394, 1999.
11. Rich J, Thierbach A, Frass M: The Combitube, self-inflating bulb, and colorimetric carbon dioxide detector to advance airway management in the first echelon of the battlefield, *Mil Med* 171(5):389-395, 2006.
12. Tyco Healthcare: Combitube, Mansfield, MA, 2005, Tyco. Text available at www.nellcor.com/_catalog/pdf/sns/dfu/10000643b_dfu_combitube.pdf. Linked from www.nellcor.com/Serv/Manuals.aspx?ID=259, retrieved June 19, 2009.
13. Tyco Healthcare: Combitube quick guide, Mansfield, MA, 2000. Tyco. Text available at www.nellcor.com/_Catalog/PDF/Product/Combitube%20QRG.pdf. Linked from www.nellcor.com/prod/Product.aspx?S1=AIR&S2=&id=259, retrieved June 19, 2009.

14. Vezina M, et al: Complications associated with esophageal-tracheal Combitube in the pre-hospital setting, *Can J Anaesth* 54(2):124-128, 2007.

Additional Readings

Agro F, et al: Current status of the Combitube: a review of the literature, *J Clin Anesth* 14:307-314, 2002.

Foley LJ, Ochroch EA: Bridges to establish an emergency airway and alternate intubating techniques, *Crit Care Clin* 16:429-444, 2000.

Gaitini LA, Vaida SJ, Agro F: The esophageal-tracheal Combitube, *Anesthesiol Clin North Am* 20:893-906, 2002.

Idris AH, Gabrielli A: Advances in airway management, *Emerg Med Clin North Am* 20:843-857, 2002.

AP Endotracheal Intubation (Perform)

P U R P O S E : Endotracheal intubation is performed to establish and maintain a patent airway, facilitate oxygenation and ventilation, reduce the risk of aspiration, and assist with the clearance of secretions.

Cynthia A. Goodrich

PREREQUISITE NURSING KNOWLEDGE

* Anatomy and physiology of the pulmonary system should be understood.
* Indications for endotracheal intubation include the following[5,12]:
  * Altered mental status (head injury, drug overdose)
  * Anticipated airway obstruction (facial burns, epiglottitis, major facial or oral trauma)
  * Upper airway obstruction (e.g., from swelling, trauma, tumor, bleeding)
  * Apnea
  * Ineffective clearance of secretions (i.e., inability to maintain or protect airway adequately)
  * High risk of aspiration
  * Respiratory distress
* Pulse oximetry should be used during intubation so that oxygen desaturation can be detected quickly.
* Preoxygenation with 100% oxygen and a self-inflating manual resuscitation bag-valve-mask device with a tight-fitting face mask should be performed for 3 to 5 minutes before intubation.

AP This procedure should be performed only by physicians, advanced practice nurses, and other healthcare professionals (including critical care nurses) with additional knowledge, skills, and demonstrated competence per professional licensure or institutional standard.

* Intubation attempts should take no longer than 15 to 20 seconds. If more than one intubation is necessary, ventilation with 100% oxygen and a self-inflating manual resuscitation bag-valve-mask device with a tight-fitting face mask should be performed for 3 to 5 minutes before each attempt. If intubation is not successful after three attempts, consider use of other airway options, such as the Combitube or King Airway.
* Application of cricoid pressure (Sellick maneuver) may increase the success of the intubation. This procedure is accomplished with applying firm downward pressure on the cricoid ring, pushing the vocal cords downward so that they are visualized more easily. *Once begun, cricoid pressure must be maintained until intubation is completed* (Fig. 2-1).
* Two types of laryngoscope blades exist: straight and curved. The straight (Miller) blade is designed so that the tip extends below the epiglottis, to lift and expose the glottic opening. The straight blade is recommended for use in obese patients, pediatric patients, and patients with short necks because their tracheas may be located more anteriorly. When a curved (Macintosh) blade is used, the tip is advanced into the vallecula (the space between the epiglottis and the base of the tongue), to expose the glottic opening.
* Laryngoscope blades are available with fiberoptic light delivery systems. These systems provide a brighter light than bulbs, which can become scratched or covered with secretions.

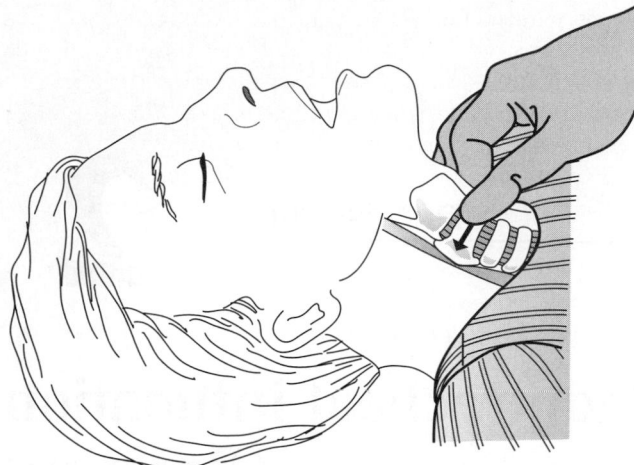

FIGURE 2-1   Cricoid pressure. Firm downward pressure on the cricoid ring pushes the vocal cords downward toward the field of vision while sealing the esophagus against the vertebral column.

- Endotracheal tube size reflects the size of the internal diameter of the tube. Tubes range in size from 2.5 mm for neonates to 9 mm for large adults. Endotracheal tubes that range in size from 7 to 7.5 mm are used for average-sized adult women, whereas endotracheal tubes that range in size from 8 to 9 mm are used for average-sized adult men (Fig. 2-2).[8,9,12] The tube with the largest clinically acceptable internal diameter should be used to minimize airway resistance and assist in suctioning.[4]
- Endotracheal intubation can be done via nasal or oral routes. The skill of the practitioner who performs the intubation and the patient's clinical condition determine the route used.
- Nasal intubation is relatively contraindicated in trauma patients with facial fractures or suspected fractures at the base of the skull and after cranial surgeries, such as transnasal hypophysectomy.
- Improper intubation technique may result in trauma to the teeth, soft tissues of the mouth or nose, vocal cords, and posterior pharynx.

- *In patients with suspected spinal cord injuries, in-line cervical immobilization of the head must be maintained during endotracheal intubation.*
- Primary and secondary confirmation of endotracheal intubation should be performed.[1,4]
  - ❖ Primary confirmation of proper endotracheal tube placement includes visualization of the tube passing through the vocal cords, absence of gurgling over the epigastric area, auscultation of bilateral breath sounds, bilateral chest rise and fall during ventilation, and mist in the tube.
  - ❖ Secondary confirmation of proper endotracheal tube placement is necessary to protect against unrecognized esophageal intubation. Methods include use of disposable end-tidal carbon dioxide (CO_2) detectors, continuous end-tidal CO_2 monitors, and esophageal detection devices.
- End-tidal CO_2 ($PetCO_2$) monitoring devices have been shown to be reliable indicators of expired CO_2 in patients with perfusing rhythms.[1,5,11,13,15] During cardiac arrest (nonperfusing rhythms), low pulmonary blood flow may cause insufficient expired CO_2.[14] CO_2 detected with an end-tidal CO_2 detector is a reliable indicator of proper tube placement.[6] If CO_2 is not detected, use of an esophageal detector device is recommended.[1,3,11,15]
- Disposable end-tidal CO_2 detectors are chemically treated with a nontoxic indicator that changes color in the presence of CO_2 and indicates that the endotracheal tube has been placed successfully into the trachea.
- Continuous end-tidal CO_2 monitors may be used to confirm proper endotracheal tube placement after intubation attempts and allow for the detection of future tube dislodgment.
- Esophageal detector devices work by creating suction at the end of the endotracheal tube with compressing a flexible bulb or pulling back on a syringe plunger. When the tube is placed correctly in the trachea, air allows for reexpansion of the bulb or movement of the syringe plunger. If the tube is located in the esophagus, no movement of the syringe plunger or reexpansion of the bulb is

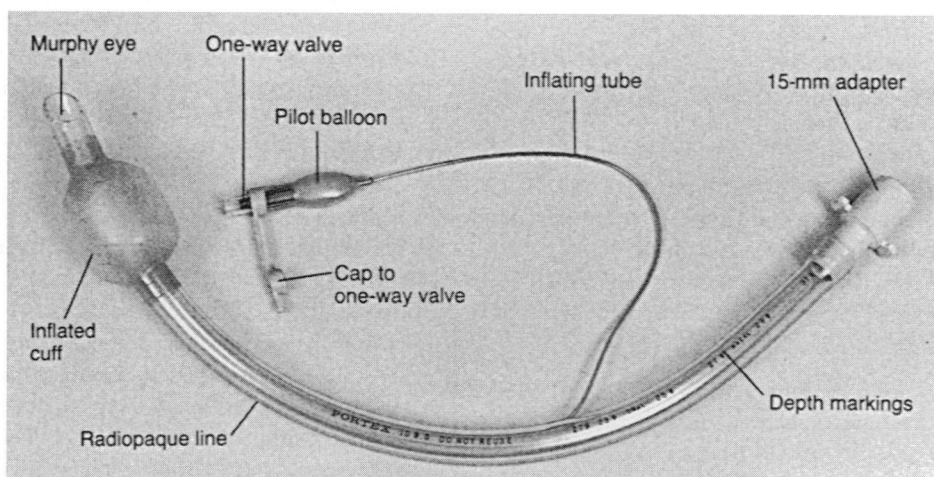

FIGURE 2-2   Parts of the endotracheal tube (soft-cuffed tube by Smiths Industries Medical Systems, Co, Valencia, Calif). *(From Kersten LD: Comprehensive respiratory nursing, Philadelphia, 1989, Saunders, 637.)*

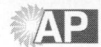

seen. These devices may be misleading in patients who are morbidly obese, patients in status asthmaticus, patients late in pregnancy, or patients with large amounts of tracheal secretions.[1]

- Double-lumen endotracheal tubes are used for independent lung ventilation in situations with bleeding of one lung or a large air leak that would impair ventilation of the good lung.
- The endotracheal tube also provides a route for the administration of emergency medications (e.g., lidocaine, epinephrine, atropine, and naloxone) when no other routes of administration are available.[4]

EQUIPMENT

- Personal protective equipment, including eye protection
- Endotracheal tube with intact cuff and 15-mm connector (women, 7-mm to 7.5-mm tube; men, 8-mm to 9-mm tube)
- Laryngoscope handle with fresh batteries
- Laryngoscope blades (straight and curved)
- Spare bulb for laryngoscope blades
- Flexible stylet
- Self-inflating manual resuscitation bag-valve-mask device with face mask connected to supplemental oxygen ($\geq$15 L/min)
- Oxygen source and connecting tubes
- Swivel adapter (for attachment to resuscitation bag or ventilator)
- Luer-tip 10-mL syringe for cuff inflation
- Water-soluble lubricant
- Rigid pharyngeal suction-tip (Yankauer) catheter
- Suction apparatus (portable or wall)
- Suction catheters
- Bite-block or oropharyngeal airway
- Endotracheal tube–securing apparatus or appropriate tape
  - ❖ Commercially available endotracheal tube holder
  - ❖ Adhesive tape (6 to 8 inches long)
  - ❖ Twill tape (cut into 30-inch lengths)
- Stethoscope
- Monitoring equipment: Continuous oxygen saturation and cardiac rhythm
- Secondary confirmation device: Disposable end-tidal CO_2 detector, continuous end-tidal CO_2 monitoring device, or esophageal detection device
- Drugs for intubation as indicated (sedation, paralyzing agents, lidocaine, atropine)

Additional equipment (to have available depending on patient need or practitioner preference) includes the following:

- Anesthetic spray (nasal approach)
- Local anesthetic jelly (nasal approach)
- Magill forceps (to remove foreign bodies obstructing the airway)
- Ventilator

PATIENT AND FAMILY EDUCATION

- Assess patient's and family's level of understanding about the condition and rationale for endotracheal intubation. ➧*Rationale:* This assessment identifies the patient's

and family's knowledge deficits concerning the patient's condition, the procedure, the expected benefits, and the potential risks. It also allows time for questions to clarify information and voice concerns. Explanations decrease patient anxiety and enhance cooperation.

- Explain the procedure and the reason for intubation, if the clinical situation permits. If not, explain the procedure and reason for the intubation after it is completed. ➧*Rationale:* This explanation enhances patient and family understanding and decreases anxiety.
- If indicated and the clinical situation permits, explain the patient's role in assisting with insertion of the endotracheal tube. ➧*Rationale:* This explanation elicits the patient's cooperation, which assists with insertion.
- Explain that the patient will be unable to speak while the endotracheal tube is in place but that other means of communication will be provided. ➧*Rationale:* This information enhances patient and family understanding and decreases anxiety.
- Explain that the patient's hands often are immobilized to prevent accidental dislodgment of the tube. ➧*Rationale:* This information enhances patient and family understanding and decreases anxiety.

PATIENT ASSESSMENT AND PREPARATION
Patient Assessment

- Verify correct patient with two identifiers. ➧*Rationale:* Prior to performing a procedure, the nurse should ensure the correct identification of the patient for the intended intervention.
- Assess immediate history of trauma with suspected spinal cord injury or cranial surgery. ➧*Rationale:* Knowledge of pertinent patient history allows for selection of the most appropriate method for intubation, which helps reduce the risk for secondary injury.
- Assess nothing-by-mouth (NPO) status, the use of a self-inflating manual resuscitation bag-valve device with mask before intubation, and signs of gastric distention. ➧*Rationale:* Increased risk of aspiration and vomiting occurs with accumulation of air (from the use of a self-inflating manual resuscitation bag-valve-mask device), food, or secretions. If a patient who has gastric distention or who has eaten recently needs to be intubated, anticipate the need to use cricoid pressure to decrease the risk of aspiration.
- Assess level of consciousness, level of anxiety, and respiratory difficulty. ➧*Rationale:* This assessment determines the need for sedation or the use of paralytic agents and the patient's ability to lie flat and supine for intubation.
- Assess oral cavity for presence of dentures, loose teeth, or other possible obstructions and remove if appropriate.
- Assess vital signs and for the following:
  - ❖ Tachypnea
  - ❖ Dyspnea
  - ❖ Shallow respirations
  - ❖ Cyanosis
  - ❖ Apnea
  - ❖ Altered level of consciousness

* ❖ Tachycardia
* ❖ Cardiac dysrhythmias
* ❖ Hypertension
* ❖ Headache
* ➣**Rationale**: Any of these conditions may indicate a problem with oxygenation or ventilation or both.
* Assess patency of nares (for nasal intubation). ➣**Rationale:** Selection of the most appropriate naris facilitates insertion and may improve patient tolerance of tube.
* Assess need for premedication. ➣**Rationale**: Various medications provide sedation or paralysis of the patient as needed.

Patient Preparation

* Perform a pre-procedure verification and time out, if nonemergent. ➣**Rational:** Ensures patient safety.
* Ensure that the patient understands preprocedural teaching, if appropriate. Answer questions as they arise, and reinforce information as needed. ➣**Rationale:** Understanding of previously taught information is evaluated and reinforced.
* Before intubation, initiate intravenous or intraosseous access. ➣**Rationale:** Readily available intravenous or intraosseous access may be necessary if the patient needs to be sedated or paralyzed or needs other medications because of a negative response to the intubation procedure.
* Position the patient appropriately.
  * ❖ Positioning of the nontrauma patient is as follows: Place the patient supine with the head in the sniffing position, in which the head is extended and the neck is flexed. Placement of a small towel under the occiput elevates it several inches, allowing for proper flexion of the neck (Fig. 2-3). ➣**Rationale:** Placement of the head in the sniffing position allows for visualization of the larynx and vocal cords by aligning the axes of the mouth, pharynx, and trachea.

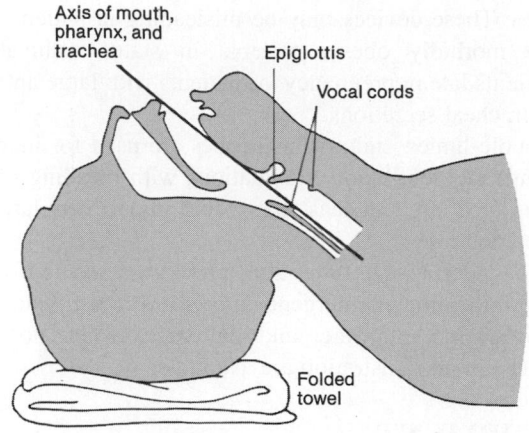

FIGURE 2-3 Neck hyperextension in the sniffing position aligns the axis of the mouth, pharynx, and trachea before endotracheal intubation. *(From Kersten LD: Comprehensive respiratory nursing, Philadelphia, 1989, Saunders, 642.)*

* ❖ Positioning of the trauma patient is as follows: Manual in-line cervical spinal immobilization must be maintained during the entire process of intubation. ➣**Rationale:** Because cervical spinal cord injury must be suspected in all trauma patients until proved otherwise, this position helps prevent secondary injury should a cervical spine injury be present.
* Premedicate as indicated. ➣**Rationale:** Appropriate premedication allows for more controlled intubation, reducing the incidence of insertion trauma, aspiration, laryngospasm, and improper tube placement.
* As appropriate, notify the respiratory therapy department of impending intubation so that a ventilator can be set up. ➣**Rationale:** The ventilator is set up before intubation.

Procedure for Performing Endotracheal Intubation

Steps	Rationale	Special Considerations
General Setup		
1. **HH**		Protective eyewear should be worn to avoid exposure to secretions.
2. **PE**		
3. Attach patient to pulse oximeter and cardiac monitor.		
4. Set up suction apparatus, and connect rigid suction-tip catheter to tubing.	Prepares for oropharyngeal suctioning as needed.	
5. Check equipment.		
A. Use 10-mL syringe to inflate cuff on tube, assessing for leaks. Completely deflate cuff.	Verifies that equipment is functional and that tube cuff is patent without leaks; prepares tube for insertion.	
B. Insert the stylet into the endotracheal tube, ensuring that the tip of the stylet does not extend past the end of the endotracheal tube.		Stylet must be recessed by at least 0.5 inch from the distal end of the tube so that it does not protrude beyond the end of the tube, resulting in damage to the vocal cords and trachea.

Procedure for Performing Endotracheal Intubation—*Continued*

Steps	Rationale	Special Considerations
C. Connect the laryngoscope blade to the handle, and check the bulb for brightness.	Verifies that the equipment is functional.	
6. Position the patient's head by flexing the neck forward and extending the head, in sniffing position (only if neck trauma is not suspected; see Fig. 2-3). If spinal trauma is suspected, request that an assistant maintain the head in a neutral position with in-line spinal immobilization.	Allows for visualization of the vocal cords with alignment of the mouth, pharynx, and trachea.	Placement of a small towel under the occiput elevates it, allowing for proper neck flexion. *Do not flex or extend neck of patient with suspected spinal cord injury; the head must be maintained in a neutral position with manual in-line cervical spine immobilization.*
7. Check the mouth for dentures and remove if present. Suction the mouth and pharynx as needed.	Dentures should be removed before oral intubation is attempted but may remain in place for nasal intubation.	
8. Insert oropharyngeal airway as indicated (see Procedure 11).	Assists in maintenance of upper airway patency.	Use only in unconscious patients.
9. Preoxygenate for 3 to 5 minutes, with 100% oxygen via a nonrebreather mask if ventilations are adequate or via a self-inflating manual resuscitation bag-valve-mask device (see Procedure 32) if ventilations are not adequate. Provide frequent and gentle breaths.	Helps prevent hypoxemia. Gentle breaths reduce incidence of air entering stomach (leading to gastric distention), decrease airway turbulence, and distribute distention, aspiration, and ventilation more evenly within the lungs.	If patient is breathing, avoid aggressive positive-pressure ventilation with a self-inflating manual resuscitation bag-valve-mask because of risk for gastric vomiting.
10. Premedicate patient as indicated. For nasotracheal intubation, **proceed to Step 32.**		
11. Remove oropharyngeal airway if present.		
Orotracheal Intubation		
12. Grasp laryngoscope (with blade in place and illuminated light on) in left hand.	Prepares for efficient blade placement.	Grasp handle as low as possible and keep wrist rigid to prevent using upper teeth as a fulcrum.
13. Use fingers of right hand to open the mouth.	Provides access to oral cavity.	
14. Slowly insert the blade into the right side of the patient's mouth, using it to push the tongue to the left (Fig. 2-4). Advance the blade inward and toward midline past the base of the tongue	Displaces the tongue to the left, increasing visualization of the glottic opening (Fig. 2-5).	Avoid pressure on the teeth and lips.
15. Request that an assistant apply cricoid pressure, if desired.	Moves the trachea toward the posterior for better visualization of the vocal cords by the practitioner.	Once cricoid pressure is applied, it must be maintained until the intubation is completed.
16. Advance the blade.		
A. With a curved blade, advance tip into vallecula and exert outward and upward gentle traction at a 45-degree angle (decreases use of teeth as a fulcrum).	Exposes the glottic opening.	Keep left arm and back straight when pulling upward, allowing for use of shoulders when lifting patient's head to the bed (Fig. 2-6).

Procedure continues on following page

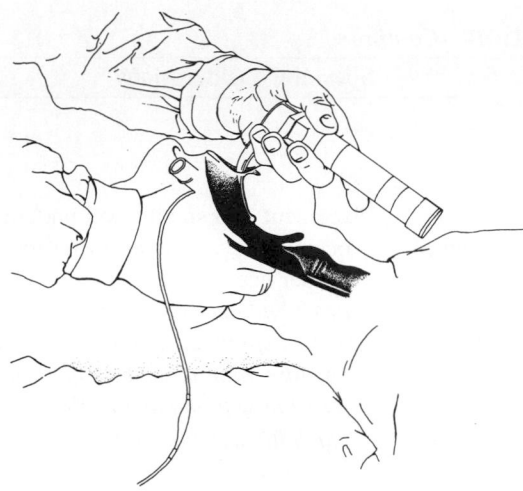

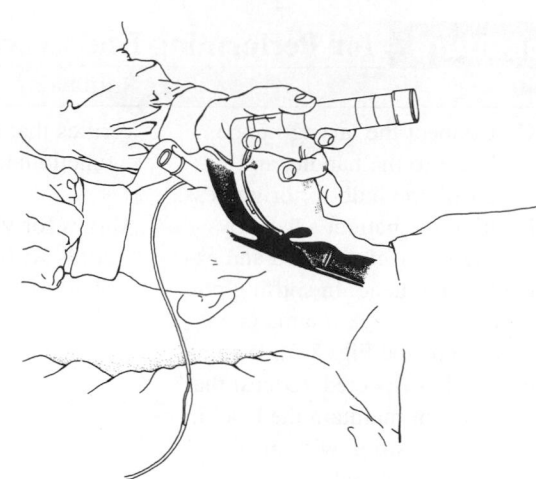

FIGURE 2-4   Technique of orotracheal intubation. The laryngo-scope blade is inserted into the oral cavity from the right, pushing the tongue to the left as it is introduced.

FIGURE 2-5   The blade is advanced into oropharynx, and the laryngoscope is lifted to expose the epiglottis.

Procedure | for Performing Endotracheal Intubation—*Continued*

Steps	Rationale	Special Considerations
B. With a straight blade, advance tip just beneath the epiglottis and exert gentle traction outward and upward at a 45-degree angle to the bed.	Exposes the glottic opening.	Keep left arm and back straight when pulling upward, allowing for use of shoulders when lifting patient's head (decreases use of teeth as a fulcrum).
17. Lift the laryngoscope handle until the vocal cords are visualized.	Allows for correct placement of tube into trachea (Fig. 2-7).	Gentle cricoid pressure (see Fig. 2-1) may assist in visualization of vocal cords and decrease risk of gastric distention and subsequent pulmonary aspiration. *When cricoid pressure is begun, it must be continued until the tube is correctly placed.*
18. Hold end of tube in right hand with the curved portion downward.	Tube is placed with the right hand.	

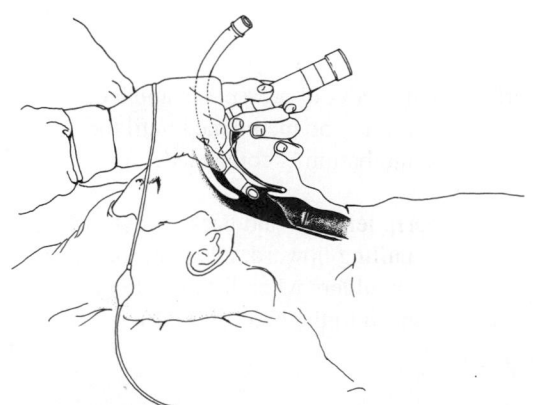

FIGURE 2-6   The tip of the blade is placed in the vallecula, and the laryngoscope is lifted further to expose the glottis. The tube is inserted through the right side of the mouth.

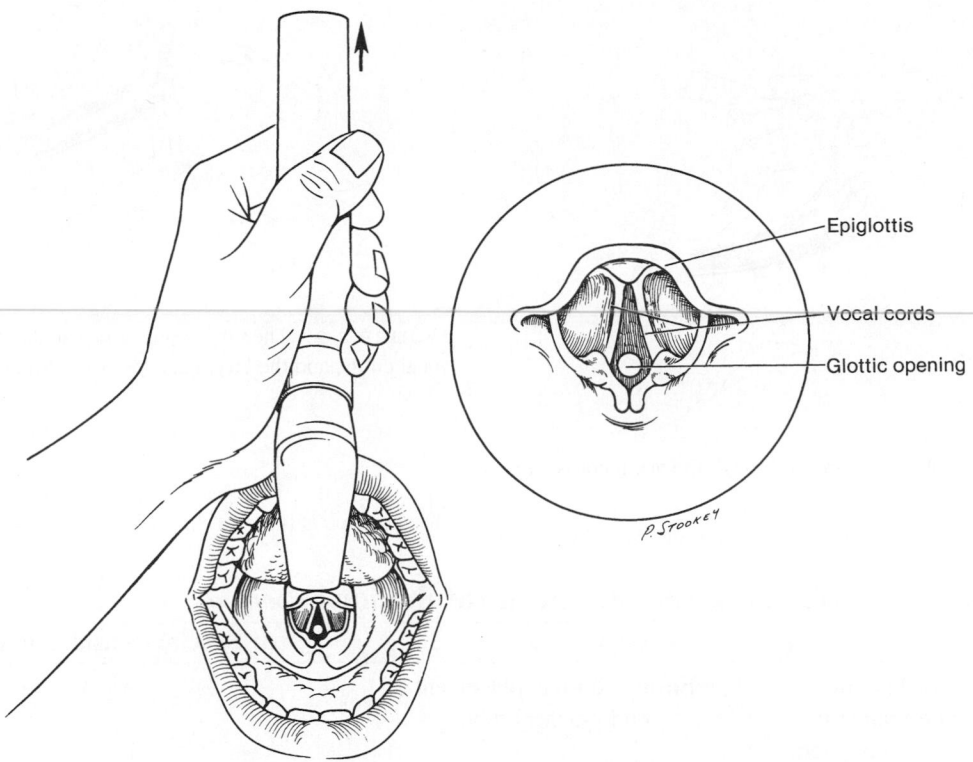

FIGURE 2-7 The endotracheal tube is passed through the vocal cords. *(From Flynn JM, Bruce NP: Introduction to critical care skills, St Louis, 1993, Mosby, 56.)*

Procedure for Performing Endotracheal Intubation—*Continued*

Steps	Rationale	Special Considerations
19. With use of direct vision, gently insert tube from right corner of mouth through the vocal cords (Fig. 2-8) until the cuff is no longer visible and has passed through the vocal cords (Fig. 2-9).	Tube must be seen passing through the vocal cords to ensure proper placement. Advance tube 1.25 to 2.5 cm farther into the trachea. When correctly positioned, the tip of the tube should be halfway between the vocal cords and the carina.[4]	The front teeth or gums should be aligned between the 19-cm and 23-cm depth markings on the tube to ensure the tip of the tube is above the carina.[4] Common tube placement at the teeth or gums is 21 cm for women and 23 cm for men.[9] If intubation is unsuccessful within 30 seconds, remove the tube. Ventilate with 100% oxygen with a bag-valve-mask device before another intubation attempt is made **(repeat Steps 12 through 18).**
20. When tube is correctly placed, continue to hold it securely in place at the lips with right hand while first withdrawing the laryngoscope blade and then the stylet with left hand.	Firmly holding tube at the lips provides stabilization and prevents inadvertent extubation.	
21. Inflate cuff with 5 to 10 mL of air depending on the manufacturer's recommendation (see Procedure 13).	Inflation volumes vary depending on manufacturer and size of tube. Keep cuff pressure between 20 and 25 mm Hg to decrease risk of aspiration and prevent ischemia and decreased blood flow.[1,4]	In adults, the minimal intracuff pressure to prevent aspiration is 25 mm Hg. Decreased mucosal capillary blood flow (ischemia) results when pressure is greater than 40 mm Hg.[4]

Procedure continues on following page

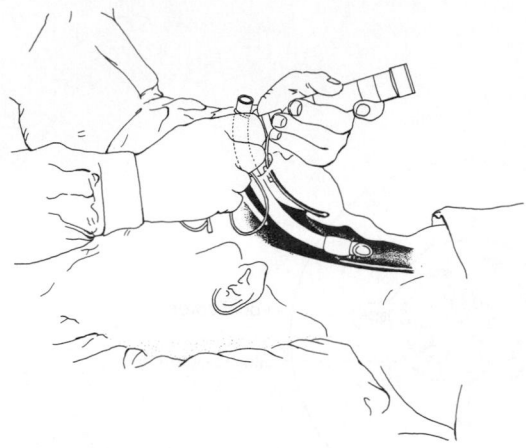

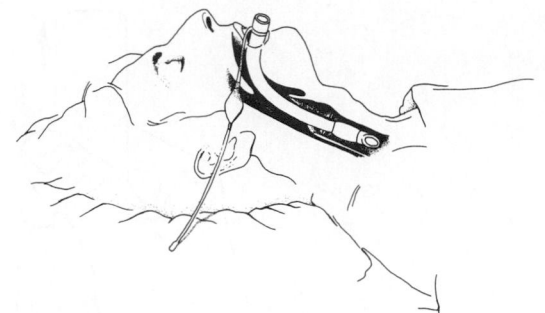

FIGURE 2-9   The tube is positioned so that the cuff is below the vocal cords, and the laryngoscope is removed.

FIGURE 2-8   The tube is advanced through the vocal cords into the trachea.

Procedure for Performing Endotracheal Intubation—*Continued*

Steps	Rationale	Special Considerations
22. Confirm endotracheal tube placement while manually bagging with 100% oxygen.	Ensures correct placement of endotracheal tube.	
A. Auscultate over epigastrium. **(Level D*)**	Allows for identification of esophageal intubation.[1,4]	If air movement or gurgling is heard, esophageal intubation has occurred. The tube must be removed and intubation reattempted. Improper insertion may result in hypoxemia, gastric distention, vomiting, and aspiration.
B. Auscultate lung bases and apices for bilateral breath sounds. **(Level D)**	Assists in verification of correct tube placement into the trachea. A right main stem bronchus intubation results in diminished left-sided breath sounds.[4]	Equal breath sounds indicate proper placement of the endotracheal tube.
C. Observe for symmetrical chest wall movement. **(Level D)**	Assists in verification of correct tube placement.[4]	Absence may indicate right main stem or esophageal intubation.
D. Attach disposable end-tidal CO_2 detector. Watch for color change, which indicates the presence of CO_2. **(Level B*)**	Disposable CO_2 detectors may be used to assist with identification of proper tube placement.[5,6,8,11,13,15] Detection of CO_2 confirms proper endotracheal tube placement into the trachea.[4]	CO_2 detectors usually are placed between the self-inflating manual resuscitation bag-valve device and the endotracheal tube. CO_2 detectors should be used in conjunction with physical assessment findings.
or Attach continuous end-tidal CO_2 monitor and watch for detection of CO_2.	During cardiac arrest (nonperfusing rhythms), low pulmonary blood flow may cause insufficient expired CO_2.[14]	
or Consider use of esophageal detection device in cardiac arrest. **(Level B)**	CO_2 detected with an end-tidal CO_2 detector is a reliable indicator of proper tube placement. If CO_2 is not detected, use of an esophageal detector device is recommended.[3,7,10,11,15]	During cardiac arrest (nonperfusing rhythms), low pulmonary blood flow may cause insufficient expired CO_2.[14]

*Level B: Well-designed, controlled studies with results that consistently support a specific action, intervention, or treatment
*Level D: Peer-reviewed professional organizational standards with clinical studies to support recommendations

Procedure for Performing Endotracheal Intubation—*Continued*

Steps	Rationale	Special Considerations
E. Evaluate oxygen saturation (SpO_2) with noninvasive pulse oximetry. (**Level D***)	SpO_2 decreases if the esophagus has been inadvertently intubated. The value may or may not change in a right main stem bronchus intubation.[1,4]	SpO_2 findings should be used in conjunction with physical assessment findings.
23. If CO_2 detection, assessment findings, or SpO_2 reveals that the tube is not correctly positioned, deflate cuff and remove tube immediately. Ventilate and hyperoxygenate with 100% oxygen for 3 to 5 minutes, then reattempt intubation, beginning with Step 12. (**Level D**)	Esophageal intubation results in gas flow diversion and hypoxemia.[1,4]	
24. If breath sounds are absent on the left, deflate the cuff and withdraw tube 1 to 2 cm. Reevaluate for correct tube placement (**Step 21**).	Absence of breath sounds on the left may indicate right main stem intubation, which is common because of the anatomic position of the right main stem bronchi. When correctly positioned, the tube tip should be halfway between the vocal cords and the carina.[3]	
25. Connect endotracheal tube to oxygen source, self-inflating manual resuscitation bag-valve device, or mechanical ventilator, using swivel adapter.	Reduces motion on tube and mouth or nares.	
26. Insert a bite-block or oropharyngeal airway (to act as a bite-block) along the endotracheal tube, with oral intubation.	Prevents the patient from biting down on the endotracheal tube.	The bite-block should be secured separately from the tube to prevent dislodgment of the tube.
27. Secure the endotracheal tube in place (according to institutional standard). (**Level D**)	Prevents inadvertent dislodgment of tube.[2,4,8]	
Use of Commercially Available Endotracheal Tube Holder		
A. Apply according to manufacturer's directions.	Allows for secure stabilization of the tube, decreasing the likelihood of inadvertent extubation.	These holders are recommended over the use of other types of endotracheal tube securing methods, such as taping and tying.[3]
Use of Twill Tape		
A. Double over a 2-ft length of twill tape; tie the tape around the tube, pulling the frayed ends of tape through the looped end; and tie where tube emerges from the lips.	Allows for secure stabilization of the tube, decreasing the likelihood of inadvertent extubation.	
B. Pull the tape ends in opposite directions around the patient's neck.		
C. Tie the two ends of the tape at the side of the patient's neck securely.	Secures tube and prevents direct pressure on back of neck.	

*Level D: Peer-reviewed professional organizational standards with clinical studies to support recommendations

Procedure continues on following page

Procedure for Performing Endotracheal Intubation—*Continued*

Steps	Rationale	Special Considerations
Use of Adhesive Tape		
A. Prepare tape as shown in Fig. 2-10.	Use of a hydrocolloid membrane (e.g., DuoDerm) on the patient's cheeks helps protect the skin.	
B. Secure tube by wrapping double-sided tape around patient's head and torn tape edges around endotracheal tube.		
28. Reevaluate for correct tube placement (**Step 21**).	Verifies that the tube was not inadvertently repositioned during the securing of the tube.	
29. Note position of tube at teeth or gums (use centimeter markings on tube).	Common tube placement at the teeth or gums is 21 cm for women and 23 cm for men.[9]	
30. Hyperoxygenate and suction endotracheal tube and pharynx (see Procedure 12 as needed).	Removes secretions that may obstruct tube or accumulate on the top of the cuff.	
31. Confirmation of correct tube position should be verified with a chest radiograph. (**Level D***)	Chest radiograph documents actual tube location (distance from the carina). Because a chest radiograph is not immediately available, it should not be used as the primary method of tube assessment.[1,4,9]	Endotracheal tubes placed bronchoscopically may not need chest radiograph verification (check institutional standard).
Nasotracheal Intubation		
32. **Follow Steps 1 through 10.**	Steps necessary to initiate nasal intubation. Dentures may be left in place for nasotracheal intubation.	
33. Spray nasal passage with anesthetic and vasoconstrictor, as indicated or ordered.	Anesthetizes and vasoconstricts nasal mucosa to decrease incidence of trauma and bleeding.	
34. Lubricate tube with local anesthetic jelly.	Allows for smooth passage of tube.	
35. Slowly insert tube into selected naris, and guide tube up from the nostril, then backward and down into the nasopharynx.	Tube is introduced into airway channel.	

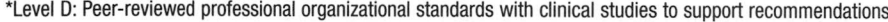

*Level D: Peer-reviewed professional organizational standards with clinical studies to support recommendations

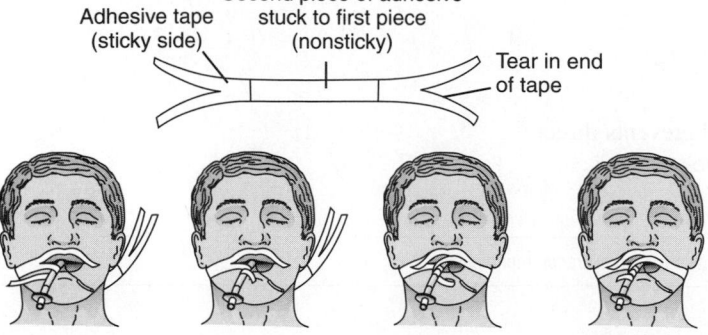

Adhesive tape (sticky side)   Second piece of adhesive stuck to first piece (nonsticky)   Tear in end of tape

FIGURE 2-10   Methods of securing adhesive tape. Example protocol for securing the endotracheal tube with adhesive tape. 1, Clean the patient's skin with mild soap and water. 2, Remove oil from the skin with alcohol and allow to dry. 3, Apply a skin adhesive product to enhance tape adherence. (When tape is removed, an adhesive remover is necessary.) 4, Place a hydrocolloid membrane over the cheeks to protect friable skin. 5, Secure with adhesive tape as shown. (*From Henneman E, Ellstrom K, St John RE: AACN protocols for practice: care of the mechanically ventilated patient series, Aliso Viejo, CA, 1999, American Association of Critical-Care Nurses, 56.*)

Procedure for Performing Endotracheal Intubation—*Continued*

Steps	Rationale	Special Considerations
36. Gently advance the tube until maximal sound of moving air is heard through the tube.	Tube is located at opening of trachea.	Breath sounds become maximal just before entering the glottis.
37. While listening, continue to advance tube during inspiration.	Facilitates movement of tube through glottic opening.	Magill forceps may assist with advancement of tube. Cricoid pressure may help align the glottic opening.
38. When endotracheal tube is placed, inflate cuff.		
39. **Follow Steps 21 through 22 and 27 through 31** to evaluate tube placement and secure tube in place.		
40. Remove protective equipment.	Reduces transmission of microorganisms and body secretions; Standard Precautions.	
41. HH		

Expected Outcomes

- Placement of patent artificial airway
- Properly positioned and secured airway
- Improved oxygenation and ventilation
- Facilitation of secretion clearance

Unexpected Outcomes

- Intubation of esophagus or right main stem bronchus (improper tube placement)
- Accidental extubation
- Cardiac dysrhythmias because of hypoxemia and vagal stimulation
- Broken or dislodged teeth
- Leaking of air from endotracheal tube cuff
- Tracheal injury at tip of tube or at cuff site
- Laryngeal edema
- Vocal cord trauma
- Suctioning of gastric contents or food from endotracheal tube (aspiration)
- Obstruction of endotracheal tube

Patient Monitoring and Care

Steps	Rationale	Reportable Conditions
		These conditions should be reported if they persist despite nursing interventions.
1. Auscultate breath sounds on insertion and every 2 to 4 hours.	Allows for detection of tube movement or dislodgment.	• Absent, decreased, or unequal breath sounds
2. Maintain tube stability, with use of specially manufactured holder, twill tape, or adhesive tape.	Prevents movement and dislodgment of tube.	• Unplanned extubation
3. Monitor and record position of tube at teeth or nose (in reference to centimeter markings on tube).	Provides for identification of tube migration.	• Tube movement from original position
4. Maintain tube cuff pressure at 20 to 25 mm Hg (see Procedure 13).	Provides adequate inflation to decrease aspiration risk and prevents overinflation of cuff to avoid tracheal damage.[1,4]	• Cuff pressure less than 20 to greater than 25 mm Hg

Procedure continues on following page

Patient Monitoring and Care —*Continued*

Steps	Rationale	Reportable Conditions
5. Hyperoxygenate and suction endotracheal tube, as needed (see Procedure 12).	Prevents obstruction of tube and resulting hypoxemia.	• Inability to pass a suction catheter • Copious, frothy, or bloody secretions • Significant change in amount or character of secretions
6. Assess for pain and/or discomfort.	Allows identification of pain and/or discomfort related to the intubation	• Pain not controlled by medications or nursing interventions
7. Inspect nares or oral cavity once per shift while patient is intubated.	Allows for the detection of skin breakdown and necrosis.	• Redness, necrosis, skin breakdown

Documentation

Documentation should include the following:

- Patient and family education
- Measurement of cuff pressure
- Vital signs before, during, and after intubation, including oxygen saturation
- Assessment of breath sounds
- Confirmation of tube placement, including chest radiograph (method of placement confirmation)
- Use of cricoid pressure
- Number of intubation attempts
- Type of intubation: Oral or nasal
- Type and size of blade used
- Occurrence of unexpected outcomes
- Use of any medications

- Nursing interventions
- Size of endotracheal tube
- Secretions
- Depth of endotracheal tube insertion centimeters at teeth, gums, or nose
- Patient response to procedure
- Size of endotracheal tube
- Secretions
- Depth of endotracheal tube insertion: Centimeters at teeth or nose
- Patient response to procedure
- Pain assessment, interventions, and effectiveness

References

1. American Heart Association: Guidelines 2005 American Heart Association guidelines for cardiopulmonary resuscitation and emergency cardiovascular care: adjuncts for airway control and ventilation, *Circulation* 112(Suppl)IV: 51-57, 2005.

CR 2. Barnason S, et al: Comparison of two endotracheal tube securement techniques on unplanned extubation, oral mucosa, and facial skin integrity, *Heart Lung* 27: 409-417, 1998.

CR 3. Bozeman WP, et al: Esophageal detector device versus detection of end-tidal carbon dioxide level in emergency intubation, *Ann Emerg Med* 27:595-599, 1996.

CR 4. Cummins RO, editor: Airway, airway adjuncts, oxygenation, and ventilation. In *ACLS: principles and practice*, Dallas, 2003, American Heart Association, 135-180.

CR 5. Goldberg JS, et al: Colorimetric end-tidal carbon dioxide monitoring for tracheal intubation, *Anesth Analg* 70: 191-194, 1990.

CR 6. Hayden SR, et al: Colorimetric end-tidal CO_2 detector for verification of endotracheal tube placement in out-of-hospital cardiac arrest, *Acad Emerg Med* 2:499-502, 1995.

CR 7. Hendey GW, et al: The esophageal detector bulb in the aeromedical setting, *J Emerg Med* 23:51-55, 2002.

CR 8. Henneman E, Ellstrom E, St John RE: Airway management. In *AACN protocols for practice: care of the mechanically ventilated patient series,* Aliso Viejo, CA, 1999, American Association of Critical-Care Nurses.

CR 9. Holleran RS: *Air and surface patient transport: principles and practice*, ed 3, St Louis, 2003, Mosby.

CR 10. Kasper CL, et al: The self-inflating bulb to detect esophageal intubation during emergency airway management, *Anesthesiology* 88:898-902, 1998.

CR 11. Schaller RJ, et al: Comparison of a colorimetric end-tidal CO_2 detector and an esophageal aspiration device for verifying endotracheal tube placement in the prehospital setting: a six-month experience, *Prehosp Disaster Med* 12:57-63, 1997.

CR 12. Stewart C: Tracheal intubation. In Stewart C, editor: *Advanced airway management*, New Jersey, 2002, Prentice Hall, 76-113.

CR 13. Takeda T, et al: The assessment of three methods to verify tracheal tube placement in the emergency setting, *Resuscitation* 56:153-157, 2003.

CR 14. Varon AJ, et al : Clinical utility of a colorimetricend-tidal CO_2 detector in cardiopulmonary resuscitation and emergency intubation, *J Clin Monit* 7:289-293, 1991.

CR 15. Zaleski L, et al: The esophageal detector device. Does it work? *Anesthesiology* 79:244-247, 1993.

Additional Readings

Committee on Trauma: *American College of Surgeons: advanced trauma life support manual,* Chicago, 2004, American College of Surgeons.

Ellis DY, Harris T, Zideman D: Cricoid pressure in the emergency department rapid sequence tracheal intubation: a risk-benefit analysis, *Ann Emerg Med* 50:653-656, 2007.

Emergency Nurses Association: *Trauma nursing core course: provider manual,* ed 6, Des Plaines, IL, 2007, Emergency Nurses Association.

National Association of Emergency Technicians: *PHTLS: basic and advanced prehospital trauma life support,* ed 5, St Louis, 2003, Mosby.

Roberts JR, Hedges JR, editors: *Clinical procedures in emergency medicine,* ed 4, Philadelphia, 2004, Saunders.

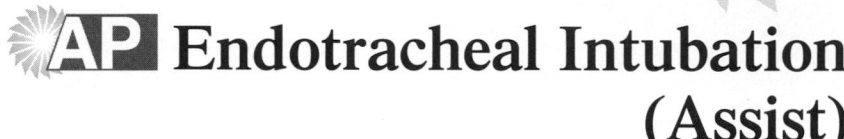

Endotracheal Intubation (Assist)

PURPOSE: Endotracheal intubation is performed to establish and maintain a patent airway, facilitate oxygenation and ventilation, reduce the risk of aspiration, and assist with the clearance of secretions.

Cynthia A. Goodrich

PREREQUISITE NURSING KNOWLEDGE

- Anatomy and physiology of the pulmonary system should be understood.
- Indications for endotracheal intubation include the following[5,12]:
  - Altered mental status (head injury, drug overdose)
  - Anticipated airway obstruction (facial burns, epiglottitis, major facial or oral trauma)
  - Upper airway obstruction (e.g., from swelling, trauma, tumor, bleeding)
  - Apnea
  - Ineffective clearance of secretions (i.e., inability to maintain or protect airway adequately)
  - High risk of aspiration
  - Respiratory distress
- Pulse oximetry should be used during intubation so that oxygen desaturation can be detected quickly.
- Preoxygenation with 100% oxygen and a self-inflating manual resuscitation bag-valve-mask device with a tight-fitting face mask should be performed for 3 to 5 minutes before intubation.

- Intubation attempts should take no longer than 15 to 20 seconds. If more than one intubation is necessary, ventilation with 100% oxygen and a self-inflating manual resuscitation bag-valve-mask device with a tight-fitting face mask should be performed for 3 to 5 minutes before each attempt. If intubation is unsuccessful after three attempts, consider use of other airway options, such as the Combitube or King Airway.
- Application of cricoid pressure (Sellick maneuver) may increase the success of the intubation. This procedure is accomplished with applying firm downward pressure on the cricoid ring, pushing the vocal cords downward so that they are visualized more easily. *Once begun, cricoid pressure must be maintained until intubation is completed* (see Fig. 2-1).
- Two types of laryngoscope blades exist: straight and curved. The straight (Miller) blade is designed so that the tip extends below the epiglottis, to lift and expose the glottic opening. The straight blade is recommended for use in obese patients, pediatric patients, and patients with short necks because their tracheas may be located more anteriorly. When a curved (Macintosh) blade is used, the tip is advanced into the vallecula (the space between the epiglottis and the base of the tongue), to expose the glottic opening.
- Laryngoscope blades are available with fiberoptic light delivery systems. These systems provide a brighter light

than bulbs, which can become scratched or covered with secretions.

- Endotracheal tube size reflects the size of the internal diameter of the tube. Tubes range in size from 2.5 mm for neonates to 9 mm for large adults. Endotracheal tubes that range in size from 7 to 7.5 mm are used for average-sized adult women, whereas endotracheal tubes that range in size from 8 to 9 mm are used for average-sized adult men (see Fig. 2-2).[8,9,12] The tube with the largest clinically acceptable internal diameter should be used to minimize airway resistance and assist in suctioning.[4]
- Endotracheal intubation can be done via nasal or oral routes. The skill of the practitioner who performs the intubation and the patient's clinical condition determine the route used.
- Nasal intubation is relatively contraindicated in trauma patients with facial fractures or suspected fractures at the base of the skull and after cranial surgeries, such as transnasal hypophysectomy.
- In patients with suspected spinal cord injuries, in-line cervical immobilization of the head must be maintained during endotracheal intubation.
- Improper intubation technique may result in trauma to the teeth, soft tissues of the mouth or nose, vocal cords, and posterior pharynx.
- Primary and secondary confirmation of endotracheal intubation should be performed.[1,4]
  - ❖ Primary confirmation of proper endotracheal tube placement includes visualization of the tube passing through the vocal cords, absence of gurgling over the epigastric area, auscultation of bilateral breath sounds, bilateral chest rise and fall during ventilation, and mist in the tube.
  - ❖ Secondary confirmation of proper endotracheal tube placement is necessary to protect against unrecognized esophageal intubation. Methods include use of disposable end-tidal carbon dioxide (CO_2) detectors, continuous end-tidal CO_2 monitors, and esophageal detection devices.
- End-tidal CO_2 ($Petco_2$) monitoring devices have been shown to be reliable indicators of expired CO_2 in patients with perfusing rhythms.[1,5,11,13,15] During cardiac arrest (nonperfusing rhythms), low pulmonary blood flow may cause insufficient expired CO_2.[14] CO_2 detected with an end-tidal CO_2 detector is a reliable indicator of proper tube placement.[6] If CO_2 is not detected, use of an esophageal detector device is recommended.[1,3,11,15]
- Disposable end-tidal CO_2 detectors are chemically treated with a nontoxic indicator that changes color in the presence of CO_2 and indicates that the endotracheal tube has been placed successfully into the trachea.
- Continuous end-tidal CO_2 monitors may be used to confirm proper endotracheal tube placement after intubation attempts and allow for the detection of future tube dislodgment.
- Esophageal detector devices work by creating suction at the end of the endotracheal tube with compressing a flexible bulb or pulling back on a syringe plunger. When the

tube is placed correctly in the trachea, air allows for reexpansion of the bulb or movement of the syringe plunger. If the tube is located in the esophagus, no movement of the syringe plunger or reexpansion of the bulb is seen. These devices may be misleading in patients who are morbidly obese, patients in status asthmaticus, patients late in pregnancy, or patients with large amounts of tracheal secretions.[1]

- Double-lumen endotracheal tubes are used for independent lung ventilation in situations with bleeding of one lung or a large air leak that would impair ventilation of the good lung.
- The endotracheal tube also provides a route for the administration of emergency medication (e.g., lidocaine, epinephrine, atropine, and naloxone), when no other routes of administration are available.[4]

EQUIPMENT

- Personal protective equipment, including eye protection
- Endotracheal tube with intact cuff and 15-mm connector (women, 7-mm to 7.5-mm tube; men, 8-mm to 9-mm tube)
- Laryngoscope handle with fresh batteries
- Laryngoscope blades (straight and curved)
- Spare bulb for laryngoscope blades
- Flexible stylet
- Self-inflating manual resuscitation bag-valve-mask device connected to supplemental oxygen ($\geq$15 L/min)
- Oxygen source and connecting tubes
- Swivel adapter (for attachment to resuscitation bag or ventilator)
- Luer-tip 10-mL syringe for cuff inflation
- Water-soluble lubricant
- Rigid pharyngeal suction-tip (Yankauer) catheter
- Suction apparatus (portable or wall)
- Suction catheters
- Bite-block or oropharyngeal airway
- Endotracheal tube–securing apparatus or appropriate tape
  - ❖ Commercially available endotracheal tube holder
  - ❖ Adhesive tape (6 to 8 inches long)
  - ❖ Twill tape (cut into 30-inch lengths)
- Stethoscope
- Monitoring equipment: continuous oxygen saturation and cardiac rhythm
- Secondary confirmation device: Disposable end-tidal CO_2 detector, continuous end-tidal CO_2 monitoring device, or esophageal detection device
- Drugs for intubation as indicated (sedation, paralyzing agents, lidocaine, atropine)
- Additional equipment, to have available as needed, includes the following:
  - ❖ Anesthetic spray (nasal approach)
  - ❖ Local anesthetic jelly (nasal approach)
  - ❖ Magill forceps (to remove foreign bodies obstructing the airway)
  - ❖ Ventilator

PATIENT AND FAMILY EDUCATION

- Assess patient's and family's level of understanding about condition and rationale for endotracheal intubation. ➤*Rationale:* This assessment identifies the patient's and family's knowledge deficits concerning the patient's condition, the procedure, the expected benefits, and the potential risks. It also allows time for questions to clarify information and voice concerns. Explanations decrease patient anxiety and enhance cooperation.
- Explain the procedure and the reason for intubation, if the clinical situation permits. If not, explain the procedure and reason for the intubation after it is completed. ➤*Rationale:* This explanation enhances patient and family understanding and decreases anxiety.
- If indicated and the clinical situation permits, explain the patient's role in assisting with insertion of endotracheal tube. ➤*Rationale:* This information elicits the patient's cooperation, which assists with insertion.
- Explain that the patient will be unable to speak while the endotracheal tube is in place but that other means of communication will be provided. ➤*Rationale:* This information enhances patient and family understanding and decreases anxiety.
- Explain that the patient's hands often are immobilized to prevent accidental dislodgment of the tube. ➤*Rationale:* This explanation enhances patient and family understanding and decreases anxiety.

PATIENT ASSESSMENT AND PREPARATION

Patient Assessment

- Verify correct patient with two identifiers. ➤*Rationale:* Prior to performing a procedure, the nurse should ensure the correct identification of the patient for the intended intervention.
- Assess immediate history of trauma with suspected spinal cord injury or cranial surgery. ➤*Rationale:* Knowledge of pertinent patient history allows for selection of the most appropriate method for intubation, which helps reduce the risk for secondary injury.
- Assess nothing-by-mouth (NPO) status, the use of a self-inflating manual resuscitation bag-valve-mask-device, and signs of gastric distention. ➤*Rationale:* Increased risk of aspiration and vomiting occurs with accumulation of air (from the use of a self-inflating manual resuscitation bag-valve-mask device), food, or secretions. If a patient who has gastric distention or who has eaten recently needs to be intubated, anticipate the need to use cricoid pressure to decrease the risk of aspiration.
- Assess level of consciousness, level of anxiety, and respiratory difficulty. ➤*Rationale:* This assessment determines need for sedation or use of paralytic agents and the patient's ability to lie flat and supine for intubation.
- Assess oral cavity for presence of dentures, loose teeth, or other possible obstructions and remove if appropriate.

- Assess vital signs and for the following:
  - ❖ Tachypnea
  - ❖ Dyspnea
  - ❖ Shallow respirations
  - ❖ Cyanosis
  - ❖ Apnea
  - ❖ Altered level of consciousness
  - ❖ Tachycardia
  - ❖ Cardiac dysrhythmias
  - ❖ Hypertension
  - ❖ Headache
- ➤*Rationale:* Any of these conditions may indicate a problem with oxygenation or ventilation or both.
- Assess patency of nares (for nasal intubation). ➤*Rationale:* Selection of the most appropriate naris facilitates insertion and may improve patient tolerance of tube.
- Assess need for premedication. ➤*Rationale:* Various medications provide sedation or paralysis of the patient as needed.

Patient Preparation

- Perform a pre-procedure verification and time out, if nonemergent. ➤*Rationale:* Ensures patient safety.
- Ensure that the patient understands preprocedural teachings, if appropriate. Answer questions as they arise, and reinforce information as needed. ➤*Rationale:* Understanding of previously taught information is evaluated and reinforced.
- Before intubation, initiate intravenous or intraosseous access. ➤*Rationale:* Readily available intravenous or intraosseous access may be necessary if the patient needs to be sedated or paralyzed or needs other medications because of a negative response to the intubation procedure.
- Position the patient appropriately.
  - ❖ Positioning of the nontrauma patient is as follows: Place the patient supine with the head in the sniffing position, in which the head is extended and the neck is flexed. Placement of a small towel under the occiput elevates it several inches, allowing for proper flexion of the neck (see Fig. 2-3). ➤*Rationale:* Placement of the head in the sniffing position allows for visualization of the larynx and vocal cords by aligning the axes of the mouth, pharynx, and trachea.
  - ❖ Positioning of the trauma patient is as follows: Manual in-line cervical spinal immobilization must be maintained during the entire process of intubation. ➤*Rationale:* Because cervical spinal cord injury must be suspected in all trauma patients until proved otherwise, this position helps prevent secondary injury should a cervical spine injury be present.
- Premedicate as indicated. ➤*Rationale:* Appropriate premedication allows for more controlled intubation, reducing the incidence of insertion trauma, aspiration, laryngospasm, and improper tube placement.
- As appropriate, notify the respiratory therapy department of impending intubation so that a ventilator can be set up. ➤*Rationale:* Ventilator is set up before intubation.

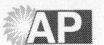

Procedure　for Performing Endotracheal Intubation

Steps	Rationale	Special Considerations
General Setup		
1. 🅷🅷		
2. 🅿🅴	Protective eyewear should be worn to avoid exposure to secretions.	
3. Attach patient to pulse oximeter and cardiac monitor.		
4. Set up suction apparatus, and connect rigid suction-tip catheter to tubing.	Prepares for oropharyngeal suctioning as needed.	
5. Check equipment.		
A. Use 10-mL syringe to inflate cuff on tube, assessing for leaks. Completely deflate cuff.	Verifies that equipment is functional and that tube cuff is patent without leaks; prepares tube for insertion.	
B. Insert the stylet into the endotracheal tube, ensuring that the tip of the stylet does not extend past the end of the endotracheal tube.		Stylet must be recessed by at least 0.5 inch from the distal end of the tube so that it does not protrude beyond the end of the tube, resulting in damage to the vocal cords and trachea.
C. Connect the laryngoscope blade to the handle, and check the bulb for brightness.	Verifies that the equipment is functional.	
6. Assist in positioning the patient's head by flexing the neck forward and extending the head in sniffing position (only if neck trauma is not suspected; see Fig. 2-3). If spinal trauma is suspected, maintain the head in a neutral position with in-line spinal immobilization.	Allows for visualization of the vocal cords by aligning the mouth, pharynx, and trachea.	Placement of a small towel under the occiput elevates it, allowing for proper neck flexion. *Do not flex or extend neck of patient with suspected spinal cord injury; the head must be maintained in a neutral position with manual in-line cervical spine immobilization.*
7. Check the mouth for dentures and remove if present. Suction the mouth and pharynx as needed.	Dentures should be removed before oral intubation is attempted but may remain in place for nasal intubation.	
8. Insert oropharyngeal airway as indicated (see Procedure 11).	Assists in maintaining upper airway patency.	Use only in unconscious patients.
9. Preoxygenate for 3 to 5 minutes, with 100% oxygen via a nonrebreather mask if ventilations are adequate or via a self-inflating manual resuscitation bag-valve-mask device (see Procedure 32 if ventilations are not adequate). Provide frequent and gentle ventilations.	Helps prevent hypoxemia. Gentle breaths reduce incidence of air entering stomach (leading to gastric distention), decrease airway turbulence, and distribute ventilation more evenly within the lungs.	If patient is breathing, avoid positive-pressure ventilation with a self-inflating manual resuscitation bag-valve-mask device because of risk for gastric distention, aspiration, and vomiting.
10. Premedicate patient as directed by the practitioner.		
11. Remove oropharyngeal airway if present.		
12. Have self-inflating manual resuscitation bag-valve-mask device connected to 100% oxygen source and face mask ready for hyperoxygenation and manual ventilation.	Intubation attempts should not take longer than 30 seconds. Patients need to be hyperoxygenated and ventilated between intubation attempts.[4]	

Procedure continues on following page

Procedure | for Performing Endotracheal Intubation—*Continued*

Steps	Rationale	Special Considerations
13. Apply cricoid pressure as directed by the practitioner who performs the intubation.	Moves the trachea toward the posterior, which provides better visualization of the vocal cords by the practitioner.	*Once cricoid pressure is applied, it must be maintained until the intubation is completed.*
14. Once tube has been correctly placed, assist with cuff inflation as directed. Inflate cuff with 5 to 10 mL of air depending on the manufacturer's recommendations.	Inflation volumes vary depending on manufacturer and size of tube. Keep cuff pressure between 20 and 25 mm Hg to decrease risk of aspiration and prevent ischemia and decreased blood flow.[1,4]	In adults, the minimal intracuff pressure to prevent aspiration is 25 mm Hg. Decreased mucosal capillary blood flow (ischemia) results when pressure is greater than 40 mm Hg.[4]
15. Once endotracheal tube has been placed, assist with tube placement confirmation while bagging with 100% oxygen.	Ensures correct placement of endotracheal tube.	
A. Auscultate over epigastrium. (**Level D***)	Allows for identification of esophageal intubation.[1,4]	If air movement or gurgling is heard, esophageal intubation has occurred. The tube must be removed and intubation reattempted. Improper insertion may result in hypoxemia, gastric distention, vomiting, and aspiration.
B. Auscultate lung bases and apices for bilateral breath sounds. (**Level D**)	Assists in verification of correct tube placement into the trachea. A right main-stem bronchus intubation results in diminished left-sided breath sounds.[4]	Equal breath sounds indicate proper placement of the endotracheal tube.
C. Observe for symmetric chest wall movement. (**Level D**)	Assists in verification of correct tube placement.[4]	Absence may indicate right main-stem or esophageal intubation.
D. Attach disposable end-tidal CO_2 detector. Watch for color change, indicating the presence of CO_2. (**Level B***)	Disposable CO_2 detectors may be used to assist with identification of proper tube placement.[4-6,11-13] Detection of CO_2 confirms proper endotracheal tube placement into the trachea.[4]	CO_2 detectors usually are placed between the self-inflating-manual resuscitation bag-valve device and the endotracheal tube. CO_2 detectors should be used in conjunction with physical assessment findings.
or Attach continuous end-tidal CO_2 monitor and watch for detection of CO_2.		During cardiac arrest (nonperfusing rhythms), low pulmonary blood flow may cause insufficient expired CO_2.[14]
or Consider use of esophageal detection device in cardiac arrest. (**Level B**)	CO_2 is detected with an end-tidal CO_2 detector is a reliable indicator of proper tube placement. If CO_2 is not detected, use of an esophageal detector device is recommended.[3,7,10,11,15]	During cardiac arrest (nonperfusing rhythms), low pulmonary blood flow may cause insufficient expired CO_2.[14]
E. Evaluate oxygen saturation (SpO_2) with noninvasive pulse oximetry. (**Level D**)	SpO_2 decreases if the esophagus has been inadvertently intubated. The value may or may not change in a right main-stem bronchus intubation.[1,4]	SpO_2 findings should be used in conjunction with physical assessment findings.

*Level B: Well-designed, controlled studies with results that consistently support a specific action, intervention, or treatment
*Level D: Peer-reviewed professional organizational standards with clinical studies to support recommendations

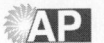

Procedure for Performing Endotracheal Intubation—*Continued*

Steps	Rationale	Special Considerations
16. If CO_2 detection, assessment findings, or Spo_2 reveals that the tube is not correctly positioned, deflate cuff and remove tube immediately. Ventilate and hyperoxygenate with 100% oxygen for 3 to 5 minutes, then reattempt intubation, beginning with Step 12. **(Level D*)**	Esophageal intubation results in gas flow diversion and hypoxemia.[1,4]	
17. If breath sounds are absent on the left, deflate the cuff and withdraw tube 1 to 2 cm. Reevaluate for correct tube placement **(Step 15)**.		Absence of breath sounds on the left may indicate right main-stem intubation, which is common because of the anatomic position of the right main-stem bronchi. When correctly positioned, the tube tip should be halfway between the vocal cords and the carina.[3]
18. Connect endotracheal tube to oxygen source, self-inflating manual resuscitation bag-valve device, or mechanical ventilator, using swivel adapter.	Reduces motion on tube and mouth or nares.	
19. Insert a bite-block or oropharyngeal airway (to act as a bite-block) along the endotracheal tube, with oral intubation.	Prevents the patient from biting down on the endotracheal tube.	The bite-block should be secured separately from the tube to prevent dislodgment of the tube.
20. Secure the endotracheal tube in place (according to institutional standard). **(Level D)**	Prevents inadvertent dislodgment of tube.[2,4,8]	Various methods are used for securing endotracheal tubes, including the use of specially manufactured tube holders, twill tape, or adhesive tape.
Use of Commercially Available Endotracheal Tube Holder		
A. Apply according to manufacturer's directions.	Allows for secure stabilization of the tube, decreasing the likelihood of inadvertent extubation.	
Use of Twill Tape		
A. Double over a 2-ft length of twill tape; tie the tape around the tube, pulling the frayed ends of tape through the looped end; and tie where tube emerges from the lips.	Allows for secure stabilization of the tube, decreasing the likelihood of inadvertent extubation.	
B. Pull the tape ends in opposite directions around the patient's neck.		
C. Tie the two ends of the tape at the side of the patient's neck securely.	Secures tube and prevents direct pressure on back of neck.	
Use of Adhesive Tape		
A. Prepare tape as shown in Fig. 2-10.	Use of a hydrocolloid membrane (e.g., DuoDerm) on the patient's cheeks helps protect the skin.	
B. Secure tube by wrapping double-sided tape around patient's head and torn tape edges around endotracheal tube.		

*Level D: Peer-reviewed professional organizational standards with clinical studies to support recommendations

Procedure continues on following page

Procedure for Performing Endotracheal Intubation—*Continued*

Steps	Rationale	Special Considerations
21. Reevaluate for correct tube placement (**Step 15**).	Verifies that the tube was not inadvertently repositioned during the securing of the tube.	
22. Note position of tube at teeth, gums, or naris (use centimeter markings on tube).		Common tube placement for oral intubation at the teeth or gums is 21 cm for women and 23 cm for men.[9]
23. Hyperoxygenate and suction endotracheal tube and pharynx (see Procedure 12) as needed.	Removes secretions that may obstruct tube or accumulate on the top of the cuff.	
24. Confirmation of correct tube position should be verified with a chest radiograph. (**Level D***)	Chest radiograph documents actual tube location (distance from the carina). Because a chest radiograph is not immediately available, it should not be used as the primary method of tube assessment.[1,4,9]	Endotracheal tubes placed bronchoscopically may not necessitate chest radiograph verification (check institutional standard).
25. Remove protective equipment.	Reduces transmission of microorganisms and body secretions; Standard Precautions.	
26. 🅷🅷		

*Level D: Peer-reviewed professional organizational standards with clinical studies to support recommendations

Expected Outcomes

• Placement of patent artificial airway

• Properly positioned and secured airway
• Improved oxygenation and ventilation

• Facilitation of secretion clearance

Unexpected Outcomes

• Intubation of esophagus or right main stem bronchus (improper tube placement)
• Accidental extubation
• Cardiac dysrhythmias because of hypoxemia and vagal stimulation
• Broken or dislodged teeth
• Leaking of air from endotracheal tube cuff
• Tracheal injury at tip of tube or at cuff site
• Laryngeal edema
• Vocal cord trauma
• Suctioning of gastric contents or food from endotracheal tube (aspiration)
• Obstruction of endotracheal tube

Patient Monitoring and Care

Steps	Rationale	Reportable Conditions
		These conditions should be reported if they persist despite nursing interventions.
1. Auscultate breath sounds on insertion and every 2 to 4 hours.	Allows for detection of tube movement or dislodgment.	Absent, decreased, or unequal breath sounds
2. Maintain tube stability, with specially manufactured holder, twill tape, or adhesive tape.	Prevents movement and dislodgment of tube.	Unplanned extubation
3. Monitor and record position of tube at teeth or nose (in reference to centimeter markings on tube).	Provides for identification of tube migration.	Tube movement from original position

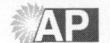

Patient Monitoring and Care —*Continued*

Steps	Rationale	Reportable Conditions
4. Maintain tube cuff pressure at 20 to 25 mm Hg (see Procedure 13).	Provides adequate inflation to decrease aspiration risk and prevents overinflation of cuff to avoid tracheal damage.[1,4]	Cuff pressure less than 20 to greater than 25 mm Hg
5. Hyperoxygenate and suction endotracheal tube, as needed (see Procedure 12).	Prevents obstruction of tube and resulting hypoxemia.	Inability to pass a suction catheter Copious, frothy, or bloody secretions Significant change in amount or character of secretions
6. Assess for pain and/or discomfort.	Allows identification of pain and/or discomfort related to the intubation	Pain not controlled by medications or nursing interventions
7. Inspect nares or oral cavity once per shift while patient is intubated.	Allows for the detection of skin breakdown and necrosis.	Redness, necrosis, skin breakdown

Documentation

Documentation should include the following:

- Patient and family education
- Measurement of cuff pressure
- Vital signs before, during, and after intubation, including oxygen saturation
- Assessment of breath sounds
- Confirmation of tube placement, including chest radiograph (method of placement confirmation)
- Use of cricoid pressure
- Number of intubation attempts
- Type of intubation: Oral or nasal

- Type and size of blade used
- Occurrence of unexpected outcomes
- Use of any medications
- Nursing interventions
- Size of endotracheal tube
- Depth of endotracheal tube insertion centimeters at teeth, gums, or nose
- Patient response to procedure
- Pain assessment, interventions, and effectiveness

References

1. American Heart Association: Guidelines 2005 American Heart Association guidelines for cardiopulmonary resuscitation and emergency cardiovascular care: adjuncts for airway control and ventilation, *Circulation* 112(Suppl)IV: 51-57, 2005.
CR 2. Barnason S, et al: Comparison of two endotracheal tube securement techniques on unplanned extubation, oral mucosa, and facial skin integrity, *Heart Lung* 27:409-417, 1998.
CR 3. Bozeman WP, et al: Esophageal detector device versus detection of end-tidal carbon dioxide level in emergency intubation, *Ann Emerg Med* 27:595-599, 1996.
CR 4. Cummins RO, editor: Airway, airway adjuncts, oxygenation, and ventilation. In *ACLS: principles and practice,* Dallas, 2003, American Heart Association, 135-180.
CR 5. Goldberg JS, et al: Colorimetric end-tidal carbon dioxide monitoring for tracheal intubation, *Anesth Analg* 70: 191-194, 1990.
CR 6. Hayden SR, et al: Colorimetric end-tidal CO₂ detector for verification of endotracheal tube placement in out-of-hospital cardiac arrest, *Acad Emerg Med* 2:499-502, 1995.
CR 7. Hendey GW, et al: The esophageal detector bulb in the aeromedical setting, *J Emerg Med* 23:51-55, 2002.

CR 8. Henneman E, Ellstrom E, St John RE: Airway management. In *AACN protocols for practice: care of the mechanically ventilated patient series,* Aliso Viejo, CA, 1999, American Association of Critical-Care Nurses.
CR 9. Holleran RS: *Air and surface patient transport: principles and practice,* ed 3, St Louis, 2003, Mosby.
CR 10. Kasper CL, et al: The self-inflating bulb to detect esophageal intubation during emergency airway management, *Anesthesiology* 88:898-902, 1998.
CR 11. Schaller RJ, et al: Comparison of a colorimetric end-tidal CO₂ detector and an esophageal aspiration device for verifying endotracheal tube placement in the prehospital setting: a six-month experience, *Prehosp Disaster Med* 12:57-63, 1997.
CR 12. Stewart C: Tracheal intubation. In: Stewart C, editor: *Advanced airway management,* NJ, 2002, Prentice Hall, 76-113.
CR 13. Takeda T, et al: The assessment of three methods to verify tracheal tube placement in the emergency setting, *Resuscitation* 56:153-157, 2003.
CR 14. Varon AJ, et al: Clinical utility of a colorimetricend-tidal CO₂ detector in cardiopulmonary resuscitation and emergency intubation, *J Clin Monit* 7:289-293, 1991.
CR 15. Zaleski L, et al: The esophageal detector device: does it work? *Anesthesiology* 79:244-247, 1993.

Additional Readings

Committee on Trauma: *American College of Surgeons: advanced trauma life support manual,* Chicago, 2004, American College of Surgeons.

Ellis DY, Harris T, Zideman D: Cricoid pressure in the emergency department rapid sequence tracheal intubation: a risk-benefit analysis, *Ann Emerg Med* 50:653-656, 2007.

Emergency Nurses Association: *Trauma nursing core course: provider manual,* ed 6, Des Plaines, IL, 2007, Emergency Nurses Association.

National Association of Emergency Technicians: *PHTLS: basic and advanced prehospital trauma life support,* ed 5, St Louis, 2003, Mosby.

Roberts JR, Hedges JR, editors: *Clinical procedures in emergency medicine,* ed 4, Philadelphia, 2004, Saunders.

Endotracheal Tube and Oral Care

PURPOSE: Endotracheal tube and oral care is performed to prevent buccal, oropharyngeal, and tracheal trauma from the tube and cuff; to provide oral hygiene; to promote ventilation; and to decrease the risk of ventilator-associated pneumonia.

Kathleen M. Vollman, Mary Lou Sole

PREREQUISITE NURSING KNOWLEDGE

- Anatomy and physiology of the pulmonary system should be understood.
- Anatomy and physiology of the oral cavity and the importance of evidence-based oral hygiene procedures on a regular basis should be understood.[1,18,21,27,49,54]
- Endotracheal (ET) tubes are used to maintain a patent airway or to facilitate mechanical ventilation. The presence of these artificial airways, especially ET tubes, prevents effective coughing and secretion removal, necessitating periodic removal of pulmonary secretions with suctioning.
- Oral care given every 2 to 4 hours appears to provide a greater improvement in oral health. If oral care is not provided for 4 to 6 hours, previous benefits are thought to be lost.[10]
- Suctioning of airways should be performed only for clinical indications and not as a routine fixed-schedule treatment (see Procedure 12). In acute care situations, suctioning is performed as a sterile procedure to prevent healthcare-acquired pneumonia.
- Adequate systemic hydration and supplemental humidification of inspired gases assist in thinning secretions for easier aspiration from airways.[20,36,37,51]

- Appropriate cuff care (see Procedure 13) helps prevent major pulmonary aspirations, prepares for tracheal extubation, decreases the risk of inadvertent extubation, provides a patent airway for ventilation and removal of secretions, and decreases the risk of iatrogenic infections.[5,15,29,37,51]
- Constant pressure from the ET tube on the mouth or nose can cause skin breakdown.
- If the patient is anxious or uncooperative, use of two caregivers for retaping or repositioning the endotracheal tube helps prevent accidental dislodgment of the tube.
- The incidence of ventilator-associated pneumonia (VAP) is increased in patients intubated for longer than 24 hours.[36,37,51]
- Nasotracheal intubation should be avoided because it increases the risk of VAP.[37,51]
- VAP is a risk factor for endotracheal intubation.
  - ❖ VAP is thought to be related to aspiration of gastric or oral secretions and colonization of the mouth related to dental plaque.[14,18,19,37,38,51]
  - ❖ VAP increases not only ventilator and intensive care unit (ICU) days and hospital length of stay, but also overall morbidity and mortality of the critically ill patient.[33,37,39,41,44,47,51,55]

EQUIPMENT

- Goggles or glasses and mask
- Bite-block or oral airway if needed
- Adhesive or twill tape; commercial endotracheal tube holder (design must ensure ability to provide oral care and suctioning)
- 2 × 2 Gauze or cotton swab for cleaning around the nares
- Normal saline solution
- Soft pediatric/adult toothbrush or suction toothbrush
- Toothettes/oral swab/oral suction swab
- Oral cleansing solution (e.g., 1.5% H_2O[2,3,18,31,44,47] chlorhexidine,[3,6,9,16,22,23,26,34,52] cetylpyridinium chloride [CPC],[3,30,43,50] toothpaste[10,24,40])

Additional equipment, to have available as needed, includes the following:

- Closed-suction setup with a catheter of appropriate size (Table 4-1)
- Sterile saline solution lavage containers for cleansing the closed suction system after use (5 to 10 mL)
- Suction catheter for oral and nasal suctioning (single-use Yankauer, covered Yankauer, disposable oral saliva ejector)
- Two sources of suction or a bifurcated connection device attached to a single suction source
- Connecting tube (4 to 6 ft)
- Nonsterile gloves
- Stethoscope

PATIENT AND FAMILY EDUCATION

- Explain the procedure to the patient and family, including the purpose of ET tube care and the importance of comprehensive oral care in prevention of infection.[1] ➦*Rationale:* This step identifies patient and family knowledge deficits concerning patient condition, procedure, expected benefits, and potential risks and allows time for questions to clarify information and voice concerns. Explanations decrease patient anxiety and enhance cooperation.
- If indicated, explain the patient's role in assisting with ET tube care. ➦*Rationale:* Eliciting the patient's cooperation assists with care.
- Explain that the patient will be unable to speak while the ET tube is in place but that other means of communication will be provided. ➦*Rationale:* This information enhances patient and family understanding and decreases anxiety.
- Explain that the patient's hands may be immobilized to prevent accidental dislodgment of the tube. ➦*Rationale:* This information enhances patient and family understanding and decreases anxiety.

PATIENT ASSESSMENT AND PREPARATION

Patient Assessment

- Verify correct patient with two identifiers. ➦*Rationale:* Prior to performing a procedure, the nurse should ensure the correct identification of the patient for the intended intervention.
- Assess for signs and symptoms that indicate that oral cavity and ET tube care is necessary.
  - ❖ Excessive secretions (oral or tracheal)
  - ❖ Dry oral mucosa
  - ❖ Debris in the oral cavity
  - ❖ Plaque buildup on teeth
  - ❖ Soiled tape or ties or commercial device
  - ❖ Patient biting or kinking tube
  - ❖ Pressure areas on nares, corner of mouth, or tongue
  - ❖ ET tube moving in and out of mouth
  - ❖ Patient able to verbalize or audible air leak around ET tube
- ➦*Rationale:* Assessment provides for early recognition that oral or ET tube care is needed.
- Assess level of consciousness and level of anxiety. ➦*Rationale:* This assessment determines the need for sedation during ET tube care and the number of care providers needed to perform the activities.

Patient Preparation

- Ensure that the patient understands preprocedural teachings. Answer questions as they arise and reinforce information as needed. ➦*Rationale:* This process evaluates and reinforces understanding of previously taught information.
- Maintain the patient in a semi-Fowler's (≥30 degrees) position during mechanical ventilation to reduce the risk of aspiration.[13,36,37,51,53] Assist the patient to a high Fowler's position or the most comfortable position for both the patient and nurse before performing the care. ➦*Rationale:* This position promotes comfort and reduces physical strain and maintains head of bed elevation to reduce risk of aspiration.[13,20,36,37,51,53]

TABLE 4-1	Guidelines for Catheter Size for Endotracheal and Tracheostomy Tube Suctioning*

Patient Age	Endotracheal Tube Size (mm)	Tracheostomy Tube Size (mm, inner diameter)	Suction Catheter Size
Small child (2 to 5 y)	4.0 to 5.0	3.5 to 5.5	6F to 8F
School-age child (6 to 12 y)	5.0 to 6.5	4.0 to 6.5	8F to 10F
Adolescent to adult	7.0 to 9.0	5.0 to 9.0	10F to 16F

*This guide should be used as an estimate only. Actual sizes depend on the size and individual needs of the patient.
(From St John RE, Seckel MA: Airway management. In AACN protocols for practice: care of the mechanically ventilated patient series, ed 2, Aliso Viejo, CA, 2002, American Association of Critical-Care Nurses.)

Procedure for Endotracheal Tube and Oral Care

Steps	Rationale	Special Considerations
1. **HH**		
2. **PE**		
3. Ensure that ET tube is connected to the ventilator with a swivel adapter.	Decreases pressure exerted by ventilator tubing on the endotracheal tube, thereby minimizing risk of pressure ulceration.	
4. Support the ET tube and tubing as needed.		
5. If suctioning is clinically indicated, hyperoxygenate before ET suction and between attempts (see Procedure 12).	Suctioning of airways should be performed only for a clinical indication and not as a routine fixed-schedule treatment. Removes secretions that may obstruct tube.	
6. If patient is nasally intubated, clean around ET tube with saline solution–soaked gauze or cotton swabs. **Proceed to Step 7.**	Removes secretions that could cause pressure and subsequent skin breakdown.	The Centers for Disease Control and Prevention (CDC) and American Thoracic Society guidelines for prevention of VAP recommend that patients intubated nasally be reintubated orally as soon as possible to reduce the risk of VAP.[40,51]
7. If patient is intubated orally, remove bite-block or oropharyngeal airway (acting as bite-block) before proceeding with oral hygiene.	The bite-block or oropharyngeal airway prevents the patient from biting down on the endotracheal tube and occluding airflow.[7]	The bite-block should be secured separately from the tube to prevent dislodgment of the ET tube. The bite-block or ET securing mechanism may be a barrier to providing good oral care.
8. Initiate oral hygiene with a pediatric or adult (soft) toothbrush, at least twice a day. Gently brush patient's teeth to clean and remove plaque from teeth. Suction oropharyngeal secretions after brushing. Use toothpaste or a cleansing solution that assists in the breakdown of debris.	Mechanical cleansing and oral hygiene reduce oropharyngeal colonization and dental plaque, which is associated with VAP.[14,17,18,24,32,37,40,42,43] Toothpaste or cleansing solution should contain additives that assist in the breakdown of mucus in the mouth. Sodium bicarbonate assists in removal of debris accumulation on oral tissue and teeth.[21]	Pediatric or soft-bristle toothbrushes may be easier to use in adult intubated patients.[33,54]
9. In addition to brushing twice daily, use oral swabs with a 1.5% hydrogen peroxide solution to clean mouth every 2 to 4 hours. Suction oropharyngeal secretions after cleansing. After each cleansing, apply a mouth moisturizer to the oral mucosa and lips to keep tissue moist. **(Level C*)**	Oral cleansing, suctioning, and moisturizing every 2 to 4 hours is a part of comprehensive oral care that has shown to improve oral health and reduce the risk of healthcare-acquired pneumonia.[10,18,44,45,47,51,54] Most studies support the safety and efficacy of greater than 1% and less than 3% H_2O_2 as a cleanser for plaque removal and maintaining overall gingival health.[31,44,45,47] Saliva serves a protective function. Mechanical ventilation causes drying of the oral mucosa, affecting salivary flow and contributing to mucositis and regions for bacterial deposits and growth.[17,18,33]	Foam swabs are effective in stimulating mucosal tissue but less effective in plaque removal.[10,29,40] Implementation of a comprehensive oral care program is recommended by the CDC to reduce VAP.[51] Use of mouthwash as a cleansing agent is not recommended.[18]

*Level C: Qualitative studies, descriptive or correlational studies, integrative reviews, systematic reviews, or randomized controlled trials with inconsistent results

Procedure continues on following page

Procedure for Endotracheal Tube and Oral Care—*Continued*

Steps	Rationale	Special Considerations
10. Suction oral cavity and pharynx frequently. (Continuous subglottic suctioning: **Level B***). (Intermittent suctioning: **Level C***)	Removes secretions that may accumulate on top of the cuff and cause microaspiration.[4,5,8,44,47] Continuous subglottic suctioning with a specially designed endotracheal tube has been shown to reduce VAP.[8,11,20,29,36,37,46,51] Intermittent deep oral cleansing with a disposable or covered catheter as a part of a comprehensive oral care program has been shown to reduce VAP in a quality improvement project.[18,44,47]	Oral suction equipment and suction tubing should be changed every 24 hours. Nondisposable, noncovered oral suction apparatus has been shown to be colonized with microorganisms present in the oral cavity.[48] Nondisposable oral suction apparatus should be rinsed with sterile isotonic sodium chloride solution after each use and placed on a paper towel if not disposable or covered.[18,44,48,51] Covered oral suction appartus should be rinsed with sterile or distilled water and cover put back in place.[18,44,48,51] Placement of tonsil suction back into the package is associated with greater colonization.[18,48,51] Disconnection of a closed suction system to provide oral suctioning may contribute to increased bacterial colonization at the point of the disconnection.[18,33,48]
11. Antiseptic oral rinses (chlorhexidine, cetylpyridinium chloride [CPC], added after brushing or done in conjunction with comprehensive oral care did achieve elimination of VAP.[28,29] **(Level B)**	Latest data show that 2% and 0.12% chlorhexidine gluconate with a twice-daily application to the oral cavity within a 2-hour time period from brushing has reduced VAP rates.[3,6,9,16,20,22,23,26,28,34,51,52] CPC has been shown to be an effective solution in the removal of plaque and prevention of gingivitis.[3,30,43,50] Mechanically ventilated patients who received a 20-fold diluted povidone-iodine swab/gargle and toothbrushing three times daily showed a significant reduction in VAP.[32]	More frequent use of antiseptics than recommended may result in greater discoloration of the teeth.[18,30,42]
12. Move oral tube to the other side of the mouth. Replace bite-block or oropharyngeal airway (to act as bite-block) along the endotracheal tube if necessary to prevent biting. If deflation of the cuff is necessary to move from one side of the mouth to the other, deep oral suctioning should be performed before deflation. **(Level C)**	Prevents or minimizes pressure areas on lips, tongue, and oral cavity. Deep oral suctioning above the cuff before deflation or position change can reduce the risk of colonized oral secretions being aspirated.[4,51]	

*Level B: Well-designed, controlled studies with results that consistently support a specific action, intervention, or treatment

*Level C: Qualitative studies, descriptive or correlational studies, integrative reviews, systematic reviews, or randomized controlled trials with inconsistent results

Procedure for Endotracheal Tube and Oral Care—*Continued*

Steps	Rationale	Special Considerations
13. After oral hygiene is completed, change the ET securing device with tape, ties, or commercial device. (**Level C***)	The securing mechanism should be changed and moved at least once daily to provide an opportunity for assessment and repositioning of the ET to reduce the risk of a pressure skin injury. If the securing mechanism loosens, more frequent change may be necessary.[25,49] When tape was compared with commercially available devices, tape was superior to three of four devices in withstanding high external forces and was the most cost effective.[2,35]	If the method to secure the endotracheal tube obstructs the ability to provide effective oral care, consider changing the method of securing.
14. Ensure proper cuff inflation (see Procedure 13) with minimal leak volume or minimal occlusion volume. (**Level C**)	Decreases risk of aspiration; ensures airflow to lungs rather than to stomach. The cuff pressure should be maintained at 20 to 30 cm of H_2O and checked on a frequent basis to ensure proper pressure is maintained.[5,15,29,37,51]	
15. Reconfirm tube placement (see Procedure 2), and note position of tube at teeth or nares.	Common tube placement at the teeth is 21 cm for women and 23 cm for men.	
16. Secure the endotracheal tube in place (according to institutional standard; see Procedure 2). (**Level C**)	Prevents inadvertent dislodgment of the tube.[15,24,25,35] Tape has shown to be a safe, cost beneficial, and effective securing mechanism to maintain position and stability of the ET tube. When compared with commercially available devices, tape was superior to three of four devices in withstanding high external forces.[2,35]	Various methods are used for securing endotracheal tubes, including use of specially manufactured tube holder, twill tape, and adhesive tape. The method for securing the endotracheal tube should not interfere with caregivers' ability to provide frequent comprehensive oral care.

*Level C: Qualitative studies, descriptive or correlational studies, integrative reviews, systematic reviews, or randomized controlled trials with inconsistent results

Expected Outcomes

- Patent airway
- Secured endotracheal tube
- Removal of oral secretions
- Intact oral and nasal mucous membranes
- Reduced oral colonization
- Moist pink oral cavity

Unexpected Outcomes

- Dislodged ET tube
- Occluded ET tube
- ET tube cuff leak
- Pressure ulcers in mouth or on the lip or nares
- Ventilator-associated pneumonia

Procedure continues on following page

Patient Monitoring and Care

Steps	Rationale	Reportable Conditions
		These conditions should be reported if they persist despite nursing interventions.
1. Keep head of bed elevated at least 30 degrees, unless contraindicated.[4,13,20,29,36,37,47,51,53,54] **(Level C*)**	Maintaining the head of the bed in an elevated position decreases the risk of aspiration. Contraindications include hemodynamic instability, decreased cerebral perfusion pressure, and patient in the prone position.	
2. Suction endotracheal tube if clinically indicated.	Maintains patent airway.	• Inability to pass suction catheter
3. Monitor amount, type, and color of secretions.		• Change in quantity or characteristics of secretions
4. If patient is nasally intubated, recommend reintubation in the oral cavity. **(Level C)**	Nasal intubation is associated with an increased risk for sinusitis and the potential development of ventilator-associated pneumonia.[20,36,37,51]	• Purulent drainage from the nares or present in the back of the throat.
5. Assess oral cavity and lips every 8 hours, and perform oral care (as outlined in **Steps 7 to 10**) every 2 to 4 hours and as needed. **(Level C)** Brush teeth and tongue every 12 hours.	If oral care is omitted for extended period, previous benefits are lost.[10,18,33,44,47] Early recognition of pressure or drainage allows for prompt intervention.	• Breakdown of lip, tongue, or oral cavity • Presence of mouth sores • Bleeding of the gums during brushing
6. With oral care, assess for buildup of plaque on teeth or potential infection related to oral abscess.	Assessment and removal of plaque decreases bacteria in the mouth.	• Continued plaque buildup on teeth, presence of an abscess
7. Avoid reusing devices unless covered or protected (i.e., in-line suction or covered Yankauer)	Apparatuses exposed to the oral cavity or secretions in the lungs then left unprotected within the environment have been shown to be colonized with bacteria in the oral cavity.[48]	
8. Reconfirm tube placement (see Procedure 2), and note position of tube at teeth or nares. Retape or secure endotracheal tube every 24 hours and as needed for soiled or loose securing devices.	Ensures secured tube.	• Tube moving in and out of mouth
9. With subglottic secretion drainage ET tube in place, if tube becomes clogged, irrigate with air per manufacturer's instructions but do not increase suction pressure beyond what is recommended by the manufacturer. **(Level D*)**	Damage to the tracheal mucosa was noted with the use of subglottic secretion drainage. In one study in pateints whose endotracheal tube was clogged, patients were reintubated and their clogged tubed was examined. In 17 of 19 subglottic suction ports, the clogging was caused by tracheal mucosa versus secretions.[12]	• Clogged subglotic suction port

*Level C: Qualitative studies, descriptive or correlational studies, integrative reviews, systematic reviews, or randomized controlled trials with inconsistent results
*Level D: Peer-reviewed professional organizational standards with clinical studies to support recommendations

Documentation

Documentation should include the following:

- Patient and family education
- Patient tolerance to suctioning
- Aspirate amount, type, and color
- Presence of nasal drainage
- Repositioning of endotracheal tube
- Retaping of endotracheal tube

- Oral care, moisturization, and oral suctioning
- Condition of lips, mouth, and tongue
- Presence of cuff leak
- Amount of air used to inflate cuff
- Centimeter mark on endotracheal tube
- Which naris endotracheal tube is in

References

1. Berry AM, Davidson PM, et al: Systematic literature review of oral hygiene practices for intensive care patients receiving mechanical ventilation, *Am J Crit Care* 16(6): 552-563, 2007.
2. Carlson J, Mayrose J, et al: Extubation force: tape versus endotracheal tube holders, *Ann Emerg Med* 50(6):686-691, 2007.
3. Chan EY, et al: Oral decontamination for prevention of pneumonia in mechanically ventilated adults: systematic review and meta-analysis, *BMJ* 334:889-893, 2007.
4. Chao YF, et al: Removal of oral secretion prior to position change can reduce the incidence of ventilator- associated pneumonia for adult ICU patients: a clinical controlled trial study, *J Clin Nurs* 18(1);22-28, 2009.
CR 5. Chendrasekhar A, Timberlake GA: Endotracheal tube cuff pressure threshold for prevention of nosocomial pneumonia, *J Applied Res* 3(3):311-314, 2003.
6. Chlebicki MP, Safdar N: Topical chlorhexidine for prevention of ventilator-associated pneumonia: a meta-analysis, *Crit Care Med* 35(2):595-602, 2007.
CR 7. Cummins RO, editor: Adjuncts for airway control, oxygenation, and ventilation, In *ACLS : principles and practice,* Dallas, 2003, American Heart Association, 167.
8. De Pew CL, et al: Subglottic secretion drainage: a literature review, *AACN Adv Crit Care* 18(4):366-379, 2007.
CR 9. DeRiso AJ II, et al: Chlorhexidine gluconate 0.12% oral rinse reduces the incidence of total nosocomial respiratory infection and nonprophylactic systemic antibiotic use in patients undergoing heart surgery, *Chest* 109:1556-15161, 1996.
CR 10. DeWalt EM: Effect of timed hygienic measures on oral mucosa in a group of elderly subjects, *Nurs Res* 24: 104-108, 1975.
11. Dezfulian C, et al: Subglottic secretion drainage for preventing ventilator-associated pneumonia: a meta-analysis, *Am J Med* 118(1):11-18, 2005.
12. Dragoumanis CK, et al: Investigating the failure to aspirate subglottic secretions with Evac endotracheal tube, *Anesth Analg* 105:1083-1085, 2007.
CR 13. Drakulovic MB, et al: Supine body position as a risk factor for nosocomial pneumonia in mechanically ventilated patients: a randomized trial, *Lancet* 354:1851-1858, 1999.
CR 14. El-Solh AA, et al: Colonization of dental plaque: a reservoir of respiratory pathogens for hospital acquired pneumonia in institutionalized elders, *Chest* 126:1575-1582, 2004.
15. Ferrer M et al: Maintenance of tracheal tube cuff pressure: where are the limits [commentary]? *Crit Care* 12:106-107, 2008.

CR 16. Ferretti GA, et al: Chlorhexidine for prophylaxis against oral infections and associated complications in patients receiving bone marrow transplants, *J Am Dent Assoc* 114:461-467, 1987.
17. Frost P, Wise MP: Tracheotomy and ventilator-associated pneumonia: the importance of oral care, *Eur Respir J* 31(1):221-222, 2008.
18. Garcia R: A review of the possible role of oral and dental colonization on the occurrence of healthcare-associated pneumonia: underappreciated risk in a call for interventions, *Am J Infect Control* 33(9):527-541, 2005.
CR 19. Garrouste-Orgeas M, et al: Oropharyngeal or gastric colonization and nosocomial pneumonia in adult intensive care unit patients: a prospective study based on genomic DNA analysis, *Am J Respir Crit Care Med* 156:1647-1655, 1997.
CR 20. Gastmeier P, Geffers C: Prevention of ventilator-associated pneumonia: analysis of studies published since 2004, *J Hosp Infect* 67(1):1-8, 2007.
CR 21. Grap MJ, et al: Oral care interventions in critical care: frequency and documentation, *Am J Crit Care* 12: 113-119, 2003.
22. Grap MJ, et al: Duration of action of a single, early oral application of chlorhexidine on oral microbial flora in mechanically ventilated patients: a pilot study, *Heart Lung* 33:83-91, 2004.
CR 23. Houston S, et al: Effectiveness of 0.12% chlorhexidine gluconate oral rinse in reducing prevalence of nosocomial pneumonia in patients undergoing heart surgery, *Am J Crit Care* 11:567-570, 2002.
24. Ishikawa A, Yoneyama T, et al: Professional oral health care reduces the number of oropharyngeal bacteria, *J Dent Res* 87(6):594-598, 2008.
CR 25. Kaplow R, Bookbinder M: A comparison of four endotracheal tube holders, *Heart Lung* 23(1):59-66, 1994.
26. Koeman M, et al: Oral decontamination with chlorhexidine reduces the incidence of ventilator associated pneumonia, *Am J Respir Crit Care Med* 173:1348-1355, 2006.
27. Labeau S, Vandijck D, et al: Evidence-based guidelines for the prevention of ventilator-associated pneumonia: results of a knowledge test among European intensive care nurses, *J Hosp Infect* 70(2):180-185, 2008.
28. Lansford T, Moncure M, et al: Efficacy of a pneumonia prevention protocol in the reduction of ventilator-associated pneumonia in trauma patients, *Surg Infect (Larchmt)* 8(5):505-10, 2007.
29. Lorente L, et al: Evidence on measures for the prevention of ventilator-associated pneumonia, *Eur Respir J* 30:1193-1207, 2007.

30. Mankodi S, et al: A 6- month clinical trial to study the effects of a cetylpyridinium chloride mouth rinse on gingivitis and plaque, *Am J Dent* 18:9A-14A, 2005.

CR 31. Marshall MV, Cancro LP, Fischman SL: Hydrogen peroxide: a review of its use in dentistry, *J Periodontol* 66: 786-796, 1995.

32. Mori H, et al: Oral care reduces incidence of ventilator associated pneumonia in ICU populations, *Intensive Care Med* 32:230-236, 2006.

CR 33. Munro CL, Grap MJ: Oral health and care in the intensive care unit: state of the science, *Am J Crit Care* 13:25-33, 2004.

34. Munro CL, et al: Chlorhexidine reduces ventilator associated pneumonia (VAP) in mechanically ventilated ICU adults, *Crit Care Med* 24,12(suppl):A1, 2006.

35. Murdoch E, Holdgate A: A comparison of tape-tying versus a tube-holding device for securing endotracheal tubes in adults, *Anaesth Intensive Care* 35(5):730-735, 2007.

36. Muscedere J, et al: Comprehensive evidence-based clinical practice guidelines for ventilator associated pneumonia: prevention, *J Crit Care* 23:126-137, 2008.

37. Niederman MS, Craven DE, et al: Guidelines for the management of adults with hospital- acquired, ventilator-associated and healthcare-associated pneumonia, *Am J Respir Crit Care Med* 171:388-416, 2005.

38. Paju S, Scannapieco FA: Oral biofilms, periodontitis, and pulmonary infections, *Oral Dis* 13(6):508-512, 2007.

39. Papadimos TJ, Hensley SJ, et al: Implementation of the "FASTHUG" concept decreases the incidence of ventilator-associated pneumonia in a surgical intensive care unit, *Patient Saf Surg* 2:3, 2008.

CR 40. Pearson LS, Hutton JL: A controlled trial to compare the ability of foam swabs and toothbrushes to remove dental plaque, *J Adv Nurs* 39:480-489, 2002.

41. Safdar N, Dezfulian C, et al: Clinical and economic consequences of ventilator-associated pneumonia: a systematic review, *Crit Care Med* 33(10):2184-2193, 2005.

42. Scannapieco FA: Pneumonia in nonambulatory patients: the role of oral bacteria and oral hygiene, *J Am Dent Assoc* 137(Suppl):21S-25S, 2006.

43. Schiffner U: Plaque and gingivitis in the elderly: a randomized, single blinded clinical trial on the outcome of intensified mechanical or anti-bacterial oral hygiene measures, *J Clin Periodontol* 34:1068-1073, 2007.

CR 44. Schleder B, Stott K, Lloyd RC: The effect of a comprehensive oral care protocol on patients at risk for ventilator-associated pneumonia, *J Advocate Health Care* 4:27-30, 2002.

CR 45. Shibly O, et al: Clinical evaluation of a hydrogen peroxide mouth rinse, sodium chlorhexidine, for prophylaxis against oral infections and associated bicarbonate dentifrice, and mouth moisturizer on oral health, *J Clin Dent* 8:145-149, 1997.

CR 46. Shorri A, O'Malley P: Continuous subglottic suctioning for the prevention of VAP: potential economic impact, *Chest* 119:228-238, 2001.

CR 47. Simmons-Trau D, et al: Reducing VAP with 6 sigma, *Nurs Manage* 35(6):41-45, 2004.

CR 48. Sole ML, Poalillo FE, et al: Bacterial growth in secretions and on suctioning equipment of orally intubated patients: a pilot study, *Am J Crit Care* 11(2):141-149, 2002.

CR 49. Sole ML, et al: A multisite survey of suctioning techniques and airway management practices, *Am J Crit Care* 12:220-232, 2003.

CR 50. Stookey GK, et al: A 6-month clinical study assessing the safety and efficacy of two cetylpyridinium chloride mouth rinses, *Am J Dent* 18:24A-28, 2005.

51. Tablan OC, Anderson LJ, et al: Guidelines for preventing health-care-associated pneumonia, 2003: recommendations of CDC and the Healthcare Infection Control Practices Advisory Committee, *MMWR Recomm Rep* 53(RR-3): 1-36, 2004.

52. Tantipong H, Morkchareonpong C, et al: Randomized controlled trial and meta-analysis of oral decontamination with 2% chlorhexidine solution for the prevention of ventilator-associated pneumonia, *Infect Control Hosp Epidemiol* 29(2):131-136, 2008.

CR 53. Torres A, et al: Pulmonary aspiration of gastric contents in patients receiving mechanical ventilation: the effect of body position, *Ann Intern Med,* 116:540-543, 1992.

54. Vollman KM: Ventilator associated pneumonia and pressure ulcer prevention as targets for quality improvement in the ICU, *Crit Care Nurs Clin North Am* 18:453:467, 2006.

55. Westwell S: Implementing a ventilator care bundle in an adult intensive care unit, *Nurs Crit Care* 13(4):203-207, 2008.

AP Extubation/Decannulation (Perform)

PURPOSE: The purpose of extubation and decannulation is to remove the artificial airway to allow the patient to breathe independently.

Kirsten N. Skillings, Bonnie L. Curtis

PREREQUISITE NURSING KNOWLEDGE

- *Extubation refers to removal of an endotracheal tube, whereas decannulation refers to removal of a tracheostomy tube.*
- Indications for extubation and decannulation include the following[3-5]:
  - ❖ The underlying condition that led to the need for an artificial airway is reversed or improved.
  - ❖ Hemodynamic stability is achieved, with no new reasons for continued artificial airway support.
  - ❖ Patient is able to effectively clear pulmonary secretions.
  - ❖ Airway problems have resolved; minimal risk for aspiration exists.
  - ❖ Mechanical ventilatory support no longer is needed.
- Most extubations or decannulations are planned. Planning allows for preparation of the patient physically and emotionally and decreases the likelihood of reintubation and hypoxic sequelae. Unintentional or unplanned extubation complicates a patient's overall recovery.[1]

AP This procedure should be performed only by physicians, advanced practice nurses, and other healthcare professionals (including critical care nurses) with additional knowledge, skills, and demonstrated competence per professional licensure or institutional standard.

- Extubation may occur in a rapid fashion when the previous indications are met, whereas decannulation generally occurs in a stepwise fashion. The patient with a tracheostomy tube may be weaned gradually from the tracheostomy tube, possibly with a combination of techniques, including downsizing the tube diameter, using tubes and inner cannulas with fenestrations, and capping the tracheostomy. The tracheostomy tube is removed when the patient is able to breathe comfortably, maintain adequate ventilation and oxygenation, and manage secretions, through the normal anatomic airway.

EQUIPMENT

- Suctioning equipment
- Personal protective equipment
- Sterile suction catheter or suction kit
- Self-inflating manual resuscitation bag-valve-device connected to 100% oxygen source
- Oxygen source and tubing
- Scissors
- Supplemental oxygen with aerosol
- 10-mL syringe
- Rigid pharyngeal suction-tip (Yankauer) catheter
- Sterile dressing for tracheal stoma

  Additional equipment, to have available as needed, includes the following:
- Endotracheal intubation supplies
- Emergency cart

PATIENT AND FAMILY EDUCATION

- Explain the procedure and the reason the endotracheal tube or tracheostomy tube is no longer needed. ➤*Rationale:* This step identifies the patient's and family's knowledge deficits concerning the patient's condition, the procedure, and the expected benefits and allows time for questions to clarify information and voice concerns. Explanations decrease patient anxiety and enhance cooperation.
- Explain the purpose and necessity of extubation or decanulation. ➤*Rationale:* Communication and explanation of therapy encourage cooperation and minimize anxiety.
- Discuss the suctioning process and the importance of coughing and deep breathing. ➤*Rationale:* Understanding therapy encourages cooperation with the follow-up procedures necessary to maintain a patent airway.
- Explain that the patient's voice may be hoarse after extubation or decannulation. With removal of a tracheostomy tube, occlusion of the stoma may be necessary to facilitate normal speech and coughing. ➤*Rationale:* Knowledge minimizes the patient's and family's fear and anxiety.
- Explain that the patient may need continued oxygen or humidification support ➤*Rationale:* Many patients continue to need oxygen support for some time after extubation. Continued humidification often helps decrease hoarseness and liquefy secretions.

PATIENT ASSESSMENT AND PREPARATION

Patient Assessment

- Desired level of consciousness has been achieved (for most patients, patient is awake and able to follow commands).[2]

- Assess the stability of the patient's respiratory status.[2,4,5]
  - ❖ Stable respiratory rate of less than 25 breaths/min
  - ❖ Absence of dyspnea
  - ❖ Absence of accessory muscle use
  - ❖ Negative inspiratory pressure less than or equal to -20 cm H_2O
  - ❖ Positive expiratory pressure greater than or equal to $+30$ cm H_2O
  - ❖ Spontaneous tidal volume greater than or equal to 5 mL/kg
  - ❖ Vital capacity greater than or equal to 10 to 15 mL/kg
  - ❖ Minute ventilation greater than or equal to 10 L/min
  - ❖ Fraction of inspired oxygen (Fio_2) less than or equal to 50%
  - ❖ Stable pulse and blood pressure and absence of serious cardiac dysrhythmias
- ➤*Rationale:* Evaluation of the patient's respiratory status identifies that intubation is no longer necessary.
- Assess patient's ability to cough. ➤*Rationale:* The ability to cough and clear secretions is important for successful airway management after extubation.

Patient Preparation

- Verify correct patient with two identifiers. ➤*Rationale:* Prior to performing a procedure, the nurse should ensure the correct identification of the patient for the intended intervention.
- Ensure that the patient understands preprocedural teachings. Answer questions as they arise, and reinforce information as needed. ➤*Rationale:* This process evaluates and reinforces understanding of previously taught information.
- Place patient in semi-Fowler's position. ➤*Rationale:* Respiratory muscles are more effective in an upright position versus a prone position. This position facilitates coughing and minimizes the risk of vomiting and consequent aspiration.

Procedure	**for Performing Extubation and Decannulation**	
Steps	**Rationale**	**Special Considerations**
1. HH		
2. PE		
3. Hyperoxygenate and suction endotracheal tube and pharynx (see Procedure 12).	Removes secretions, including those above the cuff.	
4. Cut twill tape or remove tape or securement device to free tube.		
5. Insert syringe into one-way valve of pilot balloon.	Prepares for cuff deflation.	
6. Deflate the tube cuff (if it is inflated) and instruct patient to deep breathe.	Promotes hyperinflation. Vocal cords are maximally abducted at peak inspiration.	A self-inflating manual resuscitation bag-valve-device can assist in hyperinflation (see Procedure 32).

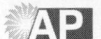

Procedure for Performing Extubation and Decannulation—*Continued*

Steps	Rationale	Special Considerations
7. Remove the tube at the peak of inspiration, while monitoring and supporting the patient.	Assists in a smooth, quick, less traumatic removal. Vocal cords are maximally abducted at peak inspiration. In addition, initial cough response expected after extubation should be more forceful if started from maximal inspiration versus expiration.[4]	Alternative methods to facilitate removal of secretions while an endotracheal tube is removed include application of positive pressure while the cuff is deflated, insertion of suction catheter 1 to 2 inches (5 cm) below distal end of tube, and application of suction while cuff is deflated and tube removed.[2]
8. Encourage the patient to deep breathe and cough.	Promotes hyperinflation; helps remove secretions.	
9. Suction the oral pharynx.	Removes secretions.	
10. Apply supplemental oxygen and aerosol, as appropriate.	Promotes warmth and moisture and prevents oxygen desaturation. Cool humidification is usually preferred after extubation to help minimize upper airway swelling.[4]	
11. Place a dry, sterile, 4 × 4 dressing over stoma when tracheostomy tube is removed.	Contains secretions that may leak out of stoma.	Tracheostomy stoma closure usually occurs within a few days.
12. Discard used supplies, remove personal protective equipment, and perform hand hygiene.	Reduces transmission of microorganisms and body secretions; Standard Precautions.	

Expected Outcomes

- Smooth atraumatic extubation or decannulation
- Stable respiratory status

Unexpected Outcomes

- Fatigue and respiratory failure
- Persistent hoarseness
- Tracheal stoma narrowing
- Aspiration
- Laryngospasm
- Trauma to soft tissue
- Upper airway obstruction
- Emergent reintubation or recannulation

Patient Monitoring and Care

Steps	Rationale	Reportable Conditions
		These conditions should be reported if they persist despite nursing interventions.
1. Monitor vital signs, respiratory status, and oxygenation immediately after extubation, within 1 hour, and per institutional standard.	Change in vital signs and oxygenation after extubation or decannulation may indicate respiratory compromise, which necessitates reintubation.	- Tachycardia - Tachypnea - Blood pressure greater than 110% baseline - Oxygen saturation (SpO_2) less than or equal to 90% - Stridor - Breathing difficulty - Chest-abdominal asynchrony
2. Promote optimal oxygenation with supplemental oxygen as needed.	Decreases incidence of oxygen desaturation immediately after extubation.	- SpO_2 less than or equal to 90%

Procedure continues on following page

Patient Monitoring and Care —*Continued*

Steps	Rationale	Reportable Conditions
3. Monitor for aspiration related to pooled secretions.	Failure to suction or ineffective suctioning of the pharynx allows accumulated secretions to advance farther into the trachea on cuff deflation.	• Patient unable to handle secretions
4. Encourage frequent coughing and deep breathing and use of an incentive spirometer.	Prevents atelectasis and secretion accumulation.	• Ineffective cough
5. Assess swallowing ability.	Presence of tube over extended periods may result in impaired swallowing ability.	• Inability to handle secretions • Inability to swallow without coughing
6. Follow institution standard for assessing pain. Administer analgesia as prescribed.	Identifies need for pain interventions.	• Continued pain despite pain interventions.

Documentation

Documentation should include the following:
- Patient and family education
- Respiratory and vital signs assessment before and after procedure
- Date and time when procedure is performed
- Patient response
- Unexpected outcomes
- Nursing interventions taken
- Pain assessment, interventions, and effectiveness

References

CR 1. O'Meade M, Guyatt G, Cook D: Weaning from mechanical ventilation: the evidence from clinical research, *Respir Care* 12:78-83, 2001.
2. Pierce L: Airway maintenance. In *Management of the mechanically ventilated patient,* ed 2, St Louis, 2007, Saunders.
3. Scales K, Pilsworth J: A practical guide to extubation, *Nurs Standard* 22(2):44-48, 2007.
4. St John RE, Seckel MA: Airway management. In Burns SM, editor: *AACN protocols for practice: care of mechanically ventilated patients,* ed 2, Sudbury, MA, 2007, Jones and Bartlett.
CR 5. Twibel R, Siela D, Mahmoodi M: Subjective perceptions in physiological variables during weaning from mechanical ventilation, *Am J Crit Care* 12:101-112, 2003.

Additional Readings

American Association for Respiratory Care: Clinical practice guideline: removal of the endotracheal tube, *Respiratory Care* 52(1):81-93, 2007.
Burns SM: Weaning from mechanical ventilation. In Burns SM, editor: *AACN protocols for practice: care of mechanically ventilated patients,* ed 2, Sudbury, MA 2007, Jones and Bartlett Publishers, 97-160.
Ead H: Post anesthesia tracheal extubation, *CACCN* 15(3): 20-25, 2004.
Henneman E: Liberating patients from mechanical ventilation: a team approach, *Crit Care Nurse* 21:25-33, 2001.

AP Extubation/Decannulation (Assist)

P U R P O S E :   The purpose of extubation and decannulation is to remove the artificial airway to allow the patient to breathe independently.

Kirsten N. Skillings, Bonnie L. Curtis

PREREQUISITE NURSING KNOWLEDGE

- *Extubation* refers to removal of an endotracheal tube, and *decannulation* refers to removal of a tracheostomy tube.
- Indications for extubation and decannulation include the following[3-5]:
  - ❖ The underlying condition that led to the need for an artificial airway is reversed or improved.
  - ❖ Hemodynamic stability is achieved, with no new reasons for continued artificial airway support.
  - ❖ The patient is able to effectively clear pulmonary secretions.
  - ❖ Airway problems have resolved; minimal risk for aspiration exists.
  - ❖ Mechanical ventilatory support is no longer needed.
- Most extubations or decannulations are planned. Planning allows for preparation of the patient physically and emotionally and decreases the likelihood of reintubation and hypoxic sequelae. Unintentional or unplanned extubation complicates a patient's overall recovery.[1]

AP   This procedure should be performed only by physicians, advanced practice nurses, and other healthcare professionals (including critical care nurses) with additional knowledge, skills, and demonstrated competence per professional licensure or institutional standard.

- Extubation may occur in a rapid fashion when the previous indications are met, whereas decannulation generally occurs in a stepwise fashion. A patient with a tracheostomy tube may be weaned gradually from the tracheostomy tube, possibly with a combination of techniques, including downsizing the tube diameter, using tubes and inner cannulas with fenestrations, and capping the tracheostomy. The tracheostomy tube is removed when the patient is able to breathe comfortably, maintain adequate ventilation and oxygenation, and manage secretions, through the normal anatomic airway.

EQUIPMENT

- Suctioning equipment
- Personal protective equipment
- Sterile suction catheter or suction kit
- Self-inflating manual resuscitation bag-valve-device connected to 100% oxygen source
- Oxygen source and tubing
- Scissors
- Supplemental oxygen with aerosol
- 10-mL syringe
- Rigid pharyngeal suction-tip (Yankauer) catheter
- Sterile dressing for tracheal stoma
  Additional equipment, to have available as needed, includes the following:
- Endotracheal intubation supplies
- Emergency cart

PATIENT AND FAMILY EDUCATION

- Explain the procedure and the reason the endotracheal tube or tracheostomy tube is no longer needed. ➤*Rationale:* This process identifies patient and family knowledge deficits concerning the patient's condition, procedure, and expected benefits and allows time for questions to clarify information and voice concerns. Explanations decrease patient anxiety and enhance cooperation.
- Explain the purpose and necessity of extubation or decannulation. ➤*Rationale:* Communication and explanation for therapy encourage cooperation and minimize anxiety.
- Discuss the suctioning process and the importance of coughing and deep breathing. ➤*Rationale:* Understanding therapy encourages cooperation with the follow-up procedures necessary to maintain a patent airway.
- Explain that the patient's voice may be hoarse after extubation or decannulation. With removal of a tracheostomy tube, occlusion of the stoma may be necessary to facilitate normal speech and coughing. ➤*Rationale:* Knowledge minimizes patient and family fear and anxiety.
- Explain that the patient may need continued oxygen or humidification support. ➤*Rationale:* Many patients continue to need oxygen support for some time after extubation. Continued humidification often helps to decrease hoarseness and liquefies secretions.

PATIENT ASSESSMENT AND PREPARATION

Patient Assessment

- Desired level of consciousness has been achieved (in most cases, the patient is awake and able to follow commands).[5]

- Assess the stability of the patient's respiratory status[2,4,5]:
- Stable respiratory rate of less than 25 breaths/min
- Absence of dyspnea
- Absence of accessory muscle use
- Negative inspiratory pressure less than or equal to -20 cm H_2O
- Positive expiratory pressure greater than or equal to $+30$ cm H_2O
- Spontaneous tidal volume greater than or equal to 5 mL/kg
- Vital capacity greater than or equal to 10 to 15 mL/kg
- Minute ventilation greater than or equal to 10 L/min
- Fraction of inspired oxygen less than or equal to 50%
- Stable pulse and blood pressure and absence of serious cardiac dysrhythmias ➤*Rationale:* Evaluation of the patient's respiratory status identifies that intubation is no longer necessary. Signs and symptoms associated with independent breathing are as follows.[2,4,5]
- Assess the patient's ability to cough. ➤*Rationale:* The ability to cough and clear secretions is important for successful airway management after extubation.

Patient Preparation

- Verify correct patient with two identifiers. ➤*Rationale:* Prior to performing a procedure, the nurse should ensure the correct identification of the patient for the intended intervention.
- Ensure that the patient understands preprocedural teachings. Answer questions as they arise, and reinforce information as needed. ➤*Rationale:* This process evaluates and reinforces understanding of previously taught information.
- Place the patient in a semi-Fowler's position. ➤*Rationale:* Respiratory muscles are more effective in an upright position versus a supine position. This position facilitates coughing and minimizes the risk of vomiting and consequent aspiration.

Procedure	for Assisting with Extubation and Decannulation	
Steps	**Rationale**	**Special Considerations**
1. HH		
2. PE		
3. Hyperoxygenate and suction endotracheal tube and pharynx (see Procedure 12).	Removes secretions, including those above the cuff.	
4. Cut twill tape, or remove tape or securement device to free tube.		
5. Insert syringe into one-way valve of pilot balloon.	Prepares for cuff deflation.	
6. Deflate the tube cuff (if it is inflated) and instruct patient to deep breathe.	Promotes hyperinflation. Vocal cords are maximally abducted at peak inspiration.	A self-inflating manual resuscitation bag-valve-device can assist in hyperinflation (see Procedure 32).

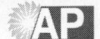

Procedure for Assisting with Extubation and Decannulation—*Continued*

Steps	Rationale	Special Considerations
7. Remove the tube at the peak of inspiration, while monitoring and supporting the patient.	Assists in a smooth, quick, less traumatic removal. Vocal cords are maximally abducted at peak inspiration. In addition, initial cough response expected after extubation should be more forceful if started from maximal inspiration versus expiration.[4]	Alternative methods to facilitate removal of secretions while an endotracheal tube is removed include application of suction while the cuff is deflated, insertion of suction catheter 1 to 2 inches (5 cm) below distal end of tube, and application of suction while cuff is deflated and tube removed.[2]
8. Encourage the patient to deep breathe and cough.	Promotes hyperinflation; helps remove secretions.	
9. Suction the oral pharynx.	Removes secretions.	
10. Apply supplemental oxygen and aerosol, as appropriate.	Promotes warmth and moisture and prevents oxygen desaturation. Cool humidification usually is preferred after extubation to help minimize upper airway swelling.[4]	
11. Place a dry, sterile 4 × 4 dressing over stoma after tracheostomy tube is removed.	Contains secretions that may leak out of stoma.	Tracheostomy stoma closure usually occurs within a few days.
12. Discard used supplies, remove personal protective equipment, and perform hand hygiene.	Reduces transmission of microorganisms and body secretions; Standard Precautions.	

Expected Outcomes

- Smooth atraumatic extubation or decannulation
- Stable respiratory status

Unexpected Outcomes

- Fatigue and respiratory failure
- Persistent hoarseness
- Tracheal stoma narrowing
- Aspiration
- Laryngospasm
- Trauma to soft tissue
- Upper airway obstruction
- Emergent reintubation or recannulation

Patient Monitoring and Care

Steps	Rationale	Reportable Conditions
		These conditions should be reported if they persist despite nursing interventions.
1. Monitor vital signs, respiratory status, and oxygenation immediately after extubation, within 1 hour, and per institutional standard.	Change in vital signs and oxygenation after extubation or decannulation may indicate respiratory compromise, which necessitates reintubation or recannulation.	• Tachycardia • Tachypnea • Blood pressure significantly higher or lower than baseline • Changes in level of consciousness • Oxygen saturation (Spo_2) less than or equal to 90% • Stridor • Breathing difficulty • Chest-abdominal asynchrony
2. Promote optimal oxygenation with supplemental oxygen as needed.	Decreases incidence of oxygen desaturation immediately after extubation.	• Spo_2 less than or equal to 90%

Procedure continues on following page

Patient Monitoring and Care —*Continued*

Steps	Rationale	Reportable Conditions
3. Monitor for aspiration related to pooled secretions.	Failure to suction or ineffective suctioning of the pharynx allows accumulated secretions to advance farther into the trachea on cuff deflation.	• Patient unable to handle secretions
4. Encourage frequent coughing and deep breathing and use of an incentive spirometer.	Prevents atelectasis and secretion accumulation.	• Ineffective cough
5. Assess swallowing ability.	Presence of tube over extended periods may result in impaired swallowing ability.	• Inability to handle secretions • Inability to swallow without coughing
6. Follow institution standard for assessing pain. Administer analgesia as prescribed.	Identifies need for pain interventions.	• Continued pain despite pain intervention

Documentation

Documentation should include the following:

- Patient and family education
- Patient response
- Respiratory and vital signs assessment before and after procedure

- Unexpected outcomes
- Date and time when procedure is performed
- Nursing interventions taken
- Pain assessment, interventions, and effectiveness

References

CR 1. O'Meade M, Guyatt G, Cook D: Weaning from mechanical ventilation: the evidence from clinical research, *Respir Care* 12:78-83, 2001.
2. Pierce L: Airway maintenance. In *Management of the mechanically ventilated patient,* ed 2, St Louis, 2007, Saunders.
3. Scales K, Pilsworth J: A practical guide to extubation, *Nurs Stand* 22(2):44-48, 2007.
4. St John RE, Seckel MA: Airway management. In Burns SM, editor: *AACN protocols for practice: care of mechanically ventilated patients,* ed 2, Sudbury, MA 2007, Jones and Bartlett Publishers, 1-57.
CR 5. Twibel R, Siela D, Mahmoodi M: Subjective perceptions in physiological variables during weaning from mechanical ventilation, *Am J Crit Care* 12:101-12, 2003.

Additional Readings

American Association for Respiratory Care: Clinical practice guideline: removal of the endotracheal tube, *Respir Care* 52(1):81-93, 2007.
Burns SM: Weaning from mechanical ventilation. In Burns SM, editor: *AACN protocols for practice: care of mechanically ventilated patients,* ed 2, Sudbury, MA 2007, Jones and Bartlett Publishers, 97-160.
Ead H: Post anesthesia tracheal extubation, *CACCN* 15(3):20-25, 2004.
Henneman E: Liberating patients from mechanical ventilation: a team approach, *Crit Care Nurse* 21:25-33, 2001.

AP Laryngeal Mask Airway

PURPOSE: A laryngeal mask airway may be used to provide an emergency airway during resuscitation of a profoundly unconscious patient who needs artificial ventilation when endotracheal intubation is not readily available or has failed in establishing an airway.[1]

Jeffrey Dawson

PREREQUISITE NURSING KNOWLEDGE

- The requirement for rapid airway management in an unconscious patient should be understood.
- The anatomy and physiology of the upper airway should be understood.
- The design of the laryngeal mask airway (LMA) available to the practitioner should be understood (Fig. 7-1):
    - An airway tube connects the mask and the 15-mm male adapter.
    - The mask's cuff, when inflated, conforms to the contours of the hypopharynx, with the opening of the air tube positioned directly over the laryngeal opening. Two aperture bars cross the opening where the tube exits into the mask.
    - An inflation line is fitted with a valve and a pilot balloon that leads to the mask's cuff.
- The final placement of an LMA in the airway should be understood (Fig. 7-2).
- The ability to ventilate an unconscious patient adequately with a mouth-to-mask or bag-valve-mask device is necessary.

- An understanding of the limitations of the LMA is needed. Limitations are as follows:
    - The LMA does *not* protect the airway from aspiration of stomach contents, and the risks of insertion and aspiration must be weighed against the need to establish an airway.[12]
    - The presence of a nasogastric tube may make regurgitation more likely because of its effect on the esophageal sphincter tone and may also prevent the LMA from properly sealing the hypopharynx.[12,13]

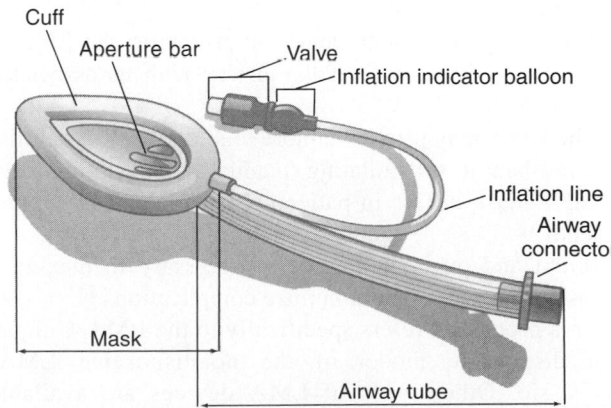

Cuff
Aperture bar
Valve
Inflation indicator balloon
Inflation line
Airway connector
Mask
Airway tube

FIGURE 7-1 Components of the laryngeal mask airway. (*From The Laryngeal Mask Company Limited: Instruction manual: LMA-Classic, San Diego, 2005, LMA.*)

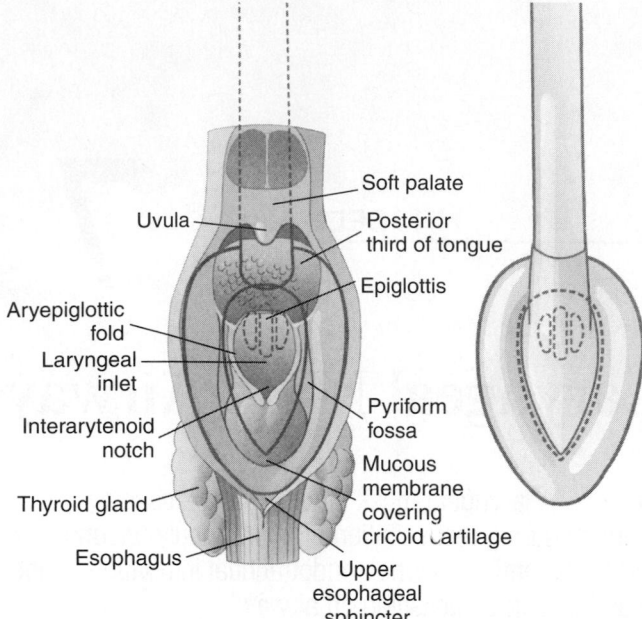

FIGURE 7-2   Dorsal view of the laryngeal mask airway showing position in relation to pharyngeal anatomy. *(From The Laryngeal Mask Company Limited: Instruction manual: LMA-Classic, San Diego, 2005, LMA.)*

- ❖ The LMA should not be used on patients who need high ventilator pressures (e.g., patients with pulmonary fibrosis, significant obesity) because the LMA provides a low-pressure seal.[12]
- ❖ The LMA should not be used in an emergency situation in which the patient is *not* profoundly unconscious and may resist insertion of the device.[12]
- ❖ The LMA should be used with caution in patients with oropharyngeal trauma, only when all other means of establishing an airway fail[1] and when the risks of insertion are weighed against the need to establish an airway.
- ❖ The LMA can cause local irritation that leads to coughing and pressure lesions, which may cause 12th cranial nerve palsy.[2]
- There are no absolute contraindications to the LMA if the alternative is loss of the airway with its associated complications.[6]
- The LMA may provide a more viable means of ventilation than a self-inflating manual resuscitation bag-valve-mask device in patients with a beard or without teeth.[11]
- Initial and ongoing training is necessary to maximize insertion success and minimize complications.[8,11]
- This procedure refers specifically to the LMA-Unique, a disposable model of the nondisposable LMA-Classic. Other types of LMA devices are available and provide additional features, such as endotracheal intubation through the LMA or gastric suctioning.
- The LMA-Unique is latex-free.[7,12]

EQUIPMENT

- Two LMA-Unique devices of the appropriate size for patient weight[3]
  - ❖ Weight ranges listed for LMA-Unique sizes are *only* approximations; the size used may need to be adjusted for individual body habitus variations (i.e., patients who are short and obese may need a smaller size). Emerging clinical data suggest that use of a larger size provides an effective seal without associated higher pharyngeal pressures.[3,7]
  - ❖ Size 3, 30 to 50 kg
  - ❖ Size 4, 50 to 70 kg
  - ❖ Size 5, 70 to 100 kg
  - ❖ Size 6, ≥100 kg
- 60-mL Luer-tip syringe
- Water-soluble lubricant
- Gloves, mask, and eye protection
- Suction equipment (suction canister with control head, tracheal suction catheters, Yankauer suction tip)
- Mouth-to-mask or self-inflating manual resuscitation bag-valve-mask device, with peak pressure manometer, attached to a high-flow oxygen source
- Bite-block, at least 3 cm thick
- Tape or commercially available tube-securing device

PATIENT AND FAMILY EDUCATION

- If time allows, provide the family with information regarding the LMA and the reason for insertion. ➥*Rationale:* This information assists the family in understanding why the procedure is necessary and decreases family anxiety.

PATIENT ASSESSMENT AND PREPARATION
Patient Assessment

- Verify correct patient with two identifiers. ➥*Rationale:* Prior to performing a procedure, the nurse should ensure the correct identification of the patient for the intended intervention.
- Assess level of consciousness and responsiveness. ➥*Rationale:* In an emergency situation, the LMA should be inserted only into a patient who is profoundly unconscious and unresponsive.[12] Laryngospasm and inability to ventilate may occur if an LMA is introduced into a conscious or semiconscious patient.
- Assess history and patient information for possibility of delayed gastric emptying (e.g., hiatal hernia, recent food ingestion, poorly controlled diabetes). ➥*Rationale:* In a patient with delayed gastric emptying, the benefits of LMA insertion must be weighed against the possibility of regurgitation.[12]
- Assess history and patient information for possibility of decreased pulmonary compliance (i.e., pulmonary fibrosis, obesity). ➥*Rationale:* The high pressures needed to ventilate a patient with decreased pulmonary compliance may override the occlusive pressure of the LMA.[12]

Patient Preparation

- Perform a pre-procedure verification and time out, if non-emergent. ➤➤*Rationale:* Ensures patient safety.
- Ensure adequate ventilation and oxygenation with either a mouth-to-mask or bag-valve-mask device. ➤➤*Rationale:* The patient is nonresponsive and apneic without assisted ventilation before the LMA insertion.

- Ensure that the suction equipment is assembled and in working order. ➤➤*Rationale:* The patient may regurgitate during the insertion or while the LMA is in place and need oropharyngeal or tracheal suctioning.
- Anything that is not permanently affixed in the patient's mouth (e.g., dentures, partials, jewelry) should be removed. ➤➤*Rationale:* Inadvertent dislodgment and aspiration might occur with the placement of the LMA.

Procedure	for Laryngeal Mask Airway (LMA-Unique) Insertion	
Steps	**Rationale**	**Special Considerations**
1. **HH**		
2. **PE**	Minimizes contamination of LMA.	
3. Ensure that a spare LMA of the same size is immediately available. **(Level M*)**	Provides for a "backup" device should the initial device fail.	
4. Remove the LMA from the package and inspect. **(Level M)**	Ensures that the device is not defective and will work as indicated.	
A. Inspect the exterior of the mask for any cuts, tears, or scratches.	Ensures that the exterior surface of the device has not been damaged in any way.	Discard the device if any evidence of damage is found, and open the backup device.
B. Inspect the interior of the airway tube for any particles.	Particles in the airway tube may be inhaled when the device is used.	Discard the device if any particles cannot be removed from the tube, and open the backup device.
C. Examine the airway opening in the mask, ensuring that the aperture bars are intact.	Broken aperture bars may allow the epiglottis to obstruct the airway.	Discard the device if the aperture bars are broken or otherwise damaged, and open the backup device.
D. Examine the 15-mm male connector at the end of the airway tube and ensure that it fits tightly into the tube.	The 15-mm male connector is essential for ventilation with a bag-valve device or ventilator.	*Do not twist the connector because this breaks the seal.*[12] Discard the device if the connector does not fit tightly into the airway tube, and open the backup device.
5. Perform the deflation and inflation tests. **(Level M)**	Ensures that the device is not defective and will work as indicated.	
A. Expel the air from the 60-mL syringe and connect it to the pilot balloon valve.	The appropriate-size syringe is needed to inflate the cuff to the proper test level.	
B. Pull back the syringe plunger to deflate the cuff fully, then examine the cuff to ensure that it remains fully deflated (Fig. 7-3).	Full deflation of the cuff helps ensure its patency.	Discard the device if the cuff does not remain fully deflated, and open the backup device.

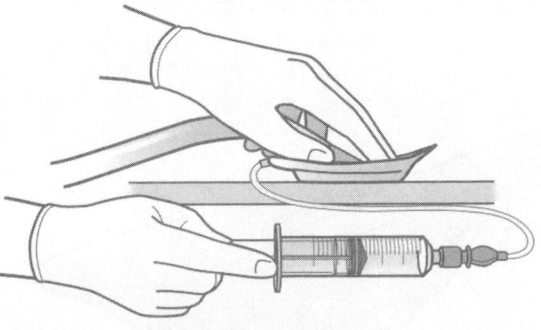

FIGURE 7-3 Method for deflating the laryngeal mask airway cuff. *(From The Laryngeal Mask Company Limited: Instruction manual: LMA-Classic, San Diego, 2005, LMA.)*

*Level M: Manufacturer's recommendations only

Procedure continues on following page

Procedure for Laryngeal Mask Airway (LMA-Unique) Insertion—*Continued*

Steps	Rationale	Special Considerations
C. Remove the syringe from the valve, pull back on the syringe to volume required for each LMA size, reattach to the valve, and inflate the cuff (Table 7-1).	Ensures that the device is not defective and will work as indicated.	
D. Examine the inflated cuff to ensure that it is symmetric without bulges.	Ensures that the device is not defective and will work as indicated.	Discard the device if the cuff bulges asymmetrically, and open the backup device.
E. Examine the pilot balloon to ensure that its inflated shape is elliptical.	Ensures that the device is not defective and will work as indicated.	Discard the device if the pilot balloon is spherical or bulges, and open the backup device.
6. Deflate the cuff by placing it, aperture side down, on a hard flat surface, smoothing out any wrinkles as air is withdrawn from the cuff with the syringe. Leave the syringe attached to the valve (see Fig. 7-3). **(Level M*)**	Facilitates smooth insertion and avoids deflection of the epiglottis.	Before insertion, the cuff should appear smooth, without wrinkles (Fig. 7-4).
7. Lubricate the posterior tip of the cuff with water-soluble lubricant. **(Level M)**	Facilitates smooth insertion.	Ensure that the lubricant does not spread to the anterior portion of the cuff because it may be aspirated.[12] Do *not* use lidocaine lubricants because they may delay the return of protective reflexes and may cause an allergic reaction.[12]
8. Place the patient's head in a sniffing position. **(Level E*)**	Facilitates smooth insertion.	The patient's head may be left in a neutral position if cervical spine injury is possible.[5]
9. Use index finger method of insertion. **(Level E)**	Ensures proper placement of the LMA.[12]	This method provides for better final placement of the LMA compared with other methods.[3]
A. Assume a position at the patient's head, and slightly lift the patient's head with the nondominant hand, maintaining upward pressure during the insertion.	Facilitates proper body position for the person inserting the device and the patient's head during insertion.	

*Level E: Multiple case reports, theory-based evidence from expert opinions, or peer-reviewed professional organizational standards without clinical studies to support recommendations

*Level M: Manufacturer's recommendations only

TABLE 7-1	Test Cuff Inflation Volumes
Laryngeal Mask Airway Size	**Air Volume for Testing *Only***
3	30 mL
4	45 mL
5	60 mL
6	75 mL

(From The Laryngeal Mask Company Limited: Instruction manual: LMA-Classic, San Diego, 2005, LMA.)

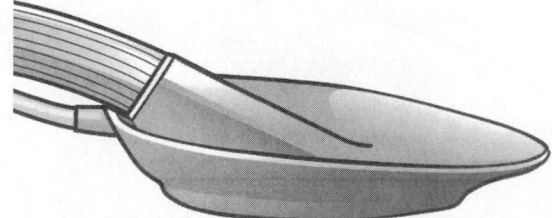

FIGURE 7-4 Laryngeal mask airway cuff properly deflated for insertion. *(From The Laryngeal Mask Company Limited: Instruction manual: LMA-Classic, San Diego, 2005, LMA.)*

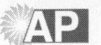

Procedure	for Laryngeal Mask Airway (LMA-Unique) Insertion—*Continued*	
Steps	**Rationale**	**Special Considerations**
B. Hold the LMA so that the dominant hand's index finger and thumb grasp the airway tube just behind the cuff (Fig. 7-5, *A*).	Facilitates proper device position for insertion.	The mask aperture must face toward the patient's feet, and the black line on the airway tube must face toward the patient's nose.
C. Insert the LMA into the patient's mouth, directing it upward toward the hard palate (Fig. 7-5, *B*).	Assists in maneuvering the LMA into the proper position.	
D. With the middle finger, open the patient's jaw and look into the mouth to ensure that the cuff is flattened against the hard palate (Fig. 7-5, *C*).	Assists in maneuvering the LMA into the proper position.	If the LMA does not flatten against the hard palate, remove and reinsert.
E. With the index finger, advance the LMA into the hypopharynx toward the hard palate, in one smooth movement (Fig. 7-5, *D*).	Moves the device into the proper position in the back of the mouth.	*Do not use force.* If the LMA does not advance, remove, reventilate, and reinsert.
F. Continue advancing the LMA until resistance is felt (Fig. 7-5, *E*).	Continues moving the LMA into the proper final position.	*Do not* hold the jaw open during this maneuver because it may cause the epiglottis or tongue to prevent advancement of the LMA. Depending on the size of the person's hand inserting the LMA and the size of the patient, the final resistance may not be met.

Procedure continues on following page

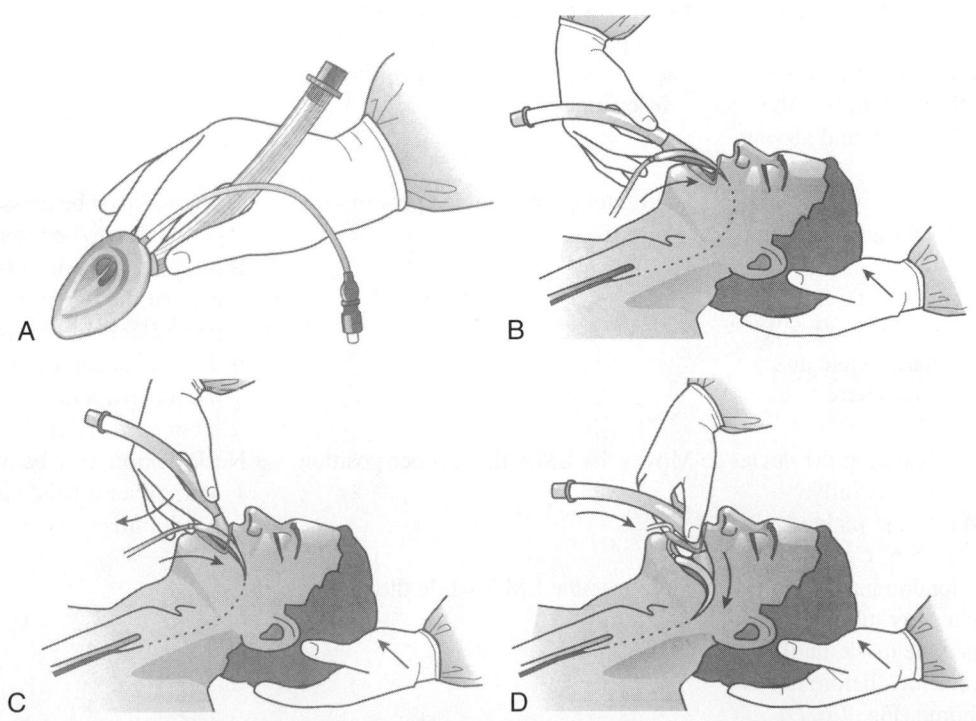

FIGURE 7-5   **A,** Method for holding the LMA for insertion. **B,** With the head extended and the neck flexed, the caregiver carefully flattens the LMA tip against the hard palate. **C,** To facilitate LMA introduction into the oral cavity, the caregiver gently presses the middle finger down on the jaw. **D,** The index finger pushes the LMA in the cranial direction following the contours of the hard and soft palates.

Continued

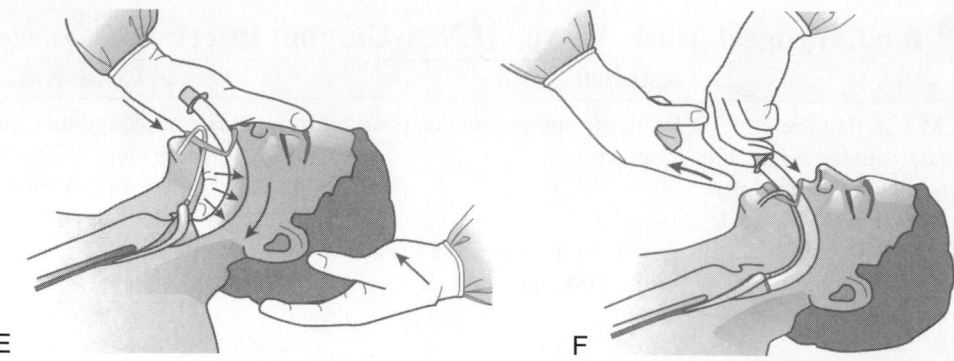

E   F

FIGURE 7-5, cont'd   **E,** Maintaining pressure with the finger in the tube in the cranial direction, the caregiver advances the LMA until definite resistance is felt at the base of the hypopharynx. Note the flexion of the wrist. **F,** The caregiver gently maintains cranial pressure with the nondominant hand while removing the index finger. *(From The Laryngeal Mask Company Limited: Instruction manual: LMA-Classic, San Diego, 2005, LMA.)*

Procedure   for Laryngeal Mask Airway (LMA-Unique) Insertion—*Continued*

Steps	Rationale	Special Considerations
G. Remove the nondominant hand from behind the patient's head and use it to stabilize the airway tube. Remove the dominant hand index finger from the patient's mouth (Fig. 7-5, *F*).	Maintains position of the LMA before the removal of the index finger.	The mask *must* be pressed up against the hard palate to be inserted correctly.[12] If the cuff curls or fails to flatten against the hard palate, remove, reventilate, and reinsert.[12] If the cuff becomes obstructed by the tonsils, a diagonal maneuver is often successful.[12]
10. Use thumb method of insertion. **(Level E*)**	May be used when accessing the patient from behind or above the head.[12]	
A. Approach the patient from the front.	Facilitates proper body position for the person inserting the device.	
B. Hold the LMA with dominant hand, with the thumb at the angle of the mask and airway tube (Fig. 7-6, *A*).	Facilitates proper device position for insertion.	
C. As the LMA is advanced into the patient's mouth, the dominant hand fingers are spread up over the patient's face, and the thumb pushes the LMA toward the hard palate and into the hypopharynx (Fig. 7-6, *B*).	Facilitates proper device position for insertion.	The mask *must* be pressed up against the hard palate to be inserted correctly.[12] If the cuff curls or fails to flatten against the hard palate, remove, reventilate, and reinsert.[12] If the cuff becomes obstructed by the tonsils, a diagonal maneuver is often successful.[12]
D. Continue advancing the device until the thumb is fully extended into the patient's mouth (Fig. 7-6, *C*).	Moves the LMA into proper position.	Neck flexion may be maintained with either a head support or the nondominant hand.
E. With the nondominant hand, grasp the airway tube and gently advance the mask, until resistance is met, before removing the thumb (Fig. 7-6, *D*).	Stabilizes the LMA while the thumb is removed.	

*Level E: Multiple case reports, theory-based evidence from expert opinions, or peer-reviewed professional organizational standards without clinical studies to support recommendations

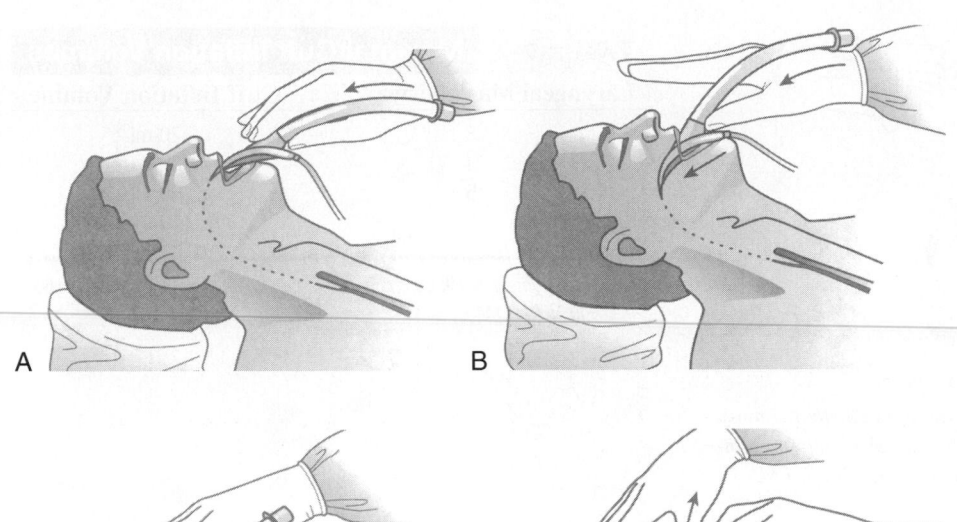

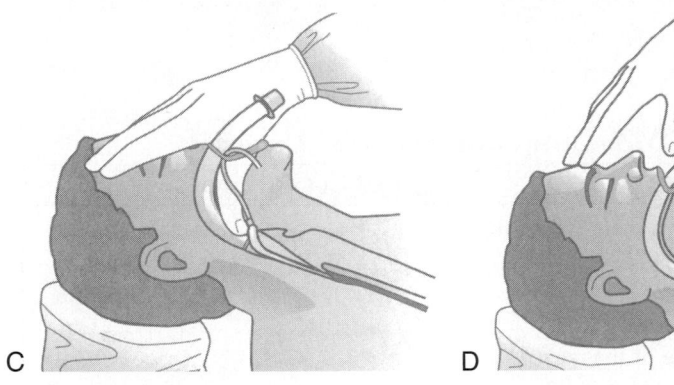

FIGURE 7-6 **A,** Method for holding the LMA for thumb insertion. **B,** With the fingers extended, press the thumb along the posterior pharynx. **C,** Advance the thumb to its fullest extent. **D,** Press LMA gently into place with the nondominant hand while removing the thumb. *(From The Laryngeal Mask Company Limited: Instruction manual: LMA-Classic, San Diego, 2005, LMA.)*

Procedure for Laryngeal Mask Airway (LMA-Unique) Insertion—*Continued*

Steps	Rationale	Special Considerations
11. Release the airway tube[2] and inflate the cuff to create a seal, with intracuff pressure approximately 60 cm H_2O (Fig. 7-7). **(Level M*)**	Releasing the airway tube during inflation allows the cuff to "seat" into the proper position during inflation.	Only one half of maximal inflation volume is necessary to create a seal (Table 7-2).[12] *Avoid overinflation of the cuff.[13]*
12. Observe for one or more signs that indicate correct placement and inflation: slight outward movement of the airway tube, slight bulging of the neck around the cricothyroid area, or no cuff visible in the mouth. **(Level M)**	Ensures correct placement and inflation of the cuff.	If *none* of these signs is observed, consider deflation of the cuff and removal of the LMA. Reventilate and insert the backup LMA.
13. Connect 15-mm male adapter to self-inflating manual resuscitation bag-valve-device and *gently* ventilate, with peak airway pressures of less than 20 cm H_2O and with tidal volumes less than or equal to 8 mL/kg of body weight.[12]	Maintenance of low ventilatory pressures prevents overriding the pressure in the cuff, creating a leak, or forcing air into the stomach.	The cuff may leak with the first few breaths as it settles into position. If the leak continues, ensure that the ventilator pressures are low.[12]
14. Confirm device placement with auscultation over the epigastrium for the absence of sounds and over the chest for bilateral breath sounds.	Confirms placement with primary assessment.	If sounds are heard in the epigastrium on auscultation, remove the device and manually ventilate the patient with a self-inflating manual resuscitation bag-valve-mask device.

*Level M: Manufacturer's recommendations only

Procedure continues on following page

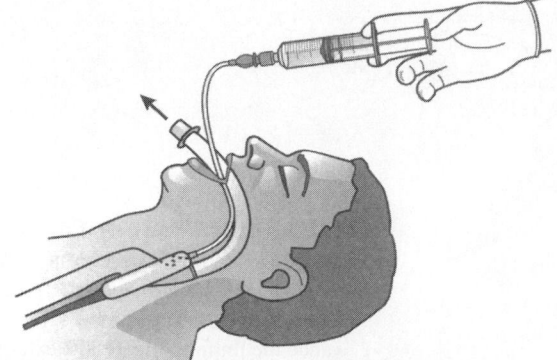

TABLE 7-2	**Maximal Cuff Inflation Volumes**
Laryngeal Mask Airway Size	**Cuff Inflation Volume**
3	20 mL
4	30 mL
5	40 mL
6	50 mL

(From The Laryngeal Mask Company Limited:Instruction manual: LMA-Classic, San Diego, 2005, LMA.)

FIGURE 7-7   Inflation without holding the tube allows the mask to seat itself optimally. *(From The Laryngeal Mask Company Limited: Instruction manual: LMA-Classic, San Diego, 2005, LMA.)*

Procedure for Laryngeal Mask Airway (LMA-Unique) Insertion—*Continued*

Steps	Rationale	Special Considerations
15. Further assess device placement with end-tidal carbon dioxide device or an esophageal detector device. **(Level M*)**	Confirms proper placement with two additional methods.[1,12]	
16. Secure the LMA. **(Level E*)**	Prevents disturbance of the correct placement.	
A. Insert an appropriately sized bite-block.	Prevents the patient from biting down on the airway tube, causing displacement of the cuff or occlusion of the airway tube.	Maintain the bite-block in place until the LMA is removed.[12]
B. Press the airway tube up toward the palate.	Secures the airway tube in position.	
C. Apply tape or commercially prepared device to hold the airway tube in place (Fig. 7-8).	Prevents movement of the airway tube and cuff.	
17. Remove the LMA as follows:	Removal, when appropriate, may prevent agitation, regurgitation, and laryngeal spasm.	
A. Gently assist with ventilations when the patient begins spontaneously breathing.	Prevents excess ventilatory pressures.	

*Level E: Multiple case reports, theory-based evidence from expert opinions, or peer-reviewed professional organizational standards without clinical studies to support recommendations
*Level M: Manufacturer's recommendations only

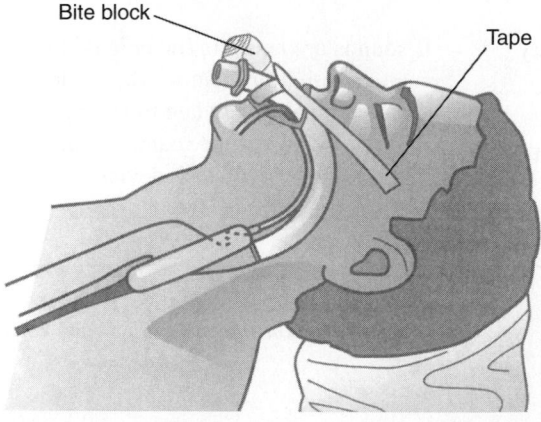

FIGURE 7-8   The bite-block and airway tube are taped together with the tube taped downward against the chin. *(From The Laryngeal Mask Company Limited: Instruction manual: LMA-Classic, San Diego, 2005, LMA.)*

Procedure   for Laryngeal Mask Airway (LMA-Unique) Insertion—*Continued*

Steps	Rationale	Special Considerations
B. Observe for signs of swallowing.	Indicates a return of some protective reflexes.	Tape or tube-securing device may be removed at this time. Leave the bite-block in place. Avoid suctioning because it may cause laryngeal spasm. The cuff should prevent aspiration.[12]
C. When the patient can open mouth to command, deflate the cuff. The LMA and bite-block are removed together.[12]	If LMA is removed before effective swallowing and coughing, secretions may enter the larynx, causing bronchospasm.	
D. Continue to assess for airway and breathing effectiveness.	Maintains monitoring of the airway and patient's ability to breathe on his or her own.	

Expected Outcomes

- Establishment of an effective airway in an emergency situation
- Maintenance of adequate ventilation
- Recovery of spontaneous ventilation

Unexpected Outcomes

- Complications related to the use of the LMA that may be related to poor insertion technique or excessive cuff pressures:
  - Regurgitation
  - Aspiration
  - Laryngospasm
  - Gagging
  - Retching
  - Trauma to tissues
  - Damage to various nerves
  - Sore or dry mouth
  - Hoarseness, stridor
  - Dysphagia, dysarthria, dysphonia
  - Cuff separation from airway tube[6]
  - Sore throat[4,10]

Patient Monitoring and Care

Steps	Rationale	Reportable Conditions
		These conditions should be reported if they persist despite nursing interventions.
1. Monitor the patient and LMA during ventilation for potential problems.	Ensures proper ventilation and airway management. Pressure-controlled and volume-controlled ventilation may be used but should be minimized or avoided because LMAs are not designed for long-term airway management. Pressure-controlled ventilation may require lower peak airway pressures.[9,12] Efforts should be made to secure a definitive airway (endotracheal intubation) as soon as possible. With mechanical ventilation, tidal volume, respiratory rate, and inspiratory-to-expiratory ratios need to be adjusted to prevent high peak airway pressures.[12]	- Inability to ventilate patient

Procedure continues on following page

Patient Monitoring and Care —*Continued*

Steps	Rationale	Reportable Conditions
A. Attach a pulse oximeter and monitor for trends.	Monitors adequate oxygenation.	• Decreased oxygen levels despite adequate oxygen delivery
B. Watch for air leaks around the cuff that may be caused by malposition. If suspected, assess for normal smooth oval swelling around cricothyroid membrane. If absent, in conjunction with prolonged expiratory phase, remove the LMA, reventilate, and reinsert.[12]	May indicate problems with the LMA position. *Do not add more air to the cuff* because it may force the soft cuff off of the larynx.[12]	• Indications of an air leak, especially with a prolonged expiratory phase or lack of normal smooth oval swelling around the cricothyroid membrane
C. If regurgitation occurs, as indicated by fluid in the airway tube, immediately tilt the patient's head down and turn body to one side, remove bag-valve device, and suction through airway tube (see Procedure 12).	Allows drainage and clearance of fluid from airway tube. If airway problems, difficulty with ventilation, or regurgitation continue, remove the LMA and establish an airway by other means.[12]	• Airway problems, difficulty with ventilation, or regurgitation
2. Follow institution standard for assessing pain. Administer analgesia as prescribed.	Identifies need for pain interventions.	• Continued pain despite pain interventions.

Documentation

Documentation should include the following:
- Initial patient assessment that indicates a need for LMA insertion
- Performance of visual inspection, inflation and deflation tests
- After insertion, assessment of end-tidal carbon dioxide and chest rise and fall
- Before removal, presence of swallowing and ability to open mouth
- Any complications while the LMA is in place (e.g., regurgitation or air leaks)
- Preoxygenation and ventilation before LMA insertion
- Insertion technique (index finger or thumb)
- Initial cuff inflation pressure
- Signs of correct placement and cuff inflation
- Placement of bite-block and securing of the LMA
- After removal, patency of airway, effectiveness of breathing, pulse oximetry and vital sign readings, patient symptoms, or signs of complications
- Pain assessment interventions and effectiveness.

References

1. American Heart Association: *Advanced cardiac life support (ACLS),* Dallas, 2006, AHA.
CR 2. Birnbaumer D, Pollack C Jr: Troubleshooting and managing the difficult airway, *Semin Respir Crit Care Med* 23(1):3-9, 2002.
CR 3. Brimacombe J, Berry A: Insertion of the laryngeal mask airway: a prospective study of four techniques, *Anaesth Intensive Care* 21:89-92, 1993.
4. Duk-Kyung K, et al: A heated humidifier does not reduce laryngo-pharyngeal complaints after brief laryngeal mask anesthesia, *Can J Anesthesia* 54:134-140, 2007.
CR 5. Hand H: Cardiopulmonary resuscitation: the laryngeal mask airway, *Emerg Nurse* 10:31-37, 2002.
CR 6. Idris AH, Gabrielli A: Advances in airway management, *Emerg Med Clin North Am* 20:843-857, 2002.
7. LMA, Inc: LMA, 2008, retrieved February 25, 2009. from www.lmana.com/faqs.php#faq06.

8. Lopez AM, et al: A clinical evaluation of four disposable laryngeal masks in adult patients, *J Clin Anesth* 20(7):508-513, 2008.
CR 9. Ocker H: A comparison of the laryngeal tube with the laryngeal mask airway during routine surgical procedures, *Anesth Analg* 95(4):1094-1097, 2002.
10. Radu AD, et al. Pharyngo-laryngeal discomfort after breast surgery: comparison between orotracheal intubation and laryngeal mask, *Breast* 17(4):407-411, 2008.
CR 11. Shuster M, Nolan J, Barnes TA: Airway and ventilation management, *Emerg Cardiovasc Care* 20:23-35, 2002.
12. The Laryngeal Mask Company Limited: *LMA instruction manual,* San Diego, 2005. LMA.
13. Ulrich-Pur H, et al: Comparison of mucosal pressures induced by cuffs of different airway devices, *Anesthesiology* 104(5):933-938, 2006.

Additional Readings

Bogetz MS: Using the laryngeal mask airway to manage the difficult airway, *Anesthesiol Clin North Am* 20:863-870, 2002.

Burns SM: Safely caring for patients with a laryngeal mask airway, *Crit Care Nurse* 21:72-74, 2001.

Gabrielli A, et al: Alternative ventilation strategies in cardiopulmonary resuscitation, *Curr Opin Crit Care* 8:199-211, 2002.

Maltby JR, Loken RG, Watson NC: The laryngeal mask airway: clinical appraisal in 250 patients, *Can J Anesth* 37:509-513, 1990.

Nolan JD: Prehospital and resuscitative airway care: should the gold standard be reassessed? *Curr Opin Crit Care* 7:413-421, 2001.

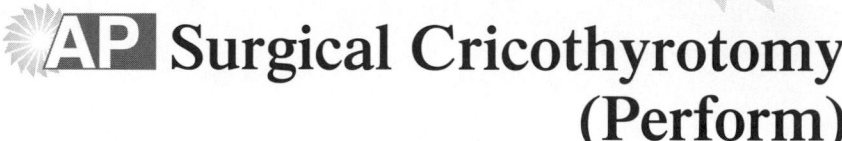

AP Surgical Cricothyrotomy (Perform)

P U R P O S E :   Surgical cricothyrotomy is an emergent procedure creating an opening in the cricothyroid membrane to facilitate placement of an endotracheal or tracheostomy tube and provide effective oxygenation and ventilation.

Patricia L. Hahn

PREREQUISITE NURSING KNOWLEDGE

- Surgical cricothyrotomy is used only when the airway cannot be obtained or maintained by standard means such as self-inflating manual resuscitation bag-valve-mask device ventilation, the use of airway adjuncts (oropharyngeal or nasopharyngeal airways), endotracheal intubation, or rescue airways (Combitube, laryngeal mask airway [LMA], or King Airway).[3,4]
- Surgical cricothyrotomy may be needed in patients with facial or neck trauma. Maintenance of the airway may be difficult in these patients because the injuries often disrupt the lower facial structures and make an adequate seal with a self-inflating manual resuscitation bag-valve device difficult to obtain. The airway may also be obstructed or disrupted, making endotracheal intubation difficult or ineffective.
- Difficulty in obtaining or maintaining an airway may result from upper airway obstruction as a result of trauma, allergic reactions with swelling and angioedema, foreign bodies, anatomic variations, and bleeding.[2]

- The need for emergent surgical cricothyrotomy must be determined quickly. This intervention is potentially life-saving, and implementation cannot be delayed.
- Surgical cricothyrotomy requires specialized training and should be performed only by highly skilled medical providers.[2]
- Commercially prepared cricothyrotomy kits are available and often use a modified Seldinger technique with a guidewire or dilator system.

Contraindications

Absolute
- Airway can be managed effectively with self-inflating manual resuscitation bag-valve-mask device, intubation, or rescue airway (Combitube, LMA, or King Airway).
- Complete transection of trachea
- Laryngotracheal disruption with retraction of distal trachea
- Fractured larynx

Relative
- Inability to identify anatomic landmarks
- Bleeding diathesis
- Children less than 12 years of age[5,6]

In young children, the airway is funnel-shaped with the narrowest portion at the cricoid ring rather than the vocal

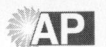

cords as in adults. This narrowing increases the risk of development of subglottic stenosis after cricothyrotomy. Percutaneous transtracheal ventilation via needle cricothyrotomy is the method of choice for surgical airway management in young children.[6]

EQUIPMENT

- Personal protective equipment (face mask, eye protection, gown, sterile gloves)
- Sterile surgical drape
- Skin antiseptic
- No. 10 or 11 blade scalpel
- 4 × 4 gauze sponges
- Suction device and suction catheter
- Curved hemostats
- Tracheal (Trousseau) dilator or nasal speculum
- 5.0 to 6.0 cuffed endotracheal tube or no. 4 tracheostomy tube
- 10-mL syringe
- Cloth tracheostomy ties
- Self-inflating manual resuscitation bag-valve-mask device with oxygen source
- Oxygen source and tubing
- Stethoscope

Additional equipment, to have available as needed, includes the following:

- Commercially prepared kit such as the Melker Emergency Cricothyrotomy Catheter (Cook Medical, Inc, Bloomington, Ind; www.cookmedical.com), which uses a specially designed airway and a modified Seldinger technique for insertion

PATIENT AND FAMILY EDUCATION

- A patient who needs emergency surgical cricothyrotomy likely is unresponsive from the inability to maintain the airway and adequate oxygenation and ventilation; therefore, patient education is not possible. If the patient is responsive, the airway and ventilatory efforts are adequate and surgical cricothyrotomy is not indicated.
- Family members should be provided with a quick and concise explanation of the emergent need to create an artificial airway. This information is often best explained by another member of the healthcare team rather than the provider performing the procedure to prevent any delay establishing the airway. If possible, obtain consent for the procedure from the family member.

PATIENT ASSESSMENT AND PREPARATION

Patient Assessment

- Assess airway patency.
  - Open the airway with a jaw-thrust or chin-lift maneuver. If traumatic injury is suspected, maintain cervical stabilization. Assess for presence of foreign bodies, secretions, or other obstructions. Use suction to clear and maintain the airway. ➻***Rationale:*** Often airway patency can be achieved and maintained with simple maneuvers such as patient positioning, use of an airway maneuver, suction, or insertion of an oral or nasal pharyngeal airway.
  - If the patient has potential for airway compromise (i.e., bleeding, swelling, or traumatic injuries) and is alert and able to maintain the airway, allow the patient to maintain a position of comfort and suction to maintain a patent airway. Do not attempt to place the patient in a supine position because this may cause significant airway compromise. ➻***Rationale:*** If the patient has the ability to maintain his or her own airway, allowing the patient to remain in an upright position, with suction provided if necessary, assists the patient in maintaining the airway. If the patient is placed in a supine position for packaging or transport, this move may cause significant airway compromise.
- Assess respiratory effort.
  - Assess rate, depth of respirations, accessory muscle use, chest wall motion, and breath sounds. If equipment is available, monitor oxygen saturation.
  - If respiratory efforts are inadequate, attempt ventilation with a self-inflating manual resuscitation bag-valve-mask device and supplemental oxygen.
  - If an airway cannot be maintained or oxygenation and ventilation with a self-inflating manual resuscitation bag-valve-mask device are inadequate, prepare for endotracheal intubation. If intubation is not possible, prepare for emergent surgical cricothyrotomy.
- ➻***Rationale:*** This process is to identify inadequate respiratory efforts quickly and determine the optimal method for oxygenation and ventilation.

Patient Preparation

- Verify correct patient with two identifiers. ➻***Rationale:*** Prior to performing a procedure, the nurse should ensure the correct identification of the patient for the intended intervention.
- Perform a pre-procedure verification and time out, if nonemergent. ➻***Rationale:*** Ensures patient safety.
- Position the patient supine and maintain cervical spine stabilization if indicated. ➻***Rationale:*** Patients who need emergent surgical cricothyrotomy often have traumatic injuries that necessitate cervical spine stabilization.
- Continue attempts to ventilate and oxygenate the patient with a self-inflating manual resuscitation bag-valve-mask device if the patient is apneic or respiratory efforts are inadequate. ➻***Rationale:*** This action can prevent further hypoxia and hypercarbia.

Procedure | for Surgical Cricothyrotomy

Steps	Rationale	Special Considerations
1. HH		
2. PE		Use of face mask and eye protection is recommended because of the increased risk of airborne blood or body fluids during this procedure.
3. Place patient in a supine position, with head and neck in neutral position.	Position the patient to expose the neck and larynx.	Maintain cervical spine stabilization if patient is at risk for cervical injury.
4. Identify the cricothyroid membrane (Fig. 8-1.) First, identify the thyroid prominence, or Adam's apple. The cricothyroid membrane is palpated at the midline, approximately one fingerbreadth below the thyroid prominence.	Identifies the correct location for incision and endotracheal tube placement. The cricothyroid membrane is preferred over the trachea because it is more anterior than the lower trachea and less thyroid and soft tissue are found between the membrane and the skin.	The incision is just inferior to the vocal cords, and superior to the thyroid gland.
5. Prepare the skin with an antiseptic solution.		
6. Spread the skin with the thumb and middle finger of the nondominant hand to make it taut and stabilize the larynx.	Allows for ease in creating an incision in the skin and keeps the larynx from shifting.	Throughout the procedure, the larynx must be immobilized.
7. Take the scalpel in the dominant hand and make a 2-cm vertical midline incision through the dermis, over the cricothyroid membrane.	Overly deep or long incisions risk damage to the larynx, cricoid cartilage, and trachea.	Some references recommend a horizontal skin incision.[1,2]

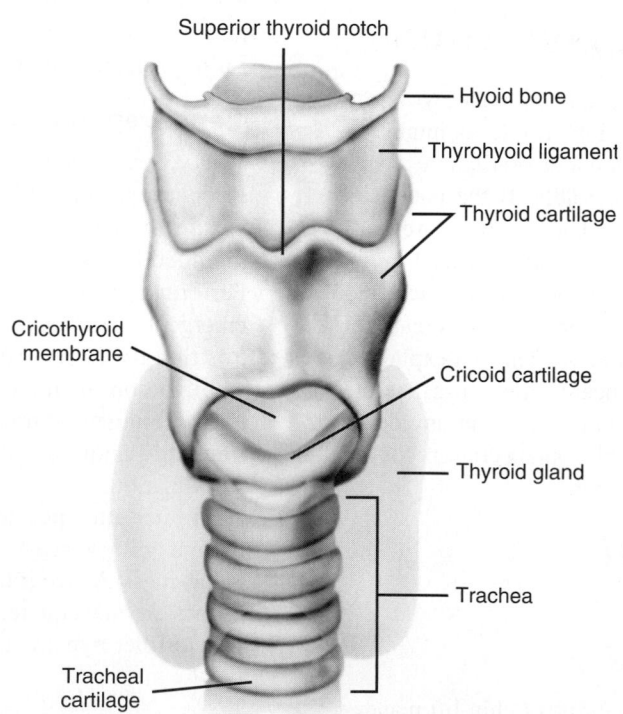

FIGURE 8-1 Anatomy of neck and location of cricothyroid membrane. *(Adapted from Patton KT, Thibodeau GA: Mosby's handbook of anatomy and physiology, St Louis, 2000, Elsevier.)*

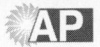

Procedure for Surgical Cricothyrotomy—*Continued*

Steps	Rationale	Special Considerations
8. Dab the wound with sterile gauze to control any bleeding from the incision. Use an assistant if available.	Use a dabbing technique to minimize further tissue trauma and bleeding.	Use an assistant, if available, to control bleeding and minimize interruptions in the procedure.
9. Identify the cricothyroid membrane. Palpate the cricothyroid membrane through the skin incision with the index finger. If necessary, use the curved hemostats to bluntly dissect through the skin to locate and visualize the cricothyroid membrane.	Blunt dissection is preferred over sharp dissection to minimize further tissue trauma and bleeding.	The index finger can be placed on the inferior aspect of the thyroid cartilage to identify the superior border of the cricothyroid membrane.
10. Make a horizontal incision in the lower half of the cricothyroid membrane with the scalpel (Fig. 8-2). The incision should be approximately 1 to 1.5 cm in length. Do not attempt to puncture the cricothyroid membrane. Use the scalpel to gently incise only the membrane. Avoid directing the scalpel toward the patient's head.	Incising the lower half of the membrane is preferred to avoid the superior cricothyroid artery and vein. The opening needs to be large enough to accommodate a 5.0 to 6.0 cuffed endotracheal or no. 4 tracheostomy tube. A puncturing motion may also puncture the posterior wall of the trachea and lacerate the esophagus and could lacerate or damage the vocal cords.	
11. Dab the wound with sterile gauze to control any bleeding from the incision. Use an assistant if available.	Use a dabbing technique to minimize further tissue trauma and bleeding.	Use an assistant, if available, to control bleeding and minimize interruptions in the procedure.
12. Insert tracheal dilator or nasal speculum into the opening in the cricothyroid membrane. Direct the tip of the speculum toward the patient's feet.	Avoids further trauma to the cricothyroid membrane or vocal cords and guides the tube into the airway.	

Procedure continues on following page

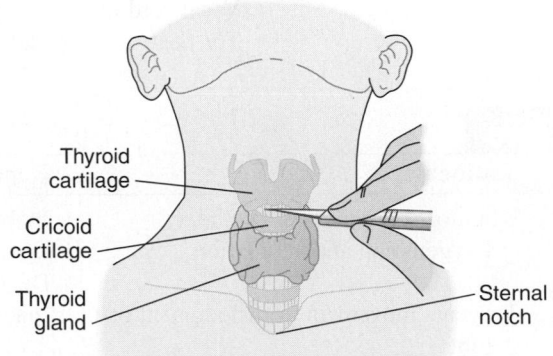

Thyroid cartilage
Cricoid cartilage
Thyroid gland
Sternal notch

FIGURE 8-2   Surgical cricothyrotomy. *(From Black JM, Hawks JH: Medical-surgical nursing: clinical management for positive outcomes, ed 8, St Louis, 2009, Elsevier.)*

Procedure   for Surgical Cricothyrotomy—*Continued*

Steps	Rationale	Special Considerations
13. Carefully spread the dilator or speculum vertically and advance the tube into the opening. If you meet resistance, do not force the tube into the opening.	The dilator or speculum enlarges the opening vertically, but use caution to avoid further trauma to the cricothyroid membrane or vocal cords. The tube should advance easily into the tracheal opening.	
14. Carefully remove the tracheal dilator or nasal speculum once the tube has been placed in the trachea.	Use caution to avoid inadvertent removal of the tube along with the dilator or speculum.	
15. Inflate the tube cuff with the syringe to a minimal occlusive pressure.	Prevents an air leak and optimizes oxygenation and ventilation.	A cuffed tube is preferred over an uncuffed tube to prevent an air leak and reduce the risk of aspiration.
16. Attach the self-inflating manual resuscitation bag-valve device to the tube and oxygenate and ventilate the patient.		
17. Auscultate for the presence of equal breath sounds and the absence of epigastric sounds with a stethoscope.	Tube position may be confirmed with the same methods as oral or nasal endotracheal tube placement.	Primary confirmation relies on physical examination techniques to confirm correct tube placement.[2]
18. Confirm correct placement with secondary means such as an exhaled CO_2 detector or monitoring device. Obtain chest radiography.	Tube position may be confirmed with the same methods as oral or nasal endotracheal tube placement.	Secondary confirmation verifies correct tube placement.[2]
19. Secure the tube with tracheostomy ties.	Prevents dislodgment or movement of tube.	Tracheostomy ties are preferred over tape. Use a square knot to secure.

Expected Outcomes

- Establishment of emergent surgical airway access
- Adequate oxygenation and ventilation
- Improved or stabilized patient condition

Unexpected Outcomes[1,2,6]

- Blood loss or hemorrhage
- Aspiration
- False passage of the endotracheal tube
- Tracheal perforation
- Esophageal perforation
- Subcutaneous emphysema
- Mediastinal emphysema
- Vocal cord injury or paralysis
- Tracheal stenosis (delayed)

Patient Monitoring and Care

Steps	Rationale	Reportable Conditions
1. Monitor breath sounds, adequacy of oxygenation and ventilation, and oxygen saturation (Spo_2).	Monitors effectiveness of airway, oxygenation and ventilation.	Inability to ventilate Decreased or absent breath sounds Decrease in Spo_2
2. Monitor endotracheal tube position.	Prevents movement or dislodgment of tube	Inadvertent dislodgment or removal of tube
3. Observe insertion site for bleeding, swelling, or subcutaneous air.	Identifies displacement of tube or significant air leak.	Excessive bleeding from the site Swelling or subcutaneous air at the insertion site
4. Follow institution standard for assessing pain. Administer analgesia as prescribed.	Identifies need for pain interventions.	Continued pain despite pain interventions.

Documentation

Documentation should include the following:

- Assessment findings to support the need for an emergent surgical airway
- Inability to obtain or maintain airway and provide oxygenation and ventilation by any other means
- Documentation of the procedure, to include date and time
- Any difficulties encountered during the procedure
- Size and type of endotracheal tube inserted and centimeter mark at skin opening
- Confirmation of proper tube placement with both primary and secondary means
- Pain assessment, interventions and effectiveness

References

CR 1. American College of Surgeons: *Airway and ventilatory management: advanced trauma life support,* ed 7, Chicago, 2004, ACS.

2. American Heart Association: *Airway, airway adjuncts, oxygenation and ventilation: advanced cardiac life support: principles and practice,* Dallas, 2006, AHA.

CR 3. McGill J, Clinton JE, Ruiz E: Cricothyrotomy in the emergency department, *Ann Emerg Med* 11:361-364, 1982.

4. Northwest MedStar, Critical Care Air Medical Transport Service: *Surgical cricothyrotomy: protocol and procedure book,* 133-134, Spokane, WA, 2008, Northwest MedStar.

CR 5. Sanders MJ: *Mosby's paramedic textbook,* ed 2, St Louis, 2001, Mosby.

CR 6. Tintinalli JE, Kelen GD, Stapczynski JS: *Emergency medicine: a comprehensive study guide,* ed 6, New York, 2004, McGraw-Hill.

Surgical Cricothyrotomy (Assist)

PURPOSE: Surgical cricothyrotomy is an emergent procedure creating an opening in the cricothyroid membrane to facilitate placement of an endotracheal or tracheostomy tube and provide effective oxygenation and ventilation.

Patricia L. Hahn

PREREQUISITE NURSING KNOWLEDGE

- Surgical cricothyrotomy is used only when the airway cannot be obtained or maintained by standard means such as self-inflating manual resuscitation bag-valve-mask device, the use of airway adjuncts (oropharyngeal or nasopharyngeal airways), endotracheal intubation, or rescue airway (Combitube, laryngeal mask airway [LMA], or King Airway).[3,4]
- Surgical cricothyrotomy may be needed in patients with facial or neck trauma. Maintenance of the airway may be difficult in these patients because the injuries often disrupt the lower facial structures and make an adequate seal with a self-inflating manual resuscitation bag-valve-mask device difficult to obtain. The airway may also be obstructed or disrupted making endotracheal intubation difficult or ineffective.
- Difficulty in obtaining or maintaining an airway may result from upper airway obstruction as a result of trauma, allergic reactions with swelling and angioedema, foreign bodies, anatomic variations, and bleeding.[2]
- The need for emergent surgical cricothyrotomy must be determined quickly. This intervention is potentially lifesaving, and implementation cannot be delayed.
- Surgical cricothyrotomy requires specialized training and should be performed only by highly skilled medical providers.[2]

- Commercially prepared cricothyrotomy kits are available and often use a modified Seldinger technique with a guidewire or dilator system.

Contraindications

Absolute
- Airway can be managed effectively with self-inflating manual resuscitation bag-valve-mask device or rescue airway (Combitube, LMA, or King Airway).
- Complete transection of trachea
- Laryngotracheal disruption with retraction of distal trachea
- Fractured larynx

Relative
- Inability to identify anatomic landmarks
- Bleeding diathesis
- Children less than 12 years of age[5,6]

In young children, the airway is funnel-shaped with the narrowest portion at the cricoid ring rather than the vocal cords as in adults. This narrowing increases the risk of development of subglottic stenosis after cricothyrotomy. Percutaneous transtracheal ventilation via needle cricothyrotomy is the method of choice for surgical airway management in young children.[6]

EQUIPMENT

- Personal protective equipment (face mask, eye protection, gown, sterile gloves)
- Sterile surgical drape
- Skin antiseptic
- No. 10 or 11 blade scalpel
- 4 × 4 gauze sponges
- Suction device and suction catheter
- Curved hemostats
- Tracheal (Trousseau) dilator or nasal speculum
- 5.0 to 6.0 cuffed endotracheal tube or no. 4 tracheostomy tube
- 10-mL syringe
- Cloth tracheostomy ties
- Self-inflating manual resuscitation bag-valve-mask device with oxygen source
- Oxygen source and tubing
- Stethoscope

Additional equipment, to have available as needed, includes the following:

- Commercially prepared kit such as the Melker Emergency Cricothyrotomy Catheter (Cook Medical, Inc, Bloomington, Ind; www.cookmedical.com), which uses a specially designed airway and a modified Seldinger technique for insertion

PATIENT AND FAMILY EDUCATION

- A patient who needs emergency surgical cricothyrotomy is likely unresponsive from the inability to maintain the airway and adequate oxygenation and ventilation; therefore, patient education is not possible. If the patient is responsive, the airway and ventilatory efforts are adequate and surgical cricothyrotomy is not indicated.
- Family members should be provided with a quick and concise explanation of the emergent need to create an artificial airway. This information is often best explained by another member of the healthcare team, rather than the provider performing the procedure, to prevent any delay in establishing the airway. If possible, obtain consent for the procedure from the family member.

PATIENT ASSESSMENT AND PREPARATION

Patient Assessment

- Assess airway patency.
  - Open the airway with a jaw-thrust or chin-lift maneuver. If traumatic injury is suspected, maintain cervical stabilization. Assess for presence of foreign bodies,

secretions, or other obstructions. Use suction to clear and maintain the airway. ➺*Rationale:* Often airway patency can be achieved and maintained with simple maneuvers such as patient positioning, use of an airway maneuver, suction, or insertion of an oral or nasal pharyngeal airway.
  - If the patient has potential for airway compromise (i.e. bleeding, swelling, or traumatic injuries) and is alert and able to maintain the airway, allow the patient to maintain a position of comfort and suction to maintain a patent airway. Do not attempt to place the patient in a supine position because this may cause significant airway compromise. ➺*Rationale:* If the patient has the ability to maintain his or her own airway, allowing the patient to remain in an upright position, with suction if necessary, assists the patient in maintaining the airway. If the patient is placed in a supine position for packaging or transport, this move may cause significant airway compromise.
- Assess respiratory effort.
  - Assess rate, depth of respirations, accessory muscle use, chest wall motion, and breath sounds. If equipment is available, monitor oxygen saturation.
  - If respiratory efforts are inadequate, attempt ventilation with a self-inflating manual resuscitation bag-valve-mask device and supplemental oxygen.
  - If an airway cannot be maintained or oxygenation and ventilation are adequate with a self-inflating manual resuscitation bag-valve-mask device, prepare for endotracheal intubation. If intubation is not possible, prepare for emergent surgical cricothyrotomy.
- ➺*Rationale:* This process is to identify inadequate respiratory efforts quickly and determine the optimal method for providing oxygenation and ventilation.

Patient Preparation

- Verify correct patient with two identifiers. ➺*Rationale:* Prior to performing a procedure, the nurse should ensure the correct identification of the patient for the intended intervention.
- Perform a pre-procedure verification and time out, if nonemergent. ➺*Rationale:* Ensures patient safety.
- Position the patient supine and maintain cervical spine stabilization if indicated. ➺*Rationale:* Patients who need emergent surgical cricothyrotomy often have traumatic injuries that require cervical spine stabilization.
- Continue attempts to ventilate and oxygenate the patient with a self-inflating manual resuscitation bag-valve-mask device if patient is apneic or respiratory efforts are inadequate. ➺*Rationale:* This action can prevent further hypoxia and hypercarbia.

Procedure for Assisting with Surgical Cricothyrotomy

Steps	Rationale	Special Considerations
1. **HH**		
2. **PE**		Use of face mask and eye protection is recommended because of the increased risk of airborne blood or body fluids during this procedure.
3. Place patient in a supine position, with head and neck in neutral position.	Position the patient to expose the neck and larynx.	Maintain cervical spine stabilization if patient is at risk for cervical injury.
4. If one assistant (assistant A) is available, continue attempts to oxygenate and ventilate the patient with a self-inflating manual resuscitation bag-valve-mask device. If a second assistant (assistant B) is available, assist the person performing the procedure.	Prevents further hypoxia and hypercarbia. Use of an assistant minimizes interruptions in the procedure.	Maintain sterile field and anticipate the needs of the person performing the procedure. Use caution when handling equipment to prevent contamination or inadvertent injury.
5. The person performing the procedure locates the cricothyroid membrane (see Fig. 8-1), prepares the skin with an antiseptic solution, and makes an incision through the skin. Assistant B anticipates need for antiseptic solution and scalpel.	Identifies the correct location for incision and tube placement. The cricothyroid membrane is preferred over the trachea because it is more anterior than the lower trachea and less thyroid and soft tissue are found between the membrane and the skin.	The incision is just inferior to the thyroid cartilage and superior to the thyroid gland.
6. Assistant B uses gauze sponges and a dabbing technique, to control any bleeding from the incision, when asked by the person performing the procedure.	A dabbing technique minimizes further tissue trauma and bleeding. Only assist with blood loss control when asked to avoid contact with the scalpel.	If a second assistant is not available, the primary assistant should continue to attempt to ventilate the patient.
7. The person performing the procedure incises the cricothyroid membrane with the scalpel. (see Fig. 8-2). Assistant B prepares the curved hemostats that may be needed to bluntly dissect the skin to locate and visualize the cricothyroid membrane. Assistant A stops ventilations just before the incision being made.	Discontinuing ventilations minimizes airborne contamination when the cricothyroid membrane is incised. Blunt dissection is preferred over sharp dissection to minimize further tissue trauma and bleeding.	
8. Assistant B controls any bleeding when requested with sterile gauze sponges and a dabbing technique.	A dabbing technique minimizes further tissue trauma and bleeding.	Use an assistant, if available, to control bleeding and minimize interruptions in the procedure.
9. Assistant B prepares the endotracheal or tracheostomy tube and tracheal dilator or nasal speculum for the person performing the procedure.	Enlarging the opening in the cricothyroid membrane allows passage of the tube.	Assistant A continues to hold ventilation attempts until the tube is placed.
10. Assistant B uses the syringe to inflate the tube cuff to a minimal occlusive pressure once the tube is placed.	Prevents an air leak and optimizes oxygenation and ventilation.	A cuffed tube is preferred over an uncuffed tube to prevent an air leak and reduce the risk of aspiration.

Procedure	**for Assisting with Surgical Cricothyrotomy**—*Continued*		
Steps	**Rationale**	**Special Considerations**	
11. Assistant A attaches the self-inflating manual resuscitation bag-valve device to the tube and oxygenates and ventilates the patient. Assistant B manually stabilizes the tube.	Prevents inadvertent movement or displacement of tube.		
12. Auscultate for the presence of equal breath sounds and the absence of epigastric sounds with a stethoscope.	Tube position may be confirmed with the same methods as oral or nasal endotracheal tube placement.	Primary confirmation relies on physical examination techniques to confirm correct tube placement.[2]	
13. Confirm correct placement with secondary means such as an exhaled CO_2 detector or monitoring device. Obtain chest radiography.	Tube position may be confirmed with the same methods as oral or nasal endotracheal tube placement.	Secondary confirmation verifies correct tube placement.[2]	
14. Secure the tube with tracheostomy ties. Dress the site with gauze and tape.	Prevent dislodgment or movement of tube.	Tracheostomy ties are preferred over tape to secure the tube. Use a square knot to secure.	

Expected Outcomes

- Establishment of emergent surgical airway access
- Provision of adequate oxygenation and ventilation
- Improved or stabilized patient condition

Unexpected Outcomes[1]

- Blood loss or hemorrhage
- Aspiration
- False passage of the endotracheal tube
- Tracheal perforation
- Esophageal perforation
- Subcutaneous emphysema
- Mediastinal emphysema
- Vocal cord injury or paralysis
- Tracheal stenosis (delayed)

Patient Monitoring and Care

Steps	**Rationale**	**Reportable Conditions**
1. Monitor breath sounds, adequacy of oxygenation and ventilation, and oxygen saturation (Spo_2).	Monitors effectiveness of airway, oxygenation, and ventilation.	• Inability to ventilate • Decreased or absent breath sounds • Decrease in Spo_2
2. Monitor endotracheal tube position.	Prevents movement or dislodgment of tube.	• Inadvertent dislodgment or removal of tube
3. Observe insertion site for bleeding, swelling, or subcutaneous air.	Identifies displacemnt of tube or significant air leak.	• Excessive bleeding from the site • Swelling or subcutaneous air at the insertion site
4. Follow institution standard for assessing pain. Administor analgesia as prescribed.	Identifies need for pain interventions.	• Continued pain despite pain interventions

Documentation

Documentation should include the following:

- Assessment findings to support the need for an emergent surgical airway
- Inability to obtain or maintain airway and provide oxygenation and ventilation by other means
- Documentation of the procedure, to include date and time
- Any difficulties encountered during the procedure
- Size and type of endotracheal tube inserted and centimeter mark at skin opening
- Confirmation of proper tube placement by both primary and secondary means
- Pain assessment, interventions and effectiveness

References

CR 1. American College of Surgeons: *Airway and ventilatory management: advanced trauma life support,* ed 7, Chicago, 2004, ACS.

2. American Heart Association: *Airway, airway adjuncts, oxygenation and ventilation: advanced cardiac life support: principles and practice,* Dallas, 2006, AHA.

CR 3. McGill J, Clinton JE, Ruiz E: Cricothyrotomy in the emergency department, *Ann Emerg Med* 11:361-364, 1982.

4. Northwest MedStar, Critical Care Air Medical Transport Service: *Surgical cricothyrotomy: protocol and procedure book,* 133-134, Spokane, WA, 2008, Northwest MedStar.

CR 5. Sanders MJ: *Mosby's paramedic textbook,* ed 2, St Louis, 2001. Mosby.

6. Tintinalli JE, Kelen GD, Stapczynski JS: *Emergency medicine: a comprehensive study guide,* ed 6, New York, 2004, McGraw-Hill.

Nasopharyngeal Airway Insertion

P U R P O S E : Nasopharyngeal airways are used to maintain a patent airway to the hypopharynx and to facilitate the removal of tracheobronchial secretions by directing the catheter and by averting tissue trauma that is associated with repeated suction attempts.[4]

Kirsten N. Skillings, Bonnie L. Curtis

PREREQUISITE NURSING KNOWLEDGE

- Nasopharyngeal airways are passed through the nose and follow the posterior nasal and oropharyngeal walls to the base of the tongue (Fig. 10-1).[3]
- The nasopharyngeal airway has three parts: the flange, cannula, and bevel or tip. The flange is the wide trumpet-like end that prevents further slippage into the airway. The hollow shaft of the cannula permits airflow into the hypopharynx. The bevel or tip is the opening at the distal end of the tube. When properly inserted, and the correct size, the tip can be seen resting posterior to the base of the tongue.
- The external diameter of the nasopharyngeal airway should be slightly smaller than the patient's external nares opening. The length of the nasopharyngeal airway is determined by measuring the distance between the naris and the tragus of the ear (Fig. 10-2).[2] Improperly sized nasopharyngeal airways may result in increased airway resistance, limited airflow (if the airway is too small), kinking and mucosal trauma, gagging, vomiting, and gastric distention (if the airway is too large). Some manufacturers provide nasopharyngeal airways shaped specifically for the right and left nares.

- The advantages of the nasopharyngeal airway include increased comfort and tolerance in a conscious patient, stable airway positioning for long periods, decreased incidence of gag reflex stimulation, and minimal incidence of mucosal trauma during frequent suctioning.

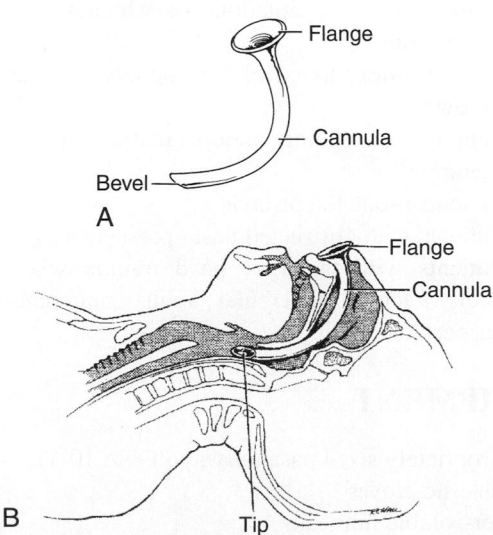

FIGURE 10-1 Nasopharyngeal airway. **A,** Airway parts. **B,** Proper placement. *(From Eubanks DH, Bone RC: Comprehensive respiratory care: a learning system, St Louis, 1990, Mosby, 518.)*

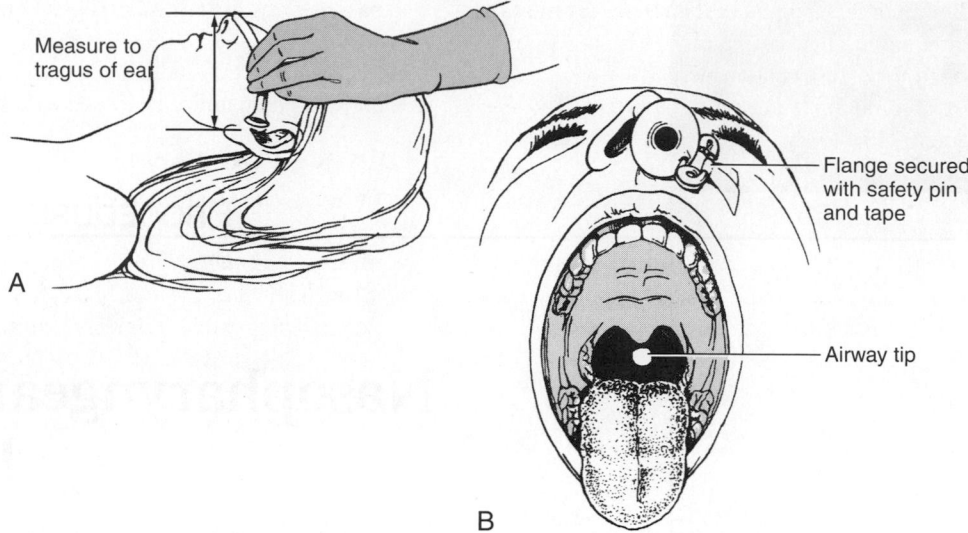

Measure to
tragus of ear

Flange secured
with safety pin
and tape

Airway tip

A

B

FIGURE 10-2 **A,** Estimating nasopharyngeal airway size. **B,** Nasopharyngeal position after insertion. *(From Eubanks DH, Bone RC: Comprehensive respiratory care: a learning system, St Louis, 1990, Mosby, 552.)*

- Nasopharyngeal airways are especially useful for relieving airway obstruction associated with mandibular-type injuries that result in jaw immobility or soft tissue obstruction. Examples of these injuries include jaw wiring, trismus, pain, edema, jaw spasms, and mechanical impairment such as temporomandibular joint fractures and zygomatic fractures. In selected patient situations, a nasopharyngeal airway may be used to facilitate the passage of a fiberoptic bronchoscope and to tamponade small bleeding blood vessels in the nasal mucosa.
- Insertion of the nasopharyngeal airway in an alert patient may stimulate the gag reflex and cause retching and vomiting.
- The nasopharyngeal airway is used most commonly in the postanesthesia recovery period to facilitate pulmonary toilets and in situations in which the patient is semiconscious.
- Contraindications to use of a nasopharyngeal airway are as follows:
  - ❖ Patients undergoing anticoagulation or antiplatelet therapy
  - ❖ Patients prone to epistaxis
  - ❖ Patients with obstructed nasal passageways
  - ❖ Patients with facial or head trauma when basilar skull fracture or cranial vault communication is suspected

EQUIPMENT

- Appropriately sized nasal airway (Table 10-1)
- Nonsterile gloves
- Water-soluble lubricant
- Suction equipment
- Flashlight
- Tongue depressor

TABLE 10-1	Nasopharyngeal Airway Sizing	
Approximate Body Weight	**Size (mm)**
Small adult	6 to 7
Medium adult	7 to 8
Large adult	8 to 9

(From Cummins RO, editor: Airway, airway adjuncts, oxygenation, and ventilation. In ACLS: principles and practice, Dallas, 2003, American Heart Association, 145-146.)

PATIENT AND FAMILY EDUCATION

- Explain the purpose of the airway and the necessity of the procedure to conscious patients or to the family of an unconscious patient. ➥*Rationale:* Communication and explanation regarding therapy are cited as important needs of patients and families to relieve anxiety and encourage communication.
- Explain the patient's role in assisting with insertion of the airway. ➥*Rationale:* Patient cooperation is elicited, and tube insertion is facilitated.
- Discuss the sensory experiences associated with nasal airway insertion, including the presence of an airway in the nose and possible gagging. ➥*Rationale:* Knowledge of anticipated sensory experiences reduces anxiety and distress.

PATIENT ASSESSMENT AND PREPARATION
Patient Assessment

- Verify correct patient with two identifiers. ➥*Rationale:* Prior to performing a procedure, the nurse should ensure the correct identification of the patient for the intended intervention.

- Assess cardiopulmonary status. ➻*Rationale:* Evaluation of the patient's cardiopulmonary status assists in determining the need for an artificial airway.
- Assess pain according to institution standard. ➻*Rationale:* This assessment identifies the need for discomfort management.
- Assess patent nasal passageway. With finger pressure, occlude one nostril; feel for air movement under the open nostril. Patency also can be assessed with inspection of each naris with a flashlight. ➻*Rationale:* Assessment of patency promotes smooth, quick, unobstructed airway insertion.
- If a difficult insertion is anticipated (e.g., with nasal polyps, septal deviation), contact the practitioner for an order to apply a topical anesthetic to coat the nasal passageway. ➻*Rationale:* Topical anesthetics with a vasoconstrictor help shrink nasal mucosa and decrease the incidence of trauma and bleeding. Vasoconstrictor property acts on capillaries to decrease bleeding.

Patient Preparation

- Ensure that the patient understands preprocedural teachings. Answer questions as they arise, and reinforce information as needed. ➻*Rationale:* This step evaluates and reinforces understanding of previously taught information.
- Position the patient. Unless contraindicated, a supine or high Fowler's position is acceptable. ➻*Rationale:* This positioning promotes patient and nurse comfort and provides easy access to the external nares.

Procedure	**for Nasopharyngeal Airway Insertion**	
Steps	**Rationale**	**Special Considerations**
1. HH		
2. PE		For copious secretions, don protective eyewear, face mask.
3. Prepare the nasopharyngeal airway.[1] **(Level D*)** A. Inspect for smooth edges. B. Generously lubricate the tip and outer cannula with water-soluble lubricant.	Decreases chances of mucosal trauma during insertion. Decreases incidence of trauma by preventing friction against dry mucosal membrane.[4]	
4. Remove excess secretions from nares.[1] **(Level D)**	Allows for visual inspection of nares; removes possible source of obstruction; removes medium for organism growth.	Nasopharyngeal and nasotracheal suction are contraindicated in patients with actual or suspected maxillofacial or skull injuries.
5. Elevate the tip of the nose and gently slide airway into nostril. Guide it medially and downward along the nasal passage.[1] **(Level D)**	Following the natural contour of the nasal passage decreases the incidence of trauma.	If resistance is encountered, rotate the tube and continue gentle forward pressure. Do not force the tube. If resistance continues, withdraw the tube and try the other nostril. During tube insertion, if the patient has increasing dyspnea or respiratory distress, consider removing the tube.
6. Ask patient to open his or her mouth, or hold the patient's mouth open, avoiding placing fingers between the patient's teeth. Control the tongue with a tongue depressor. Illuminate the oral cavity, and visualize the tip of the nasopharyngeal airway behind the uvula (see Fig. 10-2).[1] **(Level D)**	Verifying the location of the airway in the pharynx confirms proper airway positioning and allows for inspection of posterior pharynx for excessive bleeding or mucus.	
7. Verify patency of airway. Feel for air movement over the flange. Auscultate breath sounds bilaterally.[1] **(Level D)**	Optimal airway positioning allows for forward air flow, removal of secretions, and possible prevention of airway occlusion.	
8. Suction secretions as needed.[1] **(Level D)**	Maintains patent airway.	Recheck flange for proper position.

*Level D: Peer-reviewed professional organizational standards with clinical studies to support recommendations

Procedure continues on following page

Procedure | for Nasopharyngeal Airway Insertion—*Continued*

Steps	Rationale	Special Considerations
9. Reassess patient's respiratory status.[1] **(Level D*)**	Indicates effectiveness of the nasal airway.	
10. Follow institution standard for assessing pain. Administer analgesia as prescribed.[1]	Identifies need for pain interventions.	Continued pain despite pain interventions.

Expected Outcomes

- Airway patency maintained
- Effective removal of tracheobronchial secretions
- Diminished mucosal edema and trauma related to frequent suction passes

Unexpected Outcomes

- Inability to pass nasopharyngeal airway
- Airway obstruction
- Head or ear pain
- Epistaxis
- Naris and nasal mucosal ulceration

Patient Monitoring and Care

Steps	Rationale	Reportable Conditions
		These conditions should be reported if they persist despite nursing interventions.
1. Assess skin in contact with nasal airway. Remove and clean nasopharyngeal airway every 8 to 12 hours.	Consider rotating to other naris to prevent skin breakdown.	• Redness • Swelling • Drainage • Bleeding • Skin breakdown
2. Hyperoxygenate and suction as necessary, per assessment (see Procedure 12).	Retained secretions increase the potential for airway obstruction and pulmonary infections. Aging results in diminishing mucociliary clearance.	• Change in character or amount of secretions
3. Monitor respiratory status every 2 to 4 hours.	Change in respiratory status may indicate displacement of oral airway or worsening respiratory condition.	• Change in respiratory status not corrected with repositioning of airway or suctioning
4. Provide meticulous oral care every 2 to 4 hours and as needed (see Procedure 4).	Prevents secretions, encrustations, mouth infections, and airway port occlusions.	• Lacerations • Ulcerations • Areas of necrosis
5. Follow institution standard for assessing pain. Administer analgesia as prescribed.	Identifies need for pain interventions.	• Continued pain despite pain interventions

Documentation

Documentation should include the following:
- Patient and family education
- Insertion of nasopharyngeal airway
- Size of nasopharyngeal airway
- Any difficulties with insertion, including the need for ordered topical anesthetics
- Patient tolerance, including vital signs, respiratory values, and pain assessment before and after procedure
- Verification of proper placement
- Appearance and thickness of tracheal secretions, if present
- Skin integrity around tube
- Unexpected outcomes
- Nursing interventions
- Pain assessment, interventions, and effectiveness

*Level D: Peer-reviewed professional organizational standards with clinical studies to support recommendations

References

CR 1. American Association of Respiratory Care and Clinical Practice Guidelines: *Nasotracheal suctioning, revision and update,* Irving, TX, 2004, American Association of Respiratory Care.

2. Cummins RO, editor: Airway, airway adjuncts, oxygenation, and ventilation. In *ACLS: principles and practice,* Dallas, 2006, American Heart Association, 145-146.

CR 3. Eubanks DH, Bone RC: *Comprehensive respiratory care: a learning system,* St Louis, 1990, Mosby, 491-495.

4. Pierce LNB: *Management of the mechanically ventilated patient,* ed 2, St Louis, 2007, Saunders.

Additional Readings

Roberts K, Whalley H, Bleetman A: *The nasopharyngeal airway: dispelling myths and establishing the facts,* J Emerg Med 22:394-396, 2005.

St. John RE, Seckel MA: Airway management. In Burns SM: *AACN protocols for practice: care of the mechanically ventilated patient,* ed 2, Sudbury, MA, 2007, Jones and Bartlett Publishers.

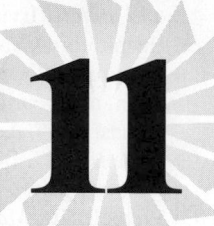

Oropharyngeal Airway Insertion

P U R P O S E :   Oropharyngeal airways are inserted to relieve airway obstruction, provide short-term maintenance of an airway, and facilitate removal of tracheobronchial secretions.

Kirsten N. Skillings, Bonnie L. Curtis

PREREQUISITE NURSING KNOWLEDGE

- Oropharyngeal airways are usually disposable and made of hard curved plastic.
- Oral airways are inserted through the open mouth with the posterior tip resting in the patient's pharynx.
- The oral airway is placed over the tongue. The curvature or body of the airway displaces the tongue forward from the posterior pharyngeal wall, a common site of airway obstruction.
- An oral airway has four parts: the flange, body, tip, and channel (Fig. 11-1). The flange, or flat surface, protruding from the mouth rests against the lips. This design protects against aspiration into the airway. The body of the airway curves over the tongue. The tip is the distal-most part of the airway toward the base of the tongue. The channel enables passage of a suction catheter.
- The Guedel airway is tubular with a flattened-oval inner diameter. A suction catheter passes through the central lumen or channel.
- The Berman airway has a channel on either side that guides the catheter along the edge of the airway into the pharyngeal space.
- Oral airways are manufactured in a variety of lengths and widths for adults, children, and infants. Sizing depends on the age and size of the patient (Table 11-1). An alternative method used to select the size of an oral airway is to measure the airway by placing the flange alongside the patient's lips and the oral airway tip alongside the angle of the jaw

(Fig. 11-2). Improperly sized airways can cause airway obstruction (if they are too small) and tongue displacement against the oropharynx (if they are too large).
- Oropharyngeal airways are used most commonly in unconscious patients because they may stimulate vomiting in a conscious or semiconscious patient.[2]
- Oral airways facilitate suctioning of the pharynx and prevent patients from biting their tongues, grinding their teeth, or occluding their endotracheal or oral gastric tubes. In addition, an oropharyngeal airway may be used in conjunction with an oral endotracheal tube to facilitate artificial ventilation, acting as a bite-block and preventing damage to the endotracheal tube, tongue, and soft tissues of the mouth.
- Improper or rough insertion techniques can result in tooth damage or loss and lacerations to the roof of the mouth. Improper lip, oral, and airway care can result in pressure sores, cracked lips, and stomatitis.
- Oropharyngeal airway placement should never be attempted in a patient who is actively seizing.

EQUIPMENT

- Appropriately sized oral airway
- Nonsterile gloves
- Tongue depressor
- Tape
  Additional equipment, to have available as needed, includes the following:
- Goggles, glasses, or face mask
- Suction equipment

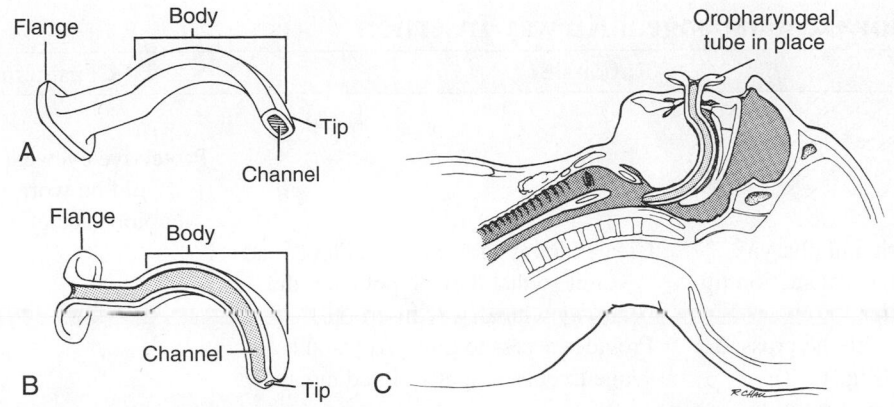

FIGURE 11-1   Oropharyngeal airways. **A,** Guedel airway. **B,** Berman airway. **C,** Properly inserted oropharyngeal tube. *(From Eubanks DH, Bone RC: Comprehensive respiratory care: a learning system, St Louis, 1990, Mosby, 518.)*

TABLE 11-1	Oral Airway Sizes	
Size of Patient	Diameter of Oral Airway (mm)	Size of Oral Airway (Guedel)
Large adult	100	5
Medium adult	90	4
Small adult	80	3

From Cummins RO, editor: Airway, airway adjuncts, oxygenation, and ventilation. In ACLS: principles and practice, Dallas, 2003, American Heart Association, 145.

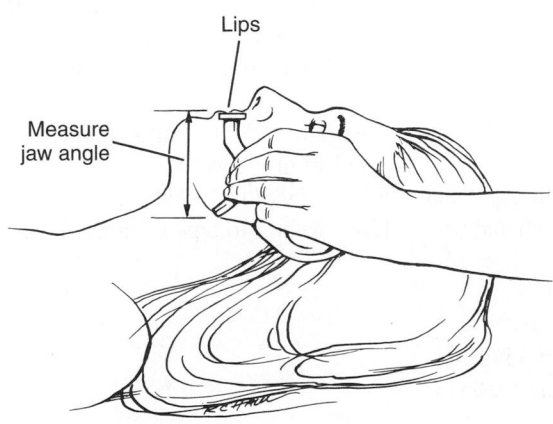

FIGURE 11-2   Alternative method for selecting size of an oro-pharyngeal airway. *(From Eubanks DH, Bone RC: Comprehensive respiratory care: a learning system, St Louis, 1990, Mosby, 552.)*

PATIENT AND FAMILY EDUCATION

- Explain the procedure to the family (if the patient's condition and time allow) and the reason for the airway insertion. ➤➤*Rationale:* This process identifies family knowledge deficits about the patient's condition, the procedure, its expected benefits, and its potential risks and allows time for questions to clarify information and voice concerns. Explanations decrease family anxiety.
- Discuss the sensory experiences associated with oral airway insertion, including the inability to clench teeth together, the presence of a hard plastic airway in the mouth, the inability to move the tongue freely, and the possibility of gagging. ➤➤*Rationale:* Knowledge of anticipated sensory experiences reduces anxiety and distress.

PATIENT ASSESSMENT AND PREPARATION

Patient Assessment

- Assess the patient's need for long-term airway maintenance. ➤➤*Rationale:* Oropharyngeal airways are generally used for temporary airway maintenance.[1-3]
- Assess condition of oral mucosa, dentition, and gums. ➤➤*Rationale:* Pre-procedural assessment provides baseline information for later comparison.
- Remove loose-fitting dentures and any foreign objects (including partial plates, tongue studs, lip rings) from the mouth. ➤➤*Rationale:* Removal ensures that objects do not advance farther into the airway during insertion.

Patient Preparation

- Verify correct patient with two identifiers. ➤➤*Rationale:* Prior to performing a procedure, the nurse should ensure the correct identification of the patient for the intended intervention.
- Ensure that patient and family understand preprocedural teachings. Answer questions as they arise, and reinforce information as needed. ➤➤*Rationale:* This step evaluates and reinforces understanding of previously taught information.
- Position the patient. A semi-Fowler's or supine position is preferred for a conscious patient. ➤➤*Rationale:* This positioning promotes patient and nurse comfort and provides easy access to the oral cavity.
- Hyperextend the patient's neck with the head-tilt chin-lift technique or the jaw-thrust technique for opening the airway of the unconscious patient. Maintain cervical stabilization in a trauma patient, using the jaw-thrust technique only. ➤➤*Rationale:* Opening the airway can prevent obstructions that result from posterior displacement of the tongue and epiglottis.

Procedure for Oropharyngeal Airway Insertion

Steps	Rationale	Special Considerations
1. **HH**		
2. **PE**		Protective eyewear or face masks should be worn in the presence of copious secretions.
3. Suction the mouth and pharynx with a rigid pharyngeal suction tip (Yankauer) catheter.	Clears airway of secretions, blood, and vomit so that they do not enter the airway with airway insertion.	
4. Open the mouth with the crossed-finger technique (Fig. 11-3). Remove dentures, if present.	Provides access to oral cavity and leverage to open a tightly closed mouth.	
5. Insert oral airway.	Provides patent upper airway and prevents posterior tongue displacement.	Remove the airway immediately if the patient gags, gasps for air, or begins breathing irregularly. A tongue depressor may assist in tongue control during insertion.
A. Insert oral airway with curved end up (Fig. 11-4, A).	Positions airway appropriately.	
B. Advance oral airway over the base of the tongue until the flange is parallel with the patient's nose.		
C. Gently rotate the tip 180 degrees to point down (see Fig. 11-4, B).	Provides for open pathway from the mouth to the pharynx.	
6. Recheck the size and position of the oral airway. Verify airway patency. **(Level D*)**	Proper placement and size are essential for securing and maintaining a patent airway.	When the oral airway is properly sized, the flange should rest against the patient's lips (see Fig. 11-2). Gagging may indicate that the airway is too long. Ensure that the lips and tongue are not between the teeth and airway.[3]
7. Consider securing the airway.	Taping is indicated to prevent expulsion of the airway. The airway should be left untaped in patients who need to be able to cough out the airway if gagging should occur because gagging may stimulate vomiting and aspiration (i.e., in a postanesthesia or semiconscious patient).	Follow institutional standards. Use care not to tape over air channel.
8. Hyperoxygenate and suction pharynx as needed (see Procedure 12).	Maintains patent airway; pooled secretions provide a medium for bacterial growth.	
9. Reassess patient's respiratory status.	Validates the effectiveness of the oral airway.	

Expected Outcomes

- Improvement of respiratory status
- Short-term patent airway

Unexpected Outcomes

- Airway obstruction
- Pulmonary aspiration
- Trauma to the lips and oral cavity
- Inability to insert oral airway because patient is combative or seizing or patient's mouth cannot be opened

*Level D: Peer-reviewed professional organizational standards with clinical studies to support recommendations.

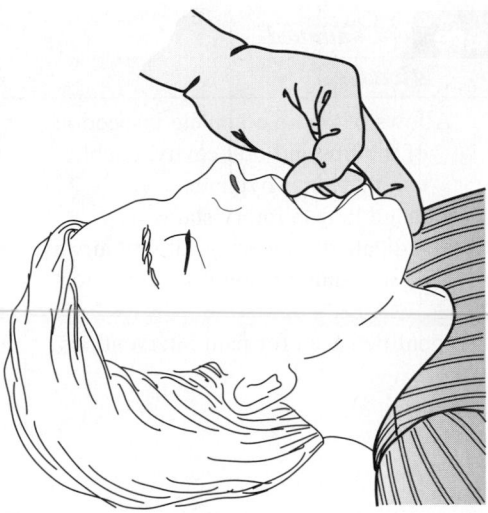

FIGURE 11-3 Crossed-finger technique for opening the mouth. *(From Eubanks DH, Bone RC: Comprehensive respiratory care: a learning system, St Louis, 1990, Mosby, 631.)*

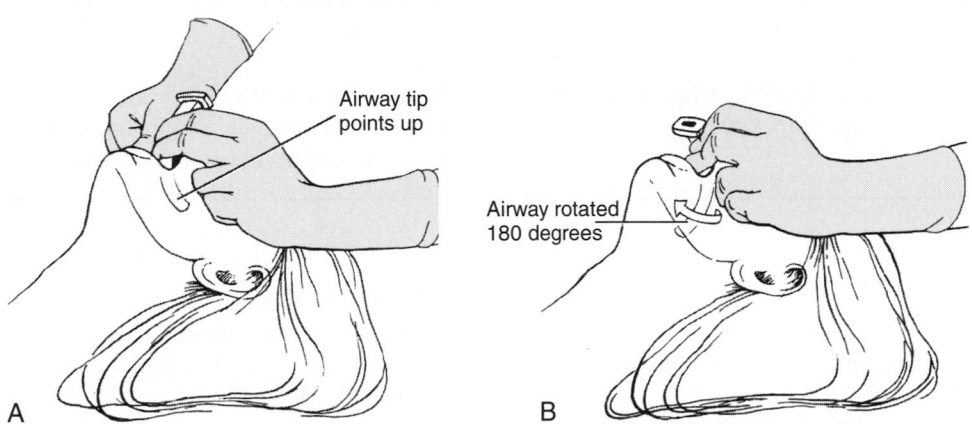

Airway tip points up

Airway rotated 180 degrees

A

B

FIGURE 11-4 Insertion of an oropharyngeal airway. **A,** Advance airway with curved end up. **B,** Rotate airway 180 degrees. *(From Eubanks DH, Bone RC: Comprehensive respiratory care: a learning system, St Louis, 1990, Mosby, 551.)*

Patient Monitoring and Care

Steps	Rationale	Reportable Conditions
		These conditions should be reported if they persist despite nursing interventions.
1. If the oropharyngeal airway is not replaced with a definitive airway, reposition the oral airway every 1 to 2 hours, assessing the lips, tongue, and mouth with each position change.	Pressure of the flange on the lips may produce ulcers and necrosis.	• Lacerations • Ulcerations • Areas of necrosis
2. Apply water-soluble gel or lip balm to the lips.	Prevents mucosal drying and cracking.	• Cracked and bleeding lips
3. Provide meticulous oral care every 2 to 4 hours and as needed (see Procedure 4).	Decreases secretions, encrustations, oral infections, and airway port occlusions.	• Lacerations • Ulcerations • Areas of necrosis • Drainage

Procedure continues on following page

Patient Monitoring and Care —*Continued*

Steps	Rationale	Reportable Conditions
4. Remove the oral airway every 8 to 12 hours or as needed. Clean airway and reinsert, as needed.	Allows for more complete inspection of the lips and oral cavity; enables complete oral hygiene.	
5. Monitor respiratory status every 2 to 4 hours.	Change in respiratory status may indicate displacement of oral airway or worsening respiratory condition.	• Stridor • Crowing • Gasping respirations • Snoring
6. Follow institution standard for assessing pain. Administer analgesia as prescribed.	Identifies need for pain interventions.	• Continued pain despite pain interventions.

Documentation

Documentation should include the following:
- Family education
- Insertion of oropharyngeal airway
- Type and size of oral airway
- Any difficulties in insertion
- Patient tolerance, including respiratory and vital signs assessments before and after procedure
- Verification of proper placement
- Appearance and thickness of tracheal or oral secretions, if present
- Oral care
- Skin integrity around tube
- Unexpected outcomes before and after procedure
- Pain assessment, interventions, and effectiveness

References

1. Cummins RO, editor: Airway, airway adjuncts, oxygenation, and ventilation. In *ACLS: principles and practice,* Dallas, 2006, American Heart Association, 145-146.
2. Dulak S: Placing an oropharyngeal airway, *RN* 68 (2):20ac1-20ac2, 2005.
3. Pierce L: *Management of the mechanically ventilated patient,* St Louis, 2007, Saunders.

Additional Reading

St John R, Seckel M: Airway management. In Burns SM, editor: *Care of mechanically ventilated patients,* ed 2, Sudbury, MA, 2007, Jones and Bartlett.

Suctioning: Endotracheal or Tracheostomy Tube

PURPOSE: Endotracheal or tracheostomy tube suctioning is performed to maintain the patency of the artificial airway and to improve gas exchange, decrease airway resistance, and reduce infection risk by removing secretions from the trachea and main-stem bronchi. Suctioning also may be performed to obtain samples of tracheal secretions for laboratory analysis.

Marianne Chulay, Maureen A. Seckel

PREREQUISITE NURSING KNOWLEDGE

- Endotracheal and tracheostomy tubes are used to maintain a patent airway and to facilitate mechanical ventilation. The presence of these artificial airways, especially endotracheal tubes, prevents effective coughing and secretion removal, necessitating periodic removal of pulmonary secretions with suctioning. In acute care situations, suctioning is always performed as a sterile procedure to prevent hospital-acquired pneumonia.
- Suctioning is performed with one of two basic methods. In the open-suction technique, after disconnection of the endotracheal or tracheostomy tube from any ventilatory tubing or oxygen sources, a single-use suction catheter is inserted into the open end of the tube. In the closed-suction technique, also referred to as in-line suctioning, a multiple-use suction catheter inside a sterile plastic sleeve is inserted through a special diaphragm attached to the end of the endotracheal or tracheostomy tube (Fig. 12-1). The closed-suction technique allows for the maintenance of oxygenation and ventilation support, which may be beneficial in patients with moderate to severe pulmonary insufficiency. In addition, the closed-suction technique

decreases the risk for aerosolization of tracheal secretions during suction-induced coughing. Use of the closed-suction technique should be considered in patients with cardiopulmonary instability during suctioning with the open technique, who have high levels of positive end-expiratory pressure (PEEP; >10 cm H_2O) or inspired oxygen (greater than 80%) or both, who have grossly bloody pulmonary secretions, or in whom airborne transmission of disease, such as active pulmonary tuberculosis, is suspected.

- Indications for suctioning include the following:
  - ❖ Secretions in the artificial airway
  - ❖ Suspected aspiration of gastric or upper airway secretions
  - ❖ Auscultation of adventitious lung sounds (rhonchi) over the trachea or main-stem bronchi or both
  - ❖ Increase in peak airway pressures when patient is on mechanical ventilation
  - ❖ Increase in respiratory rate or frequent coughing or both
  - ❖ Gradual or sudden decrease in arterial blood oxygen (Pao_2), arterial blood oxygen saturation (Sao_2), or arterial saturation via pulse oximetry (Spo_2) levels
  - ❖ Sudden onset of respiratory distress, when airway patency is questioned

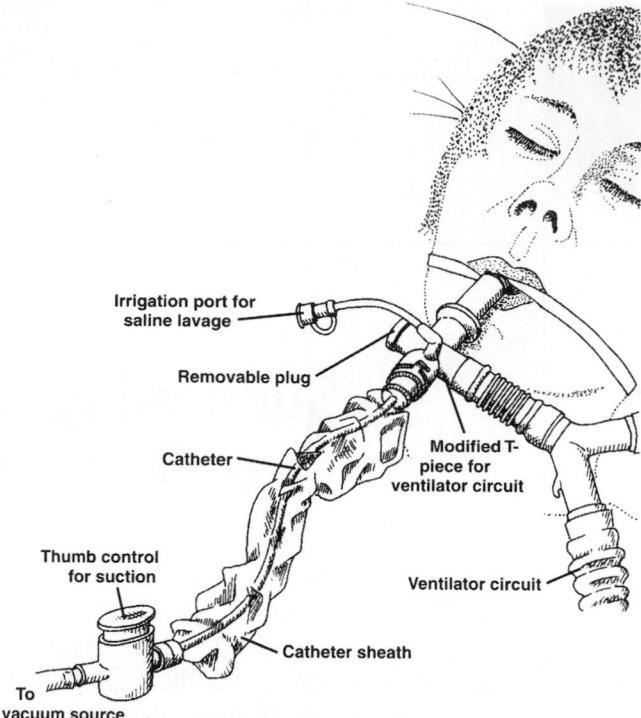

FIGURE 12-1   Closed-suction technique. *(From Sills JR: The comprehensive respiratory therapist exam review: Entry and advanced levels, St Louis, 2010, Elsevier, Mosby.)*

- Suctioning of airways should be performed only for a clinical indication and not as a routine fixed-schedule treatment.
- Hyperoxygenation always should be provided before and after each pass of the suction catheter into the endotracheal tube, whether with the open or closed suctioning method.
- Suctioning is a necessary procedure for patients with artificial airways. When clinical indicators of the need for suctioning exist, there is no absolute contraindication to suctioning. In situations in which the development of a suctioning complication would be poorly tolerated by the patient, strong evidence of a clinical need for suctioning should exist.
- Complications associated with suctioning of artificial airways include the following:
  - ❖ Hypoxemia
  - ❖ Respiratory arrest
  - ❖ Cardiac arrest
  - ❖ Cardiac dysrhythmias (premature contractions, tachycardias, bradycardias, heart blocks)
  - ❖ Hypertension or hypotension
  - ❖ Decreases in mixed venous oxygen saturation (Svo_2)
  - ❖ Increased intracranial pressure
  - ❖ Bronchospasm
  - ❖ Pulmonary hemorrhage or bleeding
  - ❖ Pain and anxiety
- Tracheal mucosal damage (epithelial denudement, hyperemia, loss of cilia, edema) occurs during suctioning when tissue is pulled into the catheter tip holes. These areas of damage increase the risk of infection and bleeding. Use of special-tipped catheters, low levels of suction pressure, or intermittent suction pressure has not been shown to decrease tracheal mucosal damage with suctioning.
- Postural drainage and percussion may improve secretion mobilization from small to large airways in diseases with large mucus production (e.g., cystic fibrosis, bronchitis).
- Adequate systemic hydration and supplemental humidification of inspired gases assist in thinning secretions for easier aspiration from airways. Instillation of a bolus of normal saline solution does not thin secretions, may cause decreases in arterial and mixed venous oxygenation, and may contribute to lower airway contamination from the mechanical dislodgment of bacteria within the artificial airway or from contamination of saline solution during instillation.[26]
- The suction catheter should not be any larger than half of the internal diameter of the endotracheal or tracheostomy tube.

EQUIPMENT

- Open technique
  - ❖ Suction catheter of appropriate size (Table 12-1)
  - ❖ Sterile saline or sterile water solution
  - ❖ Sterile gloves
  - ❖ Sterile solution container
  - ❖ Source of suction (wall mounted or portable)

TABLE 12-1	Guideline for Catheter Size for Endotracheal and Tracheostomy Tube Suctioning*			
Patient Age	**Endotracheal Tube Size (mm)**	**Tracheostomy Tube Size (mm, Inner Diameter)**	**Suction Catheter Size**	
Small child (2 to 5 y)	4.0 to 5.0	3.0 to 5.5	6F to 8F	
School-age child (6 to 12 y)	5.0 to 6.0	4.0 to 6.5	8F to 10F	
Adolescent to adult	7.0 to 9.0	5.0 to 9.0	10F to 16F	

*This guide should be used as an estimate only. Actual sizes depend on the size and individual needs of the patient. Always follow manufacturer's guidelines.

Adapted from St John RE, Seckel M: Airway management. In AACN protocols for practice: care of the mechanically ventilated patient series, Sudbury, MA, 2007, Jones & Bartlett Publishers, 41.

- ❖ Connecting tube, 4 to 6 ft
- ❖ Manual self-inflating manual resuscitation bag-valve-device connected to an oxygen flow meter, set at 15 L/min (not required with use of the ventilator to deliver hyperoxygenation breaths)
- ❖ Goggles and mask, or mask with eye shield

Additional equipment (to have available depending on patient need) includes the following:

- ❖ PEEP valve (for patients on >5 cm H_2O PEEP)
- Closed technique
  - ❖ Closed-suction setup with a catheter of appropriate size (see Table 12-1)
  - ❖ Sterile saline solution lavage containers (5 to 10 mL)
  - ❖ Suction catheter (individually packaged) for oral and nasal suctioning
  - ❖ Source of suction (wall mounted or portable)
  - ❖ Connecting tube (4 to 6 ft)
  - ❖ Nonsterile gloves
  - ❖ Goggles and mask, or mask with eye shield, and gown if necessary

PATIENT AND FAMILY EDUCATION

- Explain the procedure for endotracheal or tracheostomy tube suctioning. ➡*Rationale:* The explanation reduces anxiety.
- Explain that suctioning may be uncomfortable and could cause the patient to experience shortness of breath. ➡*Rationale:* This information reduces anxiety and elicits patient cooperation.
- Explain the patient's role in assisting with secretion removal by coughing during the procedure. ➡*Rationale:* This information encourages cooperation and facilitates removal of secretions.

PATIENT ASSESSMENT AND PREPARATION

Patient Assessment

- Assess for signs and symptoms of airway obstruction:
  - ❖ Secretions in the airway
  - ❖ Inspiratory wheezes
  - ❖ Expiratory crackles
  - ❖ Restlessness
  - ❖ Ineffective coughing

  - ❖ Decreased level of consciousness
  - ❖ Decreased breath sounds
  - ❖ Tachypnea
  - ❖ Tachycardia or bradycardia
  - ❖ Cyanosis
  - ❖ Hypertension or hypotension
  - ❖ Shallow respirations
- ➡*Rationale:* Physical signs and symptoms result from inadequate gas exchange associated with airway obstruction.
- Note peak airway pressures on the ventilator. ➡*Rationale:* These pressures indicate potential secretions in the airway, increasing resistance to gas flow.
- Evaluate Sao_2 and Spo_2 levels. ➡*Rationale:* These values indicate potential secretions in the airway, decreasing gas exchange.
- Assess signs and symptoms of inadequate breathing patterns:
  - ❖ Dyspnea
  - ❖ Shallow respirations
  - ❖ Intercostal and suprasternal retractions
  - ❖ Frequent triggering of ventilator alarms
  - ❖ Increased respiratory rate
- ➡*Rationale:* Respiratory distress is a late sign of lower airway obstruction.

Patient Preparation

- Verify correct patient with two identifiers. ➡*Rationale:* Prior to performing a procedure, the nurse should ensure the correct identification of the patient for the intended intervention.
- Ensure that the patient understands preprocedural teachings. Answer questions as they arise, and reinforce information as needed. ➡*Rationale:* This communication evaluates and reinforces understanding of previously taught information.
- Assist the patient in achieving a position that is comfortable for the patient and nurse, generally semi-Fowler's or Fowler's, with the bed elevated to the nurse's waist level. ➡*Rationale:* This positioning promotes comfort, oxygenation, and ventilation and reduces strain.
- Secure additional personnel to assist with the self-inflating manual resuscitation bag-valve-device to provide hyperoxygenation (open-suction technique only). ➡*Rationale:* Two hands are necessary to inflate the self-inflating manual resuscitation bag-valve-device for adult tidal volume levels (>600 mL).

Procedure	for Endotracheal or Tracheostomy Tube Suctioning	
Steps	**Rationale**	**Special Considerations**
1. **HH**		
2. **PE**		
3. Turn on suction apparatus and set vacuum regulator to 100 to 120 mm Hg. **(Level D*)** Follow manufacturer's directions for suction pressure levels with closed-suction catheter systems. **(Level M*)**	The amount of suction applied should be only enough to remove secretions effectively. High negative-pressure settings may increase tracheal mucosal damage.[1,30,31]	
4. Secure one end of the connecting tube to the suction source and place the other end in a convenient location within reach.	Prepares suction apparatus.	
5. Monitor patient's cardiopulmonary status before, during, and after the suctioning period. **(Level B*)**	Observes for signs and symptoms of complications: decreased arterial and mixed venous oxygen saturation, cardiac dysrhythmias, bronchospasm, respiratory distress, cyanosis, increased blood pressure or intracranial pressure, anxiety, pain, agitation, or changes in mental status.[1,4,5,14,15,22,25,29,30,31]	Development of cardiopulmonary instability, particularly cardiac dysrhythmias or arterial desaturation, necessitates immediate termination of the suctioning procedure.
6a. Open-suction technique only		
A. Open sterile catheter package on a clean surface, with the inside of the wrapping used as a sterile field.	Prepares catheter and prevents transmission of microorganisms.	
B. Depending on manufacturer, set up the sterile solution container or sterile field. Use prefilled solution container or open empty container, taking care not to touch the inside of the container. Fill with approximately 100 mL of sterile normal saline solution or sterile water.	Prepares catheter flush solution.	
C. **PE**		In the event that one sterile glove and one nonsterile glove are used, apply the nonsterile glove to the nondominant hand and the sterile glove to the dominant hand. Handle all nonsterile items with the nondominant hand.
D. Pick up suction catheter, with care to avoid touching nonsterile surfaces. With the nondominant hand, pick up the connecting tubing. Secure the suction catheter to the connecting tubing.	Maintains catheter sterility. Connects the suction catheter and connecting tubing.	The dominant hand should not come into contact with the connecting tubing. Wrapping the suction catheter around the sterile dominant hand helps prevent inadvertent contamination of the catheter.

*Level B: Well-designed, controlled studies with results that consistently support a specific action, intervention, or treatment
*Level D: Peer-reviewed professional organizational standards with clinical studies to support recommendations
*Level M: Manufacturer's recommendations only

Procedure for Endotracheal or Tracheostomy Tube Suctioning—*Continued*

Steps	Rationale	Special Considerations
E. Check equipment for proper functioning by suctioning a small amount of sterile solution from the container. Proceed to Step 7.	Ensures equipment function.	
6b. Closed-suction technique only A. Connect the suction tubing to the closed system suction port or unlock the thumb valve according to manufacturer's guidelines.		
7. Hyperoxygenate the patient for at least 30 seconds with one of the following three methods. **(Level B*)** A. Press the suction hyperoxygenation button on the ventilator with the nondominant hand. *or*	Hyperoxygenation with 100% oxygen is used to prevent a decrease in arterial oxygen levels during the suctioning procedure.[1,5,14,21,24,29,30,32]	Limited data indicate that use of a ventilator to deliver the hyperoxygenation may be more effective in increasing arterial oxygen levels.
B. Increase the baseline fraction of inspired oxygen (FiO_2) level on the mechanical ventilator. *or*		With this method, caution must be used to return the FiO_2 to baseline levels after completion of suctioning.
C. Disconnect the ventilator or gas delivery tubing from the end of the endotracheal or tracheostomy tube, attach the self-inflating manual resuscitation bag-valve-device to the tube with the nondominant hand, and administer five to six breaths over 30 seconds.	Attach a PEEP valve to the self-inflating manual resuscitation bag-valve-device for patients on greater than 5 cm H_2O PEEP. Verify 100% oxygen delivery capabilities of MRB by checking manufacturer's guidelines or with direct measurement with an in-line oxygen analyzer when baseline ventilator oxygen delivery to the patient is greater than 60%. Some models of self-inflating manual resuscitation bag-valve-device entrain room air and deliver less than 100% oxygen.	Use of a second person to deliver hyperoxygenation breaths with the self-inflating manual resuscitation bag-valve-device significantly increases tidal volume delivery. One-handed bagging rarely achieves adult tidal volume breaths (>500 mL).[10-13]
8. Remove the ventilator circuit or self-inflating manual resuscitation bag-valve-device with the nondominant hand. With the control vent of the suction catheter open to air, gently but quickly insert the catheter with the dominant hand into the artificial airway until resistance is met, then pull back 1 cm.[1,19] **(Level E*)**	Suction should be applied only as needed to remove secretions and for as short a time as possible to minimize decreases in arterial oxygen levels.	Directional or coudé catheters are available for selective right or left main stem bronchus placement. Straight catheters usually enter the right main stem bronchus.[16,19] Saline solution should not be instilled routinely into the artificial airway before suctioning.[3,6,18,24,26-30] **(Level B)**

*Level B: Well-designed, controlled studies with results that consistently support a specific action, intervention, or treatment
*Level E: Multiple case reports, theory-based evidence from expert opinions, or peer-reviewed professional organizational standards without clinical studies to support recommendations

Procedure continues on following page

Procedure for Endotracheal or Tracheostomy Tube Suctioning—*Continued*		
Steps	**Rationale**	**Special Considerations**
9. Place the nondominant thumb over the control vent of the suction catheter to apply continuous or intermittent suction. Place and maintain the catheter between the dominant thumb and forefinger as you completely withdraw the catheter for less than or equal to 10 seconds into the sterile catheter sleeve (closed-suction technique) or out of the open airway (open-suction technique).	Tracheal damage from suctioning is similar with intermittent or continuous suction.[8,17,20,23] **(Level C*)** Decreases in arterial oxygen levels during suctioning can be kept to a minimum with brief suction periods.[1,9,14,29,30] **(Level B*)**	
10. Hyperoxygenate for 30 seconds as described in **Step 7**.	Hyperoxygenation with 100% oxygen is used to prevent a decrease in arterial oxygen levels during the suctioning procedure.[1,5,14,21,24] **(Level B)**	
11. One or two more passes of the suction catheter, as delineated in **Steps 8 and 9,** may be performed if secretions remain in the airway and the patient is tolerating the procedure. Provide 30 seconds of hyperoxygenation before and after each pass of the suction catheter. **See Step 7.**	The number of suction passes should be based on the amount of secretions and the patient's clinical assessment. Arterial oxygen desaturation and cardiopulmonary complications increase with each successive pass.[14,30] **(Level E*)** Hyperoxygenation with 100% oxygen is used to prevent a decrease in arterial oxygen levels during the suctioning procedure.[1,5,14,21,24] **(Level B)**	If secretions remain in the airways after two or three suction catheter passes, allow the patient to rest before additional suctioning passes.
12. If the patient does not tolerate suctioning despite hyperoxygenation, try the following steps: A. Ensure that 100% oxygen is being delivered. B. Maintain PEEP during suctioning. Check that the PEEP valve is attached properly to the self-inflating manual resuscitation bag-valve-device with use of that method for hyperoxygenation. C. Switch to another method of suctioning (e.g., closed-suctioning technique). D. Allow longer recovery intervals between suction passes. E. Hyperventilation may be used in situations in which the patient does not tolerate suctioning with hyperoxygenation alone, with either the self-inflating manual resuscitation bag-valve-device or the ventilator.	Use of a different suctioning technique may be physiologically less demanding.[30] **(Level E)**	

*Level B: Well-designed, controlled studies with results that consistently support a specific action, intervention, or treatment

*Level C: Qualitative studies, descriptive or correlational studies, integrative reviews, systematic reviews, or randomized controlled trials with inconsistent results

*Level E: Multiple case reports, theory-based evidence from expert opinions, or peer-reviewed professional organizational standards without clinical studies to support recommendations

Procedure for Endotracheal or Tracheostomy Tube Suctioning—*Continued*		
Steps	**Rationale**	**Special Considerations**
13. When the lower airway has been cleared adequately of secretions, perform oropharyngeal suctioning. A separate suction catheter must be opened for this step with the closed-suction technique.	Suctioning of the oropharyngeal area if secretions are present may enhance patient comfort and be part of an oral hygiene program.[2] After oropharyngeal suctioning, the suction catheter is contaminated with bacteria present in the oral cavity, potentially gram-negative bacilli, and should not be used for lower airway suctioning.[7] (**Level E***)	Care should be taken to avoid oropharyngeal tissue trauma and gagging during suctioning.
14. Rinse the catheter and connecting tubing with sterile saline or sterile water solution until clear. Open suction technique: Suction up unused sterile solution until tubing is clear. Closed suction technique: Instill sterile saline or water solution into side port of in-line suction catheter, taking care not to lavage down endotracheal tube, while applying continuous suction until catheter is clear.	Removes buildup of secretions in the connecting tubing and, with the closed-suction catheter system, in the in-line suction catheter.	
15. Open-suction technique only: On completion of upper airway suctioning, wrap the catheter around the dominant hand. Pull glove off inside out. Catheter remains in glove. Pull off other glove in same fashion, and discard. Turn off suction device.	Reduces transmission of microorganisms.	
16. Suction collection tubing and canisters may remain in use for multiple suctioning episodes.	Solutions and catheters that come in direct contact with the lower airways during suctioning must be sterile to decrease the risks for hospital-acquired pneumonia. Devices that are not in direct contact with the lower airways have not been shown to increase infection risk.[7] (**Level D***)	Check institutional standards on discard of multi-use sterile solution containers and equipment removal.
17. **PE**		
18. **HH**		

*Level D: Peer-reviewed professional organizational standards with clinical studies to support recommendations
*Level E: Multiple case reports, theory-based evidence from expert opinions, or peer-reviewed professional organizational standards without clinical studies to support recommendations

Procedure continues on following page

Expected Outcomes

- Removal of secretions from the large airways
- Improved gas exchange
- Airway patency
- Amelioration of clinical signs or symptoms of need for suctioning (e.g., adventitious breath sounds, coughing, high airway pressures)
- Sample for laboratory analysis

Unexpected Outcomes

- Cardiac dysrhythmias (premature contractions, tachycardias, bradycardias, heart blocks, asystole)
- Hypoxemia
- Bronchospasm
- Excessive increases in arterial blood pressure or intracranial pressure
- Hospital-acquired infections
- Cardiopulmonary distress
- Decreased level of consciousness
- Airway obstruction

Patient Monitoring and Care

Steps	Rationale	Reportable Conditions
		These conditions should be reported if they persist despite nursing interventions.
1. Monitor patient's cardiopulmonary status before, during, and after the suctioning period. **(Level B*)**	Observes for signs and symptoms of complications.[1,4,5,14,15,22,25,29-31]	• Decreased arterial or mixed venous oxygen saturation • Cardiac dysrhythmias • Bronchospasm • Respiratory distress • Cyanosis • Increased blood pressure or intracranial pressure • Anxiety, agitation, pain, or changes in mental status • Diminished breath sounds • Decreased oxygenation • Increased peak airway pressures • Coughing • Increased work of breathing
2. Reassess patient for signs of suctioning effectiveness. **(Level E*)**		
3. Follow institution standard for assessing pain. Administer analgesia as prescribed.	Identifies need for pain interventions.	• Continued pain despite pain interventions.

Documentation

Documentation should include the following:

- Patient and family education
- Presuctioning assessment, including clinical indication for suctioning
- Suctioning of endotracheal or tracheostomy tube
- Size of endotracheal or tracheostomy tube and suction catheter
- Type of hyperoxygenation method used
- Pain assessment, interventions, and effectiveness.
- Volume, color, consistency, and odor of secretions obtained
- Any difficulties during catheter insertion or hyperoxygenation
- Tolerance of suctioning procedure, including development of any unexpected outcomes during or after the procedure
- Nursing interventions
- Postsuctioning assessment

---

*Level B: Well-designed, controlled studies with results that consistently support a specific action, intervention, or treatment

*Level E: Multiple case reports, theory-based evidence from expert opinions, or peer-reviewed professional organizational standards without clinical studies to support recommendations

References

CR 1. AARC Clinical Practice Guideline. Endotracheal suctioning of mechanically ventilated adults and children with artificial airways, *Respir Care* 38:500-504, 1993.

2. AACN Practice Alert: *Oral care in the critically ill,* 2006, retrieved August 9, 2008, from www.aacn.org/WD/Practice/Docs/Oral_Care_in_the_Critically_Ill.pdf.

CR 3. Akgul S, Akyolcu N: Effects of normal saline on endotracheal suctioning, *J Clin Nurs* 11:826-830, 2002.

4. Arroyo-Novoa CM, et al: Pain related to tracheal suctioning in awake acutely and critically ill adults: a descriptive study, *Intensive Crit Care Nurs* 24:20-27, 2007.

5. Bourgault AM, et al: Effects of endotracheal tube suctioning on arterial oxygen tension and heart rate variability, *Biol Res Nurs* 7:268-278, 2006.

6. Celik SA, Kanan N: A current conflict: use of isotonic sodium chloride solution on endotracheal suctioning in critically ill patients, *Dimens Crit Care Nurs* 25:11-14, 2006.

CR 7. Centers for Disease Control and Prevention: Guidelines for prevention of health-care-associated pneumonia, 2003: Recommendations of CDC and the Healthcare infection Control Practices Advisory Committee, *MMWR* 53(No. RR-3):1-35, 2004.

CR 8. Czarnik R, et al: Differential effects of continuous versus intermittent suction on tracheal tissue, *Heart Lung* 20:144-151, 1991.

9. Ellstrom K: The pulmonary system. In Alspach J, editor: *Core curriculum for critical care nursing,* ed 6, St Louis, 2006, Elsevier, 45-183.

CR 10. Glass C, et al: Nurse performance of hyperoxygenation, *Heart Lung* 20:299, 1991.

CR 11. Glass C, et al: Nurses' ability to achieve hyperinflation and hyperoxygenation with a manual resuscitation bag during endotracheal suctioning, *Heart Lung* 22:158-165, 1993.

CR 12. Grap MJ, et al: Endotracheal suctioning: ventilator versus manual delivery of hyperoxygenation breaths, *Am J Crit Care* 5:192-197, 1996.

CR 13. Hess D, Goff G: The effects of two-hand versus one-hand ventilation on volumes delivered during bag-valve ventilation at various resistances and compliances, *Respir Care* 32:1025-1028, 1987.

CR 14. Joanna Briggs Institute for Evidence Based Nursing and Midwifery: Tracheal suctioning of adults with an artificial airway, *Best Practice* 4:1-6, 2000.

15. Jongerden IP, et al: Open and closed endotracheal suction systems in mechanically ventilated intensive care patients: a meta-analysis, *Crit Care Med* 35:260-70, 2007.

CR 16. Kirimili B, King J, Pfaeffle H: Evaluation of tracheal bronchial suction techniques, *J Cardiovasc Surg* 59:340-344, 1970.

CR 17. Kleiber C, Krutzfield N, Rose E: Acute histologic changes in the tracheobronchial tree associated with different suction catheter insertion techniques, *Heart Lung* 17:10-14, 1988.

18. Klockare M, et al: Comparison between direct humidification and nebulization of the respiratory track at mechanical ventilation: distribution of saline solution studied by gamma camera, *J Clin Nurs* 15:301-307, 2006.

CR 19. Kubota Y, et al: Is a straight catheter necessary for selective bronchial suctioning in the adult? *Crit Care Med* 14:755-756, 1986.

CR 20. Kuzenski B: Effect of negative pressure on tracheobronchial trauma, *Nurs Res* 27:260-263, 1978.

21. Lasocki S, et al: Open and closed-circuit endotracheal suctioning in acute lung injury: efficiency and effects on gas exchange, *Anesthesiology* 104:39-47, 2006.

CR 22. McCauley C, Boller L: Bradycardiac responses to endotracheal suctioning, *Crit Care Med* 16:1165-1166, 1986.

CR 23. Ogburn-Russell L: The effect of continuous and intermittent suctioning on the tracheal mucosa of dogs, *Heart Lung* 16:297, 1987.

CR 24. Oh H, Seo W: A meta-analysis of the effects of various interventions in preventing endotracheal suctioning induced hypoxemia, *J Clin Nurs* 12:912-924, 2003.

CR 25. Puntillo KA, et al: Patients' perceptions and responses to procedural pain: results from the Thunder Project II, *Am J Crit Care* 10:238-251, 2001.

26. Rauen CA, et al: Seven evidence-based practice habits: putting some sacred cows out to pasture, *Crit Care Nurse* 28:98-124, 2008.

CR 27. Ridling DA, Martin LD, Bratton SL: Endotracheal suctioning with and without instillation of isotonic sodium chloride solutions in critically ill children, *Am J Crit Care* 12:212-219, 2003.

CR 28. Rutula W, Stiegel M, Sarubbi F: A potential infection hazard associated with the use of disposable saline vials, *Infect Control* 5:170-172, 1984.

29. St John RE: Airway and ventilator management. In Chulay M, Burns S, editors: *AACN essentials of critical care nursing,* ed 2, New York, 2006. McGraw-Hill Publishing, 111-143.

30. St John RE, Seckel MA: Airway management. In Burns SM, editor: *AACN protocol for practice: care of mechanically ventilated patients,* ed 2, Sudbury, MA, 2006. Jones and Bartlett Publishers, 1-57.

31. Subirana M, et al: Closed tracheal suction systems versus open tracheal systems for mechanically ventilated adult patients, Cochrane Database Syst Rev 4:CD004581, 2007.

CR 32. Wynne R, Botti M, Parztz J: Preoxygenation for tracheal suctioning in ventilated adults (protocol), *Cochrane Database Syst Rev* (4):CD005142, 2004.

Additional Readings

Kerr M, et al: Effect of endotracheal suctioning on cerebral oxygenation in traumatic brain-injured patients, *Crit Care Med* 27:2776-2781, 1999.

Labarca J, et al: A multistate outbreak of *Ralstonia pickettii* colonization associated with an intrinsically contaminated respiratory care solution, *Clin Infect Dis* 29:1281-1286, 1999.

Paul-Allen J, Ostrow C: Survey of nursing practices with closed-system suctioning, *Am J Crit Care* 9:9-19, 2000.

Pierce LN: *Management of the mechanically ventilated patient, ed 2,* St Louis, 2007, Elsevier.

Sole M, Byers JF, Ludy JE, et al: A multisite survey of suctioning techniques and airway management practices, *Am J Crit Care* 11:220-232, 2002.

Tracheal Tube Cuff Care

P U R P O S E :   The tracheal tube cuff helps stabilize the endotracheal or tracheal tube and maintains an adequate airway seal so that air moves through the tube into the lungs. The cuff also may decrease the risk of aspiration of large food particles, but it does not protect against aspiration of liquid.

Kirsten N. Skillings, Bonnie L. Curtis

PREREQUISITE NURSING KNOWLEDGE

- The tracheal tube cuff is an inflatable balloon that surrounds the shaft of the tracheal tube near its distal end. When inflated, the cuff presses against the tracheal wall to prevent air leakage and pressure loss from the lungs.
- Appropriate cuff care helps prevent major pulmonary aspirations, prepare for tracheal extubation, decrease the risk of inadvertent extubation, provide a patent airway for ventilation and removal of secretions, and decrease the risk of hospital-acquired infections.
- Although a variety of endotracheal and tracheal tubes exists, the most desirable tube provides a maximum airway seal with minimal tracheal wall pressure, with a high-volume low-pressure cuff (Fig. 13-1). This cuff has a relatively large inflation volume that requires lower filling pressure to obtain a seal (<25 mm Hg or 34 cm H_2O). Note: 1 mm Hg = 1.36 cm H_2O, or 1 cm H_2O = 0.74 mm Hg.
- High-volume low-pressure cuffs allow a large surface area to come into contact with the tracheal wall, distributing the pressure over a much greater area. The older cuff design (low-volume high-pressure) may require 40 mm Hg (54.4 cm H_2O) to obtain an effective seal and is undesirable.
- The amount of pressure and volume necessary to obtain a seal and prevent mucosal damage depends on tube size and design, cuff configuration, mode of ventilation, and the patient's arterial blood pressure.

- A variety of devices are available to measure cuff pressures, including bedside sphygmomanometers, special aneroid cuff manometers, and electronic cuff pressure devices. Ideally, the cuff pressures should be between 20 and 25 mm Hg and still meet the goals of cuff use. Tracheal capillary perfusion pressure is 25 to 35 mm Hg for patients with normotensive conditions. Lower cuff pressures are associated with less mucosal damage but also are associated with silent aspiration, which has been shown to be more prevalent at cuff pressures less than 20 mm Hg.[1,6,8]
- Two techniques, minimal leak technique (MLT) and minimal occlusion volume (MOV), are used to inflate and monitor air in the cuff.
  - ❖ The MLT involves air inflation of the tube cuff until any leak stops; then, a small amount of air is removed slowly until a small leak is heard on inspiration. Problems with this technique include difficulty maintaining positive end expiratory pressure (PEEP), aspiration around the cuff, and increased movement of the tube in the trachea during cuff deflation.[2,4,5,7,8] Aspiration may be prevented with deep pharyngeal suctioning before use of the MLT.
  - ❖ The MOV consists of injection of air into the cuff until no leak is heard, then withdrawal of the air until a small leak is heard on inspiration, and then addition of more air until no leak is heard on inspiration.[2,4,5,7,8]
- Each technique has distinct advantages. MLT decreases tracheal mucosal injury and assists in mobilizing secretions

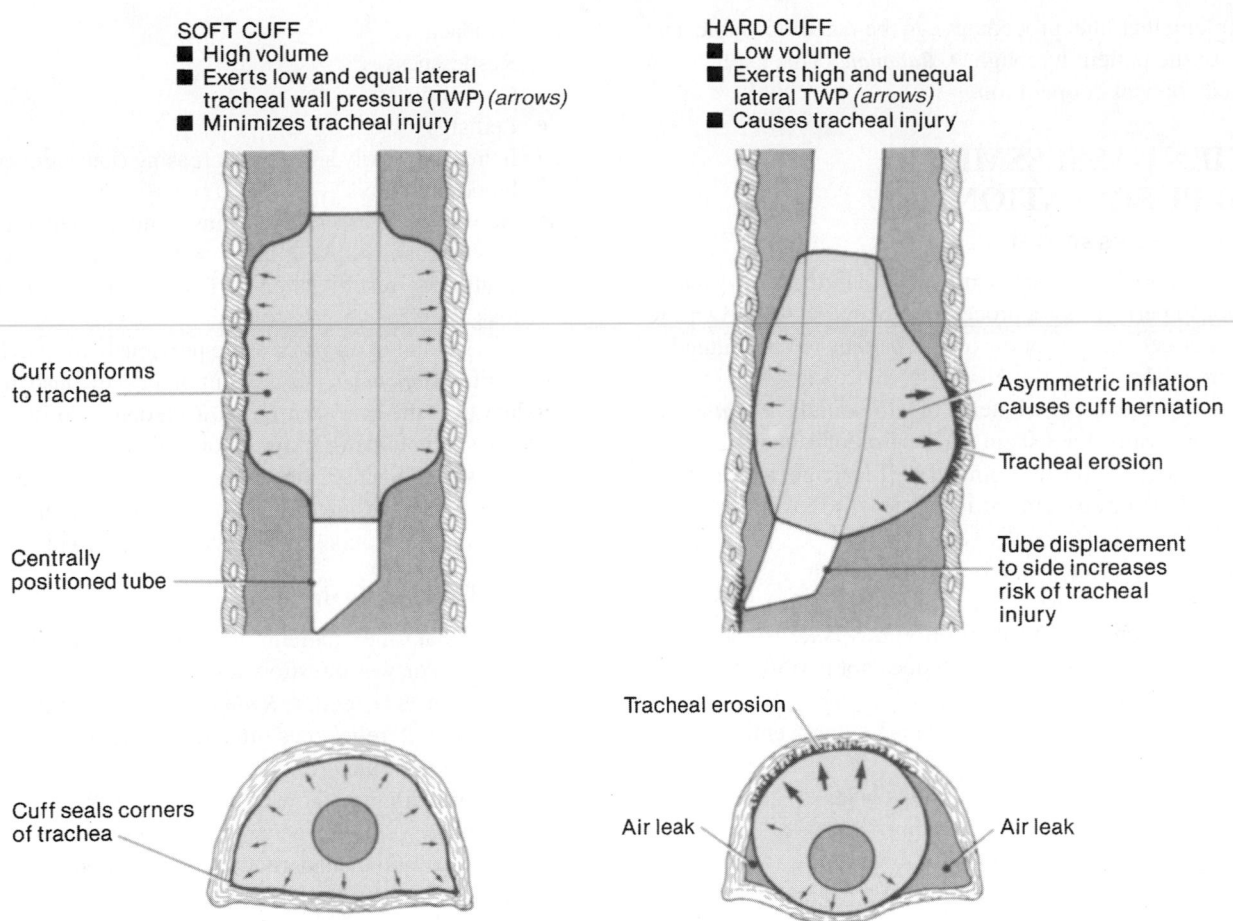

SOFT CUFF
■ High volume
■ Exerts low and equal lateral tracheal wall pressure (TWP) *(arrows)*
■ Minimizes tracheal injury

HARD CUFF
■ Low volume
■ Exerts high and unequal lateral TWP *(arrows)*
■ Causes tracheal injury

Cuff conforms to trachea

Centrally positioned tube

Asymmetric inflation causes cuff herniation

Tracheal erosion

Tube displacement to side increases risk of tracheal injury

Cuff seals corners of trachea

Tracheal erosion

Air leak

Air leak

FIGURE 13-1 Cross-sectional view in D-shaped trachea. Effects of soft and hard cuff inflation on the tracheal wall. *(From Kersten LD: Comprehensive respiratory nursing, Philadelphia 1989, Saunders, 648.)*

forward into the pharynx. MOV is used if the patient needs a seal to provide adequate ventilation or is at risk for aspiration.[4,8]

- Although rare since the use of high-volume low-pressure devices became common, the adverse effects of tracheal tube cuff inflation include tracheal stenosis, necrosis, tracheoesophageal fistulas, and tracheomalacia. These complications may be more likely to occur in conditions that adversely affect tissue response to mucosal injury, such as hypotension. Two major mechanisms are mainly responsible for airway damage: tube movement and pressure. Duration of intubation also plays a significant role.[4,8]
- Routine cuff deflation is unnecessary and is no longer recommended.[4]
- Unintentional extubation and tube manipulation can occur with ineffective patient restraint or sedation, inadequate securing of the tube, incorrect tube size and length, improper support or respiratory underinflation of endotracheal cuff, and prolonged intubation.[4]

EQUIPMENT

- 10-mL syringe
- Pressure manometer with extension line or specially designed manometer to measure cuff pressures

- Three-way stopcock
- Stethoscope
- Self-inflating manual resuscitation bag-valve device
- Oxygen source and tubing
  Additional equipment (for cuff inflation with faulty inflating device) includes the following:
- Scissors
- Padded hemostats
- Short 18-gauge or 23-gauge blunt needle
- Tongue depressor
- Tape (1 inch wide)
- Reintubation equipment, in case of accidental extubation
- Suction supplies (see Procedure 12)

PATIENT AND FAMILY EDUCATION

- Explain the procedure (if patient condition and time allow) and the reason for tracheal tube cuff care. ➥*Rationale:* This communication identifies patient and family knowledge deficits concerning the patient's condition, procedure, expected benefits, and potential risks and allows time for questions to clarify information and voice concerns. Explanations decrease patient anxiety and enhance cooperation.
- Explain the patient's role in assisting with cuff care. ➥*Rationale:* This information elicits patient cooperation.

- Explain that the procedure can be uncomfortable and cause the patient to cough. ➤*Rationale:* This explanation elicits patient cooperation.

PATIENT ASSESSMENT AND PREPARATION

Patient Assessment

- Verify correct patient with two identifiers. *Rationale:* Prior to performing a procedure, the nurse should ensure the correct identification of the patient for the intended intervention.
- Assess presence of bilateral breath sounds. ➤*Rationale:* This assessment assists in verification of tube placement.
- Assess signs and symptoms of cuff leakage, as follows:
  - ❖ Audible or auscultated inspiratory leak over larynx
  - ❖ Patient able to vocalize audibly
  - ❖ Inflation (pilot) valve balloon deflation
  - ❖ Loss of inspiratory and expiratory volume on patient with mechanical ventilation ➤*Rationale:* An adequate seal of cuff to tracheal wall does not permit air to flow past the cuff.
- Assess signs and symptoms of inadequate ventilation, as follows:
  - ❖ Rising arterial carbon dioxide tension
  - ❖ Chest-abdominal dyssynchrony
  - ❖ Patient-ventilator dyssynchrony
  - ❖ Dyspnea

- ❖ Headache
- ❖ Restlessness
- ❖ Confusion
- ❖ Lethargy
- ❖ Increasing (early sign) or decreasing (late sign) arterial blood pressure
- ❖ Activation of expiratory or inspiratory volume alarms on mechanical ventilator ➤*Rationale:* Inadequate ventilation results when cuff seal is improper or cuff leak is extensive.
- Assess amount of air or pressure previously used to inflate the cuff. ➤*Rationale:* The amount of air previously used to inflate the cuff can be used as a guideline to determine changes in volume or pressure or both.
- Assess size of tracheal tube and size of patient. ➤*Rationale:* Volume and pressure of air needed to seal the airway depend on the relationship of tube and trachea diameters.

Patient Preparation

- Ensure that the patient understands preprocedural teachings. Answer questions as they arise, and reinforce information as needed. ➤*Rationale:* This communication evaluates and reinforces understanding of previously taught information.
- Place patient in semi-Fowler's position. ➤*Rationale:* This positioning promotes general relaxation, oxygenation, and ventilation. It also reduces stimulation of the gag reflex and risk of aspiration.

Procedure | for Tracheal Tube Cuff Care

Steps	Rationale	Special Considerations
Deflation and Inflation		
1. **HH**		
2. **PE**		
3. Hyperoxygenate and suction tracheobronchial tree (see Procedure 12) and pharynx before cuff deflation.	Clears secretions in the lower airway and decreases incidence of aspiration.	If an open suction system is used, a fresh sterile catheter is needed for suctioning the tracheobronchial tree. When suctioning of the tracheobronchial tree is complete, the same catheter may be used to suction the pharynx. If a closed suction system is used in suctioning the tracheobronchial tree, a fresh sterile catheter is needed for suctioning the pharynx.
4. Remove ventilator or humidifer tubing from the endotracheal or tracheostomy tube.	Accesses tube opening.	
MOV Technique		
5. Insert air-filled 10-mL syringe tip into inflation valve (also referred to as the pilot balloon valve).	Provides a pathway between air source and cuff.	Most cuffs are sufficiently inflated with less than 10 mL of air.

Procedure | for Tracheal Tube Cuff Care—*Continued*

Steps	Rationale	Special Considerations
A. If a leak is initially present, gradually add air to the cuff until the leak is eliminated. B. If a leak is not initially present, **go to Step 6**.		
6. Ventilate the patient with a self-inflating manual resuscitation bag valve device and gradually deflate the cuff (in 0.1-mL increments) until a small leak is heard on inspiration. (**Level D***)	Prepares for measurement of cuff pressure and prevents aspiration of pharyngeal secretions.	MOV is used if the patient needs a seal to provide adequate ventilation or is at risk for aspiration.[4,8] Instruct the patient who is alert and cooperative to cough.
7. Slowly inject air on inspiration until sounds cease over larynx.	The trachea dilates during inspiration. The cuff needs to seal the airway during inspiration so that air is directed toward the lung. Cessation of air movement on auscultation indicates that the cuff is sealed against the tracheal mucosal wall.	Hazards of cuff inflation include cuff overinflation, distention, and rupture.
8. Ventilate the patient with a self-inflating manual resuscitation bag-valve-device. **Proceed to Step 12.**	The cuff is inflated when an audible leak is not heard.	The patient who is alert and cooperative may be asked to speak. If the trachea is sealed, vocalization is not possible.
Minimal Leak Test (MLT)		
9. Insert air-filled 10-mL syringe into inflation valve. A. If a leak is initially present, gradually add air to the cuff until the leak is eliminated. B. If a leak is not initially present, **go to Step 10**.	Provides a pathway between air source and cuff.	Most cuffs are sufficiently inflated with less than 10 mL of air.
10. Place a stethoscope over larynx.		
11. Slowly withdraw air (in 0.1-mL increments) from the cuff until a small leak is heard with auscultation on inspiration. (**Level D**)	Auscultation of air movement indicates air escaping through the larynx.	Intracuff pressure measurement provides an approximation of cuff-to-tracheal wall pressure.[4]
12. Remove syringe from inflation valve. (**Level D**)	Keeping a syringe on the inflation valve can cause it to become stuck in the open position, allowing air to escape and the cuff to deflate.[2]	
13. Replace any oxygen or humidity tubing. Check and secure ventilator connections, as needed.	Allows for oxygen flow and prevents oxygen desaturation.	
14. Reassess patient's airway and respiratory status.	Identifies effects of tracheal cuff care.	
15. Dispose of used supplies and equipment.		
16. Remove personal protective equipment.	Reduces transmission of microorganisms and body secretions; standard precautions.	
17. 🄷🄷		
Cuff Pressure Measurement		
18. 🄷🄷		
19. 🄿🄴		

*Level D: Peer-reviewed professional organizational standards with clinical studies to support recommendations

Procedure continues on following page

Procedure	for Tracheal Tube Cuff Care—*Continued*	
Steps	**Rationale**	**Special Considerations**
20. Connect the manometer line with a three-way stopcock (turned "off" to the patient) to the inflation valve (Fig. 13-2).	Develops an intracuff pressure-monitoring device.	This device is made easily with parts of a blood pressure cuff (e.g., aneroid manometer device). Alternatively, a specially designed manometer may be attached directly to the inflation port to measure the cuff pressure.
21. Attach an air-filled syringe to the open port of the stopcock and inject air to the tubing leading to the manometer (away from the patient) until the needle of the manometer reads between 20 and 25 mm Hg. **(Level D*)**	Measures the pressure of the air applied from the system.	Pressure should be kept at a level to maintain a seal between cuff and tracheal wall. The volume necessary to create the seal depends on tube size and cuff configuration. Contributing factors to airway damage are excessive head movement, tube size, duration of intubation, and cuff pressure.[2]
22. Turn the stopcock "off" to the port with the syringe. Read the cuff pressure now shown on the aneroid face.	The connecting channel is now between the manometer and the inflation valve, allowing evaluation of pressure in the patient's cuff.	
23. Turn the stopcock "off" to the inflation valve and disconnect the manometer line from the inflation valve.	The connecting channel to the inflation valve is removed, maintaining air in the cuff.	
24. Dispose of used supplies and equipment.		
25. Remove personal protective equipment.	Reduces transmission of microorganisms and body secretions; standard precautions.	
26. 🅷🅷		
Troubleshooting Tracheal Cuff Problems		
27. 🅷🅷		
28. 🅿🅴		
Faulty Inflation Valve		
29. Identify faulty inflation valve by determining that the cuff continually deflates, despite the addition of air to the cuff.	Determines need for repair.	When inflation valve becomes faulty and reintubation is undesirable, consider instituting an emergency cuff-inflation technique (Fig. 13-3).

*Level D: Peer-reviewed professional organizational standards with clinical studies to support recommendations

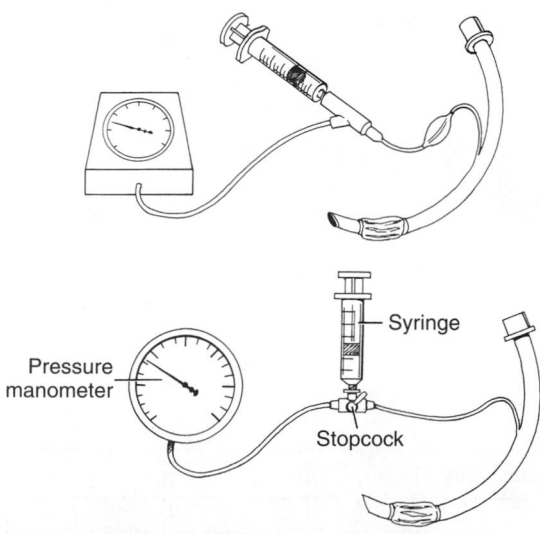

FIGURE 13-2   Measuring cuff pressure with a homemade pressure monitor. *(From Eubanks DH, Bone RC: Comprehensive respiratory care, ed 2, St Louis, 1990, Mosby.)*

Procedure for Tracheal Tube Cuff Care—*Continued*

Steps	Rationale	Special Considerations
30. Insert three-way stopcock into the inflation valve.	Provides access to cuff.	
31. Inflate the cuff with MOV technique **(Steps 5 to 8, 12)** or MLT **(Steps 9 to 12)**.	Allows for cuff inflation; restores tracheal wall and cuff seal.	
32. Clamp the inflation tube by applying a padded hemostat distal to the inflation valve.	Maintains air in cuff; provides a quick occlusion of the inflating tube.	
33. Turn the stopcock off to the inflation valve and leave in place; remove clamp.	Provides for temporary use of the tracheal tube while maintaining cuff pressure.	
Faulty Inflation Tube		
34. Identify malfunctioning of inflation tube by determining that an air leak is present in the tube.	Determines need for and method of repair.	
35. Clamp the inflation line with a padded hemostat cut off faulty end of inflation tube and valve with scissors (see Fig. 13-3).	Prepares inflation tube for repair.	
36. Insert short 18-gauge to 23-gauge blunt needle into inflation tube.	Provides inflation access.	Maintain care to avoid puncture or severing of inflation line or skin.
37. Attach three-way stopcock to a blunt needle.	Provides control of airflow in and out of inflating line.	
38. With a 10-mL syringe, inflate the cuff with air with MOV technique **(Steps 5 to 8, 12)** or MLT **(Steps 9 to 12)**.	Allows cuff inflation; restores tracheal wall and cuff seal.	
39. Turn stopcock off to the inflation tube.	Provides for temporary use of the tracheal tube while maintaining cuff pressure.	
40. Secure assembled device with tape to a tongue depressor.	Provides for stabilization and protection.	
41. Assemble equipment for tracheal tube replacement.		
42. Remove personal protective equipment.	Reduces transmission of microorganisms and body secretions; Standard Precautions.	
43. **HH**		

Procedure continues on following page

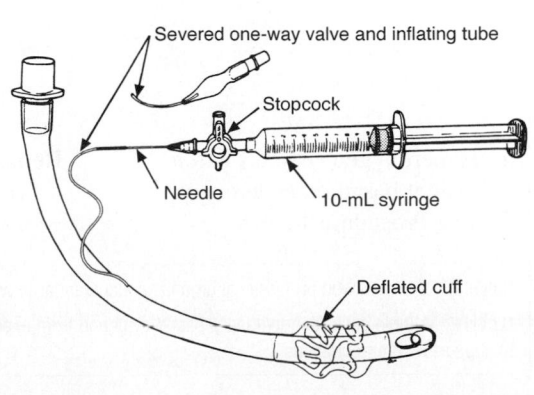

FIGURE 13-3 Attachments for emergency cuff inflation for faulty inflation line. (*From Sills J: An emergency cuff inflation technique, Respir Care 31:200, 1986.*)

Expected Outcomes

- Tracheal tube remains in correct position
- Cuff pressure is kept at a level to maintain a seal between cuff and tracheal wall (usually between 20 and 25 mm Hg)
- Cuff remains intact

Unexpected Outcomes

- Extubation or tube dislodgment
- Tracheal mucosal ischemia from cuff overinflation
- Faulty inflation valve or tube
- Cuff overinflation and distention over the end of the tube
- Cuff rupture

Patient Monitoring and Care

Steps	Rationale	Reportable Conditions
		These conditions should be reported if they persist despite nursing interventions.
1. Assess respiratory status for optimal ventilation.	Inadequate interface between tracheal cuff and tracheobronchial mucosa decreases inspiratory flow.	• Rising arterial carbon dioxide tension • Chest-abdominal dyssynchrony • Patient-ventilator dyssynchrony • Dyspnea • Headache • Restlessness • Confusion • Lethargy • Increasing (early sign) or decreasing (late sign) arterial blood pressure • Activation of expiratory or inspiratory volume alarms on the mechanical ventilator
2. Measure cuff pressure every 8 hours, or per institutional requirements, maintaining cuff pressure between 20 and 25 mm Hg.[3] **(Level E*)**[2] **(Level D*)**	Prevents tracheal injury and aspiration. Excessive cuff pressure is cited as the most frequent problem of tracheal intubation and the best predictor of tracheolaryngeal injury.[1,2] If the volume (milliliters) needed to seal the airway increases, evaluate patient for tracheal dilation with chest radiography of cuff diameter–to–tracheal diameter ratio. Increasing volumes also may indicate leak in cuff or inflation valve or tube.	• Cuff pressure less than 20 mm Hg or greater than 25 mm Hg
3. Maintain tracheal tube cuff integrity.	Manipulation of the tracheal tube increases the likelihood of cuff disruption. Cuff leak or rupture is evident when the pressure on the manometer continues to decrease.	• Inability to maintain cuff inflation • Audible air through the patient's nose or mouth • Low-pressure or low-volume alarm sounds on the mechanical ventilator • Audible or auscultated inspiratory leak over larynx • Patient able to vocalize audibly • Pilot balloon deflation • Loss of inspiratory and expiratory volume on patients with mechanical ventilation
4. Hyperoxygenate and suction patient based on assessment (see Procedure 12).	Removal of secretions reduces chance for partial or complete airway obstruction.	

*Level D: Peer-reviewed professional organizational standards with clinical studies to support recommendations

*Level E: Multiple case reports, theory-based evidence from expert opinions, or peer-reviewed professional organizational standards without clinical studies to support recommendations

Patient Monitoring and Care —*Continued*

Steps	Rationale	Reportable Conditions
5. Compare patient's cardiopulmonary status before and after tracheal tube cuff care.	Identifies the effects of tracheal tube cuff care on the cardiovascular system.	• Decreased arterial oxygen saturation • Cardiac dysrhythmias • Bronchospasm • Respiratory distress • Cyanosis • Increased blood pressure or intracranial pressure • Anxiety, agitation, or changes in level of consciousness
6. Reassess cuff pressure and volume when transporting patient from one altitude to another (i.e., air transport) or during hyperbaric therapy without environmental pressurization.	Changes in altitude change the volume of gas in the cuff; volume and pressure need to be reevaluated during and after transport.	

Documentation

Documentation should include the following:
• Patient and family education
• Cardiopulmonary and vital sign assessment before and after procedure
• Method of cuff inflation
• Cuff inflation volume and cuff pressure
• Patient's tolerance

• Appearance and characteristics of tracheal secretions, if present
• Unexpected outcomes
• Use of medications
• Use of restraints
• Date, time, and frequency with which procedure is performed
• Nursing interventions

References

1. Hess D: Tracheostomy tubes and related appliances, *Respir Care* 50(4):497-509, 2005.
2. MacIntyre N, Branson R: *Mechanical ventilation,* ed 2, Philadelphia, 2009, Saunders.
3. Morris L, Zoumalan R, Roccaforte D, et al: Monitoring tracheal tube cuff pressures in the intensive care unit: a comparison of digital palpation and manometry, *Ann Otol Rhinol Laryngol* 116(9):639-642, 2007.
4. Pierce L: Airway maintenance. In: *Management of the mechanically ventilated patient,* ed 2, St Louis, 2007, Saunders.
CR 5. Plambeck A: *Adult ventilation management,* Corexcel, Inc, 2004, retrieved April 22, 2004, from www.corexcel.com/courses/vent.htm.
6. Roman M: Tracheostomy tubes, *Medsurg Nurs* 14(2): 143-145, 2005.
7. St John R: Protocols for practice: airway management, *Crit Care Nurse* 24(2):93-96, 2004.
8. Urden L, Stacy K, Lough M, et al: *Thelan's critical care nursing: diagnosis and management,* St Louis, 2005, Mosby.

Additional Reading

Winn M, Right K: Tracheostomy: a guide to nursing care, *Austr Nurs J* 13(5):1-4, 2005.

Tracheostomy Tube Care

P U R P O S E : Tracheostomy tube care is performed to maintain airway patency and decrease infection risk by removing secretions that accumulate within the inner cannula.

Kirsten N. Skillings, Bonnie L. Curtis

PREREQUISITE NURSING KNOWLEDGE

- *Tracheotomy* refers to the surgical procedure in which an incision is made below the cricoid cartilage through the second to fourth tracheal rings (Fig. 14-1). *Tracheostomy* refers to the opening, or stoma, made by the incision. The tracheostomy tube is the artificial airway inserted into the trachea during tracheotomy (Fig. 14-2).

- Tracheostomy tubes have a variety of parts (Fig. 14-3) and are available in various sizes and styles from several manufacturers. The tubes can be metal or plastic, with

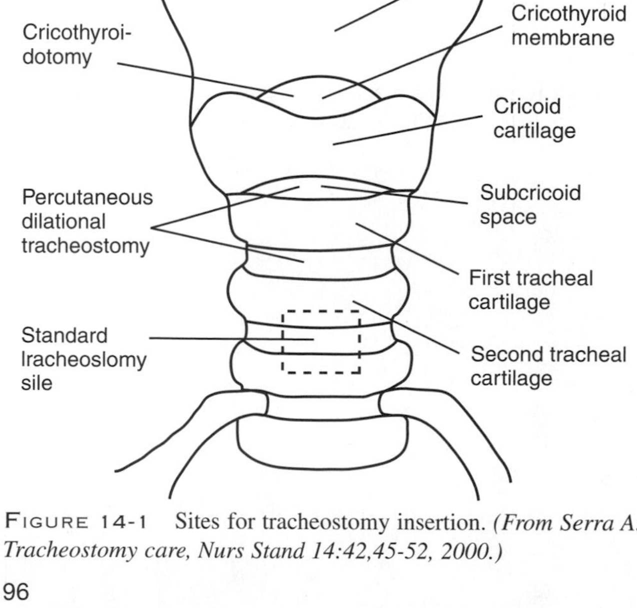

FIGURE 14-1   Sites for tracheostomy insertion. *(From Serra A: Tracheostomy care, Nurs Stand 14:42,45-52, 2000.)*

Thyroid cartilage

Cricothyroid membrane

Cricoid cartilage

Subcricoid space

First tracheal cartilage

Second tracheal cartilage

Cricothyroidotomy

Percutaneous dilational tracheostomy

Standard tracheostomy site

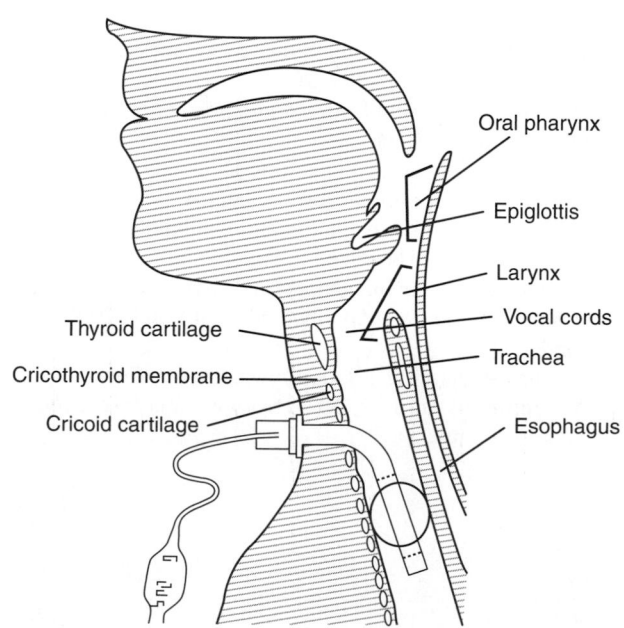

FIGURE 14-2   A tracheostomy (sometimes called a tracheotomy) is created surgically by making an opening through the skin of the neck into the trachea. *(Serra A: Tracheostomy care, Nurs Stand 14:42,45-52, 2000.)*

Oral pharynx

Epiglottis

Larynx

Vocal cords

Trachea

Esophagus

Thyroid cartilage

Cricothyroid membrane

Cricoid cartilage

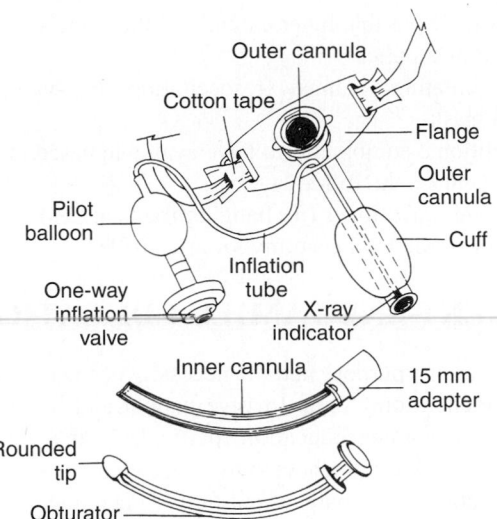

FIGURE 14-3 Parts of a tracheostomy tube. *(From Eubanks DH, Bone RC: Comprehensive respiratory care, ed 2, St Louis, 1990, Mosby, 570.)*

TABLE 14-1	**Indications for Tracheostomy**

Bypass acute upper airway obstruction
Prolonged need for artificial airway
Prophylaxis for anticipated airway problems
Reduction of anatomic dead space
Prevention of pulmonary aspiration
Retained tracheobronchial secretions
Chronic upper airway obstruction

standard or extra length. Clinicians who care for patients with tracheostomy tubes must understand the differences and select a tube that appropriately fits the patient and clinical condition. A tracheostomy tube is shorter than but similar in diameter to an endotracheal tube and has a squared-off distal tip for maximization of airflow. The outer cannula forms the body of a tracheostomy tube with a cuff. The neck flange, attached to the outer cannula, assists in stabilizing the tube in the trachea and provides the small holes necessary for proper securing of the tube. Some tracheostomy setups have an inner cannula inserted into the outer cannula. The inner cannula is removable for easy cleaning without airway compromise. The cuff is a balloon inflated with air to maintain a seal around the tube. As the air flows through the one-way inflation valve, the pilot balloon inflates, which indicates the volume of air present in the cuff.

- A cuffed tube is appropriate for use in patients who need mechanical ventilation or for whom aspiration is a problem. The cuff limits aspiration of oral and gastric secretions. Uncuffed tubes are commonly used in children, in adults with laryngectomies, and during decannulation of the tracheostomy. A fenestrated tracheostomy tube has an opening in the curvature of the posterior wall of the outer cannula. The matching fenestrated inner cannula is inserted into the outer cannula. Fenestrated tracheostomy tubes are useful for patients with smaller tracheas and during weaning.[12] With cuff deflation, options for speech are finger occlusion technique, placement of a speaking valve (Passy-Muir valve), or capping of the outer cannula; all permit air to flow through the upper airway and tracheostomy opening. Foam cuff tracheostomy tubes consist of a high-volume cuff and are composed of polyurethane foam covered with a silicone sheath. Despite the long availability of this type of tracheostomy tube, it is not commonly used and is usually reserved for patients who already have tracheal injury related to the cuff.

- A tracheotomy is performed as either an elective procedure or an emergency procedure for a variety of reasons (Table 14-1). Most often, the procedure is elective and performed in the operating room with sterile conditions. An emergency tracheotomy is performed at the bedside with aseptic technique or before arrival in the critical care unit when swelling, injury, or other upper airway obstruction prevents intubation with an endotracheal tube. Percutaneous tracheotomies also are performed at the bedside. Minimally invasive percutaneous tracheotomy was introduced recently as an alternative to the traditional surgical technique. It has gained widespread acceptance in the past decade.[5,8] This procedure consists of passing a needle into the trachea, placing a J-tipped guidewire, progressively dilating the trachea, and placing the tracheostomy tube. The percutaneous procedure has achieved outcomes comparable with outcomes with the surgical technique.[1,3]

- Protocols for emergency tracheotomy vary among institutions. Often, nurses at the bedside take an active role in assisting with tracheotomy and insertion of a tracheostomy tube; however, some institutions have surgical personnel at the bedside to assist with the procedure.

- During insertion, the obturator replaces the inner cannula. Its smooth surface protrudes from the outer cannula and minimizes tracheal trauma. When the tracheostomy tube is inserted, the obturator is removed and replaced with the inner cannula, which locks in place. The same size sterile tracheostomy tube should be available at the bedside for easy access in case of accidental decannulation.

- The decision for a tracheotomy in patients with long-term mechanical ventilation is made on the basis of the team's projection regarding length of time that mechanical ventilation or an artificial airway is required. A tracheostomy tube is the preferred method of airway maintenance in a patient who needs intubation for more than 14 to 21 days. Each case must be reviewed individually.[1,3,10,13,14] Better predictors are needed to further identify patients who can benefit from tracheotomy early in the course of mechanical ventilation.[8]

- When compared with endotracheal tubes, tracheostomy tubes provide added benefits to patients, including the following:
  - Prevention of further laryngeal injury from the translaryngeal tube
  - Improved patient comfort, acceptance, and toleration
  - Ease of oral care

- ❖ Decreased work of breathing because of less airflow resistance
- ❖ Facilitation of weaning from mechanical ventilation
- ❖ Decreased requirement for sedation
- ❖ Provision of a speech mechanism
- ❖ Enhanced communication
- ❖ Greater patient mobility
- ❖ Facilitation of removal of secretions
- ❖ Reduced risk of unintentional airway loss
- A tracheostomy tube is viewed by the body as foreign material. The body responds by increasing mucus production. Also, ciliary movement is impaired, which limits the forward movement of the mucociliary escalator. Because the tracheostomy bypasses the upper airway and its protective and hydrating mechanisms, patients are at increased risk of infection. Lack of hydration by the upper airway can lead to thick mucus, which increases the risk of airway obstruction. Tracheostomy patients should receive continuous humidified air or oxygen for this reason.[1,4]
- The tracheostomy tube creates a more stable airway, making transfer out of the critical care unit feasible when overall patient condition warrants. Also, care of the patient, such as suctioning, oral care, and ability to meet nutritional needs, is simplified.
- A stoma less than 48 hours old has not fully formed a tracheostomy tract. If the tracheostomy tube is accidentally dislodged, the tracheostomy may close and compromise the patient's airway.
- A small amount of bleeding is expected for the first few days after a tracheotomy. Bright frank bleeding or constant oozing is not expected and should be brought to the attention of the physician or advanced practice nurse.
- Consideration should be given to obtaining assistance with tracheostomy care, especially when tracheal ties are changed or a patient is agitated. An extra pair of hands can minimize the risk for accidental dislodgment.

EQUIPMENT

Some institutions may use tracheostomy care kits for cleaning a nondisposable inner cannula. Others may use disposable inner cannulas, in which case the following equipment is needed:

- Personal protective equipment
- Sterile normal saline solution (NS) or water
- Sterile cotton swabs
- Sterile 4 × 4 gauze pads
- Commericial tracheostomy tube holder
- Sterile precut tracheostomy dressing

- Sterile disposable inner cannula of the same size
- Suction supplies
- Self-inflating manual resuscitation bag-valve-device and mask

Additional equipment (to have available based on patient need) includes the following:

- Second practitioner (if changing tracheal ties)
- Extra sterile tracheostomy kit at bedside

PATIENT AND FAMILY EDUCATION

- Explain the purpose and the necessity of the tracheotomy or tracheostomy care. Involve patient and family members in ongoing education, particularly if a home discharge with the tracheostomy is anticipated. ➻*Rationale:* Education to the patient and family encourages cooperation and compliance and reduces anxiety.

PATIENT ASSESSMENT AND PREPARATION
Patient Assessment

- Assess increased production of secretions. ➻*Rationale:* Tube irritation to mucosa results in increased production of secretions.
- Assess cardiopulmonary status:
  - ❖ Decreased arterial oxygen saturation
  - ❖ Cardiac dysrhythmias
  - ❖ Bronchospasm
  - ❖ Respiratory distress
  - ❖ Cyanosis
  - ❖ Increased blood pressure or intracranial pressure
  - ❖ Anxiety, agitation, or changes in level of consciousness
- ➻*Rationale:* Evaluation of the patient's cardiopulmonary status provides valuable information about the need for and tolerance of tracheostomy tube care.

Patient Preparation

- Verify the correct patient with two identifiers. ➻*Rationale:*. Prior to performing a procedure, the nurse should ensure the correct identification of the patient for the intended intervention.
- Perform a pre-procedure verification and time out, if nonemergent. ➻*Rationale:* Ensures patient safety.
- Ensure that the patient understands preprocedural teachings. Answer questions as they arise, and reinforce information as needed. ➻*Rationale:* This communication evaluates and reinforces understanding of previously taught information.

Procedure for Tracheostomy Tube Care

Steps	Rationale	Special Considerations
1. **HH**		
2. **PE**		Protective eyewear or face mask should be worn.[9]
3. Hyperoxygenate and suction trachea and pharynx as needed (see Procedure 12).	Reduces risk of hypoxemia and arrythmias; removes secretions and diminishes patient's need to cough during the procedure.	Saline solution flushes to assist with secretion removal are not recommended. These flushes do not loosen secretions and potentiate infection.[14]
4. Remove soiled tracheostomy dressing.		
5. **HH**		
6. For disposable inner cannula: A. Open prepackaged inner cannula package. B. Apply clean gloves. C. Remove soiled inner cannula. D. Replace with prepackaged inner cannula.		
7. For nondisposable inner cannula, open prepackaged commercial tracheostomy care kit. A. Prepare sterile normal saline solution or sterile H_2O on sterile field.[12,14,18]	Reduces transmission of microorganisms; Standard Precautions.	Only sterile NS should be used for cleaning a metal tracheostomy tube because hydrogen peroxide may cause pitting of metal inner cannula.[14] Hydrogen peroxide is no longer recommended for cleaning inner cannulas or tracheostomy site.[12,14,17] Prepackaged commercial tracheostomy care kits are available.
B. Apply sterile gloves. C. Remove oxygen source and inner cannula, placing it in sterile normal saline (NS) or water.	Removes inner cannula for cleaning.	
8. Place tracheostomy collar or T tube or ventilator oxygen source over or near outer cannula. (Note: T tube and ventilator oxygen devices cannot be attached to outer cannulas when inner cannula is removed.)	Maintains oxygen supply.	If patient cannot tolerate disconnection from the ventilator for the time needed to clean the inner cannula, replace the existing inner cannula with a clean one and reattach the mechanical ventilator. Then, clean the cannula just removed from the patient and store it in a sterile container for the next time.[2]
9. Clean inner cannula with a small brush.	Assists in the removal of debris and thick secretions.	Tracheostomy care should be completed every 4 to 8 hours and as needed per volume of secretions produced.[7,11,14]
10. Rinse inner cannula by pouring NS over the cannula.		
11. Remove oxygen source from over outer cannula.	Allows access to opening of outer cannula.	
12. Insert inner cannula and lock into place.	Secures inner cannula.	
13. Reapply oxygen source to inner cannula hub.	Reestablishes oxygen supply.	

Procedure continues on following page

Procedure for Tracheostomy Tube Care—*Continued*

Steps	Rationale	Special Considerations
14. Moisten swabs and 4 × 4 gauze pads with sterile NS or water and clean stoma site, outer cannula, and neck plate surface area by wiping with cotton-tipped swabs and 4 × 4 gauze pads.	Removes debris and secretions from the stoma area.	
15. Pat dry the skin area surrounding the stoma site.	Dry surface decreases likelihood of microorganism growth and skin breakdown.	
16. Have assistant hold neck plate securely.	Decreases the incidence of tracheal tube decannulation.	Have self-inflating manual resuscitation bag-valve-device and mask available at patient bedside for emergent oxygenation source.
17. Remove current tracheostomy tube holder or cut the twill tape tie.	Prepares for application of new tracheostomy tube holder or new twill tape.	A variety of commercially tracheostomy tube holders is available. Assistant must maintain stability of the neck plate while tube holder is being exchanged. The tracheostomy tube may be sutured in place and no holder or ties used (e.g., for patients with new laryngectomy and flap).
18. Attach a new trachesotomy tube holder or twill tape. A. Tracheostomy tube holder: Connect one side of neck plate to new tracheostomy tube holder, then connect to other side of neck plate and tighten tube holder, allowing one finger under the holder to ensure it is secure. B. Twill tape: Cut a length long enough to encircle the patient's neck two times. Cut ends diagonally. Insert one end through the face plate eyelet and pull the ends even. Pass both ends of the tie around the patient's neck and insert one end through the face plate's second eyelet. Pull snugly to allow space for one finger between the tie and the patient's neck and tie the ends securely with a double square knot so that the knot rests on the side of the patient's neck. (See Fig. 14-4).	Reestablishes secure tracheal neck plate.	Some facilities may still use twill tape. Some facility policies preclude changing the tracheostomy tube holders during the first 72 hours because of the risk of rapid tracheal stoma closure.[15]
19. Apply clean precut tracheostomy dressing under neck plate.	Promotes drainage absorption.	Never cut a 4 × 4 gauze pad because cut edges fray and provide a potential source for infection.[12,14]
20. Provide appropriate oral care (see Procedure 4).		
21. Discard used supplies.		
22. Remove personal protective equipment.	Reduces the transmission of microorganisms and body secretions; Standard Precautions	
23. ▣		

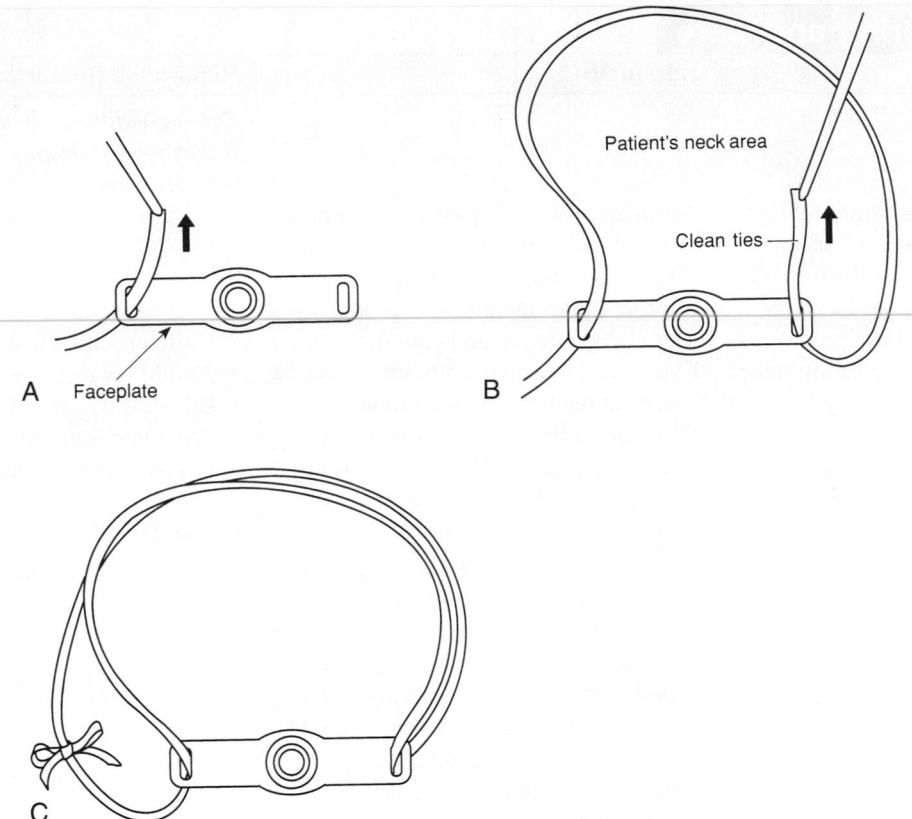

FIGURE 14-4 Placement of tracheostomy twill tape. **A,** Face plate with threading of twill tape (for prevention of decannulation, an additional person needs to stabilize face plate). **B,** Advancing of the twill tape around the back of the neck and looping through the other side of face plate. **C,** Doubling of the twill tape and securing in a knot.

Expected Outcomes

- Airway patency
- Infection prevention
- Healing promotion

Unexpected Outcomes

- Prolonged apnea, increasing hypoxemia, or cardiopulmonary arrest
- Hemorrhage
- Interstitial air: Subcutaneous emphysema, pneumothorax, pneumopericardium, and pneumoperitoneum
- Thyroid gland injury
- Cardiac dysrhythmias
- Tube-tip erosion into the tracheal innominate artery
- Skin breakdown, pressure areas, or stomatitis
- Stoma infection
- Bronchopulmonary infection
- Displacement or dislodgment out of trachea
- Excessive cuff pressure
- Leaking airway cuff
- Airway obstruction from misalignment, cuff overinflation, or dried or excessive secretions
- Tracheal stenosis, malacia, or tracheoesophageal fistula
- Tracheal ischemia, necrosis, or dilation
- Laryngeal disorders
- Dysphasia

Procedure continues on following page

Patient Monitoring and Care

Steps	Rationale	Reportable Conditions
		These conditions should be reported if they persist despite nursing interventions.
1. Provide continuous humidified air or oxygen. Warm or cool as appropriate.[7,11,14] **(Level C,* Level D*)**	Artificial airways bypass the nose and mouth, preventing normal warming, humidification, and filtering.[1,12]	
2. Auscultate lung sounds to check proper placement of tracheostomy tube and ensure tracheostomy tube is securely in place.	Improper placement may lead to inadequate ventilation and complications.	• Decreased chest wall motion
	Extra sterile tracheostomy kit should be kept at the bedside at all times.	• Unilateral breath sounds
	Displacement into the subcutaneous tissue can occur. How emergent the situation is depends on whether the upper airway is obstructed.	• Audible expiratory wheeze • Bilateral decreased breath sounds • Oxygen desaturation • Dyspnea or respiratory distress • Stridor • Ventilator alarms
	Decannulation can inadvertently occur from lack of tracheostomy tube securement. If decannulation occurs and if retention sutures are present, pull them apart to lift the trachea up and hold the tracheal stoma open. Do not cross tracheal sutures because this action will close the airway. When help arrives, a second person should reinsert the tracheostomy tube as per individual facility policy.[15]	
	If patient does not have retention sutures, open a new tracheostomy tube set, remove the inner cannula, and insert the obturator into the outer cannula and slide it into place.[15]	
3. Inspect and palpate for air under skin.	Air may escape into the incision, causing subcutaneous emphysema. *Special Note: Subcutaneous emphysema usually does not harm patients with an airway already in place. Puffiness of the soft tissue may result, however, and, if significant, can change the patient's appearance, alarming the patient and the family.*	• Subcutaneous emphysema
4. Assess for frank bleeding or constant oozing of blood.	Surgical procedures increase the risk of potential injury to adjacent tissues and structures. Stoma placement below the second and third cartilaginous rings results in an increased incidence of innominate artery erosion.	• Frank bleeding or constant oozing of blood
5. Palpate the tube for pulsation.	Pulsations felt in the tracheal tube are suggestive of impending erosion of major blood vessels.	• Pulsation of the tracheal tube
6. Follow institution standard for assessing pain. Administer analgesia as prescribed.	Identifies need for pain interventions.	• Continued pain despite pain interventions

*Level C: Qualitative studies, descriptive or correlational studies, integrative reviews, systematic reviews, or randomized controlled trials with inconsistent results,
*Level D: Peer-reviewed professional organizational standards with clinical studies to support recommendations

Patient Monitoring and Care —*Continued*

Steps	Rationale	Reportable Conditions
7. Maintain mucosal tissue integrity with appropriate cuff care procedures (see Procedure 13).	Constant pressure and irritation of the mucosal tissue can result in blood vessel and cellular damage.	• Need for increasing pressure or volume to maintain tracheal cuff seal
8. Tracheostomy care should be done every 4 to 8 hours and as needed per volume of secretions produced.[7,11,14] **(Level D*, Level E*)**	Keeps tube free of secretions, mucous, and plugs that may impede airway patency. Dry clean dressings maintain skin integrity and decrease risk of infection.	• Frequent plugs • Copious drainage • Change in characteristics or odor of drainage
9. Assess skin for signs of infection, inflammation, or pressure.	Skin irritation or breakdown may occur from neck plate, tracheostomy tube holder, or sutures, if present.	• Elevated temperature • Redness • Swelling • Excoriated or open areas • Purulent drainage
10. Monitor secretions (color, odor, amount, and consistency). Hyperoxygenate and suction (see Procedure 12) based on assessment.	Suctioning should be based on patient need rather than on a standard frequency. Change in secretion characteristics may indicate infection or inadequate hydration.	• Excessively thick secretions • Copious or purulent secretions
11. Maintain head of bed at 30 to 45 degrees and during enteral feedings.[16]	An elevated head of bed promotes oropharyngeal and nasopharyngeal drainage and minimizes the risk of aspiration Prevents ventilator-associated or hospital-acquired pneumonia.[6] Withholding enteral feeding when gastric residual volumes are high is also important in the prevention of regurgitation and pulmonary aspiration.	• High enteral residuals • Intolerance to head of bed elevation • Increased oxygen demand • Change in lung sounds • Increased quality and characteristics of secretions • Elevated temperature
12. Perform oral care every 2 to 4 hours (see Procedure 4).	Prevents bacterial overgrowth and promotes patient comfort. Prevents ventilator-associated pneumonia.	
13. Promote effective patient-provider communication (paper and pencil, letter or word boards, one-way speaking valves, if appropriate).	The patient cannot talk, which may result in fear and anxiety. Patients need an established communication mechanism. A speaking valve may be used to facilitate speech.	

*Level D: Peer-reviewed professional organizational standards with clinical studies to support recommendations
*Level E: Multiple case reports, theory-based evidence from expert opinions, or peer-reviewed professional organizational standards without clinical studies to support recommendations

Documentation

Documentation should include the following:
• Patient and family education and comprehension
• Vital signs assessed before and after procedure
• Date, time, and frequency of tracheostomy care
• Type and size of tracheostomy tube, changing of inner cannula, replacement of tracheostomy tube holder, and general condition of stoma and surrounding skin
• Nursing interventions in response to assessed complications

• Use of medications for sedation or pain and patient response
• Expected and unexpected outcomes
• Type and amount of secretions and frequency of suctioning
• Performance of oral care
• Pain assessment, interventions, and effectiveness

References

CR 1. Billau C: Suctioning. In Russell C, Matta B, editors: *Tracheostomy a multiprofessional handbook,* Cambridge, 2004, Cambridge University Press, 157-171.

CR 2. Buchfa,, VL, Fries CM: *Repiratory care in nursing procedures,* ed 3, Springhouse, PA, 2000, Springhouse Corp, 449-455.

CR 3. Burns SM, et al: Are frequent inner cannula changes necessary? A pilot study, *Heart Lung* 27:58-62, 1998.

CR 4. Henneman E, Ellstrom K, St John RE: Airway management. In *AACN protocols for practice: care of the mechanically ventilated patient series,* Aliso Viejo, CA, 1999, American Association of Critical-Care Nurses.

5. Hess D: Tracheostomy tubes and related appliances, *Respir Care* 50(4):497-509, 2005.

CR 6. Hubmayr RD, Burchardi H, Elliot M, et al: American Thoracic Society Assembly on Critical Care, European Respiratory Society, European Society of Intensive Care Medicine, Societe de Reanimation de Langue Francaise. Statement of the 4th International Consensus Conference in Critical Care on ICU-Acquired Pneumonia, Chicago, Illinois, May 2002, *Intensive Care Med* 28:1521-1536, 2002.

CR 7. McCloskey J, Bulechek G: *Nursing interventions classification,* ed 3, 2002, St Louis, Mosby.

CR 8. Mittendorf EA, et al: Early and late outcome of bedside percutaneous tracheostomy in the intensive care unit, *Am Surg* 68:342-346, 2002.

9. Potter P, Perry A: *Fundamentals of nursing,* St Louis, 2009, Mosby, 946-950.

10. Rana S, Pendem S, Pogodzinski M, et al: Tracheostomy in critically ill patients, *Mayo Clini Proce* 80(12): 1632-1638, 2005.

CR 11. Rankin N: What is optimum humidity? *Respir Care Clin North Am* 4:321-328, 1998.

12. Roman M: Tracheostomy tubes, *Medsurg Nurs* 14(2): 143-145, 2005.

13. Russell C: Providing the nurse with a guide to tracheostomy care and management, *Br J Nurs* 14(8):428-433, 2005.

CR 14. St John R: Protocols for practice: airway management, *Crit Care Nurs* 24(2):93-96, 2004.

CR 15. Seay S, Gay S, Strauss M: Tracheostomy emergencies, *Am J Nursing* 102(3):59-61, 2002.

16. Tolentino, AF, Ruppert, SD, Shiao, SY: Evidence-based practice: Use of the ventilator bundle to prevent ventilator-associated pneumonia, *Am J Crit Care,* 16(1):20-2007.

CR 17. Trundle C, Brooks R: Infection control issues in the care of a patient with a tracheostomy. In *Tracheostomy a multiprofessional handbook,* Cambridge, 2004, Cambridge University Press, 343-360.

18. Winn M, Right K: Tracheostomy: a guide to nursing care, *Austr Nurs* 13(5):1-4, 2005.

Additional Readings

Plambeck A: *Adult ventilation management, Corexcel, Inc,* 2004, retrieved 10/28/09, from www.corexcel.com/courses/vent.htm.

St John R, Seckel M: Airway management. In Burns S, editor: *Care of the mechanically ventilated patients,* ed 2, Sudbury: MA, 2007, Jones and Bartlett.

Serra A: Tracheostomy care, *Nurs Stand* 14:42,45-52, 2000.

Tamburri LM: Care of the patient with a tracheostomy, *Orthop Nurs* 19:49-58, 2000.

Thompson J, McFarland G Hirsch J, et al: Ear, nose and throat. In *Mosby's clinical nursing*, 2002, 627-630.

Continuous End-Tidal Carbon Dioxide Monitoring

P U R P O S E : End-tidal carbon dioxide provides a noninvasive continuous measurement of ventilation[12] or inhaled and exhaled carbon dioxide concentration commonly referred to as capnography. A capnograph depicts this measurement as a graphic picture or waveform tracing of each respiratory cycle. The partial pressure of end-tidal CO_2 is assumed to represent alveolar gas, which under normal ventilation/perfusion matching in the lungs closely parallels arterial levels of CO_2.

Vicki S. Good, Paul Luehrs

PREREQUISITE NURSING KNOWLEDGE

- Capnography provides the clinician with a calculation of airway respiratory rate (RR), and the combination of both end-tidal carbon dioxide ($Petco_2$) and RR can provide clinicians with one of the earliest indications that ventilation is hindered. The carbon dioxide waveform changes immediately on any degradation in quality of breathing and some of the most pertinent real-time information provided to give the caregiver an immediate alert to respiratory compromise, such as hypoventilation, airway obstruction, or cessation of breathing.[6] $Petco_2$ monitoring is the earliest indicator of airway compromise, and in the aforementioned study, abnormal $Petco_2$ findings were observed with many acute respiratory events. In another study, acute respiratory events were found to cause $Petco_2$ abnormalities seen before oxygenation desaturation or observed hypoventilation.[3]
- Capnography can be thought of as the "ventilation vital sign" because it provides breath-to-breath feedback and generates a respiratory rate that is measured at the airway. The clinician now has the ability to measure respiratory frequency and detection of respiratory depression in

patients who are not intubated sooner than with traditional monitoring techniques, which allows for safer titration of medications.[6]

- Ventilation is the bulk movement of gases into and out of the lung and is composed of two distinct processes: inspiration and expiration.
  - ❖ During inspiration, gas is delivered to the alveoli, at which time it participates in gas exchange. Oxygenation occurs when the oxygen diffuses across the alveolar membrane into the blood. CO_2 exchange occurs during this time as it diffuses across the alveolar membrane into the alveoli. Oxygenated blood is then distributed to and metabolized by the cells of muscles and organs. Oxygen saturation can be evaluated with a blood gas machine (oxygen saturation [Sao_2]) or pulse oximetry (Spo_2).
  - ❖ During expiration, alveolar gas is exhaled, which results in the elimination of CO_2. Cells produce carbon dioxide (CO_2) as a by-product of metabolism; this CO_2 is transported by the vascular system to the lungs where it is eliminated through exhalation. For exhaled CO_2 to be detected, adequate circulation must carry CO_2-laden blood from the peripheral tissues to the lungs and adequate ventilation must carry CO_2 from

the lungs to the mouth.[6] CO_2 elimination can also be evaluated with a blood gas machine (SaO_2) $PetCO_2$ monitor/capnography.

- Just as capnography cannot measure oxygenation, pulse oximetry cannot directly measure ventilation or alveolar ventilation (but SpO_2 can provide some directional reflection of ventilation changes if the patient is breathing room air). To assist in the complete monitoring of the patient's respiratory status, the two parameters must be used together: pulse oximetry to assess how well oxygen has moved across the alveolar capillary membrane into the blood to be transported to the tissues, and capnography to determine how well the patient is ventilating through the process of moving air in and out of the lungs and exhaling carbon dioxide.[6]

- For a patient who is not intubated who needs capnography, a specialized nasal cannula delivers supplemental oxygen and measures $PetCO_2$, apneic events, and respiratory rate. Placing the capnography cannula is the same as initiating a nasal cannula for supplemental oxygen. Breath samples are obtained through both nostrils, and oxygen is delivered through the nasal prongs (design depends on manufacturer). An extension in the front of the mouth can be used for patients who breathe by mouth.[6] $PetCO_2$ can be monitored in patients who are intubated; the sensor is directly connected to the ventilator circuit.

- The principles of arterial blood gas sampling (see Procedure 64) and interpretation should be understood.

- Indications for continuous end-tidal CO_2 monitoring include the following:
  - ❖ Determine a baseline CO_2 waveform and $PetCO_2$.[1,15]
  - ❖ Continuously monitor the patency of the airway and the presence of breathing.
  - ❖ Provide mechanism for early detection of changes in waveform pattern or $PetCO_2$ value that may accompany a sudden or gradual change in CO_2 production or elimination (permissive hypercapnia, hyperthermia, hypoventilation [extubation], hyperventilation therapy), or reduction in circulation (pulmonary blood flow).[1,4,11,13,15]

- Basic principles of $PetCO_2$ monitoring should be understood. The end-tidal CO_2 monitor may be a stand-alone system, a module incorporated into the patient's bedside physiologic monitor or incorporated into a mechanical ventilator. An infrared capnograph passes light through an expiratory gas sample and, with a photodetector, measures absorption of that light by the gas. The capnograph determines the amount of CO_2 in the gas sample based on the absorption properties of CO_2. The capnograph also visually graphs the pattern in which CO_2 is exhaled and provides a display called a *capnogram* or $PetCO_2$ *waveform*.[1]

- The capnograph samples exhaled CO_2 by one of two methods: aspiration (side stream) or nonaspiration (mainstream) sampling. In the side stream method, a sample of gas is transported via small-bore tubing to the bedside monitor for analysis. In the mainstream system, analysis occurs directly at the patient-ventilator circuit.[1]

- Normal $PetCO_2$ concentration in a patient with healthy lungs and airway conditions is 30 to 43 mm Hg. As the patient breathes, a characteristic waveform is created that can be divided into two segments: inspiration and expiration. Indications for $PetCO_2$ monitoring include verification of endotracheal tube (ETT) placement, CPR, procedural sedation, gastric tube placement, and endoscopic procedures.[8] The normal capnographic waveform has the following characteristics (Fig. 15-1):
  - ❖ A zero baseline represents the completion of inspiration and the beginning of exhalation of CO_2-free gas from anatomic dead space. This gas comes from the large airways, oropharynx, and nasopharynx (see Fig. 15-1, *A-B*).
  - ❖ A rapid sharp upstroke occurs as the gas from the intermediate airways, containing a mixture of fresh gas and CO_2, begins to be exhaled from the lungs (see Fig. 15-1, *B-C*).
  - ❖ A nearly flat alveolar plateau occurs as exhaled flow velocity slows and mixed gas is displaced by alveolar gas (Fig. 15-1, *C-D*). Alveolar exhalation of CO_2 is nearing completion.
  - ❖ A distance end-tidal point most closely reflects the maximal concentration of exhaled CO_2 and the end of exhalation (Fig. 15-1, *D*).
  - ❖ A rapid down stroke occurs as the patient begins the inspiration of gas that is essentially devoid of CO_2 (see Fig. 15-1, *D-E*).
  - ❖ The positively deflected limb occurs with exhalation, whereas the negatively deflected limb occurs with inhalation. This is opposite from other respiratory waveforms, including the respirogram, spirogram, and flow-volume loop. The capnogram deviates from normal whenever physiologic or mechanical disruption of the breath occurs.

EQUIPMENT

- Personal protective equipment, including goggles, mask, and gloves
- Capnograph
- Airway adapter $PetCO_2$ nasal cannula

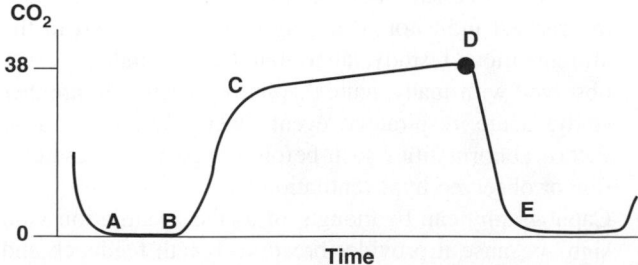

FIGURE 15-1   Essentials of the normal capnographic waveform. *(Reprinted by permission of Nellcor Puritan Bennett LLC, Boulder, CO, part of Covidien.)*

PATIENT AND FAMILY EDUCATION

- Discuss the reason for implementation of capnography. ➤*Rationale:* Discussion reduces anxiety for the patient and family associated with an additional monitor, related interventions, and unfamiliar procedures.
- If the patient is alert, explain the procedure to the patient; if the patient is not alert, explain the procedure to the family. ➤*Rationale:* This communication informs the patient and family of the purpose of monitoring, improves cooperation with interventions, and reduces anxiety.

PATIENT ASSESSMENT AND PREPARATION

Patient Assessment

- Assess indications for $PetCO_2$ monitoring[1,4,11,13,15]:
  - ❖ Acute airway obstruction or apnea (or potential for)

- ❖ Dead space ventilation (or potential for)
- ❖ Incomplete alveolar emptying (or potential for)
- ➤*Rationale:* Assessment for initiation of $PetCO_2$ monitoring ensures that patients at risk for inadequate ventilation and gas exchange receive monitoring for such occurrences, allowing for early institution of appropriate interventions.

Patient Preparation

- Verify correct patient with two identifiers. ➤*Rationale:* Prior to performing a procedure, the nurse should ensure the correct identification of the patient for the intended intervention.
- Ensure that the patient understands preprocedural teachings. Answer questions as they arise, and reinforce information as needed. ➤*Rationale:* Understanding of previously taught information is evaluated and reinforced.

Procedure	for Continuous End-Tidal Carbon Dioxide Monitoring	
Steps	**Rationale**	**Special Considerations**
1. Obtain order or follow institutional protocol for continuous $PetCO_2$ monitoring with capnography.	Order provides guideline for duration of monitoring, acceptable parameters for results, and appropriate interventions for abnormal results.	
2. Assess for proper functioning of capnograph, including electronic equipment, self-start, autocalibration, airway adapter, sensor, and display monitor; and secure connections.	Ensures reliability of $PetCO_2$ values and waveforms obtained.	
3. **HH**		
4. **PE**		
5. Connect capnograph into grounded wall outlet; connect appropriate patient cable into display monitor; turn on instrument.	Decreases incidence of electrical interference.	Check capnograph's battery capacity and charging time, if applicable.
6. Perform calibration routine. Calibration procedure should occur daily or more often when instrument is in clinical use.[1] **(Level M*)**	Accurate measurement for some devices depends on proper calibration. Improper calibration may lead to erroneous $PetCO_2$ values.	All monitors have some type of calibration procedure; see operator's manual for exact steps.
7. If patient is not intubated, apply $PetCO_2$ nasal cannula and connect to capnogroph.[1]		
8. Assemble airway adapter, sensor, and display monitor; connect to the patient's circuit as close as possible to the patient's ventilation connection.[1]	Decreases incidence of improper gas sampling.	Sampling errors and gas leaks in system are major causes of inaccurate readings. Place adapter to the patient circuit or sampling port as close as possible to the patient's airway to decrease response time to detect a change in CO_2.

*Level M: Manufacturer's recommendations only

Procedure continues on following page

Procedure for Continuous End-Tidal Carbon Dioxide Monitoring—*Continued*

Steps	Rationale	Special Considerations
9. Ensure that the light source is on top of the circuit so that condensation and secretions do not pool and obstruct the light transmission in mainstream sensor.	Decreases secretion accumulation on CO_2 port where gas is drawn for sampling.	
10. Set appropriate alarms. Alarm limits should include respiratory rate, apnea default, high and low $Petco_2$, and minimal levels of inspiratory CO_2. **(Level A*)**	Alerts the nurse to potentially life-threatening problems.[9,14]	The $Petco_2$ alarm is set 5% above and below acceptable parameter or per institutional standard. If monitor is interfaced with other equipment (electrocardiogram monitor, mechanical ventilator, pulse oximeter), ensure alarms are set consistently among all monitors.
11. **HH**		
12. **PE**		

Expected Outcomes

- Significant changes in ventilatory status are detected
- Alterations in the alveolar-arterial carbon dioxide gradient are identified

Unexpected Outcomes

- Inaccurate measurements of $Petco_2$ are displayed
- Inaccurate measurements from calibration drift or contamination of optics with moisture or secretions are displayed
- Equipment malfunction occurs
- Inadvertent extubation from weight of sensor

Patient Monitoring and Care

Steps	Rationale	Reportable Conditions
		These conditions should be reported if they persist despite nursing interventions.
1. Observe artificial airway for patency. **(Level A)**	The airway adapter often adds weight to the airway and increases the risk of dislodgment or kinking. If kinking occurs, support the airway with an artificial support or towel.[1]	• Endotracheal or tracheal tube dislodgment
2. If the patient is not intubated, check nasal cannula or mouthpiece for proper placement and ensure that it is clear of secretions.	Poor placement or occlusion of nasal cannula or mouthpiece interferes with accurate $Petco_2$ sensing.	
3. Observe waveform for quality. **(Level M*)**	If waveform is of poor quality, the numerical $Petco_2$ value should not be accepted. If the $Petco_2$ waveform is acceptable and the $Petco_2$ numerical reading is questionable, obtain arterial blood gas measurement to confirm changes in $Petco_2$.[10]	• Poor-quality waveform • Questionable $Petco_2$ reading

*Level A: Meta-analysis of quantitative studies or metasynthesis of qualitative studies with results that consistently support a specific action, intervention, or treatment

*Level M: Manufacturer's recommendations only

Patient Monitoring and Care —*Continued*

Steps	Rationale	Reportable Conditions
4. Observe waveform for gradually increasing $PetCO_2$ (Fig. 15-2). **(Level A*)**	Increasing $PetCO_2$ occurs from absorption of CO_2 from exogenous sources and increased CO_2 production.[9] Clinical conditions in which increasing $PetCO_2$ is found include increased metabolism, hyperthermia (usually indicated by a rapid rise in $PetCO_2$), sepsis, hypoventilation or inadequate minute ventilation, neuromuscular blockade, decreased alveolar ventilation, partial obstruction of the airway, use of respiratory depressant drugs, and conditions that cause metabolic alkalosis.[4,5,11,13,14]	• $PetCO_2$ increase of greater than 10% of baseline
5. Observe for a gradual increase in both baseline CO_2 and $PetCO_2$ values (Fig. 15-3). **(Level B*)**	Reflects rebreathing of previously exhaled gas. Clinical conditions in which a gradual increase in both baseline CO_2 and $PetCO_2$ levels is found include defective exhalation valve on mechanical ventilator and excessive mechanical dead space in ventilator circuit.[11,13]	• Malfunction of the ventilator
6. Observe for an exponential fall in $PetCO_2$ (Fig. 15-4). **(Level B)**	Indicates a sudden increase in dead space ventilation seen in clinical conditions such as cardiopulmonary bypass, cardiopulmonary arrest, pulmonary embolism, and severe pulmonary hypoperfusion.[2,9,15]	• Cardiopulmonary arrest • $PetCO_2$ decreased by more than 10% of baseline
7. Observe for decreased $PetCO_2$ (with a normal waveform; Fig. 15-5). **(Level B)**	Gradual decreases indicate a decrease in perfusion or a decrease in production of CO_2 and may be seen in patients with high minute volumes, hypothermia, metabolic acidosis, decreased cardiac output, and hypovolemia.[7,10]	• $PetCO_2$ decreased by more than 10% of baseline

*Level A: Meta-analysis of quantitative studies or metasynthesis of qualitative studies with results that consistently support a specific action, intervention, or treatment
*Level B: Well-designed, controlled studies with results that consistently support a specific action, intervention or treatment

Procedure continues on following page

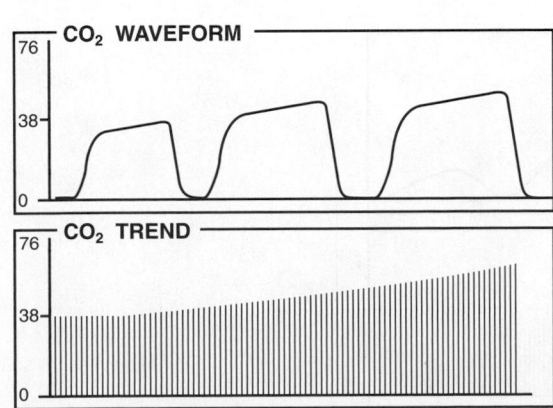

FIGURE 15-2   Gradually increasing $PetCO_2$. *(Reprinted by permission of Nellcor Puritan Bennett LLC, Boulder, CO, part of Covidien.)*

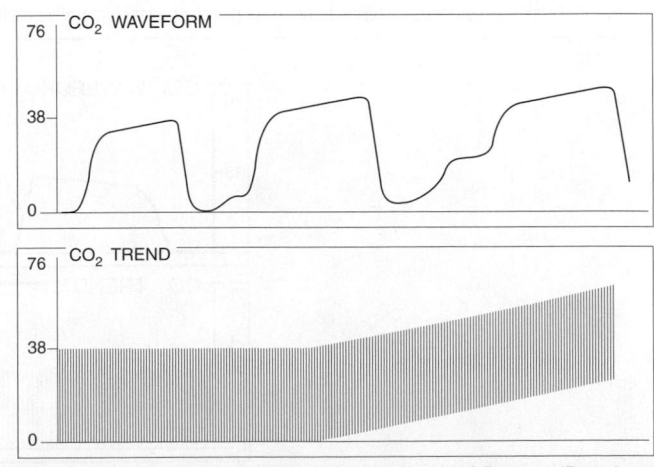

FIGURE 15-3   Gradual increase in baseline and $PetCO_2$. *(Reprinted by permission of Nellcor Puritan Bennett LLC, Boulder, CO, part of Covidien.)*

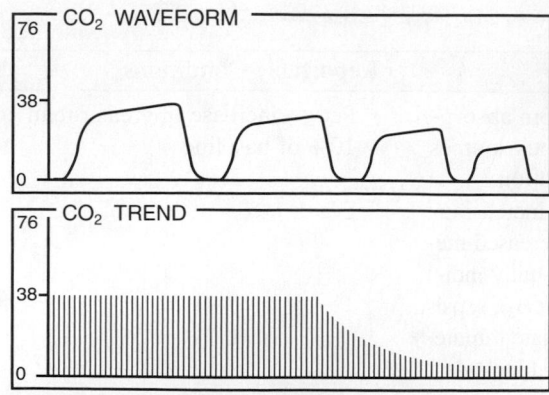

FIGURE 15-4   Exponential fall in Petco$_2$. *(Reprinted by permission of Nellcor Puritan Bennett LLC, Boulder, CO, part of Covidien.)*

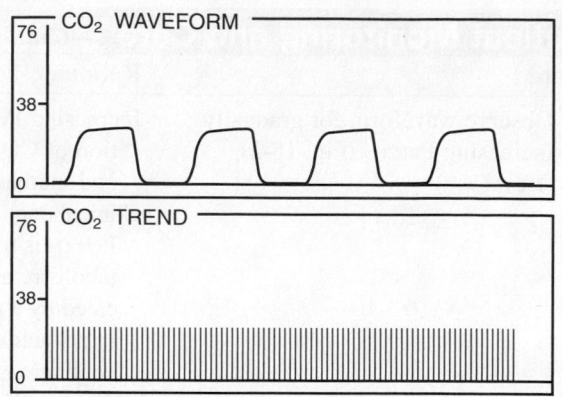

FIGURE 15-5   Decreased Petco$_2$. *(Reprinted by permission of Nellcor Puritan Bennett LLC, Boulder, CO, part of Covidien.)*

Patient Monitoring and Care —*Continued*

Steps	Rationale	Reportable Conditions
8. Observe for a sudden decrease in Petco$_2$ to low values (Fig. 15-6). **(Level B*)**	Incomplete sampling or full exhalation is not detected in the system. This may be seen in patients with a leak in the airway system, partial airway obstruction, mechanical ventilator malfunction, or partial disconnection of a ventilator circuit.[9,10,15]	• Petco$_2$ decreased by more than 10% of baseline
9. Observe for a sudden decrease in Petco$_2$ to near zero (Fig. 15-7). **(Level B)**	Drop in waveform to baseline or near baseline (baseline equals zero) implies that no respirations are present.[15] Such a drop in waveform may also occur within the case of significant ventilation/perfusion changes like pulmonary emboli.	• Dislodged endotracheal tube • Complete airway obstruction • Mechanical ventilator malfunction • Airway disconnection • Esophageal intubation
10. Observe for a sustained low Petco$_2$ without alveolar plateau (Fig. 15-8). **(Level C*)**	Sustained low Petco$_2$ values are indicative of incomplete alveolar emptying, such as in partially kinked endotracheal tube, bronchospasm, mucous plugging, improper exhaled gas sampling, or insufficient expiratory time on the ventilator.[15]	• Complete airway obstruction that necessitates reintubation • Petco$_2$ decreased greater than 10% of baseline

*Level B: Well-designed, controlled studies with results that consistently support a specific action, intervention or treatment
*Level C: Qualitative studies, descriptive or correlational studies, integrative reviews, systematic reviews, or randomized controlled trials with inconsistent results

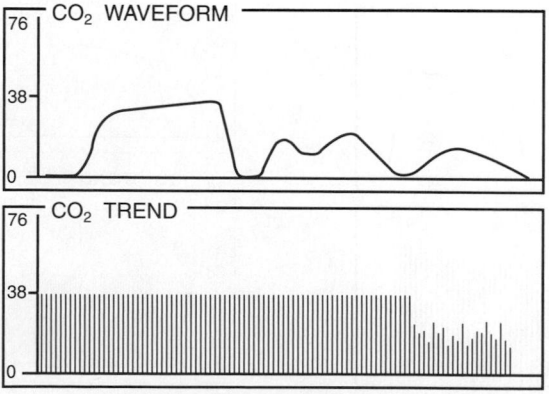

FIGURE 15-6   Sudden decrease in Petco$_2$ values. *(Reprinted by permission of Nellcor Puritan Bennett LLC, Boulder, CO, part of Covidien.)*

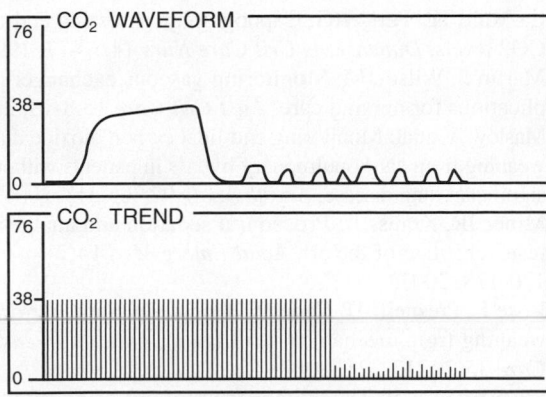

FIGURE 15-7   Sudden decrease in Petco$_2$, to near zero. *(Reprinted by permission of Nellcor Puritan Bennett LLC, Boulder, CO, part of Covidien.)*

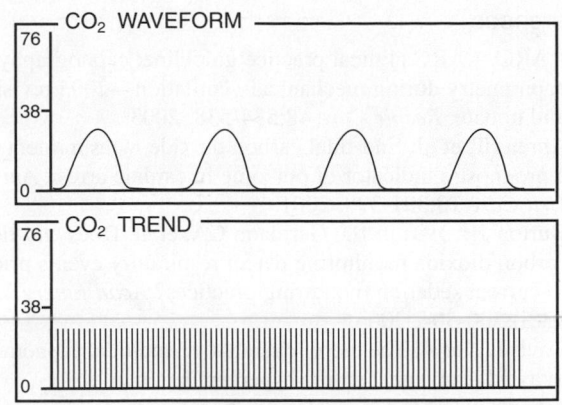

FIGURE 15-8   Low Petco$_2$, without alveolar plateau. *(Reprinted by permission of Nellcor Puritan Bennett LLC, Boulder, CO, part of Covidien.)*

Patient Monitoring and Care —*Continued*

Steps	Rationale	Reportable Conditions
11. Routinely monitor the airway adapter or sampling port for signs of obstruction.[1] **(Level M*)**	If the adapter or the port becomes obstructed, the quality of the capnographic waveform is poor and Petco$_2$ is not reliable.[1,15]	• Obstruction in the airway adapter or sampling port
12. Evaluate the patient's response to activities that may positively or negatively affect ventilation (e.g., suctioning, repositioning, change in mechanical support, nutritional supplementation, cardiopulmonary resuscitation,[3,4,10] neuromuscular blockade,[11] verification of endotracheal tube placement[4,10]). **(Level B*)**	The impact of activities (e.g., suctioning, repositioning, change in mechanical support, nutritional supplementation, cardiopulmonary resuscitation, neuromuscular blockade, verification of endotracheal tube placement) on ventilation can be evaluated with Petco$_2$ monitoring.[12]	• Petco$_2$ value decreased by more than 10% of baseline

Documentation

Documentation should include the following:
- Patient and family education
- Mechanical ventilator settings
- Petco$_2$ value and capnogram
- Paco$_2$ (partial pressure of arterial carbon dioxide) – Petco$_2$ gradient
- Arterial blood gases
- Times of calibration
- Respiratory therapies
- Medications that may affect respiratory system (e.g., neuromuscular blockers, sedatives, or bronchodilators)
- Respiratory assessment (e.g., respiratory rate, breathing patterns, adventitious sounds)
- Unexpected outcomes
- Nursing interventions

*Level B: Well-designed, controlled studies with results that consistently support a specific action, intervention or treatment
*Level M: Manufacturer's recommendations only

References

CR 1. AARC: AARC clinical practice guideline: capnography/
capnometry during mechanical ventilation—2003 revision
and update, *Respir Care* 48:534-538, 2003.

CR 2. Ahrens T, et al: End-tidal carbon dioxide measurements as
a prognostic indicator of outcome in cardiac arrest, *Am J
Crit Care* 10:391-398, 2001.

3. Burton JH, Harrah JD, Germann CA, et al: Does end-tidal
carbon dioxide monitoring detect respiratory events prior
to current sedation montoring practices? *Acad Emerg Med*
13(5):500-504, 2006.

CR 4. Davis DP, et al: The use of quantitative end-tidal capnometry
to avoid inadvertent severe hyperventilation in
patients with head injury after paramedic rapid sequence intubation, *J Trauma Inj Infect Crit Care* 56(4):808-814, 2004.

5. Delorio NM: Continuous end-tidal carbon dioxide monitoring for confirmation of endotracheal tube placement is
neither widely available nor consistently applied by
emergency physicians, *Emerg Med J* 22:490-493, 2005.

6. Eisenbacher S, Heard L: Capnography in the gastroenterology lab, *Gastroenterol Nurs* 28(2):99-106, 2005.

CR 7. Erasmus PD: The use of end-tidal carbon dioxide monitoring to confirm endotracheal tube placement in adult and
paedratic intensive care units in Australia and New
Zealand, *Anaesth Intensive Care* 32(5):672-675, 2004.

8. Hutchison R, Rodriguez L: Capnography and respiratory
depression, *Am J Nursing* 108(2):35-39, 2008.

CR 9. La-Valle TL, Perry AG: Capnography: assessing end-tidal
CO2 levels, *Dimensions Crit Care Nurs* 14:70-77, 1995.

CR 10. Martin S, Wilson M: Monitoring gaseous exchange: implications for nursing care, *Aust Crit Care* 15:8-13, 2002.

CR 11. Maslow A, et al: Monitoring end-tidal carbon dioxide during
weaning from cardiopulmonary bypass in patients without
significant lung disease, *Anesth Analg* 92:306-313, 2001.

12. Miner JR, Krauss B: Procedural sedation and analgesia
research: state of the art, *Acad Emerg Med* 14(2):
170-178, 2007.

13. Rose L, Presneill JJ, Cade JF: Update in computer-driven
weaning from mechanical ventilation, *Anaesth Intensive
Care* 35(2):213-221, 2007.

14. Silvestri S, et al: The effectiveness of out-of-hospital use
of continuous end-tidal carbon dioxide monitoring on the
rate of unrecognized misplaced intubation within a
regional emergency medical services system, *Ann Emerg
Med* 45(5):497-503, 2005.

CR 15. St John R: End-tidal carbon dioxide monitoring, *Crit
Care Nurse* 23:83-88, 2003.

Additional Readings

Gravenstein JS, Jaffe MB, Paulus DA: *Capnography: clinical
aspects,* United Kingdom, 2004, Cambridge University
Press.

Pierce LNB: *Mechanical ventilation and intensive respiratory
care,* Philadelphia, 1995, Saunders.

Continuous Venous Oxygen Saturation Monitoring

P U R P O S E : Venous oxygen saturation monitoring is performed to measure the oxygen saturation of the venous blood. The value can be obtained either from the superior vena cava or from the pulmonary artery. Continuous assessment of the balance between a patient's oxygen delivery and oxygen consumption can be monitored with a specialized fiberoptic central venous or pulmonary artery catheter and an associated computer or module.

Jan M. Headley, Karen K. Giuliano

PREREQUISITE NURSING KNOWLEDGE

- Anatomy and physiology of the cardiopulmonary system should be understood.
- Physiologic principles related to invasive hemodynamic monitoring should be understood.
- Technical aspects of central line placement and pressure monitoring should be understood.
- Technical aspects of pulmonary artery (PA) pressure monitoring should be understood.
- Physiologic concepts of oxygen delivery, oxygen demand, and tissue oxygen consumption should be understood.
- The percent of venous oxygen saturation as measured in the PA (SvO_2) is flow weighted and represents a true mixing of all venous blood: inferior vena cava (IVC), superior vena cava (SVC), and coronary sinus.
- Clinically, SvO_2 provides an index of overall oxygen balance because it is a reflection of the dynamic relationship between the patient's oxygen delivery (DO_2) and oxygen consumption (VO_2). Whenever a threat to the oxygen balance occurs, the body's primary compensatory mechanisms are to increase oxygen delivery by increasing cardiac output or to increase oxygen extraction at the tissue level.

- In a critically ill patient, if cardiac output is limited, increased extraction occurs to meet the demand for oxygen at the tissue level. The result is a decreased level of oxygen returning to the heart and a lower SvO_2 measurement. Many factors can affect the requirements for oxygen and subsequently SvO_2 (Table 16-1).[2,6,8,13]
- SvO_2 does not correlate directly with any of the determinants of oxygen delivery or oxygen consumption. Because a critically ill patient is in a dynamic state with rapidly changing oxygen demand and oxygen consumption, SvO_2 must be viewed in the light of these changing determinants and considered an index of oxygen balance.[1,2,6,8,13]
- A normal SvO_2 generally is considered to be 60% to 80%,[2,8] and a clinically significant change in SvO_2 (5% to 10%) can be an early indicator of physiologic instability.[2,8] SvO_2 values of less than 60% may result from either inadequate oxygen delivery or excess oxygen consumption. SvO_2 monitoring is used in critically ill patients for earlier detection of oxygenation instability than that obtained through traditional PA monitoring.[2,6,8,13]

TABLE 16-1	Common Conditions and Activities That Affect Venous Oxygen Saturation Values

Decreased Central and Mixed Venous Oxygen Saturation

Decreased Oxygen Delivery
Decreased cardiac output
Decreased hemoglobin
Decreased arterial oxygen saturation
Decreased arterial partial pressure of oxygen

Increased Oxygen Consumption
Fever
Pain
Shivering
Seizures
Increased work of breathing
Agitation
Infection and sepsis
Vasoactive and beta-agonist medications
Multiple organ failure
Burns
Head injury
Increased musculoskeletal activities
Numerous nursing procedures (e.g., dressing changes, suctioning, turning, and chest physiotherapy)

Increased Central and Mixed Venous Oxygen Saturation

Increased Oxygen Delivery
Increased cardiac output
Increased hemoglobin
Increased arterial oxygen saturation
Increased arterial partial pressure of oxygen

Decreased Oxygen Consumption
Hypothermia
Hypothyroidism
Pharmacologic paralysis and sedation
Anesthesia
Cellular dysfunction
Decreased work of breathing
Decreased musculoskeletal activities

- The percent of venous oxygen saturation as measured in the superior vena cava ($Scvo_2$) reflects the mixing of venous blood from the superior half of the body. It does not include blood from the IVC and coronary sinus. $Scvo_2$, right atrium (RA), and Svo_2 do not correlate absolutely. $Scvo_2$ does trend with Svo_2 in a variety of hemodynamic states. In normal conditions, $Scvo_2$ is slightly less than the RA oxygen saturation and lower than Svo_2. In septic or shock states, $Scvo_2$ is higher than Svo_2, with a difference that ranges from 5% to 7% and up to 18% in severe shock. This difference is in part because of a redistribution of blood flow caused by the various pathophysiologies. Therefore, $Scvo_2$ overestimates Svo_2 in shock conditions; a low $Scvo_2$ likely indicates an even lower Svo_2.[4,9-11]

- Small French size and shorter oximetry catheters have pediatric patient applications for assessment of venous saturation.[9]

- Some common proper setup and maintenance steps for the catheters and bedside computer or module are necessary for accurate monitoring of both $Scvo_2$ and Svo_2.

- Continuous venous saturation monitoring is performed with a three-component system (Fig. 16-1)[2,5-7]:
  - A fiberoptic central venous (CV) or PA catheter contains two fiberoptic filaments that exit at the distal lumen. One filament serves as a sending fiber for the emission of light; the other serves as a receiving fiber for the light reflected back from the blood in the vessel (Fig. 16-2).
  - The optic module houses the light-emitting diodes (LEDs), which transmit various wavelengths of light, and a photodetector, which receives light back. The light wavelengths are shone through a blood sample. Desaturated hemoglobins, saturated hemoglobins (oxyhemoglobin), and dyshemoglobins (carboxyhemoglobin, methemoglobin) have different light absorption characteristics. The ratio of hemoglobin to oxyhemoglobin is determined and reported as a percentage value.[2,5,7] All previous patient data, including calibration of saturation values and patient identification information, are stored in this component. This module should not be disconnected. If the module must be disconnected, refer to the manufacturer's instructions for a disconnection procedure that does not result in memory loss.
  - An oximeter computer, which can be a stand-alone unit or a module for a bedside monitoring system, has a microprocessor that converts the light information from the optic module into an electrical display, updated every few seconds for continuous monitoring. This information is displayed as a continuous graphic trend, a numeric display, or both, depending on the manufacturer.
  - Proper calibration of the monitor and catheter ensures accuracy of venous saturation values. The two types of

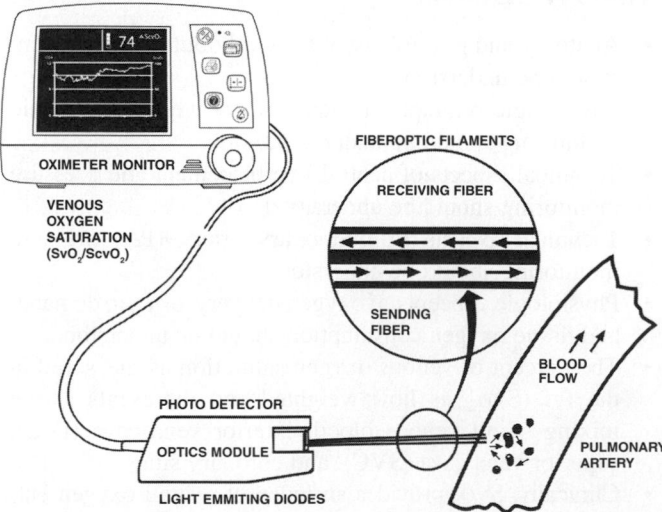

FIGURE 16-1   Oximetry system with reflectance spectrophotometry. (*From Edwards Lifesciences LLC: Understanding mixed venous oxygen saturation [Svo_2] monitoring using the Swan Ganz TD System, ed 2, Irvine, CA, 2002, Edwards Lifesciences.*)

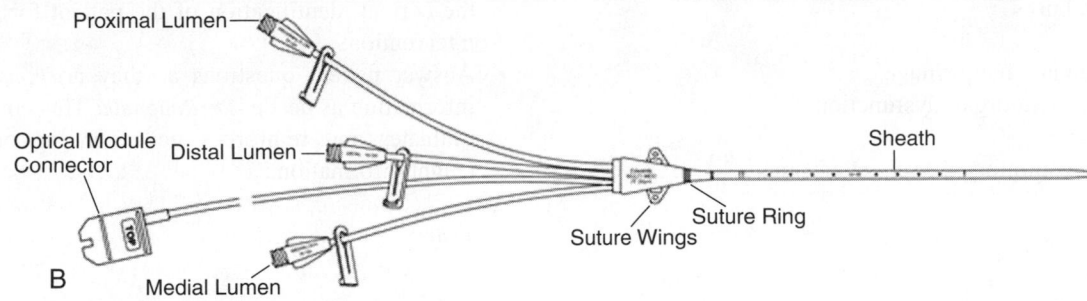

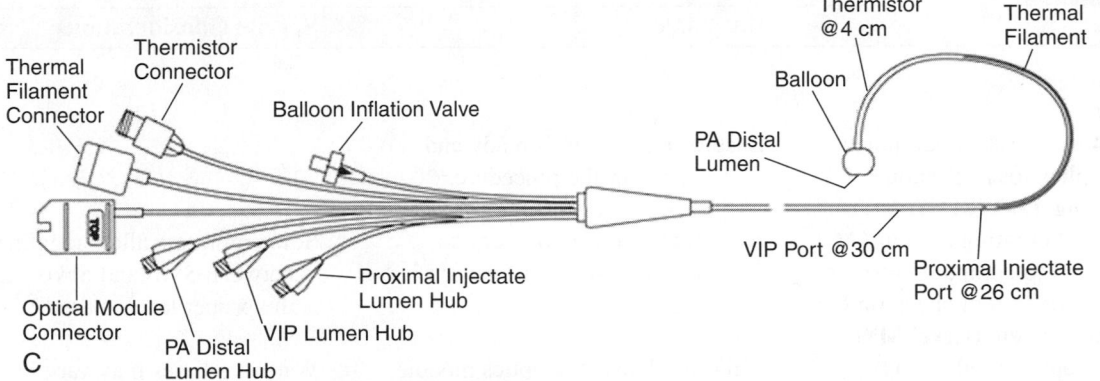

FIGURE 16-2 Oximetry catheters. **A,** Small French size for pediatric applications. **B,** Central venous catheter. **C,** Pulmonary artery catheter. *(From Edwards Lifesciences LLC, Irvine, CA, 2008.)*

calibration are in vitro, in which the catheter and optics module are calibrated before insertion; and in vivo, where the venous saturation value is compared with a laboratory co-oximeter value from a blood sample. Follow manufacturer recommendations for performing calibration procedures. Daily in vivo calibrations are recommended. In addition, proper blood sampling techniques from the distal port of the PA catheter are necessary for ensuring accurate values for calibration.[2,5,7,8]

EQUIPMENT

- Fiberoptic PA catheter for Svo_2 (various sizes, 4 Fr to 8 Fr; various lumens, 2 Fr to 7 Fr; various lengths, 25 to 110 cm)
- Fiberoptic CV catheter for $Scvo_2$ (various sizes for pediatric to adult use, 4.5 Fr to 8.5 Fr; various lengths, 5 to 20 cm; single, double, or triple lumen)
- Fiberoptic probe for $Scvo_2$
- Optic module
- Oximeter computer or bedside monitoring system module

- Equipment required for CV monitoring (see Procedure 70) or PA catheterization and pressure monitoring (see Procedure 73)

Additional equipment (to have available depending on patient need) includes the following:

- Printer

PATIENT AND FAMILY EDUCATION

- Assess patient and family understanding of the clinical benefits of venous oximetry monitoring. ➡*Rationale:* For information to be the most appropriate, assessment of the level of patient and family understanding of need for $Scvo_2$ or Svo_2 monitoring is important.
- Explain the continuous nature of this monitoring system and the significance of the alarms. ➡*Rationale:* Explanation of the procedure to the patient and family helps to alleviate fears and concerns. Additional monitors may produce increased anxiety in the patient and family.

PATIENT ASSESSMENT AND PREPARATION

Patient Assessment

- Indications for use of Scvo$_2$/Svo$_2$ monitoring include the following[1-3,5-13]:
  - ❖ High-risk cardiovascular surgery
  - ❖ Heart failure
  - ❖ Myocardial infarction
  - ❖ Respiratory failure
  - ❖ Severe burns
  - ❖ Sepsis
  - ❖ Anemia and hemorrhage
  - ❖ Multisystem organ dysfunction
  - ❖ Trauma
  - ❖ Acute respiratory distress syndrome
  - ❖ Use of positive end-expiratory pressure (PEEP)
  - ❖ As a component of early goal-directed therapy for severe sepsis and septic shock ➨*Rationale:* Scvo$_2$/Svo$_2$ monitoring is useful in the early detection of oxygenation imbalance, which can facilitate the use of early and more appropriate interventions.

Patient Preparation

- Verify correct patient with two identifiers. ➨*Rationale:* Prior to performing a procedure, the nurse should ensure the correct identification of the patient for the intended intervention.
- Answer patient questions as they arise, and reinforce information as needed. ➨*Rationale:* This communication evaluates and reinforces understanding of previously taught information.

Procedure   for Continuous Mixed Venous Oxygen Saturation Monitoring

Steps	Rationale	Special Considerations
1. **HH**		
2. **PE**		
3. Assemble necessary equipment and supplies for continuous monitoring. **(Level D*)**	Ensures equipment is ready and available for the procedure.[2,8]	
4. Connect alternating current (AC) power cord to computer, turn on, and observe system check on the computer screen. **(Level M*)**	Allows electronics to warm up; confirms component function.[5,7,8]	Some monitors allow toggling between Svo$_2$ and Scvo$_2$. Ensure the proper label is used.[5]
5. Connect optics module to computer. **(Level M)**	LEDs are housed in optics module. Approximately 5 to 20 minutes is needed to warm light source sufficiently.[5,7,8]	Warm-up times may vary by manufacturer and temperature of location of monitoring.
6. Remove outer wrap of catheter package and aseptically peel back the inner wrap portion that covers the optic connector of the catheter. **(Level M)**	Provides access to inner package. Isolates connector from catheter tip to maintain sterility during in vitro calibration.[5,7,8]	Catheter packaging may vary according to manufacturer. Follow manufacturer directions for use to ensure proper handling.
7. Firmly connect the optic connector to the optic module. **(Level M)**	Ensures connections are tight and properly aligned for light transmission.[5,7]	
8. Perform in vitro calibration or standardization. **(Level M)**	Standardizes or calibrates the light source to the catheter. Calibration is performed before catheter insertion. Catheter tip should be left in the calibration cup or container in the package during in vitro calibration.[5,7]	Catheter lumens must be dry. Do not flush catheter before performing this step or in vitro calibration is invalid.
9. Pull back remaining wrap covering catheter package with aseptic technique. **(Level M)**	Prepares catheter for insertion.[5,7]	

*Level D: Peer-reviewed professional organizational standards with clinical studies to support recommendations

*Level M: Manufacturer's recommendations only

Procedure for Continuous Mixed Venous Oxygen Saturation Monitoring—*Continued*

Steps	Rationale	Special Considerations
10. Carefully remove catheter from tray with sterile technique. Pull catheter tip up and out of the calibration cup. **(Level M*)**	Prevents the transmission of microorganisms; prevents damage to the balloon of the PA catheter.[5,7]	Fiberoptics in catheter and PA catheter balloon are fragile and may be damaged if not handled properly.
11. Attach pressure tubing, and prime lumens with flush solution (see Procedure 73).	Enables monitoring of chamber pressures during PA catheter insertion; maintains patency of lumens. Refer to institutional standards for use of heparinized flush solution.[8]	
12. Perform a pre-procedure verification and time out if non-emergent.	Ensures patient safety.	
13. Assist physician or advanced practice nurse with CV or PA catheter insertion (see Procedure 82 or 72.		
14. Observe PA waveforms during insertion (see Procedure 73).	Central PA catheter tip placement is necessary for optimal light reflection.[5,7,8]	A light intensity or signal indicator verifies adequate reflection of the light signals after the catheter tip is placed correctly.
15. Note amount of air required to inflate balloon. **(Level M)**	Inflation volume of 1.25 to 1.5 mL is recommended for proper catheter tip placement.[5,7]	Less than optimal inflation volume to obtain a wedge tracing may indicate distal catheter migration. A change in the intensity or signal indicator also may alert the clinician to this condition.
16. Set high and low alarm limits and activate alarms. **(Level D*)**	Individualizes alarm settings according to patient baseline. Audible alarms notify the clinician of significant changes in $ScvO_2/SvO_2$ values and trends.[2,8]	
17. Input patient height and weight data as per institutional standard. **(Level D)**	Allows for calculation of derived parameters.[2,5,7,8]	
18. Apply a sterile dressing to insertion site. **(Level D)**	Reduces transmission of microorganisms.[2,8]	Use institutional standard for central venous catheter dressings.
19. Firmly secure the optic module near the patient. **(Level M)**	Excessive tension on catheter or optic module may break the optic fibers.[5,7]	
20. After calibration and insertion of catheter, obtain baseline set of hemodynamic and oxygenation indices (see Procedure 72).	Provides baseline information for comparison with patient's response to interventions.[5,7]	
21. Continuously monitor PA pressure tracings and SvO_2 values. **(Level D)**	Spontaneous catheter migration may occur after insertion. As a reflection of postcapillary arterialized blood and the vessel wall, the SvO_2 value may increase.[6,8]	

*Level D: Peer-reviewed professional organizational standards with clinical studies to support recommendations
*Level M: Manufacturer's recommendations only

Procedure continues on following page

Procedure for Continuous Mixed Venous Oxygen Saturation Monitoring—*Continued*

Steps	Rationale	Special Considerations
Venous Blood Sampling Skill/In Vivo Calibration		
22. Draw mixed venous blood sample (see Procedure 65) for mixed venous blood sampling).	In vivo calibration is necessary to verify the accuracy of the computer and value displayed after insertion of the fiberoptic PA catheter. Follow specific recommendations from the manufacturer about the frequency of calibration and specific steps to implement the process. Ideally, the patient's hemodynamic and oxygenation status should be stable for optimal calibration.[2,5,8]	Mixed venous samples should be drawn only from the PA.[8,13] SVC samples should be drawn from the distal port of the CV catheter.
23. Perform a verification or in vivo calibration per institutional standard. **(Level D*)**	Typically, this is done every 24 hours or whenever the displayed value is in question. In vivo calibration verifies the accuracy of the $Scvo_2/Svo_2$ being displayed.[2,5,8]	
24. Ensure measurement is performed with a laboratory co-oximeter. **(Level D)**	Co-oximetry measures direct fractional oxyhemoglobin saturation; blood gas analyzers calculate oxygen saturation from measured partial pressure values. A calculated saturation value from a gas analyzer may not correlate with the actual patient value and, if used for calibration, may produce erroneous results.[2,8]	
25. Observe bedside monitor display for PA waveform and resume Svo_2 monitoring **(Level D)**	Reconfirms catheter tip placement in the PA.[8]	
26. Dispose of used supplies and equipment.		
27. Remove personal protective equipment.	Reduces the transmission of microorganisms and body secretions; standard precautions.	
28. **HH**		

Expected Outcomes

- Svo_2 values and trends within normal range (60% to 80%)[2,6,8]
- $Scvo_2$ values and trends greater than 70%[9-11]
- $Scvo_2/Svo_2$ trends not fluctuating greater than 5% to 10% of baseline value[2,4,10]
- Hemodynamic and oxygenation parameters optimal for patient condition

Unexpected Outcomes

- Svo_2 values less than 60% or greater than 80%
- Svo_2 value trends greater than 10% from baseline
- $Scvo_2$ value trends less than 65% to 70%[3,10,11]
- Infection from presence of an indwelling PA catheter
- PA infarction or rupture

---

*Level D: Peer-reviewed professional organizational standards with clinical studies to support recommendations

Patient Monitoring and Care

Steps	Rationale	Reportable Conditions
		These conditions should be reported if they persist despite nursing interventions.
1. Ensure that no kinks or bends are found in the catheter. **(Level D*)**	Fiberoptics are fragile and can break if not handled carefully. Overtightening of the introducer connector can cause crimping and breakage of the fiberoptics.[6,7] Subclavian or internal jugular approaches for insertion may cause kinking in the vessel if the vessel is tortuous. Sending and receiving wavelengths may show either a change in light signal or values that do not reflect the patient's status.	• Change in PA waveform or Svo_2 value that does not correlate to patient condition • Changes in RA waveforms or $Scvo_2$ value that do not correlate to patient condition
2. Monitor PA waveforms continuously. **(Level D)**	Migration of the catheter tip may reflect postcapillary arterialized blood causing an elevation in the Svo_2 value. Uncorrected catheter migration places the patient at risk for PA infarction or rupture.[8]	• Permanent wedge waveform
3. Observe Svo_2 value and trends. **(Level B*)**	Normal Svo_2 values range from 60% to 80%[3,4,8]; values outside this range may indicate an imbalance between oxygen delivery and consumption. A value change of greater than 5% to 10% may signify a clinically significant change.[4,8,10] A target value of greater than 65% in severe sepsis and septic shock is recommended.[3,4,8] If the patient's clinical presentation differs from the observed Svo_2 value or trends, recheck the accuracy of the monitoring system.	• Svo_2 values greater than 80% or less than 60%
4. Observe $Scvo_2$ value and trends. **(Level B)**	$Scvo_2$ values trend with Svo_2. A target value of greater than 70% in severe sepsis and septic shock is recommended.[4,8]	• $Scvo_2$ values less than 70%
5. Follow institution standard for assessing pain. Administer analgesia as prescribed.	Identifies need for pain interventions.	• Continued pain despite pain interventions

*Level B: Well-designed controlled studies with results that consistently support a specific action, intervention, or treatment
*Level D: Peer-reviewed professional organizational standards with clinical studies to support recommendations

Procedure continues on following page

Documentation

Documentation should include the following:
- Patient and family education
- $Scvo_2/Svo_2$ whenever the hemodynamic profile is recorded
- Additional oxygenation indices as indicated
- Specific nursing activities (e.g., suctioning, turning the patient, or titrating a vasoactive drug) and the relationship of the event with the continuous trend, especially if the event produces a marked change in the value

- Hard copy printout (as available)
- Unexpected outcomes
- Nursing interventions
- Pain assessment, interventions and effectiveness

References

CR 1. Bishop MH, et al: Prospective, randomized trial of survivor values of cardiac index, oxygen delivery, and oxygen consumption as resuscitation endpoints in severe trauma, *J Trauma* 38:780-787, 1995.

CR 2. Darovic GO: *Handbook hemodynamic monitoring,* ed 2, St Louis, 2004, Saunders.

3. Dellinger RP, Levy MM, Carlet JM, et al: Surviving sepsis campaign: international guidelines for the management of severe sepsis and septic shock: 2008. *Crit Care Med* 36:296-327, 2008.

CR 4. Edwards JD, Mayall RM: Importance of the sampling site for measurement of mixed venous oxygen saturation in shock, *Crit Care Med* 26:1356-1360, 1998.

CR 5. Edwards Lifesciences LLC: Vigilance: continuous cardiac output and Svo_2 monitoring system. In *Operations manual,* Irvine, CA, 2003, Edwards Lifesciences.

CR 6. Headley JM: Strategies to optimize the cardiorespiratory status of the critically ill, *AACN Clin Issues Crit Care Nurs* 6:121-134, 1995.

CR 7. Hospira Inc: *Q2Plus SO₂/CO computer (system operating manual,* North Chicago, 2004. Hospira.

CR 8. Jesurum JT: Svo_2 monitoring. In *AACN protocols for practice: hemodynamic monitoring,* Aliso Viejo, CA, 1998, American Association of Critical-Care Nurses.

9. Liakopoulos OJ, Ho JK, Yezbick A, et al: An experimental and clinical evaluation of a novel central venous catheter with integrated oximetry for pediatric patients undergoing cardiac surgery, *Anesth Analg* I105(6):1598-1604, 2007.

CR 10. Reinhart K, Kuhn H-J, Hartog C, et al: Continuous central venous and pulmonary artery oxygen saturation monitoring in the critically ill, *Intensive Care Med* 30:1572-1578, 2004.

11. Rivers EP, Cobra V, Whitmill M: Early goal-directed therapy in severe sepsis and septic shock: a contempory review of the literature, *Curr Opin Anesthesiol* 21:128-140, 2008.

CR 12. Vedrinne C, et al: Predictive factors for usefulness of fiberoptic pulmonary artery catheter for continuous oxygen saturation in mixed venous blood monitoring in cardiac surgery, *Anesth Analg* 85:2-10, 1997.

CR 13. White KM: Using continuous Svo_2 to assess oxygen supply/demand balance in the critically ill patient, *AACN Clin Issues Crit Care Nurs* 4:134-147, 1993.

Additional Readings

AACN: *Severe sepsis,* from www.aacn.org/WD/Practice/Docs/Severe_Sepsis_04-2006.pdf, accessed 10/01/09.

AACN: *Pulmonary artery pressure measurement,* www.aacn.org/WD/Practice/Docs/PAP_Measurement_05-2004.pdf, accessed 10/01/09.

Antonelli M, Levy M, Andrews PJD, et al: Hemodynamic monitoring in shock and implication for management, International Consensus Conference, Paris, France 27–28 April 2006, *Intensive Care Med* 33(4):1-16, 2007.

Carcillo JA, Fields AI, American College of Critical Care Medicine Task Force Committee Members: Clinical practice parameters for hemodynamic support of paediatric and neonatal patients in septic shock, *Crit Care Med* 30:1365-1378, 2002.

De Oliveira CF, de Oliveira DSF, Moura JDG, et al: ACCM/PALS haemodynamic support guidelines for paediatric septic shock: an outcomes comparison with and without monitoring central venous oxygen saturation, *Intensive Care Med* 34(6):1065-1075, 2008.

Edwards Lifesciences LLC: *Understanding continuous mixed venous oxygen saturation (Svo₂) monitoring with the Swan-Ganz oximetry TD system,* ed 2, Irvine, CA, 2002, Edwards Lifesciences.

Goodrich C: Continuous central venous oximetry monitoring, *Crit Care* Nurs Clin North Am 18:203-209, 2006.

Keckeisen M: *Pulmonary artery pressure monitoring. In AACN protocols for practice: hemodynamic monitoring,* Aliso Viejo, CA, 1998, American Association of Critical-Care Nurses.

Rivers EP, Ander DS, Powell D: Central venous oxygen saturation monitoring in the critically ill, *Curr Opin Care* 7(3):204-211, 2001.

17

Oxygen Saturation Monitoring with Pulse Oximetry

P U R P O S E : Pulse oximetry is a noninvasive monitoring technique used to estimate the measurement of arterial oxygen saturation of hemoglobin.

Sandra L. Schutz

PREREQUISITE NURSING KNOWLEDGE

- Oxygen saturation is an indicator of the percentage of hemoglobin saturated with oxygen at the time of the measurement. The reading, obtained with standard pulse oximetry, uses a light sensor that contains two sources of light (red and infrared) absorbed by hemoglobin and transmitted through tissues to a photodetector. The infrared light is absorbed by the oxyhemoglobin, and the red light is absorbed by the reduced hemoglobin. The amount and type of light transmitted through the tissue is converted to a digital value that represents the percentage of hemoglobin saturated with oxygen (Fig. 17-1).
- Oxygen saturation values obtained with pulse oximetry (SpO_2) represent one part of a complete assessment of a patient's oxygenation status and are not a substitute for measurement of arterial saturation of oxygen (SaO_2) or of ventilation (as measured with arterial partial pressure of carbon dioxide [$PaCO_2$]).
- The accuracy of SpO_2, measurements requires consideration of many physiologic variables. Patient variables include the following:
  - Hemoglobin level
  - Presence of dyshemoglobinemias (i.e., carboxyhemoglobinemia after carbon monoxide exposure)

- Arterial blood flow to the vascular bed
- Temperature of the digit or the area where the oximetry sensor is located
- Patient's oxygenation ability
- Fraction of inspired oxygen (percentage of inspired oxygen)
- Evidence of ventilation-perfusion mismatch
- Amount of ambient light seen with the sensor
- Venous return at the sensor location
- A complete assessment of oxygenation includes evaluation of oxygen content and delivery, which includes the following parameters: arterial partial pressure of oxygen (PaO_2), SaO_2 hemoglobin, cardiac output, and, when available, mixed venous oxygen saturation.
- Normal oxygen saturation values are approximately 97% to 99% in a healthy individual breathing room air. An oxygen saturation value of 95% is clinically accepted in a patient with a normal hemoglobin level. With a normal blood pH and body temperature, an oxygen saturation value of 90% is generally equated with a PaO_2 of 60 mm Hg.
- Tissue oxygenation is not reflected by arterial or oxygen saturation obtained with pulse oximetry.
- The affinity of hemoglobin with oxygen may impair or enhance oxygen release at the tissue level.
  - Oxygen is more readily released to the tissues when pH is decreased (acidosis), body temperature is increased,

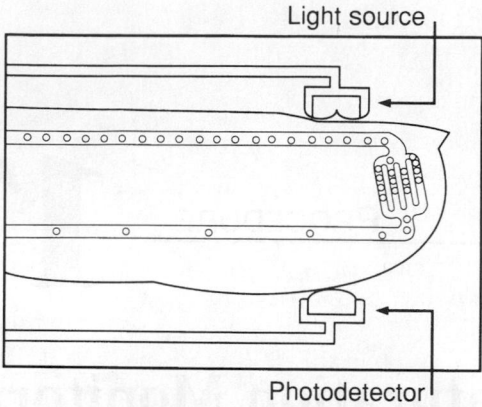

Light source

Photodetector

FIGURE 17-1   A sensor device that contains a light source and a photodetector is placed around a pulsating arteriolar bed, such as the finger, great toe, nose, or earlobe. Red and infrared wavelengths of light are used to determine arterial saturation. *(Reprinted by permission of Nellcor Puritan Bennett LLC, Boulder, CO, part of Covidien.)*

$Paco_2$, is increased, and 2,3-diphosphoglycerate levels (a by-product of glucose metabolism that facilitates the dissociation of oxygen from the hemoglobin molecule to tissue) are increased (decreased oxygen affinity).

❖ When hemoglobin has greater affinity for oxygen, less is available to the tissues (increased oxygen affinity). Conditions such as increased pH (alkalosis), decreased temperature, decreased $Paco_2$, and decreased 2,3-diphosphoglycerate (as found in stored blood products) increase oxygen binding to the hemoglobin and limit its release to the tissue.

• Oxygen saturation values may vary with the amount of oxygen usage or uptake by the tissues. In some patients, a difference is seen in Spo_2 values at rest compared with values during activity, such as ambulation or positioning.

• Oxygen saturation does not directly reflect the patient's ability to ventilate. The true measure of ventilation is determination of the $Paco_2$ in arterial blood. Use of Spo_2 in a patient with obstructive pulmonary disease may result in erroneous clinical assessments of condition. As the degree of lung disease increases, the patient's drive to breathe may shift from an increased carbon dioxide stimulus to a hypoxic stimulus. Enhancing the patient's oxygenation and increasing the Spo_2 may limit the ability to ventilate. The normal baseline Spo_2 for a patient with known severe restrictive disease and more definitive methods of determination of the effectiveness of ventilation must be assessed before consideration of interventions that enhance oxygenation.

• Any discoloration of the nail bed or obstruction of the nail bed can potentially affect the transmission of light through the digit. The impact of dark nail polish, such as blue, green, brown, or black colors,[4,5,11,17] has been reported to limit the transmission of light and thus impact the Spo_2, although a recent study showed that fingernail polish does not cause a clinically significant change in the pulse

oximeter readings in healthy individuals.[15] If the nail polish cannot be removed and is believed to be affecting the accuracy of the reading, the sensor can be placed in a lateral side-to-side position on the finger to obtain readings if no other method of sampling the arterial bed is available.[5,15] Bruising under the nail can limit the transmission of light and result in an artificially decreased Spo_2 value. Pulse oximetry has not been shown to be affected by the presence of an elevated bilirubin.[2] The presence of acrylic fingernails may impair the accuracy of the pulse oximetry reading, and removal of the nail covering may be necessary to ensure accurate measurement,[9] although unpolished acrylic nails have been proven not to affect pulse oximetry readings.[14]

• Standard pulse oximeters use two wavelengths and are unable to differentiate between oxygen and carbon monoxide bound to hemoglobin and falsely elevated Spo_2 measurements. Standard pulse oximetry equipment should never be used in suspected cases of carbon monoxide exposure. However, recent technology advancements in pulse oximetry have included the introduction of a monitor system that uses up to 12 wavelengths with a digit-based pulse oximeter sensor and that allows for measurement estimates of certain, dyshemoglobinemias (i.e., carboxyhemoglobinemia).[12] An arterial blood gas always should be obtained to determine the accurate oxygen saturation and, if a CO oximeter is available, measurement of carboxyhemoglobin and methemoglobin.[3]

• Dark skin has been suggested to possibly affect the ability of the pulse oximeter to detect arterial pulsations. One study found more frequent differences between the Spo_2 and Sao_2 in black patients when compared with lighter skinned patients[10]; another study did not find a significant difference.[13]

• Certain dyes used intravenously may interfere with the accuracy of measurements, although as a result of rapid clearance, the impact is limited. Dyes include methylene blue, indigo carmine, indocyanine green, and fluorescein.[8]

• A pulse oximeter should not be used as a predictive indicator of the actual arterial blood gas saturation.

• A pulse oximeter should never be used during a cardiac arrest situation because of the extreme limitations of blood flow during cardiopulmonary resuscitation and the pharmacologic action of vasoactive agents administered during the resuscitation effort.

• Low perfusion states such as hypotension, vasoconstriction, hypothermia, or administration of vasoconstrictive agents limit the ability of the oximeter to distinguish the true pulsatile wave form from background noise.

• In vasoconstrictive states, oxygen saturation may be measured with a finger probe, but in patients with significant shifts in hemodynamic stability, the ear or forehead has been shown to be reasonably resistant to the vasoconstrictive effects of the sympathetic nervous system.[1,16]

• Forehead sensors used in patients placed in Trendelenburg's position may require up to 20 mm Hg external pressure to achieve accurate readings, which may be accomplished with an appropriately applied headband.[1]

EQUIPMENT

- Oxygen saturation monitor
- Oxygen saturation cable and sensor, which may be disposable or nondisposable
- Manufacturer's recommended germicidal agent for cleaning the nondisposable sensor (used for cleaning between patients)

PATIENT AND FAMILY EDUCATION

- Explain the need for determination of oxygen saturation with a pulse oximeter. ➤➤*Rationale:* This explanation informs the patient of the purpose of monitoring, enhances patient cooperation, and decreases patient anxiety.
- Explain that the values displayed may vary with patient movement, amount of environmental light, patient level of consciousness (awake or asleep), and position of the sensor. ➤➤*Rationale:* This explanation decreases patient and family anxiety over the constant variability of the values.
- Explain that the use of pulse oximetry is part of a much larger assessment of respiratory status. ➤➤*Rationale:* This explanation prepares the patient and family for other possible diagnostic tests of oxygenation (e.g., arterial blood gas).
- Explain the equipment to the patient. ➤➤*Rationale:* This information facilitates patient cooperation in maintaining sensor placement.
- Explain the need for an audible alarm system for alerting clinicians of oxygen saturation values below a set acceptable limit, as determined by the clinician. Demonstrate the alarm system, alerting the patient and family to the possibility of alarms, including causes of false alarms. ➤➤*Rationale:* Provision of an understanding of the use of an alarm system and its importance in the overall management of the patient's condition and of circumstances in which a false alarm may occur assists in understanding of the SpO_2 values seen at the bedside.
- Explain the need to move or remove the sensor on a routine basis to prevent complications related to the type of sensor used and monitoring site (i.e., digit, forehead, ear). ➤➤*Rationale:* An understanding of the need to move the sensor routinely assists in patient understanding of the frequency of sensor movement.

PATIENT ASSESSMENT AND PREPARATION

Patient Assessment

- Signs and symptoms of decreased oxygenation include the following:
  - ❖ Cyanosis
  - ❖ Dyspnea
  - ❖ Tachypnea
  - ❖ Decreased level of consciousness
  - ❖ Increased work of breathing
  - ❖ Loss of protective airway (patients undergoing conscious sedation)
  - ❖ Agitation
  - ❖ Confusion
  - ❖ Disorientation
  - ❖ Tachycardia/bradycardia
- ➤➤*Rationale:* Patient assessment determines the need for continuous pulse oximetry monitoring. Anticipation of conditions in which hypoxia could be present allows earlier intervention before unfavorable outcomes occur.
- Assess the extremity (digit) or area where the sensor will be placed including the following:
  - ❖ Decreased peripheral pulses
  - ❖ Peripheral cyanosis
  - ❖ Decreased body temperature
  - ❖ Decreased blood pressure
  - ❖ Exposure to excessive environmental light sources (e.g., examination lights)
  - ❖ Excessive movement or tremor in the digit
  - ❖ Presence of dark nail polish or bruising under the nail
  - ❖ Presence of artificial nails
  - ❖ Clubbing of the digit tips
- ➤➤*Rationale:* Assessment of factors that may inhibit accuracy of the measurement of oxygenation before attempting to obtain the SpO_2 reading enhances the validity of the measurement and allows for correction of factors as possible.

Patient Preparation

- Verify the correct patient with two identifiers. ➤➤*Rationale:* Prior to performing a procedure, the nurse should ensure the correct identification of the patient for the intended intervention.
- Ensure that the patient understands preprocedural teachings. Answer questions as they arise, and reinforce information as needed. ➤➤*Rationale:* This communication evaluates and reinforces understanding of previously taught information.

Procedure for Oxygen Saturation Monitoring with Pulse Oximetry

Steps	Rationale	Special Considerations
1. **HH**		
2. **PE**		
3. Select the appropriate pulse oximeter sensor for the area with the best pulsatile vascular bed to be sampled (Fig. 17-2). The digits are the most common site because of ease of application of the sensor. Consideration of other sites may produce more accurate results in conditions of extreme peripheral vasoconstriction or decreased perfusion[1,16] **(Level C*)**	The correct sensor optimizes signal capture and minimizes artifact-related difficulties.[5,6,13,14]	Several different types of sensors are available, including disposable and nondisposable sensors, that may be applied over a variety of vascular beds, including the digit, earlobe, the nasal bridge or septum, and the forehead. The latter requires an appropriately placed headband. Do not use one manufacturer's sensors with another manufacturer's pulse oximeter unless compatibility has been verified.
4. Select desired sensor site. If digits are chosen, assess for warmth and capillary refill. Confirm the presence of an arterial blood flow to the area monitored.	Adequate arterial pulse strength is necessary for obtaining accurate SpO_2 measurements.	Avoid sites distal to indwelling arterial catheters, blood pressure cuffs, pneumatic antishock garments (PASG), or venous engorgement (e.g., arteriovenous fistulas, blood transfusions).
5. Plug oximeter power cord into grounded wall outlet if the unit is not portable. If the unit is portable, ensure sufficient battery charge by turning it on before use. Plug patient cable into monitor.	With use of electrical outlets, grounded outlets decrease the occurrence of electrical interference.	Portable systems have rechargeable batteries and depend on sufficient time plugged into an electrical outlet to maintain the proper level of battery charge. When system is used in the portable mode, always check battery capacity.
6. Apply the sensor in a manner that allows the light source (light-emitting diodes [LEDs]) to be: A. Directly opposite the light detector (photodetector). **(Level C)**	To determine a pulse oximetry value properly, the light sensors must be in opposing positions directly over the area of the sample.[6,7,18]	
B. Shielded from excessive environmental light. **(Level B*)**	Light from sources such as examination lights or overhead lights can cause falsely elevate oximetry values.[10,14,18]	If the oximeter sensor fails to detect a pulse when perfusion seems adequate, excessive environmental light (overhead examination lights, phototherapy lights, infrared warmers) may be blinding the light sensor. Troubleshoot by reapplying the sensor or shielding the sensor with a towel or blanket or moving the sensor to a different monitoring site.
C. Positioned so that all sensor-emitted light comes into contact with perfused tissue beds and is not seen by the other side of the sensor or without coming into contact with the area to be read.	If the light from the sensor's LEDs bypasses the tissue bed and is detected at the photodetector, the result is either a falsely high reading or no reading.	Known as *optical shunting,* the light bypasses the vascular bed; shielding the sensor does not eliminate this if the sensor is too large or not properly positioned.

*Level B: Well-designed, controlled studies with results that consistently support a specific action, intervention, or treatment
*Level C: Qualitative studies, descriptive or correlational studies, integrative reviews, systematic reviews, or randomized controlled trials with inconsistent results

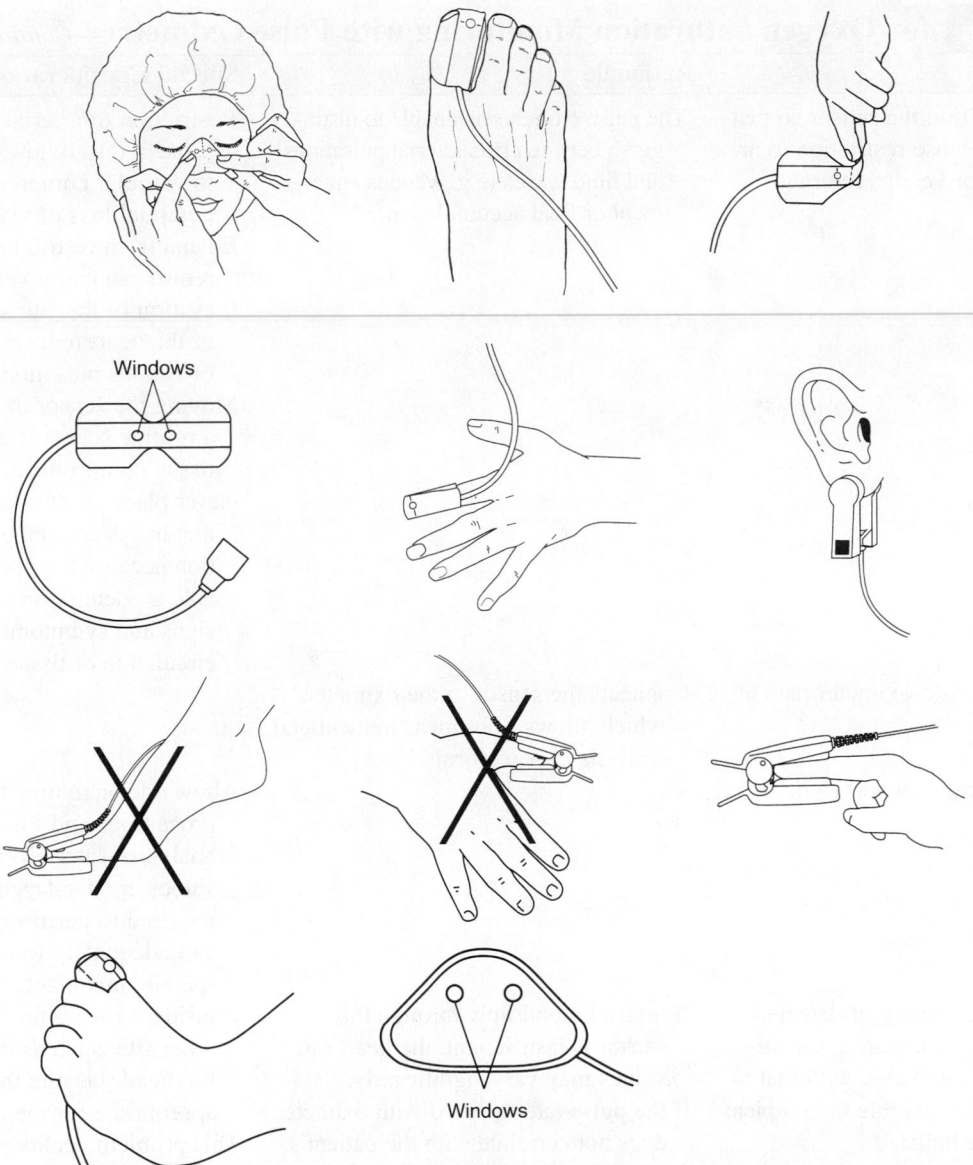

FIGURE 17-2   Sensor types and sensor sites for pulse oximetry monitoring. Use "wrap" or "clip" style sensors on the fingers (including thumb), great toe, and nose. The windows for the light source and photodetector must be placed directly opposite each other on each side of the arteriolar bed to ensure accuracy of SpO_2 measurements. Choice of the correct size of the sensor helps decrease the incidence of excess ambient light interference and optical shunting. "Clip" style sensors are appropriate for fingers (except the thumb) and the earlobe. Ensuring that the arteriolar bed is well within the clip with the windows directly opposite each other decreases the possibility of excess ambient light interference and optical shunting. *(Reprinted by permission of Nellcor Puritan Bennett LLC, Boulder, CO, part of Covidien.)*

Procedure | for Oxygen Saturation Monitoring with Pulse Oximetry—*Continued*

Steps	Rationale	Special Considerations
7. Gently position the sensor so that it does not cause restriction to arterial flow or venous return. **(Level C*)**	The pulse oximeter is unable to distinguish between true arterial pulsations and fluid waves (e.g., venous engorgement or fluid accumulation).[5,6,13.]	Restriction of arterial blood flow can cause a falsely low value and lead to vascular compromise, causing potential loss of viable tissues. Edema from restriction of venous return can cause venous pulsation. Elevation of the site above the level of the heart reduces the possibility of venous pulsation. Moving the sensor to another site on a routine schedule also reduces tissue compromise. Never place the sensor on an extremity that has decreased or absent sensation because the patient may not be able to identify discomfort or the signs and symptoms of loss of circulation or tissue compromise.
8. Plug sensor into oximeter patient cable.	Connects the sensor to the oximeter, which allows Spo$_2$ measurement and analysis of waveforms.	
9. Turn instrument power switch on.		Allow adequate time for self-testing procedures and for detection and analysis of waveforms before values are displayed. The time required to perform the self-test and adequately warm depends on specific manufacturer.
10. Determine accuracy of detected waveform by comparing the numeric heart rate value with that of a monitored heart rate or an apical heart rate or both.	If arterial blood flow through the sensor is insufficient, the heart rate values may vary significantly. If the pulse rate detected with oximeter does not correlate with the patient's heart rate, the oximeter is not detecting sufficient arterial blood flow for accurate values.	Consider moving the sensor to another site, such as the earlobe or the forehead (be sure the sensor type is appropriate for the monitoring site). This problem occurs particularly with the use of the fingers and the toes in conditions of low blood flow.
11. Set appropriate alarm limits.	Alarm limits should be set appropriate to the patient's condition.	Oxygen saturation limits should be 5% less than patient acceptable baseline. Heart rate alarms should be consistent with the cardiac monitoring limits (if monitored).
12. Remove personal protective equipment.		
13. 🅷🅷		
14. Cleanse nondisposable sensor, if used, between patients with manufacturer's recommended germicidal agent.	Reduces transmission of microorganisms to other patients.	

*Level C: Qualitative studies, descriptive or correlational studies, integrative reviews, systematic reviews, or randomized controlled trials with inconsistent results

Expected Outcomes

- All changes in oxygen saturation are detected
- The number of oxygen desaturation events is reduced
- The need for invasive techniques for monitoring oxygenation is reduced
- False-positive pulse oximeter alarms are reduced

Unexpected Outcomes

- Accurate pulse oximetry is not obtainable because of movement artifact
- Low perfusion states or excessive edema prevents accurate pulse oximetry measurements
- Disagreements occur in SaO_2 and oximeter SpO_2

Patient Monitoring and Care

Steps	Rationale	Reportable Conditions
		These conditions should be reported if they persist despite nursing interventions.
1. Evaluate laboratory data along with the patient for evidence of reduced arterial oxygen saturation or hypoxemia.	SpO_2 values are one segment of a complete evaluation of the patient's oxygenation status and supplemental oxygen therapy. Data should be integrated into a complete assessment to determine the overall status of the patient. If SpO_2 is used as an indicator of SaO_2, an arterial blood gas with CO oximetry should be done to determine whether the values correlate consistently.	• Inability to maintain oxygen saturation levels as desired
2. Evaluate sensor site every 2 to 4 hours (if a disposable sensor is used) or every 2 hours (if a reusable or nondisposable sensor is used). Rotate the site of a reusable sensor every 4 hours; replace an adhesive disposable sensor every 24 hours[13] or more frequently if the securing mechanism is compromised or soiled. Never apply additional adhesive tape to secure a sensor.	Assessment of the skin and tissues under the sensor identifies skin breakdown or loss of vascular flow, allowing appropriate interventions to be initiated. Application of additional tape may constrict blood flow at the monitoring site and result in both inaccurate monitor readings and further compromised local skin perfusion.	• Change in skin color • Loss of warmth of tissue unrelated to vasoconstriction • Loss of blood flow to the digit • Evidence of skin breakdown from the sensor • Change in color of the nail bed, which indicates compromised circulation to the nail
3. Monitor the sensor site for excessive movement, which results in motion artifact.	Excessive movement at the monitoring site may result in unreliable saturation values. Moving the sensor to a less physically active site may reduce the risk of motion artifact; use of an adhesive versus reusable sensor may also help as a result of better fit. If the digits are used, ask the patient to rest the hand on a flat or secure surface.	
4. Compare and monitor the actual heart rate with the pulse rate value from the pulse oximeter to determine accuracy of values.	The two numeric heart rate values should correlate closely. A difference in pulse rate values reported with pulse oximeter may be from excessive movement, poor peripheral perfusion at the monitoring site, or loss of pulsatile flow detection.	• Inability to correlate actual heart rate and pulse rate from oximeter

Procedure continues on following page

Documentation

Documentation should include the following:
- Patient and family education
- Indications for use of pulse oximetry
- Patient's pulse rate with Spo_2 measurements
- Fraction of inspired oxygen delivered (if patient is receiving oxygen)
- Patient clinical assessment at the time of the saturation measurement
- Sensor site
- Simultaneous arterial blood gases (if available)
- Recent hemoglobin measurement (if available)
- Skin assessment at sensor site
- Pulse oximeter monitor alarm settings
- Events precipitating acute desaturation
- Unexpected outcomes
- Nursing interventions

References

1. Agashe GS, Coakley J, Mannheimer PD: Forehead pulse oximetry, *Anesthesiology* 105:1111-1115, 2006.
CR 2. Awad AA, et al: Different responses of ear and finger pulse oximeter wave form to cold pressor test, *Anesth Analg* 92:1483-1486, 2001.
3. Barker SJ, et al: Measurement of carboxyhemoglobin and methemoglobin by pulse oximetry, *Anesthesiology* 105:892-897, 2006.
CR 4. Chan MM: What is the effect of fingernail polish on pulse oximetry? *Chest* 123: 2163-2164, 2003.
CR 5. Grap MJ: Pulse oximetry, *Crit Care Nurse* 18:94-99, 1998.
6. Grap MJ: Pulse oximetry. In *AACN protocols for practice: technology series,* Aliso Viejo, CA, 2005, American Association of Critical-Care Nurses.
CR 7. Hanowell L, Eisele JH, Downs D: Ambient light affects pulse oximeters, *Anesthesiology* 67:864-865, 1987.
CR 8. Hedges J, Baker WE, Lanoix R, et al: Pulse oximetry. In *Roberts: clinical procedures in emergency medicine,* ed 4, 32-36, 2004, Philadelphia, PA Saunders,
9. Hinkelbein J, Koehler H, Genzwuerker HV, et al: Artificial acrylic finger nails may alter pulse oximetry measurement, *Resuscitation* 74:75-82, 2006.
CR 10. Jubran A: Reliability of pulse oximetry in titrating supplemental oxygen therapy in ventilator-dependent patients, *Chest,* 97:1420-1425, 1990.
CR 11. Kelleher JF: Pulse oximetry, *J Clin Monit* 5:37-62, 1989.
12. Masimo: *Rainbow SET Pulse CO-Oximetery,* 2008, retrieved March 21, 2009, from http://www.masimo.com/Rainbow/about.htm.
CR 13. McConnell EA: Performing pulse oximetry, *Nursing* 99:11,17, 1999.
CR 14. Peters SM: The effect of acrylic nails on the measurement of oxygen saturation as determined by pulse oximetry, *AANAJ* 65:361-363, 1997.
15. Rodden AM, Spicer L, Diaz VA, et al: Does fingernail polish affect pulse oximeter readings? *Intensive Crit Care Nurs* 23:51-55, 2007.
16. Schallom L: Comparison of forehead and digit oximetry in surgical/trauma patients at risk of decreased peripheral perfusion, *Heart Lung* 36:188-194, 2007.
CR 17. Szarlarski NL, Cohen NH: Use of pulse oximetry in critically ill adults, *Heart Lung* 18:444-453, 1989.
18. Zablocki AD, Rasch DK: A simple method to prevent interference with pulse oximetry by infrared heating, *Anesth Analg* 66:915, 1987.

Additional Readings

Bianchi J, et al: Pulse oximetry index: a simple arterial assessment for patients with venous disease, *J Wound Care* 17:253-260, 2008.
Clark AP: Legal lessons: "But his O_2 sat was normal!" *Clin Nurse Specialist* 16:162-163, 2002.
Giuliano KK, et al: New-generation pulse oximetry in the care of critically ill patients, *Am J Crit Care* 14:26-39, 2005.
Witting MD, Scharf SM: Diagnostic room-air pulse oximetry: effects of smoking, race, and sex, *Am J Emerg Med* 26:131-136, 2008.

Pronation Therapy

P U R P O S E :   The prone position may be indicated in patients in whom conventional ventilator strategies have not been successful in recruiting alveoli and who continue to need maximal ventilator support with marginal oxygenation. The prone position is used in an attempt to improve oxygenation in patients with acute lung injury or acute respiratory distress syndrome. The position also may be used for mobilization of secretions as a postural drainage technique, posterior wound management that allows excellent visualization and management of the site, relief of pressure in the sacral region, positioning for operative or diagnostic procedures, and therapeutic sleep for critically ill patients who normally sleep on the abdomen at home.

Kathleen M. Vollman, Jan Powers

PREREQUISITE NURSING KNOWLEDGE

- Prone positioning is used as an adjunct short-term supportive therapy in an attempt to recruit alveoli to improve gas exchange in a critically ill patient with severely compromised lungs.
  - On the basis of numerous studies and three recent meta-analyses, patients with acute lung injury (ALI) and acute respiratory distress syndrome (ARDS) placed in the prone position significantly increase partial pressure of arterial oxygen (Pao$_2$) to fraction of inspired oxygen (Fio$_2$) when compared with the supine position. The greatest effect was seen within the first day, with continuing benefit with subsequent prone position placements up to 4 days.[1-5,7,9,10,13,18,22,24,28,30,32]
  - Two of the three meta-analyses showed no improvement in mortality with the use of the prone position.[1,28] One showed significant improvement in mortality in patients with severe ARDS and a higher severity of illness.[2]

- No significant difference was seen in number of days on mechanical ventilation with the prone position.[1,2,28] One meta-analysis showed significant reduction in the incidence of ventilator-associated pneumonia (VAP) in the prone position[28]; another showed a trend toward significance in VAP reduction of 23% ($P = 0.09$)[1]; and the third showed no difference in VAP rates between the two positions.[2]
  - Part of the variability between the analyses has to do with the inclusion criteria used to choose the studies incorporated in the meta-analysis. The analysis by Alsaghir and Martian[2] resulted in five studies that met inclusion criteria out of 63 with a total of 1316 patients. The meta-analysis preformed by Abroung and group[1] included 5 trials out of 72 with a total of 1372 patients, and the analysis by Sud and colleagues[28] included 13 trials out of 1676 studies with analysis being performed on 1559 patients.
- The last major outcomes to be examined in the meta-analyses were the presence of significant complications when the prone position was compared with the supine position. Two of the three analyses reported on

complications. One analysis showed a statistically significant higher risk for the development of pressure ulcers in the prone position,[28] and Abroung and group[1] showed no significant difference in major airway complications in the prone position. All three meta-analyses concluded that an adequately sized study optimizing the duration of proning and ventilation strategy is warranted to be able to draw definitive conclusions. A phase III trial looking at these issues has been completed but the results have not been published to date. To enhance an understanding of how prone positioning may affect gas exchange, understanding the factors that influence the distribution of ventilation and perfusion within the lung is important.

- *Distribution of ventilation:* Regional pleural pressures and local lung compliance jointly determine the volume of air distributed regionally throughout the lungs. Three major factors—gravity and weight of the lung, compliance, and heterogeneously diseased lungs—influence regional distribution. In an upright individual, the pleural pressure next to the diaphragm is less negative than at the pleural apices. The weight of the lung and the effect of gravity on the lung and its supporting structures in the upright position create this difference in regional pleural pressures. This relationship results in a higher functional residual capacity (FRC) in the nondependent zone or the apices, redirecting ventilation to the dependent zone.[8,15,35] When body position changes, changes occur in regional pleural pressures, compliance, and volume distribution. In the supine position, distribution becomes more uniform from apex to base. The ventilation of dependent lung units exceeds that of nondependent lung units, however, and a reduction in FRC is seen.[8,35] The two factors that contribute to the reduction in FRC seen in moving from the upright to the supine position include: 1, the pressure of the abdominal contents on the diaphragm[8]; and 2, the position of the heart and the relationship of the supporting structures to the lung and its influence on pleural pressure gradients.[17,20]
  - ❖ The first factor to influence pleural pressure, regional volumes, and FRC is the impact of the abdominal contents on the function of the diaphragm. In spontaneously breathing individuals in the supine position, the diaphragm acts as a shield against the pressure exerted by the abdominal contents, preventing the contents from interfering with dependent lung volume distribution. When patients are mechanically ventilated with positive-pressure breaths, sedated, or paralyzed, the active muscle tension in the diaphragm is lost, which results in a cephalad displacement of the diaphragm and allows abdominal pressures to decrease dependent lung volume inflation and FRC.[8,15] The only way to modify this influence is to change the posture to a prone position with the abdomen unsupported.[8,24]
  - ❖ The second factor to influence pleural pressure, regional volumes, FRC, and compliance is the position of the heart and supporting structures. The heart and the diaphragm extend farther dorsally and rest against a rigid spine in the supine position, squeezing the lungs beneath them. This pressure on the lungs generates more positive pleural pressures, which results in a greater propensity to collapse of the alveoli at end expiration. In the prone position, the heart and upper abdomen rest against the sternum, exerting less weight on the lung tissue. Less effect on pleural pressure occurs, which leaves the pleural pressures more negative, maintaining open alveoli.[17,21,24]

  - ❖ A third factor that contributes to the distribution of volume is heterogeneously or unevenly distributed diseased lung. The acute respiratory distress syndrome lung weight is increased twofold to threefold from normal. The increased weight is from edema and the resulting hydrostatic forces. A progressive squeezing of gas along a vertical-dorsal axis results. This decrease of regional inflation along the vertical axis results in dependent or dorsal lung collapse. In the prone position, these densities shift. The pattern almost completely reverts toward normal. The inflation gradient is less steep, and the difference results in a more homogeneous regional inflation. This inflation may be related to a redistribution of gas because of the change in hydrostatic forces caused by differences in pleural pressure, as described previously.[9,11,24]

- *Distribution of perfusion:* Similar to ventilation, regional distribution of perfusion is influenced by three factors: cardiac output, pulmonary vascular resistance, and gravity or body position.

- In an upright individual, blood flow decreases as it moves from base to apex with virtually no flow at the apex. This decrease is caused by the influence of gravity on pulmonary vascular pressures within the lung (Fig. 18-1).
  - ❖ In zone 1, near the apex, alveolar pressure exceeds arterial pressure, creating little or no flow.
  - ❖ In zone 2, the pulmonary artery pressure exceeds alveolar pressure, which exceeds the venous pressure. Blood flow in this area occurs based on the differences in pressure between the arterial and alveolar bed.
  - ❖ In zone 3, the arterial pressure is greater than the venous pressure, which is greater than the alveolar pressure. In this zone, the influence of the alveolar pressure on blood flow is reduced, resulting in freedom of flow in this region.[35,36]

- In supine and lateral positions, apical region blood flow changes. No real change is seen in basilar units, but a greater dependent versus nondependent blood flow occurs. In the prone position, a marked reduction occurs, however, in the gravitational perfusion gradient, which suggests no gravity-dependent benefit to flow in the prone position.[21]

- On the basis of the current available data as outlined here, changes in oxygenation seem to be related to differences in the regional inflation/ventilation of the lung while prone and are not related to a redistribution of blood flow.[6,17,23]

- Suggested criteria for use of the prone position include:
  - ❖ Consider use of the prone position for patients with ARDS who need potentially injurious levels of FiO_2 or plateau pressure, provided they are not put at risk from positional changes[6]

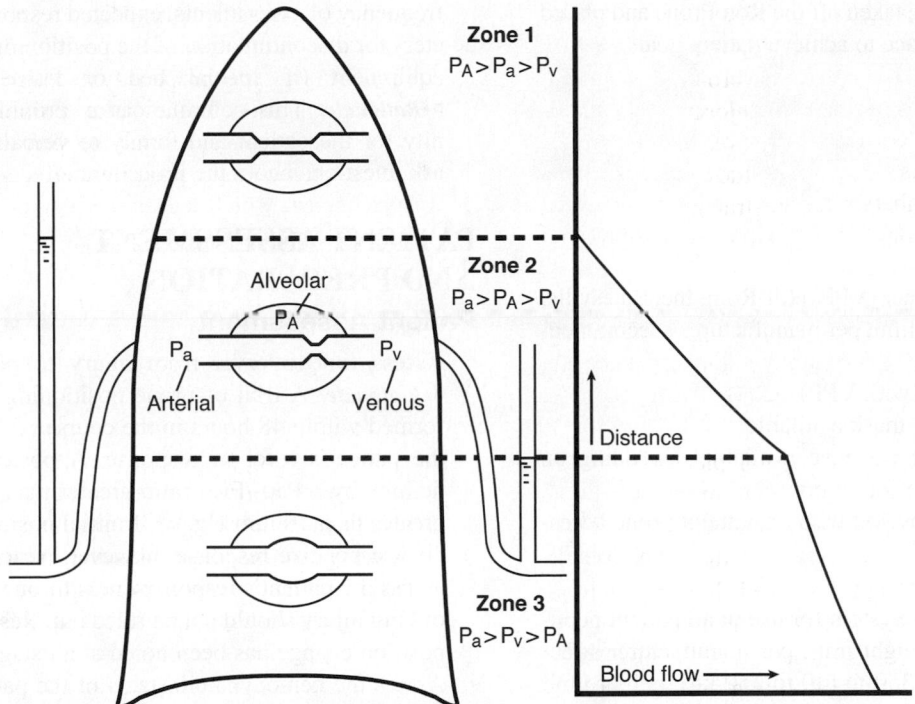

FIGURE 18-1 Zone model of the lung. Three-zone model of the lung is used to explain distribution of blood flow based on pressure variations. *(From West JB, Dollery CT, Naimark A: Distribution of blood flow in isolated lung; relation to vascular and alveolar pressures, J Appl Physiol, 19:713-724, 1964.)*

- ❖ Pao_2/Fio_2 ratio less than 200 on a Fio_2 greater than 50% with sufficient positive end-expiratory pressure used to recruit alveoli
- Contraindications and precautions to manual pronation therapy include the following[3,7,23,26,31,32]:
  - ❖ Patient unable to tolerate a head-down position
  - ❖ Increased intracranial pressure
  - ❖ Unstable spine (unless Stryker Frame [Stryker Medical], Kalamazoo, MI used)
  - ❖ Patient with hemodynamically unstable condition (as defined by a systolic blood pressure less than 90 mm Hg) with fluid and vasoactive support in place
  - ❖ With use of a support frame, patient weight greater than 135 kg
  - ❖ Weight 160 kg or greater (weigh the risk/benefit ratio for the patient and staff)
  - ❖ Extracorporeal membrane oxygenator cannula placement problems
  - ❖ Open chest or unstable chest wall
  - ❖ Bronchopleural fistula
  - ❖ Unstable pelvis
  - ❖ Facial trauma
  - ❖ Grossly distended abdomen or ischemic bowel
  - ❖ Pregnancy
  - ❖ Bifurcated endotracheal tube
- Absolute contraindications for use of Automated Prone Positioning RotoProne™ Therapy System (KCI Licensing, Inc.) include:
  - ❖ Unstable cervical, thoracic, lumbar, pelvic, skull, or facial fractures
  - ❖ Cervical or skeletal traction

- ❖ Uncontrolled intracranial pressure (ICP)
- ❖ Patient weight less than 40 kg (88 lb)
- ❖ Patient weight more than 159 kg (350 lb)
- ❖ Patient height in excess of 6 ft 6 inches
- Relative contraindications for use of Automated Prone Positioning RotoProne™ Therapy System (must weigh risk and benefits) include:
  - ❖ Hemodynamic instability
  - ❖ Severe agitation
  - ❖ Wounds at risk of dehiscence
  - ❖ Patients in prone position with open sternal wound or thoracic postsurgical incision
  - ❖ Open abdomen
  - ❖ Intolerance to face-down position
  - ❖ Any implant that potentially increases risk of skin breakdown, including, but not limited to, breast implants or penile prosthesis
  - ❖ Pregnancy
- The use of the prone position is discontinued when the patient no longer shows a positive response to the position change or mechanical ventilation support has been optimized. The literature has not clearly identified when the use of prone positioning should be discontinued. One suggestion for discontinuation is when the patient's Pao_2/Fio_2 ratio is greater than 200 on less than 50% Fio_2 and less than or equal to 10 cm of H_2O of positive end-expiratory pressure. With use of the RotoProne™ Therapy System Surface, weaning from the prone position is recommended. Increase supine time while decreasing time in the prone position until the patient is able to tolerate 24 hours in the supine position with no decrease in oxygenation response.

The patient can then be taken off the RotoProne and placed on an appropriate surface to achieve patient goals.

EQUIPMENT

- Pillows or foam blocks
- Four or five staff members
- Lift sheets
  or
- Vollman Prone Positioner (VPP; Hill-Rom, Inc, Batesville, IN; Fig. 18-2): weight limit per manufacturer's recommendation, 300 lb
- Three staff members (with VPP)
- Resuscitation bag and mask available
  Additional equipment (to have available depending on patient need) includes the following:
- Lateral rotation therapy bed with or without prone accessory kit
  or
- RotoProne™ Therapy System for use in all patient populations (Fig. 18-3): weight limit per manufacturer's recommendations, 88 to 350 lb (40 to 159 kg); height limit per manufacturer's recommendations, 54 to 78 inches (140 to 200 cm)
- Stryker Frame for use in patients with unstable spines, if available: weight limit per manufacturer's recommendations
- Capnography monitor

PATIENT AND FAMILY EDUCATION

- Explain to the patient and family the patient's lung/oxygenation problem and the reason for the use of the prone position. ➨*Rationale:* This explanation decreases patient and family anxiety by providing information and clarification.
- Explain the care procedure to the patient and family, including positioning procedure, perceived benefit,

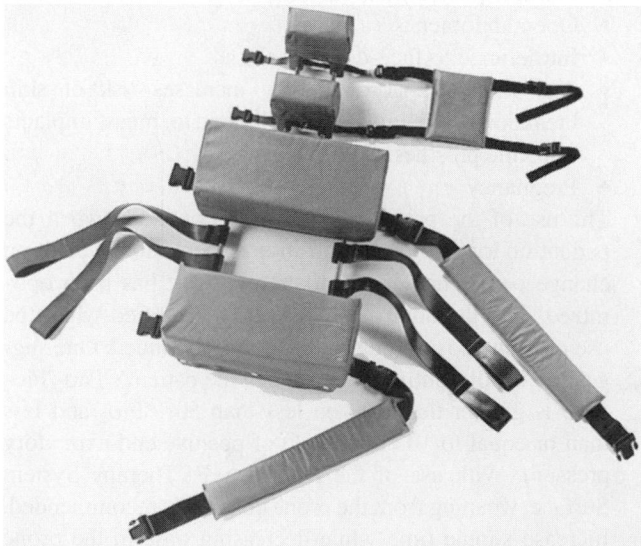

FIGURE 18-2 Diagram of Vollman Prone Positioner. *(From Hill-Rom, Inc, San Antonio, TX)*

frequency of assessments, expected response, and parameters for discontinuation of the positioning technique and equipment (if special bed or frame is initiated). ➨*Rationale:* This communication provides an opportunity for the patient and family to verbalize concerns or ask questions about the procedure.

PATIENT ASSESSMENT AND PREPARATION

Patient Assessment

- Assess time interval from injury to position change. ➨*Rationale:* A trial of prone positioning should be performed within 48 hours in the course of ARDS to assess the patient's level of response. A positive response is defined by a PaO_2/FiO_2 ratio greater than 20% or a PaO_2 greater than 10 mm Hg.[3,24] If initial positioning does not elicit a positive response, however, periodic attempts to assess the patient's responsiveness throughout the course of lung injury should not be ruled out. Response to severe position change has been noted at all stages of ARDS.
- Assess the hemodynamic status of the patient to identify the ability to tolerate a position change.[26] ➨*Rationale:* Imbalances between oxygen supply and demand must be addressed before the pronation procedure to offset any increases in oxygen demand that may be created by the physical turning. The final decision to place a patient with a hemodynamically unstable condition prone rests with the physician or advanced practice nurse who must weigh the risks against the potential benefits of the prone position.
- Assess mental status before use of the prone position. ➨*Rationale:* Agitation, whether caused by delirium, anxiety, or pain, can have a negative effect with the prone position. Nevertheless, agitation is not a contraindication for use of the prone position. The healthcare team should strive to manage the agitation effectively to provide a safe environment for the use of the prone position.
- Assess size and weight load to determine the ability to turn within the narrow critical care bed frame and to weigh the potential risk of injury to the healthcare worker. ➨*Rationale:* When manually turning a patient prone in a hospital bed, with or without a frame, one must determine whether a 180-degree turn can be accomplished within the confines of the space available. Critical care bed frames are narrow, which makes completion of the turn difficult on patients who weigh more than 160 kg. The team must consider the potential for injury to the healthcare workers when making the decision to turn morbidly obese patients prone. With use of a special bed made specifically for prone positioning, follow the weight and height limitations recommended by the manufacturer.

Patient Preparation

- Verify correct patient with two identifiers. ➨*Rationale:* Prior to performing a procedure, the nurse should ensure the correct identification of the patient for the intended intervention.

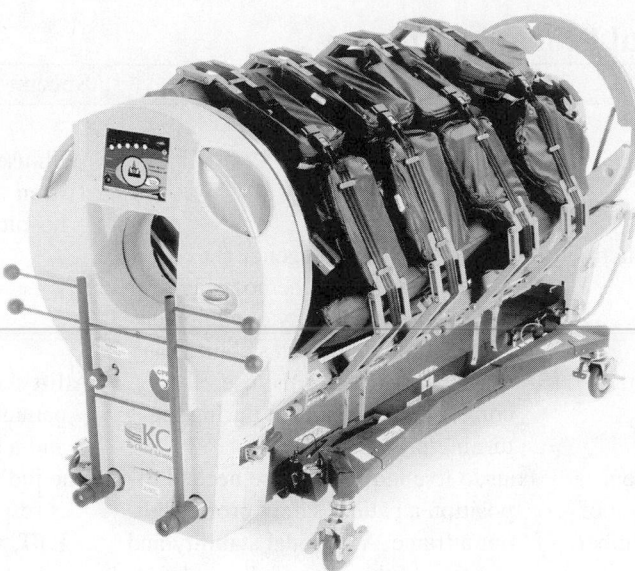

FIGURE 18-3   RotoProne™ Therapy System *(Courtesy of KCI Licensing, Inc., 2008.)*

- Ensure that the patient and family understand preprocedural teachings. Answer questions as they arise and reinforce information as needed. ➭**Rationale:** This communication evaluates and reinforces understanding of previously taught information.
- Assess patient's mental condition. ➭**Rationale:** Assessment of agitation with a reliable and valid scale and provide appropriate management before, during, and after the turn are key to accomplishing a safe procedure.
- Turn off the tube feeding 1 hour before the prone position turn. ➭**Rationale:** This action assists with gastric emptying and reduces the risk of aspiration during the turning procedure.[35] Enteral feeding can be continued during prone position[29]; use of prokinetic agents or transpyloric feedings is recommended to prevent complications associated with vomiting.[25]
- Before positioning the patient prone, the following care activities should be performed:
  - ❖ Remove electrocardiogram leads from the anterior chest wall.
  - ❖ Perform eye care, including lubrication and taping of the eyelids closed in a horizontal fashion.
  - ❖ Ensure the tongue is inside the patient's mouth. If the tongue is swollen or protruding, insert a bite-block.
  - ❖ Ensure the tape or ties of the endotracheal tube or tracheotomy tube are secure. Changing of the ties may

be necessary on return to the supine position if they are not secure. If adhesive tape is used to secure the endotracheal tube, consider double taping or wrapping completely around the head because increased salivary drainage occurs in the prone position and may loosen the adhesive.[26,32] Commercial endotracheal tube (ETT) securement devices are not recommended for use during prone positioning because of possibility of increased skin breakdown and breakdown of adhesive from increased salivary drainage.[16]
  - ❖ If a wound dressing on the anterior body is due to be changed during the prone position sequence, perform the dressing change before the turn. If saturated on return from the prone position, the dressing needs to be changed.
  - ❖ Empty ileostomy/colostomy bags before positioning. Placement of the drainage bag to gravity drainage and padding around the stoma to prevent pressure directly on stoma are recommended.
  - ❖ Capnography monitoring is suggested to help ensure proper positioning of the tube during the turning procedure and in the prone position.
- ➭**Rationale:** These activities prevent areas of pressure and potential skin breakdown; avoid complications related to injury or accidental extubation; and promote the delivery of comprehensive care before, during, and after the pronation therapy.[26,31,32,34]

Procedure   for Manual Pronation Therapy

Steps	Rationale	Special Considerations
1. HH		
2. PE		With use of the frame, ensure it has been cleaned with an appropriate hospital-approved disinfectant.
3. Ensure that emergency equipment is available.	In the event of an emergency (i.e., accidental extubation or hemodynamic instability), availability of equipment allows for rapid patient stabilization.	
4. Place a lift sheet under the patient to assist with turning.	A lift sheet allows for the use of correct body alignment during the turning procedure.[26,32]	A lift sheet is unnecessary if the patient is on a low air-loss surface and a support frame is used.
5. Without a frame: Two staff members are positioned on each side of the bed, with another staff member positioned at the head of the bed. Proceed to step 6. (**Level D***)	Four to five individuals are needed to position a patient safely prone without a frame. Additional stability and position of the personnel may be necessary, based on the size of the patient.[26,33,34]	The individual at the head of the bed is responsible for monitoring the ETT, ventilator tubing, and monitoring/intravenous lines located by the patient's head. For increased airway security, the individual at the head of the bed should hold the ETT during the turn.[26,32]
6. With a frame: One staff member is positioned on either side of the bed, with another staff member positioned at the head of the bed. (**Level C***)	Three staff members are needed for the turn: two perform the actual lifting and turning, and the third is positioned at the head of the bed.[31,32,34]	
7. Correctly position all tubes and invasive lines.	All intravenous tubing and invasive lines are adjusted to prevent kinking, disconnection, or contact with the body during the turning procedure and while the patient remains in the prone position.	If the patient is in skeletal traction, one individual needs to apply traction to the leg while the lines and weights are removed for the turn. If a skeletal pin comes into contact with the bed, a pillow needs to be placed in the correct position to alleviate pressure points.
A. Lines inserted in the upper torso are aligned with either shoulder, and the excess tubing is placed at the head of the bed. The only exception to this rule is for chest tubes or other large-bore tubes (e.g., tubes used for extracorporeal membrane oxygenation).	Disconnecting lines before the turn may help to prevent dislodgment but places the patient at an increased risk for infection.	
B. Chest tubes and lines or tubes placed in the lower torso are aligned with either leg and extend off the end of the bed.	Consider addition of an extension tube to lines that are too short to be placed at the head of bed or the end of the bed.	
C. If the patient has an open abdomen, cover with a synthetic material or vacuum dressing before positioning and identify a positioning strategy that allows the abdomen to be free of restriction.	Open abdomens are not a contraindication for use of the prone position. A cover with a synthetic material and a support such as an abdominal binder may be used effectively to secure the abdomen.[20]	
8. If on a low air-loss surface, maximally inflate.	Maximally inflating the air surface firms up the mattress, making the turn easier to perform.	

*Level C: Qualitative studies, descriptive or correlational studies, integrative reviews, systematic reviews, or randomized controlled trials with inconsistent results
*Level D: Peer-reviewed professional organizational standards with clinical studies to support recommendations

Procedure | for Manual Pronation Therapy—*Continued*

Steps	Rationale	Special Considerations

9. Always turn the patient in the direction of the mechanical ventilator.
 	
  A. Turn the patient's head so that it faces away from the ventilator. Without disconnecting the ventilator tubing from the endotracheal tube, place the portion of the tubing that extends out from the endotracheal tube on the side of the patient's face that is turned away from the ventilator.
 	
  B. Loop the remaining ventilator tubing above the patient's head (Fig. 18-4). **(Level C*)**
 	
10. If a frame is used, the straps that secure the positioner to the body are placed under the patient's head, chest (axillary area), and pelvic region at this time.		

Placing Chest/Pelvic Support or the Vollman Prone Positioner

1. When turning the patient prone without a frame and using the abdomen-unrestricted position, gather pillows at this time for manual placement under the head, upper chest, and pelvic region at a later phase in the procedure.	For lateral rotation beds with a prone position accessory kit, follow manufacturer's instructions for preparing air cushions for the prone position.	

*Level C: Qualitative studies, descriptive or correlational studies, integrative reviews, systematic reviews, or randomized controlled trials with inconsistent results

Procedure continues on following page

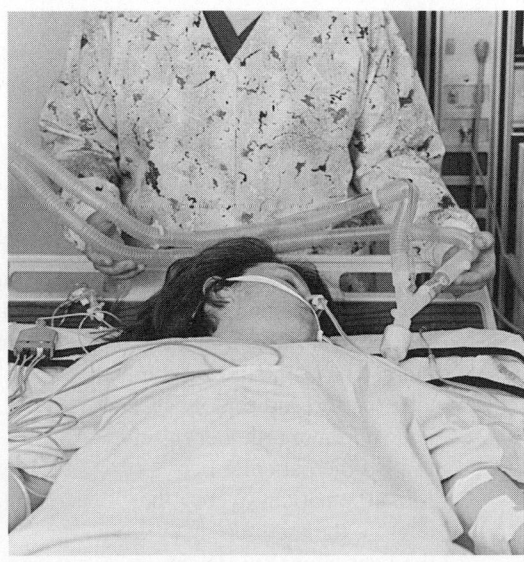

FIGURE 18-4   Positioning of ventilator tubing. *(From Hill-Rom, Inc., San Antonio, TX)*

Procedure for Manual Pronation Therapy—*Continued*

Steps	Rationale	Special Considerations
2. With the VPP: Attach the frame to the patient while the patient is in the supine position. Lay the frame gently on top of the patient. Align the chest piece to rest between the clavicle and sixth rib. (**Level C***)	The chest piece is the only nonmovable part and serves as the marker piece for proper placement and alignment of the device.[31,34]	
3. Adjust the pelvic piece to rest ½ inch above the iliac crest. (**Level C**)	This placement prevents direct pressure over bony prominences and provides sufficient distance between the chest and pelvis to allow the abdomen to be free of restriction and prevents bowing of the back.[31,34]	
4. Adjust the forehead and chin pieces to provide full facial support in a face-down or a side-lying position without interfering with the endotracheal tube.		If the patient has limited neck range of motion or a short neck, the face-down position is optimal. Because readjusting the head to relieve pressure points is difficult, moving both headpieces up to the top of the frame is recommended. Only the head cushion supports the forehead, and the chin is suspended to reduce the risk of skin breakdown from pressure.
5. Fasten the positioner to the patient with the soft adjustable straps. As the straps are tightened, the cushions compress. When fastened, lift the positioner to assess whether a secure fit has been obtained. Readjust as necessary. (**Level M***)	If the device is not secured tightly before the turn, the patient may have shear or friction injuries develop on the chest and pelvic area during the turning process.	When the device is secured correctly, it appears uncomfortable and possibly painful. As a result, the practitioner has a tendency not to fasten the device as tightly as is needed to prevent injury. When secured correctly, the device creates a feeling of pressure and a sense of security fsor the patient during the turning process.

Turning Prone with the Half-Step Technique

1. With a draw sheet, move the patient to the edge of the bed farthest away from the ventilator in preparation for the prone turn. The individual closest to the patient maintains body contact with the bed at all times, serving as a side rail to ensure a safe environment. (**Level C**)	Provides sufficient room to rotate the body safely 180 degrees within the confines of a narrow critical care bed.[31,34]	
2. Turning without a frame: Ensure a bottom sheet is under the patient. Tuck arms slightly under the buttock. Place a sheet over the patient.[32] A. Nurses on both sides of the bed take the top and bottom sheets and roll them together tightly toward the patient. B. Slide the patient over to the edge of the mattress away from the ventilator (Fig. 18-5).	Use of a wide base of support is extremely important to improve balance and prevent self-injury during the turning procedure.	

*Level C: Qualitative studies, descriptive or correlational studies, integrative reviews, systematic reviews, or randomized controlled trials with inconsistent results
*Level M: Manufacturer's recommendations only

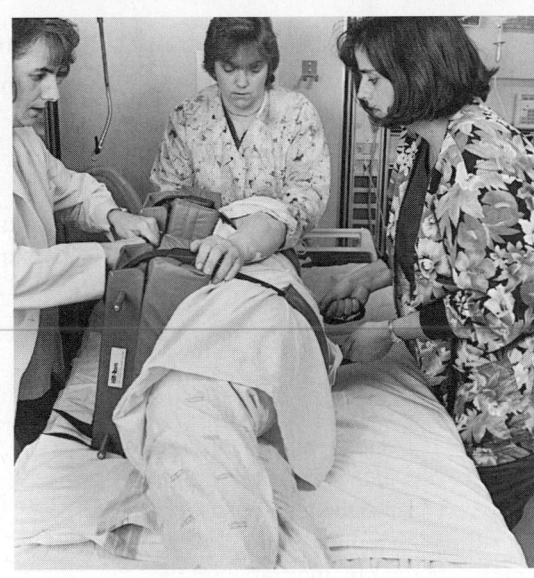

FIGURE 18-5   Turning patient prone on Vollman Prone Positioner.

Procedure	for Manual Pronation Therapy—*Continued*	
Steps	**Rationale**	**Special Considerations**
C. Tilt the patient fully onto his or her side. The patient can be placed in the abdomen-unrestricted position at this time by inserting pillows under the head, chest, and pelvic region (see Fig. 18-4).		
D. With a three count, the patient is rolled with the sheets into a prone position. The staff member at the head of the bed supports the head during the turn and ensures that all tubes and lines are secure (see Fig. 18-4).		
3. Gently rotate the arms parallel to the body, then flex them into a position of comfort so that they are lying adjacent to the head. Minor adjustments of the patient's body may be necessary to obtain correct alignment when in the prone position, whether a frame is used or not.		Many patients have range-of-motion limitations to the shoulder area that may make keeping the arms in a flexed position difficult. Many ways can be used to position the arms for comfort. The arms can be left in a side-lying position, aligned with the body, or positioned one up and one down, similar to a swimmer position.[26]
4. Turning with the VPP:		
A. Tuck the straps on the bar located between the chest and pelvic piece underneath the patient.	Helps with forward motion when the turning process begins.[31,34]	
B. Tuck the patient's arm and hand that now rest in the center of the bed under the buttocks, after position alignment with the edge of the mattress is achieved.		

Procedure continues on following page

Procedure for Manual Pronation Therapy—*Continued*

Steps	Rationale	Special Considerations
C. Cross the leg closest to the edge of the bed over the opposite leg at the ankle. **(Level C*)**		
5. Turn the patient to a 45-degree angle toward the ventilator.	Use of a wide base of support is extremely important to improve balance and prevent self-injury during the turning procedure.[31,34]	
A. The staff member on the ventilator side of the bed grips the upper steel bar.		
B. The staff member on the opposite side of the bed grasps the straps attached to the lower steel bar.		
C. With a three count, lift the patient by the frame into a prone position.		
D. During the turning procedure, the staff member at the head of the bed ensures that all tubes and lines are secure and patent (see Fig. 18-4). **(Level C)**		
6. With the VPP: Loosen the straps at this time. If the patient is unstable, keeping the straps fastened securely is recommended to facilitate a safe quick return to the supine position in the event of an emergency (Fig. 18-6).	The procedure for returning to the supine position takes less than 1 minute if the straps are fastened and a support frame is used.	
7. If on a low air-loss surface, release the maximal inflation.	A return to normal pressures on the surface helps to alleviate pressure at various bony prominences in the prone position.	If on a standard hospital mattress, the thigh-knee-calf area must be supported to minimize the risk of pressure injury and prevent discomfort.[26,31,32,34]

*Level C: Qualitative studies, descriptive or correlational studies, integrative reviews, systematic reviews, or randomized controlled trials with inconsistent results

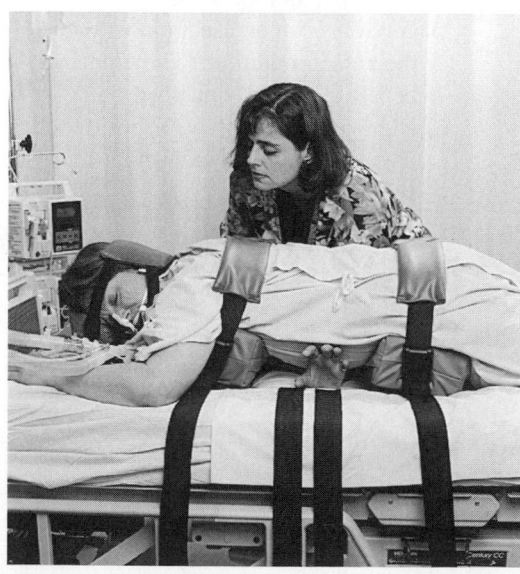

Figure 18-6 Patient lying prone on Vollman Prone Positioner. *(From Hill-Rom, Inc., San Antonio, TX)*

Procedure | for Manual Pronation Therapy—*Continued*

Steps	Rationale	Special Considerations
8. Place a support or other pillow under the ankle area.	A support in this area allows for correct body alignment and prevents tension on the tendons in the foot and ankle region.	If the patient is tall enough, dangling the feet over the edge of the mattress may be a sufficient alternative to support the ankles and feet in correct alignment.
9. Discard used supplies.		
10. Remove personal protective equipment. **HH**		
Returning to the Supine Position		
1. **HH**		
2. **PE**		
3. Align the patient with the edge of the mattress closest to the ventilator.		The patient turns toward the center of the mattress, away from the ventilator.
4. Arrange the ventilator tubing to provide sufficient mobility and length to prevent pulling during the turning procedure.	The staff member at the head of the bed is responsible for monitoring placement of the ventilator tubing, monitoring wires, and invasive lines.	
5. Straighten the patient's arms from a flexed position and bring them to rest on either side of the head. Remove leg and ankle pillow supports. If on a low air-loss surface, maximally inflate.		
6. Cross the leg closest to the edge of the bed over the opposite leg at the ankle.		
7. Without a frame: Turn the patient to a 45-degree angle with the lift sheet and the patient's body, then roll the patient onto his or her back.	Lifting and realignment in the center of the bed may be necessary when returning to the supine position if a support frame is not used.	
8. Stretch the arms parallel to the body and bring them into a downward position.		
9. With the VPP: Fasten the straps tightly before repositioning.		
10. Turn the patient to a 45-degree angle with the steel bars, then roll the patient onto his or her back (Fig. 18-7).	The steel bars on the positioning frame allow lifting as the patient is realigned into the center of the bed.	
11. Unfasten the positioner and remove from the patient. The straps may be left under the patient in preparation for the next turn.		
12. Discard used supplies.		
13. Remove personal protective equipment. **HH**		

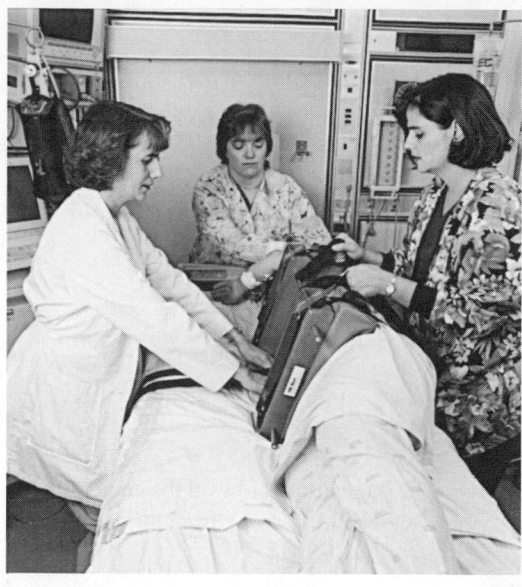

FIGURE 18-7   Patient returning to supine position. *(From Hill-Rom, Inc., San Antonio, TX)*

Procedure   for Automated Pronation Therapy (Using RotoProne™ Therapy System)

Steps	Rationale	Special Considerations
1. **HH**		
2. **PE**		
3. After removing all pieces from Roto-Prone™ Therapy System, move patient from intensive care unit (ICU) bed to RotoProne™ Therapy System.		
4. Position patient in center of the surface with head positioned in the attached head support.		Ears should be visible through ear holes on headpiece.
5. Position all tubes and invasive lines:		
A. Lines inserted in the upper torso are aligned with either shoulder and positioned at the head of the bed in tube management system.	All intravenous tubing and invasive lines are adjusted to prevent kinking, disconnection, or contact with the body during the turning procedure and while the patient remains in the prone position.	
B. Chest tubes and lines or tubes placed in the lower torso are aligned with either leg and extend through the center hole at the foot of the surface.	The addition of extension tubing to lines that are too short to be placed at the head of bed or the end of the bed may be necessary.	
C. If the patient has an open abdomen, it should be supported with some type of vacuum dressing. **(Level E*)**	Open abdominal wounds are not a contraindication for use of the prone position. A cover with a synthetic material and a support such as an abdominal binder or vacuum dressing may be used effectively to secure the abdomen.[20]	
6. Follow manufacturer's recommendations for securing patient on therapy surface. **(Level M*)**		

*Level E: Multiple case reports, theory-based evidence from expert opinions, or peer-reviewed profsessional organizational standards without clinical studies to support recommendations
*Level M: Manufacturer's recommendations only

Procedure for Automated Pronation Therapy (Using RotoProne™ Therapy System)—*Continued*		
Steps	**Rationale**	**Special Considerations**
A. Place leg piece and side packs on surface.	Ensure patient is snugly secured within side packs. If the side packs are not secured tightly before the turn, the patient may have shear or friction injuries develop during the turning process.	
B. Place abdominal support mesh over patient's abdomen.		
C. Position additional pads on patient (lower leg packs over shin, pelvic packs along iliac crests, chest pack).	All packs need to be positioned to prevent undue pressure on patient's surfaces and to avoid malposition of joints (avoid hyperextension of knees and hips in prone position).	
D. Tighten headpiece snugly around patient's head.		
E. Position all packs snugly over patient (lower leg below knees, upper leg above knees, pelvic pack over iliac crest and chest pack over chest/shoulder area).	This action prevents direct pressure over bony prominences and provides sufficient distance between the chest and pelvis to allow the abdomen to be free of restriction and prevents bowing of the back.[31,34] May need to tighten chest pads over patient last because constriction of the chest may restrict patient's ventilatory effort and increase peak airway pressures.	
F. Place face pack on patient's face and ensure top pad is above eyebrows and side pieces frame mouth.		
7. On screen at foot of bed, set therapy on RotoProne™ Therapy System to prone toward the direction of the ventilator.	These maneuvers are performed to prevent disconnection of the ventilator tubing or kinking of the ETT during the turning procedure.[26,31,32,34]	

Turning Prone with the RotoProne™ Therapy System

All steps listed below are performed on the touch screen at the foot of the surface.

1. "Check tubing," "Check airway," "Check head support" (push each button on the screen after checking).
2. Push "Rotate" button (must start rotation, before turning prone).
3. Push "Prone" button.
4. Push "Rotate and Lower" button. Press and hold button until screen changes.

Use the touch screen buttons on screen at foot of surface, following manufacturer's instructions for turning patient to prone position.

Procedure continues on following page

Procedure for Automated Pronation Therapy (Using RotoProne™ Therapy System)—*Continued*

Steps	Rationale	Special Considerations
5. "Check tubing," "Check airway," "Check head support," "Check abdominal support," "Check arm slings" (push each button on the screen after checking).		
6. Reconfirm face pack and push button on touch screen.		**Important note:** *Face pack is only piece without a safety sensor.*
7. Press "Prone." Press and hold button during entire turning procedure. (This step can also be accomplished with pushing "Prone/supine" button on hand control.)		Release button if need arises to stop the turning procedure because of kinking or pulling on tubes. An additional person may be helpful to have present during the actual turning procedure to monitor invasive lines and ventilator tubing to ensure all lines are positioned correctly. In the absence of an additional person, use of the handset at the head of the bed is recommended for turning patient so all invasive lines and tubes are visible during turning.
8. After patient is in prone position, screen shows additional buttons to "Check tubing," . . . "Check airway," "Check head support" (push each button after checking).		
9. Press "Rotate."	Patient should rotate 62 degrees to each side while in the prone position.	Degree of rotation and pause times on each side can be adjusted based on individual patient response to therapy.
10. Push "Surface position" button on screen.		
11. Place patient in "Reverse Trendelenburg" by pressing button on screen (push and hold until 11 to 12 degrees).	Reverse Trendelenburg's position is recommended to keep head of bed up to decrease edema and prevent complications associated with feeding or potential aspiration.	
12. Open back hatches in the prone position.	All hatches can be opened to allow for full chest expansion. Foot hatch should be opened and propped open to prevent undue pressure on heels.	

Procedure	**for Automated Pronation Therapy (Using RotoProne™ Therapy System)**—*Continued*	
Steps	**Rationale**	**Special Considerations**
13. Leave patient in prone position for 3 hours 15 minutes with 62-degree rotation to each side. **(Level C*)**	Recommended time to remain in the prone position is 3 hours 15 minutes alternating with 45 minutes supine to achieve a total of 19.5 hours prone time in a 24-hour period.[27] After prone time completed, position patient supine for 45 minutes as tolerated. Positioning schedule is based on whether the patient is able to sustain improvements in Pao_2 made while in the prone or supine position.	The healthcare team may decide to vary the recommended schedule based on individual patient care needs. Adjustment of time intervals and rotation times based on patient's response to therapy may be necessary. Changes to degree of rotation or pause times can be made by pushing the "therapy settings" button. If the need arises to quickly return patient to the supine position, "CPR buttons" are located on the touch screen and below the screen at the foot of the bed. Make sure all hatches are closed before returning the patient to the supine position.
14. Remove personal protective equipment. **HH**		
Turning Supine with the RotoProne™ Therapy System		
1. **HH**		
2. **PE**		
3. Close any open hatches.		
4. Push "Supine" button.		
5. Push "Rotate and Lower" button and hold until screen changes.		
6. "Check tubing," "Check airway," "Check head support" (push each button after checking).		
7. Press "Supine" and hold button during entire turning procedure. (This step can also be accomplished by pushing "Prone/ supine" button on hand control.)		Release button if need arises to stop the turning procedure because of kinking or pulling on tubes. An additional person present during the actual turning procedure may be helpful to monitor invasive lines and ventilator tubing to ensure all lines are positioned correctly. In the absence of an additional person, use of the handset at the head of the bed is recommended for turning patient so all invasive lines and tubes are visible during turning.
8. Insert locking pin after patient assumes the supine position.		
9. Open packs over patient as needed for patient care.		
10. Carefully remove face pack.		

*Level C: Qualitative studies, descriptive or correlational studies, integrative reviews, systematic reviews, or randomized controlled trials with inconsistent results

Procedure continues on following page

Procedure	**for Automated Pronation Therapy (Using RotoProne™ Therapy System)**—*Continued*	
Steps	**Rationale**	**Special Considerations**
11. Rotate patient supine as tolerated up to 45 minutes or an hour. To rotate patient supine, lower pack and either chest of pelvic pack must be secured over patient.		While patient is supine, complete all assessments and procedures scheduled. After completion, the patient may be rotated in supine position. Placement of bottom foot pack and either chest or pelvic pack is necessary for supine rotation.
		With automated prone positioning, if the patient is unable to maintain the improvement in gas exchange seen with the prone position when returned to a supine position, the patient can be returned to the prone position. If the patient tolerates supine position, the patient should optimally remain in the supine/lateral position for only 45 minutes to 1 hour before being repositioned prone.
12. Place in reverse Trendelenburg's position to get head of bed elevated to maximum 11 to 12 degrees by pushing the "Surface position" button then "Reverse Trendelenburg."		
13. Remove personal protective equipment. **HH**		

Expected Outcomes

- Increased oxygenation
- Improved secretion clearance
- Improved compliance of the lungs and alveolar recruitment

Unexpected Outcomes

- Agitation
- Disconnection or dislodgment of tubes and lines
- Peripheral arm nerve injury
- Periorbital and conjunctival edema
- Skin injuries or pressure ulcers
- Eye pressure or injury

Patient Monitoring and Care

Steps	Rationale	Reportable Conditions
		These conditions should be reported if they persist despite nursing interventions.
1. Assess patient's tolerance to the turning procedure: • Respiratory rate and effort • Heart rate and blood pressure	Oxygen saturation is not used as a measure of intolerance to the turning procedure because patients often have desaturation with a deep lateral turn; however, if the patient responds to the prone position, the condition stabilizes quickly when settled into the prone position. The lateral-turn decrease in oxygen saturation may deter the healthcare team from trying the prone position. If respiratory rate and effort, heart rate, and blood pressure do not return to normal within 10 minutes of the turn, the patient may be displaying initial signs of intolerance.[32,37]	• Failure of the respiratory rate, respiratory effort, heart rate, and blood pressure to return to normal 5 to 10 minutes after the turn
2. Assess the patient's response to the prone position: • Pulse oximetry (SpO_2) • Mixed venous oxygenation saturation (SO_2) or central mix venous oxygen saturation (ScO_2) and hemodynamics • Arterial blood gases 30 minutes after position change • PaO_2/FiO_2 ratio	Of all patients with acute lung injury turned prone, more than 70% had improvement in oxygenation.[3-5,7,10,13,18,20,22,23,32,34] A response is defined by a PaO_2/FiO_2 ratio greater than 20% or a PaO_2 greater than 10 mm Hg.[24] The time response varies among patients. Some patients immediately respond, whereas others may take 6 hours to show maximal response to the position change. Hemodynamic measurements are accurate in the prone position compared with supine as long as the zero reference point is calibrated at the phlebostatic axis.[33]	• Decrease from baseline in the SpO_2 or failure of the SO_2 or ScO_2 to return to baseline after 5 to 10 minutes
3. With manual proning, reposition the patient's head on an hourly basis in the prone position to prevent facial breakdown. While one staff member lifts the patient's head, a second staff member moves the headpieces to provide support for the head in a different position. **(Level D*)** Not necessary with automated proning.	The face and ears have minimal structural padding to reduce the risk of skin breakdown. Patients with short necks or limited neck range of motion have difficulty assuming a head side-lying position. These patients are more likely to have facial breakdown develop, making turning the patient more frequently or use of the previous technique necessary to prevent breakdown.[14,26,32]	• Skin breakdown

*Level D: Peer-reviewed professional organizational standards with clinical studies to support recommendations

Procedure continues on following page

Patient Monitoring and Care —*Continued*

Steps	Rationale	Reportable Conditions
4. Assess skin frequently for areas of nonblanchable redness or breakdown. Place a hydrocolloid dressing over areas where shearing and friction injuries are likely to occur (i.e., chest, pelvis, elbows, and knees). **(Level M*),**	Greater than 2 hours on a standard surface without changing position increases a patient's risk for breakdown. If the patient is on a pressure-reduction surface, the time remaining in a stationary position can be lengthened.[14] The use of a hydrocolloid may serve as a protective barrier, reducing the risk of shearing and friction injuries.[14,26,32] If VPP is used and a skin injury occurs on the chest or pelvis, reassess tightness of the device before the prone position turn. The injury is most often related to a loose-fitting apparatus and is likely a shear injury versus pressure.	• Nonblanchable redness • Shearing and friction injuries
5. Provide frequent oral care and suctioning of the airway as needed.	The prone position promotes postural drainage through the natural use of gravity. Drainage from the nares may be a clinical sign of an undetected sinus infection.	• Drainage from the nares • Change in amount or character of secretions
6. Maintain tube feeding as tolerated. **(Level D*)**[33] **(Level C*)**[25]	The risk for aspiration is minimal in the prone position because the patient is already in a head-down side-lying position that maximizes the use of gravity to move vomited matter safely. A reverse Trendelenburg's position changes that relationship. It may reduce the risk of microaspiration and may increase the risk of a large emesis occurring.[33] Use of prokinetic agents or transpyloric feedings is recommended to prevent complications associated with vomiting. Studies have shown increased risk of complications in the prone position in patients receiving gastric feedings. These studies recommend use of promotility agents or postpyloric feedings to reduce the risk of complications such as vomiting and enhance gastric emptying.[25]	• Evidence of tube feeding material when suctioning

*Level C: Qualitative studies, descriptive or correlational studies, integrative reviews, systematic reviews, or randomized controlled trials with inconsistent results
*Level D: Peer-reviewed professional organizational standards with clinical studies to support recommendations
*Level M: Manufacturer's recommendations only

Patient Monitoring and Care —*Continued*

Steps	Rationale	Reportable Conditions

7. Scheduling frequency: The positioning schedule is based on whether the patient is able to sustain improvements in PaO_2 made in the prone position.
A schedule of every 6 hours in the prone position is suggested.[32]
Time spent in the supine position is based on the length of time the patient is able to sustain or maintain the improvement in gas exchange that occurred while prone. Recent studies have shown 12 to 20 hours within 24 hours is the average amount of time spent in the prone position. This time may be consecutive or sequential depending on the type of apparatus used and the risk of skin injury and hemodynamic instability experienced.[3,4,10,13,18,20,22,32]
For automated proning with Roto-Prone™ Therapy System, the suggested time in the prone position is 3 hours 15 minutes prone alternating with 45 minutes as tolerated in the supine position.
  A. If the patient maintains the improvement in PaO_2 when repositioned supine, the patient can remain in the supine to lateral position for a maximum of 4 to 6 hours or return to the prone position when or if a decrease in PaO_2 is seen. **(Level C*),**
  B. With automated prone positioning, if the patient is unable to maintain the improvement in gas exchange seen with the prone position when returned to a supine position, the patient can be returned to the prone position. If the patient tolerates supine position, the patient should optimally remain in the supine/lateral position for only 45 minutes to 1 hour before being repositioned prone.
	Without a clear direction from the literature on frequency of position change, the healthcare team must weigh other physiologic factors when a patient remains in a stationary position for an extended period.
	Following the principles of pressure relief used when positioning patients laterally or supine can minimize the potential for skin injury and edema formation. Longer time spent in a single position necessitates that the support surface provide greater pressure reduction or relief than a standard hospital mattress.
	Combining the literature on the prone position and surface interface pressure, a safe suggestion for frequency of repositioning is between 4 and 6 hours.[3,4,10,13,18,20,22,30,32]
	
	Use of lateral rotation therapy in conjunction with prone positioning is suggested so that when the patient is returned to a supine position, he or she is laterally rotated. The use of continuous lateral rotation therapy has been associated with a reduction in pulmonary complications.[12,19,26,32]
		• Clinically significant decreases in oxygenation (>10 mm Hg) or oxygen saturation ($<88\%$)

*Level C: Qualitative studies, descriptive or correlational studies, integrative reviews, systematic reviews, or randomized controlled trials with inconsistent results

Procedure continues on following page

Patient Monitoring and Care —*Continued*

Steps	Rationale	Reportable Conditions
C. The use of the prone position is discontinued when the patient no longer shows a positive response to the position change or mechanical ventilation support has been optimized.	The literature has not clearly identified when the use of prone positioning should be discontinued. One suggestion for discontinuation is when the patient's Pao_2/Fio_2 ratio is greater than 200 on less than 50% Fio_2 and less than or equal to 10 cm of H_2O of positive end-expiratory pressure.	

Documentation

Documentation should include the following:

- Patient and family education
- Ability to tolerate the turning procedure
- Length of time in the prone position
- Maximal oxygenation response in the prone position
- Oxygenation response when returned to the supine position
- Positioning schedule used
- Complications noted during or after the procedure
- Use of continuous lateral rotation therapy or other devices
- Amount and type of secretions
- Unexpected outcomes
- Nursing interventions

References

1. Abroung F, et al: The effect of prone positioning in acute respiratory distress syndrome or acute lung injury: a meta-analysis: areas of uncertainty and recommendations for research, *Intensive Care Med* 34(6):1002-1011, 2008.
2. Alsaghir AH, Martian CM: Effect of prone positioning in patients with acute respiratory distress syndrome: a meta-analysis, *Crit Care Med* 36:603-609, 2008.
CR 3. Chatte G, et al: Prone position in mechanically ventilated patients with severe acute respiratory failure, *Am J Respir Crit Care Med* 155:473-478, 1997.
4. Curley MA, et al: Effect of prone positioning on clinical outcomes in children with acute lung injury: a randomized controlled trial, *JAMA* 294:229-237, 2005.
CR 5. Curley MAQ: Prone positioning of patients with acute respiratory distress syndrome: a systematic review, *Am J Crit Care* 8:397-405, 1999.
6. Dellinger PR, et al: Surviving sepsis campaign: international guidelines for management of severe sepsis and septic shock: 2008, *Crit Care Med* 36:296-327, 2008.
CR 7. Fridrich P, et al: The effects of long-term prone positioning in patients with trauma induced adult respiratory distress syndrome, *Anesth Analg* 83:1206-1211, 1996.
CR 8. Froese AB, Bryan AC: Effects of anesthesia and paralysis on diaphragmatic mechanics in man, *Anesthesiology* 41:242-255, 1974.
CR 9. Gattinoni L, et al: Body position changes redistribute lung computed tomographic density in patients with acute respiratory failure, *Anesthesiology* 74:15-23, 1991.
CR 10. Gattinoni L, et al: Effect of prone positioning on the survival of patients with acute respiratory failure, *N Engl J Med* 345:568-573, 2001.
CR 11. Gattinoni L, et al: Relationships between lung computed tomographic density, gas exchange and PEEP in acute respiratory failure, *Anesthesiology* 69:824-832, 1988.
12. Goldhill DR, Imhoff M, McLean B, et al: Rotational bed therapy to prevent and treat respiratory complications: a review and meta analysis, *Am J Crit Care* 16:50-62, 2007.
CR 13. Guerin C, et al: Effects of systematic prone positioning in hypoxemic acute respiratory failure: a randomized controlled trial, *JAMA* 292:2379-2387, 2004.
CR 14. Harcomb C: Nursing patient with ARDS in prone position, *Nurs Stand* 18(19):33-39, 2004.
CR 15. Kaneko K, et al: Regional distribution of ventilation and perfusion as a function of body position, *J Appl Physiol* 21:767-777, 1966.
16. Laux L, McGonigal M, Thieret T, et al: Use of prone positioning in a patient with acute respiratory distress syndrome, *Crit Care Nurs Q* 31(2):178-183, 2008.
17. Malbouisson LM, et al: Role of the heart in the loss of aeration characterizing lower lobes in acute respiratory distress syndrome, *Am J Respir Crit Care Med* 161:2005-2012, 2005.
18. Mancebo J, et al: A multicenter trial of prolonged prone ventilation in severe acute respiratory distress syndrome, *Am J Respir Crit Care Med* 173:1233-1239, 2006.
19. Marklew A: Body positioning and its effect on oxygenation—a literature review, *Nurs Crit Care* 11(1):16-22, 2006.
CR 20. Murray TA, Patterson LA: Prone positioning of trauma patients with acute respiratory distress syndrome and open abdominal incisions, *Crit Care Nurse* 22:52-56, 2002.

CR 21. Mutoh T, et al: Prone position alters the effect of volume overload on regional pleural pressures and improves hypoxemia in pigs in vivo, *Am Rev Respir Dis* 146:300-306, 1992.

22. Papazian L, et al: Comparison of prone positioning and high frequency oscillatory ventilation of patients with acute respiratory distress syndrome, *Crit Care Med* 33:2162-2171, 2005.

CR 23. Pappert D, et al: Influence of positioning on ventilation-perfusion relationships in severe adult respiratory distress syndrome, *Chest* 106:1511-1516, 1994.

CR 24. Pelosi P, Brazzi L, Gattinoni L: Prone position in ARDS, *Eur Respir J* 20:1017-1028, 2002.

CR 25. Reignier J, Thenoz-Jost N, Fiancette M, et al: Early enteral nutrition in mechanically ventilated patients in the prone position, *Crit Care Med* 32(1):94-99, 2004.

CR 26. Rowe C: Development of clinical guidelines for prone positioning in critically ill adults, *Nurs Crit Care* 9(2): 50-57, 2004.

27. Sebat F, Johnson D, Shoffner D, et al: Benefits, complications of prone position and utility of automated proning bed in the treatment of acute lung injury (ALI), *Chest* 132(4):572S, 2007.

28. Sud S, et al: Effect of mechanical ventilation in the prone position on clinical outcomes in patients with acute respiratory failure: a systematic review and meta-analysis, *CMAJ* 178(9):1153-1161, 2008.

CR 29. Van der Voort PH, Zandstra DF: Enteral feeding in the critically ill: comparison between supine and prone positions: a prospective crossover study in mechanically ventilated patients, *Crit Care* 5(4): 2001;.216-220

30. Voggenreiter G, et al: Prone positioning improves oxygenation in post traumatic lung injury: a prospective randomized trial, *J Trauma* 59:333-341, 2005.

CR 31. Vollman KM: *The effect of suspended prone positioning on PaO₂ and A-a gradients in adult patients with acute respiratory failure,* Master's Thesis, Long Beach, 1989, California State University.

CR 32. Vollman KM: Prone positioning in the ARDS patient: the art and science, *Crit Care Nurs Clin North Am* 16(3): 319-336, 2004.

CR 33. Vollman KM: What are the practice guidelines for prone positioning of acutely ill patients? Specifically, what are the recommendations related to hemodynamic monitoring and tube feeding? *Crit Care Nurse* 21:84-86, 2001.

CR 34. Vollman KM, Bander JJ: Improved oxygenation utilizing a prone positioner in patients with acute respiratory distress syndrome, *Intensive Care Med* 22:1105-1111, 1996.

CR 35. West JB: *Respiratory physiology: the essentials,* ed 3, Baltimore, 1985, Williams & Wilkins.

CR 36. West JB, Dollery CT, Naimark A: Distribution of blood flow in isolated lung: relation to vascular and alveolar pressures, *J Appl Physiol* 19:713-724, 1964.

CR 37. Winslow EH, et al: Effects of a lateral turn on mixed venous oxygen saturation and heart rate in critically ill adults, *Heart Lung* 19:555-561, 1990.

Thoracic Cavity Management

Autotransfusion

P U R P O S E :   Autotransfusion is the collection and filtration of blood from an active bleeding site and reinfusion of that (autologous) blood into the same patient for the maintenance of blood volume.

Robin M. Beard

PREREQUISITE NURSING KNOWLEDGE

- Understanding of transfusion and intravenous therapy and fluid balance is necessary.
- Significant blood loss, related systemic hypoperfusion, and the associated decrease in oxygen-carrying capacity, with its impact on hypoxemia, often necessitate the replacement of blood with whole blood or packed cells. In appropriate patient populations (trauma, cardiovascular, or orthopedic surgical patients), autotransfusion should be considered as the need to replace blood becomes apparent.
- Autotransfusion is commonly used for trauma victims and for patients undergoing cardiovascular and orthopedic procedures; it reduces the need for banked blood transfusions with the inherent risks of transfusion reactions and disease transmission.
- A variety of autotransfusion devices are available. An autotransfusion system may be a standard water-seal chest drainage system (see Fig. 24-1, *A*), a separate autotransfusion setup, or a modified chest drainage autotransfusion system. In addition, continuous and intermittent systems are available. A continuous system has an intravenous line connected directly from the drainage unit collection chamber to the patient. An intermittent system uses a blood collection bag in-line between the chest tube and the collection chamber.
- Many disposable systems available today have the ability to act as a reservoir for autotransfusion if the need arises. To initiate autotransfusion, the autotransfusion bag is

disconnected from the disposable system and connected to the saline solution–filled blood administration tubing. Nurses should gain familiarity with their institution's autotransfusion system and policies.
- Indications for autotransfusion in the appropriate patient populations include active bleeding (greater than 100 mL/hr) and the accumulation of greater than 300 mL of drainage in the collection chamber.
- Contraindications to autotransfusion include the following:
  ❖ Active infection or contamination of shed blood
  ❖ Malignant cells in shed blood
  ❖ Renal or hepatic insufficiency
  ❖ Established coagulopathies
  ❖ Blood that has been in the autotransfusion system for longer than institutional standards allow or as recommended by manufacturers
- Any contraindications to autotransfusion are overruled in the presence of exsanguinating hemorrhage in the absence of an adequate supply of banked blood.
- As with banked blood, patients may refuse to receive autologous blood based on religious beliefs.
- Informed consent should be obtained in nonemergency situations.

EQUIPMENT

- Personal protective equipment
- Autotransfusion collection system
- Autotransfusion system replacement bag
- Blood administration set

- 40-μm microemboli filter
- Normal saline (NS) intravenous (IV) solution

PATIENT AND FAMILY EDUCATION

- Explain the procedure to the patient, if appropriate, and the family, including the risks and benefits of using the patient's own blood. ➤*Rationale:* Information enhances patient and family understanding and decreases anxiety.

PATIENT ASSESSMENT AND PREPARATION

Patient Assessment

- Signs and symptoms of hypovolemia and associated hypoperfusion include the following:
  - ❖ Pale clammy skin
  - ❖ Hypotension
  - ❖ Tachycardia

- ❖ Dyspnea
- ❖ Decreased central venous pressure (CVP), pulmonary artery pressure (PAP), or pulmonary artery wedge pressure (PAWP)
- ❖ Decreased cardiac output or index
- ❖ Oliguria
- ❖ Decreased hemoglobin or hematocrit

Patient Preparation

- Verify correct patient using two identifiers. ➤*Rationale:* Prior to performing a procedure the nurse should ensure the correct identification of the patient for the intended intervention.
- Ensure that the patient understands preprocedural teachings. Answer questions as they arise, and reinforce information as needed. ➤*Rationale:* This communication evaluates and reinforces understanding of previously taught information.

Procedure	for Autotransfusion	
Steps	**Rationale**	**Special Considerations**
1. HH		
2. PE		
3. Assemble equipment.		
4. Set up autotransfusion unit (see manufacturer's instructions).	Suction is required to drain blood into drainage unit.	
5. If directed by physician's order, inject anticoagulant into the autotransfusion bag before collecting blood from the patient. **(Level C*)**	Several different anticoagulants may be used. Citrate phosphate dextrose (CPD) is commonly used (1 mL per 7 mL blood).[1,3]	Use of anticoagulants may be ordered by physician. Use of anticoagulants is controversial.
6. Connect the patient's drainage or chest tube to the collection bag directly or via a water-seal setup.	Allows for collection of shed blood in preparation for autotransfusion.	Autotransfusion is commonly performed with blood drained from the thoracic cavity and after orthopedic procedures.
7. Before the filled collection bag for patient infusion is disconnected, a new collection system should be prepared.	Allows for the collection of additional blood and keeps the system closed and sterile.	
8. Clamp the tubes (attached to the tubing by the manufacturer) on the new collection bag.	Clamping eliminates the risk of air entering the system.	
9. Close the clamp on the patient drainage tubing.	Stops further drainage into the bag.	
10. If the collection bag is part of the water-seal system (see Fig. 24-1), close the clamps on the tubing connected to the water-seal drainage unit.	Prepares the system for disconnection.	
11. Disconnect the filled bag from the patient system, maintaining sterility at all times.		

*Level C: Qualitative studies, descriptive or correlational studies, integrative reviews, systematic reviews, or randomized controlled trials with inconsistent results

Procedure continues on following page

Procedure | for Autotransfusion—*Continued*

Steps	Rationale	Special Considerations
12. Take the previously prepared new collection bag; attach it to the water-seal unit or to the patient's chest tube or drainage tube.	Allows for continued collection of blood.	
13. Ensure that all connections are secure; open clamps on autotransfusion bag and patient drainage tubing.	Connections must be secured to create suction for drainage.	
14. Prime the blood administration tubing with NS. Connect filled collection bag to blood administration set with microfilter. **(Level C*)**	Filters should be used to reduce the danger of microembolization.[1,3]	Do not apply pressure or use with pressure device during transfusion. A 40-mcg filter is recommended for autotransfusion.
15. Initiate infusion as prescribed	Restores blood volume.	Reinfuse blood within 6 hours (if stored at room temperature) of collection.[1]
16. Repeat procedure as needed.		
17. Discard disposable supplies with blood in infectious waste.	Prevents exposure to blood; Standard Precautions.	
18. Remove and discard personal protective equipment.	Decreases the transmission of microorganisms; Standard Precautions.	
19. **HH**		

*Level C: Qualitative studies, descriptive or correlational studies, integrative reviews, systematic reviews, or randomized controlled trials with inconsistent results

Expected Outcomes

- Patient infused with own blood in a timely manner
- Improved hemoglobin and hematocrit levels
- Improved oxygenation through increased oxygen-carrying capacity of blood
- Hemodynamic stability

Unexpected Outcomes

- Blood transfusion reaction
- Fluid overload

Patient Monitoring and Care

Steps	Rationale	Reportable Conditions
		These conditions should be reported if they persist despite nursing interventions.
1. Assess cardiopulmonary status and vital signs in 15 minutes, then hourly until 1 hour after the transfusion is completed.	Provides baseline and ongoing assessment of patient's condition.	• Tachypnea • Decreased or absent breath sounds • Hypoxemia • Tracheal deviation • Subcutaneous emphysema • Jugular vein distention • Muffled heart tones • Tachycardia • Hypotension • Dysrhythmias • Fever
2. Evaluate and maintain drainage tube patency every 2 to 4 hours.	In chest tubes, obstruction of drainage interferes with lung reexpansion.	• Inability to establish patency

Patient Monitoring and Care —*Continued*

Steps	Rationale	Reportable Conditions
3. Monitor amount and type of drainage from collection system hourly for 8 hours, then every 2 hours.	Volume loss can cause patients to become hypovolemic. Decreased or absent drainage associated with respiratory distress may indicate obstruction; decreased or absent drainage without respiratory distress may indicate lung reexpansion.	• Bloody drainage greater than 200 mL/hr • New onset of clots • Sudden decrease or absence of drainage
4. Mark the drainage level on the outside of the drainage-collection chamber in hourly or shift increments, and document in patient record.	Provides reference point for future measurements and assists in monitoring how quickly blood is accumulating for possible autotransfusion. Sudden flow of dark bloody drainage occurring with position change is often old blood that finds its way into the chest tube.	• Drainage greater than 200 mL/hr • Sudden decrease or absence of drainage • Change in characteristics of drainage
5. Monitor for blood transfusion reaction.	A patient undergoing autotransfusion is unlikely to have a blood transfusion reaction.	• Temperature increase to greater than 101°F (38.5°C)[2] • Chills • Tachycardia • Abdominal pain or back pain • Hypotension • Hematuria

Documentation

Documentation should include the following:
• Patient and family education
• Amount of drainage
• Amount of blood autotransfused
• Date and time when collection of blood started
• Date and time when transfusion started and ended

• Patient tolerance
• Unexpected outcomes
• Nursing interventions

References

CR 1. American Association of Blood Banks: *Guidelines for blood recovery and reinfusion in surgery and trauma*, Bethesda, MD, 1997, American Association of Blood Banks.
2. American Association of Blood Banks: *Technical manual*, ed 16, Bethesda, MD, 2008, American Association of Blood Banks.
CR 3. Purcell TB: Autotransfusion. In Roberts JR, Hedges JR, editors: *Clinical procedures in emergency medicine*, ed 4, Philadelphia, 2004, Saunders, 410-426.

Additional Readings

American Association of Blood Banks: *Guidance for standards for perioperative autologous blood collection and administration*, Bethesda, MD, 2002, American Association of Blood Banks.
Brown M, Whalen PK: Red blood cell transfusion in critically ill patients: emerging risks and alternatives, *Crit Care Nurse* (Suppl):1-14, Dec 2000.

Cross MH: Autotransfusion in cardiac surgery, *Perfusion* 16:391-400, 2001.
Dial S, Nguyen D, Menzies D: Autotransfusion of shed mediastinal blood: a risk factor for mediastinitis after cardiac surgery? Results of a cluster investigation, *Chest* 124(5):1847-1851, 2003.
Ley SJ: Intraoperative and postoperative blood salvage, *AACN Clin Issues* 7:238-248, 1996.
Oeltjen AM, Santrach PJ: Autologous transfusion techniques, *J Intraven Nurs* 20 :305-310, 1997.
Sirvinskas E, Veikutiene A, Benetis R, et al: Influence of early re-infusion of autologous shed mediastinal blood on clinical outcome after cardiac surgery, *Perfusion* 22(5):345-352, 2007.
Weniger J, von der Emde J, Schricker K, et al: [Autotransfusion of drainage blood after heart surgery (author's transl)], *Langenbecks Archiv Für Chirurgie* 351(4): 229-241, 1980.

AP Chest Tube Placement (Perform)

P U R P O S E : Chest tubes are placed for the removal or drainage of air, blood, or fluid from the intrapleural or mediastinal space. They also are used to introduce sclerosing agents into the pleural space to prevent a reaccumulation of fluid.

Paula A. Lusardi, Susan S. Scott, Finn Scott

PREREQUISITE NURSING KNOWLEDGE

• The thoracic cavity, in normal conditions, is a closed airspace. Any disruption results in the loss of negative pressure within the intrapleural space. Air or fluid that enters the space competes with the lung, resulting in collapse of the lung. Associated conditions are the result of disease, injury, surgery, or iatrogenic causes.

• Chest tubes are sterile flexible vinyl or silicone non-thrombogenic catheters approximately 20 inches (51 cm) long, varying in size from 12F to 40F. The size of the tube placed is determined by the condition. Chest tubes inserted for traumatic hemopneumothorax or hemothorax (blood) should be large (36F to 40F). Medium tubes (24F to 36F) should be used for fluid accumulation (pleural effusions). Tubes inserted for pneumothorax (air) should be small (12F to 24F).[2]

• Indications for chest tube insertion include the following:
  ❖ Pneumothorax (collection of air in the pleural space)
  ❖ Hemothorax (collection of blood)
  ❖ Hemopneumothorax (accumulation of air and blood in the pleural space)
  ❖ Tension pneumothorax

  ❖ Thoracotomy (e.g., open heart surgery, pneumonectomy)
  ❖ Pyothorax or empyema (collection of pus)
  ❖ Chylothorax (collection of chyle from the thoracic duct)
  ❖ Cholothorax (collection of fluid containing bile)
  ❖ Hydrothorax (collection of noninflammatory serous fluid)
  ❖ Pleural effusion

• A pneumothorax may be classified as an open, closed, or tension pneumothorax.
  ❖ *Open pneumothorax:* The chest wall and the pleural space are penetrated, which allows air to enter the pleural space, as in penetrating injury or trauma, surgical incision in the thoracic cavity (i.e., thoracotomy), or complication of surgical treatment (e.g., unintentional puncture during invasive procedures, such as thoracentesis or central venous catheter insertion).
  ❖ *Closed pneumothorax:* The pleural space is penetrated, but the chest wall is intact, which allows air to enter the pleural space from within the lung, as in spontaneous pneumothorax. A closed pneumothorax occurs without apparent injury and often is seen in individuals with chronic lung disorders (e.g., emphysema, cystic fibrosis, tuberculosis, necrotizing pneumonia); in young, tall men who have a greater than normal height-to-width chest ratio; after blunt traumatic injury; or iatrogenically, occurring as a complication of medical treatment (e.g., intermittent positive-pressure breathing [IPPB], mechanical ventilation with positive end-expiratory pressure [PEEP]).

❖ *Tension pneumothorax*: Air leaks into the pleural space through a tear in the lung and has no means to escape from the pleural cavity, creating a one-way valve effect. With each breath the patient takes, air accumulates, pressure within the pleural space increases, and the lung collapses. This condition causes the mediastinal structures (i.e., heart, great vessels, and trachea) to be compressed and shift to the opposite or unaffected side of the chest. Venous return and cardiac output are impeded, and collapse of the unaffected lung is possible. This life-threatening emergency requires prompt recognition and intervention.

❖ *Special applications*: Chest tubes can be used to instill anesthetic solutions and sclerosing agents.

• Lung that is densely adherent to the chest wall throughout the hemithorax is an absolute contraindication to chest tube therapy.[4]

• Use of chest tubes in patients with multiple adhesions, giant blebs, or coagulopathies is carefully considered; however, these relative contraindications are superseded by the need to reexpand the lung. When possible, any coagulopathy or platelet defect should be corrected before chest tube insertion. The differential diagnosis between a pneumothorax and bullous disease necessitates careful radiologic assessment.[4]

• The tube size and insertion site selected for the chest tube are determined by the indication.[4] If draining air, the tube is placed near the apex of the lung (second intercostal space); if draining fluid, the tube is placed near the base of the lung (fourth or fifth intercostal space; Fig. 20-1).

❖ When the tube is in place, the tube is sutured to the skin to prevent displacement, and an occlusive dressing is applied (see Fig. 21-1). The chest tube also is connected to a chest drainage system (see Procedure 24) to remove air and fluid from the pleural space,

which facilitates reexpansion of the collapsed lung. All connection points are secured with tape or zip ties (Parham-Martin bands) to ensure that the system remains airtight (see Fig. 21-2).

❖ The water-seal chamber should bubble gently immediately on insertion of the chest tube during expiration and with coughing. Continuous bubbling in this chamber indicates a leak within the patient or in the chest drainage system. Fluctuations in the water level in the water-seal chamber of 5 to 10 cm, rising during inhalation and falling during expiration, should be observed with spontaneous respirations. If the patient is on mechanical ventilation, the pattern of fluctuation is just the opposite. Any suction applied must be disconnected temporarily to assess correctly for fluctuations in the water-seal chamber.

❖ Mediastinal tubes generally are placed in the operating room by a surgeon after cardiac surgery.

EQUIPMENT

• Antiseptic solution or swab packets
• Caps, masks, sterile gloves, gowns, drapes
• Protective eyewear (goggles)
• Local anesthetic: 1% lidocaine solution (without epinephrine)
• Tube thoracotomy insertion tray
  ❖ Sterile towels, 4 × 4 sterile gauze
  ❖ Scalpel with no. 10 blade
  ❖ Two Kelly clamps, curved clamps
  ❖ Needle holder
  ❖ Monofilament or silk suture material with cutting needle
• Sterile basin or medicine cup
• Suture scissors
• Two hemostats
• 10-mL syringe with 20-gauge 1½-inch needle
• 5-mL syringe with 25-gauge 1-inch needle
• Thoracotomy tubes (12F to 40F, as appropriate)
• Closed chest drainage system
• Suction source
• Suction connector and connecting tubing (usually 6 feet for each tube)
• 1-inch adhesive tape or zip ties (Parham-Martin bands)
• Dressing materials
  ❖ 4 × 4 gauze pads
  ❖ Slit drain sponges
  ❖ Petrolatum gauze
  ❖ Tape
  ❖ Commercial securing device

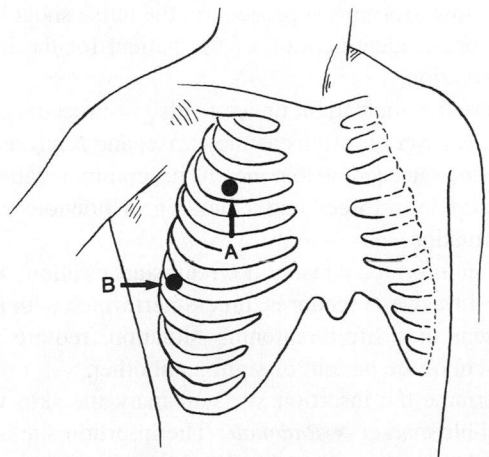

FIGURE 20-1 Standard sites for tube thoracostomy. **A,** The second intercostal space, midclavicular line. **B,** The fourth or fifth intercostal space, midaxillary line. Most clinicians prefer midaxillary line placement for all chest tubes, regardless of pathology. Placement of the tube too far posteriorly does not allow the patient to lie down comfortably. *(From Roberts JR, Hedges JR, editors: Clinicals in emergency medicine, ed 4, Philadelphia, 2004, Saunders.)*

PATIENT AND FAMILY EDUCATION

• Explain the procedure (if patient condition and circumstances allow) and the reason for the chest tube insertion.
  ➥*Rationale:* This communication identifies patient and family knowledge deficits concerning the patient's condition, expected benefits, and potential risks and allows

time for questions to clarify information and to voice concerns. Explanations decrease patient anxiety and enhance cooperation.

- Explain that the patient's participation during the procedure is to remain as immobile as possible and do relaxed breathing. ➠*Rationale:* This explanation facilitates insertion of the chest tube and prevents complications during insertion.
- After the procedure, instruct the patient to sit in a semi-Fowler's position (unless contraindicated). ➠*Rationale:* This position facilitates drainage from the lung by allowing air to rise and fluid to settle to be removed via the chest tube. This position also makes breathing easier.
- Instruct the patient to turn and change position every 2 hours. The patient may lie on the side with the chest tube but should keep the tubing free of kinks. ➠*Rationale:* Turning and changing position prevent complications related to immobility and retained pulmonary secretions. Keeping the tube free of kinks maintains patency of the tube, facilitates drainage, and prevents the accumulation of pressure within the pleural space that interferes with lung reexpansion.
- Instruct the patient to cough and deep breathe, with splinting of the affected side. ➠*Rationale:* Coughing and deep breathing increase pressure within the pleural space, facilitating drainage, promoting lung reexpansion, and preventing respiratory complications associated with retained secretions. The application of firm pressure over the chest tube insertion site (i.e., splinting) decreases pain and discomfort.
- Encourage active or passive range-of-motion exercises of the arm on the affected side. ➠*Rationale:* The patient may limit movement of the arm on the affected side to decrease the discomfort at the insertion site, which results in joint discomfort and potential joint contractures.
- Instruct the patient and family about activity as prescribed while maintaining the drainage system below the level of the chest. ➠*Rationale:* This activity facilitates gravity drainage and prevents backflow and potential infectious contamination into the pleural space.
- Instruct the patient about the availability of prescribed analgesic medication and other pain relief strategies. ➠*Rationale:* Pain relief ensures comfort and facilitates coughing, deep breathing, positioning, range of motion, and recuperation.

PATIENT ASSESSMENT AND PREPARATION

Patient Assessment

- Assess for significant medical history or injury, including chronic lung disease, spontaneous pneumothorax, hemothorax, pulmonary disease, therapeutic procedures, and mechanism of injury. ➠*Rationale:* Medical history or injury may provide the etiologic basis for the occurrence of pneumothorax, empyema, pleural effusion, or chylothorax.
- Evaluate diagnostic test results (if patient's condition does not necessitate immediate intervention), including

chest radiograph and arterial blood gases. ➠*Rationale:* Diagnostic testing confirms the presence of air or fluid in the pleural space, a collapsed lung, hypoxemia, and respiratory compromise.

- Perform hand hygiene. ➠*Rationale:* Reduces the transmission of microorganisms and body secretions (Standard Precautions).
- Assess baseline cardiopulmonary status for signs and symptoms that necessitate chest tube insertion[3]:
  - ❖ Tachypnea
  - ❖ Decreased or absent breath sounds on affected side
  - ❖ Crackles adjacent to the affected area
  - ❖ Shortness of breath, dyspnea
  - ❖ Asymmetrical chest excursion with respirations
  - ❖ Cyanosis
  - ❖ Decreased oxygen saturation
  - ❖ Hyperresonance in the affected side (pneumothorax)
  - ❖ Subcutaneous emphysema (pneumothorax)
  - ❖ Dullness or flatness in the affected side (hemothorax, pleural effusion, empyema, chylothorax)
  - ❖ Sudden, sharp chest pain
  - ❖ Anxiety, restlessness, apprehension
  - ❖ Tachycardia
  - ❖ Hypotension
  - ❖ Dysrhythmias
  - ❖ Tracheal deviation to the unaffected side (tension pneumothorax)
  - ❖ Neck vein distention (tension pneumothorax)
  - ❖ Muffled heart sounds (tension pneumothorax)

➠*Rationale:* Accurate assessment of signs and symptoms allows for prompt recognition and treatment. Baseline assessment provides comparison data for evaluation of changes and outcomes of treatment.

Patient Preparation

- Verify correct patient with two identifiers. ➠*Rationale:* Prior to performing a procedure, the nurse should ensure the correct identification of the patient for the intended intervention.
- Ensure that the patient understands pre-procedural teachings. Answer questions as they arise, and reinforce information as needed. ➠*Rationale:* This communication evaluates and reinforces understanding of previously taught information.
- Obtain informed consent if circumstances allow. ➠*Rationale:* Invasive procedures, unless performed with implied consent in a life-threatening situation, require written consent of the patient or significant other.
- Determine the insertion site and mark the skin with an indelible marker. ➠*Rationale:* The insertion site is determined by the indication for the chest tube. For air, use the second intercostal space; for fluid, use the fifth or sixth intercostal space.
- Determine the size of chest tube needed. ➠*Rationale:* Evacuation of air necessitates a smaller tube; evacuation of fluid necessitates larger tubes.
- Assist the patient to the lateral, supine (for pneumothorax), or semi-Fowler's position (for hemothorax).[6]

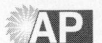

Rationale: This positioning enhances accessibility to the insertion site for positioning of the chest tube.

- Administer prescribed analgesics or sedatives as needed; follow institutional policy for moderate or procedural sedation. *Rationale:* Analgesics and sedatives reduce the discomfort and anxiety experienced and facilitate patient cooperation.

- Administer oxygen and monitor pulse oximeter or end-tidal carbon dioxide level. *Rationale:* Real-time assessment of patient's respiratory status during the procedure is provided.

- Ensure patient has a patent intravenous (IV) access. *Rationale:* This access provides a route for analgesic, sedation, and emergency medications.

Procedure for Performing Chest Tube Placement

Steps	Rationale	Special Considerations
1. Perform a preprocedure verification and time-out, if non-emergent.	Ensures patient safety.	
2. **HH**		
3. **PE**		*Chest tube insertion is a sterile procedure and requires full surgical attire, unless performed in a life-threatening situation.*
4. Have an assistant open the outer wrapper of the tube thoracotomy insertion tray, remove the tray from wrapper, and open it with sterile technique.	Reduces transmission of microorganisms.	
5. Prepare equipment. A. Check that all equipment is present. B. Have an assistant pour antiseptic solution into the sterile cup or basin with aseptic technique (or open the swab packet and stand by). C. Have an assistant open the chest tube package and empty it onto the open tray. D. Grasp suture needle with needle holder. E. Remove the trocar from the chest tube and grasp the proximal end of the chest tube with a large Kelly clamp. F. Prepare the syringe with lidocaine solution.	Facilitates insertion of the tube.	
6. Identify the insertion site and have an assistant position the patient. **(Level E*)**	Assists in preparation of area for insertion and proper placement of tube.[5]	Insertion site for air removal is right or left second intercostal space. Insertion site for fluid removal is right or left fifth or sixth intercostal space, midaxillary line. Incision site is one rib below insertion site (see Fig. 20-1).
7. Surgically prepare the skin with antiseptic solution, and drape the area surrounding the insertion site. **(Level E)**	Inhibits growth of bacteria at insertion site; maintains sterility.[5]	Prepare the area from the clavicle to the umbilicus, mid-chest to anterior axillary line.

*Level E: Multiple case reports, theory-based evidence from expert opinions, or peer-reviewed professional organizational standards without clinical studies to support recommendations

Procedure continues on following page

Procedure | for Performing Chest Tube Placement—*Continued*

Steps	Rationale	Special Considerations

8. Anesthetize the skin, subcutaneous tissue, muscle, and periosteum with 1% lidocaine solution.
  A. With a 5-mL syringe (25-gauge needle), inject a subcutaneous wheal of lidocaine at the insertion site.
  B. With a 10-mL syringe (20-gauge, 1½–inch needle), advance the needle/syringe, aspirating as you go, until air or pleural fluid is confirmed.
Inject the lidocaine deeper, and slowly withdraw the syringe, generously anesthetizing rib periosteum, subcutaneous tissue, and pleura (Fig. 20-2). **(Level D*)**
	Results in loss of sensation and decreased pain during insertion.[5]	When infiltrating with lidocaine, aspirate as you go to confirm the presence of air or fluid; 30 to 40 mL of lidocaine may be needed for anesthesia.

9. With a no. 10 blade, make a 3-cm transverse skin incision directly over the inferior aspect of the anesthetized rib below the insertion site (Fig. 20-3). **(Level E*)**	Allows for the diameter of the chest tube.[5]	When making the incision, incise down through the subcutaneous tissue; the space should be large enough to admit a finger.

*Level D: Peer-reviewed professional organizational standards with clinical studies to support recommendations

*Level E: Multiple case reports, theory-based evidence from expert opinions, or peer-reviewed professional organizational standards without clinical studies to support recommendations

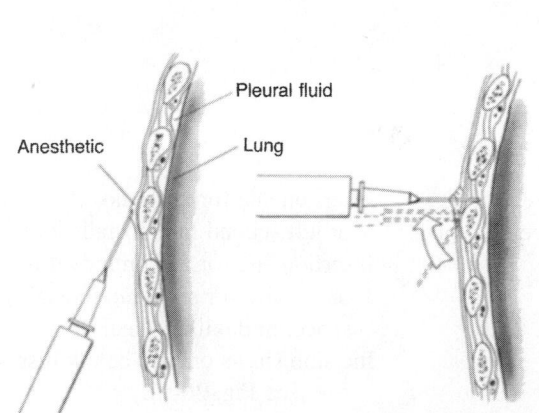

FIGURE 20-2   Insertion of a chest tube can be relatively painless with proper infiltration of the skin and pleura with local anesthetic. The liberal use of buffered 1% lidocaine without epinephrine (maximal lidocaine dose, 5 mg/kg) is recommended. *(From Roberts JR, Hedges JR, editors: Clinicals in emergency medicine, ed 4, Philadelphia, 2004, Saunders.)*

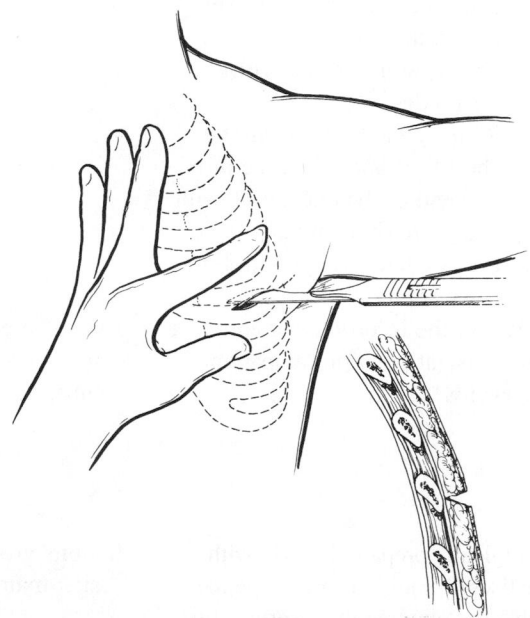

FIGURE 20-3   Transverse skin incision is made directly over the inferior aspect of the anesthetized rib down to the subcutaneous tissue. *(From Dumire SM, Paris PM: Atlas of emergency procedures, Philadelphia, 1994, Saunders.)*

Procedure for Performing Chest Tube Placement—*Continued*

Steps	Rationale	Special Considerations
10. Introduce the curved clamp through the incision, with the tips down, creating a tunnel through the subcutaneous tissue and muscle; use an opening and spreading maneuver; aim toward the superior aspect of the rib until the pleural space is reached (Fig. 20-4). **(Level E*)**	Facilitates insertion of the tube. Blunt dissection minimizes trauma to the neurovascular bundle.[5]	Additional lidocaine is infiltrated as needed. The direction of the tunnel created through the subcutaneous tissue and muscle determines the direction the chest tube takes after insertion. Be sure the clamp stays close to the ribs to avoid injury to the neurovascular bundle.
11. When the clamp is just over the superior portion of the rib, close the clamp and push it with steady pressure through the parietal pleura and into the pleural space. Widen the hole in the pleural space by spreading the clamp (Fig. 20-5). **(Level E)**	Ensures opening is large enough for the chest tube. Steady, even, controlled pressure provides control of the clamp once the pleura is perforated.[5]	This maneuver necessitates more pressure than might be anticipated. A lunging motion or use of the trocar, however, may cause a hole in lung or injury to the liver or spleen.
12. Insert the index finger to dilate the tract and hole in the pleura.	Relieves air or fluid when penetration of the space is made. Ensures entry into the pleural space and not into a space inadvertently created between the parietal pleura and chest wall.[5]	Feel for lung tissue (lung should expand and meet finger on inspiration), diaphragm, or adhesions. Break up clot, if found.

*Level E: Multiple case reports, theory-based evidence from expert opinions, or peer-reviewed professional organizational standards without clinical studies to support recommendations

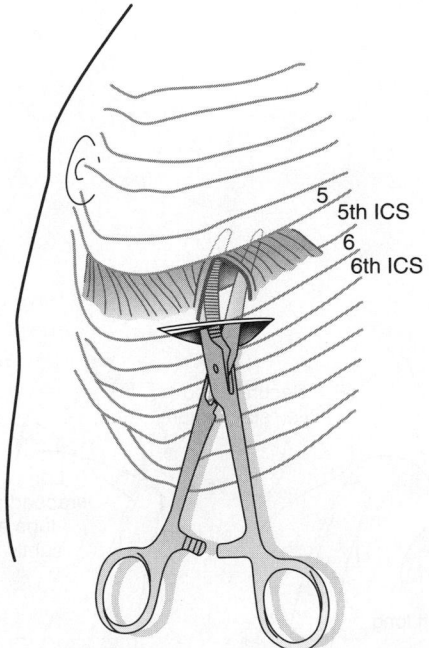

FIGURE 20-4 Blunt dissection is accomplished with forcing a closed clamp through the incision and using an opening-and-spreading maneuver to create a tunnel to the pleura. *ICS,* Intercostal space.

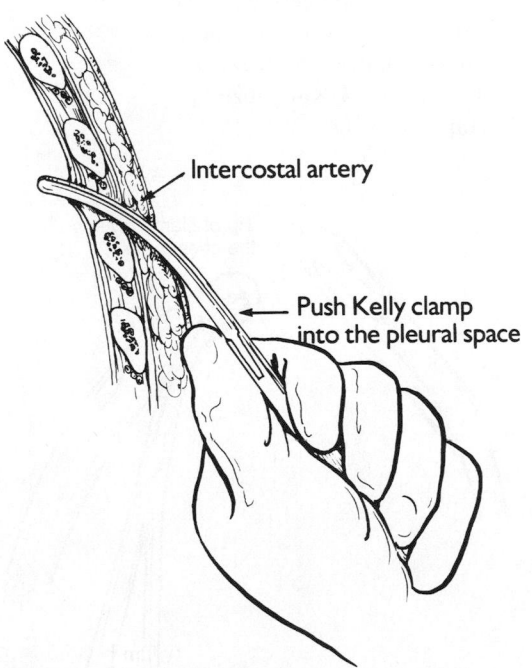

FIGURE 20-5 Just over the superior portion of the rib, close the clamp and push with steady pressure into the pleura. *(From Dumire SM, Paris PM: Atlas of emergency procedures, Philadelphia, 1994, Saunders.)*

Procedure continues on following page

Procedure for Performing Chest Tube Placement—*Continued*

Steps	Rationale	Special Considerations
13. Insert the chest tube into the chest cavity with a curved Kelly clamp, holding the proximal end to guide the tip into the pleural space (Fig. 20-6). Remove the clamp and guide the tube, in a rotating motion, through the tract and into the space. The tube is advanced until the last hole is in the pleural space. Condensation of air or fluid in the tube should be noted.	Confirms placement of the tube.	To drain air, aim the tube posteriorly and superiorly toward the apex of the lung; to drain fluid, aim the tube inferiorly and posteriorly. Do not allow any side holes of the tube to remain outside the thoracic cavity.
14. Connect the chest tube to the closed chest drainage system (see Procedure 24) and check for rise and fall (tidaling) of the H_2O column. Assistant applies ordered amount of suction.	Ensures the tube is properly positioned.	
15. Suture the tube to the chest wall. Wrap the free ends of the suture around the tube (similar to lacing a shoe). Tie the ends of the suture snugly around the top of the tube (Fig. 20-7).	Secures the position of the tube.[3] Sutures should be snug to prevent free air from passing into the subcutaneous tissue.	Type of stitch used depends on the individual; the goal is to prevent displacement of the chest tube.
16. Apply occlusive dressing. A. Petrolatum gauze is used around the chest tube, or follow institutional standards. B. Split drain sponges are placed around the chest tube, one from top, one underneath. C. Cover with 4 × 4 gauze. D. Tape dressing.	Provides airtight seal around the chest tube.[5,6]	

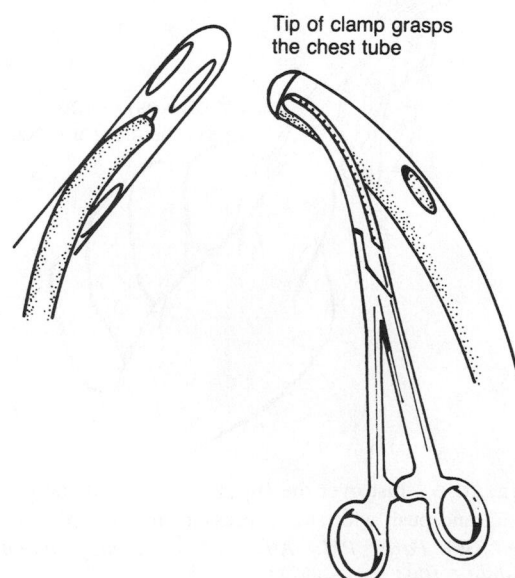

FIGURE 20-6   The tube is grasped with the curved clamp, with the tube tip protruding from the jaws. (*From Roberts JR, Hedges JR, editors: Clinicals in emergency medicine, ed 4, Philadelphia, 2004, Saunders.*)

Tip of clamp grasps the chest tube

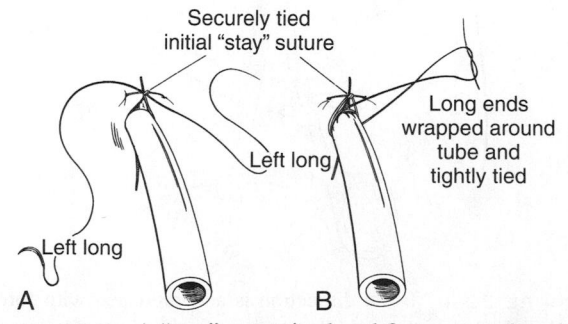

Securely tied initial "stay" suture

Left long

Left long

Long ends wrapped around tube and tightly tied

A   B

FIGURE 20-7   A "stay" suture is placed first next to the tube to close the skin incision. **A,** The knot is tied securely, and the ends, which subsequently are wrapped around the chest tube, are left long. **B,** The ends of the suture are wound twice about the tube, tightly enough to indent the tube slightly, and are tied securely. (*From Roberts JR, Hedges JR, editors: Clinicals in emergency medicine, ed 4, Philadelphia, 2004, Saunders.*)

Procedure for Performing Chest Tube Placement—*Continued*

Steps	Rationale	Special Considerations
17. Tape all connection points to the drainage system or secure with zip ties (Parham-Martin bands). **(Level E*)**	Creates an airtight system. Airtight connections prevent air leaks into the pleural space.[1,3]	Check that all tube drainage holes are in the pleural space.
18. Secure the tube below the dressing to the patient's skin with a commercial securing device or tape.	Functions as a strain relief to prevent tube and dressing dislodgment.	
19. Obtain a chest radiograph. **(Level E)**	Chest radiograph confirms placement of tube and expansion of lung and removal of fluid.[1]	Document result of chest radiograph in the patient's record.
20. Dispose of equipment.		
21. Remove personal protective equipment.	Reduces the transmission of microorganisms and body secretions; Standard Precautions.	
22. **HH**		

*Level E: Multiple case reports, theory-based evidence from expert opinions, or peer-reviewed professional organizational standards without clinical studies to support recommendations

Expected Outcomes

- Removal of air, fluid, or blood from the pleural space
- Relief of respiratory distress
- Reexpansion of the lung (validated with chest radiograph)
- Restoration of negative pressure within the pleural space

Unexpected Outcomes

- Hemorrhage or shock
- Increasing respiratory distress
- Infection
- Damage to intercostal nerve that results in neuropathy or neuritis
- Incorrect tube placement
- Chest tube kinking, clogging, or dislodgment from chest wall
- Subcutaneous emphysema

Patient Monitoring and Care

Steps	Rationale	Reportable Conditions
		These conditions should be reported if they persist despite nursing interventions.
1. Assess cardiopulmonary and vital signs every 1 to 4 hours and as needed.	Provides baseline and ongoing assessment of patient's condition. Abnormalities can indicate recurrence of the condition that necessitated chest tube insertion. On the basis of the patient's clinical condition or physician orders, vital signs may need to be checked more frequently.	Tachypnea Decreased or absent breath Hypoxemia Tracheal deviation Subcutaneous emphysema Neck vein distention Muffled heart tones Tachycardia Hypotension Dysrhythmias Fever
2. Monitor output every 1 to 4 hours, and record amount and color.	Provides data for diagnosis. Higher drainage amounts require more frequent assessment. On the basis of the patient's clinical condition or physician orders, output may need to be checked more frequently.	Bloody drainage greater than or equal to 200 mL/hr Sudden cessation of drainage Change in character of drainage

Procedure continues on following page

Patient Monitoring and Care —*Continued*

Steps	Rationale	Reportable Conditions
3. Assess for pain at the insertion site or for chest discomfort. **(Level D*)**	Pain interferes with adequate deep breathing. Pain at insertion site, particularly with inspiration, may indicate improper tube placement.[5]	Continued pain despite pain interventions.
4. Evaluate the chest drainage system for rise and fall (tidaling) in water-seal chamber. Check connections. **(Level E*)**	Water level normally rises and falls with respiration until lung is expanded. Bubbling immediately after insertion signifies that air is being removed from the pleural space; bubbling with exhalation and coughing is normal. Persistent bubbling indicates an air leak either in the patient's lung or in the chest drainage system.[8]	Absence of tidaling in water-seal chamber Persistent bubbling
5. Assess insertion site and surrounding skin with daily dressing change for presence of subcutaneous emphysema and signs of infection or inflammation.	Skin integrity is altered during insertion, which can lead to infection.[7]	Fever Redness around insertion site Purulent drainage Subcutaneous emphysema

*Level D: Peer-reviewed professional organizational standards with clinical studies to support recommendations
*Level E: Multiple case reports, theory-based evidence from expert opinions, or peer-reviewed professional organizational standards without clinical studies to support recommendations

Documentation

Documentation should include the following:
- Patient and family education
- Reason for chest tube insertion
- Respiratory and vital sign assessment before and after insertion
- Description of procedure, including tube size, date and time of insertion, insertion site, and any complications associated with procedure
- Type and amount of drainage
- Presence of fluctuation and bubbling
- Amount of suction
- Patient's tolerance to procedure
- Postinsertion chest radiograph results
- Unexpected outcomes
- Nursing interventions
- Pain assessment, interventions, and effectiveness

References

CR 1. Buchman TG, Hall BL, Bowling WM, et al: *Thoracic trauma.* In Tininalli JE, Kelen DG, Stapczynski JS, editors: *Emergency medicine: a comprehensive guide,* ed 6, New York, 2004, McGraw-Hill, 1595-1612.

2. Dev SP, Nascimiento B, Simone C, et al: Chest-tube insertion, *N Engl J Med* 357:e15, 2007.

3. Irwin RS, Rippe JM: *Intensive care medicine,* Philadelphia, 2008, Wolters Kluwer/Lippincott & Williams & Wilkins.

CR 4. Laws D, Neville E, Duffy J: BTS guidelines for insertion of a chest drain, *Thorax* 58(Suppl II):ii53-ii59, 2003.

5. May G, Bartram T: The use of intrapleural anaesthetic to reduce the pain of chest drain insertion, *Emerg Med J* 24:300-301, 2007.

CR 6. Roberts: *Clinical procedures in emergency medicine,* ed 4, Philadelphia, 2004, Saunders.

7. Sullivan B: Nursing management of patients with a chest drain, *Br J Nurs* 17(6):388-393, 2008.

CR 8. Thompson JM, McFarland GK, Hirsh JE et al: *Mosby's clinical nursing,* ed 5, St Louis, 2002, Mosby.

Additional Readings

Argall J: Seldinger technique chest drains and complication rate, *Emerg Med J* 20:169-170, 2003.

Charnock Y, Evans D: Nursing management of chest drains: a systematic review, *Aust Crit Care* 14:156-160, 2001.

Coughlin AM, Parchinsky C: Go with the flow of chest tube therapy, *Nursing* 36:36-42, 2006.

Ellis H: The applied anatomy of chest drain insertion, *Br J Hosp Med* (London) 68:M44-45, 2007.

Frankel TL, Hill PC, Stamou SC, et al: Silastic drains vs conventional chest tubes after coronary artery bypass, *Chest* 124:108-113, 2003.

Gareeboo S, Singh S: Tube thoracostomy: how to insert a chest drain, *Br J Hosp Med* (London) 67:M16-18, 2006.

Lehwaldt D, Timmins F: Nurses' knowledge of chest drain care: an exploratory descriptive survey, *Nurs Crit Care* 10:192-200, 2005.

Zgoda MA, Lunn W, Ashiku S, et al: Minimally invasive techniques: direct visual guidance for chest tube placement through a single-port thoracoscopy: a novel technique, *Chest* 127:1805-1807, 2005.

Chest Tube Placement (Assist)

P U R P O S E : Chest tubes are placed for the removal or drainage of air, blood, or fluid from the intrapleural or mediastinal space. They also are used to introduce sclerosing agents into the pleural space to prevent a reaccumulation of fluid.

Susan S. Scott, Paula A. Lusardi, Finn Scott

PREREQUISITE NURSING KNOWLEDGE

- The thoracic cavity, in normal conditions, is a closed airspace. Any disruption results in the loss of negative pressure within the intrapleural space. Air or fluid that enters the space competes with the lung, resulting in collapse of the lung. Associated conditions are the result of disease, injury, surgery, or iatrogenic causes.

- Chest tubes are sterile flexible vinyl or silicone nonthrombogenic catheters approximately 20 inches (51 cm) long, varying in size from 12F to 40F. The size of the tube placed is determined by the condition. Chest tubes inserted for traumatic hemopneumothorax or hemothorax (blood) should be large (36F to 40F). Medium tubes (24F to 36F) should be used for fluid accumulation (pleural effusions). Tubes inserted for pneumothorax (air) should be small (12F to 24F).[2]

- Indications for chest tube insertion include the following:
  - ❖ Pneumothorax (collection of air in the pleural space)
  - ❖ Hemothorax (collection of blood)
  - ❖ Hemopneumothorax (accumulation of air and blood in the pleural space)
  - ❖ Tension pneumothorax
  - ❖ Thoracotomy (e.g., open heart surgery, pneumonectomy)
  - ❖ Pyothorax or empyema (collection of pus)
  - ❖ Chylothorax (collection of chyle from the thoracic duct)
  - ❖ Cholothorax (collection of fluid containing bile)
  - ❖ Hydrothorax (collection of noninflammatory serous fluid)
  - ❖ Pleural effusion

- A pneumothorax may be classified as an open, closed, or tension pneumothorax.
  - ❖ *Open pneumothorax*: The chest wall and the pleural space are penetrated, which allows air to enter the pleural space, as in a penetrating injury or trauma; a surgical incision in the thoracic cavity (i.e., thoracotomy); or a complication of surgical treatment (e.g., unintentional puncture during invasive procedures, such as thoracentesis or central venous catheter insertion).
  - ❖ *Closed pneumothorax*: The pleural space is penetrated, but the chest wall is intact, which allows air to enter the pleural space from within the lung, as in spontaneous pneumothorax. A closed pneumothorax occurs without apparent injury and often is seen in individuals with chronic lung disorders (e.g., emphysema, cystic fibrosis, tuberculosis, necrotizing pneumonia) and in young tall men who have a greater than normal height-to-width chest ratio; after blunt traumatic injury; or iatrogenically, occurring as a complication of medical treatment (e.g., intermittent positive-pressure breathing [IPPB], mechanical ventilation with positive end-expiratory pressure [PEEP]).
  - ❖ *Tension pneumothorax:* Air leaks into the pleural space through a tear in the lung and has no means to escape from the pleural cavity, creating a one-way valve effect. With each breath the patient takes, air accumulates, pressure within the pleural space increases, and the lung collapses. This condition causes the mediastinal structures (i.e., heart, great vessels, and trachea) to be compressed and shift to the opposite or unaffected side of the chest. Venous return and cardiac output are impeded, and collapse of the unaffected lung is possible. This

life-threatening emergency requires prompt recognition and intervention.

  ❖ *Special applications*: Chest tubes can be used to instill anesthetic solutions and sclerosing agents.

• Lung that is densely adherent to the chest wall throughout the hemithorax is an absolute contraindication to chest tube therapy.

• Use of chest tubes in patients with multiple adhesions, giant blebs, or coagulopathies is carefully considered; however, these relative contraindications are superseded by the need to reexpand the lung. When possible, any coagulopathy or platelet defect should be corrected before chest tube insertion. The differential diagnosis between a pneumothorax and bullous disease necessitates careful radiologic assessment.[4]

• The tube size and insertion site selected for the chest tube are determined by the indication.[4] If draining air, the tube is placed near the apex of the lung (second intercostal space); if draining fluid, the tube is placed near the base of the lung (fifth or sixth intercostal space; see Fig. 20-1).

• When the tube is in place, the tube is sutured to the skin to prevent displacement, and an occlusive dressing is applied (Fig. 21-1). The chest tube also is connected to a chest drainage system (see Procedure 24) to remove air and fluid from the pleural space, which facilitates reexpansion of the collapsed lung. All connection points are secured with tape or zip ties (Parham-Martin bands) to ensure that the system remains airtight (Fig. 21-2).

• The water-seal chamber should bubble gently immediately on insertion of the chest tube during expiration and with coughing. Continuous bubbling in this chamber indicates a leak within the patient or in the chest drainage system. Fluctuations in the water level in the water-seal chamber of 5 to 10 cm, rising during inhalation and falling during expiration, should be observed with spontaneous respirations. If the patient is on mechanical ventilation, the pattern of fluctuation is just the opposite. Any suction applied must be disconnected temporarily to assess correctly for fluctuations in the water-seal chamber.

• Mediastinal tubes generally are placed in the operating room by a surgeon after cardiac surgery.

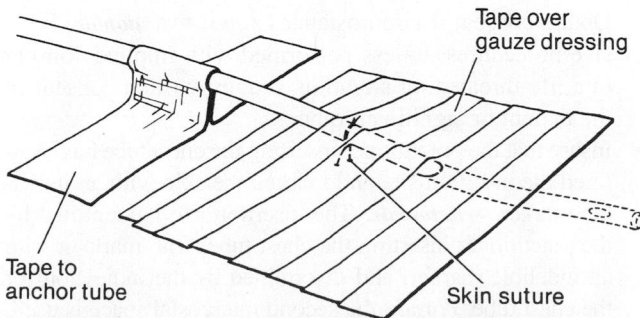

FIGURE 21-1 Occlusive chest tube dressing. *(From Kersten LD: Comprehensive respiratory nursing, Philadelphia, 1989, Saunders.)*

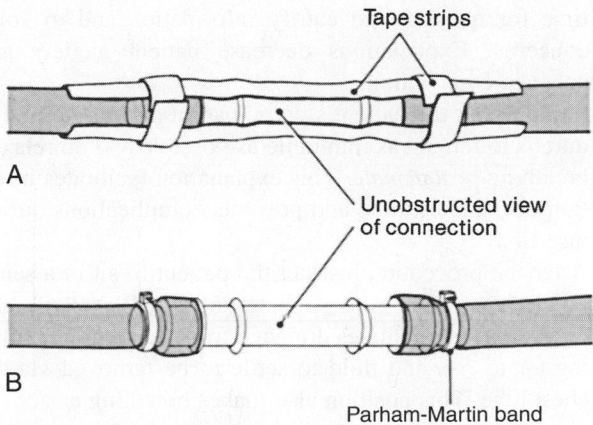

FIGURE 21-2 The securing of connection points. **A,** Tape. **B,** Parham-Martin bands. *(From Kersten LD: Comprehensive respiratory nursing, Philadelphia, 1989, Saunders.)*

EQUIPMENT

• Antiseptic solution or antiseptic swab packets
• Caps, masks, sterile gloves, gowns, drapes
• Protective eyewear (goggles)
• Local anesthetic: 1% lidocaine solution (without epinephrine)
• Tube thoracotomy tray
  ❖ Sterile towels, 4 × 4 sterile gauze
  ❖ Scalpel with no. 10 blade
  ❖ Two Kelly clamps, curved clamps
  ❖ Needle holder
  ❖ Monofilament or silk suture material with cutting needle
  ❖ Sterile basin or medicine cup
  ❖ Suture scissors
  ❖ Two hemostats
  ❖ 10-mL syringe with 20-gauge, 1½-inch needle
  ❖ 5-mL syringe with 25-gauge, 1-inch needle
• Thoracotomy tubes (12F to 40F, as appropriate)
• Closed chest drainage system
• Suction source
• Suction connector and connecting tubing (usually 6 feet for each tube)
• Y connector
• 1-inch adhesive tape or zip ties (Parham-Martin bands)
• Dressing materials
  ❖ 4 × 4 gauze pads
  ❖ Slit drain sponges
  ❖ Petrolatum gauze
  ❖ Tape
• Commercial securing device

PATIENT AND FAMILY EDUCATION

• Explain the procedure (if patient condition and circumstances allow) and the reason for the chest tube insertion.
  ➡️*Rationale:* This communication identifies patient and family knowledge deficits concerning the patient's condition, expected benefits, and potential risks and allows

time for questions to clarify information and to voice concerns. Explanations decrease patient anxiety and enhance cooperation.

- Explain that the patient's participation during the procedure is to remain as immobile as possible and do relaxed breathing. ➥*Rationale:* This explanation facilitates insertion of the chest tube and prevents complications during insertion.
- After the procedure, instruct the patient to sit in a semi-Fowler's position (unless contraindicated). ➥*Rationale:* This position facilitates drainage from the lung by allowing air to rise and fluid to settle to be removed via the chest tube. This position also makes breathing easier.
- Instruct the patient to turn and change position every 2 hours. The patient may lie on the side with the chest tube but should keep the tubing free of kinks. ➥*Rationale:* Turning and changing position prevent complications related to immobility and retained pulmonary secretions. Keeping the tube free of kinks maintains patency of the tube, facilitates drainage, and prevents the accumulation of pressure within the pleural space that interferes with lung reexpansion.
- Instruct the patient to cough and deep breathe, with splinting of the affected side. ➥*Rationale:* Coughing and deep breathing increase pressure within the pleural space, facilitating drainage, promoting lung reexpansion, and preventing respiratory complications associated with retained secretions. The application of firm pressure over the chest tube insertion site (i.e., splinting) decreases pain and discomfort.
- Encourage active or passive range-of-motion exercises of the arm on the affected side. ➥*Rationale:* The patient may limit movement of the arm on the affected side to decrease the discomfort at the insertion site, which results in joint discomfort and potential joint contractures.
- Instruct the patient and family about activity as prescribed while maintaining the drainage system below the level of the chest. ➥*Rationale:* This activity facilitates gravity drainage and prevents backflow and potential infectious contamination into the pleural space.
- Instruct the patient about the availability of prescribed analgesic medication and other pain relief strategies. ➥*Rationale:* Pain relief ensures comfort and facilitates coughing, deep breathing, positioning, range of motion, and recuperation.

PATIENT ASSESSMENT AND PREPARATION

Patient Assessment

- Assess significant medical history or injury, including chronic lung disease, spontaneous pneumothorax, hemothorax, pulmonary disease, therapeutic procedures, and mechanism of injury. ➥*Rationale:* Medical history or injury may provide the etiologic basis for the occurrence of pneumothorax, empyema, pleural effusion, or chylothorax.

- Evaluate diagnostic test results (if patient's condition does not necessitate immediate intervention), including chest radiograph and arterial blood gases. ➥*Rationale:* Diagnostic testing confirms the presence of air or fluid in the pleural space, a collapsed lung, hypoxemia, and respiratory compromise.
- Perform hand hygiene. ➥*Rationale:* Reduces the transmission of microorganisms and body secretions (Standard Precautions).
- Assess baseline cardiopulmonary status for signs and symptoms that necessitate chest tube insertion[8]:
  - ❖ Tachypnea
  - ❖ Decreased or absent breath sounds on affected side
  - ❖ Crackles adjacent to the affected area
  - ❖ Shortness of breath, dyspnea
  - ❖ Asymmetrical chest excursion with respirations
  - ❖ Cyanosis
  - ❖ Decreased oxygen saturation
  - ❖ Hyperresonance in the affected side (pneumothorax)
  - ❖ Subcutaneous emphysema (pneumothorax)
  - ❖ Dullness or flatness in the affected side (hemothorax, pleural effusion, empyema, chylothorax)
  - ❖ Sudden, sharp chest pain
  - ❖ Anxiety, restlessness, apprehension
  - ❖ Tachycardia
  - ❖ Hypotension
  - ❖ Dysrhythmias
  - ❖ Tracheal deviation to the unaffected side (tension pneumothorax)
  - ❖ Neck vein distention (tension pneumothorax)
  - ❖ Muffled heart sounds (tension pneumothorax)
  ➥*Rationale:* Accurate assessment of signs and symptoms allows for prompt recognition and treatment. Baseline assessment provides comparison data for evaluation of changes and outcomes of treatment.

Patient Preparation

- Verify correct patient with two identifiers. ➥*Rationale:* Prior to performing a procedure, the nurse should ensure the correct identification of the patient for the intended intervention.
- Ensure that the patient understands preprocedural teachings. Answer questions as they arise, and reinforce information as needed. ➥*Rationale:* This communication evaluates and reinforces understanding of previously taught information.
- Obtain consent if circumstances allow. ➥*Rationale:* Invasive procedures, unless performed with implied consent in a life-threatening situation, require written consent of the patient or significant other.
- Insure that the practitioner inserting the chest tube has identified the insertion site and marked the skin with an indelible marker. ➥*Rationale:* The insertion site is identified by the practitioner inserting the chest tube, who marks it with an indelible marker, and determined by the indication for the chest tube. For air, the second intercostal space is used; for fluid, the fifth or sixth intercostal space is used.
- Consult with the practitioner for the appropriate size chest tube to be inserted. ➥*Rationale:* Evacuation of air

necessitates a smaller tube; evacuation of fluid necessitates larger tubes.

- Assist the patient to the lateral, supine (for pneumothorax), or semi-Fowler's position (for hemothorax).[6] ➤*Rationale:* This positioning enhances accessibility to the insertion site for positioning of the chest tube.
- Administer prescribed analgesics or sedatives as needed; follow institutional policy for moderate or procedural sedation. ➤*Rationale:* Analgesics and sedatives reduce

the discomfort and anxiety experienced and facilitate patient cooperation.

- Administer oxygen and monitor pulse oximeter or end-tidal carbon dioxide level. ➤*Rationale:* Real-time assessment of patient's respiratory status during the procedure is provided.
- Ensure patient has a patent intravenous (IV) access. ➤*Rationale:* This access provides a route for analgesic, sedation, and emergency medications.

Procedure for Assisting With Chest Tube Placement

Steps	Rationale	Special Considerations
1. Perform a pre-procedure verification and time out, if nonemergent.	Ensures patient safety.	
2. **HH**		
3. **PE**		*Chest tube insertion is a sterile procedure and requires full surgical attire, unless performed in a life-threatening situation.*
4. Open the chest tube insertion tray with sterile technique.	Reduces transmission of microorganisms.	
5. Assist with preparation of the equipment.	Facilitates insertion of the tube.	
A. Check that all equipment is present.		
B. Pour antiseptic solution into basin or medicine cup with aseptic technique or open antiseptic swab packet and stand by.		
C. Open the chest tube package and empty it onto the open sterile tray.		
D. Assist to prepare a syringe with lidocaine.		
6. Assist the physician or advanced practice nurse with preparation of the insertion site.	Assists in preparation of area for insertion and proper placement of tube.[5]	Insertion site for air removal is right or left second intercostal space. Insertion site for fluid removal is right or left fifth or sixth intercostal space, midaxillary line. Incision site is one rib below insertion site (see Fig. 20-1).
7. After tube insertion, connect the chest tube to the closed chest drainage system and check for rise and fall (tidaling) of the H_2O column. Apply ordered amount of suction.	Ensures the tube is properly positioned.	
8. Assist with suturing of the tube to the chest wall.	Secures the position of the tube.[3] Sutures should be snug to prevent free air from passing into the subcutaneous tissue.	Type of stitch used depends on the individual; the goal is to prevent displacement of the chest tube.

Procedure continues on following page

Procedure | for Assisting Chest Tube Placement—*Continued*

Steps	Rationale	Special Considerations

9. Apply occlusive dressing (see Fig. 21-1).
  A. Petrolatum gauze is used around the chest tube, or follow institutional standards.
  B. Split drain sponges are placed around the chest tube, one from top, one underneath.
  C. Cover with 4 × 4 gauze.
  D. Tape dressing.
	Provides airtight seal around the chest tube.[5,6]	

10. Tape all connection points to the drainage system or secure with zip ties (Parham-Martin bands). **(Level E*)**	Creates an airtight system. Airtight connections prevent air leaks into the pleural space.[1,3]	Check that all tube drainage holes are in the pleural space.
11. Secure the tube below the dressing to the patient's skin with a commercial securing device or tape.	Functions as a strain relief to prevent tube and dressing dislodgement.	
12. Confirm tube placement with chest radiography. **(Level E)**	Chest radiograph confirms placement of tube and expansion of lung and removal of fluid.[1]	Document result of chest radiograph in the patient's record.
13. Dispose of equipment.		
14. Remove personal protective equipment.	Reduces the transmission of microorganisms and body secretions; Standard Precautions.	
15. 🅷🅷		

*Level E: Multiple case reports, theory-based evidence from expert opinions, or peer-reviewed professional organizational standards without clinical studies to support recommendations

Expected Outcomes

- Removal of air, fluid, or blood from the pleural space
- Relief of respiratory distress
- Reexpansion of the lung (validated with chest radiograph)
- Restoration of negative pressure within the pleural space

Unexpected Outcomes

- Hemorrhage or shock
- Increasing respiratory distress
- Infection
- Damage to intercostal nerve that results in neuropathy or neuritis
- Incorrect tube placement
- Chest tube kinking, clogging, or dislodgment from chest wall
- Subcutaneous emphysema

Patient Monitoring and Care

Steps	Rationale	Reportable Conditions
		These conditions should be reported if they persist despite nursing interventions.
1. Assess cardiopulmonary and vital signs every 1 to 4 hours and as needed.	Provides baseline and ongoing assessment of patient's condition. Abnormalities can indicate reoccurrence of the condition that necessitated chest tube insertion. On the basis of the patient's clinical condition or physician orders, vital signs may need to be checked more frequently.	• Tachypnea • Decreased or absent breath sounds • Hypoxemia • Tracheal deviation • Subcutaneous emphysema • Neck vein distention • Muffled heart tones • Tachycardia • Hypotension • Dysrhythmias • Fever
2. Monitor output every 1 to 4 hours, and record amount and color.	Provides data for diagnosis. Higher drainage amounts require more frequent assessment. On the basis of the patient's clinical condition or physician orders, output may need to be checked more frequently.	• Bloody drainage greater than or equal to 200 mL/hr • Sudden cessation of drainage • Change in character of drainage
3. Assess for pain at the insertion site or for chest discomfort. **(Level D*)**	Pain interferes with adequate deep breathing. Pain at insertion site, particularly with inspiration, may indicate improper tube placement.[5]	• Continued pain despite pain interventions.
4. Evaluate the chest drainage system for rise and fall (tidaling) or bubbling in water-seal chamber. Check connections. **(Level E*)**	Water level normally rises and falls with respiration until lung is expanded. Bubbling immediately after insertion signifies that air is being removed from the pleural space; bubbling with exhalation and coughing is normal. Persistent bubbling indicates an air leak either in the patient's lung or in the chest drainage system.[7]	• Absence of tidaling in water-seal chamber • Persistent bubbling
5. Assess insertion site and surrounding skin with daily dressing change for presence of subcutaneous emphysema and signs of infection or inflammation.	Skin integrity is altered during insertion, which can lead to infection.[7]	• Fever • Redness around insertion site • Purulent drainage • Subcutaneous emphysema

*Level D: Peer-reviewed professional organizational standards with clinical studies to support recommendations

*Level E: Multiple case reports, theory-based evidence from expert opinions, or peer-reviewed professional organizational standards without clinical studies to support recommendations

Documentation

Documentation should include the following:
- Patient and family education
- Reason for chest tube insertion
- Respiratory and vital sign assessment before and after insertion
- Description of procedure, including tube size, date and time of insertion, insertion site, and any complications associated with the procedure
- Type and amount of drainage
- Presence of tidaling and bubbling
- Amount of suction
- Patient's tolerance of procedure
- Postinsertion chest radiograph results
- Unexpected outcomes
- Nursing interventions
- Pain assessment, interventions, and effectiveness

References

CR 1. Buchman TG, Hall BL, Bowling WM, et al: Thoracic trauma. In Tininalli JE, Kelen DG, Stapczynski JS, editors: *Emergency medicine: a comprehensive guide,* ed 6, New York, 2004, McGraw-Hill, 1595-1612.

2. Dev SP, Nascimiento B, Simone C et al: Chest-tube insertion, *N Engl J Med* 357:e15, 2007.

3. Irwin RS, Rippe JM: *Intensive care medicine,* Philadelphia, 2008, Wolters Kluwer/Lippincott and Williams & Wilkins.

CR 4. Laws D, Neville E, Duffy J: BTS guidelines for insertion of a chest drain, *Thorax* 58(Suppl II):ii53-ii59, 2003.

5. May G, Bartram T: The use of intrapleural anaesthetic to reduce the pain of chest drain insertion, *Emerg Med J* 24:300-301, 2007.

CR 6. Roberts JR: *Clinical procedures in emergency medicine,* ed 4, Philadelphia, 2004, Saunders.

7. Sullivan B: Nursing management of patients with a chest drain, *Br J Nurs* 17(6):388-393, 2008.

CR 8. Thompson JM, McFarland GK, Hirsh JE et al: *Mosby's clinical nursing,* ed 5, St Louis, 2002, Mosby.

Additional Readings

Argall J: Seldinger technique chest drains and complication rate, *Emerg Med J* 20:169-170, 2003.

Charnock Y, Evans D: Nursing management of chest drains: a systematic review, *Aust Crit Care* 14:156-160, 2001.

Coughlin AM, Parchinsky C: Go with the flow of chest tube therapy, *Nursing* 36:36-42, 2006.

Ellis H: The applied anatomy of chest drain insertion, *Br J Hosp Med* (London) 68:M44-45, 2007.

Frankel TL, Hill PC, Stamou SC, et al: Silastic drains vs conventional chest tubes after coronary artery bypass, *Chest* 124:108-113, 2003.

Gareeboo S, Singh S: Tube thoracostomy: how to insert a chest drain, *Br J Hosp Med* (London) 67:M16-18, 2006.

Lehwaldt D, Timmins F: Nurses' knowledge of chest drain care: an exploratory descriptive survey, *Nurs Crit Care* 10:192-200, 2005.

Zgoda MA, Lunn W, Ashiku S, et al: Minimally invasive techniques: direct visual guidance for chest tube placement through a single-port thoracoscopy: a novel technique, *Chest* 127:1805-1807, 2005.

AP Chest Tube Removal (Perform)

PURPOSE: Chest tube removal is performed to discontinue a chest tube when it is no longer needed for the removal or drainage of air, blood, or fluid from the intrapleural or mediastinal space.

Peggy Kirkwood

PREREQUISITE NURSING KNOWLEDGE

- Chest tubes are placed in the pleural or mediastinal space to evacuate an abnormal collection of air or fluid or both.
- Indications for removal are based on the reason for insertion and include the following:
  - Drainage has decreased to 50 to 200 mL in prior 24 hours if tube was placed for hemothorax, empyema, or pleural effusion.
  - Research has shown that, depending on the reason for the chest tube, volumes of 200 to 450 mL/day do not adversely affect length of stay or overall costs when compared with lower threshold volumes, nor does the risk of pleural fluid reaccumulation increase.[5,21]
  - Drainage has changed from bloody to serosanguineous, no air leak is present, and amount is less than 100 mL in the past 8 hours (if tube was placed after cardiac surgery).[1,9]
  - Lungs are reexpanded (as shown on chest radiographic results).
  - Respiratory status has improved (i.e., nonlabored respirations, equal bilateral breath sounds, absence of shortness of breath, decreased use of accessory muscles, symmetrical respiratory excursion, and respiratory rate less than 24 breaths/min).
  - Fluctuations are minimal or absent in the water-seal chamber of the collection device, and the level of solution rises in the chamber.
- Air leaks have resolved for at least 24 hours (the absence of continuous bubbling in the water-seal chamber or absence of air bubbles from right to left in the air leak detector), and lung is fully reinflated on chest radiographic results.
- The air leak detector should bubble gently immediately on insertion of the chest tube during expiration and with coughing. Continuous bubbling in the air leak detector indicates a leak in the patient or the chest drainage system. Fluctuations in the water level (also known as tidaling) in the water-seal chamber of 5 to 10 cm, rising during inhalation and falling during expiration, should be observed with spontaneous respirations. If the patient is on mechanical ventilation, the pattern of fluctuation is just the opposite. Any suction applied must be disconnected temporarily to assess correctly for fluctuations in the water-seal chamber.
- Pleural tubes are placed after cardiac surgery if the pleural cavity has been entered. They typically are removed within 24 to 48 hours after surgery.[1,9]
- Mediastinal chest tubes most often are removed 24 to 36 hours after cardiac surgery.[1]
- Flexible Silastic (Blake) (Ethicon, Inc, Somerville, NJ) drains may be used in place of large-bore chest tubes in the mediastinal and pleural spaces after cardiac surgery. These tubes provide more efficient drainage and improved patient mobility with minimized tissue

trauma and pain with removal.[3,7,17] Pleural tubes placed for reasons other than postcardiac surgery necessity remain until the patient no longer needs them (i.e., no persistent air leak, stoppage of ongoing fluid leak or bleeding, or reexpansion of lung on chest radiograph).

- Chest radiographs are done periodically to determine whether the lung has reexpanded. Daily chest radiographs are not necessary while the tube is in place.[10] Reexpanded lungs, along with respiratory assessments that show improvement in the patient's respiratory status, are the basis for the decision to remove the chest tube.
- While the tubes are in place, patients may have related discomfort. Prompt removal of chest tubes encourages patients to increase ambulation and respiratory measures to improve lung expansion after surgery (e.g., coughing, deep breathing). However, removal of the chest tube may also be a painful procedure for the patient.[4,8,15,16]
- The types of sutures used to secure chest tubes vary according to the preference of the physician, the physician assistant, or the advanced practice nurse. One common type is the horizontal mattress or purse-string suture, which is threaded around and through the wound edges in a U-shape with the ends left unknotted until the chest tube is removed. Usually, one or two anchor stitches accompany the purse-string suture (Fig. 22-1).
- A primary goal of chest tube removal is removal of tubes without introduction of air or contaminants into the pleural space.

EQUIPMENT

- Suture removal set
- Antiseptic swabs (povidone-iodine, chlorhexidine gluconate with alcohol, etc)[6]
- Petrolatum gauze, as per hospital protocol
- Rubber-tipped Kelly clamps (two per chest tube) or disposable umbilical clamps

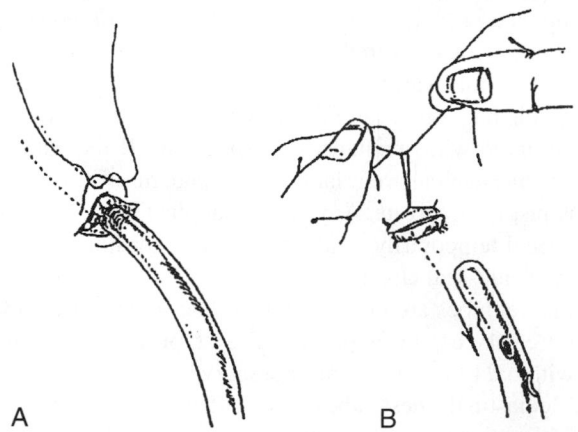

FIGURE 22-1 Purse-string suture. Removing the chest tube. **A,** First throw of a knot in the mattress suture. **B,** Removal of the chest tube and tying of purse-string suture. *(From Leonar S, Nikaidoh H: Thoracentesis and chest tube insertion. In Levin D, Morriss F, editors: Essentials of pediatric intensive care, St Louis, 1990, Quality Medical Publishing.)*

- Wide occlusive tape (2-inch)
- Elastic closure device, such as Steri-Strips (3M, St. Paul, MN)
- Dry 4 × 4 gauze sponges (two to four)
- Waterproof pad
- Personal protective equipment (goggles, sterile and nonsterile gloves, mask, gown)

Additional equipment (to have available depending on patient need) includes the following:

- Specimen collection cup (if catheter tip is to be sent to the laboratory for analysis)
- Scissors

PATIENT AND FAMILY EDUCATION

- Assess patient and family understanding of the procedure. ➤➤*Rationale:* This assessment identifies patient and family knowledge deficits concerning patient condition, procedure, expected benefits, and potential risks and allows time for questions to clarify information.
- Explain the procedure, reason for removal, and sensations to be expected.[15,19,20] The most commonly reported sensations are pulling, pain or hurting, and burning.[14] ➤➤*Rationale:* This explanation decreases patient anxiety and enhances cooperation.
- Explain the patient's role in assisting with removal. Explain that the patient should perform the Valsalva maneuver on the count of "3". Have the patient practice the maneuver before the procedure. ➤➤*Rationale:* This explanation elicits patient cooperation and facilitates removal.
- Instruct the patient to turn and reposition every 2 hours after the chest tube has been removed. ➤➤*Rationale:* This action prevents complications related to immobility and retained secretions.
- Instruct the patient to cough and deep breathe after the chest tube has been removed, with splinting of the affected side or sternum (with mediastinal tubes). ➤➤*Rationale:* This action prevents respiratory complications associated with retained secretions. The application of firm pressure over the insertion site (i.e., splinting) decreases pain and discomfort.
- Instruct the patient about the availability of prescribed analgesic medication. ➤➤*Rationale:* Analgesics alleviate pain and facilitate coughing, deep breathing, and repositioning.[8,16,20]
- Instruct the patient and family to report signs and symptoms of respiratory distress or infection immediately. ➤➤*Rationale:* Immediate reporting facilitates prompt intervention to relieve a recurrent pneumothorax or to treat an infection.

PATIENT ASSESSMENT AND PREPARATION
Patient Assessment

- Assess respiratory status:
  - ❖ Oxygen saturation within normal limits
  - ❖ Nonlabored respirations

- ❖ Absence of shortness of breath
- ❖ Decreased use of accessory muscles
- ❖ Respiratory rate of less than 24 breaths/min
- ❖ Equal bilateral breath sounds
  ➤*Rationale:* Assessment of respiratory status verifies the patient's readiness for chest tube removal.
- Assess chest tube drainage (less than 200 mL in 24 hours or less than 100 mL in 8 hours after cardiac surgery).[1,5,9,21] ➤*Rationale:* Assessment of drainage verifies patient readiness for chest tube removal.
- Assess for minimal or absence of air leak in the air leak detector zone or indicator. ➤*Rationale:* This assessment indicates whether the lung is reexpanded and whether or not air leak is present.
- Evaluate chest radiographic results. ➤*Rationale:* Lung reexpansion indicates that need for chest tube is resolved.
- Assess vital signs and (optional) arterial blood gases. ➤*Rationale:* Vital sign assessment indicates whether the patient can tolerate chest tube removal.
- Assess laboratory results for clotting capability and medications that may impact clotting. ➤*Rationale:* Low platelet levels or thrombolytic medications may precipitate excessive bleeding.[18]

Patient Preparation

- Verify correct patient with two identifiers. ➤*Rationale:* Prior to performing a procedure, the nurse should ensure the correct identification of the patient for the intended intervention.

- Ensure that the patient understands preprocedural teachings. Answer questions as they arise, and reinforce information as needed. ➤*Rationale:* This communication evaluates and reinforces understanding of previously taught information. Anticipatory preparation may prepare patients for a better experience.[15,19,20]
- Administer premedication of adequate analgesics at least 20 minutes before the procedure. Alternatively, subfascial lidocaine may be injected into the chest tube tract. Slow deep-breathing relaxation exercises in addition to opioids have also been shown to further diminish pain sensation.[8] ➤*Rationale:* Intravenous morphine 4 mg 20 minutes before or ketorolac 30 mg 60 minutes before the procedure have been shown to have substantial relief of pain without excessive analgesia.[16] Pain medication and relaxation exercises reduce the discomfort and anxiety experienced, which facilitates patient cooperation.[8,15,16]
- Time the removal procedure to occur at peak analgesic effect. ➤*Rationale:* This timing increases patient cooperation and decreases anxiety.[16]
- Place the patient in the semi-Fowler's position. Alternatively, place the patient on the unaffected side with the waterproof pad underneath the site. ➤*Rationale:* This position enhances accessibility to the insertion site of the chest tube and protects the bed from drainage.

Procedure for Performing Chest Tube Removal

Steps	Rationale	Special Considerations
1. Perform a pre-procedure verification and time out, if non-emergent.	Ensures patient safety.	
2. **HH**		
3. **PE**		
4. Open the sterile suture removal set and prepare petrolatum gauze dressing and two to four 4 × 4 gauze sponges, as per hospital protocol.	Aseptic technique is maintained to prevent contamination of the wound. Removal of pleural chest tubes should be accomplished rapidly with the simultaneous application of an occlusive dressing or closure with purse-string sutures to decrease possibility of air from entering the pleural space.	
5. Discontinue suction from chest drainage system and check for air leakage in air leak detector zone or indicator. Observe the air leak detector zone or indicator while the patient coughs.	Bubbling in the air leak detector is associated with an air leak. When an air leak is present, removal of the chest tube may cause development of a pneumothorax. Ensures a recurrent pneumothorax has not occurred.[13]	If an air leak is present, the tube should not be removed. Consult with the physician, physician assistant, or advanced practice nurse to determine appropriate action.

Procedure continues on following page

Procedure for Performing Chest Tube Removal—*Continued*

Steps	Rationale	Special Considerations
If tube was placed for a pneumothorax, institutional policies may require 6 to 24 hours of water-seal and another radiograph before the chest tube is removed.[13] **(Level C*)**		
6. Remove existing tape, and clean area around tubes with antiseptic swab.[6] Determine type of suture that secures each chest tube. Clip appropriately. If a purse-string suture is present, leave the long suture ends intact. **(Level B*)**	Allows access to the chest tube at the skin level and prepares the sutures for removal. Antiseptic swabs remove a broad spectrum of microbes quickly and provide high-level antimicrobial action for up to 6 hours after use.[6]	
7. Confirm that the tube is free from the suture and the tape.		
8. Cover pleural insertion sites with petrolatum gauze dressing and mediastinal insertion site with 4 × 4 gauze pads, as per hospital protocol.	Avoids the influx of air.	Sterile petrolatum gauze should be applied over the skin site if tube was in pleural space or if no purse-string suture is present.
9. Clamp each tube to be removed with two Kelly clamps or umbilical clamps.[12] **(Level B)**	Possibly prevents air from being introduced into the pleural space, although controversy is found in the literature.[12]	
10. Instruct the patient to perform a Valsalva maneuver at either end inspiration or end expiration.[2] A. End inspiration: Instruct patient to take a deep breath and hold it while performing the Valsalva maneuver for each tube removed. If the patient is receiving ventilator support, pause the ventilator. If the patient is receiving ventilator support and is unable to follow instructions, remove the tube during peak inspiration. B. End expiration: Instruct patient to forcibly exhale and perform the Valsalva maneuver at end expiration. C. Patients may need to hold their breath until sutures are tied. **(Level B)**	Valsalva maneuver is needed to provide positive pressure in the pleural cavity and decrease the incidence of an involuntary gasp by the patient when the tube is removed.[2]	

*Level B: Well-designed, controlled studies with results that consistently support a specific action, intervention, or treatment

*Level C: Qualitative studies, descriptive or correlational studies, integrative reviews, systematic reviews, or randomized controlled trials with inconsistent results

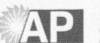
Procedure for Performing Chest Tube Removal—*Continued*

Steps	Rationale	Special Considerations
11. Remove chest tubes rapidly, smoothly, and individually while patient is performing Valsalva maneuver.	Prevents accidental entrance of air into the pleural space.	*Some resistance is expected; however, if strong resistance is encountered and rapid removal of the tube is not possible, stop the procedure and consult with the physician, physician's assistant, or advanced practice nurse immediately.*
		Resistance may indicate that the tube was inadvertently sutured during surgery or sternal closure.
A. Hold sutures in hand closer to head of patient, and apply mild pressure over exit site with folded 4 × 4 gauze pad. B. If tube was "Y" connected to another tube, cut the removed tube below the clamp to allow for easier manipulation when removing the remaining chest tubes.		
12. If a purse-string suture is present, tie it off with a square knot (see Fig. 22-1). If no purse-string was used, the site may be closed with adhesive skin closure strips.	Creates a firm closure of the chest tube site.	*Avoid pulling the suture too tight to prevent tissue necrosis at the site and to facilitate easier removal later.*
13. Secure dressing with tape.	Creates a firm closure of the chest tube site.	This action is easier with a second person to place the tape while holding pressure over the site.
14. Examine each chest tube to verify that the entire tube has been removed.	If portion of tube is not removed, surgical removal is necessary to remove it.	Consult with physician, physician assistant, or advanced practice nurse immediately if a portion of the tube remains in the patient.
15. Assess the patient's condition after the procedure, and compare the results with previous assessment results.	Ensures stable respiratory status after the procedure.	Increased work of breathing, decreased oxygen saturation, increased restlessness, symptoms of chest discomfort, and diminished breath sounds on the affected side are warning signs to be observed.
16. Obtain a chest radiograph (generally 1 to 24 hours after removal) or as clinically indicated.[10,11] **(Level B*)**	Assesses that the lung has remained expanded.[10,11]	
17. Dispose of used supplies and equipment.		
18. Remove personal protective equipment.	Standard Precautions. Decreases transmission of microorganisms.	
19. **HH**	Standard Precautions Decreases transmission of microorganisms.	

*Level B: Well-designed, controlled studies with results that consistently support a specific action, intervention, or treatment

Procedure continues on following page

Expected Outcomes

- Patient is comfortable and has no respiratory distress
- Lung remains expanded after chest tube removal
- Site remains free of infection

Unexpected Outcomes

- Pneumothorax
- Bleeding
- Skin necrosis
- Retained chest tube
- Infected chest tube insertion site

Patient Monitoring and Care

Steps	Rationale	Reportable Conditions
		These conditions should be reported if they persist despite nursing interventions.
1. Ensure adequate respiratory status. Obtain chest radiograph if difficulties arise. Specifically monitor: Oxygen saturation Work of breathing Breath sounds	Diminished respiratory status could indicate a pneumothorax. Pneumothorax could be from removal of the chest tube before all the air, fluid, or blood in the pleural space had been drained, or it may recur after removal of the chest tube if air is introduced accidentally into the pleural space through the chest tube tract.	• Decreased oxygen saturation on pulse oximetry • Increased work of breathing • Diminished breath sounds on affected side • Increased restlessness and symptoms of chest discomfort
2. Monitor insertion site for bleeding. If bleeding is found, apply pressure and place a tight occlusive dressing over site, which may be removed after 48 hours.	Persistent bleeding from insertion site could mean chest tube was against a vein or artery of chest wall before removal.	• Persistent bleeding
3. Monitor purse-string suture site for signs of skin necrosis. If seen, remove the suture and cleanse wound.	If purse-string suture was pulled too tightly closed when chest tube was removed, skin necrosis may be seen.	• Dark or inflamed skin with necrotic areas visible
4. Monitor site for signs of infection. If seen, prepare for wound cultures.	Prolonged insertion of a chest tube increases the risk that the tract created by the chest tube may become infected, or infection may occur after removal of the chest tube if the opening created by the removal becomes contaminated.	• Purulent drainage • Increased body temperature • Inflammation • Tenderness • Warmth at site
5. Monitor insertion area for development of subcutaneous emphysema.	Air may leak into the surrounding tissues and cause crepitus.	• Crepitus
6. Monitor for signs and symptoms of pericardial effusion or cardiac tamponade.	Removal of chest tubes may cause increased bleeding into pericardium. Pericardial bleeding may continue after chest tubes removed.	• Distant heart tones • Decreased blood pressure, tachycardia • Pulsus paradoxus • Narrowed pulse pressure • Equalized pulmonary artery pressures
7. Follow institution standard for assessing pain. Administer analgesia as prescribed.	Identifies need for pain interventions	• Continued pain despite pain interventions

Documentation

Documentation should include the following:
- Patient and family education
- Respiratory and vital signs assessments before and after procedure
- Date and time of procedure and by whom procedure was performed
- Amount, color, and consistency of any drainage
- Application of a sterile occlusive dressing

- Type of suture in place and what was done to it (cut and removed or tied)
- Patient's tolerance of the procedure
- Completion and results of chest radiograph
- Specimens sent to laboratory (if applicable)
- Unexpected outcomes
- Nursing interventions
- Pain assessment, interventions, and effectiveness

References

1. Abramov D, et al: Timing of chest tube removal after coronary artery bypass surgery, *J Card Surg* 20:142-146, 2005.
CR 2. Bell RL, et al: Chest tube removal: end-inspiration or end-expiration? *J Trauma* 50:674-677, 2001.
3. Bjessmo S, et al: Comparison of three different chest drainages after coronary artery bypass surgery: a randomised trial in 150 patients, *Eur J Cardiothorac Surg* 31:372-375, 2007.
4. Bruce EA, Howard RF, Franck LS: Chest drain removal pain and its management: a literature review, *J Clin Nurs* 15:145-154, 2008.
5. Cerfolio RJ, Bryant AS: Results of a prospective algorithm to remove chest tubes after pulmonary resection with high output, *J Thorac Cardiovasc Surg* 135(2): 269-273, 2008.
6. Digison MB: A review of anti-septic agents for pre-operative skin preparation, *Plast Surg Nurs* 27(4): 185-189, 2007.
CR 7. Frankel TL, et al: Silastic drains vs conventional chest tubes after coronary artery bypass, *Chest* 124:108-113, 2003.
8. Friesner SA, Curry DM, Moddeman GR: Comparison of two pain-management strategies during chest tube removal: relaxation exercise with opioids and opioids alone, *Heart Lung* 35(4):269-276, 2006.
CR 9. Gercekoglu H, et al: Effect of timing of chest tube removal on development of pericardial effusion following cardiac surgery, *J Card Surg* 18(3):217-224, 2003.
10. Hendrikse KA, et al: Low value of routine chest radiographs in a mixed medical surgical ICU, *Chest* 132(3):823-828, 2007.

11. Khan T, et al: Is routine chest radiograph following mediastinal drain removal after cardiac surgery useful? *Eur J Cardiothorac Surg* 34(3):542-544, 2008.
CR 12. Laws D, Neville E, Duffy J: British Thoracic Society guidelines for the insertion of a chest drain, *Thorax* 58(Suppl II): ii53-ii59, 2003.
CR 13. Martino K, et al: Prospective randomized trial of thoracostomy removal algorithms, *J Trauma* 46:369-371, 1999.
CR 14. Mimnaugh L, et al: Sensations experienced during removal of tubes in acute postoperative patients, *Appl Nurs Res* 12:78-85, 1999.
CR 15. Puntillo K, et al: Patients' perceptions and responses to procedural pain: results from Thunder Project II, *Am J Crit Care* 10:238-251, 2001.
CR 16. Puntillo K, Ley SJ: Appropriately timed analgesics control pain due to chest tube removal, *Am J Crit Care* 13:292-304, 2004.
17. Sakopoulos AG, et al: Efficacy of Blake drains for mediastinal and pleural drainage following cardiac operations, *J Card Surg* 20(6):574-577, 2005.
18. Sullivan B: Nursing management of patients with a chest drain, *Br J Nurs* 17(6):388-393, 2008.
CR 19. Suls J, Wan CK: Effects of sensory and procedural information on coping with stressful medical procedures and pain: a meta-analysis, *J Consult Clin Psychol* 57:372-379, 1989.
CR 20. Summer GH, Puntillo K: Management of surgical and procedural pain in a critical care setting, *Crit Care Nurs Clin North Am* 13:233-242, 2001.
CR 21. Younes RN, et al: When to remove a chest tube? A randomized study with subsequent prospective consecutive validation, *J Am Coll Surg* 195(5):658-662, 2002.

23

AP Chest Tube Removal (Assist)

P U R P O S E : Chest tube removal is performed to discontinue a chest tube when it is no longer needed for the removal or drainage of air, blood, or fluid from the intrapleural or mediastinal space.

Peggy Kirkwood

PREREQUISITE NURSING KNOWLEDGE

- Chest tubes are placed in the pleural or mediastinal space to evacuate an abnormal collection of air or fluid or both.
- Indications for removal are based on the reason for insertion and include the following:
  - ❖ Drainage has decreased to 50 to 200 mL in prior 24 hours if tube was placed for hemothorax, empyema, or pleural effusion.
  - ❖ Research has shown that, depending on the reason for the chest tube, volumes of 200 to 450 mL/day do not adversely affect length of stay or overall costs when compared with lower threshold volumes, nor does the risk of pleural fluid reaccumulation increase.[5,21]
  - ❖ Drainage has changed from bloody to serosanguineous, no air leak is present, and amount is less than 100 mL in the past 8 hours (if tube was placed after cardiac surgery).[1,9]
  - ❖ Lungs are reexpanded (as shown on chest radiographic results).
  - ❖ Respiratory status has improved (i.e., nonlabored respirations, equal bilateral breath sounds, absence of shortness of breath, decreased use of accessory muscles, symmetrical respiratory excursion, and respiratory rate less than 24 breaths/min).

- ❖ Fluctuations are minimal or absent in the water-seal chamber of the collection device, and the level of solution rises in the chamber.
- Air leaks have resolved for at least 24 hours (the absence of continuous bubbling in the water-seal chamber or absence of air bubbles from right to left in the air leak detector) and lung is fully reinflated on chest radiographic results.
- The air leak detector should bubble gently immediately on insertion of the chest tube during expiration and with coughing. Continuous bubbling in the air leak detector indicates a leak in the patient or the chest drainage system. Fluctuations in the water level (also known as tidaling) in the water-seal chamber of 5 to 10 cm, rising during inhalation and falling during expiration, should be observed with spontaneous respirations. If the patient is on mechanical ventilation, the pattern of fluctuation is just the opposite. Any suction applied must be disconnected temporarily to assess correctly for fluctuations in the water-seal chamber.
- Pleural tubes are placed after cardiac surgery if the pleural cavity has been entered. They typically are removed within 24 to 48 hours after surgery.[1,9]
- Pleural tubes placed for reasons other than postcardiac surgery necessity remain until the patient no longer needs them (i.e., no persistent air leak, stoppage of ongoing fluid leak or bleeding, or lung is reexpanded on chest radiographic results).
- Mediastinal chest tubes most often are removed 24 to 36 hours after cardiac surgery.[1]
- Flexible silastic (Blake) (Ethicon, Inc, Somervile, NJ) drains may be used in place of large-bore chest tubes in

---

AP This procedure should be performed only by physicians, advanced practice nurses, and other healthcare professionals (including critical care nurses) with additional knowledge, skills, and demonstrated competence per professional licensure or institutional standard.

the mediastinal and pleural spaces after cardiac surgery. These tubes provide more efficient drainage and improved patient mobility with minimized tissue trauma and pain with removal.[3,7,17]

- Chest tubes that remain in place for more than 7 days increase the risk of infection along the chest tube tract.
- Chest radiographs are done periodically to determine whether the lung has reexpanded. Daily chest radiographs are not necessary while the tube is in place.[10] Reexpanded lungs, along with respiratory assessments that show improvement in the patient's respiratory status, are the basis for the decision to remove the chest tube.
- While the tubes are in place, patients may have related discomfort. Prompt removal of chest tubes encourages patients to increase ambulation and respiratory measures to improve lung expansion after surgery (e.g., coughing, deep breathing). However, removal of the chest tube may also be a painful procedure for the patient.[4,8,15,16]
- The types of sutures used to secure chest tubes vary according to the preference of the physician, the physician assistant, or the advanced practice nurse. One common type is the horizontal mattress or purse-string suture, which is threaded around and through the wound edges in a U-shape with the ends left unknotted until the chest tube is removed. Usually, one or two anchor stitches accompany the purse-string suture (see Fig. 22-1).
- A primary goal of chest tube removal is removal of tubes without introduction of air or contaminants into the pleural space.

EQUIPMENT

- Suture removal set
- Antiseptic swabs (povidone-iodine, chlorhexidine gluconate with alcohol, etc)[6]
- Petrolatum gauze, per hospital policy
- Rubber-tipped Kelly clamps (two per chest tube) or disposable umbilical clamps
- Wide occlusive tape (2-inch)
- Elastic closure device, such as Steri-Strips (3M, St. Paul, MN)
- Dry 4 × 4 gauze sponges (two to four)
- Waterproof pad
- Personal protective equipment (goggles, sterile and nonsterile gloves, mask, gown)

  Additional equipment (to have available depending on patient need) includes the following:

- Specimen collection cup (if catheter tip is to be sent to the laboratory for analysis)
- Scissors

PATIENT AND FAMILY EDUCATION

- Assess patient and family understanding of the procedure. ➤*Rationale:* This assessment identifies patient and family knowledge deficits concerning patient condition,

procedure, expected benefits, and potential risks and allows time for questions to clarify information.

- Explain the procedure, reason for removal, and sensations to be expected.[15,19,20] The most commonly reported sensations are pulling, pain or hurting, and burning.[14] ➤*Rationale:* This explanation decreases patient anxiety and enhances cooperation.
- Explain the patient's role in assisting with removal. Explain that the patient should perform the Valsalva maneuver on count "3". Have the patient practice the maneuver before the procedure. ➤*Rationale:* This explanation elicits patient cooperation and facilitates removal.
- Instruct the patient to turn and reposition every 2 hours after the chest tube has been removed. ➤*Rationale:* This action prevents complications related to immobility and retained secretions.
- Instruct the patient to cough and deep breathe after the chest tube has been removed, with splinting of the affected side or sternum (with mediastinal tubes). ➤*Rationale:* This action prevents respiratory complications associated with retained secretions. The application of firm pressure over the insertion site (i.e., splinting) decreases pain and discomfort.
- Instruct the patient about the availability of prescribed analgesic medication. ➤*Rationale:* Analgesics alleviate pain and facilitate coughing, deep breathing, and repositioning.[8,16,20]
- Instruct the patient and family to report signs and symptoms of respiratory distress or infection immediately. ➤*Rationale:* Immediate reporting facilitates prompt intervention to relieve a recurrent pneumothorax or to treat an infection.

PATIENT ASSESSMENT AND PREPARATION
Patient Assessment

- Assess respiratory status:
  - ❖ Oxygen saturation within normal limits
  - ❖ Nonlabored respirations
  - ❖ Absence of shortness of breath
  - ❖ Decreased use of accessory muscles
  - ❖ Respiratory rate of less than 24 breaths/min
  - ❖ Equal bilateral breath sounds
  ➤*Rationale:* Assessment of respiratory status verifies the patient's readiness for chest tube removal.
- Assess chest tube drainage (less than 200 mL in 24 hours based on physician protocol, or less than 100 mL in 8 hours after cardiac surgery).[1,5,9,21] ➤*Rationale:* Assessment of drainage verifies patient readiness for chest tube removal.
- Assess for minimal or absence of air leak in the air leak detector zone or indicator. ➤*Rationale:* This assessment indicates whether the lung is reexpanded and whether or not air leak is present.
- Obtain chest radiographic results. ➤*Rationale:* Lung reexpansion indicates that need for chest tube is resolved.

- Assess vital signs and (optional) arterial blood gases. ➡*Rationale:* Vital sign assessment indicates whether the patient can tolerate chest tube removal.
- Assess laboratory results for clotting capability and medications that may impact clotting. ➡*Rationale:* Low platelets or thrombolytic medications may precipitate excessive bleeding.[18]

Patient Preparation

- Verify correct patient with two identifiers. ➡*Rationale:* Prior to performing a procedure, the nurse should ensure the correct identification of the patient for the intended intervention.
- Ensure that the patient understands preprocedural teachings. Answer questions as they arise, and reinforce information as needed. ➡*Rationale:* This communication evaluates and reinforces understanding of previously taught information. Anticipatory preparation may prepare patients for a better experience.[15,19,20]

- Administer premedication of adequate analgesics at least 20 minutes before procedure. Alternatively, subfascial lidocaine may be injected into the chest tube tract. Slow deep-breathing relaxation exercises in addition to opioids have also been shown to further diminish pain sensation.[8] ➡*Rationale:* Intravenous morphine 4 mg 20 minutes before or ketorolac 30 mg 60 minutes before the procedure have been shown to have substantial relief of pain without excessive analgesia.[16] Pain medication and relaxation exercises reduce the discomfort and anxiety experienced and facilitate patient cooperation.[8,15,16]
- Time the removal procedure to occur at peak analgesic effect. ➡*Rationale:* This timing increases patient cooperation and decreases anxiety.[16]
- Place the patient in the semi-Fowler's position. Alternatively, place the patient on the unaffected side with the waterproof pad underneath the site. ➡*Rationale:* This position enhances accessibility to the insertion site of the chest tube and protects the bed from drainage.

Procedure   for Performing Chest Tube Removal

Steps	Rationale	Special Considerations
1. Perform a pre-procedure verification and time out, if non-emergent.	Ensures patient safety.	
2. **HH**		
3. **PE**		
4. Open the sterile suture removal set and prepare petrolatum gauze dressing and two to four 4 × 4 gauze sponges, according to hospital protocol.	Aseptic technique is maintained to prevent contamination of the wound. Removal of pleural chest tubes must be accomplished rapidly with the simultaneous application of an occlusive dressing to prevent air from entering the pleural space.	
5. Discontinue suction from chest drainage system and check for air leakage in air leak detector zone or indicator. Observe the air leak detector zone or indicator while the patient coughs, looking for bubbling that indicates an air leak. If tube was placed for a pneumothorax, institutional policies may require 6 to 24 hours of water-seal and another radiograph before the chest tube is removed.[13] **(Level C*)**	Bubbling in air leak detector is associated with an air leak. When an air leak is present, removal of the chest tube may cause development of a pneumothorax. Ensures a recurrent pneumothorax has not occurred.[13]	If an air leak is present, the tube should not be removed. Consult with the physician, physician assistant or advanced practice nurse to determine appropriate action.

*Level C: Qualitative studies, descriptive or correlational studies, integrative reviews, systematic reviews, or randomized controlled trials with inconsistent results

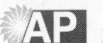

Procedure for Performing Chest Tube Removal—*Continued*

Steps	Rationale	Special Considerations
6. Remove existing tape, clean area around tubes with antiseptic swab.[6] Determine type of suture that secures each chest tube. Clip appropriately. If a purse-string suture is present, leave the long suture ends intact. **(Level B*)**	Allows access to the chest tube at the skin level and prepares the sutures for removal. Antiseptic swabs remove a broad spectrum of microbes quickly and provide high level antimicrobial action for up to 6 hours after use.[6] **(Level B)**	
7. Confirm that the tube is free from the suture and the tape.		
8. Cover pleural insertion sites with petrolatum gauze dressing and mediastinal insertion site with 4 × 4 gauze pads, according to hospital protocol.	Avoids the influx of air.	Sterile petrolatum gauze should be applied over the skin site if tube was in pleural space or if no purse-string suture is present.
9. Clamp each tube to be removed with two Kelly clamps or umbilical clamps. **(Level B)**	Possibly prevents air from being introduced into the pleural space, although controversy exists in the literature.[12]	
10. The tube is removed while patient is performing Valsalva maneuver at either end inspiration or end expiration.[2]	Valsalva maneuver is needed to provide positive pressure in the pleural cavity and decrease the incidence of an involuntary gasp by the patient when the tube is removed.[2]	
A. End inspiration: Instruct patient to take a deep breath and hold it while performing the Valsalva maneuver for each tube removed. If the patient is receiving ventilator support, pause the ventilator. If the patient is receiving ventilator support and is unable to follow instructions, remove the tube during peak inspiration phase.		
B. End expiration: Instruct patient to perform the Valsalva maneuver at end expiration.		
C. Patients may need to hold their breath until sutures are tied. **(Level B)**		
11. Secure dressing with tape.	Creates a firm closure of the chest tube site.	This action is easier with a second person to place the tape while holding pressure over the site.
12. Assess the patient's condition after the procedure, and compare the results with previous assessment results.	Ensures stable respiratory status after the procedure.	Increased work of breathing, decreased oxygen saturation, increased restlessness, symptoms of chest discomfort, and diminished breath sounds on the affected side are warning signs to be observed.

*Level B: Well-designed, controlled studies with results that consistently support a specific action, intervention, or treatment

Procedure continues on following page

Procedure | for Performing Chest Tube Removal—*Continued*

Steps	Rationale	Special Considerations
13. Obtain a chest radiograph per order or protocol (generally 1 to 24 hours after removal) or as clinically indicated.[10,11] (**Level B***)	Assesses that the lung has remained expanded.[10,11]	
14. Dispose of used supplies and equipment.		
15. Remove personal protective equipment.	Standard Precautions. Decreases transmission of microorganisms.	
16. **HH**		

*Level B: Well-designed, controlled studies with results that consistently support a specific action, intervention, or treatment

Expected Outcomes

- Patient is comfortable and has no respiratory distress
- Lung remains expanded after chest tube removal
- Site remains free of infection

Unexpected Outcomes

- Pneumothorax
- Bleeding
- Skin necrosis
- Retained chest tube
- Infected chest tube insertion site

Patient Monitoring and Care

Steps	Rationale	Reportable Conditions
		These conditions should be reported if they persist despite nursing interventions.
1. Ensure adequate respiratory status. Obtain chest radiograph if difficulties arise. Specifically monitor: Oxygen saturation Work of breathing Breath sounds	Diminished respiratory status could indicate a pneumothorax. Pneumothorax could be from removal of the chest tube before all the air, fluid, or blood in the pleural space has been drained, or it may recur after removal of the chest tube if air is introduced accidentally into the pleural space through the chest tube tract.	• Decreased oxygen saturation on pulse oximetry • Increased work of breathing • Diminished breath sounds on affected side • Increased restlessness and symptoms of chest discomfort
2. Monitor insertion site for bleeding. If bleeding is found, apply pressure and place a tight occlusive dressing over site, which may be removed after 48 hours.	Persistent bleeding from insertion site could mean chest tube was against a vein or artery of chest wall before removal.	• Persistent bleeding
3. Monitor purse-string suture site for signs of skin necrosis. If seen, remove the suture and cleanse wound.	If purse-string suture was pulled too tightly closed when chest tube was removed, skin necrosis may be seen.	• Dark or inflamed skin with necrotic areas visible
4. Monitor site for signs of infection. If seen, prepare for wound cultures.	Prolonged insertion of a chest tube increases the risk that the tract created by the chest tube may become infected, or infection may occur after removal of the chest tube if the opening created by the removal becomes contaminated.	• Purulent drainage • Increased body temperature • Inflammation • Tenderness • Warmth at site
5. Monitor insertion area for development of subcutaneous emphysema.	Air may leak into the surrounding tissues and cause crepitus.	• Crepitus

Patient Monitoring and Care —*Continued*

Steps	Rationale	Reportable Conditions
6. Monitor for signs and symptoms of pericardial effusion or cardiac tamponade.	Removal of chest tubes may cause increased bleeding into pericardium. Pericardial bleeding may continue after chest tubes removed.	• Distant heart tones • Decreased blood pressure, tachycardia • Pulsus paradoxus • Narrowed pulse pressure • Equalized pulmonary artery pressures
7. Follow institution standard for assessing pain. Administer analgesia as prescribed.	Identifies need for pain interventions	• Continued pain despite pain interventions

Documentation

Documentation should include the following:

- Patient and family education
- Respiratory and vital signs assessments before and after procedure
- Date and time of procedure and by whom procedure was performed
- Amount, color, and consistency of any drainage
- Application of a sterile occlusive dressing

- Type of suture in place and what was done to it (cut or tied)
- Patient's tolerance of the procedure
- Completion and results of chest radiograph
- Specimens sent to laboratory (if applicable)
- Unexpected outcomes
- Nursing interventions
- Pain assessment, interventions, and effectiveness

References

1. Abramov D, et al: Timing of chest tube removal after coronary artery bypass surgery, *J Card Surg* 20:142-146, 2005.
CR 2. Bell RL, et al: Chest tube removal: end-inspiration or end-expiration? *J Trauma* 50:674-677, 2001.
3. Bjessmo S, et al: Comparison of three different chest drainages after coronary artery bypass surgery: a randomised trial in 150 patients, *Eur J Cardiothorac Surg* 31:372-375, 2007.
4. Bruce EA, Howard RF, Franck LS: Chest drain removal pain and its management: a literature review, *J Clin Nurs* 15:145-154, 2008.
5. Cerfolio RJ, Bryant AS: Results of a prospective algorithm to remove chest tubes after pulmonary resection with high output, *J Thorac Cardiovasc Surg* 135(2): 269-273, 2008.
6. Digison MB: A review of anti-septic agents for pre-operative skin preparation, *Plast Surg Nurs* 27(4):185-189, 2007.
CR 7. Frankel TL, et al: Silastic drains vs conventional chest tubes after coronary artery bypass, *Chest* 124:108-113, 2003.
8. Friesner SA, Curry DM, Moddeman GR: Comparison of two pain-management strategies during chest tube removal: relaxation exercise with opioids and opioids alone, *Heart Lung* 35(4):269-276, 2006.
CR 9. Gercekoglu H, et al: Effect of timing of chest tube removal on development of pericardial effusion following cardiac surgery, *J Card Surg* 18(3):217-224, 2003.
10. Hendrikse KA, et al: Low value of routine chest radiographs in a mixed medical surgical ICU, *Chest* 132(3):823-828, 2007.

11. Khan T, et al: Is routine chest x-ray following mediastinal drain removal after cardiac surgery useful? *Eur J Cardiothorac Surg* 34(3):542-544, 2008.
CR 12. Laws D, Neville E, Duffy J: British Thoracic Society guidelines for the insertion of a chest drain, *Thorax* 58(Suppl II): ii53-ii59, 2003.
CR 13. Martino K, et al: Prospective randomized trial of thoracostomy removal algorithms, *J Trauma* 46:369-371, 1999.
CR 14. Mimnaugh L, et al: Sensations experienced during removal of tubes in acute postoperative patients, *Appl Nurs Res* 12:78-85, 1999.
CR 15. Puntillo K, et al: Patients' perceptions and responses to procedural pain: results from Thunder Project I, *Am J Crit Care* 10:238-251, 2001.
CR 16. Puntillo K, Ley SJ: Appropriately timed analgesics control pain due to chest tube removal, *Am J Crit Care* 13:292-304, 2004.
17. Sakopoulos AG, et al: Efficacy of Blakc drains for mediastinal and pleural drainage following cardiac operations, *J Card Surg* 20(6):574-577, 2005.
18. Sullivan B: Nursing management of patients with a chest drain, *Br J Nurs* 17(6):388-393, 2008.
CR 19. Suls J, Wan CK: Effects of sensory and procedural information on coping with stressful medical procedures and pain: a meta-analysis, *J Consult Clin Psychol* 57:372-379, 1989.
20. Summer GH, Puntillo K: Management of surgical and procedural pain in a critical care setting, *Crit Care Nurs Clin North Am* 13:233-242, 2001.
CR 21. Younes RN, et al: When to remove a chest tube? A randomized study with subsequent prospective consecutive validation, *J Am Coll Surg* 195(5):658-662, 2002.

Closed Chest Drainage System

P U R P O S E : Closed chest drainage systems are used to facilitate the evacuation of fluid, blood, and air from the pleural space, the mediastinum, or both; to restore negative pressure to the pleural space; and to promote reexpansion of a collapsed lung.

Joya D. Pickett

PREREQUISITE NURSING KNOWLEDGE

- Anatomy and physiology of the pulmonary system should be understood.
- Normal intrapleural pressures measure approximately -4 cm H_2O during expiration. At end inspiration, pressure decreases to -8 cm H_2O.[15]
- Closed chest drainages systems are used to facilitate the evacuation of fluid, blood, and air from the pleural space, the mediastinum, or both; to restore negative pressure to the pleural space; and to promote reexpansion of a collapsed lung.
- Closed chest drainage systems (CDSs) include:
  - ❖ Dry suction with a traditional water-seal; dry suction with a one-way valve; wet suction with a traditional water-seal; and one-bottle, two-bottle, three-bottle, and four-bottle setups
  - ❖ Gravity, suction, or both to restore negative pressure and remove air, fluid, and blood from the pleural space or the mediastinum
  - ❖ A one-way mechanism created by a water-seal that permits air and fluid to be removed and prevents backflow into the chest
  - ❖ Greater pressure within the chest than within the system; this requirement is accomplished by keeping the drainage unit at least 1 foot below the chest tube insertion site and the tubing free of dependent loops and obstructions,[1,11,13,26] which prevents siphoning of the contents back into the pleural cavity[26]
  - ❖ Differences in flow rates and in accuracy of delivered negative pressures noted in chest drainage systems that were not likely to be clinically important[6,7]

- Currently, guidelines recommend that a water-seal alone is safe for most patients with a pneumothorax or small air leak.[2-5,8,9,20,25] However, if the pneumothorax or air leak is large, expanding, or persistent, suction is recommended.[5,8,9]
- The most common amount of suction pressure ranges from -10 to -20 cm H_2O.[1,3,8,14] High suction levels may cause persistent pleural air leaks, air stealing, lung tissue entrapment, and reexpansion pulmonary edema.[14,17]
- The addition of a suction source can enhance drainage when large volumes of air or fluid must be evacuated.
  - ❖ Some systems and suction devices (e.g., Emerson pump, Cambridge, MA) contain an exit vent from the water-seal chamber that ensures the drainage unit remains vented when the suction device is off. Do not close or occlude the exit vent.[19,26] With use of CDSs without an exit vent, the drainage systems should be disconnected from suction before they are turned off.[19,26]
  - ❖ Some wall-mounted suction devices need control and pressure gauges to regulate and monitor for potential surges in suction levels.[15,19,26]
- If clinically desirable, some disposable wet suction with traditional water-seal drainage systems can provide suction levels greater than -25 cm H_2O. The suction chamber vent holes can be occluded with nonporous tape or by replacing them with the manufacturer's special pronged vent plug and connecting directly to wall regulator suction. Suction levels must be converted from prescribed levels of cm H_2O suction to mm Hg of wall suction (Table 24-1).
- Disposable CDSs:
  - ❖ Correlate to the three-bottle drainage system, with collection, water-seal, and suction control chambers

TABLE 24-1	Pressure Conversion Chart*
cm H$_2$O	mm Hg
20	15
25	18
30	22
35	26
40	30
45	33
50	37
60	44

*Approximate values.
Reprinted with permission of Atrium Medical Corporation, Hudson, NH.

positioned side by side in a molded plastic disposable unit (Fig. 24-1). These include the Pleur-Evac, Thora-Klex, Argyle, and Atrium systems.

❖ Are equipped with a positive-pressure relief valve used to prevent a tension pneumothorax if the suction tubing becomes accidentally occluded or if the suction source fails. In addition, automatic and manual pressure relief valves vent excessive negative pressure, such as may occur during deep inspiration or with milking of the chest tube.

❖ May have replaceable collection chambers, which can be removed when filled and replaced with a new one without changing the entire unit.

❖ Often have latex-free tubing.

❖ Have self-sealing ports or collection tubes for aspiration of drainage samples and removal of excess chamber fluid levels.

• Some systems have accessories that may be used to convert them to an autotransfusion unit.

• Some CDSs use dry suction with a traditional water-seal and either a regulator or a restricted orifice mechanism. Although water is added to the water-seal chamber, water does not need to be added to the suction chamber. Instead, the suction source (usually a wall regulator) is increased until an indicator appears.

• Some CDSs are waterless, referred to as dry-dry drains, and have a one-way valve, which eliminates the need to fill any chambers (except an air-leak indicator zone, as needed). A valve opens on expiration and allows patient air to exit, then closes to prevent atmospheric air from entering during inspiration. This one-way valve feature allows the system to be used in the vertical or horizontal position without loss of the seal. These systems are safe if accidentally tipped. The amount of suction delivered is regulated with an adjustable dial.

• Advantages of dry suction are ease of setup; ease of application if higher, more precise levels of suction are needed; and a quiet system.

• Some clinicians suggest use of the Emerson pump (Fig. 24-2) for patients with large bronchopleural air leaks because they are high-volume, low-resistance, portable suction devices capable of handling high airflow rates.[14,15]

• Tidaling, fluctuations that occur with inspiration and expiration, provides a continuous manometer of the pressure changes in the pleural space and indicates overall respiratory effort. Absence of fluctuations suggests obstruction of the drainage system from clots, contact with lung tissue, kinks, loss of subatmospheric pressure from fluid-filled dependent loops, or complete reexpansion of the lung.[1,10,19]

• Except for the exit vent, an airtight system is required to assist in maintaining negative pressure in the pleura and to prevent air entrapment in the pleural space.

• In general, clamping of chest tubes is contraindicated. ***Clamping a chest tube in a patient with a pleural air leak may cause a tension pneumothorax.*** The few situations in which chest tubes may be clamped briefly (i.e., less than a minute) include locating the source of an air leak, replacing the chest drainage system, determining whether a patient is ready to have the chest tube removed, and during chest tube removal.[1,14,15,21,26]

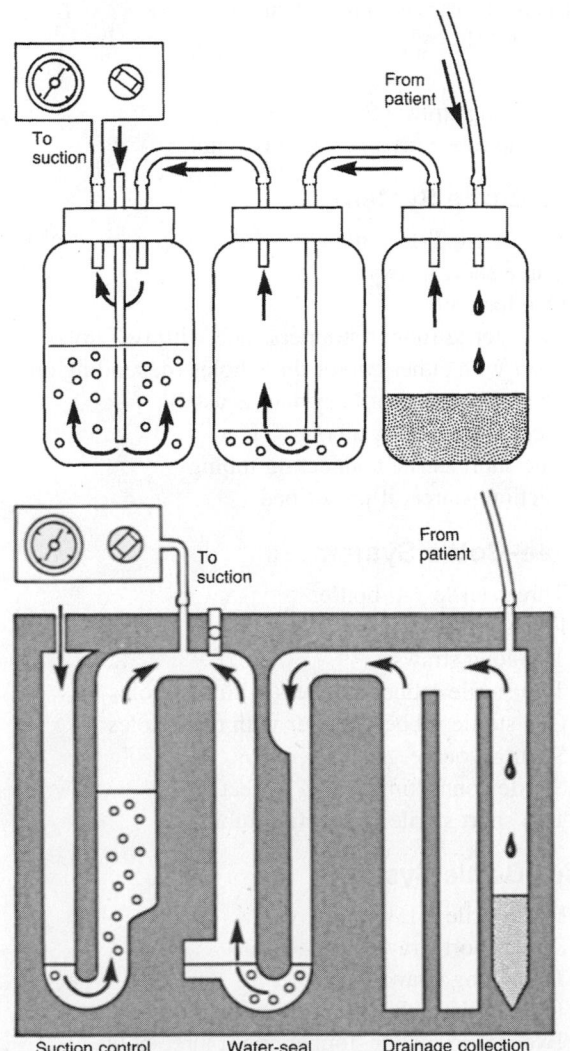

FIGURE 24-1 Disposable system correlates with three-bottle system. *(From Luce JM, Tyler ML, Pierson DJ: Intensive respiratory care, Philadelphia, 1984, Saunders.)*

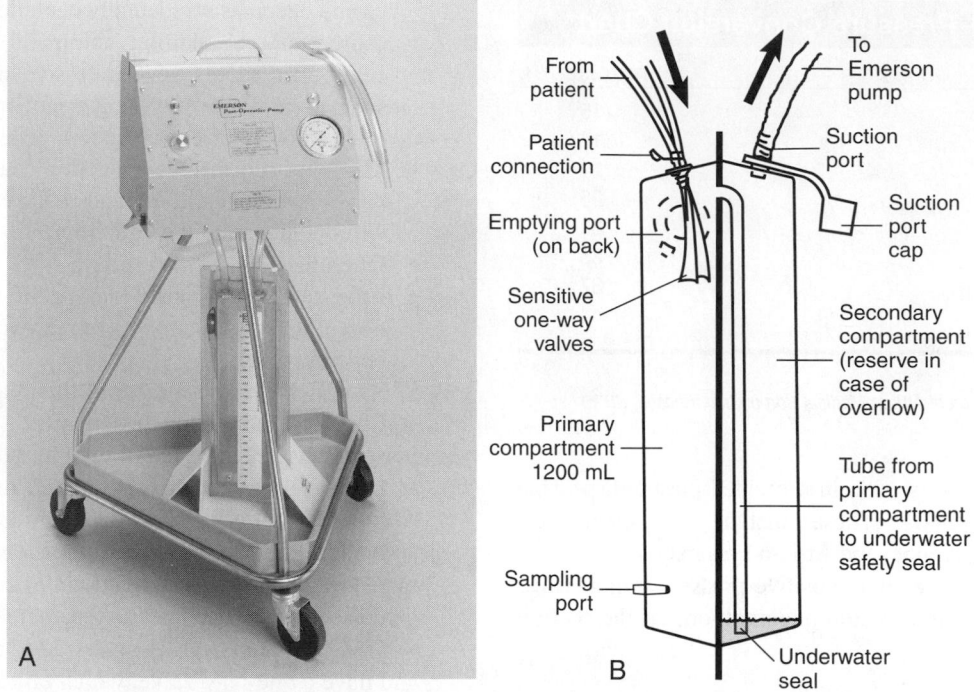

Figure 24-2 **A,** Emerson pump. **B,** Emerson disposable chest drain system. *(Courtesy J.H. Emerson, Cambridge, MA.)*

EQUIPMENT

Disposable Setup (Wet and Dry Systems)

- Disposable chest drainage unit
- Gloves
- Suction source and regulator
- Connecting tubing
- Tape (1-inch), one roll, or zip ties (Parham-Martin bands)
- 1-L bottle of sterile water or normal saline (NS) (for systems that use water)
- 50-mL Irrigation syringe (if not supplied with unit) for systems that use water

Emerson Pump (Disposable Setup)

- Disposable chest drainage unit
- Gloves
- Emerson pump
- 1-L bottle of sterile water or NS
- Flexible corrugated tubing
- Drainage tubes
- Bottle stand

All Bottle Systems

- Gloves
- Sterile water or NS
- Rack or holder for the bottles
- Tape (1-inch), one roll, or zip ties (Parham-Martin bands)

One-Bottle System

- Sterile 2-L bottle
- One short straw

- One long straw
- Sterile rubber stopper with two holes

Two-Bottle System

- Two sterile 2-L bottles
- Three short straws
- One long straw
- Two sterile rubber stoppers, one with two holes and the other with either two or three holes (depending on which type of double-bottle system is used)
- Sterile connecting tubing (6 feet)
- One short sterile connecting tubing
- Suction source, if prescribed

Three-Bottle System

- Three sterile 2-L bottles
- Five short straws
- Two long straws
- Two sterile rubber stoppers with two holes
- One sterile rubber stopper with three holes
- Suction source
- Sterile connecting tubing (6 feet)
- Two short sterile connecting tubings

Four-Bottle System

- Four sterile 2-L bottles
- Seven short straws
- Three long straws
- Two sterile rubber stoppers with two holes
- Two sterile rubber stoppers with three holes
- Sterile connecting tubing (6 feet)
- Three short sterile connecting tubings
- Suction source

PATIENT AND FAMILY EDUCATION

- Explain the procedure, the indication for the chest tube insertion, and how the closed chest drainage system works. ➤➤*Rationale:* This communication identifies patient and family knowledge deficits about the patient's condition, procedure, expected benefits, and potential risks and allows time for questions to clarify information and to voice concerns. Explanations decrease patient anxiety and enhance cooperation.

- After chest tube insertion, instruct the patient to sit in a semi-Fowler's position (unless contraindicated). ➤➤*Rationale:* Proper positioning facilitates drainage from the lung by allowing air to rise and fluid to settle, enhancing removal via the chest tube. This position also makes breathing easier.

- Instruct the patient to turn and reposition every 2 hours to facilitate drainage. The patient may lie on the side with the chest tube but should keep the tubing free of kinks. ➤➤*Rationale:* Turning and positioning prevents complications related to immobility and retained secretions. Keeping the tubing free of kinks maintains patency of the tube, facilitates drainage, and prevents the accumulation of pressure within the pleural space, which interferes with lung reexpansion.

- Instruct the patient to cough and deep breathe, with splinting of the affected side or sternum (if mediastinal tube is in place). ➤➤*Rationale:* Coughing and deep breathing increase pressure within the pleural space, facilitating drainage, promoting lung reexpansion, and preventing respiratory complications associated with retained secretions. The application of firm pressure over the chest tube insertion site (e.g., splinting) decreases pain and discomfort.

- Encourage active or passive range-of-motion exercises of the arm on the affected side. ➤➤*Rationale:* The patient may limit the movement of the arm on the affected side to decrease the discomfort at the insertion site, which results in joint discomfort and potential joint complications.

- Instruct the patient and family about activity as prescribed while maintaining the drainage system below the level of the chest. ➤➤*Rationale:* The drainage system is maintained below the level of the chest to facilitate gravity drainage and to prevent backflow into the pleural space and potential infectious contamination into the pleural space.

- Instruct the patient and family about the availability of prescribed analgesic medication and other pain relief strategies. ➤➤*Rationale:* Pain relief ensures comfort and facilitates coughing, deep breathing, positioning, and range-of-motion exercises and promotes healing.

PATIENT ASSESSMENT AND PREPARATION

Patient Assessment

- Assess significant medical history or injury, including chronic lung disease, spontaneous pneumothorax, pulmonary disease, therapeutic procedures, and mechanism of injury. ➤➤*Rationale:* Medical history or injury may provide the etiologic basis for the occurrence of pneumothorax, hemothorax, empyema, pleural effusion, or chylothorax.

- Assess baseline cardiopulmonary status, as follows:
  - ❖ Vital signs (blood pressure, heart rate, respiratory rate)
  - ❖ Shortness of breath or dyspnea
  - ❖ Anxiety, restlessness, or apprehension
  - ❖ Cyanosis
  - ❖ Decreased oxygen saturation (e.g., pulse oxymetry [SpO_2])
  - ❖ Decreased or absent breath sounds on the affected side
  - ❖ Crackles adjacent to the affected area
  - ❖ Asymmetrical chest excursion with respirations
  - ❖ Hyperresonance with percussion on the affected side (pneumothorax)
  - ❖ Dullness or flatness with percussion on the affected side (hemothorax, pleural effusion, empyema, or chylothorax)
  - ❖ Subcutaneous emphysema or crepitus (pneumothorax)
  - ❖ Sudden sharp focal chest pain
  - ❖ Tracheal deviation to the unaffected side (tension pneumothorax)
  - ❖ Neck vein distention (tension pneumothorax)
  - ❖ Muffled heart sounds (tension pneumothorax)
- ➤➤*Rationale:* Accurate assessment of signs and symptoms allows for prompt recognition and treatment. Baseline assessment provides comparison data for evaluation of changes and outcomes of treatment.

- Assess diagnostic tests (if patient's condition does not necessitate immediate intervention):
  - ❖ Chest radiograph
  - ❖ Arterial blood gases
- ➤➤*Rationale:* Diagnostic testing confirms the presence of air or fluid in the pleural space, a collapsed lung, hypoxemia, and respiratory compromise.

Patient Preparation

- Ensure the patient understands pre-procedural teachings. Answer questions as they arise, and reinforce information as needed. ➤➤*Rationale:* This communication evaluates and reinforces understanding of previously presented information.

- Verify correct patient with two identifiers. ➤➤*Rationale:* Prior to performing a procedure, the nurse should ensure the correct identification of the patient for the intended intervention.

- Administer prescribed analgesics or sedatives as needed. ➤➤*Rationale:* Analgesics and sedatives reduce the discomfort and anxiety experienced, facilitating patient cooperation and improving outcomes.

Procedure | for Using Closed Chest Drainage Systems

Steps	Rationale	Special Considerations

These steps should be followed for dry and wet disposable units, Emerson pump, and bottle units.

1. **HH**

2. **PE**

3. Open sterile packages.

Maintains aseptic technique whenever changes are made to the system.

For Disposable Dry Suction System, proceed to Step 4.

For Disposable Wet Suction System, proceed to Step 10.

For Emerson Pump Disposable Suction, proceed to Step 17.

For One-Bottle System, proceed to Step 24.

For Two-Bottle System, proceed to Step 31.

For Three-Bottle System, proceed to Step 56.

For Four-Bottle System, proceed to Step 73.

Disposable Dry Suction Chest Drainage System

Steps	Rationale	Special Considerations
4. Stabilize the unit. Some systems have a floor stand. For systems with an in-line connector, move the patient tube clamp down next to the in-line connector.	Keeping the clamp visible helps prevent inadvertent clamping.	Clamping of chest tubes can cause air trapped in the pleural space to accumulate and may cause tension pneumothorax.
5. *Dry suction with a traditional water-seal:* Remove the connector cap from the short tubing of the water-seal chamber and use the funnel provided or a 50-mL syringe to add sterile water or NS to the 2-cm level. Some systems provide prefilled sterile water containers. *Dry suction with a one-way valve:* Fill air-leak monitor zone.	Depth of solution required to establish a water-seal; the water-seal permits air and fluid to be removed from the patient and prevents the backflow of air into the chest.[1,19]	Water-seal levels greater than 2 cm increase the work of breathing; levels less than 2 cm can expose the water-seal to air and increase the risk for pneumothorax.[19]
6. Hang drainage unit from bed frame or set it on a floor stand. **(Level E*)**	Drainage unit must be kept below the level of the chest to promote gravity drainage and to prevent backflow of drainage into the pleural space, which interferes with lung expansion.[1,26]	
7. Connect the long tubing from the drainage collection chamber to the chest tube.	Creates the closed chest drainage system; avoid dependent or fluid-filled loops.	Avoid dependent or fluid-filled loops, which may create back pressure and decrease the effectiveness of suction.[13,24]
8. For gravity drainage, leave the suction control chamber open to air.	Creates the exit vent for the escape of air.	*Clamping of chest tubes can cause air trapped in the pleural space to accumulate and may cause tension pneumothorax.*

*Level E: Multiple case reports, theory-based evidence from expert opinions, or peer-reviewed professional organizational standards without clinical studies to support recommendations

Procedure   for Using Closed Chest Drainage Systems—*Continued*

Steps	Rationale	Special Considerations
9. To initiate suction, connect the CDS to the suction source and dial in the prescribed amount of suction (usually −10 to −20 cm H$_2$O), then increase suction source until indicator mark appears according to manufacturer's guidelines. **Proceed to Step 94.**	Activates suction.	Apply suction as per manufacturer's guidelines. For example, to apply −20 cm H$_2$O suction, use a minimum vacuum pressure of −80 mm Hg. Suction source vacuum should be greater than −80 mm Hg when multiple chest drains are used. For a suction level less than −20 cm H$_2$O, any observed bellows expansion across the monitor window confirms adequate suction operation. To decrease suction, set the dial, confirm patient on suction, then depress the high-negativity vent, venting to the newer lower amount.

Disposable Wet Suction Chest Drainage System

Steps	Rationale	Special Considerations
10. Stabilize the unit. Some systems have a floor stand. For systems with an in-line connector, move the patient tube clamp down next to the in-line connector.	Keeping the clamp visible helps prevent inadvertent clamping.	*Clamping of chest tubes can cause air trapped in the pleural space to accumulate and may cause tension pneumothorax.*
11. Remove the connector cap from the short tubing of the water-seal chamber and use the funnel provided or a 50-mL syringe to add sterile water or NS to the 2-cm level.	Depth of solution required to establish a water-seal; the water-seal permits air and fluid to be removed from the chest and prevents backflow of air.[1,19]	Water-seal levels greater than 2 cm increase the work of breathing; levels less than 2 cm can expose the water-seal to air and increase the risk for pneumothorax.[19]
12. For gravity drainage, leave the short tubing from the suction control chamber open to air by turning stopcock to "open" or "on" position.	Creates the exit vent for the escape of air.	Clamping or occlusion of the exit vent can cause air to remain trapped in the pleural space, which may cause tension pneumothorax.
13. For suction drainage, fill the suction control chamber with sterile water or NS to the prescribed level (usually −10 to −20 cm H$_2$O suction). Connect the short tubing from the suction control chamber to the suction source.	Suction is regulated by the height of the solution level in this chamber.	Refill the solution level as necessary to the prescribed amount to replace solution lost through evaporation. Remove excess fluid as necessary via self-sealing grommet.
14. Hang chest drainage unit from bed frame, or set it on a floor stand. **(Level E*)**	Drainage unit must be kept below the level of the chest to promote gravity drainage and to prevent backflow of drainage into the pleural space, which interferes with lung expansion.[1,26]	
15. Connect the long tubing from the drainage collection chamber to the chest tube. **(Level C*)**	Creates the drainage collection system; avoid dependent or fluid-filled loops.[13,24]	Dependent or fluid-filled loops may create back pressure and decrease the effectiveness of suction.[13,24]

*Level C: Qualitative studies, descriptive or correlational studies, integrative reviews, systematic reviews, or randomized controlled trials with inconsistent results
*Level E: Multiple case reports, theory-based evidence from expert opinions, or peer-reviewed professional organizational standards without clinical studies to support recommendations

Procedure continues on following page

Procedure for Using Closed Chest Drainage Systems—*Continued*

Steps	Rationale	Special Considerations
16. Turn on the suction source, if prescribed, to elicit gentle constant bubbling. Leave stopcock between CDS and suction source fully open and adjust force of bubbling at suction source to decrease risk for pneumothorax. **Proceed to Step 94.**	Activates suction.	Some systems have a suction control feature to maintain the desired suction level automatically despite fluctuations in the suction source. The stopcock should be kept fully in "open" or "on" position and force of bubbling should be adjusted at suction source.
Emerson Disposable Suction System Setup (see Fig. 24-2)		
17. Add sterile water or NS through the suction port into the secondary compartment (overflow compartment) up to the water-seal line.	Depth of solution required to establish a water-seal; the water-seal permits air and fluid to be removed from the chest and prevents the backflow of air.[1,19]	Water-seal levels greater than 2 cm increase the work of breathing; levels less than 2 cm can expose the water-seal to air and increase the risk for pneumothorax.[19]
18. Secure the drainage system in the Emerson pump stand with the strings supplied, or with the accessory metal hangers, suspend the drainage set from the patient's bed. **(Level E*)**	Drainage unit must be kept below the level of the chest to promote gravity drainage and to prevent backflow of drainage into the pleural space, which interferes with lung expansion.[1,26]	
19. Connect the patient tubes to the patient connection fittings. If the patient has only one chest tube, leave the second unused port fitting capped.	Helps to maintain a closed drainage system.	
20. Connect the patient's chest tubes to the patient connection tubing. **(Level C*)**	Creates the closed drainage system; avoid dependent loops.[13,24]	Dependent or fluid-filled loops may create back pressure and decrease the effectiveness of suction.[13,24]
21. For gravity drainage, leave the flexible corrugated tubing off of the suction port on the secondary compartment (overflow compartment).	Creates the exit vent for the escape of air.	***Clamping of chest tubes can cause air trapped in the pleural space to accumulate and may cause tension pneumothorax.***
22. For suction drainage, connect the flexible corrugated tube to the suction port and to the corresponding fitting in the bottom of the Emerson pump cabinet.	Creates the suction drainage system.	
23. Dial in the amount of prescribed continuous suction on the Emerson pump dial. **Proceed to Step 94.**	Activates suction.	
One-Bottle Setup (Fig. 24-3)		
24. Fill the water-seal bottle with sterile water or NS so that the bottom of the long straw is immersed approximately 2 cm.	Immersing the long straw in solution is required to establish a water-seal. The water-seal permits air and fluid to be removed from the chest and prevents the backflow of air.[1,19]	Water-seal levels greater than 2 cm increase the work of breathing; levels less than 2 cm expose the water-seal to air and increase the risk for pneumothorax.[19]

*Level C: Qualitative studies, descriptive or correlational studies, integrative reviews, systematic reviews, or randomized controlled trials with inconsistent results
*Level E: Multiple case reports, theory-based evidence from expert opinions, or peer-reviewed professional organizational standards without clinical studies to support recommendations

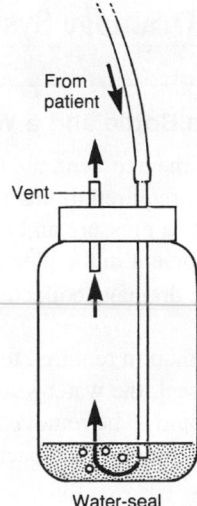

From patient

Vent

Water-seal

FIGURE 24-3 One-bottle chest drainage system. *(From Luce JM, Tyler ML, Pierson DJ: Intensive respiratory care, Philadelphia, 1984, Saunders.)*

Procedure for Using Closed Chest Drainage Systems—*Continued*

Steps	Rationale	Special Considerations
		If a large amount of drainage is anticipated, a two-bottle system is preferred, or empty the bottle whenever it is one quarter or more filled with fluid or according to institutional policy.[26]
25. Seal the bottle with the rubber stopper.	Except for the exit vent, an airtight system is required to maintain pleural negative pressure and to prevent air entrapment in the pleural space.	
26. Insert the short straw through one of the openings in the stopper and leave open to air.	The exit vent permits pleural air to escape from the system; otherwise, pressure can build up in the system, preventing further removal of pleural air and fluids.	Clamping or occlusion of the exit vent can cause air to remain trapped in the pleural space and may cause tension pneumothorax.
27. Insert the long straw through the second opening, immersing it 2 cm (less than 1 inch) beneath the surface of the solution.	Creates the water-seal.	Immersing the straw deeper than 2 cm increases the work of breathing.[19]
28. Stabilize the drainage bottle on the floor or in a special holder. **(Level E*)**	The bottle must be kept below the level of the chest to provide gravity drainage and prevent backflow of drainage into the pleural space[1,26] which interferes with lung expansion.	Disruption of the system may permit the entrance of atmospheric air into the pleural space, which may collapse the lung.
29. Connect the patient drainage tubing to the long straw of the water-seal bottle.	Creates the water-seal drainage collection bottle.	
30. Connect the patient drainage tubing to the chest tube.	Creates the closed chest drainage system.	

Proceed to Step 94.

*Level E: Multiple case reports, theory-based evidence from expert opinions, or peer-reviewed professional organizational standards without clinical studies to support recommendations

Procedure continues on following page

Procedure for Using Closed Chest Drainage Systems—*Continued*

Steps	Rationale	Special Considerations

Two-Bottle Setup With a Drainage Collection Bottle and a Water-Seal Bottle (Fig. 24-4, *A*)

Steps	Rationale	Special Considerations
31. Seal one bottle with a rubber stopper with two openings.	Except for the exit vent, an airtight system is required to maintain pleural negative pressure and to prevent air entrapment in the pleural space.	
32. Insert two short straws into the rubber stopper.	Creates the drainage collection bottle.	
33. Fill the water-seal bottle with sterile water or NS so that the bottom of the long straw is immersed approximately 2 cm.	Depth of solution required to establish a water-seal; the water-seal permits air and fluid to be removed from the chest and prevents the backflow of air.[1,19]	Water-seal levels greater than 2 cm increase the work of breathing; levels less than 2 cm expose the water-seal to air and increase the risk for pneumothorax.[19]
34. Seal the other bottle with a rubber stopper with two openings.	Except for the exit vent, an airtight system is required to maintain pleural negative pressure and to prevent air entrapment in the pleural space.	
35. Insert the short straw through one of the openings in the stopper.	Creates the exit vent for the escape of air or for connection to the suction source.	
36. Insert the long straw through the second opening, immersing it 2 cm beneath the surface of the solution.	Creates the water-seal and protects the patient from air leaks or loss of water-seal.	Immersing the straw deeper than 2 cm increases the work of breathing.[19]
37. Use the sterile tubing to connect one of the short straws of the drainage collection bottle to the long straw of the water-seal bottle.	Connects the drainage collection bottle to the water-seal bottle.	
38. Stabilize the bottles on the floor or in a special holder. **(Level E*)**	The bottles must be kept below the level of the chest to prevent backflow of drainage into the pleural space, which interferes with lung expansion.[1,26]	Disruption of the system may permit the entrance of atmospheric air into the pleural space, which may cause tension pneumothorax.
39. Connect the patient drainage tubing to the second short straw of the drainage collection bottle.	Creates a drainage avenue.	
40. Connect the patient drainage tubing to the chest tube.		
41. For gravity drainage, leave the exit vent of the water-seal bottle open to air. To apply suction, connect the suction source (i.e., Emerson pump) to the exit vent and adjust to the prescribed level (usually −10 cm to −20 cm H$_2$O suction level). **Proceed to Step 94.**	Suction increases pressure differences between the pleural space and the drainage system, which facilitates drainage from the pleural space.	Some systems have a suction control feature to maintain the desired suction level automatically despite fluctuations in the suction source. When connected to a suction system that has no exit vent, no in-flow of air equilibrates the pressure in the chamber, causing potential surges in suction. If a wall-mounted suction device is used, the exit vent of the drainage system should be disconnected if the device is turned off.[12]

*Level E: Multiple case reports, theory-based evidence from expert opinions, or peer-reviewed professional organizational standards without clinical studies to support recommendations

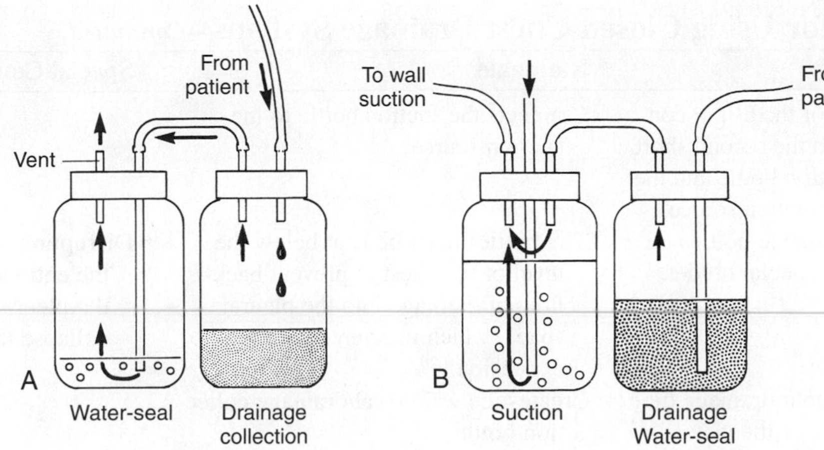

FIGURE 24-4   Two-bottle chest drainage system. **A,** Drainage collection bottle and a water-seal bottle. **B,** Water-seal/drainage collection bottle and suction control bottle. *(From Luce JM, Tyler ML, Pierson DJ: Intensive respiratory care, Philadelphia, 1984, Saunders.)*

Procedure	**for Using Closed Chest Drainage Systems**—*Continued*	
Steps	**Rationale**	**Special Considerations**
Two-Bottle Setup With a Water-Seal/Drainage Collection Bottle and a Suction Control Bottle (Fig. 24-4 *B*,)		
42. Fill the water-seal/drainage collection bottle with sterile water or NS so that the bottom of the long straw is immersed approximately 2 cm.	Depth of solution required to establish a water-seal; the water-seal permits air and fluid to be removed from the patient and prevents the backflow of air.[1,19]	
43. Seal the bottle with a rubber stopper with two openings.	Except for the exit vent, an airtight system is required to maintain pleural negative pressure and to prevent air entrapment in the pleural space.	
44. Insert the short straw through one of the openings in the stopper.	Initial step for connecting the drainage bottle to the water-seal bottle.	
45. Insert the long straw through the second opening, immersing it 2 cm beneath the surface of the solution.	Creates the water-seal and protects the patient from air leaks or loss of water-seal.	Immersing the straw deeper than 2 cm increases the work of breathing.[19]
46. Add prescribed amount of sterile water or NS to the suction bottle (usually −10 cm to −20 cm H$_2$O suction).	Creates the level of suction ordered.	The depth the straw is immersed in the solution determines the amount of suction delivered to the chest tube.[19]
47. Seal the suction bottle with the rubber stopper with three openings.	Except for the exit vent, an airtight system is required to maintain pleural negative pressure and to prevent air entrapment in the pleural space.	
48. Insert the long straw through the middle opening (leaving one end immersed in the solution and the other end open to the atmosphere).	Creates an air vent.	
49. Insert the two short straws into the remaining openings of the stopper.	Creates the setup for attachment to suction and to the overflow drainage bottle.	
50. Use the sterile tubing to connect the short straw from the water-seal/drainage collection bottle to one of the short straws of the suction bottle.	Connects the water-seal bottle to the suction source.	

Procedure continues on following page

Procedure for Using Closed Chest Drainage Systems—*Continued*

Steps	Rationale	Special Considerations
51. Attach one end of the 6-foot connecting tubing to the second short straw of the suction bottle and the other end to the suction source.	Connects the suction bottle to the suction source.	
52. Stabilize the drainage bottles on the floor or in a special holder. **(Level E*)**	The bottles must be kept below the level of the chest to prevent backflow of drainage into the pleural space, which interferes with lung expansion.[1,26]	Disruption of the system may permit the entrance of atmospheric air into the pleural space, which may collapse the lung.
53. Connect the patient drainage tube to the long straw of the water-seal/drainage collection bottle.	Creates the water-seal/drainage collection bottle.	
54. Connect the patient drainage tube to the chest tube.	Creates the chest drainage system.	The chest tube drainage system should be connected to the chest tube before suction is turned on.
55. Turn on the suction source to elicit gentle constant bubbling in the suction bottle.	Activates suction.	
Proceed to Step 94.		
Three-Bottle Setup (Fig. 24-5)		
56. Seal one of the bottles with the rubber stopper with two openings.	Except for the exit vent, an airtight system is required to maintain pleural negative pressure and to prevent air entrapment in the pleural space.	
57. Insert two short straws into the rubber stopper.	Creates the drainage collection bottle.	This bottle can be calibrated, if it is not already, by placing a piece of tape on the side so that drainage can be measured and recorded.
58. Fill the water-seal bottle with sterile water or NS so that the bottom of the long straw is immersed approximately 2 cm.	Depth of solution required to establish a water-seal; the water-seal permits air and fluid to be removed from the patient and prevents the backflow of air into the chest.[1,19]	Water-seal levels greater than 2 cm increase the work of breathing; levels less than 2 cm expose the water-seal to air and increase the risk for pneumothorax.[19]

*Level E: Multiple case reports, theory-based evidence from expert opinions, or peer-reviewed professional organizational standards without clinical studies to support recommendations

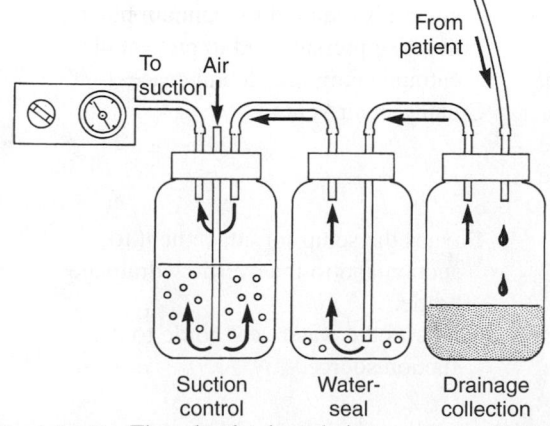

FIGURE 24-5   Three-bottle chest drainage system. (*From Luce JM, Tyler ML, Pierson DJ: Intensive respiratory care, Philadelphia, 1984, Saunders.*)

Procedure for Using Closed Chest Drainage Systems—*Continued*

Steps	Rationale	Special Considerations
59. Seal the water-seal bottle with a rubber stopper with two openings.	Except for the exit vent, an airtight system is required to maintain pleural negative pressure and to prevent air entrapment in the pleural space.	
60. Insert the short straw through one of the openings in the stopper.	Creates the exit vent for the escape of air or for connection to the suction source.	
61. Insert the long straw through the second opening, immersing it 2 cm beneath the surface of the solution.	Creates the water-seal and protects the patient from air leaks or loss of water seal.	Immersing the straw deeper than 2 cm increases the work of breathing.[19]
62. Add prescribed amount of sterile water or NS to the suction bottle (usually -10 cm to -20 cm H_2O suction).	Creates the level of suction ordered.	The depth the straw is immersed in the solution determines the amount of suction delivered to the chest tube.[19]
63. Seal the suction bottle with the rubber stopper with three openings.	Except for the exit vent, an airtight system is required to maintain pleural negative pressure and to prevent air entrapment in the pleural space.	
64. Insert the long straw through the middle opening (leaving one end immersed in the solution and the other end open to the atmosphere).	Creates the suction bottle.	
65. Insert the two short straws into the remaining openings of the stopper.	Creates the setup for attachment to suction and to the overflow drainage bottle.	
66. Use the sterile tubing to connect the short straw of the drainage collection bottle to the long straw of the water-seal bottle.	Connects the water-seal bottle to the suction bottle.	
67. Use the sterile tubing to connect the short straw from the water-seal bottle to one of the short straws of the suction bottle.	Connects the water-seal bottle to the suction bottle.	
68. Attach one end of the 6-foot connecting tubing to the second short straw of the suction bottle and the other end to the suction source.	Connects the suction bottle to the suction source.	
69. Stabilize the drainage bottles on the floor or in a special holder. **(Level E*)**	The bottles must be kept below the level of the chest to prevent backflow of drainage into the pleural space, which interferes with lung expansion.[1,26]	Disruption of the system may permit the entrance of atmospheric air into the pleural space, which may collapse the lung.
70. Connect the patient drainage tube to the short straw of the drainage collection bottle.	Provides a route for drainage to flow from the patient to the collection bottle.	
71. Connect the patient drainage tube to the chest tube.		The chest tube drainage system should be connected to the chest tube before suction is turned on.
72. Turn the suction source on to elicit gentle constant bubbling in the suction bottle.	Activates suction.	

Proceed to Step 94.
Four-Bottle Setup (Three-Bottle Setup With Vented Water-Seal Bottle; Fig. 24-6)

---

*Level E: Multiple case reports, theory-based evidence from expert opinions, or peer-reviewed professional organizational standards without clinical studies to support recommendations

Procedure continues on following page

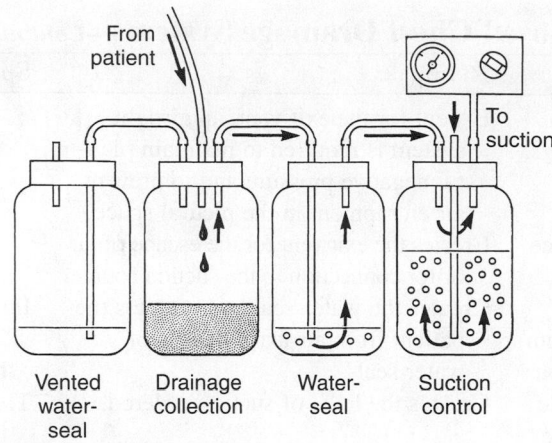

FIGURE 24-6   Four-bottle chest drainage system. *(From Luce JM, Tyler ML, Pierson DJ: Intensive respiratory care, Philadelphia, 1984, Saunders.)*

Procedure for Using Closed Chest Drainage Systems—*Continued*

Steps	Rationale	Special Considerations
73. Fill the vented water-seal bottle with sterile water or NS so that the bottom of the long straw is immersed approximately 2 cm.	Depth of solution required to establish a water-seal; the water-seal permits air and fluid to be removed from the patient and prevents the backflow of air into the chest.[1,19]	
74. Seal the bottle with a rubber stopper with two openings.	Except for the exit vent, an airtight system is required to maintain pleural negative pressure and to prevent air entrapment in the pleural space.	
75. Insert the long straw through one of the openings, immersing it 2 cm beneath the surface of the solution.	Creates the water-seal and protects the patient from air leaks or loss of water-seal.	Immersing the straw deeper than 2 cm increases the work of breathing.[19]
76. Insert a short straw through the second opening in the stopper and leave open to air.	Creates the vented water-seal that acts as a safety feature to allow the escape of positive pressure in case of problems with the suction source.	
77. Seal the drainage collection bottle with a rubber stopper with three openings.	Except for the exit vent, an airtight system is required to maintain pleural negative pressure and to prevent air entrapment in the pleural space.	
78. Insert three short straws into the rubber stopper.	Creates the drainage collection bottle.	This bottle can be calibrated, if it is not already, by placing a piece of tape on the side so that drainage can be measured and recorded.
79. Fill the water-seal bottle with sterile water or NS so that the bottom of the long straw is immersed approximately 2 cm.	Depth of solution required to establish a water-seal and to protect the patient from air leak or loss of water-seal.[1,19]	
80. Seal the bottle with a rubber stopper with two openings.	Except for the exit vent, an airtight system is required to maintain pleural negative pressure and to prevent air entrapment in the pleural space.	
81. Insert the short straw through one of the openings in the stopper.	Creates the exit vent for the escape of air for connection to the suction source.	

Procedure for Using Closed Chest Drainage Systems—*Continued*

Steps	Rationale	Special Considerations
82. Insert the long straw through the second opening, immersing it 2 cm beneath the surface of the solution.	Creates the water-seal and protects the patient from air leaks or loss of water-seal.	Immersing the straw deeper than 2 cm increases the work of breathing.[19]
83. Add prescribed amount of sterile water or NS to the suction bottle (usually −10 cm to −20 cm H$_2$O suction).	Creates the level of suction ordered.	The depth the straw is immersed in the solution determines the amount of suction delivered to the chest tube.[19]
84. Seal the suction bottle with the rubber stopper with three openings.	Except for the exit vent, an airtight system is required to maintain pleural negative pressure and to prevent air entrapment in the pleural space.	
85. Insert the long straw through the middle opening (leaving one end immersed in the solution and the other end open to the atmosphere).	Creates the manometer tube or air vent.	
86. Insert the two short straws into the remaining openings.	Creates the setup for attachment to suction and to the overflow-drainage bottle.	
87. Use the sterile tubing to connect the long straw of the vented water seal bottle to one of the short straws of the drainage collection bottle.	Provides for communication between the drainage system bottle and the vented water-seal bottle.	
88. Use the sterile tubing to connect the second straw of the drainage collection bottle to the long straw of the water-seal bottle.	Connects the drainage collection bottle to the water-seal bottle.	
89. Use the sterile tubing to connect the short straw from the water-seal bottle to one of the short straws of the suction bottle.	Connects the water-seal bottle to the suction bottle.	
90. Attach one end of the 6-foot connecting tubing to the second short straw of the suction bottle and the other end to the suction source.	Connects the suction bottle to the suction source.	
91. Stabilize the drainage bottles on the floor or in a special holder. **(Level E*)**	The bottles must be kept below the level of the chest to prevent backflow of drainage into the pleural space, which interferes with lung expansion.[1,26]	Disruption of the system may permit the entrance of atmospheric air into the pleural space, which may collapse the lung.
92. Connect the patient drainage tube to the middle short straw of the drainage collection bottle.	Provides a route for drainage to flow from the patient to the collection bottle.	
93. Connect the patient drainage tube to the chest tube.		The chest tube drainage system should be connected to the chest tube before suction is turned on.
94. Turn the suction source on to elicit gentle constant bubbling in the suction bottle.	Activates suction.	

*Level E: Multiple case reports, theory-based evidence from expert opinions, or peer-reviewed professional organizational standards without clinical studies to support recommendations

Procedure continues on following page

Procedure   for Using Closed Chest Drainage Systems—*Continued*

Steps	Rationale	Special Considerations
95. Tape all connection points in the chest drainage system (see Fig. 21- 2). A. Tape, 1-inch, is placed horizontally extending over the connections (a portion of the connector may be left unobstructed by the tape). B. Reinforce the horizontal tape with tape placed vertically so that it encircles both ends of the connector. 96. Dispose of soiled equipment and supplies. 97. Remove personal protective equipment. **HH**	Except for the exit vent, a secure and airtight system is required to avoid inadvertent disconnection that could cause air entrapment in the pleural space and decreased pleural negative pressure. This technique secures the connections but allows visualization of drainage in the connector.	Zip ties (Parham-Martin bands) may be used to secure connections instead of tape.

Expected Outcomes

- Removal of air, fluid, or blood from the chest cavity
- Fluctuation or tidaling noted in the water-seal chamber (until lung reexpanded)
- Relief of respiratory distress
- Reexpansion of the collapsed lung as validated with chest radiograph

Unexpected Outcomes

- Tension pneumothorax
- Hemorrhagic shock
- Absence of drainage and fluctuation or tidaling, or continuous bubbling in the water-seal chamber with continued respiratory distress
- No evidence of reexpansion of lung
- Fever, purulent drainage, and redness around the insertion site or purulent drainage in the chest tube

Patient Monitoring and Care

Steps	Rationale	Reportable Conditions
		These conditions should be reported if they persist despite nursing interventions.
1. Assess cardiopulmonary system and vital signs (including SpO_2) every 15 minutes 2 times, in 30 minutes 1 time, every 1 hour 4 hours after insertion. Then reassess every 2 to 4 hours and with any change in patient condition or according to institution protocol.	Provides baseline and ongoing assessment of patient's condition.	• Tachypnea • Decreased or absent breath sounds • Hypoxemia • Tachycardia • Dysrhythmias • Hypotension • Muffled heart tones • Tracheal deviation • Subcutaneous emphysema (crepitus) • Neck vein distention • Fever • Absence of fluctuations in water-seal chamber with respiratory distress

Patient Monitoring and Care —*Continued*

Steps	Rationale	Reportable Conditions
2. Monitor the amount and type of drainage by marking the drainage level on the outside of the drainage collection chamber in hourly or shift increments (depending on the amount of drainage) or in time increments established by institution policy or per practitioner orders. Monitor amount and type of drainage.	Marking container provides reference point for future measurements. Volume loss can cause patients to become hypovolemic or can signal intrapulmonary bleeding. Drainage should decrease gradually and change from bloody to pink to straw colored. Sudden flow of dark bloody drainage that occurs with position change is often old blood. Decreased or absent drainage associated with respiratory distress may indicate obstruction; decreased or absent drainage without respiratory distress may indicate lung reexpansion.	• Drainage greater than 100 mL/hr[1] • Sudden decrease or absence of drainage • Change in characteristics of drainage such as unexpectedly bloody, cloudy, or milky • New onset of clots
3. Assess patient and CDS for an air leak. If a suction source has been added, momentarily turn suction off or pinch suction tubing to accurately assess.[1] An air leak is present if air bubbles are observed in the water-seal chamber or going from right-to-left in the leak detector zone. As you assess the air-leak chamber, ask the patient to take deep breaths in and out. If you do not note an air leak ask the patient to cough.[8] When the patient's pleural space is leaking air, intermittent bubbling is seen corresponding to respirations. If bubbling is continuous, suspect an air leak in the system. To locate the source, intermittently pinch the chest tube or drainage tubing for a moment (i.e., less than a minute), beginning at the insertion site and progressing to the chest drainage unit.[1]	Assessing for an air leak is one way to determine whether the patient is experiencing a pneumothorax. Bubbling when suction is initially turned on occurs with air displaced by fluid drainage in the collection chamber, loose connections in the system, or an air leak in the pleural space.[10] With a minor air leak, bubbling may occur only with coughing when airway pressures reach their peak.[8,26] An airtight system is required to help reestablish negative pressure in the pleural space. If bubbling in the water-seal chamber stops when the chest tube is occluded at the dressing site, the air leak is inside the patient's chest or under the dressing. If a new-onset air leak, reinforce the dressing and notify the physician. If the bubbling stops when the drainage tubing is occluded along its length, the air leak is between the occlusion and the patient's chest; check to ensure all connections are airtight.[1,8] If bubbling does not stop with occlusion, replace the CDS.	• New or increasing air leaks in the chest or around the chest tube insertion site • Chest tube drainage from a mediastinal tube does not normally cause bubbling in the water-seal chamber; if noted, it may indicate communication with the pleural space; notify physician • Notify physician of system knockover and changing of the CDS (e.g., chest radiograph may be ordered)

Procedure continues on following page

Patient Monitoring and Care —*Continued*

Steps	Rationale	Reportable Conditions
4. Maintain and check chest tube and CDS patency on insertion, every 2 to 4 hours, and with a change in patient condition. Routine chest tube stripping or milking is not recommended. After careful assessment and identification of a visible clot or other obstructing drainage, gently milk (manual squeezing and releasing of small segments of tubing, or fan-folding and compressing small segments of tubing[13]) between the fingers.[10-12,16,18,22,23,27] **(Level C*)** Ensure there are no clamps on the chest tubes during milking.	Obstruction of drainage from the chest tube interferes with lung reexpansion or may cause cardiac tamponade. Stripping the entire length of the chest tube is contraindicated because it results in transient high negative pressures in the pleural space that could lead to lung entrapment.[11] No significant differences are reported in the amount of drainage when the tubing is milked as opposed to stripped.[12] Milking can cause excessive negativity. Use the high negativity relief value to restore negativity to prescribed levels **(see Step 8)**. Milking with a clamp on can result in the build-up of excessive thoracic pressure.	• Inability to establish patency • Excessive drainage
5. Maintain drainage tubing free of dependent loops (i.e., place the tube horizontally on the bed and down into the collection chamber, coiling the tubing on the bed). If a dependent loop cannot be avoided, lift and drain the tubing every 15 minutes.[13,14,24] **(Level C)**	Drainage that accumulates in dependent loops obstructs chest drainage into the collecting system and increases pressure within the lung.[10,12,13,15,22,24] Allow enough length for patient movement.	• Loops or kinks that cannot be removed
6. Monitor fluid levels in the CDS chambers by briefly turning off the suction and refill (usually every 8 hours for suction chamber and every 24 hours for water-seal) or remove solution levels as necessary to the prescribed amount.	To maintain prescribed water-seal and suction levels and to prevent complications. Water-seal levels greater than 2 cm increase the work of breathing; levels less than 2 cm expose the water-seal to air and increase the risk for pneumothorax.[1,19]	• Inability to maintain a water-seal or to keep suction at prescribed level
7. Assess for CDS patency: Note fluctuations or tidaling of fluid level in the water-seal chamber (disposable chest drainage system) or the long straw of the water-seal bottle (bottle chest drainage system) with respirations.[1,19] If a suction source has been added, momentarily turn suction off or pinch suction tubing to accurately assess for fluctuations or tidaling.	Tidaling, fluid fluctuation up and down or back and forth, indicates effective communication between the pleural space and drainage system and provides an indication of lung expansion. Fluctuations or tidaling stops when the lung is reexpanded or when the tubing is obstructed by a kink, a fluid-filled loop, the patient lying on the tubing, or a clot or tissue at the distal end.[1,10,19] Suction must be turned off to accurately assess for tidaling.	• Absence of fluctuations or tidaling

*Level C: Qualitative studies, descriptive or correlational studies, integrative reviews, systematic reviews, or randomized controlled trials with inconsistent results

Patient Monitoring and Care —*Continued*

Steps	Rationale	Reportable Conditions
8. Assess CDS equipped with a float valve for increases in the patient's negative intrathoracic pressure. Inspect water-seal chamber for increased levels (e.g., after milking of chest tube or when decreasing the amount of suction). First, ensure the chest drainage system is operating on suction. Second, temporarily depress the filtered manual vent until the float valve releases and the water column lowers.	Changes in the patient's intrathoracic pressure are reflected by the height of the water in the water-seal column. Do not lower water-seal column when suction is not operating or when patient is on gravity drainage. Resume suction while performing this operation. If suction is not operative, or operating on gravity drainage, depressing the high negative relief valve can reduce negative pressure within the collection chamber to zero (atmosphere), possibly resulting in a pneumothorax.	• Sustained increases in negative pressures
9. Assess insertion site and surrounding skin for the presence of subcutaneous emphysema (crepitus) and signs of infection or inflammation daily and with each dressing change. Dressings should be changed when soiled, per institution protocol, or when ordered by practitioner. Routine petroleum dressings are not recommended.[15] (**Level E***)	Crepitus may indicate chest tube obstruction or improper tube position. Skin integrity is altered during insertion and can lead to infection. Petroleum gauze dressing has been noted to cause skin maceration, potentiating the risk of infection.[15]	• New or increasing subcutaneous emphysema (crepitus) • Fever • Redness around insertion site • Purulent drainage
10. Monitor collection chamber for total amount of fluid. Change chest drainage system when approaching full or if system integrity is interrupted (i.e., cracked). Assess cardiopulmonary status and vital signs (including SpO_2) before and after procedure. Prepare new CDS according to manufacturer's instructions. Then, briefly (i.e., less than a minute) cross clamp the chest tube close to the patient's chest. Attach the new system, unclamp the chest tube, check connections, and assess function of drainage system.	When the patient has an air leak or pneumothorax, clamping of the chest tube may precipitate a tension pneumothorax because the air has no escape route and may accumulate in the pleural space.[1,15,17] Clamping of the chest tube should be as brief as possible.	• Respiratory distress noted during or after procedure • Changes in breath sounds after procedure • Nonfunctioning chest drainage system
11. During gravity drainage, ambulation, or transport with gravity drainage, ensure chest drain system is upright, below the chest tube insertion site, and maintain the suction control stopcock in the "on" or "open" position. Do not clamp chest tube during transport.[1,26] (**Level E**)	The suction control stopcock should always remain in the "on" or "open" position. Do not clamp or cap the suction line. Leaving the port open allows air to exit and minimizes the possibility of tension pneumothorax.	• Notify physician of inadvertent clamping or capping of the suction line

*Level E: Multiple case reports, theory-based evidence from expert opinions, or peer-reviewed professional organizational standards without clinical studies to support recommendations

Procedure continues on following page

Patient Monitoring and Care —*Continued*

Steps	Rationale	Reportable Conditions
12. Follow institution standard for assessing pain. Administer analgesia as prescribed.	Identifies need for pain interventions.	• Continued pain despite pain interventions.
13. Obtaining a drainage specimen from some disposable CDSs: Cleanse the site with alcohol and use a syringe with a smaller (e.g. 20-gauge) needle to withdraw the specimen from the self-sealing diaphragm, or self-sealing drainage tubing, as available. Momentarily forming a dependent loop in the fluid collection tubing may be necessary to obtain a specimen.	Provides a specimen for analysis.	• Inability to obtain specimen

Documentation

Documentation should include the following:

- Patient and family education
- Cardiopulmonary and vital sign assessment
- Type of drainage system used
- Amount of suction, fluctuation or tidaling, type and amount of drainage
- Air leak: Absence, presence, severity, and resolution
- Patient's tolerance of the therapy

- Respiratory, thoracic, and vital sign assessment with changes in therapy
- Completion and results of the postinsertion chest radiograph and any other ordered diagnostic tests
- Unexpected outcomes
- Nursing interventions
- Pain assessment, interventions, and effectiveness

References

CR 1. Allibone L: Nursing management of chest drains, *Nurs Stand* 17:45-56, 2003.

2. Alphonso N, et al: A prospective randomized controlled trial of suction versus non-suction to the under-water seal drains following lung resection, *Eur J Cardiothorac Surg* 27:391-394, 2005.

CR 3. Ayed AK: Suction versus water seal after thoracoscopy for primary spontaneous pneumothorax: prospective randomized study, *Ann Thorac Surg* 75:1593-1596, 2003.

4. Baumann MH: Management of spontaneous pneumothorax, *Clin Chest Med* 27:369-381, 2006.

CR 5. Baumann MH: Management of spontaneous pneumothorax: an American College of Chest Physicians Delphi consensus statement, *Chest* 119:590-602, 2001.

CR 6. Baumann MH: What size chest tube? What drainage system is ideal? And other chest tube management questions, *Curr Opin Pulm Med* 9:276-281, 2003.

CR 7. Baumann MH, et al: Comparison of function of commercially available pleural drainage units and catheters, *Chest* 123:1878-1886, 2003.

8. Cerfolio RJ: Recent advances in the treatment of air leaks, *Curr Opin Pulm Med* 11:319-323, 2005.

9. Cerfolio RJ, et al: The management of chest tubes in patients with a pneumothorax and an air leak after pulmonary resection, *Chest* 128:816-820, 2005.

CR 10. Deshpande KS, Tortolandi AJ, Kvetan V: Troubleshooting chest tube complications: how to prevent—or quickly correct—the major problems, *J Crit Ill* 18(6):275-280, 2003.

CR 11. Duncan C, Erickson R: Pressures associated with chest tube stripping, *Heart Lung* 11:166-71, 1982.

CR 12. Duncan C, Erickson R, Wiegel RM: Effect of chest tube management on drainage after cardiac surgery, *Heart Lung* 16:1-9, 1987.

CR 13. Gordon PA, et al: Positioning of chest tubes: effects on pressure and drainage, *Am J Crit Care* 6:33-38, 1997.

CR 14. Gordon PA, Norton JM, Merrell R: Redefining chest tube management: analysis of the state of practice, *Dimens Crit Care Nurs* 14:6-13, 1995.

CR 15. Gross SB: Current challenges, concepts and controversies in chest tube management, *AACN Clin Issues Crit Care Nurs* 4:260-75, 1993.

16. Halm MA: To strip or not to strip? Physiological effects of chest tube manipulation, *Am J Crit Care* 16(6): 609-612, 2007.

CR 17. Henry M, Arnold T, Harvey J: British Thoracic Society guidelines for the management of spontaneous pneumothorax, *Thorax* 58:39-52, 2003.

CR 18. Isaacson JJ, George IT, Brewer MJ: The effect of chest tube manipulation on mediastinal drainage, *Heart Lung* 15(6):601-605, 1986.

CR 19. Kam AC, O'Brien M, Kam PCA: Pleural drainage systems, *Anaesthesia* 48:154-161, 1993.

20. Kelly AM: Review of management of primary spontaneuos pneumothorax: is the best evidence clearer 15 years on? *Emerg Med Aust* 19:303-308, 2007.

21. Lehwaldt D, Timmins F: Nurses' knowledge of chest drain care: an exploratory descriptive survey, *Nurs Crit Care* 10(4):192-200, 2005.

CR 22. Lim-Levy F, et al: Is milking and stripping chest tubes really necessary? *Ann Thorac Surg* 42:77-80, 1986.

CR 23. Pierce J, Piazza D, Naftel DC: Effects of two chest tube clearance protocols on drainage in patients after myocardial revascularization surgery, *Heart Lung* 20: 125-130, 1991.

CR 24. Schmelz JO, et al: Effects of position of chest drainage tube on volume drained and pressure, *Am J Crit Care* 8:319-323, 1999.

25. Stolz AJ, et al: Predictors of prolonged air leak following pulmonary lobectomy, *Eur J Cardiothorac Surg* 334-336, 2005.

CR 26. Tang AT, Velissaris TJ, Weeden DF: An evidence-based approach to drainage of the pleural cavity: evaluation of best practice, *J Eval Clin Pract* 8:333-340, 2002.

CR 27. Wallen M, et al: Mediastinal chest drain clearance for cardiac surgery, *Cochrane Database of Systematic Review* 2:Art. No.: CD003042. DOI:10/1002/14651858. CD003042.pub2, 2004.

Additional Readings

Atrium: *Managing chest drainage,* Hudson, NH, 2007, Atrium Medical Corporation.

Atrium: *Managing dry suction chest drainage,* Hudson, NH, 2007, Atrium Medical Corporation.

Carroll PF: Ask the experts: Atrium dry suction chest drainage system, *Crit Care Nurse* 23:73-4, 2003.

AP Needle Thoracostomy (Perform)

PURPOSE: Needle thoracostomy is performed to reduce a tension pneumothorax to a simple pneumothorax in a patient with a rapidly deteriorating condition. This temporary measure is followed quickly by the insertion of a chest tube for more definitive management.

Cynthia A. Goodrich

PREREQUISITE NURSING KNOWLEDGE

- Anatomy and physiology of the pulmonary system should be understood.
- The thoracic cavity, in normal conditions, is a closed air space. Any disruption results in the loss of negative pressure within the intrapleural space. Air or fluid that enters the space competes with the lung, which results in collapse of the lung. Associated conditions are the result of disease, injury, surgery, or iatrogenic causes.
- A pneumothorax is classified as an open, closed, or tension pneumothorax. In patients with tension pneumothorax, air leaks into the pleural space through a tear in the lung and, with no means to escape from the pleural cavity, creates a one-way valve effect. With each breath the patient takes, air accumulates, pressure within the pleural space increases, and the lung collapses. As a result, the mediastinal structures (i.e., heart, great vessels, and trachea) shift to the opposite or unaffected side of the chest. Venous return and cardiac output are impeded, and the possibility of collapse of the unaffected lung exists.[1-5]
- Tension pneumothorax is a medical emergency that necessitates immediate intervention. Accurate assessment of

signs and symptoms allows for prompt recognition and treatment:
- ❖ Tracheal deviation to the unaffected side
- ❖ Neck vein distention
- ❖ Muffled heart sounds
- ❖ Tachypnea
- ❖ Decreased or absent breath sounds on the affected side
- ❖ Shortness of breath, dyspnea
- ❖ Asymmetric chest excursion with respirations
- ❖ Cyanosis
- ❖ Decreased oxygen saturation
- ❖ Subcutaneous emphysema
- ❖ Sudden sharp chest pain
- ❖ Anxiety, restlessness, apprehension
- ❖ Tachycardia
- ❖ Hypotension
- ❖ Dysrhythmias
- ❖ Pulseless electrical activity (PEA)
- Needle thoracostomy is performed with placement of a needle into the pleural space to remove air and reestablish negative pressure in a patient with an unstable condition with tension pneumothorax (Fig. 25-1).

EQUIPMENT

- Personal protective equipment
- 14- to 16-gauge hollow needle or catheter with one-way valve attached or commercially available (Heimlich) flutter valve
- Antiseptic solution

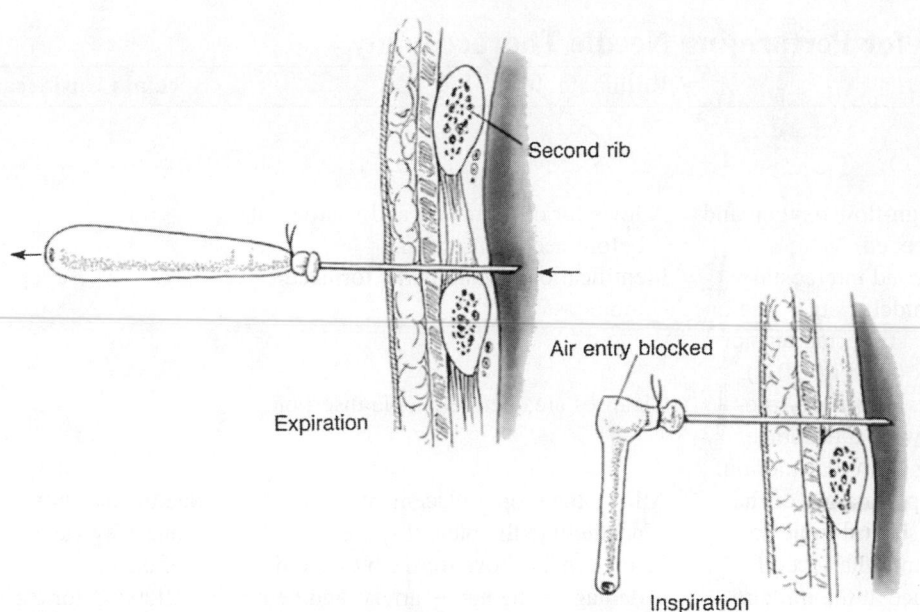

FIGURE 25-1.   Use of a needle and a sterile finger cot or a finger from a sterile glove to fashion a one-way (flutter) valve for emergency evacuation of a tension pneumothorax. A small opening is made in the free end of the glove finger to allow air to escape during expiration. *(From Cosrniff JH: An atlas of diagnostic and therapeutic procedures for emergency personnel, Philadelphia, 1978, J.B. Lippincott.)*

- 4 × 4 gauze dressing
- Tape
  Additional equipment to have available as needed includes the following:
- Oxygen
- Self-inflating manual resuscitation bag-valve-mask device
- Oxygen source and tubing
  The listed equipment can be used to create an emergency one-way valve:
  - ❖ Scissors
  - ❖ Sterile glove (powder-free)
  - ❖ Small rubber band
  Cut a finger off the glove and attach it to the needle with the rubber band.[1]

PATIENT AND FAMILY EDUCATION

- Explain the procedure and reason for needle thoracostomy. ➤*Rationale:* This communication identifies patient and family knowledge deficits concerning the patient's condition, expected benefits, and potential risks and allows time for questions to clarify information and to voice concerns. Explanations decrease patient and family's anxiety and enhance cooperation.
- If indicated, explain the patient's role in assisting with needle thoracostomy. ➤*Rationale:* Eliciting the patient's cooperation assists with insertion of a needle and flutter valve.

PATIENT ASSESSMENT AND PREPARATION
Patient Assessment

- Signs and symptoms consistent with tension pneumothorax, as noted previously. ➤*Rationale:* Accurate assessment of signs and symptoms allows for prompt recognition and treatment. Baseline assessment provides comparison data for evaluation of changes and outcomes of treatment. Tension pneumothorax is a medical emergency that necessitates immediate intervention.

Patient Preparation

- Verify correct patient with two identifiers. ➤*Rationale:* Prior to performing a procedure, the nurse should ensure the correct identification of the patient for the intended intervention.
- Ensure that the patient and family understand the emergency nature of the procedure and preprocedural teachings, if appropriate. Answer questions as they arise, and reinforce information as needed. ➤*Rationale:* This communication evaluates and reinforces understanding of previously taught information.
- Position patient in supine position with the head of the bed flat. ➤*Rationale:* This positioning allows for identification of landmarks for proper placement of needle and flutter valve.
- Perform a pre-procedure verification and time out, if nonemergent. ➤*Rationale:* Ensures patient safety.

Procedure   for Performing Needle Thoracostomy

Steps	Rationale	Special Considerations
1. 🔲 HH		
2. 🔲 PE		
3. Administer high-flow oxygen and ventilate as needed.	Allows for oxygenation and ventilation before needle insertion.	
4. Locate the second intercostal space at the midclavicular line on the side of the suspected tension pneumothorax (see Fig. 20-1).	Identification of landmarks for needle thoracostomy.	
5. If time permits, surgically prepare the skin with antiseptic solution using a circular motion.	Cleanses area before needle insertion.	
6. Locate the upper margin of the third rib with several fingers. Insert needle into the second intercostal space at the midclavicular line, pointing the needle posterior but slightly upward and sliding it over the top of the third rib.[1,2,3,4] **(Level D*)**	Allows the proper placement of the needle into the pleural space. Insert needle above third rib to avoid damaging the nerve, artery, and vein that lie just beneath each rib.	Needle and flutter valve acts as a one-way valve, preventing reentry of air into pleural space but allowing for escape of air during expiration (see Fig. 25-1).
7. Puncture the parietal pleural space. Listen for an audible escape of air as the needle enters the parietal pleural space. If a catheter over needle device is used, remove the needle.[1,2,3,4] **(Level D)**	Although an audible rush of air indicates that needle decompression has been successful, a dramatic improvement in the patient's clinical condition is the best indicator of successful intervention.	
8. Attach a flutter valve to the needle or catheter, if not already attached.[1,2,3,4] **(Level D)**	Allows air to escape the pleural space and prevents air from entering.	
9. Apply a small dressing around the needle or catheter or suture it in place.	Allows for temporary stabilization of needle or catheter until a chest tube can be inserted.	
10. Prepare for immediate chest tube insertion (see Procedures 20, 21).	Definitive treatment of tension pneumothorax.	

*Level D–Peer-reviewed professional organizational standards with clinical studies to support recommendations.

Expected Outcomes

- Removal of air from pleural space
- Reestablishment of negative intrapleural pressure
- Tension pneumothorax conversion to simple pneumothorax
- Improved oxygenation and ventilation

Unexpected Outcomes

- Resultant pneumothorax in patient without tension pneumothorax
- Damage to nerves, veins, or arteries because of improper flutter valve placement
- Local hematoma or cellulitis
- Pleural infection

Patient Monitoring and Care

Steps	Rationale	Reportable Conditions
		These conditions should be reported if they persist despite nursing interventions.
1. Stabilize the needle or catheter with dressing until chest tube is inserted.	Prevents movement and dislodgment of needle or catheter. A chest tube should be inserted as soon as practical.	• Dislodged needle or catheter
2. Constantly monitor for signs and symptoms of tension pneumothorax.[1,2,3,4] **(Level D*)**	Determines whether chest decompression has been successful and allows for early identification of new pneumothorax until chest tube has been placed.	• Tracheal deviation to the unaffected side • Neck vein distention • Muffled heart sounds • Tachypnea • Decreased or absent breath sounds on the affected side • Shortness of breath, dyspnea • Asymmetric chest excursion with respirations • Cyanosis • Decreased oxygen saturation • Subcutaneous emphysema • Sudden sharp chest pain • Anxiety, restlessness, apprehension • Tachycardia • Hypotension • Dysrhythmias
3. Follow institution standard for assessing pain. Administer analgesia as prescribed.	Identifies need for pain interventions	• Continued pain despite pain interventions

*Level D-Peer-reviewed professional organizational standards with clinical studies to support recommendations

Documentation

Documentation should include the following:

- Vital signs before and after insertion of needle or catheter, including pain, as appropriate
- Location of needle or catheter
- Size of needle or catheter used
- Response after needle or catheter placement
- Unexpected outcomes
- Nursing interventions
- Occurrence of unexpected outcomes
- Patient and family education
- Pain assessment, interventions, and effectiveness

References

1. American College of Surgeons Committee on Trauma: *Advanced trauma life support manual,* ed 7, Chicago, 2004, American College of Surgeons.
2. Emergency Nurses Association: *Trauma nursing core course: provider manual,* ed 6, Des Plaines, IL, 2007, Emergency Nurses Association.
3. Holleran RS: Air and surface patient transport: principles and practice, ed 3, St Louis, 2003, Mosby.
4. National Association of Emergency Technicians: *PHTLS: basic and advanced prehospital trauma life support,* ed 5, St Louis, 2003, Mosby.
5. Roberts JR, Hedges JR, editors: *Clinical procedures in emergency medicine,* ed 4, Philadelphia, 2004, Saunders.

AP Thoracentesis (Perform)

P U R P O S E :   Thoracentesis is performed to assist in the diagnosis and therapeutic management of patients with pleural effusions.

Susan Yeager

PREREQUISITE NURSING KNOWLEDGE

- Thoracentesis is performed with insertion of a needle or a catheter into the pleural space, which allows for removal of pleural fluid.
- Pleural effusions are defined as the accumulation of fluid in the pleural space that exceeds 10 to 20 mL and results from the overproduction of fluid or disruption in fluid reabsorption.[1]
- Thoracentesis is not used to verify the presence of pleural effusion. Diagnosis of pleural effusion is made via clinical examination, patient symptoms, and diagnostic techniques. A number of techniques can demonstrate pleural effusion with varying levels of sensitivity. Percussion requires a minimum of 300 to 400 mL for identification of a pleural effusion, whereas a standard chest radiography requires 200 to 300 mL. Lateral decubitus radiographs can be used to recognize smaller fluid amounts and highlight whether present fluid is free flowing. Ultrasound scan, computed tomography (CT) scan, and magnetic resonance imaging (MRI) technology can detect 100 mL of fluid with 100% sensitivity.[1] Therefore, initial diagnosis of pleural effusion should use imaging techniques such as chest radiographs, ultrasound scans, CT scans, or MRI combined with patient symptoms and clinical examination findings.
- Diagnostic thoracentesis is indicated for differential diagnosis for patients with pleural effusion of unknown etiology. A diagnostic thoracentesis may be repeated if initial results fail to yield a diagnosis.
- Therapeutic thoracentesis is indicated to relieve the symptoms (e.g., dyspnea, cough, hypoxemia, or chest pain) caused by a pleural effusion.
- Pleural effusions are classified as either transudative or exudative effusions.
- Exudative effusions indicate a local etiology (e.g., pulmonary embolus, infection), whereas transudative effusions usually are associated with systemic etiologies (e.g., heart failure).
- Samples of pleural fluid are analyzed and assist in distinguishing between exudative and transudative etiologies of effusion. Results of laboratory tests on pleural fluid alone do not establish a diagnosis; instead the laboratory results must be correlated with the clinical findings and serum laboratory results.
- Exudative pleural effusions meet one of the following criteria[1]:
  - Pleural fluid lactate dehydrogenase (LDH)-to-serum LDH ratio is greater than 0.6 international units/mL.
  - Pleural fluid LDH is more than two thirds of the upper limit of normal for serum LDH.
  - Pleural fluid protein-to-serum protein ratio is greater than 0.5 g/dL.
- A transudative pleural effusion is considered when none of the exudative criteria is met and is usually associated with systemic etiologies (e.g., heart failure), whereas exudative effusions indicate a local etiology (e.g., pulmonary embolus, infection, open heart surgery).
- Relative contraindications for thoracentesis include the following:
  - Patient anatomy that hinders the practitioner from clearly identifying the appropriate landmarks

---

AP   This procedure should be performed only by physicians, advanced practice nurses, and other healthcare professionals (including critical care nurses) with additional knowledge, skills, and demonstrated competence per professional licensure or institutional standard.

❖ Patients undergoing anticoagulation therapy or with an uncorrectable coagulation disorder

❖ Patients receiving positive end-expiratory pressure (PEEP) therapy

❖ Patients with splenomegaly, elevated left hemidiaphragm, or left-sided pleural effusion

❖ Patients with only one lung as a result of a previous pneumonectomy

❖ Patients with known lung disease

- Ultrasound scan–guided thoracentesis is thought to reduce complications, especially when used in the last four patient groups listed in the relative contraindications list.[3,4]

- Complications commonly associated with thoracentesis include:

  ❖ Pneumothorax

  ❖ Hemopneumothorax

  ❖ Hemorrhage

  ❖ Hypotension

  ❖ Cough

  ❖ Reexpansion pulmonary edema

- Recent studies have shown a reduction in complications with ultrasound scan–guided technique, especially when used in the last four patient groups listed in the relative contraindications list.[4-6]

- Pneumothorax is the most common postthoracentesis complication with a reported incidence rate between 3% and 30%.[11]

- Hemorrhagic complications are more likely to occur in elderly patients because of tortuosity of vessels.[8]

- Hypotension can occur as part of the vasovagal reaction during or hours after the procedure. If it occurs during the procedure, cessation of the procedure and atropine instillation may be necessary. If hypotension occurs after the procedure, it is likely the result of fluid shifting from pleural effusion reaccumulation. In this situation, the patient is likely to respond to fluid resuscitation.[11]

- Development of cough generally initiates toward the end of the procedure and should result in procedure cessation.

- Reexpansion pulmonary edema is thought to occur from overdraining of fluid too quickly. Limitation of this complication may be accomplished by minimizing fluid removal to 1000 mL,[11] but at least one study found no correlation with drainage of up to 2000 mL as long as the patient was symptom free during the procedure.[5]

EQUIPMENT

Diagnostic Thoracentesis

- Baseline diagnostic study results (i.e., lateral decubitus chest radiograph, ultrasound imaging, CT scan, or MRI)
- Completed patient informed consent form
- Functional intravenous access
- Indelible marker
- Sterile gloves
- Sterile drapes

- Sterile towels
- Adhesive bandage or adhesive strip
- Antiseptic solution
- Sterile 4 × 4 gauze pads
- Intervention medications (opioid, sedative, or hypnotic agents, local anesthetic 1% or 2% lidocaine)
- One small needle (25-gauge, ⅝-inch long)
- 5-mL syringe for local anesthetic
- Three large needles (20- to 22-gauge, 1½ to 2 inches long)
- Three-way stopcock
- Sterile 20-mL syringe
- Sterile 50-mL syringe
- Two chemistry blood tubes
- Hemostat or Kelly clamp
- Pulse oximetry equipment
- Side table
- Pillow or blanket to be placed on side table
- Available: Atropine, oxygen, thoracostomy supplies, advanced cardiac life support (ACLS) equipment
- Ultrasound scan equipment as needed

Therapeutic Thoracentesis

The following equipment is needed in addition to equipment for diagnostic thoracentesis:

- 14-gauge needle
- 16-gauge catheter
- Sterile 50-mL syringe
- Vacutainers or evacuated bottles (1- to 2-L) with pressure tubing

Additional equipment (to have available depending on patient need) includes the following:

- Two complete blood count (CBC) tubes
- One anaerobic and one aerobic media bottle for culture and sensitivity
- Sterile tubes for fungal and tuberculosis cultures

Commercially prepackaged thoracentesis kits are available in some institutions

PATIENT AND FAMILY EDUCATION

- Explain the procedure and purpose for thoracentesis, including potential complications, such as pneumothorax, pain at insertion site, cough, infection, hypoxemia, and hypovolemia. Include an explanation of the amount of fluid expected to be withdrawn, duration of time the procedure may last, and expectation of and reason for coughing during or after thoracentesis. ➥*Rationale:* This communication identifies patient and family knowledge deficits concerning patient condition, procedure, expected benefits, and potential risks and allows time for questions to clarify information and voice concerns. Explanations decrease patient anxiety and enhance cooperation.

- Explain the patient's role in thoracentesis. ➥*Rationale:* This explanation increases patient compliance, facilitates needle and catheter insertion, and enhances fluid removal.

PATIENT ASSESSMENT AND PREPARATION

Patient Assessment

- Obtain a history of symptoms, occupational exposure, and medication usage
- Assess for signs and symptoms of pleural effusion:
  - Trachea deviated away from the affected side
  - Affected side dull to flat with percussion
  - Absent or decreased breath sounds
  - Tactile fremitus
  - Pleuritic chest pain
  - Hypoxemia
  - Tachypnea
  - Dyspnea
  - Cough, weight loss, night sweats, anorexia, and malaise may also occur with pleural infection or malignancy disease[10]

  ➤*Rationale:* Although physical findings may suggest a pleural effusion, radiography or other imaging studies confirm its presence.

- Assess chest radiograph or other imaging findings. ➤*Rationale:* If at least half the hemidiaphragm is obliterated on erect anterior-posterior radiograph results, sufficient fluid is in the pleural space for a thoracentesis. Greater than 200 mL of fluid is considered abnormal in erect chest radiograph results. Lateral radiographs show blunting of the costophrenic angle with 50 mL. With a small amount of loculated fluid, however, a lateral decubitus radiograph should be obtained. Lateral decubitus radiographs assist with distinguishing between free moving fluid and pleural thickening. If the pleural effusion is measured to be greater than 10 mm deep on a lateral decubitus radiograph, a diagnostic thoracentesis can be performed. However, if the pleural effusion is measured to be less than 10 mm in diameter or loculated, ultrasound scan is necessary to distinguish between pleural effusion and pleural lesion. Ultrasound scan–guided thoracentesis may be necessary if a pleural effusion has been confirmed.[8] In the intensive care setting, supine anterior-posterior radiographs are less sensitive in the identification of pleural effusions. In this setting, hazy opacification of one lung field or minor fissure thickening may be the only clues to the presence of a pleural effusion.[10]
  - Posterior-anterior and lateral chest radiographs should be performed in all suspected pleural effusions.[7]
  - Consider ultrasound scan guidance if the effusion is small, loculated, or on the side of an elevated hemidiaphram or if the patient is on mechanical ventilation or has a bleeding diathesis.[7,8]
  - CT scans with contrast should be performed for pleural enhancement.[7]
  - In difficult drainage situations, CT scan should be used to delineate effusion size and position.[7]
- Assess medical history of pleuritic chest pain, malignancy disease, heart failure, and medication usage. ➤*Rationale:* Medical history may provide valuable clues to the cause of a patient's pleural effusion or presence of hypercoagulable states as a result of medications. Knowledge of medication usage can indicate the need for anticoagulation reversal before invasive procedure. In addition, an increasing number of medications is noted to contribute to exudative effusions. Common examples include amiodarone, phenytoin, nitrofurantoin, and methotrexate. See www.pneumotox.com for a more comprehensive listing.[7,10]
- Assess baseline vital signs, including pulse oximetry. ➤*Rationale:* Baseline assessment data provide information about patient status and allow for comparison during and after the procedure.
- Assess recent serum laboratory results, including the following:
  - Complete blood count
  - Platelet count
  - Prothrombin time/International Normalized Ratio (INR)
  - Partial thromboplastin time

  ➤*Rationale:* These studies help determine whether the patient is at increased risk for bleeding. Generally, an INR of 1.3 or less is acceptable for invasive procedures.

Patient Preparation

- Verify correct patient with two identifiers. ➤*Rationale:* Prior to performing a procedure, the nurse should ensure the correct identification of the patient for the intended intervention.
- Ensure that the patient understands preprocedural teachings. Answer questions as they arise and reinforce information. ➤*Rationale:* This communication evaluates and reinforces understanding of previously taught information.
- Obtain written informed consent for the procedure. ➤*Rationale:* Invasive procedures, unless performed with implied consent in a life-threatening situation, require written consent of the patient or significant other.
- Consider sedation or chemical paralysis. ➤*Rationale:* Sedation or chemical paralysis may be necessary to maximize positioning.
- Have atropine available. ➤*Rationale:* Bradycardia, from a vasovagal reflex, is a common occurrence during thoracentesis.
- Initiate pulse oximetry monitoring. ➤*Rationale:* Pulse oximetry provides a noninvasive means for monitoring oxygenation and heart rate at the bedside, which allows for prompt recognition and intervention should problems develop.

Procedure for Diagnostic and Therapeutic Thoracentesis

Steps	Rationale	Special Considerations
Diagnostic Thoracentesis		
1. Perform a pre-procedure verification and time out, if non-emergent.	Ensures patient safety.	
2. **HH**		
3. Assemble equipment, including intravenous access.	Ensures proper equipment is readily available throughout procedure and in emergency situations.	
4. **PE**		
5. Position patient for procedure with assistant standing in front of patient.	Positioning enhances ease of withdrawal of pleural fluid. Assuring patient is comfortable increases the chance that the procedure will be successfully completed. Having the assistant in front of the patient ensures visualization of facial cues and enables the cessation of inadvertent patient movements that might interfere with the procedure.	
A. If the patient is alert and able, position the patient on the edge of the bed with feet supported on a stool and arms resting on a pillow on an elevated bedside table (Fig. 26-1, *A*).		
B. The patient may sit on a chair backward and rest arms on a pillow on the back of the chair.		
C. If the patient is unable to sit, position the patient on the unaffected side, with the back near the edge of the bed and the arm on the affected side above the head. Elevate the head of the bed to 30 or 45 degrees, as tolerated.		
6. Percuss the affected side posteriorly to determine the highest point of the pleural effusion. Identify the intercostal space below this point and mark with a marker.	Identifies the superior border of the pleural effusion and identifies and validates the planned site for thoracentesis.	Use the posterior axillary line as the insertion point to avoid the spinal cord. If the space identified for insertion is below the eighth intercostal space (area is approximated at the posterior edge of scapula), ultrasound scan should be done to mark the fluid level and its relationship to the diaphragm, which helps identify a safe point of entry to avoid solid-organ damage.
7. Apply sterile personal protective equipment, while an assistant opens the necessary equipment onto a sterile field or opens the appropriate sterile tray with the equipment.	Reduces the transmission of microorganisms and body secretions; standard precautions.	

Procedure continues on following page

Procedure   for Diagnostic and Therapeutic Thoracentesis—*Continued*

Steps	Rationale	Special Considerations
8. Have an assistant provide preprocedural medications.	Premedication with opioid, antianxiolytic, sedative, or hypnotic assures patient comfort throughout procedure.	Know patient allergy history and have reversal medications available for the previous list of medications.
9. Prepare site with antiseptic using concentric circles from insertion site mark outward and drape area with sterile drape.	Reduces skin contaminants, which reduces the risk of infection.	
10. Anesthetize the skin with lidocaine (25-gauge, ⅝-inch needle) in the typical wheal fashion around the insertion site.	Increases comfort for patient by anesthetizing the periosteum of the rib and pleura.	
11. With 2% lidocaine and a 20- to 22-gauge, 1½- to 2-inch needle, insert the needle through the wheal. Inject the lidocaine into the deep tissue and periosteum of the underlying rib superiorly and laterally.	Anesthetizes the work area for optimal patient comfort. Insertion above the rib minimizes manipulation or laceration of the vascular bundle located beneath the rib (Fig 26-1, *B*).	Always aspirate before injecting to prevent lidocaine from entering a blood vessel or the pleural space.
12. After anesthetizing the periosteum of the underlying rib, gently advance the needle and alternately aspirate and inject lidocaine until pleural fluid is obtained in the syringe.	Anesthetizes the parietal pleura. The pleural space is identified by pleural fluid aspirate in the syringe. If air bubbles are noted, the lung tissue may have been violated or air may have been introduced by the thoracentesis system. Withdraw syringe to tissue and redirect. Withdrawal of needle minimizes manipulation of lung tissue. Familiarizing yourself with the thoracentesis equipment before the procedure also minimizes the likelihood of air introduction.[8]	

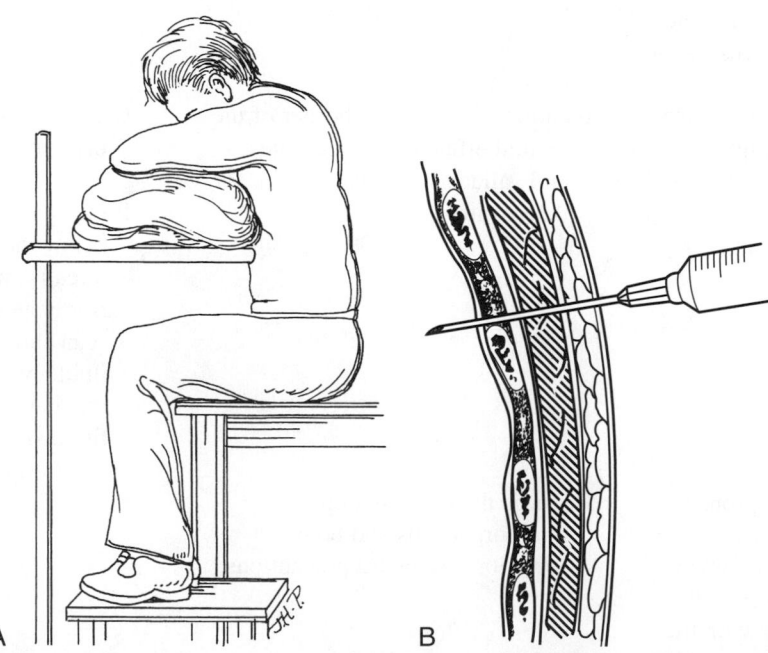

Figure 26-1   Thoracentesis. **A,** Ideal patient position for thoracentesis. **B,** Ideal placement of needle insertion.

Continued

Procedure | for Diagnostic and Therapeutic Thoracentesis—*Continued*

Steps	Rationale	Special Considerations
13. When pleural fluid is obtained, place a sterile gloved finger on the needle at the point where the needle exits the skin. Withdraw the needle and syringe. For therapeutic thoracentesis, **proceed to step 19**.	Approximates the length of insertion for the thoracentesis needle or catheter.	
14. Attach a three-way stopcock and 50-mL syringe to a 20- to 22-gauge, 1½ or 2-inch needle. Open the stopcock valve between the syringe and the needle. **(Level C*)**	The open stopcock valve allows for aspiration of pleural fluid during needle insertion and minimizes atmospheric air introduction.	Longer needles may be necessary in the obese patient.
15. Insert the selected needle via the anesthetized tract, superior to the rib, and continually aspirate until pleural fluid is obtained, filling the 50-mL syringe. Fluid should be separated into three sterile containers for microbiology, biochemistry, and cytology analysis. **(Level B*)**[7]; **(Level C)**[10]	Inserting the needle superior to the rib avoids disruption of the vascular and lymph systems. (Figure 26-1, *B*) The pleural fluid is used for laboratory testing for the differential diagnosis. A sample of 35 to 50 mL is needed for a diagnostic analysis of fluid. A change in patient position can be attempted to facilitate fluid drainage.	It is possible that no fluid is accessed (dry tap). If a dry tap occurs, ultrasound scan–guided aspiration is suggested and is successful in 97% of cases. A larger gauge needle may be needed for thick or loculated fluid, or the needle may have been inserted above or below the pleural fluid. When pleural fluid is aspirated, the needle may be stabilized with placing a hemostat or clamp on the needle at the skin site to keep the needle from advancing farther into the pleural space, preventing lung puncture. Note the appearance of the aspirated fluid because this may provide clues to the underlying etiology of effusion. Straw-colored fluid is common and typical of transudates. Blood-stained fluid is suggestive of hemothorax, malignancy disease, pulmonary infarction, trauma, or postcoronary artery bypass surgery. Pleural hematocrit of more than 50% of serum hematocrit is indicative of hemothorax. Fluid turbidity suggests empyema or chylothorax, and food particles indicates esophogeal rupture.[10]
16. Fill the specimen tubes from the pleural fluid–filled syringe by turning the stopcock "off" to the patient and allowing the tubes to fill passively by vacuum or by depressing the syringe plunger (Figure 26-1, *C*). Send the specimen tubes to the laboratory for appropriate analysis.	Analysis may aid in determining an etiology of the pleural effusion.	To interpret pleural fluid laboratory values, serum chemistry laboratory values must be obtained (e.g., pH, total protein, glucose, and LDH). Contrary to common practice, at least one study showed that immediate pH evaluation or placement of the sample on ice is not necessary if this measurement is delayed.[8]

*Level B: Well-designed, controlled studies with results that consistently support a specific action, intervention or treatment
*Level C: Qualitative studies, descriptive or correlational studies, integrative reviews, systematic reviews, or randomized controlled trials with inconsistent results

Procedure continues on following page

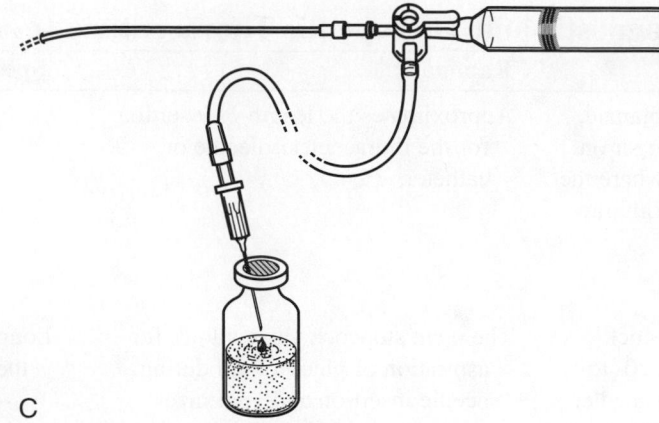

C

FIGURE 26-1, cont'd   **C,** Attach catheter to three way stopcock syringe and vacutainer. *Barton ED: Thoracentesis. In Rosen, P., Chan, T.C., Vilke, M., Sternbach, G., editors: Atlas of Emergency Procedures (pp. 36-37), St. Louis: Mosby.*

Procedure	**for Diagnostic and Therapeutic Thoracentesis**—*Continued*	
Steps	**Rationale**	**Special Considerations**
17. Evaluate patient response throughout procedure.	Monitoring patient heart rate, pulse oximetry, and clinical response throughout the procedure enables prompt intervention or cessation of procedure should complications arise.	
18. On completion of diagnostic thoracentesis, withdraw the needle. Apply pressure to the puncture site for a few minutes, then apply an adhesive strip or adhesive bandage over the puncture site. Without concrete clinical indications, a chest radiograph is not necessary after a routine thoracentesis.[2,3,5,6] **(Level C*)**		

Therapeutic Thoracentesis

19. Insert a 14-gauge needle attached to a 20-mL syringe, bevel down, into the anesthetized tract until pleural fluid is returned.	The 14-gauge needle is selected because it allows for insertion and passage of a 16-gauge catheter; a smaller sized catheter may be unstable and fold or kink on itself.	
20. When pleural fluid is obtained, remove the syringe from the needle, occluding the needle with an index finger.	Occluding the needle helps prevent the possible occurrence of a pneumothorax.	
21. Insert the 16-gauge catheter through the 14-gauge needle. Advance the catheter slowly through the needle, angling the catheter in a downward fashion toward the costodiaphragm until the catheter moves freely in the pleural space.	Advancing the catheter toward the costodiaphragm allows for optimal drainage of pleural fluid.	In therapeutic thoracentesis, a catheter is preferred over a needle because the lung is expected to reexpand. A needle could puncture the lung during reexpansion and cause a pneumothorax.

*Level C: Qualitative studies, descriptive or correlational studies, integrative reviews, systematic reviews, or randomized controlled trials with inconsistent results

Procedure for Diagnostic and Therapeutic Thoracentesis—*Continued*

Steps	Rationale	Special Considerations
22. While advancing the catheter beyond the needle tip, remove the needle and leave the catheter in the pleural space. Attach a three-way stopcock with a 50-mL syringe to the end of the catheter.	Never pull the catheter back through the needle because the catheter may be cut or sheared by the needle tip.	
23. Fill the 50-mL syringe with pleural fluid. Fill the specimen tubes from the pleural fluid–filled syringe by turning the stopcock "Off" to the patient and allowing the tubes to fill passively by vacuum or by depressing the syringe plunger (Figure 26-1, *C*). Send the specimen tubes to the laboratory for appropriate analysis. A. Amylase testing should be requested if acute pancreatitis or esophageal rupture is suspected. **(Level C*)** B. If the first pleural cytology results are negative, a second specimen should be obtained to rule out malignancy disease. **(Level B*)** C. pH tests should be performed on all nonpurulent effusions. In an infected effusion, a pH of less than 7.2 indicates the need for tube drainage.[7] **(Level B)** D. Local anesthetics (i.e., lidocaine) are acidic; therefore, care should be taken during pleural sampling to avoid contamination of sample.[10]	When changing syringes, be certain the stopcock is positioned such that air does not enter the pleural space. Analysis may aid in determining an etiology of the pleural effusion.	To interpret pleural fluid chemistry laboratory values, serum chemistry laboratory values also must be obtained (e.g., pH, total protein, glucose, LDH).
24. Attach the Vacutainer or evacuated bottles with tubing to the three-way stopcock. Open the valve to the Vacutainer and fill the Vacutainer.	The Vacutainer or evacuated bottles use negative pressure to withdraw pleural fluid from the pleural space, providing therapeutic relief. Reposition catheter or patient or both if drainage stops to determine whether fluid is still present.	Do not remove greater than 1000 to 1500 mL of pleural fluid at one time; removing more than this can cause hypovolemia, hypoxemia, or even reexpansion pulmonary edema. Reexpansion pulmonary edema is most likely to occur if a pleural effusion has been compressing the lung for more than 7 days and when more than 1.5 L of fluid is removed at one time.[8] The patient may feel the need to cough as the lung reexpands.

*Level B: Well-designed, controlled studies with results that consistently support a specific action, intervention, or treatment
*Level C: Qualitative studies, descriptive or correlational studies, integrative reviews, systematic reviews, or randomized controlled trials with inconsistent results

Procedure continues on following page

Procedure for Diagnostic and Therapeutic Thoracentesis—*Continued*

Steps	Rationale	Special Considerations
25. On completion of thoracentesis, remove the catheter. Apply pressure to the puncture site for a few minutes, then apply an adhesive strip or adhesive bandage over the puncture site. **(Level C*)**		Without concrete clinical indications, chest radiograph is not necessary after a routine thoracentesis.[3,4,6,9]
26. Reposition the patient to optimize comfort.	Patient may desire to lie down after procedure. Head of bed placement may vary if dyspnea, hypotension, or other symptoms present during procedure.	
27. Dispose of equipment.		
28. Remove personal protective equipment. **HH**		
29. Assess pain and provide interventions as needed		

*Level C: Qualitative studies, descriptive or correlational studies, integrative reviews, systematic reviews, or randomized controlled trials with inconsistent results

Expected Outcomes

- Patient is comfortable and has decreased respiratory distress
- Lung reexpansion occurs
- Site remains infection-free
- Procedure aids in diagnosis of etiology of pleural effusion

Unexpected Outcomes

- Pneumothorax
- Vasovagal response
- Dyspnea
- Hypovolemia
- Hematoma
- Hemothorax
- Liver or splenic laceration
- Reexpansion pulmonary edema

Patient Monitoring and Care

Steps	Rationale	Reportable Conditions
		These conditions should be reported if they persist despite nursing interventions.
1. Monitor vital signs and cardiopulmonary status before and after thoracentesis and as needed.	Any change in vital signs may alert the practitioner of possible unexpected outcomes. Use of supplemental oxygen may be necessary in certain patient populations.	• Tachypnea • Decreased or absent breath sounds on the affected side • Shortness of breath, dyspnea • Asymmetric chest excursion with respirations • Decreased oxygen saturation • Subcutaneous emphysema • Sudden sharp chest pain • Anxiety, restlessness, apprehension • Tachycardia • Hypotension • Dysrhythmias • Tracheal deviation to the unaffected side • Neck vein distention • Muffled heart sounds

Patient Monitoring and Care —*Continued*

Steps	Rationale	Reportable Conditions
2. If indicated, obtain a postthoracentesis expiratory chest radiograph. **(Level C*)**	A chest radiograph is used to evaluate for lung reexpansion and evidence of a possible pneumothorax or hemothorax. If a pneumothorax or hemothorax is present, a chest tube may be necessary. However, the incidence rate of pneumothorax or hemothorax has been estimated at 11%, with only 2% of patients needing chest tube placement.[8] Without concrete clinical indications, chest radiograph is not necessary after a routine thoracentesis.[3,4,6,7,9]	• Pneumothorax • Expanding pleural effusion • Catheter migration
3. Follow institution standard for assessing pain. Administer analgesia as prescribed.	Identifies need for pain interventions	• Continued pain despite pain interventions

*Level C: Qualitative studies, descriptive or correlational studies, integrative reviews, systematic reviews, or randomized controlled trials with inconsistent results

Documentation

Documentation should include the following:
- Patient and family teaching
- Consent for procedure
- Adherence to Universal Protocol
- Patient positioning and monitoring devices
- Medication administration and patient response
- Patient tolerance, including pain and pain interventions
- Insertion of catheter or needle
- Catheter or needle size used
- Any difficulties in insertion
- Patient tolerance of procedure
- Pleural fluid aspirate characteristics
- Total amount of pleural fluid aspirated
- Site assessment
- Intact catheter on withdrawal
- Occurrence of unexpected outcomes
- Postthoracentesis radiograph acquisition and results, as available
- Laboratory test ordered and results as available
- Interpretation of laboratory results
- Nursing interventions
- Pain assessment, interventions, and effectiveness

References

CR 1. Barton E: Thoracentesis. In Rosen P, Chan T, Vilke G, et al, editors: *Atlas of emergency procedures,* St Louis: 2001. Mosby.

CR 2. Colt HG, Brewer N, Barbur EB: Evaluation of patient-related and procedure-related factors contributing to pneumothorax following thoracentesis, *Chest* 116: 134-138, 1999.

CR 3. Doyle JJ, et al: Necessity of routine chest roentgenography after thoracentesis, *Ann Intern Med* 124:816-820, 1996.

CR 4. Gervais DA, et al: US-guided thoracentesis: requirement for post procedure chest radiography in patients who receive mechanical ventilation versus patients who breathe spontaneously, *Radiology* 204:503-506, 1997.

CR 5. Jones PW, et al: Ultrasound-guided thoracentesis: is it a safer method? *Chest* 123:418-423, 2003.

CR 6. Lichtenstein D, et al: Feasibility and safety of ultrasound-aided thoracentesis in mechanically ventilated patients, *Intensive Care Med* 25:955-958, 1999.

CR 7. Maskell NA, Butland RJA: BTS guidelines for the investigation of a unilateral pleural effusion in adults, *Thorax* 58:ii8, 2003.

CR 8. Parsons P, Tu Y: Thoracentesis and percutaneous pleural biopsy. In Parsons P, Heffner J, editors: *Pulmonary respiratory therapy secrets,* Philadelphia, 1997, Mosby.

CR 9. Qureshi N, Momin ZA, Brandstetter RD: Thoracentesis in clinical practice, *Heart Lung* 23:376-383, 1994.

10. Rahman N, Chapman S, Davies R: Pleural effusion: a structured approach to care, *Br Med Bull* 72(1):31-47, 2005.

CR 11. Wilson M, Irwin R: Thoracentesis. *Procedures and techniques in intensive care medicine,* Philadelphia, 2003, Lippincot & Williams & Wilkins.

Additional Readings

Antunes G, Neville E, Duffy J, et al: BTS guidelines for the management of malignant pleural effusions, *Thorax* 58(Suppl 2):ii29-38, 2003.

Davies CWH, Gleeson FV, Davies RJO: BTS guidelines for the management of pleural infection, *Thorax* 58:ii18, 2003.

Heffner JE, Brown LK, Barbieri CA: Diagnostic value of tests that discriminate between exudative and transudative pleural effusions, *Chest* 111:970-980, 1997.

Light RW, et al: Pleural effusion: the diagnostic separation of transudates and exudates, *Ann Intern Med* 77:507-513, 1992.

Loddenkemper R: Pleural effusions. In Albert R, Spiro S, Jett J, editors: *Clinical respiratory medicine,* Philadelphia, 2004, Mosby.

Mayo PH, Goltz HR, Tafreshi M, et al: Safety of ultrasound-guided thoracentesis in patients receiving mechanical ventilation, *Chest* 125(3):1059-1062, 2004.

Peterson WG, Zimmerman R: Limited utility of chest radiograph after thoracentesis, *Chest* 117:1038-1042, 2000.

Quigley RL: Thoracentesis and chest tube drainage, *Crit Care Clin* 11:111-126, 1995.

Thomsen TW, DelaPena J, Stenik GS: Thoracentesis, Videos in clinical medicine 355/e16(15) retrieved from http://content.nejm.org/cgi/content/video_preview/355/15/e16, accessed 09/14/2008.

Thoracentesis (Assist)

P U R P O S E : Thoracentesis is performed to assist in the diagnosis and therapeutic management of patients with pleural effusions.

Susan Yeager

PREREQUISITE NURSING KNOWLEDGE

- Thoracentesis is performed with insertion of a needle or a catheter into the pleural space, which allows for removal of pleural fluid.
- Pleural effusions are defined as the accumulation of fluid in the pleural space that exceeds 10 to 20 mL and results from the overproduction of fluid or disruption in fluid reabsorption.[1]
- Thoracentesis is not used to verify the presence of pleural effusion. Diagnosis of pleural effusion is made via clinical examination, patient symptoms, and diagnostic techniques. A number of techniques can demonstrate pleural effusion with varying levels of sensitivity. Percussion requires a minimum of 300 to 400 mL for identification of a pleural effusion, whereas standard chest radiography requires 200 to 300 mL. Lateral decubitus radiographs can recognize smaller fluid amounts and highlight whether present fluid is free flowing. Ultrasound scan, computed tomography (CT) scan, and magnetic resonance imaging (MRI) technology can detect 100 mL of fluid with 100% sensitivity.[1] Therefore, initial diagnosis of pleural effusion should use imaging techniques such as chest radiographs, ultrasound scan, CT scan, or MRI, combined with patient symptoms and clinical examination findings.
- Diagnostic thoracentesis is indicated for differential diagnosis for patients with pleural effusion of unknown etiology. A diagnostic thoracentesis may be repeated if initial results fail to yield a diagnosis.
- Therapeutic thoracentesis is indicated to relieve the symptoms (e.g., dyspnea, cough, hypoxemia, or chest pain) caused by a pleural effusion.
- Exudative effusions indicate a local etiology (e.g., pulmonary embolus, infection), whereas transudative effusions usually are associated with systemic etiologies (e.g., heart failure).

- Samples of pleural fluid are analyzed and assist in distinguishing between exudative and transudative etiologies of effusion. Results of laboratory tests on pleural fluid alone do not establish a diagnosis; instead, the laboratory results must be correlated with the clinical findings and serum laboratory results.
- Exudative pleural effusions meet one of the following criteria[1]:
  - ❖ Pleural fluid lactate dehydrogenase (LDH)-to-serum LDH ratio is greater than 0.6 international units/mL.
  - ❖ Pleural fluid LDH is more than two thirds of the upper limit of normal for serum LDH.
  - ❖ Pleural fluid protein-to-serum protein ratio is greater than 0.5 g/dL.
- A transudative pleural effusion is considered when none of the exudative criteria are met.
- Transudative effusions usually are associated with systemic etiologies (e.g., heart failure), whereas exudative effusions indicate a local etiology (e.g., pulmonary embolus, infection, open heart surgery).
- Relative contraindications for thoracentesis include the following:
  - ❖ Patient anatomy that hinders the practitioner from clearly identifying the appropriate landmarks
  - ❖ Patients undergoing anticoagulant therapy or having an uncorrectable coagulation disorder
  - ❖ Patients receiving positive end-expiratory pressure therapy
  - ❖ Patients with splenomegaly, elevated left hemidiaphragm, and left-sided pleural effusion
  - ❖ Patients with only one lung as a result of a previous pneumonectomy
  - ❖ Patients with known lung disease

- Ultrasound scan–guided thoracentesis is thought to reduce complications, especially when used in the last four patient groups listed in the relative contraindications list.[2,3]
- Complications commonly associated with thoracentesis include:
  - Pneumothorax
  - Hemopneumothorax
  - Hemorrhage
  - Hypotension
  - Cough
  - Reexpansion pulmonary edema

EQUIPMENT
Diagnostic Thoracentesis

- Baseline diagnostic study results (i.e., lateral decubitus chest radiograph, ultrasound scan imaging, CT scan, or MRI)
- Completed patient informed consent form
- Functional intravenous access
- Indelible marker
- Sterile gloves
- Sterile drapes
- Sterile towels
- Adhesive bandage or adhesive strip
- Antiseptic solution
- Sterile 4 × 4 gauze pads
- Intervention medications (opioid, sedative, or hypnotic agents, local anesthetic 1% or 2% lidocaine)
- One small needle (25-gauge, ⅝-inch long)
- 5-mL syringe for local anesthetic
- Three large needles (20-gauge to 22-gauge, 1½ to 2 inches long)
- Three-way stopcock
- Sterile 20-mL syringe
- Sterile 50-mL syringe
- Two chemistry blood tubes
- Hemostat or Kelly clamp
- Pulse oximetry equipment
- Side table
- Pillow or blanket to be placed on side table
- Available: Atropine, oxygen, thoracostomy supplies, advanced cardiac life support (ACLS) equipment
- Ultrasound scan equipment as needed

Therapeutic Thoracentesis

The following equipment is needed in addition to equipment for diagnostic thoracentesis:
- 14-gauge needle
- 16-gauge catheter
- Sterile 50-mL syringe
- Vacutainers or evacuated bottles (1- to 2-liter) with pressure tubing

Additional equipment (to have available depending on patient need) includes the following:
- Two complete blood count (CBC) tubes
- One anaerobic and one aerobic media bottle for culture and sensitivity

- Sterile tubes for fungal and tuberculosis cultures
Commercially prepackaged thoracentesis kits are available in some institutions.

PATIENT AND FAMILY EDUCATION

- Explain the procedure and purpose for thoracentesis, including potential complications, such as pneumothorax, pain at insertion site, cough, infection, hypoxemia, and hypovolemia. Include an explanation of the amount of fluid expected to be withdrawn, duration of time procedure may last, and expectation of and reason for coughing during or after thoracentesis. ➤➤*Rationale:* This communication identifies patient and family knowledge deficits concerning patient condition, procedure, expected benefits, and potential risks and allows time for questions to clarify information and voice concerns. Explanations decrease patient anxiety and enhance cooperation.
- Explain the patient's role in thoracentesis. ➤➤*Rationale:* This explanation increases patient compliance, facilitates needle and catheter insertion, and enhances fluid removal.

PATIENT ASSESSMENT AND PREPARATION
Patient Assessment

- Obtain a history of symptoms, occupational exposure, and medication usage.
- Signs and symptoms of pleural effusion include the following:
  - Trachea deviated away from the affected side
  - Affected side dull to flat with percussion
  - Absent or decreased breath sounds on the affected side
  - Tactile fremitus
  - Pleuritic chest pain
  - Hypoxemia
  - Tachypnea
  - Dyspnea
  - Cough, weight loss, night sweats, anorexia, and malaise may also occur with pleural infection or malignancy disease.[6]

➤➤*Rationale:* Although physical findings may suggest a pleural effusion, other imaging studies confirm its presence.
- Assess chest radiograph or other imaging findings. ➤➤*Rationale:* If at least half the hemidiaphragm is obliterated on erect anterior-posterior radiograph results, sufficient fluid is in the pleural space for a thoracentesis. Greater than 200 mL of fluid is considered abnormal in erect chest radiograph results. Lateral radiographs show blunting of the costophrenic angle with 50 mL. With a small amount of loculated fluid, however, a lateral decubitus radiograph should be obtained. Lateral decubitus radiographs assist with distinguishing between free-moving fluid and pleural thickening. If the pleural effusion is measured to be greater than 10 mm deep on a lateral decubitus radiograph, a diagnostic thoracentesis can be performed.

However, if the pleural effusion is measured to be less than 10 mm in diameter or loculated, ultrasound scan is necessary to distinguish between pleural effusion and pleural lesion. Ultrasound scan–guided thoracentesis may be necessary if a pleural effusion has been confirmed. In the intensive care setting, supine anterior-posterior radiographs are less sensitive in the identification of pleural effusions. In this setting, hazy opacification of one lung field or minor fissure thickening may be the only clues to the presence of a pleural effusion.[6]

- Assess medical history of pleuritic chest pain, cough, dyspnea, malignancy disease, heart failure, and medication usage. ➤*Rationale:* Medical history may provide valuable clues to the cause of a patient's pleural effusion or presence of hypercoagulable states. Knowledge of medication usage can indicate the need for anticoagulation reversal before an invasive procedure. In addition, an increasing number of medications is noted to contribute to exudative effusions. Common examples include amiodarone, phenytoin, nitrofurantoin, and methotrexate. See www.pneumotox.com for a more comprehensive listing.[4,6]
- Assess baseline vital signs, including pulse oximetry. ➤*Rationale:* Baseline assessment data provide information about patient status and allow for comparison during and after the procedure.
- Assess recent laboratory results, including the following:
  ❖ CBC
  ❖ Platelet count
  ❖ Prothrombin time/International Normalized Ratio (INR)
  ❖ Partial thromboplastin time
  ➤*Rationale:* These studies help determine whether the patient is at increased risk for bleeding. Generally, an INR of 1.3 or less is acceptable for invasive procedures.

Patient Preparation

- Verify correct patient with two identifiers. ➤*Rationale:* Prior to performing a procedure, the nurse should ensure the correct identification of the patient for the intended intervention.

- Ensure that the patient understands pre-procedural teachings. Answer questions as they arise and reinforce information. ➤*Rationale:* This communication evaluates and reinforces understanding of previously taught information.
- Obtain written informed consent for the procedure. ➤*Rationale:* Invasive procedures, unless performed with implied consent in a life-threatening situation, require written consent of the patient or significant other.
- Position the patient. Several alternative positions may be used, as follows:
  ❖ If the patient is alert and able, position the patient on the edge of the bed with legs supported and arms resting on a pillow on the elevated bedside table (see Fig. 26-1).
  ❖ The patient may sit on a chair backward and rest arms on a pillow on the back of the chair.
  ❖ If the patient is unable to sit, position the patient on the unaffected side, with the back near the edge of the bed and the arm on the affected side above the head. Elevate the head of the bed to 30 or 45 degrees, as tolerated.
  ➤ *Rationale:* Positioning enhances ease of withdrawal of pleural fluid.
- Have an additional member of the healthcare team positioned in front of the patient. ➤*Rationale:* This positioning reassures or comforts the patient and provides additional assistance.
- Consider sedation or paralysis. ➤*Rationale:* Sedation or paralysis may be necessary to maximize positioning.
- Have atropine available. ➤*Rationale:* Bradycardia, from a vasovagal reflex, is a common occurrence during thoracentesis.
- Initiate pulse oximetry monitoring. ➤*Rationale:* Pulse oximetry provides a noninvasive means for monitoring oxygenation and heart rate at the bedside, which allows for prompt recognition and intervention should problems occur.

Procedure	for Assisting with Diagnostic and Therapeutic Thoracentesis	
Steps	**Rationale**	**Special Considerations**
1. Perform a pre-procedure verification and time out, if non-emergent.	Ensures patient safety.	
2. **HH**		
3. **PE**		
4. Assemble equipment, including intravenous access and open procedure tray, with aseptic technique.	Ensures proper equipment is readily available throughout procedure and in emergency situations.	

Procedure continues on following page

Procedure for Assisting with Diagnostic and Therapeutic Thoracentesis—*Continued*

Steps	Rationale	Special Considerations
5. Assist with patient positioning, application of monitoring devices, and verification of intravenous access.	Positioning that optimizes patient comfort aids in patient cooperation and completion of the procedure. Application of monitoring devices, including verification of functional intravenous access, enables prompt identification and intervention should complications occur during the procedure.	
6. Assume a position in front of the patient and provide physical support for positioning, as necessary.	Having the assistant in front of the patient ensures visualization of facial cues and enables the cessation of inadvertent patient movements that might interfere with the procedure.	
7. As directed by physician or advanced practice nurse practitioner, administer procedural medications.	Premedication with opioid, antianxiolytic, sedative, or hypnotic ensures patient comfort throughout procedure.	
8. Throughout procedure, assist with providing continuous monitoring of patient vital signs and response to the procedure and interventions.	The physician or advanced practice nurse practitioner is focused on the technique required to obtain the fluid. By standing in front of the patient, facial and monitoring cues should be readily noted by the person assisting the clinician, which enables prompt identification and intervention should complications occur.	
9. As directed by physician or advanced practice nurse practitioner, assist with filling of the specimen tubes from the pleural fluid–filled syringe. Label appropriately and send the specimen tubes to the laboratory for appropriate analysis.	Analysis may aid in determining an etiology of the pleural effusion.	To interpret pleural fluid laboratory values, serum chemistry laboratory values must be obtained (e.g., pH, total protein, glucose, and LDH).
10. As directed by physician or advanced practice nurse practitioner for therapeutic thoracentesis, assist with attaching the Vacutainer or evacuated bottles with tubing to the three-way stopcock.	The physician or advanced practice nurse then turns the stopcock to the Vacutainer or evacuated bottles to withdraw fluid from the pleural space. The Vacutainer or evacuated bottles use negative pressure to withdraw pleural fluid from the pleural space, providing therapeutic relief. Reposition catheter or patient or both if drainage stops to determine whether fluid is still present.	Evacuating more than 1000 to 1500 mL of pleural fluid at one time may cause hypovolemia, hypoxemia, or reexpansion pulmonary edema. The patient may feel the need to cough as the lung reexpands.
11. On completion of thoracentesis, the physician or advanced practice nurse practitioner may apply pressure to the puncture site for a few minutes, then apply an adhesive bandage over the puncture site or may direct the assistant to do so. **(Level C*)**		Without concrete clinical indications, chest radiograph is not necessary after a routine thoracentesis.[2,3,5]

*Level C: Qualitative studies, descriptive or correlational studies, integrative reviews, systematic reviews, or randomized controlled trials with inconsistent results

Procedure for Assisting with Diagnostic and Therapeutic Thoracentesis—*Continued*

Steps	Rationale	Special Considerations
12. Reposition patient to optimize comfort.	Patient may desire to lie down after procedure. Head of bed placement may vary if dyspnea, hypotension, or other symptoms present during procedure.	
13. Dispose of soiled equipment and supplies.		
14. Remove personal protective equipment.	Reduces the transmission of microorganisms and body secretions; Standard Precautions.	
15. 🄷🄷		

Expected Outcomes

- Patient is comfortable and has decreased respiratory distress
- Lung reexpansion occurs
- Site remains infection-free
- Procedure aids in diagnosing of etiology of pleural effusion

Unexpected Outcomes

- Pneumothorax
- Vasovagal response
- Dyspnea
- Hypovolemia
- Hematoma
- Hemothorax
- Liver or splenic laceration
- Reexpansion pulmonary edema

Patient Monitoring and Care

Steps	Rationale	Reportable Conditions
		These conditions should be reported if they persist despite nursing interventions.
1. Monitor vital signs and cardiopulmonary status before and after thoracentesis and as needed.	Any change in vital signs may alert the practitioner of possible unexpected outcomes. Use of supplemental oxygen may be necessary in certain patient populations.	• Tachypnea • Decreased or absent breath sounds on the affected side • Shortness of breath, dyspnea • Asymmetric chest excursion with respirations • Decreased oxygen saturation • Subcutaneous emphysema • Sudden sharp chest pain • Anxiety, restlessness, apprehension • Tachycardia • Hypotension • Dysrhythmias • Tracheal deviation to the unaffected side • Neck vein distention • Muffled heart sounds

Procedure continues on following page

Patient Monitoring and Care —*Continued*

Steps	Rationale	Reportable Conditions
2. If indicated, obtain a postthoracentesis expiratory chest radiograph. **(Level C*)**	A chest radiograph is used to evaluate for lung reexpansion and evidence of a possible pneumothorax or hemothorax. If a pneumothorax or hemothorax is present, a chest tube may be necessary. Without concrete clinical indications, chest radiograph is not necessary after a routine thoracentesis.[2,3,5]	• Pneumothorax • Expanding pleural effusion
3. Follow institution standard for assessing pain. Administer analgesia as prescribed.	Identifies need for pain interventions	• Continued pain despite pain interventions

*Level C: Qualitative studies, descriptive or correlational studies, integrative reviews, systematic reviews, or randomized controlled trials with inconsistent results

Documentation

Documentation should include the following:
- Patient and family teaching
- Consent for procedure
- Adherence to Universal Protocol
- Patient positioning and monitoring devices
- Medication administration and patient response
- Patient tolerance, including pain and pain medications
- Pleural fluid aspirate characteristics
- Total amount of pleural fluid aspirated

- Site assessment
- Occurrence of unexpected outcomes
- Postthoracentesis radiograph acquisition and results, as available
- Laboratory test ordered and results, as available
- Nursing interventions
- Pain assessment, interventions, and effectiveness

References

CR 1. Barton E: Thoracentesis. In Rosen P, Chan T, Vilke G, et al, editors: *Atlas of emergency procedures,* St Louis, 2001. Mosby.

CR 2. Colt HG, Brewer N, Barbur EB: Evaluation of patient-related and procedure-related factors contributing to pneumothorax following thoracentesis, *Chest* 116: 134-138, 1999.

CR 3. Gervais DA, et al: US-guided thoracentesis: requirement for post procedure chest radiography in patients who receive mechanical ventilation versus patients who breathe spontaneously, *Radiology* 204:503-506, 1997.

CR 4. Maskell NA, Butland RJA: BTS guidelines for the investigation of a unilateral pleural effusion in adults, *Thorax* 58:ii8, 2003.

CR 5. Peterson WG, Zimmerman R: Limited utility of chest radiograph after thoracentesis, *Chest* 117:1038-1042, 2000.

6. Rahman N, Chapman S, Davies R: Pleural effusion: a structured approach to care, *Br Med Bull* 72(1):31-47, 2005.

Additional Readings

Antunes G, Neville E, Duffy J, et al: BTS guidelines for the management of malignant pleural effusions, *Thorax* 58(Suppl 2):ii29-38, 2003.

Davies CWH, Gleeson FV, Davies RJO: BTS guidelines for the management of pleural infection, *Thorax* 58:ii18, 2003.

Doyle JJ, et al: Necessity of routine chest roentgenography after thoracentesis, *Ann Intern Med* 124:816-820, 1996.

Heffner JE, Brown LK, Barbieri CA: Diagnostic value of tests that discriminate between exudative and transudative pleural effusions, *Chest* 111:970-980, 1997.

Light RW, et al: Pleural effusion: the diagnostic separation of transudates and exudates, *Ann Intern Med* 77:507-513, 1992.

Loddenkemper R: Pleural effusions. In Albert R, Spiro S, Jett J, editors: *Clinical respiratory medicine,* Philadelphia, 2004, Mosby.

Mayo PH, Goltz HR, Tafreshi M, et al: Safety of ultrasound-guided thoracentesis in patients receiving mechanical ventilation, *Chest* 125(3):1059-1062, 2004.

Quigley RL: Thoracentesis and chest tube drainage, *Crit Care Clin* 11:111-126, 1995.

Thomsen TW, DeLaPena J, Stenik, GS. *Thoracentesis,* Videos in Clinical Medicine, 355:e16(15) retrieved from http://content.nejm.org/cgi/content/video_preview/355/15/e16, accessed 09-14-2008 .

Wilson M, Irwin R: Thoracentesis. *Procedures and techniques in intensive care medicine,* Philadelphia, 2003, Lippincot Williams & Wilkins.

Noninvasive Positive Pressure Ventilation: Continuous Positive Airway Pressure (CPAP) and Bilevel Positive Airway Pressure (BiPAP)

P U R P O S E :   Noninvasive positive-pressure ventilation, delivered via nasal mask, pillows, or full face mask, is used to prevent airway obstruction during sleep, to maintain or improve oxygenation, to maintain or improve ventilation, and to provide respiratory muscle rest in different categories of patients in whom invasive mechanical ventilation through an artificial airway is not desired.

Suzanne M. Burns

PREREQUISITE NURSING KNOWLEDGE

- Invasive mechanical ventilation through an endotracheal tube or tracheostomy tube has been the mainstay of ventilatory support in patients with severe oxygenation and ventilation problems. However, the successful use of noninvasive positive pressure ventilation (NPPV), specifically continuous positive airway pressure (CPAP), in the 1980s to treat obstructive sleep apnea (OSA), was followed by its use to treat other chronic respiratory conditions as well.

- The addition of positive pressure ventilation in the form of bilevel positive airway pressure (BiPAP; pressure support ventilation plus positive end-expiratory pressure [PSV plus PEEP]) or conventional ventilation modes such as assist-control (A/C) provided through noninvasive ventilator-patient interfaces allowed for extension of NPPV to patients with hypercarbia and other acute and critical care applications.[1,3-5]

- NPPV is attractive for many reasons, including the avoidance of complications associated with invasive ventilation such as aspiration, pneumothorax, patient discomfort, and contamination of the airway and subsequent infection.

- However, the use of NPPV, especially in the critically ill or acutely ill patient, is time and effort intensive, especially initially when the selection of interface, mode settings, and other medical therapeutics are addressed. In addition, careful selection of patients and identification of relative and absolute contraindications to the use of NPPV are essential to avoid negative outcomes.

- Potential applications, exclusion criteria, and other aspects related to the use of NPPV are addressed subsequently and in the procedure.

Potential Applications for the Use of NPPV

- *Obstructive sleep apnea.* Traditionally, CPAP has been used in OSA to provide a pneumatic splint to the upper airway to prevent obstruction during sleep. BiPAP provides both PEEP and PSV during inspiration, both assisting with ventilation and treating hypercarbia.[1,3,4] In some patients with OSA, this method is more effective, especially in those with nighttime hypoventilation. Patients with OSA admitted to a critical care unit may need intubation and higher levels of ventilatory support than is possible to provide with NPPV. Others have conditions that may be managed on NPPV, but support levels may be higher than home NPPV settings.

- *Cardiogenic pulmonary edema.* Many studies have been accomplished that demonstrate the efficacy of NPPV in patients with congestive heart failure (CHF) and pulmonary edema.[10,11,14,16,17,19,21,24,25] In these patients, the positive pressure results in preload and afterload reduction and restoration of functional residual capacity. NPPV works synergistically with diuretics and other medical interventions, enhancing their effect. In patients with a chronic condition, such as those with OSA and CHF, treatment with CPAP for 1 month significantly decreased systolic blood pressure (BP) and improved left ventricular function.[14] Improved quality of life appears to be an additional benefit.[16] In the patient with an acute illness, studies with PSV through a face mask suggest that intubation may be prevented[10] and that its early use also accelerates improvement in partial pressure of arterial oxygen/fraction of inspired oxygen (PaO_2/FiO_2) ratio, partial pressure of arterial carbon dioxide ($PaCO_2$), dyspnea, and respiratory rate but not overall clinical outcomes.[17] Interestingly, both CPAP and BiPAP appear to be equally effective in this patient population. In an randomized controlled trial (RCT) that compared the modes, both resulted in improved vital signs and arterial blood gas values and a lower rate of endotracheal intubation without cardiac ischemic complications.[19] In the patient with an acute illness with cardiogenic pulmonary edema, the evidence supports a trial of NPPV with exception of those with extubation failure.[4,23]
- *Acute or chronic respiratory failure (i.e., chronic obstructive pulmonary disease [COPD]).* A high level of evidence supports the use of trial of NPPV in hypercapnic respiratory failure (particularly related to COPD).[4] The only exception to this recommendation is in those with extubation failure.[4] NPPV in patients with hypercapnia has been effective in reducing intubation rates[17,23] and is associated with reductions in mortality and the need for invasive mechanical ventilation but not hospital length of stay.[20]
- *Acute hypoxemic respiratory failure.* Although some studies suggest that NPPV may be effective in selected instances of acute hypoxemic respiratory failure,[2,11-13] perhaps the most compelling category for use is in patients with immunosuppression with pneumonia.[12,22] In an RCT, early initiation of NPPV in these patients was associated with significant reductions in the rates of endotracheal intubation and serious complications. In addition, an improved likelihood of survival to hospital discharge was found.[12] Unfortunately, with this exception, study findings have not conclusively supported the routine use of NPPV in hypoxemic respiratory failure patient populations.[15,23]
- *To prevent reintubation after extubation.* The use of NPPV has not been associated with prevention of need for reintubation or a reduction in mortality in patients with respiratory failure after extubation.[5,7] However, careful selection

of patients for NPPV after extubation did appear to improve outcomes in one RCT.[9] In this study, the early use of NPPV (BiPAP) in those "at risk of respiratory failure following extubation"[9] resulted in a decreased intensive care unit mortality. The risk factors included cardiac failure as cause of intubation, age more than 65 years, and increased severity of illness as identified by an Acute Physiology and Chronic Health Evaluation (APACHE) II score of more than 12 on the day of extubation.[9]

- *Failure to wean.* Although this population is underrepresented in the literature, at least one recent study suggests that the use of NPPV in patients with failure to wean successfully for three consecutive days may show better outcomes than in those weaned in a more traditional manner. In the study, BiPAP was used after early extubation and resulted in fewer days of mechanical ventilation and length of stay, less need for tracheostomy, lower incidence of complications, and improved survival.[8]
- *Invasive ventilation not desired: Palliative or end-of-life care.* In 2007, the Society of Critical Care Medicine's Palliative Noninvasive Positive Pressure Ventilation Task Force proposed recommendations for the use of NPPV for patients and families of the patients wishing to forego endotracheal intubation.[6] The recommendations focus on ensuring that patients and families understand the goals of the therapy (reduction of air hunger, etc), the criteria for determining success or failure of the NPPV, that the healthcare providers be experienced in the use of NPPV and the setting appropriate.[6] The use of the therapy for end-of-life care is controversial because some believe it unduly prolongs death and others maintain it is a means of decreasing uncomfortable symptoms such as dyspnea.

Potential Exclusions for the Use of NPPV

- *Status asthmaticus.* Because of the instability of these patient conditions and the difficulty inherent in providing ventilatory support during the acute phase (e.g., preventing hyperinflation, auto-PEEP, and barotrauma), the use of NPPV is not recommended. Few studies are available supporting its use in this category of patient condition.
- *Hemodynamic instability.* Generally, this condition refers to patients with high vasopressor requirements or other supportive therapies. These patients need full ventilatory support to ensure acid-base stability and the adequacy of oxygenation and ventilation.
- *Inadequate airway protective reflexes.* Cough and swallow are essential for airway protection. Absence of these reflexes puts the patient at risk for aspiration.
- *Encephalopathy or coma.* As noted previously, the inability to protect the airway or remove a mask (especially full face masks) when necessary puts the patient at risk for aspiration.
- *Mask fit or intolerance (claustrophobia, facial deformities, and occasionally, the absence of teeth).* Different noninvasive options are available and should be considered if intolerance of masks (nasal or full face) or other interfaces is evident.

- *Excessive secretions.* The presence of secretions necessitates that the patient be able to effectively clear the airway. When excessive secretions are present, the work associated with effective airway clearance may quickly overwhelm the patient's endurance and result in respiratory failure.
- *Severe agitation.* Agitation makes adjustment to the use of a noninvasive interface difficult. Further, leaks are increased when the interface is displaced, which makes ventilation unreliable and ineffective.
- *High FiO$_2$ requirements.* Most of the NPPV ventilators do not provide a high level of FiO$_2$ (this varies with the make, model, and manufacturer of the ventilator). In these cases, the patient may need invasive ventilation or NPPV with a conventional ventilator to ensure provision of the required FiO$_2$.

NPPV Interfaces

- Noninvasive interfaces are selected on the basis of patients' unique facial features, patient preferences, comfort, ease of use, availability, and provider experience and preference and include full face masks, nasal masks, nasal pillows, and helmets. Of these, full head helmets are the least commonly used (and not discussed further in this procedure) but may be more prevalent in the future as experience with the interfaces increases.[18] See Fig. 28-1 for NPPV interfaces.

Potential Causes of Failure of NPPV

- When NPPV fails, as evidenced by lack of improvement or further deterioration, invasive ventilation is necessary. Equipment and personnel to ensure safe intubation and application of invasive ventilation are necessary and should be ensured (see Procedures 2, 3, 35) Some potential causes of NPPV failure follow:
- *Poor patient selection.* See previous potential applications and exclusions.
- *Mask intolerance and leaks.* As noted previously, careful selection of the interface is essential to ensure success. In addition to patient facial characteristics, the actual process of applying the mask may be the reason for failure. In general, application of the mask as gently and gradually as possible is important to help the patient acclimate. Simultaneous and gradual adjustment of the mode parameters is a useful technique if the situation allows for the use of such a strategy. If mask leaks are present, patient-generated cycling may be adversely affected and result in dyssynchrony. Time-cycled modes may be helpful in these cases. Other mask complications that limit use include gastric distention and vomiting, nasal congestion, eye irritation from leaks, discomfort, claustrophobia, and nasal and facial skin breakdown.
- *Development of serious complications.* These complications include myocardial infarction, gastrointestinal bleeding, and sepsis.
- *Limitation of the ventilator.* Most NPPV ventilators do not provide for the delivery of high FiO$_2$, as noted previously. Flow capabilities may also vary and, if inadequate, result in

dyssynchrony. In one study that compared bilevel devices with standard adult critical care ventilators, the bilevel devices were found to provide superior flow delivery.[14]
- *Patient ventilator dyssynchrony.* Many reasons for dyssynchrony exist and may include both physical and mechanical reasons such as auto-PEEP, worsening condition or other complications, and ventilator limitations (e.g., CO$_2$ elimination from partial rebreathing with some NPPV circuits).

Complications of NPPV

- Complications of NPPV are similar to invasive positive pressure ventilation (PPV) and include hemodynamic changes and pulmonary barotrauma. These complications are described subsequently in this procedure.

EQUIPMENT

- Noninvasive interface (see Fig. 28-1)
- CPAP or BiPAP ventilator
- Electrocardiogram
- Pulse oximetry (oxygen saturation of hemoglobin measured with pulse oximetry: SpO$_2$)
- Self-inflating manual resuscitation bag-valve-mask device
- Oxygen source and tubing
- Suction equipment
- Intubation equipment and endotracheal tubes, should NPPV be unsuccessful (see Procedures 2, 3)
- Personal protective equipment (gloves, mask, goggles, gown, as appropriate)

PATIENT AND FAMILY EDUCATION

- Explain the procedure and the reason NPPV is being initiated to the patient and family. **➤➤Rationale:** Communication and explanations for therapy are cited as important needs of patients.
- Discuss the potential sensations the patient will experience, such as relief of dyspnea, lung inflations, noise of ventilator operation, and alarm sounds. **➤➤Rationale:** Knowledge of anticipated sensory experiences reduces anxiety and distress.
- Encourage the patient to relax. **➤➤Rationale:** This encouragement promotes general relaxation, oxygenation, and ventilation.
- Explain that the patient will be able to speak but that this should be kept to a minimum to ensure effective application of the mode. Establish a method of communication in conjunction with the patient and family before initiation of NPPV. **➤➤Rationale:** Ensuring the patient's ability to communicate is important to alleviate anxiety.
- Teach the patient and family how to use the call system and to help the patient with minor activities such as suctioning the mouth. **➤➤Rationale:** Family members have identified the need and desire to help in the patient's care.
- Provide the patient and family with information on the use of NPPV and anticipated goals of the therapy.

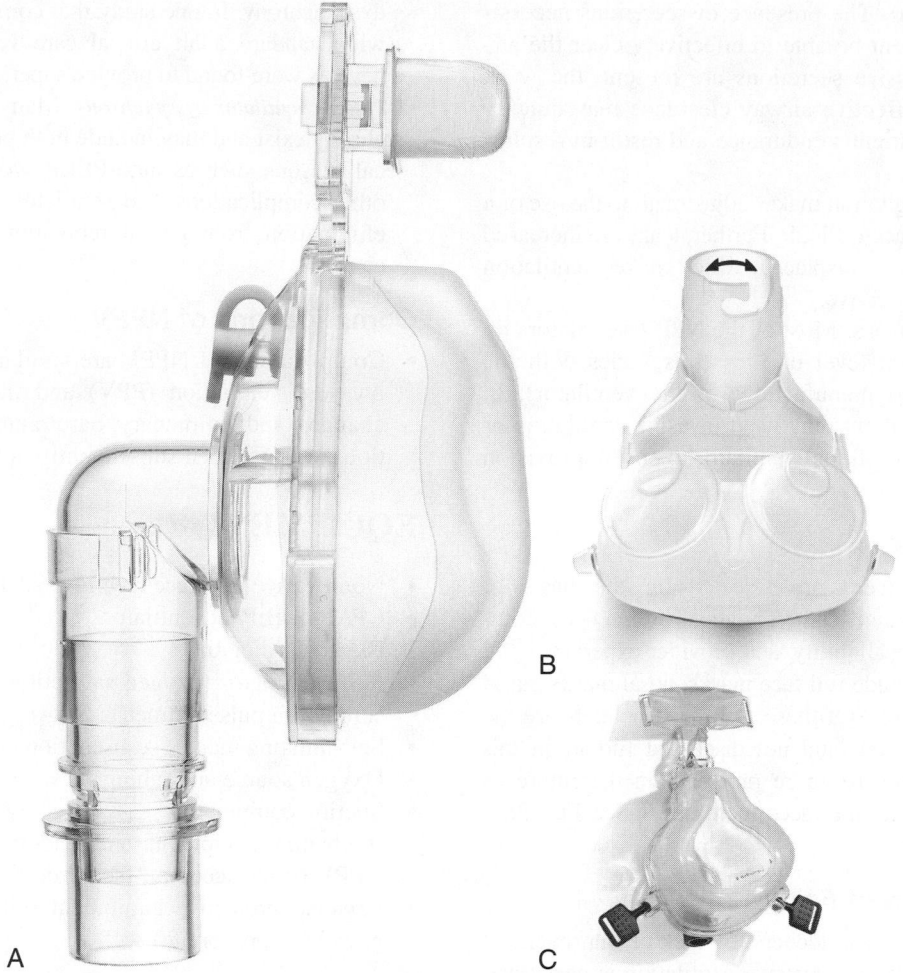

FIGURE 28-1   Noninvasive patient interfaces. **A,** Nasal mask. **B,** Nasal pillow. **C,** Full face mask. *(Images used with permission of Philips Respironics, Inc, Murrysville, PA.)*

➤➤*Rationale:* Knowledge of the prognosis, probable outcome, or chance for recovery is cited as an important need of patients and families.

- Offer the opportunity for the patient and family to ask questions about NPPV. ➤➤*Rationale:* The ability to ask questions and have questions answered honestly is cited consistently as the most important need of patients and families.

PATIENT ASSESSMENT AND PREPARATION

Patient Assessment

- Assess for the following signs and symptoms of fatigue and impending acute ventilatory failure:
  - ❖ Rising arterial carbon dioxide tension
  - ❖ Chest-abdominal dyssynchrony
  - ❖ Shallow or irregular respirations
  - ❖ Tachypnea, bradypnea, or dyspnea
  - ❖ Decreased mental status
  - ❖ Restlessness, confusion, or lethargy
  - ❖ Increasing or decreasing arterial blood pressure
  - ❖ Tachycardia
  - ❖ Atrial or ventricular dysrhythmias

➤➤*Rationale:* These signs and symptoms demonstrate failure to adequately ventilate with NPPV. If the situation is not corrected, the patient may need intubation and initiation of PPV. While PPV is considered and assembled, support ventilation via a manual self-inflating resuscitation bag, if necessary.

- Assess for the following signs and symptoms of inadequate oxygenation:
  - ❖ Decreasing arterial oxygen tension
  - ❖ Tachypnea
  - ❖ Dyspnea
  - ❖ Central cyanosis
  - ❖ Restlessness
  - ❖ Confusion
  - ❖ Agitation
  - ❖ Tachycardia
  - ❖ Bradycardia
  - ❖ Dysrhythmias
  - ❖ Intercostal and suprasternal retractions
  - ❖ Increasing or decreasing arterial blood pressure
  - ❖ Adventitious breath sounds
  - ❖ Decreasing urine output
  - ❖ Metabolic acidosis

➙*Rationale:* If hypoxemia noted by a saturation of arterial oxygen (SaO$_2$) is less than 90% or PaO$_2$ less than 60 mm Hg) cannot be immediately corrected on NPPV, the patient may need invasive PPV. While PPV is considered and assembled, provide 100% oxygen via manual resuscitation bag and mask.

- Determine pH and arterial carbon dioxide tension. ➙*Rationale:* Acute ventilatory failure is confirmed by an uncompensated respiratory acidosis. Ventilatory failure is an indication for immediate adjustment of settings and possibly invasive PPV. See previous bullet.

- Ensure that the patient understands pre-procedural teachings. Answer questions as they arise, and reinforce information as needed. ➙*Rationale:* This communication evaluates and reinforces understanding of previously taught information.
- Premedicate as needed. ➙*Rationale:* Cautious use of narcotics, sedatives, or anxiolytics may be necessary for comfort, to help allay anxiety, and to improve the patient's tolerance of NPPV. However, the use of the drugs should not adversely affect spontaneous breathing or consciousness.

Patient Preparation

- Verify correct patient with two identifiers. ➙*Rationale:* Prior to performing a procedure, the nurse should ensure the correct identification of the patient for the intended intervention.

Procedure	for Noninvasive Ventilation (CPAP and BiPAP Masks)	
Steps	**Rationale**	**Special Considerations**
1. **HH**		
2. **PE**		
Noninvasive Interface: Nasal Mask, Full Face Mask, Pillows		
1. Select noninvasive interface for use with CPAP or BiPAP (or Bi-level) (see Fig. 28-1.)	Interface device fit is essential to NPPV. The interface should be carefully selected with attention to patient preference, face and nose size, facial deformities, skin integrity, presence of nasal or oral gastric tubes, and availability.	Not all interfaces are available in hospitals for use with NPPV. The presence of a nasal or oral gastric tube does not obviate the application of NPPV. Most of the ventilators designed specifically for NPPV have leak compensation built into the system. However, a large leak may make patient-initiated cycling more difficult (described in BiPAP section) Obtunded patients and patients with excessive secretions are not good choices for NPPV. The potential for aspiration is high. Full face mask ventilation should be used cautiously. The patient should be able to remove the mask quickly if nausea and vomiting are imminent.
2. A chin strap is used if necessary to prevent excessive leaks through the mouth. Mask fit is important, as is the creative application of BiPAP. This form of therapy may be labor intensive, especially when used to prevent reintubation after extubation.		
CPAP		
1. Select mode: CPAP. This mode may be labeled CPAP or another vendor-specific name.		Refer to specific ventilator manufacturer information for specific names of the mode.

Procedure continues on following page

Procedure for Noninvasive Ventilation (CPAP and BiPAP Masks)—*Continued*		
Steps	Rationale	Special Considerations
2. Select CPAP level.	Generally, selection of a CPAP level of 3 to 5 cm/H_2O or less is adequate to begin. Increase as needed to attain goal (e.g., relief of dyspnea, improved oxygenation, comfortable breathing pattern).	
3. Select Fio_2 level.	Most CPAP ventilators provide relatively low levels of Fio_2. Often, oxygen delivery is provided by means of an oxygen flow meter in L/min and is bled into the ventilator at the patient interface or into the patient circuit. Monitoring of arterial oxygen saturation allows for adjustment as needed to attain acceptable Sao_2. If adequate oxygenation is not attained by adjusting oxygen to manufacturer specifications, a traditional ventilator may be used to supply CPAP via noninvasive interface.	There are limitations to the absolute amount of oxygen that may be bled into the system. Follow manufacturer's directions.
BiPAP (or Bilevel)		
1. Select BiPAP levels. BiPAP provides two levels of support: PSV and PEEP. Depending on the ventilator, the two levels may have different names. For example, one vendor refers to PSV as I-PAP (inspiratory positive airway pressure) and PEEP as E-PAP (expiratory positive airway pressure).	Selection of the levels of support is somewhat arbitrary, but generally, starting lower and adjusting the levels upward is a reasonable technique. The concepts and use of PSV and PEEP are described in Procedure 35 on invasive PPV.	Refer to specific ventilator manufacturer information for specific names of the modes. Generally, initiating beginning settings at low levels is reasonable (i.e., PSV of 5 cm H_2O and PEEP of 3 cm H_2O); slowly work the levels up as tolerated to attain a comfortable respiratory rate and pattern and acceptable arterial blood gas (ABG) values or other clinical parameters, such as Sao_2.

2. BiPAP options (dependent on ventilator manufacturer) include the following:
  A. A spontaneous mode, whereby the patient initiates all breaths (similar to PSV in the "stand-alone" mode).
  B. A spontaneous-timed option, which is similar to PSV with a backup rate (some vendors call this A/C).
  C. A control mode. In contrast to the spontaneous and spontaneous-timed modes, the control mode requires that a control rate and inspiratory time be selected.
	The selection of the specific BiPAP option is dependent on the patient condition and the goals of therapy.
	
	If leaks around the interface prevent patient cycling (triggering), consider a spontaneous timed option or a control option.
		Settings on specific ventilators vary. However, concepts related to the settings are the same as with invasive ventilation. See Procedure 35.

Procedure for Noninvasive Ventilation (CPAP and BiPAP Masks)—*Continued*

Steps	Rationale	Special Considerations
3. FiO_2 generally is delivered by means of an oxygen source (oxygen tubing connected to a flow meter) that is connected into the mask or in the inspiratory line at the junction of the ventilator and ventilator interface. As a result, delivery of high levels of FiO_2 is not possible. Each ventilator has specifications that dictate the maximal flows allowed.	Ventilator function may be adversely affected if the manufacturer's recommendations are not followed.	If the patient has high FiO_2 requirements, BiPAP may not be a good option. Instead, if noninvasive ventilation is still the desired intervention, consider providing the noninvasive ventilation in a traditional ventilator. If this is done, PSV may not be the best mode to use because the cycle of mechanism may be impeded by mask leaks. The A/C mode or a volume guaranteed pressure mode may be used as an alternative (exceptions exist and are ventilator specific). Refer to Procedure 35 for more on alternative modes.
4. Remove personal protective equipment. HH		

Expected Outcomes

- Maintenance of adequate pH and $PaCO_2$
- Maintenance of adequate PaO_2
- Maintenance of adequate breathing pattern
- Respiratory muscle rest
- Intact skin under mask

Unexpected Outcomes

- Unacceptable pH, $PaCO_2$, and PaO_2
- Hemodynamic instability
- Pulmonary barotrauma
- Respiratory muscle fatigue
- Skin breakdown under mask

Patient Monitoring and Care

Steps	Rationale	Reportable Conditions
		These conditions should be reported if they persist despite nursing interventions.
1. Ensure activation of available alarms.	Ensures patient safety.	• Continued activation of alarms
2. Check for stabilization and maintenance of NPPV interface.	Reduces risk of inadvertent mask removal and subsequent inadequate NPPV.	• Inability to rapidly restabilize NPPV interface and resume ventilation • Uncontrolled agitation that results in poor stabilization of NPPV interface
3. Monitor in-line thermometer to maintain inspired gas temperature (in the range 35° to 37°C [95°F to 98°F]; only applies to some ventilators).	Reduces risk of thermal injury from overheated inspired gas and risk of poor humidity from underheated inspired gas.	• Temperature less than 35°C or greater than 37°C

Procedure continues on following page

Patient Monitoring and Care —*Continued*

Steps	Rationale	Reportable Conditions
4. Keep NPPV interface and circuit clear of condensation and secretions.	Reduces risk of respiratory infection by decreasing inhalation of contaminated water droplets and secretions.	• Excessive secretions or fluid
5. Ensure availability of manual self-inflating resuscitation bag with supplemental oxygen at the head of the bed. Attach or adjust PEEP valve if the patient is on greater than 5 cm H_2O.	Provides capability for immediately delivering ventilation and oxygenation to relieve acute respiratory distress caused by hypoxemia or acidosis.	
6. Check ventilator for baseline settings and alarm activation with initial assessment and after removal and reapplication of NPPV.	Ensures that prescribed ventilator parameters are used.	• Settings different from prescribed
7. Explore any alarms to determine cause and correct.	Multiple reasons for alarms exist and may indicate mask or tubing disconnection, kinks in the tubing, or changes in the patient's condition. Always consider possibility of tension pneumothorax.	• Unexplained high or low pressure alarms
8. Change the patient's body position as often as possible but at least every 2 hours. Rotating beds may be helpful.	Frequent position changes are indicated to reduce the potential for atelectasis and pneumonia caused by secretion stasis. Promotes airway clearance.	
9. Evaluate patient-ventilator dyssynchrony.	A comfortable breathing pattern is a goal of NPPV. An inadequate breathing pattern can be corrected by adjusting the ventilator parameters or by finding and treating the underlying acute cause. Dyssynchrony may be the result of a large leak around the interface, sensitivity settings that are not sensitive enough for the patient, or auto-PEEP. Notify physician and respiratory care practitioner and assess patient with any changes in settings to assure resolution of dyssynchrony.	• Dyspnea • Chest-abdominal dyssynchrony • Rapid-shallow breathing pattern • Irregular respirations • Intercostal or suprasternal retractions
10. Observe for hemodynamic changes associated with increased CPAP, PEEP and PSV levels.	May indicate functional changes in circulating volume caused by positive intrathoracic pressure. Always consider potential for pneumothorax with acute changes. Equipment used for rapid release of tension pneumothorax should be at bedside at all times (i.e., 14-gauge needle; see Procedure 25). Chest tube insertion equipment should be readily available.	• Decreased blood pressure • Change in heart rate (increase or decrease of greater than 10% of baseline) • Decreased cardiac output • Decreased mixed venous oxygen tension • Increased arterial-venous oxygen difference (see Procedure 29)

Patient Monitoring and Care —*Continued*

Steps	Rationale	Reportable Conditions
11. Monitor for signs and symptoms of acute respiratory distress, hypoxemia, hypercarbia, and fatigue.	Respiratory distress indicates the need for changes in NPPV. While troubleshooting the difficulties, support ventilation via a self-inflating manual resuscitation bag-valve-mask-device (see Procedure 32), if necessary.	• Rising arterial carbon dioxide tension • Chest-abdominal dyssynchrony • Shallow or irregular respirations • Tachypnea, bradypnea, or dyspnea • Decreased mental status • Restlessness, confusion, lethargy • Increasing or decreasing arterial blood pressure • Increase in pulmonary capillary wedge pressure • Decreased mixed venous oxygen saturation • Tachycardia • Atrial or ventricular dysrhythmias • Significant changes in pH, PaO_2, $PaCO_2$, or SaO_2
12. Assess for signs and symptoms of pulmonary barotrauma (i.e., pneumothorax).	Early detection of pneumothorax is essential to minimize progression and the adverse effects on the patient. Tension pneumothorax requires immediate emergency decompression with a large-bore needle (i.e., 14-gauge) into the second intercostal space or midclavicular line on the affected side or immediate chest tube placement (see Procedure 25).	• Acute, increasing, or severe dyspnea • Restlessness • Agitation • Localized changes in auscultation (decreased or absent breath sounds) on the affected side • Localized hyperresonance or tympany to percussion on the affected side • Elevated chest on the affected side • Increased breathing effort • Tracheal deviation away from the side of abnormal findings • Increased peak and plateau pressures • Decreased compliance • Decreased PaO_2 or SaO_2 • Subcutaneous emphysema • Localized increased lucency with absent lung markings on chest radiograph
13. Assess skin under mask every 1 to 2 hours for pressure breakdowns.	The pressure of the mask may cause skin breakdown, which may be averted with close monitoring.	• Skin breakdowns under the mask

Documentation

Documentation should include the following:
• Patient and family education
• Date and time ventilatory assistance was instituted
• Ventilator settings, including the following: FiO_2, mode of ventilation, PSV level, respiratory frequency (total and mandatory if set), and PEEP level
• Arterial blood gas results
• SaO_2 readings
• Reason for initiating PPV

• Patient responses to NPPV (including the patient's indication of level of comfort and respiratory symptoms)
• Hemodynamic values if pulmonary artery catheter is in place
• Vital signs
• Respiratory assessment findings
• Unexpected outcomes
• Nursing interventions

References

1. Annane D, Orlikowaski D, Chevret S, et al: Nocturnal mechanical ventilation for chronic hypoventilation in patients with neuromuscular and chest wall disorders, *Cochrane Database Systematic Review* 4:CD001941, 2007.
2. Antonelli M, Conti G, Esquinas A, et al: A multiple-center survey on the use in clinical practice of noninvasive ventilation as a first-line intervention for acute respiratory distress syndrome, *Crit Care Med* 35:18-25, 2007.
3. Burns KE, Adhikar NK, Keenan SP, et al: Use of non-invasive ventilation to wean critically ill adults off invasive ventilation: meta analysis and systematic review, *BMJ* 338:b728, 2009.
4. Caples SM, Gay PC: Noninvasive positive pressure ventilation in the intensive care unit: a concise review, *Crit Care Med* 33:2651-2658, 2005.
5. Crummy F, Naughton MT: Non-invasive positive pressure ventilation for acute respiratory failure: justified or just hot air? *Intern Med J* 37:112-118, 2007.
6. Curtis JR, Cook DJ, Sinuff T, et al, the Society of Critical Care Medicine's Palliative Noninvasive Positive Pressure Ventilation Task Force: Noninvasive positive pressure ventilation I critical and palliative care settings: understanding the goals of therapy, *Crit Care Med* 35:932-939, 2007.
7. Esteban A, Frutos-Vivar F, Ferguson ND, et al: Noninvasive positive-pressure ventilation for respiratory failure after extubation, *N Engl J Med* 350:2452-2460, 2004. **CR**
8. Ferrer M, Esquinas A, Arancibia F, et al: Noninvasive ventilation during persistent weaning failure: a randomized controlled trial, *Am J Respir Crit Care Med* 168:70-76, 2003. **CR**
9. Ferrer M, Valencia M, Nicolas JM, et al: Early non-invasive ventilation averts extubation failure in patients at risk; a randomized trial, *Am J Respir Crit Care Med* 173:164-170, 2006.
10. Giacomini M, Iapichino G, Cigada M, et al: Short-term noninvasive pressure support ventilation prevents ICU admittance in patients with acute cardiogenic edema, *Chest* 123:2057-2061, 2003. **CR**
11. Gray A, Goodacre S, Newby DE, et al: Noninvasive ventilation in acute cardiogenic pulmonary edema, *N Engl J Med* 359:142-151, 2008.
12. Hilbert G, Gruson D, Vargas F, et al: Noninvasive ventilation in immunosuppressed patients with pulmonary infiltrates, fever and acute respiratory failure, *N Engl J Med* 344:481-487, 2001. **CR**
13. Honrubia T, Garcia-Lopez FJ, Franco N, et al: Noninvasive vs conventional mechanical ventilation in acute respiratory failure: a multicenter, randomized controlled trial, *Chest* 128:3790-3791, 2005.
14. Kaneko Y, Floras JS, Usui K, et al: Cardiovascular effects of continuous positive airway pressure in patients with heart failure and obstructive sleep apnea, *N Engl J Med* 348:1233-1241, 2003. **CR**
15. Keenan SP, Sinuff T, Cook DJ, et al: Does noninvasive positive pressure ventilation improve outcome in acute hypoxemic respiratory failure? A systematic review, *Crit Care Med* 32:2516-2523, 2004. **CR**
16. Mansfield DR, Golloghy NC, Kaye DM, et al: Controlled trial of continuous positive airway pressure in obstructive sleep apnea and heart failure, *Am J Respir Crit Care Med* 169:361-366, 2004. **CR**
17. Nava S, Carbone G, DiBattista N, et al: Noninvasive ventilation in cardiogenic pulmonary edema: a multicenter randomized trial, *Am J Respir Crit Care Med* 168:1432-1437, 2003. **CR**
18. Navalesi P, Costa R, Ceriana P, et al: Non-invasive ventilation in chronic obstructive pulmonary disease patients: helmet versus facial mask, *Intensive Care Med* 33:74-81, 2007.
19. Park M, Sangean MC, Volpe M de S, et al: Randomized, prospective trial of oxygen, continuous positive airway pressure, and bilevel positive airway pressure by face mask in acute cardiogenic pulmonary edema, *Crit Care Med* 32:2407-2415, 2004. **CR**
20. Peter JV, Moran JL, Phillips-Hughes J, et al: Noninvasive ventilation in acute respiratory failure: a meta-analysis update, *Crit Care Med* 30:555-562, 2002. **CR**
21. Peter JV, Moran JL, Phillips-Hughes J, et al: Effect of non-invasive positive pressure ventilation (NIPPV) on mortality in patients with acute cardiogenic pulmonary oedema: a meta-analysis, *Lancet* 367:1155-1163, 2006.
22. Rabitsch W, Staudinger T, Locker GJ, et al: Respiratory failure after stem cell transplantation: improved outcome with non-invasive ventilation, *Leuk Lymphoma* 46:1151-1157, 2005.
23. Schettino G, Altobelli N, Kacmarek RM: Noninvasive positive–pressure ventilation in acute respiratory failure outside clinical trials: experience at the Massachusetts General Hospital, *Crit Care Med* 36:441-447, 2008.
24. Vital FM, Saconato H, Ladeira MT, et al: Non-invasive positive pressure ventilation (CPAP or bilevel NPPV) for cardiogenic pulmonary edema, *Cochrane Database Systematic Review* 16:CD005351, 2008.
25. Winck JC, Azevedo LF, Costa-Pereira A, et al: Efficacy and safety of non-invasive ventilation in the treatment of acute cardiogenic pulmonary edema: a systematic review and meta-analysis, *Crit Care* 10:R69, 2006.

Additional Readings

Pierce LNB: Invasive and noninvasive modes and methods of mechanical ventilation. In Burns SM, editor: *AACN protocols for practice: care of mechanically ventilated patients,* ed 2, Boston, 2007, Jones and Bartlett Publishers.

Pierce LNB, editor: *Management of the mechanically ventilated patient,* ed 2, St Louis, 2007, Elsevier.

Tobin MJ: *Principles and practice of mechanical ventilation,* ed 2, New York, 2006, McGraw-Hill.

Arterial-Venous Oxygen Content Difference and Oxygen Transport (Delivery) and Consumption Calculations

P U R P O S E :   The arterial-venous oxygen content difference is calculated for a patient on mechanical ventilation to provide a general indication of oxygen extraction from the blood. Arterial and venous oxygen content is also used to calculate oxygen transport (delivery) and consumption (use).

Suzanne M. Burns

PREREQUISITE NURSING KNOWLEDGE

- Most oxygen carried in the blood is bound to hemoglobin and is referred to as oxygen saturation. A small percentage also is dissolved in the plasma. The total blood oxygen content is determined by adding the amount of oxygen bound to hemoglobin to that dissolved in the plasma. Oxygen content can be calculated for the arterial blood (CaO_2) and the venous blood (CO_2). By calculating the oxygen contents for arterial and venous blood and subtracting them, a rough estimate of oxygen use can be made. This value is either expressed as mL/dL or as vol %. A normal arterial-venous oxygen content difference (a-vDO_2) is 5 vol % (range, 4 to 6 vol %). In general, because the contribution of dissolved oxygen is slight, it is not used clinically to calculate CaO_2.[3,4] It is essential to remember that hemoglobin is one of the most important variables in oxygenation status.
- The partial pressure of mixed venous oxygen pressure (PO_2) and mixed venous oxygen saturation (SO_2) reflects tissue oxygenation under most conditions. When blood flow does not increase to meet higher tissue oxygen demands (as in hypodynamic conditions [e.g., shock]), more oxygen is extracted from the arterial blood, and the PO_2 and SO_2 decrease. The gradient between CaO_2 and

CO_2 widens. Conversely, when blood flow is increased (e.g., hyperdynamic flow, as in sepsis), less oxygen is extracted from the arterial blood; PO_2 and SO_2 increase, and a-vDO_2 decreases.[3,4]
- A major clinical goal of positive-pressure ventilation (PPV) and positive end-expiratory pressure (PEEP) is improved oxygenation. One potential complication of these therapies is hypotension from the effect of increased intrathoracic pressures on venous return.[1,2]
- Calculation of a-vDO_2 may reflect tissue oxygenation in some cases; however, it is not a direct measurement and can be used only for approximation. The measurement of lactic acid is thought to be a more accurate assessment of tissue hypoxia, but the formation of lactic acid occurs late in the clinical course and is often irreversible.[2] It slowly clears on improvement of the patient's condition.
- In addition to hemoglobin, one of the most important variables affecting oxygen use is cardiac output. When cardiac output is inadequate, more oxygen is extracted from the arterial blood, which lowers the CO_2.
- The product of cardiac output and CaO_2 is oxygen delivery. Oxygen consumption may be calculated by determining the product of cardiac output and a-vDO_2.[1-4]
- Measurement of cardiac output is necessary for oxygen delivery and oxygen consumption calculations (see Procedure 67).

- Normal values for oxygen delivery and consumption are approximately 1000 mL O_2/min and 250 mL O_2/min, respectively.[1-4]
- Confirmation of pulmonary artery catheter placement is necessary to ensure accuracy of measurements (see Procedure 73).[1,2]
- Calculation of the a-v difference requires the sampling of arterial blood from an indwelling arterial line or arterial puncture (see Procedures 64 and 80) and mixed venous blood from a pulmonary artery catheter (see Procedure 66).[1,2]

EQUIPMENT

- Calculator and mathematic equations
- Arterial blood gas and saturation*
- Mixed venous blood gas and saturation*
- Hemoglobin level
- Hemodynamic profile (if calculating of oxygen delivery/consumption, cardiac output is required)

  Note: To obtain accurate arterial and venous saturations, a blood sample is analyzed with a cooximeter. Calculated (versus measured) saturations from arterial and venous blood gas analysis may be used, but these are less accurate. Another widespread practice is to obtain a venous sample from a central venous catheter in lieu of a pulmonary artery catheter. Although such measurements may provide a rough approximation or estimate of venous O_2 extraction, they are often less accurate.

PATIENT AND FAMILY EDUCATION

- Inform the patient and the family of the patient's perfusion status and changes in therapy and interpret the changes. If the patient or another family member requests specific information about arterial venous oxygen content differences, explain the general relationship between a-vDO_2 and perfusion. ➤*Rationale:* Most patients and families are less concerned with the diagnostic and therapeutic details and more concerned with how the patient's condition is progressing overall or in relation to a specific physiologic function.

PATIENT ASSESSMENT AND PREPARATION

Patient Assessment

- Assess signs and symptoms of inadequate tissue oxygenation:
  - ❖ Thirst
  - ❖ Nausea
  - ❖ Anxiety
  - ❖ Apprehension
  - ❖ Skin temperature
  - ❖ Bounding pulse
  - ❖ Tachycardia
  - ❖ High cardiac output with low systemic vascular resistance
  - ❖ Cool skin
  - ❖ Weak pulse
  - ❖ Low cardiac output
  - ❖ Hypotension
  - ❖ Decreased mentation
  - ❖ Metabolic acidosis
  - ❖ Decreased pulse pressure
  - ❖ Increased systemic vascular resistance
  - ❖ Tachypnea
  - ❖ Decreased urine output
- ➤*Rationale:* Calculations of a-vDO_2 and O_2 delivery and consumption are indicated to provide a rough quantitative estimate of tissue perfusion and oxygenation.

Patient Preparation

- Verify correct patient with two identifiers. ➤*Rationale:* Prior to performing a procedure, the nurse should ensure the correct identification of the patient for the intended intervention.
- Ensure that the patient understands preprocedural teachings. Answer questions as they arise, and reinforce information as needed. ➤*Rationale:* This communication evaluates and reinforces understanding of previously taught information.

Procedure   **for Arterial-Venous Oxygen Difference Calculation**

The calculation for a-v DO$_2$ is as follows:

$Ca_{O_2}: [(1.39^* \times Hb \times Sa_{O_2}) + (0.003^* \times Pa_{O_2})] - Cv_{O_2}: [(1.39^* \times Hb \times Sv_{O_2}) + (0.003^* \times Pv_{O_2})]$

Where Ca_{O_2} *is content of arterial oxygen,* Cv_{O_2} *is content of mixed venous oxygen, Hb is hemoglobin,* Sa_{O_2} *is saturation of arterial hemoglobin with oxygen,* Pa_{O_2} *is partial pressure of arterial oxygen,* Sv_{O_2} *is saturation of mixed venous hemoglobin with oxygen,* Pv_{O_2} *is partial pressure of mixed venous oxygen.* Note: * *indicates that the number 1.39 is the maximum amount of oxygen carried by a hemoglobin molecule. The value 1.34 is also commonly used. Regardless of choice, consistency is important. The* ** *indicates the solubility coefficient for oxygen dissolved in the plasma.*

Procedure for Arterial-Venous Oxygen Difference Calculation—*Continued*

Steps	Rationale	Special Considerations
1. Obtain and analyze both arterial and mixed venous sample measurements.		
2. Determine and record the value to be used for oxygen-carrying capacity (1.39 or 1.34) so that consistency is maintained in all subsequent measurements. **(Level B*)**	The amount of oxygen carried by each gram of Hg is between 1.34 and 1.39 mL. *Use of the same oxygen carrying capacity value consistently for all a-vDo$_2$ calculations, per patient, prevents erroneous results.*[1-4]	
3. Calculate Cao$_2$ with the modified Fick equation: Cao$_2$ = 1.39 (or 1.34) × Hb × % Sao$_2$ (use decimal)	Only approximation is needed for clinical purposes.[1-4]	If using dissolved oxygen, add (0.003 × Pao$_2$); this is generally not necessary because it adds little to calculation result.
4. Calculate Cvo$_2$ with the modified Fick equation: Cvo$_2$ = 1.39 (or 1.34) × Hb × % Svo$_2$ (use decimal)	Only approximation is needed for clinical purposes.[1-4]	If using dissolved oxygen in the equation, add (0.003 × Po$_2$); this is generally not necessary because it adds little to calculation result.
5. Subtract Cvo$_2$ from Cao$_2$.	Results in a-vDo$_2$ value.[1-4]	
6. Consult with physician or advanced practice nurse if needed changes in therapy exceed therapeutic guidelines.	Large changes in a-vDo$_2$ value may indicate need for revision of the therapeutic guidelines. Provides integrated trend data to evaluate tissue oxygenation in light of pulmonary function and ventilator parameters and shows appropriate use of diagnostic and monitoring tests to evaluate or alter therapy if needed.	
7. If calculations of oxygen delivery and consumption are desired, the clinician must also determine the cardiac output. Using cardiac output (CO), the calculation for consumption is Delivery − Return = Consumption: Delivery: CO (Cao$_2$ × 10) = volume (mL) of oxygen delivered each minute to the tissues. Return: CO (Co$_2$ × 10) = volume (mL) of oxygen returned to the heart from the tissues each minute	As noted previously, changes in consumption reflect either higher O$_2$ requirements or lower O$_2$ requirements.[1-4]	All calculated results must be viewed in context with the clinical history and physical signs and symptoms.

*Level B: Well-designed, controlled studies with results that consistently support a specific action, intervention, or treatment

Expected Outcome

- Titration of PPV parameters (e.g., targeted tidal volume, mean or peak inspiratory airway pressures, PEEP, inspiratory-expiratory ratio) to maintain adequate perfusion and tissue oxygenation

Unexpected Outcome

- Hemodynamic instability

Procedure continues on following page

Patient Monitoring and Care

Steps	Rationale	Reportable Conditions
		These conditions should be reported if they persist despite nursing interventions.
1. Observe trend in a-vDo$_2$.	PPV, particularly with larger tidal volumes, PEEP, or the development of auto-PEEP, can compromise hemodynamics from increased intrathoracic pressure. A narrowing difference may indicate hyperdynamic perfusion as seen with sepsis (decreased O$_2$ extraction). A widening difference may indicate hypodynamic perfusion, such as with cardiogenic shock. The effect of PPV therapy on perfusion needs to be explored. (Unless a therapeutic plan has been predetermined, decisions related to interventions need to be made with each measurement. For example, although an increase in PEEP may be thought to have resulted in hypotension and a widened a-vDo$_2$, the intervention may be to give fluid instead of lowering PEEP.)	• Acute changes in a-vDo$_2$

Documentation

Documentation should include the following:
• Patient and family education
• The a-vDo$_2$ and arterial blood gas and hemoglobin results with which it was calculated
• The time, date, and position of the patient (e.g., supine, prone, semiprone)
• Ventilator parameters at the time the blood gas samples were drawn
• Changes in therapy based on a-vDo$_2$ value
• Patient response to interventions
• Unexpected outcomes

References

CR 1. Chulay M, Gawlinski A: *AACN protocols for practice: hemodynamic monitoring series,* Aliso Viejo, CA, 1998, American Association of Critical-Care Nurses.
2. Miller LR: Hemodynamic monitoring. In Chulay M, Burns SM, editors: *AACN essentials of critical care nursing,* New York, 2006, McGraw-Hill.
3. West JB: *Pulmonary pathophysiology: the essentials,* Baltimore, 2008, Lippincott Williams & Wilkins.
4. West JB: *Respiratory physiology: the essentials,* ed 8, Baltimore, 2008, Lippincott Williams & Wilkins.

Additional Readings

Johnson KL: Diagnostic measures to evaluate oxygenation in critically ill adults, *AACN Clin Issues* 15(4):506-524, 2005.

Auto–Positive End-Expiratory Pressure (Auto-PEEP) Calculation

P U R P O S E : An end-expiratory hold maneuver is performed to calculate auto–positive end-expiratory pressure for the patient on mechanical ventilation. The calculation of auto–positive end-expiratory pressure is necessary to assess patient risk for a variety of conditions and the need for changes in ventilator parameters.

Suzanne M. Burns

PREREQUISITE NURSING KNOWLEDGE

* Auto–positive end-expiratory pressure (Auto-PEEP) is often called occult because it is not set on the ventilator; instead, it is a result of inadequate exhalation time (Fig. 30-1).[2-11]
* Auto-PEEP is associated with high minute ventilation requirements, small-diameter endotracheal tubes, bronchospasm, long inspiratory times, high respiratory rates, and mechanical factors, such as water accumulation in the ventilator tubing.[2-11]
* Auto-PEEP may result in an increased work of breathing. The set sensitivity of the ventilator is referenced to the amount of set-PEEP selected by the clinician. Because auto-PEEP is not sensed by the ventilator, the patient has to generate a pressure equal to the set sensitivity plus auto-PEEP to "trigger" inspiratory flow or a breath from the ventilator.[2,9]
* Auto-PEEP may elevate static pressure (i.e., plateau pressure). High plateau pressures can result in barotrauma and hemodynamic compromise.[9]
* Auto-PEEP may be a desirable outcome of select ventilator settings (e.g., pressure-controlled inverse ratio ventilation). In these cases, the goal of auto-PEEP is to restore functional residual capacity and reduce shunt.
* Interventions to offset auto-PEEP include the use of large-diameter endotracheal tubes, bronchodilators, short inspiratory times, long expiratory times, lower respiratory rates, frequent emptying of ventilator circuit water

accumulation (heated circuits may eliminate this complication), and the use of sedatives and narcotics (if the patient's breathing pattern is such that it increases the minute ventilation). Occasionally the addition of set-PEEP is used to offset auto-PEEP. The addition of

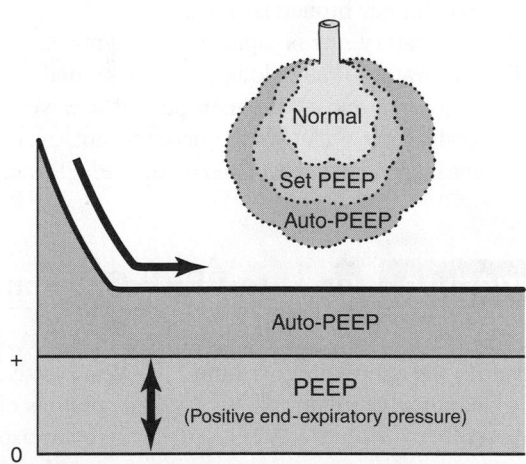

FIGURE 30-1 Auto-PEEP is PEEP over and above the set-PEEP. It can be measured by performing an end-expiratory hold maneuver and observing the airway pressure manometer or digital display. Auto-PEEP is caused by insufficient expiratory time (e.g., high rates, short expiratory times, water in the ventilator circuit, inverse respiratory ratios, bronchospasm, and high minute ventilations). Auto-PEEP can result in increased pulmonary pressures, decreased venous return, and hypotension and barotrauma. *(From Kinney M, et al: AACN clinical reference for critical care nursing, ed 4, St Louis, 1998, Mosby.)*

set-PEEP serves as a splint by keeping the airway open throughout exhalation, decreasing auto-PEEP.[2-7,11] An example of this technique is the patient with chronic obstructive pulmonary disease in whom early airway closure during exhalation results in gas trapping.

EQUIPMENT

Generally, no additional equipment is necessary because most ventilators have an end-expiratory hold button to use for determining auto-PEEP.

PATIENT AND FAMILY EDUCATION

- Inform the patient and family about the patient's respiratory status, changes in therapy, and how to interpret the changes. If the patient or family requests specific information about auto-PEEP measurements, explain the general relationship between auto-PEEP, the work of breathing, and complication risks. ➤*Rationale:* Most patients and families are less concerned with the diagnostic and therapeutic details and more concerned with how the patient's condition is progressing overall or in relation to a specific physiologic function.

PATIENT ASSESSMENT AND PREPARATION

Patient Assessment

- Assess for the presence of auto-PEEP; have a high index of suspicion if any of the following is noted:
  - ❖ Minute ventilation requirements are greater than 10 L/min.
  - ❖ The patient has chronic obstructive pulmonary disease.
  - ❖ The patient has bronchospasm.
  - ❖ The respiratory rate is rapid (i.e., ≥20/min).
  - ❖ The inspiratory time is long (i.e., >1 second).
  - ❖ Dyssynchrony exists between patient and ventilator, especially when the ventilator does not cycle with patient inspiration. ➤*Rationale:* Auto-PEEP increases

the work of breathing by increasing the threshold load to trigger inspiration. The increased work of breathing may cause fatigue.

- ❖ Auto-PEEP is present (when any of the previously listed criteria is present) and the patient is hypotensive or shows signs of barotrauma.
- ❖ Patients in status asthmaticus are at high risk for auto-PEEP. Consider the presence of auto-PEEP as the result of vigorous bagging, high ventilator rates, or large tidal volumes, especially if hypotension is present. ➤*Rationale:* Auto-PEEP, similar to intentional PEEP, puts the patient at risk for barotrauma from increased intra-alveolar pressures. In patients with asthma, lung compliance is good, but airway resistance is high, which encourages dynamic hyperinflation (alveolar overdistention) and potential barotrauma. Hemodynamic compromise occurs when the increased alveolar pressure results in compression of the corresponding capillaries; decreased venous return and hypotension result.

- Auto-PEEP may not be detected in some patients with severe asthma despite its presence. This situation may occur if the end-expiratory hold maneuver is too short to allow complete equilibration of pressures and with airway obstruction. In addition, if airways are noncommunicating, as in the case of obstruction from mucus or severe bronchospasm, auto-PEEP is not able to be measured. Assume auto-PEEP in these cases. Monitoring of plateau pressure may be a better method of assessment of hyperinflation (see Procedure 31).[5-7]

Patient Preparation

- Verify correct patient with two identifiers. ➤*Rationale:* Prior to performing a procedure, the nurse should ensure the correct identification of the patient for the intended intervention.
- Ensure that the patient understands preprocedural teachings. Answer questions as they arise, and reinforce information as needed. ➤*Rationale:* This communication evaluates and reinforces understanding of previously taught information.

Procedure	for Auto-PEEP Calculation	
Steps	**Rationale**	**Special Considerations**
1. Identify the end-expiratory hold button on the ventilator.[1,3-10] **(Level B*)**	When activated end-expiratory hold buttons close the ventilator systems to atmospheric pressure at end exhalation. The presence and level of auto-PEEP can be measured during an end-expiratory hold maneuver because the pressure in the system equilibrates.	Normally, the pressure in the ventilator is exposed to atmospheric pressure during exhalation, and the airway pressure manometer or readout drops to 0 or the set-PEEP level.

*Level B: Well-designed, controlled studies with results that consistently support a specific action, intervention, or treatment

Procedure	**for Noninvasive Ventilation (CPAP and BiPAP Masks)**—*Continued*	
Steps	**Rationale**	**Special Considerations**
2. Push the end-expiratory hold button at the end of exhalation (right before the next inspiration).[8-10] **(Level B*)**	Auto-PEEP is the level of PEEP between set-PEEP and the highest level (total PEEP) noted during this maneuver. Generally, this action is done for only a few seconds until the final expiratory level (reflecting the total PEEP) is detected. However, in some patients it may take longer. Observe the patient during the maneuver to assure tolerance.	In patients with rapid respiratory rates and in agitated patients, auto-PEEP is difficult to measure accurately. Use of sedatives, muscle relaxants, or both may be necessary.
A. Observe the baseline pressure level on the airway pressure manometer or on the digital readout. B. If auto-PEEP is present, the baseline (0 or set-PEEP level) increases to the level of auto-PEEP.		In patients with asthma, an end-expiratory hold may not exhibit auto-PEEP despite the presence of significant dynamic hyperinflation. This may be the result of noncommunicating airways (obstructed, etc). In these cases, assumption of the presence of auto-PEEP is prudent. Plateau pressure may be a better measure to assess the results of therapeutic interventions in these cases. In addition, some suggest the addition of set-PEEP in increments to open noncommunicating airways. If the additional PEEP results in more distention, the plateau pressure increases. If it contributes to enhanced alveolar emptying, the plateau pressure decreases (or stays the same).
C. Record the total PEEP over the set-PEEP level. 3. **HH** 4. Consult physician, advanced practice nurse, or respiratory therapist as needed for changes in therapy.		

Expected Outcomes

- Auto-PEEP is identified, monitored, and eliminated (if undesirable)
- Therapy is titrated, if possible, to minimize or eliminate auto-PEEP

Unexpected Outcomes

- Pulmonary barotrauma
- Cardiovascular compromise

*Level B: Well-designed, controlled studies with results that consistently support a specific action, intervention, or treatment

Procedure continues on following page

Patient Monitoring and Care

Steps	Rationale	Reportable Conditions
		These conditions should be reported if they persist despite nursing interventions.
1. Evaluate the presence of auto-PEEP in the conditions noted in patient assessment.	Prevent complications by determining the presence of auto-PEEP and intervening appropriately; this is especially important in patients with profound hyperinflation (i.e., status asthmaticus). Interventions may need to be aggressive; the patient may need paralytics and sedatives so that ventilatory support can be reduced to allow for more complete exhalation. With reduction of ventilatory support (i.e., decrease in tidal volume [Vt], rate, and minute ventilation), hypercarbia ensues and is anticipated, which is referred to as permissive hypercarbia.[1] The clinical goal is to reduce dynamic hyperinflation and potential lung injury.	• Presence of auto-PEEP
2. Assess for signs and symptoms of barotrauma, hemodynamic compromise, or both.	Barotrauma is a potential complication of auto-PEEP. Hemodynamic compromise is the result of "capillary squeeze" from the high intrathoracic pressure.	• Decreased breath sounds or absent breath sounds • Respiratory distress • Unexplained vital sign changes (i.e., hypotension, tachycardia)

Documentation

Documentation should include the following:
• Patient and family education
• Presence and level of auto-PEEP
• Any changes in ventilator parameters
• Unexpected outcomes
• Nursing interventions taken

References

CR 1. Bidani A, Tzouanakis AE, Carenas VJ, et al: Permissive hypercapnia in acute respiratory failure, *JAMA* 272: 957-962, 1994.

2. Burns SM: Ventilating patients with acute severe asthma: what do we really know? *AACN Advanced Crit Care* 17:188-193, 2006.

CR 3. Coussa ML, Guerin C, Eissa NT, et al: Partitioning of work of breathing in mechanically ventilated COPD patients, *J Appl Physiol* 75(4):1711-1719, 1993.

CR 4. Georgopoulos D, Giannouli E, Patakas D: Effects of extrinsic positive end-expiratory pressure on mechanically ventilated patients with chronic obstructive pulmonary disease and dynamic hyperinflation, *Intensive Care Med* 19:197-203, 1993.

CR 5. Leatherman JW, McArthur C, Shapiro RS: Effect of prolongation of expiratory time on dynamic hyperinflation in mechanically ventilated patients with severe asthma, *Crit Care Med* 32:1542-1545, 2004.

CR 6. Leatherman JW, Ravenscraft SA: Low-measured auto-positive end-expiratory pressure during mechanical ventilation of patients with severe asthma: hidden auto-positive end expiratory pressure, *Crit Care Med* 24:541-546, 1996.

CR 7. MacIntyre NR, Cheng KC, McConnell R: Applied PEEP during pressure support reduces inspiratory threshold of intrinsic PEEP, *Chest* 111:188-193, 1997.

CR 8. Pepe PE, Marini JJ: Occult positive end-expiratory pressure in mechanically ventilated patients with airflow obstruction, *Am Rev Respir Dis* 126:166-173, 1994.

CR 9. Rossi A, Gottfried SB, Zocchi L, et al: Measurement of static compliance of the total respiratory system in patients with acute respiratory failure during mechanical ventilation: the effect of intrinsic positive end-expiratory pressure, *Am Rev Respir Dis* 131(5):672-677, 1985.

CR 10. Smith TC, Marini JJ: Impact of PEEP on lung mechanics and work of breathing in severe airflow obstruction, *J Appl Physiol* 65:1488-1499, 1988.

11. Tobin MJ, Alex CA, Fahey PJ: Fighting the ventilator. In Tobin MJ, editor: *Principles and practice of mechanical ventilation,* New York, 2006, McGraw-Hill.

Additional Readings

Burns S: Mechanical ventilation and weaning. In Carlson KK, editor: *AACN advanced critical care nursing,* St Louis, 2009, Elsevier.

Pierce LNB: Invasive and noninvasive modes and methods of mechanical ventilation. In Burns SM, editor: *AACN protocols for practice: care of mechanically ventilated patients,* ed 2, Boston, 2007, Jones and Bartlett.

Pierce LNB: Mechanical ventilation: indications, ventilator performance of the respiratory cycle, and inititation. In Pierce LNB, editor: *Management of the mechanically ventilated patient,* ed 2, St Louis, 2007, Elsevier.

Compliance and Resistance Measurement

P U R P O S E :   Clinical measurements of compliance and resistance are performed to assess trends in respiratory status, determine the effectiveness of therapy, and titrate therapy.

Suzanne M. Burns

PREREQUISITE NURSING KNOWLEDGE

- *Compliance* is a measure of lung (and chest wall) distensibility. Conditions that decrease compliance include acute lung injury (ALI), acute respiratory distress syndrome (ARDS), pulmonary edema, atelectasis, pneumonia, obesity, pulmonary fibrosis, and kyphoscoliosis. Compliance increases with emphysema.[2,5]
- *Resistance* is a measure of how easily gases move down the airways. Conditions that adversely affect resistance include bronchospasm, secretions, and endotracheal tube size.[2,5]
- Compliance and resistance are reflected in the patient on mechanical ventilation by changes in peak inspiratory and plateau pressures (i.e., volume modes) and by changes in volume (i.e., pressure modes). With monitoring of changes in volume per unit change in pressure (mL/cm H_2O), trends can be measured and therapies adjusted.[2,5]
- Although spirometry or plethysmography are required for the exact measurement of airway flow resistance and lung compliance, two clinical measurements are frequently used to estimate the contributions of each in a patient on mechanical ventilation: dynamic compliance (C_{dyn}), which is more accurately called dynamic characteristic, and static compliance (C_{stat}).
    - ❖ The measurements of C_{dyn} and C_{stat} are obtained while the patient is on a volume mode of ventilation. C_{dyn} requires that the delivered volume be divided by the peak inspiratory pressure (PIP) minus positive end-expiratory pressure (PEEP). PIP reflects both the contribution of airway resistance (how easily gases flow down the airways) and lung compliance (dispensability

of the lung). Thus the measurement of C_{dyn}, which does not separate resistance and compliance is a measure of the overall state of the lung (inclusive of compliance and resistance). For this reason, *dynamic characteristic* is a more accurate term for this measurement than is *dynamic compliance*.[2,3,5]

- ❖ C_{stat} is measured during a breath-hold maneuver (i.e., end inspiration). By stopping gas flow, the pressure in the system equilibrates, and the resultant pressure reflects the pressure required to distend the lungs separate from the pressure needed to move gases down the airways. The pressure measured during the breath hold is called *static pressure* (also called *plateau, alveolar,* or *distending pressure*). By also subtracting PEEP, this number becomes the denominator for the calculation of C_{stat} (i.e., tidal volume ÷ [plateau pressure − PEEP]). The normal gradient between PIP and plateau pressure is 10 to 15 cm H_2O. In comparison of the difference between the two, the contribution of airway resistance is easily noted. Although PIP and plateau pressure are helpful in monitoring clinical trends, calculation of C_{dyn} and C_{stat} is most useful for quantifying the degree of improvement or compromise over time.[2,5]

- Static pressure is especially helpful to monitor when the lung is stiff (e.g., ALI or ARDS) and when great potential exists for barotrauma (e.g., pneumothorax) or volutrauma (e.g., alveolar injury).[1,2,4] In a randomized controlled trial by the ARDS Network, patients ventilated with low-volume ventilation (i.e., 6 mL/kg) had a lower mortality rate than patients ventilated at larger "traditional" volumes (i.e., 12 mL/kg).[4] The plateau pressures associated with the low-volume ventilation were less than 30 cm H_2O. The clinical goal for patients with ARDS is to ensure a tidal volume (Vt) of 6 mL/kg and, with both volume and pressure ventilation; plateau pressure should be less than 30 cm H_2O (see Procedure 35).[4]

- Measuring static pressure may increase the risk of barotrauma or cardiovascular compromise; this risk is low, however, because the measurement should take only a few seconds to accomplish.

EQUIPMENT

- Calculator
- Ventilator measurements: Vt, PIP, static pressure, PEEP, (see Procedure 35) and auto-PEEP, if present (see Procedure 30)

PATIENT AND FAMILY EDUCATION

- Inform the patent and family about the patient's respiratory status, changes in therapy, and how to interpret the changes. If the patient or a family member requests specific information about C_{dyn} or C_{stat}, explain the relationship between the measurements and the ability to get air into the lungs and down the airway. ➤➤*Rationale:* Most patients and families are less concerned with diagnostic and therapeutic details and more concerned with how the patient's condition is progressing overall.

PATIENT ASSESSMENT AND PREPARATION

Patient Assessment

- Verify correct patient with two identifiers. ➤➤*Rationale:* Prior to performing a procedure, the nurse should ensure the correct identification of the patient for the intended intervention.
- If the patient is on a volume mode, monitor PIP for gradual or acute airway or compliance changes. ➤➤*Rationale:* Given a constant tidal volume, a change in PIP indicates a change in airway resistance or lung compliance.
- If the patient is on a pressure mode, monitor tidal volume for gradual or acute airway or compliance changes. ➤➤*Rationale:* With pressure modes of ventilation, the pressure is stable. Thus, a change in tidal volume (or rate if the patient is breathing spontaneously) is indicative of a change in compliance or resistance.

Patient Preparation

- Ensure that the patient understands pre-procedural teachings. Answer questions as they arise, and reinforce information as needed. ➤➤*Rationale:* This communication evaluates and reinforces understanding of previously taught information.
- Premedicate as needed. ➤➤*Rationale:* This measurement may be extremely difficult in a patient who is breathing rapidly or is agitated. Sedation and paralytics are sometimes necessary.

Procedure for Compliance and Resistance Measurement

Steps	Rationale	Special Considerations
1. 🅷🅷		
Dynamic Compliance (C_{dyn}) (Level B*)		
C_{dyn} and C_{stat} *have been extensively tested at bedside in many patient populations.*[1-5]		
2. Identify the PIP.	PIP is used as a rough estimate of the mechanical properties of the lung and chest wall and of airway resistance.	
3. Identify the delivered exhaled tidal volume.	Data collection for calculation.	Air leaks around the artificial airway or through chest tubes prevent an accurate measurement of C_{dyn}. Ensure that any cuff leak is minimal. Exhaled tidal volume differs from inspired tidal volume with large leaks.
4. Identify the amount of PEEP and auto-PEEP.	Data collection for calculation.	If auto-PEEP is present, add to PEEP as total PEEP to ensure accurate calculation (see Procedure 30). If auto-PEEP is not anticipated or desired, work on strategies to eliminate it. (see Procedure 30).
5. Record PIP, tidal volume, and total PEEP (i.e., PEEP plus auto- PEEP).	Data collection for calculation.	
6. Subtract total PEEP from PIP.	Reflects PIP without PEEP.	

*Level B: Well-designed, controlled studies with results that consistently support a specific action, intervention, or treatment

Procedure continues on following page

Procedure | for Compliance and Resistance Measurement—*Continued*

Steps	Rationale	Special Considerations
7. Divide tidal volume by the number obtained in **Step 6**. The result equals the C_{dyn} as expressed in mL/cm H_2O. 8. **HH**	Compliance is defined as the unit change in volume per unit change in pressure.	
Static Compliance (C_{stat})		
1. **HH**		
2. Observe several ventilator respiratory cycles.	Allows for determination of exhaled tidal volume	Air leaks around the artificial airway or through chest tubes prevent an accurate measurement of Cdyn. Ensure that any cuff leak is minimal. Exhaled tidal volume differs from inspired tidal volume with large leaks.
3. Identify initiation of the ventilator inspiratory cycle.	Determines timing of the beginning of inspiration.	
4. At the end of inspiration, activate the inspiratory pause (inflation hold) while watching the airway pressure manometer or the digital readout. Note the drop and plateau of the PIP level (plateau pressure) and immediately deactivate the inspiratory pause, allowing exhalation.	At this point, the flow of gas through the airway stops, the gases in the system equilibrate (static, no gas flow either way in the airways), and the resultant lower pressure is the static pressure (also called *plateau, alveolar,* and *distending pressure*).	This measurement may be extremely difficult in a patient who is breathing rapidly or agitated. Administration of sedation and paralytics is sometimes necessary to perform the maneuver.
5. Record the static pressure.	Data collection for calculation.	
6. Subtract total PEEP (PEEP plus auto-PEEP) from plateau pressure.	Reflects pressure plateau without PEEP.	
7. Divide tidal volume by the number obtained in step 6. The result equals the C_{stat} and is expressed in mL/cm H_2O. 8. **HH**	C_{stat} is the relationship of the tidal volume to the plateau (static) pressure.	Air leaks around the artificial airway or through chest tubes prevent an accurate measurement of static compliance. Ensure an intact cuff.

Expected Outcome

- Therapy titrated to patient response

Unexpected Outcomes

- Pulmonary barotrauma
- Cardiovascular compromise

Patient Monitoring and Care

Steps	Rationale	Reportable Conditions
		These conditions should be reported if they persist despite nursing interventions.
1. Observe trends in C_{dyn} and C_{stat}.	Increasing values with a constant tidal volume indicate improvement in underlying disease process and effectiveness of interventions (improved compliance and decreased resistance).	- Bradycardia - Tachycardia - Decrease in saturation to less than or equal to 90%

Patient Monitoring and Care —*Continued*

Steps	Rationale	Reportable Conditions
	Decreasing values with constant tidal volume indicate increased airway resistance or decreased compliance from progression of underlying disease process and ineffective interventions.	• Changes or trends • Increasing PIP or plateau pressure

Documentation

Documentation should include the following:
- Patient and family education
- C_{dyn} (mL/cm H_2O) and C_{stat} (mL/cm H_2O) calculations
- Patient tolerance
- Nursing interventions
- Unexpected outcomes

References

1. Dreyfuss D, et al: High inflation pressure pulmonary edema: respective effects of high airway pressure, high tidal volume, and positive end-expiratory pressure, *Am Rev Respir Dis* 137:1159-1164, 1988.
2. Marini JJ: Lung mechanics determinations at the bedside: instrumentation and clinical applications, *Respir Care* 35:669, 1990.
3. Pepe PE, Marini JJ: Occult positive end-expiratory pressure in mechanically ventilated patients with airflow obstruction, *Am Rev Respir Dis* 126:166-170, 1982.
4. The Acute Respiratory Distress Syndrome Network: Ventilation with lower tidal volumes as compared with traditional tidal volumes for acute lung injury and the acute respiratory distress syndrome, *N Engl J Med* 342:1301-1307, 2000.
5. West JB: *Respiratory physiology: the essentials,* ed 8, Baltimore, 2008, Lippincott Williams & Wilkins.

Additional Readings

Burns S: Mechanical ventilation and weaning. In Carlson KK, editor: *AACN advanced critical care nursing*, St Louis, 2009, Elsevier.
Pierce LNB: Practical physiology of the pulmonary system. In Pierce LNB, editor: *Management of the mechanically ventilated patient*, ed 2, St Louis 2007, Elsevier.
West JB: *Pulmonary pathophysiology: the essentials*, Baltimore, 2008, Lippincott Williams & Wilkins.

Manual Self-Inflating Resuscitation Bag-Valve Device

PURPOSE: The manual self-inflating resuscitation bag-valve device is used to provide ventilation and oxygenation with or without an artificial airway in place and is referred to as "bagging."

Suzanne M. Burns

PREREQUISITE NURSING KNOWLEDGE

- Bagging is an essential skill used in emergency situations, such as cardiopulmonary arrest. Bagging also is indicated for the following:
  - ❖ To provide oxygenation and ventilation before and after suctioning airway procedures and during patient transports
  - ❖ To assess airway patency and proper airway device placement
  - ❖ To evaluate the interaction of patient and ventilator
  - ❖ To alter the ventilatory pattern
  - ❖ Bagging should result in chest movement and auscultatory evidence of bilateral air entry.
  - ❖ In patients without an artificial airway in place, effective bagging requires an unobstructed airway, slight head and neck hyperextension (i.e., the same technique used for mouth-to-mouth ventilation), and firm placement of the face mask over the nose and mouth (Fig. 32-1). An exception to this technique is with known or suspected cervical spine injury, in which the patient's airway is opened with the chin-lift method (without neck hyperextension). Effective bagging is best accomplished with two people: one to secure the mask and ensure head and neck placement and one to bag.[1] In patients with artificial airways, such as endotracheal or nasotracheal tubes or tracheostomies, the nurse must understand the components of artificial airways and their relationship to the upper airway anatomy (see Procedures 1, 2, 3, 7, 8, 9, 12, 13, 14, 18).

- ❖ **When signs and symptoms of respiratory distress are noted in a patient on mechanical ventilation, the patient should be bagged on 100% oxygen if troubleshooting the ventilator does not immediately solve the problem.** Large bagged breaths or rapid rates during bagging may result in dynamic hyperinflation and resultant hypotension.[2,3] Hyperinflation occurs when exhalation time is inadequate, which results in auto–positive end-expiratory pressure (auto-PEEP) and decreased venous return (see Procedure 30), with the resultant hypotension. Dynamic hyperinflation is most commonly associated with bronchospasm and chronic obstructive pulmonary disease.[2] A high index of suspicion for the presence of dynamic hyperinflation is

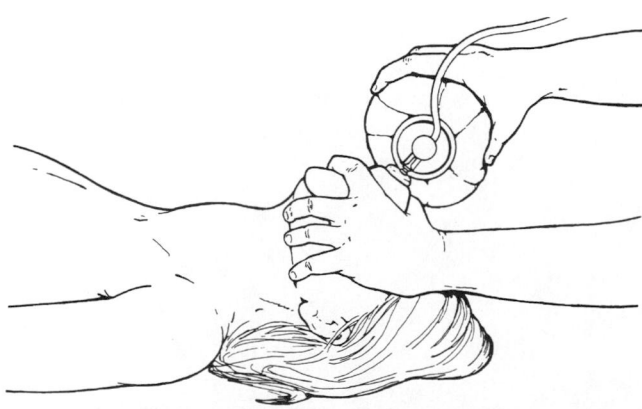

FIGURE 32-1   Proper technique of ventilation with manual self-inflating resuscitation bag-valve device and face mask. *(From Wilkins RL, Stoller JK, Kacmarek RM: Egan's fundamentals of respiratory care, ed 8, St Louis, 2008, Mosby.)*

necessary if hypotension occurs with bagging. A brief disconnection from the bag or the provision of longer exhalation times or both results in a rapid increase in blood pressure. Bagging is resumed at a slower rate and with longer expiratory times.

EQUIPMENT

- Manual self-inflating resuscitation bag-valve device (of appropriate size) (Fig. 32-2) and appropriately sized mask
- Oxygen source, flow regulator, and tubing
- PEEP valve or PEEP attachment (if patient on greater than 10 cm H_2O of PEEP)
- Personal protective equipment (i.e., gloves, mask, goggles, gown, as appropriate)
- Additional equipment to have available depending on patient need:
  - Oxygen analyzer when specific fraction (i.e., lower than 100%) of inspired oxygen (Fio_2) is desired
  - Portable respirometer if accurate tidal volume delivery on a breath-to-breath basis is required (e.g., during patient transports)

PATIENT AND FAMILY EDUCATION

- Inform the patient and family that the patient needs assisted breathing and, if currently on a ventilator, the patient will be disconnected from the ventilator and bagging will be performed. Describe the reason (e.g., suctioning, transporting, patient comfort) for bagging and explain that if the patient is dyspneic or otherwise distressed, bagging must be done immediately. ➤*Rationale:* Information about the patient's therapy is an important need of patients and family members. Dyspnea is uncomfortable and frightening. It leads to anxiety, fear, and distrust. Failure to diagnose promptly and alleviate the cause of respiratory distress puts the patient at risk for further decompensation.
- Inform the patient and family that the patient may be in different positions during bagging (i.e., side-lying, prone, supine, Trendelenburg's, reverse Trendelenburg's, semi-Fowler). Bagging may be more difficult, however, if the diaphragm and abdominal contents are in positions that resist lung inflation. ➤*Rationale:* Positioning is not an impediment to bagging as long as an intact airway is in place. Bagging may be more difficult in some positions.

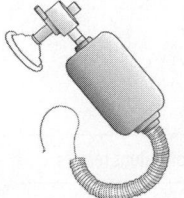 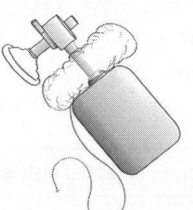 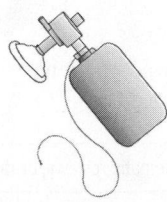

Bag-valve assembly with rear bag reservoir   Bag-valve assembly with collar reservoir   Bag-valve assembly without reservoir

FIGURE 32-2 Manual self-inflating bags: bag-valve assembly with and without reservoir.

- Discuss the sensory experience associated with bagging. ➤*Rationale:* Knowledge of anticipated sensory experiences decreases anxiety and distress.
- Instruct the patient to communicate discomfort with breathing during bagging. ➤*Rationale:* The bagging technique can be altered to produce a comfortable breathing pattern.
- Offer the opportunity for the patient and family to ask questions about bagging. ➤*Rationale:* The ability to ask questions and have questions answered honestly is cited consistently as the most important need of patients and families.

PATIENT ASSESSMENT AND PREPARATION

Patient Assessment

- Verify correct patient with two identifiers. ➤*Rationale:* Prior to performing a procedure, the nurse should ensure the correct identification of the patient for the intended intervention.
- Determine oxygenation and ventilation status and observe for the following signs:
  - Sudden decrease in arterial oxygen saturation (Sao_2)
  - Sudden decrease in pulse oximetry saturation (Spo_2)
  - Sudden change in mental status
  - Tachycardia
  - Tachypnea
  - Respiratory distress
  - Diaphoresis
  - Agitation

  ➤*Rationale:* Any acute change in patient status may indicate that bagging is necessary.
  - Rapid response with 100% Fio_2 protects the patient and allows for rapid evaluation of airway resistance, placement and function of artificial airway, and interaction of patient and ventilator.
- Determine airway resistance (how easily air moves down the airways) and lung compliance (how easily the lungs and chest wall distend). ➤*Rationale:* Airway resistance and lung compliance can be assessed by bagging the patient with breaths that are similar in volume and rate to the breaths provided by the ventilator. Focus on the degree of ease (or difficulty) with which the bag is compressed during inspiration. **If bagging the patient is difficult, look for causes of high airway resistance (e.g., obstructed airway, bronchospasm) or low lung compliance (e.g., mucus obstruction, pulmonary edema, pneumonia, acute respiratory distress syndrome, pneumothorax).** Compare findings with findings after interventions, such as suctioning and bronchodilator use. Changes in resistance and compliance can be confirmed by evaluating dynamic characteristic and static compliance when the patient is placed back on the ventilator (see Procedure 31).
- Ensure proper placement and function of the artificial airway (see Procedures 1, 2, 3, 7, 8, 9, 12, 13, 14). ➤*Rationale:* The positioning and patency of the airway are ensured.

- Evaluate interaction of patient and ventilator and specifically note dyssynchrony of patient and ventilator by observing for the following:
  - ❖ Breathing pattern not in synchrony with ventilator breaths
  - ❖ Wheezing
  - ❖ Restlessness
  - ❖ Dyspnea
  - ❖ Altered level of consciousness
  - ❖ Agitation
  - ❖ Decreased or unequal breath sounds
  - ❖ Tachycardia or bradycardia
  - ❖ Dysrhythmias
  - ❖ Cyanosis
  - ❖ Hypertension or hypotension
  - ❖ Diaphoresis
- ➡*Rationale:* Bagging may aid in the return of a synchronous breathing pattern and recognition of the cause (e.g., obstruction). If signs and symptoms persist despite bagging, other causes (e.g., pulmonary embolus) should be considered. Therapeutic interventions to ensure synchrony and effective oxygenation and ventilation may be necessary and may include administration of medications such as sedatives, narcotics, and bronchodilators. Additional diagnostic evaluations also may be needed (e.g., bronchoscopy, ventilation-perfusion scans, computed tomography–pulmonary angiography [CT-PA]).

Patient Preparation

- Ensure that the patient understands pre-procedural teachings, or if the patient's condition precludes teaching, assure the patient that bagging will help with less shortness of breath. Answer questions as they arise, and reinforce information as needed. ➡*Rationale:* This communication evaluates and reinforces understanding of previously taught information.

Procedure	for Manual Self-Inflating Resuscitation Bag

Steps	Rationale	Special Considerations
Using the Manual Self-Inflating Bag-Valve Device for Respiratory Distress or Evaluation of Pulmonary Status		
1. **HH**		
2. **PE**		
3. Check that the bag is attached to an oxygen source that is turned on. Attach a PEEP valve or adjust the PEEP level on the bag if the patient is on a ventilator with a PEEP of 10 cm H_2O or more.	Safety precaution. Provides direct route for oxygen to flow into the bag. The PEEP valve maintains PEEP during bagging.	Some bags are directly attached to the gas source and fill with the source gas with every breath (when bag is released after inspiration).
4. If the patient is on mechanical ventilation, disconnect patient from the ventilator. Activate alarm silence. Connect bag to artificial airway.	Allows for manual ventilation.	
5. Observe patient's breathing pattern and rate. Attempt to synchronize manual breaths with the patient's spontaneous effort. Because larger breaths are more difficult to provide with manual ventilation compared with breaths provided by the ventilator, a higher manual rate may be required initially.[1] **(Level C*)**	Helps patient gain control over breathing by ensuring ventilation and adequate oxygenation.[1]	
6. Encourage patient to relax as manual breaths are provided.	Provides synchrony between patient breaths and manual breaths.	

*Level C: Qualitative studies, descriptive or correlational studies, integrative reviews, systematic reviews, or randomized controlled trials with inconsistent results

Procedure for Manual Self-Inflating Resuscitation Bag—*Continued*

Steps	Rationale	Special Considerations
7. Gradually slow the rate of manual breaths to approximate the ventilator frequency or to a rate that meets the patient's demand.	Reestablishes synchrony. When respiratory distress is relieved with a rate and volume comparable with that delivered by the ventilator, the patient can be reconnected. If the patient is on a low rate (e.g., intermittent mandatory ventilation of 4) or low-pressure support level, common during weaning, the distress may be the result of fatigue. A return to higher ventilator support settings may be necessary after bagging.	
8. Ascertain whether the patient is comfortable with the manual breaths. Assess the ease or difficulty with which the bag is deflated.	Promotes comfort.	
A. If signs and symptoms of distress are absent the patient can be reconnected to the ventilator.	Indicates that respiratory distress is relieved.	If the patient becomes distressed after reconnection, consider further assessment to determine etiology and potential interventions. Additional steps are as follows: Call for assistance while bagging and look for additional confirmatory physical assessment findings, such as tympanic percussion (i.e., pneumothorax), diminished breath sounds with consolidation (i.e., atelectasis, pneumonia), or crackles (i.e., pulmonary edema), to determine etiology of acute distress.
B. If distress is not eliminated with bagging, consider the following steps: Provide higher level of ventilator support if distress is evident on lower levels as in weaning trials; hyperoxygenate and suction (see Procedure 12); assess for the presence of bilateral breath sounds and symmetrical chest expansion; assess the ease (or difficulty) with which the bag can be inflated; evaluate ventilator functioning; obtain assistance (respiratory care or experienced nurse) to determine adequacy of ventilator function; consider anxiety and discomfort as potential causes of dyspnea.	Indicates respiratory distress cannot be relieved with bagging. Further assessment is needed. Distress may be a result of fatigue. Suction provides information related to the presence of secretions or airway obstruction. By auscultating the lungs during bagging, essential information related to tube placement (e.g., migration to right main stem) or patient status (e.g., bronchospasm, pulmonary edema) may be obtained. Asymmetrical chest expansion may be the result of a displaced artificial airway, pneumothorax, or obstruction. A change in ease of bagging provides gross data about increasing (improved) or decreasing (deteriorating) lung compliance.	These data should correlate with changes in peak inspiratory pressure (volume ventilation) or tidal volume or respiratory rate (pressure ventilation) on the ventilator. In some situations, such as pulmonary embolus, no distinct physical assessment findings may be immediately evident. Whether or not distress is alleviated with bagging and returns with reconnection, the ventilator may be malfunctioning or the settings may be inadequate for the patient's acute change in physical status. Support the patient until appropriate interventions are accomplished.

Procedure continues on following page

Procedure | for Manual Self-Inflating Resuscitation Bag—*Continued*

Steps	Rationale	Special Considerations
	Alarms should deactivate automatically, unless the problem has not been adequately addressed. A leak or other malfunction results in patient distress and inadequate oxygenation and ventilation. Although psychologic reasons for respiratory distress are possible, rule out physiologic causes first.	The use of anxiolytics or analgesics or both may be appropriate to decrease anxiety and pain. However, a thorough evaluation of the cause of distress must be undertaken both before and after administration.
9. Return patient to ventilator when respiratory distress is relieved. Reactivate and check ventilator alarms and settings. Observe breathing pattern, patient ventilator synchrony, peak inspiratory pressure (volume ventilation), and tidal volume and respiratory frequency (patient initiated). Check that call system is within patient's reach, if appropriate.	Safety precautions. Ensures nurse is alerted to actual or potential life-threatening problems.	
10. **PE**	Standard Precautions; reduces the risk of transmission of microorganisms and body secretions.	

Maintenance Ventilation Such As With Patient Transport

Portable ventilators are highly recommended for use during transport instead of manual bagging. Regardless, bagging may possibly be required for long intervals, such as during patient transport. The following procedure is designed to provide a ventilatory pattern similar to that provided by the ventilator. Procedures may vary depending on institutional standards.		
1. **HH**		
2. **PE**		
3. Check that bag is attached to oxygen source that is turned on. Attach a PEEP valve or adjust the PEEP level on the bag if the patient is on a ventilator with a PEEP of 10 cm H_2O or more.	Safety precaution. Provides direct route for oxygen to flow into the bag. The PEEP valve maintains PEEP during bagging.	Some bags are directly attached to the gas source and fill with the source gas with every breath (when bag is released after inspiration).
4. Disconnect patient from ventilator. Silence ventilator alarms.	Because the nurse is at the bedside and no problem exists with the patient or ventilator, the alarms are not needed to summon help or disturb other patients.	
5. Insert portable respirometer between bag and artificial airway.	Ensures that tidal volume and PEEP approximate that provided by ventilator.	
6. Bag patient at approximate rate depth and pattern as ventilator breaths.	Maintains ventilation pattern similar to that provided by ventilator.	

Procedure for Manual Self-Inflating Resuscitation Bag—*Continued*

Steps	Rationale	Special Considerations
7. Analyze average tidal volume delivered manually. Adjust bag compressions as necessary to produce tidal volume that approximates ventilator tidal volume. Repeat until approximate tidal volume is reproducible.	Achieves reproducible manual breaths.	
8. Remove portable respirometer, and insert portable oxygen analyzer between bag and artificial airway or use 1.0 Fio_2.	Allows Fio_2 to be analyzed.	Policies vary among institutions. Generally, 1.0 Fio_2 is used during patient transports, and analysis of oxygen level is not necessary.
9. Analyze Fio_2 delivered. Adjust liter flow of oxygen to produce same Fio_2 as ventilator breaths or to maintain Sao_2 at desired level.	Prevents hypoxia and maintains prescribed Fio_2.	Fio_2 delivered with bag depends on delivered oxygen liter flow and the type of manual resuscitation bag used. Reservoir tubing may be needed to ensure desired oxygen in some cases. Most current bags have reservoirs.
10. Remove oxygen analyzer and manually ventilate patient at tidal volume, ventilator frequency, and Fio_2 that approximate ventilator settings.	Approximates baseline ventilation and oxygenation.	
11. Periodically ascertain that the patient is comfortable with the bagging technique. Adjustments may be needed to maintain patient comfort with manual ventilation.	Promotes patient comfort.	The patient who is being ambulated may need larger minute ventilation than usual to match cardiac output, increased carbon dioxide production, and oxygen consumption during activity.
12. Reconnect patient to ventilator. Reactivate ventilator alarms. Ensure that call bell is within patient reach.	Safety precautions. Ensures that the nurse is alerted to actual or potential life-threatening problems.	
13. **HH** **PE**	Standard precautions; reduces the risk of transmission of microorganisms and body secretions.	

Expected Outcomes

- Maintenance of adequate oxygenation and ventilation
- Resolution of acute respiratory distress

Unexpected Outcomes

- Hemodynamic instability from dynamic hyperinflation
- Pulmonary barotrauma (e.g., pneumothorax)
- Inability to restore adequate ventilation and oxygenation with bagging
- Inadvertent extubation during bagging
- Equipment failure and inability to bag

Procedure continues on following page

Patient Monitoring and Care

Steps	Rationale	Reportable Conditions
		These conditions should be reported if they persist despite nursing interventions.
1. Evaluate trends or sudden changes in lung compliance or airway resistance.	Improvement or deterioration in lung function can be approximated with evaluation of patient's response to bagging.	• Difficulty bagging (stiff) • No observable chest movement • Agitation • Diaphoresis • Hypertension or hypotension • Tachycardia or bradycardia
2. Observe for signs and symptoms of obstructed upper and lower airways, including comfortable appearance; stable or improved level of consciousness; synchrony of patient and ventilator; symmetrical breath sounds; stable heart rate, rhythm, and blood pressure; and absence of rhonchi, wheezes, and dyspnea.	Proper technique results in a comfortable synchronous breathing pattern.	• Dyssynchronous breathing
3. Observe the patient during bagging. The patient should look comfortable. The chest should rise and fall evenly with bagging deflations and inflations.	Proper technique results in a comfortable synchronous breathing pattern.	• Dyssynchronous breathing
4. Monitor Spo_2 for maintenance of adequate oxygenation during bagging. End-tidal carbon dioxide tension ($Petco_2$) may be used to monitor adequacy of ventilation (e.g., carbon dioxide with acceptable limits).	If adequate oxygen is being delivered and ventilation is adequate, Spo_2 and $Petco_2$ should be unchanged or improve with bagging.	• Decrease in Spo_2 greater than 10% • Increase of $Petco_2$ greater than 10%

Documentation

Documentation should include the following:
- Patient and family education
- Reason for bagging (e.g., to suction during transport)
- Frequency
- Response of the procedure
- Unexpected outcomes
- Nursing interventions

References

CR 1. Grap MJ, et al: Endotracheal suctioning: ventilator vs manual delivery of hyperoxygenation breaths, *Am J Crit Care* 5:192-197, 1996.

CR 2. Pepe PE, Marini JJ: Occult positive end-expiratory pressure in mechanically ventilated patients with airflow obstruction, *Am Rev Respir Dis* 126:166-170, 1982.

3. Pierce LNB: Administration of oxygen humidification, and aerosol therapy. In editor? *Management of the mechanically ventilated patient,* ed 2, St Louis, 2007, Elsevier.

Additional Readings

Guidelines Committee of the American College of Critical Care Medicine; Society of Critical Care Medicine and American Association of Critical-Care Nurses Transfer Guidelines Task Force. Guidelines for the transfer of critically ill patients, *Crit Care Med* 1994 Jul;22(7): 1203-4.

Indices of Oxygenation

P U R P O S E : Alveolar-arterial oxygen difference, arterial partial pressure of oxygen–to–fraction of inspired oxygen ratio, arterial partial pressure of oxygen–to–alveolar partial pressure of oxygen ratio, and blood flow shunted–to–blood flow total ratio are calculated for identification of shunt as the primary mechanism of hypoxemia, assessment of trends in oxygenation, and determination of effectiveness and titration of therapies.

Suzanne M. Burns

PREREQUISITE NURSING KNOWLEDGE

- Arterial partial pressure of oxygen (Pao_2) is primarily determined by the concentration of inspired oxygen and the amount of carbon dioxide in the alveolus.[1-3]
- In healthy lungs, alveolar oxygen diffuses rapidly into the pulmonary capillaries, and arterial oxygenation approximates that of the alveolus. The normal alveolar-arterial oxygen difference ($A\text{-}aDo_2$) in a patient breathing 21% oxygen is 10 to 20 mm Hg (i.e., Pao_2 [100], Pao_2 [80]). When 100% oxygen is inspired, the normal gradient is 50 to 70 mm Hg.[1-3]
- Trends in alveolar-arterial (A-a) gradient are evaluated most accurately when the Pao_2 and Pao_2 are measured on room air or after inspiration of 100% oxygen for 15 minutes.[1-3]
- Other clinical indices of oxygenation that are commonly used include the $Pao_2 : Pao_2$ (a:A) ratio and the ratio of Pao_2 to fraction of inspired oxygen (Fio_2; P:F). These indices all are relatively easy to use and are helpful in estimates of trends in hypoxemia.[1,4,5]
- The advantage of the a:A and P:F ratios is that a more constant value, despite changes in Fio_2, can be calculated. A normal a:A ratio is 0.8 to 1. The smaller the number, the higher the degree of shunt. The normal value for P:F ratio is greater than 300. A smaller P:F ratio reflects a higher degree of shunt. A P:F ratio of 200 to 300

is used to define acute lung injury (ALI), whereas a P:F ratio of less than 200 is associated with acute respiratory distress syndrome (ARDS).[4,5]

- In patients with shunt (perfusion to unventilated lung units), venous blood is shunted past the closed alveoli without becoming oxygenated. Although Pao_2 may be "normal" because of an increase in Fio_2, a shunt exists. The A-a gradient increases. A-a gradient is considered a useful, albeit crude, clinical estimate of shunt. The A-a gradient value is helpful to trend changes in oxygenation status, the effect of therapies and other interventions.
- Concepts related to shunt and the refractory nature of shunt to increasing Fio_2 are inherent in all the indices (i.e., shunt is not responsive to oxygen). Although other reasons for hypoxemia exist in addition to shunt (i.e., hypoventilation on room air, diffusion block, ventilation to perfusion [V/Q] mismatch), the indices are generally most often used in the most severe pulmonary conditions that affect oxygenation. In these conditions (e.g., ARDS), quantification of the degree of shunt is helpful to trend the progress of the disease, determine the efficacy of therapies, and aid in prognosis.[1-3,5]
- The gold standard for quantifying shunt is calculation of shunted blood flow–to–total blood flow ratio (Qs:Qt). Calculation of Qs:Qt requires analysis of a mixed venous sample (from a pulmonary artery catheter or venous oxygen saturation [Svo_2] catheter); calculations of A-a

gradient, $Pao_2:Fio_2$, and $Pao_2:Pao_2$ do not. The measurement of Qs:Qt is detailed in Procedure 34.[2,3,5]
- Accurate interpretation of arterial and mixed venous blood gas analysis is necessary.

EQUIPMENT

- Arterial blood gas (ABG) results (after 15 minutes of 100% Fio_2) for calculation of A-aDo_2; if other indices are used (e.g., a:A ratio, P:F ratio), record the Fio_2 level when the ABG is drawn
- Calculator

PATIENT AND FAMILY EDUCATION

- Verify correct patient with two identifiers. **➤Rationale:** Prior to performing a procedure, the nurse should ensure the correct identification of the patient for the intended intervention.
- Inform the patient and family about the patient's oxygenation status and the rationale and implications for changes in therapy. If the patient or a family member requests specific information about oxygenation studies, explain the rationale for measurement. **➤Rationale:** Most patients and families are less concerned with the diagnostic and therapeutic details and more concerned with how the patient's condition is progressing overall.

PATIENT ASSESSMENT AND PREPARATION
Patient Assessment

- Assess for signs and symptoms of inadequate oxygenation:
  - Decreasing arterial oxygen tension
  - Tachypnea
  - Dyspnea
  - Central cyanosis
  - Restlessness
  - Confusion
  - Agitation
  - Tachycardia
  - Bradycardia
  - Dysrhythmias
  - Intercostal and suprasternal retractions
  - Increasing or decreasing arterial blood pressure
  - Adventitious breath sounds
  - Decreasing urine output
  - Metabolic acidosis
- **➤Rationale:** Clinical findings may indicate problems with oxygenation.
- Determine arterial oxygen tension or saturation. **➤Rationale:** Hypoxemia is confirmed by a decreasing Pao_2 or saturation of arterial oxygen (Sao_2) or an absolute Pao_2 of less than 60 mm Hg or absolute Sao_2 of less than 90%.
- Determine trend of indices and therapies. **➤Rationale:** Improvement or deterioration can be quantified by monitoring indices over time.

Procedure	**for Oxygenation Indices**	
Steps	Rationale	Special Considerations

Calculation of Oxygenation Indices

When calculating A-aDo_2, adjust the Fio_2 to 1.0 for 15 minutes before drawing the ABG. For calculation of the a:A ratio and P:F ratio, ABGs may be drawn without adjustment to the Fio_2.[1-5] **(Level B*)**

1. Use the equation in Table 33-1 for calculation of A-aDo_2.

TABLE 33-1	**Calculation of A-aDo_2**

$Pao_2 = Fio_2 (P_{Bar} - PH_2O) - (Paco_2/RQ)$

$Pao_2 - Pao_2 = A\text{-}aDo_2$

P_{Bar}, Barometric pressure (760 mm Hg); *PH_2O,* pressure of water vapor (47 mm Hg); *RQ,* respiratory quotient (0.8).

2. Use the equation in Table 33-2 for calculation of a:A ratio.

TABLE 33-2	**Equation for Calculation of Arterial:Alveolar Ratio**

Pao_2 (obtained from arterial blood gas) $= Pao_2$

See Table 33-1 for calculation of Pao_2.

---

*Level B: Well-designed, controlled studies with results that consistently support a specific action, intervention, or treatment

Procedure for Oxygenation Indices—*Continued*

Steps	Rationale	Special Considerations
3. Use the equation in Table 33-3 for calculation of P:F ratio.		

TABLE 33-3 Equation for Calculation of Pao_2:Fio_2 (P:F) Ratio

Pao_2 (obtained from arterial blood gas) $\div$ Fio_2 (expressed as a decimal)

Steps	Rationale	Special Considerations
4. Document indices in patient record with the following data: A. ABG results. B. Ventilator parameters, including Fio_2 at the time ABGs were drawn. C. Position of patient at the time the blood was drawn. D. Date and time ABGs were drawn. E. Changes in therapy, if any, based on indices.	All data viewed together are needed for decision making regarding changes in therapy. Positioning (e.g., patient in prone position) may be used as a means to improve shunt.	
5. On the basis of the calculation, consult with physician, advanced practice nurse, or respiratory therapist as needed for changes in therapy.		

Expected Outcomes

- Maintenance of adequate oxygenation (i.e., Sao_2, Pao_2)
- Timely decrease in Fio_2 and titration of positive end-expiratory pressure

Unexpected Outcomes

- Hemodynamic instability
- Pulmonary barotrauma
- Oxygen toxicity

Patient Monitoring and Care

Steps	Rationale	Reportable Conditions
		These conditions should be reported if they persist despite nursing interventions.
1. Observe trends in oxygenation indices.	Oxygenation indices reflect the approximate degree of shunting as a mechanism of hypoxemia. Changes may reflect status of disease process and effectiveness of therapy.	• Significant change in indices
2. Observe for increasing Pao_2 or Sao_2. Monitoring of the indices is less helpful when Pao_2 is greater than 60 mm Hg or Sao_2 is less than 90% on an Fio_2 of less than 0.4.	Shunting, as a mechanism of hypoxemia, requires high oxygen concentrations to maintain marginal oxygenation. Shunting is not contributing significantly to hypoxemia if the patient has an adequate arterial oxygen tension on Fio_2 of less than 0.40.	• Acceptable Pao_2 or Sao_2 with Fio_2 less than 0.40

Procedure continues on following page

Documentation

Documentation should include the following:
- Patient and family education
- Oxygenation index value, ABG results, FiO_2, and ventilator parameters at time blood was drawn
- Time, date, and position of patient (e.g., supine or left lateral)

- Changes in therapy based on the $A\text{-}aDO_2$
- Patient response to interventions
- Unexpected outcomes
- Nursing interventions

References

1. West JB: *Respiratory physiology: the essentials,* ed 8, Baltimore, 2008, Lippincott Williams & Wilkins.
2. West JB: *Pulmonary pathophysiology: the essentials,* Baltimore, 2008, Lippincott Williams & Wilkins.
CR 3. Covelli HD, Nessan VJ, Tuttle WK: Oxygen derived variables in acute respiratory failure, *Crit Care Med* 11:646-649, 1983.
CR 4. The Acute Respiratory Distress Syndrome Network: Ventilation with lower tidal volumes as compared with traditional tidal volumes for acute lung injury and the acute respiratory distress syndrome, *N Engl J Med* 342:1301-1307, 2000.
5. Theodore AC, Jefferson LS: Oxygenation and mechanisms of hypoxemia, *UpToDate Online* 16.2: 2008.

Additional Reading

Johnson KL: Diagnostic measures to evaluate oxygenation in critically ill adults, *AACN Clini Issues* 15(4): 506-524, 2005.

Shunt Calculation

P U R P O S E : Shunt calculation is performed to differentiate shunting from other mechanisms of hypoxemia, to quantify the shunt, to assess trends in progression or improvement of shunt, and to determine the effectiveness and duration of therapy.

Suzanne M. Burns

PREREQUISITE NURSING KNOWLEDGE

- Right-to-left intrapulmonary shunting (also referred to as physiologic shunting, wasted blood flow, and venous admixture) is the pathologic phenomenon whereby venous blood is shunted past the alveoli without taking up oxygen. This blood then returns to the left side of the heart as venous blood with a low oxygen tension.[1,2]
- Right-to-left intrapulmonary shunting is expressed as a fraction or percentage of shunted blood flow (Qs) to total blood flow (Qt) as expressed by the equation (Qs/Qt). The normal physiologic shunt is less than 5% and is caused by venous blood from the bronchial and coronary veins returning to the left side of the heart as desaturated blood.[1,2]
- Shunting of blood past the alveoli means that a certain percentage of the blood flows through an area of lung that receives no ventilation. Examples of conditions in which shunt is present include acute respiratory distress syndrome, acute lung injury, atelectasis, pneumonia, and pulmonary edema with fluid-filled alveoli.
- As the percentage of the shunted cardiac output increases, the mixture of venous shunted blood with arterial blood increases with a concomitant decrease in the arterial oxygen tension. The extent of the hypoxemia depends on the amount of the lung parenchyma that is not ventilated.
- The hallmark of right-to-left intrapulmonary shunting is persistent hypoxemia despite high concentrations of inspired oxygen (called refractory hypoxemia).[1,2]
- For evaluation of shunt, heparinized* arterial and mixed venous blood samples are analyzed with a cooximeter to determine saturation. Use of the calculated saturation obtained in conjunction with blood gas analysis or with pulse oximetry is not as accurate.[1,2]

EQUIPMENT

- Calculator
- Qs/Qt equation
- Mixed venous and arterial blood gas and saturation measurements
- Pulmonary artery catheter, for drawing mixed venous blood samples, or venous oxygen saturation (Svo_2) catheter. If an Svo_2 catheter is used, the mixed venous saturation recorded on the monitor can be used for the calculation (as long as in vitro and in vivo calibrations have been done according to manufacturer's recommendations)

PATIENT AND FAMILY EDUCATION

- Keep the patient and family informed about the patient's oxygenation status. Inform them of changes in therapy and how to interpret the changes. If the patient or a family member requests specific information about intrapulmonary shunting, explain the general relationship between Qs/Qt and hypoxemia. ➨*Rationale:* Most patients and families are less concerned with the diagnostic and therapeutic details and more concerned with how the patient's condition is progressing overall or in relation to a specific physiologic function.

---

*The use of heparin is not universal. Refer to critical care unit policy. It is avoided in those with potential for or acquired heparin-induced thrombocytopenia.

PATIENT ASSESSMENT AND PREPARATION

Patient Assessment

- Signs and symptoms of inadequate oxygenation include the following:
  - Decreasing arterial oxygen tension and saturation
  - Tachypnea
  - Dyspnea
  - Central cyanosis
  - Restlessness
  - Confusion
  - Agitation
  - Tachycardia
  - Bradycardia
  - Dysrhythmias
  - Intercostal and suprasternal retractions
  - Increasing or decreasing arterial blood pressure
  - Adventitious breath sounds
  - Decreasing urine output
  - End-organ failure or metabolic acidosis or both
- ➤*Rationale:* Calculation of Qs/Qt is indicated to help differentiate between the mechanisms of hypoxemia, to determine the degree of shunt for trending, and to evaluate the effectiveness of therapies.

Patient Preparation

- Verify correct patient with two identifiers. ➤*Rationale:* Prior to performing a procedure, the nurse should ensure the correct identification of the patient for the intended intervention.
- Determine arterial oxygen tension or saturation. ➤*Rationale:* Hypoxemia is confirmed by a decreasing arterial partial pressure of oxygen (Pao_2), decreasing arterial oxygen saturation (Sao_2), an absolute Pao_2 of less than 60 mm Hg, or an absolute Sao_2 of less than 90%. A low Pao_2 and a low Sao_2 with increasing supplemental oxygen confirm hypoxemia caused by right-to-left intrapulmonary shunting.
- Determine Qs/Qt trends with therapies and interventions. ➤*Rationale:* Calculation of Qs/Qt is indicated to help differentiate mechanisms of hypoxemia and to provide appropriate interventions. The effect of therapies such as positive end-expiratory pressure (PEEP), selected ventilator modes (e.g., pressure release ventilation, inverse ratio), and prone positioning on shunting and oxygenation can be quantified.

Procedure for Shunt Calculation

Steps	Rationale	Special Considerations
1. **HH**		
2. **PE**		
3. Draw heparinized blood sample slowly from distal port of the pulmonary artery catheter or obtain the Svo_2 reading from the Svo_2 monitor or module. Be sure to discard the first 3 mL because it contains flush solution.[1,2] **(Level B*)**	If sample is drawn too rapidly, aspiration of arterialized blood from the capillary bed is possible; calculation of Qs/Qt will be inaccurate. The calculation of Qs/Qt has been used as the gold standard for clinical shunt measurement.[1,2]	
4. Draw arterial blood sample simultaneously or within a few minutes of drawing mixed venous sample.	Ensures accuracy.	
5. Send the samples to be analyzed. Analysis of saturation is best done with cooximeter.	Use of calculated saturation obtained via blood gas analysis is less accurate.	
6. Remove personal protective equipment.	Standard Precautions; prevents transmission of microorganisms and body substances.	
7. **HH**		
8. Obtain Qs/Qt with the equation in Table 34-1.		

Expected Outcomes

- Maintenance of adequate Pao_2
- Timely titration of PEEP and fraction of inspired oxygen (Fio_2) and the application of other ventilatory therapies or positioning, as appropriate

Unexpected Outcomes

- Severe hypoxemia
- Hemodynamic instability

*Level B: Well-designed, controlled studies with results that consistently support a specific action, intervention, or treatment

TABLE 34-1	Qs/Qt Calculation

$Qs/Qt = (Cc_{O_2} - Ca_{O_2})/(Cc_{O_2} - Cv_{O_2})$

$Cc_{O_2} = (Hgb \times 1.39^* \times Sat^\dagger [1.0]) + (Pa_{O_2}^\ddagger \times 0.003)$

$Ca_{O_2} = (Hgb \times 1.39^* \times Sa_{O_2}) + (Pa_{O_2} \times 0.003)$

$Cv_{O_2} = (Hgb \times 1.39^* \times Sv_{O_2}) + (Pv_{O_2} \times 0.003)$

Cc_{O_2}, This is the oxygen content in mL/l00 ml (Volumes %) of blood that is reflective of a "model" alveolar/capillary unit (blood flow and alveolar ventilation are matched); Ca_{O_2}, arterial oxygen content in mL/100 mL of blood; $C\bar{v}_{O_2}$, mixed venous oxygen content in mL/100 mL of blood; Hgb, hemoglobin; Sat, saturation of hemoglobin; $P\bar{v}_{O_2}$, partial pressure of mixed venous oxygen.

For ease of calculation, the portion of the equation that determines the O_2 dissolved in plasma may be eliminated because the contribution of the dissolved portion of O_2 to O_2 content is extremely small. For continuity purposes, this should be determined by unit policy.

*Depending on institutional policy, standards between 1.39 and 1.34 are used.

†In the equation for calculation of $C\bar{c}_{O_2}$, saturation is assumed to be 100% as in an "ideal" capillary with no shunt.

Patient Monitoring and Care

Steps	Rationale	Reportable Conditions
		These conditions should be reported if they persist despite nursing interventions.
1. Observe trend in Qs/Qt.	An increasing shunt indicates worsening of the disease process or ineffective therapy. A decreasing shunt indicates improving disease process or effective therapy. The greater the blood flow past unoxygenated alveoli, the greater the shunt and the greater the hypoxemia.	• A change in Qs/Qt of greater than 5%
2. Observe for increasing Pa_{O_2} or Sa_{O_2} in conjunction with Fi_{O_2} and PEEP levels.	Shunt, as a mechanism of hypoxemia, requires high oxygen concentrations to maintain marginal oxygenation. Shunting is not contributing significantly to hypoxemia if the patient has adequate arterial oxygen tension on Fi_{O_2} of less than or equal to 0.40. When Pa_{O_2} is greater than 60 mm Hg or Sa_{O_2} is greater than 90% on Fi_{O_2} of less than or equal to 0.45, monitoring of Qs/Qt is no longer necessary	• Pa_{O_2} less than 60 mm Hg • Sa_{O_2} less than 90%

Documentation

Documentation should include the following:

• Patient and family education
• Qs/Qt percent
• Date and time Qs/Qt was performed
• Arterial and mixed venous blood gas results calculated
• Time, date, position of patient (e.g., supine or left lateral)

• Fi_{O_2} and ventilator parameters at the time blood gases were drawn
• Changes in therapy based on the calculated Qs/Qt
• Patient response to interventions
• Unexpected outcomes
• Nursing interventions

References

1. West JB: *Pulmonary pathophysiology: the essentials,* Baltimore, 2008, Lippincott Williams & Wilkins.
2. West JB: *Respiratory physiology: the essentials,* ed 8, Baltimore, 2008, Lippincott Williams & Wilkins.

Invasive Mechanical Ventilation (Through an Artificial Airway): Volume and Pressure Modes

P U R P O S E : Initiation and maintenance of positive-pressure ventilation through an artificial airway are accomplished to maintain or improve oxygenation and ventilation and to provide respiratory muscle rest. Selection of volume or pressure modes is dependent on the available evidence, clinical goals, availability of modes, and practitioner preference.

Suzanne M. Burns

PREREQUISITE NURSING KNOWLEDGE

- Indications for the initiation of mechanical ventilation include the following:
  - Apnea (e.g., neuromuscular or cardiopulmonary collapse)
  - Acute ventilatory failure, which is generally defined as a pH of less than or equal to 7.25 with an arterial partial pressure of carbon dioxide ($PaCO_2$) greater than or equal to 50 mm Hg
  - Impending ventilatory failure (serial decrement of arterial blood gas [ABG] values or progressive increase in signs and symptoms of increased work of breathing)
  - Severe hypoxemia: An arterial partial pressure of oxygen (PaO_2) of less than or equal to 50 mm Hg on room air indicates a critical level of oxygen in the blood. Although oxygen delivery devices may be used before intubation, the refractory nature of shunt (perfusion without ventilation) may necessitate that positive pressure be applied to reexpand closed alveoli. Restoration of functional residual capacity (FRC; lung volume that remains at the end of a passive exhalation) is the goal.

- Respiratory muscle fatigue: The muscles of respiration can become fatigued if they are made to contract repetitively at high workloads.[87] Fatigue occurs when muscle energy stores become depleted. Weakness, hypermetabolic states, and chronic lung disease are examples of conditions in which patients are especially prone to fatigue. When fatigue occurs, the muscles no longer contract optimally and hypercarbia results.[8,20] Twelve to 24 hours of rest are typically needed to rest the muscles. Respiratory muscle rest requires that the workload of the muscles (or muscle loading) be offset so that mitochondrial energy stores can be repleted.[8,20] Respiratory work and rest vary with different modes and the application of the same. In general, when hypercarbia is present, mechanical ventilation is necessary to relieve the work of breathing. Muscle unloading is accomplished differently and depends on patient-ventilator interaction and the mode.[13,14,55,57,61,68]

- Ventilators are categorized as either negative or positive pressure. Although negative-pressure ventilation (i.e., the iron lung) was used extensively in the 1940s, introduction of the cuffed endotracheal tube resulted in the dominance of positive-pressure ventilation (PPV) in clinical practice during the second half of the 20th century.

Although sporadic interest in negative-pressure ventilation continues, the cumbersome nature of the ventilators and the lack of airway protection associated with this form of ventilation preclude a serious resurgence of this mode of ventilation.

❖ Positive pressure ventilation: Positive-pressure modes of ventilation have traditionally been categorized into volume and pressure. However, with the advent of microprocessor technology, sophisticated iterations of traditional volume and pressure modes of ventilation have evolved.[69] Many of the modes have names that are different from traditional volume and pressure modes, but they are similar in many cases. Little data exist to show that the newer modes improve outcomes.[17,69] A wide variety of modes described in this procedure are actually a combination of volume and pressure but for ease of learning are classified into specific categories.

❖ Volume ventilation has traditionally been the most popular form of PPV, largely because tidal volume (Vt) and minute ventilation (MV) are ensured, which is an essential goal in the patient with acute illness. With volume ventilation, a predetermined Vt is delivered with each breath regardless of resistance and compliance. Vt is stable from breath to breath, but airway pressure may vary. To rest the respiratory muscles with volume ventilation, the ventilator rate must be increased until spontaneous respiratory effort ceases. When spontaneous effort is present, such as with initiation of an assist/control (A/C) breath, respiratory muscle work continues throughout the breath.[61]

❖ With traditional *pressure ventilation,* the practitioner selects the desired pressure level and the Vt is determined by the selected pressure level, resistance, and compliance. This characteristic is important to note in caring for a patient with an unstable condition on a pressure mode of ventilation. Careful attention to Vt is necessary to prevent inadvertent hyperventilation or hypoventilation. To ensure respiratory muscle rest on pressure-support ventilation (PSV), workload must be offset with the appropriate adjustment of the pressure-support (PS) level. To accomplish this adjustment, the PS level is increased to lower the spontaneous respiratory rate to less than or equal to 20 breaths/min and to attain a Vt of 6 to 10 mm/kg.[13,14,55]

❖ *Pressure* ventilation provides for an augmented inspiration (pressure is maintained throughout inspiration). The flow pattern (speed of the gas) is described as decelerating; that is, gas flow delivery is high at the beginning of the breath and tapers off toward the end of the breath. This pattern is in contrast to volume ventilation, in which the flow rate is typically more consistent during inspiration (i.e., the same at the beginning of the breath as at the end of the breath). The decelerating flow pattern associated with pressure ventilation is thought to provide better gas distribution and more efficient ventilation.[14,55,56]

❖ Increasingly sophisticated ventilator technology has resulted in the development of volume-assured pressure modes of ventilation. Ventilator manufacturers have responded rapidly to the request of practitioners that pressure modes of ventilation be designed in such a way that volume be guaranteed on a breath-to-breath basis. The potential value of such modes is obvious. The more desirable decelerating flow pattern may be provided and plateau pressures controlled, with ensured Vt and MV.

❖ Additional modes of ventilation have been promoted for use in patients with acute respiratory distress syndrome (ARDS), including high-frequency oscillation, pressure-release ventilation, and other ventilator-specific modes, such as biphasic, adaptive support and proportional assist ventilation. Although some data exist that suggest the modes may be beneficial in patients with ARDS, to date no change in mortality rate has been noted, although positive trends have been demonstrated in some variables of interest such as oxygenation.[12,18,19,24,27,38,39,41,59,66,73,75,79-82,84,90]

• Summary descriptions of modes, mode parameters, and ventilator alarms are provided within this procedure and in Tables 35-1, 35-2, and 35-3.

• Complications of PPV include volume-pressure trauma, hemodynamic changes, and pulmonary barotrauma.

❖ Volume-pressure trauma, in contrast to barotrauma (or air leak disease), was first described in animals with stiff noncompliant lungs who were ventilated with traditional lung volumes (range, 10 to 12 mL/kg). The investigators noted that the large volumes translated into high plateau pressures (also known as static, distending, or alveolar pressure) and subsequent acute lung injury. The lung injury was described as a loss of alveolar integrity (i.e., alveolar fractures) and movement of fluids and proteins into the alveolar space (sometimes called non-ARDS-ARDS).[28,29,37,70,93] Plateau pressures of 30 cm H_2O or more for greater than 48 to 72 hours were associated with the injury.[28]

❖ Studies in humans followed the recognition that large Vts may be associated with lung injury.[42,86] The ARDS Network conducted randomized controlled trial (RCTs) of adult patients with ARDS that compared low lung volume ventilation (6 mL/kg) with more traditional volumes (i.e., 12 mL/kg). The results showed that the lower volume ventilation resulted in a lower mortality rate.[86] As a result, current recommendations are to limit volumes (and lower pressures) in patients with stiff lungs. With pressure ventilation, pressure is limited by definition; however, until additional evidence emerges on the efficacy of controlling pressures versus volumes in ARDS, a goal should be to ensure a Vt in the 6 mL/kg range. Another lung protective strategy is that of is that of "recruitment" and the prevention of "derecruitment." Investigators showed that stiff noncompliant lungs were at risk of trauma from the repetitive opening associated with tidal breaths. The application of higher levels of

TABLE 35-1 Traditional Modes of Mechanical Ventilation (on All Ventilators)

Volume Modes

Control Ventilation (CV) or Controlled Mandatory Ventilation (CMV)

Description: With this mode, the ventilator provides all of the patient's minute ventilation. The clinician sets the rate, Vt, inspiratory time, and PEEP. Generally, this term is used to describe situations in which the patient is chemically relaxed or is paralyzed from a spinal cord or neuromuscular disease and is unable to initiate spontaneous breaths. The ventilator mode setting may be set on CMV, assist/control (A/C), or synchronized intermittent mandatory ventilation (SIMV) because all these options provide volume breaths at the clinician-selected rate.

Assist/Control (A/C) or Assisted Mandatory Ventilation (AMV)

Description: This option requires that a rate, Vt, inspiratory time, and PEEP be set for the patient. The ventilator sensitivity also is set, and when the patient initiates a spontaneous breath, a full-volume breath is delivered.

Synchronized Intermittent Mandatory Ventilation (SIMV)

Description: This mode requires that rate, Vt, inspiratory time, sensitivity, and PEEP are set by the clinician. In between mandatory breaths, patients can spontaneously breathe at their own rates and Vt. With SIMV, the ventilator synchronizes the mandatory breaths with the patient's own inspirations.

Pressure Modes

Pressure Support Ventilation (PSV)

Description: This mode provides an augmented inspiration to a patient who is spontaneously breathing. With PS, the clinician selects an inspiratory pressure level, PEEP, and sensitivity. When the patient initiates a breath, a high flow of gas is delivered to the preselected pressure level, and pressure is maintained throughout inspiration. The patient determines the parameters of Vt, rate, and inspiratory time.

Pressure-Controlled/Inverse Ratio Ventilation (PC/IRV)

Description: This mode combines pressure-limited ventilation with an inverse ratio of inspiration to expiration. The clinician selects the pressure level, rate, inspiratory time (1:1, 2:1, 3:1, 4:1), and PEEP level. With prolonged inspiratory times, auto-PEEP may result. The auto-PEEP may be a desirable outcome of the inverse ratios. Some clinicians use PC without IRV. Conventional inspiratory times are used, and rate, pressure level, and PEEP are selected.

Positive End-Expiratory Pressure (PEEP) and Continuous Positive Airway Pressure (CPAP)

Description: This ventilatory option creates positive pressure at end exhalation. PEEP restores FRC. The term PEEP is used when end-expiratory pressure is provided during ventilator positive pressure breaths.

TABLE 35-2 Volume and Pressure Modes and Corresponding Ventilator Parameters

Mode Name and Description	Main Parameters	Comments
Assist Control (A/C)	Vt RR Ti Sensitivity Fio_2 PEEP	Generally considered a support mode. Must switch to another mode or method for weaning.
Synchronized Mandatory Ventilation (SIMV)	Vt RR Ti Sensitivity Fio_2 PEEP	Originally used as a weaning mode; however, work of breathing is high at low IMV rates. Often used in conjunction with PSV.
Pressure Support Ventilation (PSV)	PS level Sensitivity Fio_2 PEEP	Often pressure is arbitrarily selected (e.g., 10 to 20 cm H_2O) then adjusted up or down to attain the desired tidal volume. Some use the plateau pressure if transitioning from volume ventilation as a starting point.
Pressure Control Ventilation (PCV)	IPL fx Ti Sensitivity Fio_2 PEEP	Variants of PCV include Volume Assured Pressure Options and some other modes such as Airway Pressure Release Ventilation and Bilevel Ventilation. They are listed below.
Pressure Controlled–Inverse Ratio Ventilation	As for PCV, but an inverse inspiratory:expiratory (I:E) ratio is attained by lengthening the Ti. Inverse ratios include 1:1, 2:1, 3:1, and 4:1.	Some ventilators allow for the I:E ratio to be selected.

TABLE 35-2 | **Volume and Pressure Modes and Corresponding Ventilator Parameters—*cont'd***

Mode Name and Description	Main Parameters	Comments
Examples of Ventilator-Specific Mode Options	*Parameter names vary with specific ventilator.*	*The modes listed below are available on only select ventilators. Examples of these are included but may not be comprehensive.*
Airway Pressure Release Ventilation	Pressure high (P_{HIGH}): high CPAP level. Pressure low (P_{LOW}) is generally 0 to 5 cm H_2O. Time high (T_{HIGH}). Time low (T_{LOW}). Fio_2.	Generally, the CPAP level is adjusted to ensure adequate oxygenation while the fx of the releases are increased or decreased to meet ventilation goals. Vt is variable dependent on the CPAP level, compliance and resistance of the patient, and patient spontaneous effort.
Volume Assured Pressure Modes (1 to 5 below)	These modes provide pressure breaths with a volume guarantee.	These modes are ventilator specific. Although the similarities are greater than the differences, they are called different names. Often the names suggest that the mode is a volume mode, yet a decelerating flow pattern (associated with pressure ventilation) is always provided.
1. Volume Support (VS)	Vt Sensitivity Fio_2 PEEP	The pressure level is automatically adjusted to attain the desired Vt. If control of pressure is desired it must be carefully monitored.
2. Pressure Regulated Control (PRVC)	fx and Ti set in addition to those set for volume support (VS).	As with VS. The difference is that this is a control mode. Spontaneous breaths, however, may also occur.
3. Volume Support (VS)	Vt Sensitivity Fio_2 PEEP	This mode is one option in a category called Volume Ventilation Plus. This is the spontaneous breathing option in this category and is similar to VS above.
4. Volume Control Plus (VC+)	fx and Ti are set in addition to those set for VS.	This mode is also a mode option listed in the category called Volume Ventilation Plus. To access this mode, the user selects the SIMV or Assist/Control (both control modes) then selects VC+. For some clinicians, this is confusing because it appears that the patient is on two different modes versus VC+.
BiLevel Positive Airway Pressure (Bi-level or BiPAP)	$PEEP_H$ $PEEP_L$ fx and Ti	If additional support is desired for patient initiated breathing, pressure support in BiLevel mode (Psupp) may be selected as well. Attention to Vt is important because the patient can augment Vt significantly with supported spontaneous breaths.
Adaptive Support Ventilation (ASV)	Body weight %MinVol (minute volume), high pressure limit	Once basic settings are selected, ASV is started and %MinVol is adjusted if indicated. Spontaneous breathing is automatically encouraged, and when the inspiratory pressure (Pinsp) is consistently 0 and fx control (rate) is 0, extubation may be considered.
Proportional Assist Ventilation (PAV)	Proportional Pressure Support (PPS_{TM}): PEEP, Fio_2, percent volume assist and flow assist Proportional Assist Plus: PAV+: PEEP, Fio_2, percent support	Depending on the ventilator, the amount of assist that is provided is determined by the clinician and different parameters are selected to do so. Default percent support numbers are recommended, but the clinician must determine the timing of reductions of same.
Automatic Tube Compensation (ATC)	Endotracheal tube internal diameter Percent compensation	This is not a mode but rather a pressure option to offset the work associated with tube resistance. It can be combined with other modes or used alone as in a CPAP weaning trial.

Adapted with permission from Burns S: Pressure modes of mechanical ventilation: the good, bad and the ugly, AACN Adv Crit Care 19:399-411, 2008.

TABLE 35-3	Ventilator Alarms

Disconnect Alarms (Low-Pressure or Low-Volume Alarms)

When disconnection occurs, the clinician must be immediately notified. Generally, this alarm is a continuous one and is triggered when a preselected inspiratory pressure level or minute ventilation is not sensed. With circuit leaks, this same alarm may be activated even though the patient may still be receiving a portion of the preset breath. Physical assessment, digital displays, and manometers are helpful in troubleshooting the cause of the alarms.

Pressure Alarms

High-pressure alarms are set with volume modes of ventilation to ensure notification of pressures that exceed the selected threshold. These alarms are usually set 10 to 15 cm H_2O above the usual peak inspiratory pressure (PIP). Some causes for alarm activation (generally an intermittent alarm) include secretions, condensate in the tubing, biting on the endotracheal tubing, increased resistance (i.e., bronchospasm), decreased compliance (e.g., pulmonary edema, pneumothorax), and tubing compression.

Low-pressure alarms are used to sense disconnection, circuit leaks, and changing compliance and resistance. They are generally set 5 to 10 cm H_2O below the usual PIP or 1 to 2 cm H_2O below the PEEP level or both.

Minute ventilation alarms may be used to sense disconnection or changes in breathing pattern (rate and volume). Generally, low–minute ventilation and high–minute ventilation alarms are set (usually 5 to 10 L/min above and below usual minute ventilation). When stand-alone pressure support ventilation (PSV) is in use, this alarm may be the only audible alarm available on some ventilators.

Fio_2 alarms are provided on most new ventilators and are set 5 to 10 mm Hg above and below the selected Fio_2 level.

Alarm silence or pause options are built in by ventilator manufacturers so that clinicians can temporarily silence alarms for short periods (i.e., 20 seconds) because alarms must stay activated at all times. The ventilators reset the alarms automatically.

Alarms provide important protection for patients on ventilation. However, inappropriate threshold settings decrease usefulness. When threshold gradients are set too narrowly, alarms occur needlessly and frequently. Conversely, alarms that are set too loosely (wide gradients) do not allow for accurate and timely assessments.

From Burns SM: Mechanical ventilation and weaning. In Kinney MR, et al, editors: AACN clinical reference for critical care nursing, ed 4, St Louis, 1998, Mosby.

positive end-expiratory pressure (PEEP) was associated with better recruitment and resulted in improved mortality rates.[3,4,73]

❖ The extent of hemodynamic changes associated with PPV depends on the level of applied positive pressure, the duration of positive pressure during different phases of the breathing cycle, the amount of pressure transmitted to the vascular structures, the patient's intravascular volume, and the adequacy of hemodynamic compensatory mechanisms. PPV can reduce venous return, shift the intraventricular septum to the left, and increase right ventricular afterload as a result of increased pulmonary vascular resistance.[1,50] The hemodynamic effects of PPV may be prevented or corrected by optimizing filling pressures to accommodate the PPV-induced changes in intrathoracic pressures; by minimizing the peak pressure, plateau pressure, and PEEP; and by optimizing the inspiratory-to-expiratory (I:E) ratio.

❖ Pulmonary barotrauma (i.e., air leak disease) is damage to the lung from extrapulmonary air that may result from changes in intrathoracic pressures during PPV. Barotrauma is manifested by pneumothorax, pneumomediastinum, pneumopericardium, pneumoperitoneum, and subcutaneous emphysema. The risk of barotrauma in a patient receiving PPV is increased with preexisting lung lesions (e.g., localized infections, blebs), high inflation pressures (i.e., large Vt, PEEP, main-stem bronchus intubation, patient-ventilator asynchrony), and invasive thoracic procedures (e.g., subclavian catheter insertion, bronchoscopy, thoracentesis). Barotrauma from PPV may be prevented by controlling peak and plateau pressures,

optimizing PEEP, preventing auto-PEEP, ensuring patient-ventilator synchrony, and ensuring proper artificial airway position.

❖ Auto-PEEP is a common complication of mechanical ventilation and can result in hemodynamic compromise and even death. Because increased intrathoracic pressures are transmitted to the adjacent capillaries, venous return is decreased and the effect can be profound. Auto-PEEP and dynamic hyperinflation should be assumed in the patient on ventilation with acute severe asthma whose condition is hemodynamically compromised, and a brief cessation of mechanical ventilation or decrease in rate and shortening of inspiratory time should be accomplished.[54,71] Auto-PEEP is caused by inadequate expiratory time relative to the patient's lung condition. Auto-PEEP is associated with prolonged inspiratory times, short expiratory times, high minute ventilation requirements, bronchospasm, low elastic recoil, mucus hypersecretion, increased wall thickness, airway closure or collapse, and mechanical factors (e.g., water in the ventilator circuit, pinched ventilator tubing).[54,71] Correcting these factors reduces auto-PEEP. In some cases, adding set PEEP results in reduction of the inspiratory trigger threshold and thus improvement of patient triggering.[15,58]

• Associated complications of PPV include ventilator-associated pneumonia (VAP)[6], deep vein thrombosis (and subsequent pulmonary embolus), and gastrointestinal bleeding. Although all the associated complications are important and require that appropriate evidence-based prophylaxis regimens are initiated, only VAP is discussed. Please refer to other system-specific chapters in this manual for information on the others.

❖ VAP occurs after 3 to 5 days of mechanical ventilation and accounts for one third of all healthcare-associated infections and between 50% and 83% of infections in the patient with MV.[6,26,52,78,91]

❖ Modifiable risk factors to the aspiration of colonized organisms in the patient on ventilation include interventions such as proper endotracheal tube cuff inflation (secretions that collect above the cuff of the endotracheal or tracheostomy tube and leak past the cuff into the lungs), use of continuous aspiration subglottic suctioning (CASS) tubes, decreased ventilator tubing changes, use of heat and moisture exchangers (HMEs), stringent hand washing, backrest elevation (BRE) of greater than 30 degrees, and when possible, the use of noninvasive ventilation (especially in patients with immunocompromise).[5,6,10,16,22,26,32,43,45,51,64,72,83]

❖ Other interventions with a lower level of evidence supporting their use include oral care techniques such as mouth care and oral decontamination with agents such as chlorhexidine or oral antibiotics.[45] Of interest, gastric residual volumes have not been found to be consistently associated with VAP.[46,65] Table 35-4 lists the top recommendations of authoritative professional organizations for the prevention of VAP.

EQUIPMENT

• Endotracheal or tracheostomy tube (see Procedures 2 and 14)
• Electrocardiogram and pulse oximetry
• Manual self-inflating resuscitation bag-valve device (with PEEP adjusted to patient baseline level or with a PEEP valve)
• Appropriately sized resuscitation face mask
• Ventilator
• Suction equipment
• End-tidal carbon dioxide detector, with a colorimetric CO_2 detector or continuous monitor: The colorimetric detectors are used to ensure proper endotracheal tube placement and are a standard of care for intubation in many institutions. The continuous monitors are used in assessment of patients on ventilation on an ongoing basis.

PATIENT AND FAMILY EDUCATION

• Explain the procedure and the reasons for PPV to the patient and family.[6] ➤**Rationale:** Communication and explanations for therapy are cited as important needs of patients and families.

• Discuss the potential sensations the patient will experience, such as relief of dyspnea, lung inflations, noise of ventilator operation, and alarm sounds. ➤**Rationale:** Knowledge of anticipated sensory experiences reduces anxiety and distress.

• Encourage the patient to relax. ➤**Rationale:** This encouragement promotes general relaxation, oxygenation, and ventilation.

• Explain that the patient will be unable to speak. Establish a method of communication in conjunction with the patient and family before initiating mechanical ventilation, if necessary. ➤**Rationale:** Ensuring the patient's ability to communicate is important to alleviate anxiety.

• Teach the family how to perform desired and appropriate activities of direct patient care, such as pharyngeal suction with the tonsil-tip suction device, range-of-motion exercises, and reconnection to ventilator if inadvertent disconnection occurs. Demonstrate use of call bell. ➤**Rationale:** Family members have identified the need and desire to help in the patient's care.

• Provide the patient and family with information on the critical nature of the patient's dependence on PPV. ➤**Rationale:** Knowledge of the prognosis, probable outcome, or chance for recovery is cited as an important need of patients and families.

• Offer the opportunity for the patient and family to ask questions about PPV. ➤**Rationale:** Asking questions and having questions answered honestly are cited consistently as the most important need of patients and families.

TABLE 35-4	**Top Modifiable VAP Prevention Interventions: Guidelines by Authoritative Professional Organizations.**

Top Guideline Recommendations by Professional Associations*
BRE (>30 to 45 degrees)
CASS tubes
Cuff inflation
Hand washing and aseptic technique
HMEs
No routine ventilator circuit change
Noninvasive ventilation when possible

*Professional Associations: American Thoracic Society (ATS), American Association of Critical-Care Nurses (AACN), Centers for Disease Control and Prevention (CDC), and Canadian Critical Care Trials Group and the Canadian Critical Care Society (CCCT/CCCS).

PATIENT ASSESSMENT AND PREPARATION
Patient Assessment

- Assess for signs and symptoms of acute ventilatory failure and fatigue:
  - Rising arterial carbon dioxide tension
  - Chest-abdominal dyssynchrony
  - Shallow or irregular respirations
  - Tachypnea, bradypnea, or dyspnea
  - Decreased mental status
  - Restlessness, confusion, or lethargy
  - Increasing or decreasing arterial blood pressure
  - Tachycardia
  - Atrial or ventricular dysrhythmias

  ➻*Rationale:* Ventilatory failure indicates the need for initiation of PPV. While PPV is being considered and assembled, support ventilation via a self-inflating manual resuscitation bag-valve-mask, if necessary.

- Determine arterial pH and carbon dioxide tension.
  ➻*Rationale:* Acute ventilatory failure is confirmed by an uncompensated respiratory acidosis. Ventilatory failure is an indication for PPV.

- Assess for signs and symptoms of inadequate oxygenation:
  - Decreasing arterial oxygen tension
  - Tachypnea
  - Dyspnea
  - Central cyanosis
  - Alterations in level of consciousness
  - Restlessness
  - Confusion
  - Agitation
  - Tachycardia
  - Bradycardia
  - Dysrhythmias
  - Intercostal and suprasternal retractions
  - Increasing or decreasing arterial blood pressure
  - Adventitious breath sounds
  - Decreasing urine output
  - Metabolic acidosis

  ➻*Rationale:* Hypoxemia may indicate the need for PPV. While PPV is being considered and assembled, provide 100% oxygen via manual resuscitation bag and mask or via an oxygen delivery device, such as a nonrebreather mask.

- Determine Pao_2 or arterial oxygen saturation (Sao_2).
  ➻*Rationale:* Hypoxemia is confirmed by Pao_2 of less than 60 mm Hg or Sao_2 of less than 90% on supplemental oxygen. Hypoxemia may indicate the need for PPV.

- Assess for signs and symptoms of inadequate breathing patterns:
  - Dyspnea
  - Chest-abdominal dyssynchrony
  - Rapid-shallow breathing pattern
  - Irregular respirations
  - Intercostal or suprasternal retractions
  - Inability to say a whole sentence

  ➻*Rationale:* Respiratory distress is an indication for PPV. A comfortable breathing pattern is a goal of PPV. An inadequate breathing pattern on ventilatory support can be corrected by determining and treating the underlying acute cause such as pulmonary edema or by fixing a mechanical problem such as a malpositioned endotracheal tube. Adjustment of the ventilator parameters in these cases may be necessary.

- Assess for signs of atelectasis:
  - Localized changes in auscultation (increased or bronchial breath sounds)
  - Localized dullness to percussion
  - Increased breathing effort
  - Tracheal deviation toward the side of abnormal findings
  - Increased peak and plateau pressures
  - Decreased compliance
  - Decreased Pao_2 or Sao_2 (with constant ventilator parameters)
  - Localized consolidation ("whiteout," opacity) on chest radiograph

  ➻*Rationale:* Early detection of atelectasis indicates the need for alteration of interventions to promote resolution (e.g., hyperinflation techniques, PEEP adjustments).

- Assess for signs and symptoms of pulmonary barotrauma (i.e., pneumothorax):
  - Acute, increasing, or severe dyspnea
  - Restlessness
  - Agitation
  - Localized changes in auscultation (decreased or absent breath sounds) on the affected side
  - Localized hyperresonance or tympany to percussion on the affected side
  - Elevated chest on the affected side
  - Increased breathing effort
  - Tracheal deviation away from the side of abnormal findings
  - Increased peak and plateau pressures
  - Decreased compliance
  - Decreased Pao_2 or Sao_2
  - Subcutaneous emphysema
  - Localized increased lucency with absent lung markings on chest radiograph

  ➻*Rationale:* Early detection of pneumothorax is essential to minimize progression to cardiac tamponade and death. Tension pneumothorax requires immediate emergency decompression with a large-bore needle (i.e., 14-gauge) into the second intercostal space, midclavicular line on the affected side, or immediate chest tube placement (see Procedure 20).

- Assess for signs of volume-pressure trauma that are consistent with ARDS:
  - Acute, increasing, or severe dyspnea
  - Restlessness
  - Agitation
  - Generalized crackles, especially in the dependent portions of the lung
  - Refractory hypoxemia

- Increased peak and plateau pressures
- Decreased compliance
- Decreased PaO_2 or SaO_2
- Bilateral diffuse whiteout with chest radiograph
- PaO_2:fraction of inspired oxygen (FiO_2) [P:F ratio] of less than 200
- A noncardiac etiology for the "wet" lung

➤**Rationale:** Volume-pressure trauma is assumed if the patient has the last three criteria noted. Ventilatory management should focus on ensuring that lung protective strategies are in place so that additional injury does not ensue. Some examples include Vt of 6 mL/kg and lung recruitment with PEEP. In general, these strategies result in hypercarbia because ventilation is not efficient.

- Assess for signs of cardiovascular depression (particularly after an increase in Vt, PEEP, or continuous positive airway pressure [CPAP] or with other hyperinflation maneuvers):
  - Acute or gradual decrease in arterial blood pressure
  - Tachycardia, bradycardia, or dysrhythmias
  - Weak peripheral pulses, pulsus paradoxus, or decreased pulse pressure
  - Acute or gradual increase in pulmonary capillary wedge pressure
  - Decreased mixed venous oxygen tension

➤**Rationale:** PPV can cause decreased venous return and afterload because of the increase in intrathoracic pressure. This mechanism often manifests immediately after initiation of mechanical ventilation and with large Vt, increases in PEEP or CPAP levels, and manual hyperinflation techniques. Cardiovascular depression associated with manual or periodic ventilator hyperinflation is immediately reversible with cessation of hyperinflation. Decreases in blood pressure with PPV also may be seen with hypovolemia.

- Assess for signs and symptoms of inadvertent extubation:
  - Vocalization
  - Activated ventilator alarms
  - Low pressure
  - Low minute ventilation
  - Inability to deliver preset pressure
  - Decreased or absent breath sounds
  - Gastric distention
  - Changes in endotracheal tube (ETT) depth
  - Signs and symptoms of inadequate ventilation, oxygenation, and breathing pattern

➤**Rationale:** Inadvertent extubation is sometimes obvious (e.g., the endotracheal tube is in the patient's hand).

Often, the tip of the endotracheal tube is in the hypopharynx or in the esophagus, however, and inadvertent extubation may not be immediately apparent. Reintubation may be necessary, although some patients may not need reintubation. If reintubation is necessary, ventilation and oxygenation are assisted with a manual self-inflating resuscitation bag-valve device and face mask.

- Assess for signs and symptoms of a malpositioned endotracheal tube:
  - Dyspnea
  - Restlessness or agitation
  - Unilateral decreased or absent breath sounds
  - Unilateral dullness to percussion
  - Increased breathing effort
  - Asymmetric chest expansion
  - Increased peak inspiratory pressure (PIP)
  - Changes in ETT depth
  - Radiographic evidence of malposition

➤**Rationale:** Early detection and correction of a malpositioned endotracheal tube can prevent inadvertent extubation, atelectasis, barotrauma, and problems with gas exchange.

- Evaluate the patient's need for long-term mechanical ventilation. ➤**Rationale:** This evaluation allows the nurse to anticipate patient and family needs for the patient's discharge to an extended care facility, rehabilitation center, or home on PPV.

Patient Preparation

- Verify correct patient with two identifiers. ➤**Rationale:** Prior to performing a procedure, the nurse should ensure the correct identification of the patient for the intended intervention.
- Perform a pre-procedure verification and time out, if nonemergent. ➤**Rationale:** Ensures patient safety.
- Ensure that the patient understands preprocedural teachings. Answer questions as they arise, and reinforce information as needed. ➤**Rationale:** This communication evaluates and reinforces understanding of previously taught information.
- Premedicate as needed. ➤**Rationale:** Administration of sedatives, narcotics, or muscle relaxants may be necessary to provide adequate oxygenation and ventilation in some patients.
- Ensure patient is positioned properly for optimum ventilation. ➤**Rationale:** Placement of the patient in a head of bed elevation of at least 30 degrees enhances diaphragmatic excursion, decreases intrathoracic pressure and helps prevent aspiration and VAP.

Procedure	for Invasive Mechanical Ventilation (Through an Artificial Airway): Volume and Pressure Modes	
Steps	**Rationale**	**Special Considerations**

1. **VP**
2. **HH**
3. **PE**

Volume Modes

Steps	Rationale	Special Considerations
4. Select mode (see Tables 35-1 and 35-2). **(Level B*)** This level is representative of the three traditional volume modes and mode settings (control, synchronized intermittent mandatory ventilation [SIMV] and A/C). Control ventilation: The intent of control ventilation is to have volume and rate ensured. As with all modes of ventilation, the patient is never completely "locked out" and can breathe between the control breaths, which is ensured by setting the sensitivity or flow triggers **(see Step 8)**. However, should control over ventilation be desired, sedation and often paralytic agents are provided to ensure the goal. SIMV: With this mode, a rate (fx) and tidal volume (Vt) are set and are delivered in synchrony with the patient's respiratory effort. Between mandatory breaths, the patient may initiate breaths at a patient-determined volume and rate. A/C: Ventilation ensures that a control rate and volume are set. Patient-initiated breaths are delivered at the predetermined volume selected for the control breaths.	Mode selection varies depending on the clinical goal and clinician preference. Traditional volume modes that may provide total ventilatory support include control, SIMV and A/C. With IMV and A/C the ventilator rate must be high enough or the patient sedated so that spontaneous effort is not present.[61,62,77] Other modes may also provide complete support depending on the settings. Remember that the goal is to offset the patient's work of breathing. See subsequent description of other modes and their application.	IMV is often used in conjunction with PSV (to overcome circuit resistance and to decrease the work of breathing associated with spontaneous effort).[33] The use of IMV plus PSV has been associated with prolonged weaning times.[31] If respiratory muscle rest is the goal with IMV plus PSV, the level of PSV should be high enough to provide a Vt of 6 to 12 mL/kg and to maintain a total rate (IMV plus PSV breaths) of less than or equal to 20 breaths/min.[13,14,55,77]
5. Set Vt between 6 and 12 mL/kg. In patients with ARDS, Vt should be set at 6 mL/kg.	Vt is selected in conjunction with rate (fx) to attain a MV 5 to 10 L/min with a $Paco_2$ 35 to 45 mm Hg. Large Vt values (12 mL/kg) have been associated with lung injury in patients with ARDS.[28,29,37,70,93]	When lower Vt values are used in an attempt to reduce lung injury, the patient needs heavy sedation and often muscle relaxants to prevent spontaneous effort; hypercarbia is an expected outcome of low Vt values.[9,42] Permissive hypercarbia is generally well tolerated in patients if the pH is reduced gradually (over 24 to 48 hours); pH around 7.2 is cited as an end point if tolerated.

*Level B: Well-designed, controlled studies with results that consistently support a specific action, intervention, or treatment

Procedure	**for Invasive Mechanical Ventilation (Through an Artificial Airway): Volume and Pressure Modes—*Continued***	
Steps	**Rationale**	**Special Considerations**
		Occasionally, bicarbonate infusions are used to keep the pH within an acceptable range. However, this temporizing maneuver may result in a higher $PaCO_2$ because bicarbonate is metabolized into CO_2 and H_2O.
		Permissive hypercarbia should not be attempted in patients with elevated intracranial pressure or patients with myocardial ischemia, myocardial injury, or dysrhythmias.
		Patients who are allowed to become hypercarbic may need sedation and often muscle relaxants (paralytic agents) to control ventilation.
6. Select respiratory frequency between 10 and 20 breaths/min.	Vt and fx are selected to maintain an acceptable $PaCO_2$ with a MV between 5 and 10 L/min. Generally, once Vt is selected, fx is the parameter adjusted to attain a desired $PaCO_2$; the rate selected depends on whether or not the clinical goal is to rest or work the respiratory muscles.	When low Vts are used, as in ARDS, a higher fx may be necessary to maintain pH and $PaCO_2$ at acceptable levels because smaller Vts provide less efficient ventilation; the result is higher CO_2 and lower pH.[9,28,29,37,42,70,93]
7. For I:E times, select inspiratory time (this parameter name is different depending on the ventilator). Examples include percent inspiratory time, inspiratory time, flow rate, and peak flow. I:E ratios are usually 1:2 or 1:3. A typical inspiratory time for an adult is in the range of 0.75 to 1 second. Adjust flow as necessary to attain patient ventilator synchrony.	Inspiratory flow refers to the speed with which Vt is delivered during inspiration. Increasing the flow rate shortens the inspiratory time. Conversely, slowing the flow rate lengthens the inspiratory time. Achieves the desired I:E ratio and comfortable breathing patterns.	Generally, flow rates of approximately 50 L/min are used initially and adjusted to provide an inspiratory time that synchronizes with patient effort. Short inspiratory times and long expiratory times are necessary in patients with obstructive lung diseases (e.g., emphysema, asthma).[15,71] In contrast, patients with restrictive diseases, such as ARDS, have noncompliant lungs. Longer inspiratory times enhance recruitment and prevent derecruitment.[4,86]
8. Set the sensitivity (trigger sensitivity) between −1 and −2 cm H_2O pressure. Most ventilators have pressure-sensing sensitivity mechanisms that trigger flow, which means that the patient must generate a decrease in the system pressure with an inspiratory effort. When the ventilator senses the drop in pressure, flow (or a breath) is delivered.	The more negative the number, the less sensitive the ventilator is to patient effort, which increases the patient respiratory workload and may lead to dyssynchrony.[7]	When auto-PEEP is present, the patient has to generate a negative pressure equal to the set sensitivity plus the level of auto-PEEP.[58,71] Auto-PEEP is common in patients with asthma, chronic obstructive pulmonary disease, and high respiratory rates and minute ventilation. This additional work may fatigue the patient. Patient ventilator dyssynchrony is likely.[58,71]

Procedure continues on following page

Procedure	for Invasive Mechanical Ventilation (Through an Artificial Airway): Volume and Pressure Modes—*Continued*	
Steps	**Rationale**	**Special Considerations**
If the ventilator has a flow-triggering option, select the flow trigger in L/min. The smaller the number, the more sensitive the ventilator. Flow triggering is set in conjunction with a base flow (flow in L/min that is provided between ventilator breaths). Flow rate is monitored in the expiratory limb of the ventilator. When flow is disrupted during a spontaneous breath, a decrease in flow downstream is sensed; additional flow or a breath is delivered.	Flow triggering has been associated with faster ventilator response times and less work of breathing than pressure sensing.[7]	
9. Set Fio_2 to 0.60 to 1.0 (60% to 100%) if Pao_2 is unknown. Adjust Fio_2 downward as tolerated by monitoring Sao_2 and arterial blood gas values.	Initiation of PPV with maximal oxygen concentration avoids hypoxemia while optimal ventilator settings are being determined and evaluated. In addition, it permits measurement of the percentage of venous admixture (shunt), which provides an estimate of the severity of the gas-exchange abnormality (see Procedures 29 and 34). The goal is an Fio_2 less than or equal to 0.5; high levels of Fio_2 result in increased risk of oxygen toxicity, absorption atelectasis, and reduction of surfactant synthesis.[23,34,44]	
10. Select PEEP level. Initial setting is often 5 cm H_2O. PEEP may be adjusted as needed after evaluation of tolerance (e.g., Sao_2, Pao_2, physical assessment). PEEP levels are increased to restore FRC and allow for reduction of Fio_2 to safe levels (i.e., less than or equal to 0.5) to decrease the risk of oxygen toxicity.	A PEEP level of 5 cm H_2O is considered physiologic (essentially the amount of pressure at end exhalation normally provided by the glottis).	High levels of PEEP greater than or equal to 10 cm H_2O rarely should be interrupted because reestablishment of FRC (and Pao_2) may take hours. Prevention of this derecruitment in the patient with ARDS is especially important.[3,4] Super-PEEP levels (i.e., greater than or equal to 20 cm H_2O) may be necessary in patients with noncompliant lungs (e.g., patients with ARDS) to prevent lung injury. The repetitive opening and closing of stiff alveoli is thought to result in alveolar damage; to that end, the use of high PEEP levels to maintain alveolar distention and to prevent injury during PPV is considered a protective lung strategy.[2,28,29,53,74] In general, when high PEEP levels are used, Vt values are lower than normal and subsequent hypercarbia may be anticipated. Use of muscle relaxants, sedatives, and narcotics is often necessary to prevent patient spontaneous breathing.

Procedure	for Invasive Mechanical Ventilation (Through an Artificial Airway): Volume and Pressure Modes—*Continued*	
Steps	**Rationale**	**Special Considerations**
11. Continuous positive airway pressure (CPAP) is often referred to as PEEP without the positive pressure breaths. CPAP is a spontaneous breathing mode that provides continuous pressure throughout the ventilatory cycle. It is commonly used as a mode for spontaneous breathing weaning trials (see Procedure 28). A traditional application of CPAP is for obstructive sleep apnea (OSA) through a noninvasive mask or prongs. When used for OSA, the mode provides a pneumatic splint to the airways to prevent obstruction during sleep (see Procedure 28).		Generally, the pressure levels of CPAP are relatively low but vary with individual patient conditions.
Pressure Modes (Invasive)		
1. Select mode: PSV, pressure-controlled/inverse ratio ventilation (PC/IRV), volume-assured pressure support option (VAPS), airway pressure release ventilation (APRV), adaptive support ventilation (ASV), proportional assist ventilation (PAV), automatic tube compensation (ATC) or high-frequency oscillation (HFO).	Mode selection depends on clinical goals, mode availability (these vary widely with different ventilators), and clinician preference. To date, no mode has emerged as superior.[17,69] Modes include those designed for spontaneous breathing and those for control or partial control of ventilation.	Many new modes that use microprocessor technology are available on specific ventilators. Although many are similar to traditional modes, others are not. Parameter names also vary. The reader is encouraged to refer to specific ventilator operating manuals and websites for details not contained in this procedure.
2. PSV augments spontaneous respirations with a clinician-selected pressure level. Adjust the PSV level to attain a Vt between 8 and 12 mL/kg with a spontaneous respiratory rate (RR) less than or equal to 20 breaths/min (if respiratory muscle rest is desired; this is called PSVmax). Decrease PSV level during weaning trials as tolerated by patient. Tolerance criteria for trials may be predetermined by protocols or on an individual basis. Often during trials, Vt values are allowed to be lower (i.e., 5 to 8 mL/kg) and RR higher (i.e., 25 to 30 breaths/min) than when rest is the goal. However, these parameters are always evaluated in conjunction with other signs and symptoms of fatigue and intolerance.[13,14,33,55,56,92] **(Level B*)**	Pressure level in conjunction with compliance and resistance determines delivered Vt.	PSV sometimes is used between IMV breaths to offset the work of breathing associated with artificial airways and circuits during spontaneous breathing.[13,14,33,55,56] PSV generally is considered a weaning mode of ventilation, which necessitates stability of patient condition. PSV may be used in patients with less stable conditions provided that close attention is given to changes in Vt and RR.[92] High levels of PSV may provide respiratory muscle unloading.

*Level B: Well-designed, controlled studies with results that consistently support a specific action, intervention, or treatment

Procedure continues on following page

Procedure for Invasive Mechanical Ventilation (Through an Artificial Airway): Volume and Pressure Modes —*Continued*

Steps	Rationale	Special Considerations
Select PSV level (as previously). Set sensitivity (as with volume ventilation). Set PEEP (as with volume ventilation). Set Fio$_2$ (as with volume ventilation).		
3. Pressure control (PC) and pressure control inverse ratio ventilation (PC/IRV) are both control modes of ventilation. With these modes, a pressure level is selected; the rate and inspiratory time are selected as well. They were originally used to manage patients with ARDS in whom the goal was to limit the pressure level. In addition, the decelerating flow pattern of the modes was considered desirable. PC/IRV was used to enhance lung recruitment by prolonging inspiration. Expiration was shortened, thereby decreasing the potential for derecruitment.	Absolute pressure level is the sum of the inspiratory pressure level (IPL) and PEEP.	If the clinical goal is to ensure a plateau pressure of less than or equal to 30 cm H$_2$O, the pressure level may be lowered gradually over 24 to 48 hours to prevent sudden changes in Paco$_2$ and pH.[1,85]
A. Select inspiratory pressure level (IPL). With this pressure mode, the level of pressure support is often identified as IPL versus PSV.	Rate and IPL determine MV.	
B. Select rate.		
C. Select inspiratory time or inverse I:E ratio (ventilators vary).	I:E ratios are set at 1:1, 2:1, 3:1, or 4:1 by selecting the appropriate inspiratory time. Ratios are adjusted upward to improve shunt and oxygenation. Blood pressure may be adversely affected. Rate is usually relatively high (e.g., 20 to 25 breaths/min).	Generally, clinicians start with 1:1 ratios and increase as necessary to improve oxygenation. A limiting factor related to prolonged inspiratory times is hemodynamic compromise and hypotension, which is generally why the use of ratios greater than 2:1 rarely is seen clinically. Auto-PEEP is common and may be a desired outcome of PC/IRV.[21,49]
D. Select PEEP level. When transitioning from volume ventilation to PC/IRV, the PEEP initially is maintained at the level used previously until the effect of the IRV is assessed.	Because IRV may result in auto-PEEP, evaluation of the total amount of PEEP present is important.	
E. Select Fio$_2$ (as with volume ventilation).		

Procedure	for Invasive Mechanical Ventilation (Through an Artificial Airway): Volume and Pressure Modes—*Continued*

Steps	Rationale	Special Considerations
F. Set sensitivity (as with volume ventilation). **(Level B*)**	The goal of PC/IRV is to improve oxygenation and allow for reduction of Fio_2 to less than or equal to 0.5.[21,40,85] This is done in conjunction with the addition of PEEP. Always set sensitivity so that the patient can get a breath if needed.	If controlled ventilation is the goal, chemical relaxation may be necessary in conjunction with sedatives and narcotics. Patient tolerance of IRV (i.e., the prolonged inspiratory times) is unlikely without such interventions. Remember that IRV may result in auto-PEEP (which may be a desirable outcome of the mode). Regardless, auto-PEEP should be anticipated and measured regularly.

4. Volume-guaranteed pressure options are pressure modes that guarantee a volume. The breath delivery varies with the specific mode. For volume-guaranteed pressure support options, parameter selection (i.e., pressure, volume, rate) is specific to the ventilator; however, selection of desired (or guaranteed) Vt is required. Some ventilators also require selection of the pressure level. Spontaneous breathing modes and controlled modes are available.
  A. For volume-guaranteed pressure options, please see specific ventilator manual for parameter setting.
  B. PEEP, Fio_2 and sensitivity are set as per volume ventilation, as are rate and inspiratory time if the mode is a control mode. However, the desired Vt must be selected as well.
	Specific names vary depending on ventilator manufacturer. Examples include Pressure Augmentation (Bear Medical Systems, Riverside, CA) and Volume Support and Pressure Regulated Volume Control (Siemens Medical, Iselin, NJ)[1]; similar modes are available on other manufacturer's ventilators. **(Level C*)**
	See Table 35-3 parameters for volume-guaranteed pressure options.
		Few studies have been accomplished that show the superiority of these modes. In addition, many modes are available only on specific ventilators.
		These modes are complex; concurrent use of pressure, flow, and volume waveform displays may be necessary to assess the modes accurately. Refer to specific ventilator operating manuals or websites for additional information.

5. APRV and biphasic ventilation are relatively new modes that appear on selected ventilators. Used most commonly for patients with ARDS, the modes use relatively high levels of pressure to recruit the lung (restore FRC).[18,19,27,38,41,75,80]	Although the modes appear to be safe and effective, randomized controlled trials are not available. Regardless, one big advantage to these modes is that they do not require that the patient be heavily sedated or paralyzed. Spontaneous breathing is expected. Generally, the patient's breathing pattern is rapid.	Few studies have been accomplished that show the superiority of these modes. In addition, many modes are available on specific ventilators. These ventilatory modes require a steep learning curve on the part of the practitioners and clinicians who care for the patients; as with most new forms of ventilation, education of staff should occur before the mode is used. Although the appeal of APRV and Bi-Phasic ventilation is in part because the patient may breath spontaneously, it is unclear whether the associated work load is advantageous.[73]

*Level B: Well-designed, controlled studies with results that consistently support a specific action, intervention, or treatment
*Level C: Qualitative studies, descriptive or correlation studies, integrative reviews, systematic reviews, or randomized controlled trials with inconsistent results

Procedure continues on following page

Procedure	**for Invasive Mechanical Ventilation (Through an Artificial Airway): Volume and Pressure Modes**—*Continued*	
Steps	**Rationale**	**Special Considerations**
A. With APRV, a high level of CPAP is selected, and brief expiratory "releases" are provided at set intervals (similar to setting a RR); the releases are very brief (less than or equal to 1.5 seconds).	The high level of CPAP helps "recruit" the lung. Alveolar filling and emptying time constants in the ARDS lung vary; the brief expiratory releases provided with APRV allow for more uniform emptying throughout the lung and ultimately improved gas distribution.[35,36] An additional benefit of periodic airway pressure releases is that they may decrease the potential negative effect of the high CPAP level on venous return.[35,36,50] **(Level C*)**	
B. With the biphasic mode, two different levels of PEEP are selected and are called Hi-PEEP and Low-PEEP. This is really an interaction of traditional PC ventilation. A rate is set, and the cycles look similar to PC or PC/IRV ventilation (depending on the I:E ratio). The major difference is that flow is available to the patient for spontaneous breathing at both pressure levels. In addition, PS may be added to assist in decreasing the work associated with spontaneous breathing.	The theoretical advantage of this mode over traditional PC/IRV is that the mode may fully support lung recruitment while still allowing for spontaneous breathing at the two pressure levels. In contrast to traditional PC/IRV, the patient receives additional flow adequate to meet inspiratory demands throughout the ventilatory cycle. Deterioration with spontaneous effort is less likely; as a result, heavy sedation and paralytics may be avoided.	
C. For APRV and Bi-Phasic mode options, please see specific ventilator manual for parameter settings.		
D. FiO_2 and sensitivity are basic to both modes.		

E. Specific APRV settings:
  i. Pressure high (P_{HIGH}), which is the high CPAP level.
  ii. Pressure low (P_{LOW}), which is generally 0 to 5 cm H_2O.
  iii. Time high (T_{HIGH}).
  iv. Time low (T_{LOW}).		

F. Specific Bi-Phasic settings:
  i. PEEP High ($PEEP_H$).
  ii. PEEP Low ($PEEP_L$).
  iii. fx.
  iv. Inspiratory time (Ti).		

*Level C: Qualitative studies, descriptive or correlation studies, integrative reviews, systematic reviews, or randomized controlled trials with inconsistent results

| Procedure | for Invasive Mechanical Ventilation (Through an Artificial Airway): Volume and Pressure Modes—*Continued* | |

Steps	Rationale	Special Considerations
6. Adaptive support ventilation (ASV): The mode is referred to by the ventilator manufacturer as "intelligent ventilation" and is designed to assess lung mechanics on a breath-to-breath basis (controlled loop ventilation) for spontaneous and control settings.[82,84] It achieves an optimal Vt by automatically adjusting mandatory respiratory fx and inspiratory pressure. Built into the mode are algorithms that are "lung protective." The protective strategies are designed to minimize auto-PEEP and prevent apnea, tachypnea, excessive dead space, and excessively large breaths.[82,84] Parameters to set include body weight, minute volume (%MinVol), and high pressure limit in addition to Fio$_2$. **(Level C*)**	The working concept with this mode is that the patient will breathe at fx and Vt that minimize elastic and resistive loads. In all modes, the opportunity for spontaneous breathing is promoted (the user does not have to switch back and forth from one mode to another to encourage spontaneous breathing because this is automatically done). Thus, the interactions required by the clinician are few.	The higher the %MinVol, the higher the level of support provided to the patient.
7. Proportional assist ventilation (PAV): The concept with this pressure mode is to prevent fatiguing workloads while still allowing the patient to spontaneously breathe. Current PAV modes take measurements throughout the inspiratory cycle and automatically adjust the pressure, flow, and volume proportionally to offset the resistance and elastance of the system with each inspiration (patient and circuit). Different names for the modes are provided by specific manufacturers, and parameters that require adjustment vary somewhat between the ventilators. Parameter settings include: PEEP, Fio$_2$, percent volume assist, and percent flow assist	PAV may provide a more physiologic breathing pattern.[12,39,90] The modes recognize that patient effort reflects work and demand and base the adjustments accordingly. **(Level C)** The percent of assist is adjusted to higher percent if less work is desired and lower percent if more work is necessary.	Few studies have been accomplished that show the superiority of this mode. In addition, many modes are available on specific ventilators.
8. Automatic tube compensation (ATC) is a ventilatory adjunct rather than a mode and is available on many current ventilators. It is designed to overcome the work of breathing imposed by the artificial airway. Parameters include internal diameter size of the endotracheal tube and the desired percent of compensation.[89]	ATC adjusts the pressure (proportional to tube resistance) needed to provide a variable fast inspiratory flow during spontaneous breathing.	ATC is increased during inspiration and lowered during expiration, thus decreasing the work of breathing as a result of tube resistance. In some patients, the use of ATC has resulted in auto-PEEP.[30] **(Level C)**

*Level C: Qualitative studies, descriptive or correlation studies, integrative reviews, systematic reviews, or randomized controlled trials with inconsistent results

Procedure continues on following page

Procedure for Invasive Mechanical Ventilation (Through an Artificial Airway): Volume and Pressure Modes—*Continued*

Steps	Rationale	Special Considerations
9. High-frequency oscillation (HFO) differs significantly from conventional ventilator modes or mode options. HFO does not require bulk movement of volume in and out of the lungs; rather, a bias flow of gases is provided, and an oscillator disperses the gases throughout the lung in what has been called augmented dispersion at high frequencies.[24,59]	The method achieves oscillation of the lung around a constant airway pressure (essentially opening the lung and keeping it open).[24,59,76] **(Level C*)**	Studies to date have not shown the superiority of this mode over traditional modes in adults with ARDS. The mode is safe if appropriately applied; however, it is not easily understood by practitioners and clinicians. Especially of concern is the fact that patients on the mode often need sedation and neuromuscular blockade.
The parameters for HFO are different from conventional ventilation.[76]		
A. Bias flow: Flow in L/min (somewhere around 40 to 50 L/min).	The bias flow combined with the oscillatory activity (extremely rapid pulses in a back and forth motion) results in the constant infusion of fresh gases and evacuation of old gases.	
B. Oscillatory frequency (fx): In Hz (5 Hz is cited in one study as a starting point).[11]		
C. Mean airway pressure: Generally slightly greater than conventional ventilation initially.		
D. ΔP: The change in pressure or pressure amplitude (generally adjusted to achieve chest wall vibration).	ΔP and fx are adjusted to achieve $Paco_2$ within a target range.	
E. Fio_2 level and PEEP level: As in conventional ventilation (generally PEEP is greater than 10).		
F. Percent inspiratory time: Controls the percentage of time the oscillator spends in the inspiratory phase. A starting place is 33%.		
10. Remove personal protective equipment. **PE** **HH**		
11. Ensure activation of alarms (see Table 35-3).	Safety of the patient is paramount.	
Humidity		
Humidity is essential to prevent the drying effect of the gases provided by the ventilator.	Inspired gases may be humidified with the use of standard cascade or high-volume humidifiers. Many institutions use disposable heat and moisture exchanges (HMEs) in place of conventional humidifiers.	HMEs are popular because they decrease the risk of infection and are inexpensive.

*Level C: Qualitative studies, descriptive or correlation studies, integrative reviews, systematic reviews, or randomized controlled trials with inconsistent results

Procedure for Invasive Mechanical Ventilation (Through an Artificial Airway): Volume and Pressure Modes—*Continued*

Steps	Rationale	Special Considerations
1. For conventional humidifiers, ensure that the humidifier has adequate fluid (sterile distilled water) and that the thermostat setting is adjusted according to manufacturer's recommendations.	Gases generally are humidified before entering the artificial airway. Temperature is measured at the patient's airway; temperatures between 35°C and 37°C (95° and 98°F) are considered optimal.[63]	Cool circuits may be tolerated well in patients without secretions. In patients with thick or tenacious secretions, attention to inspired temperature is important to prevent mucus plugging; circuit temperatures may need to be closer to body temperature (37°C versus 35°C) in these cases.
2. HMEs are placed between the airway and the ventilator circuit.	The moisture in warmed exhaled gases passes through the vast surface area of the HME and condenses. With inspiration, dry gases pass through the HME and become humidified. The use of HMEs has been associated with decreased incidence of ventilator-associated pneumonias in patients on ventilation.[11,25,47,88] **(Level B*)**	
A. Change HMEs per manufacturer's instructions.	The longer the HME is in line, the more efficient the humidification; however, inspiratory resistance increases over time. HMEs are often changed every 2 to 3 days (refer to manufacturer's instructions). In patients undergoing weaning, the additional resistive load added by these humidifiers may preclude their use.[47,48,60,67]	
B. Do not use if secretions are copious or bloody.	Obstruction is possible, and HMEs are not indicated in these conditions.	

Expected Outcomes

- Maintenance of adequate pH and $Paco_2$
- Maintenance of adequate Pao_2
- Maintenance of adequate breathing pattern
- Respiratory muscle rest

Unexpected Outcomes

- Unacceptable pH, $Paco_2$, and Pao_2
- Hemodynamic instability
- Pulmonary barotrauma
- Inadvertent extubation
- Malpositioned endotracheal tube
- Nosocomial lung infection
- Acid-base disturbance
- Respiratory muscle fatigue

Patient Monitoring and Care

Steps	Rationale	Reportable Conditions
		These conditions should be reported if they persist despite nursing interventions.
1. Ensure activation of all alarms each shift (see Table 35-3).	Ensures patient safety.	- Continued activation of alarms

*Level B: Well-designed, controlled studies with results that consistently support a specific action, intervention, or treatment

Procedure continues on following page

Patient Monitoring and Care —*Continued*

Steps	Rationale	Reportable Conditions
2. Check for secure stabilization and maintenance of endotracheal tube (see Procedure 4).	Reduces risk of inadvertent extubation.	• Unplanned extubation • Dislodgment of airway
3. Monitor in-line thermometer to maintain inspired gas temperature (in the range 35° to 37°C [95° to 98°F]).	Reduces risk of thermal injury from overheated inspired gas and risk of poor humidity from underheated inspired gas.	• Temperature less than 35°C or greater than 37°C
4. Keep ventilator tubing clear of condensation (drain tubing from clean to dirty).	Reduces risk of respiratory infection by decreasing inhalation of contaminated water droplets.	• Continued condensation
5. Ensure availability of self-inflating manual resuscitation bag-valve device attached to supplemental oxygen at the head of the bed. Attach or adjust PEEP valve if the patient is on greater than 5 cm H_2O.	Provides capability for immediate delivering of ventilation and oxygenation to relieve acute respiratory distress caused by hypoxemia or acidosis.	
6. Check ventilator for baseline Fio_2, PIP, Vt, fx, and alarm activation with initial assessment and after removal of ventilator from patient for suctioning, bagging, or draining ventilator tubing.	Ensures that prescribed ventilator parameters are used (e.g., 100% oxygen used for suctioning is not inadvertently delivered after suctioning procedure), provides diagnostic data to evaluate interventions (e.g., PIP is reduced after suctioning or bagging), and ensures that the monitoring and warning functions of the ventilator are functional (i.e., alarms).	• Fio_2, PIP, Vt, or fx settings different from prescribed
7. Explore any changes in peak inspiratory pressure greater than 4 cm H_2O or decreased (sustained) Vt on PSV. Immediately explore the cause of high-pressure alarms.	Acute changes in PIP or Vt may indicate mechanical malfunction, such as tubing disconnection, cuff or connector leaks, tubing or airway kinks, or changes in resistance and compliance. Always consider possibility of tension pneumothorax. Have equipment readily available (see Procedure 20).	• Unexplained high-pressure alarms
8. Place bite-block between the teeth if the patient is biting on the oral endotracheal tube (see Procedure 4).	An oral airway serves the same purpose but may not be tolerated as well as the bite-block because it may induce gagging.	• Biting on tube
9. Change the patient's body position as often as possible, but at least every 2 hours.	Frequent position changes are indicated to reduce the potential for atelectasis and pneumonia caused by secretion stasis. Promotes airway clearance. One of the most modifiable factors related to VAP.	
A. Continuous lateral rotation therapy may be helpful.		
B. Maintain backrest elevation (BRE) of 30 to 45 degrees.		

Patient Monitoring and Care —*Continued*

Steps	Rationale	Reportable Conditions
10. Evaluate patient-ventilator dyssynchrony by manually ventilating the patient with a self-inflating manual resuscitation bag-valve device (see Procedure 32).	By taking the patient off the ventilator for manual ventilation, synchrony may be accomplished more quickly than on the ventilator. This intervention may reduce risk of barotrauma and cardiovascular depression. If patient breathes in synchrony with bagging, consider changes in ventilatory parameters. If patient does not breathe synchronously with bagging, explore differential diagnoses of problems distal to the airway. Respiratory care practitioner, nurse practitioner, or physician consultation may be necessary.	• Patient-ventilator dyssynchrony
11. Observe for hemodynamic changes associated with increased Vt or PEEP.	May indicate functional changes in circulating volume caused by positive intrathoracic pressure. Always consider potential for pneumothorax with acute changes. Equipment used for rapid release of tension pneumothorax should be at bedside at all times (i.e., 14-gauge needle; see Procedure 25). Chest tube insertion equipment should be readily available.	• Decreased blood pressure • Change in heart rate (increase or decrease of greater than 10% of baseline) • Decreased cardiac output • Decreased mixed venous oxygen tension • Increased arterial-venous oxygen difference (see Procedure 29)
12. Monitor for signs and symptoms of acute respiratory distress, hypoxemia, hypercarbia, and fatigue.	Respiratory distress indicates the need for changes in PPV. While troubleshooting the difficulties, support ventilation via a manual self-inflating resuscitation bag (see Procedure 32), if necessary.	• Chest-abdominal dyssynchrony • Shallow or irregular respirations • Tachypnea, bradypnea, or dyspnea • Decreased mental status • Restlessness, confusion, lethargy • Increasing or decreasing arterial blood pressure • Tachycardia • Atrial or ventricular dysrhythmias • Significant changes in arterial pH, PaO_2, $PaCO_2$, or SaO_2

Documentation

Documentation should include the following:
• Patient and family education
• Date and time ventilatory assistance was instituted
• Ventilator settings, including the following: mode, FiO_2, mode of ventilation, Vt, respiratory frequency (total and mandatory), PEEP level, I:E ratio or inspiratory time, PIP, dynamic compliance (C_{dyn}), and static compliance (C_{stat})
• Arterial blood gas results
• SaO_2 readings
• Reason for initiation of PPV

• Patient responses to PPV (including the patient's indication of level of comfort and respiratory symptoms)
• Hemodynamic values
• Vital signs
• Respiratory assessment findings
• Unexpected outcomes
• Nursing interventions
• Degree of backrest elevation
• Humidifier change maintenance

References

1. Abraham E, Yoshira G: Cardiorespiratory effects of pressure controlled ventilation in severe respiratory failure, *Chest* 98:1445-1449, 1990.

2. Amato MBP, et al: Volume-assured, pressure support ventilation (VAPSV): a new approach for reducing muscle workload during acute respiratory failure, *Chest* 102:1225-1234, 1992.

3. Amato MBP, et al: Beneficial effects of the "open lung approach" with low distending pressures in acute respiratory distress syndrome, *Am J Respir Crit Care Med* 152:1835-1846, 1995.

4. Amato MBP, Barbas CSV, Medeiros DM, et al: Effect of a protective-ventilation strategy on mortality in the acute respiratory distress syndrome, *N Engl J Med* 338:347-354, 1998.

5. American Association of Critical-Care Nurses: *AACN practice alert: ventilator-associated pneumonia,* 2004, retrieved from www.aacn.org/WD/Practice/Docs/Ventilator_Associated_Pneumonia_1-2008.pdf accessed 9/15/09

6. American Thoracic Society and the Infectious Diseases Society of America: Guidelines for the management of adults with hospital acquired, ventilator-associated and healthcare associated pneumonia, *Am Rev Respir Crit Care Med* 171:388-416, 2005.

7. Banner MJ, Blanch PB, Kirby RR: Imposed work of breathing and methods of triggering a demand-flow continuous positive airway system, *Crit Care Med* 21:183-190, 1993.

8. Bellemare F, Grassino A: Evaluation of human diaphragm fatigue, *J Appl Physiol* 53:1196-1206, 1982.

9. Bidani A, et al: Permissive hypercapnia in acute respiratory failure, *JAMA* 272:957-962, 1994.

10. Bonten MJ, Kollef MH, Hall JB: Risk factors for ventilator-associated pneumonia: from epidemiology to patient management, *Clin Infect Dis* 38:1141-1149, 2004.

11. Boots RJ, et al: Clinical utility of hygroscopic heat and moisture exchanges in intensive care patients, *Crit Care Med* 25:1707-1712, 1997.

12. Bosma K, Ferreyra G, Ambrogio C, et al: Patient-ventilator interaction and sleep in mechanicalliy ventilated patients: pressure support versus proportional assist ventilation, *Crit Care Med* 35:1048-1054, 2007.

13. Brochard L, et al: Inspiratory pressure support prevents diaphragmatic fatigue during weaning from mechanical ventilation, *Am Rev Respir Dis* 139:513-521, 1989.

14. Brochard L, Pluskwa F, Lemaire R: Improved efficacy of spontaneous breathing with inspiratory pressure support, *Am Rev Respir Dis* 136:411-415, 1987.

15. Burns SM: Ventilating patients with acute severe asthma: what do we really know? *AACN Adv Crit Care* 17:188-193, 2006.

16. Burns SM: Prevention of aspiration pneumonia in the enterally fed critically ill ventilated patient: keeping the head up takes a village! *Pract Gastroenterol* 31:63-72, 2007.

17. Burns SM: Pressure modes of mechanical ventilation: the good, the bad and the ugly, *AACN Adv Crit Care* 19:399-411, 2008.

18. Calzia E, Lindner KH, Witt S, et al: Pressure time product and work of breathing during biphasic continuous positive airway pressure and assisted spontaneous breathing, *Am J Respir Crit Care Med* 150:904-910, 1994.

19. Cane RD, Peruzzi WT, Shapiro BA: Airway pressure release ventilation in severe acute respiratory failure, *Chest* 100:460-463, 1991.

20. Cohen CA, et al: Clinical manifestations of inspiratory muscle fatigue, *Am J Med* 73:308-316, 1982.

21. Cole AGH, Weller SF, Sykes MK: Inverse ratio ventilation compared with PEEP in adult respiratory failure, *Intensive Care Med* 10:227-232, 1984.

22. Craven DE, Kunches LM, Kilinsky V, et al: Risk factors for pneumonia and fatality in patients receiving continuous mechanical ventilation, *Am Rev Respir Dis* 133:792-796, 1986.

23. Davis WB, et al: Pulmonary oxygen toxicity: early reversible changes in human alveolar structures induced by hyperoxia, *N Engl J Med* 309:878-883, 1983.

24. Derak S, et al, and the Multicenter Oscillatory Ventilation for Acute Respiratory Distress Syndrome Trial (MOAT) Study Investigators: High-frequency oscillatory ventilation for acute respiratory distress syndrome in adults: a randomized controlled trial, *Am J Respir Crit Care Med* 166:801-808, 2002.

25. Djedaini K, et al: Changing heat and moisture exchanges every 48 hours rather than 24 hours does not alter their efficacy and the incidence of nosocomial pneumonia, *Am J Respir Crit Care Med* 152:1562-1569, 1995.

26. Dodek P, Keenan S, Cook D, et al, for the Canadian Critical Care Trials Group and the Canadian Critical Care Society: Evidence-Based Clinical Practice Guidelines for the Prevention of Ventilator-Associated Pneumonia, *Ann Intern Med* 141:305-313, 2004.

27. Downs JB, Stock MC: Airway pressure release ventilation: a new concept of ventilatory support, *Crit Care Med* 15:459-461, 1987.

28. Dreyfuss D, et al: High inflation pressure pulmonary edema: respective effects of high airway pressure, high Vt, and positive end-expiratory pressure, *Am Rev Respir Dis* 137:1159-1164, 1988.

29. Dreyfuss D, Saumon G: The role of Vt, FRC, and end-inspiratory volume in the development of pulmonary edema following mechanical ventilation, *Am Rev Respir Dis* 148:1194-1203, 1993.

30. Elsasser S, Guttmann J, Stocker R, et al: Accuracy of automatic tube compensation in new-generation mechanical ventilators, *Crit Care Med* 31:2619-2626, 2003.

31. Esteban A, Alia I, Ibanez J, et al: Modes of mechanical ventilation and weaning a national survey of Spanish hospital, *Chest* 106:1188-1193, 1994.

32. Fagon J, Chastre J, Vuagnat A, et al: Nosocomial pneumonia and mortality among patients in intensive care units, *JAMA* 275:866-869, 1996.

33. Fiastro JF, Habib MP, Quan SF: Pressure support compensation for respiratory work due to endotracheal tubes and demand continuous positive airway pressure, *Chest* 93:499-505, 1998.

34. Fisher AB: Oxygen therapy: side effects and toxicity, *Am Rev Respir Dis* 122:61-69, 1980.

35. Frawley PM, Habashi N: Airway pressure release ventilation: theory and practice, *AACN Clin Issues* 12:234-246, 2001.

36. Frawley PM, Habashi NM: Airway pressure release ventilation and pediatrics: theory and practice, *Crit Care Nurs Clin North Am* 16:337-348, 2004.

37. Fu Z, et al: High lung volume increases stress failure in pulmonary capillaries, *J Appl Physiol* 73:123-133, 1992.

38. Garner W, Downs JB, Stock MC, et al: Airway pressure release ventilation (APRV): a human trial, *Chest* 94: 779-781, 1998.

39. Giannouli E, Webster K, Roberts D, et al: Response of ventilator-dependent patients to different levels of pressure support and proportional assist, *Am J Respir Crit Care Med* 159:1716-1725, 1999.

40. Gurevich MJ, Van Dyke J, Young ES, et al: Improved oxygenation and lower peak airway pressure in serve adult respiratory distress syndrome: treatment with inverse ratio ventilation, *Chest* 89:211-213, 1986.

41. Habashi NM: Other approaches to open-lung ventilation: airway pressure release ventilation, *Crit Care Med* 33:S228-S240, 2005.

42. Hickling KG, et al: Low mortality rate in acute respiratory distress syndrome using low volume, pressure limited ventilation with permissive hypercapnia: a prospective study. *Crit Care Med* 22:1568-1578, 1994.

43. Hilbert G, et al: Noninvasive ventilation in immunosuppressed patients with pulmonary infiltrates, fever and acute respiratory failure, *N Engl J Med* 344:481-487, 2001.

44. Holm BA, et al: Pulmonary physiological and surfactant changes during injury and recovery from hyperoxia, *J Appl Physiol* 59:1402-1409, 1985.

45. Hospital Infections Program, National Center for Infectious Diseases, CDC: Public health focus: surveillance, prevention and control of nosocomial pneumonia, *MMWR* 41:783-787, 1992.

46. Ibanez J, Penafiel A, Raurich JM, et al: Gastroesophageal reflux in intubated patients receiving enteral nutrition: effect of supine and semi-recumbent positions, *J Parenter Enteral Nutr* 16:419-422, 1992.

47. Iotti GA, et al: Unfavorable mechanical effects of heat and moisture exchangers in ventilated patients, *Intensive Care Med* 23:399-405, 1997.

48. Johnson PA, Raper RF, Fisher M: The impact of heat and moisture exchanging humidifiers on work of breathing, *Anaesth Intensive Care* 23:697-701, 1995.

49. Kacmarek RM, Hess D: Editorial: pressure-controlled inverse-ratio ventilation: panacea or auto-PEEP? *Respiratory Care* 35:945-948, 1990.

50. Kaplan LJ, Bailey H, Formosa V: Airway pressure release ventilation increases cardiac performance in patients with acute lung injury/adult respiratory distress syndrome, *Crit Care* 5:221-226, 2001.

51. Kollef M: Ventilator–associated pneumonia: a multivariate analysis, *JAMA* 270:1965-1970, 1993.

52. Kollef MH, Shorr A, Tabak YP, et al: Epidemiology and outcomes of health-care-associated pneumonia: results from a large US database of a culture-positive pneumonia, *Chest* 128:3854-3862, 2005.

53. Lachman B: Open up the lung and keep the lung open, *Intensive Care Med* 18:319-321, 1992.

54. Leatherman J, Ravenscraft SA: Low measured auto-positive end expiratory pressure during mechanical ventilation of patients with severe asthma: hidden auto-positive end-expiratory pressure, *Crit Care Med* 24:541-546, 1996.

55. MacIntyre NR: Respiratory function during pressure support ventilation, *Chest* 89:677-683, 1986.

56. MacIntyre NR: Effects of initial flow rate and breath termination criteria on pressure support ventilation, *Chest* 99:134-138, 1991.

57. MacIntyre NR: Ventilatory muscles and mechanical ventilatory support, *Crit Care Med* 25:1106-1107, 1997.

58. MacIntyre NR, Cheng K-CG, McConnell R: Applied PEEP during pressure support reduces the inspiratory threshold load of intrinsic PEEP, *Chest* 111:188-193, 1997.

59. MacIntyre NR: High-frequency ventilation [editorial], *Crit Care Med* 26:1955-1956, 1998.

60. Manthous CA, Schmidt GA: Resistive pressure of a condenser humidifier in mechanically ventilated patients, *Crit Care Med* 22:1792-1795, 1994.

61. Marini JJ, Rodriguez M, Lamb V: The inspiratory workload of patient-initiated mechanical ventilation, *Am Rev Respir Dis* 134:902-909, 1986.

62. Marini JJ, Smith TC, Lamb VJ: External work output and force generation during synchronized intermittent mechanical ventilation: effect of machine assistance on breath effort, *Am Rev Respir Dis* 138:1169-1179, 1998.

63. McEvoy MT, Carey TJ: Shivering and rewarming after cardiac surgery: comparison of ventilator circuits with humidifier and heated wires to heat and moisture exchangers, *Am J Crit Care* 4:293-299, 1995.

64. Mehta S, Hill NS: State of the art: non-invasive ventilation, *Am J Respir Crit Care Med* 163:540-577, 2001.

65. Metheny NA, Schallom L, Oliver DA, et al: Gastric residual volume and aspiration in crucially ill patens receiving gastric feedings, *Am J Crit Care* 17:512-520, 2008.

66. Mols G, von Ungern-Sternberg B, Rohr E, et al: Respiratory comfort and breathing pattern during volume proportional assist ventilation and pressure support ventilation: a study on volunteers with artificially reduced compliance, *Crit Care Med* 28:1940-1946, 2000.

67. Nishimara M, et al: Comparison of flow-resistive work load due to humidifying devices, *Chest* 97:600-604, 1990.

68. O'Kroy JA, Coast JR: Effects of flow and resistive training on respiratory muscle endurance and strength, *Respiration* 60:279-283, 1993.

69. Orlando R: Editorial: ventilators: how clever, how complex? *Crit Care Med* 2704-2705, 2003.

70. Parker JC, Hernandez LA, Peevy KJ: Mechanisms of ventilator-induced lung injury, *Crit Care Med* 21:131-143, 1993.

71. Pepe PE, Marini JJ: Occult positive end-expiratory pressure in mechanically ventilated patients with airflow obstruction, *Am Rev Respir Dis* 126:166-173, 1994.

72. Peter JV, et al: Noninvasive ventilation in acute respiratory failure: a meta analysis update, *Crit Care Med* 30:555-562, 2002.

73. Putensen C, et al: Long-term effects of spontaneous breathing during ventilatory support in patients with acute lung injury, *Am J Respir Crit Care Med* 164:43-49, 2001.

74. Ranieri VM, et al: Effects of positive end-expiratory pressure on alveolar recruitment and gas exchange in patients with the adult respiratory distress syndrome, *Am Rev Respir Dis* 144:544-551, 1991.

75. Rathgeber J, Schorn B, Falk V, et al: The influence of controlled mandatory ventilation (CMV), intermittent mandatory ventilation (IMV) and biphasic intermittent positive airway pressure (BIPAP) on duration of intubation and consumption of analgesics and sedatives: a prospective analysis in 596 patients following adult cardiac surgery, *Eur J Anaesth* 14:576-582, 1997.

76. Rose L: High-frequency oscillatory ventilation in adults: clinical considerations and management priorities, *AACN Adv Crit Care* 19:412-420, 2008.

CR 77. Sassoon CSH, et al: Inspiratory muscle work of breathing during flow-by, demand-flow and continuous-flow systems in patients with chronic obstructive pulmonary disease, *Am Rev Respir Dis* 143:860-866, 1993.

78. Shorr AF, Kollef MH: Ventilator-associated pneumonia: insights from recent clinical trials, *Chest* 128:583-591, 2005.

CR 79. Slutsky AS: Consensus Conference on Mechanical Ventilation, January 28-30, 1993. at Northbrook, IL, USA: parts 1 and 2, *Intensive Care Med* 20:64-79, 150-62, 1994.

CR 80. Staudinger T, Kordova H, Roggla M, et al: Comparison of oxygen cost of breathing with pressure support ventilation and biphasic intermittent positive airway pressure ventilation, *Crit Care Med* 26:1518-1522, 1998.

CR 81. Stock M, Downs JB: Airway pressure release ventilation: a new approach to ventilatory support during acute lung injury, *Respir Care* 32:517-524, 1987.

CR 82. Sulzer CF, Chiolero R, Chassot PG, et al: Adaptive support ventilation for fast tracheal extubation after cardiac surgery: a randomized controlled study, *Anesthesiology* 95:1339-1345, 2001.

CR 83. Tablan OC, Anderson LJ, Besser R, et al: Guidelines for preventing health-care–associated pneumonia, recommendations of CDC and the Healthcare Infection Control Practices Advisory Committee March 26, 2004. MMWR 53(RR03):1-36, 2004. Available at www.cdc.gov/mmwr/preview/mmwrhtml/rr5303a1.htm.

CR 84. Tassaux D, Dalmas E, Gratadour P, et al: Patient-ventilator interactions during partial ventilatory support: a preliminary study comparing the effects of adaptive support ventilation with synchronized intermittent mandatory ventilation plus inspiratory pressure support, *Crit Care Med* 30:801-807, 2002.

CR 85. Tharratt RS, Allen RP, Albertson TE: Pressure controlled inverse ratio ventilation in severe adult respiratory failure, *Chest* 94:755-762, 1998.

CR 86. The Acute Respiratory Distress Syndrome Network: Ventilation with lower tidal volumes as compared with traditional tidal volumes for acute lung injury and the acute respiratory distress syndrome, *N Engl J Med* 342:1301-1307, 2000.

CR 87. Tobin MJ, et al: Konno-Mead analysis of ribcage-abdominal motion during successful and unsuccessful trials of weaning from mechanical ventilation, *Am Rev Respir Dis* 135:1320-1328, 1987.

CR 88. Unal N, et al: A novel method of evaluation of three heat-moisture exchangers in six different ventilator settings, *Intensive Care Med* 24:138-146, 1998.

89. Unoki T, Serita A, Grap MJ: Automatic tube compensation during weaning form mechanical ventilation; evidence and clinical implications, *Crit Care Nurse* 28:34-42, 2008.

90. Varelmann D, Wrigge H, Zinserling J, et al: Proportional assist versus pressure support ventilation in patients with acute respiratory failure: cardiorespiratory responses to artificially increased ventilatory demand, *Crit Care Med* 33:1968-1975, 2005.

CR 91. Vincent JL, Bihari DJ. Suter PM, et al: The prevalence of nosocomial pneumonia in intensive care units in Europe (EPIC), *JAMA* 274:639-644, 1995.

CR 92. Vittacca M, Bianchi L, Zanotti E, et al: Assessment of physiologic variables and subjective comfort under different levels of pressure support ventilation, *Chest* 126: 851-859, 2004.

CR 93. West JB, et al: Stress fracture in pulmonary capillaries. *J Appl Physiol* 70:1731-1742, 1991.

Additional Readings

Burns S: Mechanical ventilation and weaning. In Carlson KK, editor: *AACN advanced critical care nursing*, St Louis, 2009, Elsevier.

Pierce LNB: Invasive and noninvasive modes and methods of mechanical ventilation. In Burns SM, editor: *AACN protocols for practice: care of mechanically ventilated patients*, ed 2, Boston, 2007, Jones and Bartlett.

Pierce LNB, editor: *Management of the mechanically ventilated patient*, ed 2, St Louis, 2007, Elsevier.

Tobin MJ: *Principles and practice of mechanical ventilation*, ed 2, New York, 2006, McGraw-Hill.

West JB: *Respiratory physiology: the essentials*, ed 8, Baltimore, 2008, Lippincott Williams & Wilkins.

West JB: *Pulmonary pathophysiology: the essentials*, Baltimore, 2008, Lippincott Williams & Wilkins.

Selected Manufacturers' Websites

Avea: retrieved September 15, 2009, from www.viasyshealthcare.com/prod_serv/downloads/284_Avea_Comp_Spec_Sheet.pdf.

Drager: retrieved September 15, 2009 from www.draeger.com/MT/internet/pdf/CareAreas/CriticalCare/cc_bipap_book_en.pdf and www.draeger.com/MT/internet/pdf/CareAreas/CriticalCare/cc_evita_atcpps_br_en.pdf.

Hamilton Medical: retrieved November 17, 2008, from www.med1online.com/documents/Hamilton_Products_Galileo_Classic_Specs.pdf; and retrieved January 2, 2008, from www.hamilton-medical.com/GALILEO-ventilators.37.0.html

Maquet: retrieved November 16, 2008, from www.maquet.com/productPage.aspx?m1=112599774495&m2=112808545902&m3=105584076919&productGroupID=112808545902&productConfigID=105584076919&languageID=1&titleCountryID=224.

Puritan Bennett: retrieved November 16, 2008, from www.puritanbennett.com/prod/Product.aspx?S1=VEN&S2=&id=289.

Standard Weaning Criteria: Negative Inspiratory Force or Pressure, Positive Expiratory Pressure, Spontaneous Tidal Volume, Vital Capacity, and Rapid Shallow Breathing Index

P U R P O S E : Weaning criteria are measured to evaluate respiratory muscle strength (negative inspiratory force or pressure and positive expiratory pressure) and endurance (spontaneous tidal volume and vital capacity). Another index, the rapid shallow breathing index, has been developed to identify a breathing pattern associated with unsuccessful weaning. The results of these criteria may help determine the need for intubation, the ability of the patient to tolerate weaning trials, the presence of respiratory muscle fatigue, and extubation potential.

Suzanne M. Burns

PREREQUISITE NURSING KNOWLEDGE

- Weaning criteria emerged in the late 1970s in an attempt to identify patient potential for successful extubation. Although these "standard weaning criteria," which included negative inspiratory force or pressure (NIF or NIP), positive expiratory pressure (PEP), spontaneous tidal volume (SVt), and vital capacity (VC), were used widely over the years to test weaning readiness, they gradually grew out of favor because they did not perform well as predictors, especially in disparate categories of patient conditions.[2] Two systematic reviews evaluated the weaning process and concluded that weaning criteria (also known as predictors or indices) did not predict weaning.[4,8] They were found to be good negative predictors (i.e., that the weaning attempt would be unsuccessful) but poor positive predictors (i.e., that the weaning attempt would be successful).[1,9,11,12]

Regardless, the criteria do provide information about respiratory muscle strength and endurance and may be especially helpful in following trends in gains in strength and endurance in patients with debilitated weak conditions or in patients with myopathies. The criteria also may help in evaluation of respiratory muscle fatigue (see Procedure 37).

- Negative inspiratory force (NIF) also is called *negative inspiratory pressure* (NIP) or sometimes *maximal inspiratory pressure* (MIP). The measurement of NIF is *effort independent* (the patient does not have to actively cooperate) and is considered the most reliable of the standard weaning criteria (SWC). NIF is a measure of inspiratory respiratory muscle strength. It is a strong negative predictor but a poor positive predictor.[1,4,12] The most common threshold cited for NIF is less than or equal to -20 cm H_2O. Because this measurement is non–effort dependent, with good technique (see the procedure), the value is reliable unless central drive is impaired. For example, with sedation, a cuff leak, or respiratory muscle fatigue, the value may be adversely affected.

- Positive expiratory pressure (PEP) is effort dependent and requires that the patient cooperate fully to obtain a reliable value. PEP is a measure of expiratory muscle strength and ability to cough. The threshold for PEP is greater than or equal to $+30$ cm H_2O.

- Spontaneous tidal volume (SVt) is a measure of respiratory muscle endurance. The threshold for SVt is greater than or equal to 5 mL/kg of body weight. When muscles fatigue, the compensatory breathing pattern is rapid and shallow. As a result, investigators have combined SVt and spontaneous respiratory rate (fx) in a ratio called the rapid shallow breathing index (fx/Vt).[13]

- The fx/Vt index threshold associated with success is less than or equal to 105. This threshold is calculated by obtaining the spontaneous respiratory rate and dividing it by the Vt in liters.[13] In elderly medical patients, the threshold is less than or equal to 130.[7]

- Vital capacity (VC) is also a measure of respiratory muscle endurance or reserve or both. A fatigued patient is unable to triple or even double the size of a breath. The threshold for VC is greater than or equal to 10 to 15 mL/kg (at least two to three times SVt).

- Vital capacity may be especially helpful in patients with neurologic conditions like myasthenia or Guillain-Barré syndrome. In these patients, a decrease in the VC suggests loss of reserve and impending respiratory muscle failure.[3]

- All SWC are best used in combination with other assessment data to determine the appropriateness of weaning trials or extubation.[2,4,8,11,12]

- Randomized controlled trials (RCTs) were conducted to determine when and how best to wean patients from mechanical ventilatory support. The studies showed the efficacy and safety of multidisciplinary protocols with use of a "wean screen" (a set of discrete criteria that suggest stability, such as a fraction of inspired oxygen [FiO_2] less than 0.50, positive end-expiratory pressure [PEEP] less than 8 cm H_2O, no vasopressor use, etc.) followed by a carefully monitored spontaneous breathing trial (SBT) in attaining positive outcomes.[5,6,10] These study results have greatly obviated reliance on traditional weaning criteria as predictive tools.

EQUIPMENT*

- An aneroid pressure manometer (also called a force meter)
- A respirometer, to measure volumes or monitor spontaneous volumes on the ventilator
- Appropriate adapters and one-way valves
- Self-inflating manual resuscitation bag-valve device, connected to an oxygen source

---

*Some ventilators allow for measurement of these parameters while the patient is on the ventilator. Refer to specific ventilator guidelines for measurement.

PATIENT AND FAMILY EDUCATION

- Inform the patient and family about the patient's respiratory status, changes in therapy, and how to interpret the changes. If the patient or a family member requests specific information about the measurements, explain the relationship between these measurements and respiratory muscle strength and endurance. ➤*Rationale:* Most patients and families are less concerned with the diagnostic and therapeutic details and more concerned with how the patient's condition is progressing overall. However, patients and families readily grasp the concepts of muscle strength and endurance. They may wish to follow the patient's progress by monitoring the results of the tests over time. If appropriate, the family can be recruited to help encourage the patient to provide a maximal effort during measurements.

- Discuss the sensations the patient may experience, such as transient shortness of breath and fatigue. ➤*Rationale:* Knowledge of anticipated sensory experiences reduces anxiety and distress.

- Explain to the patient the importance of cooperation and maximal effort to achieve valid and reliable measurements. ➤*Rationale:* Information about the patient's therapy, including the rationale, is cited consistently as an important need of patients and family members.

PATIENT ASSESSMENT AND PREPARATION
Patient Assessment

- Assess for the signs and symptoms of inadequate ventilation:
  - Increasing carbon dioxide tension in expired air or arterial blood
  - Chest-abdominal dyssynchrony
  - Shallow or irregular respirations
  - Tachypnea or bradypnea
  - Dyspnea
  - Restlessness, confusion, lethargy
  - Increasing or decreasing arterial blood pressure beyond a predetermined threshold level
  - Tachycardia or bradycardia beyond an predetermined threshold level
  - New onset atrial or ventricular dysrhythmias
  - ➤*Rationale:* Inadequate ventilation may indicate the need for positive-pressure ventilation. If signs and symptoms suggest inadequate ventilation, measurement of SWC may be helpful in determining respiratory muscle strength and endurance and the potential need for positive-pressure ventilation. Conversely, if no signs and symptoms of inadequate ventilation are present in a patient on positive-pressure ventilation, SWC measurements (in conjunction with other patient data) are useful to determine the patient's ability to tolerate weaning trials and possibly extubation.

- Assess patient's need for a long-term artificial airway and mechanical ventilatory assistance. ➤*Rationale:* Consistently low measurements in conjunction with overall patient status (e.g., mental status, hemodynamics, fluid and electrolyte balance, comfort, mobility) may suggest the need for permanent full-time or part-time ventilator support.

Patient Preparation

- Verify correct patient with two identifiers. ➡*Rationale*: Prior to performing a procedure, the nurse should ensure the correct identification of the patient for the intended intervention.

- Ensure that the patient understands pre-procedural teachings. Answer questions as they arise, and reinforce information as needed. ➡*Rationale*: This communication evaluates and reinforces understanding of previously taught information.
- Consider positioning the patient in a high semi-Fowler's position, if the patient's condition allows. ➡*Rationale*: Placing the patient in a high semi-Fowler's position, if possible, enables the patient to use the force of gravity during measurements.

Procedure for Weaning Criteria

Steps	Rationale	Special Considerations
Steps 1- 11 (Level B*)[1-13]		
1. VP		
2. HH		
3. PE		
4. Attach portable respirometer to airway via adapter and series of one-way valves. Note: If patient is on positive pressure ventilation, place patient back on ventilator (or manually ventilate) to rest for a few minutes between all measurements.	Respirometer is used to measure SVt and VC. Depending on institutional standard and specific ventilator, volumes and pressures may be measured while patient is on the ventilator.	Generally, a series of one-way valves are used for attachment of the respirometer and aneroid manometer. If patient is on positive pressure ventilation (PPV), place patient back on ventilator (or manually ventilate) to rest for a few minutes between all measurements. Ensure that a large cuff leak is not present because it will adversely affect the measurements.
5. Measure SVt: Instruct the patient to breathe normally for 1 minute. Count the respiratory rate and record the minute ventilation. Divide minute ventilation by fx to obtain average SVt.		If patient's oxygen saturation decreases to less than 90% *(this may vary with the individual patient and thresholds set by the healthcare team)* or other signs of intolerance of the procedure emerge, the test is aborted or may be done for a shorter interval (i.e., test for 15 seconds and multiply result by 4 for calculation of full minute).
6. Measure VC: Instruct the patient to inhale as deeply as possible, zero respirometer, and instruct patient to exhale as completely as possible. The VC may be tested more than once to obtain the best effort.	A good VC effort mandates a maximal inspiration followed by a maximal expiration.	
7. Measure NIF as follows: A. The inspiratory one-way valve should be closed or capped to ensure a closed system for measurement of inspiratory effort. Attach pressure manometer to airway with adapter and one-way valves.	Ensures best effort and evaluation reproducibility. Pressure manometer is used to measure NIF. Some ventilators allow for the measurement to be accomplished with the patient on the ventilator.	The pressure manometer is usually attached to the airway via a series of one-way valves (Fig. 36-1). The valves (one for inspiration, and one for expiration) are capped as necessary to ensure a closed system and a clean measurement device for attachment to the patient's artificial airway.

*Level B: Well-designed, controlled studies with results that consistently support a specific action, intervention, or treatment

Procedure continues on following page

Negative Inspiratory Pressure

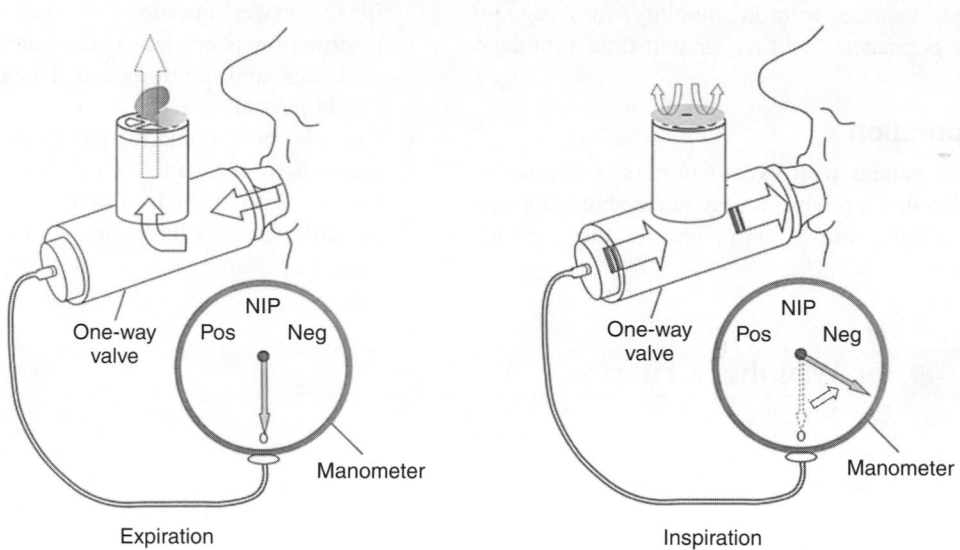

Positive Expiratory Pressure

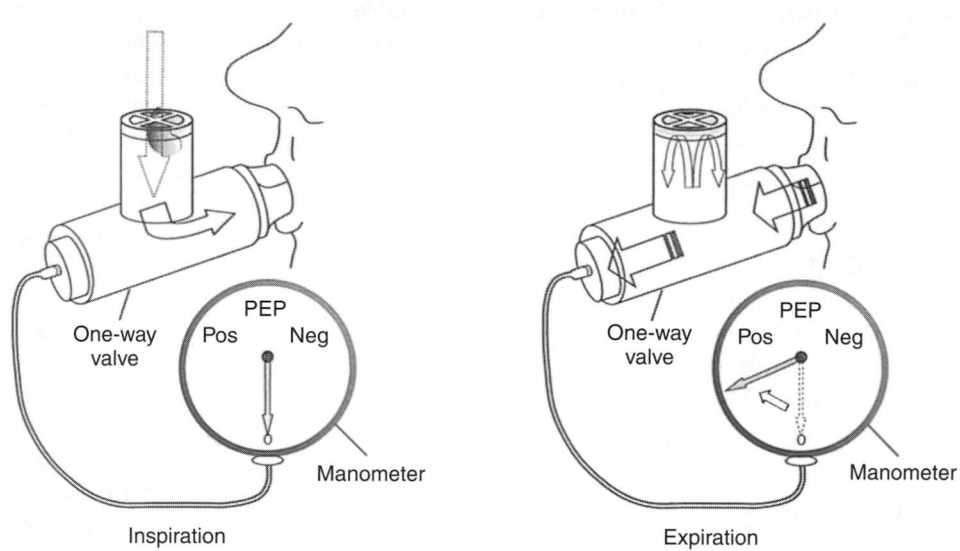

FIGURE 36-1   Measurement of negative inspiratory pressure (NIP) and positive expiratory pressure (PEP).

Procedure for Weaning Criteria—*Continued*

Steps	Rationale	Special Considerations
B. Instruct the patient to inhale as deeply as possible. Observe the manometer needle during inspiration. This test can be done for 20 seconds (and sometimes longer) with multiple attempts by patient (2 or 3 attempts in a row are common).	The goal is to obtain the patient's best effort. However, this test may be done even if the patient is not able to participate actively. After a few seconds attached to the closed system manometer, the patient initiates a series of breaths and generates a negative pressure. The exception is a when central respiratory drive is absent.	NIF can be frightening for patients because getting a breath during the maneuver is impossible. Coaching should include warning the patient that this test renders him or her temporarily unable to take a breath.

Procedure for Weaning Criteria—*Continued*

Steps	Rationale	Special Considerations
		Watch the manometer with each inspiratory maneuver. during the 20 seconds. Stop the procedure after the best NIF measurement, when 20 seconds elapses, or if the patient does not tolerate the procedure (e.g., experiences agitation, bradycardia, significant oxygen desaturation).
8. Measure PEP as follows: A. The expiratory valve should be closed or capped to ensure that the patient is able to take in a breath but must exhale against a closed system. Attach the pressure manometer to the airway via adapter and one-way valves.		
B. Instruct the patient to exhale forcefully after taking a deep breath. Do this a number of times (not to exceed 20 seconds). Take the greatest positive number.	Obtains patient's best effort.	As with NIF, any deterioration of the patient's condition indicates that the test should be aborted.
9. Encourage the patient throughout all measurements.	Provides incentive.	
10. Remove personal protective equipment. **HH**		
11. Discuss the results with team.	Decisions related to weaning trials, intubation, or extubation are made with the results of these tests in conjunction with others.	

Expected Outcome

- Valid and reliable measurements

Unexpected Outcomes

- Invalid and unreliable measurements
- Untoward physical, emotional, or hemodynamic changes

Patient Monitoring and Care

Steps	Rationale	Reportable Conditions
		These conditions should be reported if they persist despite nursing interventions.
1. Compare the SWC measurements with the desired patient goals.	If the measurements do not meet anticipated levels, the patient may need either initiation of positive pressure ventilation or continuance of mechanical ventilation.	• NIF more positive than -20 cm H_2O (e.g., -10 cm H_2O) • PEP less positive than $+30$ cm H_2O (e.g., $+10$ cm H_2O) • SVt less than 5 mL/kg

Procedure continues on following page

Patient Monitoring and Care —*Continued*

Steps	Rationale	Reportable Conditions
	If the measurements equal or exceed the goals, initiation of weaning trials or extubation may be possible.	• VC less than 10 mL/kg • Any deterioration of patient's condition during measurements that does not immediately respond by returning to mechanical ventilator or bagging

Documentation

Documentation should include the following:
- Patient and family education
- Best values obtained
- Patient's tolerance for the tests

- Unexpected outcomes
- Nursing interventions

References

1. Burns SM, Burns JE, Truwit JD: Comparison of five clinical weaning indices, *Am J Crit Care* 3:342-352, 1994.
2. Burns SM: The science of weaning: when and how? *Crit Care Clin North Am* 16:379-386, 2004.
3. Chevrolet J, Deleamont P: Repeated vital capacity measurements as predictive parameters of mechanical ventilation need and weaning success in the Guillain-Barre syndrome, *Am Rev Respir Dis* 144:814-818, 1991.
4. Cook D, et al: Evidence report on criteria for weaning from mechanical ventilation: contract no. 290-97-0017, Rockville, MD, 1999, Agency for Health Care Policy and Research.
5. Ely EW, et al: Effect on the duration of mechanical ventilation of identifying patients capable of breathing spontaneously, *N Engl J Med* 335:1964-1969, 1996.
6. Kollef MH, et al: A randomized controlled trial of protocol directed versus physician directed weaning from mechanical ventilation, *Crit Care Med* 25:567-574, 1997.
7. Krieger BP, et al: Serial measurements of the rapid shallow breathing index as a predictor of weaning outcome in elderly medical patients, *Chest* 112:1029-1034, 1997.
8. MacIntyre, NR, et al: Evidence-based guidelines for weaning and discontinuing ventilatory support: a collective task force facilitated by the American College of Chest Physicians; the American Association for Respiratory Care; and the American College of Critical Care Medicine, *Chest* 120(6 Suppl):375S-395S, 2001.
9. Mador MJ: Weaning parameters: are they clinically useful? *Chest* 102:1642, 1992.
10. Marelich GP, et al: Protocol weaning of mechanical ventilation in medical and surgical patients by respiratory care practitioners and nurses: effect on weaning time and incidence of ventilator associated pneumonia, *Chest* 118:459-467, 2000.
11. Meade M, Guyett G, Cook D, et al: Predicting success in weaning from mechanical ventilation, *Chest* 120(6S): 400-424, 2001.
12. Yang KL: Reproducibility of weaning parameters: a need for standardization, *Chest* 102:1829-1832, 1992.
13. Yang KL, Tobin MJ: A prospective study of indexes predicting the outcome of trials of weaning from mechanical ventilation, *N Engl J Med* 324:1445-1450, 1991.

Additional Readings

Burns SM: Mechanical ventilation and weaning. In Carlson KK, editor: *AACN advanced critical care nursing,* St Louis 2009, Elsevier.

Burns SM: Weaning from mechanical ventilation. In Burns SM, editor: *AACN protocols for practice: care of mechanically ventilated patients,* ed 2, Boston, 2007, Jones and Bartlett.

Mahanes D, Lewis R: Ventilatory management. *AACN-AANN protocols for practice: monitoring technologies in critically ill neuroscience patients,* Publishers, Boston, 2009, Jones and Bartlett.

Weaning Process

P U R P O S E : The purpose of the weaning process is to liberate patients from mechanical ventilation. Removal of the artificial airway is a desirable outcome of the weaning process but is not essential for liberation from ventilatory support.

Suzanne M. Burns

PREREQUISITE NURSING KNOWLEDGE

- Knowledge and skills related to the care of patients on mechanical ventilation (e.g., airway management, suctioning, mechanical ventilator modes, blood gas interpretation) are necessary.

Short-Term versus Long-Term Mechanical Ventilation

- Short- versus long-term weaning is not clearly defined in the literature. Further, definitions vary in studies, which makes comparisons difficult. Regardless, patients who need mechanical ventilation for longer than 3 consecutive days clearly are at risk of needing mechanical ventilation for 12 to 14 days or longer.[13] As duration of ventilation increases, the risk of iatrogenic (i.e., hospital-acquired) complications increases, all of which lengthen time on the ventilator. To that end, appropriate prophylaxis regimens, interventions designed to improve clinical factors that impede weaning, early assessment of weaning readiness, and protocol-directed weaning trials are essential to good outcomes.

Timing of Tracheostomy Tube Placement

- In some patients, especially those with anticipated long stays on the ventilator (spinal cord injury, progressive neurologic disorders, etc), a tracheostomy tube is placed early in the hospitalization. Other patients may also receive a tracheostomy, especially if they have had multiple unsuccessful attempts at weaning. These patients often have long stays on the ventilator, and weaning trials tend to be accomplished with progressively longer tracheostomy collar trials in comparison with other methods, as described subsequently.

- A recent randomized controlled trial (RCT) suggests that patients with early tracheostomy placement who are considered at risk of 2 weeks of mechanical ventilation have better outcomes if provided with a tracheostomy on day 2 of mechanical ventilation.[40] Although the results are intriguing, they may be attributable to the fact that less sedation is necessary in patients with tracheostomies than in those with endotracheal tubes.[37] As described subsequently, the use of sedation infusions is linked to prolonged ventilator times.

Weaning Assessment

- In the past, the assessment of weaning readiness was accomplished by determining whether or not the patient's condition was stable, the reason for mechanical ventilation was resolved or improving, and the results of selected weaning criteria (or weaning indices) met threshold levels (Tables 37-1 and 37-2; see Procedure 36).[10,41,50] Experts also noted that before weaning trials were initiated, attention to other clinical factors was essential.[12,32] Clinical tools and checklists that ensure systematic attention to these factors help ensure good outcomes, an example of which is found in Table 37-3. In addition, prophylaxis regimes are necessary to prevent complications in patients on ventilation. These complications include ventilator-associated pneumonia (VAP), deep vein thrombosis, gastrointestinal bleeding, and sinusitis. Refer to Procedure 35 for a discussion of VAP prophylaxis and system-specific chapters for the others.

- Unfortunately, weaning indices have proven to be disappointing predictors of a patient's ability to wean.[12,32,35,45]

TABLE 37-1	**Standard Weaning Criteria**

Negative inspiratory pressure, ≤-20 cm H_2O
Positive expiratory pressure, $\geq+30$ cm H_2O
Spontaneous tidal volume, ≥5 mL/kg
Vital capacity, ≥10 to 15 mL/kg
Fraction of inspired oxygen, $\leq50\%$
Minute ventilation, ≤10 L/min

Modified from Burns SM: Mechanical ventilation and weaning. In Kinney MR, et al, editors: AACN clinical reference for critical care nursing, ed 4, St Louis, 1998, Mosby.

TABLE 37-2	**Rapid Shallow Breathing**

fx/Vt

Spontaneous respiratory frequency in 1 minute divided by Vt in liters
fx/Vt > 105 = weaning success
fx/Vt < 105 = weaning failure

fx, Frequency; Vt, tidal volume.
Data from Yang KL, Tobin JM: A prospective study of indexes predicting the outcome of trials of weaning from mechanical ventilation, N Engl J Med 324:1445-50, 1991.

TABLE 37-3	**Burns Weaning Assessment Program (BWAP)***

Patient name _____
Patient history number _____

Yes	No	Not Assessed	
			General Assessment
___	___	___	1. Hemodynamically stable (pulse rate, cardiac output)?
___	___	___	2. Free from factors that increase or decrease metabolic rate (seizures, temperature, sepsis, bacteremia, hypothyroid, hyperthyroid)?
___	___	___	3. Hematocrit $\geq25\%$ (or baseline)?
___	___	___	4. Systemically hydrated (weight at or near baseline, balanced intake and output)?
___	___	___	5. Nourished (albumin 2.5, parenteral/enteral feedings maximized)? (If albumin is low and anasarca or third spacing is present, score for hydration should be "No.")
___	___	___	6. Electrolytes within normal limits (including Ca^{++}, Mg^+, PO_4)? Correct Ca^{++} for albumin level.
___	___	___	7. Pain controlled? (Subjective determination.)
___	___	___	8. Adequate sleep/rest? (Subjective determination.)
___	___	___	9. Appropriate level of anxiety and nervousness? (Subjective determination.)
___	___	___	10. Absence of bowel problems (diarrhea, constipation, ileus)?
___	___	___	11. Improved general body strength/endurance (i.e., out of bed in chair, progressive activity program)?
___	___	___	12. Chest roentgenogram improving?
			Respiratory Assessment
			Gas Flow and Work of Breathing
___	___	___	13. Eupneic respiratory rate and pattern (spontaneous respiratory rate 25, without dyspnea, absence of accessory muscle use). This may be assessed off the ventilator while measuring 20 to 23.
___	___	___	14. Absence of adventitious breath sounds (rhonchi, rales, wheezing)?
___	___	___	15. Secretions thin and minimal?
___	___	___	16. Absence of neuromuscular disease/deformity?
___	___	___	17. Absence of abdominal distention/obesity/ascites?
___	___	___	18. Oral endotracheal tube 7.5 ID or tracheotomy 6.0 ID.
			Airway Clearance
___	___	___	19. Cough and swallow reflexes adequate?
			Strength
___	___	___	20. Negative inspiratory pressure ≤ -20 cm H2O
___	___	___	21. Positive expiratory pressure $\geq + 30$ cm H2O
			Endurance
___	___	___	22. Spontaneous tidal volume ≥5 mL/kg?
___	___	___	23. Vital capacity ≥10 to 15 mL/kg?
			Arterial Blood Gases
___	___	___	24. pH 7.30 to 7.45
___	___	___	25. $Paco_2$ approximately 40 mm Hg (or baseline) with minute ventilation ≤10 L/min (evaluated while on ventilator)
___	___	___	26. Pao_2 60 or Fio_2 $\leq40\%$

*To score the BWAP: Divide the number of "Yes" responses by 26.
Ca^{++}, Calcium; Mg^+, magnesium; *ID,* inside diameter; PO_4, phosphate.
Copyright Burns SM, 1990.

Most predictors focus on pulmonary-specific factors. Some investigators have combined indices and pulmonary factors to enhance the comprehensive nature of the indices and their predictive potential. In general, the indices are poor positive predictors (they do not tell us the patient *will* wean), but they are good negative predictors (they tell us the patient *will not* wean).[13,32,35,45] Thus, use of the indices is not widespread. In fact, the various weaning indices are best used to evaluate the components from which they are designed (breathing pattern, respiratory muscle strength, etc.).

Weaning Process: Weaning Trial Protocols

- The weaning process has changed dramatically as a result of a number of RCTs published in the late 1990s and early 2000s.[7,14,19,26,34,48] The studies showed that protocol-directed spontaneous breathing trials greatly reduced ventilator duration. Additional studies with protocols linked tight glucose control and aggressive sedation management to ventilator duration, intensive care unit (ICU) length of stay (LOS), hospital LOS, and mortality.[4,27,28,47] These protocols are briefly described.

- Protocol-directed multidisciplinary weaning with "weaning screens" and short duration spontaneous breathing trials (SBTs) have been shown to be superior to "individualized" weaning processes.[7,14,19,34,48] The use of the protocols decreases practice variation, perhaps the major reason for their effectiveness. Key to the success of the protocols is the use of the weaning screen, which requires that a minimum of clinical factor thresholds (e.g., hemodynamic stability, fraction of inspired oxygen [Fio_2], positive end-expiratory pressure [PEEP] level) is met.[14] This requirement ensures early and aggressive testing of patient readiness. Once the screen is passed, the patient is placed on a SBT for a short duration. One hour is generally adequate. If signs of intolerance emerge, the patient is returned to ventilatory support and a trial is reattempted at a later time as predetermined by the protocol. See Table 37-4 for an example of a protocol.

Weaning Process: Other Key Elements

- The association between sedation infusion use and negative clinical outcomes of patients on ventilation resulted in studies that tested the efficacy of methods to reduce the use of sedatives in these patients. Two RCTs used nurse-managed methods.[4,27] In a study by Brook and colleagues,[4] a sedation algorithm was used to direct sedation use. Kress and colleagues[27] performed a daily sedation interruption. Both methods resulted in improved outcomes. Concerns about the potential negative impact of abrupt withdrawal of sedation in the critically ill were addressed. One study showed that those who had a daily interruption of sedation sustained significantly less psychologic harm and fewer complications than those who were not provided a daily sedation interruption.[28,43] Additional studies linked sedation use (specifically benzodiazepines) to delirium and subsequent cognitive dysfunction in ICU patients on ventilation.[16-18,39] Current

TABLE 37-4	Example CPAP Protocol

A. Mode
CPAP (0, or low level)

B. Wean Screen
Hemodynamically stable (no vasopressor use or maintenance inotropes only)
Fio_2 less than or equal to 0.5
PEEP less than or equal to 8 cm H_2O

C. Protocol Steps
1. Ensure complete rest the previous night and until the trial begins. (Complete respiratory muscle rest is defined as total cessation of respiratory effort when in assist-control or IMV modes; respiratory rate less than 20 breaths/min with inspiratory Vt of 6 to 10 mL/kg in PSV mode.)
2. Place the patient on selected CPAP level at the same Fio_2 as when ventilated.
3. Trial is from ½ hour to 1 hour (as determined by team).
4. If signs of intolerance develop at any time during the trial, place the patient back on the previous ventilator settings. Make adjustments as necessary to achieve respiratory muscle rest.
5. If the patient tolerates the trial, consider extubation.

D. Intolerance Criteria
1. Respiratory rate increase to 30 breaths/min (sustained).
2. Heart rate increase by 20% (sustained).
3. Oxygen saturation decreases to less than 90% (sustained).
4. Systolic blood pressure > 180 mm Hg or < 90 mm Hg.
5. Agitation.
6. Diaphoresis.
7. Anxiety.
8. Vt less than 5 mL/kg (sustained).
9. Excessive dyspnea (new or unrelated to intermittent activity)
10. Patients are also "rested" and the weaning process held if any of the following conditions apply:
    a. During acute events (e.g., hypotension, bronchospasm)
    b. Intrahospital transports
    c. Temperature spikes
    d. Trendelenburg's position required (e.g., for line placement or other procedures).

Adapted from University of Virginia Protocols.

guidelines on sedation use in critical care incorporate these elements in recommendations for management of both sedation and delirium.[25]

- Another RCT focused on the management of blood glucose in a surgical (mostly cardiac) patient population. In this study, a glucose level maintained at or below 110 g/dL (or 6.1 μmol/L) resulted in decreased sternal wound infections, shortened weaning times, and decreased ICU and hospital LOS. It also significantly reduced in-hospital mortality rates.[47]

- Recently, a multicenter RCT was accomplished that combined sedation interruption with a "wake-up and breathe" trial (i.e., SBT). In this study, patients assigned to the intervention (sedation interruption and wake up) had significantly more days of spontaneous breathing, earlier discharge from the ICU and hospital, and better 1-year survival rates than those in the control group.[22]

See Table 37-5 for summary of protocols for weaning and sedation use.

Adherence to Protocols

- Although the RCTs described show the importance of wean screens, SBTs, sedation management, and tight glucose control to weaning outcomes, studies on the adherence with the same are not encouraging. Adherence studies show that acceptance is low and that the protocols may not be realistic for use in everyday practice[33, 36,38,49]. Given the increasing complexity of the clinical setting and the increasing shortage of ICU nurses and other healthcare professionals, rigorous protocols designed and implemented by study investigators are unlikely to be easily duplicated. We have much to learn in this area.

Modes for Weaning

- We have learned much about methods for weaning, but no specific weaning modes have emerged as superior.[10,12, 19,32,48] As previously noted, SBTs appear to be the best method; most of these use breathing through a T-piece or on the ventilator (with or without the addition of continuous positive airway pressure [CPAP] or other flow mechanisms, such as automatic tube compensation).[14] Regardless, advocates of other modes such as pressure support ventilation (PSV) suggest they may be equally as effective. Although RCTs do not exist to support these hypotheses, evidence-based data exist that may provide rationale for the application of these modes.

Respiratory Muscle Fatigue, Work, Rest, and Conditioning

- The concept of respiratory muscle fatigue must be understood if it is to be prevented in the patient weaning from ventilation. All muscles may fatigue if work exceeds energy stores. Signs and symptoms of impending fatigue include dyspnea, tachypnea, chest-abdominal asynchrony, and increasing arterial partial pressure of carbon dioxide ($Paco_2$, a late sign).[2,11,46] Generally, fatigue may be prevented by avoiding premature or excessively long or difficult weaning trials.

- The concepts of work, rest, and conditioning are useful to consider when selecting weaning modes and methods. Two classifications—high-pressure low-volume work

and low-pressure high-volume work—are essential to the understanding of these three categories.

- ❖ High-pressure low-volume work is associated with the use of a T-piece, CPAP, and low intermittent mandatory ventilation (IMV) rates. Generally, any method that requires that the patient breathe spontaneously (without inspiratory support) results in high-pressure low-volume work. This form of muscle conditioning is thought to build sarcomeres because it uses maximal muscle loading.[30] Conditioning episodes are generally of short duration with full muscle rest between episodes. This type of conditioning is referred to as strengthening training.

- ❖ Low-pressure high-volume work is found with the use of PSV, in which inspiration is augmented. For any given pressure level, workload is less than if the patient were breathing spontaneously. At high levels of PSV, little work occurs, but as the level is reduced, muscle workload increases. Conditioning with PSV often is referred to as endurance conditioning; muscles are not worked to maximal effort. Instead, training focuses on gradual reductions of the level and maintenance of a specific level of work for progressively longer intervals.[5,6,29-31]

- With both types of conditioning, the goal is to progress the trials without inducing fatigue. To that end, rest is that level of ventilatory support that "unloads" the respiratory muscles. The level of support needed may differ with each patient; however, two basic concepts may be useful: 1, when signs of intolerance emerge, the trial is stopped and the patient is rested; and 2, application of rest varies with the weaning mode. For example, if the mode is PSV, then the PSV is increased to that level necessary to decrease the spontaneous rate (e.g., <20/min) and result in a synchronous comfortable breathing pattern. With high-pressure low-volume modes such as CPAP, the patient is returned to full ventilatory support.

Multidisciplinary Approaches

- Weaning is the process of gradual reduction of ventilatory support. To that end, a plan for weaning is determined by the multidisciplinary team and is applied and monitored carefully.[8,9,14,15,23,24,34,44] The plan, whether it uses a protocol or consists of a more individualized

TABLE 37-5	Effect of Protocols for Weaning and Sedation on Selected Outcomes by Author			
Author (Type of Protocol)	**Vent Duration**	**ICU LOS**	**Hospital LOS**	**Mortality**
Kollef et al[26] (weaning protocol)	Yes*	Not reported	No	No
Ely et al[14] (weaning protocol)	Yes*	No	No	No
Marelich et al[34] (weaning protocol)	Yes*	Not reported	Not reported	No
Kress et al[27] (sedation protocol)	Yes*	Yes*	No	No
Brook et al[4] (sedation protocol)	Yes*	Yes*	Yes*	No
Girard et al[22]	Yes*	Yes*	Yes*	1 year survival*

*Statistically significant.

written plan, should be available to all healthcare workers involved in the weaning process. Assessment of weaning potential may include checklists of factors important to weaning, such as the Burns Weaning Assessment Program (BWAP[8-10]; Table 37-3). In addition, prophylaxis for VAP and other potential complications associated with mechanical ventilation must be ensured.
- Outcomes of system initiatives designed to ensure the comprehensive implementation of evidence-based interventions are promising. Advanced practice nurses were used to manage and monitor the conditions of patients in their care.[8,9,24,44] The results suggest that use of such models of care are to be encouraged, but few have been developed, tested, and published (Table 37-6). Further, they tend to compare retrospective with prospective data elements, thus limiting the strength of the evidence. Unfortunately, RCTs of such system initiatives are unlikely to be accomplished in the future.

EQUIPMENT

- Weaning through the ventilator (e.g. CPAP, flow-by, automatic tube compensation ATC) requires that the digital readout of tidal volume and respiratory rate be assessable to the clinician for monitoring purposes
- If T-piece or tracheotomy collar setup is needed, a flow meter with a functional heated aerosol humidifier for the trials is necessary; the setup should have an in-line thermometer and a water trap
- Tracheotomy collar or T-piece adapters
- Personal protective equipment, as appropriate
  - Nonsterile gloves
  - Mask
  - Goggles
  - Gown
- Pressure manometers
- Weaning protocol or wean plan
- Extubation equipment (see Procedures 5 and 6)

PATIENT AND FAMILY EDUCATION

- Explain the procedures and reason for initiation of weaning. **➛Rationale:** Anxiety is reduced when patients are prepared for the sensations they may experience during procedures.
- Reassure the patient of the nurse's or the therapist's presence during initiation of weaning. **➛Rationale:** Assurance of the caregiver's support and monitoring decreases anxiety.
- Discuss the sensations the patient may experience, such as smaller lung inflations, dyspnea, and change or absence of ventilator sounds. Describe that weaning trials are a form of conditioning and do require effort. Some dyspnea is to be expected. **➛Rationale:** Patients (in particular, patients who have been on prolonged positive-pressure ventilation [PPV] support) may report discomfort with resumption of spontaneous breathing.
- Encourage the patient to relax and breathe comfortably. **➛Rationale:** Relaxation decreases muscle tension.
- Assure the patient and family that rapid return to ventilatory support will be accomplished if the patient becomes excessively dyspneic, becomes anxious, or exhibits untoward physiologic changes (e.g., desaturation; blood pressure, heart rate, and rhythm changes; diaphoresis). **➛Rationale:** For trust to develop, the patient and family must believe that the nurse will not allow the trials to harm the patient.

PATIENT ASSESSMENT AND PREPARATION

Patient Assessment

- Regular evaluation of factors that impede weaning in conjunction with factors that measure respiratory muscle strength, endurance, and gas exchange is necessary to ensure that all factors are being addressed appropriately (see Tables 37-1, 37-2, and 37-3). **➛Rationale:** Improvement of factors that impede weaning is essential to the attainment of positive outcomes.
- Assess progress toward achievement of individual short-term goals frequently. **➛Rationale:** Successful weaning may be achieved within a short time (1/2 to 2 hours) if patient response is monitored closely and interventions are applied in tandem with patient response.
- In patients who need mechanical ventilation for very long times (and often need a tracheostomy), assessment of daily progress toward achievement of individual long-term goals is important, in collaboration with the physician, respiratory therapist, patient, and family, as appropriate. **➛Rationale:** Successful weaning may be achieved

TABLE 37-6 Effect of System Initiatives, by Author, on Outcome Variables*

Author/Population/Design	Vent Time	ICU LOS	Hospital LOS	Mortality	Cost
Henneman et al[24] (MICU, pre-post design)	Yes*	Yes*	No	No	No
Smyrnios et al[44] (MICU/SICU/CCU, prospective)	Yes*	Yes*	Yes*	No	Yes
Burns et al[8] (MICU, STICU, TCV-ICU, CCU, NICU, prospective)	Yes*	Yes*	Yes*	Yes*	Yes

*Statistically significant).
MICU, Medical ICU; *SICU,* surgical ICU; *CCU,* coronary care unit; *STICU,* surgical-trauma ICU; *NICU,* neuroscience ICU *TCV:* thoracic-cardiovascular ICU

within days to weeks in these patients if patient response is methodically evaluated and interventions are applied in tandem with patient response.

- Observe breathing pattern and note symptoms of dyspnea in response to decrements in PPV support. Other signs of fatigue include the following:
  - ❖ Accessory muscle use
  - ❖ Chest or abdominal asynchrony
  - ❖ Retractions
  - ❖ Rapid shallow breathing pattern
  - ➥*Rationale:* These are signs and symptoms of potential or actual respiratory muscle fatigue. Interventions to offset the work of breathing are necessary.
- Note whether the patient experiences changes in level of consciousness or nonverbal behavior and has symptoms of dyspnea or fatigue. ➥*Rationale:* Work of breathing may be such that the patient is maintaining an adequate breathing pattern and gas exchange at the moment but does not have sufficient reserves to continue expending energy to breathe. Patient exhaustion during weaning results in psychologic and physiologic delays in the weaning progress.
- Assess arterial blood gases as needed. ➥*Rationale:* Although frequent arterial blood gas assessments are rarely necessary during weaning if active attention is paid to signs and symptoms of intolerance, arterial blood gases are the only definitive method of evaluating efficiency of gas exchange. Evaluate of $Paco_2$ is especially important with spontaneous breathing if rapid return to increased ventilatory settings is not part of the plan or if dramatic changes in the patient's condition are seen. $Paco_2$ is the definitive indicator of the adequacy of ventilation. $Paco_2$ (and pH) within the patient's normal physiologic range indicates that the patient's spontaneous ventilation is adequate. Weaning protocols are extremely helpful in that they identify intolerance criteria so that if they should emerge, return to ventilatory support may be prompt.
- Assess end-tidal carbon dioxide ($Petco_2$) levels. ➥*Rationale:* $Petco_2$ levels are best used to trend CO_2 levels. It is important to know the $Paco_2$ level that corresponds to the $Petco_2$ level to use the $Petco_2$ values most efficiently. Remember that the $Petco_2$ values vary depending on the size of the breath. Larger tidal volume breaths provide more accurate values; the $Paco_2$ $Petco_2$-difference is less than when the tidal volumes are small. With small tidal volumes, there is more dead space ventilation and the $Paco_2$ $Petco_2$- difference is larger, which makes accurate trending difficult. This is especially the case during a spontaneous breathing trial when breath size varies. See Procedure 15 on $Petco_2$ for more in-depth information.

- Assess oxygenation indices (see Procedure 33) during trials: arterial oxygen saturation (Sao_2) or arterial partial pressure of oxygen (Pao_2). ➥*Rationale:* Sao_2 is a real-time continuous indicator of oxygenation during weaning trials and should be monitored continually. A saturation of greater than or equal to 90% generally indicates oxygenation adequacy. Pao_2 is the definitive indicator of the adequacy of oxygenation and, in some cases, is required. A Pao_2 within the patient's normal physiologic range indicates that the patient's oxygenation is adequate with spontaneous breathing. Generally, Pao_2 greater than 60 mm Hg and Sao_2 greater than or equal to 90% on a fraction of inspired oxygen (Fio_2) of less than or equal to 0.4 is acceptable during trials.
- Assess patient anxiety level. ➥*Rationale:* Resumption of spontaneous breathing may cause anxiety, particularly in patients who have been on prolonged PPV support. Encouragement is necessary, in addition to assurance that prompt return to ventilatory support will be accomplished, if the patient becomes excessively tired, anxious, or otherwise distressed. Patients must trust that the healthcare workers will address their concerns competently and rapidly during weaning trials.

Patient Preparation

- Verify correct patient with two identifiers. ➥*Rationale:* Prior to performing a procedure, the nurse should ensure the correct identification of the patient for the intended intervention.
- Ensure that the patient understands preprocedural teachings. Answer questions as they arise, and reinforce information as needed. ➥*Rationale:* This communication evaluates and reinforces understanding of previously taught information.
- Address factors that are impeding wean potential. These factors may include pH level, hemodynamic stability, electrolytes, strength, endurance, mobility, nutrition, and fluid status, to name a few. A systematic approach with use of a checklist helps avoid variation in practice. ➥*Rationale:* Weaning has been associated with the correction of a myriad of physiologic factors. Weaning is not solely dependent on respiratory muscle strength and endurance.
- Establish weaning screen criteria. ➥*Rationale:* Weaning screen criteria are essential for the rapid and safe assessment of weaning trial readiness.
- Wean trial duration should be set before beginning the trial. ➥*Rationale:* Prolonged SBTs may fatigue the patient and result in poor outcomes. All key bedside caregivers must be aware of the limits of the trial and when to stop should signs of intolerance emerge.

Procedure for Weaning Trial

Steps	Rationale	Special Considerations
1. VP		
2. HH		
3. PE		
4. Position the patient for optimal ventilation.		
5. Communicate with the patient and family throughout the weaning process.	Attention is given to the patient's subjective response to weaning. The clinician remains with the patient (especially at the beginning of the trial); monitors frequently during trials; coaches the patient; reinforces the goals and desired outcomes; reminds the patient that talking, eating, self-care activities, and mobilization are facilitated by successful weaning and extubation; and celebrates weaning progress with the patient and family.	

T-Piece or Tracheotomy Collar Trials

Steps	Rationale	Special Considerations
1. Connect patient to heated aerosol via T-piece or tracheostomy collar. Inform the patient that the trial will feel different than when on the ventilator and to try to breathe normally. Monitor respiratory frequency, breathing pattern, heart rate, cardiac rhythm, SaO_2, and general appearance of patient.	Heated aerosol replaces water that normally would be added by the upper airway if it were not bypassed by the endotracheal or tracheostomy tube. This method of weaning uses high-pressure low-volume work. High-volume low-pressure work is best accomplished in short duration trials (i.e., 1 hour). Longer trials may unduly tire the patient. Signs and symptoms of tolerance must be heeded if respiratory muscle fatigue is to be prevented.[5,11]	Abort weaning for any signs of patient intolerance and place patient back on PPV support. Patients with tracheostomies may be those who have been tested repeatedly but in whom the short trials have been unsuccessful. In these patients who are *chronically critically ill* and on ventilation, tracheostomy trials are lengthened gradually over days or even weeks. A common method of weaning includes gradually longer spontaneous breathing trials during the day with rest periods between trials. Once the spontaneous breathing trial is successful for 10 to 12 consecutive hours, extension of the trials may progress to nighttime hours. Other factors that focus on rehabilitation (mobility, etc.) are addressed concomitantly.
2. After a predetermined time interval or with the emergence of signs of intolerance, place patient back on resting ventilator settings. **(Level B*)**	To ensure respiratory muscle conditioning and forward progress during weaning trials, the work of breathing must not be excessive; do not exceed predetermined wean trial duration. Adequate rest between trials and at night offsets fatigue and encourages effective respiratory muscle conditioning. Patient is placed back on the ventilator to rest until all data regarding weaning response can be assessed.[5,11]	

*Level B: Well-designed, controlled studies with results that consistently support a specific action, intervention, or treatment

Procedure continues on following page

Procedure for Weaning Trial—*Continued*

Steps	Rationale	Special Considerations
3. If patient successfully meets full trial criteria, notify physician or advanced practice nurse and team regarding patient's response, and consider extubation. If a protocol is in place, extubation may be the next step and may not require such notification.		

CPAP Trials (Levels 0 to 10 cm H_2O)

Steps	Rationale	Special Considerations
1. Explain purpose and procedure to patient and family, and switch patient from resting settings to CPAP level. Instruct the patient to breathe normally, and monitor for signs and symptoms of intolerance (described previously). With use of protocol, refer to specific criteria. **(Level B*)**	As with the T-piece, this method uses high-pressure low-volume work. Prompt return to the ventilator is necessary if excessive work and fatigue are to be prevented.[1,3,5,11,21,42,46]	An advantage of CPAP over T-piece trials is that tidal volume (Vt) and respiratory rate are monitored easily throughout the trial by means of the digital display on the ventilator. Alarms, such as a low minute ventilation alarm, may be set with a CPAP trial.
2. After predetermined time interval on CPAP or with signs or symptoms of intolerance, place patient back on resting ventilator settings. **(Level B)**	Do not exceed predetermined wean trial duration. Adequate rest between trials and at night offsets fatigue and encourages effective respiratory muscle conditioning. The patient is placed back on the ventilator to rest until all data regarding weaning response can be assessed.[5,11,14,46]	
3. Notify the physician, advanced practice nurse, or team of results of trials. If last step of wean plan or protocol has been attained, extubation should be considered. (If protocol is used, this step may be automatic.)		

Synchronized Intermittent Mandatory Ventilation Weaning Method

Steps	Rationale	Special Considerations
1. Gradually and progressively decrease synchronized intermittent mandatory ventilation (SIMV) breaths. **(Level B)**	This method of weaning provides a gradual reduction of ventilator support. The preset breaths are progressively decreased as the patient assumes a greater proportion of the minute volume with spontaneous breathing.	Some SIMV demand valves offer high resistance to spontaneous breathing. Work of breathing may be greatly increased and fatigue may ensue, especially at low IMV rates (e.g. 4/min).[1,3,21,42] To avoid this, PSV is commonly used between IMV breaths to offset the work associated with small tube sizes, circuit resistance, and high breathing rates.[6,30] This method of weaning has been associated with prolonged weaning trial duration in at least one study.[20]

*Level B: Well-designed, controlled studies with results that consistently support a specific action, intervention, or treatment

Procedure   for **Weaning Trial**—*Continued*

Steps	Rationale	Special Considerations
		The method has largely been replaced with SBTs with T-piece or CPAP because they are easier to accomplish. This decreases variation in practice. If this mode is used, a plan must be in place for progressive weaning and a clinical end point must be predetermined.
2. Assess the patient for signs and symptoms of fatigue, inadequate gas exchange, and impaired breathing pattern with decreases in SIMV rate. **(Level B*)**	Determines patient response to weaning. A plan that clearly describes the end point of this method is essential.[8-10,12,14,23,24,26]	Lower levels of IMV (i.e., less than or equal to 4/min), when not used with PSV, are similar to strength-conditioning trials. Adequate rest times should be ensured between trials and especially at night.
Pressure Support Weaning Method		
1. Start at pressure support maximum (PSVmax) and decrease level according to the protocol or as clinically indicated (i.e., no signs of intolerance). **(Level B)**	This weaning method provides for endurance conditioning; to that end, the level is decreased gradually as patient's endurance increases. PSVmax is the level that attains a spontaneous respiratory rate of less than or equal to 20 breaths/min, absence of accessory muscle use, and a Vt of 6 to 10 mL/kg.[5,6,29] Higher respiratory rates and smaller Vt values are generally acceptable during trials. Because the mode uses low-pressure high-volume work, weaning intervals may be longer than with strengthening modes.[5,6,29] Regardless, full support should be ensured at night and for rest, especially early in the weaning stage.	Work is increased gradually by lowering the level of PSV in increments. Caution with high levels of PSV should be used with patients who have obstructive lung conditions because the higher levels may promote overdistention and air trapping.
2. Monitor patient responses to weaning. Return to full ventilatory support if signs of intolerance occur and when intended duration of trial has been reached. **(Level B)**	PSV, despite requiring spontaneous effort, reduces the work of breathing associated with circuits, endotracheal tubes, and high breathing rates.[29] Fatigue is possible if the level is not appropriately selected.[5,6] PSV at higher levels can unload the respiratory muscles and provide respiratory muscle rest.[5,6,29]	An incompletely inflated artificial airway cuff can create a leak that prevents the PSV cycle-off mechanism from activating (i.e., the ventilator cycles off when it senses that flow is one fourth the original flow). If this decrement of flow is not recognized, the result is an inappropriately long inspiratory time.
3. When the clinical goal for PSV wean is accomplished, extubation is discussed with the physician, advanced practice nurse, and team.	If protocol is used, the next step may be automatic.	
4. Remove personal protective equipment. HH		

*Level B: Well-designed, controlled studies with results that consistently support a specific action, intervention, or treatment

Procedure continues on following page

Expected Outcomes

- Timely and successful discontinuance of PPV
- Comfortable and adequate breathing pattern during the weaning process

Unexpected Outcomes

- Tracheal injury
- Pulmonary barotrauma
- Cardiovascular depression
- Fatigue
- Hypoxemia
- Hypercapnia
- Dyspnea
- Unsuccessful, demoralizing weaning trials

Patient Monitoring and Care

Steps	Rationale	Reportable Conditions
		These conditions should be reported if they persist despite nursing interventions.
1. Evaluate overall patient stability (i.e., physiologic, psychologic, and mechanical) in a systematic manner. Frequency of evaluation may vary depending on how long the patient has been on the ventilator and the patient's psychologic and physiologic stability. A multidisciplinary approach is encouraged.	Patient stability and overall condition must be considered before initiating active weaning trials. A weaning screen is used as a minimum threshold for attempting a trial. Premature attempts may be a harmful and frustrating for all involved, yet delayed weaning results in negative outcomes. Thus, use of a weaning screen helps identify potential early in the process and should be used. A multidisciplinary team approach ensures active attention to the diverse factors that affect weaning readiness. See Tables 37-1, 37-2, and 37-3.	• Changes that suggest physiologic instability should result in a return to ventilatory support until the patient's condition is stable
2. During weaning trials, pay particular attention to signs and symptoms of intolerance and respiratory muscle fatigue. If signs of intolerance occur, prompt return to PPV is necessary.	Trials continued despite emergence of signs of intolerance lead to fatigue and failure. Cardiopulmonary failure and collapse are potential outcomes.	• Signs of weaning trial intolerance (tachypnea, dyspnea, chest and abdominal asynchrony) • Agitation • Mental status changes • Significant decrease in Sao_2 (Sao_2 less than 90% or 10% decrease) • Changes in pulse rate or rhythm • Blood pressure increase or decrease
3. If no signs of intolerance occur during trials, continue until the patient successfully achieves the trial criteria and report results to the physician, advanced practice nurse, and team so that additional planning can occur (e.g., extubation) or follow protocol steps to extubation.		

Documentation

Documentation should include the following:

- Patient and family education
- Individualized goals for weaning
- Procedure used for weaning (e.g., T-piece, decreasing IMV/SIMV support, pressure support)
- Parameters used to assess patient readiness to wean and weaning trial tolerance, including a wide variety of clinical indicators (discussed previously)

- Patient response to decrements in mechanical ventilation support
- Mode or method of weaning
- Duration of trial
- Level of support (if appropriate, as in PSV, flow-by, or CPAP)
- Unexpected outcomes

References

CR 1. Banner MJ, Blanch PB, Kirby RR: Imposed work of breathing and methods of triggering a demand-flow continuous positive airway system, *Crit Care Med* 21: 183-190, 1993.

CR 2. Bellemare F, Grassino A: Evaluation of human diaphragm fatigue, *J Appl Physiol* 53:1196-206, 1982.

3. Beydon L, et al: Inspiratory work of breathing during spontaneous ventilation using demand valves and continuous flow systems, *Am Rev Respir Dis* 138:300-304, 1988.

CR 4. Brook AD, Ahrens TS, Schaff R, et al: Effect of a nursing-implemented sedation protocol on the duration of mechanical ventilation, *Crit Care Med* 27:2609-2615, 1999.

CR 5. Brochard L, et al: Inspiratory pressure support prevents diaphragmatic fatigue during weaning from mechanical ventilation, *Am Rev Respir Dis* 139:513-521, 1989.

CR 6. Brochard L, Pluskwa F, Lemaire F: Improved efficacy of spontaneous breathing with inspiratory pressure support, *Am Rev Respir Dis* 136:411-415, 1987.

CR 7. Brochard L, et al: Comparison of three methods of gradual withdrawal from ventilatory support during weaning from mechanical ventilation, *Am J Respir Crit Care* 150:896-903, 1994.

CR 8. Burns SM, et al: Implementation of an institutional program to improve clinical and financial outcomes of patients requiring mechanical ventilation: one year outcomes and lessons learned, *Crit Care Med* 31: 2752-2763, 2003.

CR 9. Burns SM, et al: Design, testing and results of an outcomes-managed approach to patients requiring prolonged ventilation, *Am J Crit Care* 7:45-47, 1998.

10. Burns SM: The science of weaning: when and how? *Crit Care Nurs Clin North Am* 16:379-386, 2004.

CR 11. Cohen CA, et al: Clinical manifestations of inspiratory muscle fatigue, *Am J Med* 73:308-316, 1982.

CR 12. Cook D, et al: *Evidence report on criteria for weaning from mechanical ventilation: contract no. 290-97-0017,* Rockville, MD, 1999, Agency for Health Care Policy and Research.

CR 13. Douglas SL, Daly BJ, Gordon N, et al: Survival and quality of life: short-term versus long-term ventilator patients, *Crit Care Med* 30:2655-2662, 2002.

CR 14. Ely EW, et al: Effect on the duration of mechanical ventilation of identifying patients capable of breathing spontaneously, *N Engl J Med* 335:1864-1869, 1998.

CR 15. Ely EW, Bennett PA, Bowton DL, et al: Large scale implementation of a respiratory therapist-driven protocol for ventilator weaning, *Am J Respir Crit Care Med* 159:439-446, 1999.

CR 16. Ely EW, Margolin R, Francis J, et al: Evaluation of delirium in critically ill patients: validation of the Confusion Assessment Method for the Intensive Care Unit (CAM-ICU), *Crit Care Med* 29:1370-1379, 2001.

CR 17. Ely EW, Gautam S, Margolin R, et al: The impact of delirium in the intensive care unit on hospital length of stay, *Intensive Care Med* 27:1892-1900, 2001.

CR 18. Ely EW, Shintani A, Truman B, et al: Delirium as a predictor of mortality in mechanically ventilated patients in the intensive care unit, *JAMA* 291:1753-1762, 2004.

CR 19. Esteban A, et al: A comparison of four methods of weaning patients from mechanical ventilation, *N Engl J Med* 332:345-350, 1995.

CR 20. Esteban A, et al, and the Spanish Lung Failure Collaborative Group: Modes of mechanical ventilation and weaning: a national survey of Spanish hospitals, *Chest* 106: 1188-1193, 1994.

CR 21. Gibney NRT, Wilson RS, Pontoppidan H: Comparison of work of breathing on high gas flow and demand valve continuous positive airway pressure systems, *Chest* 82: 1982.

22. Girard TD, Kress JP, Fuchs BD, et al: Efficacy and safety of a paired sedation and ventilator weaning protocol for mechanically ventilated patients in intensive care (Awakening and Breathing Controlled trial): a randomised controlled trial, *Lancet* 371:126-134, 2008.

CR 23. Grap MJ, Strickland D, Tormay L, et al: Collaborative practice: development, implementation, and evaluation of a weaning protocol for patients receiving mechanical ventilation, *Am J Crit Care* 12:454-460, 2003.

CR 24. Henneman E, et al: Using a collaborative weaning plan to decrease duration of mechanical ventilation and length of stay in the intensive care unit for patients receiving long-term mechanical ventilation, *Am J Crit Care* 11: 132-140, 2002.

CR 25. Jacobi J, Fraser GL, Coursin DB, et al: Clinical practice guidelines for the sustained use of sedatives and analgesics in the critically ill adult, *Crit Care Med* 30:119-141, 2002.

CR 26. Kollef MH, et al: A randomized, controlled trial of protocol-directed versus physician-directed weaning from mechanical ventilation, *Crit Care Med* 25:557-574, 1997.

CR 27. Kress JP, Pohlman AS, O'Conner MF, et al: Daily interruption of sedative infusions in critically ill patients undergoing mechanical ventilation, *N Engl J Med* 342:1471-1477, 2000.

CR 28. Kress JP, Gehlbach B, Lacy M, et al: The long-term psychological effects of daily sedative interruption on critically ill patients, *Am J Respir Crit Care Med* 168:1457-1461, 2003.

CR 29. MacIntyre NR: Respiratory function during pressure support ventilation, *Chest* 89:677-683, 1986.

CR 30. MacIntyre NR: Weaning from mechanical ventilatory support: volume-assisting intermittent breaths versus pressure assisting every breath, *Respir Care* 33:121-125, 1988.

CR 31. MacIntyre NR: Ventilatory modes and mechanical ventilatory support, *Crit Care Med* 25:1106-1107, 1997.

CR 32. MacIntyre NR, et al: Evidence-based guidelines for weaning and discontinuing ventilatory support: a collective task force facilitated by the American College of Chest Physicians; the American Association for Respiratory Care; and the American College of Critical Care Medicine, *Chest* 120(6 Suppl):375S-395S, 2001.

33. Malesker MA, Foral PA, McPhillips AC, et al: An efficiency evaluation of protocols for tight glycemic control in intensive care units, *Am J Crit Care* 16:589-598, 2007.

CR 34. Marelich GP, Murin S, Battistela F, et al: Protocol weaning of mechanical ventilation in medical and surgical patients by respiratory care practitioners and nurses: effect on weaning time and ventilator associated pneumonia, *Chest* 118:459-467, 2000.

CR 35. Meade M, Guyatt G, Cook D, et al: Predicting success in weaning from mechanical ventilation, *Chest* 120(6 Suppl):400S-424S, 2001.

36. Metha S, Burry L, Fischer S, et al: Canadian survey of the use of sedatives, analgesics, and neuromuscular blocking agents in critically ill patients, *Crit Care Med* 34:374-380, 2006.

37. Nieszkowska A, Combes A, Luyt C, et al: Impact of tracheotomy on sedative administration, sedation level, and comfort of mechanically ventilated intensive care unit patients, *Crit Care Med* 33:2527-2533, 2005.

38. Oeyen SG, Hoste EA, Roosens CD, et al: Adherence to and efficacy and safety of an insulin protocol in the critically ill: a prospective observational study, *AJCC* 16:599-608, 2007.

39. Pandharipande P, Shintani A, Peterson J, et al: Lorazepam is an independent risk factor for transitioning to delirium in intensive care unit patients, *Anesthesiology* 104:21-26, 2006.

CR 40. Rumbak MJ, Newton M, Truncale T, et al: A prospective, randomized study comparing early percutaneous dilational tracheotomy to prolonged translaryngeal intubation (delayed tracheotomy) in critically ill medical patients, *Crit Care Med* 32:1689-1694, 2004.

CR 41. Sahn SA, Lakshminarayan S: Bedside criteria for discontinuation of mechanical ventilation, *Chest* 63:1002-1005, 1973.

CR 42. Sassoon CSH, et al: Inspiratory muscle work of breathing during flow-by, demand-flow, and continuous-flow systems in patients with chronic obstructive pulmonary disease, *Am Rev Respir Dis* 145:1219-1222, 1992.

CR 43. Schweickert WD, Gehlbach BK, Pohlman AS, et al: Daily interruptions of sedative infusions and complications of critical illness in mechanically ventilated patients, *Crit Care Med* 32:1272-1276, 2004.

CR 44. Smyrnios NA, et al: Effects of a multifaceted, multidisciplinary, hospital-wide quality improvement program on weaning from mechanical ventilation, *Crit Care Med* 30:1224-1230, 2002.

45. Tanios MA, Nevins ML, Hendra KP, et al: A randomized controlled trial of the role of weaning predictors in clinical decision making, *Crit Care Med* 34:2530-2535, 2006.

CR 46. Tobin MJ, et al: Konno-Mead analysis of ribcage-abdominal motion during successful and unsuccessful trials of weaning from mechanical ventilation, *Am Rev Respir Dis* 135:1320-1328, 1987.

CR 47. Van den Berghe G, Wouters P, Weekers F, et al: Intensive insulin therapy in critically ill patients, *N Engl J Med* 354:1359-1367, 2001.

CR 48. Vitacca M, Vianello A, Colombo D, et al: Comparison of two methods for weaning COPD patients requiring mechanical ventilation for more than 15 days, *Am J Respir Crit Care Med* 164: 225-230, 2001.

49. Weinert CR, Calvin AD: Epidemiology of sedation and sedation adequacy for mechanically ventilated patients in a medical and surgical intensive care unit, *Crit Care Med* 35:393-401, 2007.

CR 50. Yang KL, Tobin JM: A prospective study of indexes predicting the outcome of trials of weaning from mechanical ventilation, *N Engl J Med* 324:1445-1450, 1994.

Additional Readings

Burns SM: Mechanical ventilation and weaning. In Carlson K, editor: *AACN's advanced critical care nursing,* St Louis, 2009, Elsevier.

Burns SM: Practice protocol: weaning from mechanical ventilation. In Burns S, editor: *AACN protocols for practice series: care of the mechanically ventilated patient,* ed 2, Sudbury, 2007, Jones and Bartlett.

Burns SM: Weaning from mechanical ventilation. In Pierce LNB, editor: *Management of the mechanically ventilated patient,* ed 2, St Louis, 2007, Elsevier.

Pierce LNB, editor: *Management of the mechanically ventilated patient,* ed 2, St Louis, 2007, Elsevier.

Tobin MJ: *Principles and practice of mechanical ventilation,* ed 2, New York, 2006, McGraw-Hill.

Peripheral Nerve Stimulators

P U R P O S E : Peripheral nerve stimulators are used in association with the administration of neuromuscular blocking drugs to assess nerve impulse transmission at the neuromuscular junction of select skeletal muscles.

Janet G. Whetstone Foster

PREREQUISITE NURSING KNOWLEDGE

- Peripheral nerve stimulators (PNSs) are used in association with the administration of neuromuscular blocking drugs (NMBDs) to block skeletal muscle activity.
- NMBDs are given in the intensive care unit, along with sedatives and opioids, most commonly to coordinate contemporary modes of mechanical ventilation with breathing in patients with severe lung injury. Neuromuscular blocking agents are also used to assist with the management of increased intracranial pressure after a head injury; for severe muscle spasms associated with seizures, tetanus, and drug overdose; to reduce intraabdominal hypertension[1]; in hypothermia protocols for cardiac arrest[6]; and for preservation of delicate reconstructive surgery.
- NMBDs do not affect sensation or level of consciousness. Because NMBDs lack amnesic, sedative, and analgesic properties, sedatives and analgesics should *always* be given concurrently to minimize the patient's awareness of blocked muscle activity and discomfort. Sedatives and analgesics should be initiated *before* NMBDs because neuromuscular blockade hinders the assessment of anxiety and pain.[5]
- Numerous medications, such as aminoglycosides and other antibiotics, beta blockers, calcium channel blockers, corticosteroids, and anesthetics, and conditions, such as acidosis and various electrolyte imbalances, potentiate the effects of neuromuscular blocking agents. Thus, the level of blockade is subject to variation, which necessitates vigilant monitoring with a PNS and titration of the NMBD.[6]

- The muscle twitch response to a small electrical stimulus delivered by the PNS corresponds to an estimated number of nerve receptors blocked by the NMBDs and assists the clinician in the assessment and titration of the medication dosage. The level of blockade is estimated by observing the muscle twitch after stimulating the appropriate nerve with a small electrical current delivered by the PNS.
- The train-of-four (TOF) method of stimulation is most commonly used for ongoing monitoring of NMBD use. After delivery of four successive stimulating currents to a select peripheral nerve with the PNS, in the absence of significant neuromuscular blockade, four muscle twitches follow. The four twitches signify that 75% or fewer of the receptors are blocked. Three twitches correspond to approximately 80% blockade, and two to one twitches in response to four stimulating currents correlate with approximately 85% to 90% blockade of the neuromuscular junction receptors.[9] One to two twitches is the recommended level of block, although the appropriate level has not yet been determined through research in the critically ill population.[5] Absence of twitches may indicate that 100% of receptors are blocked, which exceeds the desired level of blockade (Table 38-1).
- The stimulating current is measured in milliamperes (mA). The usual range of mA required to stimulate a peripheral nerve and elicit a muscle twitch is 20 to 50 mA, although increasing the current to 70 or 80 mA may be necessary, especially in the obese patient.[9]
- Some stimulators do not indicate the mA. Instead, digital or dialed numbers ranging from 1 to 10 represent the range of mA from 20 to 80 mA. With use of these instruments, the usual setting is 2 to 5, although a setting of 10 is sometimes necessary. Other stimulators (with and without digital

TABLE 38-1	Train-of-Four Stimulation as a Correlation of Blocked Nerve Receptors
TOF (No. of Twitches)	Percent of Receptors Blocked (Approximately)[7]
0/4	100
1/4	90
2/4	85
3/4	80
4/4	75 or less

Nagelhout JJ, Naglaniczny KL: Nurse anesthesia, ed 3, Philadelphia, 2004, Saunders.

displays) automatically adjust the voltage output relative to resistance and deliver the current accordingly.[10]

- The ulnar nerve in the wrist is recommended for testing, although the facial and the posterior tibial nerves may also be used.
- Peripheral nerve monitoring is used in conjunction with the assessment of clinical goals, and *clinical decisions should never be made solely on the basis of the twitch response.*
- Titration of the drugs according to clinical assessment and muscle twitch response may help provide a sufficient level of blockade without overshooting the goal. Overshooting the level of blockade with use of excessive doses of NMBDs is of special concern in the critically ill patient because it may predispose the patient to prolonged paralysis and muscle weakness, reported extensively in the literature.[6] Monitoring with a PNS during the administration of NMBDs results in the use of less medication, hastens recovery of spontaneous ventilation, and accelerates restoration of neuromuscular transmission (NMT),[2] which is necessary for resumption of muscle activity. Although some patients have severe muscle weakness after neuromuscular blockade, peripheral nerve monitoring during NMBD therapy facilitates prompt recovery of NMT when therapy is terminated.[2]

EQUIPMENT

- Peripheral nerve stimulator
- Two pre-gelled electrode pads (the same as is used for electrocardiography monitoring)
- Two lead wires packaged with the peripheral nerve stimulator
- Alcohol pads for skin degreasing and cleansing
  Additional equipment, as needed, includes the following:
- A bipolar touch stimulator probe may be substituted for the pre-gelled electrodes and lead wires
- Scissors or clippers if hair removal is necessary

PATIENT AND FAMILY EDUCATION

- Explain the purpose of peripheral nerve monitoring, for example, assessing the effect and guiding the dosage of drug. ➤➤*Rationale:* This explanation may decrease anxiety.

- Describe the equipment to be used. ➤➤*Rationale:* This description may decrease anxiety.
- Reassure the patient and family that medications for sedation and analgesia are provided throughout this therapy so the patient is comfortable while paralyzed. ➤➤*Rationale:* Reassurance that the patient's pain and anxiety will be treated during therapy is provided.
- Describe the experience of the stimuli as a slight prickly sensation. ➤➤*Rationale:* The use of sensation descriptors is effective in reducing anxiety.
- Explain that the electrodes require periodic changing, which feels like removing an adhesive-backed bandage. ➤➤*Rationale:* This explanation may elicit decreased anxiety.

PATIENT ASSESSMENT AND PREPARATION

Patient Assessment

- Verify correct patient with two identifiers. ➤➤*Rationale:* Prior to performing a procedure, the nurse should ensure the correct identification of the patient for the intended intervention.
- Assess the patient for the best location for electrode placement. Consider criteria such as edema, fat, hair, diaphoresis, wounds, dressings, and arterial and venous catheters. ➤➤*Rationale:* This assessment improves conduction of stimulating current through dermal tissue.
- Assess the patient for history or presence of hemiplegia, hemiparesis, or peripheral neuropathy. ➤➤*Rationale:* Motor response to nerve stimulation of the affected limb may be diminished; receptors may be resistant to NMBDs and lead to excess doses.[9]
- Assess whether burns are present or whether topical ointments are being used. ➤➤*Rationale:* In patients with burns or topical ointments, for whom electrode adherence is difficult, a bipolar touch probe may be more effective than the electrode pads and lead wires. Poor electrode adherence interferes with the conduction of the stimulating current.

Patient Preparation

- Ensure that the patient and family understand pre-procedural teachings. Answer questions as they arise and reinforce information as needed. ➤➤*Rationale:* Evaluates and reinforces understanding of previously taught information.
- Clip hair at the electrode placement sites if necessary. ➤➤*Rationale:* This action improves electrode contact, which facilitates current flow to the nerve.
- Cleanse skin and degrease with alcohol. ➤➤*Rationale:* Cleansing improves electrode contact, which facilitates current flow to the nerve
- Apply the electrodes and test the TOF response to determine the adequacy of the location before initiating administration of an NMBD. In an emergent situation, testing the TOF response before the administration of an NMBD may not be possible. ➤➤*Rationale:* Testing improves the reliability of the interpretation of the TOF response.

- Whenever possible, determine the supramaximal stimulation (SMS) level before initiating NMBDs. The SMS is the level at which additional stimulating current elicits no further increase in the intensity of the four twitches. In an emergent situation, determination of the SMS level before the administration of an NMBD may not be possible. →*Rationale:* This determination helps establish adequate stimulating current and improves reliability of testing.

Procedures for Peripheral Nerve Stimulators

Steps	Rationale	Special Considerations
Testing the Ulnar Nerve		
1. **HH**		
2. **PE**		
3. Extend the arm, palm up, in a relaxed position; cleanse with alcohol pad (Fig. 38-1).	The ulnar nerve is superficial and easy to locate; degreasing increases conduction.	
4. Apply two pre-gelled electrodes over the path of the ulnar nerve (see Fig. 38-1). Place the distal electrode on the skin at the flexor crease on the ulnar surface of the wrist, as close to the nerve as possible. Place the second electrode approximately 1 to 2 cm proximal to the first, parallel to the flexor carpi ulnaris tendon. **(Level E*)**	Enables stimulation of the ulnar nerve. Skin resistance causes the greatest impediment to current flow, which can be reduced through clean dry skin and secure electrodes. The electrode gel enhances conduction. Maintaining the electrodes as close as possible in alignment with the nerve minimizes artifact from direct muscle stimulation.[9]	Ensure that the patient's wrist is clean and dry.
5. Use caution in selecting the site of the electrode placement to avoid direct stimulation of the muscle rather than the nerve. **(Level E)**	Direct muscle stimulation elicits a response similar to the TOF, which makes evaluation of blocked nerve impulse transmission difficult.	In patients with hemiplegia, place the electrodes on the unaffected limb because resistance to NMBDs on the affected side may lead to excess doses.[9] In patients with limbs immobilized from orthopedic casts, use the unaffected limb because possible resistance to some NMBDs on the affected limb may lead to excess doses.[4]
6. Plug the lead wires into the nerve stimulator, matching the negative (black) and positive (red) leads to the black and red connection sites.	Necessary for the conduction of electrical current.	
7. Attach the lead wires to the electrodes. Connect the negative (black) lead to the distal electrode over the crease in the palmar aspect of the wrist. Connect the positive (red) lead to the proximal electrode.	Prepares the equipment.	
8. Turn on the PNS and select the current determined by the SMS or, if not performed, a low current (10 to 20 mA is typical).	Excessive current results in overstimulation and can cause repetitive nerve firing.	Patients with diabetes mellitus may need higher stimulating current than patients without diabetes because of impaired motor nerve fibers and nerve endings.[8]

*Level E: Multiple case reports, theory-based evidence from expert opinions, or peer-reviewed professional organizational standards without clinical studies to support recommendations

Procedure continues on following page

Procedures | for Peripheral Nerve Stimulators—*Continued*

Steps	Rationale	Special Considerations
9. Depress the TOF key; through tactile assessment, determine twitching of the thumb and count the number of twitches. Do not count finger movements, only the thumb.	Finger movements result from direct muscle stimulation. The quality of the twitches may be subtle and decrease in amplitude with increasing edema; detection with tactile methods increases sensitivity and accuracy.	Placing the operator's hand over the fingers helps reduce interpretation of artifactual movement. Use the dominant hand for tactile assessment because it may more accurately detect the TOF response.
10. Maintain a consistent current with each stimulation.	Increases reliability and validity in the quality of the twitch response.	
11. Discard used supplies.		
12. Remove gloves and perform hand hygiene.	Reduces the transmission of microorganisms; Standard Precautions.	

Testing the Facial Nerve

1. Place one electrode on the face at the outer canthus of the eye and the second electrode approximately 2 cm below, parallel with the tragus of the ear (Fig. 38-2).	Stimulates the facial nerve. Maintaining the electrodes as close as possible in alignment with the nerve minimizes artifact from direct muscle stimulation.[9]	Ensure that the patient's face is clean and dry. When wounds, edema, invasive lines, and other factors interfere with ulnar nerve testing, the facial or posterior tibial nerves may be substituted. The risk for direct muscle stimulation is greater, however, with resulting underestimation of blockade. Also, the alternate nerves correlate less well with blockade of the diaphragm.[7] **(Level C*)**
2. Plug the lead wires into the nerve stimulator, matching the black and red leads to the black and red connection sites.	Necessary for conduction of the electrical current.	

*Level C: Qualitative studies, descriptive or correlational studies, integrative reviews, systematic reviews, or randomized controlled trials with inconsistent results

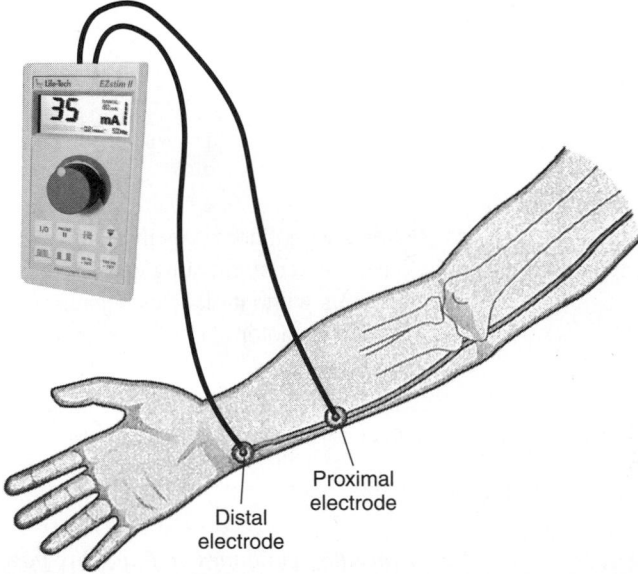

FIGURE 38-1   Placement of electrodes along the ulnar nerve.

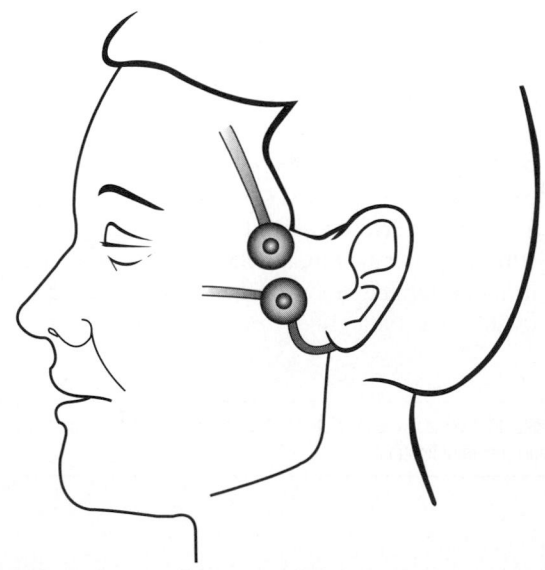

FIGURE 38-2   Placement of electrodes along the facial nerve.

Procedures · Peripheral Nerve Stimulators—*Continued*

Steps	Rationale	Special Considerations
3. Attach the lead wires to the electrodes. Connect the negative (black) lead to the distal electrode at the tragus of the ear. Connect the positive (red) lead to the proximal electrode at the outer canthus of the eye.	Prepares the equipment.	
4. Turn on the PNS and select the current determined by the SMS or, if not performed, a low current (10 to 20 mA is typical).	Excessive current results in overstimulation and can cause repetitive nerve firing.	
5. Depress the TOF key; through tactile assessment, determine twitching of the muscle above the eyebrow and count the number of twitches.	Determines the neuromuscular blockade at the junction between a branch of the facial nerve and orbicularis muscle.	
6. Discard used supplies.		
7. Remove gloves and perform hand hygiene.	Reduces the transmission of microorganisms; standard precautions.	

Testing the Posterior Tibial Nerve

1. Place one electrode approximately 2 cm posterior to the medial malleolus (Fig. 38-3). **(Level E*)**	Stimulates the posterior tibial nerve. Maintaining the electrodes as close as possible in alignment with the nerve minimizes artifact from direct muscle stimulation.[9]	Ensure that the patient's skin is clean and dry.
2. Place the second electrode approximately 2 cm above the first (see Fig. 38-3).		

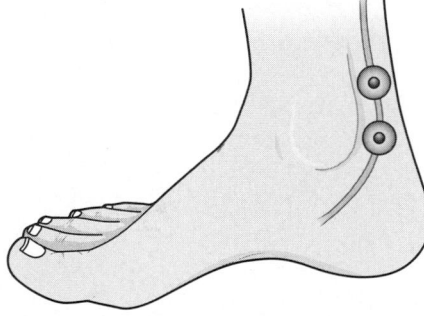

FIGURE 38-3   Placement of electrodes along the posterior tibial nerve.

3. Plug the lead wires into the nerve stimulator, matching the black and red leads to the black and red connection sites.	Necessary for conduction of the electrical current.	
4. Attach the lead wires to the electrodes. Connect the negative (black) lead to the distal electrode 2 cm posterior to the medial malleolus. Connect the positive (red) lead to the proximal electrode 2 cm above the medial malleolus.	Prepares the equipment.	

*Level E: Multiple case reports, theory-based evidence from expert opinions, or peer-reviewed professional organizational standards without clinical studies to support recommendations

Procedure continues on following page

Procedures Peripheral Nerve Stimulators—*Continued*

Steps	Rationale	Special Considerations
5. Turn on the PNS and select the current determined by the SMS or, if not performed, a low current (10 to 20 mA is typical).	Excessive current results in overstimulation and can cause repetitive nerve firing.	
6. Depress the TOF key; through tactile assessment of plantar flexion of the great toe, count the number of twitches.	Determines the neuromuscular blockade at the junction between the posterior tibial nerve and the flexor hallucis brevis muscle.	
7. Discard used supplies.		
8. 🅷🅷		

Determine the Supramaximal Stimulation (SMS)

1. Beginning at 5 mA, increase the mA in increments of 5 mA until four twitches are observed.		
2. Note the amount of current (in mAs) that corresponds to four vigorous twitches. Administer one to two more TOF stimuli to confirm the response. This current level is then used in TOF testing, for that site.	If no increase in intensity of the muscle twitch is found when the mA is increased, the SMS is the level at which four vigorous twitches were observed.	For example, if a strong response is observed at 30 mA, raise the current to 35 mA. If no increase is seen in intensity of the twitch, the SMS is 30 mA. If an increase is seen, raise the mA to 40 mA. If an additional increase is seen in twitch intensity, raise it to 45 mA. If the intensity shows no further increase, the SMS is 40 mA.

Determine the TOF Response During NMBD Infusion

1. Retest the TOF 10 to 15 minutes after a bolus dose or when continuous infusion of NMBD is given/initiated/changed.	Evaluates the level of blockade provided.	Always assess electrode condition and placement before testing.
2. If more than one or two twitches occur and neuromuscular blockade is unsatisfactory for clinical goals, increase the infusion rate as prescribed or according to hospital protocol and retest in 10 to 15 minutes.	Signifies that less than 85% to 90% of receptors are blocked.	
3. Retest every 4 to 8 hours after a clinically stable and satisfactory level of blockade is achieved.	Evaluates the level of blockade and avoids underestimation and overestimation of blockade.	

Troubleshooting with Zero Twitches

1. Change the electrodes and ensure that the patient's skin is clean and dry. **(Level E*)**	Drying of the gel or poor contact from moisture or soiling compromises conduction.[10]	
2. Check the lead connections and the PNS for mechanical failure and change the battery if needed. **(Level E)**	One of the most common causes of PNS malfunction is low battery voltage.[9]	
3. Increase the stimulating current. **(Level E)**	The current may be inadequate to stimulate the nerve, especially for increasingly edematous patients.[9]	
4. Retest another nerve (the other ulnar nerve or facial or posterior tibial nerves).	Avoids overestimating the level of blockade with false zero twitch responses.	

*Level E: Multiple case reports, theory-based evidence from expert opinions, or peer-reviewed professional organizational standards without clinical studies to support recommendations

Procedures | Peripheral Nerve Stimulators—*Continued*

Steps	Rationale	Special Considerations
5. If no other explanations are found for a zero response, check the NMBD infusion for the rate, dose, and concentration. Reduce the infusion rate of the NMBD as prescribed or according to hospital protocol. **(Level E*)**	Excessive neuromuscular blockade produces absence of a twitch response and, if allowed to persist, may contribute to prolonged paralysis or severe weakness.[6] Peripheral hypothermia causes a decrease in twitch response and may require a decrease in NMBD by 80%.[9]	

Expected Outcomes

- Slight discomfort during the TOF test
- The muscles of the thumb twitch, rather than the fingers, when the ulnar nerve is stimulated
- The twitch response approximates the number of blocked peripheral nerve receptors; for example, four twitches before initiating the NMBD infusion and one to two twitches when a desired level of blockade is achieved
- The NMBD dosage is titrated according to the TOF test and clinical goals
- Resumption of four twitches occurs within 2 hours when the NMBD is discontinued[7]

Unexpected Outcomes

- Moderate to severe discomfort from the TOF test
- Impaired skin integrity when the electrodes are removed
- The fingers twitch when the ulnar nerve is stimulated as a result of artifact; if the thumb does not twitch, this signifies direct muscle rather than ulnar nerve stimulation
- Resumption of four twitches does not occur within 2 hours of discontinuation of NMBD[7]

Patient Monitoring and Care

Steps	Rationale	Reportable Conditions
		These conditions should be reported if they persist despite nursing interventions.
1. Cleanse and thoroughly dry the skin before applying electrodes.	Improves the electrode adherence.	
2. Change the electrodes every 24 hours or whenever they are loose or when the gel becomes dry.	Optimizes conduction of the stimulating current.	
3. Select the most accessible site with the smallest degree of edema and hair and with no wounds, catheters, or dressings that impede accurate electrode placement over the selected nerve.	Facilitates ease in testing, electrode adherence, and the conduction of current.	
4. Never use the Single Twitch, Tetany, or Double Burst settings, if available on the PNS.	These methods are designed for profound neuromuscular blockade and may cause extreme discomfort.[10] **(Level E)**	
5. Assess the patient's oxygenation and ventilation, neurologic function, and tissue perfusion before increasing the rate of the NMBD infusion.	The patient may have subtle movement of the extremities with an acceptable TOF response. Clinical decisions should never be made solely on the TOF test results.	- Excessive patient movement despite acceptable TOF - Change in vital signs - Decreased oxygenation (e.g., measured via arterial blood gas or pulse oximetry) - Change in neurologic function

*Level E: Multiple case reports, theory-based evidence from expert opinions, or peer-reviewed professional organizational standards without clinical studies to support recommendations

Procedure continues on following page

Patient Monitoring and Care —*Continued*

Steps	Rationale	Reportable Conditions
6. Extreme caution must be exercised to prevent the PNS lead wires from contacting an external pacing catheter or pacing lead wires.	Direct electrical current can be conducted from the PNS through the pacing wires to the heart.	• Cardiac dysrhythmias or change in patient condition
7. Perform the TOF testing every 4 to 8 hours during NMBD infusion after the patient's condition is clinically stable and a satisfactory level of neuromuscular blockade is achieved.	Determines an effective dose of NMBD.	• Abnormal TOF results
8. Consider objective methods of sedation monitoring, such as bispectral index monitoring (see Procedure 86) or evoked potentials, during NMBD therapy.[3] **(Level E*)**	Muscle paralysis during therapy with NMBDs hinders sedation assessment with subjective instruments.	
9. Remove the electrodes, lead wires, and PNS from the patient for magnetic resonance imaging (MRI) or exposure to any magnetic field.	Metal objects are attracted to the magnetic field.	
10. Follow institution standard for assessing pain. Administer analgesia as prescribed.	Identifies need for pain interventions	Continued pain despite pain interventions

*Level E: Multiple case reports, theory-based evidence from expert opinions, or peer-reviewed professional organizational standards without clinical studies to support recommendations

Documentation

Documentation should include the following:
- Patient and family education
- The time, baseline SMS mA, most recent mA, TOF twitch response, and the nerve site tested
- The TOF response as 0/4, 1/4, 2/4, 3/4, or 4/4
- Dosage of NMBD

- Assessment data (e.g., neurologic, pulmonary, cardiovascular)
- Unexpected outcomes
- Troubleshooting attempts
- Additional interventions
- Pain assessment, interventions, and effectiveness

References

1. De Laet I, Hoste E, Verholen E, et al: The effect of neuromuscular blockers in patients with intra-abdominal hypertension, *Intensive Care Med* 33(10):1811-1814, 2007. Epub June 27, 2007.
2. Foster J, Clark AP: Functional recovery after neuromuscular blockade in mechanically ventilated critically ill patients, *Heart Lung* 35(3):178-189, 2006.
3. Jacobi J, et al: Clinical practice guidelines for the sustained use of sedatives and analgesics in the critically ill adult, *Crit Care Med* 30:119-140, 2002.
4. Kim KS, et al: The duration of immobilization causes the changing pharmacodynamics of mivacurium and rocuronium in rabbits, *Anesth Analg* 96:438-442, 2003.
5. Murray M, et al: Clinical guidelines for sustained neuromuscular blockade in the adult critically ill patient, *Crit Care Med* 30:142-156, 2002.
6. Murray MJ, Brull SJ, Bolton CF: Brief review: nondepolarizing neuromuscular blocking drugs and critical illness myopathy, *Can J Anaesth* 53(11):1148-1156, 2006.
7. Nagelhout JJ, Naglaniczny KL: *Nurse anesthesia,* ed 3, Philadelphia, 2004, Saunders.
8. Saitoh Y, et al: Monitoring of neuromuscular block after administration of vecuronium in patients with diabetes mellitus, *Br J Anaesth* 90:480-486, 2003.

9. Thompson C: *Monitoring the neuromuscular junction,* retrieved August 5, 2008, from www.usyd.edu.au/su/anaes/lectures/nmj_monitoring_clt/nmjonitoring.html.

10. Viamed: *Operator's Manual Microstim,* retrieved August 4, 2008, from www.viamed.co.uk/products/microstim/microstim.htm.

Additional Reading

Arbor R: Continuous nervous system monitoring, EEG, the bispectral index, and neuromuscular transmission, *AACN Clin Issues* 14:185-207, 2003.

PROCEDURE **39**

Automated External Defibrillation

P U R P O S E :   An automated external defibrillator is a defibrillator that, with use of a computerized detection system, analyzes cardiac rhythms, distinguishes between rhythms that require defibrillation and rhythms that do not, and delivers a series of preprogrammed electrical shocks. The automated external defibrillator is designed to allow early defibrillation by providers who have minimal or no training in rhythm recognition or manual defibrillation.

Charlotte A. Green

PREREQUISITE NURSING KNOWLEDGE

- Defibrillation is the therapeutic use of an electrical shock that temporarily stops or stuns an irregularly beating heart and allows the spontaneously repolarizing pacemaking cells within the heart to recover and resume more normal electrical activity. Ventricular fibrillation (VF) and ventricular tachycardia (VT) are the only two rhythms recognized as shockable by an automated external defibrillator (AED) (Fig. 39-1).

- Time is the major determining factor in the success rates of defibrillation. For every minute defibrillation is delayed, the chance of success decreases by 7% to 10%.[1,2,5] When used in conjunction with effective CPR, the decrease in the likelihood of success is more gradual and averages 3% to 4% per minute.[1,2,5]

- Although defibrillation is the definitive treatment for VF and pulseless VT, the use of the AED is not a standalone skill; it is used in conjunction with CPR. CPR should be started as soon as the patient is found to be pulseless and not stopped until the AED has been turned

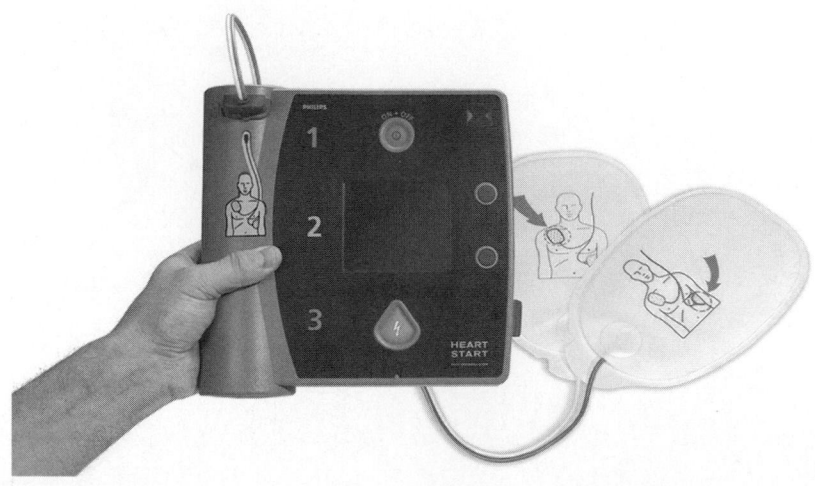

FIGURE 39-1 Automated external defibrillator device. *(Courtesy Philips Medical Systems.)*

on, the pads have been attached, and the machine is prompting the provider to "stand clear" or "don't touch the patient."[1,2,5] Immediate postshock CPR starting with compressions has been documented to lead to increased return of spontaneous circulation and increased cerebral survival,[4,5] which is why time is not taken to check for a rhythm or pulse after defibrillation.

- Ventricular fibrillation depletes the cardiac energy stores of adenosine triphosphate (ATP) more rapidly than a normal rhythm. The longer a heart goes without circulation, the more depleted its energy stores. In a heart with depleted energy stores, defibrillation is more likely to result in asystole because no fuel remains to support spontaneous depolarization or myocardial contraction. Effective CPR can supply the needed oxygen and energy substrates to the heart cells and allow them to return to a perfusing rhythm.[4,5]

- Three stages of VF are seen in cardiac arrest. The first phase is the electrical phase. During this phase, which is considered the first 4 to 5 minutes of VF, defibrillation is most likely to be effective, and the sooner the shock can be delivered the more likely it is to work. During the next 5 to 10 minutes after VF occurs, the hemodynamic or circulatory phase, a brief period of CPR may "prime the pump" and provide oxygen and energy substrate to the myocardial cells, improving the effectiveness of the defibrillation. If the patient is found during this phase, or if CPR is not ongoing when the defibrillator arrives, effective CPR needs to be administered for approximately 2 minutes, or five cycles of 30 compressions to two ventilations, before the shock. The metabolic phase starts 10 minutes after VF. During this phase, the cardiac cells have experienced global ischemia and energy depletion if no CPR has been initiated. CPR before defibrillation is more likely to be successful and needs to be used in conjunction with advanced cardiac life support (ACLS) therapies.[4,5]

- The AED is attached to the patient with adhesive electrode pads. Through these pads, the rhythm is analyzed and a shock delivered, if indicated. If the AED recognizes VF or VT, visual and verbal prompts guide the operator to deliver a shock to the patient. The AED, not the operator, makes the decision about whether the rhythm is appropriate for defibrillation.

- The chance of the AED shocking inappropriately is minimal.[1,5,7] The AED should be applied only to unresponsive, nonbreathing, pulseless patients. To keep artifact interference to a minimum, the patient should not be touched or moved during the analysis time.

- The mnemonic "PAAD" makes it easy for the rescuer to remember the steps of operation of the AED: "P" for Power on, "A" for Attach the pads, "A" for clear to Analyze, and "D" for clear to Defibrillate.

- Although AEDs are simple to use, healthcare personnel should be familiar with and technically competent in use of their AED.

- The AED is recommended for use in children ages 1 through 8 years if the child shows no signs of circulation. Approximately 5% to 15% of children in arrest have initial VF.[1,5,6] Primary VF in children rapidly changes to asystole; rhythm detection and rapid defibrillation in children is most effective. It is best if the defibrillator has a pediatric switch or pediatric pads, which have an attenuator in the cord that decreases the amount of energy delivered. If pediatric pads are not available, adult pads should be used.[1-3,5,7] With use of adult pads, ensure that they do not touch each other because this may cause electrical arcing and skin burns and divert defibrillation energy. The pads should be at least 1 inch apart. If the pads cannot be fit on the child's chest in a lead two position, an anterior-posterior pad placement should be used.[1-3,5,7,9] Never use pediatric pads on an adult or large child because the reduced energy levels delivered by these electrodes may not be effective for treatment of VF.

- The use of AEDs in prehospital settings has increased the success of defibrillation. The goal in the hospital should be to have the ability to defibrillate any person in cardiac arrest within 3 minutes or less of discovery. Placement of AED units in nonmonitored patient units and in public use areas of a hospital increases patient chances of survival.[2,5,6,8,10,11] AEDs are also recommended to be placed in freestanding or ambulatory care settings.

- Many manual defibrillators that can be purchased have analysis capability that allows a tiered response (i.e., individuals with different skill levels can use the same defibrillator).

- Most AEDs in use in emergency response systems (EMS) or in the hospital have a method of recording the event, in the form of rhythm strip printouts, audio and event recording devices, data cards, or computer chips that can print an event summary.

- AEDs can be purchased with and without monitor screens. AEDs with screens may allow the provider with rhythm recognition skills to override the AED's analysis and recommendations.

- An important safety issue an AED operator must address is the possibility of inadvertently shocking a bystander or other provider at the scene. The operator must clear the patient verbally and visibly, by looking at the patient from head to toe, before and during the discharge of the energy to the patient.

- All defibrillation programs need to include training for the potential operators. Training should include psychomotor skills, troubleshooting, equipment maintenance, and how to interface with ACLS providers. Providers have the responsibility to be familiar with the machine they will use.

- When a resuscitation team (e.g., 911 responders, code team, ACLS providers) arrives, the team assumes responsibility for monitoring and treating the patient.

EQUIPMENT

- AED
- Nonsterile gloves
- Barrier device or airway management equipment (bag-valve device with mask and oxygen)
- Hand towel

- At least two sets of adult defibrillation pads and potentially one set of child defibrillation pads

Additional equipment to have available as needed includes the following:
- Trauma shears (with ability to cut through underwires)
- Clippers or scissors
- Extra electrocardiographic (ECG) paper
- Spare data card
- Backboard

PATIENT AND FAMILY EDUCATION

- AEDs are used in emergency situations with limited or no time to educate the family about the equipment or the procedure. If family is present in the room during the arrest, a staff member should be assigned to keep the family informed of the procedures taking place and to offer support. ➤➤*Rationale:* Information provides education and support.
- Occasionally, after a sudden cardiac event, a patient may be discharged from an institution with an AED. In these situations, patient and family education is essential and should include information regarding performing CPR and technical competence with the AED. ➤➤*Rationale:* Education prepares the family for potential future emergencies.

PATIENT ASSESSMENT AND PREPARATION

Patient Assessment

- Establish that the patient is unresponsive, nonbreathing, and pulseless. ➤➤*Rationale:* AEDs are indicated for the treatment of patients in cardiac arrest.

Patient Preparation

- Remove clothing from the patient's chest and ensure that the skin is dry where the AED electrodes will be placed. ➤➤*Rationale:* This action prepares the patient for placement of the AED electrodes and minimizes the risk of electrical burns.

Procedure for Automated External Defibrillation		
Steps	**Rationale**	**Special Considerations**
1. HH		
2. PE		
3. Establish that patient is unresponsive, not breathing, and pulseless.	AEDs are indicated for the treatment of patients in cardiac arrest.	
4. Call for or obtain the AED; activate emergency response procedures for your settings.	Defibrillation is the definitive treatment for VF and pulseless VT.	Knowledge of how to activate the emergency response team in your setting is vital.
5. Perform CPR until the AED is available, turned on, attached to the patient, and prompts you to clear the patient.	CPR helps keep the patient in a shockable rhythm longer, increasing the chance that defibrillation will be effective.	Personal protective equipment should be used in all settings, including gloves and a bag-valve device with mask, a barrier device, or a bag-valve device with a mask connected to oxygen. Place a backboard under the patient who is in bed.
6. The person in charge of the AED should: A. Open the AED. B. Press the "on" button. C. Proceed with the next steps as instructed by the AED.	When the AED is on, the prompts remind you of what to do.	Some AEDs automatically turn on when they are opened. CPR should continue during the next few steps.
7. Attach the electrode pads to the patient's bare, dry chest:	Moisture under the pads can decrease the effectiveness of the contact of the electrode pads.	
A. Place one pad below the right clavicle to the right of the sternum and the other to the left of the left nipple or slightly lower than the nipple line with the center of the electrode pad on the midaxillary line. The electrode pads have pictures that indicate where to place them. Refer to Figure 39-1.	This placement ensures that the heart is between the two electrode pads, maximizing the current flow through the heart.	Placing an electrode pad on the sternum decreases effectiveness. Bone blocks some of the energy. Even with proper placement, only 4% to 25% of the delivered current actually passes through the heart, so proper pad placement is crucial.[5]

Procedure	for Automated External Defibrillation—*Continued*	
Steps	**Rationale**	**Special Considerations**
		Frequently electrode pads are not placed properly; they are placed too close together with both on the top of the chest.[5]
		Polarity of the electrode pads is interchangeable for defibrillation purposes. However, if ECG monitoring is being done, the QRS complex is inverted if the positive and negative pads are reversed.
B. An alternative electrode pad position is anterior-posterior placement, where one pad is anterior over the left apex and the other is posterior behind the heart in the infrascapular location.	This placement also ensures that the heart is between the two electrode pads.	Ensure that the electrode pads are directly above and below each other.
8. Connect the cables from the electrode pads to the AED.	Prepares equipment.	
9. Place the electrode pads firmly to eliminate air pockets and to form a complete seal.	The AED uses the electrode pads to monitor and to shock. Good contact must be ensured to defibrillate most effectively; air pockets under the electrode can cause electrical sparks and skin burns.	
A. Do not place the electrode pads over any medication or monitoring patches. Remove any medication pads from the chest and wipe the chest clean.	Defibrillating over medication patches can cause burns and block the transfer of energy from the electrode pad to the heart.	
B. For the patient with an implantable cardioverter defibrillator (ICD) or pacemaker, recommendations are to keep the electrode pads 3 inches from the device generator. When possible for these patients, anterior-posterior placement is preferred. Other acceptable placement options are on the lateral chest wall on the right and left sides (biaxillary) or placement of the left pad in the standard apical position and the other pad on the right or left upper back.[5]	Placement of electrode pads directly over an implanted device can divert energy away from the heart and can damage the device.	Some manufacturers recommend placing electrode pads 6 inches away from the device generators if possible. The ICD or pacemaker should be checked for possible damage to the device after defibrillation. Try to place the pads without interrupting CPR. Pad placement should not delay defibrillation.[5]
10. Once the electrode pads are in place and plugged in, most AEDs sense an electrical pattern and tell the operator to make sure no one is touching the patient ("stand clear" or "don't touch the patient").	The machine needs to analyze the rhythm to determine whether defibrillation is needed, and touching the patient or doing CPR may give the machine a false message or delay the ability of the AED to analyze the rhythm.	CPR must be stopped at this point. No one should be touching the patient when the AED is analyzing.

Procedure continues on following page

Procedure for Automated External Defibrillation—*Continued*

Steps	Rationale	Special Considerations
11. Wait for the AED to analyze the patient's rhythm:		
A. If a shock is advised, clear the patient visually and verbally.	The AED has determined that the rhythm is either VF or VT; defibrillation is needed. Maintain safety for everyone around the patient. Anyone touching the patient or any conductive apparatus that is in contact with the patient (e.g., stretcher frame, intubation stylet) when the energy is discharged receives some of that shock.	Use a mnemonic such as "I'm clear, you're clear, we're all clear," and look at the patient while talking to ensure that no one is touching the patient. Another mnemonic is "Shocking on three. One, I am clear. Two, you are clear. Three, we are all clear. Shocking now."
B. If no shock is advised, restart CPR.	If the patient is not in a shockable rhythm and was pulseless, the only treatment is CPR until the ACLS team arrives.	
12. Push the shock button or buttons, as prompted while looking at the patient.	Delivering the shock quickly is the best way to convert the fatal rhythm. Most AEDs discharge the energy into the machine if the shock button is not pushed within a preset time frame, usually about 10 to 15 seconds.	The energy levels for AEDs are preset to an energy level recommended by the manufacturer. Some AEDs are fully automatic and deliver a shock if needed without user interaction. In this case, the AED warns the user to stand clear before delivering the shock.
13. Immediately restart CPR, beginning with compressions. Continue CPR for 2 minutes, approximately five cycles of 30 compressions to two breaths. (**Level B***)	Providing immediate postshock compressions increases the probability of return of spontaneous circulation.[1,2,4,5]	Change compressors every 2 minutes to ensure effectiveness of CPR. Performing chest compressions is tiring, and effectiveness decreases after 2 minutes.[1,2,5]
14. After 2 minutes, the AED prompts the providers "stand clear" or "don't touch the patient" to allow it to analyze the rhythm, determining whether the rhythm remains shockable.	Checks to see whether the initial shock was effective or whether the patient needs to be defibrillated again.	Ensure that no one touches the patient during the analysis. A good time to change compressors is during the analysis pause.
15. **Repeat steps 10 to 14,** if prompted to shock again.	If the patient remains in a shockable rhythm, CPR and defibrillation are most likely to be effective in return of spontaneous circulation.	Be sure to clear the patient for analysis and shocking.
16. If you receive a "no shock advised" message, resume CPR until the ACLS team arrives and the rhythm can be checked.	Continues emergency intervention.	If a change occurs in the patient's condition, check a pulse. If a pulse is found, check for adequate breathing. If adequate breathing is not found and the patient has a pulse, provide rescue breaths at a rate of one every 5 to 6 seconds with a bag-valve device with mask and oxygen if available.
17. Once the patient has a pulse, obtain vital signs and assess level of consciousness.	Determines the patient's response to CPR and use of the AED.	

*Level B: Well-designed, controlled studies with results that consistently support a specific action, intervention, or treatment

Procedure for Automated External Defibrillation—*Continued*

Steps	Rationale	Special Considerations
18. Transfer the patient to a critical care unit.	Continues assessment and medical intervention.	
19. Ensure that AED is cleaned and electrodes are replaced.	Prepares emergency equipment for future use.	
20. Discard used supplies in appropriate receptacle.	Reduces the transmission of micro-organisms; standard precautions.	
21. ▥		

Expected Outcomes

- Restoration of perfusing rhythm
- Restoration of spontaneous respirations
- Transfer to a critical care unit for postresuscitation care.

Unexpected Outcomes

- Operator or bystander shocked
- Skin burns
- Pain
- Unsuccessful resuscitation; death

Patient Monitoring and Care

Steps	Rationale	Reportable Conditions
		These conditions should be reported if they persist despite nursing interventions.
1. Monitor vital signs at least every 15 minutes until stable.	Determines hemodynamic stability.	• Abnormal vital signs • Dysrhythmias
2. Monitor ECG rate and rhythm.	A patient with VF or VT is at risk for additional dysrhythmias.	• Dysrhythmias
3. Administer antidysrhythmia medications.	Antidysrhythmic medications may prevent the risk of additional dysrhythmias.	• Dysrhythmias
4. Follow institution standard for assessing pain. Administer analgesia as prescribed.	Identifies need for pain interventions	• Continued pain despite pain interventions

Documentation

Documentation should include the following:
- Type of arrest (witnessed or not witnessed)
- Time from patient collapse to first shock (only if witnessed)
- CPR information (including start and stop times)
- CPR performed before AED application: yes/no
- Time of application of AED
- Time from activation of AED to first shock
- Number of times patient was defibrillated
- Preshock and postshock rhythms
- Any complications
- Assessment after resuscitation (if applicable)
- Pain assessment, interventions and effectiveness
- Unexpected outcomes
- Nursing interventions
- Patient and family education

References

CR 1. American Heart Association: Guidelines for cardiopulmonary resuscitation and emergency cardiovascular care, part 4: adult basic life support, *Circulation* 112(Suppl IV): IV-35-46, 2005.
2. American Heart Association: *Health care provider basic life support provider manual,* Dallas, 2006, American Heart Association.
CR 3. Atkinson E, et al: Specificity and sensitivity of automated external defibrillator rhythm analysis in infant and children, *Ann Emerg Med* 42:185-196, 2003.
4. Berg RA, 0: Immediate post-shock chest compressions improve outcome from prolonged ventricular fibrillation, *Resuscitation* 78:71-76, 2008.
5. Field JM, editor: *ACLS resource text: for instructors and experienced providers,* Dallas, 2008, American Heart Association.

6. Gombotz H, Weh B, Mitterndorfer W, et al: In-hospital cardiac resuscitation outside the ICU by nursing staff equipped with automated external defibrillators: the first 500 cases, *Resuscitation* 70:416-422, 2006.

7. Markenson D, Pyles L, Neish S, and the Committee on Pediatric Emergency Medicine and Section on Cardiology and Cardiac Surgery: Ventricular fibrillation and the use of automated external defibrillators on children, *Pediatrics* 120:1368-1379, 2007.

CR 8. Martinez-Rubio A, et al: Advances for treating in-hospital cardiac arrest: safety and effectiveness of a new automatic external cardioverter-defibrillator, *J Am Coll Cardiol* 41(4):627-632, 2003.

CR 9. Samson R, Berg R, Bingham R, and PALS Task Force: Use of automated external defibrillators for children: an update; an advisory statement from the Pediatric Advanced Life Support Task Force, International Liaison Committee on Resuscitation, *Resuscitation* 57:237-243, 2003.

10. Sandroni C, Nolan J, Cavallaro F, et al: In-hospital cardiac arrest: incidence, prognosis and possible measures to improve survival, *Intensive Care Med* 33:237-245, 2007.

CR 11. Zafari M, et al: A program encouraging early defibrillation results in improved in-hospital resuscitation efficacy, *J Am Coll Cardiol* 44(4):846-852, 2004.

Cardioversion

P U R P O S E :   Cardioversion is the therapy of choice for termination of hemodynamically unstable tachydysrhythmias. It also may be used to convert hemodynamically stable atrial fibrillation or atrial flutter into normal sinus rhythm.

Cynthia Hambach

PREREQUISITE NURSING KNOWLEDGE

- Understanding of the anatomy and physiology of the cardiovascular system, principles of cardiac conduction, basic dysrhythmia interpretation, and electrical safety is needed.
- Basic and advanced cardiac life support knowledge and skills are essential.
- Clinical and technical competence in the use of the defibrillator is important.
- Synchronized cardioversion is recommended for termination of those dysrhythmias that result from a reentrant circuit, which include unstable supraventricular tachycardia, atrial fibrillation, atrial flutter, and unstable monomorphic ventricular tachycardia with a pulse.[3,6] Because ventricular tachycardia is often a precursor to ventricular fibrillation, cardioversion has the potential to prevent this life-threatening dysrhythmia.
- The electrical current delivered with cardioversion depolarizes the myocardial tissue involved in the reentrant circuit. This depolarization renders the tissue refractory; thus, it is no longer able to initiate or sustain reentry.[3,6] A countershock synchronized to the QRS complex allows for the electrical current to be delivered outside the heart's vulnerable period in which a shock can precipitate ventricular fibrillation.[2,3,5-7] This synchronization occurs a few milliseconds after the highest part of the R wave but before the vulnerable period associated with the T wave.[3,5,6]
- Cardioversion may be implemented in the patient with an emergent condition. The aforementioned dysrhythmias are converted with synchronized cardioversion when the patient develops symptoms from the rapid ventricular response. Symptoms may include hypotension, chest pressure, shortness of breath, dyspnea on exertion,

decreased level of consciousness, pulmonary edema, crackles, rhonchi, jugular vein distention, peripheral edema, and ischemic electrocardiogram (ECG) changes.[5]
- Elective cardioversion may be used to convert hemodynamically stable atrial fibrillation or atrial flutter into normal sinus rhythm.[1,2,7] With use to convert atrial fibrillation or atrial flutter, anticoagulation therapy is considered for 3 weeks before cardioversion to decrease the risk of thromboembolism.[2,7,9] Anticoagulation therapy may not be necessary if atrial fibrillation or atrial flutter has been present for less than 48 hours.[2,7] A physician or advanced practice nurse may choose to perform a transesophageal echocardiogram to exclude the possibility of an atrial thrombus before cardioversion for patients at high risk for thromboembolism. The patient is started on intravenous heparin, and the cardioversion is performed within 24 to 48 hours.[1,2,7,9] Anticoagulation therapy should be continued for 4 weeks after cardioversion because of the possibility of delayed embolism.[1,2,7,9]
- Elective cardioversion also may be used in patients with hemodynamically stable ventricular or supraventricular tachydysrhythmias unresponsive to medication therapy.[1]
- If time and clinical condition permit, the patient should be given a combination of analgesia and sedation to minimize discomfort.[2,3,5-7]
- Defibrillators deliver energy or current in waveform patterns. Delivered energy levels may differ among the various defibrillators and waveforms. Various types of monophasic waveforms are used in older defibrillators. Biphasic waveforms have been designed more recently and are used in implantable defibrillators, automatic external defibrillators, and most manual defibrillators.
  - ❖ Monophasic waveforms deliver energy in one direction. The energy travels through the heart from one paddle or pad to the other.[3,6,10]

❖ Biphasic waveforms deliver energy in two directions. The energy travels through the heart in a positive direction then reverses itself and flows back through the heart in a negative direction.[3,6,10] Biphasic waveform technology is able to decrease the amount of current needed to terminate the dysrhythmia, decreasing the amount of potential damage to the myocardium.[3] In more recent studies, atrial fibrillation was successfully cardioverted with biphasic waveform shocks that ranged from 100 to 120 J.[3,11,12,14] More research is needed to determine a specific recommendation for biphasic waveform cardioversion.[3] For that reason, the American Heart Association states that biphasic waveform shocks are acceptable if documented as clinically equivalent to reports of monophasic shocks.[3,5]

• Biphasic defibrillators measure and compensate for transthoracic impedance before the delivery of the shock, which allows the defibrillator to deliver the actual amount of energy selected by the rescuer.[3,6]

EQUIPMENT

• Defibrillator/monitor with ECG oscilloscope/recorder capable of delivering a synchronized shock
• ECG cable
• Conductive gel or paste, prepackaged gelled conduction pads or self-adhesive defibrillation pads connected directly to the defibrillator
• Intravenous sedative or analgesic pharmacologic agents as prescribed
• Bag-valve device with mask and oxygen delivery
• Flow meter for oxygen administration, oxygen source
• Emergency suction and intubation equipment
• Blood pressure monitoring equipment
• Pulse oximeter
• Intravenous infusion pumps
Additional equipment to have available as needed includes the following:
• Cardiac board
• Emergency medications
• Emergency pacing equipment

PATIENT AND FAMILY EDUCATION

• Assess patient and family understanding of the etiology of the dysrhythmia. ➦*Rationale:* This assessment determines the patient and family understanding of the condition and additional educational needs.
• Explain the procedure to the patient and family. ➦*Rationale:* This explanation decreases anxiety and promotes patient cooperation.
• Explain the signs and symptoms of hemodynamic compromise associated with the preexisting cardiac dysrhythmias to the patient and family. ➦*Rationale:* This explanation enables the patient and family to recognize when the patient needs to notify the nurse or physician.
• Evaluate and discuss with the patient the need for long-term pharmacologic support. ➦*Rationale:* This

discussion allows the nurse to anticipate educational needs of the patient and family regarding specific discharge medications.
• Assess and discuss with the patient the need for lifestyle changes. ➦*Rationale:* The underlying pathophysiology may necessitate alterations in the patient's current lifestyle and require a plan for behavioral changes.

PATIENT ASSESSMENT AND PREPARATION

Patient Assessment

• Assess the patient's ECG results for tachydysrhythmias, including paroxysmal supraventricular tachycardia, atrial fibrillation, atrial flutter, and ventricular tachycardia, which could require synchronized cardioversion. ➦*Rationale:* Tachydysrhythmias may precipitate deterioration of hemodynamic stability.[3,5]
• Assess the patient's vital signs and any associated symptoms of hemodynamic compromise with each significant change in ECG rate and rhythm. ➦*Rationale:* Deterioration of vital signs or the presence of associated symptoms indicates hemodynamic compromise that could become life-threatening.[3,5]
• Assess for the presence or absence of peripheral pulses and the patient's level of consciousness. ➦*Rationale:* This baseline determination assists in the detection of cardioversion-induced peripheral embolization.[2,6,7,9]
• Obtain the patient's serum potassium, magnesium, and digitalis levels and arterial blood gas results. ➦*Rationale:* Electrolyte imbalances, acid-base disturbances, and digitalis toxicity significantly contribute to electrical instability and may potentiate postconversion dysrhythmias.[2] Hypokalemia should be corrected to prevent postconversion dysrhythmias. Although cardioversion is considered a safe practice in patients taking digitalis glycosides, they are generally held on the day of cardioversion.

Patient Preparation

• Verify correct patient with two identifiers. ➦*Rationale:* Prior to performing a procedure, the nurse should ensure the correct identification of the patient for the intended intervention.
• Ensure that the patient and family understand preprocedural teaching. Answer questions as they arise, and reinforce information as needed. ➦*Rationale:* This communication evaluates and reinforces understanding of previously taught information.
• Ensure that informed consent is obtained. ➦*Rationale:* Informed consent protects the rights of the patient and makes competent decision-making possible for the patient, however, in emergency circumstances, time may not allow for the consent form to be signed.
• Perform a pre-procedure verification and time out if nonemergent. ➦*Rationale:* Ensures patient safety.
• Obtain 12 lead ECG. ➦*Rationale:* Provides baseline data.
• Give the patient nothing by mouth per institution policy. ➦*Rationale:* Decreases the risk of aspiration.

- Establish a patent intravenous access. ➤*Rationale:* Medication administration may be necessary.[3,5]
- Assist the patient to a supine position. ➤*Rationale:* Supine positioning provides the best access for procedure initiation, intervention, and management of possible adverse effects.
- Remove all metallic objects from the patient. ➤*Rationale:* Metallic objects are excellent conductors of electrical current and could result in burns.
- Remove transdermal medication patches from the patient's chest or ensure the defibrillator pads or paddles do not touch patches. ➤*Rationale:* Transdermal medication patches may block the transfer of energy from the pads or paddles to the patient and may produce a chest burn when the pads or paddles are placed over it.[3,5,10]
- Ensure that the patient is in a dry environment, and dry the patient's chest, if it is wet. ➤*Rationale:* Water is a conductor of electricity. If the patient and rescuer are in contact with water, the rescuer may receive a shock or the patient may receive a skin burn. Also, if the patient's chest is wet, the current may travel from one paddle across the water to the other, resulting in a decreased amount of energy to the myocardium.[3,5]

- If the patient has a hairy chest, clipping or removing the hair from the chest (if time is available) may be necessary. ➤*Rationale:* This action allows the electrodes to adhere to the chest.[3,5] Chest hair has been known to increase transthoracic impedance in patients.[13,15]
- Remove loose-fitting dentures, partial plates, or other mouth prostheses. ➤*Rationale:* Removal decreases the risk of airway obstruction during the procedure. Evaluate each individual situation (e.g., dentures may facilitate a tighter seal for airway management).
- Preoxygenate the patient as prescribed and appropriate to the condition. ➤*Rationale:* Adequate oxygenation of cardiac tissue diminishes the risk of cerebral and cardiac complications.[5]
- Maintain a patent airway with oxygenation throughout the procedure. ➤*Rationale:* Respiratory depression and hypoventilation can occur after administration of sedatives and analgesics.
- If time allows, consider administration of sedation and analgesia as prescribed. ➤*Rationale:* These medications provide amnesia and decrease anxiety and pain during the procedure.[2,3,5-7]

Procedure for Cardioversion

Steps	Rationale	Special Considerations
1. **HH**		
2. **PE**		
3. Connect the patient to the monitoring lead wires on the defibrillator.	The R wave must be sensed by the defibrillator to achieve synchronization for cardioversion.[5]	
4. Select a monitor lead that displays an R wave of sufficient amplitude to activate the synchronization mode of the defibrillator. In most models, synchronization is achieved when the monitoring lead produces a tall R wave. **(Level M*)**	Synchronized cardioversion must sense the R wave to deliver the current outside the heart's vulnerable period.[2,3,5,7] Lead II generally produces a large R wave.	If a combination defibrillator/monitor is not being used, a converter cable must connect the monitor to the defibrillator to achieve synchronization.
5. Place the defibrillator in the synchronization mode. Ensure that the patient's QRS complexes appear with a marker to signify correct synchronization of the defibrillator with the patient's ECG rhythm (Fig. 40-1). To confirm that the synchronization has been achieved, observe for visual flashing on the screen or listen for auditory beeps. If necessary, adjust the R wave gain until the synchronization marker appears on each R wave. **(Level D*)**	Synchronization prevents the random delivery of an electrical charge, which may cause ventricular fibrillation.[2,3,5,7]	

*Level D: Peer-reviewed professional organizational standards with clinical studies to support recommendations
*Level M: Manufacturer's recommendations only

Procedure continues on following page

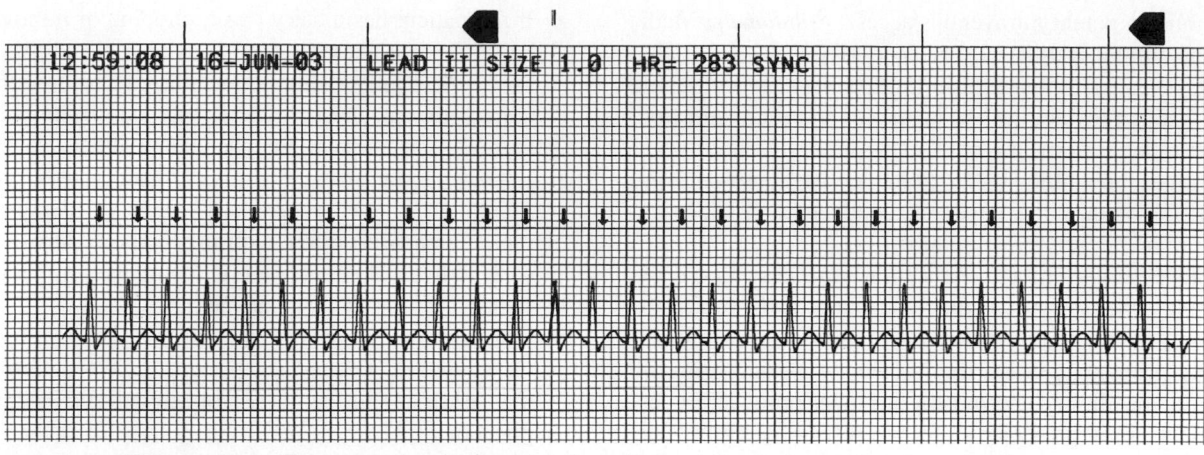

12:59:08   16-JUN-03   LEAD II SIZE 1.0   HR= 283 SYNC

FIGURE 40-1   R wave synchronization. Note the vertical synchronization marker above each R wave.

Procedure	**for Cardioversion**—*Continued*	
Steps	**Rationale**	**Special Considerations**
6. If the defibrillator is unable to distinguish between the peak of the QRS complex and the peak of the T wave, as in polymorphic ventricular tachycardia, proceed with unsynchronized defibrillation (see Procedure 41).	Avoids a delay or failure of shock delivery in the synchronized mode.[3,5]	
7. Prepare the patient or paddles or both with the proper conductive agent. **(Level D*)**	Reduces transthoracic resistance, enhancing electrical conduction through subcutaneous tissue.[3,5-7]	Self-adhesive defibrillation pads connected directly to the defibrillator have been found to be as effective as paddles.[3,5] Advantages of hands-free cardioversion are safety and convenience of use in any of the appropriate locations. These devices can be used for monitoring, and they allow for rapid delivery of a shock if necessary. For that reason, they are recommended for routine use instead of standard paddles.[3,5] Prepackaged gelled conductive pads are available for placement in the area of each paddle.[3] Gel pads should be replaced if they appear to be drying out or after three countershocks. Never use alcohol-soaked pads because they are combustible when in contact with electrical current. Conductive gel should be evenly dispersed on the defibrillator paddles and should adequately cover the surface; be careful not to smear gel between paddles because current may follow through the alternate pathway over the chest wall and avoid the heart.[3,10]

*Level D: Peer-reviewed professional organizational standards with clinical studies to support recommendations

Procedure	for Cardioversion—*Continued*	
Steps	**Rationale**	**Special Considerations**
		Do not use inappropriate gel (i.e., ultrasound scan gel) because it increases the transthoracic resistance and decreases the current given to the patient[3]; it also may cause burns or sparks, which can increase the risk of fire.[10]
8. Ensure that the defibrillator cables are positioned to allow for adequate access to the patient.	Allows cardioversion to occur without excessive tension on the cables.	
9. Turn on the ECG recorder for a continuous printout.	Establishes a visual recording of the patient's current ECG status and response to intervention. Provides a permanent record of the patient response to intervention.	
10. Follow these steps for pad or paddle placement:	Cardioversion is achieved by passing an electrical current through the cardiac muscle mass to restore a single source of impulse generation; this pathway maximizes current flow through the myocardium.[3,5,10]	Most pads or paddles are 8 to 12 cm in diameter.[3]
A. Place one pad or paddle at the heart's apex, just to the left of the nipple at the midaxillary line. Place the other pad or paddle just below the right clavicle to the right of the sternum (Fig. 40-2).	Prepares for cardioversion.	Avoid placing pads or paddles over lead wires.[3]

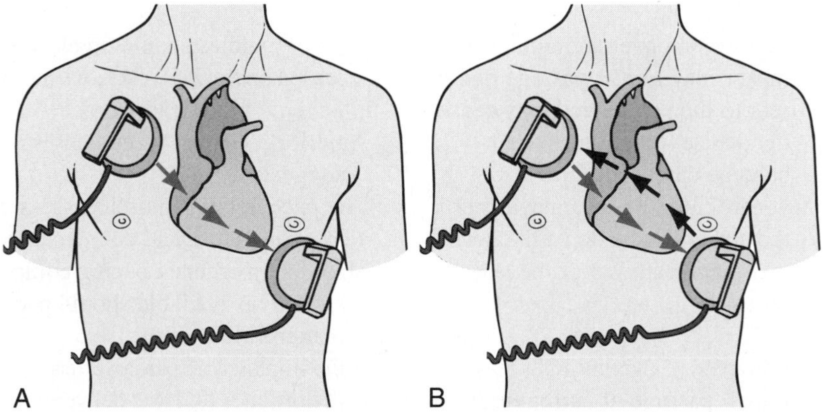

FIGURE 40-2 Paddle placement and current flow in **A,** monophasic defibrillation and **B,** biphasic defibrillation. *(From Lewis SL, et al: Medical-surgical nursing: assessment and management of clinical problems, ed 7, St Louis, 2007, Mosby.)*

B. In women, the apex pad or paddle is placed at the fifth to sixth intercostal space with the center of the pad or paddle at the midaxillary line.	Placement over a woman's breast should be avoided to reduce transthoracic resistance.	

Procedure continues on following page

Procedure	**for Cardioversion**—*Continued*	
Steps	**Rationale**	**Special Considerations**

C. Anterior-posterior placement also may be used.
  1. Self-adhesive defibrillation pads are used for this approach.
  2. The anterior pad is placed in the anterior left precordial area (Fig. 40-3).
  3. The posterior pad is placed posteriorly behind the heart in the right or left infrascapular area (see Fig. 40-3).
	All methods of pad or paddle placement are effective.[3]
	Some investigators have found the anterior-posterior placement to be more effective.[4,8]	

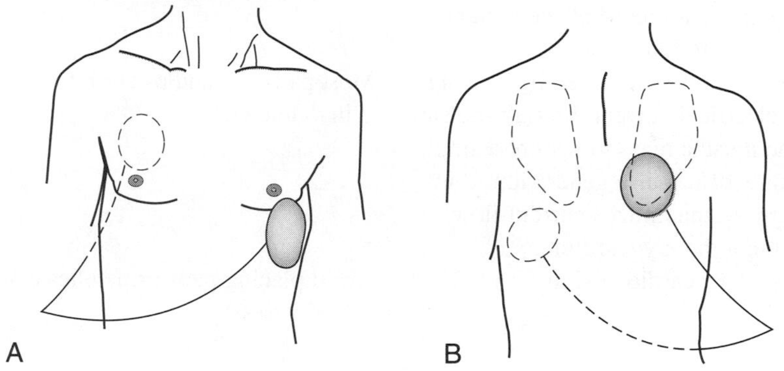

A

B

FIGURE 40-3 Anterior-posterior placement of self-adhesive defibrillation pads. **A,** Anterior pad placed over the left precordium. **B,** Posterior pad placed under the right scapula.

4. An alternative approach is to place the anterior pad in the right infraclavicular area and the posterior pad in the left infrascapular position.		
D. In a patient with a permanent pacemaker, do not place pads or paddles directly over the pulse generator.	Cardioversion over an implanted pacemaker may impair passage of current to the patient and may cause the device to malfunction or become damaged.[2,3,5,7,10] Myocardial injury also may occur if the current flows down the lower resistance pathway of the lead wires.[2,7]	Pads or paddles should be placed at least 1 inch (2.5 cm) from the pulse generator and lead wires.[3,5] Anterior-posterior placement is also suggested.[7] The pacemaker should be assessed after any electrical countershock.[3,7] Standby emergency pacing equipment should be available should pacemaker failure occur.
E. Pad or paddle placement in the patient with an ICD is the same as standard paddle placement for cardioversion (see Fig. 40-2). Pads or paddles should not be placed over the device. **(Level D*)**	Cardioversion over an ICD may impair passage of current to the patient and cause the device to malfunction or become damaged.[2,3,5,10]	If the implantable cardioverter-defibrillator (ICD) is delivering shocks to the patient, wait 30 to 60 seconds before cardioverting the patient with the manual defibrillator.[5] The ICD should be checked after external countershock.[3]
11. Charge the defibrillator as prescribed or in accordance with the recommendations of the American Heart Association (Table 40-1). **(Level D)**	The defibrillator is charged with the lowest energy level necessary to convert the tachydysrhythmia.[3]	

*Level D: Peer-reviewed professional organizational standards with clinical studies to support recommendations

TABLE 40-1	American Heart Association Energy Level Recommendations for Treatment of Tachydysrhythmias			
Stable Monomorphic Ventricular Tachycardia With a Pulse	**Supraventricular Tachycardia**	**Atrial Fibrillation**	**Atrial Flutter**	
First Attempt Cardiovert with 100 J	Cardiovert with 50 J	Cardiovert with 100 to 200 J	Cardiovert with 50 J	
Second Attempt Cardiovert with 200 J	Cardiovert with 100 J	Cardiovert with 300 J	Cardiovert with 100 J	
Subsequent Attempts Cardiovert with 300 J, then 360 J	Cardiovert with 200 J, then 300 J, then 360 J	Cardiovert with 360 J	Cardiovert with 200 J, then 300 J, then 360 J	

Note: These recommendations are for monophasic energy dose. Use of clinically equivalent biphasic energy dose is acceptable. Polymorphic ventricular tachycardia should be treated as ventricular fibrillation. With elective cardioversion of atrial fibrillation, an initial biphasic dose of 100 J to 120 J may be followed with escalation as needed. Also, consult the device manufacturer for specific recommendations.
(From Field JM: Advanced cardiac life support provider manual, Dallas, 2006, American Heart Association.)

Procedure for Cardioversion—*Continued*

Steps	Rationale	Special Considerations
12. Disconnect the oxygen source during actual cardioversion.	Decreases the risk of combustion in the presence of electrical current.[3,10]	Arcing of electrical current in the presence of oxygen could precipitate an explosion and subsequent fire hazard.[3,10]
13. Apply pressure to each paddle against the chest wall.	Firm paddle pressure decreases transthoracic resistance, improving the flow of current across the axis of the heart.[3,15]	This application of pressure is not necessary for defibrillator models with hands-free and automatic transthoracic impedance sensing/correction options built in.
14. State "all clear" or similar wording three times, and visually verify that everyone is clear of contact with the patient, bed, and equipment.	Maintains safety to caregivers because electrical current can be conducted from the patient to another individual if contact occurs.	Use a mnemonic such as "I'm clear, you're clear, we're all clear," and look at the patient while talking to ensure that no one is touching or is in contact with the patient. When using hands-free cardioversion, take special care to clear other personnel from patient contact because they do not have the visual cue of the paddles being placed on the patient's chest.
15. Verify that the defibrillator is in the synchronization mode and that the patient's QRS complexes appear with a marker to signify correct synchronization of the defibrillator with the patient's ECG rhythm (see Fig. 40-1). **(Level D*)**	Synchronization prevents the random delivery of an electrical charge, which may potentiate ventricular fibrillation.[2,3,5,7]	
16. Depress both buttons on the paddles simultaneously, and hold until the defibrillator fires. In the synchronized mode, a delay occurs before the charge is released, which allows the sensing mechanism to detect the QRS complex.	Depolarizes the cardiac muscle.	If self-adhesive, hands-free defibrillation pads are used, the charge is delivered by depressing the discharge button on the defibrillator.

*Level D: Peer-reviewed professional organizational standards with clinical studies to support recommendations

Procedure continues on following page

Procedure   for Cardioversion—*Continued*

Steps	Rationale	Special Considerations
17. Observe the monitor for conversion of the tachydysrhythmia, and assess the patient's pulse. If a pulse is noted, assess the patient's vital signs and level of consciousness.	Simultaneous depolarization of the myocardial muscle cells should re-establish a single source of impulse generation.	If unsuccessful in converting the rhythm, proceed with repeated energy recommendations (see Table 40-1). Ensure that the defibrillator is still in the synchronization mode; many defibrillators revert back to the unsynchronized mode after cardioversion. Ventricular fibrillation may develop after cardioversion. If so, deactivate the synchronizer and follow the procedure for defibrillation (see Procedure 41).[5]
18. Clean the defibrillator, and remove any gel from the paddles.	Conductive gel accumulated on the defibrillator paddles impedes surface contact and increases transthoracic resistance.	
19. If self-adhesive defibrillation pads were used, evaluate the placement and integrity of pads.	Self-adhesive defibrillation pads may crimp, crack, or fold with loss of adhesiveness.	Loss of adhesive integrity in self-adhesive defibrillation pads may occur in restless or diaphoretic patients.
20. Discard used supplies in appropriate receptacle.	Reduces the transmission of microorganisms; standard precautions.	
21. 🅗🅗		

Expected Outcomes

- Reestablishment of a single source of impulse generation for the cardiac muscle
- Hemodynamic stability

Unexpected Outcomes

- Continued tachydysrhythmias
- Ventricular fibrillation that progresses to cardiopulmonary arrest
- Bradycardia
- Asystole
- Pulmonary edema
- Systemic embolization
- Respiratory complications
- Hypotension
- Pacemaker or ICD dysfunction
- Skin burns
- Pain

Patient Monitoring and Care

Steps	Rationale	Reportable Conditions
		These conditions should be reported if they persist despite nursing interventions.
1. Evaluate neurologic status before and after cardioversion. Reorient as needed to person, place, and time.	An altered level of consciousness may occur after hemodynamically unstable dysrhythmias.[3,5] Cerebral emboli may develop as a postprocedural complication.[2,6,7,9]	• Change in level of consciousness • Sensory or motor changes
2. Monitor pulmonary status before and after cardioversion.	Hemodynamically unstable tachydysrhythmias may cause respiratory complications, such as pulmonary edema.[3,5]	• Dyspnea • Crackles • Rhonchi

Patient Monitoring and Care —*Continued*

Steps	Rationale	Reportable Conditions
3. Monitor cardiovascular status (blood pressure, heart rate, and rhythm) before and after cardioversion.	Respiratory depression and hypoventilation can occur after administration of sedatives and analgesics. Dysrhythmias may develop after cardioversion.[1,2,7]	• Slow shallow respirations • Decrease in oxygen saturation as measured with pulse oximetry • Hypotension • Supraventricular dysrhythmias • Ventricular dysrhythmias • Bradycardia
4. Prepare for administration of intravenous antidysrhythmic medications as prescribed.	Dysrhythmias may develop after cardioversion.[1,2,7]	• Asystole • Supraventricular dysrhythmias • Ventricular dysrhythmias • Bradycardia • Asystole
5. Evaluate for burns.	Erythema at the electrode sites may be seen from local hyperemia in the current pathway. Skin burns may be minimized with use of gel pads or applying appropriate paste or gel to the paddles.	• Skin burns
6. Follow institution standard for assessing pain. Administer analgesia as prescribed.	Identifies need for pain interventions.	• Continued pain despite pain interventions

Documentation

Documentation should include the following:
- Patient and family education
- Signed informed consent
- Universal Protocol requirements, if nonemergent
- Neurologic, pulmonary, and cardiovascular assessment before and after cardioversion
- Interventions to prepare the patient for cardioversion
- The joules used and the number of cardioversion attempts made
- Pain assessment, interventions and effectiveness
- Printout of the ECG tracing depicting the cardiac rhythm before and after cardioversion (before and after each attempt if more than one attempt is used)
- Condition of the skin of the chest wall
- Unexpected outcomes and nursing interventions
- Serum electrolytes, digoxin level, and coagulation laboratory results

References

1. American College of Cardiology/American Heart Association/American College of Physicians Task Force on Clinical Competence and Training: American College of Cardiology/American Heart Association 2006 update of the clinical competence statement on invasive electrophysiology studies, catheter ablation and cardioversion, *Circulation* 114:1654-1668, 2006.
2. American College of Cardiology/American Heart Association Task Force on Practice Guidelines and the European Society of Cardiology Committee for Practice Guidelines: American College of Cardiology/American Heart Association/European Society of Cardiology 2006 guidelines for the management of atrial fibrillation, *Circulation* 114:e257-354, 2006.
3. **CR** American Heart Association: 2005 Guidelines for cardiopulmonary resuscitation and emergency cardiovascular care, circulation, part 5: electrical therapies: automated external defibrillators, defibrillation, cardioversion, and pacing, *Circulation* 112(Suppl IV):IV-35-46, 2005.
4. **CR** Botto GI, et al: External cardioversion of atrial fibrillation: role of paddle position on technical efficacy and energy requirements, *Heart* 82:726-730, 1999.
5. Field JM, editor: *Advanced cardiac life support provider manual,* Dallas, 2006, American Heart Association.
6. Gowda SA, et al: Cardioversion of atrial fibrillation, *Prog Cardiovasc Dis* 48(2):88-107, 2005.
7. **CR** Kim SS, Knight BP: Electrical and pharmacologic cardioversion for atrial fibrillation, *Med Clin North Am* 92: 101-120, 2008.
8. **CR** Kirchhof P, et al: Anterior-posterior versus anterior-lateral electrode positions for external cardioversion of atrial fibrillation: a randomized trial, *Lancet* 360:1275-1279, 2002.
9. Klein AL, et al: Efficacy of transesophageal echocardiography-guided cardioversion of patients with atrial fibrillation at 6 months: a randomized controlled trial, *Am Heart J* 151:380-389, 2006.
10. **CR** Mair M: Monophasic and biphasic defibrillators: the evolving technology of cardiac defibrillation, *Am J Nurs* 103:58-60, 2003.

CR 11. Marinsek M, et al: Efficacy and impact of monophasic versus biphasic countershocks for transthoracic cardioversion of persistent atrial fibrillation, *Am J Cardiol* 92: 988-991, 2003.

CR 12. Page RL, et al: Biphasic versus monophasic shock waveform for conversion of atrial fibrillation, *J Am Coll Cardiol* 39:1956-1963, 2002.

CR 13. Sado DM, et al: Comparison of the effects of removal of chest hair with not doing so before external defibrillation on transthoracic impedance, *Am J Cardiol* 93:98-100, 2004.

CR 14. Scholten M, et al: Comparison of monophasic and biphasic shocks for transthoracic cardioversion of atrial fibrillation, *Heart* 89:1032-1034, 2003.

CR 15. White RD, et al: Transthoracic impedance does not affect defibrillation, resuscitation or survival in patients with out-of-hospital cardiac arrest treated with non-escalating biphasic waveform defibrillator, *Resuscitation* 64:63-69, 2005.

Defibrillation (External)

PURPOSE: External defibrillation is performed to eradicate life-threatening ventricular fibrillation or pulseless ventricular tachycardia. The goal for defibrillation is to restore coordinated cardiac electrical and mechanical pumping action, resulting in restored cardiac output, tissue perfusion, and oxygenation.

Cynthia Hambach

PREREQUISITE NURSING KNOWLEDGE

- Understanding of the anatomy and physiology of the cardiovascular system, principles of cardiac conduction, basic dysrhythmia interpretation, and electrical safety is needed.
- Basic and advanced cardiac life support (ACLS) knowledge and skills are necessary.
- Clinical and technical competence in the use of the defibrillator is needed.
- Ventricular fibrillation and pulseless ventricular tachycardia are lethal dysrhythmias. Early emergent defibrillation is the treatment of choice to restore normal electrical activity and coordinated contractile activity within the heart.[2,8]
- The electrical current delivered with defibrillation depolarizes the myocardium, terminating all electrical activity and allowing the heart's normal pacemaker to resume electrical activity within the heart.[2,8] Defibrillator paddles or pads placed over the patient's chest wall surface in the anterior-apex or anterior-posterior position maximize the current flow through the myocardium.[2]
- Defibrillators deliver energy or current in waveform patterns. Delivered energy levels may differ between different defibrillators and waveforms. Various types of monophasic waveforms are used in older defibrillators. Biphasic waveforms have been designed more recently and are used currently in implantable cardioverter defibrillators (ICDs), automatic external defibrillators, and most manual defibrillators.
- Monophasic waveforms deliver energy in one direction. The energy travels through the heart from one paddle or pad to the other.[2]

- Biphasic waveforms deliver energy in two directions. The energy travels through the heart in a positive direction and then reverses itself and flows back through the heart in a negative direction.[10] Researchers have found that biphasic waveform technology is able to decrease the amount of current needed to terminate the dysrhythmia (less than or equal to 200 J), decreasing the amount of potential damage to the myocardium.[7,13] Researchers also found that 115- to 130-J biphasic waveform shocks achieved the same first shock success rate as 200-J monophasic waveform shocks and these shocks also produced less ST-segment change than the monophasic shocks.[1,7] Investigators from in-hospital and out-of-hospital studies concluded that repetitive lower energy biphasic waveform shocks had equal or higher success rates for eradicating ventricular fibrillation than defibrillators that increase the current with each shock (200 J, 300 J, 360 J).[1,2] More research is needed to determine a specific recommendation for the optimal energy level for biphasic waveform defibrillation.[1,2,7] Biphasic energy recommendations are device specific. Biphasic defibrillators use one of two waveforms. Devices with a biphasic truncated exponential waveform are effective with 150 to 200 J of energy, whereas devices with a rectilinear waveform are effective with 120 J of energy. If the operator is unaware of the effective biphasic dose, the American Heart Association (AHA) recommends delivery of 200 J for the first shock, followed by equal or higher doses for subsequent shocks.[2,8] This energy level was chosen because it falls within the reported ranges of effective doses for first and subsequent biphasic shocks.[2,8]
- Biphasic defibrillators measure and compensate for transthoracic impedance before the delivery of the shock,

329

which allows the defibrillator to deliver the actual amount of energy selected by the rescuer.[1,2]

- A wearable cardioverter defibrillator (WCD) has recently been developed for patients at high risk for sudden cardiac death. Patient populations may include those who do not meet the current guidelines for an ICD implantation but who are at risk; those who are unable to receive an ICD because of infection; and those patients at high risk who are awaiting cardiac transplant. This wearable defibrillator has the ability to detect and treat life-threatening tachy-dysrhythmias without bystander support and allows the patient to ambulate freely. The initial defibrillators were programmed to provide a monophasic waveform for shocks. Preliminary results have shown that WCD is a safe and effective method to terminate life-threatening dysrhythmias in this high-risk patient population. The next generation devices use biphasic shocks, which are also proving to be successful in terminating ventricular fibrillation.[11]

EQUIPMENT

- Defibrillator with electrocardiogram (ECG) oscilloscope/recorder
- ECG cable
- Conductive gel, paste, or prepackaged gelled conduction pads or self-adhesive defibrillation pads connected directly to the defibrillator
- Bag-valve device with mask and oxygen delivery
- Flow meter for oxygen administration, oxygen source
- Emergency suction and intubation equipment
- Blood pressure monitoring equipment
- Pulse oximeter
- Intravenous infusion pumps

  Additional equipment to have available as needed includes the following:
- Cardiac board
- Emergency medications
- Emergency pacing equipment

PATIENT AND FAMILY EDUCATION

- Teaching may need to be performed after the procedure. ➵*Rationale:* If emergent defibrillation is performed in the face of hemodynamic collapse, education may be impossible until after the procedure has been performed.
- Assess patient and family understanding of the etiology of the dysrhythmia. ➵*Rationale:* This assessment determines the patient and family understanding of the condition and guides additional educational needs.
- Explain the procedure to the patient and the family. ➵*Rationale:* This explanation decreases anxiety and promotes understanding.
- Explain to the patient and the family the signs and symptoms of hemodynamic compromise associated with pre-existing cardiac dysrhythmias. ➵*Rationale:* This explanation enables the patient and the family to recognize when to contact the nurse or physician.

- Evaluate and discuss with the patient the need for long-term pharmacologic support. ➵*Rationale:* This evaluation and discussion allows the nurse to anticipate educational needs of the patient and family regarding specific discharge medications.
- Assess and discuss with the patient the need for lifestyle changes. ➵*Rationale:* Underlying pathophysiology may necessitate alterations in the patient's current lifestyle and require a plan for behavioral changes.
- Assess and discuss with the patient the need as applicable for an ICD. ➵*Rationale:* Life-threatening dysrhythmias may persist after initial defibrillation and pharmacologic interventions.[4]
- Assess and discuss with the patient the need as applicable for an emergency communication system. ➵*Rationale:* People with recurrent life-threatening dysrhythmias are at risk for cardiac arrest.[4]

PATIENT ASSESSMENT AND PREPARATION
Patient Assessment

- Assess the ECG results for tachydysrhythmias, including paroxysmal supraventricular tachycardia, atrial fibrillation, atrial flutter, atrial tachycardia, and ventricular tachycardia. ➵*Rationale:* Tachydysrhythmias often precede ventricular fibrillation, can be life-threatening, and can precipitate deterioration of hemodynamic stability.[2]
- Assess the ECG results for ventricular fibrillation. ➵*Rationale:* Ventricular fibrillation is life-threatening; if not terminated immediately, death ensues.[2]
- Assess vital signs. ➵*Rationale:* Blood pressure and pulse are absent in the presence of ventricular fibrillation because of the loss of cardiac output.[2]

Patient Preparation

- Verify correct patient with two identifiers. ➵*Rationale:* Prior to performing a procedure, the nurse should ensure the correct identification of the patient for the intended intervention.
- Ensure that the patient and family understand preprocedural teachings (if time is available). Answer questions as they arise, and reinforce information as needed. ➵*Rationale:* This communication evaluates and reinforces understanding of previously taught information.
- If possible, ask a member of pastoral care or another designated healthcare provider to provide support for family members during the procedure. ➵*Rationale:* Pastoral care team members or the clergy may provide support to ease family members' anxiety during the procedure.
- Remove all metallic objects from the patient. ➵*Rationale:* Metallic objects are excellent conductors of electrical current and could result in burns.
- Remove transdermal medication patches from the patient's chest or ensure the defibrillator pad or paddle does not touch the patch. ➵*Rationale:* Transdermal medication patches may block the transfer of energy from the pad or paddle to the patient and produce a chest burn when the pad or paddle is placed over it.[2,8]

- Ensure that the patient is in a dry environment, and dry the patient's chest, if it is wet. ➥*Rationale:* Water is a conductor of electricity. If the patient and rescuer are in contact with water, the rescuer may receive a shock or the patient may receive a skin burn. Also, if the patient's chest is wet, the current may travel from one paddle across the water to the other, resulting in a decreased amount of energy to the myocardium.[2,8]
- If the patient has a hairy chest, clipping or removing the hair from the chest (if time is available) may be necessary. ➥*Rationale:* This action allows the electrodes to adhere to the chest.[2,8] Chest hair has been known to increase transthoracic impedance in patients.[12,14]

- Initiate basic life support (BLS) if immediate defibrillation is not available. ➥*Rationale:* Basic life support maintains cardiac output to diminish irreversible organ and tissue damage.[2]
- Oxygenate the patient with a bag-valve device with mask and 100% oxygen. ➥*Rationale:* Adequate oxygenation diminishes the risk of cerebral and cardiac complications.[3,8]
- Place the defibrillator in the defibrillation mode. ➥*Rationale:* The defibrillation mode must be set to disperse the electrical charge randomly because the synchronization mode does not fire in the absence of a QRS complex.

Procedure for Defibrillation (External)

Steps	Rationale	Special Considerations
1. **HH**		
2. **PE**		
3. Prepare the patient or paddles or both with proper conductive agent. **(Level D*)**	Reduces transthoracic resistance, thus enhancing electrical conduction through subcutaneous tissue.[2] Minimizes erythema from the electrical current.[9]	Self-adhesive defibrillation pads connected directly to the defibrillator have been found to be as effective as paddles. Advantages of hands-free defibrillation are safety and convenience of use.[2,8] Defibrillation pads can be used for monitoring, and they allow for fast delivery of a shock if necessary. For that reason, the pads are recommended for routine use instead of standard paddles.[2,8] Prepackaged gelled conductive pads are available for placement in the area of the defibrillation paddles.[2,8] Gel pads should be replaced if they appear to be drying out or after three countershocks. Never use alcohol-soaked pads because they are combustible when in contact with electrical current. Conductive gel should be evenly dispersed on the defibrillator paddles and should adequately cover the surface. Do not use inappropriate gel (e.g., ultrasound scan gel) because it increases the transthoracic resistance and decreases the current given to the patient.[2] It may also cause burns or sparks, which can increase the risk of fire.[10] Be careful not to smear gel between paddles because current may follow an alternate pathway over the chest wall and avoid the heart.[2]

*Level D: Peer-reviewed professional organizational standards with clinical studies to support recommendations

Procedure continues on following page

Procedure   **for Defibrillation (External)**—*Continued*

Steps	Rationale	Special Considerations
4. Ensure that the defibrillator cables are positioned to allow for adequate access to the patient.	Allows defibrillation to occur without excessive tension on cables.	
5. Turn on the ECG recorder for continuous printout.	Establishes a visual recording of the patient's current ECG, verifies response to intervention, and provides a permanent record of the response to defibrillation.	
6. Follow these steps for pad or paddle placement:		
A. Place one pad or paddle at the heart's apex, just to the left of the nipple at the midaxillary line. Place the other pad or paddle below the right clavicle to the right of the sternum (see Fig. 40-2).	Defibrillation is achieved by passing an electrical current through the cardiac muscle mass to restore a single source of impulse generation. This pathway maximizes current flow through the myocardium.[2]	Most pads or paddles range from 8 to 12 cm in diameter and are effective.[2] Avoid placing pads or paddles over lead wires.[2]
B. In women, the apex pad or paddle is placed at the fifth to sixth intercostal space with the center of the pad or paddle at the midaxillary line.	Placement over a woman's breast should be avoided to reduce transthoracic resistance.	
C. Anterior-posterior placement may also be used.	All methods of pad placement are effective.[2]	
1. Self-adhesive defibrillation pads are used for this approach.		
2. The anterior pad is placed in the anterior left precordial area, and the posterior pad is placed posteriorly behind the heart in the right or left infrascapular area (see Fig. 40-3).		
3. An alternative approach is to place the anterior pad in the right infraclavicular area and the posterior pad in the left infrascapular position.		
D. If the patient has a permanent pacemaker, do not place pads or paddles directly over the pulse generator.	Defibrillation over an implanted pacemaker may impair passage of current to the patient and may cause the device to malfunction or become damaged.[2,8]	Place the paddle or pad at least 1 inch (2.5 cm) from the pulse generator and lead wire.[2,8] Anterior-posterior placement is also suggested. The pacemaker should be assessed after any electrical countershock.[2] Standby emergency pacing equipment should be available in case the patient's permanent pacemaker does not function appropriately.

Procedure for Defibrillation (External)—*Continued*

Steps	Rationale	Special Considerations
E. Pad or paddle placement in the patient with an ICD is the same as standard placement for defibrillation (see Fig. 40-2). Pads or paddles should not be placed over the device. **(Level D*)**	Defibrillation over an implanted ICD may impair passage of current to the patient and cause the device to malfunction or become damaged.[2,8]	The ICD should be checked after external countershock.[2] If the ICD is delivering shocks to the patient, wait 30 to 60 seconds before defibrillating the patient with the manual defibrillator.[2,8]
7. Charge the defibrillator as prescribed or in accordance with AHA recommendations. **(Level D)**	The defibrillator is charged with the lowest energy level needed to convert ventricular fibrillation or pulseless ventricular tachycardia.[2]	AHA monophasic energy recommendations for adults are for a 360-J shock.[2,8] Biphasic energy recommendations are device specific. Devices with a biphasic truncated exponential waveform are effective with 150 to 200 J, whereas devices with a rectilinear waveform are effective with 120 J. If the operator is unaware of the effective biphasic dose, AHA recommends delivering 200 J for the first shock, followed by equal or higher doses for subsequent shocks. This energy level was chosen because it falls within the reported ranges of effective doses for first and subsequent biphasic shocks.[2,8]
8. Disconnect the oxygen source during actual defibrillation.	Decreases the risk of combustion in the presence of electrical current.[2]	Arcing of electrical current in the presence of oxygen could precipitate an explosion and subsequent fire hazard.[2]
9. Apply pressure to each paddle against the chest wall.	Firm paddle pressure decreases transthoracic resistance, thus improving the flow of electrical current across the axis of the heart.[2]	This application of pressure is not necessary for defibrillator models with hands-free and automatic transthoracic impedance sensing/correction options built in.
10. State "all clear" or similar wording three times and visually verify that all personnel are clear of contact with the patient, bed, and equipment.	Maximizes safety to self and caregivers because electrical current can be conducted from the patient to another person if contact occurs.	Use a mnemonic such as "I'm clear, you're clear, we're all clear," and look at the patient while talking to ensure that no one is touching or is in contact with the patient. With use of a hands-free defibrillation, take special care to clear other personnel from patient contact because they do not have the visual cue of the paddles being placed on the patient's chest.
11. Verify that the patient is still in ventricular fibrillation or pulseless ventricular tachycardia (VT).	Ensures that defibrillation is necessary.	

*Level D: Peer-reviewed professional organizational standards with clinical studies to support recommendations

Procedure continues on following page

Procedure for Defibrillation (External)—*Continued*

Steps	Rationale	Special Considerations
12. Depress both buttons on the paddles simultaneously and hold until the defibrillator fires. In the defibrillation mode, an immediate release of the electrical charge occurs.	Depolarizes the cardiac muscle.[2]	If self-adhesive hands-free defibrillation pads are used, the charge is delivered by depressing the discharge button on the defibrillator.
13. Administer 2 minutes (approximately five cycles) of CPR. **(Level D*)**	CPR is needed for 2 minutes to provide some coronary and cerebral perfusion until adequate heart function resumes.[2,8]	
14. Observe the monitor for conversion of the dysrhythmia. If a stable rhythm is noted, assess for the presence of a carotid pulse. If a pulse is palpated, assess vital signs and level of consciousness.	Simultaneous depolarization of the myocardial muscle cells should reestablish a single source of impulse generation.[4]	
15. If the patient is still in ventricular fibrillation or pulseless VT, continue CPR and immediately charge the paddles to 360 J (monophasic) or device-specific value (same as first shock or higher; biphasic) and repeat Steps 8 to 14. **(Level D)**	Immediate action increases the chance of successful subsequent depolarization of cardiac muscle.[4]	A vasopressive medication such as epinephrine or vasopressin may be given during CPR to increase cerebral and coronary perfusion.[4,8]
16. If the second attempt is unsuccessful, continue CPR and immediately charge the paddles to 360 J (monophasic) or device-specific value (same as first shock or higher; biphasic) and repeat Steps 8 to 14. **(Level D)**	Immediate action increases the chance of successful subsequent depolarization of cardiac muscle.[4]	An antidysrhythmic medication such as amiodarone or lidocaine may be given during CPR to assist in terminating the dysrhythmia.[4]
17. If the third attempt is unsuccessful, continue with ACLS. **(Level D)**	Actions necessary to maintain the delivery of oxygenated blood to vital organs.[4]	BLS must be continued throughout resuscitation.[4,8]
18. Obtain vital signs and assess level of consciousness.	Determines patient response to defibrillation.	
19. Transfer patient to a critical care unit (if not in a critical care unit).	Continues assessment and medical intervention.	
20. After the emergency has ended, clean the defibrillator and remove the gel.	Prepares emergency equipment for future use.	
21. If the self-adhesive defibrillation pads were used, evaluate the placement and integrity of the pads.	Self-adhesive defibrillation pads may crimp, crack, or fold with loss of adhesiveness.	Loss of adhesive integrity in self-adhesive defibrillator pads can occur in restless or diaphoretic patients.
22. Discard used supplies in appropriate receptacle.	Reduces transmission of microorganisms; standard precautions.	
23. **HH**		

*Level D: Peer-reviewed professional organizational standards with clinical studies to support recommendations

Expected Outcomes

- Reestablishment of a single source of impulse generation for the cardiac muscle
- Hemodynamic stability

Unexpected Outcomes

- Continued ventricular fibrillation
- Cardiopulmonary arrest
- Asystole
- Respiratory complications
- Cerebral anoxia and brain death
- Systemic embolization
- Hypotension
- Pacemaker or ICD dysfunction
- Skin burns
- Pain

Patient Monitoring and Care

Steps	Rationale	Reportable Conditions
		These conditions should be reported if they persist despite nursing interventions.
1. Evaluate neurologic status before and after defibrillation. Reorient as necessary to person, place, and time.	Altered level of consciousness may occur after cardiac arrest.[6,8]	• Change in level of consciousness
2. Monitor the patient's airway and pulmonary status after defibrillation.	Goal is to support cardiac and pulmonary function to optimize tissue perfusion to vital organs, especially the brain.[6,8]	• Change in respirations • Change in breath sounds • Decreased oxygen saturation as measured with pulse oximetry • Abnormal arterial blood gas measurement
3. Monitor vital signs immediately after defibrillation and at least every 15 minutes until stable.	Vital signs should stabilize after achieving a normal heart rate and rhythm.	• Hypotension • Hypertension • Tachycardia • Bradycardia
4. Administer intravenous fluids or medications to maintain normal blood pressure.	Goal is to support cardiac and pulmonary function to optimize tissue perfusion to vital organs, especially the brain.[5]	• Hypotension • Hypertension
5. Continue to monitor the ECG after defibrillation.	Postdefibrillation dysrhythmias may occur.[4]	• Dysrhythmias
6. Initiate intravenous antidysrhythmic pharmacologic therapy as prescribed.	Ventricular fibrillation is indicative of the myocardium's state of irritability. If antidysrhythmic therapy is not administered, recurrence of ventricular fibrillation is probable.[4]	• Dysrhythmias despite antidysrhythmic therapy
7. Assess for burns.	Erythema at electrode sites may be seen from local hyperemia in the current pathway. Skin burns may be minimized with use of gel pads or placement of appropriate paste or gel on the paddles.	• Skin burns
8. Monitor electrolyte levels.	Abnormal electrolyte levels may have contributed to the development of ventricular dysrhythmias.[6]	• Abnormal electrolyte results
9. Consider other possible causes for ventricular fibrillation or pulseless ventricular tachycardia.	Interventions may be aimed at correcting underlying pathophysiology and preventing recurrence of lethal dysrhythmias.[6]	

Procedure continues on following page

Patient Monitoring and Care —*Continued*

Steps	Rationale	Reportable Conditions
10. Follow institution standard for assessing pain. Administer analgesia as prescribed.	Identifies need for pain interventions.	• Continued pain despite pain interventions

Documentation

Documentation should include the following:

- Neurologic, pulmonary, and cardiovascular assessments before and after defibrillation
- Interventions to prepare the patient for defibrillation
- The joules (J) used and the number of defibrillation attempts made
- Printout of ECG tracings that depict the cardiac rhythm before and after defibrillation
- Pain assessment, interventions and effectiveness

- Patient response to defibrillation
- Condition of skin of the chest wall
- Unexpected outcomes and nursing interventions
- Patient and family education

References

CR 1. AHA: Low-energy biphasic waveform defibrillation: evidence-based review applied to emergency cardiovascular care guidelines; a statement for healthcare professionals from the American Heart Association Committee on Emergency Cardiovascular Care and the Subcommittees on Basic Life Support, Advanced Cardiac Life Support and Pediatric Resuscitation, *Circulation* 97:1654-1667, 1998.

CR 2. American Heart Association: 2005 Guidelines for cardiopulmonary resuscitation and emergency cardiovascular care, part 5: electrical therapies: automated external defibrillators, defibrillation, cardioversion, and pacing, *Circulation* 112(Suppl IV): IV-35-46, 2005.

CR 3. American Heart Association: 2005 Guidelines for cardiopulmonary resuscitation and emergency cardiovascular care, part 7.1: adjuncts for airway control and ventilation, *Circulation* 112(Suppl IV): IV-51-57, 2005.

CR 4. American Heart Association: 2005 Guidelines for cardiopulmonary resuscitation and emergency cardiovascular care, part 7.2: management of cardiac arrest, *Circulation* 112(Suppl IV): IV-58-66, 2005.

CR 5. American Heart Association: 2005 Guidelines for cardiopulmonary resuscitation and emergency cardiovascular care, part 7.4: monitoring and medications, *Circulation* 112(Suppl IV):IV-78-83, 2005.

CR 6. American Heart Association: 2005 Guidelines for cardiopulmonary resuscitation and emergency cardiovascular care, part 7.5: postresuscitation support, *Circulation* 112(Suppl IV):IV-84-88, 2005.

CR 7. Faddy SC, et al: Biphasic and monophasic shocks for transthoracic defibrillation: a meta analysis of randomized controlled trials, *Resuscitation* 58:9-16, 2003.

8. Field JM, editor: *Advanced cardiac life support provider manual,* Dallas, 2006, American Heart Association.

CR 9. Graham-Garcia J, et al: Defibrillation and biphasic shocks: implications for perianesthesia nursing, *J Perianesth Nurs* 20(1):23-34, 2005.

CR 10. Mair M: Monophasic and biphasic defibrillators: the evolving technology of cardiac defibrillation, *Am J Nurs* 103(8):58-60, 2003.

CR 11. Reek S, et al: Clinical efficacy of a wearable defibrillator in acutely terminating episodes of ventricular fibrillation using biphasic shocks, *PACE* 26:2016-2022, 2003.

CR 12. Sado DM, et al: Comparison of the effects of removal of chest hair with not doing so before external defibrillation on transthoracic impedance, *Am J Cardiol* 93:98-100, 2004.

CR 13. White RD: New concepts in transthoracic defibrillation, *Emerg Med Clin North Am* 20:785-807, 2002.

CR 14. White RD, et al: Transthoracic impedance does not affect defibrillation, resuscitation or survival in patients with out-of-hospital cardiac arrest treated with non-escalating biphasic waveform defibrillator, *Resuscitation* 64:63-69, 2005.

Additional Readings

Tough J: Elective and emergency defibrillation, *Nurs Stand* 22(38):49-57, 2008.

AP Defibrillation (Internal)

PURPOSE: Internal defibrillation is the delivery of an electrical current directly to the myocardial surface via special paddles placed through an open sternotomy or thoracotomy.

Linda Schakenbach

PREREQUISITE NURSING KNOWLEDGE

- Understanding is needed of cardiovascular anatomy and physiology, principles of cardiac conduction, dysrhythmia interpretation, and electrical safety.
- Advanced cardiac life support knowledge and skills are needed.
- Clinical and technical competence in the use of the defibrillator is needed.
- Knowledge of aseptic and sterile technique is necessary.
- Knowledge of internal paddle placement and energy requirements for internal defibrillation is needed.
- Emergent open sternotomy or thoracotomy precedes internal defibrillation (see Procedures 43 and 44).
- Internal paddle placement should ensure that the axis of the heart is situated between the sources of current.
- Energy requirements for internal defibrillation usually range from 5 to 20 J for biphasic shocks and 10 to 40 J for monophasic shocks.[3,4]

EQUIPMENT

- Surgical head cover, mask, eye protection, sterile gown, sterile gloves
- Open sternotomy or thoracotomy tray
- Sterile internal paddles (ensure compatibility with the defibrillator)
- Defibrillator with electrocardiogram (ECG) oscilloscope and recorder

- Antiseptic solution (e.g., 2% chlorhexidine-based preparation)
- Large sterile suction catheter, tubing, suction canisters, suction regulator, and suction source
- Flow meter for oxygen administration
- Bag-valve device with mask capable of delivering 100% oxygen and at least 500-mL volumes
- Intubation equipment
- Intravenous access and IV fluids (e.g., 500 mL of normal saline)
  Additional equipment as needed includes the following:
- Emergency medications
- Emergency pacemaker equipment

PATIENT AND FAMILY EDUCATION

- Teaching may need to be performed after the procedure. ➥*Rationale:* Internal defibrillation usually is performed in the face of sudden hemodynamic collapse.
- Explain to the family the need for internal defibrillation. ➥*Rationale:* This information keeps the family informed.
- Discuss with the patient and family the need for follow-up electrophysiologic studies (EPS), as applicable. ➥*Rationale:* This discussion enables the patient and family to understand the importance of EPS for diagnosis and treatment of the dysrhythmia and monitoring both the effects of the dysrhythmia and efficacy of the treatment plan.
- Explain to the patient and family the underlying disease pathology. ➥*Rationale:* This explanation assists the patient and family with understanding the cause of the symptoms and the rationale for diagnostics, treatments, ongoing monitoring, and both expected and unexpected outcomes.

AP This procedure should be performed only by physicians, advanced practice nurses, and other healthcare professionals (including critical care nurses) with additional knowledge, skills, and demonstrated competence per professional licensure or institutional standard.

- Explain to the patient and family the signs and symptoms of hemodynamic compromise associated with the cardiac dysrhythmia. ➤➤*Rationale:* This explanation helps the patient and family to recognize when the patient needs to contact healthcare providers.

PATIENT ASSESSMENT AND PREPARATION

Patient Assessment

- Assess for dysrhythmias, especially ventricular ectopy. ➤➤*Rationale:* Ventricular dysrhythmias may precede ventricular tachycardia and ventricular fibrillation.
- Assess vital signs when dysrhythmias occur. ➤➤*Rationale:* This assessment provides data about the patient's response to dysrhythmias.
- Assess for pulseless ventricular tachycardia or ventricular fibrillation. ➤➤*Rationale:* Assessment determines the need for resuscitation, which may include internal cardiac defibrillation. If immediate intervention is not initiated, return of circulation may not be possible.

Patient Preparation

- Verify correct patient with two identifiers. ➤➤*Rationale:* Prior to performing a procedure, the nurse should ensure the correct identification of the patient for the intended intervention.
- Place the patient in a flat supine position. ➤➤*Rationale:* This position provides the best access during the procedure and during intervention for management of adverse effects.
- Remove all metallic objects from the patient. ➤➤*Rationale:* Metallic objects are conductors of electrical current and may cause burns.
- Prepare the patient's skin with antibacterial solution and drape the patient. ➤➤*Rationale:* This preparation decreases the potential for infection.
- Administer sedation and analgesia as prescribed. ➤➤*Rationale:* Promotes patient comfort during the procedure.
- Assist with maintaining an airway and ventilation before the initiation of the procedure. ➤➤*Rationale:* The patient's airway is protected and maintained, and a means for adequate ventilation and oxygenation is provided.

Procedure | for Defibrillation Internal

Steps	Rationale	Special Considerations
1. 🅷🅷		
2. 🅷🅷		
3. Initiate basic and advanced cardiac life support.[3] **(Level D*)**	Life-saving interventions are necessary.	External defibrillation should be attempted first whenever possible (see Procedure 41).
4. Assist the physician, advanced practice nurse, or other healthcare provider performing the procedure with applying personal protective and sterile equipment (e.g., head cover, mask, eye protection, sterile gown, sterile gloves).	Assists with preparation. May decrease the risk of patient infection. Decreases the risk of healthcare provider exposure to the patient's blood and body fluids.	The provider performing the procedure should perform hand antisepsis and hand scrub.[1,2]
5. Assist as needed with opening the patient's chest and fully draping the patient with exposure of the chest (see Procedures 43 and 44).	Prepares for the procedure.	
6. Set up a sterile suction system and turn on the system.	Fluid may need to be evacuated from the mediastinum before defibrillation.	
7. If necessary, ensure that the defibrillator is plugged into a grounded electrical wall outlet.	Provides power source.	Some defibrillators run on battery and thus do not need to be plugged into an electrical wall outlet.
8. Set the defibrillator to the defibrillation mode.	The defibrillation mode must be selected to deliver the electrical charge immediately.	The defibrillation mode is usually the default setting of the defibrillator, but confirm the setting.
9. Ensure that the defibrillator is positioned close to the patient.	Facilitates access to the defibrillator.	The defibrillator cannot touch the patient, field, or healthcare providers but must be close enough to treat the patient.

*Level D: Peer-reviewed professional organizational standards with clinical studies to support recommendations

Procedure for Defibrillation Internal—*Continued*

Steps	Rationale	Special Considerations
10. Connect the internal paddle cable to the defibrillator when the healthcare provider performing the procedure hands the cable to you.	Prepares the equipment.	Maintain asepsis by not touching the healthcare provider handing off the paddle cable. Use caution when pulling the connector to the defibrillator so that objects on the sterile field are not dislodged or entangled.
11. Turn on the ECG recorder for a continuous printout.	Provides a recording of the patient's ECG before, during, and after defibrillation.	
12. Charge the defibrillator as prescribed by the healthcare provider performing the procedure (usually 5 to 20 J for biphasic shocks, 10 to 40 J for monophasic shocks).[3,4] (**Level D***)	The defibrillator is charged with the lowest energy level necessary to convert the pulseless rhythm to one with a pulse and minimize damage to the myocardium.	One paddle is placed over the right atrium or right ventricle; the other paddle is placed over the apex (Fig. 42-1). Biphasic shocks of 5 to 20 J usually are sufficient to convert pulseless rhythms.[3] Refer to the defibrillator manufacturer's operation guidelines for specific recommendations.
13. Ensure that the healthcare provider delivering the shock states "all clear" three times and visually verifies that all personnel are clear of contact with the patient, bed, and equipment.	Electrical current can be conducted from the patient to another person if contact occurs.	Use a mnemonic such as "I'm clear, you're clear, we're all clear," and look at the patient while talking to ensure that no one is touching or is in contact with the patient.

*Level D: Peer-reviewed professional organizational standards with clinical studies to support recommendations

Procedure continues on following page

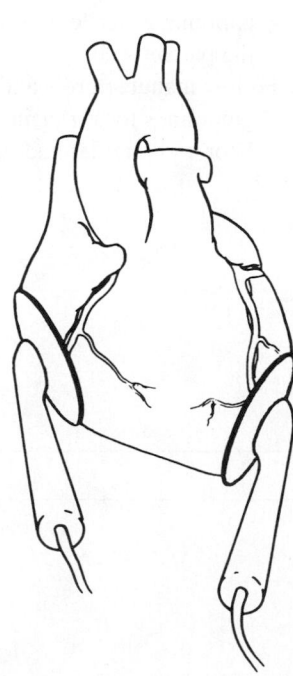

FIGURE 42-1 Paddle placement for internal defibrillation. (*From Kinkade S, Lohrman JE: Critical care nursing procedures: a team approach, Philadelphia, 1990, BC Decker.*)

Procedure for Defibrillation Internal—*Continued*

Steps	Rationale	Special Considerations
14. The healthcare provider delivering the shock simultaneously depresses and holds the buttons on each paddle until the defibrillator discharges. **(Level M*)**	In the defibrillation mode, an immediate release of the electrical charge depolarizes cardiac muscle. Simultaneous depolarization of the myocardial muscle cells may result in simultaneous repolarization of enough myocardial cells to reestablish a single cardiac impulse.	Follow manufacturer's recommendations. The charge also may be delivered by depressing the discharge button on the defibrillator until the charge is delivered. Some internal paddles can be discharged only by depressing the discharge button on the defibrillator.
15. Assess the patient's response to defibrillation:		
A. If the first defibrillation is not successful, assist the team with additional defibrillations as prescribed.	Continues emergency treatment.	Open-chest cardiac compression may be initiated if internal defibrillation is not successful.
B. If defibrillation is successful, obtain vital signs and assess the patient.	Aids in determining whether additional interventions are needed.	Provide additional supportive therapies as needed. Epicardial pacing may be needed if the patient's ECG rhythm converts to asystole or bradycardia. Vasoactive agents may also be prescribed.
16. Prepare the patient for transfer to the operating room or assist as needed with closing the patient's chest at the bedside.	Additional surgical exploration may be necessary and the chest needs to be closed.	Notify the operating room staff before transporting the patient. Cover the patient's chest with a sterile drape or dressing before transporting the patient to the operating room. Coordinate patient transport with other healthcare providers (e.g., respiratory therapy, anesthesiology). If the healthcare provider performing the procedure determines the incision cannot be closed, assist with applying a sterile dressing to cover the patient's chest.
17. Ensure that the defibrillator is cleaned with a cleansing solution. Place the internal paddles in the appropriate bag or container and send it for decontamination, disinfection, and sterilization. Obtain sterile internal paddles to restock emergency supplies.	Reduces the transmission of microorganisms and prepares for another emergency.	Follow manufacture's and institutional guidelines for cleansing the defibrillator and internal paddles.
18. Discard used supplies in appropriate receptacles.	Reduces the transmission of microorganisms; Standard Precautions.	
19. 🅷🅷		

*Level M: Manufacturer's recommendations only

Expected Outcomes

- Reestablishment of a single origin of the cardiac impulse
- Hemodynamic stability

Unexpected Outcomes

- Inability to resuscitate; death
- Cerebral anoxia, brain impairment
- Infection
- Myocardial injury (e.g., from hypoxia, defibrillation, sternotomy/thoracotomy, internal compressions)
- Pain

Patient Monitoring and Care

Steps	Rationale	Reportable Conditions
		These conditions should be reported if they persist despite nursing interventions.
1. Continue to monitor the patient's cardiac rate and rhythm after defibrillation.	Dysrhythmias may develop.	• Dysrhythmias
2. Assess the patient's neurologic status after defibrillation. Reorient as necessary.	Determines patient's neurologic status after arrest and defibrillation.	• Change in level of consciousness
3. Monitor the patient's pulmonary status after defibrillation and assisted ventilation.	Determines function of the patient's respiratory center after arrest and defibrillation.	• Change in respirations • Decrease in oxygen saturation • Abnormal arterial blood gas results
4. Monitor the patient's vital signs immediately after defibrillation and at least every 15 minutes until stable.	Determines the patient's hemodynamic stability.	• Abnormal vital signs
5. Initiate intravenous antidysrhythmic medications as prescribed.	Antidysrhythmic medications may be prescribed to prevent or control dysrhythmias.	• Dysrhythmias
6. Administer blood replacement products if prescribed.	Replaces blood that may have been lost during the procedure.	
7. Monitor electrolyte levels.	Abnormal electrolyte levels may contribute to the development of ventricular dysrhythmias.	• Abnormal electrolyte results
8. Monitor for signs and symptoms of infection.	Disruption of skin integrity and introduction of foreign material into the thoracic cavity predisposes the patient to the risk of infection.	• Elevated white blood cell count or band neutrophils • Elevated temperature • Pain at incision site • Erythema • Drainage from the incision site
9. Follow institution standard for assessing pain. Administer analgesia as prescribed.	Identifies need for pain interventions.	• Continued pain despite pain interventions

Documentation

Documentation should include the following:
- Cardiovascular, respiratory, and neurologic assessments before and after defibrillation
- Each defibrillation and joules used
- Printout of ECG tracings with cardiac events before, during, and after each defibrillation
- Patient response to defibrillation
- Pain assessment, interventions and effectiveness
- Any unexpected outcomes and interventions taken
- Amount of chest drainage
- Time chest was closed or when the patient was transferred to the operating room
- Patient and family education

References

1. AORN (Association of periOperative Registered Nurses): *Perioperative standards and recommended practices,* Denver, 2008, AORN.
2. Phillips N: *Berry & Kohn's operating room technique,* ed 11, St Louis, 2007, Mosby.
CR 3. Soar J, et al: European Resuscitation Council guidelines for resuscitation 2005 section 7: cardiac arrest in special circumstances, *Resuscitation* 67(Suppl 1):S135-S170, 2005.
CR 4. Winterhalter M, et al: Effectiveness and safety of internal rectilinear biphasic versus monophasic defibrillation in patients undergoing cardiac surgery, *J Cardiothorac Vasc Anesth* 19(6):739-745, 2005.

Additional Readings

CR American Heart Association: 2005 AHA guidelines for cardio-pulmonary resuscitation and emergency cardiovascular care, *Circulation* 112(24 Suppl): 2005.
CR Boyce JM, Pittet D: Guidelines for hand hygiene in health-care settings, *MMWR* 51(RR16):1-44, 2002.

AP Emergent Open Sternotomy (Perform)

PURPOSE: Emergent open sternotomy for a patient after cardiac surgery is performed to identify and eliminate areas of persistent hemorrhage, relieve pericardial tamponade, and provide access for open cardiac massage and internal defibrillation.

Linda Schakenbach

PREREQUISITE NURSING KNOWLEDGE

- Knowledge of anatomy and physiology of the cardiovascular system is necessary.
- Advanced cardiac life support knowledge and skills are needed
- Understanding of the signs and symptoms of cardiac tamponade is necessary.
- Emergency open sternotomy is performed for patients who have undergone a median sternotomy, usually within the first 2 weeks of cardiac surgery.
- Emergent open sternotomy is indicated for exsanguinating hemorrhage or cardiac tamponade with imminent cardiac arrest.[6,7]
  - ❖ The goal of mediastinal exploration for persistent hemorrhage is to stop the bleeding and retain circulating blood volume. The requirement for homologous blood transfusion and incidence of wound infection associated with an undrained mediastinal hematoma may be decreased.[3]
  - ❖ The goal of mediastinal exploration for cardiac tamponade is to relieve the pressure on the ventricles during diastole. The decreased pressure allows the ventricles to fill during diastole, which should increase contractility, stroke volume, and cardiac output to improve systemic perfusion.

- Knowledge and skills related to aseptic and sterile technique, surgical instrumentation, sternal opening, sternal exploration, sternal closure, and suturing are needed.[1,4-6]
- Paralytic agents may be a necessary adjunct to sedation to improve oxygenation, diminish muscle activity, and enhance visualization.
- Internal defibrillation may be necessary if life-threatening dysrhythmias occur (see Procedure 42).

EQUIPMENT

- Antiseptic solution (e.g., 2% chlorhexidine-based preparation)
- Head cover, masks, eye protection, sterile gown, sterile gloves, sterile drapes
- Sterile open-chest set and sternotomy tray
  - ❖ Wire cutter
  - ❖ Rib spreader
  - ❖ Kelly clamps and skin snaps
  - ❖ Knife handle
  - ❖ Scissors
- Electrocautery equipment: Generator, cautery, electrical dispersing pad (e.g., grounding pad)
- Large sterile suction catheter (e.g., Yankauer)
- Suction containers, tubing, regulator, and suction source
- Radiopaque gauze or other surgical sponge materials
- Polypropylene (Prolene) suture (cutting needle) and other suture material according to preference
- Clip applicator and clips
- Syringes: 3 ml, 5 ml, 10 ml, and 20 ml
- Knife blades: Nos. 10, 11, 15
- Sternal wires or bands

- Sterile stapler or sutures
- Sterile dressing supplies
- Emergency medication and resuscitation equipment, including internal defibrillation paddles and external defibrillation pads or paddles
  Additional equipment as needed includes the following:
- Prescribed analgesia or sedation
- Prescribed blood products and intravenous solutions
- Sterile staple remover
- Defibrillator and compatible internal defibrillation paddles
- Warm saline solution with or without an antibiotic, as prescribed
- Chest tubes and chest tube drainage system
- Epicardial wires
- Intra-aortic balloon pump or other mechanical assist device
- Peripheral nerve stimulator (used if paralytic agents are administered)

PATIENT AND FAMILY EDUCATION

- Teaching may not be provided until after the procedure. ➥*Rationale:* When an emergent sternotomy is performed for rapid hemodynamic collapse, education of the patient and family may not be possible prior to the procedure.
- Explain the reason that the open sternotomy procedure was performed and its outcome or anticipated outcome. ➥*Rationale:* This explanation provides information and encourages the patient and family to ask questions and clarify details about the patient and procedure.

PATIENT ASSESSMENT AND PREPARATION

Patient Assessment

- Assess hemodynamic and neurologic status. ➥*Rationale:* This assessment identifies baseline data that may indicate the need for emergent open sternotomy and provides comparison data.
- Assess the patient's medical history, specifically for coagulation disorders, renal disease with coexistent uremia, and functional status of the right and left ventricle. ➥*Rationale:* Baseline data are obtained.
- Assess current laboratory data, specifically complete blood cell count, platelet count, international normalized ratio, activated partial thromboplastin time, and fibrinogen. ➥*Rationale:* Near-normal baseline coagulation study results decrease the likelihood of coagulopathy as a possible cause for ongoing hemorrhage.
- Assess for signs and symptoms of cardiac tamponade:
  - ❖ Sudden decrease or cessation in chest tube drainage
  - ❖ Hypotension (mean arterial blood pressure, <60 mm Hg)
  - ❖ Altered mental status
  - ❖ Apical heart rate greater than 110 beats/min
  - ❖ Narrowing of pulse pressure
  - ❖ Distended neck veins
  - ❖ Distant heart sounds
  - ❖ Equalization of intracardiac pressures, with right atrial, pulmonary artery diastolic, pulmonary artery occlusion, and (if measured) left atrial pressures
  - ❖ Decreased cardiac output and cardiac index
  - ❖ Pulsus paradoxus
  - ➥*Rationale:* The presence of some or all of these signs and symptoms assists the healthcare provider to decide whether an emergent open sternotomy is necessary.
- Assess for excessive chest tube drainage. ➥*Rationale:* Presence of bleeding assists with the determination of the need for mediastinal exploration. Follow institution guidelines regarding determination of the timing of mediastinal exploration. One recommendation is when chest tube drainage continues at equal to or greater than 3 mL/kg/hr for at least 3 hours.[2]

Patient Preparation

- Verify correct patient with two identifiers. ➥*Rationale:* Prior to performing a procedure, the nurse should ensure the correct identification of the patient for the intended intervention.
- Ensure that the patient and family understand procedural teaching (if time is available). Answer questions as they arise and reinforce information as needed. ➥*Rationale:* Understanding of the information provided is evaluated and reinforced.
- Obtain informed consent (may not be possible if the procedure is an emergency). ➥*Rationale:* Informed consent protects the rights of the patient and ensures a competent decision for the patient and the family.
- Perform a pre-procedure verification and time out, if nonemergent. ➥*Rationale:* Ensures patient safety.
- If time allows, obtain a transthoracic echocardiogram in an attempt to identify mediastinal fluid or clot and ventricular filling and wall motion. ➥*Rationale:* An echocardiogram aids in the diagnosis of effusion or tamponade and confirms the necessity for an open sternotomy.
- Ensure the patient's airway is protected and that supplemental oxygen is delivered. ➥*Rationale:* The probability that the patient's ventilatory needs will be met is enhanced.
- Position the patient in the supine position with the head of the bed flat. ➥*Rationale:* This position ensures visualization of the chest and enhances hemodynamic stability.
- Prescribe and ensure that an analgesic or sedative is administered. ➥*Rationale:* Promotes patient comfort.

Procedure　for Performing Emergent Open Sternotomy

Steps	Rationale	Special Considerations
1. Call the physician and operative team.	The physician can assess the need for further surgical intervention. The operative team may be needed to assist at the bedside or to prepare the operating room if further exploration is needed.	Follow institution standard.
2. **HH**		
3. Prepare the electrocautery device for possible use: Apply the electrical dispersing pad (i.e., grounding pad) to the patient's dry skin and attach the grounding cable to the device.[1] **(Level D*)**	Electrocautery is used to terminate capillary oozing or bleeding.	Grounding is essential to avoid burning the patient and possible electrical shock to the healthcare providers.
4. Ensure that a new sterile suction system is set up.	Suction within the mediastinum is necessary during the procedure.	
5. **PE**		
6. Remove the sternal dressing and cleanse the chest with an antiseptic solution (e.g., 2% chlorhexidine solution). Remove gloves when cleansing is completed.	Inhibits microorganism transmission.	Prepare the skin beginning at the incision line, extending outward to include the area from the chin to the midabdomen (caudal to the umbilicus) and to include the area out to one anterior axillary line and then outward to the opposite anterior axillary line. Minimize solution from running off of the surgical site, dripping, pooling, and soaking fabric and the patient's hair. Ensure alcohol-based preparation agents have not wet the patient's hair or bedding nor pooled in skinfolds or the umbilicus because the risk of fire is increased (nonflammable preparations eliminate the risk of fire).[1]
7. Don personal protective equipment and sterile equipment: 　A. Surgical head cover, mask, and eye protection 　B. Perform hand antisepsis/hand scrub 　C. Sterile gown and sterile gloves	Removes debris and transient microorganisms.[1] Inhibits rebound microorganism growth.[1]	All personnel in the room must don caps and masks.
8. Open the sternotomy tray on a clean dry surface.	Prepares equipment.	
9. Fully drape the patient with exposure of only the surgical site.[1,2,4] **(Level D)**	A large sterile field minimizes the risk of infection and provides space to maintain asepsis of instruments and supplies during the procedure.	Allows good view of the incision.

*Level D: Peer-reviewed professional organizational standards with clinical studies to support recommendations

Procedure continues on following page

Procedure for Performing Emergent Open Sternotomy—*Continued*

Steps	Rationale	Special Considerations
10. Hand off the distal end of the electrocautery cable (active electrode) to the critical care nurse or assisting healthcare provider.	Cautery is used to stop bleeding from small vessels.	The cautery control is not sterile. The connection must be handed off of the sterile field without the healthcare provider performing the procedure and the assisting personnel touching each other.
11. Open the incision down to the sternum with the staple remover or scalpel, exposing the sternal wires or bands.	Ensures visualization of the sternal wires or bands.	Remove staples with a staple remover; cut sutures and tissue with a scalpel.
12. Cauterize oozing and bleeding sites as needed.	Minimizes blood loss and enhances visualization of the surgical field.	
13. Cut the sternal wires (or bands) from the top to the bottom with the wire cutter, or untwist the wires with the heavy needle holder.	Provides access to the mediastinum. The sternal wires fatigue and break when untwisted with the heavy needle holders.	Use care when removing the sternal wires to minimize damage to the heart, underlying equipment (e.g., epicardial pacing wires, chest tubes), and coronary artery bypass grafts and injury to the healthcare provider.
14. With your hands, gently separate the sternum.	Caution must be taken to separate the sternum gently because the heart, bypass grafts, and pacing wires rest just under the sternal bone.	
15. Place the sternal retractor under the sternal bone. Slowly crank it open while feeling along the edge of the retractor blades and observing the mediastinal cavity and heart for anything caught in the retractor.	Exposes the heart and mediastinum.	Sternal retractor blades can trap and tear bypass grafts and pacing wires if caught and pulled apart when the retractor is cranked open.
16. For bleeding, apply pressure with a finger over any bleeding site and suction the remainder of the chest, evacuating any clots.	Pressure on the bleeding site may minimize blood loss.	Resuscitate with intravenous fluids, inotropic medications, and blood products as necessary.
17. Control and ligate bleeding sites, enhance the sternal retraction, and provide suctioning and electrocautery as needed.	May eliminate the need for further exploration and assists with better visualization of the surgical field.	The physician determines whether the patient needs to be transferred to the operating room for further surgical intervention.
18. If pulseless ventricular tachycardia or ventricular fibrillation occurs, internal defibrillation is needed.	Emergency intervention is needed.	
19. Insert or assist with insertion of chest tubes or epicardial pacing wires as needed (see Procedure 42).	Chest tubes and epicardial pacing wires can be displaced during sternal retraction or mediastinal exploration.	
20. Warm saline solution with or without an antibiotic may be used to flush the chest cavity before closing the incision.	May decrease the incidence of infection.	
21. Assist with the placement of mechanical assist devices if needed.	Cardiac tamponade may conceal right or left ventricular dysfunction; mechanical assistance may be necessary to improve cardiac output.	

Procedure for Performing Emergent Open Sternotomy—*Continued*

Steps	Rationale	Special Considerations
22. Assist with patient transport to the operating room if necessary.	The patient may need further exploration; surgical repair of coronary artery bypass grafts, cardiac valves, or the myocardium; or insertion of an assist device (e.g., intra-aortic balloon pump, ventricular assist device).	Ensure that the patient's chest is covered with sterile drapes or with a dressing during transportation.
23. If the patient does not need to return to the operating room, assist the physician with reinsertion of sternal wires as follows: A. Grasp the sternal wire with the needle holder. B. From under the sternum, push one end of the wire up between two ribs at the sternal border. C. Repeat step B with the other end of the wire on the opposite side of the sternum (same intercostal space). D. Pull the sternum together with the wire and twist the edges of the wires together with the needle holder. E. Cut off the excess wire and bend the twisted edges flat against the sternum. F. Repeat with additional wires every two to three ribs until the sternum is closed.	Ensures sternal closure.	Caution must be taken not to penetrate the heart, pericostal vessels, lungs, or bypass grafts with the sternal wires. Multiple wiring techniques can be used for sternal wound closure; the advanced practice nurse or physician performing the procedure may use an alternate method or use sternal bands to close the sternum.
24. Assist the physician with tissue and skin closure according to preference (staples or sutures).	Promotes wound healing.	The patient's chest may be left open and covered with a sterile occlusive dressing if severe tissue swelling or ventricular dysfunction exists.
25. Apply an occlusive dressing to the sternal incision, epicardial pacing wires, and chest tube sites.	Dressings provide a physical barrier to external sources of contamination and cushion from physical contact and trauma; they absorb drainage, maintain a moist environment at body temperature to enhance wound healing, and are used for aesthetics.	
26. Dispose of sharps per facility standard.[1,5]	Minimizes risk of sharps injury.	A chest radiograph may be prescribed to rule out the presence of any retained surgical sponges, needles, or instruments.
27. Remove and package instruments for sterilization, discard used supplies in appropriate receptacles, and remove and discard personal protective equipment.	Reduces the transmission of microorganisms and body secretions; standard precautions; prepares equipment.	
28. **HH**		

Procedure continues on following page

Expected Outcomes

- Resolution of the condition that necessitated the emergent open sternotomy
- Increased cardiac output
- Increased tissue perfusion, including cerebral, renal, and peripheral perfusion
- Standard chest tube drainage
- Decreased need for blood transfusions

Unexpected Outcomes

- Severe right or left ventricular dysfunction
- Continued dysrhythmias, bleeding, or coagulation disorders
- Myocardial, aortic, coronary artery, or coronary artery bypass graft perforation
- Cardiac arrest
- Pneumothorax
- Myocardial infection
- Atrial and ventricular dysrhythmias
- Pain
- Infection

Patient Monitoring and Care

Steps	Rationale	Reportable Conditions
		These conditions should be reported if they persist despite nursing interventions.
1. Perform cardiovascular, hemodynamic, and peripheral vascular assessments every 15 to 30 minutes as patient status requires (including vital signs, pulmonary artery pressures, cardiac index, level of consciousness, and urine output).	Determines hemodynamic stability and volume status; recurrent tamponade or dysrhythmias may develop during and after sternotomy. Determines the adequacy of cerebral perfusion; hemodynamic instability can lead to cerebral anoxia. Determines adequate perfusion to the kidneys.	• Mean arterial blood pressure less than 60 mm Hg • Abnormal changes in heart rate • Decrease in cardiac index • Abnormal pulmonary artery pressures • Urine output less than 0.5 mL/kg/hr • Equalizing pulmonary artery pressures • Change in level of consciousness
2. Assess heart and lung sounds every 2 hours and as needed.	Abnormal heart and lung sounds may indicate the need for additional treatment.	• Distant heart sounds or additional changes in heart and lung sounds
3. Monitor coagulation, hematologic, and electrolyte laboratory blood study results.	Coagulation and hematologic profiles provide data that indicate the risk of bleeding and indicate the need for additional treatment. Electrolyte studies provide data regarding the risk for dysrhythmias and decreased contractility.	• Abnormal hemoglobin and hematocrit, activated partial thromboplastin time, international normalized ratio, platelets, fibrinogen, calcium, magnesium, or potassium
4. Closely monitor chest tube drainage.	Determines functioning of the chest tube drainage system and the amount of chest drainage.	• Cessation of chest tube drainage • Increased chest tube drainage • Clots in the chest tube drainage system
5. Follow institution standard for assessing pain. Administer analgesia as prescribed.	Identifies need for pain interventions.	• Continued pain despite pain interventions

Documentation

Documentation should include the following:
- Patient and family education
- Signed informed consent, if non-emergent
- Universal Protocol requirement, if non-emergent
- Pain assessment, interventions and effectiveness
- Indications for the procedure and the procedure performed
- Amount of blood collected from chest suctioning
- Estimated blood loss
- Patient therapies and response, including hemodynamics, inotropic or vasopressor agents, analgesia, sedation, ventilation, and neurologic status
- Additional interventions
- Unexpected outcomes

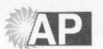
References

1. AORN (Association of periOperative Registered Nurses): *Perioperative standards and recommended practices,* Denver, 2008, AORN.
2. Chikwe J, Beddow E, Glenville B: *Cardiothoracic surgery,* New York, 2006, Oxford University Press Inc.
CR 3. Mason RJ, Broaddus VC, Murray JF, et al: *Murray & Nadel's textbook of respiratory medicine,* ed 4, St Louis, 2005, Saunders.
4. Phillips N: *Berry & Kohn's operating room technique,* ed 11, St Louis, 2007, Mosby.
5. Rothrock JC: *Alexander's care of the patient in surgery,* ed 13, St Louis, 2007, Mosby.
6. Sethares K, Seifert PC, Smith H: Care of patients undergoing cardiac surgery. In Moser DK, Riegel B, editors: *Cardiac nursing: a companion to Braunwald's heart disease,* St Louis, 2008, Saunders.
CR 7. Soar J, et al: European Resuscitation Council guidelines for resuscitation 2005 section 7: cardiac arrest in special circumstances, *Resuscitation* 67(Suppl 1):S135-S170, 2005.

Additional Readings

CR Boyce JM, Pittet D: Guidelines for hand hygiene in health-care settings, *MMWR* 51(RR16):1-44, 2002.
Christie SL, Sawatzky JV: Acute cardiac tamponade: anticipate the complication, *CACCN* 19:13-17, 2008.
CR Currey J, Botti M: The haemodynamic status of cardiac surgical patients in the initial 2-h recovery period, *Eur J Cardiovasc Nurs* 4:207-214, 2005.
CR Finkelmeier BA: Cardiothoracic surgical nursing, ed 2. Philadelphia, Lippincott, 2000.

Emergent Open Sternotomy (Assist)

P U R P O S E :   Emergent open sternotomy for a patient after cardiac surgery is performed to identify and eliminate areas of persistent hemorrhage, relieve pericardial tamponade, and provide access for open cardiac massage and internal defibrillation.

Linda Schakenbach

PREREQUISITE NURSING KNOWLEDGE

- Knowledge of the anatomy and physiology of the cardiovascular system is necessary.
- Advanced cardiac life support knowledge and skills are needed.
- Understanding of signs and symptoms of cardiac tamponade is necessary.
- Emergency open sternotomy is performed for patients who have undergone a median sternotomy, usually within the first 2 weeks of cardiac surgery.
- Emergent open sternotomy is indicated for exsanguinating hemorrhage or cardiac tamponade with imminent cardiac arrest.[5,6]
  - ❖ The goal of mediastinal exploration for persistent hemorrhage is to stop the bleeding and retain circulating blood volume. The requirement for homologous blood transfusion and incidence of wound infection associated with an undrained mediastinal hematoma[3] may be decreased.
  - ❖ The goal of mediastinal exploration for cardiac tamponade is to relieve the pressure on the ventricles during diastole. The decreased pressure allows the ventricles to fill during diastole, which should increase contractility, stroke volume, and cardiac output to improve systemic perfusion.
- Knowledge and skills related to aseptic and sterile technique are needed.
- Internal defibrillation may be necessary if life-threatening dysrhythmias occur (see Procedure 42).

EQUIPMENT

- Antiseptic solution (e.g., 2% chlorhexidine-based preparation)
- Head cover, masks, eye protection, sterile gown, sterile gloves, sterile drapes
- Sterile open-chest set and sternotomy tray
  - ❖ Wire cutter
  - ❖ Rib spreader
  - ❖ Kelly clamps and skin snaps
  - ❖ Knife handle
  - ❖ Scissors
- Electrocautery equipment: Generator, cautery, electrical dispersing pad (e.g., grounding pad)
- Large sterile suction catheter (e.g., Yankauer)
- Suction containers, tubing, regulator, and suction source
- Radiopaque gauze or other surgical sponge materials
- Polypropylene (Prolene) suture (cutting needle), other suture material according to preference
- Clip applicator and clips
- Syringes: 3 ml, 5 ml, 10 ml, and 20 ml
- Knife blades: Nos. 10, 11, 15
- Sternal wires or bands
- Sterile stapler or sutures
- Sterile dressing supplies
- Emergency medication and resuscitation equipment
  Additional equipment as needed includes the following:
- Prescribed analgesia and sedation
- Blood products and intravenous solutions as prescribed

- Sterile staple remover
- Defibrillator and compatible internal defibrillation paddles
- Warm saline solution with or without an antibiotic, as prescribed
- Chest tubes and chest tube drainage system
- Epicardial wires
- Intra-aortic balloon pump or other mechanical assist device
- Peripheral nerve stimulator (used if paralytic agents are administered)

PATIENT AND FAMILY EDUCATION

- Teaching may not be provided until after the procedure. ➼*Rationale:* Internal defibrillation usually is performed in the face of sudden hemodynamic collapse.
- Explain the reason that the open sternotomy procedure was performed and its outcome or anticipated outcome. ➼*Rationale:* This explanation provides information and encourages the patient and family to ask questions and clarify details about the patient and procedure.

PATIENT ASSESSMENT AND PREPARATION

Patient Assessment

- Assess hemodynamic and neurologic status. ➼*Rationale:* This assessment identifies baseline data that may indicate the need for emergent open sternotomy and provides comparison data.
- Assess the patient's medical history, specifically for coagulation disorders, renal disease with coexistent uremia, and functional status of the right and left ventricles. ➼*Rationale:* Baseline data are obtained.
- Assess current laboratory data, specifically complete blood cell count, platelet count, international normalized ratio, activated partial thromboplastin time, and fibrinogen. ➼*Rationale:* Near-normal baseline coagulation study results decrease the likelihood of coagulopathy as a possible cause for ongoing hemorrhage.
- Assess for signs and symptoms of cardiac tamponade:
  - ❖ Sudden decrease or cessation in chest tube drainage
  - ❖ Hypotension (mean arterial blood pressure, <60 mm Hg)
  - ❖ Altered mental status
  - ❖ Apical heart rate greater than 110 beats/min

- ❖ Narrowing of pulse pressure
- ❖ Distended neck veins
- ❖ Distant heart sounds
- ❖ Equilibrium of intracardiac pressures, with right atrial, pulmonary artery diastolic, pulmonary artery occlusion, and (if measured) left atrial pressures
- ❖ Decreased cardiac output and cardiac index
- ❖ Pulsus paradoxus
  ➼*Rationale:* The presence of some or all of these signs and symptoms assists the healthcare team to decide whether an emergent open sternotomy is necessary.
- Assess for excessive chest tube drainage. ➼*Rationale:* Presence of bleeding assists with the determination of the need for mediastinal exploration. Follow institution guidelines regarding determination of the timing of mediastinal exploration. One recommendation is when chest tube drainage continues at equal to or greater than 3 mL/kg/hr for at least 3 hours.[2]

Patient Preparation

- Verify correct patient with two identifiers. ➼*Rationale:* Prior to performing a procedure, the nurse should ensure the correct identification of the patient for the intended intervention.
- Ensure that the patient and family understand procedural teachings (if time available). Answer questions as they arise, and reinforce information as needed. ➼*Rationale:* Understanding of the information provided is evaluated and reinforced.
- Ensure that informed consent was obtained (may not be possible if the procedure is an emergency). ➼*Rationale:* Informed consent protects the rights of the patient and ensures a competent decision for the patient and the family.
- Perform a pre-procedure verification and time out, if nonemergent. ➼*Rationale:* Ensures patient safety.
- Ensure the patient's airway is protected and that supplemental oxygen is delivered. ➼*Rationale:* Ensures adequate ventilation and oxygenation.
- Position the patient in the supine position with the head of the bed flat. ➼*Rationale:* This position ensures visualization of the chest and enhances hemodynamic stability.
- Provide analgesics and/or sedatives as prescribed. ➼*Rationale:* Promotes patient comfort.

Procedure | for Assisting with Emergent Open Sternotomy

Steps	Rationale	Special Considerations
1. Assist as needed with calling the patient's physician and operative team.	The physician can reassess the need for further surgical intervention. The operative team may be needed to assist at the bedside or to prepare the operating room if further exploration is needed.	Follow institution standard.

Procedure continues on following page

Procedure   for Assisting with Emergent Open Sternotomy—*Continued*

Steps	Rationale	Special Considerations
2. **HH**		
3. Assist with preparation of the electrocautery device for possible use: A. Apply the electrical dispersing pad (i.e., grounding pad) to the patient's dry skin. B. Attach the grounding cable to the electrocautery device.[1] **(Level D*)**	Used to terminate capillary oozing or bleeding.	Grounding is essential to avoid burning the patient and possible electrical shock to the healthcare providers.
4. Assist with setting up a new sterile suction system.	Suction within the mediastinum is necessary during the procedure.	
5. **HH** **PE**		
6. Assist if needed with removing the sternal dressing.	Prepares for the procedure.	Assist if needed with preparation for cleansing the patient's chest (see Procedure 43.
7. If needed, assist the physician, advanced practice nurse, or other healthcare provider performing the procedure with: A. Donning surgical head cover, mask, and eye protection. B. Donning sterile gown and sterile gloves.	Inhibits rebound microorganism growth.[1]	All personnel in the room must don head covers and masks.
8. Assist as needed, with opening the sternotomy tray on a clean dry surface.	Prepares equipment.	
9. Assist as needed with fully draping the patient with exposure of only the surgical site.[1,2,4] **(Level D)**	A large sterile field minimizes the risk of infection and provides space to maintain asepsis of instruments and supplies during the procedure.	Allows good view of the incision.
10. Assist as needed with setting up the electrocautery system (e.g. adjusting the controls).	Cautery is used to stop bleeding from small vessels.	The cautery control is not sterile. The connection must be handed off of the sterile field without the healthcare provider performing the procedure and the assisting personnel touching each other.
11. Assist as needed with providing supplies, so that the healthcare provider can open the patient's chest, and with removing sharp objects (e.g., cut wires) from the surgical field.	Assists with procedure and ensures that removed wires are safely discarded.	
12. Assist with suctioning as needed.	Clears blood from the field.	
13. If pulseless ventricular tachycardia or ventricular fibrillation occurs, assist with obtaining equipment for internal defibrillation (see Procedure 42).	Provides emergent intervention.	

*Level D: Peer-reviewed professional organizational standards with clinical studies to support recommendations

Procedure for Assisting with Emergent Open Sternotomy—*Continued*

Steps	Rationale	Special Considerations
14. Assist with the placement of chest tubes or epicardial pacing wires as needed.	Epicardial pacing wires and chest tubes can be displaced during sternal retraction.	
15. Assist as needed with flushing the chest cavity with warm saline solution with or without an antibiotic.	May decrease the incidence of infection.	
16. Assist with placement of mechanical assist devices if needed.	Cardiac tamponade can conceal right or left ventricular dysfunction; mechanical assistance may be necessary to improve cardiac output.	
17. Assist with transporting the patient to the operating room if necessary.	The patient may need further exploration or surgical repair of coronary artery bypass grafts, cardiac valves, the myocardium, or placement of an assist device (e.g., intra-aortic balloon pump, ventricular assist device).	Ensure that the patient's chest is covered with sterile drapes or with a dressing during transportation.
18. If the patient does not return to the operating room, assist the healthcare provider performing the procedure by providing supplies for reinsertion of the sternal wires as needed.	Ensures sternal closure.	
19. Assist as needed by providing supplies for tissue and skin closure.	Ensures closure of the sternal incision.	
20. Assist or apply an occlusive dressing to the sternal incision, epicardial pacing wires, and chest tube sites.	Dressings provide a physical barrier to external sources of contamination and cushion from physical contact and trauma; they absorb drainage, maintain a moist environment at body temperature to enhance wound healing, and are used for aesthetics.	The patient's chest may be left open and covered with a sterile occlusive surgical dressing if severe ventricular dysfunction exists.
21. Discard used supplies, and remove and discard personal protective equipment.	Reduces the transmission of microorganisms and body secretions; Standard Precautions.	A chest radiograph may be ordered to rule out the presence of any retained surgical sponges, needles, or instruments.
22. HH		
23. Assist if needed with packaging used instruments for sterilization.	Prepares equipment.	

Expected Outcomes

- Resolution of the condition that necessitated the emergent open sternotomy
- Increased cardiac output
- Increased tissue perfusion, including cerebral, renal, and peripheral perfusion
- Standard chest tube drainage
- Decreased need for blood transfusions

Unexpected Outcomes

- Severe right or left ventricular dysfunction
- Continued dysrhythmias, bleeding, or coagulation disorders
- Myocardial, aortic, coronary artery, or coronary artery bypass graft perforation
- Cardiac arrest
- Pneumothorax
- Myocardial infarction
- Atrial and ventricular dysrhythmias
- Pain
- Infection

Procedure continues on following page

Patient Monitoring and Care

Steps	Rationale	Reportable Conditions
		These conditions should be reported if they persist despite nursing interventions.
1. Perform cardiovascular, hemodynamic, and peripheral vascular assessments every 15 to 30 minutes as patient status requires (including vital signs, pulmonary artery pressures, cardiac index, level of consciousness, and urine output).	Evaluate hemodynamic stability and volume status; recurrent tamponade or dysrhythmias may develop during and after sternotomy. Assess the adequacy of cerebral perfusion; hemodynamic instability can lead to cerebral anoxia. Determines perfusion to the kidneys.	• Mean arterial blood pressures less than 60 mm Hg • Abnormal changes in heart rate • Decrease in cardiac index • Abnormal pulmonary artery pressures • Urine output less than 0.5 mL/kg/h • Abnormal or equalizing pulmonary artery pressures • Change in levels of consciousness
2. Assess heart and lung sounds every 2 hours and as needed.	Abnormal heart and lung sounds may indicate the need for additional treatment.	• Distant heart sounds or additional changes in heart and lung sounds
3. Monitor coagulation, hematologic, and electrolyte laboratory blood study results.	Coagulation and hematologic profiles provide data that indicate the risk of bleeding and indicate the need for additional treatment. Electrolyte studies provide data regarding the risk for dysrhythmias and decreased contractility.	• Abnormal hemoglobin and hematocrit, activated partial thromboplastin time, international normalized ratio, platelets, fibrinogen, calcium, magnesium, or potassium levels
4. Monitor chest tube drainage.	Determines functioning of the chest tube drainage system and the amount of chest drainage.	• Cessation of chest tube drainage • Increased chest tube drainage • Clots in chest tube drainage system
5. Follow institution standard for assessing pain. Administer analgesia as prescribed.	Identifies need for pain interventions.	• Continued pain despite pain interventions

Documentation

Documentation should include the following:
• Patient and family education
• Signed informed consent, if non-emergent
• Universal Protocol requirement, if non-emergent
• Indications for procedure and the procedure performed
• Amount of blood collected from chest suctioning
• Estimated blood loss
• Patient therapies and response, including hemodynamic values, inotropic or vasopressor agents, ventilation, and neurologic status
• Additional interventions
• Unexpected outcomes
• Pain assessment, interventions and effectiveness

References

1. AORN (Association of periOperative Registered Nurses): *Perioperative standards and recommended practices,* Denver, 2008, AORN.
2. Chikwe J, Beddow E, Glenville B: *Cardiothoracic surgery,* New York, 2006, Oxford University Press Inc.
CR 3. Mason RJ, Broaddus VC, Murray JF, et al: *Murray & Nadel's textbook of respiratory medicine,* ed 4, St Louis, 2005, Saunders.
4. Phillips N: *Berry & Kohn's operating room technique,* ed 11, St Louis, 2007, Mosby.
5. Sethares K, Seifert PC, Smith H: Care of patients undergoing cardiac surgery. In Moser DK, Riegel B, editors: *Cardiac nursing: a companion to Braunwald's heart disease,* St Louis, 2008, Saunders.

CR 6. Soar J, et al: European Resuscitation Council guidelines for resuscitation 2005 section 7: cardiac arrest in special circumstances, *Resuscitation* 67(Suppl 1):S135-S170, 2005.

Additional Readings

CR Boyce JM, Pittet D: Guidelines for hand hygiene in healthcare settings, *MMWR* 51(RR16):1-44, 2002.
Christie SL, Sawatzky JV: Acute cardiac tamponade: anticipate the complication, *CACCN* 19:13-17, 2008.
CR Currey J, Botti M: The haemodynamic status of cardiac surgical patients in the initial 2-h recovery period, *Eur J Cardiovasc Nurs* 4:207-214, 2005.
Finkelmeier BA: *Cardiothoracic surgical nursing,* ed 2, Philadelphia, 2000, Lippincott.
CR Rothrock JC: *Alexander's care of the patient in surgery,* ed 13, St Louis, 2007, Mosby.

AP Pericardiocentesis (Perform)

PURPOSE: Pericardiocentesis is performed for removal of fluid from the pericardial sac, analysis of this fluid for identification of the etiology of pericardial effusion, and prevention or treatment of cardiac tamponade. Cardiac output usually is improved after pericardiocentesis.

Deborah E. Becker

PREREQUISITE NURSING KNOWLEDGE

- Advanced cardiac life support knowledge and skills are needed.
- Knowledge of sterile technique is required.
- Clinical and technical competence in the performance of pericardiocentesis is necessary.
- Knowledge of cardiovascular anatomy and physiology is needed.
- Pericardial effusion is the abnormal accumulation of greater than 50 mL of serosanguineous fluid within the pericardial sac.
- A pericardial effusion can be noncompressive or compressive. With a compressive effusion, increased pressure is found within the pericardial sac, which may result in cardiac tamponade and resistance to cardiac filling.
- The presentation of acute and chronic fluid accumulation varies. A rapid collection of fluid (over minutes to hours) may result in hemodynamic compromise with volumes of less than 250 mL. Chronically developing effusions (over days to weeks) allow for hypertrophy and distention of the fibrous parietal membrane.[2] Patients with chronic

effusions may accumulate greater than or equal to 2000 mL of fluid before exhibiting symptoms of hemodynamic compromise.[1-4]

- Symptoms of cardiac tamponade are not specific. Patients may have signs and symptoms of an associated disease. With a decrease in cardiac output, the patient often has development of tachycardia, tachypnea, pallor, cyanosis, impaired cerebral and renal function, diaphoresis, hypotension, neck vein distention, distant or faint heart sounds, and pulsus paradoxus.[1-3]
- The amount of fluid in the pericardium is evaluated through chest radiograph, two-dimensional echocardiogram, and clinical findings.
- When cardiac tamponade or a large enough effusion to warrant drainage is verified, a pericardiocentesis is performed to remove fluid from the pericardial sac. An acute tamponade resulting in hemodynamic instability necessitates an emergency procedure. Blind pericardiocentesis should be performed only in extreme emergency situations.[4]
- Pericardiocentesis commonly is performed via a subxiphoid approach.
- Two-dimensional echocardiography is recommended to assist in guiding the needle during the pericardiocentesis.[8]
- This procedure may be performed in the cardiac catheterization laboratory with fluoroscopy.
- Inability to obtain pericardial drainage, reaccumulation of pericardial fluid, or cardiac injury may progress into cardiac tamponade, which necessitates urgent or emergent chest exploration.

EQUIPMENT

- Pericardiocentesis tray (or thoracentesis tray)
- 16-gauge or 18-gauge, 3-inch cardiac needle or catheter over the needle
- Antiseptic solution (e.g., 2% chlorhexidine-based preparation)
- Two packs of 4×4 gauze sponges
- No. 11 knife blade with handle (scalpel)
- Sterile 50-mL to 60-mL, 10-mL, 5-mL, and 3-mL syringes
- Sterile drapes and towels
- Masks, goggles or face shields, surgical head covers, sterile gowns, and gloves
- Two three-way stopcocks
- 1% Lidocaine (injectable)
- 12-lead ECG machine
- Culture bottles and specimen tubes for fluid analysis
- 2-inch and 3-inch tape
  Additional equipment as needed includes the following:
- Emergency cart (defibrillator, emergency respiratory equipment, emergency cardiac medications, and temporary pacemaker)
- Two-dimensional echocardiography equipment
- Sterile marker
- Echocardiogram contrast medium
- Suture supplies
- If continuous drainage is necessary:
  - ❖ J guidewire, 0.035 diameter
  - ❖ Vessel dilator, 7 Fr
  - ❖ Pigtail catheter, 7 Fr
  - ❖ Tubing and drainage bag or bottle
  - ❖ Three-way stopcock and nonvented caps

PATIENT AND FAMILY EDUCATION

- Instruct the patient and family regarding the reason the pericardiocentesis is needed; describe the procedure; and explain expected outcomes, alternatives, and possible complications. ➵**Rationale:** This communication helps the patient and family to understand the procedure. Information about the procedure reduces anxiety and apprehension.
- Instruct the patient and family about potential signs and symptoms of recurrent pericardial effusion (e.g., dyspnea, dull ache or pressure within the chest, dysphagia, cough, tachypnea, hoarseness, hiccups, or nausea).[2,3] ➵**Rationale:** Early detection of pericardial effusion may prevent complications from cardiac compression.
- Instruct the patient and family about the patient's risk for recurrent pericardial effusion. ➵**Rationale:** Prediction of pericardial effusion may allow early detection of a potentially life-threatening problem.

PATIENT ASSESSMENT AND PREPARATION

Patient Assessment

- Determine the history of the present illness and mechanism of injury (if applicable), medical history, and current medical therapies. ➵**Rationale:** The history is needed to determine the patient's present health, to identify potential risk factors, and to provide an opportunity for the nurse to establish a relationship with the patient.
- Assess the patient's heart rate, cardiac rhythm, heart sounds (S_1, S_2, rubs), venous pressure (noninvasive or invasive), blood pressure, pulse pressure, oxygen saturation via pulse oximetry (SpO_2), respiratory status, and neurologic status. ➵**Rationale:** These data are needed to compare baseline data to assess for changes during or after the procedure.
- Assess current laboratory values, including the complete blood cell count, electrolytes, and coagulation profile. ➵**Rationale:** These data are needed to identify the potential for cardiac dysrhythmias or abnormal bleeding. If the international normalized ratio or partial thromboplastin time or both are elevated, consider reversing the level of anticoagulation therapy before performing the procedure or defer the procedure until the levels indicate a reduced possibility of bleeding.

Patient Preparation

- Ensure that the patient and family understand preprocedural teaching. Answer questions as they arise, and reinforce information as needed. ➵**Rationale:** This communication evaluates and reinforces understanding of previously taught information.
- Verify correct patient with two identifiers. ➵**Rationale:** Prior to performing a procedure, the nurse should ensure the correct identification of the patient for the intended intervention.
- Obtain informed consent (may not be possible if the procedure is an emergency). ➵**Rationale:** Informed consent protects the rights of the patient and ensures a competent decision for the patient and the family.
- Perform a pre-procedure verification and time out, if nonemergent. ➵**Rationale:** Ensures patient safety.
- Coordinate the procedure with the echocardiogram technician to assist with the two-dimensional echocardiogram if this approach is being taken. ➵**Rationale:** Echocardiogram-directed pericardiocentesis allows for more precise localization of the effusion and may help to prevent complications.[1,2,7]
- If tolerated, position the patient comfortably in the supine position with the head of the bed elevated 30 to 60 degrees. ➵**Rationale:** This position facilitates the aspiration of pericardial fluids and the ease of breathing.
- Prescribe and ensure that an analgesic or sedative is administered. ➵**Rationale:** Analgesia and sedation reduce anxiety and promote comfort.
- Apply the limb leads and connect the leads to the cardiac bedside monitoring system or to the 12-lead ECG machine. ➵**Rationale:** The ECG is analyzed during and after the procedure to monitor the patient for changes that may indicate cardiac injury.

Procedure for Performing Pericardiocentesis

Steps	Rationale	Special Considerations
1. **HH**		
2. **PE**		
3. Open the pericardiocentesis tray and supplies with aseptic technique.	Minimizes the potential for infection.	
4. As tolerated, ensure that the patient is positioned comfortably in the supine position (with the head of the bed elevated 30 to 60 degrees).	Facilitates aspiration of fluids and ease of breathing.	
5. Cleanse the skin with antiseptic solution (e.g., 2% chlorhexidine-based preparation).	Minimizes the potential for infection.	Clipping the hair may be necessary before applying antiseptic solution.
6. If two-dimensional echocardio-gram is being used, **skip to step 14.**		
7. Apply mask, goggles, or face shield, surgical cap, sterile gown, and sterile gloves. Fully drape the patient with exposure of only the surgical site.	Minimizes the risk of infection; maintains aseptic and sterile precautions	
8. Attach a three-way stopcock to a 3-inch cardiac needle, and attach to a 50-mL to 60-mL syringe.	Provides the mechanism to aspirate fluid.	
9. Attach a syringe with 1% lidocaine to one side of the stopcock.	Reduces patient discomfort.	As the needle is introduced, the provider may insert a small amount of 1% lidocaine to add analgesic effect.
10. Continuously monitor the bedside ECG or 12-lead ECG, vital signs, Spo$_2$, and venous pressure during needle aspiration and fluid withdrawal.[1-3]	Determines patient response during the procedure.	
11. Subxiphoid approach to pericardi-ocentesis: (see Figure 45-1) A. Slowly insert the needle (while aspirating with the 50-mL to 60-mL syringe) into the skin just under the xiphoid at a 30-degree angle. B. The needle is inserted into the left xiphocostal angle perpendicular to the skin and 3 to 4 mm below the left costal margin. C. After the needle is advanced to the inner aspect of the rib cage, the needle's hub is depressed so that the needle points toward the patient's left shoulder. D. The needle is advanced 5-10 mm until fluid is aspirated. E. Remove the needle and maintain the sheath in the fluid space while draining the effusion.[4]	Minimizes the risk of cardiac injury.	The movement of the heart usually defibrinates blood in the pericardial space so that it cannot clot. Clotting usually indicates penetration of the heart chamber and blood obtained from within a ventricle or atrium.[1,3] If clotting occurs with the fluid obtained, withdraw the needle and reinsert slowly in a different direction.

Procedure continues on following page

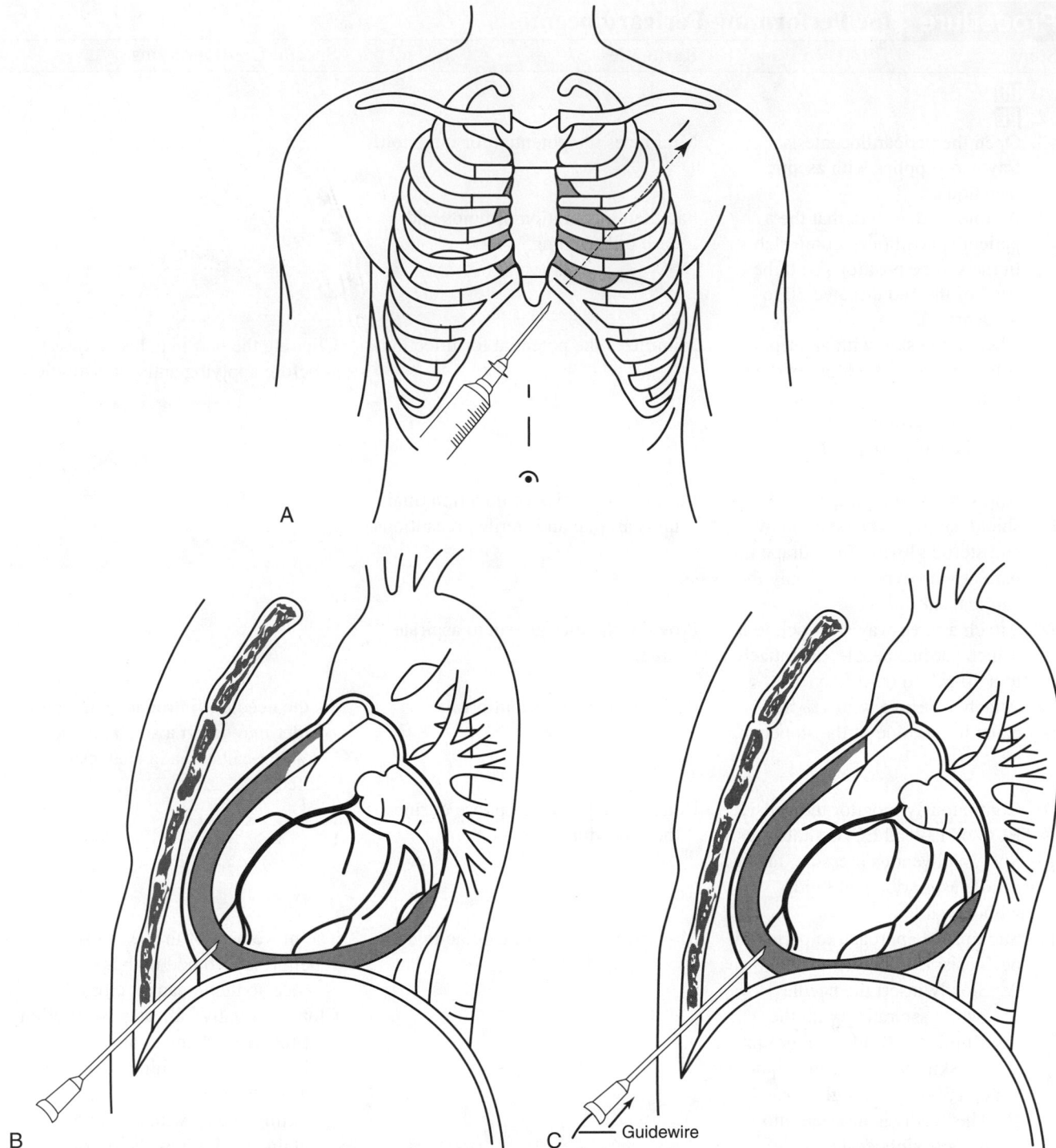

FIGURE 45-1   Subxiphoid approach to catheter placement into pericordial space. **A,** A short needle (16-gauge or 18-gauge) is inserted into the left xiphocostal angle perpendicular to the skin and 3 to 4 mm below the left costal margin. **B,** After the needle is advanced to the inner aspect of the rib cage, the needle's hub is depressed so that the needle points toward the patient's left shoulder. The needle is then cautiously advanced about 5 to 10 mm until fluid is reached. The fingers may sense a distinct "give" when the needle penetrates the parietal pericardium. Successful removal of fluid confirms the needle's position. **C,** The syringe is then disconnected from the needle, and the flexible tip of the guidewire is advanced into the pericardial space. The needle is withdrawn and replaced with a soft multihole pigtail catheter (no. 6F to 8F) with use of the Seldinger technique.

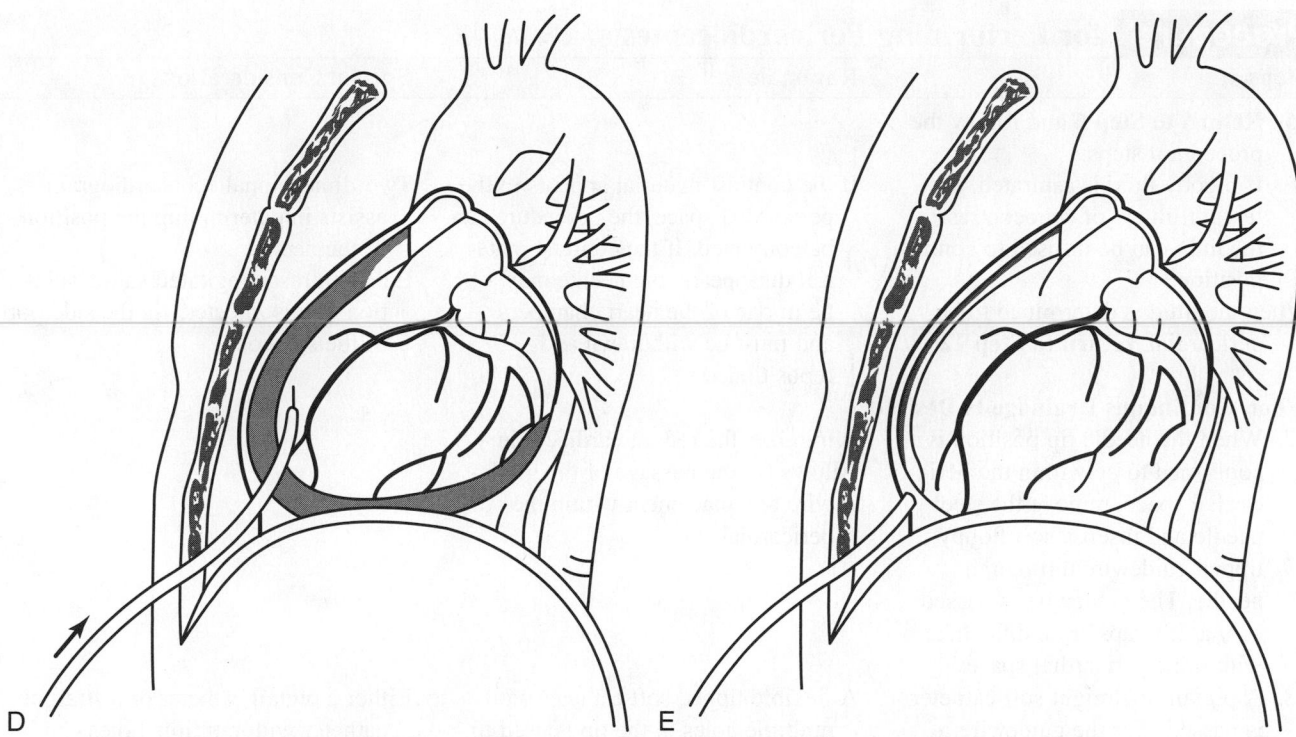

FIGURE 45-1, cont'd **D,** After dilation of the needle tract, the catheter is advanced over the guide-wire into the pericardial space. **E,** Once the catheter is properly positioned, aspiration of fluid should result in rapid improvement in blood pressure and cardiac output, a decrease in atrial and pericardial pressures, and a decrease in the degree of any paradoxical pulse. Electrical alternans, if present, also decreases or disappears. *(From Spodick DH: The technique of pericardiocentesis, J Crit Ill 2:91, 1987.)*

Procedure | for Performing Pericardiocentesis—*Continued*

Steps	Rationale	Special Considerations
12. When the needle position is confirmed, obtain the fluid samples and remove the needle. No more than 50 to 150 mL of pericardial fluid should be removed at one time.[5] **(Level E*)** If continuous drainage is needed, go **to step 17. If** not, **go to step 22.**	Provides diagnosis of the organism involved in the pericardial effusion.	Usual tests include body fluid cytology, cell count, electrolytes, routine aerobic and anaerobic cultures, acid-fast bacilli cultures, and other tests as indicated.
13. Label the specimen and send the specimen to the laboratory.	Prepares the sample for analysis.	
When Two-Dimensional Echocardiogram Is Used		
14. If available, perform a two-dimensional echocardiogram (or have a technician perform one). Determine the location and size of the effusion and the ideal entry site and needle trajectory for the pericardiocentesis.	Two-dimensional echocardiogram allows for more accurate identification of the location and size of the pericardial effusion. The ideal entry site is the point where the effusion is closest to the transducer and fluid accumulation is maximal.[1,3,8]	A straight trajectory that best avoids vital structures, including the liver, myocardium, and lung, should be chosen. The internal mammary artery also should be avoided. Mark the skin with a sterile marker to assist in guiding the needle and to make note of the trajectory to be taken.[1,3]

*Level E: Multiple case reports, theory-based evidence from expert opinions, or peer-reviewed professional organizational standards without clinical studies to support recommendations

Procedure continues on following page

Procedure for Performing Pericardiocentesis—*Continued*

Steps	Rationale	Special Considerations
15. **Return to Step 6** and follow the procedural steps.		
16. If bloody fluid is aspirated, a few milliliters of echocontrast medium can be infused to confirm position.[1,3,8] When the fluid is determined to be pericardial, **return to Step 12**.	If the contrast material appears in the pericardial space, the procedure can be continued. If the contrast material disappears, the needle may be in one of the heart chambers and must be withdrawn and repositioned.	Two-dimensional echocardiogram assists in determining the position of the needle. Echocontrast is agitated saline solution that is injected via the side port of the stopcock.[7]
When Continuous Drainage Is Desired		
17. When the needle tip position is confirmed to be within the pericardial space, remove the steel needle and insert a soft floppy-tipped guidewire through the needle. The guidewire is passed so that it wraps around the heart within the pericardial space.[1,3]	Minimizes the risk of cardiac injury. Allows for the passage of the guidewire and placement within the pericardial space.	
18. A pigtail or straight soft catheter is passed over the guidewire.	A flexible-tipped soft catheter with multiple holes in the tip is used to facilitate drainage of the effusion. Use of a soft-tipped catheter reduces the chances of causing myocardial injury and dysrhythmias during the procedure.[1]	Either a pigtail catheter or a straight catheter with multiple holes can be used for better drainage.
19. Remove the guidewire and connect the end of the catheter to the three-way stopcock and the drainage collection bag.[1,3]	Maintains asepsis; allows for continual drainage of the effusion.	If the effusion is small, when fluid is drained, remove the catheter.
20. If an indwelling catheter is placed to continuously drain a large pericardial effusion, attach the catheter to the sterile bag or bottle using aseptic technique (see Procedure 78).	Facilitates fluid drainage; minimizes the potential for infection.	
21. If an indwelling catheter is to remain in place, secure the catheter by suturing the catheter securely to the patient's chest wall.	Prevents dislodging or accidental discontinuation of drainage.	
22. Cleanse the area around the catheter with an antiseptic solution and apply an occlusive sterile dressing.	May reduce the risk of infection.	
23. Continue bedside ECG monitoring, and discontinue 12-lead ECG (if used).	Allows monitoring of cardiac rate and rhythm.	
24. Dispose of used supplies in appropriate receptacles.	Reduces the transmission of microorganisms; Standard Precautions.	
25. HH		
26. If an indwelling catheter is placed, consider prescribing antibiotics.	May reduce the risk of infection.	

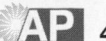

Expected Outcomes

- Fluid removed from the pericardial sac
- Relief of pain, discomfort, or other symptoms that indicated need for the procedure
- Improved cardiac output
- Patient's blood pressure, venous pressure, heart sounds, pulse pressure, and cardiac rhythm within normal limits

Unexpected Outcomes

- Decrease in blood pressure, increase in venous pressure, cardiac dysrhythmias, or excessive bleeding
- Hemodynamic instability
- ST-segment depression
- PR-segment elevation
- Cardiac tamponade
- Pain

Patient Monitoring and Care

Steps	Rationale	Reportable Conditions
		These conditions should be reported if they persist despite nursing interventions.
1. Continuously monitor ECG; assess venous pressure, blood pressure, SpO$_2$, and neurologic status during and every 15 minutes after the procedure until stable (if available, continuously monitor cardiac index and systemic vascular resistance).	A change in these signs may indicate cardiac tamponade, cardiac injury, or hemodynamic instability.	• Increasing venous pressure • Decreasing arterial pressure • Change in level of consciousness • Pulsus paradoxus • Decreased cardiac index • Abnormal systemic vascular resistance
2. Treat dysrhythmias if they occur.	Dysrhythmias may lead to cardiac decompensation.	• Persistent dysrhythmias despite appropriate intervention
3. Auscultate heart and lung sounds immediately after the procedure.	Evaluates potential fluid reaccumulation or puncture of the lung.	• Asymmetric breath sounds • Dyspnea • Tachypnea • Decreased SpO$_2$ • Distant or faint heart sounds
4. Obtain a portable chest radiograph immediately after the procedure.	Assesses for pneumothorax and hemothorax.	• Pneumothorax • Hemothorax
5. Obtain a two-dimensional echocardiogram within several hours after the procedure.	Determines the effectiveness of the pericardial drainage.	• Pericardial effusion
6. Monitor the pericardiocentesis site for bleeding every 15 minutes after the procedure is completed until the patient's condition is stable, then every 4 hours for 24 hours. If an indwelling catheter is present, continue to monitor the site every 4 hours until the catheter has been removed.	Assesses for postprocedural hemostasis and possible drainage.	• Bleeding or hematoma at site
7. Monitor hemoglobin, hematocrit, and coagulation studies every 8 hours after the procedure for 24 hours and then as indicated.	Assesses for potential of effusion recurrence or bleeding at the site.	• Bleeding or hematoma at site • Decrease in hemoglobin or hematocrit values • Changes in coagulation study results
8. Assess pericardiocentesis site every day.	Determines the presence of infection.	• Erythema • Edema • Purulent drainage • Foul odor • Temperature greater than 100.5°F (>38°C)

Procedure continues on following page

Patient Monitoring and Care —*Continued*

Steps	Rationale	Reportable Conditions
9. Prescribe site care: A. Cleanse the area surrounding the pericardial catheter with an antiseptic solution (e.g., 2% chlorhexidine-based preparation).	May reduce infection. The Centers for Disease Control and Prevention (CDC) do not have a specific recommendation for care of pericardial catheters or site care.	
B. Apply a dry sterile gauze or transparent dressing with the date and time of the dressing change.	The CDC recommends replacing intravascular catheter dressings when the dressing becomes damp, loosened, or soiled or when inspection of the site is necessary.[6]	
10. Evaluate the size of the effusion within 24 hours of the indwelling catheter placement with the use of a two-dimensional echocardiogram.	Records how effective drainage was and whether the need for the indwelling catheter continues to exist.	• Increased size of the effusion
11. Remove the indwelling catheter when no longer needed with use of aseptic technique.	Minimizes the potential for infection.	
12. Be prepared for chest exploration if deterioration in the patient's condition occurs.	Deterioration may indicate development of further cardiac tamponade.	• Decreased blood pressure • Presence of dysrhythmias • Increased venous pressure • Change in mental or respiratory status • Diaphoresis • Distant heart sounds
13. Provide emotional support to the patient throughout the procedure.	Minimizes apprehension and anxiety.	
14. Keep the patient and family informed about the patient's condition. Be available to answer patient's and family's questions and facilitate meeting their needs as appropriate.	The unknown increases the anxiety and apprehension of the patient and family.	
15. Follow institution standard for assessing pain. Administer analgesia as prescribed.	Identifies need for pain interventions.	• Continued pain despite pain interventions

Documentation

Documentation should include the following:
- Pre-procedure instruction and patient's and family's response
- Universal Protocol requirement, if non-emergent
- Signed informed consent form
- Pre-procedure and post-procedure blood pressure; venous pressures; pulmonary arterial pressures; cardiac index, cardiac output, systemic vascular resistance, if available; heart sounds; level of consciousness; respiratory status; cardiac rhythm
- Pre-procedure and post-procedure hemoglobin, hematocrit, and coagulation results, if performed
- Medications administered
- Placement of indwelling catheter, if used
- Removal of indwelling catheter, if used
- Assessment of pericardiocentesis fluid
- Amount and consistency of post-procedure drainage
- Occurrence of unexpected outcomes
- Pain assessment, interventions and effectiveness
- Pre-procedural and post-procedural evaluation and location of effusion with two-dimensional echocardiogram, if used
- ECG rhythm strips
- Emergency interventions necessary
- Specimens sent to the laboratory

References

1. Becker RC: Pericardiocentesis. In Irwin RS et al: *Procedures and techniques in intensive care medicine,* ed 6, Philadelphia, 2008, Lippincott Williams & Wilkins.
CR 2. Belenkie I: Pericardial disease. In Hall JB, et al, editor: *Principles of critical care,* ed 3, Quebec, 2005.
CR 3. Harper RJ: Pericardiocentesis. In Roberts JR, et al, editors: *Clinical procedures in emergency medicine,* ed 4, Philadelphia, 2004, Elsevier.
CR 4. Hoit BD: Management of effusive and constrictive pericardial heart disease, *Circulation* 105:2939-2942, 2002.
5. LeWinter MM: Pericardial diseases. In Libby P, et al: *Braunwald's heart disease: a textbook of cardiovascular medicine,* ed 8, Philadelphia, 2008, Saunders.
CR 6. O'Grady NP, et al: Guidelines for the prevention of intravascular catheter-related infections, *Am J Infect Control* 30(8):476-489, 2002.
CR 7. Rifkin RD, Mernoff DB: Noninvasive evaluation of pericardial effusion composition by computed tomography, *Am Heart J,* 149:1120-1127, 2005.
CR 8. Tsang TS, et al: Echocardiographically guided pericardiocentesis: evolution and state-of-the-art technique, *Mayo Clin Proc* 73:647-652, 1998.

Additional Readings

Kuhn B, Peters J, Marx GR, et al: Etiology, management and outcome of pediatric pericardial effusions, *Pediatr Cardiol* 29:90-94, 2008.
CR Mavroukakis S, Stine A: Nursing management of adults with disorders of the coronary arteries, myocardium,or pericardium. In Beare PG, Myers JL, editors: *Adult health nursing,* St Louis, 1998, Mosby.

Pericardiocentesis (Assist)

P U R P O S E :   Pericardiocentesis is performed for removal of fluid from the pericardial sac, analysis of this fluid for identification of the etiology of pericardial effusion, and prevention or treatment of cardiac tamponade. Cardiac output usually is improved after pericardiocentesis.

Deborah E. Becker

PREREQUISITE NURSING KNOWLEDGE

- Advanced cardiac life support knowledge and skills are needed.
- Knowledge of sterile technique is necessary.
- Knowledge of cardiovascular anatomy and physiology is needed.
- Pericardial effusion is the abnormal accumulation of greater than 50 mL of serosanguineous fluid within the pericardial sac.
- A pericardial effusion can be noncompressive or compressive. With a compressive effusion, increased pressure is found within the pericardial sac, which may result in cardiac tamponade and resistance to cardiac filling.
- The presentation of acute and chronic fluid accumulation varies. A rapid collection of fluid (over minutes to hours) may result in hemodynamic compromise with volumes of less than 250 mL. Chronically developing effusions (over days to weeks) allow for hypertrophy and distention of the fibrous parietal membrane.[2] Patients with chronic effusions may accumulate greater than or equal to 2000 mL of fluid before exhibiting symptoms of hemodynamic compromise.[1,2]
- Symptoms of cardiac tamponade are not specific. Patients may have signs and symptoms of an associated disease. With a decrease in cardiac output, the patient often has development of tachycardia, tachypnea, pallor, cyanosis, impaired cerebral and renal function, sweating, hypotension, neck vein distention, distant or faint heart sounds, and pulsus paradoxus.[1-3]

- The amount of fluid in the pericardium is evaluated through chest radiograph, two-dimensional echocardiogram, and clinical findings.
- When cardiac tamponade or a large enough effusion to warrant drainage is verified, a pericardiocentesis is performed to remove fluid from the pericardial sac. An acute tamponade that results in hemodynamic instability necessitates an emergency procedure. Blind pericardiocentesis should be performed only in extreme emergency situations. The use of electrocardiographic (ECG) monitoring from the needle tip with an alligator clip is not recommended.[4]
- Pericardiocentesis commonly is performed via a subxiphoid approach.
- Two-dimensional echocardiography is recommended to assist in guiding the needle during the pericardiocentesis.[7]
- This procedure may be performed in the cardiac catheterization laboratory with fluroscopy.
- Inability to obtain pericardial drainage, reaccumulation of pericardial fluid, or cardiac injury may progress into cardiac tamponade that necessitates urgent or emergent chest exploration.

EQUIPMENT

- Pericardiocentesis tray (or thoracentesis tray)
- 16-gauge or 18-gauge, 3-inch cardiac needle or catheter over the needle
- Antiseptic solution (e.g., 2% chlorhexidine-based preparation)
- Two packs of 4 × 4 gauze sponges

- No. 11 knife blade with handle (scalpel)
- Sterile 50-mL to 60-mL, 10-mL, 5-mL, and 3-mL syringes
- Sterile drapes and towels
- Masks, goggles or face shields, surgical head covers, sterile gowns, and gloves for all personnel
- Two three-way stopcocks
- 1% lidocaine (injectable)
- 12-lead ECG machine
- Culture bottles and specimen tubes for fluid analysis
- 2-inch and 3-inch tape
  Additional equipment as needed includes the following:
- Emergency cart (defibrillator, emergency respiratory equipment, emergency cardiac medications, and temporary pacemaker)
- Two-dimensional echocardiography equipment
- Sterile marker
- Echocardiogram contrast medium
- Suture supplies
- If continuous drainage is necessary:
  - ❖ J guidewire, 0.035 diameter
  - ❖ Vessel dilator, 7 Fr
  - ❖ Pigtail catheter, 7 Fr
  - ❖ Tubing and drainage bag or bottle
  - ❖ Three-way stopcock and nonvented caps

PATIENT AND FAMILY EDUCATION

- Instruct the patient and family regarding the reason the pericardiocentesis is needed; describe the procedure; and explain the expected outcomes, alternatives, and possible complications. ➥*Rationale:* This communication helps the patient and family to understand the procedure. Information about the procedure reduces anxiety and apprehension.
- Instruct the patient and family about potential signs and symptoms of recurrent pericardial effusion (e.g., dyspnea, dull ache or pressure within the chest, dysphagia, cough, tachypnea, hoarseness, hiccups, or nausea).[2,3] ➥*Rationale:* Early detection of pericardial effusion may prevent complications from cardiac compression.
- Instruct the patient and family about the patient's risk for recurrent pericardial effusion. ➥*Rationale:* Prediction of pericardial effusion may allow early detection of a potentially life-threatening problem.

PATIENT ASSESSMENT AND PREPARATION

Patient Assessment

- Determine the history of the present illness and mechanism of injury (if applicable), medical history, and current medical therapies. ➥*Rationale:* The history is needed to determine the patient's present health, to identify

potential risk factors, and to provide an opportunity for the nurse to establish a relationship with the patient.
- Assess the patient's heart rate, cardiac rhythm, heart sounds (S_1, S_2, rubs), venous pressure (noninvasive or invasive), blood pressure, pulse pressure, oxygen saturation with pulse oximetry (SpO_2), respiratory status, and neurologic status. ➥*Rationale:* These data are needed to compare baseline data to assess for changes during or after the procedure.
- Assess the current laboratory values, including the complete blood cell count, electrolyte levels, and coagulation profile. ➥*Rationale:* These data are needed to identify the potential for cardiac dysrhythmias or abnormal bleeding. If the international normalized ratio or partial thromboplastin time or both are elevated, the level of anticoagulation therapy may be reversed before the procedure or the procedure may be deferred until the levels indicate a reduced possibility of bleeding.

Patient Preparation

- Ensure that the patient and family understand preprocedural teachings. Answer questions as they arise, and reinforce information as needed. ➥*Rationale:* This communication evaluates and reinforces understanding of previously taught information.
- Verify correct patient with two identifiers. ➥*Rationale:* Prior to performing a procedure, the nurse should ensure the correct identification of the patient for the intended intervention.
- Ensure that informed consent is obtained. ➥*Rationale:* Informed consent protects the rights of the patient and makes competent decision making possible for the patient; however, in emergency circumstances, time may not allow for the consent form to be signed.
- Perform a pre-procedure verification and time out, if non-emergent. ➥*Rationale:* Ensures patient safety.
- Assist if needed with coordinating the procedure with the echocardiogram technician if the two-dimensional echocardiogram approach will be used. ➥*Rationale:* The echocardiogram technician locates the fluid accumulation, which makes performing the pericardiocentesis easier for the provider.[1,2,6]
- If tolerated, position the patient comfortably in the supine position with the head of bed elevated 30 to 60 degrees. ➥*Rationale:* The supine position facilitates aspiration of pericardial fluids and ease of breathing.
- Administer analgesics or sedatives as prescribed. ➥*Rationale:* Analgesia and sedation reduce anxiety and promote comfort.
- Apply the limb leads and connect the patient to the cardiac bedside monitoring system or to the 12-lead ECG machine. ➥*Rationale:* The ECG is analyzed during and after the procedure to monitor the patient for changes that may indicate cardiac injury.

Procedure for Assisting with Pericardiocentesis

Steps	Rationale	Special Considerations
1. **HH**		
2. **PE**		
3. Assist as needed with opening the pericardiocentesis tray and the appropriate supplies with use of aseptic technique (other supplies are opened as needed).	Minimizes the potential for infection.	
4. If tolerated, ensure that the patient is positioned comfortably in the supine position (with the head of the bed elevated 30 to 60 degrees).	Facilitates the aspiration of fluids and ease of breathing.	
5. Assist the physician, advance practice nurse, or healthcare provider if needed with cleansing the patient's skin with antiseptic solution (e.g., 2% chlorhexidine-based preparation).	Minimizes the potential for infection.	Clipping hair from the area may be necessary before applying the antiseptic solution.
6. If two-dimensional echocardiogram is being used, **skip to Step 14**.		
7. Assist personnel as needed with applying personal protective and sterile equipment (e.g., masks, head covers, sterile gowns, and sterile gloves). Assist as needed with fully draping the patient with exposure of only the surgical site.	Protects provider and maintains aseptic and sterile technique.	
8. Assist if needed with attaching a three-way stopcock to a 3-inch cardiac needle and attach to a 50-mL to 60-mL syringe.	Provides the mechanism to aspirate fluid.	
9. Assist with preparing a syringe with 1% lidocaine.	Reduces patient's discomfort.	As the needle is introduced, the provider may insert a small amount of 1% lidocaine to add analgesic effect.
10. Continuously monitor the bedside ECG or 12-lead ECG, vital signs, SpO$_2$, and venous pressure during needle aspiration and fluid withdrawal.[1-3]	Determines patient response during the procedure.	Emergent chest exploration may be necessary if aspiration is unsuccessful, pericardial fluid repeatedly accumulates, or complications develop.[1,3]
11. Continuously monitor the patient as the healthcare provider slowly inserts the needle. If two-dimensional echocardiogram is used, **Go to step 14**.	Assists with the procedure.	The movement of the heart usually defibrinates blood in the pericardial space so that it cannot clot. Clotting usually indicates penetration of the heart chamber and blood obtained from within a ventricle or atrium.[1,3]
12. Assist if needed with obtaining pericardial fluid samples. If continuous drainage is used, **go to step 17**. **If not, go to step 22**.	Provides diagnosis of organism involved in pericardial effusion.	Usual tests include body fluid cytology, cell count, electrolytes, routine aerobic and anaerobic cultures, acid-fast bacilli cultures, and other tests as indicated.
13. Assist if needed with labeling the specimens and send the specimens to the laboratory.	Prepares the samples for analysis.	

Procedure for Assisting with Pericardiocentesis—*Continued*

Steps	Rationale	Special Considerations
When Two-Dimensional Echocardiogram Is Used		
14. Assist the healthcare provider and the echocardiogram technician as needed in performing a two-dimensional echocardiogram.	Two-dimensional echocardiogram allows for more accurate identification of the location and the size of the pericardial effusion. The ideal entry site is the point where the effusion is closest to the transducer and fluid accumulation is maximal.[1,3,7]	Assist if needed with marking the skin with a sterile marker.
15. **Return to Step 7** and proceed.		
16. If bloody fluid is aspirated, be prepared to assist the healthcare provider in infusing a few milliliters of echocontrast medium into the space where the needle is to confirm position.[1,3,7] When this is determined to be pericardial fluid, return to step 12.	If contrast material appears in the pericardial space, the procedure can be continued. If the contrast material disappears, the needle may be in one of the heart chambers and must be withdrawn and repositioned.	Two-dimensional echocardiogram assists in determining the position of the needle. Echocontrast is agitated saline solution that is injected via the side port of the stopcock.[6]
When Continuous Drainage Is Desired		
17. When the needle tip position is confirmed to be within the pericardial space, assist the healthcare provider if needed as he or she removes the steel needle and inserts a soft floppy-tipped guidewire through the needle. The guidewire is passed so that it wraps around the heart within the pericardial space.[1,3]	Minimizes the risk of cardiac injury. Allows for the passage of the guide wire and placement within the pericardial space.	
18. Assist the healthcare provider with removing the guidewire and connecting the end of the catheter to the three-way stopcock and the drainage collection bag.[1,3]	Maintains asepsis; allows for continual drainage of the effusion.[1]	
19. If an indwelling catheter is placed to continuously drain a large pericardial effusion, assist the healthcare provider with attaching the sterile bag or bottle with aseptic technique (see Procedure 78).	Facilitates fluid drainage; minimizes the potential for infection.	
20. If an indwelling catheter is in place, assist the provider if needed by providing suture supplies.	Prevents dislodging or accidental discontinuation of the drainage.	
21. Assist if needed with cleansing the area around the catheter with antiseptic solution and apply an occlusive sterile dressing.	May reduce the risk of infection.	
22. Continue bedside ECG monitoring, and discontinue the 12-lead ECG (if used).	Allows monitoring of cardiac rate and rhythm.	
23. Dispose of used supplies in appropriate receptacles.	Reduces the transmission of microorganisms; Standard Precautions.	
24. **HH**		
25. Administer antibiotics as prescribed.	May reduce the risk of infection.	

Procedure continues on following page

Expected Outcomes

- Fluid removed from the pericardial sac
- Relief of pain, discomfort, or other symptoms that indicated the need for the procedure
- Improved cardiac output
- Patient's blood pressure, venous pressure, heart sounds, pulse pressure, and cardiac rhythm within normal limits

Unexpected Outcomes

- Decrease in blood pressure, rise in venous pressure, cardiac dysrhythmias, or excessive bleeding
- Hemodynamic instability
- ST-segment depression
- PR-segment elevation
- Cardiac tamponade
- Pain

Patient Monitoring and Care

Steps	Rationale	Reportable Conditions
		These conditions should be reported if they persist despite nursing interventions.
1. Continuously monitor the patient's ECG; evaluate venous pressure, systemic blood pressure, heart sounds, SpO_2, and neurologic status during and every 15 minutes after the procedure until stable (if available, continuously monitor cardiac index and systemic vascular resistance).	A change in these signs may indicate cardiac tamponade, cardiac injury, or hemodynamic instability.	• Increasing venous pressure • Decreasing arterial pressure • Decrease in intensity of heart sounds • Change in level of consciousness • Pulsus paradoxus • Decreased cardiac index • Decreased systemic vascular resistance
2. Treat dysrhythmias as prescribed.	Dysrhythmias may lead to cardiac decompensation.	• Persistent dysrhythmias despite appropriate intervention
3. Auscultate heart and lung sounds immediately before and after the procedure.	Evaluates potential fluid reaccumulation or puncture of the lung.	• Asymmetric breath sounds • Dyspnea • Tachypnea • Decreased SpO_2 • Distant or faint heart sounds
4. Ensure a portable chest radiograph is obtained immediately after the procedure.	Assesses for pneumothorax and hemothorax.	• Pneumothorax • Hemothorax
5. Ensure a two-dimensional echocardiogram is obtained within several hours after the procedure.	Shows the effectiveness of the pericardial drainage.	• Pericardial effusion
6. Monitor the pericardiocentesis site for bleeding every 15 minutes after the procedure is completed until the patient's condition is stable, then every 4 hours for 24 hours. If an indwelling catheter is present, continue to monitor the site every 4 hours until the catheter has been removed.	Assesses for post-procedural hemostasis and possible drainage.	• Bleeding or hematoma at the site • Drainage at the insertion site
7. Monitor hemoglobin, hematocrit, and coagulation levels as prescribed (e.g., every 8 hours after the procedure for 24 hours and then as indicated).	Assesses for the potential of effusion recurrence or bleeding at the site.	• Bleeding or hematoma at site • Decrease in hemoglobin or hematocrit • Changes in coagulation study results
8. Assess the pericardiocentesis site every day.	Determines the presence of infection.	• Erythema • Edema • Purulent drainage • Foul odor • Temperature greater than 100.5°F (>38°C)

Patient Monitoring and Care —*Continued*

Steps	Rationale	Reportable Considerations
9. Perform site care as prescribed or according to institution standard:		• Signs and symptoms of infection
A. Cleanse the area surrounding the pericardial catheter with an antiseptic solution (e.g., 2% chlorhexidine-based preparation).	Reduces infection. The Centers for Disease Control and Prevention (CDC) do not have a specific recommendation for care of pericardial catheters or site care.	
B. Apply a dry sterile gauze or transparent dressing with the date and time of the dressing change. Follow institution standard **(Level E)**.	The CDC recommends replacing intravascular catheter dressings when the dressing becomes damp, loosened, or soiled or when inspection of the site is necessary.[5]	
10. Be prepared for chest exploration if the patient's status deteriorates.	Deterioration in the patient's hemodynamic status may indicate an increasing effusion and the need for immediate surgical intervention.	• Decreased blood pressure • Dysrhythmias • Increased venous pressure • Change in mental or respiratory status • Diaphoresis • Distant or faint heart sounds
11. Provide emotional support to the patient throughout and after the procedure.	Minimizes apprehension and anxiety.	
12. Keep the patient and family informed about the patient's condition. Be available to answer patient's and family's questions and facilitate meeting their needs as appropriate.	The unknown increases the anxiety and apprehension of the patient and family.	
13. Follow institution standard for assessing pain. Administer analgesia as prescribed.	Identifies need for pain interventions.	• Continued pain despite pain interventions

*Level E: Multiple case reports, theory-based evidence from expert opinions, or peer-reviewed professional organizational standards without clinical studies to support recommendations

Documentation

Documentation should include the following:
- Preprocedure instruction and patient's and family's response
- Signed informed consent
- Universal Protocol requirement, if non-emergent
- Pre-procedure and post-procedure blood pressure; venous pressures; pulmonary arterial pressures; cardiac index, cardiac output, and systemic vascular resistance, if available; heart sounds; level of consciousness; respiratory status; cardiac rhythm
- Pre-procedure and post-procedure hemoglobin, hematocrit, and coagulation results, if performed
- Medications administered
- Placement of the indwelling catheter, if used

- Removal of the indwelling catheter, if used
- Assessment of pericardiocentesis fluid
- Amount and consistency of post-procedure drainage
- Occurrence of unexpected outcomes
- Pain assessment, interventions, and effectiveness
- ECG rhythm strips
- Emergency interventions necessary
- Specimens sent to the laboratory

References

1. Becker RC: Pericardiocentesis. In Irwin RS, et al, editors: *Procedures and techniques in intensive care medicine,* ed 6, Philadelphia, 2008, Lippincott Williams & Wilkins.
2. **CR** Belenkie I: Pericardial disease. In Hall JB, et al: *Principles of critical care,* ed 3, Quebec, 2005, McGraw-Hill.
3. **CR** Harper RJ: Pericardiocentesis. In Roberts JR, et al, editors: *Clinical procedures in emergency medicine,* ed 4, Philadelphia, 2004, Elsevier.
4. **CR** Hoit BD: Management of effusive and constrictive pericardial heart disease, *Circulation* 105:2939-2942, 2002.
5. **CR** O'Grady NP, et al: Guidelines for the prevention of intravascular catheter-related infections, *Am J Infect Control* 30(8):476-489, 2002.
6. **CR** Rifkin RD, Mernoff DB: Noninvasive evaluation of pericardial effusion composition by computed tomography, *Am Heart J* 149:1120-1127, 2005.
7. **CR** Tsang TS et al, : Echocardiographically guided pericardiocentesis: evolution and state-of-the-art technique, *Mayo Clin Proc* 73:647-652, 1998.

Additional Readings

Kuhn B, Peters J, Marx GR, et al: Etiology, management and outcome of pediatric pericardial effusions, *Pediatr Cardiol* 29:90-94, 2008.

CR Mavroukakis S, Stine A: Nursing management of adults with disorders of the coronary arteries, myocardium, or pericardium. In Beare PG, Myers JL, editors: *Adult health nursing,* St Louis, 1998, Mosby.

Atrial Electrogram

P U R P O S E : An atrial electrogram is obtained to determine the presence of atrial activity in a dysrhythmia or to identify the relationship between atrial and ventricular depolarizations.

Teresa Preuss, Debra Lynn-McHale Wiegand

PREREQUISITE NURSING KNOWLEDGE

- Understanding of the anatomy and physiology of the cardiovascular system, principles of cardiac conduction, and basic dysrhythmia interpretation is necessary.
- Principles of general electrical safety apply with use of temporary invasive pacing. Gloves should always be worn when handling pacing electrodes to prevent microshock because even small amounts of electrical current can cause serious dysrhythmias if transmitted to the heart.
- Advanced cardiac life support knowledge and skills are needed.
- Atrial electrograms (AEGs) offer a more definitive means for assessing and interpreting rhythm abnormalities.[4]
- The American Heart Association Practice Standards for Electrocardiographic Monitoring in Hospital Settings recommend recording an AEG whenever tachycardia of unknown origin develops in a patient after cardiac surgery.[2,4]
- Indications for AEG are as follows:
  - ❖ When atrial activity is not clearly detected on electrocardiographic (ECG) monitoring
  - ❖ For determination of the relationship between atrial and ventricular activity
  - ❖ For differentiation of wide-complex rhythms (i.e., ventricular tachycardia and supraventricular tachycardia with aberrant ventricular conduction)
  - ❖ For differentiation of narrow-complex supraventricular tachycardias (i.e., sinus tachycardia, atrial tachycardia, paroxysmal supraventricular tachycardia, atrial flutter, atrial fibrillation with relatively regular RR intervals, or junctional tachycardia)

- AEGs can be performed with multichannel telemetry or a bedside ECG monitor that allows for simultaneous display of the AEG along with the surface ECG. A 12-lead ECG machine also can be used to obtain an AEG.
- AEG is a method of recording electrical activity that originates from the atria with use of temporary atrial epicardial wires placed during cardiac surgery. Standard ECG monitoring records electrical events from the heart with electrodes located on the surface of the patient's body, which is a considerable distance from the myocardium. One limitation of ECG monitoring may be its inability to detect P waves effectively.
- AEGs detect electrical events directly from the atria, which provides a greatly enhanced tracing of atrial activity. This enhanced tracing allows for comparison of atrial events with ventricular events and determination of the relationship between the two.
- Accurate identification of the epicardial atrial pacing wire or wires is important.
- The two types of AEGs that can be obtained from epicardial pacing wires are unipolar and bipolar.
  - ❖ A unipolar electrogram measures electrical activity between one atrial epicardial wire and a surface ECG electrode. The unipolar AEG detects atrial and ventricular activity.
  - ❖ A bipolar electrogram detects electrical activity between the two atrial epicardial wires. The bipolar AEG predominantly detects atrial activity because both electrodes are attached to the atria.

EQUIPMENT

- Nonsterile gloves
- Temporary atrial epicardial pacing wires placed during cardiac surgery

- Multichannel ECG monitor and recorder or 12-lead ECG machine (ensure that biomedical safety standards are met and machine is safe for use with epicardial wires)
- Sterile dressings and materials needed for site care Additional equipment as needed:
- ECG electrodes

PATIENT AND FAMILY EDUCATION

- Provide information about the normal conduction system, normal and abnormal heart rhythms, and symptoms of abnormal heart rhythms. ➡️*Rationale:* This information helps the patient and family to understand the patient's condition and encourages the patient and family to ask questions.
- Provide information about the AEG and the reason for the AEG and explanation of the equipment. ➡️*Rationale:* This communication decreases patient anxiety and helps the patient and family to understand the procedure, why it is needed, and how it will help the patient.
- Explain the patient's expected participation during the procedure. ➡️*Rationale:* This explanation encourages patient assistance.

PATIENT ASSESSMENT AND PREPARATION

Patient Assessment

- Assess the patient's cardiac rhythm for the presence of atrial activity in more than one lead from the multichannel ECG monitor or 12-lead ECG. ➡️*Rationale:* This

assessment determines the presence or absence of P waves and the potential need for an AEG.
- Assess the patient's cardiac rhythm for the relationship between atrial and ventricular activity. ➡️*Rationale:* This assessment determines the relationship between P waves and QRS complexes and the potential need for an AEG.
- Assess for dysrhythmias. ➡️*Rationale:* This assessment determines the patient's baseline cardiac rhythm.
- Assess the patient's hemodynamic status (e.g., systolic, diastolic and mean arterial pressure, level of consciousness, dizziness, shortness of breath, nausea, vomiting, cool or clammy skin, and chest pain). ➡️*Rationale:* Hemodynamic status and need for immediate intervention are determined.

Patient Preparation

- Verify correct patient with two identifiers. ➡️*Rationale:* Prior to performing a procedure, the nurse should ensure the correct identification of the patient for the intended intervention.
- Ensure that the patient understands pre-procedure teaching. Answer questions as they arise, and reinforce information as needed. ➡️*Rationale:* This communication evaluates and reinforces understanding of previously taught information.
- Expose the patient's chest and identify the epicardial pacing wires. ➡️*Rationale:* This action provides access to the atrial pacing wires.

Procedure	**for Atrial Electrogram**	
Steps	**Rationale**	**Special Considerations**
1. [HH]		
2. [PE]		Use of gloves prevents microshocks with handling of epicardial wires.
3. Expose and identify the atrial epicardial pacing wires.	Differentiation of the atrial from the ventricular wires is important to ensure that the appropriate epicardial wires are used.	Typically the atrial wires exit the chest to the right of the patient's sternum and the ventricular wires exit to the left of the patient's sternum (Fig. 47-1).
Obtaining a Unipolar AEG with Multichannel Telemetry or Bedside ECG Monitor: Lead V		
1. Detach the V lead wire from the electrode on the patient's chest.	Prepares equipment.	Determine that the ECG monitoring system meets all safety requirements.
2. Place the tip of one of the atrial epicardial wires in direct contact with: A. The metal on the end of the V lead wire.[2] **(Level D*)** (Fig. 47-2) *or*	Electrical activity is transmitted from the epicardial wire to the ECG monitoring system.	A lead wire with alligator clips at both ends also can be used to connect the epicardial pacing wire to the monitor.

*Level D: Peer-reviewed professional organizational standards with clinical studies to support recommendations

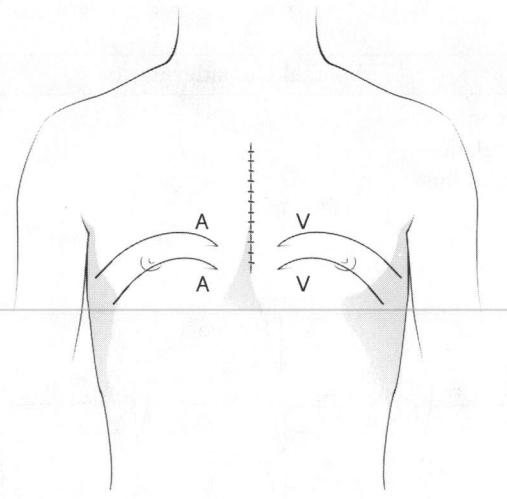

FIGURE 47-1   Atrial wires exit the chest to the right of the patient's sternum. Ventricular wires exit the chest to the left of the patient's sternum. *(Drawing by Todd Sargood.)*

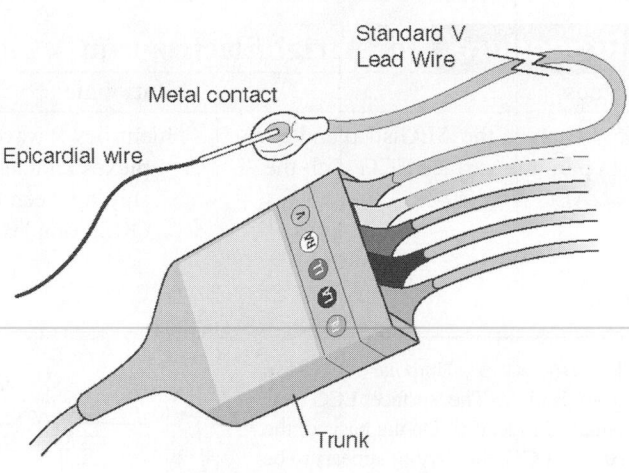

ECG Bedside Monitor Cable

FIGURE 47-2   Tip of atrial epicardial wire in direct contact with the metal on the end of the V lead wire. *(Drawing by Paul W. Schiffmacher, Thomas Jefferson University, Philadelphia.)*

Procedure   for Atrial Electrogram—*Continued*

Steps	Rationale	Special Considerations
B. The conductive gel on the adhesive side of the electrode attached to the V lead wire.[3] (Fig. 47-3).		The electrode can be wrapped around the atrial wire if continued monitoring is indicated to diagnose an unknown intermittent rhythm.[3] (Fig. 47-4).
3. Select lead V on the ECG monitor and a surface ECG lead.	Use of the precordial lead allows for detection of atrial electrical activity between the lead V and an indifferent limb lead in a unipolar configuration.	
4. Record a dual-channel strip.	Displays the AEG simultaneously with a surface ECG lead.	

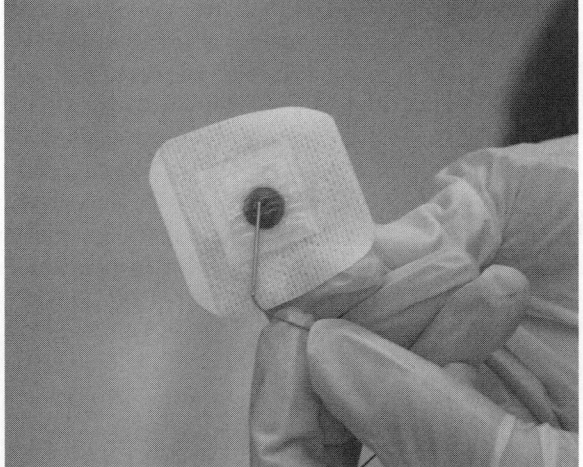

FIGURE 47-3   The tip of the atrial epicardial wire in direct contact with the conductive gel on the adhesive side of the electrode. *(Kern LS , McRae ME, Funk M: ECG monitoring after cardiac surgery: post-opeative atrial fibrillation and the atrial electrogram, AACN Adv Crit Care 18[3]:298, 2007.)*

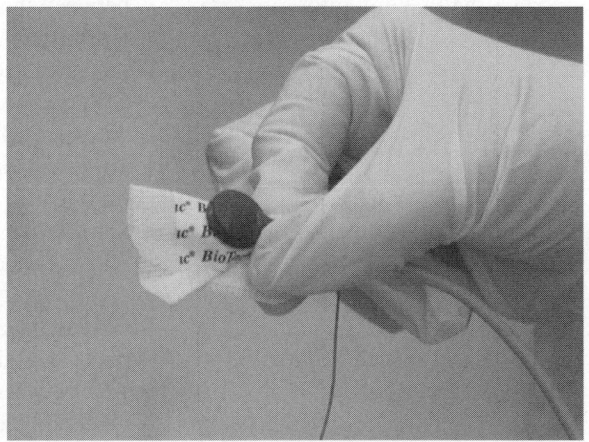

FIGURE 47-4   An electrode wrapped around the tip of the atrial epicardial wire. *(Kern LS, McRae ME, Funk M: ECG monitoring after cardiac surgery: postoperative atrial fibrillation and the atrial electrogram, AACN Adv Crit Care 18[3]:299, 2007.)*

Procedure continues on following page

Procedure | for Atrial Electrogram—*Continued*

Steps	Rationale	Special Considerations
5. Analyze the AEG strip and compare the surface ECG with the AEG (Fig. 47-5).	Identifies P waves and QRS complexes and determines the relationship between the P waves and the QRS complexes.	

FIGURE 47-5   Unipolar AEG strip from lead V. The surface ECG was obtained in lead II. On the basis of the surface ECG, the rhythm appears to be junctional with no evidence of P waves or atrial activity. The unipolar AEG shows retrograde P waves that follow the QRS complex, confirming the junctional rhythm interpretation.

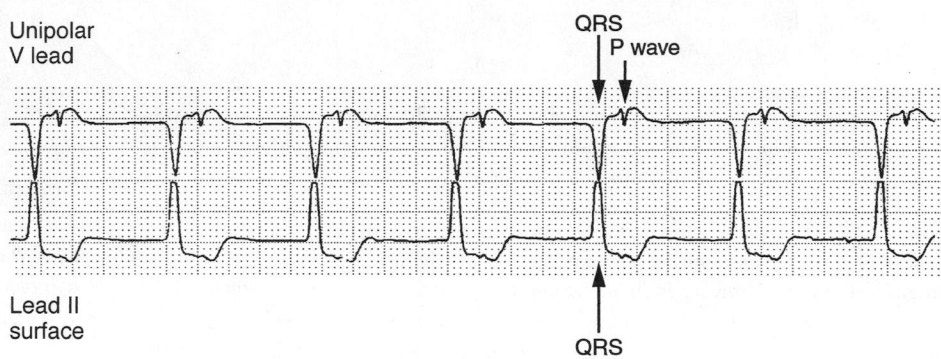

Obtaining a Unipolar AEG with Multichannel Telemetry or Bedside ECG Monitor: Lead I

1. Detach the right arm (RA) lead wire from the electrode on the patient's chest.	Prepares equipment.	Determine that the ECG bedside monitoring system meets all safety requirements.

2. Place the tip of one of the atrial epicardial wires in direct contact with:
   A. The metal on the end of the RA lead wire.[2] **(Level D*)**
or
   B. The conductive gel on the adhesive side of the electrode attached to the RA lead wire.[3] (see Fig. 47-3)
	Electrical activity is transmitted from the epicardial wire to the ECG monitoring system.	A lead wire with alligator clips at both ends also can be used to connect the epicardial pacing wire to the monitor.
		
		The electrode can be wrapped around the atrial wire if continued monitoring is indicated to diagnose an unknown intermittent rhythm.[3] (see Fig. 47-4)

3. Select lead I and a surface ECG lead on the ECG monitor.	Lead I detects electrical activity between the RA limb lead and the left arm (LA) limb lead. Because the atrial pacing wire is in contact with the RA lead, lead I detects the electrical activity between the atrial wire and the surface LA limb lead.	
4. Record a dual-channel strip.	Displays the AEG simultaneously with a surface ECG lead.	A dual-channel recorder permits the comparison of the surface ECG with the AEG.
5. Analyze the AEG strip and compare the surface ECG with the AEG (Fig. 47-6).	Identifies P waves and QRS complexes and determines the relationship between the P waves and the QRS complexes.	

*Level D: Peer-reviewed professional organizational standards with clinical studies to support recommendations

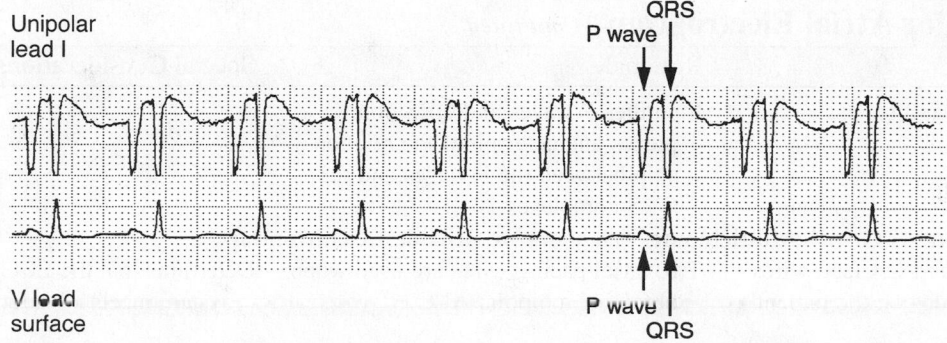

FIGURE 47-6   Unipolar AEG strip from lead I. The surface ECG was obtained in lead V. The unipolar AEG was obtained in lead I. The atrial activity is magnified in lead I.

Procedure   for Atrial Electrogram—*Continued*

Steps	Rationale	Special Considerations

Obtaining a Unipolar AEG with a 12-Lead ECG Machine

1. Connect the patient to the 12-lead ECG machine (see Procedure 60).	Provides another method of obtaining an AEG.	Determine that the 12-lead ECG machine meets all safety requirements.
2. Attach one atrial epicardial pacing wire to the clip of the RA lead wire of the 12-lead ECG machine (Fig. 47-7).	Prepares for the AEG.	

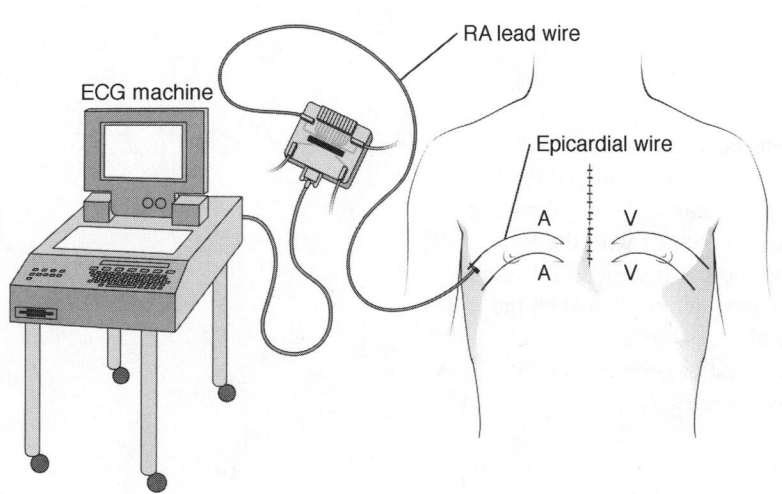

FIGURE 47-7   Attach 12-lead ECG per procedure except that the RA lead wire connects to one of the atrial-epicardial pacing wires. *(Drawing by Todd Sargood.)*

3. Run a 12-lead ECG.	Lead I measures the electrical activity between the RA and LA. Because the atrial pacing wire is connected to the RA lead, lead I detects the electrical activity between the atrial wire and the surface LA limb lead. Lead II measures the electrical activity between the RA and left leg (LL). Because the atrial pacing wire is connected to the RA lead, lead II detects the electrical activity between the atrial wire and the surface LL lead.	

Procedure continues on following page

Procedure for Atrial Electrogram—*Continued*

Steps	Rationale	Special Considerations
4. Analyze leads I and II.	Identifies P waves and QRS complexes and determines the relationship between the P waves and the QRS complexes.	

Obtaining a Bipolar AEG with Multichannel Telemetry or Bedside ECG Monitor

1. Detach the RA and LA lead wires from the electrodes on the patient's chest.	Two atrial pacing wires are used when obtaining a bipolar AEG.	Determine that the ECG monitoring system meets all safety requirements.
2. Atrial pacing wires:		
A. Place the tip of one atrial epicardial pacing wire to the metal on the end of the RA lead wire and limb lead and place the tip of the other atrial epicardial pacing wire to the metal on the end of the LA lead wire and limb lead.	Connection to the limb leads of the ECG machine allows for the detection and recording of atrial electrical activity.	A lead wire with alligator clips at both ends also can be used to connect the epicardial pacing wires to the monitor.
or		
B. Place the tip of one atrial epicardial pacing wire to the conductive gel on the adhesive side of the electrode attached to the RA lead wire and limb lead and place the tip of the other atrial epicardial pacing wire to the conductive gel on the adhesive side of the electrode attached to the LA lead wire and limb lead (see Fig. 47-3)		The electrodes can be wrapped around the atrial wires if continued monitoring is indicated to diagnose an unknown intermittent rhythm.[3] (see Fig. 47-4)
3. Select lead I on the bedside ECG monitor (Fig. 47-8).	Lead I detects electrical activity between the RA limb lead and the LA limb lead. Because the atrial pacing wires are in contact with the RA lead and the LA lead, lead I detects the electrical activity between the two atrial wires.	
4. Record a dual-channel strip.	Displays the AEG simultaneously with a surface ECG.	

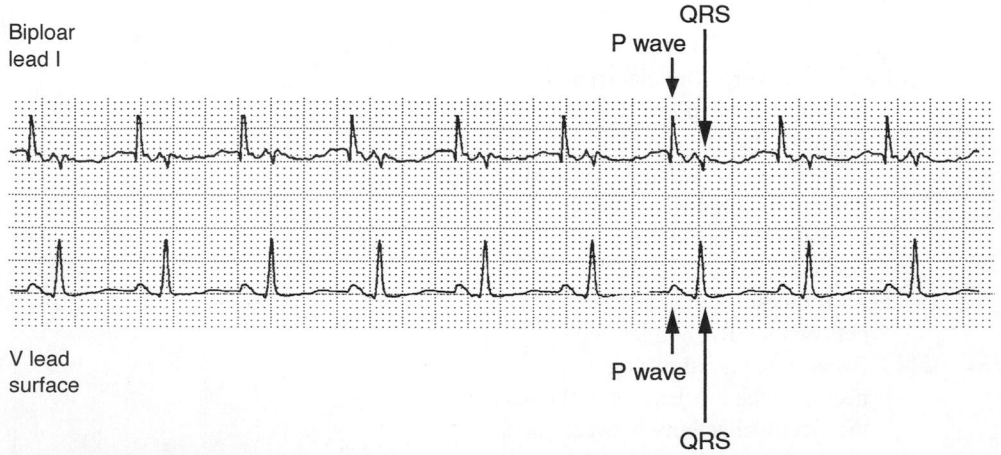

FIGURE 47-8 Bipolar AEG strip from lead I. The surface ECG was obtained in lead V. The bipolar AEG was obtained in lead I. The atrial activity is magnified in lead I. Also note how small the ventricular activity is in lead I.

Procedure for Atrial Electrogram—*Continued*

Steps	Rationale	Special Considerations
5. Analyze the AEG strip.	Identifies P waves and QRS complexes; determines the relationship between the P waves and the QRS complexes.	

Obtaining a Bipolar AEG with a 12-Lead ECG Machine

Steps	Rationale	Special Considerations
1. Connect the patient to the 12-lead ECG machine (see Procedure 60).	Provides another method of obtaining an AEG.	Determine that the 12-lead ECG machine meets all safety requirements.
2. Attach one atrial epicardial pacing wire to the RA limb lead and the other atrial epicardial pacing wire to the LA limb lead of the 12-lead ECG machine.	Connection to the limb leads of the ECG machine allows for the detection and recording of atrial electrical activity.	A bipolar AEG cannot be performed if the patient only has one atrial wire.
3. Run a 12-lead ECG (Fig. 47-9).	Lead I measures the electrical activity between the RA and LA limb leads, which sense atrial activity from both epicardial wires, to provide a bipolar tracing.	
4. Analyze lead I (see Fig. 47-9).	Displays bipolar AEG for analysis. Identifies P waves and QRS complexes and determines the relationship between the P waves and the QRS complexes.	Bipolar tracings usually magnify atrial activity and minimize ventricular activity. With this method, unipolar AEGs also are obtained in lead II and lead III.

Procedure continues on following page

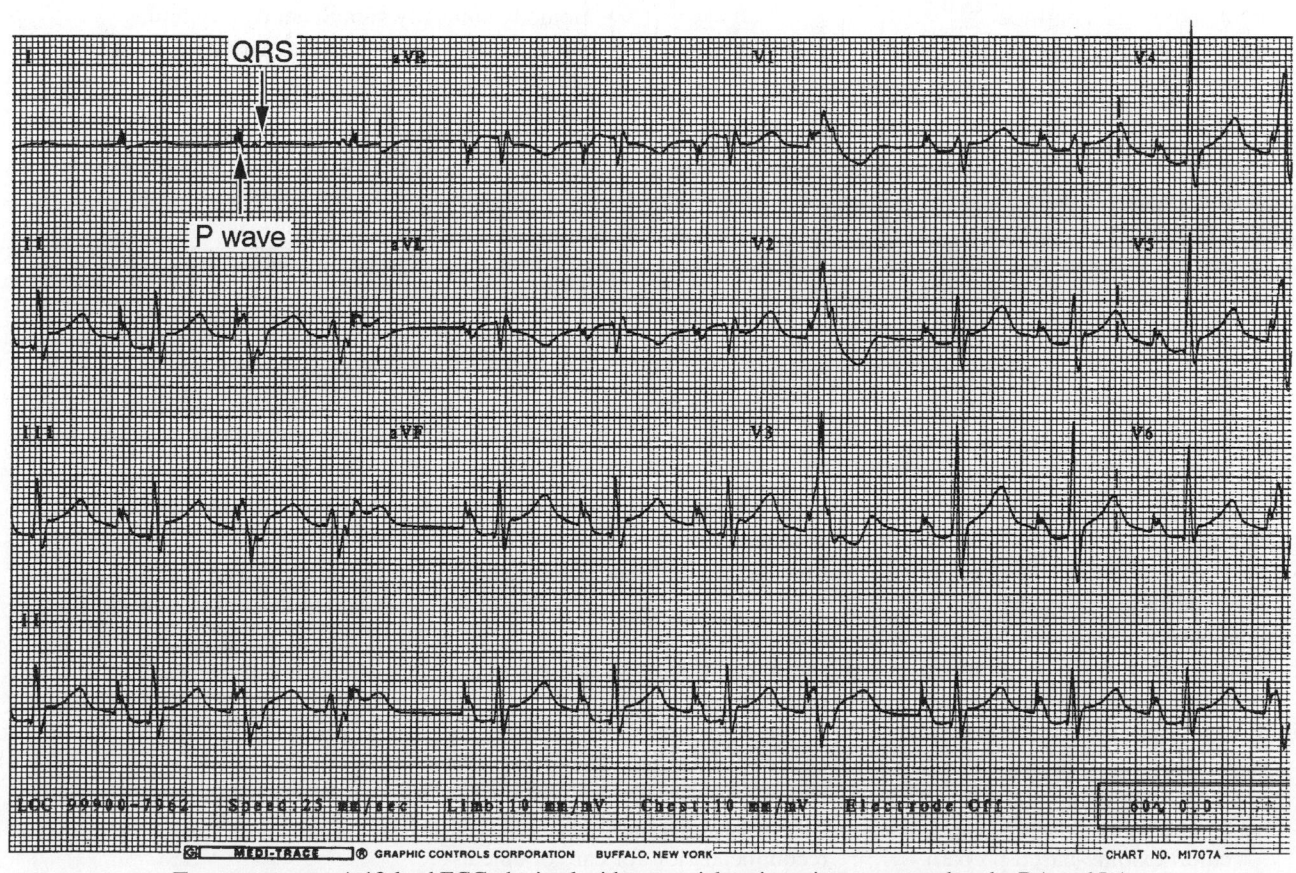

FIGURE 47-9   A 12-lead ECG obtained with two atrial pacing wires connected to the RA and LA lead wires. Lead I shows a bipolar AEG. The P wave is greater in size than the QRS complex. Leads II and III show unipolar AEGs. In leads II and III, atrial activity is enhanced. Throughout, the 12-lead ECG atrial activity is enhanced.

Procedure for Atrial Electrogram—*Continued*

Steps	Rationale	Special Considerations
After AEG Is Obtained		
1. Disconnect the atrial wires:		
A. With telemetry or a bedside monitoring system: Reconnect the ECG lead wire(s) to the electrode(s) on the patient's chest.	Reestablishes continuous ECG monitoring.	
B. With the 12-lead ECG system: Disconnect the atrial epicardial wires from the ECG lead wire clips.	Removes equipment used for obtaining the AEG.	
2. Apply a dry sterile dressing to the epicardial wire exit sites.	Reduces the transmission of microorganisms; Standard Precautions.	Follow institution guidelines for site care.
3. Place the uninsulated portion of the epicardial wires in an insulated material.[1,5]	Prevents microshock.	
4. Discard used supplies in appropriate receptacle.		
5. **HH**		
6. Label the dual channel strip with AEG next to the AEG recording and the surface lead next to the surface lead recording.	Reduces the transmission of microorganisms; Standard Precautions.	

Expected Outcomes

- Atrial activity is identified
- The relationship between atrial and ventricular activity is determined

Unexpected Outcomes

- Hemodynamically significant dysrhythmias
- Dysrhythmias in which atrial activity is unclear or the relationship between atrial and ventricular activity is unclear
- Microshocks that cause dysrhythmias

Patient Monitoring and Care

Steps	Rationale	Reportable Conditions
		These conditions should be reported if they persist despite nursing interventions.
1. Evaluate the AEG for the presence of atrial activity and its relationship to ventricular activity. Compare with the surface ECG for interpretation.	AEG determines the presence or absence of atrial activity.	• Inability to identify atrial activity
2. Monitor the ECG rhythm for changes.	The underlying dysrhythmia may change during the AEG.	• Altered hemodynamic status caused by change in ECG rhythm
3. Monitor vital signs and level of consciousness during the AEG and as needed.	Ensures adequate tissue perfusion.	• Hemodynamic instability • Change in level of consciousness
4. Assess and treat dysrhythmias.	Identifies dysrhythmias that need intervention.	• Return of rhythm stability • Change in cardiac rate or rhythm • Any signs or symptoms of infection
5. Site care should be as follows:		
A. Cleanse the area surrounding the epicardial pacing wires with an antiseptic solution (e.g., 2% chlorhexidine-based preparation). **(Level E*)**	May reduce infection. The Centers for Disease Control and Prevention (CDC) does not have a specific recommendation for care of epicardial pacing wires or site care.[6]	

Patient Monitoring and Care —*Continued*

Steps	Rationale	Reportable Considerations
B. Apply a dry sterile dressing with the date and time of the dressing change. Institution standard should be followed for frequency and type of dressing.	The CDC recommends replacing the dressing when it becomes damp, loosened, or soiled or when inspection of the site is necessary.[6]	
C. Protect the exposed uninsulated portion of the epicardial pacing wires in an insulated environment according to institution standards (e.g., closed container, finger cots, insulated gloves).	Prevents microshocks and potentially lethal dysrhythmias.	

*Level E: Multiple case reports, theory-based evidence from expert opinions, or peer-reviewed professional organizational standards without clinical studies to support recommendations[4]

Documentation

Documentation should include the following:

- Patient and family education
- ECG tracings before, during, and after the AEG
- AEG tracing with interpretation

- Hemodynamic status and level of consciousness
- Patient tolerance of the procedure
- Occurrence of unexpected outcome

References

1. Batra AS, Balaji S: Postoperative temporary epicardial pacing: when, how and why? *Ann Ped Cardiol* 1(2):120-125, 2008.
CR 2. Drew BJ, et al: Practice standards for electrocardiographic monitoring in hospital settings: an American Heart Association Scientific Statement from the Councils on Cardiovascular Nursing, Clinical Cardiology, and Cardiovascular Disease in the Young, *Circulation* 110:2721-2746, 2004.
3. Kern LS, McRae ME, Funk M: ECG monitoring after cardiac surgery: postopeative atrial fibrillation and the atrial electrogram, *AACN Adv Crit Care* 18:294-304, 2007.
4. Miller JN, Drew BJ: Atrial electrogrms after cardiac surgery: survey of clinical practice, *Am J Crit Care* 16:350-359, 2007.

5. Overbay D, Criddle L: Mastering temporary invasive cardiac pacing, *Crit Care Nurs* 24(3):25-32, 2004.
6. O'Grady NP, et al: Guidelines for prevention of intravascular catheter-related infections, *Am J Infect Control* 30:476-489, 2002.

Additional Readings

CR Waldo AL, Henthorn RW, Plumb VJ: Temporary epicardial wire electrodes in the diagnosis and treatment of arrhythmias after open heart surgery, *Am J Surg* 148:275-283, 1984.
CR Waldo AL, et al: Use of temporarily placed epicardial atrial wire electrodes for the diagnosis and treatment of cardiac arrhythmias following open-heart surgery, *J Thorac Cardiovasc Surg* 76:500-506, 1978.

AP Atrial Overdrive Pacing (Perform)

P U R P O S E :   Atrial overdrive pacing is used to terminate reentrant atrial dysrhythmias, especially atrial flutter, and allow restoration of sinus rhythm. Sinus rhythm enhances cardiac output by allowing atrial contraction to contribute to ventricular filling.

Linda Schakenbach

PREREQUISITE NURSING KNOWLEDGE

- Knowledge of the anatomy and physiology of the cardiovascular system, principles of cardiac conduction, and basic and advanced dysrhythmia interpretation is necessary.
- Knowledge of pacemaker function and patient response to pacemaker therapy is needed.
- Principles of general electrical safety need to be applied with use of temporary invasive pacing.
- Gloves always should be worn when handling pacemaker electrodes to prevent microshock because even small amounts of electrical current can cause serious dysrhythmias if they are transmitted to the heart.
- Clinical and technical competence related to the use of a temporary atrial pacemaker pulse generator and the rapid atrial pacing feature is needed (Fig. 48-1).
- Advanced cardiac life support knowledge and skills are necessary.
- Supraventricular dysrhythmias (e.g., atrial flutter, reentrant atrial tachycardia, atrioventricular [AV] nodal reentry tachycardia, reentrant tachycardias that use an accessory pathway, such as Wolff-Parkinson-White

[WPW] syndrome) sometimes can be terminated by overdrive atrial pacing.
- Atrial fibrillation occasionally terminates with overdrive atrial pacing, but this is not a reliable therapy for atrial fibrillation.
- Overdrive atrial pacing is performed most commonly with epicardial atrial pacing wires placed during cardiac surgery. A transvenous atrial pacing lead with an active fixation tip to help keep the lead in the atrium also can be used.
- Overdrive atrial pacing involves the delivery of short bursts of rapid pacing stimuli through an epicardial atrial pacing wire or a transvenous lead in the atrium. The physician or advanced practice nurse determines the duration and rate of the burst.
  - ❖ One approach to overdrive pacing is to atrial pace the heart with 20 milliampere (mA) at a rate 20% to 30% faster than the intrinsic atrial rate for 30 seconds, then stop pacing. An alternate approach is to initiate atrial pacing at a rate 20 beats/min faster than the intrinsic atrial rate; if 1:1 capture does not occur after 30 seconds, the paced rate can be increased by 20 beats/min; repeat every 30 seconds until 1:1 capture is achieved. Continue pacing until the heart rate decreases from AV block (e.g., 2:1, 3:1) or 1 to 2 minutes of 1:1 pacing have occurred, then stop pacing.[6]
  - ❖ Successive bursts usually are performed at gradually increasing rates (maximal capability of the pulse generator for overdrive atrial pacing is 800 pulses/min) and may be delivered for up to 2 minutes.[7]

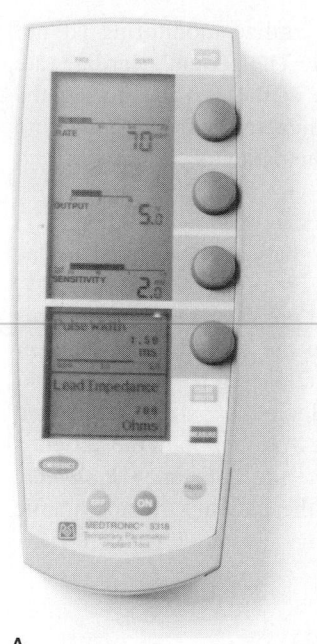
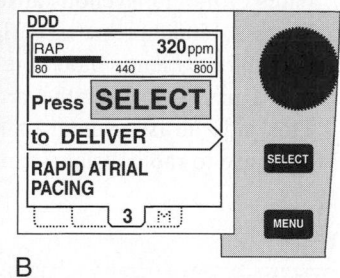

FIGURE 48-1 **A,** Temporary dual-chamber pulse generator with overdrive atrial pacing capability. **B,** Enlargement of lower screen on the pacemaker showing rapid atrial pacing controls. *(Courtesy Medtronic, Inc.)*

- The atrial pacing wire or atrial pacing lead needs to be accurately identified with initiation of overdrive pacing because pacing the ventricle at rapid rates may result in ventricular tachycardia or ventricular fibrillation.
- Rapid atrial pacing may result in degeneration of the atrial rhythm to atrial fibrillation with a rapid ventricular response. This pacemaker-induced atrial fibrillation usually does not sustain itself for more than a few minutes before it converts to normal sinus rhythm.[6]
- If an accessory pathway is present, rapid atrial pacing can result in conduction to the ventricles over the accessory pathway, leading to ventricular fibrillation.
- Overdrive suppression of the sinus node may result in periods of bradycardia, asystole, junctional or ventricular escape rhythms, or polymorphic ventricular tachycardia on termination of the atrial overdrive pacing and the atrial tachydysrhythmia.
- Conversion of an atrial tachydysrhythmia can result in dislodgment of atrial thrombus and embolization of clots to the pulmonary or systemic circulation.

EQUIPMENT

- Nonsterile gloves
- External pulse generator capable of rapid atrial pacing
- Connecting cable (between the pulse generator and the patient's pacemaker leads)
- Cardiac monitor and recorder
- Electrocardiogram (ECG) electrodes
- Double alligator clip or wire with connector pins (if needed to create a ground wire)

- Materials for epicardial pacing wire site care:
  - ❖ Antiseptic pads or swab sticks (e.g., 2% chlorhexidine-based preparation)
  - ❖ Gauze pads
  - ❖ Tape
- Insulating material for epicardial pacing wires or transvenous pacing electrode connector pins (e.g., finger cots, glove, needle caps)
- Blood pressure monitoring system
  Additional equipment to have available as needed includes the following:
- Defibrillator
- Emergency medications
- Airway management equipment
- Standard pulse generator or transcutaneous pacemaker and equipment

PATIENT AND FAMILY EDUCATION

- Explain the procedure and its purpose to the patient and family. ➤➤*Rationale:* This explanation decreases patient and family anxiety and promotes cooperation with the procedure.
- Reassure the patient that atrial pacing usually cannot be felt and that any sensation most likely will be a "fluttering" feeling in the chest. ➤➤*Rationale:* This reassurance prepares the patient and may decrease the patient's anxiety.

PATIENT ASSESSMENT AND PREPARATION

Patient Assessment

- Assess the patient's ECG rhythm and intervals, noting atrial and ventricular rates. ➤➤*Rationale:* This assessment determines baseline cardiac conduction.
- Assess the patient's vital signs and hemodynamic parameters. ➤➤*Rationale:* This assessment determines baseline cardiovascular function.
- Assess for signs and symptoms that might be caused by the dysrhythmia (e.g., shortness of breath, dizziness, nausea, chest pain, signs of poor peripheral perfusion). ➤➤*Rationale:* The patient's response to the dysrhythmia is determined.
- Assess the patency of the intravenous access. ➤➤*Rationale:* Intravenous access is needed for possible administration of fluids and medications.
- Note any medications that might have an effect on the patient's cardiac rhythm or hemodynamic parameters (e.g., beta blockers, calcium channel blockers, antidysrhythmics, digoxin). ➤➤*Rationale:* Knowledge of medication therapy can alert the healthcare providers to potential cardiac rhythms (e.g., bradycardia or atrioventricular block) after termination of the atrial dysrhythmia.
- Review the patient's coagulation study results. ➤➤*Rationale:* Therapeutic coagulation levels may decrease the risk of embolization.[2,4,6,7]

Patient Preparation

- Verify correct patient with two identifiers. ➤➤*Rationale:* Prior to performing a procedure, the nurse should ensure the correct identification of the patient for the intended intervention.
- Obtain informed consent (may not be possible in an emergency). ➤➤*Rationale:* Informed consent protects the rights of the patient and makes a competent decision possible for the patient.
- Ensure that the patient and family understand pre-procedural teaching. Answer questions as they arise and reinforce information as needed. ➤➤*Rationale:* This communication evaluates and reinforces understanding of previously taught information.
- Perform a pre-procedure verification and time out, if non-emergent. ➤➤*Rationale:* Ensures patient safety.

- Initiate continuous bedside cardiac monitoring (if not already in place). ➤➤*Rationale:* The patient's cardiac rate and rhythm must be visible at the bedside during the procedure to determine atrial capture during pacing and to evaluate the response of the patient's cardiac rate and rhythm after pacing.
- Obtain a 12-lead ECG as needed. ➤➤*Rationale:* The ECG may aid in determining the patient's baseline cardiac rhythm.
- Assist the patient to a supine position. ➤➤*Rationale:* This position facilitates access to the epicardial pacemaker wires or the transvenous atrial pacing lead wire.
- Place a blood pressure cuff on the patient's arm and obtain the patient's blood pressure or obtain the patient's blood pressure from the arterial catheter. ➤➤*Rationale:* This aids in assessment of the patient's hemodynamic response to rapid atrial pacing.

Procedure   for Performing Atrial Overdrive Pacing

Steps	Rationale	Special Considerations
1. **HH**		
2. **PE**		Gloves protect the patient from microshock while pacemaker wires are being handled.[5,6]
3. Attach the connecting cable to the external pulse generator, making sure that the positive (+) pole of the cable is connected to the (+) terminal of the pulse generator and the negative (−) pole of the cable is connected to the (−) terminal.	The connecting cable provides extra length so that the pulse generator does not have to be placed on the patient's chest or abdomen.	
4. For epicardial atrial pacing:		
A. Expose the atrial epicardial pacing wires.	The atrial epicardial wires usually exit the chest to the right of the patient's sternum (see Fig. 47-1).	The atrial epicardial pacing wires can be verified by performing an atrial electrocardiogram (see Procedure 47).
B. Connect an atrial epicardial pacing wire to the negative terminal of the connecting cable.	The pacing current is delivered through the negative terminal of the pulse generator; an epicardial pacing wire on the atrium must be connected to the negative terminal for the atrium to receive pacing impulses.	
C. Connect a second epicardial pacing wire or a ground wire to the positive terminal of the connecting cable.	The pacing circuit is completed as energy reaches the positive electrode.	If only one atrial pacing wire is present, additional options for a ground wire include an ECG monitoring electrode on the chest near the epicardial pacing wire exit site or a subcutaneous needle in the tissue on the chest. The positive terminal of the connecting cable is connected to the metal snap of the monitoring electrode or the subcutaneous needle hub with a double alligator clip.
5. For transvenous atrial pacing:		
A. Identify the proximal and the distal electrode connector pins on the external portion of the atrial pacing lead.	The pacing stimulus travels from the pulse generator to the negative terminal and energy returns to the pulse generator via the positive terminal.	

Procedure for Performing Atrial Overdrive Pacing—*Continued*

Steps	Rationale	Special Considerations
B. Connect the distal (negative) electrode connector pin to the negative terminal of the connecting cable.	Energy from the pulse generator is directed to the distal electrode in contact with the atrium.	
C. Connect the proximal (positive) electrode connecting pin to the positive terminal of the connecting cable.	The pacing circuit is completed as energy reaches the positive electrode.	
6. Set the rate and the milliampere (mA/output) controls on the pulse generator.	The settings are based on the characteristics of the patient's dysrhythmia and the threshold needed for atrial capture.	
7. Initiate atrial overdrive pacing. Pace the atrium for a brief period of 30 seconds to 2 minutes, then abruptly terminate pacing (Figs. 48-2 and 48-3).	Short bursts of pacing stimuli at a rapid rate are intended to create refractory tissue in the atrium and interrupt the reentry circuit responsible for the tachydysrhythmia.	Bursts can be repeated at faster rates and for longer intervals until the dysrhythmia terminates or changes.
A. Pace the heart with 20 mA at a rate 20% to 30% faster than the intrinsic atrial rate for 30 seconds, then stop pacing.[6]		Refer to the pulse generator's technical manual for instructions on how to initiate rapid atrial pacing.

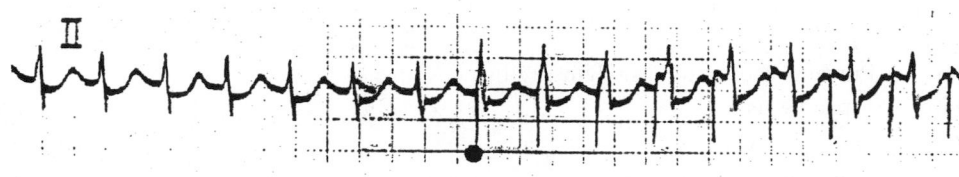

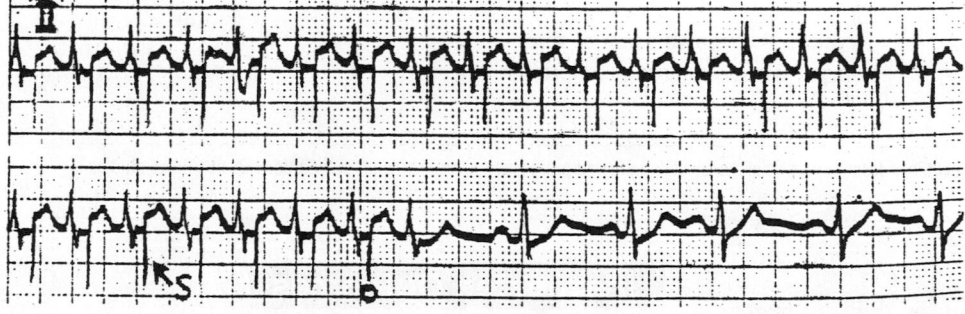

FIGURE 48-2 The *top trace* shows ECG lead II recorded during an episode of paroxysmal atrial tachycardia at a rate of 150 beats/min. Beginning with the eighth beat in this trace (*black dot*), rapid atrial pacing at a rate of 165 beats/min was initiated. In the *middle trace,* which begins 12 seconds after the top trace, atrial capture is shown clearly. In the *bottom trace,* which is continuous with the middle trace, sinus rhythm appears when atrial pacing is terminated abruptly (*open circle*). Paper recording speed was 25 mm/s. *S,* Stimulus artifact. (*From Cooper TB, MacLean WAH, Waldo AL: Overdrive pacing for supraventricular tachycardia: a review of theoretical implications and therapeutic techniques, Pacing Clin Electrophysiol 1:200, 1978.*)

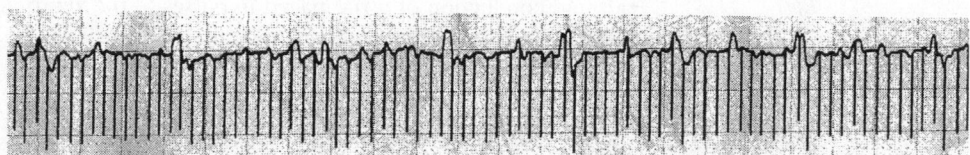

FIGURE 48-3 Rhythm strip shows rapid atrial pacing in an attempt to terminate atrial flutter.

Procedure continues on following page

Procedure for Performing Atrial Overdrive Pacing—*Continued*

Steps	Rationale	Special Considerations
B. An alternate approach is to initiate atrial pacing at a rate 20 beats/min faster than the intrinsic atrial rate; if 1:1 capture does not occur after 30 seconds, increase the paced rate by 20 beats/min; repeat every 30 seconds until 1:1 capture is achieved. Continue pacing until the heart rate decreases from AV block (e.g., 2:1, 3:1) or 1 to 2 minutes of 1: 1 pacing have occurred, then stop pacing.[6] **(Level E*)**		On termination of the dysrhythmia, the sinus node may be suppressed for a period, resulting in bradycardia, asystole, junctional or ventricular escape rhythms, or ventricular tachycardia. Initiation of temporary atrial, ventricular, or transcutaneous pacing may be necessary until normal sinus function returns.
8. When atrial pacing is completed, disconnect the connecting cable from the epicardial pacing wires or from the transvenous pacing electrode connector pins.	Removes the rapid atrial pacemaker.	Standard pacemaker therapy can be initiated if necessary.
9. Apply a sterile occlusive dressing to the pacemaker site if not already in place.	May reduce the incidence of infection.	
10. Protect the exposed pacemaker electrode connector pins or epicardial pacemaker wires with an insulating material (e.g., finger cots, needle covers).[1,5] **(Level E)**	Prevents microshock, which can result in symptomatic dysrhythmias.	
11. Coil the epicardial wires on top of the gauze dressing, cover with another piece of gauze, and tape in place.	Prevents accidental dislodgment of pacing wires.	
12. Label each epicardial pacemaker wire or dressing to identify atrial and ventricular pacing wires.	Aids identification of the epicardial pacemaker wires.	
13. Discard used supplies in appropriate receptacles.	Reduces the transmission of microorganisms; standard precautions.	
14. **HH**		

*Level E: Multiple case reports, theory-based evidence from expert opinions, or peer-reviewed professional organizational standards without clinical studies to support recommendations

Expected Outcomes

- Return to normal sinus rhythm
- Stable or improved hemodynamic status

Unexpected Outcomes

- Continuation of the tachydysrhythmia
- Conversion to atrial fibrillation
- Prolonged period of bradycardia or asystole after termination of the tachydysrhythmia
- Rapid conduction of atrial paced impulses to the ventricle through an accessory pathway, resulting in ventricular tachycardia or ventricular fibrillation
- Emergence of a slow junctional or ventricular escape rhythm or ventricular tachycardia after termination of the tachydysrhythmia
- Microshock that results in ventricular tachycardia or fibrillation
- Pain

Patient Monitoring and Care

Steps	Rationale	Reportable Conditions
		These conditions should be reported if they persist despite nursing interventions.
1. Monitor the patient's cardiac rhythm continuously at the bedside during the procedure and after the procedure.	Allows for immediate recognition of rhythm changes or return of the initial tachydysrhythmia.	• Rhythm changes • Return of initial tachydysrhythmia • Any significant or hemodynamically unstable dysrhythmia • Need for additional temporary pacing to maintain adequate heart rate after conversion of the tachydysrhythmia
2. Monitor the patient's vital signs before initiating overdrive pacing, every 5 to 10 minutes during attempts to overdrive pace, with any significant rhythm change during the procedure, and on termination of the procedure. If the patient's condition is not hemodynamically stable after the procedure, monitor vital signs every 5 to 10 minutes until stable. Monitor vital signs per unit standard if the patient's condition is stable after the procedure.	Changes in vital signs may indicate significant change in patient's condition. Blood pressure often improves with cessation of the tachydysrhythmia or restoration of normal sinus rhythm; blood pressure may deteriorate if the ventricular rate accelerates because of overdrive pacing. If the patient is receiving antidysrhythmic medications, changes in vital signs may indicate an adverse medication reaction.	• Abnormal vital signs
3. Replace gauze dressings every 2 days and transparent dressings at least every 7 days.[3] Cleanse the site with an antiseptic solution (e.g., 2% chlorhexidine-based solution). Follow institution standard. (**Level E***)	Although guidelines specific to epicardial wires and transvenous pacemaker sites do not exist, the Centers for Disease Control and Prevention (CDC) recommend replacing dressings on intravascular catheters when the dressing becomes damp, loosened, or soiled or when inspection of the site is necessary.[3]	• Redness or exudate around site • Increased white blood cell count, increased band neutrophil values • Elevated temperature
4. Monitor the patient's response to antidysrhythmic medications.	Antidysrhythmic medications may be necessary to prevent recurrence of the initial tachydysrhythmia or to control the ventricular rate.	• Prolongation of QT interval • Rhythm changes
5. Follow institution standard for assessing pain. Administer analgesia as prescribed.	Identifies need for pain interventions.	• Continued pain despite pain interventions

*Level E: Multiple case reports, theory-based evidence from expert opinions, or peer-reviewed professional organizational standards without clinical studies to support recommendations

Documentation

Documentation should include the following:
- Signed informed consent, if non-emergent
- Universal Protocol requirements, if non-emergent
- Patient and family education provided and an evaluation of their understanding of the procedure
- Rhythm strip documenting initial cardiac rate and rhythm
- Initial vital signs
- Pacemaker settings for each attempt of overdrive pacing: rate, mA, duration
- Rhythm strip documenting each overdrive pacing burst
- Number of pacing attempts
- Patient's response to the procedure (e.g., anxiety, pain)
- Pain assessment, interventions and effectiveness
- Postprocedure rhythm strip
- Postprocedure vital signs
- Any medications given during procedure
- Any unexpected outcomes
- Additional interventions

References

1. Batra AS, Balaji S: Post operative temporary epicardial pacing: when, how and why? *Ann Pediatr Cardiol* 1(2):120-125, 2008.
2. Blomström-Lundqvist C, et al: ACC/AHA/ESC guidelines for the management of patients with supraventricular arrhythmias: executive summary: a report of the American College of Cardiology/American Heart Association Task Force on Practice Guidelines and the European Society of Cardiology Committee for Practice Guidelines (Writing Committee to Develop Guidelines for the Management of Patients With Supraventricular Arrhythmias), *J Am Coll Cardiol* 42:1493-1531, 2008.
CR 3. O'Grady NP, et al: Guidelines for the prevention of intravascular catheter-related infections, *Am J Infect Control* 30:476-489, 2002.
4. Oligin JE, Zipes DP: Specific arrhythmias: diagnosis and treatment. In Libby P, et al, editors: *Braunwald's heart disease: a textbook of cardiovascular medicine,* ed 8, Philadelphia, 2008, Saunders/Elsevier.
CR 5. Overbay D, Criddle L: Mastering temporary invasive cardiac pacing, *Crit Care Nurs* 24(3):25-32, 2004.
6. Palazzo MO: Atrial fibrillation and postoperative cardiac surgery patient, *Crit Care Nurs Clin North Am* 19:395-402, 2007.
7. Smith W, Hood M: Arrhythmias. In Sidebotham D, et al, editors: *Cardiothoracic critical care,* Philadelphia, 2007, Butterworth-Heinemann.

Additional Reading

CR American Heart Association: 2005 AHA guidelines for cardiopulmonary resuscitation and emergency cardiovascular care, *Circulation* 112(24 Suppl), 2005.

AP Epicardial Pacing Wire Removal

P U R P O S E : Temporary epicardial pacing wires are inserted into the epicardium during cardiac surgery and are removed when pacing therapy is no longer needed.

Linda Schakenbach

PREREQUISITE NURSING KNOWLEDGE

* Knowledge of the cardiovascular anatomy and physiology is necessary.
* Knowledge of principles of aseptic technique is needed.[1,4,6,7]
* Knowledge of placement and function of epicardial pacing wires is necessary.
* Advanced cardiac life support knowledge and skills are needed.
* Principles of general electrical safety need to be applied with use of temporary epicardial pacemaker wires.
* Gloves always should be worn when handling epicardial pacemaker electrodes to prevent microshock because even small amounts of electrical current can cause serious dysrhythmias if they are transmitted to the heart.
* Knowledge of cardiac dysrhythmias and treatment of life-threatening dysrhythmias is necessary.
* Relative contraindications to epicardial pacing wire removal include bleeding, abnormal coagulation study results, presence of dysrhythmias that necessitate pacing assistance, and compromised hemodynamic status.
* Knowledge of signs and symptoms of cardiac tamponade is needed (e.g., hemodynamic instability, dyspnea, muffled heart sounds, diaphoresis, equalizing pulmonary artery pressures, jugular venous distention, pulsus paradoxus, altered level of consciousness).

EQUIPMENT

* Gown, goggles or face shield with mask, nonsterile gloves
* Antiseptic solution (e.g., 2% chlorhexidine-based solution)
* Suture removal kit
* Sterile gauze
  Additional equipment that may be needed includes the following:
* Emergency equipment
* Temporary transcutaneous or transvenous pacing equipment

PATIENT AND FAMILY EDUCATION

* Assess patient and family readiness to learn, and identify factors that affect learning. ➤*Rationale:* This assessment allows the nurse to individualize teaching.
* Provide information about the epicardial pacing wires, the reason for their removal, and an explanation of the procedure. ➤*Rationale:* This information helps the patient and family to understand the procedure and why it is needed and may decrease anxiety.
* Explain the patient's expected participation during and after the procedure. ➤*Rationale:* Encourages patient participation in the treatment plan and may decrease anxiety.
* Explain that the patient may feel mild pain and a burning or pulling sensation during the procedure.[2,5] ➤*Rationale:* This explanation prepares the patient for the procedure.

AP This procedure should be performed only by physicians, advanced practice nurses, and other healthcare professionals (including critical care nurses) with additional knowledge, skills, and demonstrated competence per professional licensure or institutional standard.

PATIENT ASSESSMENT AND PREPARATION

Patient Assessment

- Assess the patient's baseline cardiovascular, hemodynamic, and peripheral vascular status. ➡*Rationale:* This assessment provides data that can be used for comparison with pos-removal assessment data and hemodynamic values.
- Assess the patient's current laboratory data, including electrolyte and coagulation study results. ➡*Rationale:* This assessment identifies laboratory abnormalities. Baseline coagulation studies are helpful in determining the patient's risk for bleeding. Electrolyte abnormalities may increase cardiac irritability.
- Ensure that the patient is not receiving anticoagulation therapy. ➡*Rationale:* Epicardial pacing wires are not usually discontinued while the patient is receiving anticoagulation therapy; follow physician prescription.

Patient Preparation

- Verify correct patient with two patient identifiers. ➡*Rationale:* Prior to performing a procedure, the nurse should ensure the correct identification of the patient for the intended intervention.

- Ensure that the patient and family understand preprocedural teaching. Answer questions as they arise, and reinforce information as needed. ➡*Rationale:* Evaluates and reinforces understanding of previously taught information.
- Remove epicardial pacing wires at least the day before discharge (approximately 24 hours or longer).[3,6,9] ➡*Rationale:* Removal at this time provides time for observation for potential complications.
- Administer prescribed analgesic medication before removing the epicardial pacing wires.[8] ➡*Rationale:* Analgesics may minimize discomfort during epicardial pacing wire removal.
- Determine the patency of an intravenous (IV) catheter. ➡*Rationale:* A patent IV is necessary should emergency fluids or medications be needed.
- Ensure that patient has electrocardiographic (ECG) monitoring. ➡*Rationale:* ECG monitoring provides assessment for the presence of potential dysrhythmias during epicardial wire removal.

Procedure | for Epicardial Pacing Wire Removal

Steps	Rationale	Special Considerations
1. [HH]		
2. [PE]		Gloves minimize the possibility of microshock when in contact with the epicardial pacing wires.
3. Assist the patient into the supine position.	The supine position provides the best access during the procedure.	Epicardial pacing wires are removed with the patient lying in bed.
4. Remove the dressing and tape over the epicardial wires.	Exposes the epicardial wire exit sites.	
5. Cleanse each of the epicardial pacing wire exit sites with an antiseptic solution (e.g., 2% chlorhexidine solution).	May reduce the risk of infection.	Cleanse at least a 3-inch area around each of the exit sites.
6. Untie or cut the suture first knot of each of the epicardial pacing wires at the skin.	Prepares for epicardial pacing wire removal.	
7. Remove each epicardial pacing wire by pulling with a steady, slow, gentle tension.	Steady, slow, gentle tension uncoils the pacing lead from the epicardial surface of the heart.	Obtain an ECG strip and observe the patient's ECG monitor while removing the epicardial wires. Dysrhythmias are common during epicardial pacemaker wire removal.[2] If steady, slow, gentle tension does not remove the wires, stop the procedure and notify the physician.

Procedure | for Epicardial Pacing Wire Removal—*Continued*

Steps	Rationale	Special Considerations
8. Inspect each epicardial pacing wire to ensure that each wire is intact and to assess for the presence of tissue.[3,9] (**Level E***)	Ensures that each epicardial wire extracted is completely intact.	If bleeding occurs at the epicardial pacing wire site, apply direct pressure until bleeding stops. If tissue is noted on the epicardial wire(s) observe the patient for hemodynamic instability. Notify the physician if bleeding or oozing continues. Notify the physician if tissue is present on any of the epicardial wires removed.
9. Apply a sterile occlusive dressing over the epicardial exit sites.	May decrease the risk of infection until the exit sites heal.	
10. Discard used supplies in appropriate receptacle.	Reduces the transmission of microorganisms and body secretions; Standard Precautions.	
11. 🖐		

Expected Outcomes

- Removal of the epicardial pacing wires
- Stable cardiac rate and rhythm
- Stable vital signs

Unexpected Outcomes

- Dysrhythmias
- Hemodynamic instability
- Pain
- Hemorrhage
- Cardiac tamponade
- Hematoma
- Infection

Patient Monitoring and Care

Steps	Rationale	Reportable Conditions
		These conditions should be reported if they persist despite nursing interventions.
1. After the procedure, obtain the patient's vital signs 15 minutes × 4, every 30 minutes × 2, and every 1 hour × 2, or as recommended by institutional standard.	Determines the patient's hemodynamic status.	• Abnormal vital signs
2. Continue ECG monitoring (telemetry or other) for at least 24 hours after removal of epicardial pacing wires.[6] (**Level E**)	Provides assessment of possible dysrhythmias.	• Dysrhythmias • ECG changes
3. Maintain bed rest for at least 1 hour after removal of epicardial pacemaker wires.[6] (**Level E**)	Prepares patient for emergency intervention if needed.	• Abnormal vital signs • Bleeding • Dysrhythmias

*Level E: Multiple case reports, theory-based evidence from expert opinions, or peer-reviewed professional organizational standards without clinical studies to support recommendations

Procedure continues on following page

Patient Monitoring and Care —*Continued*

Steps	Rationale	Reportable Considerations
4. When obtaining vital signs, assess for signs and symptoms of cardiac tamponade.	Early detection is important because cardiac tamponade is a potentially fatal complication.	• Hypotension and tachycardia • Pulsus paradoxus • Beck's triad (jugular venous distention, hypotension, and muffled heart sounds) • Altered level of consciousness • Cyanosis
5. Follow institution standard for assessing pain. Administer analgesia as prescribed.	Identifies need for pain interventions.	• Continued pain despite pain interventions

Documentation

Documentation should include the following:
• Patient and family education
• Removal of epicardial pacing wires
• Patient tolerance of the procedure
• Pain assessment, interventions, and effectiveness

• Site assessment
• Vital signs and ECG strip
• Occurrence of unexpected outcomes and interventions

References

1. AORN (Association of periOperative Registered Nurses): *Perioperative standards and recommended practices,* Denver, 2008, AORN.

CR 2. Carroll KC, Reeves LM, Andersen G, et al: Risks associated with removal of ventricular epicardial pacing wires after cardiac surgery, *Am J Crit Care* 7(6):444-449, 1998.

3. Clark L: Bedside nurses removing epicardial pacer wires: from concept to practice, *Can J Cardiovascr Nurs* 17(1):27-30, 2007.

4. Conte JV, et al: *The Johns Hopkins manual of cardiac surgical care,* ed 2, Philadelphia, 2008, Mosby.

5. Mullin MH, Roschkov S, Jensen L, et al: Sensations during removal of epidural pacing wires after coronary artery bypass graft surgery, *Heart Lung* 38(5):337-381, 2009.

6. Pennsylvania Patient Safety Authority: Minimizing complications from temporary epicardial pacing wires after cardiac surgery, *PA-PSRS Patient Safe Advis* 3(1):1-6, 2006.

7. Phillips N: *Berry & Kohn's operating room technique,* ed 11, St Louis, 2007, Mosby.

8. Roschkov S, Jensen L: Coronary artery bypass graft patients' pain perception during epicardial pacing wire removal, *Can J Cardiovasc Nurs* 14:2004.

CR 9. Wollan DL: Removal of epicardial pacing wires: an expanded role for nurses, *Prog Cardiovasc Nurs* 10(4): 21-26, 1995.

Additional Readings

CR Gentry WH, Hassan AA: Complications of retained epicardial pacing wires: an unusual bronchial foreign body, *Ann Thorac Surg* 56(6):1391-1393, 1993.

Hornig GS, Ashley E, Balsam L, et al: Progressive dyspnea after CABG: complication of retained epicardial pacing wires, *Ann Thorac Surg* 86:1352-1354, 2008.

CR Matwiyoff GN, McKinlay JR: Transepidermal migration of external cardiac pacing wire presenting as a cutaneous nodule, *J Am Acad Dermatol* 42(5): 2000.

CR Meier DJ, Tamirisa KP, Eitzman DT: Ventricular tachycardia associated with transmyocardial migration of an epicardial pacing wire, *Ann Thorac Surg* 77:1077-1079, 2004.

Rothrock JC: *Alexander's care of the patient in surgery,* ed 13, St Louis, 2007, Mosby.

Implantable Cardioverter-Defibrillator

PURPOSE: The implantable cardioverter-defibrillator is a device that is used to prevent sudden cardiac death from malignant ventricular dysrhythmias. The implantable cardioverter-defibrillator continuously monitors a patient's rhythm and attempts to convert ventricular tachycardia or ventricular fibrillation via antitachycardia pacing, cardioversion, defibrillation, or some combination of these. The implantable cardioverter-defibrillator has the capability for backup bradycardia pacing.

Carol A. Offutt, Sharon R. Josephson-Keeven

PREREQUISITE NURSING KNOWLEDGE

- Knowledge of the anatomy and physiology of the cardiovascular system, principles of cardiac conduction, and basic dysrhythmia interpretation is needed.
- Knowledge of basic functioning of implantable cardioverter-defibrillators (ICDs) and patient response to ICD therapy is needed.
- Knowledge of principles of defibrillation threshold, antidysrhthmia medications, alteration in electrolytes, and effect on the defibrillation threshold is necessary.
- Advanced cardiac life support (ACLS) knowledge and skills are needed.
- Clinical and technical competence related to use of the external defibrillator is necessary.
- Indications for ICD implantation, based on the 2008 American College of Cardiology (ACC)/American Heart Association (AHA)/ Heart Rhythm Society (HRS) guidelines[6]:
  - ❖ Class I: Indicated in:
    - ○ Survivors of cardiac arrest as a result of ventricular fibrillation (VF) or sustained unstable ventricular tachycardia (VT)
    - ○ Patients with structural heart disease and sustained VT
  - ○ Patients with syncope of undetermined origin with hemodynamically significant VT or VF at electrophysiology study (EPS)
  - ○ Patients with nonischemic dilated cardiomyopathy (DCM) with left ventricular ejection fraction (LVEF) less than or equal to 35%, New York Heart Association (NYHA) functional class II or III
  - ○ Patients with LVEF less than 35% as a result of prior myocardial infarction (MI; more than 40 days after MI), NYHA class II or III; or LVEF less than 30%, NYHA function class I
  - ○ Patients with nonsustained VT as a result of prior MI, LVEF less than 40%, with inducible VF or sustained VT at EPS
  - ❖ Class IIa: Reasonable for:
    - ○ Patients with unexplained syncope, significant left ventricular (LV) dysfunction, nonischemic DCM
    - ○ Patients with sustained VT with normal or near-normal ventricular function
    - ○ Patients with hypertrophic cardiomyopathy (HCM) or arrhythmogenic right ventricular dysplasia (ARVD), with one or more major risk factors for sudden cardiac death (SCD)
    - ○ Patients with long QT syndrome who are having syncope or VT while receiving beta blockers

391

- ○ Patients who are not hospitalized and await transplantation
- ○ Patients with Brugada syndrome, with either syncope or with documented VT that has not resulted in cardiac arrest
- ○ Patients with catecholaminergic polymorphic VT with syncope or documented sustained VT on beta blocker therapy
- ○ Patients with cardiac sarcoidosis, giant cell myocarditis, or Chagas' disease
- ❖ Class IIb: May be considered in:
  - ○ Patients with nonischemic cardiomyopathy with LVEF less than or equal to 35%, NYHA functional class I
  - ○ Patients with long QT syndrome and risk factors for SCD
  - ○ Patients with syncope and advanced structural heart disease in whom thorough invasive and noninvasive investigations have failed to define a cause
  - ○ Patients with familial cardiomyopathy associated with SCD
- The ICD system is composed of a pulse generator and a lead system. The pulse generator is titanium and contains the capacitors, circuitry, and a lithium battery (Fig. 50-1).
- Battery longevity may be greater than 6 years, depending on the number of times therapies are delivered and the frequency of pacing.[5] The pulse generator is typically located in a pectoral subcutaneous pocket.
- The leads are insulated wires that sense the patient's intrinsic rhythm and can pace or deliver therapies (Fig. 50-2). Leads are classified as atrial or ventricular, endocardial (transvenous) or epicardial (myocardial), unipolar or bipolar, and active or passive fixation.[8] The lead systems may be single, double, or multiple.
- Leads may be attached to the heart via active or passive fixation. Active fixation leads use a screw, barb, or hook at the tip that is embedded into the myocardium to ensure stability of the lead. Passive fixation leads use tines or fins at the tip that allow the lead to attach to trabeculae of the myocardium.

- Most leads are endocardial (transvenous) leads and are inserted transvenously through the subclavian, cephalic, or axillary veins.
- Epicardial leads are less common but are used in special circumstances. Epicardial pacing leads may be placed on the outside of the left ventricular to provide biventricular pacing when coronary sinus placement of the LV lead has been unsuccessful. Epicardial patches may be placed on the outside of the heart, both anteriorly and posterior. Epicardial patches provide a greater surface area for defibrillation (See Fig. 50-2).
- All leads have a cathode (negative pole) and an anode (positive pole). A unipolar lead uses one conductor wire, with a distal electrode as cathode and the metal can as the anode. This configuration produces a large electrical circuit and a large pacing artifact on electrocardiography (ECG). Because of the large area covered, this configuration is susceptible to stimulation of chest muscles and also to electromagnetic interference. A bipolar lead uses two electrodes on the distal end of the lead to form the circuit. The cathode is located at the distal tip, and the anode several millimeters proximal to the tip. Because of the closer circuitry, a smaller pacing artifact is seen on ECG.
- All ICDs function as pacemakers. Some ICDs are also biventricular pacemakers. Cardiac resynchronization therapy (CRT) paces the right and left ventricles to-

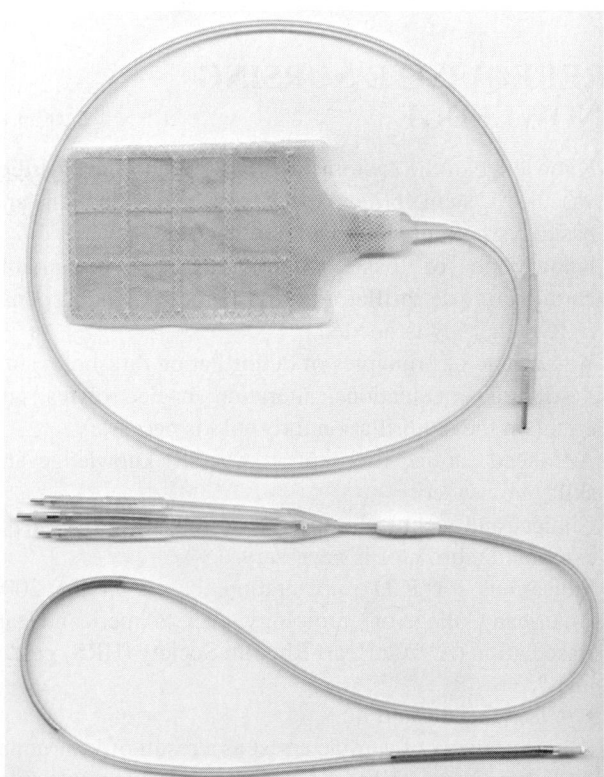

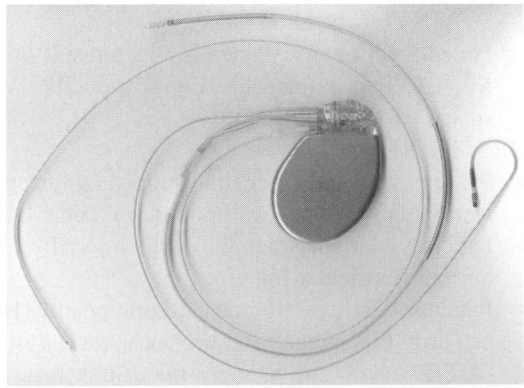

FIGURE 50-1 ICD and lead system (including superior vena cava lead, right ventricular lead, and coronary sinus lead). *(Courtesy Boston Scientific Corporatio, Natick, MA.)*

FIGURE 50-2 *Top,* ICD patch that is placed on the right ventricle. *Bottom,* Superior vena cava lead. *(Courtesy Boston Scientific Corporation, Natick, MA.)*

gether to establish synchrony in an effort to improve LV function. CRT is considered for patients with symptomatic heart failure, optimized medical therapy, LVEF less than 35%, and prolonged QRS duration of greater than 120 milliseconds.[1] Biventricular pacing must be as close to 100% as possible for the greatest benefit. Biventricular pacing leads are placed in the right atrium, the right ventricle, and an epicardial vein on the surface of the left ventricle accessed through the coronary sinus.

- The ICD detects tachydysrhythmias, delivers antitachycardia pacing (ATP) or electrical therapy (shock), and provides bradycardia pacing. ATP attempts to convert monomorphic VT by pacing at a rate faster than the VT rate, thereby terminating the dysrhythmia. ATP is a painless way of treating VT, sometimes avoiding shock therapy altogether. The PainFree II trial demonstrated that compared with shocks, empirical ATP for fast VT was highly effective, equally safe, and, improved quality of life.[17] Cardioversion is generally referred to as synchronized electrical therapy. Defibrillation is not synchronized and is generally used to convert ventricular dysrhythmias.
- The ICD therapies may be programmed from one to three zones. Typically, the zones are labeled as 1, VT, usually at slower VT rates of 140 to180 beats per minute (varies according to physician preference and patient situation); 2, fast VT, usually at rates in the range of 180 to 220 beats per minute or higher; and 3, VF for rates usually greater than 220 beats per minute. VT zones may be programmed for sequential therapies of ATP followed by electrical defibrillation if ATP is unsuccessful.
- A defibrillator code was developed in 1993 by the North American Society of Pacing and Electrophysiology and the British Pacing and Electrophysiology Group to describe the capabilities and operation of ICDs. The defibrillator code is patterned after the pacemaker code; however, it has some important differences (Table 50-1).[2] The defibrillator code offers less information about the ICD's antibradycardia pacing function but more specific information about the shock functions.
- A magnet applied over an ICD disables the device therapies of ATP and electrical cardioversion/defibrillation but

does not affect pacemaker function. The magnet is used during procedures that may cause electromagnetic interference (EMI). EMI from cautery devices, for example, may be improperly sensed as a tachydysrhythmia, causing inappropriate device shock. In most models, removal of the magnet restores normal ICD function. Some models, however, do not resume previous settings once the magnet is removed.[9] Checking with the manufacturer before magnet use is best to determine the specific recommendations for each ICD. If a device programmer and trained personnel are available, device tachydysrhythmia detection and therapies can be disabled through the programmer for the duration of the procedure.

- Emotional adjustments vary with each patient and family. Patients may experience depression, anxiety, fear, and anger. Some patients view the device as an activity restriction, and others see it as a life-saving device that allows normal life to resume. Preimplantation psychologic variables, such as degree of optimism or pessimism, and an anxious personality style may place patients at a higher level of risk for difficulty adjusting to the ICD.[13] Support groups may serve a vital role for ICD recipients who are anxious and for patients who may need additional support.[10] Interventions to reduce psychologic distress and improve quality of life may reduce morbidity and mortality in these patients.[3,11,12,15]
- The option of ICD deactivation should be discussed before the device is implanted.[18] Early discussions of device deactivation facilitate later discussions and are an important part of the informed consent process.

EQUIPMENT

- ECG monitor and recorder
- ECG electrodes

Additional equipment to have available as needed includes the following:

- ICD programmer (commonly obtained from the electrophysiology department or specific manufacturer)
- Magnet (doughnut or bar type)
- 12-lead ECG machine

TABLE 50-1	NASPE/BPEG Defibrillator Code		
Position I	Position II	Position III	Position IV
Shock Chamber	*Antitachycardia Pacing Chamber*	*Tachycardia Detection*	*Antibradycardia Pacing Chamber*
O = None	O = None	E = Electrogram	O = None
A = Atrium	A = Atrium	H = Hemodynamic	A = Atrium
V = Ventricle	V = Ventricle		V = Ventricle
D = Dual (A + V)	D = Dual (A + V)		D = Dual (A + V)

NASPE/BPEG, North American Society of Pacing and Electrophysiology/British Pacing and Electrophysiology Group.
From Bernstein AD, et al., 1993. The NASPE/BPEG defibrillator code (NBD code). Pacing Clin Electrophysiol, 16, 1776, 1993.

- Analgesia and sedation as prescribed
- Emergency medications and resuscitation equipment
- Antidysrhythmia medications as prescribed

PATIENT AND FAMILY EDUCATION

- Assess learning needs, readiness to learn, and factors that influence learning. ➤*Rationale:* This assessment allows the nurse to individualize teaching in a meaningful manner.
- Assess patient and family understanding of ICD therapy and the reason for its use. ➤*Rationale:* This assessment provides information regarding knowledge level and necessity of additional teaching.
- Provide information about the normal conduction system, such as structure of the conduction system, source of the heartbeat, normal and abnormal heart rhythms, symptoms of abnormal heart rhythms, and the potentially life-threatening nature of VT and VF. ➤*Rationale:* Understanding of the conduction system and dangerous dysrhythmias assists the patient and family in recognizing the seriousness of the patient's condition and the need for ICD therapy.
- Provide information about ICD therapy, including the reason for the ICD, device operation, location of the device, types of therapy given by the device, risks and benefits of the device, and follow-up. ➤*Rationale:* Understanding of ICD functioning assists the patient and family in developing realistic perceptions of ICD therapy.
- Discuss postimplant incision care, including inspection of the incision and pocket. The incision is kept dry for several days after the procedure. ➤*Rationale:* The nurse or physician needs to know whether any of the following signs or symptoms of infection appear: redness, edema, warmth, drainage, and/or fever.
- Discuss postoperative activity. For the first 4 to 6 weeks after implant: 1, no lifting of the arm on the side of the ICD above the shoulder or extending the arm to back (including activities such as swimming, golfing, and bowling); 2, no lifting of items heavier than 10 lb; and 3, no excessive pushing, pulling, or twisting. ➤*Rationale:* The activity restrictions help to prevent new leads from dislodgment.
- Provide patients with an identification card (temporary cards are usually given to patients at the time of implant, and permanent cards are sent to patients by the manufacturer several weeks later). Encourage the patient to wear Medic Alert identification and to carry the identification card at all times. ➤*Rationale:* This identification ensures that appropriate information is available to anyone caring for the patient.
- If patients are prescribed antidysrhythmic medication, stress the importance of continuing the medication. ➤*Rationale:* Antidysrhythmic medications suppress dysrhythmias and may limit potential ICD shocks.

- Discuss the need for patients to keep a current list of medications in their wallets. ➤*Rationale:* The patient or other family members should be prepared to provide necessary information to healthcare providers in an emergency situation.
- In select circumstances, the healthcare team may recommend that family members learn CPR. ➤*Rationale:* Family members may be more prepared for an emergency situation (e.g., if the ICD does not convert a life-threatening rhythm or the ICD malfunctions).
- Educate patients and families about what to do for a device shock. The shock varies in intensity from mild to severe pain. If patients have received an isolated shock and are asymptomatic afterward, they should call their healthcare provider to determine further action (usually an appointment for device interrogation). If patients have received multiple shocks in a short period of time (within minutes to hours), or if they have had one shock and do not feel well, they should activate the emergency medical services (EMS) system by calling 911 to seek emergency evaluation at an emergency room.[14] ➤*Rationale:* Repeated shocks may indicate conditions that necessitate prompt treatment, such as electrolyte imbalance or ischemia. They may also indicate malfunction of the device sensing, which may occur with lead fracture.
- Inform patients to call their healthcare provider if they hear an audible tone emitted from the device. An audible tone may indicate battery depletion or signal device parameter alerts (such as lead impedance out of normal range). Some devices use vibratory alerts in place of audible tones to signal an alert condition. ➤*Rationale:* The ICD should be interrogated to determine the reason for the tone and to ensure safe device function.
- Inform patients and families that family members are not harmed if they touch the patient when a shock is delivered. ➤*Rationale:* This information prepares the patient and family and may decrease anxiety.
- Driving restrictions vary from state to state and among physicians. Each patient should discuss plans for long trips and driving restrictions with the physician. Current guidelines prohibit anyone with an ICD from obtaining a commercial driver's license.[7] ➤*Rationale:* These restrictions are intended to prevent motor vehicle accidents from sudden loss of consciousness while driving.
- Educate patients and families that the terms "elective replacement indicated" (ERI) and "end of life" (EOL) are used to describe the status of the battery. At ERI, the battery is able to function for approximately another 2 to 3 months. A generator change is done as soon as possible during that time period. At EOL, the generator must be changed promptly. ➤*Rationale:* This teaching prepares patients and families for generator changes, alleviates misunderstanding, and may decrease anxiety.

- Inform patients and family members about follow-up device checks or "interrogations." Stress the importance of keeping these appointments. Devices are checked every 3 to 6 months (but may be more frequent if any issues arise that necessitate monitoring). Many follow-up checks are now done remotely, through internet-based systems. A transmitter device is mailed to the patient from the device manufacturer. ➤*Rationale:* Routine interrogation maintains optimal functioning of the ICD and alerts providers of dysrhythmias.
- Inform the patient and family of potential sources of EMI to the ICD. In the hospital, EMI include magnetic resonance imaging, diathermy, computed tomography, lithotripsy, electrocautery, radiation therapy, and nerve stimulators. Outside the hospital, these include handheld wands used by airport security, arc welders, large transformers or motors, antitheft devices at stores or libraries, cellular phones less than 6 inches away from the pulse generator, the antenna of an operating citizens' band or ham radio, improperly grounded electrical equipment, and handheld tools less than 12 inches away from the pulse generator. Cellular phones should be positioned on the opposite side of device.[16] ➤*Rationale:* EMI can deactivate ICD therapies.
- Explore the patient's feelings about having an ICD. Approximately 30% to 50% of patients experience a degree of psychologic stress after implant.[13] ICD support groups have been helpful to many. ➤*Rationale:* Acknowledging these stressors may alleviate the most common psychologic disturbances after ICD implantation, which include stress, anxiety, depression, and fear.
- Inform patients to notify their physicians if the device begins to wear through the skin or the device site becomes reddened, warm, painful, or has discharge. ➤*Rationale:* These signs and symptoms identify problems (e.g., infection) that need additional medical care.

PATIENT ASSESSMENT AND PREPARATION

Patient Assessment

- Assess the patient's cardiac rate and rhythm. ➤*Rationale:* This assessment establishes baseline data.
- Presurgical instructions usually include withholding anticoagulation therapy as prescribed for several days before the procedure, maintaining nothing by mouth (NPO) for at least 8 hours before the procedure, and obtaining complete blood cell count (CBC), chemistries, prothrombin time (PT), and partial thromboplastin time (PTT) for baseline data. ➤*Rationale:* All these actions ensure patient safety to prevent complications such as excessive bleeding and aspiration.
- Assess the patency of the patient's intravenous access. ➤*Rationale:* Intravenous access should be ensured for administration of prescribed medications.
- Administer antibiotics as prescribed. ➤*Rationale:* Antibiotics are administered to reduce infection from skin microorganisms such as *Staphylococcus aureus* (cause of early infection) and *Staphylococcus epidermidis* (cause of later infection).[9]
- Identify the manufacturer of the ICD and how it is programmed. ➤*Rationale:* Interrogation of the device provides important information: battery voltage and impedance, charge time, dysrhythmias detected by device (logbook) and any therapies given (ATP or shock), pacing and sensing thresholds, and impedances for all leads, percent of pacing and sensing in each chamber, and review of programmed parameters.[19] Interrogation usually also reveals device and lead information (models and serial numbers), implant date, and implanting physician information. See Figure 50-3 for an example of an ICD interrogation report.

Patient Preparation

- Verify correct patient with two identifiers. ➤*Rationale:* Prior to performing a procedure, the nurse should ensure the correct identification of the patient for the intended intervention.
- Ensure that the patient and family understand preprocedural teaching. Answer questions as they arise, and reinforce information as needed. ➤*Rationale:* Understanding of previously taught information is evaluated and reinforced.
- Ensure that informed consent has been obtained (before ICD insertion). ➤*Rationale:* Informed consent protects the rights of the patient and makes a competent decision possible for the patient.
- Perform a pre-procedure verification and time out (before ICD insertion). ➤*Rationale:* Ensures patient safety.
- Provide analgesia or sedatives as prescribed and needed. ➤*Rationale:* Analgesia and sedatives promote comfort and may decrease anxiety.

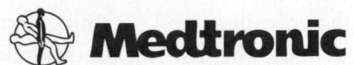 **Medtronic**   **Quick Look**

Device: En Trust	Serial Number:	Date of Interrogation:	**-Feb-2007 16:08:52**
Patient:		Physician:	

1	**Device Status (Implanted: 13-Jun-2006)**			**Measured on:**
	Battery Voltage (ERI=2.61 V)	3.17 V		24-Feb-2007
	Last Full Energy Charge	7.9 sec		13-Dec-2006

2		**Atrial(5076)**	**RV**	
	Pacing Impedance	488 ohms	504 ohms	24-Feb-2007
	Defibrillation Impedance		RV=76 ohms	24-Feb-2007
	Programmed Amplitude/Pulse Width	3 V / 0.4 ms	3 V / 0.4 ms	

3	Measured P/R Wave	3 mV	20 mV	24-Feb-2007
	Programmed Sensitivity	0.3 mV	0.45 mV	

4	**Parameter Summary**					
	Mode AAI<=>DDD	Lower Rate	60 bpm	Paced AV	180 ms
	Mode Switch 171 bpm	Upper Track	130 bpm	Sensed AV	150 ms
		Upper Sensor	130 bpm		

5	**Detection**		**Rates**	**Therapies**
	AT/AF	Monitor	>171 bpm	All Rx Off
	VF	On	>200 bpm	ATP During Charging, 25J, 35J × 5
	FVT	OFF		All Rx Off
	VT	On	171-200 bpm	Burst(3), Ramp(3), 20J, 35J × 3

Enhancements On: AF/All, Sinus Tach

Clinical Status	**Since 24-Oct-2006**	**Cardiac Compass Trends (Jun-2006 to Feb-2007)**

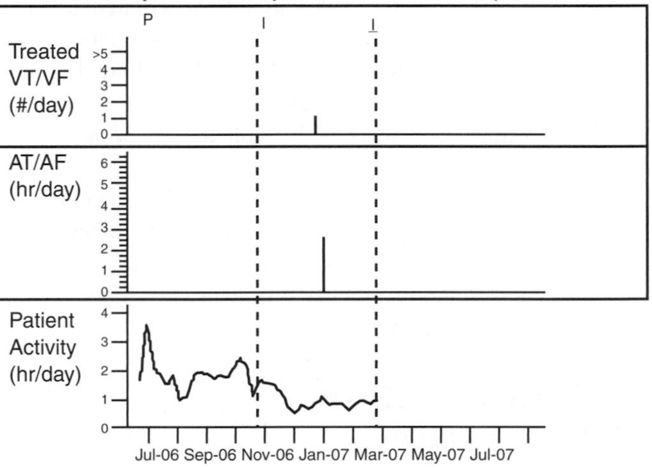

6	**Treated**		Treated
	VF	0	VT/VF
	FVT (Off)		(#/day)
	VT	1	
	AT/AF (Monitor)		

7	**Monitored**		AT/AF
	VT (Off)		(hr/day)
	VT-NS (>4 beats, >171 bpm)	3	
	SVT: VT/VF Rx Withheld	0	
	AT/AF	1	

	Time in AT/AF	<0.1 hr/day (<0.1%)	Patient
	Longest AT/AF	2 hours	Activity (hr/day)

	Functional	**Last Week**
	Patient Activity	0.9 hr/day

Jul-06 Sep-06 Nov-06 Jan-07 Mar-07 May-07 Jul-07

9	**Therapy Summary**	**VT/VF**	**AT/AF**	**Pacing**	**(% of Time Since 24-Oct-2006)**	8
	Pace-Terminated Episodes	1 of 1	0	AS-VS	44.5%	
	Shock-Terminated Episodes	0	0	AS-VP	<0.1%	
	Total Shocks	0	0	AP-VS	55.4%	
	Aborted Charges	0	0	AP-VP	<0.1%	
				MVP	On	

10	**OBSERVATIONS (1)**
	Patient Activity less than 2 hr/day for 17 weeks.

FIGURE 50-3   **A,** Printout from an ICD interrogation.

1	Are the battery voltage and charge time OK?

2	How are the leads performing?

3	Is sensing OK? Are the sensitivity settings appropriate?

4	What are the pacing parameters? Do they look appropriate for the patient?

5	What are the detection and therapy parameters? Do they look appropriate for the patient?

6	Has the device treated any VT/VF episodes?

7	Has the device detected any AT/AF, SVT, or nonsustained episodes?

8	Have you minimized unnecessary right ventricular pacing?

9	Were therapies successful? Assess any episodes using EGMs, Interval Plots, and Episode Texts.

10	Are there any observations?

FIGURE 50-3, cont'd **B,** Questions to consider during ICD interrogation. Health care providers trained at interpretation of results can gather this type of information from an ICD device check.

Procedure for Implantable Cardioverter-Defibrillator

Steps	Rationale	Special Considerations
1. **HH**		
2. Cleanse the skin for application of the ECG electrodes with cleansing pads or soap and water (see Procedure 57).	Proper skin preparation is essential to maintain appropriate skin-to-electrode contact.	Clipping of chest hair may be necessary to ensure good skin contact with the electrodes.
3. Attach the ECG leads to the electrodes, place the electrodes on the patient's chest, and record the ECG.	Assesses cardiac rhythm.	
4. If the patient experiences VT or VF:		Run a continuous ECG strip of the dysrhythmia from the bedside monitor if possible; record a 12-lead ECG if possible. Note: The device may not detect VT/VF if the rate of the VT is below the programmed detection rate.[4]

Procedure continues on following page

Procedure   for Implantable Cardioverter-Defibrillator—*Continued*

Steps	Rationale	Special Considerations
A. Assess and stay with the patient.	Ensures patient safety and provides an opportunity to assess the patient's response to the dysrhythmia.	
B. Wait for the device to function: antitachycardia pacing or shock therapy.	The ICD requires a brief period (8 to 30 seconds) to assess the VT or VF and to initiate therapy.	
C. If the dysrhythmia continues, wait for the ICD to recharge and shock again if indicated.	The ICD reassesses the cardiac rhythm, recharges, and shocks again as preprogrammed.	
D. If the ICD has been functioning as preprogrammed and still does not convert the dysrhythmia, initiate ACLS.	Provides emergency care.	Assess the patient's response to VT; the patient's condition may be hemodynamically stable or unstable. Follow ACLS standards. Notify the physician or advanced practice nurse immediately and prepare emergency equipment.
E. Apply defibrillation electrodes (patches) or paddles in one of the two following ways:		
1. Place one electrode or paddle at the heart's apex just to the left of the nipple in the midaxillary line (at fifth to sixth intercostal space) and place the other electrode or paddle just below the right clavicle to the right of the sternum.	The electrical current passes through the cardiac muscle.	Defibrillator paddles and defibrillation electrodes should not be placed over medication patches or the ICD generator. The paddles and electrodes should be a minimum of 2 inches away from the generator when external shocks are delivered.
or		
2. Apply anterior-posterior defibrillation electrodes or paddles. The anterior electrode or paddle is placed in the anterior left precordial area, and the posterior electrode or paddle is placed posteriorly behind the heart in the left infrascapular area.		
F. If the ICD does not convert VT/VF and the patient's condition is hemodynamically unstable, externally defibrillate the patient according to ACLS guidelines.	Provides emergency treatment.	ICDs have preprogrammed pacing capability; cardiac pacing is initiated by the ICD if the result of defibrillation is bradycardia or asystole. If external defibrillation is needed, the ICD should be interrogated to assess for potential damage to the device.
5. Deactivation of the ICD:	The ICD may need to be deactivated if it is defibrillating a cardiac rhythm that is not VT or VF, such as atrial fibrillation with a rapid ventricular response. The device also is temporarily deactivated during surgical procedures where EMI may interfere with appropriate device function. If the device is functioning inappropriately, deactivation may be necessary to prevent harm to the patient.	Follow institution standards regarding personnel who can deactivate an ICD. The following circumstances may necessitate ICD deactivation: lead dislodgment, lead migration, lead fracture, inappropriate identification of the rhythm, and inappropriate defibrillation threshold. Consider connecting the patient to an external defibrillator as indicated and desired.

Procedure for Implantable Cardioverter-Defibrillator—*Continued*

Steps	Rationale	Special Considerations
	The ICD may be deactivated if therapy is no longer effective or needed or is not desired.[18]	
A. Follow physician prescription.		
B. The ICD may be deprogrammed by personnel trained in use of the ICD programmer.	Ensures that the device is deprogrammed as prescribed.	Follow institution standards regarding personnel who can deactivate the ICD with use of the programmer.

C. If the ICD programmer is unavailable, a magnet may be used to deactivate the device:
  1. Place a bar or doughnut magnet over the ICD generator.
  2. Follow manufacturer's guidelines regarding removing the magnet or taping the magnet in place. (**Level M***)
	Deactivation response to a magnet varies among manufacturers.
	Some ICDs are deactivated when the magnet is placed on the skin above the generator, and then the magnet can be removed. Other ICDs are deactivated only when the magnet remains on the skin over the generator.
		Follow institution standards regarding personnel who can deactivate the ICD with a magnet.
		A magnet applied over an ICD disables the device therapies of ATP and electrical cardioversion/defibrillation, but it does not turn off pacemaker function. The magnet may initiate asynchronous pacing.
		If information about a patient's ICD model and magnet features is unknown or is not clear, contact the personnel responsible for ICDs in your institution or contact the manufacturer to determine this information.
		Some ICDs emit a synchronous tone that occurs with each R wave when the device is activated and a constant tone when the ICD is deactivated. Knowledge of which manufacturers have this ability and whether the feature is turned on is important; not all devices emit a synchronous tone.

6. Reactivation of an ICD: A. Follow physician prescription. B. The ICD may be reprogrammed by personnel trained in use of the ICD programmer.	Returns the ICD to preprogrammed settings.	Follow institution standards regarding personnel who can reactivate the ICD with use of the programmer.

C. If the ICD programmer is not available:
  1. Place a bar or doughnut magnet over the ICD generator.
  2. Remove the magnet.
  (**Level M**)
	When the magnet is removed, most ICDs automatically reactivate.	Follow the manufacturer's recommendations regarding magnet features.
		Some ICDs emit a synchronous tone that occurs with each R wave when the device is activated and a constant tone when the ICD is deactivated. Knowledge of which manufacturers have this ability and whether the feature is turned on is important; not all devices emit a synchronous tone.

7. Discard used supplies in appropriate receptacle. 8. **HH**	Reduces the transmission of microorganisms; standard precautions.	

*Level M: Manufacturer's recommendations only

Procedure continues on following page

Expected Outcomes

- ICD detects life-threatening VT or VF
- ICD delivers appropriate therapy, including antitachycardia pacing and defibrillation as necessary
- Cardiac rhythm is converted to a hemodynamically stable rhythm
- ICD provides bradycardia pacing as needed

Unexpected Outcomes

- Failure of the ICD to detect VT or VF
- Failure of the ICD to convert life-threatening dysrhythmia despite appropriate therapy and defibrillation attempts
- Failure of the backup pacing system to pace if bradycardia or asystole is the result of defibrillation
- Inappropriate defibrillation
- Infection at the ICD pulse generator site, leads, or myocardium
- Lead fracture or migration
- Pulse generator migration
- Pulse generator pocket hematoma
- Loosened set screw in device header (this screw holds the lead circuitry in place in the device header); loose set screws usually manifest as improper device function and occur generally immediately after implant
- Air embolism
- Venous thrombosis
- Cardiac tamponade
- Skin erosion
- Pneumothorax
- Frozen shoulder on operative side
- Twiddler's syndrome (manipulation of the device in the device pocket by a patient, either intentionally or unintentionally, which may lead to dislodgement)

Patient Monitoring and Care

Steps	Rationale	Reportable Conditions
		These conditions should be reported if they persist despite nursing interventions.
1. Monitor the ECG continuously.	Detects dysrhythmias.	• Dysrhythmias
2. Monitor the ICD for antitachycardia pacing, cardioversion, and defibrillation.	Detects functioning of the ICD.	• Ventricular dysrhythmias • ICD therapy • Defibrillation • ICD malfunction
3. Assess the patient's response to ICD defibrillation, including cardiac rate and rhythm, level of consciousness, and vital signs.	Determines patient status and necessity for additional treatment.	• Cardiac rate and rhythm before and after defibrillation • Level of consciousness • Vital signs
4. Follow institution standard for assessing pain. Administer analgesia as prescribed.	Identifies need for pain interventions.	• Continued pain despite pain interventions
5. Monitor for signs and symptoms of infection.	Placement of an invasive device may result in infection.	• Redness • Edema • Drainage • Increased white blood cell count • Increased temperature
6. Monitor for signs of bleeding and hematoma at ICD insertion site.	Placement of an invasive device may result in untoward bleeding.	• Bleeding at incision • Edema around ICD site

Documentation

Documentation should include the following:
- Device interrogation information: battery voltage and charge time, dysrhythmias detected by device and any therapies given, status of leads, programmed parameters (see Figs. 50-3, *A* and 50-3, *B*)
- Patient and family education
- Adjustment to device
- All rhythm strip recordings

- Patient response to ICD therapy
- Pain assessment, interventions, and effectiveness
- Anxiety assessment, interventions, and effectiveness
- Occurrence of any unexpected outcomes
- Additional interventions

References

1. Abraham WT, Yancy CW: Cardiac resynchronization therapy: a practical guide for device optimization, part I, *CHF* 12:169-173, 2006.
2. Bernstein AD, et al: The NASPE/BPEG defibrillator code (NBD code), *Pacing Clin Electrophysiol* 16:1776, 1993.
3. Bostwick JM, Sola CL: An updated review of implantable cardioverter/defibrillators, induced anxiety, and quality of life, *Psychiatr Clin North Am* 30(4):677-688, 2007.
4. Bubien RS, et al: *Defibrillation and resynchronization, AACN Clin Issues* 15(3):340-361, 2004.
5. Ellenbogen KA, Wood MA: *Cardiac pacing & ICDs,* ed 5, Oxford, 2008, Blackwell Publishing.
6. Epstein AE, et al: ACC/AHA/HRS 2008 guidelines for device-based therapy of cardiac rhythm abnormalities: a report of the American College of Cardiology/American Heart Association Task Force on Practice Guidelines (Writing Committee to Revise the ACC/AHA/NASPE 2002 Guideline Update for Implantation of Cardiac Pacemakers and Antitachydysrhythmia Devices) developed in collaboration with the American Association for Thoracic Surgery and Society of Thoracic Surgeons, *J Am Coll Cardiol* 51(21):e1-e61, 2008.
7. Esptein AE, et al: Addendum to "Personal and Public Safety Issues Related to Tachydysrhthmias That May Affect Consciousness: Implications for Regulation and Physician Recommendations: A Medical/Scientific Statement From the American Heart Association and the North American Society of Pacing and Electrophysiology" Public Safety Issues in Patients with Implantable Defibrillators: a scientific statement from the American Heart Association and the Heart Rhythm Society, *Circulation* 115:1170-1176, 2007.
8. Hayes DL, Asirvatham SJ: *Dictionary of cardiac pacing, defibrillation, resynchronization, and arrythmias,* Minneapolis, MN, ed 2, Cardiotext Publishing, 2007.
9. McMullan J, et al: Care of the pacemaker/implantable cardioverter-defibrillator patient in the ED, *Am J Emerg Med* 25(7):1-13, 2007.
10. Myers GM, James GD: Social support, anxiety, and support group participation in patients with an implantable cardioverter defibrillator, *Prog Cardiovasc Nurs* 23(4):160-167, 2008.
11. Sears SF, et al: Effective management of ICD patients psychosocial issues and patient critical events, *J Cardiovasc Electrophysiol*, epublication at printing/ahead of print, 2009.
12. Sears SF, et al: State-of-the-art: anxiety management of patient with implantable cardioverter-defibrillators, *Stress Health* 24(3):239-248, 2008.
13. Shea J, et al: Quality of life issues in patients with implantable cardioverter defibrillators: driving, occupation, and recreation, *AACN Clini Issues* 15(3):478-89, 2004.
14. Stevenson WG, et al: Clinical assessment and management of patients with implanted cardioverter-defibrillators presenting to nonelectrophysiologists, *Circulation* 110:3866-3869, 2004.
15. Thomas SA, et al: Quality of life and psychological status of patients with implantable cardioverter defibrillators, *Am J Crit Care* 15(4):389-398, 2006.
16. Trupp RJ, Bubien RS: Care of patients with implanted cardiac rhythm management devices. In Moser DK, Riegel B, editors: *Cardiac nursing: a companion to Braunwald's heart disease,* St Louis, 2008, Elsevier.
17. Wathen MS, et al: Prospective randomized multicenter trial of empirical antitachycardia pacing versus shocks for spontaneous rapid ventricular tachycardia in patients with implantable cardioverter-defibrillators: Pacing Fast Ventricular Tachycardia Reduces Shock Therapies (PainFREE Rx II) trial results, *Circulation* 110(17):2591-2596, 2004.
18. Wiegand DL, Kalowes, P; Withdrawal of cardiac medications and devices, *AACN Adv Criti Care* 18(4):415-425, 2007.
19. Wilkoff BL, et al: HRS/EHRA expert consensus on the monitoring of cardiovascular implantable electronic devices (CIEDs): description of techniques, indications, personnel, frequency and ethical considerations, *Heart Rhythm* 5(6): 2008.

Additional Readings

Abraham WT, et al, for the MIRACLE Study Group: Cardiac resynchronization in chronic heart failure, *N Engl J Med* 346:1845-1853, 2002.

Bardy GH, Lee KL, Mark DB, et al, for the Sudden Death in Heart Failure Trial (SCD-HeFT) investigators: Amiodarone or an implantable cardioverter-defibrillator for congestive heart failure, *N Engl J Med* 352:225-237, 2005.

Bristow MR, Saxon LA, Boehmer J, et al: Comparison of Medical Therapy, Pacing, and Defibrillation in Heart Failure (COMPANION) investigators: cardiac-resynchronization therapy with or without an implantable defibrillator in advanced chronic heart failure, *N Engl J Med* 350(21):2140-2150, 2004.

CR Buxton AE, et al, for the Multicenter Unsustained Tachycardia Trial investigators: a randomized study of the prevention of sudden death in patients with coronary artery disease, *N Engl J Med* 341:1882-1890, 1999.

CR Gura MT, et al: North American Society of Pacing and Electrophysiology standards of professional practice for the allied professional in pacing and electrophysiology, *PACE* 26:127-131, 2003.

CR Kadish A, Dyer A, et al: Prophylactic defibrillator implantation in patients with nonischemic dilated cardiomyopathy, *N Engl J Med* 350:2151- 2158, 2004.

CR Moss AJ, Zareba W, et al: Prophylactic implantation of a defibrillator in patients with myocardial infarction and reduced ejection fraction, *N Engl J Med* 346:877-883, 2002.

CR Moss AJ, et al: Improved survival with an implanted defibrillator in patients with coronary disease at high risk for ventricular tachydysrhthmia: Multicenter Automatic Defibrillator Implantation Trial investigators, *N Engl J Med* 335:1933-1940, 1996.

CR Mushlin A, Jackson Hall WJ, Zwanziger J, et al, for the MADIT investigators: The cost-effectiveness of automatic implantable cardiac defibrillators: results from MADIT, *Circulation* 97:2129-2135, 1998.

Sears SF, et al: Quality of death and ICDs, *PACE* 29: 637-642, 2006.

CR St John Sutton MG, et al: Effect of cardiac resynchronization therapy on left ventricular size and function in chronic heart failure, *Circulation* 107(15):1985-1990, 2003.

CR Young JB, Abraham WT, Smith AL, et al: Combined cardiac resynchronization and implantable cardioversion defibrillation in advanced chronic heart failure: the MIRACLE ICD trial, *JAMA* 289:2685-2694, 2003.

Wingate S, Wiegand D: End of life care in the critical care unit for patients with heart failure, *Crit Care Nurse* 28(2):84-96, 2008.

Permanent Pacemaker (Assessing Function)

P U R P O S E : The purpose of permanent pacing is to electrically stimulate myocardial contraction, and to restore and maintain an appropriate heart rate or ventricular synchrony when a chronic conduction or impulse formation disturbance exists in the cardiac conduction system. Assessment of the permanent pacemaker is important in maintaining proper function.

Carol A. Offutt

PREREQUISITE NURSING KNOWLEDGE

- Knowledge of the normal anatomy and physiology of the cardiovascular system, cardiac conduction, and basic dysrhythmia interpretation is necessary.
- Knowledge of pacemaker function and patient response to pacemaker therapy is needed.
- Advanced cardiac life support knowledge and skills are needed.
- Permanent pacing is indicated for the following clinical conditions[5]:
  - Symptomatic sinus node dysfunction
  - Acquired atrioventricular (AV) block in adults
  - Chronic bifascicular and trifascicular block
  - AV block associated with acute myocardial infarction
  - Hypersensitive carotid sinus and neurocardiogenic syncope
  - Specific conditions related to cardiac transplantation, neuromuscular diseases, sleep apnea syndromes, or infiltrative and inflammatory diseases such as cardiac sarcoidosis
  - Prevention and termination of supraventricular tachycardia via pacing
  - Hypertrophic cardiomyopathy with sinus node dysfunction or AV block
  - Certain congenital heart defects
  - Left ventricular dysfunction, to restore ventricular synchrony (cardiac resynchronization therapy [CRT])[1,3,8]

- Relative contraindications to permanent pacemakers include the following:
  - Active infection (e.g., endocarditis, positive blood culture results)
  - Bleeding with abnormal coagulation laboratory results
- Components of the pacemaker are the pulse generator and the leads. The pulse generator weighs about 1 oz and is typically implanted subcutaneously in a pectoral pocket. The outer casing is made of titanium and contains the electronic components and the battery necessary to sustain pacing for years (Fig. 51-1). Typical battery life is 5 to 10 years and is dependent on variables such as output values, impedance, and percentage pacing. A transvenous

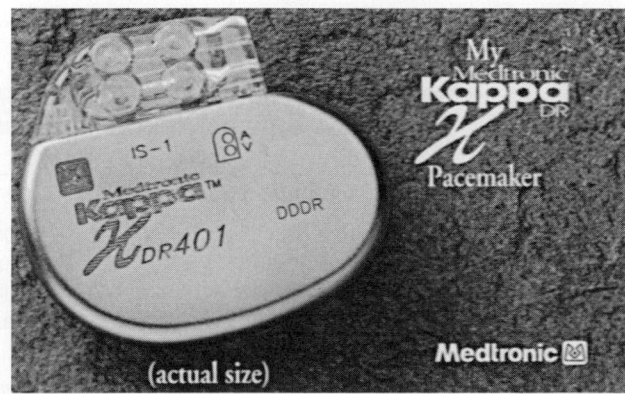

FIGURE 51-1   Permanent pacemaker pulse generator. (*Courtesy of Medtronic, Inc., Minneapolis, MN.*)

pacing lead may be positioned in the right atrium, the right ventricle, or the left ventricle (or a combination of these), depending on the type of pacing needed.

- Unipolar pacing involves a relatively large electrical circuit. The distal tip of the pacing lead is the negative electrode and is in contact with the myocardium. The positive electrode encompasses the metallic pacemaker case, located in the soft tissue. Energy is delivered from the negative electrode to the positive electrode, causing myocardial depolarization. The electrocardiogram (ECG) tracing shows a large, easily visible spike.

- Bipolar pacing uses a smaller electrical circuit in which the distal tip of the pacing lead is the negative electrode in contact with the myocardium. The pacing lead has a second positive electrode that is located within 1 cm of the negative electrode. Energy is delivered from the negative electrode to the positive electrode, causing myocardial depolarization. The ECG tracing may show small spikes, or the spikes may not be visible on a surface ECG.

- Basic principles of cardiac pacing include sensing, pulse generation, capture, and impedance (Table 51-1 lists definitions).

- Depending on the type of pacemaker, the pacemaker lead may be placed in the atrium, the right ventricle, or the left ventricle. A standard code exists to describe pacemakers (Table 51-2).[2] The nurse must know the programmed mode with the pacemaker code to determine whether the device is functioning appropriately. Refer to Table 51-3 to review different programmed modes for pacemakers.

- Dual-chamber or DDD pacemakers contain pacing leads that are located in the atrium and the ventricle. Pacing and sensing occur in both chambers. Pacing is inhibited by sensed atrial or ventricular activity. Sensed or paced atrial activity triggers a ventricular paced response in the absence

---

TABLE 51-1　Pertinent Definitions Related to Pacemakers

Sensing	Ability of the pacemaker to detect intrinsic myocardial electrical activity. The pacemaker is either inhibited from delivering a stimulus or initiates an electrical impulse based on the programmed response.
Pulse generation	Occurs when the pacemaker produces a programmed electrical current for a programmed duration. This energy travels through the transvenous lead wires to the myocardium. The electrical impulse is seen as a line or spike on the ECG recording (pacemaker spikes are shown in Fig. 51-4).
Capture	Successful stimulation of the myocardium by the pacemaker impulse that results in depolarization. Two settings are used to ensure capture: amplitude and pulse width. Evidenced on the ECG by a pacemaker spike/stimulus followed by either an atrial or ventricular complex, depending on the chambers being paced (see Fig. 51-4).
Lead impedance	Opposition to flow of electrical current by the leads, electrodes, the electrode-myocardial interface, and body tissues.[6] Measured in ohms, normally between 200 and 1200 ohms. A lead insulation break can cause impedance to fall below 200 ohms. A lead fracture can cause impedance to exceed 2000 ohms.
Failure of pulse generation	The pacemaker does not discharge a pacing stimulus to the myocardium at its programmed time. Evidenced by the absence of a pacemaker spike on the ECG where expected (see Fig. 51-5).
Failure to sense	The pacemaker has either detected extraneous signals that mimic intrinsic cardiac activity (oversensing) or has not accurately identified intrinsic activity (undersensing). Oversensing is recognized on the ECG by pauses where paced beats were expected and prolongation of the interval between paced beats (see Fig. 51-6). Oversensing leads to underpacing. Undersensing is recognized on the ECG by inappropriate pacemaker spikes relative to the intrinsic electrical activity (pacemaker spikes occurring within the P wave, QRS complex, or T wave) and shortened distances between paced beats (see Fig. 51-7). Undersensing leads to overpacing.
Failure to capture	Pacemaker has delivered a pacing stimulus that was unable to initiate depolarization and contraction of the myocardium. Evidenced on the ECG by pacemaker spikes that are not followed by a P wave for atrial pacing or spikes not followed by a QRS complex for ventricular pacing (see Fig. 51-8).

TABLE 51-2　Revised NASPE/BPEG Generic Code for Antibradycardia Pacing[*]

I	II	III	IV	V
Chambers Paced	*Chambers Sensed*	*Response to Sensing*	*Rate Modulation*	*Multisite Pacing*
0 = None	0 = None	0 = None	0 = None	0 = None
A = Atrium	A = Atrium	T = Triggered	R = Rate modulation	A = Atrium
V = Ventricle	V = Ventricle	I = Inhibited		V = Ventricle
D = Dual (A + V)	D = Dual (A + V)	D = Dual (T + I)		D = Dual (A + V)
S = Single (A or V)[†]	S = Single (A or V)[†]			

[†]Manufacturer's designation only. *NASPE*, North American Society of Pacing and Electrophysiology; *BPEG*, British Pacing and Electrophysiology Group.
(From Bernstein AD, et al: The revised NASPE/BPEG generic code for antibradycardia, adaptive-rate, and multisite pacing, Pacing Clin Electrophysiol *25:261, 2002.)*

TABLE 51-3	Programmed Pacing Modes
Pacemaker Code	**Pacemaker Response**
A00	Atrial pacing; no sensing; asynchronous mode→paces atria at fixed, preprogrammed rate.
AAI	Atrial pacing, atrial sensing and inhibition; intrinsic P waves inhibit atrial pacing; if no sensed atrial events→paces in atria at preprogrammed rate.
AAIR	Atrial pacing; atrial sensing; intrinsic P waves inhibit atrial pacing; if no sensed atrial events→paces in atria; rate response to patient's activity.
V00	Ventricular pacing; no sensing; asynchronous mode→paces ventricle at fixed, preprogrammed rate.
VVI	Ventricular pacing: ventricular sensing; intrinsic QRS inhibits ventricular pacing; if no sensed events→paces in ventricle at preprogrammed rate.
VVIR	Ventricular pacing: ventricular sensing; intrinsic QRS inhibits ventricular pacing; if no sensed events→paces in ventricle; rate response to patient's activity.
D00	Atrial and ventricular pacing: no sensing; asynchronous mode→paces atria and ventricles at fixed, preprogrammed rate.
DDI	Atrial and ventricular pacing; atria and ventricular sensing; no tracking of atria: sensed atrial events inhibit atrial pacing/do not trigger a ventricular pacing pulse; sensed atrial events with absent ventricular event inhibit atrial pacing but do pace ventricle at preprogrammed rate; if both atrial and ventricular events absent→AV sequential pacing results at preprogrammed rate.
DDIR	Atrial and ventricular pacing; atrial and ventricular sensing; no tracking of atria (as described previously in DDI); AV sequential rate modulation.
DDD	Atrial and ventricular pacing; atrial and ventricular sensing; intrinsic P wave and intrinsic QRS can inhibit pacing; intrinsic P wave can trigger a paced QRS (tracks the atrium).
	May see four possible combinations in DDD mode: 1, atrial sensed/ventricular sensed; 2, atrial sensed/ventricular paced; 3, atrial paced/ventricular sensed; 4, atrial paced/ventricular paced.
DDDR	Atrial and ventricular pacing; atrial and ventricular sensing; tracks the atrium: intrinsic P wave and intrinsic QRS can inhibit pacing, intrinsic P wave can trigger a paced QRS; AV sequential rate modulation.

of intrinsic ventricular activity within a programmed AV interval.[4]

- Biventricular pacemakers (CRT) contain leads in the right atrium and the right ventricle and on the surface of the left ventricles and simultaneously pace the right and left ventricle (Fig. 51-2).
- Some pacemaker systems also include an implantable cardioverter-defibrillator (ICD; see Procedure 50).
- Some pacemakers can be programmed to switch modes (e.g., DDD mode to VVI mode) to avoid pacing at the upper rate in patients who experience intermittent atrial dysrhythmias in which rapid atrial rates are generated.

- Certain pacemakers can be programmed with pacing therapies for atrial dysrhythmias. This programming is called antitachycardia pacing, in which the device paces faster than a patient's heart rate in an attempt to convert the rhythm.
- Rate-responsive pacemakers include a sensor and are designed to mimic normal changes in heart rate based on physiologic needs. Most commonly, the sensor reacts to motion and vibration or respirations and initiates an appropriate change in the pacing rate, depending on metabolic activity. These patients have a set pacemaker rate range.
- Inappropriate pacemaker function includes failure of pulse generation, failure to sense, and failure to capture (see Table 51-1 for definitions).
- Electromagnetic interference (EMI) may interfere with pacemaker function and includes electrocautery, cardioversion and defibrillation, magnetic resonance imaging (which is contraindicated for patients on pacemakers), diathermy, and transcutaneous nerve stimulators. Other outside causes of EMI include welding equipment less than 24 inches from the device, electrical motors, chain saws, battery-powered cordless power tools and drills less than 12 inches from device, magnetic mattresses and chairs, and airport wands for security checks. Household appliances such as microwave ovens rarely cause EMI. Cell phones may cause EMI and should be used on the ear opposite the device. The cell phone should be carried on the opposite side of the body, with at least 6 inches maintained between the cell phone and the device.[10]

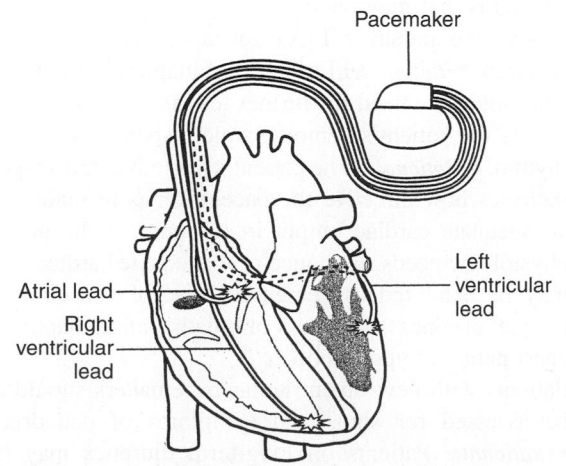

FIGURE 51-2 Biventricular pacemaker (cardiac resynchronization therapy). (*Courtesy Medtronic, Inc, Minneapolis, MN.*)

Patients who are pacemaker-dependent may experience dizziness, lightheadedness, near syncope, or syncope if EMI inhibits proper sensing and therefore inhibits pacing.

- A pacemaker programmer appropriate for the pacemaker make and model is required for a device check or "interrogation." Note that some situations may require notification of the device manufacturer to obtain the proper interrogation equipment (the device programmer). Manufacturer information can be found on the patient's pacemaker identification card.

EQUIPMENT

- ECG monitor and recorder with paper
- ECG cable and electrodes

Additional equipment to have available as needed includes the following:

- Pacemaker magnet
- Pacemaker programmer appropriate for the pacemaker manufacturer and model

PATIENT AND FAMILY EDUCATION

- Assess learning needs, readiness to learn, and factors that influence learning. ➤➤*Rationale:* This assessment allows the nurse to individualize teaching in a meaningful manner.
- Provide information about the normal conduction system, such as structure of the conduction system, source of heartbeat, normal and abnormal heart rhythms, and symptoms of abnormal heart rhythms. Patients with cardiomyopathy and heart failure need further information about ventricular dyssynchrony. ➤➤*Rationale:* Understanding of the normal conduction system and pumping function assists the patient and family in recognizing the need for permanent pacemaker therapy.
- Provide information about permanent pacing, including the reason for pacing; explanation of the equipment; what to expect during permanent pacing; precautions and restrictions in activities of daily living; signs and symptoms of complications; instructions on when to call the physician, advanced practice nurse, or pacemaker clinic; and information on expected follow-up. ➤➤*Rationale:* Understanding of pacemaker functioning and expectations after discharge assists the patient and family in developing realistic perceptions of permanent pacing therapy. Information may improve compliance with restrictions and promote effective lifestyle management after discharge.
- Provide information about required device follow-up, including in-clinic evaluation, transtelephonic monitoring, or remote monitoring. ➤➤*Rationale:* Periodic pacemaker checks are essential for routine device monitoring and evaluation of changes in patient condition related to the pacemaker. Current guidelines[12] recommend the following minimum frequency of routine device checks within 72 hours of device implant (in-clinic), 2 to 12 weeks after implant (in-clinic), followed by every 3 to 12 months

(in-clinic or remote), and then every 1 to 3 months at signs of battery depletion (in-clinic or remote). Devices may be checked more frequently as needed (e.g., if a change occurs in antidysrhythmia medications or heart failure therapies).

- Instruct patients to carry their identification card at all times. Patients receive identification cards from the manufacturer at the time of implant. These cards identify the model of pacemaker used. Also encourage patients to wear Medic Alert information, especially if admitted to the hospital. ➤➤*Rationale:* This instruction ensures that appropriate identifying information is available to other healthcare providers, if needed.

PATIENT ASSESSMENT AND PREPARATION

Patient Assessment

- Identify the manufacturer of the pacemaker. This information may be found on the patient's identification card. If no card is available, the make of the device may be identified on chest radiography. ➤➤*Rationale:* Identification of the manufacturer ensures that the correct programmer is used to review the programmed pacemaker parameters.
- Identify the programmed mode of the pacemaker. ➤➤*Rationale:* Knowledge of how the pacemaker is intended to respond is necessary to detect appropriate and inappropriate function.
- Identify the reason for permanent pacemaker support. ➤➤*Rationale:* Knowledge of the clinical indication (e.g., complete heart block) provides the nurse with baseline data, such as pacemaker dependency, when evaluating pacemaker function and patient response.
- Determine the patient's pacemaker history: date of insertion; last battery change; most recent pacemaker check; any problems with the pacemaker or pacemaker site; and any unexpected symptoms such as dizziness, chest pain, shortness of breath, palpitations, or activity intolerance. ➤➤*Rationale:* The pacemaker history provides information useful in determination of any problems that may occur.
- Assess the patient's ECG for appropriate pacemaker function. ➤➤*Rationale:* Evidence of inappropriate function determines the need for further testing.
- Assess the patient's hemodynamic response to the paced rhythm. ➤➤*Rationale:* The patient's hemodynamic response indicates how effective the pacemaker is in maintaining an adequate cardiac output in response to the patient's physiologic needs. Evidence of inadequate cardiac output may be exhibited as decreased level of consciousness, fatigue, dizziness, shortness of breath, pallor, diaphoresis, chest pain, or hypotension.
- Patients with new biventricular pacemakers should also be assessed for signs and symptoms of dehydration. ➤➤*Rationale:* Patients on long-term diuretics may have overdiuresis after pacemaker implantation as a result of improved circulation and hemodynamics.

Patient Preparation

- Verify the correct patient with two patient identifiers. ➤➤*Rationale:* Prior to performing a procedure, the nurse should ensure the correct identification of the patient for the intended intervention.
- Ensure that the patient and family understand teaching. Answer questions as they arise, and reinforce informa-tion as needed. ➤➤*Rationale:* This communication evalu-ates and reinforces understanding of previously taught information.
- Pacemaker interrogation may be performed with the patient either sitting or in supine position. ➤➤*Rationale:* This position prepares the patient for pacemaker interrogation.

Procedure	for Assessing Function of Permanent Pacemaker	
Steps	**Rationale**	**Special Considerations**
1. **HH**		
2. **PE**		
3. Prepare skin with cleansing pads or soap and water for the applica-tion of ECG electrodes.	Proper skin preparation is essential to maintain appropriate skin-to-electrode contact.	
4. Attach the ECG leads to the electrodes, and place the electrodes on the patient's chest (see Procedure 57).	Attaching the leads to the electrodes first and then placing the electrodes on the chest produces less discomfort.	
5. Record an ECG rhythm strip.	Allows for evaluation of the patient's intrinsic rhythm and aids in assess-ment of pacemaker function.	

6. Follow institution standard for recording a rhythm strip with a magnet placed over the pacemaker:
  A. Place the pacemaker magnet on top of the pacemaker generator.
  B. Record the ECG rhythm strip.
  C. Remove the magnet.
 	
  D. Assess the ECG rhythm.
	A magnet placed over the pacemaker causes the pacemaker to pace at the preprogrammed parameters.
	
	After the magnet is removed, the ECG rhythm represents the patient's cur-rent status (intrinsic rhythm, paced rhythm, or a combination).
		Follow institution standard to ensure that a nurse can use the pacemaker magnet.

7. Inspect the ECG rhythm strip for pacemaker spikes, and evaluate for evidence of failure to sense or failure to capture (Figs. 51-3 through 51-8). A. Identify atrial activity. Is the pacemaker programmed to detect atrial activity? Was the atrial activity sensed? What is the pacemaker programmed to do when atrial activity is sensed? If the pacemaker is programmed to trigger ventricular pacing with sensed atrial activity, is a ventricular paced complex seen at the programmed AV interval? If not, did an intrinsic QRS complex occur before the programmed AV interval?	Determines whether the pacemaker is functioning adequately and assesses electrical activity of the atria and ventricles. Determines the presence of atrial activity in response to the pacemaker settings.	Depending on the type of lead and programming, pacemaker spikes may be difficult to detect on the surface ECG.

Procedure continues on following page

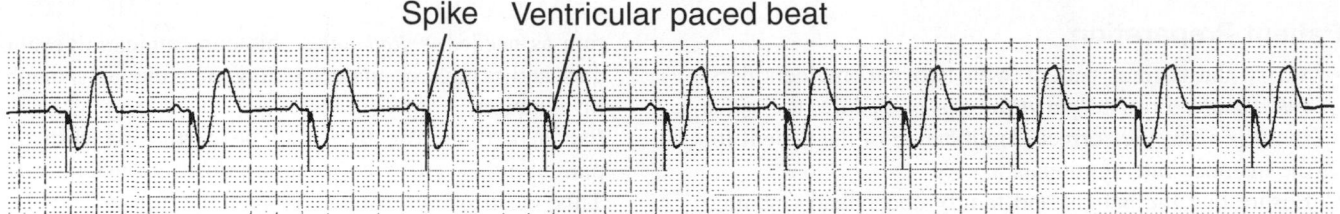

Spike   Ventricular paced beat

FIGURE 51-3   DDD pacing, normal operation: atrial activity sensed, ventricle paced.

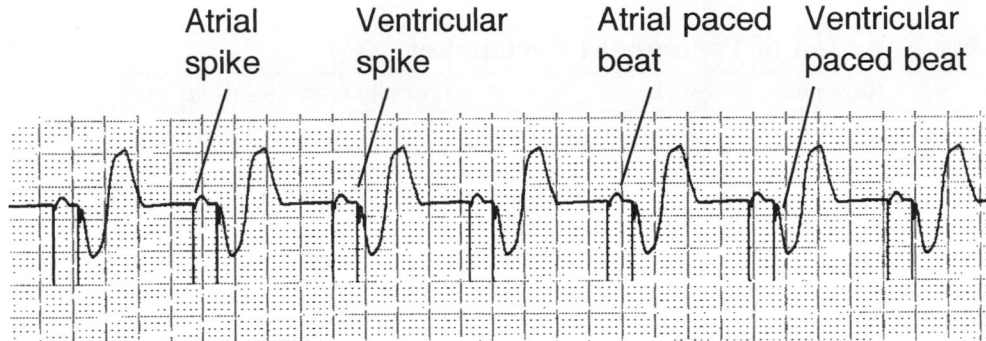

Atrial spike   Ventricular spike   Atrial paced beat   Ventricular paced beat

FIGURE 51-4   Dual-chamber DDD pacing, normal operation: atrial paced, ventricle paced.

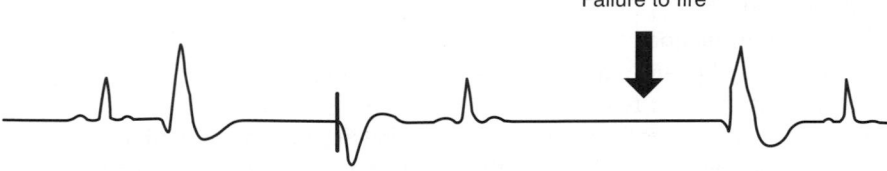

Failure to fire

FIGURE 51-5   Failure of pulse generation.

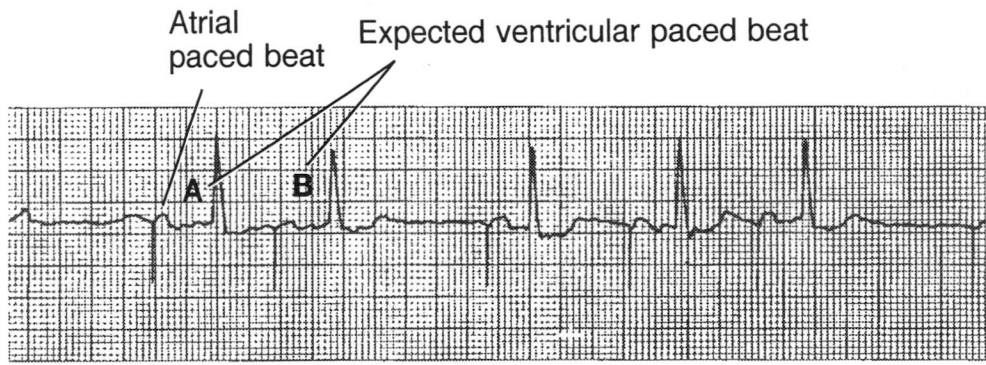

Atrial paced beat   Expected ventricular paced beat

A   B

FIGURE 51-6   Ventricular oversensing and possibly ventricular pulse generation failure. Ventricular spike expected at 150 ms. Ventricular spike and corresponding ventricular depolarization did not occur at points *A* and *B*. Also, atrial timing reset by oversensed ventricular activity resulted in erratic atrial pacing (suspicious for fracture of ventricular lead).

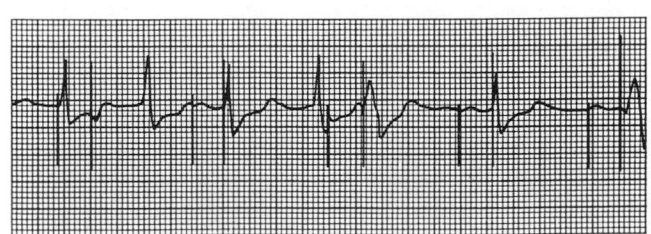

FIGURE 51-7   Ventricular undersensing. Pacemaker appears to be firing asynchronously. The third and sixth ventricular complexes represent concurrent intrinsic ventricular depolarization overlaid by inappropriate pacemaker fire.

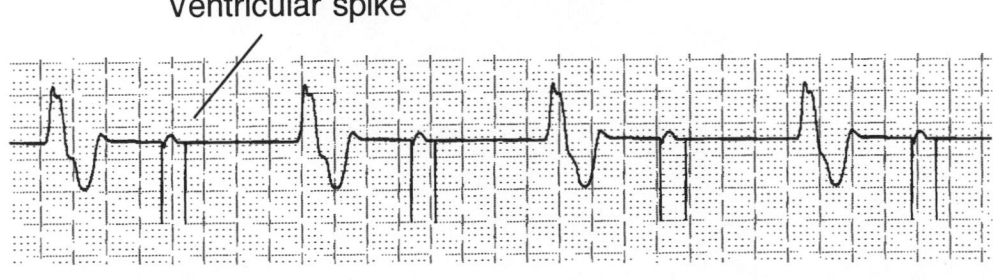

Ventricular spike

FIGURE 51-8   DDD system with failure to capture or sense ventricular activity. All ventricular spikes show absence of corresponding ventricular depolarization. No timing circuit reset by intrinsic ventricular complexes.

Procedure for Assessing Function of Permanent Pacemaker—*Continued*

Steps	Rationale	Special Considerations
B. If no intrinsic atrial activity is present, determine whether the pacemaker is programmed to pace the atrium. If atrial pacing should be occurring, determine the lower rate limit at which the pacemaker stimulates atrial activity. Evaluate whether the pacemaker is firing at this rate.		If a pacemaker spike is present but evidence of atrial capture is not present, attempt to assess the presence of atrial contraction by: 1. Looking for the *"a" wave* in the central venous pressure (or right atrial pressure) waveform (if available). 2. Changing the ECG lead. 3. Listening to the heart sounds (S_1 becomes softer in the absence of atrial contraction because left ventricular contractility affects the loudness of S_1).[3]
C. Identify ventricular activity. Is the pacemaker programmed to detect intrinsic activity? Is it sensed appropriately? What is the pacemaker programmed to do when ventricular activity is sensed? Does inhibition of ventricular pacing occur?	Determines the presence of ventricular activity in response to the pacemaker settings.	Failure of ventricular capture can be a life-threatening situation. With biventricular pacing, the loss of capture in one ventricle may be seen only by a change in the patient's condition or a change in the QRS width or appearance.
D. If no intrinsic ventricular activity is found, determine whether the pacemaker is programmed to pace the ventricles. If pacing should occur, identify the lower rate limit and determine whether ventricular pacing spikes are occurring at this rate. If ventricular pacing spikes are occurring at intervals that are longer than the lower rate limit, evaluate for oversensing of unwanted signals. If ventricular pacing spikes are occurring at intervals that are shorter than the lower rate limit, is the pacemaker in a rate-responsive mode? Is hidden atrial activity triggering a ventricular output? Is atrial oversensing found? Determine whether each ventricular pacing spike is followed by a QRS complex. If the pacemaker has an upper rate limit, determine whether the patient is being paced appropriately when that limit has been reached.	Determines the presence of ventricular activity in response to the pacemaker settings.	
E. If antitachycardia pacing is programmed, determine whether the tachycardia detection criterion has been met and whether the pacemaker intervened appropriately.	Determines appropriate pacemaker function.	

Procedure continues on following page

Steps	Rationale	Special Considerations
F. If the patient has a biventricular pacemaker, verify that the ventricles are consistently paced.[7,9]	The purpose of biventricular pacing is to pace both ventricles simultaneously to restore ventricular synchrony. If the patient is not consistently being paced in the ventricles, the system is not working properly.	Detailed interrogation of function is needed because a surface ECG rhythm strip does not provide enough information to assess proper function adequately. Figure 51-9 illustrates various aspects of biventricular pacing.
8. Perform a check of the pacemaker with use of the manufacturer's programmer (only done by trained personnel), when available and as prescribed:	Determines appropriate pacemaker function.	Follow institution standard regarding training required before use of the pacemaker programmer. Pacemaker device check with the programmer provides the following information[11,12]:
A. Place the wand attached to the programmer over the patient's pacemaker.	The wand retrieves and transmits the programmed information.	• Battery voltage (and impedance) • Magnet rate (varies by manufacturer) • Pacing and sensing thresholds for atrium and right ventricle, and pacing threshold for left ventricle
B. Perform testing of sensing, capture thresholds, and lead impedances.	Allows for determination of pacemaker function, programmed parameters, dysrhythmias, and alerts.	• Pacing lead impedance for all leads • Dysrhythmias detected by the device (e.g. mode switches, high ventricular rate episodes) • Percentage of pacing in each chamber • Review of programmed parameters • Review of any "safety" or automatic device alerts • Review of hemodynamic measurements or recordings of any other programmed parameters (e.g., heart rate variability, activity level), depending on type of device.

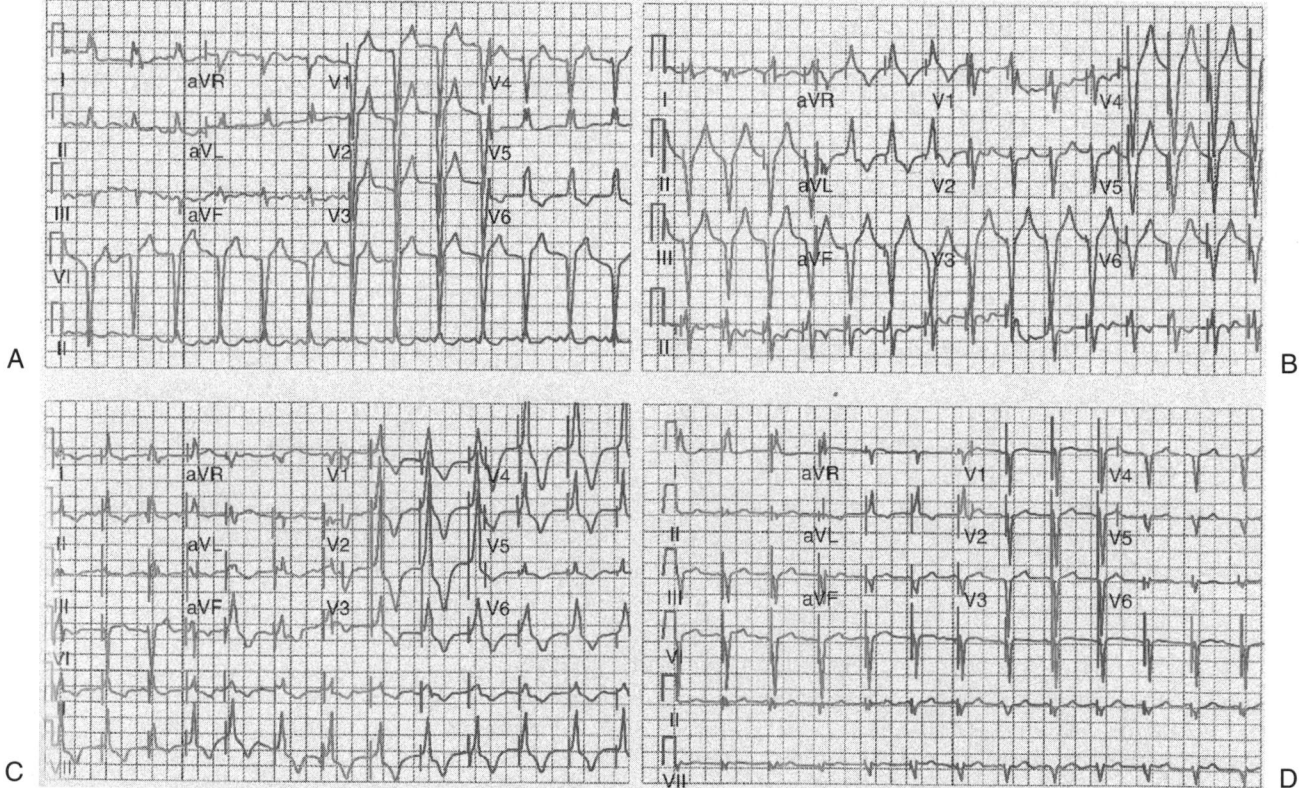

FIGURE 51-9 Biventricular pacing. A, Intrinsic ventricular activation (left bundle branch block).
B, Right ventricular pacing. C, Left ventricular pacing. D, Biventricular pacing. (*Used with permission.
Ellenbogen KA, Wood MA: Cardiac pacing & ICDs, ed 5, Oxford, 2008, Blackwell Publishing, 1095.*)

Procedure for Assessing Function of Permanent Pacemaker—*Continued*

Steps	Rationale	Special Considerations
C. Determine whether the pacemaker needs to be reprogrammed.	Ensures proper programming.	
9. Assess the patient's vital signs and hemodynamic response.	The patient may have the electrical activity of pacing without the associated mechanical activity of cardiac contraction (e.g., pulseless electrical activity).	
10. If inappropriate pacemaker function is detected, notify the physician or advanced practice nurse immediately and implement basic life support and advanced cardiac life support as needed.	Inappropriate pacemaker function may compromise cardiac output and necessitate immediate adjustment of settings or replacement of malfunctioning components.	
11. Discard used supplies in appropriate receptacle.	Reduces the transmission of microorganisms; Standard Precautions.	
12. 🖐		

Expected Outcomes

- Appropriate pacemaker functioning with appropriate pacemaker functioning
- Adequate systemic tissue perfusion and cardiac output as evidenced by patient being alert and oriented and normotensive, with no dizziness, shortness of breath, chest discomfort, or lightheadedness
- No discomfort
- No signs or symptoms of fluid or infection at the incision

Unexpected Outcomes

- Failure to sense (e.g., oversensing, undersensing) or failure to capture; failure to sense or capture in the immediate postimplant period may indicate lead dislodgment
- Lead perforation of the myocardium may occur within the first 24 hours of implant; signs and symptoms may include intermittent failure of pacing or sensing, distant heart sounds, pericardial rub, and in extreme cases, hemodynamic instability
- Diaphragmatic stimulation may occur if high voltage outputs are needed to pace the ventricles
- Hematoma
- Wound infection
- Venous thrombus
- Pain

Patient Monitoring and Care

Steps	Rationale	Reportable Conditions
		These conditions should be reported if they persist despite nursing interventions.
1. Monitor the ECG continuously.	Determines whether the patient's cardiac rate and rhythm are consistent with the programmed pacemaker parameters.	• Failure of the pacemaker to perform as programmed • Oversensing • Undersensing • Failure to capture
2. Monitor the patient's vital signs and hemodynamic status.	Determines the patient's response to pacemaker therapy.	• Abnormal vital signs • Hemodynamic instability
3. Assess the pacemaker pocket in the acute postimplant phase for evidence of hematoma.	Determines the presence of bleeding.	• Bleeding at incision • Edema around pacemaker site

Procedure continues on following page

Patient Monitoring and Care —*Continued*

Steps	Rationale	Reportable Conditions
4. Assess for signs and symptoms of infection.	Identifies infection.	• Redness • Edema • Drainage • Elevated white blood cell count • Elevated temperature
5. Follow institution standard for assessing pain. Administer analgesia as prescribed.	Identifies need for pain interventions.	• Continued pain despite pain interventions

Documentation

Documentation should include the following:
- Device indications and device type
- Patient education and evaluation of patient and family understanding
- Programmed parameters
- ECG rhythm strip recordings
- Evaluation of pacemaker function

- Physical assessment, including vital signs and hemodynamic response
- Unexpected outcomes
- Interventions needed and evaluation of interventions
- Pain assessment, interventions and effectiveness

References

CR 1. Abraham WT, et al, for the MIRACLE Study Group: Cardiac resynchronization in chronic heart failure, *N Engl J Med* 346:1845-1853, 2002.

CR 2. Bernstein AD, et al: The revised NASPE/BPEG generic code for antibradycardia, adaptive-rate, and multisite pacing, *Pacing Clin Electrophysiol* 25:261, 2002.

CR 3. Bristow MR, et al: Cardiac-resynchronization therapy with or without an implantable defibrillator in advanced chronic heart failure, *N Engl J Med* 350:2140-2150, 2004.

4. Ellenbogen KA, Wood MA: *Cardiac pacing & ICDs*, ed 5, Oxford, 2008, Blackwell Publishing.

5. Epstein AE, et al: ACC/AHA/HRS 2008 guidelines for device-based therapy of cardiac rhythm abnormalities, *JACC* 51(21):e1-e61, 2008.

6. Hayes DL, Asirvatham SJ: *Dictionary of cardiac pacing, defibrillation, resynchronization, and arrhythmias*, Minneapolis, 2007, Cardiotext.

7. Scheibly K, Tsiperfal A: ECG evidence of biventricular capture, *Progress Cardiovasc Nurs* Summer:177-179, 2007.

CR 8. St John Sutton MG, et al: Effect of cardiac resynchronization therapy on left ventricular size and function in chronic heart failure, *Circulation* 107(15):1985-1990, 2003.

9. Sweeney MO: Programming and follow-up of cardiac resynchronization devices. In Ellenbogan KA, et al: *Clinical cardiac pacing, defibrillation, and resynchronization therapy*, Philadelphia, 2007, Elsevier.

10. Trupp RJ, Bubien RS: Care of patients with implanted cardiac rhythm management devices. In Moser DK, Riegel B, editors: *Cardiac nursing: a companion to Braunwald's heart disease*, St Louis, 2008, Elsevier.

11. Wilkoff BL: *Pacemaker remote follow-up evaluation and review: results of the PREFER trial: late-breaking clinical trial session*, Heart Rhythm Society Sessions, May 14, 2008, San Francisco.

12. Wilkoff BL, et al: HRS/EHRA expert consensus on the monitoring of cardiovascular implantable electronic devices (CIEDs): description of techniques, indications, personnel, frequency and ethical considerations, *Heart Rhythm* 5(6): 2008.

Additional Readings

CR Albert NM: Cardiac resynchronization therapy through biventricular pacing in patients with heart failure and ventricular dyssynchrony, *Crit Care Nurse* 23(3 Suppl):2-13, 2003.

Czarnecki R: Biventricular pacing: when one or two leads aren't enough, *Cardiac Insider* Spring:7-10, 2007.

Epstein LM: Practical considerations for remote monitoring, *Congest Heart Fail* 14(5 Suppl):25-28, 2008.

Germany R: The use of device-based diagnostics to manage patients with heart failure, *Congest Heart Fail* 14(5 Suppl):19-24, 2008.

CR Gura MT, et al: North American Society of Pacing Electrophysiology: standards of professional practice for the allied professional in pacing and electrophysiology, *Pacing Clin Electrophysiol* 26:127-31, 2003.

CR Herbst MC: Permanent pacemakers. In Davis L, editor: *Cardiovascular nursing secrets*, St Louis, 2004, Elsevier.

CR Hesselson AB: *Simplified interpretation of pacemaker ECGs*, Baltimore, 2003, Futura/Blackwell Publications.

CR Kenny T: *The nuts and bolts of cardiac pacing*, Malden, MA, 2005, Blackwell Publishing.

Kenny T: *The nuts and bolts of cardiac resynchronization therapy*, Malden, MA, 2007, Blackwell Publishing.

CR Majorowicz K: Persons requiring permanent pacemakers. In *Continuing education for nurses 2003*, Sacramento, 2003, CME Resource.

Sauer WH, Bristow MR: The comparison of medical therapy, pacing, and defibrillation in heart failure (COMPANION) trial in perspective, *J Interv Card Electrophysiol* 21(1): 3-11, 2008.

Temporary Transcutaneous (External) Pacing

P U R P O S E : Transcutaneous or external pacing stimulates myocardial depolarization through the chest wall. External pacing is used as a temporary measure when normal cardiac conduction fails to produce myocardial contraction and the patient experiences hemodynamic instability.

Valerie Spotts

PREREQUISITE NURSING KNOWLEDGE

- Knowledge of cardiac anatomy and physiology is needed.
- Knowledge of cardiac monitoring (see Procedure 57) is necessary.
- The ability to interpret basic dysrhythmias is needed.
- Knowledge of temporary pacemaker function and expected patient responses to pacemaker therapy is needed.
- Clinical and technical competence in the use of the external pacing equipment is necessary.
- Indications for transcutaneous pacing are as follows[1,6]:
  - ❖ Symptomatic bradycardia unresponsive to medications
  - ❖ In standby mode for the following rhythms in acute myocardial infarction setting[4]:
    - ○ Symptomatic sinus node dysfunction
    - ○ Mobitz type II second-degree heart block
    - ○ Third-degree heart block
    - ○ Newly acquired left, right, or alternating bundle-branch block or bifascicular block
- Temporary transvenous pacing is indicated when prolonged pacing is needed.
- Contraindications for transcutaneous pacing are as follows[2,6]:
  - ❖ Severe hypothermia
  - ❖ Asystole (as presenting rhythm)
- Pacing is contraindicated in severe hypothermia because cold ventricles are more prone to ventricular fibrillation and are more resistant to defibrillation.[6] Transcutaneous pacing for an asystolic arrest is no longer recommended in the 2005

Advanced cardiac life support (ACLS) guidelines because of a lack of evidence that it improves survival rates.[2]
- External cardiac pacing is a temporary method of stimulating ventricular myocardial depolarization through the chest wall via two large pacing electrodes (patches). The electrodes are placed on the anterior and posterior chest wall and are attached by a cable to an external pulse generator (Fig. 52-1). The external pulse generator delivers energy (milliamps) to the myocardium based on the set pacing rate, output, and sensitivity. Some models of external pulse generators are combined with an external defibrillator, and the electrodes of these models may be used for pacing and defibrillation.
- *Sensitivity* refers to the ability of the pacemaker to detect intrinsic myocardial activity.
- In the nondemand or asynchronous mode, pacing occurs at the set rate regardless of the patient's intrinsic rate. In the demand or synchronous mode, the pacemaker senses intrinsic myocardial activity and paces when the intrinsic cardiac rate is lower than the set rate on the external pulse generator.
- *Pacing* occurs when the external pulse generator delivers enough energy through the pacing electrodes to the myocardium, which is known as pacemaker firing and is represented as a spike on the electrocardiographic (ECG) tracing (Fig. 52-2).
- *Electrical capture* occurs when the pacemaker delivers enough energy to the myocardium so that depolarization occurs. Capture is seen on the ECG with a pacemaker spike followed by a ventricular complex. The ventricular complex occurs after the pacemaker spike, and the QRS is

413

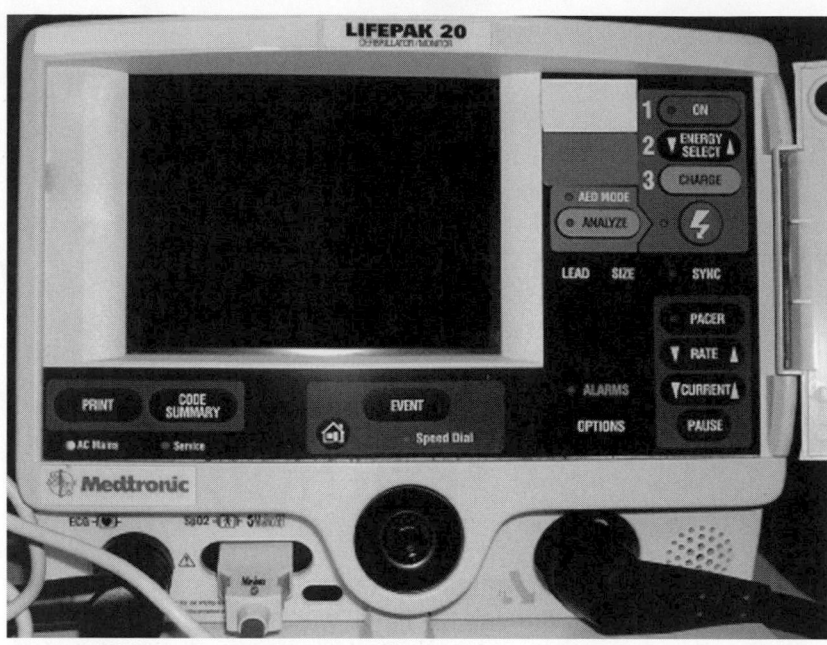

FIGURE 52-1 LIFEPAK 20: Provides defibrillation, monitoring, and external pacing. *(Reproduced with permission of Medtronic, USA, Inc, Minneapolis, MN.)*

wide, with the initial and terminal deflections in opposite directions. In Fig. 52-2, complexes 2 and 3 begin with a downward (negative) deflection and end with an upward (positive) direction. *Mechanical capture* occurs when a paced QRS complex results in a palpable pulse.

- *Standby pacing* is when the pacing electrodes are applied in anticipation of possible use but pacing is not needed at the time.

EQUIPMENT

- Blood pressure monitoring equipment
- External pulse generator
- Pacing cable
- Pacemaker electrodes (patches)
- ECG electrodes
- ECG monitor
- ECG cable

Additional equipment to have available as needed includes the following:

- Emergency cart with medications and other equipment
- Scissors
- Transvenous pacing equipment

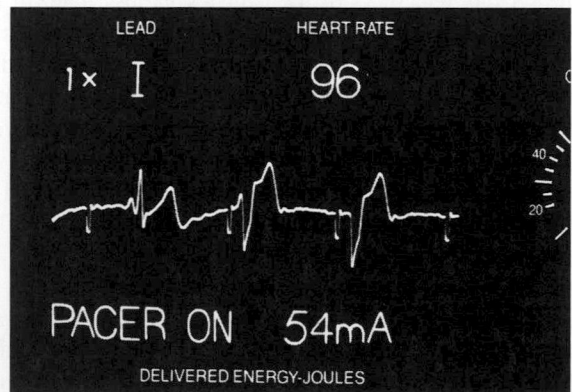

FIGURE 52-2 ECG tracing of external pacing. *(From Zoll Medical Corporation, Burlington, MA.)*

PATIENT AND FAMILY EDUCATION

- Assess learning needs, readiness to learn, and factors that influence learning. ↠*Rationale:* This assessment reveals the patient's and family's knowledge so that teaching can be individualized to be meaningful to the patient and family.
- Discuss basic facts about the normal conduction system, the reason external cardiac pacing is indicated, and what happens to the patient when pacing occurs. ↠*Rationale:* This discussion assists the patient and family in recognizing the need for external pacing and what to expect when pacing occurs.
- Discuss interventions to alleviate discomfort. ↠*Rationale:* This discussion provides the patient with an opportunity to validate perceptions. It gives the patient and family knowledge that interventions are used to minimize the level of discomfort.
- If indicated, inform the patient and family of the possibility of the need for transvenous or permanent pacing support. ↠*Rationale:* This information prepares the patient and family for the possibility of additional therapy. If permanent pacing is necessary, the patient and family need further instruction about possible lifestyle modifications and follow-up visits and information about the pacemaker to be implanted.

PATIENT ASSESSMENT AND PREPARATION

Patient Assessment

- Assess the patient's cardiac rate and rhythm for the presence of dysrhythmias that indicate the need for external cardiac pacing. ↠*Rationale:* Recognition of a dysrhythmia is the first step in determining the need for external cardiac pacing or placing the external pacemaker on standby.
- Determine the patient's hemodynamic response to the dysrhythmia, such as the presence or absence of a pulse; presence of hypotension, altered level of consciousness;

dizziness; shortness of breath; nausea and vomiting; cool, clammy, diaphoretic skin; or the development of chest pain. ➛*Rationale:* The decision to initiate pacing depends on the effect of the dysrhythmia on the patient's cardiac output.

Patient Preparation

- Verify correct patient with two identifiers. ➛*Rationale:* Prior to performing a procedure, the nurse should ensure the correct identification of the patient for the intended intervention.
- Ensure that the patient and family understand preprocedural teaching. Answer questions as they arise, and reinforce information as needed. ➛*Rationale:* This communication evaluates and reinforces understanding of previously taught information.
- Maintain bedside ECG monitoring. ➛*Rationale:* External pacing units do not provide central monitoring or dysrhythmia detection.
- Administer sedative or analgesic medication as prescribed to a conscious patient before initiation of pacing. ➛*Rationale:* External cardiac pacing is uncomfortable.
- Assist the patient to the supine position and expose the patient's torso while maintaining modesty. ➛*Rationale:* This positioning prepares for electrode (patch) placement.

Procedure for Temporary Transcutaneous (External) Pacing

Steps	Rationale	Special Considerations
1. HH		
2. PE		
3. Administer sedation or analgesic as prescribed. **(Level D*)**	Decreases discomfort associated with external cardiac pacing.[3,6,7,9]	Not indicated for patients who are unconscious with hemodynamically unstable conditions. Not indicated for standby because pacing may not be needed.
4. Turn on the pulse generator and monitor. **(Level M*)**	Provides power source.	Many devices work on battery or alternating current (AC) power.
5. Prepare the skin on the patient's chest and back by washing with nonemollient soap and water.	Removal of skin oils, lotion, and moisture improves electrode adherence and maximizes delivery of energy through the chest wall.	Optional step in an emergency. Dry thoroughly. Trim body hair with scissors, if necessary. Avoid use of flammable liquids to prepare the skin (e.g., alcohol, benzoin) because of increased potential for burns. Avoid shaving chest hair because the presence of nicks in the skin under the pacing electrodes can increase patient discomfort. Remove any medication patches applied to the chest area.
6. Apply the ECG electrodes to the ECG leads.	Prepares equipment.	
7. Connect the ECG cable to the monitor inlet of the pulse generator.	Prepares equipment.	Follow manufacturer's recommendations Attachment of the ECG electrodes to the ECG leads and the ECG cable to the pacemaker monitor is optional for some manufacturers in an emergency. If the ECG leads are not placed, the pacemaker may function in the asynchronous mode. The pacemaker may not function unless both the ECG monitoring connection and the pacing electrode connection are both connected to the pacemaker.

*Level D: Peer-reviewed professional organizational standards with clinical studies to support recommendations
*Level M: Manufacturer's recommendations only

Procedure continues on following page

Procedure **for Temporary Transcutaneous (External) Pacing**—*Continued*		
Steps	Rationale	Special Considerations
8. Apply the ECG electrodes to the patient (see Procedure 57).	Displays the patient's intrinsic rhythm on the monitor.	Follow manufacturer's recommendations.
9. Adjust the ECG lead and size to the maximum R wave size. Look for an indicator that the pacemaker is sensing the QRS complexes on the intrinsic rhythm, usually seen as a marker above each native QRS complex.	Detection of the intrinsic rhythm is necessary for the demand mode of pacing.	Lead II usually provides the most prominent R wave.
10. Apply the back (posterior, +) pacing electrode between the spine and left scapula at the level of the heart (Fig. 52-3). **(Level M*)**	Placement of the pacing electrodes in the recommended anatomic location enhances the potential for successful pacing.	Avoid placing the pacing electrodes over bone because this increases the level of energy needed to pace, increases patient discomfort, and increases the possibility of noncapture.
11. Apply the front (anterior, −) pacing electrode at the left, fourth intercostal space, midclavicular line (Fig. 52-4). **(Level M)**	Placement of the pacing electrodes in the recommended anatomic location enhances the potential for successful pacing.	For women, adjust the position of the pacing electrode below and lateral to breast tissue to ensure optimal adherence. Avoid placement of the pacing electrodes over the bedside monitor ECG electrodes and permanently placed devices, such as implantable cardioverter-defibrillators or permanent pacemakers.
12. If the patient's condition is hemodynamically unstable, the back (posterior) electrode may be placed over the patient's right sternal area at the second or third intercostal space. The front (anterior) electrode is maintained at the apex (fourth or fifth intercostal space, midclavicular line; Fig. 52-5). **(Level M)**	Facilitates ease of electrode placement for emergent pacing.	Pacing may be less effective with this method of electrode placement.[8,9]

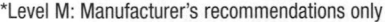

*Level M: Manufacturer's recommendations only

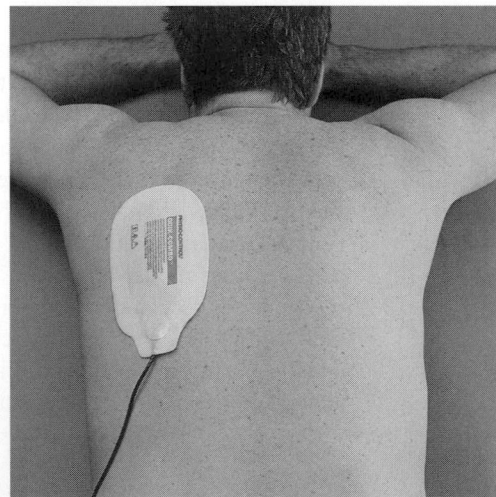

FIGURE 52-3   Location of the posterior (back) pacing electrode. *(Aehlert B: ACLS study guide, ed 3, St Louis, 2007, Mosby, 229.)*

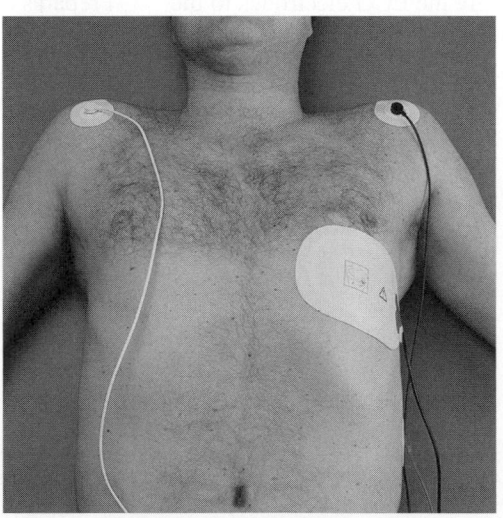

FIGURE 52-4   Location of the anterior (front) pacing electrode. *(Aehlert B: ACLS study guide, ed 3, St Louis, 2007, Mosby, 229.)*

Procedure for Temporary Transcutaneous (External) Pacing—*Continued*

Steps	Rationale	Special Considerations
13. Connect the pacing electrodes to the pacemaker cable and connect the pacemaker cable to the external pulse generator. **(Level M*)**	Necessary for the delivery of electrical energy.	
14. Set the pacemaker rate, level of energy (output, mA) (Fig. 52-6).	Each patient needs different pacemaker settings to provide safe and effective external pacing.	Follow institution standards to ensure that a nurse can initiate external cardiac pacing.
		The demand mode is used as long as the ECG leads are attached to the pacemaker monitor
A. Set the demand or synchronous mode.	The demand mode is used to prevent competition from the patient's intrinsic rhythm.	In the asynchronous mode, the pacemaker fires regardless of the intrinsic rhythm and rate.
B. Set the rate.	Pacing should be at a rate that maintains adequate cardiac output but does not induce ischemia.	The pacemaker may have a default setting (e.g., 80 bpm) that can be adjusted as needed.
C. Set the mA. 1. Slowly increase the mA setting (output) until capture is present. **(Level M)**	Use the lowest amount of energy that consistently results in myocardial capture and contraction to minimize discomfort.[1]	The pacemaker may have a default setting (e.g., 70 mA) that can be adjusted as needed.
2. Set the mA slightly higher than the capture threshold (an additional 2 mA).[1,6] **(Level E*)**		The average adult usually can be paced with a current of 40 to 70 mA.

*Level E: Multiple case reports, theory-based evidence from expert opinions, or peer-reviewed professional organizational standards without clinical studies to support recommendations
*Level M: Manufacturer's recommendations only

Procedure continues on following page

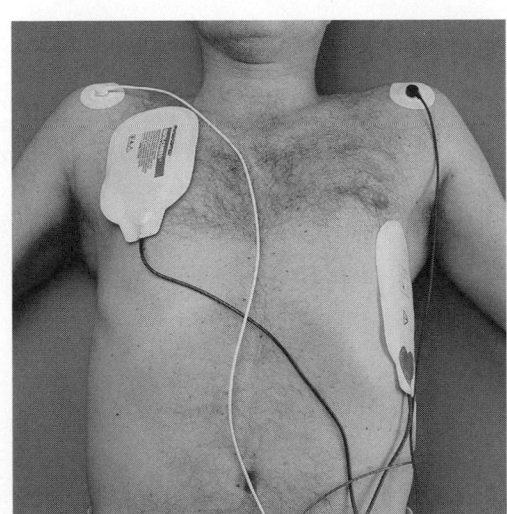

FIGURE 52-5 Location of anterior-lateral pacing electrodes. *(Aehlert B: ACLS study guide, ed 3, St Louis, 2007, Mosby, 229.)*

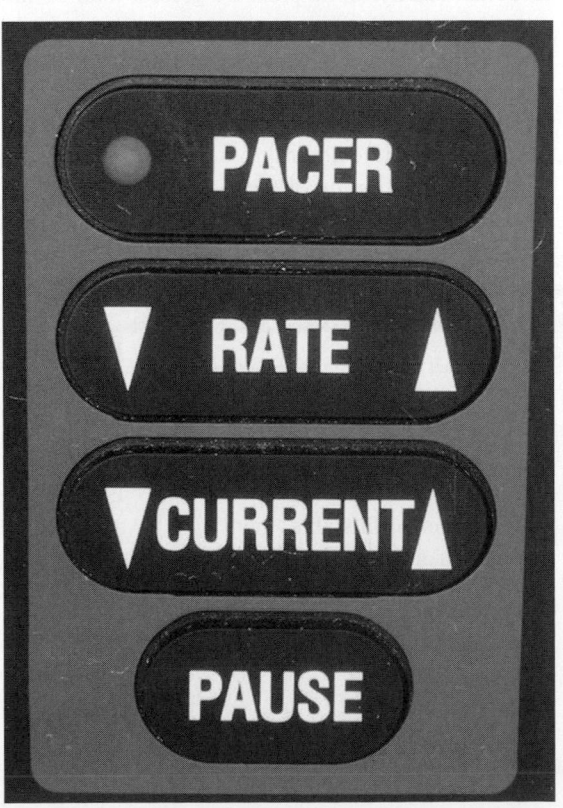

FIGURE 52-6 Controls for external pacemaker settings.

Procedure for Temporary Transcutaneous (External) Pacing—*Continued*

Steps	Rationale	Special Considerations
15. When the pacemaker fires, observe that each pacemaker spike is followed by a wide ventricular complex and a T wave in the opposite deflection of the QRS. (Refer to Fig. 52-2.)	Identifies appropriate functioning of the pacemaker.	If a pacemaker spike occurs and is not followed by a ventricular complex, slowly increase the energy (mA) level. Artifact from skeletal muscle twitching may make an ECG tracing difficult to interpret. Skeletal muscle twitching occurs at lower mA settings, before capture of the myocardium.[1,6,8]
16. Palpate the patient's pulse (e.g., femoral pulse, right brachial pulse, radial pulse).	Ensures adequate blood flow with paced complexes.	The carotid pulses usually are not palpated because the electrical stimulation from the pacemaker may mimic a pulse.[1,6]
17. Evaluate the patient's vital signs and hemodynamic response to pacing.	The patient's hemodynamic response should improve with pacing if symptoms were related to bradycardia.[1,3,6]	If symptoms do not improve with pacing, assess for other causes. Acidosis and electrolyte abnormalities need to be corrected for an effective response to pacing.
18. Evaluate the patient's response to the initial dose of prescribed sedative or analgesic.	Pacing may not be tolerated by the patient.[1,6]	Administer additional prescribed sedatives or analgesics as needed.
19. Discard used supplies in appropriate receptacle.	Reduces the transmission of microorganisms; Standard Precautions.	
20. 🖐		

Expected Outcomes

- Adequate systemic tissue perfusion and cardiac output as evidenced by blood pressure greater than 90 mm Hg systolic (or resolution of hypotension), return to baseline mental status, absence of dizziness or syncope, absence of shortness of breath, absence of nausea and vomiting, and absence of ischemic chest pain
- Stable cardiac rate and rhythm
- Adequate functioning of the pacemaker

Unexpected Outcomes

- Failure of the pacemaker to sense the patient's underlying rhythm with the possibility of R-on-T phenomenon (initiation of ventricular tachydysrhythmias as a result of an improperly timed spike on the T wave)
- Failure of the pacemaker to capture the myocardium
- Failure of the pacemaker to pace
- Discomfort, including skin burns from the delivery of high levels of energy through the chest wall, painful sensations, and skeletal muscle twitching

Patient Monitoring and Care

Steps	Rationale	Reportable Conditions
		These conditions should be reported if they persist despite nursing interventions.
1. Monitor vital signs every 15 minutes until stable, then hourly or more frequently as needed.	Ensures adequate tissue perfusion with paced beats. Adjustments in the pacing rate may need to be made based on vital signs.	- Change in vital signs - Hemodynamic instability

Patient Monitoring and Care —*Continued*

Steps	Rationale	Reportable Conditions
2. Continue to monitor the patient's cardiac rate and rhythm through the central monitoring system. The pacing spike may obscure or mimic the QRS complex, making ventricular capture difficult to see.[5] Select a lead that minimizes the size of the pacing spike and maximizes the QRS complex.[5] Set the pacemaker option on the central monitoring system.	Provides an alarm system. Of note, if ECG leads are disconnected from the pacemaker monitor, pacing reverts to asynchronous, which could compete with the native rhythm.	• Changes in capture or sensing • Dysrhythmias

3. Monitor level of comfort and sedation level:
  A. Assess the patient's level of comfort and sedation level following institution standard.
  B. Administer prescribed analgesic and sedative medications as needed.
  C. Adjust the level of energy to the lowest level for capture.
  D. Evaluate the patient's response to interventions.
	The external delivery of energy through the chest wall may cause varying degrees of discomfort.[1,3,6,9]	• Continued pain despite interventions to alleviate pain
		• Patient intolerance of the prescribed medications (e.g., severe nausea, hypotension, decreased respirations)

4. Obtain an ECG recording strip to document pacing function on initiation of pacing and every 4 to 8 hours and as needed or according to institution standard.	Documents cardiac rate, rhythm, and pacemaker activity.	• Failure to capture • Failure to pace
5. Evaluate pacemaker function (capturing and sensing) with any change in patient condition or vital signs.	Ensures continued functioning of the pacemaker. Introduction of other variables, such as electrolyte imbalance or metabolic changes, may alter the level of energy needed to pace effectively.	• Inability to maintain appropriate sensing and capture • Changes in patient condition that affect appropriate pacemaker function

6. Monitor the patient's cardiac rate and rhythm for resolution of the dysrhythmia that necessitates pacemaker intervention.
  A. This monitoring may necessitate turning the pacemaker off if prescribed to assess the patient's underlying rate and rhythm. Do not turn the pacemaker off if the patient is 100% paced.
  B. When assessing the patient's intrinsic rate and rhythm, reduce the pacing rate slowly.
	Determines whether the dysrhythmia has subsided.
	
	A sudden cessation of pacing can lead to asystole because the intrinsic rate and rhythm may be suppressed by continuous pacing.[8]
		• Worsening of the baseline cardiac rate and rhythm (e.g., change from symptomatic second-degree heart block to complete heart block)

7. Check the adherence of the pacing electrodes to the skin at least every 4 hours. If pacing is not occurring, assess the skin integrity under the pacing electrodes.	Changes in skin integrity caused by burns or skin breaks significantly alters the patient's level of comfort and exposes the patient to possible infection.	• Changes in skin integrity • Burns

Procedure continues on following page

Patient Monitoring and Care —*Continued*

Steps	Rationale	Reportable Conditions
Change the electrodes at least every 24 hours or after 8 hours of continuous pacing.[8] **(Level M*)**	Pacing electrodes should not be used once they have been out of the package for 24 hours.[8]	

*Level M: Manufacturer's recommendations only

Documentation

Documentation should include the following:

- Patient and family education
- Patient preparation
- Date and time external cardiac pacing is initiated
- Description of events that warranted intervention
- Vital signs and physical assessment before and after external cardiac pacing
- ECG recordings before and after pacing
- Pain assessment, interventions and effectiveness

- Medications administered
- Pacing rate, mode, mA
- Percentage of the time the patient is paced if in the demand mode
- Status of skin integrity when the pacing electrodes are changed
- Unexpected outcomes
- Additional interventions

References

1. Aehlert B: *ACLS study guide,* ed 3, St Louis, 2007, Mosby.
CR 2. American Heart Association: Guidelines for cardiopulmonary resuscitation and emergency cardiovascular care: part 5: electrical therapies: automated external defibrillators, defibrillation, cardioversion, and pacing, *Circulation* 112(Suppl IV):IV-35-IV-45, 2005.
CR 3. American Heart Association: Guidelines for cardiopulmonary resuscitation and emergency cardiovascular care: part 7.3: management of symptomatic bradycardia and tachycardia, *Circulation* 112(Suppl IV):IV-67-IV-77, 2005.
CR 4. Antman EM, et al: ACC/AHA guidelines for management of patients with ST-elevation myocardial infarction: a report of the American College of Cardiology/American Heart Association Task Force on Practice Guidelines, *Circulation* 100:e82-e293, 2004.
CR 5. Drew B, et al: Practice standards for electrocardiographic monitoring in hospital settings: an American Heart Association scientific statement from the Councils on Cardiovascular Nursing, Clinical Cardiology, and Cardiovascular Disease in the Young: endorsed by the International Society of Computerized Electrocardiology and the American Association of Critical-Care Nurses, *Circulation* 110: 2721-2746, 2004.

6. Field J, editor: Part 4: *ACLS core cases, bradycardia case in advanced cardiac life support provider manual,* Dallas, 2006, American Heart Association.
7. Gibson T: A practical guide to external cardiac pacing, *Nursing Standard* 22:20,45-48, 2008.
8. Medtronic Physio-Control Corp: *LIFEPAK 20 defibrillator/ monitor operating instructions,* Physio-Control, Inc. Redmond, WA, 2008.
CR 9. Zoll P: Noninvasive temporary cardiac pacing, *J Electrophys* 1:2,156-161, 1987.

Additional Readings

CR Doukky R, et al: Using transcutaneous cardiac pacing to best advantage: how to ensure successful capture and avoid complications, *J Crit Illness* 5:219-25, 2003.
Jacobson C, Marzlin K, Webner C: Chapter 17. In *Electrical management of arrhythmias in cardiovascular nursing practice,* Burien, WA, 2007, Cardiovascular Nursing Education Associates.

AP Temporary Transvenous Pacemaker Insertion (Perform)

P U R P O S E : The purpose of temporary cardiac pacing is to ensure or restore an adequate heart rate and rhythm. A transvenous pacemaker is inserted as a temporary measure when the normal conduction system of the heart fails to produce or conduct an electrical impulse, resulting in hemodynamic compromise or other debilitating symptoms.

Deborah E. Becker

PREREQUISITE NURSING KNOWLEDGE

- Knowledge of the normal anatomy and physiology of the cardiovascular system, principles of cardiac conduction, and basic and advanced dysrhythmia interpretation is needed.
- Knowledge of temporary pacemaker function and expected patient responses to pacemaker therapy is necessary.
- Clinical and technical competence in central line insertion, temporary transvenous pacemaker insertion, and suturing is needed.
- Clinical and technical competence related to use of temporary pacemakers is necessary.
- Competence in chest radiograph interpretation is needed.
- Advanced cardiac life support knowledge and skills are needed.
- Principles of general electrical safety apply with use of temporary invasive pacing methods. Gloves always should be worn when handling electrodes to prevent microshock.

AP This procedure should be performed only by physicians, advanced practice nurses, and other healthcare professionals (including critical care nurses) with additional knowledge, skills, and demonstrated competence per professional licensure or institutional standard.

- The insertion of a temporary transvenous pacemaker is performed in emergency and elective clinical situations. Temporary transvenous pacing may be used to:
  - Stimulate the myocardium to contract in the absence of an intrinsic rhythm
  - Establish adequate cardiac output and blood pressure
  - Ensure tissue perfusion to vital organs
  - Reduce the possibility of ventricular dysrhythmias in the presence of bradycardia
  - Supplement an inadequate rhythm, such as when transient decreases in heart rate occur (e.g., chronotropic incompetence in shock)
  - Allow the administration of medications that may cause a rhythm or conduction abnormality (e.g., beta blockers) in the symptomatic bradycardia, complete heart block, new bundle-branch block with transient complete heart block, alternating bundle-branch block)
- Temporary transvenous pacing is indicated for the following:
  - Third-degree atrioventricular (AV) block
  - Type II AV block
  - Dysrhythmias that are complicating acute myocardial infarction (e.g., symptomatic bradycardia, complete heart block, new bundle-branch block with transient complete heart block, alternating bundle-branch block)
  - Sinus node dysfunction (e.g., symptomatic bradydysrhythmias, treatment of bradycardia-tachycardia syndromes, sick sinus syndrome)

- ❖ Ventricular standstill or cardiac arrest
- ❖ Long QT syndrome with ventricular dysrhythmias
- ❖ Drug toxicity
- ❖ Postoperative cardiac surgery
- ❖ Prophylaxis with cardiac diagnostic or interventional procedures
- ❖ Chronotropic incompetence in the setting of cardiogenic shock
- When temporary transvenous pacing is used, the pulse generator is attached externally to a pacing lead wire that is inserted through a vein into the right atrium or right ventricle.
- Veins used for the insertion of a transvenous pacing lead wire are the subclavian, femoral, brachial, internal jugular, or external jugular.
- Single-chamber ventricular pacing is the most appropriate method in an emergency because the goal is to establish a heart rate as quickly as possible.
- The transvenous pacing lead is an insulated wire with one or two electrodes at the tip of the wire (Fig. 53-1).
- The pacing lead can be a hard-tipped or a balloon-tipped pacing catheter that is placed in direct contact with the endocardium. Most temporary leads are bipolar with the distal tip electrode (seen as a metal ring) separated from the proximal electrode by 1 to 2 cm of pacing catheter (also seen as a metal ring; see Fig. 53-1).
- Basic principles of cardiac pacing include sensing, pacing, and capture.
- Sensing refers to the ability of the pacemaker device to detect intrinsic myocardial electrical activity. Sensing occurs if the pulse generator is in the synchronous or demand mode. The pacemaker either is inhibited from delivering a stimulus or initiates an electrical impulse.
- Pacing occurs when the temporary pulse generator is activated and the programmed level of energy travels from the pulse generator through the temporary pacing lead wire to the endocardium, which is known as pacemaker

firing and is represented as a vertical line or spike on the electrocardiogram (ECG) recording.

- Capture refers to the successful conduction of the pacemaker impulse through the myocardium, resulting in depolarization. Capture is evidenced on the ECG by a pacemaker spike followed by either an atrial or a ventricular complex, depending on the chamber being paced. The healthcare provider can assess whether the electrical depolarization resulted in mechanical activity by observing the right atrial pressure, left atrial pressure, or pulmonary artery or arterial pressure waveforms or whether the ventricle is paced by palpating a pulse.
- Temporary pulse generator features include the following:
  - ❖ The temporary pulse generator houses the controls and the energy source for pacing.
  - ❖ Pulse generators can be used for single-chamber pacing with one set of terminals at the top of the pulse generator, into which the pacing wires are inserted (via connecting cable).
  - ❖ A dual-chamber pacemaker requires two sets of terminals, one each for the atrial and ventricular wires.
  - ❖ Different models of pacemakers use either dials or touch pads for changing the settings.
  - ❖ The pacing rate is determined by the rate set by the dial or rate pad.
  - ❖ The AV interval dial or pad on a dual-chamber pacemaker controls the amount of time between atrial and ventricular stimulation (electronic PR interval).
  - ❖ The energy delivered to the endocardium is determined by setting the output (milliamperage [mA]) dial or pad on the pulse generator.
  - ❖ Dual-chamber pacing requires that mA are set for the atria and the ventricle.
- The ability of the pacemaker to detect the patient's intrinsic rhythm is determined by the pacing mode. In the asynchronous mode, the pacemaker functions as a fixed-rate pacemaker and is not able to sense any of the

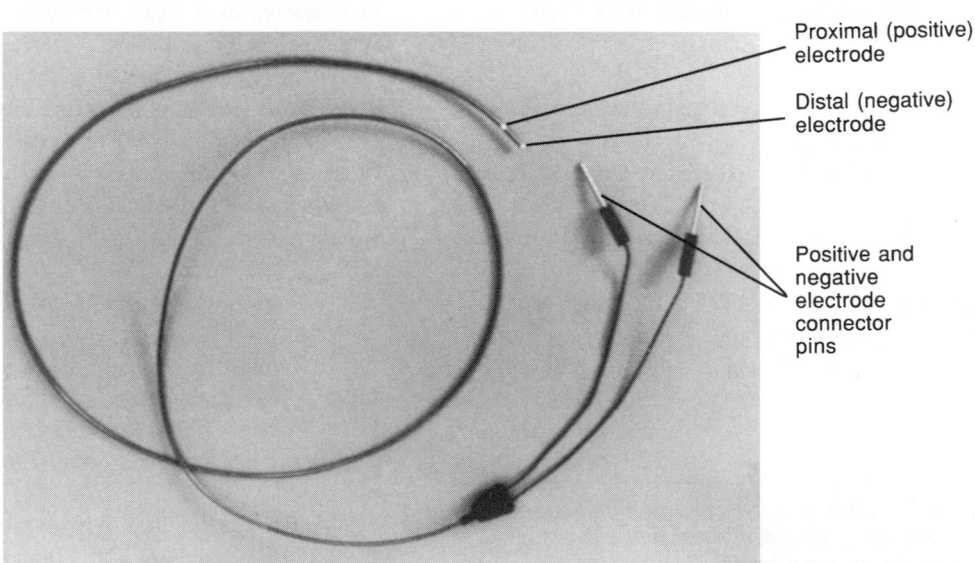

FIGURE 53-1   Bipolar lead wire.

Proximal (positive) electrode

Distal (negative) electrode

Positive and negative electrode connector pins

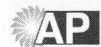

patient's inherent cardiac electrical activity. In the synchronous mode, the pacemaker is able to sense the patient's inherent cardiac electrical activity.

- The ability of the pacemaker to depolarize the myocardium depends on many variables: position of the electrode and degree of contact with viable endocardial tissue; level of energy delivered through the pacing wire; presence of hypoxia, acidosis, or electrolyte imbalances; fibrosis around the tip of the catheter; and concomitant medication therapy.[2,4]
- All electrical equipment in the patient's room must be properly grounded to prevent interference from occurring.

EQUIPMENT

- Antiseptic skin preparation solution (e.g., 2% chlorhexidine-based solution)
- Sterile drapes, towels, masks, head cover, goggles or face shields, gowns, gloves, and dressings
- Balloon-tipped pacing catheter and insertion tray
- Pacing lead wire (if balloon-tipped catheter is unavailable)
- Pulse generator
- 9-V battery for pulse generator
- Connecting cables
- Alligator clips or wires with connecting pins
- ECG monitor and recorder
- Supplies for dressing at insertion site
  Additional equipment as needed includes the following:
- Local anesthetic
- Percutaneous introducer needle or 14-gauge needle
- Introducer sheath with dilator
- Guidewire (per physician or advanced practice nurse choice)
- Suture with needle, syringes, needles, and scalpel
- Emergency equipment
- Portable ultrasound scan equipment
- Fluoroscopy
- Lead aprons or shields
- 12-lead ECG machine

PATIENT AND FAMILY EDUCATION

- Assess learning needs, readiness to learn, and factors that influence learning. ➟*Rationale:* This assessment enables teaching to be individualized in a manner that is meaningful to the patient and the family.
- Discuss basic facts about the normal conduction system, such as structure and function of the conduction system, normal and abnormal heart rhythms, and symptoms and significance of abnormal heart rhythms. ➟*Rationale:* The patient and family should understand the conduction system, why the procedure is necessary, and what potential risks and benefits are associated with this invasive procedure.
- Provide a basic description of the temporary transvenous pacemaker insertion procedure. ➟*Rationale:* The patient and family should be informed of the invasive nature of the procedure and any risks associated with the procedure.

An understanding of the procedure may reduce anxiety associated with the procedure.

- Describe the precautions and restrictions required while the temporary pacemaker is in place, such as limitation of movement, avoiding handling the pacemaker or touching exposed portions of the electrodes, and situations in which the nurse should be notified (e.g., if the dressing becomes damp, if the patient experiences dizziness). ➟*Rationale:* Understanding potential limitations may improve the patient's cooperation with restrictions and precautions.

PATIENT ASSESSMENT AND PREPARATION
Patient Assessment

- Assess the patient's cardiac rhythm for the presence of the dysrhythmia that necessitates the initiation of temporary cardiac pacing. ➟*Rationale:* This assessment determines the need for invasive cardiac pacing.
- Assess the patient's hemodynamic response to the dysrhythmia. Rhythm disturbances may reduce cardiac output significantly, with detrimental effects on perfusion of vital organs. ➟*Rationale:* This assessment determines the urgency of the procedure. It may indicate the need for temporizing measures (e.g., vasopressors or transcutaneous pacing).
- Review current medications. ➟*Rationale:* Medications may be implicated as a cause of the dysrhythmia that led to the need for pacemaker therapy, or medications may need to be held as a result of concomitant effect. Other medications, such as antidysrhythmics, may alter the pacing threshold.
- Review the patient's current laboratory study results, including chemistry, electrolyte profile, arterial blood gases, coagulation profile, platelet count, and cardioactive medication levels. ➟*Rationale:* This review assists in determining whether inserting the pacemaker was precipitated by metabolic disturbances or medication toxicity and establishes the pacing milieu. The review provides the healthcare provider with information regarding the risk for abnormal bleeding during or after the procedure is performed.
- Assess the presence and position of the central venous access. ➟*Rationale:* The temporary transvenous pacing catheter is advanced through the central venous circulation. If access already is established, proper placement must be ensured before the pacing catheter can be advanced through the circulatory system.

Patient Preparation

- Verify correct patient using two identifiers. ➟*Rationale:* Prior to performing a procedure, the nurse should ensure the correct identification of the patient for the intended intervention.
- Ensure that the patient and family understand preprocedural teaching. Answer questions as they arise and reinforce information as needed. ➟*Rationale:* Evaluates

and reinforces understanding of previously taught information.
- Obtain informed consent. ➤➤*Rationale:* Informed consent protects the rights of the patient and makes a competent decision possible for the patient; however, in emergency circumstances, time may not allow a consent form to be signed.
- Perform a pre-procedure verification and time out, if non-emergent. ➤➤*Rationale:* Ensures patient safety.
- Connect the patient to a 5-lead monitoring system or to a 12-lead ECG machine. ➤➤*Rationale:* This monitoring

facilitates the placement of the balloon-tipped catheter by indicating the position of the catheter during its placement. Also, it allows for monitoring of the patient's cardiac rhythm during the procedure.
- Prescribe and ensure that pain medication and/or sedation is administered. ➤➤*Rationale:* Medication may be indicated depending on the patient's level of anxiety and pain. Sedation or pain medication may not be possible if the patient's condition is hemodynamically unstable.

Procedure	**for Performing Temporary Transvenous Pacemaker Insertion**	
Steps	**Rationale**	**Special Considerations**
1. **HH**		
2. **PE**		
3. Connect the patient to the bedside monitoring system, and monitor the ECG continuously (see Procedure 57).	Monitors the patient's intrinsic heart rate and rhythm during and after the procedure to evaluate for adequate rate and pacemaker function.	If the monitoring system is not a 5-lead system, also connect the patient to the 12-lead ECG machine (see Procedure 60).
4. Assess pacemaker functioning, and insert a new battery into the pulse generator if needed (see Fig. 54-9).	Ensures a functional pacemaker pulse generator.	Different ways to assess battery function depend on the model and manufacturer; check manufacturer's recommendations for specific instructions.
5. Attach the connecting cable to the pulse generator, connecting the "positive" on the cable to the "positive" on the pulse generator and the "negative" on the cable to the "negative" on the pulse generator.	Prepares the pacing system; the pacing stimulus travels from the pulse generator to the negative terminal, and energy returns to the pulse generator via the positive terminal.	Some lead wires are labeled distal and proximal; distal connects to negative, and proximal connects to positive. Some lead wires may not have negative and positive marked on them. Polarity is established when the wires are placed in the connecting cable. Two connecting cables are needed with both atrial and ventricular pacing.
6. Check the placement of the central venous access with chest radiography before starting the procedure.	Central venous access is needed as the transvenous pacing catheter is passed through the central venous system.	If central venous access is needed, refer to Procedure 81.
7. All personnel performing and assisting with the procedure should apply personal protective and sterile equipment (e.g., masks, head covers, goggles or face shields, sterile gowns, and gloves).	Minimizes the risk of infection and maintains standard and sterile precautions.	Gloves should be worn whenever the pacing electrodes are handled to prevent microshock.[6]
8. Cleanse the site with antiseptic solution (e.g., 2% chlorhexidine-based preparation).	Minimizes the risk of infection.	
9. Drape the site with the sterile drapes.	Provides a sterile field and reduces the transmission of microorganisms.	
10. Insert the balloon-tipped pacing catheter through the introducer, and advance the pacing lead.	The transvenous pacing catheter is threaded through the central venous system.	

Procedure for Performing Temporary Transvenous Pacemaker Insertion—*Continued*

Steps	Rationale	Special Considerations
11. Inflate the balloon when the tip of the pacing lead is in the vena cava.	The air-filled balloon allows the blood flow to carry the catheter tip into the desired position in the right ventricle.	
12. Transcutaneous ultrasound scan of the chest during the insertion procedure may assist in ensuring proper placement.[5] **(Level E*)**	Ultrasound scan visualization of the pacing catheter as it is being passed through the central venous system may ensure a quicker and more accurate placement of the pacing electrode within the endocardium of the right ventricle.[1,3,5]	Fluoroscopy may be needed to permit direct visualization of the pacing electrode. If fluoroscopy is used, all personnel must be shielded from the radiation with lead aprons or be positioned behind lead shields. Drape the patient below the waist with a lead sheet or apron.
13. Slowly advance the pacing lead. If transcutaneous ultrasound is not used to guide catheter placement, lead placement can be verified by: A. Use the V lead of the bedside monitoring system or the 12-lead ECG machine. B. Connect the patient to the limb leads. C. Use an alligator clip or a wire with connector pins if needed (Fig. 53-2).	For transvenous, ventricular pacing, the negative pacing electrode is positioned in the endocardium (at the apex) of the right ventricle. The ECG is derived directly from the pacing electrode, and the position of the catheter tip is verified by the internal electrical recording that shows ST-segment elevation indicating contact with the endocardium.	If premature ventricular contractions or runs of ventricular tachycardia occur, deflate the balloon and withdraw the catheter a little; reposition the pacing lead with the balloon deflated.

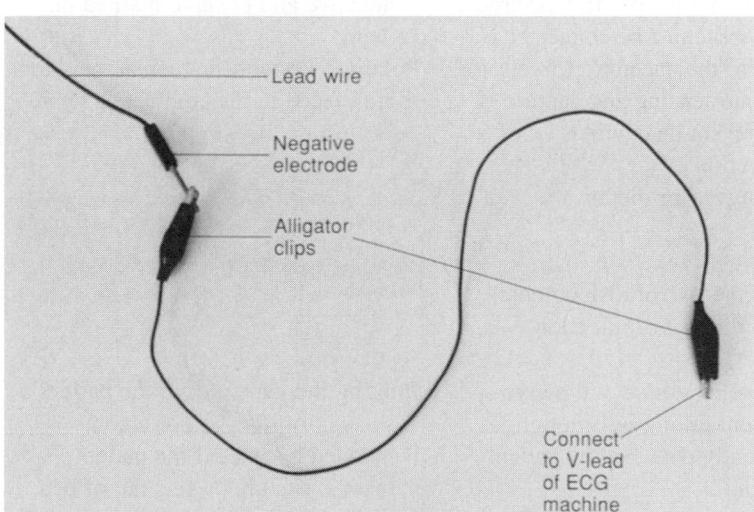

FIGURE 53-2 Alligator clips. *ECG,* electrocardiogram.

D. Attach the V lead of the ECG monitoring system or the 12-lead ECG machine to the negative electrode connector pin (distal pin) of the pacing lead wire.

*Level E: Multiple case reports, theory-based evidence from expert opinions, or peer-reviewed professional organizational standards without clinical studies to support recommendations

Procedure continues on following page

Procedure	**for Performing Temporary Transvenous Pacemaker Insertion—*Continued***	
Steps	**Rationale**	**Special Considerations**

E. Set the monitoring system to record the V lead continuously.

F. Observe the ECG for ST-segment elevation in the V lead recording (Fig. 53-3).

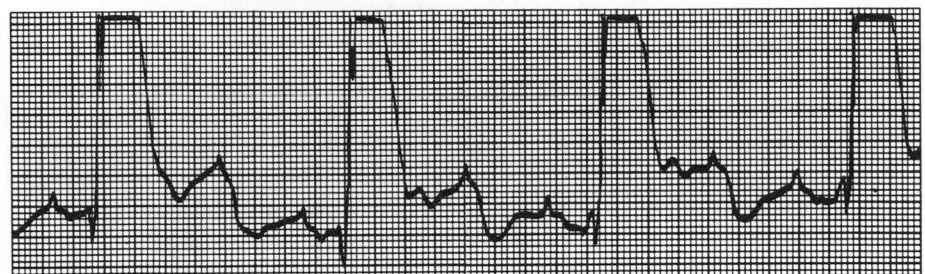

FIGURE 53-3   ECG rhythm recorded in the right ventricle; elevated ST segments when the pacing electrode is wedged against the endocardial wall of the right ventricle. *(From Meltzer LE, Pinneo R, Kitchell JR: Intensive coronary care, ed 4, Bowie, MD, 1983, Robert J. Brady Co.)*

Steps	**Rationale**	**Special Considerations**
G. Observe for left bundle-branch block pattern and left axis deviation that usually can be identified.	As a result of the temporary pacing catheter transmission of impulses from within the right ventricle, conduction of the impulse throughout the ventricles occurs via cellular conduction of the impulse rather than transmission down the bundle branches.	
14. After the electrodes are properly positioned, deflate the balloon, and connect the external electrode pins to the pulse generator via the connecting cables. Ensure that the positive and negative electrodes are connected to the respective positive and negative terminals on the pulse generator via the connecting cables.	Energy from the pulse generator is directed to the negative electrode in contact with the ventricle. The pacing circuit is completed as energy reaches the positive electrode. The lead wires must be connected securely to the pacemaker to ensure appropriate sensing and capture and to prevent inadvertent disconnection.	A bridging connecting cable is recommended for use between the pacing wires and the pulse generator. Some lead wires may not have negative and positive marked on them. Polarity is established when the wires are placed in the connecting cable.
15. Set pacemaker settings and initiate pacing (refer to Procedure 54).	Initiates pacemaker therapy.	
16. Suture the pacing lead in place.	Minimizes the risk of dislodgment.	
17. Apply a sterile occlusive dressing over the site.	Minimizes the risk of infection.	
18. Secure necessary equipment to provide some stability for the pacemaker, such as hanging the pulse generator on an intravenous pole, strapping the pulse generator to the patient's torso, or hanging the pulse generator from a carrying device.	The pulse generator should be protected from falling or becoming inadvertently detached by patient movement. Disconnection or tension on the pacing electrodes may lead to pacemaker malfunction.	Pinning the generator to the patient's sheets or pillow is not recommended because if the patient moves, sits up, or gets out of bed, the pacing lead may be inadvertently disconnected. Keep the pulse generator in clear view so that all are aware it is in use.
19. Discard used supplies in appropriate receptacles.		
20. **HH**	Reduces the transmission of microorganisms; standard precautions	
21. Obtain a chest radiograph.	In the absence of fluoroscopy, a chest radiograph is essential to detect potential complications associated with insertion and to visualize lead position.	

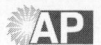

Expected Outcomes

- Paced rhythm on ECG consistent with parameters set on the pacemaker, as evidenced by appropriate heart rate, proper sensing, and proper capture
- Patient exhibits hemodynamic stability, as evidenced by systolic blood pressure greater than 90 mm Hg, mean arterial blood pressure greater than 60 mm Hg, alert and oriented condition, and no syncope or ischemia
- Pacemaker leads are securely connected to the pulse generator

Unexpected Outcomes

- Inability to achieve proper placement of the pacing catheter
- Failure of the pacemaker to sense, causing competition between the pacemaker-initiated impulses and the patient's intrinsic cardiac rhythm
- Failure of the pacemaker to capture the myocardium
- Pacemaker oversensing that causes the pacemaker to be inappropriately inhibited
- Stimulation of the diaphragm that causes hiccupping, possibly related to pacing the phrenic nerve, perforation, wire dislodgment, or excessively high pacemaker mA setting
- Development of phlebitis, thrombosis, embolism, or bacteremia
- Ventricular dysrhythmias from manipulation within the cardiac chamber
- Pneumothorax, hemothorax, pneumomediastinum, or development of subcutaneous emphysema from the insertion procedure[2,4]
- Myocardial perforation, cardiac tamponade, or post-pericardiotomy syndrome from the insertion procedure and electrode placement
- Air embolism
- Lead dislodgment
- Pain

Patient Monitoring and Care

Steps	Rationale	Reportable Conditions
		These conditions should be reported if they persist despite nursing interventions.
1. Monitor vital signs and hemodynamic response to pacing following institution standard and as often as the patient's condition warrants.	The goal of cardiac pacing is to improve cardiac output by increasing heart rate or by overriding life-threatening dysrhythmias.	• Change in vital signs associated with signs and symptoms of hemodynamic deterioration
2. Evaluate the ECG for the presence of the paced rhythm or resolution of the initiating dysrhythmia.	Proper pacemaker functioning is assessed by observing the ECG for pacemaker activity consistent with the parameters set.	• Inability to obtain capture may be a result of oversensing, undersensing, or poor lead contact with the endocardium
3. Follow institution standard, for assessing pain. Administer analgesia as prescribed.	Identifies need for pain interventions.	• Continual hiccups (may indicate wire perforation)
		• Continued pain despite pain interventions
4. Check and document sensitivity and threshold at least every 24 hours. Threshold may be checked by physicians in patients at high risk (e.g., if pacemaker dependent).	Ensures proper pacemaker functioning. Prevents unnecessarily high levels of energy delivery to the myocardium. Threshold may be checked more frequently if the patient's condition changes or pacemaker function is questioned.	• Problems with sensitivity or threshold

Procedure continues on following page

Patient Monitoring and Care —*Continued*

Steps	Rationale	Reportable Conditions
5. Change the dressing as determined by institutional policy depending on the type of dressing used. A. Cleanse the surrounding area with antiseptic solution, such as a 2% chlorhexidine-based preparation. B. Apply dry sterile dressing. C. Record the date and the time of the dressing change.	Decreases the potential for infection. Although guidelines do not exist specific to pacing wires, the Centers for Disease Control and Prevention (CDC) recommend replacing dressings on intravascular catheters when the dressing becomes damp, loosened, or soiled or when inspection of the site is necessary.[7]	• Increased temperature • Increased white blood cell count • Purulent drainage at the insertion site • Warmth, redness, discoloration, or pain at the site
6. Monitor for other complications.	Early recognition leads to prompt treatment.	• Embolus • Thrombosis • Perforation of the myocardium • Pneumothorax • Hemothorax • Phlebitis
7. Monitor electrolyte levels.	Electrolyte imbalances may precipitate dysrhythmias.	• Abnormal electrolyte values
8. Ensure that all pacemaker connections are secure.	Maintenance of tight connections is necessary to ensure proper sensing, to ensure impulse conduction, and to minimize the risk of microshock conduction to the heart.	• Inability to maintain tight connections with available equipment, jeopardizing pacing therapy

Documentation

Documentation should include the following:

• Description of the events that warranted intervention
• Patient and family education and response to education
• Signed informed consent form
• Universal Protocol requirements
• Date and time of insertion
• Date and time of initiation of pacing
• Type of pacing wire inserted and location of insertion
• Pacemaker settings: mode, rate, output, sensitivity setting, threshold measurements, and whether pacemaker is on or off

• ECG monitoring strip recording before and after pacemaker insertion, with interpretation
• Vital signs and hemodynamic parameters before, during, and after the procedure
• Proper placement confirmed with chest radiography
• Patient response to procedure
• Complications and interventions
• Occurrence of unexpected outcomes and interventions taken
• Pain assessment, interventions and patient response to medication
• Date and time pacing was discontinued

References

1. Dahlberg ST: Temporary cardiac pacing. In Irwin RS, et al: *Procedures and techniques in intensive care medicine,* ed 6, Philadelphia, 2008, Lippincott Williams & Wilkins.
CR 2. Espiritu JD, Keller CA: Pneumomediastinum and subcutaneous emphysema from pacemaker placement, *Pacing Clin Electrophysiol* 24:1041-1042, 2001.
3. Harrigan RA, Chan TC, Moonblatt S, et al: Temporary transvenous pacemaker placement in the emergency department, *J Emerg Med* 32:105-111, 2007.
4. Huysmans W, Budts W: Late free atrial wall rupture after percutaneous atrial septal defect closure and transvenous pacemaker implantation, *Catheter Cardiovasc Interv* 72:286-288, 2008.
CR 5. Macedo W Jr, et al: Ultrasonographic guidance of transvenous pacemaker insertion in the emergency department: a report of three cases, *J Emerg Med* 17:491-496, 1999.
CR 6. Norman EM: Critical care extra: critical questions: avoiding electrical hazards, temporary pacing wires, *Am J Nurs* 98:16GG-HH, 1998.
CR 7. O'Grady NP, et al: Guidelines for the prevention of intravascular catheter-related infections, *Am J Infect Control* 30:476-489, 2002.

Temporary Transvenous and Epicardial Pacing

P U R P O S E : The purpose of temporary cardiac pacing is to ensure or restore an adequate heart rate and rhythm. Transvenous and epicardial pacing are initiated as temporary measures when a failure of the normal conduction system of the heart to produce an electrical impulse results in hemodynamic compromise.

Valerie Spotts

PREREQUISITE NURSING KNOWLEDGE

- Knowledge of the normal anatomy and physiology of the cardiovascular system, principles of cardiac conduction, and basic dysrhythmia interpretation is necessary.
- Understanding of temporary pacemakers is needed to evaluate pacemaker function and the patient's response to pacemaker therapy.
- Clinical and technical competence related to use of temporary pacemakers is needed.
- Advanced cardiac life support knowledge and skills are necessary.
- Basic principles of hemodynamic monitoring are essential in assessment of the efficacy of temporary pacing therapy.
- Knowledge of the pulmonary artery (PA) catheter function and its use relative to hemodynamic monitoring is a necessity with use of a PA catheter with pacing function (see Procedure 73).
- Knowledge of the care of the patient with central venous catheters (see Procedure 70) is needed.
- Principles of general electrical safety apply with use of temporary invasive pacing methods. Gloves always should be worn when handling electrodes to prevent microshock. In addition, the exposed proximal ends of the pacing wires should be insulated when not in use to prevent microshock.[9-11]
- The insertion of a temporary pacemaker is performed in emergent and elective clinical situations.

- Temporary pacing may be used to stimulate the myocardium to contract in the absence of an intrinsic rhythm, establish an adequate cardiac output and blood pressure to ensure tissue perfusion to vital organs, reduce the possibility of ventricular dysrhythmias in the presence of bradycardia, supplement an inadequate rhythm with transient decreases in heart rate (e.g., chronotropic incompetence in shock), or allow the administration of medications (e.g., beta blockers) to treat ischemia or tachydysrhythmias in the presence of conduction system dysfunction or bradycardia.
- Temporary invasive pacing is indicated for the following[4,6,8]:
  - ❖ Symptomatic third-degree atrioventricular (AV) block
  - ❖ Symptomatic second-degree heart block
  - ❖ Dysrhythmias that complicate acute myocardial infarction
  - ❖ Symptomatic bradycardia or bradydysrhythmias
  - ❖ New bundle-branch block with transient complete heart block
  - ❖ Alternating bundle-branch block
  - ❖ Symptomatic sinus node dysfunction
  - ❖ Treatment of bradycardia-tachycardia syndrome (sick sinus syndrome)
  - ❖ Ventricular standstill or cardiac arrest
  - ❖ Long QT syndrome with ventricular dysrhythmias
  - ❖ Medication toxicity or adverse effects of a medication
  - ❖ Postoperative cardiac surgery
  - ❖ Low cardiac output states

- ❖ Prophylaxis with cardiac diagnostic or interventional procedures
- ❖ Chronotropic incompetence in the setting of cardiogenic shock
- The three primary methods of invasive temporary pacing are: transvenous endocardial pacing, pacing via a PA catheter, and epicardial pacing.
- Transvenous pacing:
  - ❖ In temporary transvenous pacing, the pulse generator is externally attached to a pacing lead that is inserted through a vein into the right atrium or ventricle.
  - ❖ Veins used for insertion of the pacing lead are the subclavian, femoral, brachial, internal jugular, or external jugular veins.
  - ❖ Single-chamber ventricular pacing is the most common method used in an emergency because the goal is to establish a heart rate as quickly as possible.
  - ❖ Temporary atrial or dual-chamber pacing can be initiated if the patient needs atrial contraction for improvement in hemodynamics.
  - ❖ The pacing lead is an insulated wire with one or two electrodes at the tip of the wire (Fig. 54-1).
  - ❖ The pacing lead can be a hard-tipped or balloon-tipped pacing catheter that is placed in direct contact with the endocardium. Most temporary leads are bipolar, with the distal tip electrode separated from the proximal ring by 1 to 2 cm (see Fig. 53-1).
  - ❖ An external temporary pulse generator is connected to the transvenous pacing wire via a bridging or connecting cable.
- Pacing via a PA catheter:
  - ❖ Temporary atrial or ventricular pacing via a thermodilution PA catheter can be done with combination catheters that are specifically designed for temporary pacing.
  - ❖ PA pacing catheters feature atrial and ventricular ports for the introduction of the pacing lead wires (Fig. 54-2).
  - ❖ Use of a PA catheter combines the capabilities of PA pressure monitoring, thermodilution cardiac output measurement, fluid infusion, mixed venous oxygen sampling, and temporary pacing.
  - ❖ One limitation of these multifunction catheters is that the simultaneous measurement of pulmonary artery occlusion pressure (PAOP) and pacing is usually not possible. Balloon inflation can cause repositioning of the pacing electrode with catheter movement; measurement of the PAOP may cause pacing to become intermittent.[8]
- Temporary epicardial pacing
  - ❖ Temporary epicardial pacing is a method of stimulating the myocardium through the use of polytetrafluoroethylene (PTFE)-coated, unipolar or bipolar stainless steel wires that are sutured loosely to the epicardium after cardiac surgery (Fig. 54-3).

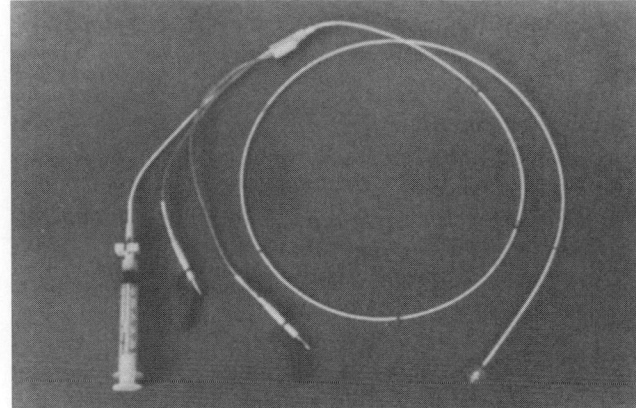

FIGURE 54-1   Balloon-tipped bipolar lead wire for transvenous pacing.

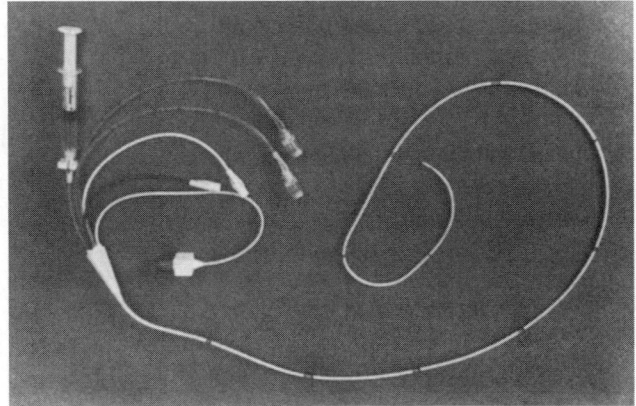

FIGURE 54-2   Pulmonary artery catheter with atrial and ventricular pacing lumens.

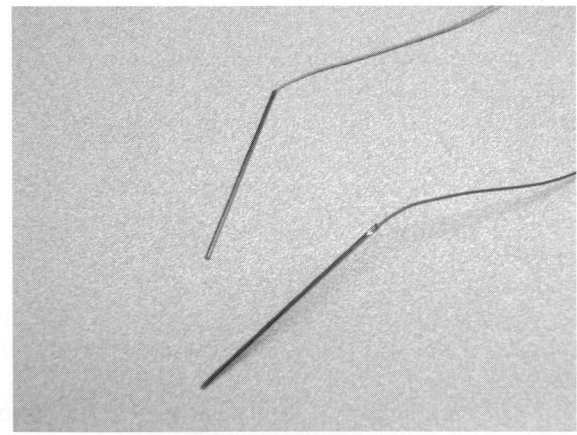

FIGURE 54-3   Epicardial wires.

- ❖ The epicardial wires may be attached to the right atrium for atrial pacing, the right ventricle for ventricular pacing, or both for AV pacing.
- ❖ Each pacing wire is brought through the chest wall before the chest is closed.

❖ Typically, the atrial wires are located on the right of the sternum, and the ventricular wires exit to the left of the sternum (Fig. 54-4)

❖ An external temporary pulse generator (Figs. 54-5 and 54-6) is connected to the epicardial pacing wires via a bridging or connecting cable (Figs. 54-7).

• Basic principles of cardiac pacing include sensing, pacing, and capture.

• Sensing refers to the ability of the pacemaker device to detect intrinsic myocardial electrical activity. Sensing occurs if the pulse generator is in the synchronous or demand mode. The pacemaker either is inhibited from delivering a stimulus or initiates an electrical impulse.

• Pacing occurs when the temporary pulse generator is activated and the requisite level of energy travels from the pulse generator through the temporary wires to the myocardium, which is known as pacemaker firing and is represented as a line or spike on the electrocardiogram (ECG) recording.

• Capture refers to the successful stimulation of the myocardium by the pacemaker, resulting in depolarization.

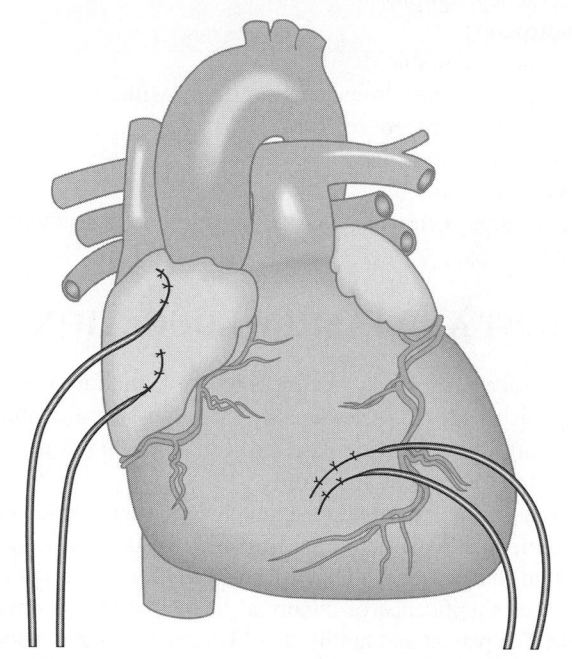

Two atrial wires   Two ventricular wires

FIGURE 54-4   Location of atrial and ventricular epicardial lead wires.

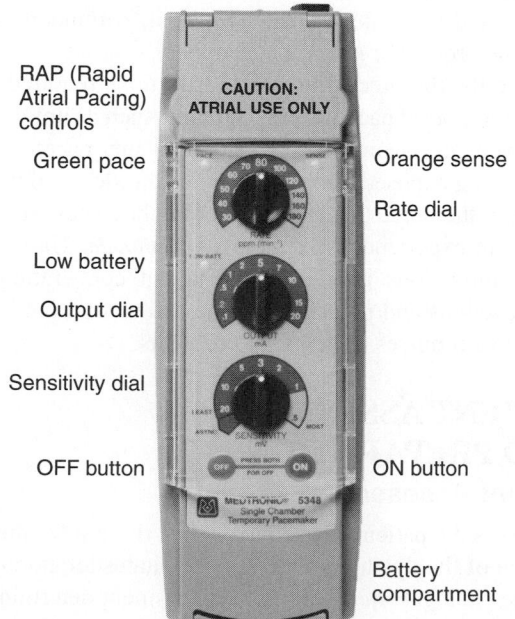

RAP (Rapid Atrial Pacing) controls

CAUTION: ATRIAL USE ONLY

Green pace

Orange sense

Rate dial

Low battery

Output dial

Sensitivity dial

OFF button

ON button

Battery compartment

FIGURE 54-5   Single-chamber temporary pulse generator. *(Courtesy Medtronic USA, Inc., Minneapolis, MN)*

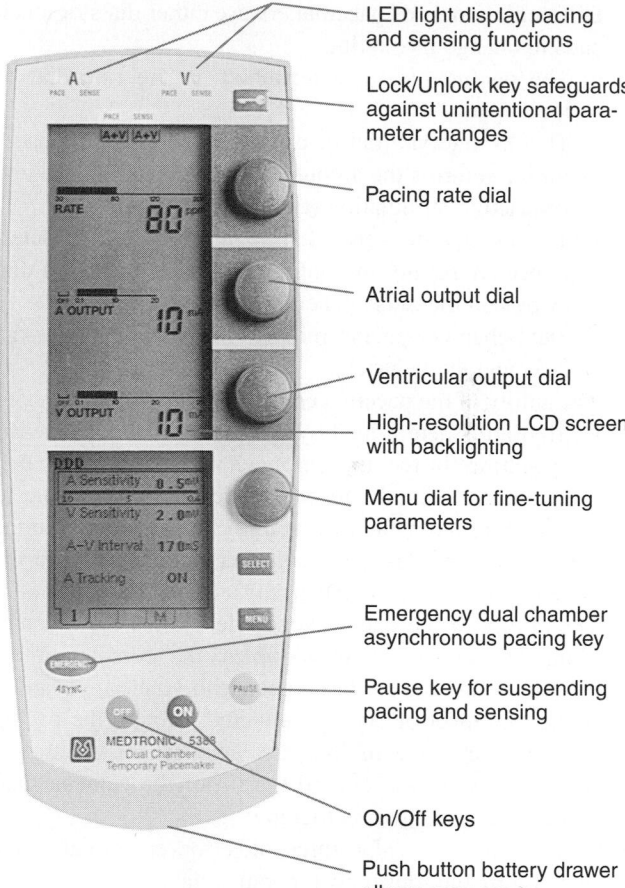

LED light display pacing and sensing functions

Lock/Unlock key safeguards against unintentional parameter changes

Pacing rate dial

Atrial output dial

Ventricular output dial

High-resolution LCD screen with backlighting

Menu dial for fine-tuning parameters

Emergency dual chamber asynchronous pacing key

Pause key for suspending pacing and sensing

On/Off keys

Push button battery drawer allows easy access

FIGURE 54-6   Dual-chamber temporary pulse generator. *LED-light-emitting diode; LCD-liquid crystal display, (Courtesy Medtronic USA, Inc., Minneapolis, MN).*

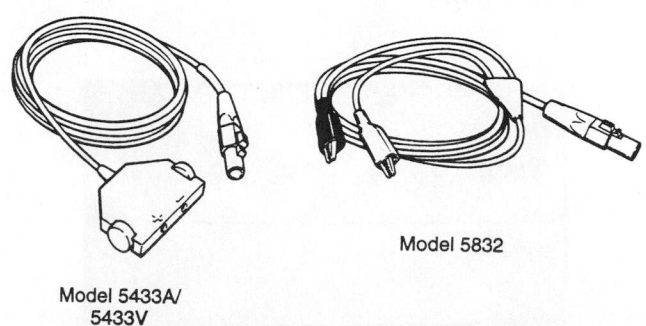

Model 5433A/ 5433V

Model 5832

FIGURE 54-7   Connecting cables. *(Courtesy Medtronic USA, Inc., Minneapolis, MN)*

Capture is evidenced on the ECG as an atrial or ventricular complex following the pacemaker spike, depending on the chamber being paced.

- Temporary pulse generator:
  - ❖ The temporary pulse generator houses the controls and energy source for pacing.
  - ❖ Some pulse generators can be used for single-chamber pacing and have one set of terminals at the top of the pulse generator into which the pacing wires are inserted (via connecting cable; see Fig. 54-5).
- A dual-chamber pacemaker requires two sets of terminals for the atrial and ventricular wires (see Figs. 54-6 and 54-8).
- Different models of pacemakers use either dials or touch pads to change the settings.
  - ❖ The pacing rate is determined by the rate dial or touch pad.
  - ❖ The AV interval dial or pad on a dual-chamber pacemaker controls the amount of time between atrial and ventricular stimulation (electronic PR interval).
  - ❖ The energy delivered to the myocardium is determined by setting the output (milliampere [mA]) dial or pad on the pulse generator.
  - ❖ Dual-chamber pacing requires that mA be set for the atria and the ventricle.
- The ability of the pacemaker to detect the patient's intrinsic rhythm is determined by the pacing mode and sensitivity setting. In the asynchronous mode, the pacemaker functions as a fixed-rate pacemaker and is not able to sense any of the patient's inherent cardiac activity. In the synchronous mode, the pacemaker is able to sense the patient's inherent cardiac activity.
- The ability of the pacemaker to depolarize the myocardium depends on many variables: the position of the electrodes and degree of contact with viable myocardial tissue; the level of energy delivered through the pacing wire; the presence of hypoxia, acidosis, or electrolyte imbalances; fibrosis around the tip of the catheter; and concomitant medication therapy.[8,10]
- Atrial and ventricular thresholds for epicardial wires increase by the fourth postoperative day.[3]

EQUIPMENT

- Antiseptic solution (e.g., 2% chlorhexidine-based preparation)
- Nonsterile gloves

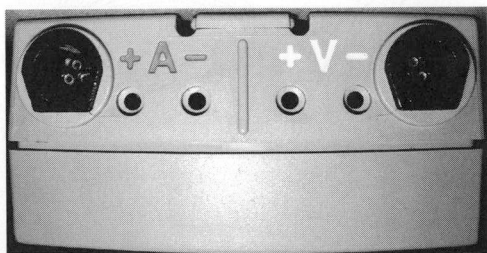

FIGURE 54-8　Pulse generator terminals to connect cables from atrial and ventricular leads.

- Pacing lead wires
- Pulse generator
- 9-V battery for pulse generator
- Connecting cables
- ECG monitoring equipment
- Dressing supplies
  Additional equipment to have available includes:
- Central venous catheter insertion supplies (see Procedure 81)
- Alligator clips or wire with connector pins
- Suture, needles, syringes
- Emergency equipment
- Fluoroscopy
- Lead aprons or shields
- Multiple-pressure transducer system, with use of PA catheter (see Procedure 76)
- 12-lead ECG machine
- Local anesthetic
- Sterile drapes, towels, masks, goggles or face shields, gowns, caps

PATIENT AND FAMILY EDUCATION

- Assess learning needs, readiness to learn, and factors that influence learning. ➤➤*Rationale:* This assessment enables teaching to be individualized in a manner that is meaningful to the patient and family.
- Discuss basic information about the normal conduction system, such as structure and function of the conduction system, normal and abnormal heart rhythms, and symptoms or significance of abnormal heart rhythms. ➤➤*Rationale:* The patient and family should understand the conduction system and why the procedure is necessary.
- Provide a basic description of the temporary pacemaker insertion procedure. ➤➤*Rationale:* The patient and family should be informed of the invasive nature of the procedure and any risks associated with it. An understanding of the procedure may reduce anxiety.
- Describe the precautions and restrictions required while the temporary pacemaker is in place, such as limitation of movement, avoidance of handling the pacemaker or touching exposed portions of the electrodes, and when to notify the nurse (e.g., if the dressing becomes wet, if the patient experiences dizziness). ➤➤*Rationale:* Understanding limitations may improve patient cooperation with restrictions and precautions. The patient and family also will alert nurses to potential problems.

PATIENT ASSESSMENT AND PREPARATION

Patient Assessment

- Assess the patient's baseline cardiac rhythm for the presence of the dysrhythmia that necessitates temporary cardiac pacing. ➤➤*Rationale:* This assessment determines the need for invasive cardiac pacing.
- Assess the patient's hemodynamic response to the dysrhythmia. Rhythm disturbances may reduce cardiac output

significantly with detrimental effects on perfusion to vital organs. ➡*Rationale:* This assessment determines the urgency of the procedure. It may indicate the need for temporizing measures, such as vasopressors or transcutaneous pacing.

- Review the patient's current medications. ➡*Rationale:* Medications may be a cause of the dysrhythmia that led to the need for pacemaker therapy, or medications may need to be held because of concomitant effect. Other medications, such as antidysrhythmics, may alter the pacing threshold.
- Review the patient's current laboratory study results, including chemistry or electrolyte profile, arterial blood gases, or cardioactive medication levels. ➡*Rationale:* This review assists in determining whether the need for pacing was precipitated by metabolic disturbances or medication toxicity and establishes the pacing milieu.

Patient Preparation

- Verify correct patient using two identifiers. ➡*Rationale:* Prior to performing a procedure, the nurse should ensure the correct identification of the patient for the intended intervention.
- Ensure that the patient and family understand preprocedural teaching. Answer questions as they arise, and reinforce information as needed. ➡*Rationale:* This communication evaluates and reinforces understanding of previously taught information.
- Confirm that informed consent has been obtained. ➡*Rationale:* Informed consent protects the rights of the patient and makes a competent decision possible for the patient; however, in emergency circumstances, time may not allow the consent form to be signed.
- Perform a pre-procedure verification and time out, if nonemergent. ➡*Rationale:* Ensures patient safety.

Procedure | for Temporary Transvenous and Epicardial Pacing

Steps	Rationale	Special Considerations
Initiating Temporary Pacing		
1. **HH**		
2. **PE**		
3. Connect the patient to the bedside monitoring system and monitor the ECG continuously (see Procedure 57).	Monitors the patient's intrinsic rhythm and the patient's rhythm during and after the procedure to evaluate for adequate pacemaker function.	Skin preparations may be needed to remove oils to improve impulse transmission.[2]
4. Assess pacemaker functioning and insert a new battery into the pulse generator if needed (Fig. 54-9).	Ensures a functional pacemaker pulse generator.	Different ways to assess battery function depend on the model and manufacturer; check manufacturer recommendations for specific instructions.
5. Attach the connecting cable to the pulse generator, connecting the "positive" on the cable to the "positive" on the pulse generator and the "negative" on the cable to the "negative" on the pulse generator.	Prepares the pacing system; the pacing stimulus travels from the pulse generator to the negative terminal, and energy returns to the pulse generator via the positive terminal.	Some lead wires are labeled distal and proximal; distal connects to negative, and proximal connects to positive. Some lead wires may not have negative and positive marked on them. Polarity is established when the wires are placed in the connecting cable. Two connecting cables are needed with both atrial and ventricular pacing.

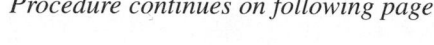

Procedure continues on following page

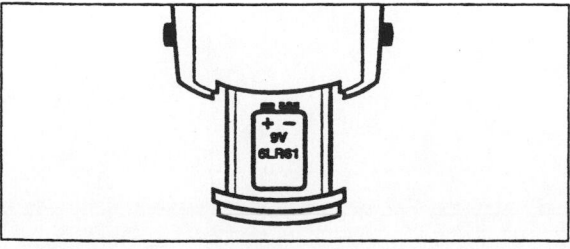

FIGURE 54-9 Placement of the new battery. Insert the new battery, close the compartment, and press the "on" button. (*Courtesy Medtronic USA, Inc., Minneapolis, MN*)

Procedure **for Temporary Transvenous and Epicardial Pacing**—*Continued*		
Steps	Rationale	Special Considerations

Assisting with Initiation of Temporary Transvenous Pacing

Steps	Rationale	Special Considerations
1. Follow **Steps 1 through 5** in Initiating Temporary Pacing.		
2. If a central venous catheter is not in place, assist as needed with catheter insertion (see Procedure 82).	A central line is needed for transvenous pacing.	
3. Assist as needed with insertion of the transvenous pacing lead wire.	Provides needed assistance.	
4. All personnel performing and assisting with the procedure should apply personal protective and sterile equipment (e.g., masks, head covers, goggles or face shields, sterile gowns, and sterile gloves).[7]	Minimizes the risk of infection, maintains sterility, and maintains standard and sterile precautions.	
5. Assist as needed with cleansing the insertion site with antiseptic solution (e.g., 2% chlorhexidine-based preparation).	Minimizes the risk of infection.	Gloves should be worn whenever handling the pacing electrodes to prevent microshock.[9-11]
6. Assist as needed with draping the insertion site.	Provides a sterile field and reduces the transmission of microorganisms.	
7. Assist as needed as the pacing lead is passed through the introducer.	Facilitates the insertion process.	If a balloon-tipped pacing lead is used, balloon inflation occurs when the tip of the pacing lead is in the vena cava. The air-filled balloon allows the blood flow to carry the catheter tip into the desired position in the right ventricle.
8. Assist with verifying the position of the transvenous pacing lead wire:	For transvenous, ventricular pacing, the negative pacing electrode is positioned in the endocardium (at the apex) of the right ventricle.	
A. Ultrasound scan.	Ultrasound may assist with insertion of the pacing electrode.	The pacing catheter may be inserted with transcutaneous ultrasound scan.
B. Fluoroscopy.	Fluoroscopy allows direct visualization of the pacing electrode.	If fluoroscopy is used, all personnel must be shielded from the radiation with lead aprons or be positioned behind lead shields.
C. Chest radiography.		

Procedure for Temporary Transvenous and Epicardial Pacing—*Continued*

Steps	Rationale	Special Considerations

D. Bedside monitoring system or 12-lead ECG machine.
  1. Connect the patient to the limb leads.
  2. Attach the V lead of the ECG monitoring system or the 12 lead ECG machine to the negative electrode connector pin (distal pin) of the pacing lead wire (an alligator clip or wire with connector pins may be needed). (see Fig. 53-2).
  3. Set the monitoring system to record the V lead continuously.
  4. Observe the ECG for ST-segment elevation in the V lead recording (see Fig. 53-3).
  5. Observe for left bundle-branch block pattern and left axis deviation that usually can be identified.
	The ECG is derived directly from the pacing electrode, and the position of the catheter tip is verified by the internal electrical recording, which shows ST-segment elevation when in contact with the myocardium.
	
	As a result of the temporary pacing catheter transmission of impulses from within the right ventricle, conduction of the impulse throughout the ventricles occurs via cellular conduction of the impulse rather than transmission down the bundle branches.	

9. After the pacing lead wire is properly positioned, connect the external electrode pins to the pulse generator via the connecting cables. Ensure that the positive and negative electrode connector pins are connected to the respective positive and negative terminals on the pulse generator (see Fig. 54-8) via the connecting cables (Fig. 54-10).	Energy from the pulse generator is directed to the negative electrode in contact with the ventricle. The pacing circuit is completed as energy reaches the positive electrode. The lead wires must be connected securely to the pacemaker to ensure appropriate sensing and capture and to prevent inadvertent disconnection.	A connecting cable is recommended for use between the pacing wires and the pulse generator. Some lead wires are labeled distal and proximal; distal connects to negative, and proximal connects to positive. Some lead wires may not have negative and positive marked on them. Polarity is established when the wires are placed in the connecting cable. Ensure all connections are secure.

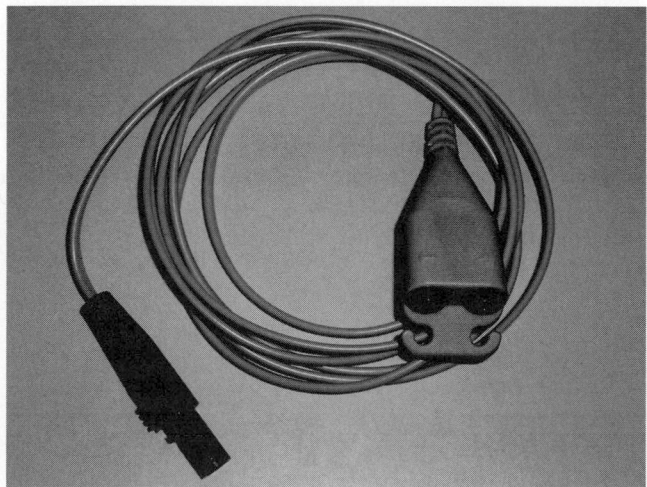

FIGURE 54-10 Transvenous cable that connects to transvenous pacemaker leads with shrouded pins. *(Courtesy Medtronic USA, Inc., Minneapolis, MN.)*

Procedure continues on following page

Procedure | for Temporary Transvenous and Epicardial Pacing—*Continued*

Steps	Rationale	Special Considerations
10. For AV demand pacing, when an atrial lead is placed in addition to a ventricular lead, connect the atrial electrodes to the atrial terminals and the ventricular electrodes to the ventricular terminals. Attach the connecting cable(s) to the pulse generator for each chamber that is being paced (atrium or ventricle) (see Fig. 54-8)	Ensures that the atrial electrodes and ventricular electrodes are connected correctly to the pulse generator. Secure connections are essential for proper sensing and conduction of pacemaker energy. The pacing stimulus travels from the pulse generator to the negative terminal, and energy returns to the pulse generator via the positive terminal.	Some pacemaker models require that the positive on the connecting cable is connected to the positive on the pulse generator and that the negative on the connecting cable is connected to the negative on the pulse generator. Transvenous temporary atrial leads may be placed short term for procedures and then removed.

Assisting With Initiating Temporary Pacing via a Pulmonary Artery Catheter

Steps	Rationale	Special Considerations
1. Follow **Steps 1 through 5** in Initiating Temporary Pacing.	Prepares equipment.	
2. Assist the physician or advanced practice nurse with insertion of the PA catheter (see Procedure 73).	Provides assistance as needed.	Pacing electrodes may be inserted at the time of PA catheter insertion, or they may be inserted at a later time, when temporary pacing is needed because of a change in patient condition.
3. Obtain the appropriate pacing lead for insertion.	Only probes specifically manufactured for use with the PA catheter should be used; check specific manufacturer's recommendations.	Continuous monitoring of the right ventricular pressure waveform via the pacing lumen is recommended before insertion of the electrode to ensure correct placement of the right ventricular port 1 to 2 cm distal to the tricuspid valve.
4. Assist the physician or advanced practice nurse with insertion of the pacing lead wire.	Close monitoring of the ECG during insertion of the pacing lead is necessary to detect dysrhythmias.	Follow specific manufacturer's instructions regarding pacing lead insertion and securing the pacing lead in place within the catheter lumen.
5. After the electrodes are properly positioned, connect the positive and negative electrode connector pins to the pulse generator via the connecting cable. Ensure that the positive and negative electrodes are connected to the respective positive and negative terminals on the pulse generator via the connecting cable.	Energy from the pulse generator is directed to the negative electrode. The pacing circuit is completed as energy reaches the positive electrode. The electrodes must be connected securely to the pulse generator to ensure appropriate sensing and capture and to prevent inadvertent disconnection.	Gloves should be worn whenever handling the pacing electrodes to prevent microshock.[9-11]
6. Check institutional policy or obtain specific physician prescription regarding not wedging the PA catheter.	Intermittent capture has been noted during the wedging procedure as a result of movement of the electrode with catheter migration into the wedge position.[5]	Usually, the PA catheter is not wedged during pacing therapy.[5]

Epicardial Pacing

Steps	Rationale	Special Considerations
1. Follow **Steps 1 through 5** in Initiating Temporary Pacing.		
2. Apply nonsterile gloves.	Gloves should be worn whenever handling the epicardial wires to prevent microshock.[9-11]	

Procedure for Temporary Transvenous and Epicardial Pacing—*Continued*

Steps	Rationale	Special Considerations
3. Expose the epicardial pacing wires, and identify the chamber of origin. Epicardial wires that exit to the right of the sternum are atrial in origin. Epicardial wires that exit to the left of the sternum are ventricular in origin (see Fig. 54-3).	Identifies the correct chamber for pacing.	
4. Connect the epicardial wires to the pulse generator via the connecting cable. Ensure that the positive and negative electrodes are connected to the respective positive and negative terminals on the pulse generator via the connecting cable.	The epicardial wires must be connected securely to the pulse generator to ensure appropriate sensing and capture and to prevent inadvertent disconnection. Use of a unipolar or bipolar configuration needs to be established; this depends on where the epicardial wires are located. In a unipolar pacing system, only one electrode is in contact with the chamber being paced (the negative electrode). The positive, or indifferent (ground), electrode may be an ECG electrode patch, may be an epicardial wire sewn to the subcutaneous tissue of the chest wall, or may be a subcutaneous needle inserted into the chest wall. With bipolar pacing, both electrodes are in direct contact with the myocardial tissue of the chamber being paced.	The epicardial wire connected to the negative terminal determines where the energy is delivered. The wire connected to the positive terminal determines how the energy returns to the pulse generator. With AV demand pacing, both atrial epicardial wires are connected to the atrium (via cable) and the ventricular epicardial wires are connected to the terminal labeled ventricle (via cable). With bipolar pacing, either wire can be the negative electrode.[4] With unipolar pacing (one electrode in contact with the heart), the epicardial wire must be the negative electrode, and the ECG patch, skin wire, or subcutaneous needle is the positive electrode.

All Methods of Temporary Pacing

Steps	Rationale	Special Considerations
1. Determine the mode of pacing desired.	The pacing mode chosen should be the one that best achieves the goal of pacing therapy. Possibilities include atrial, ventricular, or AV asynchronous (fixed rate) pacing or atrial, ventricular, or AV synchronous (demand) pacing.	Asynchronous pacing in the presence of an intrinsic rhythm may result in R-on-T phenomenon, leading to a lethal dysrhythmia, and should be used only in the absence of an intrinsic rhythm.[5,6,8]
2. Set the pacemaker mode, pacemaker rate, and level of energy (output or mA) as prescribed or as determined by sensitivity and stimulation threshold testing (see subsequent **Steps 3, 4, and 5**).	Prepares pacemaker equipment.	Follow institution standard regarding whether critical care nurses can set the pacemaker mode and energy level and test the sensitivity and stimulation threshold levels. The demand or the synchronous mode is recommended to avoid competition between the pacemaker-initiated beats and the patient's intrinsic rhythm. Output is set to ensure capture of the myocardium. In AV demand pacing, separate output settings are used to ensure capture of the atrium and the ventricle.

Procedure continues on following page

Procedure	for Temporary Transvenous and Epicardial Pacing—*Continued*	
Steps	**Rationale**	**Special Considerations**
3. Depending on the pulse generator, turn all settings to the lowest level, then turn on the pulse generator. **(Level M*)**	Prepares the equipment.	Follow manufacturer's recommendations. Settings cannot be adjusted on some pulse generators until after the pulse generator is turned on. Additional pulse generators turn on at default settings, after a self-test, and the settings can be adjusted at that time.
4. Determine the sensitivity threshold (for each chamber as appropriate). Set the rate for 10 beats/min below the patient's intrinsic rate.[1,6,11] **(Level M)**	Sensitivity threshold is the level at which intrinsic myocardial activity is recognized by the sensing electrodes. Setting the pacemaker rate lower than the intrinsic rate avoids competition between the pacemaker and the patient's intrinsic rhythm. For demand pacing, the sensitivity must be measured and set.	This step is omitted if the patient has no intrinsic rhythm. In determination of sensitivity threshold, the mA should be turned to the lowest level to avoid the possibility of a pacemaker stimulus falling on the T wave (R-on-T phenomenon) and inducing a potentially lethal dysrhythmia.[4] After the sensitivity threshold is determined, some physicians and advanced practice nurses prefer to set sensitivity settings all the way to the demand mode (most sensitive), regardless of the sensitivity threshold. Follow institution standard. If the sensitivity is set to the most sensitive, the pacemaker may be inappropriately inhibited because it may detect and interpret extra-myocardial activity (e.g., muscle movement, artifact) as actual myocardial activity.
A. Gradually turn the sensitivity dial counterclockwise (or to a higher numeric setting) and observe the sense indicator light for flashing. The sense indicator light stops flashing when the device is unable to sense the patient's intrinsic rhythm.		
B. Slowly turn the sensitivity dial clockwise (or to a lower numeric setting) until the sense indicator light flashes with each complex and the pace indicator light stops. This value is the sensing threshold.		
C. Set the sensitivity dial to the number that was half the sensing threshold to provide a 2:1 safety margin.[1,6,11]		
5. Determine the stimulation threshold (for each chamber as necessary).[1,6,11]	The output dial regulates the amount of electrical current (mA) that is delivered to the myocardium to initiate depolarization. The output (mA) is set at least two times above the stimulation threshold to allow for increases in the stimulation threshold without loss of capture.[1,6,11]	This step should be performed by a physician or advanced practice nurse in a patient who is pacemaker-dependent for bradydysrhythmia. Individual institutional policies govern when threshold determination should be done and whether a nurse may test the stimulation threshold; thresholds may not be determined if sensitivity is poor or if the patient's inherent heart rate is greater than 90 beats/min. Threshold may increase or decrease within hours of electrode placement as a result of fibrosis at the tip of the catheter, medication administration (e.g., some antidysrhythmics), alteration of position, or underlying pathology.[1,4,6,8]

*Level M: Manufacturer's recommendations only

Procedure	for Temporary Transvenous and Epicardial Pacing—*Continued*	
Steps	**Rationale**	**Special Considerations**
		In the case of dual-chamber pacing, the threshold for each chamber is assessed. Pacing rates vary depending on the indication for pacing.
A. Set the pacing rate approximately 10 beats/min above the patient's intrinsic rate. B. Gradually decrease the output from 20 mA until capture is lost. C. Gradually increase the mA until 1:1 capture is established. This is the stimulation threshold. The pace light will be flashing. D. Set the mA at least two times higher than the stimulation threshold.[1,6,11] This output setting is sometimes referred to as the maintenance threshold. 6. Set the prescribed pacemaker rate. 7. Assess the cardiac rate and rhythm for appropriate pacemaker function: A. Capture: Is there a QRS complex for every ventricular pacing stimulus? Is there also a P wave for every atrial pacing stimulus (Fig. 54-11)? B. Rate: Is the rate at or above the pacemaker rate if in the demand mode? C. Sensing: Does the sense light indicate that every QRS complex is sensed?	Ensures adequate cardiac output. The ECG tracing should reflect appropriate response to the pacemaker settings if functioning properly. Sometimes atrial activity may not be visible because of low-voltage amplitude. If the patient is solely paced via atrial pacing, ventricular tracking and response should follow the atrial rate setting.	

Procedure continues on following page

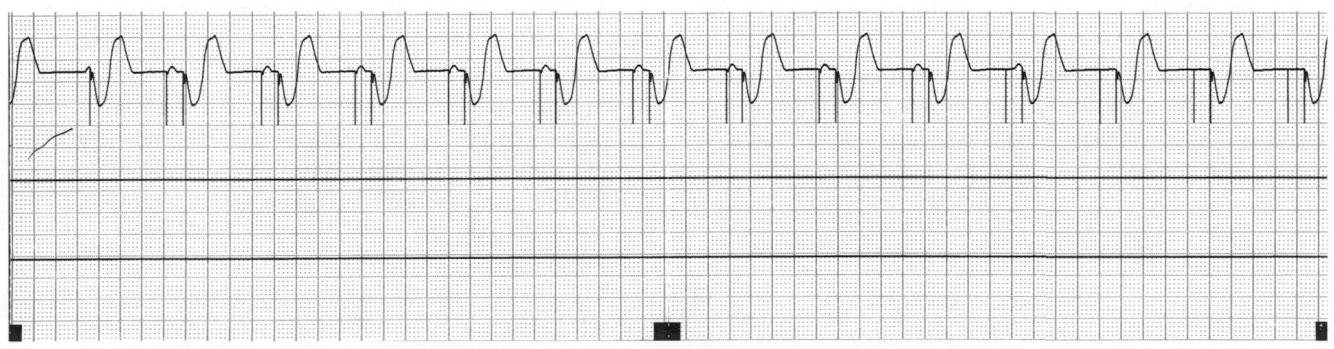

FIGURE 54-11 Pacemaker ECG strip of atrioventricular pacing. Note the atrial pacing spike before each P wave and the ventricular pacing spike before each QRS complex.

Procedure   for Temporary Transvenous and Epicardial Pacing—*Continued*

Steps	Rationale	Special Considerations
8. After the settings are adjusted for optimal patient response, place the protective plastic cover over the pacemaker controls, or place the controls in the locked position.	Pacemaker settings may be inadvertently altered by patient movement or handling if the controls are not covered or locked.	The patient may need to be reminded not to touch the pulse generator.
9. Assess patient response to pacing, including blood pressure, level of consciousness, heart rhythm, and other hemodynamic parameters.	Pacemaker settings are determined by patient response.	
10. Apply a sterile occlusive dressing over the insertion site.	Prevents infection.	The epicardial electrodes and the insertion sites may be covered with a 4 × 4-inch dressing and taped to the chest.[4,11] The wires may be placed over the dressing and covered with gauze.
11. Secure the necessary equipment to provide some stability for the pacemaker, such as hanging the pulse generator on an intravenous pole, strapping the pulse generator to the patient's torso, hanging the pulse generator around the patient's neck, or securing the pulse generator under a draw sheet.	The pulse generator should be protected from falling or becoming inadvertently detached by patient movement.	Exposed wires should be secured in an insulated material (e.g., finger cots, glove, plastic cap).[9-11]
12. Discard used supplies in appropriate receptacles.	Reduces the transmission of microorganisms; Standard Precautions.	
13. 🅷🅷		
14. Obtain a chest radiograph as prescribed.	In the absence of fluoroscopy, a radiograph is essential to detect potential complications associated with insertion and to visualize lead position.	Not necessary for epicardial pacing.
15. Selectively restrict patient mobility depending on the insertion site.	Prevents electrode dislodgment.	Follow institution policy regarding ambulation for the patient with a temporary pacemaker.

Expected Outcomes

- Paced rhythm on ECG consistent with parameters set on the pacemaker, as evidenced by appropriate heart rate, sensing, and capture
- Patient exhibits hemodynamic stability, as evidenced by a systolic blood pressure greater than 90 mm Hg, a mean arterial blood pressure greater than 60 mm Hg, baseline mental status, and no syncope or ischemia
- Epicardial pacemaker wires are securely connected to the pulse generator

Unexpected Outcomes

- Failure of the pacemaker to sense, causing competition between the pacemaker-initiated impulses and the patient's intrinsic cardiac rhythm
- Failure of the pacemaker to capture the myocardium
- Pacemaker oversensing that causes the pacemaker to be inappropriately inhibited
- Stimulation of the diaphragm that causes hiccupping may be related to pacing the phrenic nerve, perforation, wire dislodgment, or an excessively high pacemaker mA setting
- Phlebitis, thrombosis, embolism, or bacteremia
- Ventricular dysrhythmias
- Pneumothorax or hemothorax
- Myocardial perforation and cardiac tamponade
- Air embolism
- Lead dislodgment
- Pacemaker syndrome as a result of loss of AV synchrony
- Continual hiccups (may indicate wire perforation)
- Pain

Patient Monitoring and Care

Steps	Rationale	Reportable Conditions
		These conditions should be reported if they persist despite nursing interventions.
1. Monitor vital signs and hemodynamic response to pacing following institution standard and as often as the patient condition warrants.	The goal of cardiac pacing is to improve cardiac output by increasing heart rate or by overriding life-threatening dysrhythmias.	• Abnormal vital signs associated with signs and symptoms of hemodynamic deterioration
2. Evaluate the ECG for the presence of the paced rhythm or resolution of the initiating dysrhythmia.	Proper pacemaker functioning is assessed by observing the ECG for pacemaker activity consistent with the parameters set.	• Inability to obtain a paced rhythm (loss of capture or failure to capture) • Oversensing • Undersensing
3. Follow institution standard for assessing pain. Administer analgesia as prescribed.	Identifies need for pain interventions.	• Continued pain despite pain interventions • Continual hiccups
4. Check and document sensitivity and stimulation threshold according to institution standard (e.g., usually at least every 24 hours).[8,9] Threshold may be checked by physicians in patients at high risk (e.g., if pacemaker dependent).	Ensures proper pacemaker functioning and prevents high levels of energy delivery to the myocardium. Threshold may be checked more frequently if the patient's condition changes or pacemaker function is questioned.	• Problems with sensitivity or threshold

5. Change the dressing as determined by institutional policy, depending on the type of dressing used.
  A. Cleanse the pacemaker lead site(s) with antiseptic solution (e.g., 2% chlorhexidine-based preparation).
  B. Apply dry sterile dressing and tape.
  C. Record date of dressing change.
	Decreases the potential for infection. Although guidelines do not exist specific to pacing wires, the Centers for Disease Control and Prevention (CDC) recommends replacing dressings on intravascular catheters when the dressing becomes damp, loosened, or soiled or when inspection of the site is necessary.[7]	• Increased temperature
		• Increased white blood cell count
		• Drainage at the insertion site
		• Warmth or pain at the insertion site

6. Monitor for other complications.	Early recognition leads to prompt treatment.	• Embolus • Thrombosis • Perforation of the myocardium • Pneumothorax • Hemothorax • Phlebitis
7. Monitor electrolyte levels as prescribed.	Electrolyte imbalances may precipitate dysrhythmias.	• Abnormal electrolyte values
8. Ensure that all connections are secure and low battery indicator is not present.	Maintenance of tight connections is necessary to ensure proper pacemaker functioning. Battery life varies with the amount of pacing energy needed.	• Inability to maintain tight connections with available equipment, jeopardizing pacing therapy
9. If the pulse generator is no longer needed for a patient with epicardial pacing wires, isolate and contain the tips to avoid microshocks.[9-11]	Microshocks can lead to lethal dysrhythmias. Epicardial wires are often left in place after pacing is no longer needed (generator is disconnected).	• Microshocks

Procedure continues on following page

Documentation

Documentation should include the following:
- Patient and family education
- Signed informed consent form
- Universal Protocol requirements
- Date and time of initiation of pacing
- Description of events that warranted intervention
- Vital signs and hemodynamic parameters before, during, and after the procedure
- ECG monitoring strip recording before and after pacemaker insertion
- Type of pacemaker wire inserted and location

- Pacemaker settings: mode, rate, output, sensitivity setting, threshold measurements, and whether the pacemaker is on or off
- Patient response to the procedure
- Complications and interventions
- Medications administered and patient response to the medication
- Pain assessment, interventions, and patient response to medication
- Date and time pacing was discontinued
- Adjustment to monitoring system settings to ensure detection of paced rhythms

References

1. Abate E, Kusumoto FM, Goldschlager NF: Techniques for temporary pacing. In Kusumoto FM, Goldschlager NF, editors: *Cardiac pacing for the clinician,* ed 2, New York, 2007, Springer-Verlag.
CR 2. Drew B: Practice standards for electrocardiographic monitoring in hospital settings: an American Heart Association scientific statement from the Councils on Cardiovascular Nursing, Clinical Cardiology, and Cardiovascular Disease in the Young: endorsed by the International Society of Computerized Electrocardiology and the American Association of Critical-Care Nurses, *Circulation* 110: 2721-2746, 2004.
CR 3. Elmi F, Tullo NG, Khalighi K: Natural history and predictors of temporary epicardial pacemaker wire function in patients after open heart surgery, *Cardiology* 98:175-180, 2002.
CR 4. Finkelmeier BA: *Temporary pacing and defibrillation in cardiothoracic surgical nursing,* Philadelphia, 2000, Lippincott.
CR 5. Gammage MD: Temporary cardiac pacing, *Heart* 83: 715-720, 2000.
6. Medtronic Corp: *Model 5388 dual chamber temporary pacemaker technical manual,* Minneapolis, 2007, Medtronic.
CR 7. O'Grady NP, et al: Guidelines for the prevention of intravascular catheter-related infections, *Am J Infect Control* 30:476-489, 2002.
8. Overbay D, Criddle L: Mastering temporary invasive cardiac pacing, *Crit Care Nurse* 24(3):25-32, 2004.
CR 9. Reade MC: Temporary epicardial pacing after cardiac surgery: a practical review: part 1: general considerations in the management of epicardial pacing, *Anaesthesia* 62:264-271, 2007.
CR 10. Timothy PR, Rodeman BJ: Temporary pacemakers in critically ill patients: assessment and management strategies, *AACN Clin Issues* 15:305-325, 2004.
CR 11. Woods SL, Froelicher ES, Adams S, et al, editors: Pacemakers and implantable defibrillators. In *Cardiac nursing,* ed 5, Philadelphia, 2005, Lippincott Williams and Wilkins.

Additional Readings

Batra AS, Balaji S: Post operative temporary epicardial pacing: when, how and why? *Ann Pediatr Card* 1(2): 120-125, 2008.
CR Conover M: Chapter 33. In *Electrical stimulation therapies in understanding electrocardiography*, ed 8, St Louis, 2003, Mosby.
CR Conover M: Chapter 34. In *Pacemaker therapies for bradyarrhythmias in understanding electrocardiography*, ed 8, St Louis, 2003, Mosby.
Hongo RH, Goldschlager NF: Cardiac pacing in the critical care setting. In Kusumoto FM, Goldschlager NF, editors: *Cardiac pacing for the clinician*, ed 2, New York, 2007, Springer-Verlag.

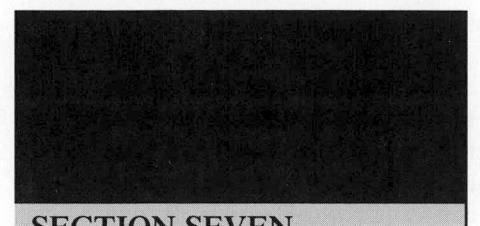

Circulatory Assist Devices

PROCEDURE **55**

Intraaortic Balloon Pump Management

P U R P O S E : Intraaortic balloon pump therapy is designed to increase coronary artery perfusion, increase systemic perfusion, decrease myocardial workload, and decrease afterload.

Deborah Castellucci

PREREQUISITE NURSING KNOWLEDGE

- Knowledge of the anatomy and physiology of the cardio-vascular system is needed.
- Understanding of the principles of hemodynamic monitoring, electrophysiology, dysrhythmias, and coagulation is necessary.
- Clinical and technical competence related to the use of the intra-aortic balloon pump (IABP) is needed.
- Advanced cardiac life support knowledge and skills are necessary.
- Indications for IABP therapy are as follows:
  - ❖ Cardiogenic shock
  - ❖ Refractory unstable angina
  - ❖ Acute myocardial infarction (MI) complicated by left ventricular failure[3,12,26,28]
  - ❖ Refractory unstable angina
  - ❖ Recurrent ventricular dysrhythmias as a result of ischemia[16]
  - ❖ Support before, during, and after coronary artery bypass graft surgery[2,29]
  - ❖ Support before, during, and after coronary artery angioplasty or additional interventional cardiology procedures for patients at high risk[4,11]
  - ❖ Mechanical complications of acute MI, including aortic stenosis, mitral stenosis, mitral valvuloplasty, mitral insufficiency, ventricular septal defect, and left ventricular aneurysm
  - ❖ Intractable ventricular dysrhythmias[13,18]
  - ❖ Bridge to cardiac transplantation, ventricular assist devices, or total artificial hearts

- ❖ Cardiac injury, including contusion and coronary artery tears
- ❖ Septic shock
- ❖ Patient at high risk undergoing noncardiac surgery[18,29]
- Contraindications to IABP therapy are as follows:
  - ❖ Moderate to severe aortic insufficiency
  - ❖ Thoracic and abdominal aortic aneurysms
- The relative value of IABP therapy in the presence of severe aortoiliac disease, major coagulopathies, and terminal disease should be evaluated individually.
- IABP therapy is an acute short-term therapy for patients with reversible left ventricular failure or an adjunct to other therapies for irreversible heart failure. Cardiac assistance with the IABP is performed to improve myocardial oxygen supply and reduce cardiac workload. Intra-aortic balloon (IAB) pumping is based on the principles of counterpulsation (Fig. 55-1).
- The events of the cardiac cycle provide the stimulus for balloon function, and the movement of helium gas between the balloon and the control console gas source produces inflation and deflation of the balloon.
- Recognition of the R wave or the QRS complex on the electrocardiogram (ECG) is the most commonly used trigger source.
- Inflation occurs during ventricular diastole and causes an increase in aortic pressure. This increased pressure displaces blood proximally to the coronary arteries and distally to the rest of the body. The result is an increase in myocardial oxygen supply and subsequent improvement in cardiac output.

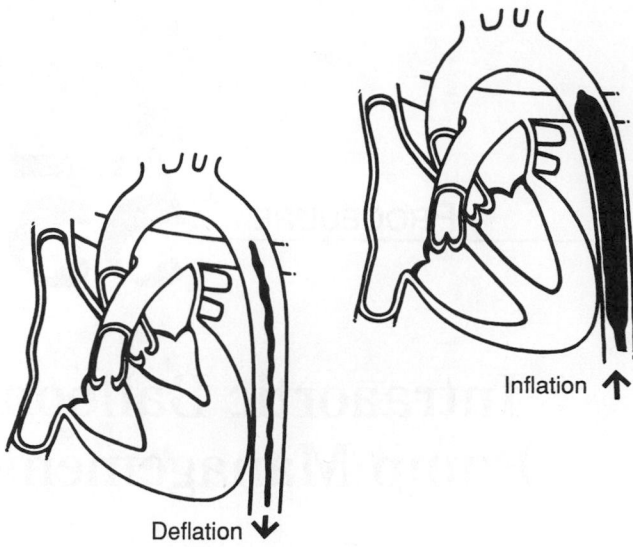

FIGURE 55-1   Counterpulsation. *(Courtesy Datascope Corp, Montvale, NJ.)*

- Deflation occurs just before ventricular systole or ejection, which decreases the pressure within the aortic root, reducing afterload and cardiac workload.
- Insertion and placement verification:
  - ❖ The IAB catheter is commonly placed in the femoral artery via percutaneous puncture or arteriotomy.
  - ❖ The IAB catheter can also be placed via a transthoracic approach.[15]
  - ❖ The IAB catheter lies approximately 2 cm inferior to the left subclavian artery and superior to the renal arteries. This position allows for maximum balloon effect without occlusion of other arterial supplies (Fig. 55-2).
  - ❖ The IAB should not fully occlude the aorta during inflation. It should be 85% to 90% occlusive.
  - ❖ Fluoroscopy may be used to aid in IAB catheter positioning, especially for patients with a tortuous aorta.
  - ❖ Correct catheter position is verified via radiography if fluoroscopy is not used during catheter insertion. The visibility of the IAB catheter tip may be enhanced when the IABP is temporarily placed on standby (follow manufacturer's guidelines).
  - ❖ The central lumen of many IAB catheters provides a means for monitoring aortic pressure.
  - ❖ Some IAB catheters use fiberoptic technology. These catheters have a fiberoptic sensor located at the tip of the IAB catheter. The sensor transmits the pressure signal to the IAB console.
- Timing methods of IABP therapy vary slightly from manufacturer to manufacturer. With the traditional or conventional method, the IAB deflates at the QRS complex, before isovolumetric contraction. The IAB also deflates at the QRS complex with the real-time method. An important principle of real timing is the duration of the balloon deflation during cardiac systole. During real timing, the IAB is timed to deflate at the onset of each QRS complex and to remain deflated throughout systole. A

constant diastolic interval is not necessary for real timing.[5,6,19,22]
- The mechanics of the IABP control console vary from manufacturer to manufacturer.
- Specific information concerning controls, alarms, troubleshooting, and safety features is available from each manufacturer and should be read thoroughly by the nurse before use of the equipment.

EQUIPMENT

- IABP, gas supply
- ECG and arterial pressure monitoring supplies
- IAB catheter (size range, 7 Fr to 10 Fr for adults; balloon catheters vary in balloon volumes, 25 to 50 mL)
- IAB catheter insertion kit
- Antiseptic solution (e.g., 2% chlorhexidine-based preparation)
- Caps, goggles or face shields, masks, sterile gowns, gloves, and drapes
- Sterile dressing supplies

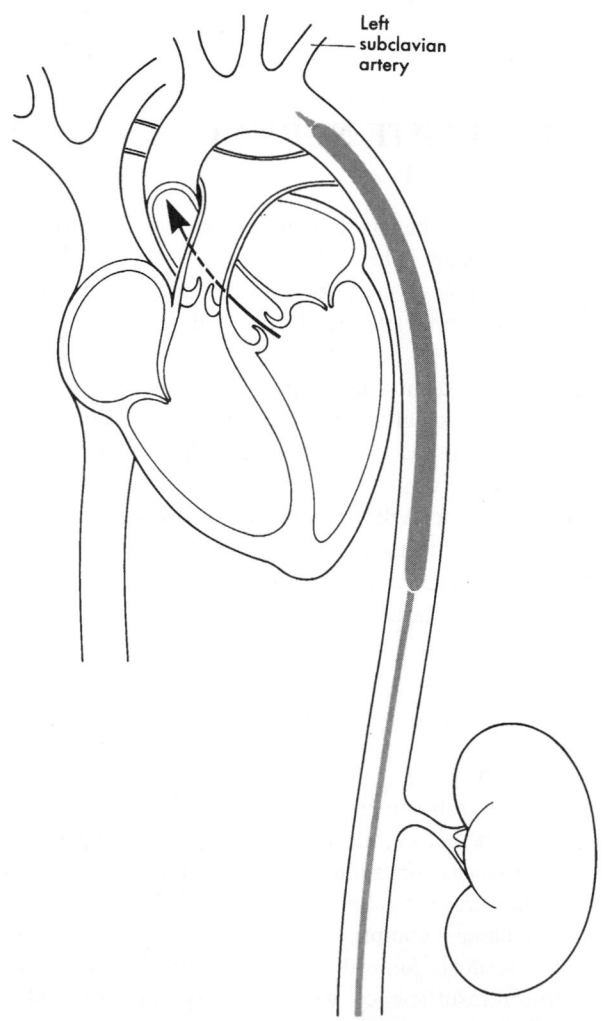

FIGURE 55-2   Intra-aortic balloon positioned in the descending thoracic aorta, just below the left subclavian artery but above the renal artery. *(From Quaal SJ: Comprehensive intraaortic balloon counterpulsation, ed 2, St Louis, 1993, Mosby.)*

- O-silk suture on a cutting needle or a sutureless securement device
- No. 11 scalpel, used for skin entry
- 1% Lidocaine without epinephrine, one 30-mL vial
- Stopcocks, one two-way and one three-way
- One Luer-Lok plug
- 500 mL of normal saline flush solution (refer to institution standards or physician prescription regarding use of a heparin flush solution)
- Single-pressure transducer system (see Procedure 76)

Additional equipment to have available depending on patient status includes the following:
- Analgesics and sedatives as prescribed
- Lead apron (needed if procedure is performed with fluoroscopy)
- Prescribed intravenous (IV) solutions
- Emergency medications and resuscitation equipment
- Vasopressors as prescribed
- Antibiotics as prescribed
- Heparin infusion or dextran if prescribed

PATIENT AND FAMILY EDUCATION

- Assess patient and family understanding of IABP therapy and the reason for its use. ➥*Rationale:* Clarification or reinforcement of information is an expressed family need during times of stress and anxiety.
- Explain the standard care to the patient and family, including the insertion procedure, IABP sounds, frequency of assessment, alarms, dressings, need for immobility of the affected extremity, expected length of therapy, and parameters for discontinuation of therapy. ➥*Rationale:* This explanation encourages the patient and family to ask questions and prepares the patient and family for what to expect.
- After catheter removal, instruct the patient to report any warm or wet feeling on the leg and any dizziness or lightheadedness. ➥*Rationale:* These feelings may be indicative of bleeding at the insertion site.

PATIENT ASSESSMENT AND PREPARATION

Patient Assessment

- Assess the patient's medical history, specifically related to competency of the aortic valve, aortic disease, or peripheral vascular disease. ➥*Rationale:* This assessment provides baseline data regarding cardiac functioning and identifies contraindications to IABP therapy.
- Assess the patient's cardiovascular, hemodynamic, peripheral vascular, and neurovascular status. ➥*Rationale:* This assessment provides baseline data.
- Assess the extremity for the intended IAB catheter placement for the quality and strength of the femoral, popliteal, dorsalis pedal, and posterior tibial pulses.[7,27]
- Assess the ankle/arm index as follows:
  ❖ Record the brachial systolic pressure with a Doppler scan signal.

- ❖ Locate the posterior tibial or dorsalis pedalis pulse with a Doppler scan signal.
- ❖ Apply the blood pressure cuff around the ankle, above the malleolus.
- ❖ Inflate the cuff to 20 mm Hg above the brachial systolic pressure.
- ❖ Note the reappearance of the Doppler scan signal as the cuff deflates.
- ❖ Divide the ankle systolic pressure by the brachial systolic pressure to determine the ankle/arm index (normal range, 0.8 to 1.2).
  ➥*Rationale:* The IAB catheter is inserted into the vasculature of the extremity that exhibits the best perfusion. Also, this assessment provides baseline data related to peripheral blood flow, which may be compromised by the IAB.
- Assess the patient's current laboratory profile, including complete blood count (CBC), platelet count, prothrombin time (PT), partial thromboplastin time (PTT), bleeding time, and international normalized ratio (INR). ➥*Rationale:* Provides baseline data. Baseline coagulation studies are helpful in determining the risk for bleeding. Platelet function may be affected by the mechanical trauma from balloon inflation and deflation.
- Assess for signs and symptoms of cardiac failure that necessitate IABP therapy, including the following:
  ❖ Unstable angina[4]
  ❖ Altered mental status
  ❖ Heart rate greater than 110 beats/min
  ❖ Dysrhythmias
  ❖ Systolic blood pressure less than 90 mm Hg
  ❖ Mean arterial pressure (MAP) less than 70 mm Hg with vasopressor support
  ❖ Cardiac index less than 2.4[3]
  ❖ Pulmonary artery occlusion pressure (pulmonary artery wedge pressure) greater than 18 mm Hg
  ❖ Decreased mixed venous oxygen saturation (Svo_2)
  ❖ Inadequate peripheral perfusion
  ❖ Urine output less than 0.5 mL/kg/hr
  ➥*Rationale:* Physical signs and symptoms result from the heart's inability to adequately contract and from inadequate coronary or systemic perfusion.

Patient Preparation

- Verify correct patient with two identifiers. ➥*Rationale:* Prior to performing a procedure, the nurse should ensure the correct identification of the patient for the intended intervention.
- Ensure that the patient and family understand preprocedural teaching. Answer questions as they arise, and reinforce information as needed. ➥*Rationale:* Understanding of previously taught information is evaluated and reinforced.
- Validate that the informed consent form has been signed. ➥*Rationale:* Informed consent protects the rights of the patient and makes a competent decision possible for the patient; however, in emergency circumstances, time may not allow the form to be signed.

- Perform a pre-procedure verification and time out, if non-emergent. ➤**Rationale:** Ensures patient safety.
- Validate the patency of central and peripheral intravenous access. ➤**Rationale:** Central access is needed for vasopressor administration; peripheral access is needed for fluid administration.

- Place the patient in a supine position and prepare the intended insertion site with an antiseptic solution. ➤**Rationale:** Prepares the intended access site and positions the patient for IAB insertion.

Procedure | for Assisting with IAB Catheter Insertion

Steps	Rationale	Special Considerations
1. HH		
2. PE		
3. Turn on the IABP console and the helium gas.	Provides power source and activates the gas that drives the IABP.	Follow the manufacturer's recommendations.
4. Sedate the patient as prescribed and as needed; the affected extremity may need to be restrained.	Movement of the lower extremity may inhibit insertion of the catheter or contribute to catheter kinking once the IAB is in place.	A knee immobilizer or a sheet placed over the affected leg and tucked in may minimize movement of the affected leg.
5. Establish ECG input to the IABP console and obtain an ECG configuration with optimal R wave amplitude and absence of artifact. Indirect ECG input can be obtained via "slave" of the bedside ECG to the IABP console.	The R wave is the preferred trigger signal from which the IABP can reference systole and diastole and therefore establish inflation and deflation points.	Usually, one set of ECG electrodes connects to the bedside monitoring system and the second set of ECG electrodes connects to the IABP console. With use of a slave signal, refer to the bedside monitor manufacturer instructions for optimizing the ECG and pacemaker recognition.
6. Assist with placement of hemodynamic monitoring lines if they are not already present (refer to Procedure 73).	Hemodynamic monitoring aids in the assessment and management of the patient who needs IABP therapy.	A radial arterial catheter is commonly inserted.[25]
7. Complete the IABP console preparation. Refer to the instruction manual.	Ensures adequate functioning of the IABP device.	Models of the pump console vary. Review of manufacturer instructions is recommended.
8. All personnel performing and assisting with the procedure should apply personal and protective sterile equipment (e.g., masks, head covers, goggles or face shields, sterile gowns, and gloves).	Minimizes the risk of infection and maintains standard and sterile precautions.	
9. Drape the intended insertion site with the sterile drapes.	Provides a sterile field and reduces the transmission of microorganisms.	
10. Assist as needed with removing the IAB catheter from the sterile packing and place the catheter and insertion tray on the sterile field.	Makes supplies available and maintains sterility.	Catheters vary in balloon volumes. An adequate volume is necessary to achieve optimal hemodynamic effects from IABP therapy. Patient height may be used as a guideline for selection of balloon volume. Clinical judgment and patient factors, such as patient torso length, are considered.[11]
11. Administer a heparin bolus before arterial puncture, if clinically indicated and prescribed.	Anticoagulation therapy may decrease the incidence of thromboemboli related to the indwelling IAB catheter.	Systemic anticoagulation therapy may not be used in all patients.[30]

Procedure for Assisting with IAB Catheter Insertion—*Continued*

Steps	Rationale	Special Considerations
12. Attach the supplied one-way valve to the Luer-tip of the distal end of the balloon helium lumen.	Creates a device for removing air from the balloon catheter.	
13. Pull back slowly on the syringe until all the air is aspirated.	Removes air from the balloon, creating a vacuum.	Maintains the wrap of the balloon for insertion.
14. Disconnect the syringe only, leaving the one-way valve in place.	Prevents air entry back into the balloon.	
15. Follow the manufacturer recommendations for lubricating the catheter before insertion. **(Level M*)**	May decrease the drag on the catheter during insertion.	Not all IAB catheters need lubrication. Review manufacturer instructions.
16. Flush the inner lumen of the IAB catheter before insertion.	Removes air from the central lumen.	If the catheter is not flushed before insertion, allow the backflow of arterial blood before connection to the flush system.[23] Follow institution policy or physician prescription regarding the use of heparinized normal saline solution.
17. Assist as needed with the introducer sheath or dilator assembly and insertion.	Prepares for balloon catheter entry.	Some IABs are inserted without a sheath. If the IAB is inserted via the sheathless method, only the dilator is used.[9,10]
18. Assist with balloon catheter insertion.	Catheter placement is a necessary part of IAB setup.	Some fiberoptic IABP catheters need to be calibrated before insertion. Follow manufacturer's guidelines.
19. Assist with removal of the one-way valve according to the manufacturer's recommendations.	Releases the vacuum and readies the balloon for counterpulsation.	
20. If the inner lumen of a double-lumen catheter is used to monitor arterial pressure, attach a three-way stopcock with a single-pressure transducer system (see Procedure 76) connected to the monitor and set the alarms.	Monitors the arterial pressure.	Follow institution policy or physician prescription regarding the use of heparinized normal saline solution. The inner lumen, if used, must be attached to an alarm system because undetected disconnection could result in life-threatening hemorrhage. The proximal tip of the inner lumen used for arterial pressure monitoring is at the level of the left subclavian artery, not at the aortic arch; therefore, this location is not the same as a central line placed at the aortic root.[23,24]
21. Avoid fast flush and blood sampling from the central aortic lumen.	Air may enter the system during fast flush and also during blood sampling, resulting in air emboli.	Some manufacturers and institutions recommend hourly fast flush of central lumen lines. If fast flush is required and prescribed, ensure that the IABP is on standby (not pumping) during the flush. However, the risk of air embolus entry or dislodging a thrombus at the lumen tip is a major concern. Refer to institutional policy in regard to fast flush of central lumen catheters.

*Level M: Manufacturer's recommendations only

Procedure continues on following page

Procedure	for Assisting with IAB Catheter Insertion—*Continued*	
Steps	**Rationale**	**Special Considerations**
22. Attach the helium tubing to the balloon helium lumen and connect the helium tubing to the IABP console.	Attachment is necessary to initiate therapy.	The helium tubing is packaged with the IAB.
23. Follow the steps for timing, troubleshooting, and patient monitoring.	Provides for appropriate operation of counterpulsation.	Many IABP consoles have features for automatic timing. Refer to specific manufacturer's instructions.
24. Conventional IAB: A. Level the air-fluid interface of the stopcock. B. Zero the hemodynamic monitoring system.	Ensures accurate arterial pressure measurement.	
Fiberoptic IAB: A. Calibrate the system. B. Follow the manufacturer's instructions for calibration.[21,25]		Refer to specific manufacturer instructions for fiberoptic IAB catheters. Some fiberoptic IAB catheters self-calibrate.
25. Obtain a portable chest radiograph as soon as possible. Temporarily place the IABP on standby while obtaining the chest radiograph.	Correct IAB catheter position must be confirmed to prevent complications associated with the interference of the arterial blood supply. Placing the IABP on standby enhances the visibility of the balloon on the radiograph.	If fluoroscopy is used for insertion of the catheter, a radiograph immediately after placement is not necessary. Some patients may have hemodynamic instability when the IABP is on standby for more than a few seconds; assess each patient's hemodynamic response to IABP therapy.
26. Ensure that the IAB is secured to the patient's skin.	Maintains optimal position and reduces the risk of IAB catheter migration.	The IAB catheter may be sutured or a sutureless securement device may be used to secure the catheter.
27. Apply a sterile dressing to the catheter insertion site.	Minimizes the risk of infection.	
28. Discard personal protective equipment in appropriate receptacle.	Reduces the transmission of microorganisms; Standard Precautions.	
29. **HH**		

Procedure	for Timing of the IABP	
Steps	**Rationale**	**Special Considerations**
1. Select an ECG lead that optimizes the R wave. **(Level M*)**	The R wave of the ECG is the preferred trigger source for identifying the cardiac cycle.	Refer to manufacturer instructions for trigger options.
2. Assess the timing of the IABP with the arterial waveform.	The arterial waveform assists in identification of accurate IAB inflation and deflation.[21,23,24]	Refer to specific manufacturer instructions for automatic timing.
3. Set the IABP to the auto-time mode.	The IABP console automatically adjusts timing of inflation and deflation.	Some IABP consoles have this feature.
4. Timing can be checked by setting the IABP frequency to the every-other-beat setting (1:2 or 50%; Fig. 55-3).	Comparison can be made between the assisted and unassisted arterial waveforms.	

*Level M: Manufacturer's recommendations only

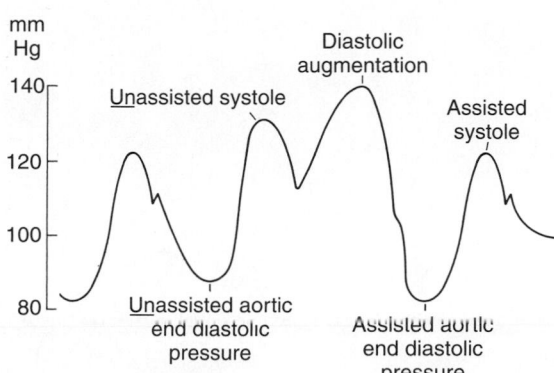

mm Hg

140

120

100

80

Diastolic augmentation

Unassisted systole

Assisted systole

Unassisted aortic end diastolic pressure

Assisted aortic end diastolic pressure

FIGURE 55-3 Intra-aortic balloon pump frequency of 1:2. *(Courtesy Datascope Corp, Fairfield, NJ.)*

Procedure | for Timing of the IABP—*Continued*

Steps	Rationale	Special Considerations
5. Inflation:	The dicrotic notch represents closure of the aortic valve.	
A. Identify the dicrotic notch of the assisted systolic waveform (see Fig. 55-3).		
B. Adjust inflation later to expose the dicrotic notch.	Identifies the landmark for accurate inflation.	
C. Slowly adjust inflation earlier until the dicrotic notch disappears and a sharp V wave forms (see Fig. 55-3).	Balloon augmentation should occur after the aortic valve closes.[5,22]	A sharp V wave may not be seen in patients with low systemic vascular resistance.
D. Compare the augmented pressure with the patient's unassisted systolic pressure.	Balloon augmentation ideally is equal to or greater than the patient's unassisted systolic blood pressure.[11]	If balloon augmentation is less than the patient's systolic pressure, consider the possibility that the patient is hypovolemic or tachycardic, the balloon is positioned too low, or the balloon volume is set too low.[25] Low volume may also be the result of an inadequate fill volume or an IAB catheter that is too small for the patient.
E. Adjust inflation if needed.	Necessary to achieve optimal diastolic augmentation.	Timing of inflation varies slightly depending on the location of the arterial catheter and resulting physiologic delays.[22,24] Radial: Inflate 40 to 50 ms before the dicrotic notch. Femoral: Inflate 120 ms before the dicrotic notch (Fig. 55-4). The radial artery is recommended for use for pressure monitoring for IABP timing.[22,24]
6. Deflation:		
A. Identify the assisted and unassisted aortic end-diastolic pressures and the assisted and unassisted systolic pressures (see Fig. 55-3).[5,6]	These landmarks are important in determination of accurate IAB deflation.	IABP frequency is set at 1:2 (50%).

Procedure continues on following page

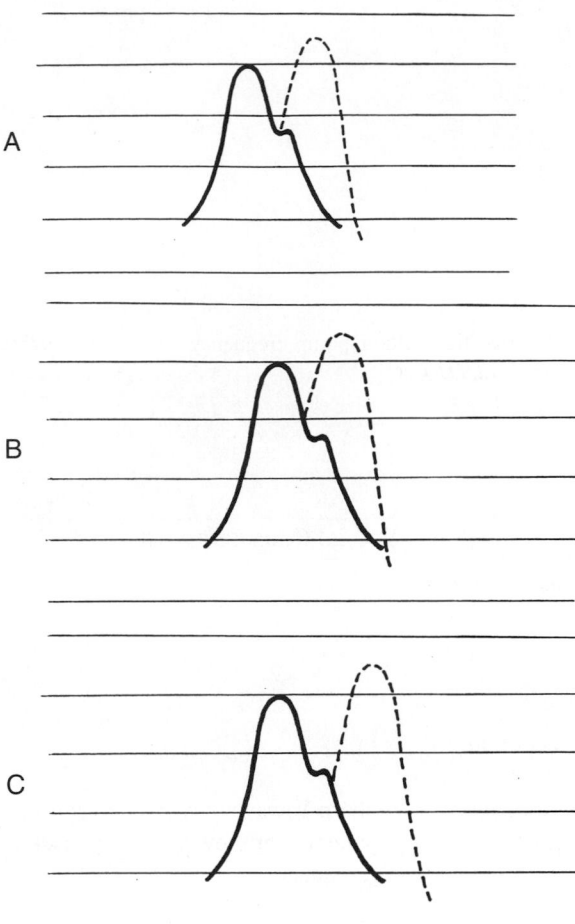

FIGURE 55-4   IABP inflation. **A,** Radial. **B,** Femoral. **C,** Central aortic.

Procedure   for Timing of the IABP—*Continued*

Steps	Rationale	Special Considerations
B. Set the balloon to deflate so that the assisted aortic end-diastolic pressure is as low as possible (lower than the patient's unassisted diastolic pressure) while still maintaining optimal diastolic augmentation and not impeding on the next systole (the assisted systole).	The assisted systolic pressure is less than the unassisted systolic pressure as a result of a decrease in afterload, thus reducing the myocardial workload.[22]	Reduction of afterload decreases the energy required by the heart during systole. Afterload reduction without diminishment of diastolic augmentation is important to achieve.
7. Set the IABP frequency to 1:1 (100%; Fig. 55-5).	Ensures that each heartbeat is assisted.	
8. Assess timing every hour, whenever the heart rate changes by more than 10 beats/min, and when the rhythm changes.	Inappropriate timing prevents effective IABP therapy.	Many IABP models use algorithms to automatically adjust timing for changes in heart rate and rhythm. Refer to the specific manufacturer guidelines for a description of automatic timing modes and their specific features.
9. Assess and intervene to correct inappropriate timing.	Ensures accurate timing and optimal functioning of the IABP.	

1:1 IABP Frequency

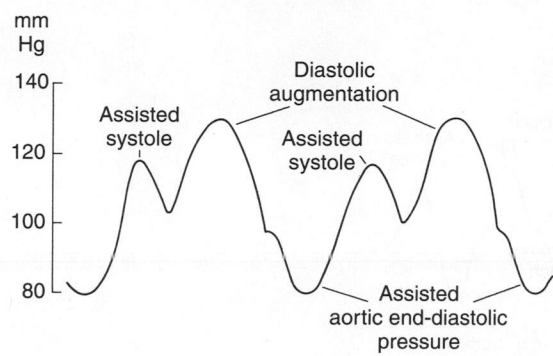

FIGURE 55-5 Correct intra-aortic balloon pump timing (1:1). *(Courtesy Datascope Corp, Fairfield, NJ.)*

Timing Errors
Early Inflation

Inflation of the IAB prior to aortic valve closure

Waveform Characteristics:
• Inflation of IAB prior to dicrotic notch
• Diastolic augmentation encroaches onto systole (may be unable to distinguish)

Physiologic Effects:
• Potential premature closure of aortic valve
• Potential increased in LVEDV and LVEDP or PCWP
• Increased left ventricular wall stress or afterload
• Aortic regurgitation
• Increased MVo$_2$ demand

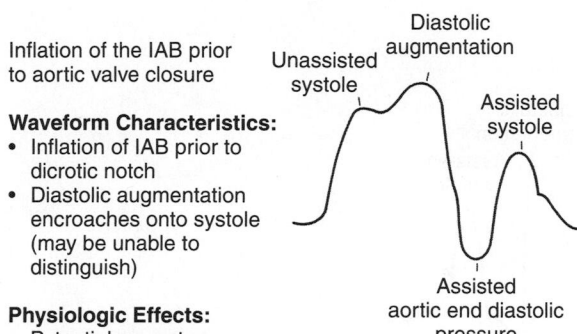

FIGURE 55-6 Early inflation. *(Courtesy Datascope Corp, Fairfield, NJ.)*

Procedure	for Timing of the IABP—*Continued*	
Steps	**Rationale**	**Special Considerations**
A. Problem: Early inflation (Fig. 55-6). Intervention: Move inflation later.	Inflation occurs before closure of the aortic valve, leading to premature aortic valve closure, increased left ventricular volume, and decreased stroke volume.	
B. Problem: Late inflation (Fig. 55-7). Intervention: Adjust inflation earlier.	A delay in inflation leads to a decrease in coronary artery perfusion.	
C. Problem: Early deflation (Fig. 55-8). Intervention: Adjust deflation later.	Deflation occurs before the aortic valve opens, leading to decreased balloon augmentation and less or no afterload reduction; coronary artery perfusion may also be decreased.	Note the sharp diastolic wave after augmentation and the increase in the assisted systolic pressure.

Procedure continues on following page

Timing Errors
Late Inflation

Inflation of the IAB markedly
after closure of the aortic valve

Waveform Characteristics:
• Inflation of the IAB after
  the dicrotic notch
• Absence of sharp V
• Suboptimal diastolic
  augmentation

Physiologic Effects:
• Suboptimal coronary artery
  perfusion

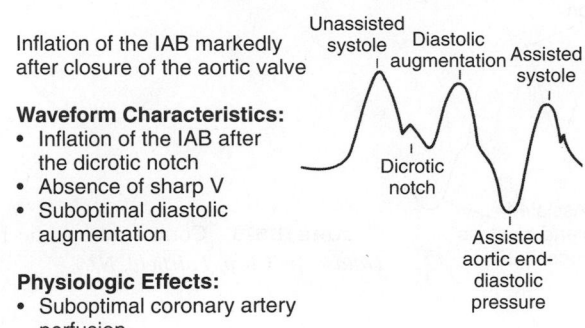

FIGURE 55-7   Late inflation. *(Courtesy Datascope Corp, Fairfield, NJ.)*

Timing Errors
Early Deflation

Premature deflation of the IAB
during the diastolic phase

Waveform Characteristics:
• Deflation of IAB is seen as a
  sharp drop following diastolic
  augmentation
• Suboptimal diastolic
  augmentation
• Assisted aortic end diastolic
  pressure may be equal to
  or less than the unassisted
  aortic end diastolic pressure
• Assisted systolic pressure
  may rise

Physiologic Effects:
• Suboptimal coronary perfusion
• Potential for retrograde coronary
  and carotid blood flow
• Angina may occur as a result of retrograde
  coronary blood flow
• Suboptimal afterload reduction
• Increased MVO$_2$ demand

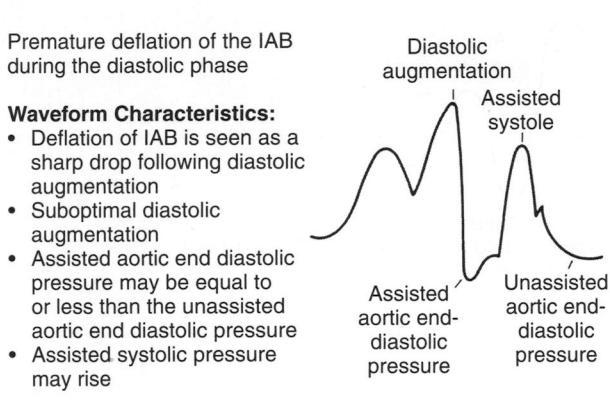

FIGURE 55-8   Early deflation. *(Courtesy Datascope Corp, Fairfield, NJ.)*

Procedure	for Timing of the IABP—*Continued*	
Steps	**Rationale**	**Special Considerations**
D. Problem: Late deflation (Fig. 55-9). Intervention: Adjust deflation earlier.	Deflation occurs after the aortic valve has opened, leading to an increase in the aortic end-diastolic pressure and an increase in afterload.	Note the delayed diastolic wave after augmentation and the diminished assisted systole. Late deflation is identified by a diminished assisted systolic pressure, an increase in heart rate, an increase in filling pressures, a decrease in cardiac output and cardiac index, and an increased afterload. Maintaining a reliable trigger minimizes the risk of late deflation.[5,6,11,21]

Timing Errors
Late Deflation

Deflation of the IAB late in diastolic phase as aortic valve is beginning to open

Waveform Characteristics:
- Assisted aortic end-diastolic pressure may be equal to or greater than the unassisted aortic end diastolic pressure
- Rate of rise of assisted systole is prolonged
- Diastolic augmentation may appear widened

Physiologic Effects:
- Afterload reduction is essentially absent
- Increased MVO$_2$ consumption due to the left ventricle ejecting against a greater resistance and a prolonged isovolumetric contraction phase
- IAB may impede left ventricular ejection and increase the afterload

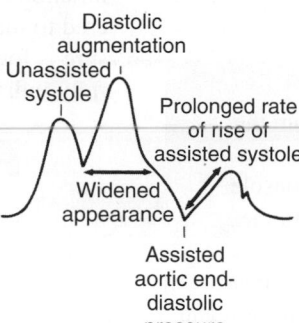

FIGURE 55-9 Late deflation. (*Courtesy Datascope Corp, Fairfield, NJ.*)

Procedure for Balloon Pressure Waveform

Steps	Rationale	Special Considerations
1. Determine whether the IABP console has a balloon pressure waveform.	Helium is shuttled in and out of the IAB catheter, and the balloon pressure waveform represents this movement.	Refer to the specific manufacturer instructions regarding the balloon pressure waveform.
2. Assess the balloon pressure waveform.	Reflects pressure that is in the IAB.	
3. Determine whether the balloon pressure waveform is normal (Fig. 55-10). A normal balloon pressure waveform:	A normal balloon pressure waveform reflects that the IAB is inflating and deflating properly.[20]	

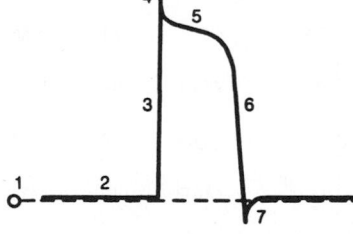

FIGURE 55-10 Normal balloon gas waveform. *1*, zero baseline; *2*, fill pressure; *3*, rapid inflation; *4*, peak inflation artifact; *5*, plateau pressure or inflation plateau pressure; *6*, rapid deflation; *7*, peak deflation pressure and return to fill pressure. (*Courtesy* Arrow International.)

A. Has a fill pressure (baseline pressure) slightly above zero.	Reflects pressure in the tubing between the IAB and the IABP driving mechanism.	
B. Has a sharp upstroke.	Occurs as gas inflates the IAB catheter.	
C. Has peak inflation artifact.	This overshoot pressure artifact is caused by gas pressure in the pneumatic line.[1]	

Procedure continues on following page

Procedure | for Balloon Pressure Waveform—*Continued*

Steps	Rationale	Special Considerations
D. Has a pressure plateau.	This plateau is created as the IAB remains inflated during diastole.	The plateau indicates the length of time of inflation and whether full inflation (volume) has been delivered to the IAB. If no plateau pressure is found, the IAB may not be fully inflated.
E. Has a rapid deflation.	Gas is quickly shuttled from the IAB.	
F. Has a negative deflection below baseline and then returns to baseline.	Gas returns to the IABP console and then stabilizes within the system.	
4. Compare the balloon pressure waveform with the arterial pressure waveform (Fig. 55-11). Note the similarity in the width of the balloon pressure waveform and the augmented arterial waveform.[16]	Demonstrates the relationship between the balloon pressure waveform and the arterial waveform. Reflects the effect of the balloon on the augmented arterial pressure.	
5. Determine whether the balloon pressure waveform meets the previous description.	Abnormal balloon pressure waveforms may indicate restriction to helium shuttle.	Refer to the specific manufacturer's instructions regarding troubleshooting abnormal balloon pressure waveforms.

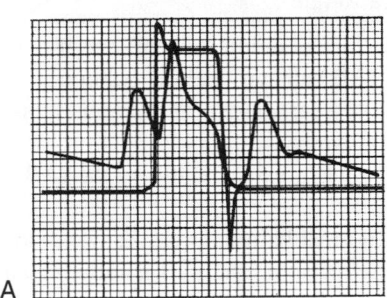

A

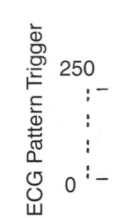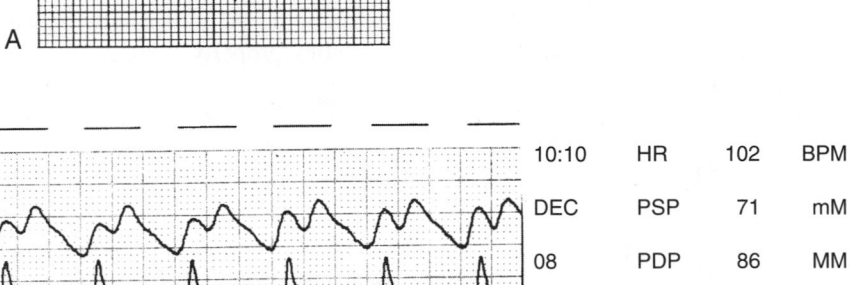

10:10	HR	102	BPM
DEC	PSP	71	mM
08	PDP	86	MM
	EDP	39	MM
	MAP	49	MM

FIGURE 55-11   **A,** Balloon pressure waveform superimposed on the arterial pressure waveform. **B,** Actual recording of an arterial pressure waveform *(top)* and balloon gas waveform *(bottom)* from a patient with balloon pump. *(Courtesy Arrow International.)*

Procedure for Troubleshooting

Steps	Rationale	Special Considerations

1. Atrial fibrillation:
  A. Assess and treat the underlying cause.
  B. Set the IABP to inflate and deflate most of the patient's beats.
	The underlying cause of the dysrhythmia should be treated.	Inflation of the IAB should correspond to the diastolic interval of each cardiac cycle.
		The IAB automatically deflates on the R wave.

C. Refer to manufacturer's instructions for the appropriate IABP console settings for atrial fibrillation (e.g., the atrial fibrillation trigger mode).	Select a mode on the IABP console for optimal R wave tracking.	The real-time method of timing may track dysrhythmias better than traditional or conventional IABP timing.[20]

2. Tachycardia:
  A. Assess and treat the underlying cause.
  B. Set the timing and the frequency of the IABP to optimize hemodynamic response.
	The underlying cause of the tachycardia should be treated.
	IAB timing and frequency should be set to optimize coronary perfusion and afterload reduction.
		Because diastole is shortened during tachycardia, the IAB inflation time also is shortened.
		The IABP may need to be changed to a 1:2 frequency. Pumping every other beat may improve the patient's hemodynamic status.
		Some IABPs with automatic timing can track rates as high as 220 beats/min.

3. Asystole:
  A. Switch the trigger to arterial pressure.
 	
  B. If the IABP console is not in the auto-operation mode:
    1. Set inflation to provide diastolic augmentation.
    2. Set deflation to occur before the upstroke of the next systole.
	This trigger can be used if an arterial pressure is generated from chest compressions.
	Sets the IABP timing.
		Follow Advanced Cardiac Life Support (ACLS) standards for emergency care.
		Refer to manufacturer's manual.
		Preliminary research suggests that when used during cardiopulmonary resuscitation, IAB counterpulsation increases cerebral and coronary perfusion.[2,11]

C. If chest compressions do not provide an adequate trigger:
    1. Turn or push the control to internal trigger.
 	
    2. Set the rate at 60 to 80 beats/min.
    3. Set the IABP frequency to 1:2.
 	
    4. Turn the balloon augmentation down to 50%.
  D. If the IABP console is in the auto-timing mode, the console automatically attempts to self-time if an arterial pressure is generated or switches to an internal trigger.
	The internal trigger keeps the IAB catheter moving so that clot formation is minimized.[20]
	Maintains consistent movement of IAB catheter.
	A 1:2 frequency is adequate to prevent thrombus formation on the IAB catheter.
	Slight inflation and deflation of the IAB catheter prevents clot formation.
	Sets the IABP timing and maintains consistent movement of the IAB catheter.
		Refer to manufacturer's guidelines for recommendations for minimal balloon volume.

Procedure continues on following page

Procedure for Troubleshooting—*Continued*

Steps	Rationale	Special Considerations
4. Ventricular tachycardia or ventricular fibrillation:		
A. Assess and treat the underlying cause.	The underlying cause of the tachycardia should be treated.	
B. Cardiovert or defibrillate as necessary (see Procedures 40 and 41).	Attempts to convert the dysrhythmia.	Follow ACLS standards for emergency care. Ensure that personnel are cleared from the patient and equipment before cardioversion or defibrillation. The IABP console is electrically isolated.
5. Loss of vacuum or IABP failure:		
A. Check and tighten the connections on the pneumatic tubing.	A loose connection may contribute to a loss of vacuum.	
B. Check the compressor power source.	Ensures that power is available to drive the helium.	
C. Hand inflate and deflate the balloon every 5 minutes if necessary. **(Level M*)**	Prevents clot formation along the dormant balloon.	Refer to specific manufacturer's guidelines for manually inflating and deflating the IAB. Ensure that the correct syringe is kept with the IABP console for this emergency; check manufacturer's guidelines for frequency of hand inflation.
D. Change the IAB console. **(Level M)**	Establishes a power source and effective IABP therapy.	
6. Suspected balloon perforation:		
A. Observe for loss of augmentation.	Helium may be gradually leaking from the balloon catheter.	Set the alarm limits so the alarms sound with a drop of 10 mm Hg in diastolic augmentation.
B. Check for blood in the catheter tubing.	Blood or any discoloration in the helium tubing indicates that the balloon has perforated and that arterial blood is present.	It is possible for a balloon leak to be self-sealing as a result of the surface tension between the inside and the outside of the IAB membrane. This may be evidenced by the presence of dried blood in the catheter tubing. The dried blood may appear as a brownish, coffee-ground–like substance.
C. Assess for changes or lack of a normal balloon pressure waveform.	The balloon pressure waveform may be absent if the balloon is unable to retain gas, or the pressure plateau may gradually decrease if the IAB is leaking gas.	
7. Balloon perforation:		
A. Place the IABP on standby.	Prevents further IAB pumping and continued gas exchange.	Some IABP consoles automatically shut off if a leak is detected. The IAB catheter should be removed within 15 to 30 minutes.[8]
B. Clamp the IAB catheter.	Prevents arterial blood backup.	
C. Disconnect the IAB catheter from the IABP console.	Prevents blood from backing up into the IABP console.	
D. Notify the physician.	The IAB catheter needs to be removed or replaced immediately.	If the IAB leak has sealed itself off, this may result in entrapment of the IAB in the vasculature. Surgical removal may be necessary.

*Level M: Manufacturer's recommendations only

Procedure for Troubleshooting—*Continued*

Steps	Rationale	Special Considerations
E. Prepare for IAB catheter removal or replacement.	The IAB catheter should not lie dormant for longer than 30 minutes.	Do not manually inflate and deflate the IAB if balloon perforation is suspected. Perforation of a balloon membrane may indicate that the patient's vascular condition may induce abrasion or perforation in subsequent balloon membranes.
F. Discontinue anticoagulation therapy as prescribed.	Clotting occurs more readily if anticoagulation therapy is stopped (necessary if removing the catheter).	

Procedure for Weaning and IAB Catheter Removal

Steps	Rationale	Special Considerations
1. 🅷🅷		
2. Assess clinical readiness for weaning.	Optimal clinical and hemodynamic parameters validate readiness for weaning.	Patient hemodynamic status should be optimal before weaning from IABP therapy. Signs of clinical readiness include the following: no angina, heart rate less than 110 beats/min, absence of unstable dysrhythmias, MAP greater than 70 mm Hg with minimal or no vasopressor support, pulmonary artery occlusion pressure (PAOP) less than 18 mm Hg, cardiac index greater than 2.4, mixed venous oxygen saturation between 60% and 80%, capillary refill less than 2 seconds, and urine output greater than 0.5 mL/kg/hr.
3. Change the assist ratio to 1:2 (50%), and monitor the patient's response for 1 to 6 hours, as prescribed, or per institution's protocol.	The length of time required to wean from IABP therapy depends on the hemodynamic response of the patient and the length of time the patient has received IABP therapy.[12,27]	Follow physician prescription or institution policy on IABP weaning.
4. If hemodynamic parameters remain stable, further change the ratio (depending on the patient and the balloon console assist frequencies, or as prescribed).	IABP consoles vary in assist ratios.	Follow physician prescription or institution policy on IABP weaning.
5. Discontinue heparin or dextran 4 to 6 hours before IAB catheter removal, or reverse heparin with protamine (as prescribed) just before catheter removal.	Decreases the likelihood of bleeding after balloon removal.	
6. Turn the IABP to standby or off and disconnect the IAB from the console.	Ensures deflation of the IAB catheter.	The patient's arterial pressure collapses the balloon membrane for withdrawal.
7. Assist with removing sutures or the sutureless securement device.	Prepares for IAB removal.	
8. Assist the physician or advanced practice nurse with removal of the percutaneous balloon.	Facilitates removal.	The IAB catheter is not withdrawn into the sheath but removed as an entire unit to avoid shearing the balloon.

Procedure continues on following page

Procedure for Weaning and IAB Catheter Removal—*Continued*

Steps	Rationale	Special Considerations
9. Ensure that pressure is held on the insertion site for 30 to 45 minutes after the IAB catheter is withdrawn.	Ensures that hemostasis is obtained and decreases the incidence of bleeding and hematoma formation.	A femoral compression system can be used to achieve hemostasis (see Procedure 77). Pressure may be needed for a longer period of time if the patient has been receiving anticoagulant therapy of if coagulation study results are abnormal.
10. Assess the insertion site for signs of bleeding or hematoma formation before application of a sterile pressure dressing.	Assists in the detection of bleeding.	
11. Apply a pressure dressing to the insertion site for 2 to 4 hours.	Minimizes bleeding from the insertion site.	
12. Obtain vital signs and hemodynamic parameters every 15 minutes $\times$ 4, every 30 minutes $\times$ 2, then every hour as the patient's condition warrants.	Determines patient stability or instability.	
13. Assess the quality of perfusion to the decannulated extremity immediately after removal and every 1 hour $\times$ 2, then every 2 hours or as prescribed.	Removal of the IAB catheter may dislodge thrombi on the catheter and lead to arterial occlusion.	
14. Maintain immobility of the decannulated extremity and maintain bed rest with the head of the bed no greater than 30 degrees for 8 hours, as prescribed or according to institution protocol.	Promotes healing and decreases stress at the insertion site.	
15. Discard used supplies in appropriate receptacle.	Reduces the transmission of microorganisms and body secretions; standard precautions.	
16. 🅷🅷		

Expected Outcomes

- Increased myocardial oxygen supply
- Decreased myocardial oxygen demand
- Increased cardiac output
- Increased tissue perfusion, including cerebral, renal, and peripheral circulation

Unexpected Outcomes

- Impaired perfusion to the extremity with the IAB catheter in place
- Balloon perforation
- Inappropriate IAB placement
- Pain
- Bleeding or coagulation disorders
- Aortic dissection
- Infection

Patient Monitoring and Care

Steps	Rationale	Reportable Conditions
		These conditions should be reported if they persist despite nursing interventions.
1. Perform systematic cardiovascular, peripheral vascular, and hemodynamic assessments every 15 to 60 minutes as patient status requires.		

Patient Monitoring and Care —*Continued*

Steps	Rationale	Reportable Conditions
A. Level of consciousness.	Assesses for adequate cerebral perfusion; thrombi may develop and dislodge during IABP therapy; the IAB may migrate, decreasing blood flow to the carotid arteries.	• Change in level of consciousness
B. Vital signs and pulmonary artery pressures.	Demonstrates effectiveness of IABP therapy.	• Unstable vital signs • Significant changes in hemodynamic pressures • Lack of response to IABP therapy
C. Arterial and balloon pressure.	Ensures effectiveness of IABP timing and therapy.	• Difficulty achieving effective IABP therapy
D. Cardiac output, cardiac index, and systemic vascular resistance determinations.	Demonstrates effectiveness of IABP therapy.	• Abnormal cardiac output, cardiac index, and systemic vascular resistance values
E. Circulation to extremities.	Determines peripheral perfusion. If reportable conditions are found, they may indicate catheter or embolus obstruction of perfusion to the extremity. Specifically, decreased perfusion to the left arm may indicate misplacement of the IAB catheter.[2,8,14,27]	• Capillary refill greater than 2 seconds • Diminished or absent pulses (e.g., antecubital, radial, popliteal, tibial, pedal) • Color pale, mottled, or cyanotic • Diminished or absent sensation • Pain • Diminished or absent movement • Cool or cold to touch
F. Urine output.	Determines perfusion to the kidneys.	• Urine output less than 0.5 mL/kg/hr
2. Assess heart and lung sounds every 4 hours and as needed.	Abnormal heart and lung sounds may indicate the need for additional treatment. Special note: When the patient's condition permits, place the IABP on standby to accurately auscultate heart and lung sounds because IABP therapy creates extraneous sounds and impairs heart and lung sound assessment.	• Abnormal heart and lung sounds
3. Maintain the head of bed at less than 45 degrees.	Prevents kinking of the IAB catheter and migration of the catheter.	
4. Monitor for signs of balloon perforation by assessing the helium tubing on a regular basis for evidence of discoloration or blood in the tubing.	In the event of balloon perforation, a very small amount of helium could be released into the aorta, potentially causing an embolic event. Because of pressure gradients in the aorta, blood is more likely to enter the balloon membrane and be dehydrated by the helium.	• Blood or brown flecks in tubing • Loss of IABP augmentation • Control console alarm activation (e.g., gas loss)
5. Maintain accurate IABP timing.	If timing is not accurate, cardiac output may decrease rather than increase.	• Signs and symptoms of hemodynamic instability

Procedure continues on following page

Patient Monitoring and Care —*Continued*

Steps	Rationale	Reportable Conditions
6. Log-roll the patient every 2 hours. Prop pillows to support the patient and to maintain alignment. Consider use of pressure-relief devices. **(Level E*)**	Promotes comfort and skin integrity and prevents kinking of the IAB catheter. Special note: Log-rolling may not be tolerated in patients with severe hemodynamic compromise; low-pressure beds are necessary for these patients. Low-pressure beds can decrease the occurrence of pressure ulcers in patients who need IABP therapy.[4,23]	
7. Immobilize the cannulated extremity with a draw sheet tucked under the mattress or with a soft ankle restraint or a knee immobilizer.	Prevents dislodgment and migration of the IAB catheter. Special note: Assess skin integrity and perfusion distal to the restraint every hour.	
8. Initiate passive and active range-of-motion exercises every 2 hours to extremities that can be mobilized.	Prevents venous stasis and muscle atrophy.	
9. Assess the area around the IAB catheter insertion site every 2 hours and as needed for evidence of hematoma or bleeding.	IAB catheter inflation and deflation traumatize red blood cells and platelets. Anticoagulation therapy may alter hemoglobin and hematocrit and coagulation values.[30]	• Bleeding at insertion site • Hematoma at insertion site
10. Maintain anticoagulation therapy as prescribed; monitor coagulation studies.	Prophylactic anticoagulation therapy may be used to prevent thrombi and emboli development.	• Abnormal coagulation study results
11. Monitor patient for systemic evidence of bleeding or coagulation disorders.	Hematologic and coagulation profiles may be altered as a result of blood loss during balloon insertion, anticoagulation, and platelet dysfunction as a result of mechanical trauma by balloon inflation and deflation.[30]	• Bleeding from IAB insertion site • Bleeding from incisions or mucous membranes • Petechiae or ecchymoses • Guaiac-positive nasogastric aspirate or stool • Hematuria • Decreased hemoglobin or hematocrit • Decreased filling pressures • Increased heart rate • Retroperitoneal hematoma • Pain in the lower abdomen, flank, thigh, or lower extremity
12. Follow institution standard for assessing pain. Administer analgesia as prescribed.	Promotes comfort.	• Continued pain despite pain interventions

*Level E: Multiple case reports, theory-based evidence from expert opinions, or peer-reviewed professional organizational standards without clinical studies to support recommendations

Patient Monitoring and Care —*Continued*

Steps	Rationale	Reportable Conditions
13. Replace gauze dressings at the IAB catheter site every 2 days and transparent dressings at least every 7 days. Cleanse the site with an antiseptic solution (e.g., 2% chlorhexidine solution). **(Level D*)**	Decreases the incidence of infection and allows an opportunity for site assessment. Although guidelines do not exist specifically for IAB site dressings, the Centers for Disease Control and Prevention (CDC)[17] recommend replacing invasive line dressings when the dressing becomes damp, loosened, or soiled or when inspection of the site is necessary.	• Signs or symptoms of infection
14. Assess for balloon migration.	The IAB should be positioned 2 cm below the left subclavian artery and just above the renal arteries. If the IAB migrates proximally, it may occlude the subclavian or carotid arteries. If the IAB migrates too low, it could occlude the renal or mesenteric arteries.	• Signs of possible subclavian artery occlusion: unequal or absent radial pulse and dampening or loss of the arterial pressure waveform in the ipsilateral radial artery (radial artery on the same side as the IAB catheter) • Signs of possible carotid artery occlusion include change in level of consciousness and orientation or unilateral neurologic deficit • Signs of renal artery occlusion: oliguria or anuria, back or flank pain, nausea, and anorexia • Signs of mesenteric occlusion: abdominal pain, diarrhea, nausea, and decreased bowel sounds
15. Identify parameters that demonstrate clinical readiness to wean from IABP therapy.	Close observation of the patient's tolerance to weaning procedures is necessary to ensure that the body's oxygen demands can be met. The presence of these reportable conditions indicates that consideration should be given to weaning the patient from the IABP.	• No angina • Heart rate less than 110 beats/min • Absence of unstable dysrhythmias • MAP greater than 70 mm Hg with little or no vasopressor support • PAOP less than 18 mm Hg • Cardiac index greater than 2.4 • Svo_2 between 60% and 80% • Capillary refill less than 2 seconds • Urine output greater than 0.5 mL/kg/hr

*Level D: Peer-reviewed professional organizational standards with clinical studies to support recommendations

Documentation

Documentation should include the following:
- Patient and family education
- Informed consent
- Universal protocol requirements
- Insertion of the IAB catheter (including size of catheter used and balloon volume)
- Peripheral pulses and neurovascular assessment of the affected extremity
- Any difficulties with insertion
- IABP frequency
- Patient response to the procedure and to IABP therapy
- Assessment of pain, interventions and response to interventions
- Confirmation of placement (e.g., chest radiograph)
- Insertion site assessment
- Hemodynamic status
- IABP pressures (unassisted end-diastolic pressure, unassisted systolic pressure, balloon augmented pressure, assisted systolic pressure, assisted end-diastolic pressure, and MAP)
- Occurrence of unexpected outcomes
- Additional nursing interventions taken

References

CR 1. Arafa OE, et al: Intra-aortic balloon pumping for predominantly right ventricular failure after heart transplantation, *Ann Thoracic Surg* 70:1587-1593, 2000.

CR 2. Arafa OE, et al: Vascular complications of the intra-aortic balloon pump in patients undergoing open heart operations: 15-year experience, *Ann Thoracic Surg* 67:645-651, 1999.

CR 3. Barron HV, Every NR, Parson LS, et al: The use of intraaortic balloon counterpulsation in patients with cardiogenic shock complicating acute myocardial infarction: data from national registry of myocardial infarction, *Am Heart J* 141:933-939, 2001.

CR 4. Brodie BR, et al: Intra-aortic balloon counterpulsation before primary percutaneous transluminal coronary angioplasty reduces catheterization laboratory events in high-risk patients with acute myocardial infarction, *Am J Cardiol* 84:18-23, 1999.

CR 5. Cadwell CA, Tyson G: Real timing. In Quaal S, editor: *Comprehensive intraaortic balloon counterpulsation,* ed 2, St Louis, 1993, Mosby.

CR 6. Cadwell CA, Hobson KS, Petis S: Clinical observations with real timing, *Crit Care Nurs Clin North Am* 8: 357-370, 1996.

7. Christenson JT, Sierra J, Romand JA, et al: Long intraaortic balloon treatment time leads to more vascular complications, *Asian Cardiovasc Thoracic Ann* 15(5):408-412, 2007.

CR 8. Cook L, et al: Intra-aortic balloon pump complications: a five-year retrospective study of 283 patients, *Heart Lung* 28:195-202, 1999.

CR 9. Diver D: Sheathless balloon insertion. In Quaal SJ, editor: *Comprehensive intra-aortic balloon counterpulsation,* St Louis, 1993, Mosby.

10. Erdogan HB, Goksedef D, Erentug V, et al: In which patients should sheathless IABP be used? An analysis of vascular complications in 1211 cases, *J Cardiac Surg* July(4):342-346, 2006.

CR 11. Ferguson JJ, Cohen M, Freedman RJ Jr, et al: The current practice of intraaortic balloon counterpulsation: results from the benchmark registry, *J Am Coll Cardiol* 38: 1456-1462, 2001.

CR 12. Hochman JS, et al: Cardiogenic shock complicating acute myocardial infarction-etiologies: management and outcome: a report from the SHOCK trial registry: should we emergently revascularize occluded coronaries for cardiogenic shock? *J Am Coll Cardiol* 36(3A):1663-1610, 2000.

CR 13. Kang N, Edwards M, Larbalestier R: Preoperative intra-aortic balloon pumps in high risk patients undergoing open heart surgery, *Ann Thoracic Surg* 72:54-57, 2001.

14. Klein AJ, Messenger JC, Casserly IP: Endovascular treatment of intraaortic balloon pump-induced acute limb ischemia, *Catheter Cardiovasc Interv* 70(1):138-142, 2007.

15. Marcu CB, Donohue TJ, Ferneini A, et al: Intraaortic balloon pump insertion through the subclavian artery: subclavain artery insertion of IABP, *Heart Lung Circ* 15(2):148-150, 2006.

CR 16. Nordhaug D, Steensrud T, Muller S, et al: Intraaortic balloon pumping improves hemodynamic and right ventricular efficiency in acute ischemic right ventricular failure, *Ann Thoracic Surg* 78(4):1426-1432, 2004.

CR 17. O'Grady NP, et al: Guidelines for the prevention of intravascular catheter-related infections, *Am J Infect Control* 30:476-489, 2002.

CR 18. Prunler F, et al: *Intra-aortic balloon counterpulsation (IABP) in high-risk acute myocardial infarction [abstract],* presented at First World Conference on Intra-Aortic Balloon Counterpulsation, Athens, 2000.

CR 19. Quaal SJ: Conventional timing using the arterial pressure waveform. In Quaal SJ, editor: *Comprehensive intra-aortic balloon counterpulsation,* ed 2, St Louis, 2000, Mosby.

CR 20. Quaal SJ: Caring for the intra-aortic balloon pump patient: most frequently asked questions, *Crit Care Nurs Clin North Am* 8:471-476, 1996.

CR 21. Quaal SJ: Interactive hemodynamics of IABC. In Quaal SJ, editor: *Comprehensive intra-aortic balloon counterpulsation,* St Louis, 1993, Mosby.

CR 22. Quaal SJ: Intra-aortic balloon pumping timing: an overview, *Crit Care Int* Jan-Feb:12-14, 1997.

CR 23. Quaal SJ: Nursing care of the intra-aortic balloon catheter's inner lumen, *Prog Cardiovasc Nurs* 14:11-13, 1999.

CR 24. Quaal SJ: Interpreting the arterial pressure waveform in the intra-aortic balloon pumped patient, *Prog Cardiovasc Nurs* 15:116-118, 2001.

CR 25. Quaal SJ: Physiological and clinical analysis of the arterial pressure waveform in the IABP patient, *Can Perfusion Canadienne* 10:6-13, 2000.

CR 26. Sanborn T, Sleeper LA, Bates ER, et al: Impact of thrombolysis, intraaortic balloon pump counterpulsation and their combination in cardiogenic shock complicating acute myocardial infarction: a report from the SHOCK Trial registry, *J Am Coll Cardiol* 36(3):1123-1129, 2000.

27. Sice A: Intraaortic balloon counterpulsation complicated by limb ischemia, a reflective commentary, *Nurs Crit Care* 11(6):297-304, 2006.

CR 28. Sleeper LA, Ramanathan K, Picard MH, et al: Functional status and quality of life after emergency revascularization for cardiogenic shock complicating acute myocardial infarction, *J Am Coll Cardiol* 46(2):266-273, 2005.

CR 29. Torchiana DF, et al: Intra-aortic balloon pumping for cardiac support; trends in practice and outcome, *J Thoracic Cardiovasc Surg* 114:758-764, 1997.

CR 30. Vanderheide RH, Thadhani R, Kufer DJ: Association of thrombocytopenia with the use of intra-aortic balloon pumps, *Am J Med* 105:27-32, 1998.

Additional Readings

CR Bates ER, et al: The use of intra-aortic balloon counterpulsation as an adjunct to reperfusion therapy in cardiogenic shock, *J Cardiol* 65(Suppl 1):S37-S42, 1998.

CR Berger PB, et al: Impact of an aggressive invasive catheterization and revascularization strategy on mortality in patients with cardiogenic shock in the Global Utilization of Streptokinase and Tissue Plasminogen Activator for Occluded Coronary Arteries (GUSTO-I) trial: an observational study, *Circulation* 96:122-127, 1997.

CR Blusch T, et al: Vascular complications related to intra-aortic balloon counterpulsation: an analysis of ten years experience, *Thorac Cardiovasc Surg* 45:55-59, 1997.

Bream-Rouwenhorst HR, Hobbs RA, Horwitz PA: Thrombocytopenia in patients treated with heparin, combination antiplatelet therapy, and intra-aortic balloon pump counterpulsation, *J Interv Cardiol* 21(4):350-356, 2008.

CR Christenson JT, et al: Evaluation of preoperative intra-aortic balloon pump support in high risk coronary patients, *Eur J Cardiothoracic Surg* 11:1097-1103, 1997.

CR Christenson JT, Schmuziber M, Simonet F: Effective surgical management of high-risk coronary patients using preoperative intra-aortic balloon counterpulsation therapy, *Cardiovasc Surg* 9:383-390, 2001.

Field ML, Rengarajan A, Khan O, et al: Preoperative intra aortic balloon pumps in patients undergoing coronary artery bypass grafting, *Cochrane Database Syst Rev* 1: 2007.

CR Garrett K, Grady KL: Intra-aortic balloon pumping through the common iliac artery: management of the ambulatory intra-aortic balloon pump patient, *Prog Cardiovasc Nurs* 15:14-20, 2000.

CR Kovak PJ, et al: Thrombolysis plus aortic counterpulsation improved survival of patients who present to the community hospital with cardiogenic shock, *J Am Coll Cardiol* 29:454-458, 1997.

CR Low R: Intra-aortic balloon counterpulsation in acute myocardial infarction: too few or too many? *JACC* 41:1946-1947, 2003.

CR Mertlich GB, et al: Effect of increased intra-aortic balloon pressure on catheter volume: relationship to changing attitude, *Crit Care Med* 20:297-303, 1992.

Mishra S, et al: Role of prophylactic intra-aortic balloon pump in high-risk patients undergoing percutaneous intervention, *Am J Cardiol* 98(5):608-612, 2006.

CR Ohman E, Hochman J: Aortic counterpulsion in acute myocardial infarction: physiologically important, but does the patient benefit? *Am Heart J* 141:889-892, 2001.

Osentowski MK, Holt DW: Evaluating the efficacy of intra-aortic balloon pump timing using the auto-timing mode of operation with the Datascope CS100, *J Extracorp Technol* 39(2):87-90, 2007.

Reid MB, Cottrell D: Nursing care of patients receiving intra-aortic balloon counterpulsation, *Crit Care Nurse* 25(5): 40-49, 2005.

Santa-Cruz RA, Cohen RA, Ohman EM: Aortic counterpulsation: a review of the hemodynamic effects and indications for use, *Catheter Cardiovasc Interv* 67(1):68-77, 2006.

CR Stone GW, Ohman E, Miller M: Contemporary utilization and outcomes of intra-aortic balloon counterpulsation in acute myocardial infarction, *JACC* 41:1940-1947, 2003.

CR Talley JD, Ohman EM, Mark OB: Economic implications of the prophylactic use of intra-aortic balloon counterpulsation in the setting of acute myocardial infarction: the Randomized IABP Study Group, *Am J Cardiol* 79:S90-S94, 1997.

AP Ventricular Assist Devices

P U R P O S E : Ventricular assist devices are used for cardiogenic shock and postcardiotomy support to allow for myocardial recovery, for bridge to cardiac transplantation, and for destination therapy (permanent implantation) in patients with New York Heart Association class IIIB or IV heart failure who are on optimal medical therapy and are not eligible for cardiac transplant.[3-6,9,14]

Desiree A. Fleck, Mark Puhlman

PREREQUISITE NURSING KNOWLEDGE

- Understanding of the normal anatomy and physiology of the cardiovascular, peripheral vascular, and pulmonary systems is important.
- Understanding of the management of heart failure is essential.
- Knowledge of the principles of hemodynamic monitoring, cardiopulmonary bypass, electrophysiology and dysrhythmias, and coagulation is needed.
- Clinical and technical competence related to use of ventricular assist devices (VADs) is necessary.
- Advanced cardiac life support knowledge and skills are needed.
- Complications of VAD therapy include, but are not limited to, bleeding, cardiac tamponade, right ventricular failure with univentricular support, hepatic dysfunction, pulmonary dysfunction, renal dysfunction, infection, cerebral infarcts, thrombosis, embolism, and VAD malfunction.[3,6]
- Effective cardiac assistance with the VAD is affected greatly by preload, afterload, right ventricular failure, cardiac tamponade, and cardiac dysrhythmias; the interaction between the patient and the device requires close monitoring.

AP This procedure should be performed only by physicians, advanced practice nurses, and other healthcare professionals (including critical care nurses) with additional knowledge, skills, and demonstrated competence per professional licensure or institutional standard.

- The device is implanted surgically in the operating room. Specific information concerning controls, alarms, troubleshooting, and safety features is available from each manufacturer and should be read thoroughly by the nurse before use of the equipment. Please refer to the operator's manual for all systems for more detail.
- Indications for VAD therapy include the following[4,6, 9,10, 14]:
  - ❖ Inability to wean from cardiopulmonary bypass
  - ❖ Bridge to cardiac transplant
  - ❖ New York Heart Association class IIIB or IV status in a patient whose condition does not respond to optimal medical therapy and who is not a transplant candidate
  - ❖ Bridge to myocardial recovery
- Relative contraindications of VAD therapy include the following:
  - ❖ Body surface area (BSA) less than 1.3 m² (ABIOMED BVS 5000 or AB 5000 ventricle; Abiomed Inc, Danvers, MA)[1-3]
  - ❖ BSA less than 1.5 m² (HeartMate XVE left ventricular assist device [LVAD; Thoratec Corporation, Pleasanton, CA][11,12])
  - ❖ BSA less than 1.2 m² (HeartMate II left ventricular assist device [LVAD; Thoratec Corporation, Pleasanton, CA][11,12])
  - ❖ Renal or liver failure unrelated to cardiac incident
  - ❖ Comorbidity that limits life expectancy to less than 3 years
- Psychosocial and cognitive conditions may limit the use of a VAD except in bridge to recovery because the patient needs to have the cognitive skills to manage the VAD.

- Ventricular assist devices are pulsatile or nonpulsatile.
- ABIOMED BVS 5000 circulatory support system (Fig. 56-1)[2]:
  - ❖ The ABIOMED BVS 5000 is an extracorporeal, pneumatically driven pump capable of delivering short-term (less than 3 weeks) left, right, or biventricular support.
  - ❖ The drive console controls systole by delivering air into the lower rigid plastic pumping chamber, displacing blood from the blood sac. Blood drains passively from the patient's atrium into the atrial chamber of the blood pump. When the atrial chamber of the blood pump is full and the pressure inside the atrial chamber exceeds the pressure inside the ventricular chamber, the trileaflet valve opens, allowing blood to flow into the ventricular chamber of the blood pump. Blood pump diastole is completed as soon as the ventricular chamber is filled with 100 mL. The diastolic filling time is adjusted automatically to changes in the patient's preload to ensure the ventricular chamber is filled to capacity (100 mL).
  - ❖ The vertically aligned pneumatic blood pumps are adjusted to optimize flow. The blood flow from the patient to the blood pump depends on the console used. The BVS 5000t (transport) console and the AB 5000 console allow for vacuum-assisted filling of the chamber. Filling of the pumps depends solely on gravity when the BVS 5000 or BVS 5000i (high-flow) consoles are used. The top of the blood pump should be between 0 and 10 inches below the level of the patient's atria when a 42 Fr atrial cannula is used and 4 to 14 inches when a 32 Fr or 36 Fr atrial cannula is used (see Fig. 56-1). Moving the pump above or below this level can affect flow. Adjusting the height of

the blood pump alters filling of the blood chambers. It is important to allow 2 minutes for the system to adjust before making additional changes.
  - ❖ Outflow from the BVS is used in place of cardiac output for calculations such as systemic vascular resistance, pulmonary vascular resistance, and cardiac index.
  - ❖ External heat is not applied to the blood pump, tubing, or cannulas.
  - ❖ ABIOMED tubing insulators are used to retain heat in the tubing.
  - ❖ Anticoagulation therapy with heparin is necessary.
- ABIOMED AB 5000 ventricle[1] (Fig. 56-2):
  - ❖ The AB 5000 ventricle is a pulsatile, pneumatically driven blood pump approved for short-term (less than 3 weeks) support to allow time for myocardial recovery. It can provide support for one or both ventricles and must be used in conjunction with the AB 5000 circulatory support system console. The ventricle holds approximately 100 mL of blood. Cannulas exit the skin, and the ventricle lies on the patient's abdomen. Filling of the ventricle is facilitated with a vacuum within the console and is not affected by height. The ventricle is made partially of aluminum and plastic and has inflow and outflow valves to ensure unidirectional blood flow.
  - ❖ The following items must never come into contact with the ventricle because they could damage the plastic within the ventricle: ketones, such as acetone; aromatic hydrocarbons, such as gasoline; halogenated hydrocarbon–based anesthetic agents; other hydrocarbonated hydrocarbons, such as chloroform; and highly alkaline chemicals, such as sodium hydroxide.
  - ❖ Anticoagulation therapy with heparin initially followed by warfarin (Coumadin) is necessary.

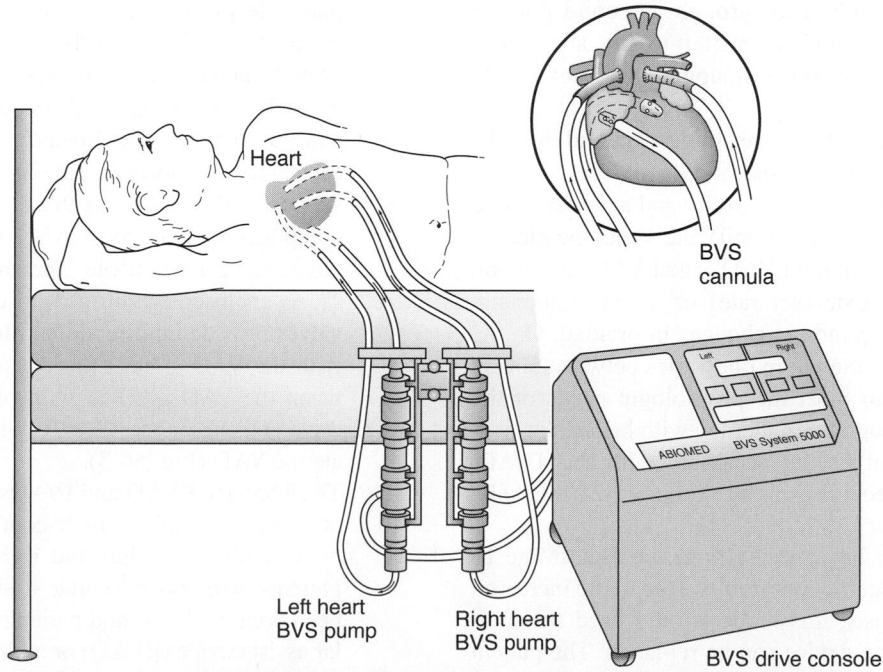

Heart

BVS cannula

Left heart BVS pump **Right heart BVS pump** **BVS drive console**

FIGURE 56-1 ABIOMED BVS 5000 System. *(From Dixon JF, Farris DD: The ABIOMED BVS 5000 system, AACN Clin Issues Crit Care Nurs 2:552-561, 1991.)*

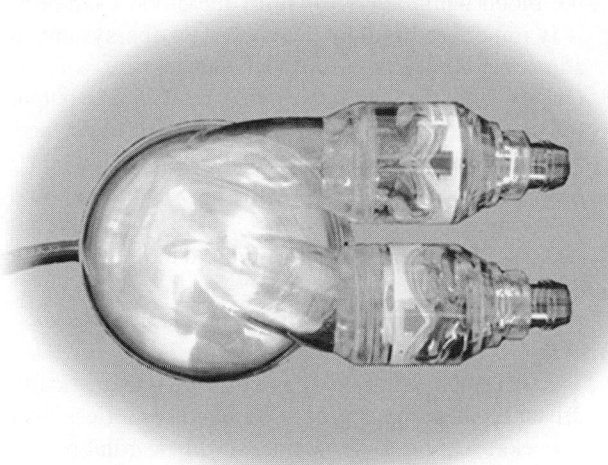

FIGURE 56-2 ABIOMED AB 5000 ventricle. *(Courtesy Abiomed, Inc, Danvers, MA.)*

- HeartMate XVE (extended lead vented electric) left ventricular assist system (LVAS):[17]
  - ❖ Thoratec Corporation offers an implantable VAD for left ventricular assistance, the HeartMate XVE LVAD.
  - ❖ This VAD is used for long-term support.
  - ❖ The LVAD may be implanted intra-abdominally or preperitoneally in a rectus muscle pocket.
  - ❖ The HeartMate XVE LVAD is made of titanium, holds 83 mL of blood, and weighs approximately 3 lb. Blood flows through a small tube placed in the left ventricular apex through a porcine inflow valve into the pump. When the pump fills with blood, a sensor inside the device starts the electric motor. Blood is pumped through a second porcine outflow valve through a graft into the aorta. The LVAD is placed in the left upper quadrant of the abdomen.
  - ❖ A driveline is passed underneath the skin and exits the right upper quadrant of the abdomen. The driveline connects the LVAD to a controller and a power source (batteries or a power base unit) and vents the electric motor that is within the LVAD. The LVAD can run on the fixed rate mode (set rate) or on the automatic mode, which responds to changes in preload. On the automatic mode, the pump rate varies between 50 and 120 beats/min to meet the physiologic needs of the patients. Anticoagulation therapy with heparin or warfarin (Coumadin) is not necessary with this LVAD. Most patients receive aspirin, 81 mg or 325 mg daily, however.
  - ❖ The device can be operated with the HeartMate IP console if the electric motor fails. Due to the increased risk of thrombosis, this mode is only used for short duration until the device can be replaced. The patient will also be anticoagulated with heparin or warfarin during this mode of operation.

- Thoratec Paracoporeal Ventricular Assist Device (PVAD):[18]
  - ❖ The Thoratec Paracorporeal VAD (PVAD) is made of polyurethane and is pneumatically driven. A flexible polyurethane diaphragm divides the blood chamber. An influx of pressurized air (through the pneumatic tubing and into the VAD) drives the flexible diaphragm against the blood chamber, pushing blood from the VAD to the patient, and controls the duration of systole. Mechanical valves provide unidirectional blood flow. When the pneumatic drive is used, the pump can only be run in a fixed mode (asynchronous) or auto mode (volume) for right, left, or biventricular support
  - ❖ The Thoratec PVAD is approved for use as a bridge to transplant and post-cardiotomy recovery.
  - ❖ The Thoratec PVAD is connected via the driveline and a cable to the dual-drive console (DDC), which controls pump function. The console is plugged into an electrical outlet when the patient is not ambulating. This VAD is primarily for short-term and intermediate use. The VADs may also be connected to the smaller TLC-II driver giving the patient 2 hours of battery life and a smaller 20 pound driver to push rather than the 500-pound dual-drive hospital driver (DDC).
  - ❖ The Thoratec PVAD may be used in smaller patients.
  - ❖ The three major components of the system are the blood pump, cannulas, and drive console. The smooth, seamless blood sac is enclosed within a rigid case. Small bubbles in a silicone oil lubricant may be seen during use. A small magnetic switch (called the Hall effect switch) is mounted in the upper case. When the PVAD is full of blood, a switch is tripped sending a signal to the console to eject blood.
- Thoratec IVAD[18]:
  - ❖ The Thoratec IVAD (Thoratec Corporation) is an implantable pneumatic system approved for postcardiotomy use and as a bridge to transplantation. It can provide univentricular or biventricular support. It is the only device approved for long-term (greater than 3 weeks if necessary) biventricular support. It is also the device of choice in patients who need ventricular support with a BSA less than 1.5 m². The three major components of the system are the blood pump, cannulas, and drive console. The smooth, seamless blood sac is enclosed within a rigid case. Two mechanical valves provide unidirectional blood flow. A fill switch with the VAD signals the console to eject the blood when the VAD is filled with blood. Either the dual-drive console or the TLC-II portable driver can operate the VAD (Fig. 56-3).
  - ❖ The Thoratec PVAD and IVADs[18] are both driven by a dual-drive console, which contains two independent drive modules for left and right ventricular support. Patients with biventricular assist devices (BiVADs) need both modules, and patients with a right ventricular assist device (RVAD) or a LVAD need one module. When only one module is being used, the other module can serve as a backup if pump failure occurs. The

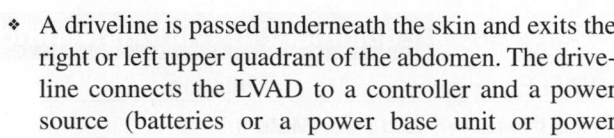

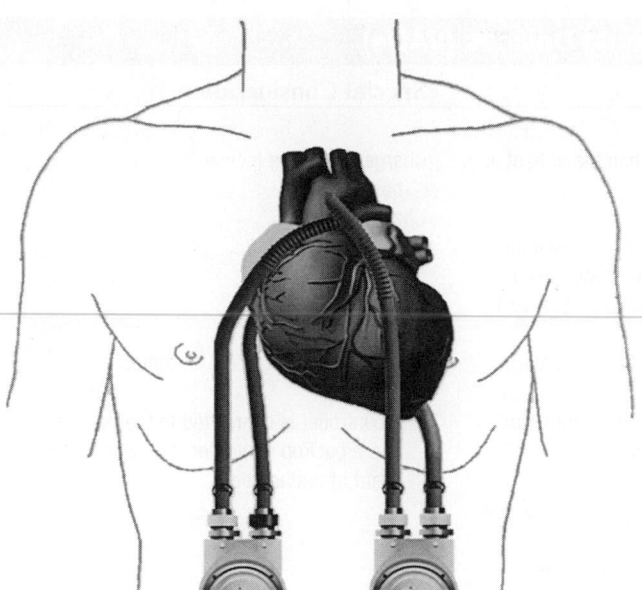

FIGURE 56-3 Thoratec biventricular assist device. *(Courtesy Thoratec Corporation, Pleasanton, CA.)*

console supplies air pressure to eject blood from the pump into the arterial system and vacuum to assist pump filling. A full 65-mL stroke volume is possible from 20 to 110 beats/min, providing cardiac outputs of 1.2 to 7.2 L/min.

* ❖ The recommended control modes for operation include asynchronous/fixed or volume/automatic. A fixed rate allows the operator to choose a VAD rate that is asynchronous with the patient's intrinsic heart rate. The automatic mode also is asynchronous to the patient's intrinsic heart rate but responds to changes in physiologic conditions.
* ❖ Anticoagulation therapy with heparin initially followed by warfarin is needed.
* The HeartMate II LVAS[16]:
  * ❖ The HeartMate II left ventricular assist system (Thoratec Corp) HeartMate II LVAS (left ventricular assist system)[16] is a continuous flow pump and is approved as a bridge to transplant and destination therapy in patients with advanced heart failure.
  * ❖ The LVAD may be implanted intra-abdominally or preperitoneally in a rectus muscle pocket.
  * ❖ The HeartMate II is made of titanium and weighs approximately 1.5 lb. Blood flows from the left ventricle through the pump and back to the patient's circulation via the outflow graft.
  * ❖ Continuous flow is generated by a small rotor inside the pump. The speed of the pump is set by the LVAD team and does not change in response to preload.
  * ❖ The LVAD is placed in the left upper quadrant of the abdomen.

* ❖ A driveline is passed underneath the skin and exits the right or left upper quadrant of the abdomen. The driveline connects the LVAD to a controller and a power source (batteries or a power base unit or power module).
* ❖ Anticoagulation therapy with heparin or warfarin is necessary with this LVAD with a goal INR range of 1.8 to 2.5. Most patients receive aspirin, 81 mg or 325 mg daily in addition to warfarin.
* The Impella LP 2.5 and LP 5.0:
  * ❖ The Impella LP 2.5 and 5.0 systems (Abiomed Inc) are nonpulsatile microaxial flow devices that deliver 2.5 L (Impella LP 2.5) or 5.0 L (Impella LP 5.0) of blood flow.[10]
  * ❖ The pumps are implanted percutaneously in the cardiac catheterization laboratory. A surgical cut down to expose the femoral artery is necessary for the Impella LP 5.0.
  * ❖ The Impella 5.0 can also be implanted directly via sternotomy.
  * ❖ When positioned properly, the Impella sits across the aortic valve, with the inlet area in the left ventricle and the outlet area in the ascending aorta.
  * ❖ Transesophageal echocardiography is needed to confirm proper placement.
  * ❖ The console continuously monitors pump placement and alerts the operator to catheter displacement and other alarm states.
* The TandemHeart (CardiacAssist, Pittsburgh, PA):[11,12]
  * ❖ The TandemHeart is a continuous centrifugal flow device that delivers up to 4 L of blood flow.[11,12] This is a left atrial to femoral bypass system for short-term use.
  * ❖ The pumps are implanted via a percutaneous approach in the cardiac catheterization laboratory.
  * ❖ There is a 21 Fr cannula that is inserted to the left atrium via a transseptal cannulation from the right atrium and blood is ejected to the centrifugal pump and returned via the femoral artery.
  * ❖ The TandemHeart operates via an electromagnetic rotor that operates at a range of 3000 to 7500 rpm.[11,12]
  * ❖ The pump is driven by a microprocessor controller
  * ❖ The TandemHeart has a dual-chamber pump. The upper housing allows for the movement of blood. The lower housing communicates with the controller and contains a continuous flow of saline with heparin to decrease the risk of thrombus formation and provide lubrication.[11,12]

EQUIPMENT

* VAD drive console/unit or monitor (Table 56-1)
* Connection cables (specific to device; see Table 56-1)
* Backup drive console/unit/monitor, batteries, and controller (see Table 56-1)
* Emergency pump device (hand crank, foot pump, hand pump or bulb, depending on device; see Table 56-1)
* Vent filters (HeartMate XVE)

TABLE 56-1   Equipment for Various Ventricular Assist Devices (VADs)

VAD Equipment	Function	Special Consideration
HeartMate XVE and HeartMate II [17]		
Power base unit (power module) with cable	Provides electrical power for the LVAD when the patient is attached.	Charges batteries (power base unit)
Battery charger	Used in conjunction with power module	Chages batteries
System monitor	Displays the VAD rate, stroke volume, and flow. Used initially in the operating room and early postoperative period to monitor LVAD flow, alarms, change modes, and program fixed rate.	
Display module	Displays VAD rate, stroke volume, mode, flow, and alarm status.	Used in the hospital and at home.
Controller	"Brains" of the system. Computer software programmed to run the LVAD and provide safety alarms is housed in the controller.	One controller is connected to the patient, and a backup controller is available in the event of malfunction.
Controller cell: One in the controller and a backup	Powers the controller so that in the event of disconnection of all power to the LVAD, an alarm sounds.	
Vent filter (XVE only)	Filters air that is shuffled back and forth through the driveline during a cycle.	
Large batteries	Two batteries are used to power the LVAD to allow for patient ambulation. Batteries are carried in a shoulder holster or fanny pack. Battery life is checked every 30 to 60 minutes by pushing down the alarm silence button. Batteries are fully charged when four green lights appear. Batteries are changed when one green light is lit.	Two batteries last approximately 4 hours. Lithium/hydride batteries can give up to 10 hours per pair
Battery clips	Used to hold batteries for portable operation.	
Hand pump (XVE only)	Used for a backup emergency.	The hand pump always must be with the patient in the event that the pump stops and cannot be started.
24-Hour emergency battery (outpatient use)	Provides backup energy source.	Each patient is given at least a 24-hour battery in the event that electrical power is lost for an extended period.
Thoratec Paracoporeal and Ventricular Assist Device [18]		
Thoratec IVAD: The smooth, seamless blood sac is enclosed within a rigid case	Two mechanical valves provide unidirectional blood flow. A fill switch within the VAD signals the console to eject the blood when the VAD is filled with blood.	
Dual-drive console	Contains two independent drive modules for left or right ventricular support.	Set rate: 50 to 60 beats/min.
Asynchronous: Rate set by healthcare provider	The console supplies air pressure to eject blood from the pump into the arterial system and supplies the vacuum to assist with VAD filling. This should always be kept plugged in except during patient transport/ambulation.	
Volume	VAD ejects when the electrical lead senses that the VAD is full. The rate and flows change depending on volume status and other physiologic changes.	
Set rate	Actual rate in asynchronous mode, volume mode: uses backup rate.	
Set % of systole	% of systole: pump ejection time 25% to 30% (1/2 of set rate, 300 ms).	
Drive pressure	Ejects blood from the VAD. LVAD: 230 to 245 mm Hg. RVAD: 140 to 160 mm Hg.	
Vacuum: −25 to −40 mm Hg	Assists with VAD filling.	
Hand pump	Can be used to run a VAD manually in the event of console failure until a backup console can be connected.	Always keep hand pumps with the console.
Electrical lead	On volume/automatic mode, the electrical lead senses when the VAD is full and communicates to the console to empty the VAD.	
Pneumatic lead	The console delivers pressurized air through the pneumatic lead to cause collapse of the blood sac and ejection of the blood into the circulation.	

TABLE 56-1 **Equipment for Various Ventricular Assist Devices (VADs)—cont'd**

VAD Equipment	Function	Special Consideration
TLC-II System Components[18]		
TLC-II driver with carrying case (the carrying case is kept over the driver for protection)	The portable driver is a lightweight, portable, pneumatic VAD driver powered by batteries or external power.	Designed to provide portable pneumatic drive power for ambulatory patients supported with the Thoratec VAD.
Mobility cart	The driver can be strapped to the cart for easy patient ambulation.	
AC adapter	Connects the portable driver to a wall outlet to allow the VAD to be run off of electrical power instead of battery when the patient is not ambulating to conserve battery strength.	
Li-ion rechargeable batteries	Provides at least 55 minutes (BiVAD support) to 80 minutes (RVAD or LVAD support).	
TLC-II battery charger	Can fully recharge one or two batteries in approximately 2 hours.	
Docking station-HeartTouch computer	Runs an interface-monitoring program that is specially designed to communicate with the TLC-II driver.	Required only for start-up and diagnostic procedures.
TLC-II Output Range		
VAD modes: Automatic or fixed	Automatic mode allows for more physiologic use of the VAD.	
VAD rate: 30 to 110 beats/min	Allows for changes in preload.	
Ejection time: 230 to 370 ms		
Peak drive pressure:		
LVAD: 240 mm Hg.		
RVAD: 160 mm Hg.		
Vacuum: −25 to −40 mm Hg		

- Dressing supplies:
  - Sterile normal saline solution
  - 4 × 4 sterile gauze pads
  - Tape, 1-inch and 2-inch
  - Sterile gloves
  - Head covers
  - Masks
  - Sterile gowns
  - Sterile drapes
  - Ace wrap (6-inch)
  - 6 × 6 bordered gauze
- Suture removal kit
  Additional equipment as needed includes the following:
- Emergency equipment and medications
- Flashlight
- Intravenous pole
- Four smooth chest clamps
- Blood pump set

PATIENT AND FAMILY EDUCATION

- Assess patient and family understanding of VAD therapy and the reason for its use. ➤*Rationale:* Clarification or reinforcement of information is an expressed patient and family need during times of stress and anxiety.
- Explain the environment and planned care to the patient and family, including the frequency of assessment, sounds and function of equipment, placement of the device, explanation of alarms, dressings and therapy, decreased or assisted mobility, and parameters for discontinuation of therapy. Before surgery, a meeting with another patient on a VAD may be helpful for the patient and family, if both patients are agreeable. ➤*Rationale:* This communication provides information and encourages the patient and family to ask questions or voice concerns or fears related to the therapy. Meeting with another patient with a VAD provides social support.
- If appropriate, begin discharge teaching to include operation of VAD, dressing changes, battery changes, placement of self on and off of the battery and the power base unit or monitor, changing of the controller, and appropriate bathing techniques with use of shower equipment. ➤*Rationale:* This teaching provides information and ensures that the patient will be safe at home. It also allows the patient and family to ask questions as needed.

PATIENT ASSESSMENT AND PREPARATION

Patient Assessment

- Assess the patient's medical history, history of heart failure, height, weight, body surface area (BSA) specifically related to the competency of the aortic/pulmonic valves, competency of the mitral/tricuspid valves, pulmonary hypertension, right ventricular function, left ventricular function, and peripheral vascular disease. ➤*Rationale:* This assessment provides baseline data regarding cardiac functioning and facilitates decision making regarding insertion of the appropriate device and postoperative management.

- Perform cardiovascular, hemodynamic, peripheral vascular, neurovascular, and psychosocial assessment and assessment of body mass index and BSA. ➤*Rationale:* These assessments provide baseline data and help with determination of the type of device to use.
- Assess the current laboratory profile, including the complete blood cell count, platelet count, prothrombin time, partial thromboplastin time (PTT), international normalized ratio (INR), blood chemistry, liver profile, protein, and albumin levels. ➤*Rationale:* This assessment provides baseline data and may indicate end-organ dysfunction related to low-flow state. It also may be used to predict the patient's risk of bleeding.

Patient Preparation

- Verify correct patient with two identifiers. ➤ *Rationale:* Prior to performing a procedure, the nurse should ensure the correct identification of the patient for the intended intervention.
- Ensure that the patient and family understand preoperative teaching. Answer questions as they arise, and reinforce information as needed. ➤*Rationale:* This communication evaluates and reinforces understanding of previously taught information.
- Ensure that informed consent has been signed (if it is known before surgery that the VAD will be placed). ➤*Rationale:* Informed consent protects the rights of the patient and makes a competent decision possible for the patient and family.
- Perform a pre-procedure verification and time out, if nonemergent. ➤*Rationale:* Ensures patient safety.
- Provide emotional support to the patient and family. ➤*Rationale:* The patient and family are under an extreme amount of stress.

Procedure for Ventricular Assist Devices

Steps	Rationale	Special Considerations
Abiomed BVS 5000 VAD (Level M*)		
1. 🔲HH		
2. Obtain the needed equipment: A. Abiomed BVS 5000 blood chambers. B. Abiomed BVS 5000, 5000i, or 5000t console; Abiomed AB 5000 console.		
3. Ensure that the console is plugged into a three-pronged outlet with emergency generator backup.	Provides the power source.	The battery life is approximately 1 hour.
4. Adjust the level of the blood pump between 0 and 10 inches below the level of the patient's atria when a 42 Fr atrial cannula is used and 4 to 14 inches when a 32 Fr or 36 Fr atrial cannula is used, for optimal filling.	The level of the pump is important in assisting with gravity filling of the atrial chamber of the blood pumps, especially with use of the BVS 5000 or 5000i console.	
5. Inspect the blood chambers for complete filling and emptying.	Ensures adequate VAD output.	Optimize blood pump filling by: • Lowering the blood pump. • Administering intravenous fluids or blood products as prescribed. • Assessing for cardiac tamponade. • Administering inotropes (e.g., milrinone, dobutamine) as necessary to optimize right ventricular function when the patient has only LVAD support.

*Level M: Manufacturer's recommendations only

Procedure **for Ventricular Assist Devices**—*Continued*

Steps	Rationale	Special Considerations
6. Inspect the valves within the blood pump chamber at least every 2 hours for thrombus formation. Use a flashlight to assist in visualization.	Thrombus formation can lead to pulmonary embolism or stroke.	Administer a heparin infusion to maintain a PTT of 2 to 2.5 times the laboratory's normal value or an activated coagulation time (ACT) of 180 to 200 seconds or as prescribed. A heparin bolus is not recommended unless specifically prescribed; heparin is usually started after mediastinal drainage is less than 50 to 75 mL/hr × 3 hours. PTT or ACT should be monitored hourly until therapeutic and then every 2 hours. For unresolved atrial or ventricular dysrhythmias, the ACT may be increased to 250 to 300 seconds or the PTT may be increased to 2.5 to 3 times normal.
7. Ensure the connection between the cannula and tubing is secured.	Disconnection of the cannula or tubing can result in exsanguination.	Tie bands should be applied in the operating room. When transporting a patient, a team member (e.g., nurse, perfusionist, physician) must be responsible for monitoring the tubing and blood chambers.
Abiomed AB 5000 Ventricle (Level M*) 1. 🔲 2. Obtain the needed equipment: A. AB 5000 ventricle. B. AB 5000 console.		
3. Ensure that the AB 5000 console is plugged into a three-pronged outlet with emergency generator backup.	The AB 5000 ventricle can be used only with the AB 5000 console.	The battery life is approximately 1 hour.
4. Inspect the valves within the ventricle at least every 8 hours for thrombus formation. Use a flashlight to assist in visualization.	Thrombus formation can lead to pulmonary embolism or stroke.	Administer a heparin infusion to maintain a PTT of 2 to 2.5 times the laboratory's normal value or an ACT of 180 to 200 seconds or as prescribed. A heparin bolus is not recommended unless specifically prescribed; heparin is usually started after mediastinal drainage is less than 50 to 75 mL/hr × 3 hours. PTT or ACT should be monitored hourly until therapeutic and then every 2 hours. For unresolved atrial or ventricular dysrhythmias, the ACT may be increased to 250 to 300 seconds or the PTT may be increased to 2.5 to 3 times normal.

*Level M: Manufacturer's recommendations only

Procedure continues on following page

Procedure	for Ventricular Assist Devices—*Continued*	
Steps	**Rationale**	**Special Considerations**
5. Troubleshooting Abiomed BVS 5000 and AB 5000 console alarms:	Alarms must be addressed promptly to prevent complications.	
A. Low flow:	Inadequate VAD output and decreased organ perfusion may result from:	
• Assess for obstruction of lines, and correct the problem if present.	Obstruction of blood lines.	
• Lower the blood pump chamber (BVS 5000 only).	Blood pump placed too high (BVS 5000 only).	
• Administer fluids or blood products as prescribed.	Inadequate blood volume.	
• Provide inotropic support or pulmonary vasodilators or both to improve right ventricular function for patients with only LVAD support.	Right ventricular failure.	
B. High pressure/low flow:	Inadequate VAD output and decreased organ perfusion may result from:	
• Check tubing and cannula for kinks.	Cannula or blood pump tubing kinked or occluded.	
• Decrease systemic vascular resistance; keep systolic blood pressure less than 140 mm Hg or as prescribed.	Increased systemic vascular resistance.	
C. Low pressure/low flow:	If tubing disconnects from the console, the VAD stops, which can lead to death.	Check lines; reconnect driveline to resume flow. If BiVAD support is needed with the Abiomed system, ensure that left-sided flow is higher than right-sided flow to avoid pulmonary edema.
• Ensure the tubing is connected to the console.	Disconnection of the tubing from the console.	
• Check the tubing for leaks and replace the tubing if needed.	Leak in the tubing.	
D. Low battery:	Potential for VAD stoppage.	The battery life is approximately 1 hour.
• Ensure that the console is plugged into a three-pronged outlet with emergency generator backup.	The battery has less than 10 minutes of power.	
E. Continuous audible alarm:	VAD failure.	Remove the foot pump.
• Use the foot pump (BVS 5000, 5000i, 5000t) or hand pump (AB 5000) to operate the VAD.		Move the transfer level to the vertical position.
• Call for help and change the console.		
F. Complete console failure:	VAD failure.	Remove the foot pump.
• Use the foot pump (BVS 5000, 5000i, 5000t) or hand pump (AB 5000) to operate the VAD.		
• Call for help to change the console.		

HeartMate XVE[17] and HeartMate II[16] LVAS

1. **HH**

2. Changing from the power base unit or power module to batteries.	Ensures that the battery is charged.	Batteries are fully charged when four green lights appear.

Procedure for Ventricular Assist Devices—*Continued*

Steps	Rationale	Special Considerations
A. Check the battery life every 30 to 60 minutes by pushing down the alarm silence button.		Batteries are changed when two green lights are lit.
B. Place a battery into each battery clip by lining up the arrow on the large battery and battery clip and inserting until the battery clicks securely into the holder.	Allows patient ambulation.	Ensure location of hand pump.
C. Disconnect the white controller cable from the power base unit (power module) cable by loosening the white nut and then pulling them apart.	An alarm sounds once per second, and a yellow wrench lights (XVE) or the green dot flashes (HM-II), indicating disconnection from the power base unit (power module).	Do not disconnect both power sources at the same time or the VAD loses power and may stop.
D. Connect the white controller cable to the battery clip.	The alarm is resolved.	
E. Disconnect the black controller cable from the power base unit (power module) cable by loosening the black nut and then pulling them apart.	An alarm sounds once per second, and a yellow wrench lights (XVE) or the green dot flashes (HM-II), indicating disconnection from the power base unit. The alarm resolves after the cable is connected properly.	HeartMate XVE is represented by XVE and the HeartMate II is represented by HM-II.
3. Changing from batteries to power base unit (power module).		Patients are attached to the power base unit (power module) at night.
A. Disconnect the white controller cable from the battery clip.		An alarm sounds once per second, and a yellow wrench lights (XVE) or the green dot flashes (HM-II), indicating disconnection from the battery. Do not disconnect both cables at the same time because power failure occurs.
B. Connect the white controller cable to the white power base unit (power module) cable connection.	Patient data return to the personal or display monitor.	The alarm is resolved.
C. Disconnect the black controller cable from the battery clip.	Allows the power to be returned to the power base unit (XVE) or the green dot flashes (HM-II).	An alarm sounds once per second, and a yellow wrench lights (XVE) or the green dot flashes (HM-II), indicating disconnection from the battery.
D. Connect the black controller cable to the black power base unit (power module).	Returns the power to the power base unit (power module).	The alarm is resolved.
E. Remove the batteries from the clips and place the batteries back into the power base unit (battery charging unit).	Allows the batteries to recharge.	
4. Changing modes (XVE only).		Some physicians prefer the fixed mode for the initial 24 hours of insertion and on select patients.
A. Touch the mode button (cloud/swirl picture) on the controller.	In the fixed mode, the pump runs at a predetermined set rate; the factory set rate is 50 and is adjusted specific to the patient's needs.	One beep indicates that the mode changed to fixed; two beeps indicate that the mode changed to automatic.

Procedure continues on following page

Procedure for Ventricular Assist Devices—*Continued*

Steps	Rationale	Special Considerations
B. Adjust the rate while in the fixed mode as needed or prescribed.	In the automatic mode, the pump rate adjusts between 50 and 120 beats/min based on preload and right ventricular function.	
5. Self-test.		
A. Place the patient on the power base unit (power module), then hold down the mode button until all the lights on the controller light and a loud alarm sounds.	A self-test is done each day to check the function of the pump, controller, and controller cell strength.	If the controller cell is low, the red battery light goes on and then off, then flashes for the duration of the self-test; at the end of the self-test, a yellow wrench lights (XVE) or yellow dot flashes (HM-II) and the display screen reads "controller cell low."
B. Observe the battery picture on the right top corner of the controller to assess battery strength.	A controller cell battery usually lasts 3 to 6 months.	The patient should be in a sitting or lying position. The pump slows to 40 beats/min during the self-test.
6. Changing the controller.		
A. Place the controller cell (small round black) battery in the new controller.	Provides power to the controller.	The patient should be in a sitting or lying position.
B. Lay out the new controller next to the old controller.	Eases the transition and changing of the controllers.	
C. Ensure the hand pump is available (XVE only).	The hand pump nearby allows easy use in the event of the inability to connect the new controller.	
D. Disconnect the white cable from the battery or power base (power module).	Allows for the controller change.	The controller alarms once a second, and a yellow wrench lights (XVE) or green dot flashes (HM-II).
E. Disconnect the black cable from the battery or power base (power module).	Allows for the controller change.	The controller alarms continuously; the pump stops.
F. XVE only: Push down the black release button, and disconnect the controller from the driveline. HM-II only: Twist the release lever guard and push down the silver release lever and disconnect the controller from the driveline.	Allows for the controller change.	The controller stops alarming.
G. Line up the "black triangles (XVE only) or black lines (HM-II only)," and connect the new controller.	Eases the transition when connecting the new controller.	The controller starts alarming.
H. Connect the new white cable to a battery or power base (power module) cable.	Allows the patient data to be displayed and the power to be restored.	The pump starts at a fixed rate of 50; it alarms once per second, and a yellow wrench lights (XVE only). The pump starts at the preset rate of the controller (HM-II only)
I. Connect the new black cable to a battery or power base (power module) cable.	Restores power.	The controller stops alarming.

Procedure for Ventricular Assist Devices—*Continued*

Steps	Rationale	Special Considerations
J. XVE only: Switch the mode to automatic by touching the swirl/cloud mode button on the controller.	The pump turns on in the fixed mode at a rate of 50. The automatic mode is considered to be more physiologic.	The fixed rate can be adjusted at a later time if needed.
7. Hand pumping (XVE only).	Used when the VAD fails.	Never hand pump if the LVAD is still pumping. The controller continues to alarm until disconnected or the controller battery cell is removed.
A. Remove the vent filter, disconnect VAD from the controller, and connect the hand pump.	Allows for hand pumping	
B. Push in the white button (purge valve) and hold.	Purges the air.	
C. Push in the black ball and hold.	Provides vacuum.	
D. Release the white button.	Allows for reinflation of the ball.	
E. Release the black ball.	The ball inflates.	
F. Count to 10 slowly.	Allows for adequate vacuum.	
G. Press the white button	Allows the ball to fill all the way	
H. Swing the handles around and pump 60 to 90 times a minute.	Allows for adequate VAD pumping and flow.	Ensure that the black ball is fully depressed during pumping and fills completely.
8. Switching from hand pumping to the pneumatic console (XVE only).	Used when the VAD fails.	Hand pumping must be done before changing the patient to the pneumatic console.
A. Ensure that the stroke volume limiter is attached to the pneumatic connection on the back of the console, and ensure that the console is plugged into the AC outlet.	The stroke volume limiter is required to shuttle air back and forth between the VAD and the console.	
B. Turn on the pneumatic console.	Supplies the power.	The button is located on the front of the console on the far left.
C. Disconnect the hand pump from the vent port of the driveline and connect it to the stroke volume limiter.	The patient could become unresponsive.	The LVAD is stopped for approximately 1 minute. Ensure the patient is lying down. Maintain a patent airway and proceed.
D. Ensure the vent clip on the stroke volume limiter is open.	Allows for adequate pumping.	
E. Push the vent button.	The system reads "vent cycle activated" when it is venting. When the cycle is complete, the message disappears.	The system vents itself; this takes about 10 seconds.
F. Close the vent clip on the stroke volume limiter before the vent cycle is complete.	Allows for the VAD to function.	
G. Push the fixed button. Gradually, over the next few minutes, increase the rate to the patient's normal rate.	The pump starts at a rate of 72.	The pump runs only on fixed. Record the rate. Flows are not displayed.

Procedure continues on following page

Procedure for Ventricular Assist Devices—*Continued*

Steps	Rationale	Special Considerations
H. The pump must be vented every 4 hours by: 1. Opening the vent clip 2. Pushing the vent button 3. When the cycle is complete, close the vent clip. 4. Pumping resumes.	Assess the stroke volume limiter for movement of the diaphragm and buildup of moisture.	Ensure the patient is lying down throughout the entire procedure.
9. Troubleshooting HeartMate XVE[10] alarms (alarm symbol):		Always check the patient, then check connections from patient to controller and then from controller to patient. If patient is on the monitor, the alarm is visible on the monitor.
A. Alarm: Red heart: • Check whether the LVAD is still pumping by listening for the sound and feeling over the abdomen. • Check that the controller is connected securely to the driveline. • Change the power source. (change batteries or, if on the power base unit (power module). • Remove the vent filter. • If the device still fails to operate, disconnect the system controller power connections and begin manual pumping with the HeartMate hand pump. • Seek additional help.	The VAD may not be functioning adequately.	Emits a steady tone. Can occur if the LVAD flow is less than 1.5 L/min. Give intravenous fluids and treat dysrhythmias as prescribed.
B. Alarm: yellow wrench: • Check the connections. • Check that the batteries are in the battery clips properly. • Prepare to change the controller. • Call the VAD coordinator before changing the controller.	The VAD may not be functioning adequately.	Emits 1 beep per second.
C. Alarm: 1/2 yellow wrench: • Call for help. • Replace the system controller.	The VAD may not be functioning adequately.	Emits 1 beep per second.
D. Alarm: Red battery: • Immediately replace the batteries, or change to an alternate power source. The LVAD automatically goes into the Power Saver Mode (50 beats/min).	Less than 5 minutes of battery power remains.	Emits a steady tone.
E. Alarm: Yellow battery: • Change to an alternate power source.	Less than 15 minutes of battery power remains.	Emits 1 beep per second.

Procedure for Ventricular Assist Devices—*Continued*

Steps	Rationale	Special Considerations
F. Alarm: Yellow battery, flashing: • Replace the system controller battery cell. • Perform a system controller self test to clear the alarm.		Does not emit an audio sound.
G. Power base (power module) unit alarm: **AC fail:** • Change the power sources. Switch from the power base unit (power module) to batteries or emergency power pack. • Ensure that the power base unit (power module) is plugged into an outlet with emergency power backup. • If all batteries are used up before electrical power is restored, use the emergency power pack or prepare to hand pump.	External power to the power base unit (power module) is off. The power base unit internal battery powers the pump for 45 minutes.	Emits a steady tone.
H. Power base unit (power module) alarm: **Lo batt:** • Change the power sources. Switch from the power base unit to (power module) to batteries. • If all batteries are used up before the electrical power is restored, use the emergency power pack or prepare to hand pump.	The power base unit (power module) internal battery is almost depleted.	This alarm is a steady tone.
I. Power base unit (power module) Alarm: **Alarm reset:** • Press the alarm reset switch. • The AC fail alarm is silenced and does not come back on.	Used to silence the power base unit AC (power module) fail alarm.	If the patient is connected to the power base unit (power module), all alarms sound at the power base unit (power module) and controller; both need to be silenced.
10. Troubleshooting HeartMate II alarms (alarm symbol):		Always check the patient, then check connections from patient to controller and then from controller to patient. If patient is on the monitor, the alarm is visible on the monitor.
A. Alarm: Red heart: • Check whether the LVAD is still pumping by listening for the sound with a stethoscope. • Check that the controller is connected securely to the driveline. • Change the power source. (Change batteries or, if on the power base unit (power module).	The VAD may not be functioning adequately. If VAD is running, check patient for hypovolemia, lethal dysrhythmias, hypertension or right heart failure If device is not running, perform procedures to left.	Emits a steady tone. Can occur if the LVAD flow is less than 1.5 L/min. Give intravenous fluids and treat dysrhythmias as prescribed.

Procedure continues on following page

Procedure   for Ventricular Assist Devices—*Continued*

Steps	Rationale	Special Considerations
• If the device still fails to operate, disconnect the system controller power connections and prepare to change system controller. Consult the VAD coordinator immediately and change system controller. DO NOT GO BACK TO POWER BASE (POWER MODULE). Remain on batteries. • Seek additional help.		
B. Alarm: Green dot flashing: • Check the connections. • Check that the batteries are in the battery clips properly. • Prepare to change the controller. • Call the VAD coordinator before changing the controller.	The VAD may not be functioning adequately.	Emits 1 beep per second.
C. Alarm: Red battery: Immediately replace the batteries, or change to an alternate power source. The LVAD automatically goes into the Power Saver Mode	Less than 5 minutes of battery power remains.	Emits a steady tone.
D. Alarm: Yellow battery: Change to an alternate power source.	Less than 15 minutes of battery power remains.	Emits 1 beep per second.
E. Alarm: Yellow battery, flashing: • Replace the system controller battery cell. • Perform a system controller self test to clear the alarm.		Does not emit an audio sound.
F. Power base (power module) unit alarm: AC fail: • Change the power sources. Switch from the power base unit (power module) to batteries or emergency power pack. • Ensure that the power base unit (power module) is plugged into an outlet with emergency power backup. • If all batteries are used up before electrical power is restored, use the emergency power pack.	External power to the power base unit (power module) is off. The power base unit internal battery powers the pump for 45 minutes.	Emits a steady tone.

Thoratec Dual Driver and TLC-II[18]

1. **HH**
2. Dual driver console: switching to the dual driver console.

Procedure for Ventricular Assist Devices—*Continued*

Steps	Rationale	Special Considerations
A. Open the back door of the console.	Allows access to some of the controls.	
B. Turn on the top and bottom module using the toggle switch.	Allows use in the biventricular mode.	
C. Turn on the top and the bottom compressor by switching the "light" switches on.	Turns on the power to both VADs.	
D. Place the emergency valve on the back inside console door to the center "normal" position.	Allows for emergency protection.	
E. Adjust the set rate to the previous setting.	Allows for optimal use of VADs.	
F. Adjust the set % systole to the previous setting.	Allows for optimal emptying and filling.	
G. Adjust the pressure to the previous setting.	Optimal setting is determined in the operating room.	
H. Adjust the vacuum to the previous setting.	Optimal setting is determined in the operating room.	
I. Connect the pneumatic lines; change the LVAD (red) line first, then the RVAD (blue) line.	Allows the VADs to function.	
J. Connect the electric leads.	Provides data input.	
K. Place on the volume mode.	Provides for better cardiac output or VAD flow.	
L. Assess for VAD filling and emptying.	Ensures adequate filling and emptying.	
M. Readjust pressure and the vacuum as needed.	Optimizes filling and emptying.	Do not exceed a pressure of 250 mm Hg or a vacuum of 50 mm Hg.
3. Assessment of VAD filling.		
A. Check the green fill light on the console.	The green light flashes with each VAD ejection.	
B. Visually inspect the VAD to ensure that the blood sac is filling completely.	Ensures adequate filling.	
C. Incomplete VAD filling: Correct as needed: • Volume load. • Coagulopathies. • Medications to improve right ventricular output as prescribed. • Increase pharmacologic support as prescribed.	Incomplete VAD filling may occur for physiologic reasons, including hypovolemia, bleeding, right ventricular failure (LVAD only), ventricular recovery, cardiac tamponade, or inadequate pharmacologic support.	
D. Incomplete VAD filling: Correct as needed: • Increase vacuum. • Decrease set rate. • Decrease set % systole.	Mechanical reasons for incomplete VAD filling may occur because of a kinked cannula or pneumatic hose, insufficient vacuum, set rate too high, or eject time too long.	
4. Assessment of VAD ejection.		
A. Flash test is done by shining the light from a flashlight at an angle through the VAD housing and assessing for a flash of light on the opposite side.	If the flash of light is seen, the blood sac is emptying completely.	If the VAD is not ejecting completely, the displayed VAD flows are not accurate.

Procedure continues on following page

Procedure for Ventricular Assist Devices—*Continued*

Steps	Rationale	Special Considerations
B. Incomplete VAD emptying: • Increase the drive pressure (should be at least 100 mm Hg higher than the pulmonary artery systolic pressure for a RVAD and 100 mm Hg higher than the systolic blood pressure for a LVAD). • Lower the systolic blood pressure (goal, less than <140 mm Hg). • Increase the set % systole.	VAD drive pressures too low. Systolic pulmonary artery or systemic blood pressure too high. Outflow cannula kinked. Set % systole too low.	
5. Start up procedure for TLC-II. A. Place the driver in the docking station. B. Connect the power, and turn it on. C. Connect the power cable (yellow) and the computer cable (green). D. Place the two charged batteries in the holders. E. Use the setup plugs to eliminate pressure alarms during setup.		
F. Turn on the key switch, remove the key, and place it in the pocket of the carrying case on the key chain.	Ensures VAD functioning and maintains key location.	
G. Press the "Silence" button.	Silences the alarm for 30 seconds.	

H. On the HeartTouch computer, touch the VAD settings, press initialize, and confirm the following parameters or adjust to the individual patient:
• VAD configuration: BiVAD or LVAD
• Mode: Automatic or fixed
• Low rate: 50 beats/min
• LVAD beat rate: 80 beats/min (default rate on fixed mode)
• RVAD beat rate: 70 beats/min
• Eject time: 300 msec
• Accumulator pressure:
  - BiVAD: 250 mm Hg
  - LVAD: 250 mm Hg
  - RVAD: 220 mm Hg
	Ensures adequate use and function of the VAD system.	

I. Enter the patient's name and identification number.	Maintains the settings for the patient.	
J. Verify that the patient is connected to the appropriate pneumatic and electrical lines.	Ensures adequate VAD function.	The 5-foot section comes from the VAD, and the 7-foot section from the console; they connect together to form a 12-foot line. The lines are color coded; red is LVAD and blue is RVAD.

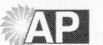

Procedure for Ventricular Assist Devices—*Continued*

Steps	Rationale	Special Considerations
K. Connect the patient to the TLC-II driver. Connect the pneumatic LVAD line to the console first by separating the 12-foot line. Connect the 5-foot section to the console. Next, connect the RVAD pneumatic line.		Always change the LVAD lead first, then the RVAD.
L. Connect the "fill" electric cable(s) next. The 5-foot section connects to the console.		
M. Switch to the automatic mode.	Allows for more physiologic use of the VAD.	
N. Adjust the vacuum regulator.	Allows for more efficient use of the VAD. Ensure that the VADs are filling properly.	
6. Troubleshooting Thoratec [17,18] alarms:		
A. Pressure alarm: Drive pressure less than 100 mm Hg or greater than 250 mm Hg. • Adjust pressure to recommended settings, and assess VAD emptying. • Ensure pneumatic line is connected (low pressure). • Change pneumatic line if leaking. • Change to backup console.	The pressure may be high or low because of VAD rate change, pressure changed by a healthcare provider, pneumatic leak, transducer failure or calibration incorrect, or compressor or uninterruptible power supply failure.	
B. Low battery alarm: • Plug the console into a wall outlet.	Module batteries have less than 30 minutes power; uninterruptible power supply has less than 5 minutes of power.	Uninterruptible power supply battery time is 40 minutes; the status panel is on the lower front console indicated by 4 four green lights, which disappear one at a time. Keep the console plugged in at all times except when the patient is ambulating or being transported to another department.
C. Synch alarm (-E- instead of VAD output): • Treat the physiologic causes. • Adjust the pressure and the vacuum to the recommended settings, and change the console. • Change the gray electrical lead.	The synch alarm may result from no fill signal, poor VAD filling, fill cable (gray electric lead) malfunction, drive pressure less than 100 mm Hg or greater than 250 mm Hg, eject time less than 250 msec, set rate too high, set % systole too high, fill cable disconnection, fill switch failure (extremely rare; —VAD functions only on asynch mode), or module failure.	

Procedure continues on following page

Procedure for Ventricular Assist Devices—*Continued*

Steps	Rationale	Special Considerations
7. Troubleshooting TLC-II[18] Alarms:		
A. Low batteries:.	The battery needs to be replaced because there is less than 10 minutes of battery life left.	
• Replace the battery packs immediately; replace the indicated battery first: change battery A or B.		
• Switch to backup driver immediately.		
• Then change the emergency battery in the initial driver.		
B. Loss of full signal: No L or R full signal, check the cable.	Loss of full signal may result from poor VAD filling, electric lead malfunction or disconnection, full switch failure in the VAD, pneumatic lead disconnected, or driver malfunction.	
• Check the VAD for filling; fill the cable, pneumatic lead, and all connections.		
• Change the fill cable if the VAD is filling completely.		
• Administer volume if not filling completely.		
C. High pressure: High L or R pressure.	Pneumatic lead occlusion, cannula kinked or occluded, or transducer failure.	
• Check the VAD cannula and the pneumatic leads.		
D. Low pressure: Low L or R pressure, check, replace.	Pneumatic line disconnection, compressor failure, or system air leak.	
• Check VAD, pneumatic lines, and for system leak.		
• Replace with backup driver.		
E. High vacuum: High L or R vacuum; replace.	A high-vacuum alarm may result from a transducer error or failure or because of a compressor or vacuum relief valve occlusion.	
• Verify the VAD is working.		
• Adjust the vacuum regulator to reduce vacuum; if not corrected, replace the driver.		
F. Low vacuum: Low L or R vacuum; replace.	A low-vacuum alarm may result from compressor failure, solenoid failure, or a system leak.	
• Check the VAD.		
• Adjust the vacuum regulator; if not corrected, replace the driver.		
G. Occlusion alarms: RVAD or LVAD occlusion;, check lines and VAD.	Occlusion alarms may result from pneumatic line occlusion or cannula occluded or kinked.	
• Check the pneumatic lines, cannula, and VAD.		
• Call for assistance.		
H. High temperature: High temperature; replace.	The high-temperature alarm may result from a blocked air vent.	
• Check the air vent, clear the air intake filter if necessary, replace.		

Procedure for Ventricular Assist Devices—*Continued*

Steps	Rationale	Special Considerations
I. Low temperature: Low temperature; wait. • Wait until the driver warms up.	The driver may be too cold.	
J. Service interval: Service interval; replace. • Replace with backup; return to Thoratec for service.	Preset at 1500 hours (62 days of continuous use).	
K. Internal alarm: Alarm 18 to 22; replace. • Replace immediately. • Notify the team.	A problem exists within the driver electronics.	
L. Emergency backup: No message or emergency system on. • Message display off: Check whether the driver has power before replacing.	All power sources have been removed, solenoid drive electronics fail, motor electronics fail to deliver sufficient pressure, or microprocessor fails.	

M. Complete mechanical failure
  1. Assess the patient; determine the need for cardiopulmonary resuscitation (CPR).
  2. Observe the VAD/console/blood pumps and identify the alarm.
  3. If the pumps have stopped, connect the hand pump(s) to the driveline(s) and squeeze at 60 beats/min.
  4. If the patient is on the dual-driver console and only one module fails, the VAD(s) can be driven temporarily by the module that is working by placing the emergency selector valve into the appropriate position.
 	
  5. Change to the backup console.
  6. Notify the cardiac transplant VAD surgeon. Consider CPR.
	Provides a source of power.
	
	If VAD(s) are not restarted, patient death may result.
		Do not hand pump the RVAD greater than the LVAD.
		Keep the hand pump with the patient at all times.
		The emergency selector valve is located on the inside of the console back door; this has three positions.
		The center position is "normal," and the driver modules operate independently.
		The "out" position allows the top module to drive both VADs.
		The "in" position allows the bottom module to drive both VADs.

Expected Outcomes

• Increased myocardial oxygen supply and decreased myocardial oxygen demand
• Increased cardiac output
• Increased tissue perfusion
• Safe bridge to heart transplant or recovery
• Improved exercise tolerance and quality of life

Unexpected Outcomes

• Device failure
• VAD infection
• Systemic infection
• Neurologic dysfunction
• Bleeding and coagulation disorders
• Multisystem organ failure
• Thrombotic event
• Pain

Procedure continues on following page

Patient Monitoring and Care

Steps	Rationale	Reportable Conditions
		These conditions should be reported if they persist despite nursing interventions.
1. Perform systematic cardiovascular, respiratory, peripheral vascular, and hemodynamic assessment every 60 minutes and as patient status necessitates. Follow institution standard.		
A. Level of consciousness.	Assesses for the adequacy of cerebral perfusion; thrombi may develop and dislodge during VAD therapy.	• Change in level of consciousness, increased agitation or confusion
B. Vital signs and pulmonary artery pressures.	Demonstrates the effectiveness of VAD therapy and evaluates ventricular function.	• Unstable vital signs and abnormal hemodynamic pressures • Lack of response to VAD therapy
C. VAD flow and mixed venous oxygen saturation.	Demonstrates the effectiveness of VAD therapy.	• Abnormal values
D. Circulation to the extremities.	Demonstrates adequate peripheral perfusion. If reportable conditions are found, they may indicate thrombotic or embolic obstruction of perfusion to an extremity.	• Capillary refill greater than 2 seconds • Diminished or absent pulses (radial, popliteal, tibial, pedal) • Color pale, mottled, or cyanotic • Diminished or absent sensation • Pain • Diminished or absent movement • Cool or cold to touch
E. Urine output.	Demonstrates adequate perfusion to the kidneys.	• Urine output less than 0.5 mL/kg/hr
2. Assess VAD, heart, and lung sounds every 4 hours and as needed. Follow institution standard.	Abnormal VAD, heart, and lung sounds may indicate the need for additional treatment.	• Abnormal VAD sounds, such as such as grinding, sputtering • Diastolic murmur • Crackles or rhonchi
3. Monitor for signs of inadequate filling and emptying.	Adequate VAD function depends on an appropriate volume status. See each section for more detail. Abiomed BVS 5000: Atrial and ventricular chambers expand and collapse completely when adequate filling and emptying occurs. Thoratec: Absence of a "flash" indicates incomplete emptying; absence of green fill light indicates incomplete filling.	• Inadequate filling or emptying
4. Logroll the patient every 2 hours until hemodynamic stability is obtained (XVE, HM-II, Thoratec PVAD and IVAD) then advance activity as tolerated. TandemHeart, Impella and BVS 5000 patients should remain on bedrest for the duration of their support. Prop pillows to support the patient and to maintain alignment. Consider specialty beds for high-risk skin.	Promotes comfort and skin integrity, and prevents kinking of the VAD drivelines. Note: This step is for hemodynamically stable conditions only.	• Disruption of skin integrity

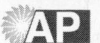

Patient Monitoring and Care —*Continued*

Steps	Rationale	Reportable Conditions
5. Initiate passive and active range-of-motion exercises every 2 hours.	Prevents venous stasis and muscle atrophy.	• Contractures
6. Assess the area around the VAD cannulas/drivelines exit site(s) every 2 hours and as needed for evidence of bleeding. Ensure that each driveline is positioned properly and secured. Use of a VAD stabilizer belt[17] may help.	Anticoagulation therapy increases the risk of bleeding.	• Bleeding at exit/driveline site
7. Assess coagulation studies: A. Monitor complete blood cell count, platelet, prothrombin time, PTT, and INR as prescribed. B. Anticoagulation guidelines (per hospital policy as prescribed for each individual patient). C. Monitor haptoglobin and plasma-free hemoglobin for signs of hemolysis as prescribed.	All VADs except the HeartMate XVE require prophylactic anticoagulation therapy to prevent thrombi and emboli development.	• Abnormal values of complete blood cell count, platelet, prothrombin time, PTT, and INR

Abiomed BVS 5000 and AB 5000 Ventricle[1,2]

   A. Initiate heparin as prescribed when mediastinal drainage is 50 to 75 mL/hr for 3 consecutive hours.

   B. Heparin bolus is not recommended.

   C. Initiate heparin infusion as prescribed, but usually not greater than 16 hours after surgery.

   D. Initial heparin infusion 10 to 15 units/kg/hr or as prescribed.

   E. Monitor activated PTT or ACT every hour until therapeutic, then every 2 hours.

   F. Goal activated PTT: 2 to 2.5 × laboratory normal value or as prescribed.

   G. Goal ACT: 180 to 200 seconds or as prescribed.

   H. ACT: Increased to 250 to 300 seconds or activated PTT 2.5 to 3 × normal for atrial or ventricular fibrillation or VAD flows less than 3 L/min or as prescribed.

Procedure continues on following page

Patient Monitoring and Care —*Continued*

Steps	Rationale	Reportable Conditions

Thoratec PVAD/IVAD[18]
  A. Initiate heparin as prescribed when mediastinal drainage is 50 to 75 mL/hr for 3 consecutive hours.
  B. Initiate heparin infusion as prescribed, but usually not greater than 16 hours after surgery.
  C. Heparin bolus is not recommended.
  D. Initiate heparin at 10 units/kg/hr or as prescribed.
  E. Goal activated PTT: 1.5 to 2 × control or as prescribed.
  F. Monitor activated PTT 2 hours after change, and when condition is stable, every 4 hours.
  G. Start warfarin when condition is stable, and administer orally as prescribed.
  H. INR goal 3 to 3.5 or as prescribed.		

8. Monitor the patient for systemic evidence of bleeding or coagulation disorders.	Hematologic and coagulation profiles may be altered as a result of blood loss during VAD insertion, anticoagulation therapy, platelet dysfunction, and hemolysis.	• Bleeding from the VAD insertion site • Bleeding from incisions or mucous membranes • Petechiae/ecchymosis • Guaiac-positive nasogastric aspirate or stool • Hematuria • Decreased hemoglobin/hematocrit • Decreased filling volumes • Increased heart rate • Decreased VAD flow
9. Change the VAD site dressing every 24 hours and as needed. Do not use prophylactic topical agents because they may increase maceration and increase the risk of resistant microorganisms.[4,7,19]	Decreases the incidence of infection and allows an opportunity for site assessment. Special note: Most manufacturers do not recommend use of povidone-iodine because of degradation of the drivelines. Also, no acetone should be in the patient's room. Patients with an open sternotomy may need a physician at the bedside during dressing changes.	• Signs and symptoms of infection
10. Change the air filter weekly (HeartMate XVE LVAD) and as needed.	Decreases the risk of overheating the VAD.	• Any signs of fluid or black dust in the driveline or filter
11. Follow institution standard for assessing pain. Administer analgesia as prescribed.	Identifies need for pain interventions. The patient may experience pain from VAD placement, limited mobility, or carrying the equipment.	• Continued pain despite pain interventions

Patient Monitoring and Care —*Continued*

Steps	Rationale	Reportable Conditions
12. Early ambulation is essential to patient rehabilitation. When the patient's condition is hemodynamically stable, ambulate the patient progressively. Use of an interdisciplinary rehabilitation team is essential.[4]	Prevents the hazards of immobility and begins rehabilitation. Ensure the VAD is secured when the patient is ambulating.	• Postural hypotension • Decrease in VAD flow with position changes • Unrelieved dizziness • Prolonged deconditioning • Signs of transient ischemic attack or cerebrovascular accident
13. Identify parameters that demonstrate clinical readiness to wean from VAD therapy (postcardiotomy support, Abiomed or Thoratec PVAD, IVAD).[8,15] Most frequently this is done in the operating room and requires additional anticoagulation therapy. ACT is usually greater than 300 seconds when VAD flow is less than 3 L/min. Weaning is done only with the surgeon present.	Determines hemodynamic readiness for weaning and stability during weaning; short-term support after cardiotomy or for cardiogenic shock is usually 5 to 14 days.	• Signs and symptoms of infection or hemodynamic instability

Before weaning:

   A. Absence of lethal or unstable dysrhythmia.

   B. Mean arterial pressure greater than 70 mm Hg with little or no vasopressor support.

   C. Pulmonary artery occlusion pressure less than 18 mm Hg.

   D. Mixed venous oxygen saturation 60% to 80%.

   E. Capillary refill less than 2 seconds.

   F. Urine output greater than 0.5 mL/kg/hr.

   G. Return of native aortic valve opening and closing on the arterial waveform on minimal support.

   H. Return of heart sounds.

   I. Return of native tricuspid valve opening and closing on the pulmonary artery waveform.

During weaning:

   A. Ability to maintain normal LVAD flow when the RVAD is weaned off.

   B. Ability to maintain normal blood pressure and pulmonary artery pressures with the LVAD weaned off.

Procedure continues on following page

Patient Monitoring and Care —*Continued*

Steps	Rationale	Reportable Conditions
14. Begin patient and family education as early as possible.[4,9,13]	Before discharge, patients and families must show adequate knowledge and understanding regarding the mechanics and alarms of the device (HeartMate and Thoratec VADs).	

Documentation

Documentation should include the following:
- Patient and family education
- Universal protocol requirements
- Informed consent
- Patient response to the VAD
- Confirmation of placement
- Hemodynamic status
- Pain assessment, interventions, and effectiveness
- Activity level
- Unexpected outcomes
- Additional interventions

- Abiomed: Level of pump (BVS 5000), complete filling and emptying, flow
- Thoratec PVAD or IVAD: Mode, set rate, set % systole, LVAD and RVAD drive pressures, complete filling and emptying
- HeartMate XVE: Flow, rate and stroke volume, mode
- HeartMate II: Pump speed, flow, motor power and pulse index
- Driveline site
- Backup drive console and emergency pump device
- Dressing changes and site assessments
- Skin integrity
- Patient tolerance
- Complete filling/emptying

References

CR 1. ABIOMED, Inc: *AB 5000 ventricle training guide,* Danvers, MA, 2003, Abiomed.

CR 2. ABIOMED, Inc: *Clinical reference manual,* Danvers, MA, 2003, Abiomed.

CR 3. Chillocott S, Atkins P, Adamson R: Left ventricular assist as a viable alternative for cardiac transplantation, *Crit Care Nurs Q* 20:64-69, 1998.

4. Drews T, Jurmann M, Michael D, et al: Differences in pulsatile and non-pulsatile mechanical circulatory support in long-term use, *J Heart Lung Transplantation* 27:1096-1101, 2008.

CR 5. Frazier OH: Prologue: ventricular assist devices and total artificial hearts: a historical perspective, *Cardiol Clin* 21:1-13, 2003.

CR 6. Holmes EA: Outpatient management of long-term assist devices, *Cardiol Clin* 21:93-99, 2003.

CR 7. Hravnak M, George E, Kormos RL: Management of chronic left ventricular assist device percutaneous lead insertion sites, *J Heart Lung Transplant* 12(5): 856-863, 1993.

CR 8. Konstam MA, Czerska B, Bohm M, et al: Continuous aortic flow augmentation: a pilot study of hemodynamic and renal responses to a novel percutaneous intervention in decompensated heart failure, *Circulation* 2002; 112:3107.

CR 9. Kukuy EL, et al: Devices as destination therapy, *Cardiol Clin* 21:67-73, 2003.

10. LaRocca GM, Shimbo D, Rodriguez CJ, et al: The Impella Recover LP 5.0 left ventricular assist device: a bridge to coronary artery bypass grafting and cardiac transplantation, *J Am Soc Echocardiogr* 19:468.e5-7, 2006.

11. Lee, MS, Makkar, RR: Percutaneous left ventricular assist devices. *Cardiol Clini* 24 265-275, 2006.

CR 12. Lemos PA, Cummins P. and Lee CH et al: Usefulness of percutaneous left ventricular assistance to support high-risk percutaneous coronary interventions, *Am J Cardiol* 91:479-481, 2003.

13. Long et al: Improving outcomes with long-term destination therapy using left ventricular assist devices, *J Thorac Cardiovasc Surg* 135:1353-1361, 2008.

CR 14. Rose EA, et al: Long-term mechanical left ventricular assistance for end stage heart failure, *N Engl J Med* 345:1435-1443, 2001.

CR 15. Thiele, H, Lauer, B, Hambrecht et al: Reversal of cardiogenic shock by percutaneous left atrial-to-femoral atrial bypass assistance, *Circulation* 104: 2917-2922, 2001.

16. Thoratec Corporation: *Thoratec HeartMate II LVAS clinical operation and patient management,* Pleasanton, CA, 2008, Thoratec.

CR 17. Thoratec Corporation: *HeartMate XVE LVAS operating manual,* Pleasanton, CA, 2003, Thoratec.

CR 18. Thoratec Corporation: *Thoratec VAD and IVAD clinical operation and patient management,* Pleasanton, CA, 2004, Thoratec.

Additional Readings

CR Arabia F, et al: Biventricular cannulation for the Thoratec ventricular assist device, *Ann Thorac Surg* 66:2119-2120, 1998.

CR Bond AE, et al: The left ventricular assist device, *Am J Nurs* 103:32-41, 2003.

CR DeRose J, et al: Implantable left ventricular assist devices provide an excellent outpatient bridge to transplantation and recovery, *J Am Coll Cardiol* 30:1773-1777, 1997.

CR Dixon JF, Farris DD: The ABIOMED BVS 5000 system, *AACN Clin Issues Crit Care Nurs* 2:552-561, 1991.

CR Goldstein DJ, Oz MC: *Cardiac assist devices,* New York, 2000, Futura Publishing.

John R, et al: Low thromboembolic risk for patients with the Heartmate II left ventricular assist device, *J Thorac Cardiovasc Surg* 136:1318-1323, 2008.

CR Livinston E, et al: Increased activation of the coagulation and fibrinolytic systems leads to hemorrhagic complications during left ventricular assist implantation, *Circulation* 94(Suppl II):II227-II234, 1996.

CR McCarthy P, et al: One hundred patients with the HeartMate left ventricular assist device: evolving concepts and technology, *J Thorac Cardiovasc Surg* 115:904-912, 1998.

McGee E Ci J r , McCarthy P Mi , Moazami N i . Temporary Mechanical Circulatory Support. Cohn Lh, ed. *Cardiac Surgery in the Adult,* 507-534, New York, 2008, McGraw-Hill.

Miller L, Pagani F, Russell S, et al: Use of a continuous-flow device in patients awaiting heart transplantation, *N Engl J Med* 357:885-896, 2007.

CR Mussivand T, et al: Critical anatomic dimensions for intrathoracic circulatory assist devices, *Artif Organs* 16:281-285, 1992.

Pitsis AA, Visouli AN: Update on ventricular assist device management in the ICU, *Curr Opin Crit Care* 14(5): 569-578, 2008.

CR Schakenbach LH: Care of the patient with a ventricular assist device. In *Protocols for practice,* Aliso Viejo, CA, 2002, American Association of Critical-Care Nurses.

Wiegand DL, Kalowes PG: Withdrawal of cardiac medications and devices, *AACN Adv Crit Care* 18(4):415-425, 2007.

Windecker S: Percutaneous left ventricular assist devices for treatment of patients with cardiogenic shock, *Curr Opin Crit Care* 13:521-527, 2007.

PROCEDURE **57**

Electrocardiographic Leads and Cardiac Monitoring

P U R P O S E : Continuous electrophysiologic monitoring is performed routinely for most patients with acute and critical illnesses. A key component of electrophysiologic monitoring is the electrocardiogram. The electrocardiogram provides a continuous graphic picture of cardiac electrical activity. The electrocardiogram can be used for diagnostic, documentation, and treatment purposes.

Mary G. McKinley

PREREQUISITE NURSING KNOWLEDGE

- Knowledge of the anatomy and physiology of the cardiovascular system, principles of cardiac conduction, principles of electrophysiology, electrocardiogram (ECG) lead placement, basic dysrhythmia interpretation, and electrical safety is necessary.
- Advanced cardiac life support knowledge and skills are needed.
- Electrophysiologic monitoring with hardwire and telemetry is indicated for all patients in critical care units and for patients in selected acute care settings, postanesthesia areas, operating rooms, and emergency departments.
- Electrophysiologic monitoring is designed to give a graphic display of the electrical activity in the heart generated by depolarization and repolarization of cardiac tissue.
- Hardwire ECG monitors have electrodes and lead wires that are attached directly to the patient. Impulses are transmitted directly from the patient to the monitor (Fig. 57-1).
- Telemetry systems have electrodes and lead wires that are attached from the patient to a battery pack and transmit impulses to the monitor via radio wave transmission (Fig. 57-2).
- Telemetry is useful in progressive ambulation and evaluation of activity tolerance. A disadvantage to telemetry is that ambulation and activity can increase distortion of the ECG pattern.

- Specific areas of the chest are used for electrode placement to obtain a view of the electrical activity in a particular area of the heart (commonly called a lead).
- ECG monitors use a three-lead or five-lead wire system to provide different views (leads) of the heart's electrical activity. Most acute and critical care units use a five-lead system for continuous bedside monitoring or telemetry.
- Standardized placement of leads is important so that information obtained is assessed within a common frame of reference and so that appropriate judgments can be made on the patient's cardiac status. Alterations of electrode position may distort the appearance of the waveform significantly and can lead to misdiagnosis or mistreatment.
- The two major factors that determine the views of the ECG deflection on the monitor are the location of the electrodes on the body and the direction of the cardiac impulse in relation to the position of the electrode.
- A basic rule of electrocardiography is the rule of electrical flow. This rule notes that if electricity flows toward the positive electrode, an upright pattern is produced on the monitor or graph paper. If the electricity flows away from the positive electrode (or toward the negative electrode), a downward pattern or deflection is produced on the monitor or graph paper. Lead wires attached to the patient are coded (+, P [positive]; or –, N [negative]; RA [right arm]; RL [right leg]; LA [left arm]; LL [left leg]; V or C [V or precordial vector and C or chest lead] in some way for ease in correct placement. Placement of the

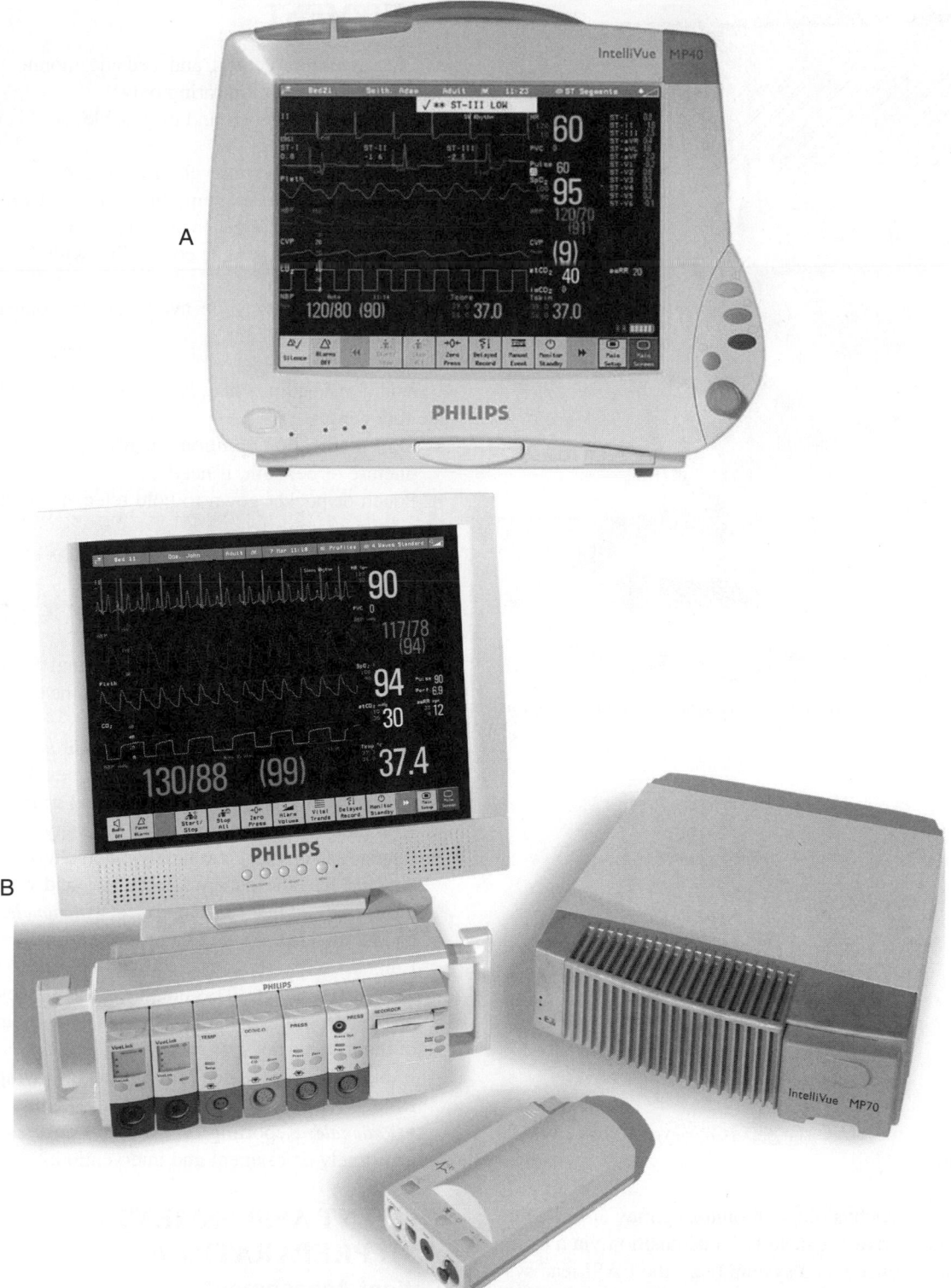

FIGURE 57-1   **A,** Bedside monitoring system. **B,** Networked patient monitor with portal technology for critical and intermediate care. *(Courtesy Philips Medical System, Andover, MA.)*

leads gives different views of the electrical conduction through the heart.

- Information from the bedside via hardwire or telemetry can be transferred to a central monitor, where it can be printed, stored, and analyzed (Fig. 57-3).

- Five-lead bedside monitoring systems provide a continuous readout of two or more leads simultaneously. This readout provides more information and a comparison of the ECG patterns. Optimal lead selection is based on the goals of monitoring for each patient's clinical situation.

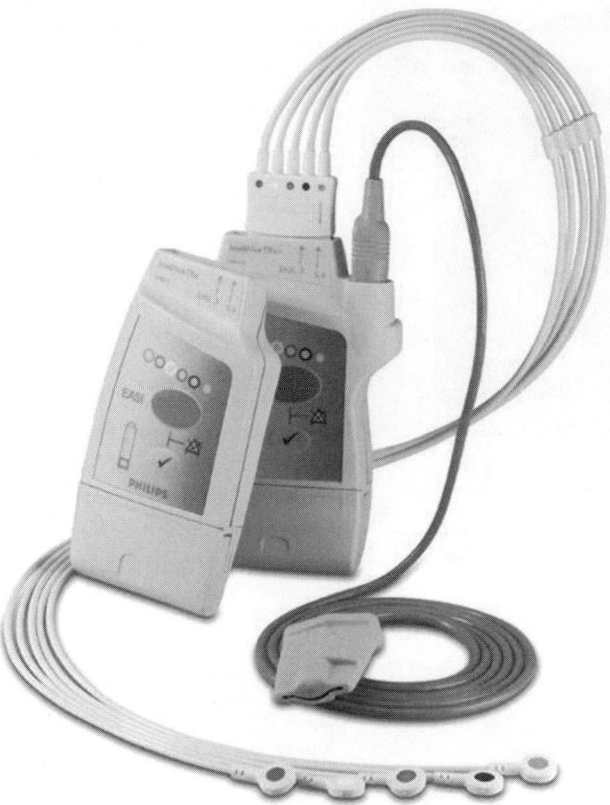

FIGURE 57-2   Telemetry monitoring system. *(Courtesy Philips Medical Systems, Andover, MA.)*

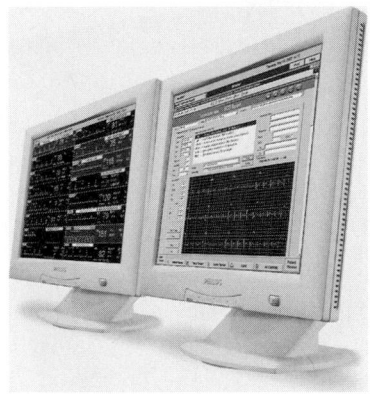

FIGURE 57-3   Central station. *(Courtesy Philips Medical Systems, Andover, MA.)*

- Bedside electrophysiologic monitoring may also provide continuous derived 12-lead ECG acquisition via a torso-positioned reduced lead system (e.g., the EASI lead system; Philips Monitoring, Andover, MA). In this application, the reduced lead configuration varies according to the manufacturer and the device but provides the availability of a continuous 12-lead ECG, which can be accessed for information over a predetermined time (commonly 24 to 48 hours). This application greatly expands the information available from bedside monitors and requires accurate and consistent lead placement based on the manufacturer's requirements. Derived ECGs are not equivalent to standard 12-lead ECGs and are not recommended as a substitute.[1]

EQUIPMENT

- ECG monitor (central and bedside monitor) or battery pack (telemetry monitoring only)
- Electrodes, pregelled and disposable
- Nonsterile gloves
- Dry gauze pads or terrycloth washcloth
- Cleansing pads or nonemollient soap and water
- Lead wires (no longer than 18 inches)
- Patient cable (should be compatible with the monitor and the lead wires)
- ECG calipers (may be available electronically via the central monitor)
- Alcohol pads
  Additional equipment to have available as needed includes the following:
- Skin preparation solution, such as skin barrier wipe or tincture of benzoin, if needed
- Pouch or pocket gown to hold telemetry unit (telemetry monitoring only)
- Clippers or scissors to clip hair from the chest as needed

PATIENT AND FAMILY EDUCATION

- Assess the readiness of the patient and family to learn. ➧*Rationale:* Anxiety and concerns of the patient and family may inhibit the ability to learn.
- Provide explanations of the equipment and alarms to the patient and family. ➧*Rationale:* These explanations assist in making the patient and family feel more comfortable with monitoring and may reduce anxiety.
- Reassure the patient and family that monitoring is continuous and that the patient's heart rate and rhythm will be monitored and treated as indicated. ➧*Rationale:* The patient and family are reassured that immediate care is available.
- Emphasize that the patient should feel free to move about in bed. ➧*Rationale:* This emphasis encourages movement on the part of the patient and allays fears about disruption of the monitoring system.
- Explain the importance of reporting any symptoms, such as pain, dizziness, palpitations, or chest discomfort. ➧*Rationale:* Reporting of symptoms ensures appropriate and timely assessment and intervention.

PATIENT ASSESSMENT AND PREPARATION
Patient Assessment

- Assess the patient's peripheral pulses, vital signs, heart sounds, level of consciousness, lung sounds, neck vein distention, presence of chest pain or palpitations, and any peripheral circulatory disorders (i.e., decreased pulses, clubbing, cyanosis, and dependent edema). ➧*Rationale:* This assessment provides baseline assessment data.
- Assess whether the patient has a history of cardiac dysrhythmias or cardiac problems. ➧*Rationale:* The history provides baseline data and may guide selection of monitoring leads.

- Assess landmarks for identification of correct placement of electrodes. ➤➤*Rationale:* This assessment ensures accurate placement of leads for accurate interpretation.

Patient Preparation

- Verify correct patient with two identifiers. ➤➤*Rationale:* Prior to performing a procedure, the nurse should ensure the correct identification of the patient for the intended intervention.
- Ensure that the patient and family understand preprocedural teaching. Answer questions as they arise, and reinforce information as needed. ➤➤*Rationale:* This communication evaluates and reinforces the understanding of previously taught information.
- Assist the patient to the supine position. ➤➤*Rationale:* This position enables easy access to the chest for electrode placement.
- Assist the patient in removing clothing that covers the chest while providing for the patient's privacy. ➤➤*Rationale:* Clothing removal provides a clear view of the chest and allows for identification of landmarks and proper placement of leads while the patient's privacy is maintained.

Procedure for Electrophysiologic Monitoring: Hardwire and Telemetry

Steps	Rationale	Special Considerations
1. ▦		
2. Turn on the computerized central monitoring system.	When activated, the central monitoring system alarm sounds to notify the nurse of problems with the ECG for interpretation and attention.	The nurse must assess the patient to confirm findings, verify patterns, and evaluate computer interpretations.
3. For telemetry monitoring, insert a battery into the telemetry unit, matching polarity markings on the transmitter.	Batteries can fail if left sitting on the shelf or in the unit. Polarity must match for proper functioning of the unit.	Refer to manufacturer recommendations about battery storage and replacement.
4. Ensure that the monitor is plugged into a grounded alternating current (AC) wall outlet.	Maintains electrical safety.	
5. Turn on the bedside monitor.	Provides the power source to the monitor.	The equipment may require self-test and warm-up time.
6. Identify whether a three-lead or a five-lead wire system is available.	Assists in determining possible placement of electrodes and leads that can be viewed.	Optimal lead selection should be based on the type of lead system available and the goals of monitoring for each patient's clinical situation.
7. Check the cable and lead wires for fraying, broken wires, or discoloration.	Detects conditions that may give an inaccurate ECG trace.	Safety must be maintained; if equipment is damaged, obtain alternative equipment and notify the biomedical engineer for repair.
8. Plug the patient cable into the monitoring system.	Hardware systems require a direct connection to the bedside monitoring system.	
9. Check that the lead wires are plugged into the patient cable correctly and securely.	Reduces the chance of disconnection, distortion, or outside interference with the ECG tracing.	Manufacturers code the lead connections so that the correct attachments can be made; often these are color coded, but they may be letter or symbol coded.
A. Three-lead system (Fig. 57-4): The negative wire plugs into the opening marked *N*, −, or *RA*. The positive wire plugs into the opening marked *P*, +, *LL*, or *LA*. The ground wire plugs into the opening marked *G* (Ground), *Neutral*, or *RL*.		The three-lead system is the oldest and simplest of all cardiac monitoring lead systems. Only one lead can be displayed. This system is often used in portable monitor defibrillators.[2]

Procedure continues on following page

Procedure for Electrophysiologic Monitoring: Hardwire and Telemetry—*Continued*

Steps	Rationale	Special Considerations

B. Five-lead system (Fig. 57-5):
  The right arm wire plugs into the opening marked *RA*.
  The left arm wire plugs into the opening marked *LA*.
  The left leg wire plugs into the opening marked *LL*.
  The right leg wire plugs into the opening marked *RL*.
  The chest wire plugs into the opening marked *C* or *V*.
		Commonly used in most hospitals today. Provides views from the six limb leads (I, II, III, augmented vector right [aVR,] augmented vector left [aVL], augmented vector foot or [aVF]) plus one precordial (V) lead.[2]

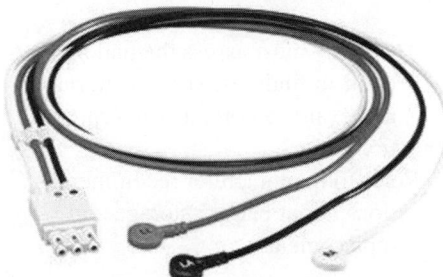

FIGURE 57-4 Three-lead wire system. (*Courtesy Philips Medical Systems, Andover, MA.*)

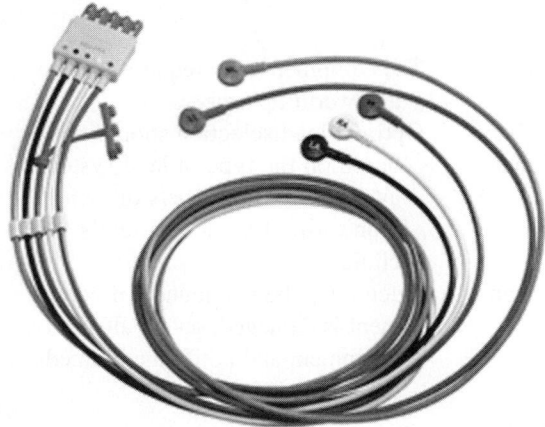

FIGURE 57-5 Five-lead wire system. (*Courtesy Philips Medical Systems, Andover, MA.*)

Steps	Rationale	Special Considerations
10. Connect the electrodes to the lead wires before placing the electrodes on the patient.	Prepares the monitoring system.	Placing electrodes on the chest and then attaching the lead wires can be uncomfortable for the patient and can contribute to the development of air bubbles in the electrode gel, which can decrease conduction distorting the ECG image.

11. Choose electrode placement:
  A. Three-lead system:
   • Lead I
   • Lead II
   • Lead III
   • Modified chest lead 1 (MCL_1)
   • MCL_6
	Choice is based on constraints on chest wall space (dressings or injury sites) and type of information needed or desired.
	Leads that can be monitored with this system are lead I, lead II, lead III, or a modified chest lead, such as MCL_1 or MCL_6.
		Select the limb leads appropriate for the clinical situation[1,3]:
		1. Atrial flutter: II, III, or aVF.
		2. Inferior myocardial infarction (MI): II, III, or aVF; select the lead with maximal elevation of ST segment on the 12-lead ECG.

Procedure for Electrophysiologic Monitoring: Hardwire and Telemetry—*Continued*

Steps	Rationale	Special Considerations
	The goals of bipolar monitoring (with a three-lead system) include tracking heart rate, detecting R waves for synchronized direct-current shock in electrocardioversion, and detecting ventricular fibrillation.	3. Anterior MI: Select the lead with maximal elevation of ST segment on the 12-lead ECG. 4. After angioplasty: Select III or aVF, whichever has the tallest R wave. 5. If three channels are available, use $V_1 + I + aVF$.[1] 6. Use lead II to diagnose atrial activity and measure heart rate or V_1 to diagnose wide QRS complex.[2]
B. Five-lead system: • First choice: Select V_1 and the limb lead appropriate for the clinical situation (see Special Considerations) • Second choice: Substitute V_6 for V_1 when the patient cannot have an electrode at the sternal border or when the QRS complex amplitude is not adequate for optimized computerized monitoring **(Level E*)**	One limb lead and one precordial lead can be displayed simultaneously with a two-channel system. V_1 is the precordial lead recommended.[2] V_1 is an excellent lead for diagnosis of dysrhythmias with a wide QRS complex (e.g. bundle-branch blocks, ventricular pacemaker rhythms, and wide QRS tachycardias).[2]	
12. **PE**		
13. Identify the sternal notch or angle of Louis.	The sternal notch identifies the second rib and assists in locating the fourth intercostal space (ICS) so that accurate placement may be achieved.	
A. Palpate the upper sternum to identify where the clavicle joins the sternum (suprasternal notch). B. Slide fingers down the center of the sternum to the obvious bony prominence. This is the sternal notch, which identifies the second rib and provides a landmark for noting the fourth ICS. C. Locate the fourth ICS.		
14. Clean the area for the application of electrodes with cleansing pads or soap and water and dry thoroughly. **(Level E)**	Provides for adequate transmission of electrical impulses. Moist skin is not conducive to electrode adherence.[2] Failure to properly prepare the skin may cause inappropriate monitoring alarms.[2]	Clipping of chest hair may be necessary to ensure good skin contact with the electrodes.
15. Clean the intended sites with alcohol pads. Consider use of skin preparation solutions. **(Level E)**	Alcohol or skin preparations may be needed to remove oils to improve impulse transmission.[2]	Skin preparation solutions should not be applied to the area of the skin that will be in direct contact with the electrode gel because transmission of impulses may be decreased.
16. Abrade the skin with a washcloth or gauze pad.	Removes dead skin cells, promoting impulse transmission.	

*Level E: Multiple case reports, theory-based evidence from expert opinions, or peer-reviewed professional organizational standards without clinical studies to support recommendations

Procedure continues on following page

Procedure   for Electrophysiologic Monitoring: Hardwire and Telemetry—*Continued*

Steps	Rationale	Special Considerations
17. Remove the backing from the pregelled electrodes and test the center of the pads for moistness.	Gel can dry out in storage; gel should be moist to allow for impulse transmission.	
18. Apply electrodes to the sites, ensuring a seal. Avoid pushing on the gel pads.	Electrodes must be placed tightly to prevent external influences from affecting the ECG. Pressing on the gel pad can cause the gel to leak onto the adhesive surfaces and may interfere with transmission.	

19. Place electrodes as follows:
A. Three-lead system: MCL_1 and MCL_6 (Fig. 57-6):
  • Apply right arm (RA) electrode to the patient's left shoulder.
  • Apply left arm (LA) electrode at fourth ICS right sternal border.
  • Apply left leg (LL) electrode to the fifth ICS at midaxillary line.
  • Select lead I to obtain MCL_1 and lead II to obtain MCL_6.
	Proper positioning is essential to ensure a correct view of the leads.[1,4]	Lead selection is based on chest wall constraints and the clinical situation.

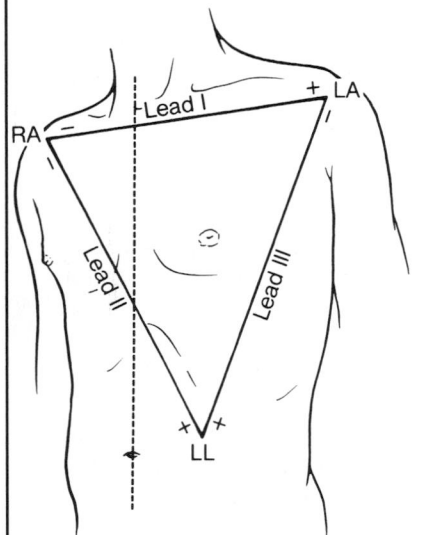

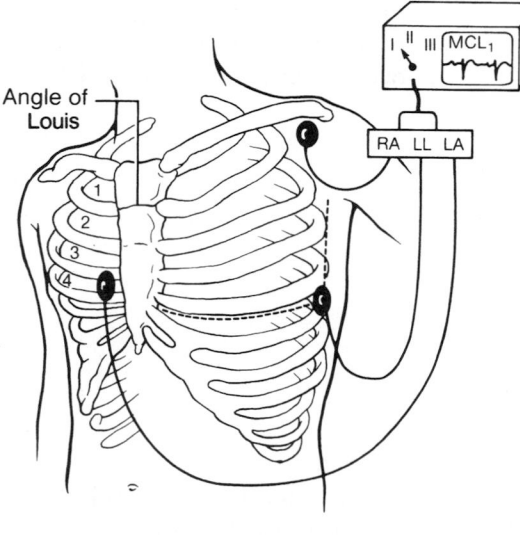

FIGURE 57-6   Three-lead application. *(From Drew B: Bedside electrocardiographic monitoring, AACN Clin Issues Crit Care 4:28, 1993.)*

| B. Lewis lead (Fig. 57-7):
  • Apply right arm (RA) electrode at first ICS right sternal border.
  • Apply left arm (LA) electrode to fourth ICS right sternal border.
  • Apply left leg (LL) electrode to fourth ICS left sternal border
  • Set the lead selector to lead I. | Lewis lead offers the best visualization of P waves for patients with atrial dysrhythmias. | |

Angle of Louis

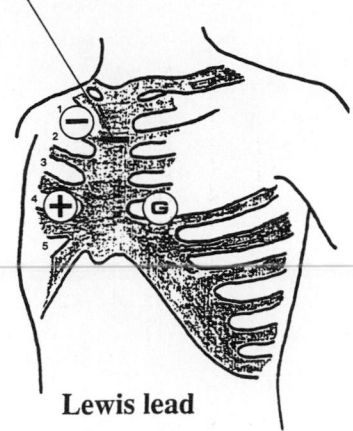

Lewis lead

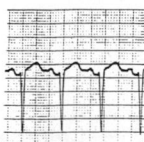

FIGURE 57-7 Three-lead system with Lewis lead.

Procedure for Electrophysiologic Monitoring: Hardwire and Telemetry—*Continued*		
Steps	**Rationale**	**Special Considerations**
C. Five-lead system (Fig. 57-8): • Apply right arm (RA) electrode to the right shoulder close to the junction of the right arm and torso. • Apply left arm (LA) electrode to the left shoulder close to the junction of the left arm and torso. • Apply right leg (RL) electrode at the level of the lowest rib, on the right abdominal region, or on the hip. • Apply left leg (LL) electrode at the level of the lowest rib, on the left abdominal region, or on the hip.	Arm electrodes that are placed under the clavicle or leg electrodes that are placed too high on the ribs can alter the point of view of the leads and result in inaccurate recording.[2,4]	
• Apply the chest lead electrode on the selected site: V_1, fourth ICS right sternal border; or V_6, fifth ICS midaxillary line. • Set the lead selector or monitor the appropriate leads.	Only one precordial lead can be displayed; placement of the electrode identifies the lead used.	
20. Reduce tension on the lead wires and cables.	Decreases tension on the lead wires to alleviate undue stress, which can cause interference or faulty recordings.	
A. For hardwire monitoring, fasten the lead wire and patient cable to the patient's gown, making a loop.	Minimizes pulling on the electrodes, which can be uncomfortable for the patient.	

Procedure continues on following page

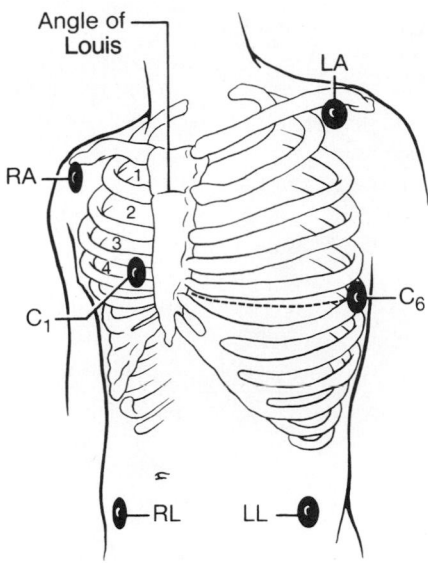

Angle of
Louis

LA

RA

1
2
3
4

C₁

C₆

RL   LL

FIGURE 57-8   Five-lead application. *(From Drew B: Bedside electro-cardiographic monitoring, AACN Clin Issues Crit Care 4:26, 1993.)*

Procedure	**for Electrophysiologic Monitoring: Hardwire and Telemetry**—*Continued*	
Steps	**Rationale**	**Special Considerations**
B. For telemetry monitoring, secure the transmitter in a pouch or pocket in the patient's gown.	The transmitter must be secure so that it is not dropped or damaged.	
21. Examine the ECG tracing on the monitor for the size of the R waves and T waves.	The R wave should be approximately twice the height of the other components of the ECG to ensure proper detection by the heart rate counter in the equipment. The accuracy of the alarm system often depends on the R wave. If the T wave is nearly equal to the R wave, double counting can occur, resulting in false alarms.	Manufacturers provide for calibration of the ECG to 1 mV, and monitors have size adjustments that can be used to increase or decrease the size of the ECG.
22. Obtain an ECG strip (Fig. 57-9) and interpret it for rhythm, rate, presence and configuration of P waves, length of PR interval, length of QRS complexes, presence and configuration of T waves, length of QT interval, presence of extra waves (e.g., U waves), and presence of dysrhythmias.	Reviews the normal conduction sequence and identifies abnormalities that may necessitate further evaluation or treatment.	

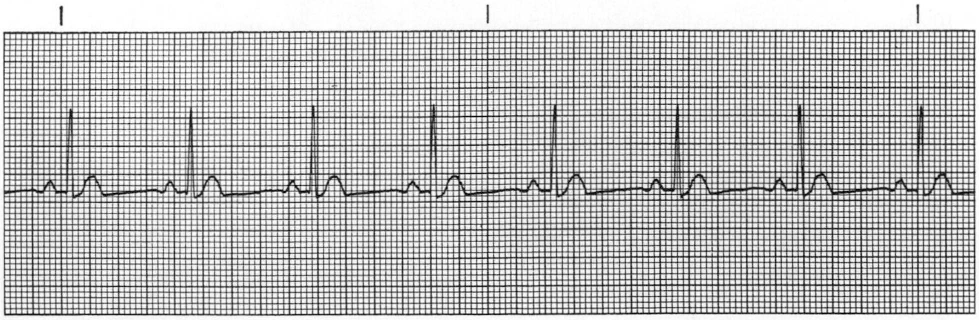

FIGURE 57-9   Monitor strip of clear ECG pattern.

Procedure for Electrophysiologic Monitoring: Hardwire and Telemetry—*Continued*

Steps	Rationale	Special Considerations
23. Set the alarms. Upper and lower alarm limits are set on the basis of the patient's current clinical status and heart rate.	Activates the bedside or telemetry monitor alarm system.	Monitoring systems allow for setting and adjusting alarms at the bedside or the central console. The types of alarms may include rate (high or low), abnormal rhythms or complexes, pacemaker recognition, and others, depending on the manufacturer. Caution: Never turn off bedside monitor alarms, except in specific circumstances (i.e., anticipated end of life). Alarms should be adjusted according to the known clinical status of the patient.
24. Set ST segment parameters (see Procedure 59).		
25. Discard used supplies in appropriate receptacles.	Reduces the transmission of microorganisms; standard precautions.	
26. 🅷🅷		

Expected Outcomes

- Properly applied electrodes
- A clear ECG monitor tracing displayed (see Fig. 57-9)
- Alarms set appropriate to the patient's clinical status
- Prompt identification and treatment of dysrhythmias

Unexpected Outcomes

- Altered skin integrity
- AC interference, also called 60-cycle interference (Fig. 57-10)
- Wandering baseline (Fig. 57-11)
- False alarms
- Artifact or waveform interference (Fig. 57-12)
- Microshock

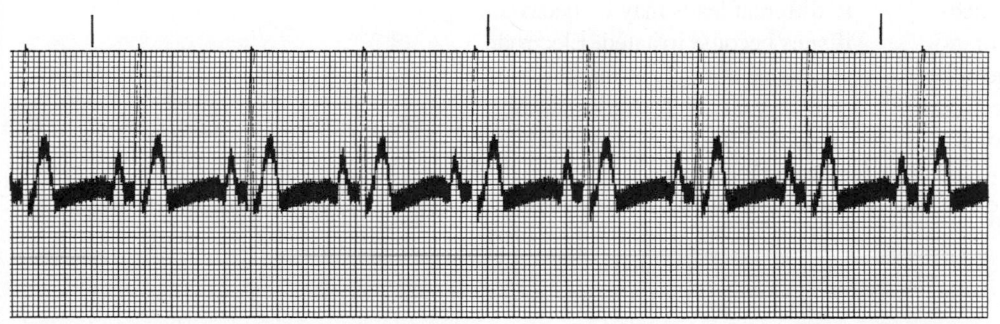

FIGURE 57-10   Monitor strip with 60-cycle interference.

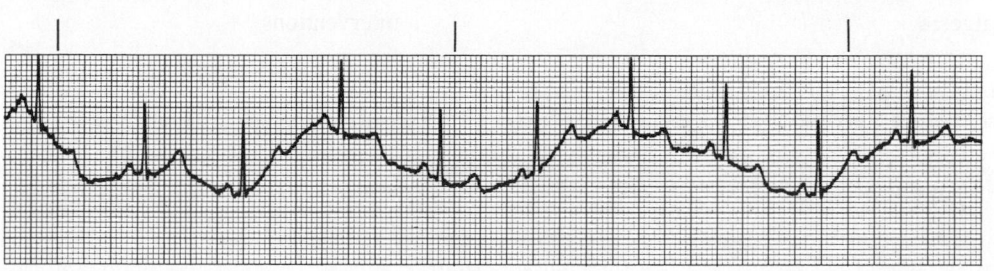

FIGURE 57-11   Monitor strip with erratic baseline.

Procedure continues on following page

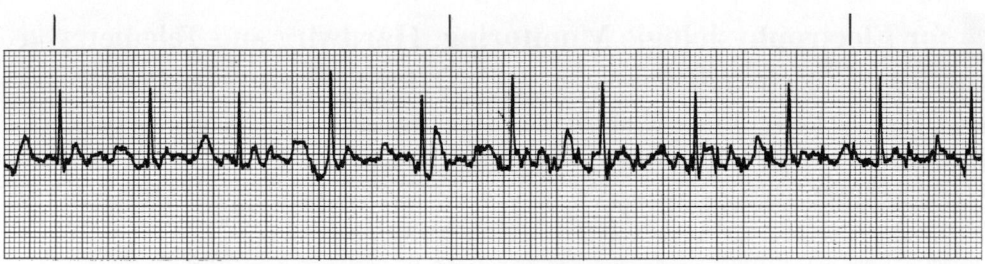

FIGURE 57-12   Monitor strip with interference.

Patient Monitoring and Care

Steps	Rationale	Reportable Conditions
		These conditions should be reported if they persist despite nursing interventions.
1. Evaluate the ECG monitor pattern for the presence of P waves, QRS complexes, a clear baseline, and absence of artifact or distortion. Obtain a rhythm strip on admission, at every shift (as per institution protocol), and with rhythm changes.	A clear pattern is needed to make accurate judgments about the patient's status and treatment.[2]	• Abnormal cardiac ECG complexes, rate, and rhythm
2. Evaluate the ECG pattern continually for dysrhythmias, assess patient tolerance of the changes, and provide prompt nursing intervention.	Changes in the ECG pattern may indicate significant problems for the patient and may necessitate immediate intervention or additional diagnostic tests, such as a 12-lead ECG.	• Abnormal cardiac rate and rhythm • Hemodynamic instability
3. Evaluate skin integrity around the electrodes on a daily basis, and change the electrodes every 24 to 48 hours or according to institution standard. Rotate sites when changing electrodes. Monitor the skin for any allergic reaction to the adhesive or gel. Change all electrodes if a problem occurs with one. **(Level E*)**	Skin integrity must be maintained to have a clear picture of the ECG. Replacing electrodes every 48 hours prevents drying of the gel and may prevent skin breakdown. A change to different leads may be necessary if sites become irritated. Electrode resistance changes as the gel dries, so changing all electrodes at once prevents differences in resistance between electrodes.[2]	• Alteration in skin integrity
4. Check electrode placement every shift.	Accurate interpretation of many dysrhythmias depends on proper placement of the electrodes and knowledge of which lead is being viewed.	
5. Follow institution standard for assessing pain. Administer analgesia and nitrates as prescribed.	Identifies need for pain interventions.	• Continued pain despite pain interventions

*Level E: Multiple case reports, theory-based evidence from expert opinions, or peer-reviewed professional organizational standards without clinical studies to support recommendations

Documentation

Documentation should include the following:
- Patient and family education
- An initial or baseline ECG strip, with the lead, interpretation, dysrhythmias, and treatments noted
- Routine ECG strips according to institution protocol
- Assessment of pain, interventions, and response to interventions

- An ECG strip should be recorded whenever a change is found in cardiac rate or rhythm, the patient experiences chest pain, a change in lead placement occurs, or the effect of antidysrhythmic agents is evaluated
- Unexpected outcomes
- Additional nursing interventions

References

1. AACN: *AACN practice alert, dysrhythmia monitoring,* Aliso Viejo, CA, 2008, American Association of Critical Care.
CR 2. Drew BJ, et al: Practice standards for electrocardiographic monitoring in hospital settings: an American Heart Association scientific statement from the Councils on Cardiovascular Nursing, Clinical Cardiology, and Cardiovascular Disease in the Young, *Circulation* 110:2721-2746, 2004.
3. Kligfield P, et al: Recommendations for the standardization and interpretation of the electrocardiogram: part 1: the electrocardiogram and its technology: a scientific statement from the American Heart Association Electrocardiography and Arrhythmias Committee, Council on Clinical Cardiology: The American College of Cardiology Foundation; and the Heart Rhythm Society, *Circulation* 115:1306-1324, 2007.
CR 4. Leeper B: Continuous ST-segment monitoring, *AACN Clin Issues* 14:145-154, 2003.

Additional Readings

Alspach J: *Core curriculum for critical care nursing,* Philadelphia, 2006, Saunders.
Donnely MP, et al: Lead selection: old and new methods for locating the most electrocardiogram information, *J Electrocardiol* 41:257-263, 2008.
Drew BJ, Kingfield P: Standardizing electrocardiograpic leads: introduction to a symposium, *J Electrocardiol* 41:187-189, 2008.
Drew BJ: Putting it all together: case studies on ECG monitoring, *AACN Adv Crit Care* 18:305-317, 2007.
Drew BJ: Pitfalls and artifacts in electrocardiography, *Cardiol Clin,* 24:309-315, 2006.
Drew BJ, et al: Practice standards for ECG monitoring in hosptial settings: executive summary and guide for implementation, *Crit Care Nurs Clin North Am* 18:157-168, 2006.
CR Jahrsdoerfer M, et al: Clinical usefulness of the EASI 12-continuous electrographic monitoring system, *Crit Care Nurse* 25:28-38, 2005.
CR Sole M, Klein D, Moseley M: *Introduction to critical care nursing,* ed 4, Philadelphia, 2004, Saunders.

Extra Electrocardiographic Leads: Right Precordial and Left Posterior Leads

P U R P O S E : Extra electrocardiographic leads are used in conjunction with the standard 12-lead electrocardiogram to provide additional diagnostic information.

Shu-Fen Wung, Barbara J. Drew

PREREQUISITE NURSING KNOWLEDGE

- Understanding of the anatomy and physiology of the cardiovascular system, basic rhythm interpretation, and electrical safety is necessary.
- Advanced cardiac life support knowledge and skills are needed.
- Familiarity with principles of electrophysiology is needed.
- The right ventricular (RV) leads V_{1R} through V_{6R} and left posterior leads V_7 through V_9 are unipolar leads in which the chest electrode serves as the "exploring" electrode or positive pole of the lead. These precordial leads view the heart from the vantage point of their electrode positions on the chest, similar to the standard precordial leads V_1 through V_6.
- For recordings of RV or left posterior leads, the three limb electrodes (right arm [RA], left arm [LA], left leg [LL]) also are required to create a central terminal (negative pole); one limb electrode (right leg [RL]) serves as the ground lead and is used to stabilize the electrocardiographic (ECG) recording.
- Accuracy in identification of anatomic landmarks for location of electrode sites and knowledge of the importance of accurate electrode placement are needed. Nurses must locate accurately the electrode positions for the standard 12-lead ECG because the same anatomic landmarks are used to locate the RV and left posterior leads. Accurate ECG interpretation is possible only when the recording electrodes are placed in the proper positions.

Slight alterations of the electrode positions may distort significantly the appearance of the ECG waveforms and can lead to misdiagnosis.[9] Reliable comparison of serial (more than two ECGs recorded at different times) ECG recordings relies on accurate and consistent electrode placement. An indelible marker is recommended for use with clear identification of the electrode locations to ensure that the same electrode locations are selected when serial ECGs are recorded.

- Nurses should be aware of body positional changes that can alter ECG recordings. Serial ECGs should be recorded with the patient in a supine position to ensure that all recordings are done in a consistent manner. Side-lying positions and elevation of the torso may change the position of the heart within the chest and can change the waveforms on the ECG recording.[2,3] If a position other than supine is clinically necessary, notation of the altered position should be made on the tracing.
- Right precordial leads are useful in diagnosis of a RV myocardial infarction (MI).
  - ❖ These RV leads are important because they enable clinicians to identify patients with an acute MI who are at high risk of atrioventricular (AV) conduction disturbances,[4] to predict the site of coronary artery occlusion, and to guide appropriate hemodynamic monitoring and interventions. Left posterior leads are used to aid in the detection of posterior wall MI and to facilitate timely reperfusion treatment. Recording of left posterior leads also can help in the differential diagnosis of tall R waves in lead V_1 and V_2.[6]

- Nurses should be able to operate the 12-lead ECG machine. Calibration of 1 mV equals 10 mm and paper speed of 25 mm/s are standards used in clinical practice. For ST-segment analysis, filter settings of 0.05 to 100 Hz are recommended by the American Heart Association.[12] Any variation used for particular clinical purposes should be noted on the tracing. Specific information regarding configuring the ECG machine, troubleshooting, and safety features is available from the manufacturer and should be read before use of the equipment.

- Nurses should be able to interpret recorded ECGs for the presence or absence of myocardial ischemia, MI, and dysrhythmias so that patients can be treated appropriately. Patients with an acute inferior MI and RV involvement, determined by ST-segment elevation in the right precordial leads, are at high risk for high-degree AV block. Nurses should monitor patients closely for conduction disturbances and anticipate the need for temporary pacing. Patients with RV infarction are prone to hypotension and shock that responds to treatment with fluid resuscitation.

- Indications for recording a right precordial ECG are as follows:
  - ❖ Evaluation and treatment of suspected acute MI, especially patients with inferior wall MI (ST-segment elevation in leads II, III, and augmented vector foot or aVF)
  - ❖ Evaluation of the risk for AV node conduction disturbances and anticipation of treatment plans
  - ❖ Prediction of the site of coronary artery occlusion (RV infarction occurs with proximal right coronary artery [RCA] occlusion)
  - ❖ Determination of the risk of "volume-responsive" shock, in which case fluid resuscitation is warranted and vasodilators (e.g., nitroglycerin) are contraindicated

- Indications for recording a left posterior ECG are as follows:
  - ❖ Evaluation and treatment of acute or suspected MI, especially patients with isolated ST-segment depression in the precordial leads V_1 through V_3 and patients with a nondiagnostic ECG
  - ❖ Presence of chest pain or anginal-equivalent symptoms (e.g., jaw, left shoulder or arm discomfort, or shortness of breath) or ST-segment depression in the left precordial leads V_1 through V_3 after percutaneous coronary interventions of the left circumflex artery
  - ❖ Any of these ECG characteristics indicative of posterior MI in lead V_1: R waves greater than or equal to 6 mm in height, R wave greater than or equal to 40 ms in duration, R/S ratio (R wave amplitude in mm over S wave amplitude in mm) greater than or equal to 1, or S wave less than or equal to 3 mm. In lead V_2: R wave greater than or equal to 15 mm in height, R wave greater than or equal to 50 ms in duration, R/S ratio greater than or equal to 1.5, or S wave less than or equal to 4 mm.[11]

  - ❖ Differentiation of true posterior MI from other conditions that can cause tall R waves in lead V_1, such as RV hypertrophy, right bundle-branch block, Wolff-Parkinson-White syndrome, and ventricular septal hypertrophy

- In patients with RV infarction who exhibit shock, volume expansion is used to provide adequate RV and left ventricular filling pressures and to restore arterial pressure and peripheral blood flow. Positive inotropic agents also may be indicated to augment the residual contractile force of the damaged RV. Use of vasodilators (e.g., nitroglycerin) should generally be avoided because they cause venous dilation and reduced preload. Use of diuretics (e.g., furosemide). Diuretics should be avoided because they reduce preload and left ventricular filling.[7]

EQUIPMENT

- Dry gauze pads or terrycloth washcloth
- Nonsterile gloves
- Cleansing pads or nonemollient soap and water
- Alcohol pads
- Indelible marker
- 12-lead ECG machine with attached patient cable and lead wires
- ECG electrodes
  Additional equipment to have available as needed includes the following:
- Hair clipper or scissors to clip hair from chest if needed
- Skin preparation solution, such as skin barrier wipe or tincture of benzoin

PATIENT AND FAMILY EDUCATION

- Describe the procedure and reasons for obtaining extra ECG leads. Reassure the patient that the procedure is painless. ➤➤*Rationale:* This communication clarifies information, reduces anxiety, and gains cooperation from the patient.
- Explain the patient's role in assisting with the ECG recording and emphasize actions that improve the quality of the ECG tracing, such as relaxing, avoiding conversation and body movement, and breathing normally. ➤➤*Rationale:* This explanation ensures the patient's cooperation to improve the quality of the tracing and avoids unnecessary repeating of ECGs because of muscle artifact.

PATIENT ASSESSMENT AND PREPARATION
Patient Assessment

- Interpret previously recorded ECGs. ➤➤*Rationale:* Each patient has an individual baseline ECG. Previous ECG recordings can help clinicians determine whether a change is acute or chronic.
- Assess for the presence of anginal symptoms, such as chest pain, pressure, tightness, heaviness, fullness, or squeezing sensation; radiated pain; shortness of breath,

nausea, and extreme fatigue. ➤➤*Rationale:* This evaluation correlates ECG changes with patient symptoms.

- Assess the patient's medical history of cardiac diseases, such as MI and medications. ➤➤*Rationale:* Knowledge about the patient's cardiac history and medications can help in interpretation of ECG recordings (Fig. 58-1). For example, digitalis therapy causes chronic ST-segment depression that does not indicate ischemia. A normal-looking isoelectric ST segment in a patient on digitalis therapy may indicate acute ischemia. Patients with a prior posterior MI might have abnormal Q waves in the left posterior leads.
- Interpret the patient's standard 12-lead ECG for any signs of myocardial ischemia or MI and dysrhythmias. ➤➤*Rationale:* Nurses should be able to evaluate the standard 12-lead ECG for the location of ischemia or infarction and assess the possibility of RV and posterior involvement (Fig. 58-2).

Patient Preparation

- Verify correct patient with two identifiers. ➤➤*Rationale:* Prior to performing a procedure, the nurse should ensure the correct identification of the patient for the intended intervention.
- Ensure that the patient and family understand preprocedural teaching. Answer questions as they arise, and reinforce information as needed. ➤➤*Rationale:* This communication evaluates and reinforces the understanding of previously taught information.
- Assist the patient to the supine position and expose the patient's torso while maintaining the patient's modesty. ➤➤*Rationale:* This position enables the recording of a standard 12-lead ECG and allows comparison of serial ECGs and comparison with standard waveforms. Body positional changes, such as elevation and rotation, can change recorded amplitudes and axes.

Pre-PTCA

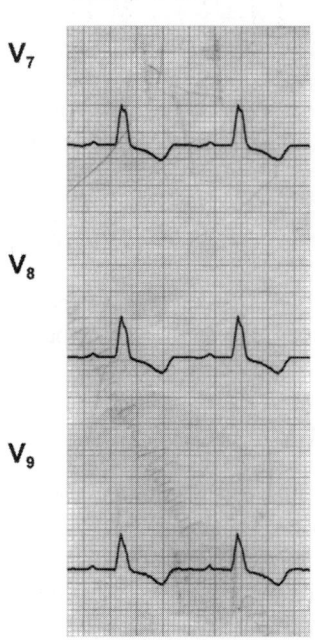

LCX Occlusion

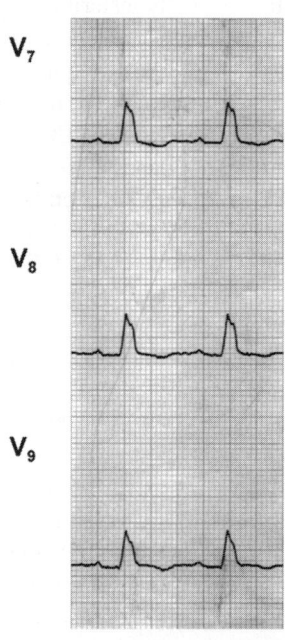

FIGURE 58-1   Baseline ST-segment deviation as a result of left bundle-branch block before percutaneous coronary intervention *(left panel,* before angioplasty). During angioplasty balloon inflation of the proximal left circumflex (LCX) coronary artery *(right panel,* LCX occlusion), the patient developed myocardial ischemia with chest pain radiating to the left arm. ST segments in the left posterior leads (V₇, V₈, and V₉) became elevated compared with the baseline preangioplasty tracing to produce a normal-looking, isoelectric ST segment. This pseudonormalization of the ST segment during ischemia can be misinterpreted as normal without assessment of the baseline ECG.

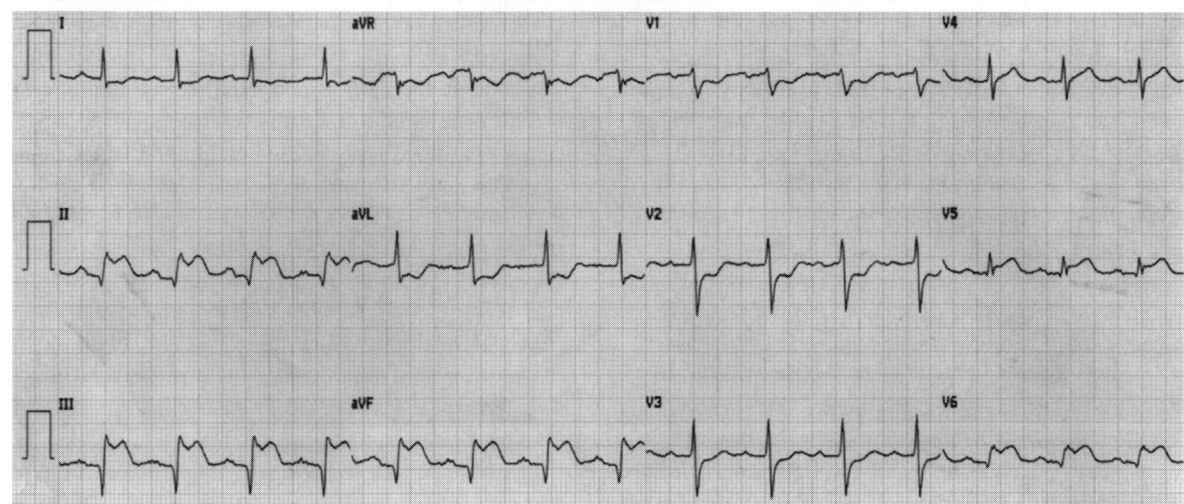

FIGURE 58-2   Initial ECG in a patient admitted to the emergency department with an acute inferior MI (elevated ST segments and Q waves in leads II, III, and aVF) with apical involvement (elevated ST segment in leads V₄, V₅, and V₆). ST-segment depression in leads V₁, V₂, and V₃ suggests posterior involvement. Left posterior and right precordial leads should be recorded to assess posterior and RV involvement.

Procedure for Extra Electrocardiographic Leads

Steps	Rationale	Special Considerations
1. **HH**		
2. **PE**		
3. Check the patient cable and lead wires for fraying or broken wires.	Detects any condition that might cause the ECG recording to be incomplete or inaccurate.	If the equipment is damaged, obtain alternative equipment and notify a biomedical engineer for repair.
4. Check the lead wires for accurate labels.	Obtains accurate ECG recordings and proper placement of leads.	
5. Plug the ECG machine into a grounded wall outlet.	Maintains electrical safety.	Follow manufacturer's recommendations and institution protocol on electrical safety per biomedical department.
6. Turn the ECG machine on and program the ECG machine: paper speed, 25 mm/s; calibration, 10 mm/mV; filter settings, 0.05 to 100 Hz. **(Level E*)**	Prepares equipment. In accordance with clinical practice and recommendation for ST-segment analysis by the American Heart Association (AHA).[12]	Follow the manufacturer's recommendation in configuring the ECG machine.
7. Place the patient in a supine position. **(Level B*)**	Body position changes can cause ST-segment deviation and QRS waveform alteration.[1,3,13,14]	ECGs should be recorded in the same body position to ensure ECG changes are not caused by a change in body position. If another position is clinically necessary, note the altered position on the ECG recording.
8. Expose the body parts for electrode placement.	Overexposing of body parts may cause shivering and lack of privacy.	
9. Identify the electrode sites and mark with an indelible marker.	When multiple ECG recordings are needed, minimization of ECG changes caused by altered electrode placement is important.[9]	After accurate identification of the locations, an indelible marker should be used to mark the electrode sites.
Limb Leads		
• Right arm (RA): Inside right forearm. • Left arm (LA): Inside left forearm. • Right leg (RL): Anywhere on the body; by convention, usually on the right ankle or inner aspect of the calf. • Left leg (LL): Left ankle or inner aspect of the calf.	Accurate electrode placement is essential for obtaining valid and reliable data for ECG recordings. RL electrode is a ground electrode that does not contribute to the ECG tracings.	The limb leads are placed in the same way as when recording a standard 12-lead ECG (see Procedure 60).
Right Precordial Leads (Fig. 58-3)		
• V_{1R}: Fourth intercostal space (ICS) at the left sternal border (same as V_2). • V_{2R}: Fourth ICS at the right sternal border (same as V_1). • V_{3R}: Halfway between V_{2R} and V_{4R}.	All patients with an acute inferior wall MI should have right precordial leads recorded in addition to precordial leads V_1 through V_6.	These right precordial leads are placed across the right precordium with the same landmarks that are used for the precordial leads.[12]

*Level B: Well-designed controlled studies with results that consistently support a specific action, intervention, or treatment
*Level E: Multiple case reports, theory-based evidence from expert opinions, or peer-reviewed professional organizational standards without clinical studies to support recommendations

Procedure continues on following page

Right Precordial Leads

Midclavicular line

Anterior axillary line

Midaxillary line

Angle of Louis

V_{1R}: 4th intercostal space (ICS) at left sternal border

(same as V_2)

V_{2R}: 4th ICS at right sternal border (same as V_1)

V_{3R}: halfway between V_{2R} and V_{4R}

V_{4R}: right midclavicular line in the 5th ICS

V_{5R}: right anterior axillary line at the same horizontal

level as V_{4R}

V_{6R}: right midaxillary line at the same horizontal

level as V_{4R}

V_{6R} V_{5R} V_{4R} V_{3R} V_{2R} V_{1R}

FIGURE 58-3   Electrode locations for recording a right precordial ECG. *(From Drew BJ, Ide B: Right ventricular infarction, Prog Cardiovasc Nurs 10:46, 1995.)*

Procedure for Extra Electrocardiographic Leads—*Continued*

Steps	Rationale	Special Considerations
• V_{4R}: Right midclavicular line in the fifth ICS. • V_{5R}: Right anterior axillary line at the same horizontal level as V_{4R}. • V_{6R}: Right midaxillary line at the same horizontal level as V_{4R}.	Slight alterations in the position of one precordial electrode may distort significantly the appearance of the cardiac waveforms and can have a significant impact on the diagnosis.[8]	V_{1R} is at the same location as V_2, and V_{2R} is at the same location as V_1 in the standard 12-lead ECG (Fig. 58-4). The redundancy of V_1 (or V_{2R}) and V_2 (or V_{1R}) can be used to ensure that the ECGs are recorded accurately. Identify the sternal notch and move downward to locate the angle of Louis; the second ICS is located right below the angle of Louis.

Conventional 12-Lead ECG

Right Precordial Leads

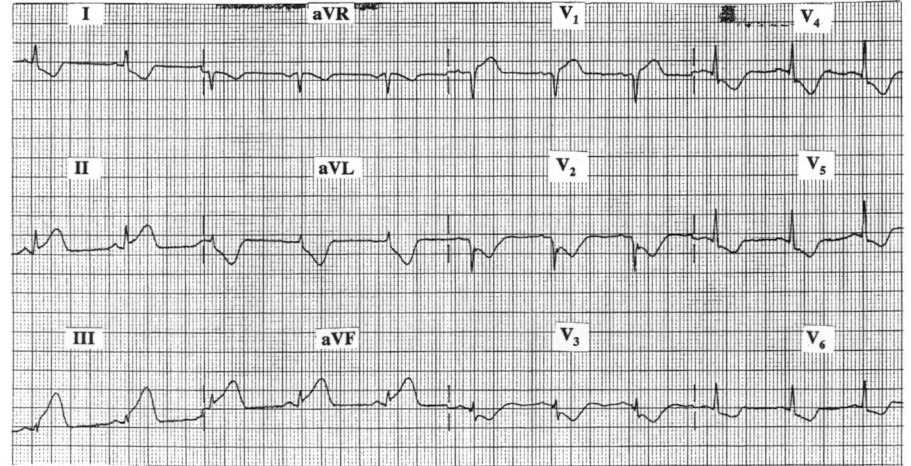

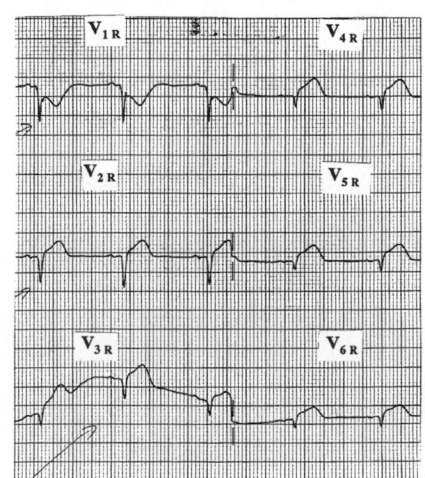

FIGURE 58-4   ST-segment elevation in leads II, III, and aVF indicates acute inferior wall MI. These characteristics on the standard 12-lead ECG *(left panel)* suggest RV infarction: diagnosis of an inferior MI; ST-segment elevation in lead III exceeding that of lead II; ST-segment elevation confined to V_1 without elevation in the remaining precordial leads; and ST depression in lead aVL.[15] Definitive diagnosis of RV infarction is made by observing ST-segment elevation greater than or equal to 1 mm in one or more of the right precordial leads. In the *right panel*, ST-segment elevation is seen in V_{2R} (V_1) through V_{6R}. *(From Drew BJ, Ide B: Right ventricular infarction, Prog Cardiovasc Nurs 10:46, 1995.)*

Procedure for Extra Electrocardiographic Leads—*Continued*

Steps	Rationale	Special Considerations
Left Posterior Leads (Fig. 58-5)		
• V_7: Posterior axillary line at the same level as V_4 through V_6. • V_8: Halfway between V_7 and V_9. • V_9: Left paraspinal line at the same level as V_4 through V_6.	Left posterior leads are placed to view the posterior wall of the left ventricle. Left posterior leads should be recorded in patients admitted with a suspected posterior MI or known to have left circumflex artery disease.	Help the patient turn to the right side to expose the left side of the back. Ensure the patient is safely turned. Leads V_4 through V_6 are located at the midclavicular line in the fifth ICS; leads V_7 through V_9 are at the same horizontal level as V_4 through V_6
10. Clean the area for the application of electrodes with cleansing pads or soap and water and dry thoroughly. **(Level E*)**	Provides for adequate transmission of electrical impulses, reducing noise and improving quality of the signal.[12] Moist skin is not conducive to electrode adherence.[10]	Poor electrode contact may produce instability of the recording, causing baseline wander.

Left Posterior Leads

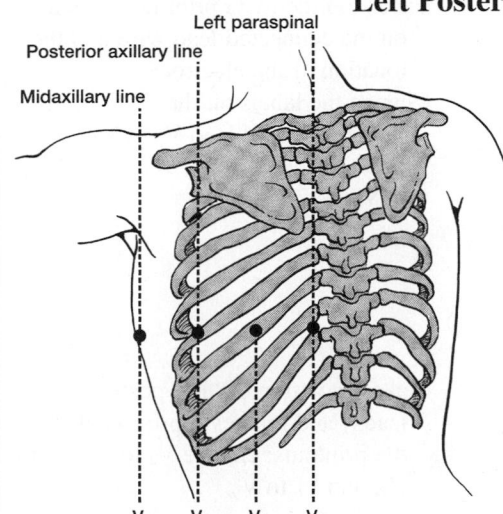

V_7: posterior axillary line at the same level as V_{4-6}

V_8: halfway between V_7 and V_9

V_9: left paraspinal line at the same level as V_{4-6}

FIGURE 58-5 Electrode locations for recording a left posterior ECG.

11. Clean the intended sites with alcohol pads. Consider use of skin preparation solutions. **(Level E)**	Alcohol or skin preparations may be needed to remove oils to improve impulse transmission.[10]	Clip hair if necessary.
12. Abrade the skin with a gauze pad or a terrycloth washcloth.	Removes dead skin cells and may promote impulse transmission.	
13. Place the electrodes on the marked locations.	Secure the electrodes to obtain quality ECG recordings.	If limb plate electrodes are used, do not overtighten to minimize discomfort.

*Level E: Multiple case reports, theory-based evidence from expert opinions, or peer-reviewed professional organizational standards without clinical studies to support recommendations

Procedure continues on following page

Procedure for Extra Electrocardiographic Leads—*Continued*

Steps	Rationale	Special Considerations
14. Identify the number of available ECG channels for simultaneous recording in the ECG machine.	Newer multiple-channel machines can record 16 leads at a time, which allows simultaneous recording of a standard 12-lead ECG and four channels of RV leads V_{3R} through V_{6R} or three channels of left posterior leads V_7 through V_9.	If the ECG machine can record only 12 leads, record three separate ECGs: (1) standard 12-lead with precordial leads; (2) RV leads; and (3) left posterior leads. Some newer generation ECG machines may allow recording more than 12 leads. If the machine can record 16 leads, you can record two ECGs: (1) standard 12-lead plus RV leads (V_{3R} through V_{6R}), then (2) standard 12-lead plus left posterior leads (V_7 through V_9). Follow institution protocol for recording these extra leads so that a consistent method is used to avoid confusion.
15. Connect the lead wires to the electrodes and record the ECG. Correctly label the ECG tracings, with the extra leads noted.	Identifies RV and posterior leads.	Make a notation on the ECG tracing that these are RV leads or posterior leads. Labels on the ECG printout depend on the connected lead wire and the location of the electrode.
A. For recording RV leads with a 12-lead ECG machine, connect as follows: V_1 wire to electrode V_{1R} V_2 wire to electrode V_{2R} V_3 wire to electrode V_{3R} V_4 wire to electrode V_{4R} V_5 wire to electrode V_{5R} V_6 wire to electrode V_{6R}	When the unipolar precordial lead wires V_1 through V_6 are connected to the RV or left posterior electrodes, the ECG machine records signals from where the electrodes are placed.	Change the labels on the ECG printouts from V_1 to V_{1R}, V_2 to V_{2R}, V_3 to V_{3R}, V_4 to V_{4R}, V_5 to V_{5R}, and V_6 to V_{6R}.
B. For recording of left posterior leads with a 12-lead ECG machine, connect as follows: V_4 wire to electrode V_7 V_5 wire to electrode V_8 V_6 wire to electrode V_9		Make a notation of "left posterior leads" and relabel appropriately on the printouts: change V_4 to V_7, V_5 to V_8, and V_6 to V_9.
16. Assess the quality of the tracing.	Ensures a clear tracing is obtained and no lead is off.	
17. Discard used supplies in appropriate receptacles.	Reduces the transmission of microorganisms; Standard Precautions.	
18. **HH**		

Expected Outcomes

- Clear and accurate recording of ECG tracings that allows clinicians to diagnose dysrhythmias and ischemia
- Institution protocol should be developed for recording the extra posterior and RV leads according to the availability and type of ECG machine so that the recording method is consistent

Unexpected Outcomes

- Inaccurate lead placement: electrode misplacement or incorrect lead connection
- Failure to identify the recordings as either RV or left posterior ECGs and to change the ECG leads to their correct labels; this could lead to misdiagnosis
- Poor ECG tracing caused by electrical artifact from external or internal sources

Expected Outcomes	Unexpected Outcomes *—Continued*
	• External artifact introduced by line current (60-cycle interference) may be minimized by disconnecting nearby electrical devices, unplugging the ECG machine and operating on battery, improving grounding, or replacing lead wires • Internal artifact may result from body movement, shivering, muscle tremors, and hiccups

Patient Monitoring and Care

Steps	Rationale	Reportable Conditions
		These conditions should be reported if they persist despite nursing interventions.
1. Evaluate the ECG recordings for acute RV or posterior myocardial ischemia or infarction (Fig. 58-6). Record whether the patient has chest pain on the ECG tracing. Use 0 to 10 score to quantify pain severity (e.g., 8/10 chest pain).	Promptly initiates appropriate interventions, such as reperfusion treatment or vasodilators.	• Abnormal ST-segment deviation (elevation or depression) may indicate acute myocardial ischemia, injury, or infarction.
2. Assess the presence of chest pain or anginal equivalent symptoms (e.g., jaw, left shoulder or arm discomfort, or shortness of breath).	Ischemia caused by decreased coronary blood flow or increased myocardial oxygen demand may produce anginal symptoms.	• Angina
3. Evaluate the patient's ECG for signs of AV node conduction disturbances in patients with RV infarction (e.g., second-degree or third-degree AV block).	The RCA supplies blood to the AV node in 90% of patients. Occlusion of the RCA proximal to the RV branch decreases the blood supply to the AV nodal artery.	• Patients with an acute MI with RV involvement, as evidenced by a QRS pattern or ST-segment elevation greater than or equal to 1 mm in the right precordial leads[5]

Procedure continues on following page

Standard 12-Lead ECG   **Left Posterior Leads**

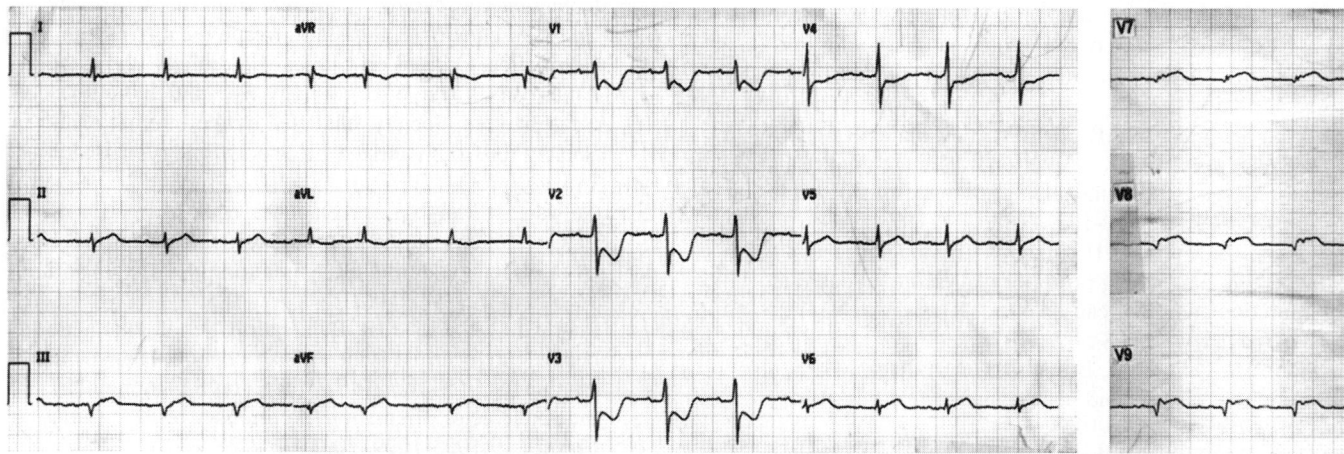

FIGURE 58-6 An ECG recorded in a 76-year-old patient with diabetes during occlusion of the left circumflex artery. ST-segment depression is observed in precordial leads V_1 to V_4, which suggests a posterior MI *(left panel)*. Left posterior leads V_7 to V_9 are helpful in recording ST-segment elevation that confirms posterior myocardial ischemia *(right panel)*. Observing ST-segment elevation in the contiguous posterior leads allows patients with an acute MI to benefit from thrombolytic therapy, which would be denied based on analysis of the standard 12-lead ECG alone.

Patient Monitoring and Care —*Continued*

Steps	Rationale	Reportable Conditions
4. Assess the patient's hemodynamic status	The incidence rate of high-degree AV block in patients with inferior MI with RV involvement is significantly higher (48%) than in patients without RV MI (13%).[4] Hypotension and reduced cardiac output in patients with RV infarction could be attributed to inadequate left ventricular filling.[7]	• Cardiovascular and hemodynamic changes associated with RV ischemia, injury, or infarction (e.g., elevated mean atrial pressure, reduced cardiac output, hypotension, and prominent venous engorgement).

Documentation

Documentation should include the following:
• Patient and family education
• The reason the extra leads are recorded (e.g., suspected RV infarction, posterior MI)
• Description of associated symptoms
• Interpretation of the ECGs recorded

• Interventions as indicated from the recorded ECG
• Occurrence of unexpected outcomes
• Assessment of pain, interventions and response to interventions
• Additional interventions

References

CR 1. Adams MG, Drew BJ: Body position effects on the ECG: implication for ischemia monitoring, *J Electrocardiol* 30:285-291, 1997.

CR 2. Adams-Hamoda MG, Caldwell MA, Stotts NA, et al: Factors to consider when analyzing 12-lead electrocardiograms for evidence of acute myocardial ischemia, *Am J Crit Care* 12:9-18, 2003.

3. Baevsky RH, Haber MD, Blank FS, et al: Supine vs semi-recumbent and upright 12-lead electrocardiogram: does change in body position alter the electrocardiographic interpretation for ischemia? *Am J Emerg Med* 25:753-756, 2007.

CR 4. Braat SH, Brugada P, den Dulk K, et al: Value of lead V4R for recognition of the infarct coronary artery in acute inferior myocardial infarction, *Am J Cardiol* 53:1538-1541, 1984.

CR 5. Braat SH, Gorgels AP, Bar FW, et al: Value of the ST-T segment in lead V4R in inferior wall acute myocardial infarction to predict the site of coronary arterial occlusion, *Am J Cardiol* 62:140-142, 1988.

CR 6. Casas RE, Marriott HJ, Glancy DL: Value of leads V7-V9 in diagnosing posterior wall acute myocardial infarction and other causes of tall R waves in V1-V2, *Am J Cardiol* 80:508-509, 1997.

CR 7. Cohn JN, Guiha NH, Broder MI, et al: Right ventricular infarction: clinical and hemodynamic features, *Am J Cardiol* 33:209-214, 1974.

8. Drew BJ: Pitfalls and artifacts in electrocardiography, *Cardiol Clin* 24:309-315, vii, 2006.

9. Drew BJ: Pseudo myocardial injury patterns because of nonstandard electrocardiogram electrode placement, *J Electrocardiol* 41:202-204, 2008.

CR 10. Drew BJ, et al: Practice standards for electrocardiographic monitoring in hospital settings: an American Heart Association Scientific Statement from the Councils on Cardiovascular Nursing, Clinical Cardiology, and Cardiovascular Disease in the Young, *Circulation* 110:2721-2746, 2004.

CR 11. Haisty WK Jr, Pahlm O, Wagner NB, et al: Performance of the automated complete Selvester QRS scoring system in normal subjects and patients with single and multiple myocardial infarctions, *J Am Coll Cardiol* 19:341-346 1992.

12. Kligfield P, Gettes LS, Bailey JJ, et al: Recommendations for the standardization and interpretation of the electrocardiogram: part I: the electrocardiogram and its technology: a scientific statement from the American Heart Association Electrocardiography and Arrhythmias Committee, Council on Clinical Cardiology; the American College of Cardiology Foundation; and the Heart Rhythm Society: endorsed by the International Society for Computerized Electrocardiology, *Circulation* 115:1306-1324, 2007.

CR 13. Nelwan SP, Meij SH, van Dam TB, et al: Correction of ECG variations caused by body position changes and electrode placement during ST-T monitoring, *J Electrocardiol* 34(Suppl):213-216, 2001.

CR 14. Pharand C, Nasmith JB, Rajaonah JC, et al. Distinction between myocardial ischemia and postural changes in continuous ECG monitoring based on ST-segment amplitude and vector orientation: preliminary results, *Can J Cardiol* 19:1023-1029, 2003.

15. Wung SF: Discriminating between right coronary artery and circumflex artery occlusion by using a noninvasive 18-lead electrocardiogram, *Am J Crit Care* 16:63-71, 2007.

Continuous ST-Segment Monitoring

PURPOSE: Bedside ST-segment monitoring provides ongoing surveillance for detection of transient myocardial ischemia. This technology should be applied to patients who are being evaluated or are diagnosed with acute coronary syndrome, including acute myocardial infarction and unstable angina.[2,3,8,13,16] For these patients, continuous ST-segment monitoring is valuable in determining the success of thrombolytic therapy and percutaneous coronary intervention and detecting recurrent or transient ischemia. The goal of continuous ST-segment monitoring is to detect new or recurrent myocardial ischemia.

Michele M. Pelter, Mary G. Carey

PREREQUISITE NURSING KNOWLEDGE

- Understanding of the anatomy and physiology of the cardiovascular system, principles of cardiac conduction, electrocardiogram (ECG) lead placement, basic dysrhythmia interpretation, and electrical safety is needed.
- Advanced cardiac life support knowledge and skills are necessary.
- Continuous monitoring of the ECG for ischemic ST-segment changes is more reliable than patient symptoms because more than three quarters of ECG-detected ischemic events are clinically silent.[2,8,13,16] Patients who have transient ischemia detected with continuous ST-segment monitoring are more likely to have unfavorable outcomes, including myocardial infarction (MI) and death, compared with patients without such events.[2,3,8,10,11,13,16]
- Because of the dynamic, unpredictable, and silent nature of myocardial ischemia, continuous monitoring of patients for ischemia is essential. Clinicians should monitor the trend of the ST segments over time and evaluate any ST-segment changes (elevation or depression) for possible myocardial ischemia (Fig. 59-1).
- Other nonischemic causes for a change in the ST-segment trend are movement of the skin electrodes, dysrhythmias,

intermittent bundle-branch block pattern, body position changes, and ventricular paced rhythms.[8,12]

- The first type of ischemia seen in patients with acute coronary syndrome (ACS) is supply-related ischemia from coronary occlusion. Coronary occlusion is brought on by disruption of an atherosclerotic plaque followed by cycles of plaque rupture, platelet stimulation, coronary vasospasm, and thrombus formation.[5,6,14,19] Because this type of ischemia threatens the entire thickness of the myocardium, immediate treatment to reestablish blood flow to the heart is essential. The typical ECG manifestation of total coronary occlusion is ST-segment elevation visible in the ECG leads that lie directly over the ischemic myocardial zone. Occlusion of the right coronary artery (RCA) typically produces ST-segment elevation in leads II, III, and augmented vector foot or aVF (Fig. 59-2). Occlusion of the left anterior descending (LAD) coronary artery typically produces ST-segment elevation in leads V_2, V_3, and V_4 (Fig. 59-3). Diagnosis of total coronary occlusion of the left circumflex coronary artery (LCX) is more complex because placement of the standard ECG electrodes is on the anterior chest, opposite the wall that this coronary artery supplies. Occlusion of the LCX may produce ST-segment depression in leads V_1, V_2, or V_3, which reflects the reciprocal, or mirror image,

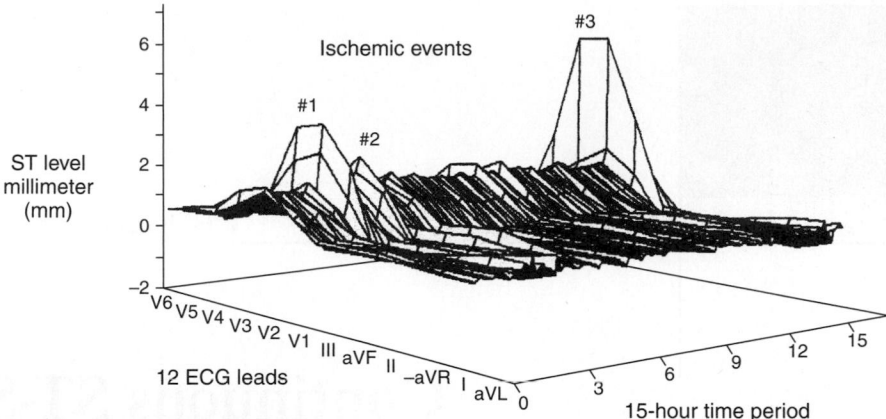

FIGURE 59-1   The importance of assessing the trend of the ST segments over time. The three-dimensional image illustrates ST-segment deviation in millimeters *(Y-axis)* in all 12 ECG leads *(X-axis)* over a 15-hour period *(Z-axis)*. Illustrated are three separate ischemic events, characterized by ST-segment elevation, in leads V_3 to V_5. *(Adapted from Pelter MM, Adams MG, Drew BJ: Transient myocardial ischemia is an independent predictor of adverse in-hospital outcomes in patients with acute coronary syndromes treated in the telemetry unit, Heart Lung 32:71-78, 2003.)*

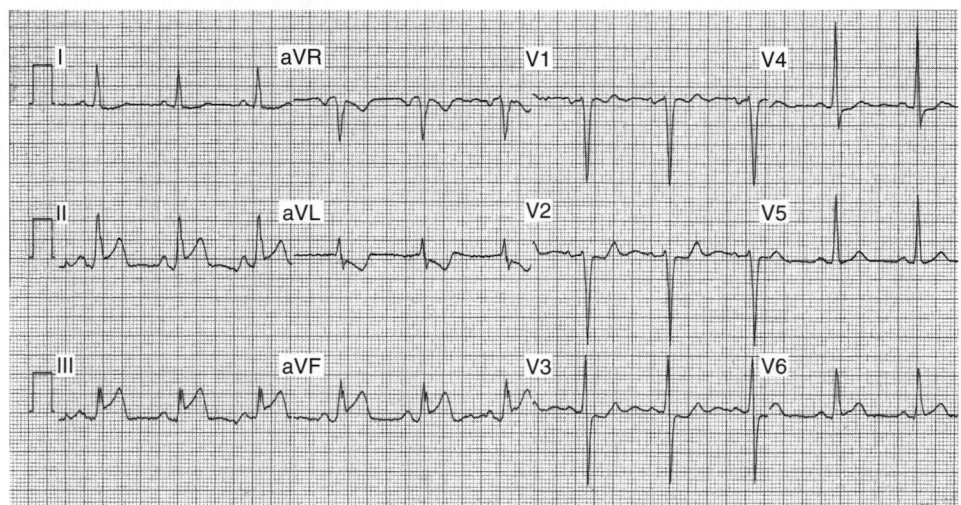

FIGURE 59-2   The typical ST-segment pattern of supply-related ischemia in the inferior wall. The RCA is likely occluded, resulting in ST-segment elevation in leads II, III, and aVF.

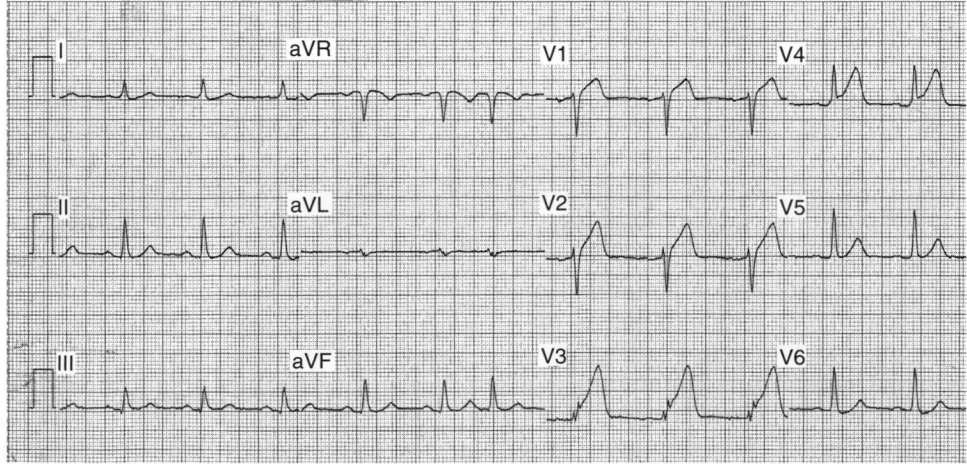

FIGURE 59-3   The typical ST-segment pattern of supply-related ischemia in the anterior wall. The LAD artery is likely occluded, resulting in ST-segment elevation in leads V_2 to V_4.

ST-segment elevation occurring in the posterior wall of the myocardium.

- A second type of ischemia for which patients with ACS or stable angina are at risk is demand-related ischemia. This type of ischemia may occur when the demand for oxygen (i.e., exercise, tachycardia, or stress) exceeds the flow capabilities of a coronary artery with a stable atherosclerotic plaque. The ST-segment pattern of demand-related ischemia is depression, often appearing in several ECG leads (Fig. 59-4).

- Diagnosis of myocardial ischemia necessitates continuous monitoring of all 12 ECG leads because the mechanism of ischemia may vary (i.e., occlusion versus demand-related ischemia), resulting in distinctly different ST-segment patterns (e.g., elevation or depression). If only two ECG leads are available, however, the best two are leads III and V_3.[8] Patient-specific monitoring also may be done if a prior 12-lead ECG was obtained during acute ischemia (i.e., ST-segment elevation MI, percutaneous coronary intervention [PCI], or treadmill test). In this scenario, the ECG lead or leads showing maximal ST-segment deviation should be selected for continuous monitoring to detect recurrent ischemia.

- According to current consensus statements,[8,9] multilead ST-segment monitoring is indicated in most patients with the following diagnoses:
  - ❖ Early phase of acute MI (ST elevation, non-ST elevation, "rule-out")
  - ❖ Chest pain (or anginal equivalent) that prompts a visit to the emergency department
  - ❖ After nonurgent PCI procedures with suboptimal results
  - ❖ Variant angina resulting from coronary vasospasm

- According to these same guidelines,[8,9] ST-segment monitoring may be of benefit for the following cases:
  - ❖ Postacute MI
  - ❖ After nonurgent uncomplicated PCI
  - ❖ With high risk for ischemia after cardiac or noncardiac surgery

- ST-segment monitoring may not be appropriate for certain patient groups because current software cannot reliably interpret ST-segment changes resulting from myocardial ischemia.[8,9] Specifically, it may not be suitable to monitor patients with:
  - ❖ Left bundle-branch block
  - ❖ Ventricular paced rhythm
  - ❖ Confounding dysrhythmias that obscure the ST segment
  - ❖ Agitation causing excessive artifact

- A variety of bedside and telemetry cardiac monitors are currently available for use in clinical practice. Not all monitoring systems are equipped with ST-segment monitoring software, however. Clinicians must determine whether their cardiac monitoring system has ST-segment monitoring capabilities.

EQUIPMENT

- Electrodes, pregelled and disposable
- Cardiac monitor with ST-segment monitoring capability and patient cable
- Nonsterile gloves
- Gauze pads or terrycloth washcloth
- Cleansing pads or nonemollient soap and water
- Alcohol pads
- ECG calipers

  Additional equipment to have available as needed includes the following:
- Clippers or scissors to clip hair from chest if needed
- Indelible marker
- 12-lead ECG machine

PATIENT AND FAMILY EDUCATION

- Explain the purpose of ST-segment monitoring. ➤*Rationale:* This explanation decreases patient and family anxiety.
- Encourage the patient to report any symptoms of chest pain or anginal equivalent (e.g., arm pain, jaw pain,

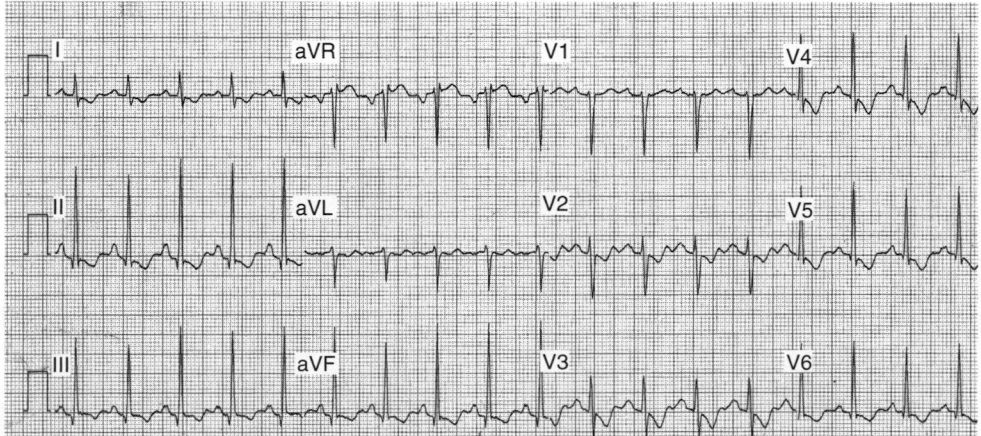

FIGURE 59-4   The typical ST-segment pattern of demand-related ischemia. Note the ST-segment depression appearing in nearly every ECG lead, with the exception of V_1 and aVR. Note also that this patient is experiencing tachycardia, a common cause of demand-related ischemia.

shortness of breath, or nausea). ➤*Rationale:* This education heightens the patient's awareness of cardiac sensations and encourages communication of anginal symptoms.

PATIENT ASSESSMENT AND PREPARATION

Patient Assessment

- Identify patients at risk for ischemia.[8] ➤*Rationale:* Patients at risk for myocardial ischemia need to be identified.
- Assess the patient's cardiac rhythm. ➤*Rationale:* This assessment provides baseline data and ensures the patient has a cardiac rhythm suitable for ST-segment monitoring.
- Identify the patient's baseline ST-segment levels before initiating ST-segment monitoring. ➤*Rationale:* The

patient's baseline ST-segment level is identified for comparison with subsequent changes.

Patient Preparation

- Verify correct patient with two identifiers. ➤*Rationale:* Prior to performing a procedure, the nurse should ensure the correct identification of the patient for the intended intervention.
- Ensure that the patient and family understand preprocedural teaching. Answer questions as they arise, and reinforce information as needed. ➤*Rationale:* This communication evaluates and reinforces understanding of previously taught information.
- Place the patient in a resting supine position in bed, and expose the patient's torso while maintaining modesty. ➤*Rationale:* This preparation provides access to the patient's chest for electrode placement and ensures that an artifact-free ECG is obtained.

Procedure | for Continuous ST-Segment Monitoring

Steps	Rationale	Special Considerations
1. **HH**		
2. **PE**		
3. Identify accurate electrode placement (Fig. 59-5; see also Procedures 57 and 60).	Ensures accurate ECG data.[8]	Electrodes (V_3 to V_5) should be placed immediately below a pendulous breast so that the breast lies on top of the electrode, preventing motion artifact.
4. Clean the area for the application of electrodes with cleansing pads or soap and water and dry thoroughly. **(Level E*)**	Provides for adequate transmission of electrical impulses. Moist skin is not conducive to electrode adherence.[8] Failure to properly prepare the skin may cause inappropriate monitoring alarms.[8]	Chest hair may need clipping with scissors to ensure good skin contact with the electrodes.

*Level E: Multiple case reports, theory-based evidence from expert opinions, or peer-reviewed professional organizational standards without clinical studies to support recommendations

---

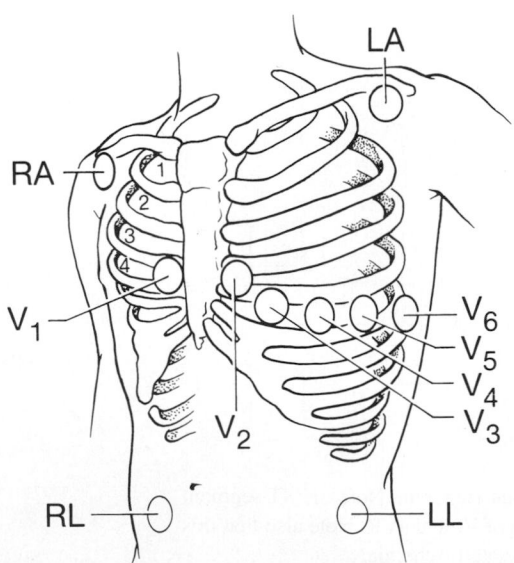

FIGURE 59-5   Correct lead placement for 12-lead ST-segment monitoring. Limb electrodes must be located as close as possible to the junction to the limb and the torso. To ensure an inferior view of the myocardium, the left leg *(LL)* electrode must be placed well below the level of the umbilicus. For V_1, the electrode is located at the fourth intercostal space to the right of the sternum. V_2 is in the same fourth intercostal space just to the left of the sternum, and V_4 is in the fifth intercostal space on the midclavicular line. Placement of lead V_3 is halfway on a straight line between leads V_2 and V_4. Leads V_5 and V_6 are positioned on a straight line from V_4, with V_5 in the anterior axillary line and V_6 in the midaxillary line. *RA*, Right arm; *LA*, left arm; *RL*, right leg.

Procedure for Continuous ST-Segment Monitoring—*Continued*

Steps	Rationale	Special Considerations
5. Clean the intended sites with alcohol pads. Consider use of skin preparation solutions. (**Level E***)	Alcohol or skin preparations may be needed to remove oils and dead skin cells to improve impulse transmission.[4,8,15] Moist skin is not conducive to electrode adherence.[4,8,15]	
6. Abrade the skin with a washcloth or gauze pad.	Removes dead skin cells, promoting impulse transmission.	
7. If possible, mark any precordial location with a black indelible marker.	Prevents inaccurate electrode placement after bathing or inadvertent removal of the electrodes.	Continuous ST-segment monitoring trends depend on stable electrode placement. Sudden changes in ST-segment trends often indicate electrode movement.
8. Remove the backing from the pregelled electrodes and test the center of the pads for moistness.	Gel can dry out in storage; gel should be moist to allow for impulse transmission.	
9. Connect the ECG leads to the electrodes before placing the electrodes on the patient (see Procedure 57).	Prepares the monitoring system and prevents unnecessary pressure on the patient's chest when connecting the lead wires to the electrodes.	
10. Select the monitoring leads.	Although any ECG lead can be used for ST-segment monitoring, monitoring of all 12 ECG leads or the selection of a lead(s) based on the myocardial zone at risk is desirable (e.g., inferior or anterior).[8]	If continuous 12-lead ECG monitoring is unavailable, lead-specific ischemia monitoring is encouraged. Lead III is sensitive to inferior ischemia, and V_3 is sensitive to anterior or posterior ischemia.[8,9]
11. If required by the bedside monitor manufacturer, identify the ECG complex landmarks and select the J point + 60-ms landmark.[8,9] (**Level M***)	Prepares the monitoring system and ensures accurate monitoring.	Refer to manufacturer's recommendations.
12. Set the ST-segment alarm.	Maximizes the sensitivity and specificity of ST-segment monitoring and may reduce unnecessary false alarms.	For bedside cardiac monitoring, the alarm threshold should be set 1 to 2 mm above and below the patient's baseline ST-segment level (Fig. 59-6).[8,9] Establishing a patient-specific ST-segment level, rather than an isoelectric ST-segment level is important because the patient's baseline ST-segment level is rarely isoelectric.[8,9,12]
13. Discard used supplies in appropriate receptacles.	Reduces the transmission of microorganisms; Standard Precautions.	
14. HH		
15. Print the baseline ECG tracing to evaluate the quality of the signal and secure for future reference.	Ensures a quality baseline ECG for comparing subsequent changes because ST-segment monitoring is based on continuous trending.	Verify that lead wires are not reversed, especially the limb leads.

*Level E: Multiple case reports, theory-based evidence from expert opinions, or peer-reviewed professional organizational standards without clinical studies to support recommendations
*Level M: Manufacturer's recommendations only

Procedure continues on following page

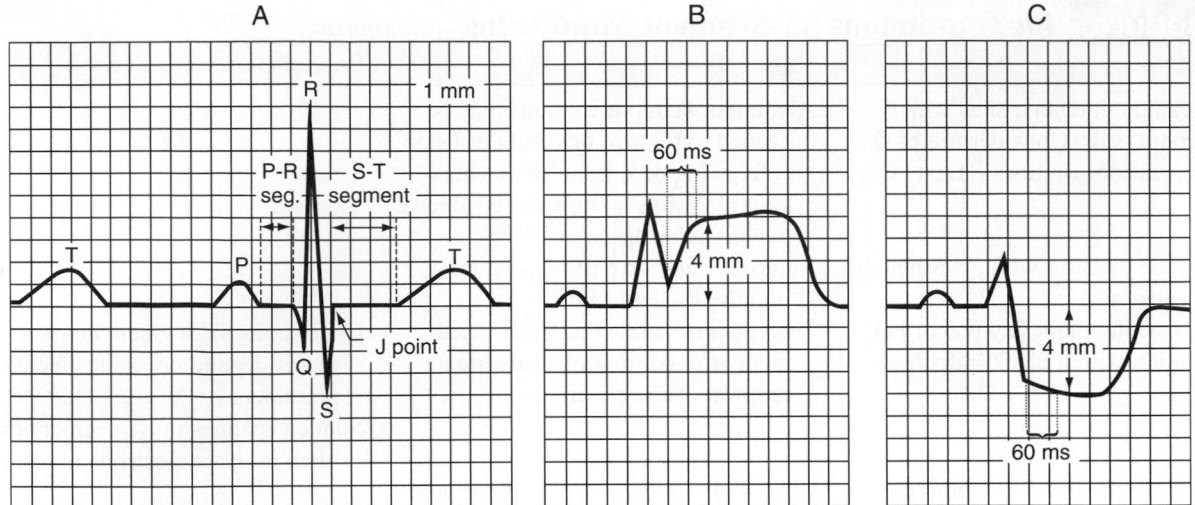

FIGURE 59-6   **A,** Normal ECG complex. Measurement points used in ST-segment analysis are indicated. The PR segment is used to identify the isoelectric line. The ST segment begins at the J point, which is the end of the QRS complex. The ST-segment measurement point can be measured at 60 or 80 ms past the J point. **B,** ST-segment elevation. The ST segment shown measures +4 mm. **C,** ST-segment depression. The ST segment shown measures –4 mm. *(Adapted from Tisdale LA, Drew BJ: ST segment monitoring for myocardial ischemia, AACN Clin Issues Crit Care Nurs 4:36, 1993.)*

Procedure for Continuous ST-Segment Monitoring—*Continued*

Steps	Rationale	Special Considerations
16. If possible, obtain an ECG with the patient in right and left side-lying positions and secure these for future reference.	Comparison of side-lying ECGs with ECGs from subsequent alarms may prevent interpreting as ischemia false-positive ST-segment deviations caused by changes in body position.[1,7,17]	

Expected Outcomes

- Accurate ECG monitoring that allows clinicians to interpret ST-segment changes
- Timely detection of myocardial ischemia
- An increase in the number of bedside alarms when the ST-segment software is initiated. These may be caused by actual ischemia, body position changes, transient dysrhythmias, heart rate changes, artifact, lead misplacement[12]

Unexpected Outcomes

- Skin sensitivity to electrodes
- Inappropriate diagnosis of ischemia in nonischemic conditions (i.e., bundle-branch block, early repolarization)[18]
- Inappropriate intervention based on a false ST-segment alarm[7]
- Pain assessment, interventions, and effectiveness

Patient Monitoring and Care

Steps	Rationale	Reportable Conditions
		These conditions should be reported if they persist despite nursing interventions.
1. Check electrode placement every shift	Enhances the quality of ST-segment monitoring.	
2. Evaluate ST-segment trends routinely while obtaining vital signs.	Ensures that no significant deviations in the ST-segment trend occur.	• ST-segment trend changes

Patient Monitoring and Care —*Continued*

Steps	Rationale	Special Considerations
3 Interpret all ST-segment alarms and determine the cause. If actual ischemia is noted, assess the patient for signs and symptoms that suggest acute ischemia, anginal equivalents, hemodynamic changes, or dysrhythmias and then obtain a 12-lead ECG.	Ensures accurate interpretation A 12-lead ECG assists with determining ischemia location and type (i.e., supply versus demand). Determines the patient's response to ischemia.	• ST-segment changes • Onset of symptoms or anginal equivalent
4. Assess the patient for signs and symptoms that suggest acute ischemia, even if no new ST-segment changes are identified, and obtain a 12-lead ECG as needed.	Determines the presence of ischemia. Because ischemia can be clinically silent, a 12-lead ECG assists with determining ischemia location and type (i.e., supply versus demand)	• ST-segment changes • Onset of symptoms or anginal equivalent
5. Follow institution standard for assessing pain. Administer analgesia and nitrates as prescribed.	Identifies need for pain interventions.	• Continued pain despite pain interventions

Documentation

Documentation should include the following:
• Patient and family education
• Initiation of ST-segment bedside monitoring
• Initial ECG strip with baseline ST segment
• Any ST-segment changes or any symptoms that suggest acute ischemia

• Presence and intensity of chest pain or anginal equivalent, interventions, and effectiveness
• Additional interventions taken
• Unexpected outcomes

References

CR 1. Adams MG, Drew BJ: Body position effects on the ECG: implication for ischemia monitoring, *J Electrocardiol* 30(4):285-291, 1997.

CR 2. Adams MG, Pelter MM, Wung SF, et al: Frequency of silent myocardial ischemia with 12-lead ST segment monitoring in the coronary care unit: are there sex-related differences? *Heart Lung* 28(2):81-86, 1999.

CR 3. Akkerhuis KM, Klootwijk PA, Lindeboom W, et al: Recurrent ischaemia during continuous multilead ST-segment monitoring identifies patients with acute coronary syndromes at high risk of adverse cardiac events; meta-analysis of three studies involving 995 patients, *Eur Heart J* 22(21):1997-2006, 2001.

CR 4. Clochesy JM, Cifani L, Howe K: Electrode site preparation techniques: a follow-up study, *Heart Lung* 20(1):27-30, 1991.

5. Cura FA, Escudero AG, Berrocal D0, et al: Protection of distal embolization in high-risk patients with acute ST-segment elevation myocardial infarction (PREMIAR), *Am J Cardiol* 99(3):357-363, 2007.

CR 6. DeWood MA, Spores J, Notske R, et al: Prevalence of total coronary occlusion during the early hours of transmural myocardial infarction, *N Engl J Med* 303(16):897-902, 1980.

CR 7. Drew BJ, Adams MG: Clinical consequences of ST-segment changes caused by body position mimicking transient myocardial ischemia: hazards of ST-segment monitoring? *J Electrocardiol* 34(3):261-264, 2001.

CR 8. Drew BJ, Califf RM, Funk M, et al: AHA scientific statement: practice standards for electrocardiographic monitoring in hospital settings: an American Heart Association Scientific Statement from the Councils on Cardiovascular Nursing, Clinical Cardiology, and Cardiovascular Disease in the Young: endorsed by the International Society of Computerized electrocardiology and the American Association of Critical-Care Nurses, *J Cardiovasc Nurs* 20(2):76-106, 2005.

CR 9. Drew BJ, Krucoff MW: Multilead ST-segment monitoring in patients with acute coronary syndromes: a consensus statement for healthcare professionals: ST-Segment Monitoring Practice Guideline International Working Group, *Am J Crit Care* 8(6):372-388, 1999.

CR 10. Drew BJ, Pelter MM, Adams MG: Frequency, characteristics, and clinical significance of transient ST segment elevation in patients with acute coronary syndromes, *Eur Heart J* 23(12):941-947, 2002.

CR 11. Drew BJ, Pelter MM, Lee E, et al: Designing prehospital ECG systems for acute coronary syndromes: lessons learned from clinical trials involving 12-lead ST-segment monitoring, *J Electrocardiol* 38(4 Suppl):180-185, 2005.

CR 12. Drew BJ, Wung SF, Adams MG, et al: Bedside diagnosis of myocardial ischemia with ST-segment monitoring technology: measurement issues for real-time clinical decision making and trial designs, *J Electrocardiol* 30(Suppl):157-165, 1998.

CR 13. Gottlieb SO, Weisfeldt ML, Ouyang P, et al: Silent ischemia as a marker for early unfavorable outcomes in patients with unstable angina, *N Engl J Med* 314(19):1214-1219, 1986.

CR 14. Krucoff MW, Croll MA, Pope JE, et al: Continuously updated 12-lead ST-segment recovery analysis for myocardial infarct artery patency assessment and its correlation with multiple simultaneous early angiographic observations, *Am J Cardiol* 71(2):145-151, 1993.

CR 15. Medina V, Clochesy JM, Omery A: Comparison of electrode site preparation techniques, *Heart Lung* 18(5):456-460, 1989.

CR 16. Pelter MM, Adams MG, Drew BJ: Transient myocardial ischemia is an independent predictor of adverse in-hospital outcomes in patients with acute coronary syndromes treated in the telemetry unit, *Heart Lung* 32(2):71-78, 2003.

17. Shusterman V, Goldberg A, Schindler DM, et al: Dynamic tracking of ischemia in the surface electrocardiogram, *J Electrocardiol* 40(6 Suppl):S179-S186, 2007.

18. Stephens KE, Anderson H, Carey MG, et al: Interpreting 12-lead electrocardiograms for acute ST-elevation myocardial infarction: what nurses know, *J Cardiovasc Nurs* 22(3):186-193, 2007.

CR 19. Stone GW, Webb J, Cox DA, et al: Distal microcirculatory protection during percutaneous coronary intervention in acute ST-segment elevation myocardial infarction: a randomized controlled trial, *JAMA* 293(9):1063-1072, 2005.

Additional Readings

CR Adams MG, Pelter MM: In hospital cardiac monitoring. In Conover M, editor: *Understanding electrocardiography,* ed 8, St Louis, 2003, Mosby, 431-443.

CR Adams-Hamoda MG, et al: Factors to consider when analyzing 12-lead electrocardiograms for evidence of acute myocardial ischemia, *Am J Crit Care* 12, 9-18, 2003.

Wagner GS: *Marriott's practical electrocardiology,* ed 11, Philadelphia, 2008, Lippincott Williams & Wilkins.

PROCEDURE **60**

Twelve-Lead Electrocardiogram

PURPOSE: A 12-lead electrocardiogram provides information about the electrical system of the heart from 12 different views or leads. The electrocardiogram is the most commonly conducted cardiovascular diagnostic procedure.[3] Common uses of a 12-lead electrocardiogram include diagnosis of acute coronary syndromes, identification of dysrhythmias and conduction disturbances, and determination of the effects of medications or electrolytes on the electrical system of the heart.

Mary G. McKinley

PREREQUISITE NURSING KNOWLEDGE

- Understanding of the anatomy and physiology of the cardiovascular system, principles of cardiac conduction, the cardiac cycle, properties of cardiac tissue (automaticity, excitability, conductivity, and refractoriness), principles of electrophysiology, electrocardiographic (ECG) lead placement, basic dysrhythmia interpretation, and electrical safety is necessary.
- Advanced cardiac life support knowledge and skills are needed.
- Clinical and technical competence in the use of the 12-lead ECG machine and recorder is necessary.
- A 12-lead ECG provides different views or leads of the electrical activity of the heart. The leads are standard limb leads (I, II, III), augmented limb leads (Augmented Vector Right or aVR, Augmented Vector Foot or aVF, and Augmented vector Left or aVL), and six chest leads (V_1 to V_6).
- The standard and augmented leads view the heart from the vertical or frontal plane (Fig. 60-1), and the chest leads view the heart from the horizontal plane (Fig. 60-2).
- The graphic display consists of the P, Q, R, S, and T waves, which represent electrical activity within the heart.

- Serial 12-lead ECGs (more than two ECGs recorded at different times) may be obtained. The accuracy of interpretation relies on consistent electrode placement. Indelible markers can be used to identify the electrode locations to ensure that the same lead placement is used when serial ECGs are recorded.
- Advances in technology have allowed for online or wireless transmission, networking capabilities, and computerized interpretation of the 12-lead ECG (Fig. 60-3). The 12-lead ECG cable is attached to a processing device that

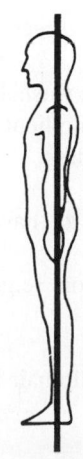

FIGURE 60-1   Vertical plane leads: I, II, III, aVR, aVL, aVF.

519

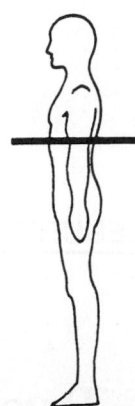

FIGURE 60-2   Horizontal plane leads: V_1 to V_6.

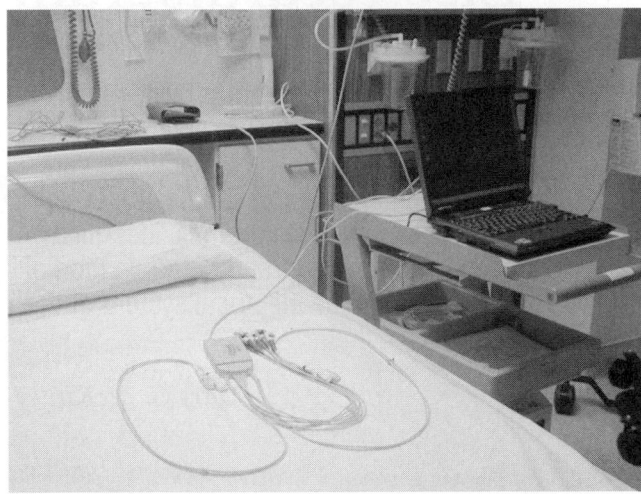

FIGURE 60-3   Example of a wireless ECG device. The 12-lead cable is attached to a processing device that can then be transmitted to the medical record.

digitizes the 12-lead ECG recording and transfers the information to the wireless device, which transmits the information to the medical record. This increases access to the 12-lead ECG for review and can assist with rapid interpretation and treatment of the patient.

EQUIPMENT

- 12-lead ECG machine and recorder
- Electrodes
- Gauze pads or terrycloth washcloth
- Cleansing pads or nonemollient soap and water
- Patient cable and lead wires
- Alcohol pads
  Additional equipment to have available as needed includes the following:
- Skin preparation solution (e.g., skin barrier wipe or tincture of benzoin)
- Indelible marker
- Clippers or scissors to clip hair from chest if needed

PATIENT AND FAMILY EDUCATION

- Assess the readiness of the patient and family to learn. ➡️*Rationale:* Anxiety and concerns of the patient and family may inhibit the ability to learn.
- Provide explanations of the equipment and procedure to the patient and family. ➡️*Rationale:* Information may decrease anxiety.
- Emphasize that the patient should not talk but should relax, lie still, and breathe normally. ➡️*Rationale:* Chest movement can distort the ECG picture.
- Reassure the patient and family that the 12-lead ECG will be reviewed and that any alterations or problems will be addressed. ➡️*Rationale:* Patients and families need to be reassured that immediate care is available if it is needed.

PATIENT ASSESSMENT AND PREPARATION

Patient Assessment

- Assess the patient's peripheral pulses, vital signs, heart sounds, level of consciousness, lung sounds, neck vein distention, presence of chest pain or palpitations, and peripheral circulatory disorders (e.g., clubbing, cyanosis, and dependent edema). ➡️*Rationale:* Physical signs and symptoms may result from alterations in performance of the cardiovascular system.
- Assess the patient's history of cardiac dysrhythmias or cardiac problems. ➡️*Rationale:* This assessment provides baseline data.
- Assess patient medications. ➡️*Rationale:* This assessment provides baseline data.
- Assess previous 12-lead ECGs. ➡️*Rationale:* Previous ECGs provide baseline data.

Patient Preparation

- Verify correct patient with two identifiers. ➡️*Rationale:* Prior to performing a procedure, the nurse should ensure the correct identification of the patient for the intended intervention.
- Ensure that the patient and family understand preprocedural teaching. Answer questions as they arise, and reinforce information as needed. ➡️*Rationale:* This information evaluates and reinforces understanding of previously taught information.
- Assist the patient to a supine position. ➡️*Rationale:* This position allows easy access to the chest for electrode placement; changes in body position may affect the accuracy of the ECG recording.
- Assist the patient in removing clothing that covers the chest while providing for the patient's privacy. ➡️*Rationale:* Removal of clothing provides a clear view of the chest and allows for identification of landmarks and proper placement of leads while maintaining the patient's privacy.

Procedure for 12-Lead Electrocardiogram

Steps	Rationale	Special Considerations
1. **HH**		
2. Check cables and lead wires for fraying, broken wires, or discoloration.	Detects conditions that can give an inaccurate ECG trace.	If equipment is damaged, obtain alternative equipment and notify the biomedical engineer for repair.
3. Plug the ECG machine into a grounded alternating current (AC) wall outlet or ensure functioning if battery operated.	Maintains electrical safety.	
4. Turn the ECG machine on and input the information required.	Equipment may require self-test and warm-up time. Multichannel machines may require input of information (e.g., data about the patient) to store the ECG appropriately.	Follow the manufacturer's recommendations and requirements regarding input of information and warm-up time.
5. **PE**		
6. Ensure that the patient is in the supine position and is not touching the bedrails or footboard.	Provides adequate support for limbs so that muscle activity is minimal. Touching the bedrails or footboard may increase the chance of distortion of the ECG tracing. Body position changes can cause alterations in the ECG tracing.	The supine position is best, but Fowler's position or other positions may be used for comfort. ECGs should be recorded in the same position to ensure that tracing changes are not caused by changes in body position. If another position is clinically necessary, note the position on the tracing or in the comments of the machine input.
7. Expose only the necessary parts of the patient's legs, arms, and chest.	Provides privacy and warmth, which reduces shivering.	Ensuring privacy may reduce anxiety, which can alter the ECG reading. Shivering interferes with the recording.
8. Identify lead sites:	Ensures the accuracy of the lead placement.	Mark the sites with an indelible marker if serial ECGs are anticipated.
A. Limb leads (Fig. 60-4).	Promotes correct positioning of the limb leads. Ensures an accurate tracing of the heart from a view in the vertical and frontal planes.	Limb leads should be placed in fleshy areas; bony prominences should be avoided. The limb leads need to be placed equidistant from the heart and should be positioned in approximately the same place on each limb.

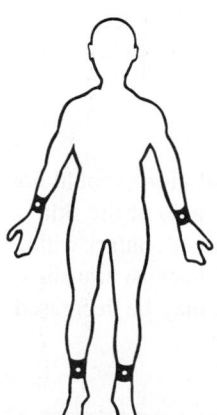

FIGURE 60-4   Limb lead placement in 12-lead ECG.

Procedure continues on following page

Procedure for 12-Lead Electrocardiogram—*Continued*

Steps	Rationale	Special Considerations
B. Chest leads (Fig. 60-5), as follows: Identify the angle of Louis or the sternal notch. Palpate the upper sternum to identify where the clavicle joins the sternum (suprasternal notch). Slide fingers down the center of the sternum to the obvious bony prominence. This is the sternal notch, which identifies the second rib and provides a landmark for noting the fourth intercostal space (ICS). When the fourth ICS is located, place the V leads: V_1 at the fourth ICS right sternal border; V_2 at the fourth ICS left sternal border; V_3 equidistant between V_2 and V_4; V_4 at the fifth ICS midclavicular line; V_5 horizontal level to V_4 at the anterior axillary line; and V_6 horizontal level to V_4 at the midaxillary line.	The angle of Louis or the sternal notch assists with identifying the second rib for correct placement of precordial leads in the appropriate intercostal space. Accurate placement ensures the correct electrical tracing of the heart from the horizontal plane. Slight alterations in the position of any of the precordial leads may alter the ECG significantly and can affect diagnosis and treatment.[2]	Variation in precordial lead placement of as little as 2 cm can result in important diagnostic errors, particularly in anteroseptal infarction and ventricular hypertrophy.[3] If precordial leads cannot be accurately placed because of chest wounds, placement of defibrillator pads, or other reasons, the alternative site should be clearly documented on the ECG.[1] Electrodes should be placed under the breast in women.[3]

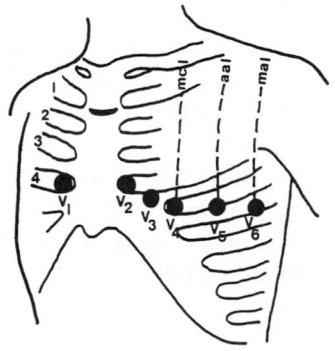

FIGURE 60-5   Precordial or chest lead placement.

Steps	Rationale	Special Considerations
9. Cleanse the area for the application of electrodes with cleansing pads or soap and water, and dry thoroughly. (**Level E***)	Provides for adequate transmission of electrical impulses, reducing noise and improving quality of the signal.[3] Moist skin is not conducive to electrode adherence.[2]	Clipping of hair may be necessary to ensure good skin contact with the electrode.
10. Clean the intended sites with alcohol pads. Consider use of skin preparation solutions. (**Level E**)	Alcohol or skin preparations may be needed to remove oils to improve impulse transmission.[2]	Skin preparation solutions should not be applied to the area of the skin that will be in direct contact with the electrode gel because transmission of impulses may be decreased.
11. Abrade the skin with a washcloth or gauze pad.	Removes dead skin cells, promoting impulse transmission.	

*Level E: Multiple case reports, theory-based evidence from expert opinions, or peer-reviewed professional organizational standards without clinical studies to support recommendations

Procedure for 12-Lead Electrocardiogram—*Continued*

Steps	Rationale	Special Considerations
12. For pregelled electrodes, remove the backing and test for moistness. For adhesive electrodes, remove the backing and check each adhesive pad, as each should be sticky or moist.	Allows for appropriate conduction of impulses.	Gel must be moist. If pregelled electrodes are not moist or adhesive electrodes are not sticky, replace the electrodes.
13. Apply the electrodes securely.	Electrodes must be secure to prevent external influences from affecting the ECG.	
14. Fasten the lead wires to the limb electrodes, avoiding bending or strain on the wires, and use the correct lead-to-electrode connection.	Provides for correct lead-to-limb connection.	
15. Identify the multiple-channel machine recording setting (Fig. 60-6).	Multiple-channel machines run several leads simultaneously and can be set to run leads in different configurations.	Obtain the tracing that is needed for the clinical situation.

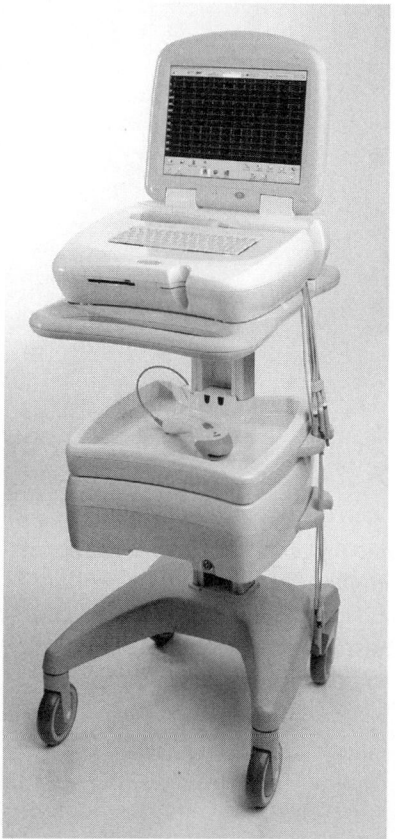

FIGURE 60-6 Multiple-channel ECG machine. (*Courtesy Philips Medical Systems, Andover, MA.*)

16. Turn the ECG machine on and program the ECG machine: paper speed, 25 mm/s; calibration, 10 mm/mV; filter settings, 0.05 to 100 Hz. (**Level E***)	Ensures an accurate trace within standard limits for proper interpretation.[3]	Manufacturers provide a calibration check in the machine to identify the sensitivity setting. Most machines have automatic settings.

*Level E: Multiple case reports, theory-based evidence from expert opinions, or peer-reviewed professional organizational standards without clinical studies to support recommendations

Procedure continues on following page

Procedure for 12-Lead Electrocardiogram—*Continued*

Steps	Rationale	Special Considerations
17. Obtain a 12-lead ECG recording. Most systems record each lead for 3 to 6 seconds and automatically mark the correct lead.	The ECG must be marked accurately and have a clear baseline without artifact for correct interpretation. Three to 6 seconds is all that is needed for a permanent record; a longer strip may be obtained if a rhythm strip is needed. A rhythm strip is a long recording of a lead; lead II is commonly used.	
18. Record the chest leads as previously described. Note: A multiple-channel machine runs the limb and chest leads simultaneously.	The chest leads may be set up and done automatically by the machine. The 12-lead ECG tracing should be free of respiratory artifact.	Respiratory artifact can be common in the chest leads and may require position changes to ensure a good baseline. If sequential ECGs are to be obtained, lead sites should be marked to ensure that the same sites are used in subsequent ECGs.
19. Examine the 12-lead ECG tracing to see whether it is clear; repeat the ECG if it is not.	While the patient is still connected to the machine, the nurse should examine the ECG to see whether any leads need to be repeated.	
20. Interpret the recording for rhythm, rate, presence and configuration of P waves, length of PR intervals, length of QRS complexes, configuration and deviation of the ST segments, presence and configuration of T waves, length of QT intervals, presence of extra waves (e.g., U waves), and identification of dysrhythmias.	Reviews the normal conduction sequence and identifies abnormalities that may necessitate further evaluation or treatment.	
21. Evaluate the 12-lead ECG for any signs of ischemia, injury, or infarct and other significant myocardial alterations.	Identifies pathophysiologic processes that may necessitate further evaluation or treatment.	
22. Disconnect the equipment; clean the gel off the patient (if necessary) and prepare the equipment for future use.	Increases patient comfort.	Some pregelled electrodes can be left in place for repeat ECGs. Follow the manufacturer's directions and hospital policy for electrode use and removal in these cases.
23. Discard used supplies in appropriate receptacles.	Reduces the transmission of microorganisms; Standard Precautions.	
24. **HH**		

Expected Outcomes

- A clear 12-lead ECG recording obtained (Fig. 60-7)
- Prompt identification of abnormalities

Unexpected Outcomes

- Altered skin integrity
- Inaccurate lead placement or limb lead reversal (Fig. 60-8)
- AC interference, also called 60-cycle interference (see Fig. 57-10)
- Wandering baseline (see Fig. 57-11)
- Artifact or waveform interference (see Fig. 57-12)

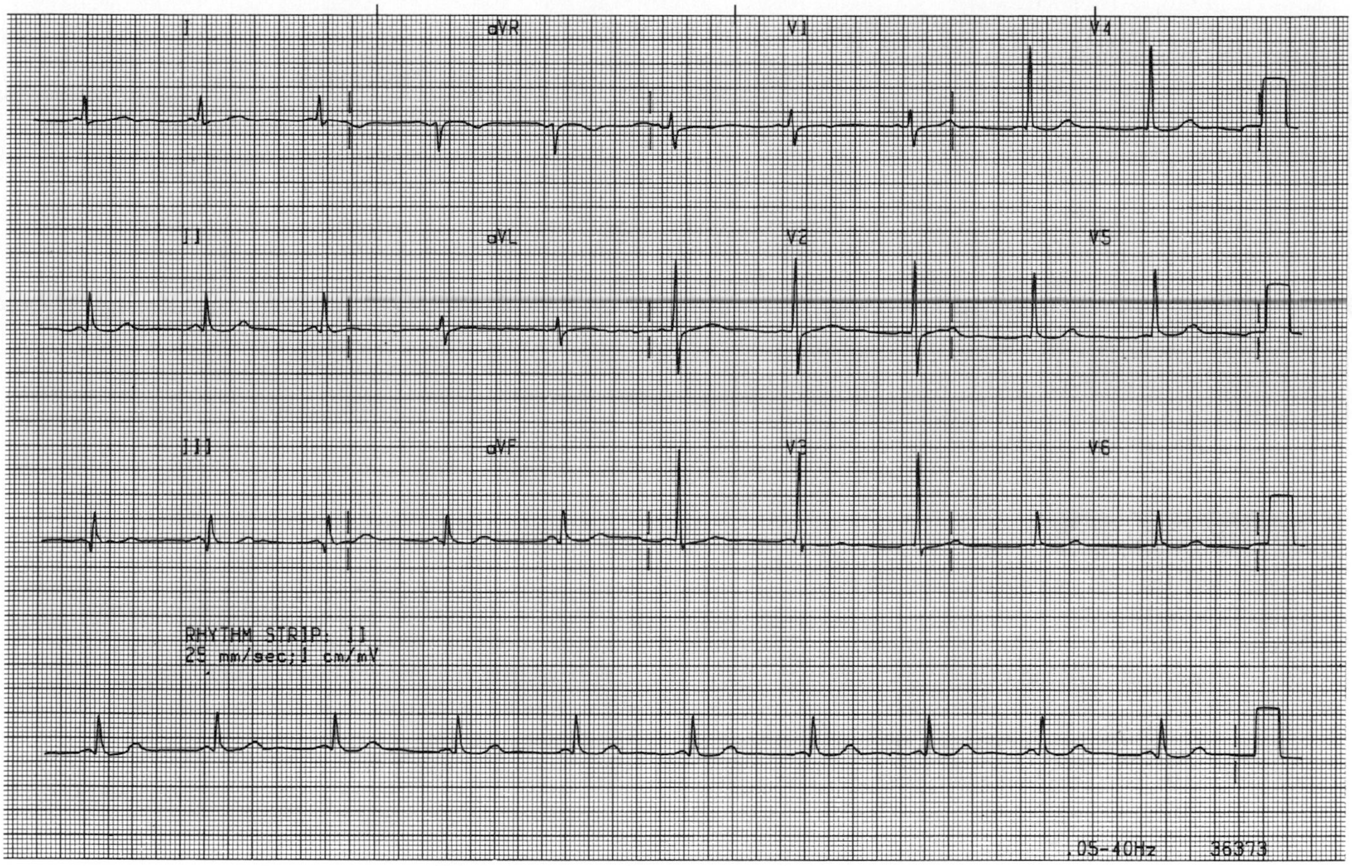

FIGURE 60-7   Clear 12-lead ECG recording.

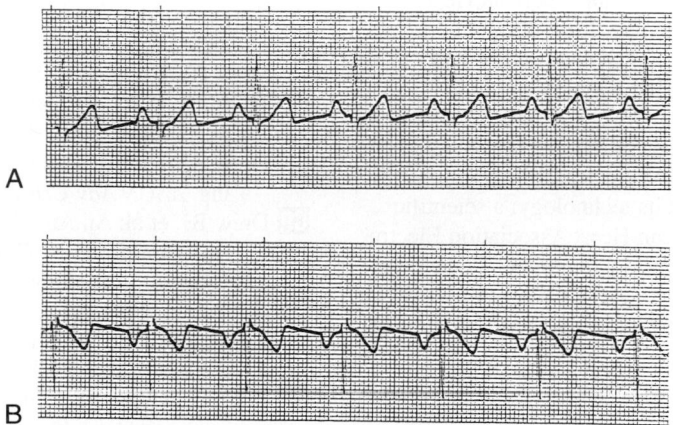

FIGURE 60-8   Limb lead reversal on 12-lead ECG in lead I. **A,** Correct placement. **B,** Incorrect placement.

Patient Monitoring and Care

Steps	Rationale	Reportable Conditions
1. Obtain a 12-lead ECG as prescribed and as needed (e.g., for angina or dysrhythmias). 2. Compare the 12-lead ECG with the previous 12-lead ECGs. 3. Follow institution standard for assessing pain. Administer analgesia and nitrates as prescribed.	Provides determination of myocardial ischemia, injury, and infarction. Aids in diagnosis of dysrhythmias. Determines normal and abnormal findings. Promotes comfort.	*These conditions should be reported if they persist despite nursing interventions.* • Angina • Dysrhythmias • Abnormal 12-lead ECG • Any abnormal changes in the 12-lead ECG • Continued pain despite pain interventions

Documentation

Documentation should include the following:
• Patient and family education
• The fact that a 12-lead ECG was obtained
• The reason for the 12-lead ECG
• Any altered lead placement and reason
• Symptoms that the patient experienced (e.g., chest pain, syncope, dizziness, or palpitations)

• Pain assessment, interventions and patient response to interventions
• Follow-up to the 12-lead ECG, as indicated
• Unexpected outcomes
• Additional nursing interventions

References

1. Drew BJ: Pitfalls and artifacts in electrocardiography, *Cardiol Clin* 24:309-315, 2006.
CR 2. Drew BJ, et al: Practice standards for electrocardiographic monitoring in hospital settings: an American Heart Association Scientific Statement from the Councils on Cardiovascular Nursing, Clinical Cardiology, and Cardiovascular Disease in the Young, *Circulation* 110:2721-2746, 2004.
3. Kligfield P, et al: Recommendations for the standardization and interpretation of the electrocardiogram: part 1: the electrocardiogram and its technology: a scientific statement from the American Heart Association Electrocardiography and Arrhythmias Committee, Council on Clinical Cardiology: The American College of Cardiology Foundation; and the Heart Rhythm Society, *Circulation* 115:1306-1324, 2007.

Additional Readings

CR Adams-Hamoda MG, et al: Factors to consider when analyzing 12-lead electrocardiograms for evidence of acute myocardial ischemia, *Am J Crit Care* 12:9-16, 2003.

CR Adams-Hamoda MG, Pelter M: Interpreting a postoperative 12-lead ECG waveform, *Am J Crit Care* 12:267-268, 2003.
Alspach J: *Core curriculum for critical care nursing,* Philadelphia, 2006, Saunders.
Donnely MP, et al: Lead selection: old and new methods for locating the most electrocardiogram information, *J Electrocardiol* 41:257-263, 2008.
Drew BJ, Kligfield P: Standardizing electrocardiographic leads: introduction to a symposium, *J Electrocardiol* 41:187-189, 2008.
Drew BJ: Putting it all together: case studies on ECG monitoring, *AACN Adv Crit Care* 18:305-317, 2007.
CR Drew BJ, et al: An American Heart Association scientific statement from the Councils on Cardiovascular Nursing, Clinical Cardiology, and Cardiovascular Disease in the Young, *Circulation* 110:2721-2746, 2004.
Gregg RE, et al: What is inside the electrocardiograph? *J Electrocardiol* 41:8-14, 2008.
CR Jefferies P, Woolf S, Linde B: Technology-based vs. traditional instruction: a comparison of two methods for teaching the skill of performing a 12-lead ECG, *Nurs Educ Perspect* 24:70-74, 2003.

PROCEDURE

61

AP Arterial Catheter Insertion (Perform)

P U R P O S E : Arterial catheters are used for continuous monitoring of blood pressure and frequent arterial blood gas and laboratory sampling.

Deborah E. Becker

PREREQUISITE NURSING KNOWLEDGE

- Knowledge of anatomy and physiology of the vasculature and adjacent structures is needed.
- Nurses must be adequately prepared to insert arterial catheters. This preparation should include specific educational content about arterial catheter insertion and opportunities to demonstrate clinical competency.
- Understanding of the principles of hemodynamic monitoring is necessary.
- Clinical competence in suturing is needed.
- Conditions that warrant the use of arterial pressure monitoring include patients with the following:
  - ❖ Acute hypotension or hypertension (hypertensive crisis)
  - ❖ Hemodynamic instability or circulatory collapse
  - ❖ Cardiac arrest
  - ❖ Hemorrhage
  - ❖ Shock from any cause
  - ❖ Continuous infusion of vasoactive medications
  - ❖ Frequent arterial blood gas measurements
  - ❖ Nonpulsatile blood flow (i.e., use of nonpulsatile ventricular assist devices or extracorporeal membrane oxygenation)
  - ❖ Intraaortic balloon pump therapy

- ❖ Neurologic injury
- ❖ Coronary interventional procedures
- ❖ Major surgical procedures
- ❖ Multiple trauma
- ❖ Respiratory failure
- ❖ Sepsis
- ❖ Obstetric emergencies
- Noninvasive indirect blood pressure measurements determined with auscultation of Korotkoff sounds distal to an occluding cuff consistently average 10 to 20 mm Hg lower than simultaneous direct measurement.[13]
- Arterial waveform inspection can help with rapid diagnosis of the presence of valvular disorders, and determine the effects of dysrhythmias on perfusion, the effects of the respiratory cycle on blood pressure, and the effects of intraaortic balloon pump therapy or ventricular assist device therapy on blood pressure.
- The preferred artery for arterial catheter insertion is the radial artery (see Fig. 80-1). Although this artery is smaller than the ulnar artery, it is more superficial and can be more easily stabilized during the procedure.[9] The brachial artery is a safe and reliable alternative site for arterial puncture and line placement.[18]
- At times, the femoral artery may be used for arterial catheter insertion. The use of this artery can be technically difficult because of the proximity of the femoral artery to the femoral vein (see Fig. 80-2).
- The most common complications associated with arterial puncture include pain, vasospasm, hematoma formation, infection, hemorrhage, and neurovascular compromise.[3,8,19]

AP This procedure should be performed only by physicians, advanced practice nurses, and other healthcare professionals (including critical care nurses) with additional knowledge, skills, and demonstrated competence per professional licensure or institution standard.

- Causes of failure to cannulate the artery include a tangential approach to the artery, tortuosity of the artery or arterial spasm, or impingement of the needle tip on the posterior wall.[20]
- Site selection is as follows:
  - Use the radial artery as the first choice. Conduct a modified Allen's test before performing an arterial puncture on the radial artery (see Fig. 80-3). Normal palmar blushing is complete before 7 seconds, indicating a positive result; 8 to 14 seconds is considered equivocal; and 15 or more seconds indicates a negative test result. Doppler flow studies or plethysmography can also be performed to ensure the presence of collateral flow. Research shows these studies to be more reliable than the modified Allen's test.[1,20] Thrombosis of the arterial cannula is a common complication. Ensuring collateral flow distal to the puncture site is important for prevention of ischemia. Puncture of both the radial and ulnar arteries on the same hand is never recommended, to prevent compromising blood supply to the hand.[4,10,14,16]
  - Use the brachial artery as the second choice, except in the presence of poor pulsation caused by shock, obesity, or a sclerotic vessel (e.g., because of previous cardiac catheterization). The brachial artery is larger than the radial artery. Hemostasis after arterial cannulation is enhanced by its proximity to the bone if the entry point is approximately 1.5 inches above the antecubital fossa.
  - Use the femoral artery in the case of cardiopulmonary arrest or altered perfusion to the upper extremities. The femoral artery is a large superficial artery located in the groin. It is easily palpated and punctured. Complications related to femoral artery puncture include hemorrhage and hematoma formation (because bleeding can be difficult to control), inadvertent puncture of the femoral vein (because of its close proximity to the artery), infection (because aseptic technique is difficult to maintain in the groin area), and limb ischemia (if the femoral artery is damaged).

EQUIPMENT

- 2-inch, 20-gauge, nontapered Teflon cannula-over-needle; or prepackaged kit that includes a 6-inch, 18-gauge, Teflon catheter with appropriate introducer and guidewire
- Single-pressure transducer system (see Procedure 76)
- Monitoring equipment consisting of a connecting cable, monitor, oscilloscope display screen, and recorder
- Nonsterile gloves, head covering, goggles
- Sterile gloves and gown
- Antiseptic solution (e.g., 2% chlorhexidine-based preparation)
- Sterile 4 × 4 gauze pads
- Suture material
- 1% lidocaine without epinephrine, 1 to 2 mL
- 3-mL syringe with 25-gauge needle
- Sheet protector

- Sterile drape
- 2-inch tape
- Chlorhexidine-impregnated sponge

Additional supplies to have available as needed include the following:
- Bath towel
- Small wrist board
- Sutureless securement device

PATIENT AND FAMILY EDUCATION

- Explain the procedure and the purpose of the arterial catheter. ➤*Rationale:* This explanation decreases patient and family anxiety.
- Explain to the patient that the procedure may be uncomfortable but that a local anesthetic will be used first to alleviate most of the discomfort. ➤*Rationale:* Patient cooperation is elicited, and insertion is facilitated.
- Explain the patient's role in assisting with catheter insertion. ➤*Rationale:* This explanation elicits patient cooperation and facilitates insertion.

PATIENT ASSESSMENT AND PREPARATION

Patient Assessment

- Obtain the patient's medical history, including history of diabetes, hypertension, peripheral vascular disease, vascular grafts, arterial vasospasm, thrombosis, or embolism. Obtain the patient's history of coronary artery bypass graft surgery in which radial arteries were removed for use as conduits or presence of arteriovenous (AV) fistulas or shunts. ➤*Rationale:* Extremities with any of these problems should be avoided as sites for cannulation because of the potential for complications. Patients with diabetes mellitus or hypertension are at higher risk for arterial or venous insufficiency. Previously removed radial arteries are a contraindication for ulnar artery cannulation.
- Assess the patient's medical history of coagulopathies, use of anticoagulant therapy, vascular abnormalities, or peripheral neuropathies. ➤*Rationale:* This assessment assists in determining safety of the procedure and aids in site selection.
- Assess the patient's allergy history (e.g., allergy to lidocaine, topical anesthetic cream, antiseptic solutions, or tape). ➤*Rationale:* This assessment decreases the risk for allergic reactions.
- Assess the patient's current anticoagulation therapy, known blood dyscrasias, and pertinent laboratory values (e.g., platelet levels, partial thromboplastin time [PTT], prothrombin time [PT], and International normalized ratio [INR]) before the procedure. ➤*Rationale:* Anticoagulation therapy, blood dyscrasias, or alterations in coagulation studies could increase the risk for hematoma formation or hemorrhage.
- Assess the intended insertion site for the presence of a strong pulse. ➤*Rationale:* Identification and localization of the pulse increases the chance of a successful arterial cannulation.

- Presence of collateral flow to the area distal to the arterial catheter should be evaluated before the artery is cannulated. For radial arterial lines, a modified Allen's test should be performed. ➤➤*Rationale:* This assessment determines the presence of collateral flow to the hand to reduce vascular complications.
- If available, assess the intended artery with a Doppler ultrasound scan. ➤➤*Rationale:* This assessment aids in determination of the patency of the artery and blood flow.[1,2,16] Identification and localization of the artery to be cannulated increases the chance of a successful cannulization and reduces the complication rate and need for multiple attempts at placement.[19]

Patient Preparation

- Verify correct patient with two identifiers. ➤➤*Rationale:* Prior to performing a procedure, the nurse should ensure the correct identification of the patient for the intended intervention.
- Perform a pre-procedure verification and time out, if non-emergent. ➤➤*Rationale:* Ensures patient safety.
- Ensure that the patient and family understand preprocedural teaching. Answer questions as they arise and reinforce information as needed. ➤➤*Rationale:* Understanding of previously taught information is evaluated and reinforced.
- Obtain informed consent. ➤➤*Rationale:* Informed consent protects the rights of the patient and makes a competent decision possible for the patient; however, in emergency circumstances, time may not allow the form to be signed.
- Place the patient supine with the head of the bed at a comfortable position. The limb into which the arterial catheter will be inserted should be resting comfortably on the bed. ➤➤*Rationale:* This placement provides patient comfort and facilitates insertion.
- Place a towel under the back of the wrist to hyperextend the wrist and tape it in place or have someone hold it (if the radial artery is being used). ➤➤*Rationale:* This placement positions the arm and brings the artery closer to the surface.
- Elevate and hyperextend the patient's arm. Support the arm with a pillow (when using the brachial artery). ➤➤*Rationale:* This action increases accessibility of the artery.
- When the femoral artery is used, position the patient supine with the head of the bed at a comfortable angle. The patient's leg should be straight with the femoral area easily accessible. ➤➤*Rationale:* This position is the best for localizing the femoral artery pulse.

Procedure for Performing Arterial Catheter Insertion

Steps	Rationale	Special Considerations
1. 🄷🄷		
2. Prepare a single pressure transducer system (see Procedure 76).	Prepares equipment.	
3. If the radial artery is to be used, the modified Allen's test should be performed before arterial catheter insertion (see Fig. 80-3). **(Level C*)**	Although evidence is found in support of and against the use of the modified Allen's test, the test can be performed before a radial artery puncture in an attempt to assess the patency of the ulnar artery and to assess for an intact superficial palmar arch.[3,4,6,7,9,14,16,17]	The modified Allen's test does not always ensure adequate flow through the ulnar artery. A Doppler ultrasound flow indicator can also be used to further verify blood flow. [1,6,16]
A. With the patient's hand held overhead, instruct the patient to open and close the hand several times.	Forces the blood from the hand.	If the patient is unconscious or unable to perform the procedure, clench the fist passively for the patient.
B. With the patient's fist clenched, apply direct pressure on both the radial and the ulnar arteries.	Obstructs the flow of blood to the hand.	
C. Instruct the patient to lower and open the hand.	Allows observation for pallor.	Performed passively if the patient is unconscious or unable to assist.

*Level C: Qualitative studies, descriptive or correlational studies, integrative reviews, systematic reviews, or randomized controlled trials with inconsistent results

Procedure continues on following page

Procedure for Performing Arterial Catheter Insertion—*Continued*

Steps	Rationale	Special Considerations
D. While maintaining pressure on the radial artery, release the pressure over the ulnar artery and observe the hand for the return of color.	Return of color within 7 seconds indicates patency of the ulnar artery and an intact superficial palmar arch; this is interpreted as normal Allen's test results. If color returns between 8 and 14 seconds, the test is considered equivocal and the healthcare provider must consider the risk and benefits of continuing with performing this procedure. If 15 or more seconds are needed for color to return, test results are considered abnormal and another site should be considered.	If the test results are abnormal, the modified Allen's test should be performed on the opposite hand. If results for both hands are abnormal, consider use of a site other than the radial arteries.
4. **HH**		
5. **PE**		
6. Prepare the site with the antiseptic solution (e.g., 2% chlorhexidine-based preparation).[5]	Limits the introduction of potentially infectious skin flora into the vessel during the puncture.	
A. Cleanse the site with a back-and-forth motion while applying friction for 30 seconds.		
B. Allow the antiseptic solution to dry.		
7. **HH**		
8. Apply sterile gown and gloves.	Reduces the transmission of microorganisms; sterile precautions.	
9. Drape the area around the site with sterile drapes.	Provides a sterile field and minimizes the transmission of organisms.	
10. Locally anesthetize the puncture site.[4,7,9,11,12,16] **(Level C*)**	Provides local anesthesia for the arterial puncture.	Most patients experience pain during arterial puncture.[7,9]
A. Use a 1-mL syringe with a 25-gauge needle to draw up 0.5 mL of 1% lidocaine without epinephrine.	Minimizes vessel trauma. Absence of epinephrine decreases the risk for peripheral vasoconstriction.	Recent research exploring the efficacy of lidocaine ointment as an alternative to intradermal lidocaine shows promising results.[12,15,18] If this method is used, manufacturer's recommendations should be followed.
B. Aspirate before injecting the local anesthetic.	Determines whether or not a blood vessel has been inadvertently entered.	
C. Inject intradermally and then with full infiltration around the intended arterial insertion site. Use approximately 0.2 to 0.3 mL for an adult.	Decreases the incidence of localized pain during injection of all skin layers. Patients report reduced pain when a local intradermal anesthetic agent is used before arterial puncture.[7]	
11. Perform the percutaneous puncture of the selected artery.	Increases the likelihood of correctly locating the artery and decreases the chance of the vessel rolling.	
A. Palpate and stabilize the artery with the index and middle fingers of the nondominant hand.		

*Level C: Qualitative studies, descriptive or correlational studies, integrative reviews, systematic reviews, or randomized controlled trials with inconsistent results

Procedure for Performing Arterial Catheter Insertion—*Continued*

Steps	Rationale	Special Considerations
B. With the needle bevel-up and the syringe at a 30-degree to 60-degree angle to the radial or brachial artery, puncture the skin slowly.[21] Adjust the angle to a 60-degree to 90-degree angle to the femoral artery.	A slow gradual thrust promotes entry into the artery without inadvertently passing through the posterior wall.	
12. Advance the needle and the cannula until a blood return is noted in the hub, then slowly advance the catheter about ¼ to ½ inch farther to ensure that the cannula is in the artery.	Advancing the cannula farther ensures that the entire cannula is in the artery and not just the tip of the stylet.	
13. If, on initial insertion, a blood return is not noted, a 3-mL syringe may be placed at the end of the cannula. While advancing the catheter, gentle withdrawing of the syringe plunger may be performed in an effort to determine proper placement in the artery.	Some arteries may vasospasm as a result of sudden insertion of the catheter. Taking the time to place a syringe on the catheter and withdrawing slightly during insertion may allow the artery to relax and help to determine whether proper placement within the artery has been achieved.	
14. Level the catheter to the skin; then continue to advance the cannula to its hub with a steady rotary action.	The rotary action helps to advance the catheter through the skin.	
15. Correct positioning is confirmed by the presence of pulsatile blood return on the removal of the stylet.	Arterial blood is pulsatile, which confirms intraarterial placement.	
16. Once positioning is confirmed, remove the stylet and connect the catheter to the single-pressure transducer system and flush the system.	Maintains catheter patency and prepares the system for arterial blood pressure monitoring.	
17. Level the air-fluid interface (zeroing stopcock) to the phlebostatic axis, zero the monitoring system, verify the arterial waveform, and activate the alarm system (see Procedure 62).	Prepares the monitoring system; provides notification of abnormal blood pressure parameters and system disconnections.	
18. Suture the arterial catheter in place.	Maintains arterial catheter positioning; reduces the chance of accidental dislodgment.	A sutureless securement device may be used to secure the catheter.
19. Apply a chlorhexidine-impregnated sponge and an occlusive sterile dressing and label the insertion information (see Procedure 62).	Provides a sterile environment; reduces the risk for infection.	
20. Discard used supplies in appropriate receptacles; dispose of needles and other sharp objects in appropriate containers.	Reduces the transmission of microorganisms; Standard Precautions. Safely removes sharp objects.	
21. **HH**		

Procedure continues on following page

Expected Outcomes

- Successful cannulation of the artery
- Ability to obtain blood samples from the arterial catheter
- Peripheral vascular and neurovascular systems intact
- Alterations in hemodynamic stability identified and treated accordingly

Unexpected Outcomes

- Pain or severe discomfort during the insertion procedure
- Complications of puncture or vasospasm
- Complications after puncture, such as: change in color, temperature, or sensation; movement of the extremity used for insertion; or hematoma, hemorrhage, infection, or clot at the insertion site
- Inability to cannulate the artery

Patient Monitoring and Care

Steps	Rationale	Reportable Conditions
		These conditions should be reported if they persist despite nursing interventions.
1. Observe the insertion site for signs of hemostasis after the procedure.	Postinsertion bleeding can occur in any patient but is more likely to occur in patients with coagulopathies or patients undergoing anticoagulation therapy.	• Excessive bleeding • Hematoma • Changes in vital signs
2. Assess the arterial catheter insertion site and involved extremity for signs of postinsertion complications.[13]	Arterial catheter insertion can result in peripheral vascular and neurovascular compromise of the extremity distal to the puncture site.	• Changes in pulse, color, size, temperature, sensation, or movement in the extremity used for the arterial catheter insertion
3. Assess the arterial catheter insertion site for signs or symptoms of infection.	Determines necessity for catheter removal and further treatment.	• Erythema, warmth, hardness, tenderness, or pain at the arterial line insertion site • Presence of purulent drainage from the arterial line insertion site
4. Follow institution standard for assessing pain. Administer analgesia as prescribed.	Identifies need for pain interventions.	• Continued pain despite pain interventions

Documentation

Documentation should include the following:
- Patient and family education
- Performance of the modified Allen's test before insertion and its results (when using the radial artery)
- Preprocedure verifications and time out
- Signed consent form
- Arterial site used
- Insertion of the arterial catheter (date, time, and initials marked on the dressing itself)
- Size of cannula-over-needle catheter used
- Any difficulties in the insertion
- Patient tolerance of the procedure
- Pain assessment, interventions, and effectiveness
- Appearance of the site
- Appearance of the limb, color, pulse, sensation, movement, capillary refill time, and temperature of the extremity after insertion is complete
- Occurrence of unexpected outcomes
- Nursing interventions taken

References

CR 1. Abu-Omar Y, et al: Duplex ultrasonography predicts safety of radial artery harvest in the presence of an abnormal Allen test, *Ann Thorac Surg* 77:116-119, 2004.

2. Barone JE, Madlinger RV: Should an Allen test be performed before artery cannulation? *J Trauma* 61:468-470, 2006.

CR 3. Buffington S: Specimen collection and testing. In Nattina, Sandra M, editor: *Lippincott's nursing procedures,* ed 2, Springhouse, PA, 1996, Springhouse Corp, 145-147.

4. Celenski SA, Seneff MG: Arterial line placement and care. In Irwin RS, et al, editors: *Procedures and techniques in intensive care medicine,* ed 6, Philadelphia, 2008, Lippincott Williams & Wilkins, 38-46.

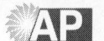

5. Centers for Disease Control and Prevention: Guidelines for the prevention of intravascular catheter-related infections, *MMWR* 51(RR-10):1-31, 2002.

6. Chernecky CC, Berger BJ, editors: *Laboratory tests and diagnostic procedures,* ed 5, St Louis, 2008, Saunders Elsevier.

7. Clarke S: Arterial lines: an analysis of good practice, *J Child Healthcare* 3:22-27, 1999.

8. Cummins RO, editor: *Advanced cardiac life support,* Dallas, 1997, American Heart Association, 13.9-13.10.

9. Giner J, et al. Pain during arterial puncture, *Chest* 110:1443-1445, 1996.

10. Gomella LG, Haist SA: Bedside procedures. In Gomella LG, Haist SA, editors: *Clinician's pocket reference: the scut monkey,* ed 11, 2007, available at www.accessmedicine.com/content.aspx?aID=2694363.

11. Hudson TL, Dukes SF, Reilly K: Use of local anesthesia for arterial punctures, *Am J Crit Care* 15:595-599, 2006.

12. Hussey VM, Poulin MV, Fain JA: Effectiveness of lidocaine hydrochloride on venipuncture sites, *AORN J* 66:472-475, 1997.

13. Imperial-Perez F, McRae M: *Protocols for practice: hemodynamic monitoring series. arterial pressure monitoring,* Aliso Viejo, CA, 1998, American Association of Critical-Care Nurses.

14. Intravenous Nurses Society: Infusion nursing standards of practice, *J Infusion Nurs* 2006, Jan-Feb;29(1 Suppl):S1-92.

15. Martin C, et al: Long-term arterial cannulation in ICU patients using the radial artery or dorsalis pedis artery, *Chest* 119:901-906, 2001.

16. National Committee for Clinical Laboratory Standards: *Procedures for the collection of arterial blood specimens: approved standards H11-A4,* ed 4, Wayne, PA, 2004, National Committee for Clinical Laboratory Standards.

17. Oettle AC, et al: Evaluation of Allen's test in both arms and arteries of left and right-handed people, *Surg Radiol Anat* 28:3-6, 2006.

18. Okeson GC, Wulbrecht PH: The safety of brachial artery puncture for arterial blood sampling, *Chest* 114:748-751, 1998.

19. Qvist J, Peterfreund R, Perlmutter G: Transient compartment syndrome of the forearm after attempted radial artery cannulation, *Anesth Anal* 83:183-185, 1996.

20. Shiver S, Blaivas M, Lyon M: A prospective comparison of ultrasound-guided and blindly placed radial arterial catheters, *Acad Emerg Med* 13:1275-1279, 2006.

21. Williams DJ, Ahmed ST, Latto IP: A survey of venous and arterial cannulation techniques used for routine adult coronary artery bypass grafting, *Internet J Anesthesiol* 6:12, 2003.

Arterial Catheter Insertion (Assist), Care, and Removal

P U R P O S E : Arterial catheters are used to continuously monitor blood pressure, to titrate vasoactive agents, and to obtain serial blood gases or other laboratory specimens in patients with critical illnesses.

Rose B. Shaffer

PREREQUISITE NURSING KNOWLEDGE

- Knowledge of the anatomy and physiology of the vasculature and adjacent structures is needed.
- Knowledge of the principles of hemodynamic monitoring is necessary.
- Understanding of the principles of aseptic technique is needed.
- Conditions that warrant the use of arterial pressure monitoring include patients with:
  - Hemodynamic instability (e.g., acute hypotension, hypertensive crisis)
  - Cardiac arrest
  - Shock from any cause (e.g., hemorrhagic, septic)
  - Continuous infusion of vasoactive medications
  - Frequent arterial blood gas measurements (e.g., patients who need ventilatory support, patients with acute critical illnesses)
  - Nonpulsatile blood flow (e.g., those patients with ventricular assist device therapy or extracorporeal membrane oxygenation therapy)
  - Intraaortic balloon pump therapy
  - Coronary interventional procedures
  - Major surgical procedures (e.g., neurologic, abdominal, cardiac, thoracic, vascular, trauma)
  - Obstetric emergencies
- Arterial pressure represents the forcible ejection of blood from the left ventricle into the aorta and out into the arterial system. During ventricular systole, blood is ejected into the aorta, generating a pressure wave. Because of the

intermittent pumping action of the heart, this arterial pressure wave is generated in a pulsatile manner (Fig. 62-1). The ascending limb of the aortic pressure wave (anacrotic limb) represents an increase in pressure because of left ventricular ejection. The peak of this ejection is the peak systolic pressure, which should be less than 120 mm Hg in adults.[18] After reaching this peak, the ventricular pressure declines to a level below aortic

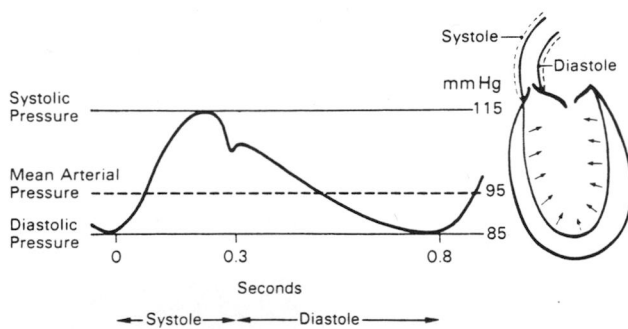

FIGURE 62-1 The generation of a pulsatile waveform. This is an aortic pressure curve. During systole, the ejected volume distends the aorta and aortic pressure rises. The peak pressure is known as the aortic systolic pressure. After the peak ejection, the ventricular pressure falls; when it drops below the aortic pressure, the aortic valve closes, which is marked by the dicrotic notch, the end of the systole. During diastole, the pressure continues to decline and the aortic wall recoils, pushing blood toward the periphery. The trough of the pressure wave is the diastolic pressure. The difference between the systolic and diastolic pressure is the pulse pressure. *(From Smith JJ, Kampine JP: Circulating physiology, Baltimore, 1980, Williams & Wilkins, 55.)*

pressure and the aortic valve closes, marking the end of ventricular systole. The closure of the aortic valve produces a small rebound wave that creates a notch known as the dicrotic notch. The descending limb of the curve (diastolic downslope) represents diastole and is characterized by a long declining pressure wave, during which the aortic wall recoils and propels blood into the arterial network. The diastolic pressure is measured as the lowest point of the diastolic downslope, which should be less than 80 mm Hg in adults.[18]

- The difference between the systolic and diastolic pressures is the pulse pressure, with a normal value of about 40 mm Hg.
- Arterial pressure is determined by the relationship between blood flow through the vessels (cardiac output) and the resistance of the vessel walls (systemic vascular resistance). The arterial pressure is therefore affected by any factors that change either cardiac output or systemic vascular resistance.
- The average arterial pressure during a cardiac cycle is called the mean arterial pressure (MAP). MAP is not the average of the systolic plus the diastolic pressures because during the cardiac cycle, the pressure remains closer to diastole than to systole for a longer period (at normal heart rates). The MAP is calculated automatically by most patient monitoring systems; however, it can be calculated with the following formula:

$$MAP = \frac{(systolic\ pressure) + (diastolic\ pressure \times 2)}{3}$$

- MAP represents the driving force (perfusion pressure) for blood flow through the cardiovascular system. MAP is at its highest point in the aorta. As blood travels through the circulatory system, systolic pressure increases and diastolic pressure decreases, with an overall decline in the MAP (Fig. 62-2).
- The location of arterial catheter placement depends on the condition of the arterial vessels and the presence of other catheters (i.e., the presence of a dialysis shunt is a contraindication for placement of an arterial catheter in the same extremity). Once inserted, the arterial catheter causes little or no discomfort to the patient and allows continuous blood pressure assessment and intermittent blood sampling. If intraaortic balloon pump therapy is necessary, arterial pressure may be directly monitored from the tip of the balloon in the aorta.
- The radial artery is the most common site for arterial pressure monitoring. When arterial pulse waveforms are recorded from a peripheral site (instead of a central site), the waveform morphology changes. The anacrotic limb becomes more peaked and narrowed, with increased amplitude; therefore, the systolic pressure in peripheral sites is higher than the systolic pressure recorded from a more central site (see Fig. 62-2). In addition, the diastolic pressure decreases, the diastolic downslope may show a secondary wave, and the dicrotic notch becomes less prominent from distal sites.

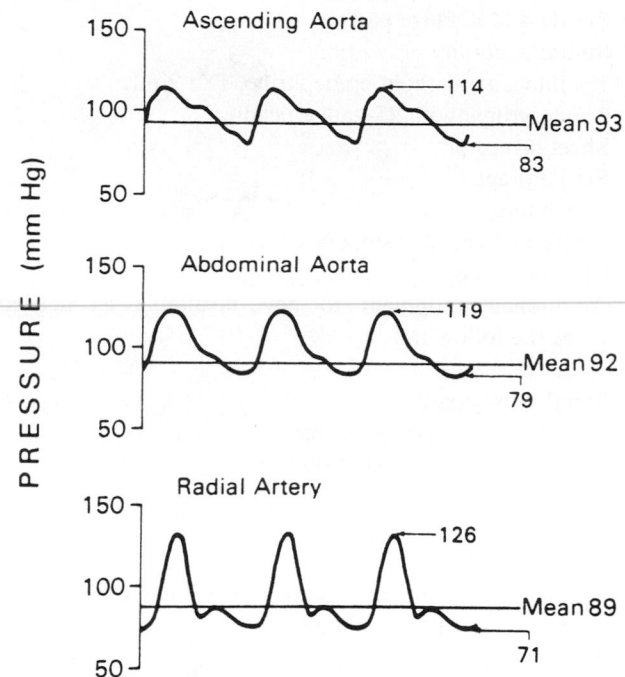

FIGURE 62-2   Arterial pressure from different sites in the arterial tree. The arterial pressure waveform varies in configuration, depending on the location of the catheter. With transmission of the pressure wave into the distal aorta and large arteries, the systolic pressure increases and the diastolic pressure decreases; with a resulting heightening of the pulse, pressure declines steadily. *(From Smith JJ, Kampine JP: Circulating physiology, Baltimore, 1980, Williams & Wilkins, 57.)*

- Vasodilators and vasoconstrictors may change the appearance of the waveforms from distal sites. Vasodilators may cause the waveform to take on a more central appearance. Vasoconstrictors may cause the systolic pressure to become more exaggerated because of enhanced resistance in the peripheral arteries.
- Several potential complications are associated with arterial pressure monitoring. Infection at the insertion site can develop and cause sepsis. Clot formation in the catheter can lead to arterial embolization. The catheter can cause vessel perforation with extravasation of blood and flush solution into the surrounding tissue. Finally, the distal extremity can develop circulatory or neurovascular impairment.

EQUIPMENT

- 1- to 2-inch (2.5- to 5-cm) over-the-needle catheter (14-gauge to 20-gauge for adults) or prepackaged kit with catheter, introducer, and guidewire
- Single-pressure transducer system (see Procedure 76)
- Monitoring equipment consisting of a connecting cable, monitor, oscilloscope display screen, and recorder
- Nonsterile gloves, head coverings, goggles
- Sterile gloves and gowns
- Antiseptic solution (e.g., 2% chlorhexidine-based preparation)

- Sterile 4 × 4 gauze pads
- Suture materials
- 1% lidocaine without epinephrine, 1 to 2 mL
- 3-mL syringe with 25-gauge needle
- Sheet protector
- Sterile drape
- 2-inch tape
- Nonvented caps for stopcock
- Chlorhexidine-impregnated sponge

  Additional equipment to have available as needed includes the following:
- Bath towel
- Small wrist board
- Sutureless securement device
- Blood-conserving closed system
- Arm board
- Transparent dressing
- Suture removal kit
- Transducer holder, intravenous pole, and carpenter or laser level (for pole mounts)
- 70% alcohol

PATIENT AND FAMILY EDUCATION

- Explain the procedure and the purpose of the arterial catheter. ➥*Rationale:* This explanation decreases patient and family anxiety.
- Explain the standard of care to the patient and family, including insertion procedure, alarms, dressings, and length of time the catheter is expected to be in place. ➥*Rationale:* This explanation encourages the patient and family to ask questions and voice concerns about the procedure and decreases patient and family anxiety.
- Explain the patient's expected participation during the procedure. ➥*Rationale:* Patient cooperation during insertion is encouraged.
- Explain the importance of keeping the affected extremity immobile. ➥*Rationale:* This explanation encourages patient cooperation to prevent catheter dislodgment and ensures a more accurate waveform.
- Instruct the patient to report any warmth, redness, pain, or wet feeling at the insertion site at any time, including after catheter removal. ➥*Rationale:* These symptoms may indicate infection, bleeding, or disconnection of the tubing or catheter.

PATIENT ASSESSMENT AND PREPARATION
Patient Assessment

- Obtain the patient's medical history, including a history of diabetes and hypertension. ➥*Rationale:* Patients with diabetes mellitus or hypertension are at higher risk for arterial or venous insufficiency.

- Obtain the patient's medical history for peripheral arterial disease, vascular grafts, arteriovenous (AV) fistulas or shunts, arterial vasospasm, thrombosis, or embolism. In addition, obtain the patient's history of coronary artery bypass graft surgery in which radial arteries were removed for use as conduits. ➥*Rationale:* Extremities with any of these problems should be avoided as sites for cannulation because of the potential for complications.
- Assess the patient's current anticoagulation therapy, history of blood dyscrasias, and pertinent laboratory values (prothrombin time [PT], international normalized ratio [INR], partial thromboplastin time [PTT], and platelets) before the procedure. ➥*Rationale:* Anticoagulation therapy, blood dyscrasias, or alterations in coagulation studies could increase the risk of hematoma formation or hemorrhage.
- Assess the patient's allergy history (e.g., allergy to heparin, lidocaine, antiseptic solutions, or adhesive tape). ➥*Rationale:* This assessment decreases the risk for allergic reactions. Patients with heparin-induced thrombocytopenia should not receive heparin in the flush solution.
- Assess the neurovascular and peripheral vascular status of the extremity to be used for the arterial cannulation, including color, temperature, presence and fullness of pulses, capillary refill, presence of bruit (in larger arteries such as the femoral artery), and motor and sensory function (as compared with the opposite extremity). Note: A modified Allen's test should be performed before cannulation of the radial artery (see Fig. 80-3). ➥*Rationale:* This assessment may help identify any neurovascular or circulatory impairment before cannulation to avoid potential complications.

Patient Preparation

- Verify correct patient with two identifiers. ➥*Rationale:* Prior to performing a procedure, the nurse should ensure the correct identification of the patient for the intended intervention.
- Ensure that the patient and family understand preprocedural teaching. Answer questions as they arise, and reinforce information as needed. ➥*Rationale:* Understanding of previously taught information is evaluated and reinforced.
- Ensure that informed consent is obtained. ➥*Rationale:* Informed consent protects the rights of the patient and allows a competent decision to be made by the patient; however, in emergency circumstances, time may not allow the form to be signed.
- Perform a pre-procedure verification and time out, if nonemergent. ➥*Rationale:* Ensures patient safety.
- Place the patient's extremity in the appropriate position with adequate lighting of the insertion site. ➥*Rationale:* This placement prepares the site for cannulation and facilitates an accurate insertion.

Procedure	**for Assisting with Insertion of an Arterial Catheter**	
Steps	**Rationale**	**Special Considerations**
1. 🄷🄷		
2. If the radial artery is to be used, the modified Allen's test is recommended before arterial catheter insertion (see Fig. 80-3). **(Level C*)**	Although evidence is found in support of and against the use of the modified Allen's test, it can be performed before radial artery puncture in an attempt to assess the patency of the ulnar artery and to assess for an intact superficial palmar arch.[2,5,17]	
3. Prepare the flush solution (see Procedure 76). Follow institution standard for adding heparin to the intravenous (IV) bag, if heparin is not contraindicated. **(Level B*)**	Heparinized flush solutions are commonly used to minimize thrombi and fibrin deposits on the catheter. Catheters flushed with heparinized saline solution are more likely than those flushed with nonheparinized saline solution to remain patent.[1,14,20]	Other factors that promote patency of the arterial line besides heparinized saline solution include the following: male gender, longer arterial catheters, larger vessels cannulated, patients receiving other anticoagulants or thrombolytics, and short-term use of the catheter.[1] Dextrose solutions are not used because they support the growth of microorganisms.[11] Although heparin may prevent thrombosis,[11,14] it has been associated with thrombocytopenia and other hematologic complications.[3]
4. Consider use of a blood conservation arterial line system. **(Level B)**	Reduces the risk of nosocomial anemia.[4,8,13,15,16]	
Assisting with Insertion		
1. 🄷🄷		
2. 🄿🄴		
3. Prime or flush the entire single-pressure transducer system (see Procedure 76).	Removes air bubbles. Air bubbles within the tubing dampen the waveform. Air bubbles introduced into the patient's circulation can cause an air embolism.	Air is more easily removed from the hemodynamic tubing when the system is not under pressure.
4. Assist with immobilizing the extremity during catheter insertion.	Facilitates insertion.	Administer sedation as prescribed if the patient is restless. If a radial catheter is being inserted, consider placing a rolled bath towel under the wrist to assist with positioning the arm.
5. Assist with skin preparation and catheter insertion, if needed.	Facilitates insertion.	
6. Once the catheter is positioned, connect the primed tubing to the arterial catheter.	Provides a secure attachment.	The catheter must be held in place while the connections are made.

*Level B: Well-designed, controlled studies with results that consistently support a specific action, intervention, or treatment
*Level C: Qualitative studies, descriptive or correlational studies, integrative reviews, systematic reviews, or randomized controlled trials with inconsistent results

Procedure continues on following page

Procedure   for Assisting with Insertion of an Arterial Catheter—*Continued*

Steps	Rationale	Special Considerations
7. Connect the pressure cable from the arterial transducer to the bedside monitor.	Connects the arterial catheter to the bedside monitoring system.	
8. Set the scale.	Permits waveform analysis.	The scale for the arterial pressure is set based on the patient's blood pressure.
9. Level the arterial air-fluid interface (zeroing stopcock) to the phlebostatic axis (see Figs. 76-7 and 76-9).	Leveling ensures the air-fluid interface of the monitoring system is level with a reference point on the body. The phlebostatic axis reflects central arterial pressure.[10]	Use a pole mount or patient mount according to institution protocol (see Procedure 76). The tip of the arterial catheter is not used as the reference point because it measures transmural pressure of a specific area in the arterial tree, which may be increased by hydrostatic pressure.[10]
10. Zero the system connected to the arterial catheter by turning the stopcock off to the patient, opening it to air, and zeroing the monitoring system (see Procedure 76).	Prepares the monitoring system so that arterial pressures can accurately be obtained.	
11. Turn the stopcock off to the top port of the stopcock. Place a sterile cap or a needleless cap on the top port of the stopcock.	Prepares the system for monitoring.	
12. Observe the waveform and perform a dynamic response test (square wave test; Fig. 62-3).	Determines whether the system is damped.	
13. Assist with securing or suturing the catheter in place.	Prevents dislodgement and loss of access.	
14. If needed, assist with applying a chlorhexidine-impregnated sponge to the arterial catheter site.[9,11,19] **(Level D*)**	Reduces the transmission of microorganisms.	A sutureless securement device can be used to stabilice the arterial catheter.
15. Apply a sterile occlusive dressing.	Provides a sterile environment.	The Centers for Disease Control and Prevention (CDC) does not recommend the routine application of topical antimicrobial ointment to the insertion site of intravascular catheters.[11]
16. Document date and time the dressing was applied the external dressing.	Determines when the dressing was applied.	
17. Apply an arm board, if necessary.	Ensures the correct position of the extremity for an optimal waveform.	
18. Set the alarm parameters according to the patient's current blood pressure.	Activates the bedside and central alarm system.	
19. Discard used supplies in appropriate receptacles; dispose of needles and other sharp objects in appropriate containers.	Reduces the transmission of microorganisms; Standard Precautions. Safely removes sharp objects.	
20. **HH**		

*Level D: Peer-reviewed professional organizational standards with clinical studies to support recommendations

When the fast flush of the continuous flush system is activated and quickly released, a sharp upstroke terminates in a flat line at the maximal indicator on the monitor and hard copy. This is then followed by an immediate rapid downstroke extending below baseline with just 1 or 2 oscillations within 0.12 second (minimal ringing) and a quick return to baseline. The patient's pressure waveform is also clearly defined with all components of the waveform, such as the dicrotic notch on an arterial waveform, clearly visible.

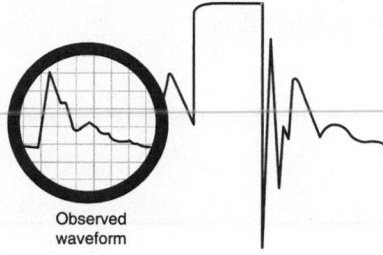

Square wave test configuration

A

Observed waveform

Intervention

There is no adjustment in the monitoring system required.

The upstroke of the square wave appears somewhat slurred, the waveform does not extend below the baseline after the fast flush and there is no ringing after the flush. The patient's waveform displays a falsely decreased systolic pressure and false high diastolic pressure as well as poorly defined components of the pressure tracing such as a diminished or absent dicrotic notch on arterial waveforms.

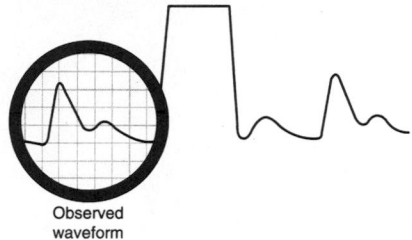

Square wave test configuration

B

Observed waveform

Intervention

To correct for the problem:
1. Check for the presence of blood clots, blood left in the catheter following blood sampling, or air bubbles at any point from the catheter tip to the transducer diaphragm and eliminate these as necessary.
2. Use low compliance (rigid), short (less than 3 to 4 feet) monitoring tubing.
3. Connect all line components securely.
4. Check for kinks in the line.

The waveform is characterized by numerous amplified oscillations above and below the baseline following the fast flush. The monitored pressure wave displays false high systolic pressures (overshoot), possibly false low diastolic pressures, and "ringing" artifacts on the waveform.

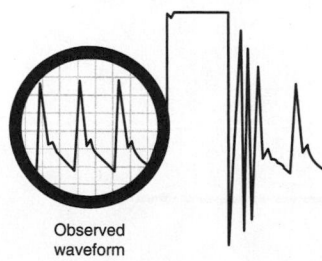

Square wave test configuration

C

Observed waveform

Intervention

To correct the problem, remove all air bubbles (particularly pinpoint air bubbles) in the fluid system, use large-bore, shorter tubing, or use a damping device.

FIGURE 62-3 Dynamic response test (square wave test) using the fast flush system. **A,** Optimally damped system. **B,** Overdamped system. **C,** Underdamped system. *(From Darovic GO, Zbilut JP: Fluid-filled monitoring systems. In Hemodynamic monitoring, ed 3, Philadelphia, 2002, Saunders, 122.)*

Procedure	for Assisting with Insertion of an Arterial Catheter—*Continued*	
Steps	**Rationale**	**Special Considerations**
21. Run a waveform strip and record the patient's baseline arterial pressures.	Obtains baseline data.	Digital values are not used because they are averaged calculations.
22. Record the manual (noninvasive) blood pressure and compare with the arterial (invasive) blood pressure.	Obtains baseline data.	No direct relationship exists between noninvasive and invasive blood pressures because noninvasive techniques measure blood flow and invasive techniques measure pressure.[10]

Procedure	for Troubleshooting an Overdamped Waveform	
Steps	**Rationale**	**Special Considerations**
1. **HH**		
2. **PE**		
3. Identify the overdamped waveform (Fig. 62-4).	Identifies the problem.	An overdamped waveform results in a falsely low systolic pressure and a falsely high diastolic pressure.

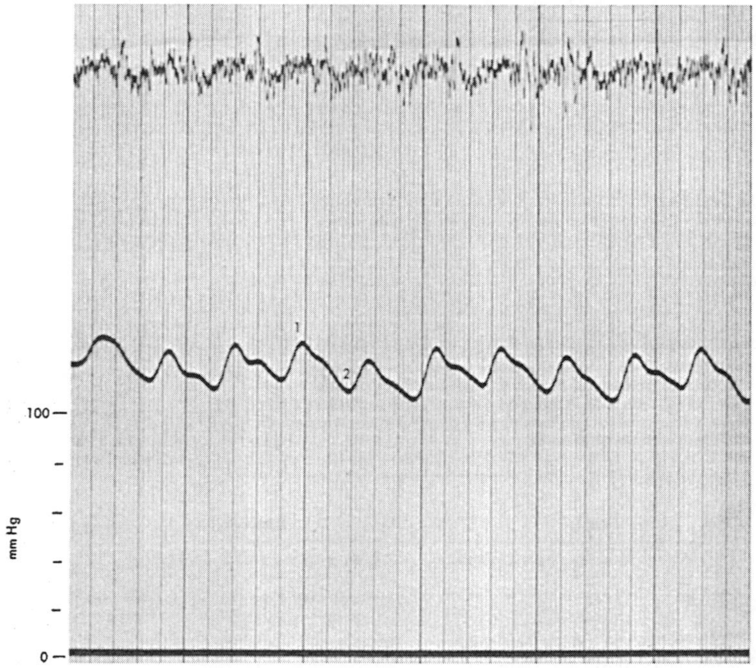

FIGURE 62-4   Overdamped arterial waveform (*1*, systole; *2*, diastole). (*From Daily EK, Schroeder JS: Hemodynamic waveforms, St Louis, 1990, Mosby, 110.*)

4. Check the patient.	A sudden hypotensive episode can look like an overdamped waveform (Fig. 62-5).	
5. Perform a dynamic response test if the arterial waveform seems to be overdamped (see Fig. 62-3).	Overdamping should be assessed immediately to ensure waveform accuracy and to prevent clotting of the catheter.	

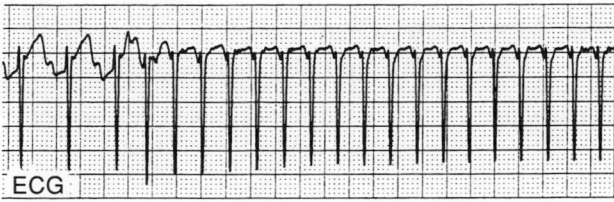

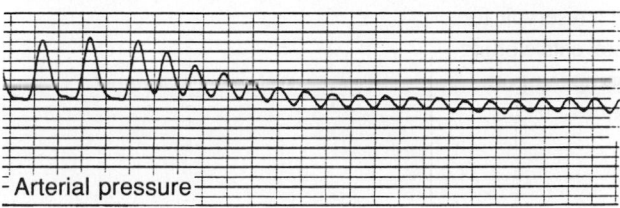

FIGURE 62-5 Patient developed supraventricular tachycardia *(SVT)* with a fall in arterial pressure. Note how the arterial waveform appears overdamped but is in fact reflecting a severe hypotensive episode associated with the tachycardia.

Procedure for Troubleshooting an Overdamped Waveform—*Continued*

Steps	Rationale	Special Considerations
6. If the waveform is overdamped, follow these steps:		
A. Check the arterial line insertion site for catheter positioning.	Wrist movement in the radial site or leg flexion in the femoral site can cause catheter kinking or dislodgment, resulting in an overdamped waveform.	
B. Check the system for air bubbles and eliminate them if they are found.	Air bubbles can be a cause of an overdamped system; air bubbles can also cause emboli.	
C. Check the tubing system for leaks or disconnections and correct the problem if it is found.	Ensures all connections are tight.	
D. Check the flush bag to ensure fluid is present in the bag and that pressure is maintained at 300 mm Hg.	An empty flush bag or a pressure of less than 300 mm Hg may result in an overdamped system.	
E. A catheter with an overdamped waveform should always be aspirated before flushing.	Use of the fast-flush device or flushing with a syringe first may force a clot at the catheter tip into the arterial circulation.	
Attempt to aspirate and flush the catheter as follows:	Assists with the withdrawal of air in the tubing or clots that may be at the catheter tip.	
• Using the stopcock closest to the patient, remove the non-vented cap from the blood sampling port and attach a 5- or 10-mL syringe to the top port of the stopcock (see Fig. 66-1).	A 5-mL syringe generates less pressure and may prevent arterial spasm in smaller arteries (e.g., radial artery).	A 10-mL syringe may be needed for larger arteries (e.g., femoral artery). A needleless system can also be used.
• Turn the stopcock off to the flush solution (see Fig. 66-2).	Opens the system from the patient to the syringe.	
• Gently attempt to aspirate; if resistance is felt, reposition the extremity and reattempt aspiration. If resistance is still felt, stop and notify the physician or advanced practice nurse.	Assesses catheter patency. Normally, blood should be aspirated into the syringe without difficulty.	

Procedure continues on following page

Procedure	for Troubleshooting an Overdamped Waveform—*Continued*	
Steps	**Rationale**	**Special Considerations**
• If blood is aspirated, remove 3 mL, turn the stopcock off to the patient, and discard the 3-mL sample.	Removes any clotted material within the catheter.	All blood wastes should be disposed using standard precautions.
• Fast-flush the remaining blood from the stopcock onto a sterile gauze pad or into another syringe and remove the syringe.	Removes blood residue from the stopcock, where it could be a reservoir for bacterial growth, and prevents clotting of blood in the blood sampling port.	
• Turn the stopcock off to the blood sampling port (see Fig. 66-1) and place a new sterile nonvented cap on the port.	Maintains sterility and a closed system.	
• Use the fast-flush device to clear the line of blood.	Prevents the arterial line from clotting.	
7. Discard used supplies in the appropriate receptacles.	Reduces the transmission of microorganisms; Standard Precautions.	
8. **HH**		

Procedure	for Troubleshooting an Underdamped Waveform	
Steps	**Rationale**	**Special Considerations**
1. **HH**		
2. **PE**		
3. Identify the underdamped waveform and perform a dynamic response test (see Fig. 62-3).	Identifies the problem.	An underdamped waveform results in a falsely high systolic pressure and a falsely low diastolic pressure.
4. Check the system for air bubbles and eliminate them if they are found.	Air bubbles can contribute to underdamping; air bubbles can also cause emboli.	
5. Check the length of the pressurized tubing system.	Ensures that the tubing length is minimized.	
6. Discard used supplies in appropriate receptacles.	Reduces the transmission of microorganisms; Standard Precautions.	
7. **HH**		

Procedure	for Arterial Catheter Dressing Change	
Steps	**Rationale**	**Special Considerations**
1. **HH**		
2. **PE**		
3. Gently remove the dressing and chlorhexidine-impregnated sponge, with care not to place tension on the arterial catheter.	Removes the previous dressing.	
4. Observe for signs of infection.	Determines whether the catheter needs to be changed.	
5. Cleanse the insertion site with antiseptic solution (e.g., 2% chlorhexidine-based preparation).[11]	Decreases the risk for bacterial growth at the insertion site.	Allow time for the solution to air dry.

Procedure	for Arterial Line Dressing Change—*Continued*	
Steps	Rationale	Special Considerations
6. Apply a new chlorhexidine impregnated sponge to site.[9,11,19] **(Level D*)**	Decreases the risk for bacterial growth at the insertion site.	
7. Apply a sterile occlusive dressing.	Provides a sterile environment.	
8. Document date and time of the dressing change on the external dressing.	Determines when the dressing was changed.	
9. Discard used supplies in appropriate receptacle.	Reduces the transmission of microorganisms; Standard Precautions.	
10. ⬛ HH		

*Level D: Peer-reviewed professional organizational standards with clinical studies to support recommendations

Procedure	for Removal of the Arterial Catheter	
Steps	Rationale	Special Considerations
1. Assess the patient's coagulation profile (PT, INR, PTT, platelets) before removal of the arterial catheter.	Elevated PT, INR, PTT, and decreased platelets affect time to hemostasis.	If laboratory values are abnormal, pressure needs to be applied for a longer period to achieve hemostasis.
2. ⬛ HH		
3. ⬛ PE		
4. Turn off the arterial monitoring alarms.	Alarm system is no longer needed.	
5. Remove the dressing and the chlorhexidine-impregnated sponge.	Prepares for catheter removal.	
6. Clip the sutures or remove the stabilizing device.	Prepares for catheter removal.	
7. Turn the stopcock off to the flush solution (see Fig. 66-2).	Prepares for removal.	Shut off the arterial pressure alarm.
8. Apply pressure 1 to 2 finger widths above the insertion site.	The arterial puncture site is above the skin puncture site because the catheter enters the skin at an angle.	
9. Remove the arterial catheter and place a sterile 4 × 4 gauze pad over the catheter site.	Prevents splashing of blood.	
10. Continue to hold proximal pressure and immediately apply firm pressure over the insertion site as the catheter is removed.	Prevents bleeding.	
11. Continue to apply pressure for a minimum of 5 minutes for the radial artery.	Achieves hemostasis.	Follow institution standard. Longer periods of direct pressure may be needed to achieve hemostasis (e.g., patients receiving systemic heparin or thrombolytics, patients with catheters in larger arteries such as the femoral artery, or patients with abnormal coagulation values).

Procedure continues on following page

Procedure for Removal of the Arterial Catheter—*Continued*

Steps	Rationale	Special Considerations
12. Apply a pressure dressing to the insertion site.	A pressure dressing helps prevent rebleeding.	The dressing should not encircle the extremity (prevents ischemia of the extremity).
13. Discard used supplies in an appropriate receptacle.	Reduces the transmission of micro-organisms; Standard Precautions.	
14. **HH**		

Expected Outcomes

- Minimal discomfort from the arterial catheter
- Maintenance of baseline hemoglobin and hematocrit levels
- Adequate circulation to the involved extremity
- Adequate sensory and motor function of the extremity
- Maintenance of catheter site without infection

Unexpected Outcomes

- Pain or discomfort from the arterial catheter insertion site
- Decreased hemoglobin and hematocrit values
- Catheter disconnection with significant blood loss
- Impaired peripheral tissue perfusion (e.g., edema, coolness, pain, paleness, or slow capillary refill of fingers or toes of cannulated extremity)
- Presence of a new bruit
- Impaired sensory or motor function of the extremity
- Fluid volume overload or deficit
- Elevated temperature or elevated white blood cell count
- Redness, warmth, edema, or drainage at or from the insertion site

Patient Monitoring and Care

Steps	Rationale	Reportable Conditions
		These conditions should be reported if they persist despite nursing interventions.
1. Assess the neurovascular and peripheral vascular status of the cannulated extremity immediately after catheter insertion and every 4 hours, or more often if warranted, according to institution standard.	Validates adequate peripheral vascular and neurovascular integrity. Changes in sensation, motor function, pulses, color, temperature, or capillary refill may indicate ischemia, arterial spasm, or neurovascular compromise.	- Diminished or absent pulses - Pale, mottled, or cyanotic appearance of the extremity - Extremity that is cool or cold to the touch - Capillary refill time of more than 2 seconds - Diminished or absent sensation - Diminished or absent motor function

2. Check the arterial line flush system every 4 hours to ensure the following:
  • Pressure bag or device is inflated to 300 mm Hg.
  • Fluid is present in the flush solution.
	Ensures that approximately 1 to 3 mL/hr of flush solution is delivered through the catheter, thus maintaining patency and preventing backflow of blood into the catheter and tubing.
	The catheter clots off if fluid is not continuously infusing	

Patient Monitoring and Care —*Continued*

Steps	Rationale	Reportable Conditions
3. Monitor for overdamped or under-damped waveforms. An overdamped waveform is characterized by a flattened waveform, a diminished or absent dicrotic notch, or a waveform that does not fall to baseline (see Fig. 62-4). An underdamped waveform is characterized by catheter fling (see Fig. 62-3,*C*).	An optimally damped system provides an adequate waveform with appropriate blood pressure readings. With an overdamped waveform, the patient's systolic pressure may be read inaccurately low. Common causes of an overdamped waveform include air bubbles in the system, use of compliant tubing, loose connections in the system, too many stopcocks in the system, cracked tubing or stopcock, arterial cannula occlusion, catheter tip against the arterial wall, blood in the transducer, and insufficient pressure of the flush solution. With an underdamped waveform, systolic pressures may be read inaccurately high. Common causes of an underdamped waveform include: excessive tubing length, movement of the catheter in the artery, patient movement, and air bubbles in the system.	• Overdamped or underdamped wave-form that cannot be corrected with troubleshooting procedures
4. Perform a dynamic response test every 8 to 12 hours, when the system is opened to air, or when the accuracy of readings is in question (see Fig. 62-3).	An optimally damped system provides an accurate waveform.	• Overdamped or underdamped wave-form that cannot be corrected with troubleshooting procedures
5. Zero the transducer during the initial setup and before insertion, if disconnection occurs between the transducer and the monitoring cable, if disconnection occurs between the monitoring cable and the monitor, and when the values obtained do not fit the clinical picture. Follow manufacturer recommendations for disposable systems.	Ensures accuracy of the hemodynamic monitoring system.	
6. Recheck leveling whenever patient position changes (see Procedure 76).	Ensures accurate reference point for the phlebostatic axis.	
7. Observe the insertion site for signs and symptoms of infection.	Infected catheters must be removed as soon as possible to prevent bacteremia. The CDC does not recommend routinely replacing peripheral arterial catheters to prevent catheter-related infections.[11]	• Redness at the site • Purulent drainage • Tenderness or pain at the insertion site • Elevated temperature • Elevated white blood cell count
8. Change the hemodynamic monitoring system (flush solution, pressure tubing, transducers, and stopcocks) every 96 hours. (**Level B***) The flush solution may need to be changed more frequently.	The CDC[11] and research findings[7,12] recommend that the hemodynamic flush system can be used safely for 96 hours. This recommendation is based on research conducted with disposable pressure monitoring systems used for peripheral and central lines.	

*Level B: Well-designed, controlled studies with results that consistently support a specific action, intervention, or treatment

Procedure continues on following page

Patient Monitoring and Care —*Continued*

Steps	Rationale	Reportable Conditions
9. Run an arterial pressure strip and obtain measurement of the arterial pressures during end expiration.	Eliminates the effect of the respiratory cycle on the arterial pressure waveform.	
10. Obtain an arterial waveform strip to place on the patient's chart at the start of each shift and whenever a change is found in the waveform.	The printed waveform allows assessment of the adequacy of the waveform, damping, or respiratory variation.	
11. Monitor hemoglobin or hematocrit values daily or as prescribed.	Allows assessment of nosocomial anemia.	• Abnormal hemoglobin values • Abnormal hematocrit values
12. Replace gauze dressings every 2 days and transparent dressings at least every 7 days.[6,7] **(Level D*)**	Decreases the risk for infection at the catheter site. The CDC recommends replacing the dressing when the dressing becomes damp, loosened, or soiled or when inspection of the site is necessary.[11]	
13. Follow institution standard for assessing pain. Administer analgesia as prescribed.	Identifies need for pain interventions.	• Continued pain despite pain interventions

*Level D: Peer-reviewed professional organizational standards with clinical studies to support recommendations

Documentation

Documentation should include the following:

- Informed consent obtained
- Patient and family education
- Preprocedure verifications and time out
- Peripheral vascular and neurovascular assessment before and after the procedure and after the catheter is removed
- Date and time of insertion with the size of the catheter placed and the site of placement
- Assessment of the insertion site
- Patient response to the insertion procedure

- Status of the patient alarms and their parameters
- Pain assessment, interventions, and effectiveness
- Type of flush solution used
- Intake of flush solution (e.g., 3 mL/hr) on intake and output sheet
- Initial insertion waveform (recorded), labeled with the date, time, and systolic and diastolic pressures
- Time of arterial catheter removal
- Unexpected outcomes
- Additional nursing interventions

References

CR 1. American Association of Critical-Care Nurses: Evaluation of the effects of heparinized and nonheparinized flush solutions on the patency of arterial pressure monitoring lines: the AACN Thunder Project, *Am J Crit Care* 2:3-15, 1993.

2. Barone J, Madlinger RV: Should an Allen test be performed before radial artery cannulation? *J Trauma* 6:468-470, 2006.

CR 3. Chong BH: Heparin-induced thrombocytopenia, *Br J Haematol* 89:431-439, 1995.

CR 4. Gleason E, Grossman S, Campbell C: Minimizing diagnostic blood loss in critically ill patients, *Am J Crit Care* 1:85-90, 1992.

CR 5. Greenwood MJ, et al: Vascular communications of the hand in patients being considered for transradial coronary angiography: is the Allen's test accurate? *J Am Coll Cardiol* 46:2013-2017, 2005.

6. Infusion Nurses Society: Infusion nursing standards of practice, *J Infusion Nurs* 29:S1-S92, 2006.

CR 7. Luskin RL, et al: Extended use of disposable pressure transducers: a bacteriologic evaluation, *JAMA* 255:916-920, 1986.

CR 8. MacIsaac CM, et al: The influence of a blood conserving device on anaemia in intensive care patients, *Anaesth Intensive Care* 31:653-657, 2003.

CR 9. Maki DG, Narans LL, Knasinski V, et al: Prospective, randomized, investigator-masked trial of novel chlohexidine-impregnated disk (Biopatch) on central venous and arterial catheters [abstract], *Infect Control Hosp Epidemiol* 21:96, 2000.

CR 10. McGhee BH, Bridges MEJ: Monitoring arterial blood pressure: what you may not know, *Crit Care Nurse* 22:60-79, 2002.

CR 11. O'Grady NP, et al: Guidelines for the prevention of intravascular catheter-related infections, Centers for Disease Control and Prevention, *MMWR* 51(RR-10):1-36, 2002.

CR 12. O'Malley MK, et al: Value of routine pressure monitoring system changes after 72 hours of continuous use, *Crit Care Med* 22:1424-1430, 1994.

CR 13. Peruzzi WT, et al: A clinical evaluation of a blood conservation device in medical intensive care unit patients, *Crit Care Med* 21:501-506, 1993.

CR 14. Randolph AG, et al: Benefit of heparin in peripheral venous and arterial catheters: systematic review and meta-analysis of randomised controlled trials, *BMJ* 316:969-975, 1998.

CR 15. Silver MJ, et al: Evaluation of a new blood-conserving arterial line system for patients in intensive care units, *Crit Care Med* 21:507-511, 1993.

CR 16. Silver MJ, et al: Reduction of blood loss from diagnostic sampling in critically ill patients using a blood-conserving arterial line system, *Chest* 104:1711-1715, 1993.

CR 17. Slogoff S, Keats AS, Arlund C: On the safety of radial artery cannulation, *Anesthesiology* 59:42-47, 1983.

CR 18. US Department of Health and Human Services, National Institutes of Health, National Heart, Lung, and Blood Institute, National High Blood Pressure Education Program: *The seventh report of the joint national committee on prevention, detection, evaluation and treatment of high blood pressure,* 2004, retrieved July 27, 2009, from Publication No. 04-5230, www.nhlbi.nih.gov/guidelines/hypertension/jnc7full.pdf.

19. Timsit J, et al: Chlorhexidine-impregnated sponges and less frequent dressing changes for prevention of catheter-related infections in critically ill adults, *JAMA* 310:1231-1241, 2009.

CR 20. Zevola DR, Dioso J, Moggio R: Comparison of heparinized solutions for maintaining patency of arterial and pulmonary artery catheters, *Am J Crit Care* 6:52-55, 1997.

Additional Readings

Barbeito A, Mark JB: Arterial and central venous pressure monitoring, *Anesthesiol Clin* 24:717-735, 2006.

CR Bridges EJ, et al: Ask the experts, *Crit Care Nurse* 17:96-97,101-102, 1997.

CR Chulay M, Holland S: Ask the experts: where should the transducer be leveled for radial or femoral arterial pressure monitoring? *Crit Care Nurse* 16:103-107, 1996.

CR Darovic GO: Arterial pressure monitoring. *In: Hemodynamic monitoring: invasive and noninvasive clinical application,* ed 3, Philadelphia, 2002, Saunders.

CR Foster B: Continuing discussion on transducer placement. . . ask the experts column of the December issue 1996. . . zero referencing arterial lines, *Crit Care Nurse* 17:18, 1997.

CR Gorny DA: Arterial blood pressure measurement technique, *AACN Clin Issues* 4:66-80, 1993.

Halm MS: Flushing hemodynamic catheters: what does the science tell us? *Am J Crit Care* 17:73-76, 2008.

CR Imperial-Perez F, McRae M: Protocols for practice: applying research at the bedside: arterial pressure monitoring, *Crit Care Nurse* 22:70-72, 2002.

CR Imperial-Perez F, McRae M: *Protocols for practice: hemodynamic monitoring series: arterial pressure monitoring,* Aliso Viejo, CA, 1998, American Association of Critical-Care Nurses.

Lapum JL: Patency of arterial catheters with heparinized solutions versus non-heparinized solutions: a review of the literature, *Can J Cardiovasc Nurs* 16:64-67, 2006.

Leeper B: Ask the experts: what is the standard regarding isotonic sodium chloride solution versus heparin in pressure monitoring systems? *Crit Care Nurse* 26:137-138, 2006.

CR O'Grady NP, et al: Patient safety and the science of prevention: the time for implementing the guidelines for the prevention of intravascular catheter-related infections is now, *Crit Care Med* 31:291-292, 2003.

Shaffer C: Diagnostic blood loss in mechanically ventilated patients, *Heart Lung* 36:217-222, 2007.

CR Tuncali BE, et al: A comparison of the efficacy of heparinized and nonheparinized solutions for maintenance of perioperative radial arterial catheter patency and subsequent occlusion, *Anesth Analg* 100:1117-1121, 2005.

Arterial Pressure-Based Cardiac Output Monitoring

P U R P O S E : Arterial pressure-based cardiac output monitoring is a minimally invasive technology that can be used to obtain hemodynamic data on a continuous basis.

Mary Ellen Kern

PREREQUISITE NURSING KNOWLEDGE

- Knowledge of the anatomy and physiology of the cardiovascular system is necessary.
- Knowledge of the anatomy and physiology of the vasculature and adjacent structures is needed.
- Understanding of the pathophysiologic changes that occur in heart disease and affect flow dynamics is necessary.
- Understanding of aseptic technique is needed.
- Understanding of the hemodynamic effects of vasoactive medications is needed.
- Understanding of the principles involved in hemodynamic monitoring is necessary.
- Knowledge of invasive cardiac output monitoring is needed.
- Knowledge of arterial waveform interpretation is needed.
- Knowledge of definitions and norms for cardiac output, cardiac index, systemic vascular resistance, stroke volume, stroke index, preload, afterload, and contractility and stroke volume variation is necessary.
- Arterial pressure represents the forcible ejection of blood from the left ventricle into the aorta and out into the arterial system. During ventricular systole, blood is ejected into the aorta, generating a pressure wave. Because of the intermittent pumping action of the heart, this arterial pressure wave is generated in a pulsatile manner (see Fig. 62-1). The ascending limb of the aortic pressure wave (anacrotic limb) represents an increase in pressure because of left ventricular ejection. The peak of this ejection is the peak systolic pressure,

which is normally 100 to 140 mm Hg in adults. After reaching this peak, the ventricular pressure declines to a level below aortic pressure and the aortic valve closes, marking the end of ventricular systole. The closure of the aortic valve produces a small rebound wave that creates a notch known as the dicrotic notch. The descending limb of the curve (diastolic downslope) represents diastole and is characterized by a long declining pressure wave, during which the aortic wall recoils and propels blood into the arterial network. The diastolic pressure is measured as the lowest point of the diastolic downslope and is normally 60 to 80 mm Hg.

- The difference between the systolic and diastolic pressures is called the pulse pressure, with a normal value of 40 mm Hg.[9]
- Arterial pressure is determined by the relationship between blood flow through the vessels (cardiac output), the compliance of the aorta and larger vessels and the resistance of the more peripheral vessel walls (systemic vascular resistance). The arterial pressure is therefore affected by any factors that change either cardiac output, compliance or systemic vascular resistance.
- The average arterial pressure during a cardiac cycle is called the mean arterial pressure (MAP). It is not the average of the systolic plus the diastolic pressures, because at normal heart rates, systole accounts for 1/3 of the cardiac cycle and diastole accounts for 2/3 of the cardiac cycle. The MAP is calculated automatically by most patient monitoring systems; however,

it can be calculated roughly by using the following formula:

$$MAP = \frac{(\text{systolic pressure}) + (\text{diastolic pressure} \times 2)}{3}$$

- MAP represents the driving force (perfusion pressure) for blood flow through the cardiovascular system. MAP is at its highest point in the aorta. As blood travels through the circulatory system, systolic pressure increases and diastolic pressure decreases, with an overall decline in the MAP (see Fig. 62-2).
- Arterial pressure-based cardiac output (APCO) is obtained from an arterial catheter.[3,5,11]
- APCO technology measures the rate of flow (cardiac output).
- Stroke volume and heart rate are key determinants of cardiac output.
- Although systemic vascular resistance affects cardiac output, the location of that effect is global and not limited by location of that measurement because cardiac output is flow per minute throughout the body. Manufacturers of the arterial pressure-based cardiac output systems have factored in variance for both radial artery catheters and femoral artery catheters.[3]

EQUIPMENT

- Invasive arterial catheter and insertion kit
- Specialized sterile transducer and sensor kit (manufacturer-specific)
- Intravenous (IV) pole and cartridge holder (manufacturer-specific)
- Pressure transducer system, including flush solution recommended according to institution standard, a pressure bag or device, pressure tubing with transducer, and flush device
- Pressure module and cable for interface with the monitor
- Monitoring system (central and bedside monitor)
- Special monitor to interface with the bedside monitor for trending and display of hemodynamic values (manufacturer-specific)
- Dual-channel recorder
- Indelible marker
- Nonvented caps
- Leveling device (low-intensity laser or carpenter level)
- Sterile and nonsterile gloves
  Additional equipment as needed includes the following:
- Heparin
- 3-mL syringe
- 4 × 4 gauze pads or hydrocolloid gel pad
- Tape

PATIENT AND FAMILY EDUCATION

- Explain the rationale for arterial line insertion, including how the arterial pressure is displayed on the bedside monitor. ➤➤*Rationale:* This explanation may decrease patient and family anxiety.
- Explain the standard of care to the patient and family, including insertion procedure, alarms, dressings, and length of time the catheter is expected to be in place. ➤➤*Rationale:* This explanation encourages the patient and family to ask questions and voice concerns about the procedure and decreases patient and family anxiety.
- Explain the patient's expected participation during the procedure. ➤➤*Rationale:* Patient cooperation during insertion is encouraged.
- Explain the importance of keeping the affected extremity immobile. ➤➤*Rationale:* This explanation encourages patient cooperation to prevent catheter dislodgment and ensures a more accurate waveform.
- Instruct the patient to report any warmth, redness, pain, or wet feeling at the insertion site at any time, including after catheter removal. ➤➤*Rationale:* These symptoms may indicate infection, bleeding, or disconnection of the tubing or catheter.

PATIENT ASSESSMENT AND PREPARATION

Patient Assessment

- Obtain the patient's medical history, including a history of diabetes and hypertension. ➤➤*Rationale:* Patients with diabetes mellitus or hypertension are at higher risk for arterial or venous insufficiency.
- Obtain the patient's medical history for peripheral vascular disease, vascular grafts, arteriovenous (AV) fistulas or shunts, arterial vasospasm, thrombosis, or embolism. In addition, obtain the patient's history of coronary artery bypass graft surgery in which radial arteries were removed for use as conduits. ➤➤*Rationale:* Extremities with any of these problems should be avoided as sites for cannulation because of the potential for complications.
- Assess the neurovascular and peripheral vascular status of the extremity to be used for the arterial cannulation, including color, temperature, presence and fullness of pulses, capillary refill, presence of bruit, and motor and sensory function (as compared with the opposite extremity). Note: A modified Allen's test should be performed before cannulation of the radial artery (see Fig. 80-3). ➤➤*Rationale:* This assessment identifies any neurovascular or circulatory impairment before cannulation to avoid potential complications.
- Assess the patient's vital signs and compliance factors (e.g., age, gender, height, weight). ➤➤*Rationale:* This assessment provides baseline data. The compliance factors allow for the individual variables that ultimately dictate pulse pressure and its relevance (proportionality) to stroke volume.

Patient Preparation

- Verify correct patient with two identifiers. ➤➤*Rationale:* Prior to performing a procedure, the nurse should ensure the correct identification of the patient for the intended intervention.
- Ensure that the patient and family understand preprocedural teaching. Answer questions as they arise, and reinforce

information as needed. ➤➤**Rationale:** Understanding of previously taught information is evaluated and reinforced.

- Ensure that informed consent has been obtained. ➤➤**Rationale:** Informed consent protects the rights of the patient and makes a competent decision possible for the patient.
- Perform a pre-procedure verification and time out, if non-emergent. ➤➤**Rationale:** Ensures patient safety.

- Validate the patency of the peripheral IV line. ➤➤**Rationale:** Access may be needed for administration of emergency medications or fluids.
- Place the patient's extremity in the appropriate position with adequate lighting of the insertion site. ➤➤**Rationale:** This placement prepares the site for cannulation and facilitates an accurate insertion.

Procedure	**for Arterial Pressure-Based Cardiac Output Monitoring**	
Steps	**Rationale**	**Special Considerations**
Initiating the Procedure		
1. HH		
2. PE		
3. If a catheter is to be inserted in the radial artery, a modified Allen's test is recommended before arterial cannulation (see Fig. 80-3). **(Level C*)**	Ensures the adequacy of collateral blood flow of the extremity to be cannulated.[2,8,13]	
4. Prepare the flush solution (see Procedure 76). Follow institution standard for adding heparin to the intravenous (IV) bag, if heparin is not contraindicated. **(Level B*)**	Heparinized flush solutions are commonly used to minimize thrombi and fibrin deposits on the catheter. Catheters flushed with heparinized saline solution are more likely than those flushed with nonheparinized saline solution to remain patent.[1,12,14]	Other factors that promote patency of the arterial line besides heparinized saline solution include: male gender, longer arterial catheters, larger vessels cannulated, patients receiving other anticoagulants or thrombolytics, and short-term use of the catheter.[1] Although heparin may prevent thrombosis,[6,12] it has been associated with thrombocytopenia and other hematologic complications.[6]
5. Gather the equipment needed for obtaining an arterial pressure-based cardiac output.	Prepares supplies.	Refer to the specific manufacturer for additional required equipment for set-up and maintenance. Some technologies require additional calibration procedures and equipment.[3-5,7,9]
6. Obtain the patient's baseline compliance factors (e.g., age, gender, height, weight). **(Level M*)**	This information is needed to allow for the individual variables that ultimately dictate pulse pressure and its relevance (proportionality) to stroke volume.	Follow manufacturer guidelines. Some manufacturers require calibration. Manufacturers that do not require calibration use age, gender, height, and weight to determine vascular compliance. An accurate weight reflecting perfused tissue is important in the determination of body surface area (BSA) and cardiac index.

*Level B: Well-designed, controlled studies with results that consistently support a specific action, intervention, or treatment
*Level C: Qualitative studies, descriptive or correlational studies, integrative reviews, systematic reviews, or randomized controlled trials with inconsistent results
*Level M: Manufacturer's recommendations only

Procedure	for Arterial Pressure-Based Cardiac Output Monitoring—*Continued*	
Steps	**Rationale**	**Special Considerations**
		Fluid weight gain often is discounted because it is not perfused tissue. Medications are generally based on perfused weight in the case of morbidly obese patients. Because adipose tissue is highly vascular, actual weight and height are necessary to determine body surface area. This is particularly important for calculating cardiac index.

Setting up the Arterial Pressure-Based Cardiac Output (APCO) System

1. **HH**		
2. **PE**		
3. Open the APCO sensor kit.	Prepares equipment.	Follow manufacturer recommendations.
4. Secure all connections.	Tight connections ensure the integrity of the system.	Vented caps are standard with transducer sets and kits and allow for initial priming of the system.
5. Insert the APCO sensor into the mounting plate that is secured on the IV pole next to the patient.	Stabilizes the sensor.	
6. Level the vent port near the sensor with the phlebostatic axis of the patient.	The reference point is the phlebostatic axis because it accurately reflects central arterial pressure.	
7. Prime or flush the entire APCO system:	Removes air bubbles.	Priming of the system must be by gravity to avoid small bubbles from entering the tubing and interfering with accurate signal transmission.
A. Pull the flush tab to deliver the flush solution through the sensor and out through the vent port.	Air interferes with an accurate signal.	
B. Close the vent port by turning the stopcock to the neutral position.		
C. Place a sterile nonvented cap on the top of the stopcock.	Maintains a closed sterile system.	
D. Hold the pressure tubing in an upright position and pull the flush tab to purge air from the remaining part of the line through the end of the tubing.	Removes remaining air from the system.	
8. Inflate the pressure bag or device to 300 mm Hg.	Inflating the pressure bag to 300 mm Hg allows approximately 1 to 3 mL/hr of flush solution to be delivered through the catheter, thus maintaining catheter patency and minimizing clot formation.	
9. Assist with insertion of the arterial catheter (see Procedure 62).	Provides needed assistance.	
10. Connect the bedside monitor cable to the APCO sensor (Fig. 63-1).	Information can then be transferred from the sensor to the monitor.	Follow manufacturer guidelines. (Some cables are color coded.)

Procedure continues on following page

Procedure for Arterial Pressure-Based Cardiac Output Monitoring—*Continued*

Steps	Rationale	Special Considerations
11. Enter the patient's gender, age, height, and weight.	This information is needed to allow for the individual variables that ultimately dictate pulse pressure and its relevance (proportionality) to stroke volume. The result is stroke volume variability.	Follow manufacturer guidelines. Some manufacturers require calibration.
12. Set up the monitor (see Fig. 63-1):		Follow the manufacturer's guidelines as the set up may vary.
A. Turn the knob on the monitor to "CO," for cardiac output.	Prepares the equipment.	
B. Press the knob and the CO menu opens.	Pressing the knob is equivalent to enter.	
C. Rotate the knob until the "zero the arterial pressure" is highlighted, and press the knob.	Begins the zeroing process.	
D. Open the stopcock positioned on the mounted sensor to air.	Allows the monitor to use atmospheric pressure as a reference for zero.	
E. Select "zero the arterial pressures" and press "zero."	Zeroing negates the effects of atmospheric pressure.	
F. Zero the arterial module on the patient's bedside monitor.	Zeroing negates the effects of atmospheric pressure.	
G. Return the stopcock to the neutral position and place a sterile nonvented cap on the top of the stopcock.	Closes the system, maintains sterility of the system, and initiates monitoring.	Both the bedside monitor and the APCO monitor should display the patient's arterial pressure waveform.
13. Observe the CO display.	Provides assessment data.	The cardiac output value is updated every 20 seconds.
14. Set the alarm parameters according to the patient's current blood pressure.	Activates the bedside and central alarm system.	Follow manufacturer guidelines.
15. Dispose of used supplies in appropriate receptacles.	Reduces the transmission of microorganisms; Standard Precautions.	
16. **HH**		

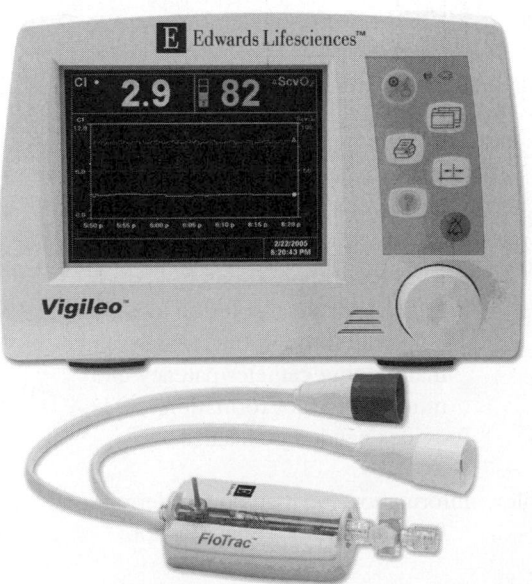

FIGURE 63-1   FloTrac sensor and Vigileo monitor. *(Courtesy of Edwards Lifesciences, LLC, 2009.)*

Expected Outcomes

- Accurate measurement of CO
- Minimal discomfort from the arterial catheter
- Maintenance of baseline hemoglobin and hematocrit levels
- Adequate circulation to the involved extremity
- Adequate sensory and motor function of the extremity
- Maintenance of the catheter site without infection

Unexpected Outcomes

- Inability to accurately measure CO
- Infection
- Impaired peripheral tissue perfusion (e.g., edema, coolness, pain, paleness, or slow capillary refill of the fingers of the cannulated extremity)
- Perforated or lacerated artery
- Pain or discomfort from the arterial catheter insertion site
- Decreased hemoglobin and hematocrit values
- Catheter disconnection with significant blood loss

Patient Monitoring and Care

Steps	Rationale	Reportable Conditions
		These conditions should be reported if they persist despite nursing interventions.
1. Assess the neurovascular and peripheral vascular status of the cannulated extremity immediately after catheter insertion and every 4 hours, or more often if warranted, according to institution standard.	Validates adequate peripheral vascular and neurovascular integrity. Changes in sensation, motor function, pulses, color, temperature, or capillary refill may indicate ischemia, arterial spasm, or neurovascular compromise.	• Diminished or absent pulses • Pale, mottled, or cyanotic appearance of the extremity • Extremity that is cool or cold to the touch • Capillary refill time of more than 2 seconds • Diminished or absent sensation • Diminished or absent motor function
2. Assess the arterial catheter insertion site for signs and symptoms of infection.	Identifies the possibility of site infection.	• Redness at the site • Purulent drainage • Tenderness or pain at the insertion site • Elevated temperature • Elevated white blood cell count
3. Continuously monitor heart rate, blood pressure, and cardiac indices. Document parameters hourly and as necessary with condition changes.	Provides assessment of patient status.	• Abnormal vital signs • Abnormal cardiac output • Abnormal cardiac index
4. Follow institution standard for assessing pain. Administer analgesia as prescribed.	Identifies need for pain interventions.	• Continued pain despite pain interventions
5. Assess the patient's response to prescribed interventions.	The hemodynamic management of the patient requires close monitoring and interventions based on the parameters obtained from the APCO data.	• Abnormal cardiac output • Abnormal cardiac index • Abnormal vital signs
6. Replace gauze dressings every 2 days and transparent dressings at least every 7 days. **(Level D*)**	Decreases the risk for infection at the catheter site. The CDC recommends replacing the dressing when the dressing becomes damp, loosened, or soiled, or when inspection of the site is necessary.[10]	• Abnormal hemoglobin values

*Level D: Peer-reviewed professional organizational standards with clinical studies to support recommendations

Procedure continues on following page

Documentation

Documentation should include the following:

- Patient and family education
- Informed consent
- Pre-procedure verification and time out
- Patient tolerance of the procedure
- Peripheral vascular and neurovascular assessment before and after the procedure
- Assessment of the insertion site
- Patient response to the insertion procedure
- Status of the patient alarms
- Pain assessment, interventions, and effectiveness

- Type of flush used
- Intake of flush solution on intake and output record
- Vital signs, cardiac output, cardiac index, and other hemodynamic parameters
- Positive flow by modified Allen's test if the radial artery is used
- Site assessment
- Unexpected outcomes
- Additional nursing interventions

References

CR 1. American Association of Critical-Care Nurses: Evaluation of the effects of heparinized and nonheparinized flush solutions on the patency of arterial pressure monitoring lines: the AACN Thunder Project, *Am J Crit Care* 2:3-15, 1993.

2. Barone J, Madlinger RV: Should an Allen test be performed before radial artery cannulation? *J Trauma* 6: 468-470, 2006.

3. Button D, Weibel L, Reuthebuch O, et al: Clinical evaluation of the FloTrac/Vigileo system and two established continuous cardiac output monitoring devices in patients undergoing cardiac surgery, *Br J Anaesth* 99(3): 329-336, 2007.

4. Cecconi M, Wilson J, Rhodes A: Pulse pressure analysis. In Vincent JL, editor: *Yearbook of intensive care and emergency medicine*, Brussels, 2006, Springer-Verlag, 176-184.

5. Chakravarthy M, Patil TA, Jayaprakash K, et al: Comparison of simultaneous estimation of cardiac output by four techniques in patients undergoing off-pump coronary artery bypass surgery: a prospective observational study, *Ann Cardiac Anaesth* 10(2):121-126, 2007.

CR 6. Chong BH: Heparin-induced thrombocytopenia, *Br J Haematol* 89:431-439, 1995.

7. de Waal E, Kalkma C, Rex S, et al: Validation of a new arterial pulse contour-based cardiac output device, *Crit Care Med* 35(8):1904-1909, 2007.

CR 8. Greenwood MJ, et al: Vascular communications of the hand in patients being considered for transradial coronary angiography: is the Allen's test accurate? *J Am Coll Cardiol* 46:2013-2017, 2005.

9. Headley JM: Clinically relevant monitoring using arterial pressure-based technologies and stroke volume variation to assess fluid responsiveness, *NTI News Online* 20/21: 1-6, 2007.

CR 10. O'Grady NP, et al: Guidelines for the prevention of intravascular catheter-related infections, Centers for Disease Control and Prevention, *MMWR* 51(RR-10):1-36, 2002.

11. Prasser C, Bele S, Keyl C, et al: Evaluation of a new arterial pressure-based cardiac output device requiring no external calibration, *BMC Anesthesiol* 7(186):1471-2253,7-9, 2007.

CR 12. Randolph AG, et al: Benefit of heparin in peripheral venous and arterial catheters: systematic review and meta-analysis of randomised controlled trials, *BMJ* 316:969-975, 1998.

CR 13. Slogoff S, Keats AS, Arlund C: On the safety of radial artery cannulation, *Anesthesiology* 59:42-47, 1983.

CR 14. Zevola DR, Dioso J, Moggio R: Comparison of heparinized solutions for maintaining patency of arterial and pulmonary artery catheters, *Am J Crit Care* 6:52-55, 1997.

Additional Reading

McGee WT, Malloux P, Jodka P, et al: The pulmonary artery catheter in critical care, *Semin Dial* 19:480-491, 2006.

Blood Sampling from an Arterial Catheter

P U R P O S E : Blood sampling from an arterial catheter is performed to obtain blood specimens for arterial blood gas analysis or other laboratory testing.

Rose B. Shaffer

PREREQUISITE NURSING KNOWLEDGE

- Knowledge of aseptic and sterile technique is necessary.
- Knowledge of the vascular anatomy and physiology is needed.
- Understanding of gas exchange and acid-base balance is necessary.
- Technique for specimen collection and labeling should be understood.
- Principles of hemodynamic monitoring are necessary.
- Knowledge about the care of patients with arterial catheters (see Procedure 62) and stopcock manipulation (see Procedure 76) is needed.
- Understanding of the closed arterial line blood sampling system is necessary.
- Closed blood sampling systems provide the opportunity to reinfuse the blood to the patient after the laboratory sample is obtained to help reduce the risk of nosocomial anemia.[3,7,10,14,15]

EQUIPMENT

- Nonsterile gloves
- Sterile 4 × 4 gauze pads
- Appropriate blood specimen tubes (or arterial blood gas [ABG] kit)
- Labels with the patient's name and appropriate identifying data
- Laboratory form and specimen labels
- Goggles or fluid shield face mask
- Needleless blood sampling access device

- Extra blood specimen tube (for discard)
- Sterile nonvented cap or needleless cap
- Antiseptic solution
  Additional equipment as needed includes the following:
- Bag of ice
- Syringes, 5- and 10-mL
- Needleless cannula (for closed arterial blood sampling system)

PATIENT AND FAMILY EDUCATION

- Explain the procedure to the patient and family. **➤➤***Rationale:* Teaching provides information and may reduce anxiety and fear.
- Explain the importance of keeping the affected extremity immobile. **➤➤***Rationale:* This explanation encourages patient cooperation during blood withdrawal.

PATIENT ASSESSMENT AND PREPARATION

Patient Assessment

- Assess the patency of the arterial catheter. **➤➤***Rationale:* This ensures a functional arterial catheter.
- Assess the patient's previous laboratory results. **➤➤***Rationale:* This assessment provides data for comparison.

Patient Preparation

- Verify correct patient with two identifiers. **➤➤***Rationale:* Prior to performing a procedure, the nurse should ensure the correct identification of the patient for the intended intervention.

- Ensure that the patient and family understand preprocedural teaching. Answer questions as they arise, and reinforce information as needed. ➤*Rationale:* Understanding of previously taught information is evaluated and reinforced.

- Expose the stopcock to be used for blood sampling, and position the patient's extremity so that the site can easily be accessed. ➤*Rationale:* This prepares the site for blood withdrawal.

Procedure	**for Blood Sampling from an Arterial Catheter**	
Steps	**Rationale**	**Special Considerations**
1. ▮HH▮		
2. ▮PE▮		
3. When obtaining an ABG sample, open the ABG kit and use the plunger to rid the excess heparin and air from the syringe.	Prepares the ABG syringe.	Heparin is usually in powdered form. If prepackaged ABG kits are not available, draw 0.5 mL of a 1:1000 dilution of heparin in a 3-mL syringe. Pull back on the plunger to coat the inside of the syringe and the needle. Rid the excess heparin and air from the syringe.[2]
4. Temporarily suspend the arterial alarms.	Prevents the alarm from sounding as the pressure waveform is lost during the blood draw.	

Blood Sampling with a Needleless Blood Sampling Access Device or a Syringe

1. Arterial stopcock:		
A. Remove the nonvented cap from the port of the three-way stopcock closest to the patient and attach the needleless blood sampling access device (Figs. 64-1 and 64-2, *A*) or syringe (Fig. 64-2, *B*) to the stopcock. *Or*	Prepares for blood sampling.	
B. Cleanse the needleless cap at the top of the stopcock closest to the patient with an antiseptic solution.[1,9] **(Level B*)** Attach the needleless blood sampling access device (see Fig. 65-1).		Chlorhexidine and povidone-iodine solutions may be more effective than alcohol in reducing external microbial contamination.[1]

*Level B: Well-designed controlled studies with results that consistently support a specific action, intervention, or treatment

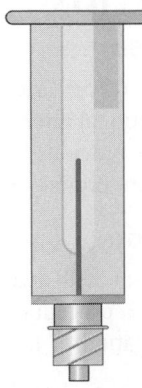

Figure 64-1   Needleless blood sampling access device. (*Drawing by Paul W. Schiffmacher, Thomas Jefferson University Hospital, Philadelphia, PA.*)

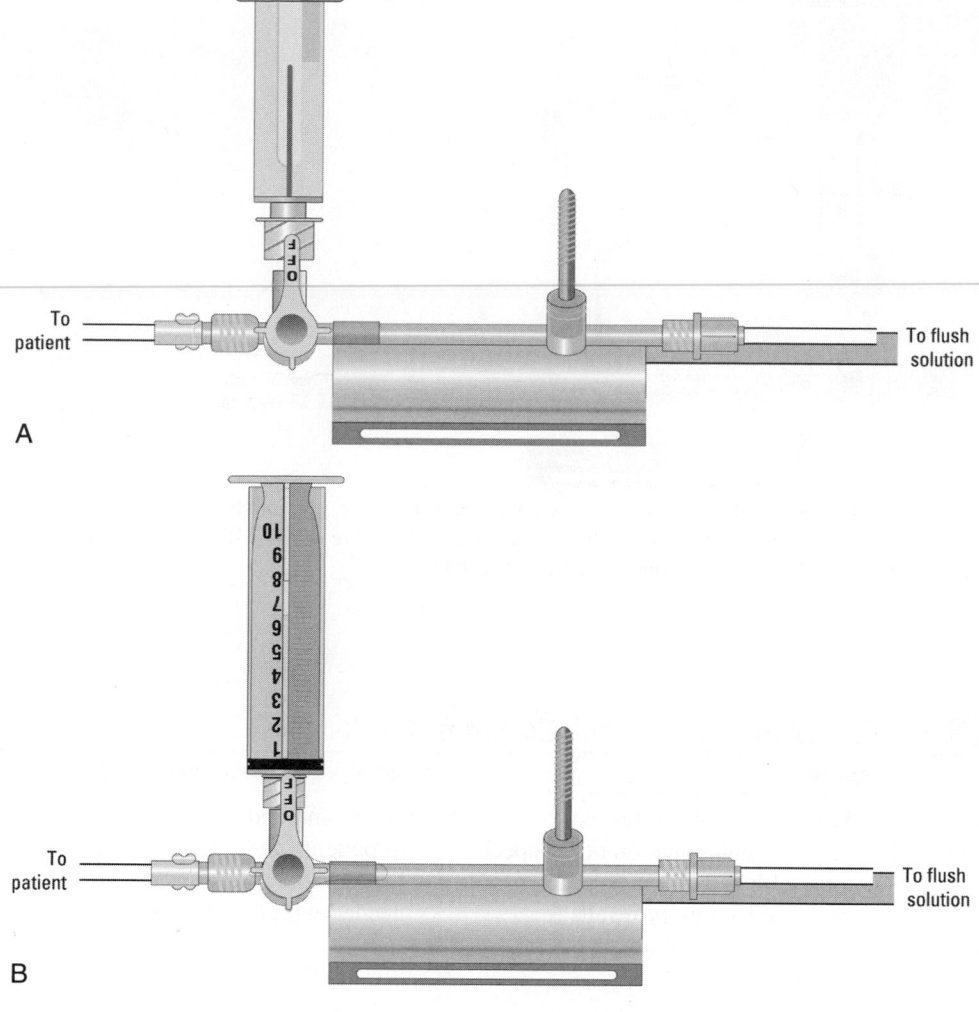

FIGURE 64-2 **A,** The needle-less blood sampling access device attached to the port of the three-way stopcock. The stopcock is turned "off" to the port of the stop-cock. **B,** A syringe attached to the port of the three-way stopcock. The stopcock is turned "off" to the port of the stopcock). *(Drawing by Paul W. Schiffmacher, Thomas Jefferson University Hospital, Philadelphia, PA.)*

Procedure	for Blood Sampling from an Arterial Catheter—*Continued*		
Steps	**Rationale**	**Special Considerations**
2. Turn the stopcock off to the flush solution (see Fig. 64-3 or 65-2).	The needleless blood sampling access device or syringe is then in direct contact with the blood in the arterial catheter.	
3. When using a needleless blood sampling access device, engage the blood specimen tube to obtain the discard volume or, if using a syringe, slowly and gently aspirate the discard volume.	Clears the catheter of flush solution.	
A. When obtaining blood for an ABG sample, discard a blood sample that is two times the dead-space volume. **(Level B*)**	The discard volume includes the dead space and the blood diluted by the flush solution (e.g., dead space of 0.8 mL = 1.6 mL discard).[11,12]	The dead space is the space between the tip of the arterial catheter to the top port of the stop cock.

*Level B: Well-designed controlled studies with results that consistently support a specific action, intervention, or treatment

Procedure continues on following page

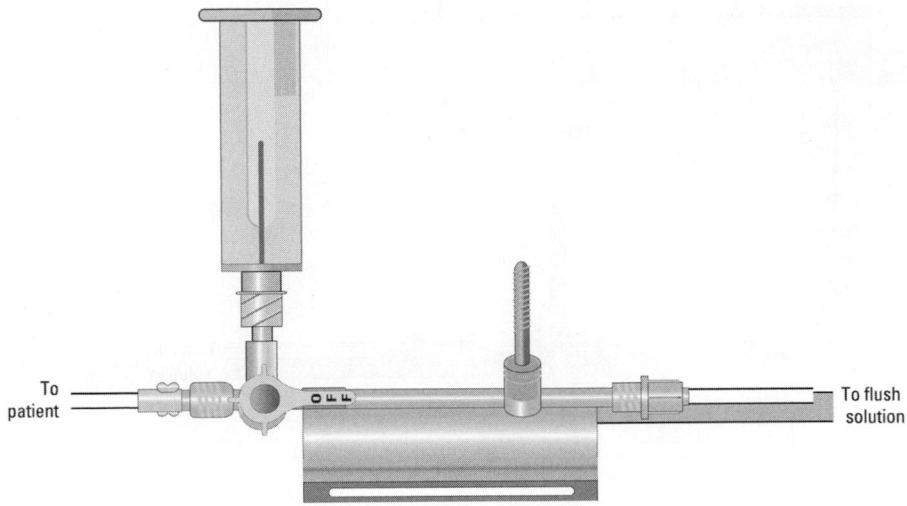

FIGURE 64-3   The needleless blood sampling access device attached to the port of the three-way stopcock. The stopcock is turned "off" to the flush solution. *(Drawing by Paul W. Schiffmacher, Thomas Jefferson University Hospital, Philadelphia, PA)*

Procedure | for Blood Sampling from an Arterial Catheter—*Continued*

Steps	Rationale	Special Considerations
B. When obtaining blood for coagulation studies (particularly activated partial thromboplastin time [aPTT]) from a heparinized arterial line, use a discard volume of six times the dead-space volume. **(Level B*)**	Additional discard is needed to prevent contamination of the specimen with heparin in order to ensure accurate laboratory results (e.g., dead space of 0.8 mL = 4.8 mL discard).[4-6,8,13]	This recommendation does not apply to patients undergoing systemic heparin therapy. More research is needed with this patient population.
4. Turn the stopcock off to the syringe.	Stops blood flow and closes the top port of the stopcock.	Not necessary if using a needleless blood sampling device.
5. Remove the syringe or the blood specimen tube and discard in the appropriate receptacle.	Removes and safely disposes of the discard.	If unable to dispose of the discard specimen immediately, place it away from the field so it is not mistaken for the actual blood specimen(s) for laboratory analysis.
6. Obtain the blood sample:	Obtains the appropriate blood specimens.	If obtaining laboratory specimens in addition to an ABG and coagulation studies, obtain the routine laboratory studies first and then obtain the ABG and coagulation studies to minimize the heparin effect.
A. If using the needleless system, the stopcock should remain off to the flush solution as each blood specimen tube is engaged.	The needleless blood sampling access device is a nonvented system, so no backflow of arterial blood from the patient occurs.	

*Level B: Well-designed controlled studies with results that consistently support a specific action, intervention, or treatment

Procedure for Blood Sampling from an Arterial Catheter—*Continued*

Steps	Rationale	Special Considerations
B. If using syringes to obtain blood specimens: Turn the stopcock off to the patient before changing each syringe (Figs. 64-4, *A*). After each new syringe is attached to the blood sampling port, turn the stopcock off to the flush solution (Figs. 64-4, *B*).	Prevents backflow of arterial blood through the open blood sampling port. Opens the arterial line from the patient to the syringe.	
C. When obtaining an ABG sample, turn the stopcock off to the patient and attach the ABG syringe directly to the top port of the stopcock or place the ABG syringe inside of the needleless access device.	Prepares for connection of the ABG syringe.	

Procedure continues on following page

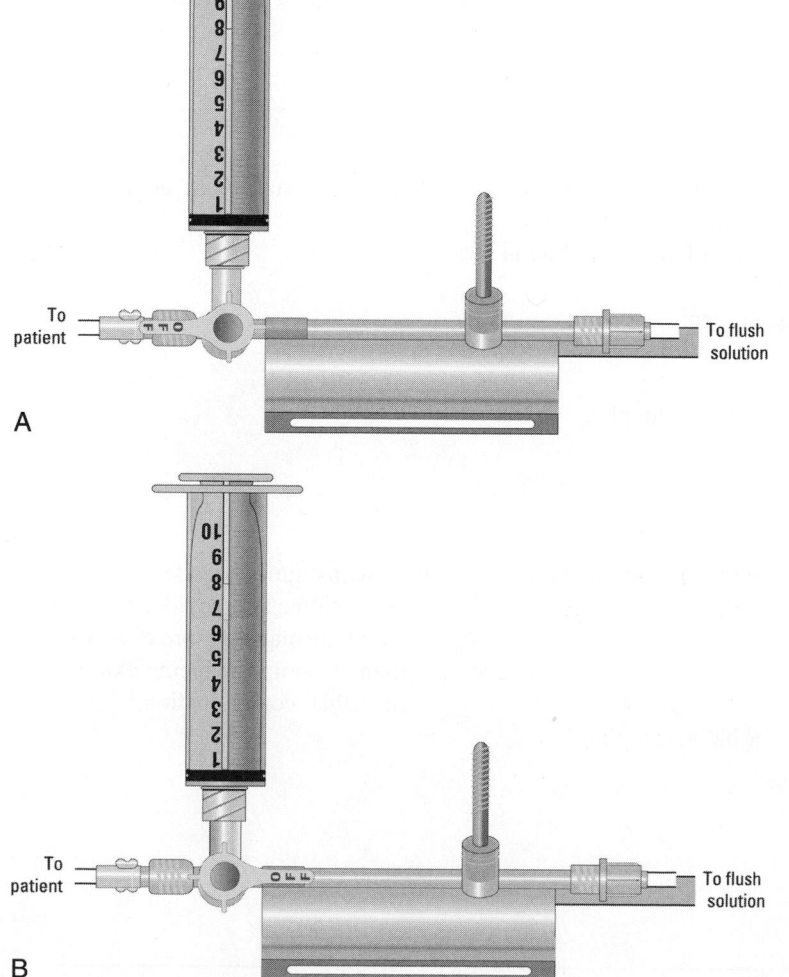

FIGURE 64-4 **A,** A syringe attached to the port of the three-way stopcock. The stopcock is turned "off" to the patient. **B,** A syringe attached to the top of the three-way stopcock. The stopcock is turned "off" to the flush solution. (*Drawing by Paul W. Schiffmacher, Thomas Jefferson University Hospital, Philadelphia, PA.*)

Procedure for Blood Sampling from an Arterial Catheter—*Continued*

Steps	Rationale	Special Considerations
D. Turn the stopcock off to the flush solution.	Opens the arterial line to the ABG syringe.	
E. Gently aspirate the ABG sample.	Obtains the ABG sample while minimizing vessel trauma.	
F. Turn the stopcock off to the patient before removing the ABG syringe.	Prevents the backflow of arterial blood.	
G. Expel any air bubbles from the ABG syringe and cap the syringe.	Ensures accuracy of the ABG results.	
7. After the last specimen is obtained, turn the stopcock off to the patient.	Detaches the specimen and ensures no backflow of arterial blood from the patient.	
8. Using the fast flush device, flush the remaining blood from the top port of the stopcock onto a sterile gauze pad, into a discard syringe, or into a blood specimen tube.	Clears blood from the system.	Follow institution standard.
9. Turn the stopcock off to the top port of the stopcock.	Opens the system up for continuous arterial pressure monitoring.	Remove the needleless blood sampling access device if used.
10. Place a new, sterile, nonvented cap or a needleless cap to the top port of the stopcock.	Maintains a closed sterile system.	
11. Using the fast flush device, flush the remaining blood in the arterial catheter back into the patient.	Promotes patency of the arterial catheter.	
Blood Sampling with a Closed Arterial Blood Sampling System		
1. Slowly and gently pull back on the blood withdrawal reservoir plunger until it fills to the full capacity (Fig. 64-5).	Withdraws and stores blood from the patient until it is ready to be reinfused after blood sampling is complete.	Temporarily silence the arterial alarm.
2. Close the stopcock by turning it perpendicular to the tubing (Fig. 64-6).	Closes the system.	
3. Attach a needleless cannula (Fig. 64-7) to the needleless blood sampling access device (Fig. 64-8, *A*) or a syringe (Fig. 64-8, *B*).	Prepares for blood sampling.	
4. Cleanse the blood sampling port with an antiseptic solution.[1,9] **(Level B*)**	Prepares for blood sampling and reduces the risk for infection.	Follow institution standard. Chlorhexidine and povidone-iodine solutions may be more effective than alcohol in reducing external microbial contamination.[1]
5. While holding the base of the blood sampling port, engage (push) the needleless cannula (with the attached needleless blood sampling access device or syringe) into the blood sampling port (Fig. 64-9).	Prepares for blood sampling.	

*Level B: Well-designed controlled studies with results that consistently support a specific action, intervention, or treatment

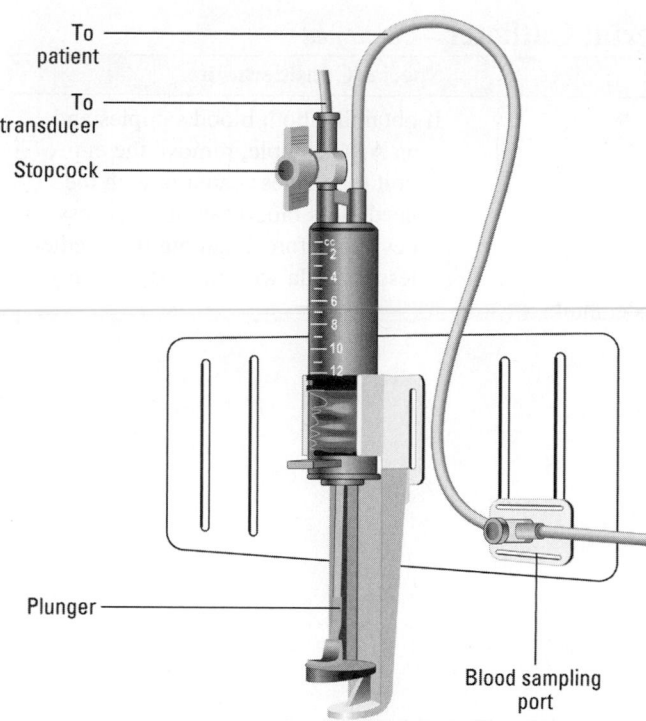

To patient

To transducer

Stopcock

Plunger

Blood sampling port

FIGURE 64-5 Closed blood sampling system. *(Drawing by Paul W. Schiffmacher, Thomas Jefferson University Hospital, Philadelphia, PA.)*

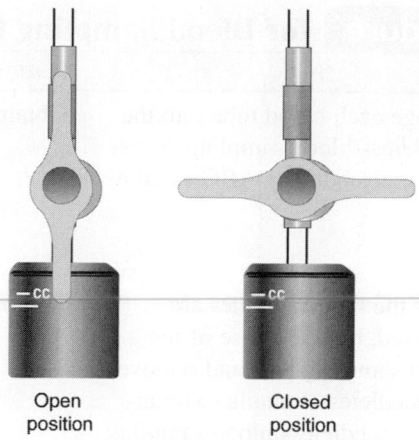

Open position

Closed position

FIGURE 64-6 The stopcock of the closed blood sampling system in the open and closed position. *(Drawing by Paul W. Schiffmacher, Thomas Jefferson University Hospital, Philadelphia, PA.)*

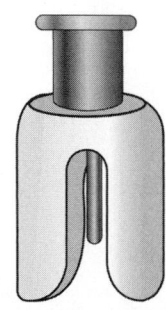

FIGURE 64-7 The needleless cannula for the closed blood sampling system. *(Drawing by Paul W. Schiffmacher, Thomas Jefferson University Hospital, Philadelphia, PA.)*

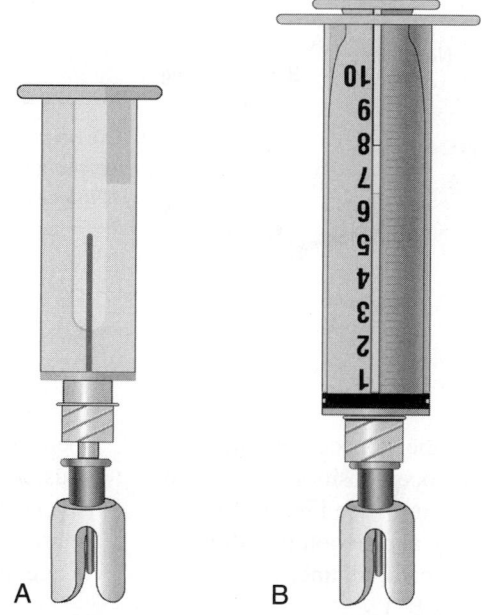

A   B

FIGURE 64-8 **A,** The needleless cannula attached to a needleless blood sampling access device. **B,** The needleless cannula attached to a syringe. *(Drawing by Paul W. Schiffmacher, Thomas Jefferson University Hospital, Philadelphia, PA.)*

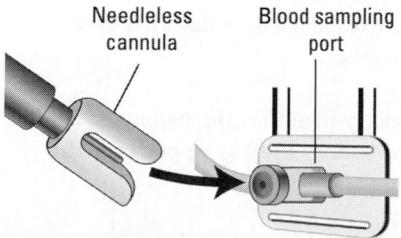

Needleless cannula

Blood sampling port

FIGURE 64-9 Attachment of the needleless cannula into the blood sampling port of the closed blood sampling system. *(Drawing by Paul W. Schiffmacher, Thomas Jefferson University Hospital, Philadelphia, PA.)*

Procedure   for Blood Sampling from an Arterial Catheter—*Continued*

Steps	Rationale	Special Considerations
6. Engage each blood tube into the needleless blood sampling access device or obtain an ABG sample.	Obtains the sample.	If obtaining both blood samples and an ABG sample, remove the entire unit (needleless cannula with the needleless blood sampling access device) before engaging the needleless cannula with the ABG syringe.
7. After the blood samples are obtained, hold the base of the blood sampling port and remove the needleless cannula (with attached needleless blood sampling access device or ABG syringe) from the sampling port by pulling it straight out (Fig. 64-10).	Removes the needleless cannula.	

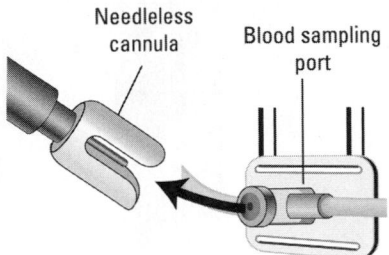

Needleless cannula   Blood sampling port

FIGURE 64-10   Removal of the needleless cannula from the blood sampling port of the closed blood sampling system. *(Drawing by Paul W. Schiffmacher, Thomas Jefferson University Hospital, Philadelphia, PA.)*

Steps	Rationale	Special Considerations
8. Open the stopcock by turning it to the open position (parallel to the tubing) (see Fig. 64-6).	Opens the system to prepare for reinfusion of the stored withdrawn blood sample.	
9. Slowly and smoothly reinfuse the discard volume.[3,7,10,14,15] **(Level B*)**	Returns blood to the patient to help reduce the risk of nosocomial anemia.	
10. Swab the blood sampling port with antiseptic solution.	Removes excess blood and fluid from the sampling port to prevent bacterial growth.	
11. Flush the system with the fast flush device.	Promotes the patency of the arterial catheter.	
After Blood Specimens Are Obtained		
1. Turn the alarms on and ensure that the waveform returns.	Provides accurate waveform and safe blood pressure monitoring.	
2. Discard used supplies in appropriate receptacles.	Removes and safely discards used supplies.	
3. 🄷🄷		
4. Label the specimens and complete the laboratory form per institution protocol.	Properly identifies the patient and laboratory tests to be performed.	For ABG samples, note the time the specimen was drawn and the percentage of oxygen therapy and any other data required by institution protocol.
5. Send the specimen for analysis.	Needed for analysis.	Follow institution standard regarding the use of ice for ABG samples.

*Level B: Well-designed controlled studies with results that consistently support a specific action, intervention, or treatment

Expected Outcomes

- Adequate blood sample with minimal blood loss
- No hemolysis of specimens
- No arterial spasm
- Arterial line patency maintained

Unexpected Outcomes

- Inadequate blood sample
- Hemolysis of specimens
- Arterial spasm
- Dilution of specimens that causes inaccurate laboratory results
- Anemia
- Clotting of the arterial catheter

Patient Monitoring and Care

Steps	Rationale	Reportable Conditions
		These conditions should be reported if they persist despite nursing interventions.
1. Use the minimal volume of blood discard.	Helps prevent nosocomial anemia.	• Decrease in hemoglobin or hematocrit levels
2. Monitor hemoglobin or hematocrit daily or as prescribed.	Allows early detection of nosocomial anemia.	• Decrease in hemoglobin or hematocrit levels
3. Attempt to group blood draws together whenever possible.	Diminishes the number of times the system is entered to help minimize the risk for infection.	• Signs of catheter-related infection
4. Before and after the blood withdrawal, assess and evaluate the arterial waveform.	Ensures accurate arterial pressure monitoring.	
5. Turn on arterial blood pressure alarms after blood withdrawal and review parameters.	Ensures safe arterial pressure monitoring.	
6. Obtain laboratory specimen results.	Monitors test results.	• Abnormal specimen results

Documentation

Documentation should include the following:
- Patient and family education
- Date, time, and type of specimen drawn
- Unexpected outcomes
- Additional nursing interventions
- Results of laboratory tests, when available

References

CR 1. Casey AL, et al: A randomized, prospective clinical trial to assess the potential infection risk associated with the PosiFlow needleless connector, *J Hosp Infection* 54:288-293, 2003.

CR 2. Darovic GO: Arterial pressure monitoring. In *Hemodynamic monitoring: invasive and noninvasive clinical application,* ed 3, Philadelphia, 2002, Saunders.

CR 3. Gleason E, Grossman S, Campbell C: Minimizing diagnostic blood loss in critically ill patients, *Am J Crit Care* 1:85-90, 1992.

CR 4. Gregersen RA, et al: Accurate coagulation studies from heparinized radial artery catheters, *Heart Lung* 16(6): 686-692, 1987.

CR 5. Harper J: Use of intraarterial lines to obtain coagulation samples, *Focus Crit Care* 15:51-55, 1988.

CR 6. Laxson CJ, Titler MG: Drawing coagulation studies from arterial lines: an integrative literature review, *Am J Crit Care* 3:16-24, 1994.

CR 7. MacIsaac CM, et al: The influence of a blood conserving device on anaemia in intensive care patients, *Anaesth Intensive Care* 31:653-657, 2003.

CR 8. Molyneaux RD, Papciak B, Rorem DA: Coagulation studies and the indwelling heparinized catheter, *Heart Lung* 16:20-23, 1987.

CR 9. O'Grady NP, et al: Guidelines for the prevention of intravascular catheter-related infections: Centers for Disease Control and Prevention, *MMWR Rec Rep* 51(RR-10): 1-29, 2002.

CR 10. Peruzzi WT, et al: A clinical evaluation of a blood conservation device in medical intensive care unit patients, *Crit Care Med* 21:501-506, 1993.

CR 11. Preusser BA, et al: Quantifying the minimum discard sample required for accurate arterial blood gases, *Nurs Res* 38:276-279, 1989.

CR 12. Rickard CM, et al: A discard volume of twice the dead-space ensures clinically accurate arterial blood gases and electrolytes and prevents unnecessary blood loss, *Crit Care Med* 31:1654-1658, 2003.

CR 13. Rudisill PT, Moore LA: Relationship between arterial and venous activated partial thromboplastin time values in patients after percutaneous transluminal coronary angioplasty, *Heart Lung* 18:514-519, 1989.

CR 14. Silver MJ, et al: Evaluation of a new blood-conserving arterial line system for patients in intensive care units, *Crit Care Med* 21:507-511, 1993.

CR 15. Silver MJ, et al: Reduction of blood loss from diagnostic sampling in critically ill patients using a blood-conserving arterial line system, *Chest* 104:1711-1715, 1993.

Additional Readings

CR Alzetani A, Vohra HA, Patel RL: Can we rely on arterial line sampling in performing activated plasma thrombo-plastin time after cardiac surgery? *Eur J Anaesthesiol* 21:384-388, 2004.

CR Andrews T, Waterman H, Hillier V: Blood gas analysis: a study of blood loss in intensive care, *J Adv Nurs* 30: 851-857, 1999.

CR Cannon K, Mitchell KA, Fabian TC: Prospective randomized evaluation of two methods of drawing coagulation studies from heparinized arterial lines, *Heart Lung* 14:392-395, 1985.

CR Dirks JL: Innovations in technology: continuous intra-arterial blood gas monitoring, *Crit Care Nurs* 15:19-29, 1995.

CR Heap MJ, et al: Are coagulation studies on blood sampled from arterial lines valid? *Anaesthesia* 52: 640-645, 1997.

CR Hoste EAJ, et al: Significant increase of activated partial thromboplastin time by heparinization of the radial artery catheter flush solution with a closed arterial system, *Crit Care Med* 30:1030-1034, 2002.

CR Imperial-Perez F, McRae M: *Protocols for practice: hemody-namic monitoring series: arterial pressure monitoring,* Aliso Viejo, CA, 1998, American Association of Critical-Care Nurses.

CR Kaplow R: Comparison of two techniques for obtaining samples for coagulation studies: venipuncture and intraarte-rial, *Heart Lung* 17:651-653, 1988.

CR Kajs M: Comparison of coagulation values obtained by tradi-tional venipuncture and intra-arterial line methods, *Heart Lung* 15:622-627, 1986.

CR Martinez JA, et al: Clinical utility of blood cultures drawn from central venous or arterial catheters in critically ill surgical patients, *Crit Care Med* 30:7-13, 2002.

CR Reinhardt AC, et al: Minimum discard volume from arterial catheters to obtain coagulation studies free from heparin effect, *Heart Lung* 16:699-705, 1987.

CR Richiuso N: Accuracy of aPTT values drawn from heparinized arterial lines in children, *DCCN* 17:14-19, 1998.

CR Templin K, Shively M, Riley J: Accuracy of drawing coagula-tion samples from heparinized arterial lines, *Am J Crit Care* 2:88-95, 1993.

PROCEDURE 65

Blood Sampling from a Central Venous Catheter

PURPOSE: To obtain blood from the central venous catheter for laboratory analysis.

Teresa Preuss, Debra Lynn-McHale Wiegand

PREREQUISITE NURSING KNOWLEDGE

- Knowledge of anatomy and physiology of the cardiovascular system is needed.
- Understanding of principles of sterile and aseptic technique and infection control is necessary.
- The technique for specimen collection and labeling should be understood.
- Signs and symptoms of catheter-related infection and sepsis should be known.
- Infection has been identified as a potentially life-threatening complication of central venous catheterization, with an associated estimated mortality rate of 10% to 25% for each infection.[4,6,10,12]
- Knowledge of strategies to prevent catheter-related infections is essential.[7,8,11]
- Knowledge regarding the care of patients with central venous catheters (CVCs) is needed (see Procedure 82).
- Understanding of the principles of hemodynamic monitoring is necessary.
- The effect of heparin and hemolysis on various blood tests and appropriate discard volumes should be understood.
- Although blood can be withdrawn from CVCs, alternate routes of blood withdrawal (e.g., venipuncture, arterial catheters) should be considered first to minimize the risk of central venous catheter-related bloodstream infections.
- A needleless system should be used for capping and accessing CVC ports. Study results show that needleless systems not only reduce needle-stick injuries and the resultant risk for transmission of blood-borne infection to healthcare workers[8] but also may reduce central venous catheter-related bloodstream infections.[1,3]

EQUIPMENT

- Nonsterile gloves
- Goggles or fluid shield face mask
- Antiseptic solution (e.g., 2% chlorexidine-based solution)
- Needleless blood sampling access device
- Blood specimen tubes
- 10-mL syringe
- Sterile normal saline solution for injection
- Extra blood specimen tube for discard
- Laboratory form and patient identification specimen labels

Additional equipment to have available as needed includes the following:

- 4 × 4 gauze pad
- Needleless caps

PATIENT AND FAMILY EDUCATION

- Explain the purpose for blood sampling to the patient and family. ➤➤***Rationale:*** Teaching provides information and decreases anxiety and fear.
- Explain the patient's expected participation during the procedure. ➤➤***Rationale:*** This explanation increases patient cooperation and assistance.

PATIENT ASSESSMENT AND PREPARATION

Patient Assessment

- Assess the patency of the CVC. **➤Rationale:** This ensures a functional CVC catheter. If the CVC is clotted, blood sampling cannot be performed.
- Assess previous laboratory results. **➤Rationale:** These results provide baseline data andv data for comparison.
- Assess whether intravenous solutions or medications are infusing through the CVC. **➤Rationale:** Intravenous solutions and medication need to be stopped temporarily before blood sampling.

Patient Preparation

- Verify correct patient with two identifiers. **➤Rationale:** Prior to performing a procedure, the nurse should ensure the correct identification of the patient for the intended intervention.
- Ensure that the patient and family understand preprocedural teaching. Answer questions as they arise, and reinforce information as needed. **➤Rationale:** Understanding of previously taught information is evaluated and reinforced.
- Position the patient so that the blood sampling port is exposed. **➤Rationale:** This positioning improves the ease of obtaining the blood sample and minimizes the contamination of the stopcock.

Procedure	**for Blood Sampling from Central Venous Catheters**	
Steps	**Rationale**	**Special Considerations**

1. **HH**
2. **PE**

Blood Sampling from the CVC Hemodynamic Monitoring System

Steps	Rationale	Special Considerations
1. Cleanse the needleless cap at the top of the stopcock of the hemodynamic monitoring system with an antiseptic solution.[3,8] **(Level B*)**	Reduces the risk for infection.	Follow institution standard. Chlorhexidine and povidone-iodine solutions may be more effective than alcohol in reducing external microbial contamination.[3]
2. Attach the needleless blood sampling device to the capped stopcock of the CVC hemodynamic monitoring system (Fig. 65-1).	Prepares for blood sampling.	
3. Suspend the right atrial pressure/central venous pressure (RAP/CVP) monitoring alarm.	Prevents the alarm from sounding because the RAP/CVP waveform is lost during the blood sampling.	
4. Turn the stopcock off to the monitoring system and flush solution (Fig. 65-2).	The needleless blood sampling device is now in contact with the central venous blood.	
5. Insert a blood specimen tube into the blood sampling device to obtain the discard volume. **(Level B)**	Clears the catheter of flush solution. The discard volume includes the dead space (from the tip of the lumen to the top port of the needleless capped stopcock) and the blood diluted by the flush solution (e.g., 3.5 mL).[2,5,9]	Dead space information for a catheter is usually listed in the information that comes with the catheter.
6. Remove the discard blood specimen tube and discard in appropriate receptacle.	Removes discard safely.	
7. Insert the blood specimen tube into the blood sampling device to obtain the specimen.	Obtains the blood specimen.	
8. After obtaining the specimen, detach the blood sampling device from the capped stopcock and discard it in the appropriate receptacle.	Removes and safely discards equipment.	The blood in the needleless cap can be cleared by fast flushing the blood into a blood specimen tube or syringe (Fig 65-3).

---

*Level B: Well-designed controlled studies with results that consistently support a specific action, intervention, or treatment

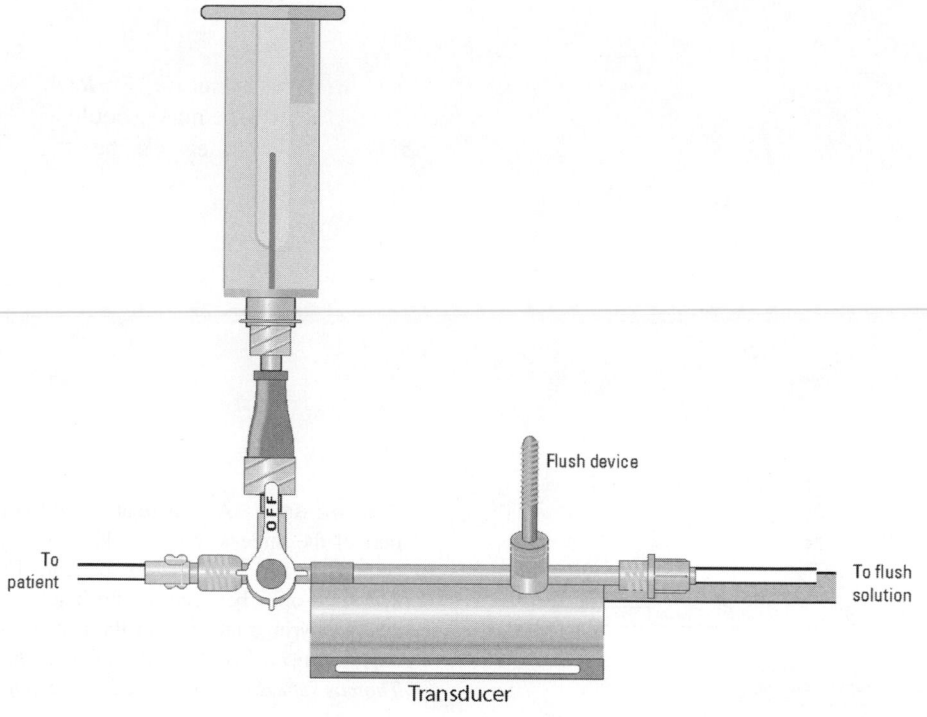

FIGURE 65-1 Needleless blood sampling device attached to the needleless capped stopcock of the hemodynamic monitoring system. The stopcock is open to the transducer system. *(Drawing by Paul W. Schiffmacher, Thomas Jefferson University, Philadelphia, PA.)*

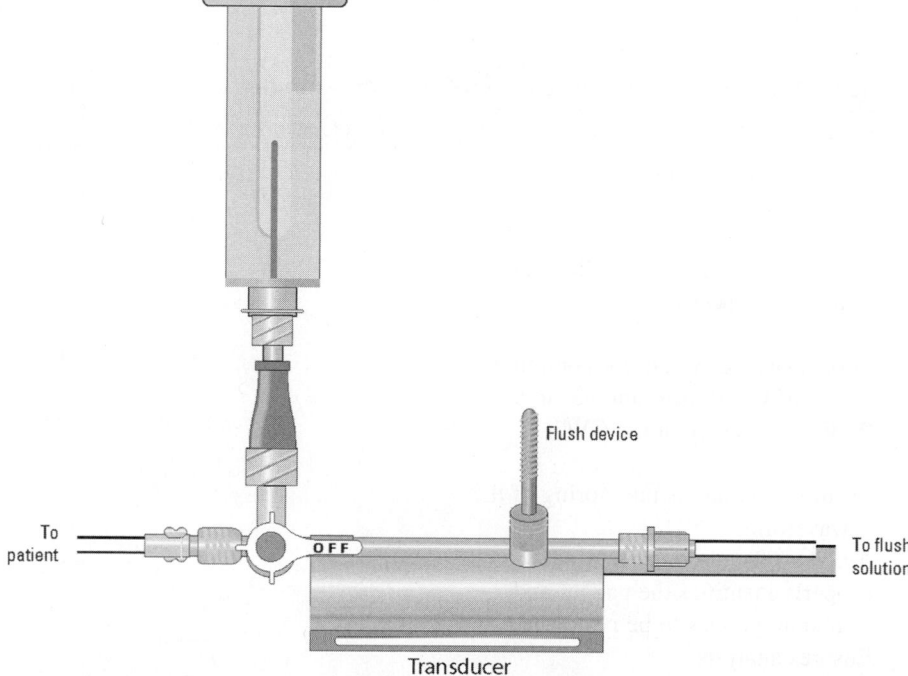

FIGURE 65-2 Needleless blood sampling device attached to the needleless capped stopcock of the hemodynamic monitoring system. The stopcock is turned "off" to the monitoring system and flush solution. *(Drawing by Paul W. Schiffmacher, Thomas Jefferson University, Philadelphia, PA.)*

Procedure for Blood Sampling from Central Venous Catheters—*Continued*

Steps	Rationale	Special Considerations
9. Cleanse the needleless cap at the top of the stopcock with an antiseptic solution.[3,8] **(Level B*)**	Reduces the risk for infection.	Follow institution standard. Chlorhexidine and povidone-iodine solutions may be more effective than alcohol in reducing external microbial contamination.[3]

*Level B: Well-designed controlled studies with results that consistently support a specific action, intervention, or treatment

Procedure continues on following page

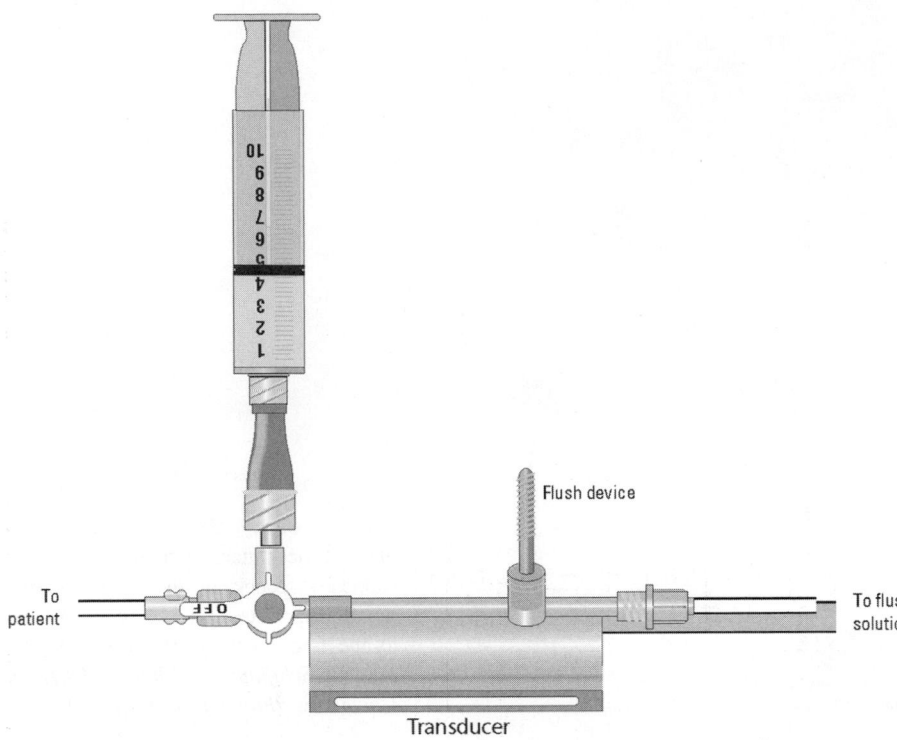

FIGURE 65-3 A syringe attached to the port of the three-way stopcock. The stopcock is turned "off" to the patient. The system is open between the flush solution and the syringe attached to the needleless cap. *(Drawing by Paul W. Schiffmacher, Thomas Jefferson University, Philadelphia, PA.)*

Procedure   for Blood Sampling from Central Venous Catheters—*Continued*

Steps	Rationale	Special Considerations
10. Attach a 10-mL syringe filled with sterile normal saline solution to the needleless capped stopcock.	Prepares flush solution.	
11. Gently flush the normal saline solution into the needleless cap (see Fig. 65-4).	Clears blood from the needleless cap and the stopcock.	
12. Turn the stopcock off to the blood sampling device.	This opens the system for continuous RAP/CVP pressure monitoring.	
13. Fast flush the remaining blood in the CVC back into the patient.	Promotes patency of the CVC.	
14. Observe the monitor for return of the RAP/CVP waveform.	Ensures continuous monitoring of the waveform.	
15. Turn the alarms back on.	Activates the alarm system.	
16. Label the specimen and laboratory form.	Properly identifies the patient and laboratory tests to be performed.	
17. Send the specimen for analysis.	Ensures analysis.	
18. Discard used supplies in appropriate receptacles.	Removes and safely discards used supplies.	
19. 🄷🄷		
Blood Sampling from a Single CVC Port That Is Not Monitored		
1. Stop intravenous solutions and medications before blood sampling.	Minimizes the risk of diluting the blood specimen, which may affect the accuracy of the laboratory results.	If the blood sample is obtained from a multiple-lumen catheter (e.g., triple lumen), stop intravenous and medication infusions from all of the CVC ports. Ensure that temporarily stopping intravenous medications does not affect hemodynamic stability.

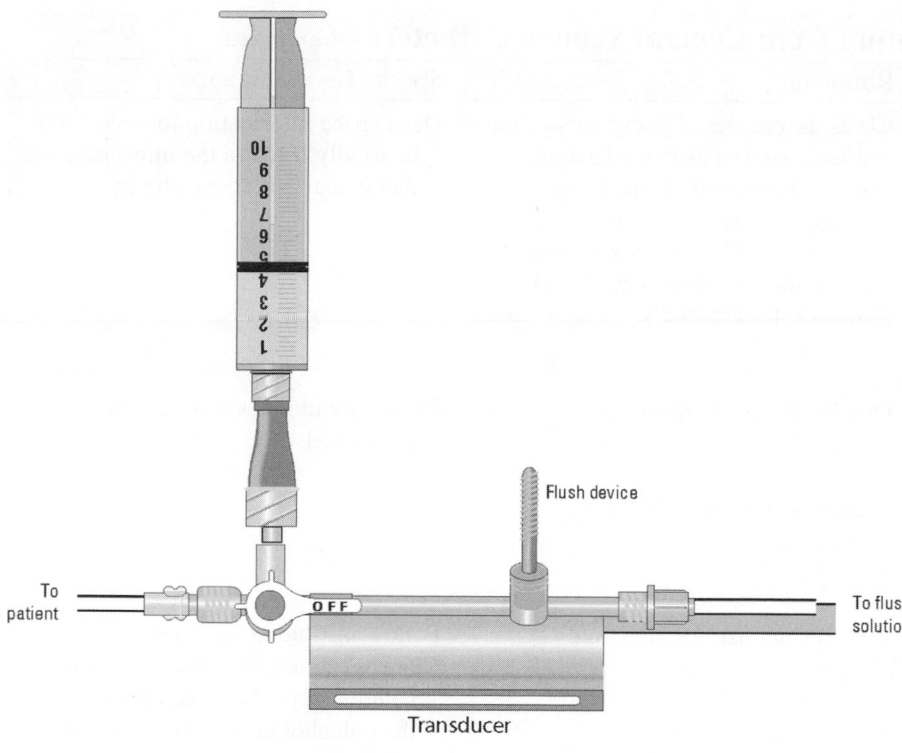

FIGURE 65-4 A syringe attached to the port of the three-way stopcock. The stopcock is turned "off" to the monitoring system and flush solution. The system is open between the patient and the syringe attached to the needless cap. (*Drawing by Paul W. Schiffmacher, Thomas Jefferson University, Philadelphia, PA.*)

Procedure	**for Blood Sampling from Central Venous Catheters**—*Continued*	
Steps	**Rationale**	**Special Considerations**
2. Remove and cap the intravenous solution infusing through the intended blood sampling port.	Prepares equipment and maintains asepsis of the intravenous system.	
3. Cleanse the needleless cap at the end of the CVC sampling port with an antiseptic solution.[3,8] **(Level B*)**	Reduces the risk for infection.	Follow institution standard. Chlorhexidine and povidone-iodine solutions may be more effective than alcohol in reducing external microbial contamination.[3] If the blood sample is being obtained from a multiple-lumen catheter, the blood sample should be obtained from the distal lumen.
4. Attach the needleless blood sampling device to the needleless cap of the CVC port (Fig. 65-5).	Prepares for blood sampling.	

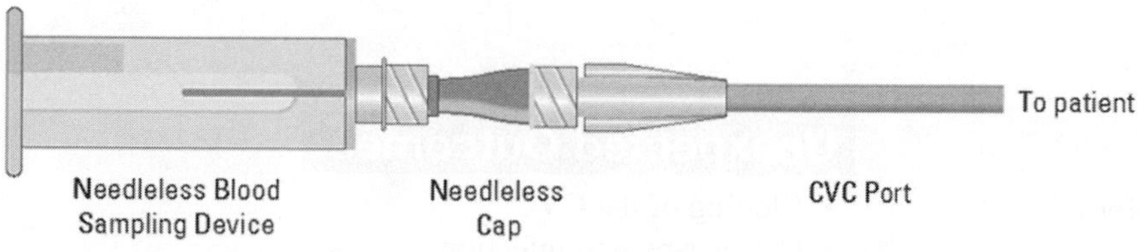

Needleless Blood Sampling Device   Needleless Cap   CVC Port   To patient

FIGURE 65-5 The needleless blood sampling device attached to the needleless cap of the CVC port. (*Drawing by Paul W. Schiffmacher, Thomas Jefferson University, Philadelphia, PA.*)

*Level B: Well-designed controlled studies with results that consistently support a specific action, intervention, or treatment

Procedure continues on following page

Procedure for Blood Sampling from Central Venous Catheters—*Continued*

Steps	Rationale	Special Considerations
5. Insert a blood specimen tube into the blood sampling device to obtain the discard volume.	Clears the catheter of flush solution. The discard volume includes the dead space (from the tip of the lumen through the needleless cap) and the blood diluted by the intravenous and medication solutions (e.g., 3.5 mL).[2,5,9]	Dead space information for a catheter is usually listed in the information that comes with the catheter.
6. Remove the discard blood specimen tube and discard in the appropriate receptacle.	Removes discard safely.	
7. Insert the blood specimen tube into the blood sampling device to obtain the specimen.	Obtains the blood specimen.	Obtain additional specimens as prescribed.
8. After obtaining the specimen, detach the blood sampling device from the capped stopcock and discard it in the appropriate receptacle.	Removes and safely discards equipment.	
9. Cleanse the needleless cap of the CVC port with an antiseptic solution.[3,8] (**Level B***)	Reduces the risk for infection.	Follow institution standard. Chlorhexidine and povidone-iodine solutions may be more effective than alcohol in reducing external microbial contamination.[3]
10. Attach a 10-mL syringe filled with sterile normal saline solution to the needleless cap of the CVC port.	Prepares flush solution.	
11. Gently flush the normal saline solution into the needleless cap.	Clears blood from the needleless cap and the CVC port.	
12. Remove the normal saline solution syringe and discard it in the appropriate receptacle.	Removes and safely discards equipment.	
13. Cleanse the needleless cap of the CVC port with an antiseptic solution. [3,8] (**Level B**)	Reduces the risk for infection.	Follow institution standard. Chlorhexidine and povidone-iodine solutions may be more effective than alcohol in reducing external microbial contamination.[3]
14. Reattach and resume the intravenous solution or medication infusion.	Continues treatment.	
15. Label the specimen and laboratory form.	Properly identifies the patient and laboratory tests to be performed.	
16. Send the specimen for analysis.	Ensures analysis.	
17. Discard used supplies in appropriate receptacles.	Removes and safely discards used supplies.	
18. 🅷🅷		

Expected Outcomes

- Catheter remains patent with good waveform if monitoring system is used
- Catheter site remains free from infection
- Adequate blood sample with minimal blood loss
- No hemolysis of the specimen

Unexpected Outcomes

- Clotting of the CVC
- Catheter-related infection
- Inability to obtain blood sample
- Hemolysis of specimens
- Dilution of specimens that causes inaccurate laboratory results

*Level B: Well-designed controlled studies with results that consistently support a specific action, intervention, or treatment

Patient Monitoring and Care

Steps	Rationale	Reportable Conditions
		These conditions should be reported if they persist despite nursing interventions.
1. Use the minimal volume of blood discard.	Helps prevent nosocomial anemia.	• Decreased hemoglobin level and hematocrit level
2. Monitor hemoglobin and hematocrit values if frequent blood sampling is needed.	Allows early detection of nosocomial anemia.	• Decreased hemoglobin level and hematocrit level
3. Attempt to obtain all blood samples at one time when possible.	Diminishes the number of times the system is entered to help minimize the risk of infection.	• Signs of catheter-related sepsis
4. Before and after the blood withdrawal, assess and evaluate the RAP/CVP waveform if monitored.	Ensures accurate RAP/CVP monitoring.	• Abnormal RAP/CVP values and trends
5. Obtain laboratory specimen results.	Assesses patient condition.	• Abnormal specimen results

Documentation

Documentation should include the following:
- Patient and family education
- Time and type of specimen drawn
- Results of laboratory tests when available
- Unexpected outcomes
- Inability to obtain sample

References

CR 1. Bouza E, et al: A needleless closed system device (CLAVE) protects from intravascular catheter tip and hub colonization: a prospective randomized study, *J Hosp Infection* 54:279-287, 2003.

CR 2. Carlson KK, et al: Obtaining reliable plasma sodium and glucose determinations from pulmonary artery catheters, *Heart Lung* 19:613-619, 1990.

CR 3. Casey AL, et al: A randomized, prospective clinical trial to assess the potential infection risk associated with the PosiFlow needleless connector, *J Hosp Infection* 54:288-293, 2003.

CR 4. Kluger DM, Maki DG: The relative risk of intravascular device related bloodstream infections in adults [abstract]. *In Abstracts of the 39th Interscience Conference on Antimicrobial Agents and Chemotherapy,* San Francisco, CA, 1999, American Society for Microbiology, 514.

CR 5. Krueger KE, et al: The reliability of laboratory data from blood samples collected through pulmonary artery catheters, *Arch Pathol Lab Med* 105:343-344, 1981.

CR 6. Maki DG: Pathogenesis, prevention and management of infections due to intravascular devices used for infusion therapy. In Bison AL, Waldvogel F, editors: *Infections associated with indwelling medical devices,* Washington, DC, 1989, American Society for Microbiology, 161-177.

CR 7. Mermel LA: Prevention of central venous catheter-related infections: what works other than impregnated or coated catheters? *J Hosp Infection* 65(Supp 2):30-33, 2007.

CR 8. O'Grady NP, et al: Guidelines for the prevention of intravascular catheter-related infections, *Am J Infect Control* 30:476-489, 2002.

CR 9. Palermo LM, Andrews RW, Ellison N: Avoidance of heparin contamination in coagulation studies drawn from indwelling lines, *Anesth Analg* 59:222-224, 1980.

CR 10. Pittet D, Tarara D, Wenzel RP: Noscomial bloodstream infection in critically ill patients: excess length of stay, extra costs and attributable mortality, *JAMA* 271:1598-1601, 1994.

CR 11. Safdar N, Kluger DM, Maki DG: A review of risk factors for catheter-related bloodstream infection caused by percutaneously inserted, noncuffed central venous catheters, *Medicine* 81:466-479, 2002.

CR 12. Smith RL, Meixler SM, Simberkoff MS: Excess mortality in critically ill patients with nosocomial bloodstream infections, *Chest* 100:164-167, 1991.

Additional Readings

CR Beutz M, et al: Clinical utility of blood cultures drawn from central vein catheters and peripheral venipuncture in critically ill medical patients, *Chest* 123:854-861, 2003.

Maki DG, et al: The risk of bloodstream infection in adults with different intravascular devices: a systematic review of 200 published prospective studies, *Mayo Clin Proc* 81:1159-1171, 2006.

Shapey IM, et al: Central venous catheter-related bloodstream infections: improving post-insertion catheter care, *J Hosp Infection* 71:117-122, 2009.

Blood Sampling from a Pulmonary Artery Catheter

P U R P O S E :   Blood is removed from the pulmonary artery catheter for determination of mixed venous oxygen saturation.

Teresa Preuss, Debra Lynn-McHale Wiegand

PREREQUISITE NURSING KNOWLEDGE

- Knowledge of sterile technique is needed.
- Knowledge of cardiovascular and pulmonary anatomy and physiology is necessary.
- Gas exchange and acid-base balance should be understood.
- Technique for specimen collection and labeling should be known.
- Principles of hemodynamic monitoring need to be understood.
- Knowledge about the care of patients with pulmonary artery catheters (see Procedure 73) and stopcock manipulation (see Procedure 76) is needed.
- The most frequent blood specimen obtained from the pulmonary artery is one for mixed venous oxygen saturation (Svo_2) analysis.
- Svo_2 measures the oxygen saturation of the venous blood in the pulmonary artery (see Procedure 16).
- Svo_2 samples are obtained to calibrate the equipment when continuously monitoring Svo_2 values.
- Routine blood sampling from the pulmonary artery catheter is not recommended because entry into the sterile system may increase the incidence of catheter-related infection.

EQUIPMENT

- Nonsterile gloves
- Goggles or fluid shield face mask
- Antiseptic solution
- Needleless blood sampling access device

- Two 10-mL syringes
- Blood specimen tubes
- Blood gas sampling syringe
- Needleless cap or nonvented cap
- Laboratory form and specimen label
  Additional equipment to have available as needed includes the following:
- Bag of ice
- Sterile 4 × 4 gauze pad

PATIENT AND FAMILY EDUCATION

- Explain the purpose for blood sampling. **➡*Rationale:*** Teaching provides information and may reduce anxiety and fear.
- Explain the patient's expected participation during the procedure. **➡*Rationale:*** This explanation encourages patient assistance.

PATIENT ASSESSMENT AND PREPARATION

Patient Assessment

- Assess the patient's cardiopulmonary and hemodynamic status, including abnormal lung sounds, respiratory distress, dysrhythmias, decreased mentation, agitation, and skin color changes. **➡*Rationale:*** These signs and symptoms could necessitate blood sampling for venous oxygenation.
- Assess for a decrease in cardiac output related to changes in preload, afterload, or contractility. **➡*Rationale:*** Mixed venous blood samples are used to evaluate changes in cardiopulmonary function.

Patient Preparation

- Verify correct patient with two identifiers. ➤➤*Rationale:* Prior to performing a procedure, the nurse should ensure the correct identification of the patient for the intended intervention.
- Ensure that the patient understands preprocedural teaching. Answer questions as they arise, and reinforce information as needed. ➤➤*Rationale:* Understanding of previously taught information is evaluated and reinforced.
- Position the patient so that the stopcock for blood sampling is exposed. ➤➤*Rationale:* This positioning improves the ease of obtaining the blood sample and minimizes the contamination of the stopcock.

Procedure	**for Blood Sampling from a Pulmonary Artery Catheter**	
Steps	**Rationale**	**Special Considerations**
1. ▣ HH		
2. ▣ PE		
3. When drawing a mixed venous oxygen (Svo₂) sample, open the arterial blood gas (ABG) kit and expel the excess air and heparin from the syringe.	Prepares the ABG syringe.	Heparin is usually in powdered form.
4. Temporarily suspend the pulmonary artery (PA) alarms.	Prevents the alarm from sounding because the PA waveform is lost during the blood draw.	
5. PA distal stopcock: A. Remove the nonvented cap from the stopcock of the distal lumen of the PA catheter. *or*	Prepares the line for blood sampling.	
B. Cleanse the needleless cap at the top of the stopcock of the distal lumen of the PA catheter with an antiseptic solution.[2,4] **(Level B*)**	Prepares the line for blood sampling and reduces the risk for infection.	Follow institution standard. Chlorhexidine and povidone-iodine solutions may be more effective than alcohol in reducing external microbial contamination.[2]
6. Place a sterile syringe or a needleless blood sampling access device into the top port of the stopcock of the distal lumen of the PA catheter (see Figs. 65-1 and 66-1).	Prepares for blood sampling.	
7. Turn the stopcock off to the flush solution. (see Figs. 65-2 and 66-2).	The syringe or needleless blood sampling access device is then in direct contact with the blood in the PA.	
8. With a syringe, slowly and gently aspirate the discard volume or, if using a needleless blood sampling access device, engage the blood specimen tube to obtain the discard volume. **(Level B)**	Clears the catheter of flush solution. The discard volume includes the dead space (from the tip of the distal lumen to the top port of the stopcock) and the blood diluted by the flush solution (e.g., 3.5 mL).[1,3,5]	If additional laboratory studies are needed, larger discard volumes may be necessary for accurate results.[1,5]
9. Turn the stopcock off to the syringe or the needleless blood sampling access device (see Figs. 65-1 and 66-1).	Stops blood flow and closes the top port of the stopcock.	
10. Remove the syringe or the blood specimen tube and discard in the appropriate receptacle.	Removes and safely disposes of the discard.	

*Level B: Well-designed, controlled studies with results that consistently support a specific action, intervention, or treatment

Procedure continues on following page

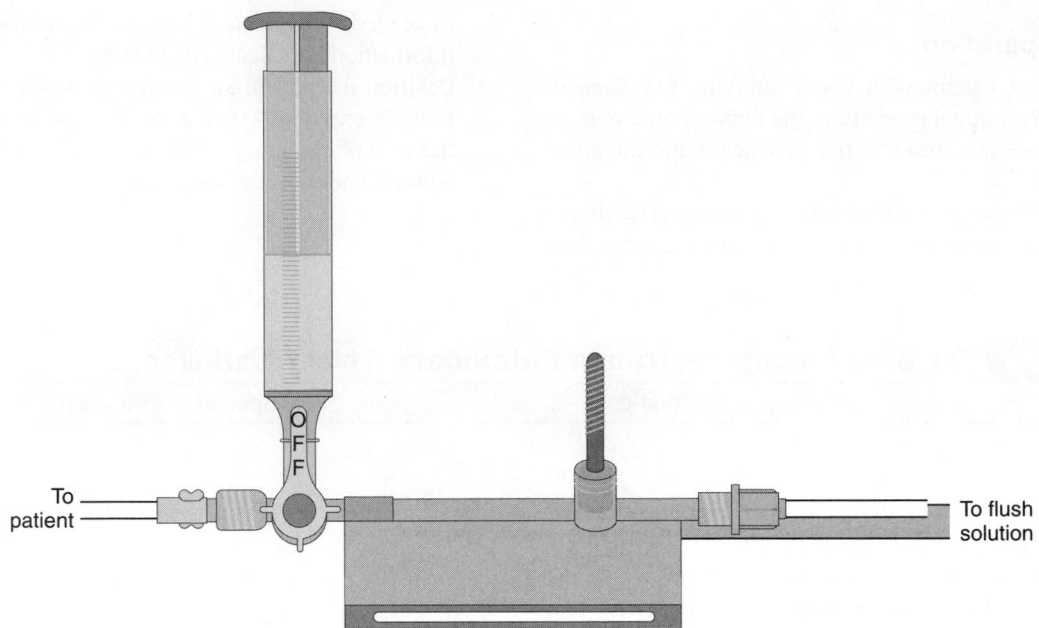

FIGURE 66-1   A syringe attached to the port of the three-way stopcock. The stopcock is turned "off" to the port of the stopcock. *(Drawing by Paul W. Schiffmacher, Thomas Jefferson University, Philadelphia, PA.)*

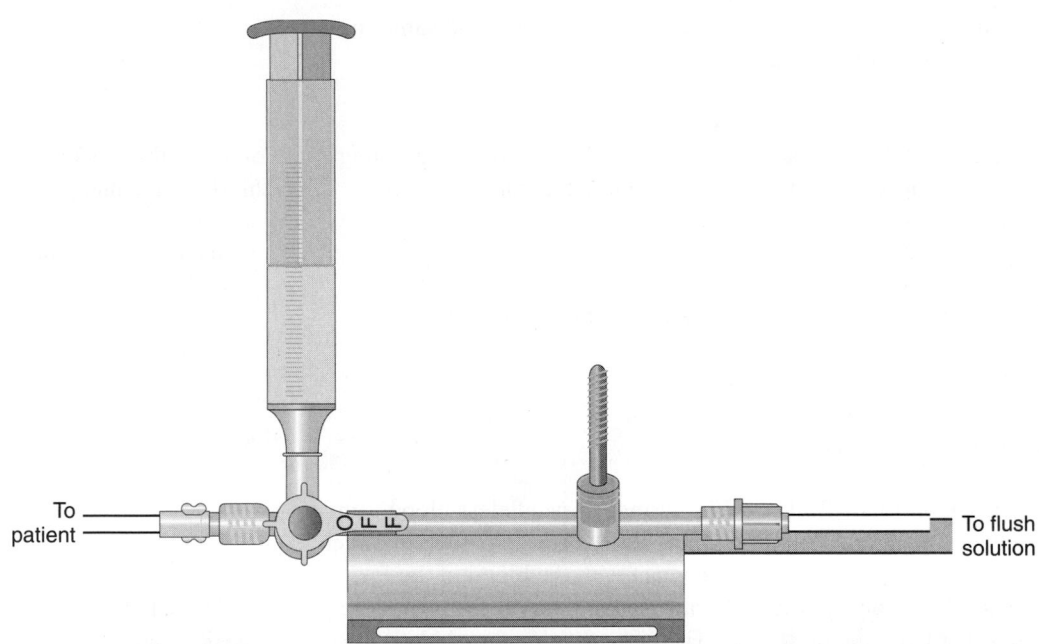

FIGURE 66-2   A syringe attached to the port of the three-way stopcock. The stopcock is turned "off" to flush solution. *(Drawing by Paul W. Schiffmacher, Thomas Jefferson University, Philadelphia, PA.)*

Procedure	**for Blood Sampling from a Pulmonary Artery Catheter—***Continued*	
Steps	**Rationale**	**Special Considerations**
11. Insert an ABG syringe into the stopcock or insert the ABG syringe into the needleless blood sampling access device.	Prepares for removal of a blood sample.	
12. Turn the stopcock off to the flush system (see Figs. 65-2 and 66-2).	Prepares for blood sampling.	

Procedure for Blood Sampling from a Pulmonary Artery Catheter—*Continued*

Steps	Rationale	Special Considerations
13. Slowly aspirate the Svo₂ sample (e.g., 1 mL).	Slow aspiration is important to prevent contamination of the mixed venous sample with arterial blood from the pulmonary capillaries, which will falsely elevate the Svo₂ value.	
14. Turn the stopcock off to the syringe or the needleless blood sampling access device (see Figs. 65-1 and 66-1).	Prevents bleeding.	
15. Remove the ABG syringe.	Detaches the specimen.	
16. Expel any air bubbles from the ABG syringe and cap the syringe.	Ensures the accuracy of the Svo₂ results.	
17. Turn the stopcock off to the patient.	Prepares the system.	
18. Fast flush the remaining blood from the top port of the stopcock onto a sterile gauze pad (after removing the needleless or nonvented cap), into a discard syringe, or into a blood specimen tube.	Clears blood from the system.	
19. Turn the stopcock off to the top port of the stopcock (see Figs. 65-1 and 66-1).	Opens the system up for continuous PA pressure monitoring.	Remove the needleless blood sampling access device if used.
20. Attach a new sterile nonvented cap or a needleless cap to the top port of the stopcock.	Maintains a closed sterile system.	
21. Flush the remaining blood in the PA catheter back into the patient.	Promotes patency of the PA catheter.	
22. Turn the alarms back on.	Activates the alarm system.	
23. Observe the monitor for return of the PA waveform.	Ensures continuous monitoring of the PA waveform.	
24. Label the specimen and laboratory form.	Properly identifies the patient and laboratory tests to be performed.	Label the blood-gas laboratory slip as a mixed venous sample.
25. Send the specimen for analysis.	Needed for ABG analysis.	Follow institution policy regarding use of ice for ABG samples.
26. Discard used supplies in appropriate receptacle.	Removes and safely discards used supplies.	
27. 🄷🄷		

Expected Outcomes

- Adequate blood sample with minimal blood loss
- PA catheter patency maintained
- Svo₂ value and trends within normal range (60% to 80%)

Unexpected Outcomes

- Inability to obtain Svo₂ sample
- Clotting of the PA catheter
- Arterial sample obtained as a result of rapid withdrawal of blood from the pulmonary capillaries instead of mixed venous oxygen sample for blood-gas analysis

Procedure continues on following page

Patient Monitoring and Care

Steps	Rationale	Reportable Conditions
		These conditions should be reported if they persist despite nursing interventions. Abnormal PA waveforms or values
1. Before and after the blood withdrawal, assess and evaluate the PA waveform.	Ensures that the PA catheter is properly positioned.	
2. Correlate the Svo_2 results with the measured cardiac output.	Changes in the Svo_2 indicate changes in cardiac output and hemodynamic status.	• Abnormal mixed venous oxygen saturation, preload, afterload, cardiac output, and cardiac index
3. Correlate the Svo_2 results with the clinical assessment data.	Svo_2 decreases with: • increased oxygen consumption • decreased oxygen delivery Svo_2 increases with: • decreased tissue oxygen consumption • increased oxygen delivery	• Fever • Shivering • Seizures • Agitation • Pain • Decreased cardiac output • Decreased hemoglobin • Decreased arterial oxygen saturation • Hypothermia • Late sepsis • Increased cardiac output

Documentation

Documentation should include the following:
- Patient and family education
- Time and date of the Svo_2 sample
- Svo_2 results

- Any difficulties with PA catheter blood sampling
- Nursing interventions performed
- Unexpected outcomes

References

CR 1. Carlson KK, et al: Obtaining reliable plasma sodium and glucose determinations from pulmonary artery catheters, *Heart Lung* 19:613-619, 1990.

CR 2. Casey AL, et al: A randomized, prospective clinical trial to assess the potential infection risk associated with the PosiFlow needleless connector, *J Hosp Infection* 54:288-293, 2003.

CR 3. Krueger KE, et al: The reliability of laboratory data from blood samples collected through pulmonary artery catheters, *Arch Pathol Lab Med* 105:343-344, 1981.

CR 4. O'Grady NP, et al: Guidelines for the prevention of intravascular catheter-related infections, *Am J Infect Control* 30(8):476-489, 2002.

CR 5. Palermo LM, Andrews RW, Ellison N: Avoidance of heparin contamination in coagulation studies drawn from indwelling lines, *Anesth Analg* 59:222-224, 1980.

Additional Readings

CR Darovic GO: *Hemodynamic monitoring: invasive and noninvasive clinical application,* ed 3, Philadelphia, 2002, Saunders.

CR Goodrich C: Continous central venous oximetry monitoring, *Crit Care Nurs North Am* 18:203-209, 2006.

Cardiac Output Measurement Techniques (Invasive)

P U R P O S E : Cardiac output measurements are performed for assessment and monitoring of cardiovascular status. Cardiac output measurements are used in evaluation of patient responses to clinical interventions, mechanical assist devices, and vasoactive and inotropic medications. When a pulmonary artery catheter is in place, cardiac output measurements provide useful initial and trend data that may improve care for critically ill patients with hemodynamic instability.

Deborah G. Klein

PREREQUISITE NURSING KNOWLEDGE

- Understanding of normal anatomy and physiology of the cardiovascular system and pulmonary system is necessary.
- Understanding of basic dysrhythmia recognition and treatment of life-threatening dysrhythmias is needed.
- Pathophysiologic changes associated with structural heart disease (e.g., ventricular dysfunction from myocardial infarction, diastolic or systolic changes and valve dysfunction) should be understood.
- Understanding of the principles of aseptic technique is necessary.
- Understanding of the pulmonary artery (PA) catheter (see Fig. 73-1), lumens and ports, and the location of the PA catheter in the heart and PA (see Fig. 73-2) is needed.
- Multiple pressure transducer systems (see Procedure 76) should be understood.
- Competence in the use and clinical application of hemodynamic waveforms and values obtained with a PA catheter is necessary. Hemodynamic waveform interpretation of right atrial pressure (RAP) or central venous pressure (CVP), pulmonary artery pressure (PAP), and pulmonary artery occlusion pressure (PAOP) or pulmonary artery wedge pressure (PAWP) provides confirmation of proper catheter placement.

- Knowledge of vasoactive and inotropic medications and their effects on cardiac function, ventricular function, coronary vessels, and vascular smooth muscles is needed.
- Cardiac output (CO) is defined as the amount of blood ejected by the left ventricle per minute and is the product of stroke volume (SV) and heart rate (HR). It is measured in liters per minute.

$$CO = SV \times HR$$

- Normal CO is 4 to 8 L/min. The four physiologic factors that affect CO are preload, afterload, contractility, and heart rate.
- Stroke volume is the amount of blood volume ejected from either ventricle during one beat. Left ventricular stroke volume is the difference between left ventricular end-diastolic volume and left ventricular end-systolic volume. Left ventricular stroke volume is normally 60 to 100 mL/beat. Major factors that influence stroke volume are preload, afterload, and contractility.
- Right heart preload refers to the amount of blood in the right ventricle (RV) at the end of diastole and is measured by the RAP or CVP. Elevations in left heart filling pressures may be accompanied by parallel changes in RAP, especially in patients with left systolic ventricular dysfunction. Other factors that affect RAP are venous return, intravascular volume, vascular capacity, and pulmonary pressure. Right heart preload is increased in right

heart failure, right ventricular infarction, pericardial tamponade, tension pneumothorax, tricuspid regurgitation, and fluid overload. Right heart preload is decreased in hypovolemic states.

- Left heart preload refers to the amount of blood in the left ventricle (LV) at the end of diastole and is measured by the PAOP or PAWP. When LV preload or end-diastolic volume increases, the muscle fibers are stretched. The increased tension or force of contraction that accompanies an increase in diastolic filling is called the Frank-Starling law. The Frank-Starling law allows the heart to adjust its pumping ability to accommodate various levels of venous return. Note: In patients with advanced chronic LV dysfunction and remodeled hearts (spherical or globular-shaped LV instead of the normal elliptical-shaped LV), the Frank-Starling law does not apply. In these patients, muscle fibers of the heart are already maximally lengthened; as a result, the heart cannot respond significantly to increased filling or stretch with increased force of contraction.

- Afterload refers to the force the ventricular myocardial fibers must overcome to shorten or contract. It is the force that resists contraction. The amount of force the LV must overcome influences the amount of blood ejected into the systemic circulation. Afterload is influenced by peripheral vascular resistance (the force opposing blood flow within the vessels), systolic blood pressure, systolic stress, and systolic impedance. Peripheral resistance is affected by the length and radius of the blood vessel, arterial blood pressure, and venous constriction or dilation. The systolic force

of the heart is increased in conditions that cause vasoconstriction (increased afterload), including aortic stenosis, hypertension, or hyperviscosity of blood (e.g., polycythemia). The systolic force of the heart is decreased in conditions that cause vasodilation or decrease the viscosity of blood (e.g., anemia). Right ventricular afterload is measured as pulmonary vascular resistance. Left ventricular afterload is measured as systemic vascular resistance.

- Contractility is defined as the ability of the myocardium to contract and eject blood into the pulmonary or systemic vasculature. Contractility is increased by sympathetic neural stimulation, the release of calcium, and norepinephrine and decreased by parasympathetic neural stimulation, acidosis, and hyperkalemia. Contractility and HR can be influenced by neural, humoral, and pharmacologic factors.

- In addition to stroke volume, CO is affected by heart rate. Normally, nerves of the parasympathetic and sympathetic nervous system regulate heart rate through specialized cardiac electrical cells. Heart rate and rhythm are influenced by neural, humoral, and pharmacologic factors. Decreased HR can be the result of increased parasympathetic neural stimulation, decreased sympathetic neural stimulation, or decreased body temperature. Increased HR can be triggered by exercise, catecholamine release, or hypotension. At HRs greater than 180 beats/min, there may be inadequate time for diastolic filling, resulting in decreased CO. Because multiple factors regulate cardiac performance and impact CO, these factors must be assessed (Fig. 67-1).

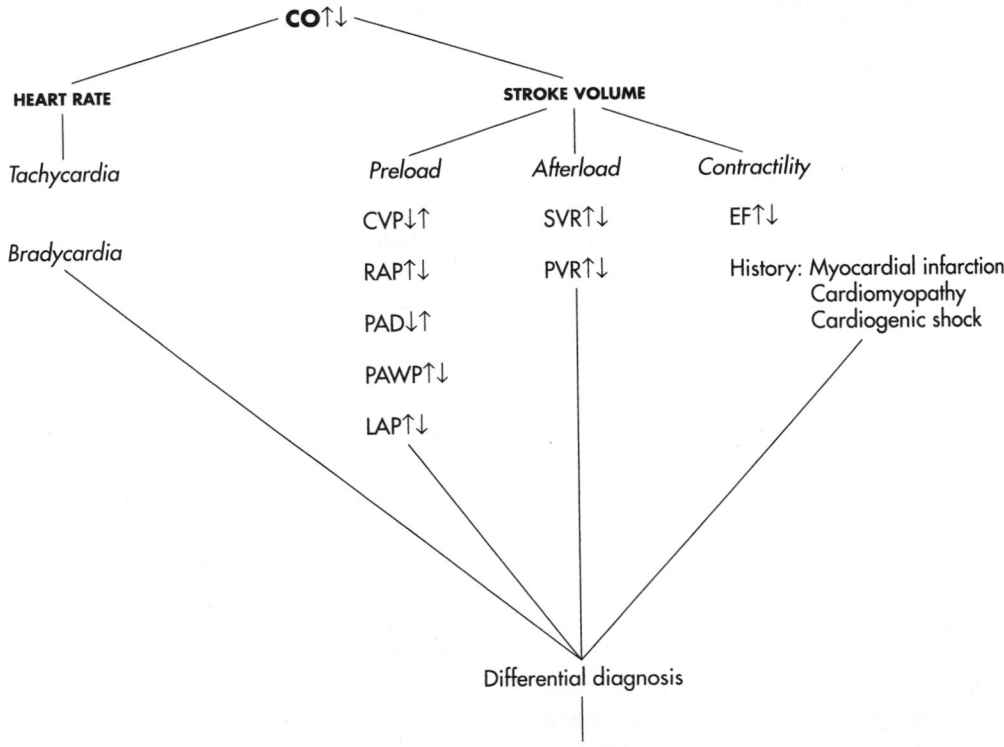

FIGURE 67-1   Systematic assessment of the determinants of cardiac output may assist the clinician in defining the etiologic factors of cardiac output alteration more precisely. *(From Whalen DA, Keller R: Cardiovascular patient assessment. In Kinney MR, et al, editors: AACN clinical reference for critical care nurse, ed 4, St Louis, 1998, Mosby, 227-319.)*

- Cardiac index adjusts the CO to an individual's body size (square meter of body surface area). It is a more precise measurement of cardiac performance than CO.
- Refer to Table 67-1 for normal hemodynamic values and calculations.
- At the bedside, cardiac output measurements are obtained through a PA catheter via the intermittent bolus thermodilution CO method (TDCO) or the continuous CO (CCO) method.
- The TDCO method proceeds as follows:
  - ❖ An injectate (5% dextrose in water) of a known volume (10 mL) and temperature (room or cold temperature) is injected into the right atrium (RA) through the proximal port of the PA catheter. This injectate exits in the RA, where it mixes with blood and flows through the right ventricle to the PA. A thermistor located at the tip of the PA catheter senses the change in blood temperature as the blood passes

the tip of the catheter in the PA. The CO is calculated as the difference in temperatures on a time versus temperature curve.
- CO can be calculated from PA catheters with two types of thermistors:
  - ❖ A single thermistor has one inline temperature sensor near the tip of the catheter that lies in the PA when in proper position.
  - ❖ A dual thermistor has two inline temperature sensors, one in the right atrium/superior caval vein (immediately above the injectate port opening) and one near the tip of the catheter (same position as single thermistor). Because a temperature sensor is located in the right atrium, there is no need to enter a "correction factor" or "computation constant" into the computer to account for the loss in thermal indicator (heat) from the hub of the RA injectate port to the RA. Investigators found that the second thermistor improved accuracy when compared with Fick CO measurements and also improved precision or

TABLE 67-1 Hemodynamic Parameters

Parameters	Calculations	Normal Value
Body surface area (BSA)	*Weight (kg) × height (cm) × 0.007184*	*Varies with size (range = 0.58 to 2.9 m²)*
CO	HR × SV	4-8 L/min
Stroke volume (SV)	CO × 1000 ÷ HR	60-100 mL/beat
Stroke volume index (SVI)	SV ÷ BSA	30-65 mL/beat/m²
Cardiac index (CI)	CO ÷ BSA	2.5-4.5 L/min/m²
Heart rate (HR)		60-100 beats/min
Preload		
Central venous pressure (CVP) or RAP		2-6 mm Hg
Left atrial pressure (LAP)		4-12 mm Hg
Pulmonary artery diastolic pressure (PADP)		5-15 mm Hg
PAOP		4-12 mm Hg
RVEDP		0-8 mm Hg
LVEDP		4-10 mm Hg
Afterload		
Systemic vascular resistance (SVR)	MAP − CVP/RAP × 80 ÷ CO	900-1400 dynes/s/cm⁻⁵
SVR index (SVRI)	MAP − CVP/RAP × 80 ÷ CI	2000-2400 dynes/s/cm⁻⁵/m²
Pulmonary vascular resistance (PVR)	PAMP − PAOP × 80 ÷ CO	100-250 dynes/s/cm⁻⁵
PVR index (PVRI)	PAMP − PAOP × 80 ÷ CI	255-315 dynes/s/cm⁻⁵/m²
Systolic blood pressure		100-130 mm Hg
Contractility		
Ejection fraction (EF):		
Left	LVEDV × 100 ÷ SV	60%-75%
Right	RVEDV × 100 ÷ SV	45%-50%
Stroke work index:		
Left	SVI (MAP − PAOP) × 0.0136	50-62 g-m/m²/beat
Right	SVI (MAP − CVP) × 0.0136	5-10 g-m/m²/beat
Pressures:		
MAP	DBP + ⅓ (SBP − DBP)	70-105 mm Hg
PAMP	PADP + ⅓ (PASP − PADP)	9-16 mm Hg

DBP, Diastolic blood pressure; *MAP,* mean arterial pressure; *LVEDP,* left ventricular end-diastolic pressure; *RVEDP,* right ventricular end-diastolic pressure; *PAMP,* pulmonary artery mean pressure; *PAOP,* pulmonary artery occlusion pressure; *LVEDV,* left ventricular end-diastolic volume; *RVEDV,* right ventricular end-diastolic volume; *PASP,* pulmonary artery systolic pressure; *PADP,* pulmonary artery diastolic pressure; *SBP,* systolic blood pressure.
Adapted from Tuggle D: Optimizing hemodynamics: strategies for fluid and medication titration in shock. In Carlson K, editor: AACN advanced critical care nursing, St Louis, 2009, Saunders, 1106; and Ahrens T: Hemodynamic monitoring, Crit Care Nurs Clin N Am 11:19-31, 1999.

repeatability of CO measurements in both cold and room temperature.[4,24] In one study, cold injectate had excellent precision with the standard single-thermistor PA catheter. Researchers concluded that the dual-thermistor PA catheter provided the greatest benefit in decreasing measurement variability when room temperature injections were used to measure CO.[4]

- The change in temperature over time is plotted as a curve and displayed on the bedside monitor screen. CO is mathematically calculated from the area under the curve and is displayed digitally and graphically on the monitor screen (Fig. 67-2). The area under the curve is inversely proportional to the rate of blood flow. Thus, a high CO is associated with a small area under the curve, whereas a low CO is associated with a large area under the curve (Fig. 67-3, *A*).

- The thermistor near the distal tip of the catheter detects the temperature change and sends a signal to the CO computer and bedside monitor. The computer calculates the CO with the modified Stewart Hamilton equation, and the CO number is displayed on the monitor screen. The average result of three to five measurements is used to determine CO.

- Accuracy of TDCO is dependent on adequate mixing of blood and injectate, forward blood flow, steady baseline temperature in the PA, and appropriate procedural technique.[3,16,19] In addition, loss of thermal indicator (heat), respiratory artifact, and hemodynamic instability can cause variability from one injection to another.[19,29]

- Commercially available closed system delivery sets (CO-Set, Edwards Lifesciences, LLC, Irvine, CA) can be used with both cold and room temperature injectate (Figs. 67-4 and 67-5).

- The CCO method proceeds as follows:
  ❖ CO can be obtained with a heat-exchange CO catheter. This catheter has a membrane that allows for heat to exchange with blood in the right atrium. Continuous measurement of CO can be performed without the need for injected fluid.
  ❖ The PA catheter with CCO capability contains a 10-cm thermal filament located close to the injection port (15 to 25 cm from the tip of the catheter, near the proximal lumen port). When a PA catheter is properly placed, the thermal filament section of the catheter is located in the right ventricle. This filament emits a pulsed low heat energy signal in a

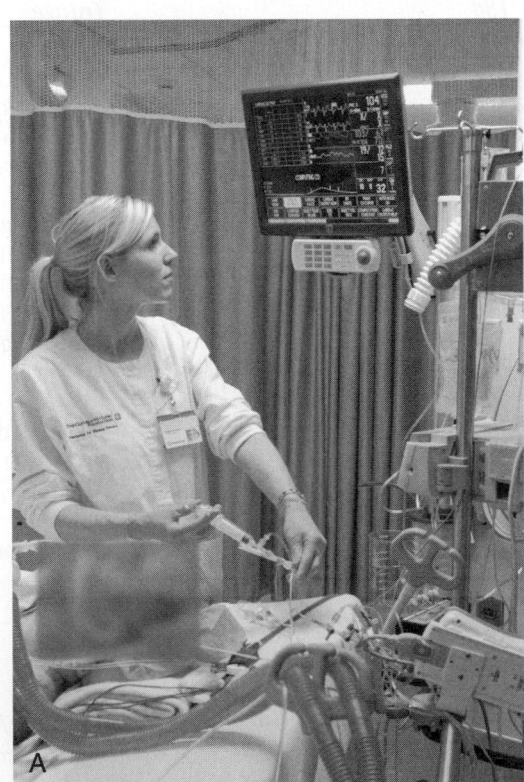

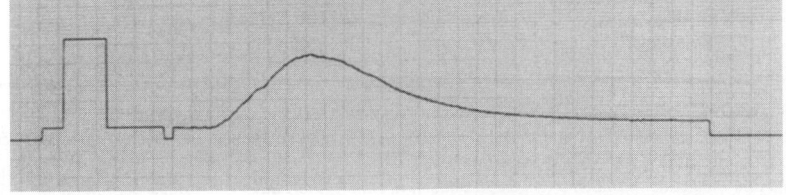

FIGURE 67-2 **A,** Examining cardiac output curves to establish reliability of values. **B,** Normal cardiac output curve with rapid upstroke and smooth progressive decrease in temperature sensing. *(B: From Ahrens T: Hemodynamic monitoring, Crit Care Nurs Clin North Am 11[1]:28, 1999.)*

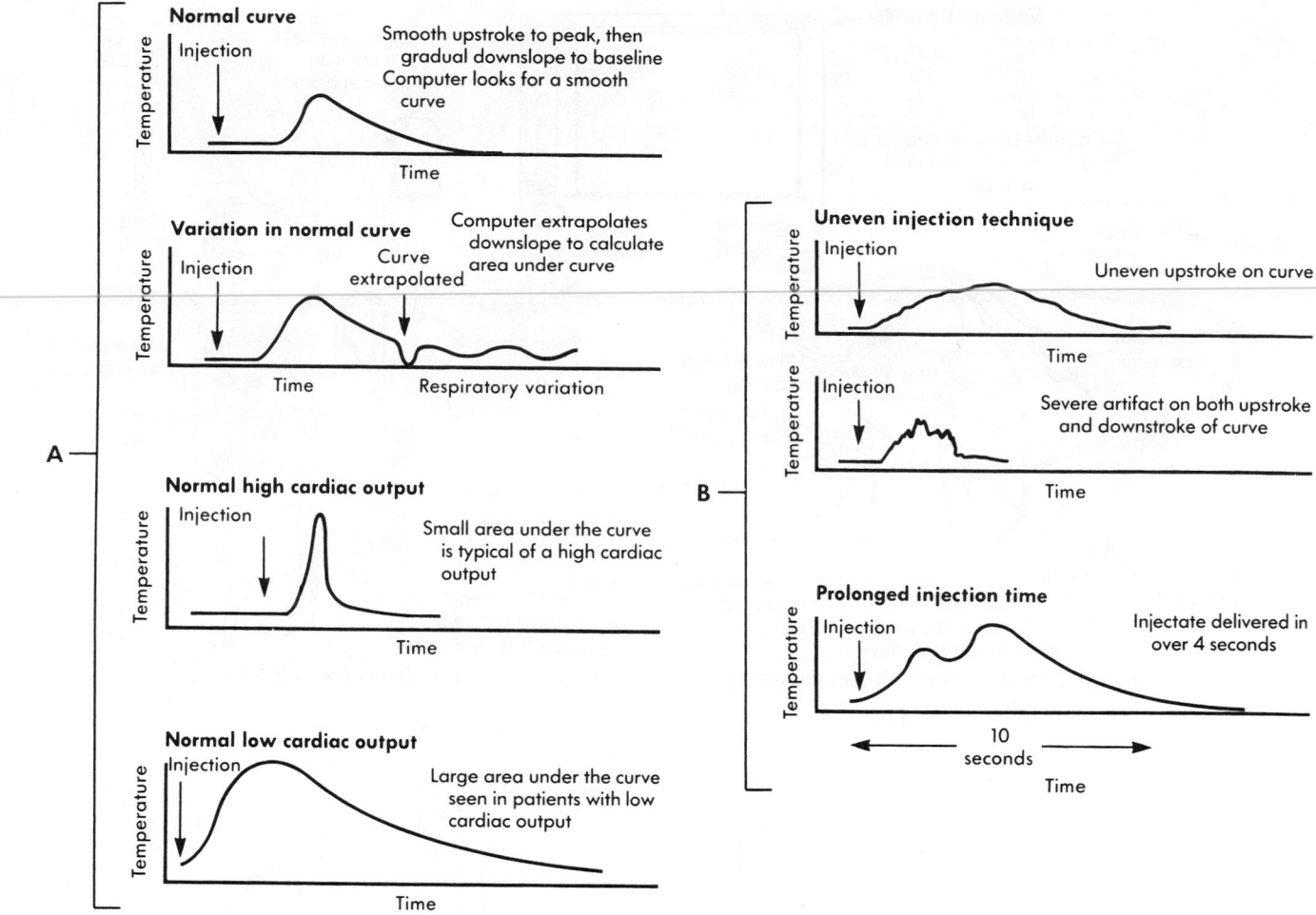

FIGURE 67-3 **A,** Variations in the normal cardiac output curve seen in certain clinical conditions. **B,** Abnormal cardiac output curves that produce an erroneous cardiac output value. *(From Urden LD, Stacy KM, Lough ME: Critical care nursing: diagnosis and management, ed 6, St Louis, 2010, Mosby.)*

30- to 60-second pseudorandom binary (on/off) sequence,[2] which allows blood to be heated and the heat signal adequately processed over time as blood passes through the ventricle. A bedside computer constructs thermodilution curves detected from the pseudorandom heat impulses and measures CO automatically. The computer screen displays digital readings updated every 30 to 60 seconds, reflecting the average CO of the preceding 3 to 6 minutes. The CCO eliminates the need for fluid boluses, reduces contamination risk, and provides a continuous CO trend.[1,2,29]

❖ Because the CCO computer constantly displays and frequently updates the CO, treatment decisions can be expedited. Derived hemodynamic calculations (e.g., cardiac index and systemic vascular resistance) can be obtained with greater frequency, thereby providing up-to-time information in assessment of response to therapies that affect hemodynamics.[1]

• CCO has been compared with TDCO, transesophageal Doppler scan technique, and aortic transpulmonary technique to determine its precision. Study results all show small bias, limits of agreement, and 95% confidence limits, reflecting that CCO provides accurate measurement of CO and is a reliable method.[1,2,6,21,29,36,48]

• Adequate mixing of blood and indicator (heat) is necessary for accurate CCO measurements. Conditions that prevent appropriate mixing or directional flow of the indicator or blood include intracardiac shunts or tricuspid regurgitation.

• The CCO method is based on the same physiologic principle as the TDCO method (indicator-dilution technique). The TDCO method uses a bolus of injectate as the indicator for measurement of CO. The CCO method uses heat signals produced by the thermal filament as the indicator. The CCO computer provides a time-averaged rather than instantaneous CO reading. CCO values are influenced by the same principles as TDCO.

• The heated thermal filament has a temperature limit to a maximum of 44°C (111.2° F). When calibrated by the manufacturer, CCO computers produce reliable calculations within a temperature range of 30°C to 40°C (86° F

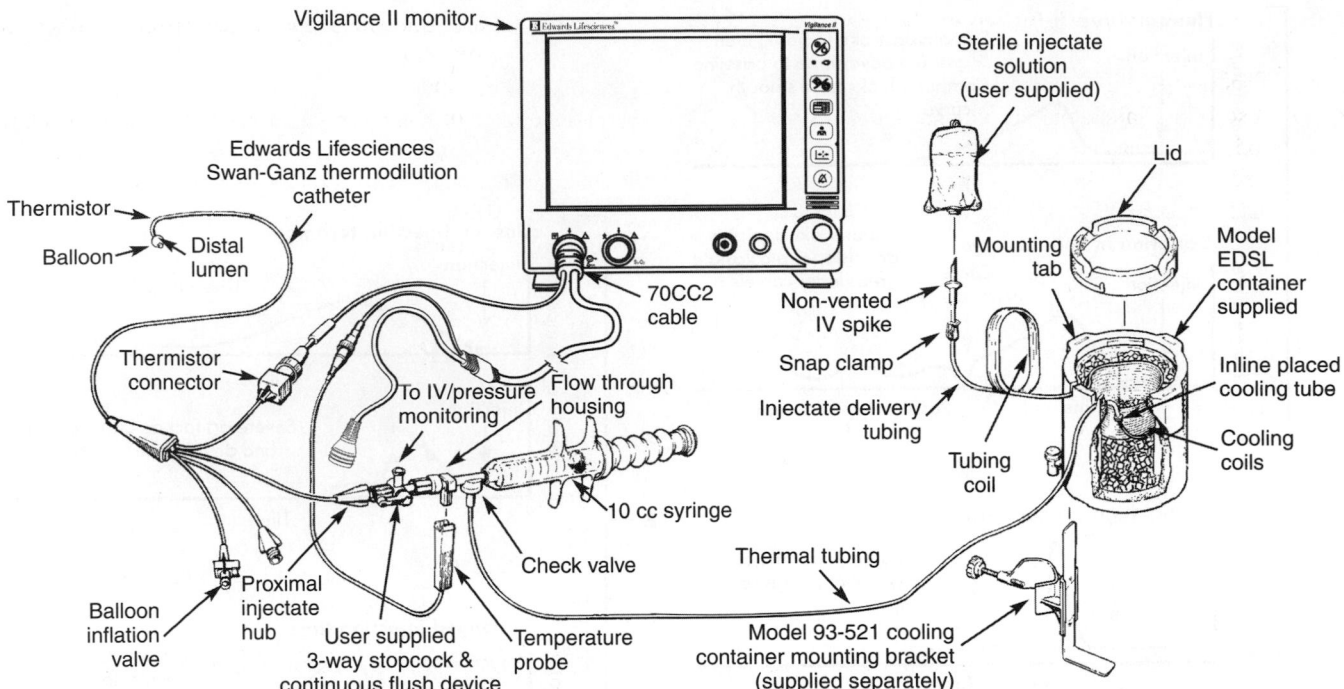

FIGURE 67-4   Closed injectate delivery system. Cold temperature injectate. (*From Edwards Lifesciences, LLC, Irvine, CA.*)

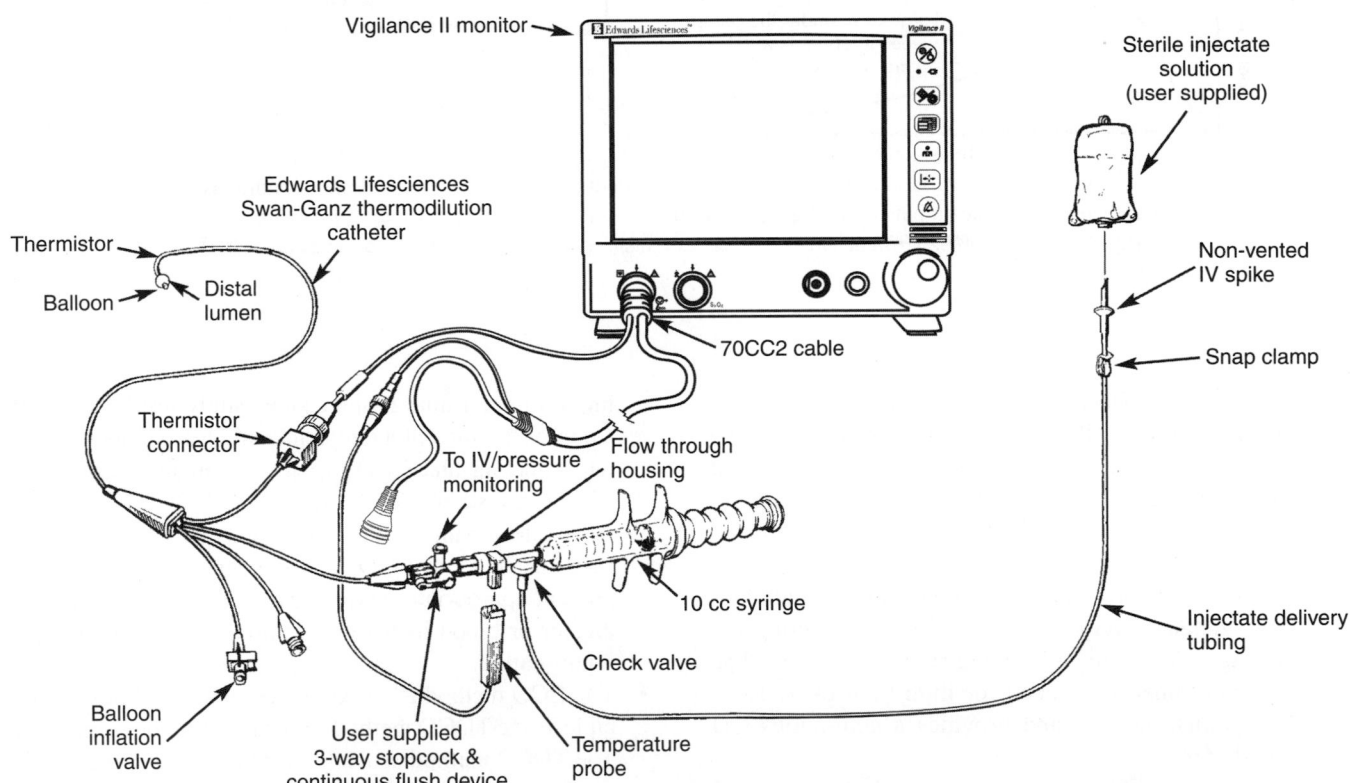

FIGURE 67-5   Closed injectate delivery system. Room temperature injectate. (*From Edwards Lifesciences, LLC, Irvine, CA.*)

to 104° F) or 31° C to 43° C (87.8° F to 109.4° F). An error message appears if the temperature in the PA is out of range.

- Infusions through proximal lumens should be limited to maintenance of patency of the lumen. Concomitant infusions through the proximal lumen can theoretically affect CCO measurements by altering the pulmonary artery temperature. Studies have shown that such infusions can cause variations in TDCO measurements.[18,45] To date, no published data describing the effect of concurrent central line infusions on the accuracy of CCO measurements are available, but large infusions of fluid are discouraged.[8,15]

- Because bolus injections are not needed with the CCO method, the prevalence of user error is theoretically reduced.[14]
- The CCO catheter can be used to obtain both CCO and TDCO measurements.
- The CCO does not reflect acute changes in CO values because the updated value on the monitor display is an average of 3 to 6 minutes of data. A delay of approximately 10 or more minutes to detect a change of 1 L/min in CO may occur. When monitoring a patient with an unstable condition that is being aggressively treated with medication or other therapies, one should be aware of the delay in data displayed.

EQUIPMENT

- Nonsterile gloves
- Cardiac monitor
- Hemodynamic monitoring system (see Procedure 76)
- PA catheter (in place)
- CO computer or module
- Connecting cables
- Injectate temperature probe
- Injectate solution
  Additional equipment as needed includes the following:
- Bolus thermodilution
  - ❖ Four 10-mL D_5W syringes (prefilled or empty with cold or room temperature solution)*
  - ❖ D_5W injectate solution bag with intravenous (IV) tubing and three-way Luer-Lok stopcock*
  - ❖ Ice (for cold injectate only)
  - ❖ Nonvented caps for stopcocks
- Setup for CCO
- Syringe holder or automatic injector device
- Printer
- Dispensing port

PATIENT AND FAMILY EDUCATION

- Explain the procedure for CO and the reason for its measurement. Include expectations related to sensations during the procedure (the patient should not experience pain or discomfort). ➥*Rationale:* Explanation decreases patient and family anxiety. Preparatory information of sensations decreases patient fear of the impending procedure.
- Explain the monitoring equipment involved, the frequency of measurements, and the goals of therapy. ➥*Rationale:* Explanation encourages the patient and family to ask questions and voice specific concerns about the procedure.
- Explain any potential variations in temperature the patient may or may not experience if a cold injectate is used. ➥*Rationale:* This explanation acknowledges the varying physical responses to the injectate and the possible perception of cold solution and may decrease anxiety associated with the procedure.

PATIENT ASSESSMENT AND PREPARATION
Patient Assessment

- Assess the patient's history of medication therapy, including medication allergies, recent bolus therapies, and current medication regime. ➥*Rationale:* Medications can influence CO measurements.
- Assess the patient's medical history for the presence of coronary artery disease, valvular heart disease, and left or right ventricular dysfunction. ➥*Rationale:* Medical history provides baseline information regarding cardiovascular performance.
- Assess current intracardiac pressures and PAP, RAP, and PAOP waveforms. ➥*Rationale:* This assessment ensures the PA catheter is positioned properly with a free-floating thermistor sensor and provides useful information about the presence and severity of mitral and tricuspid valve regurgitation.
- Assess the patient's vital signs, fluid balance, heart and lung sounds, skin color, temperature, mentation, peripheral pulses, cardiac rate and rhythm, and hemodynamic values. In patients with advanced systolic heart failure, assess for pulsus alternans (alternating strong and weak pulses). ➥*Rationale:* Clinical information provides data regarding blood flow and tissue perfusion. Abnormalities can influence the variability of CO measurements.

Patient Preparation

- Verify correct patient with two identifiers. ➥*Rationale:* Prior to performing a procedure, the nurse should ensure the correct identification of the patient for the intended intervention.
- Ensure that the patient and family understand preprocedural teaching. Answer questions as they arise, and reinforce information as needed. ➥*Rationale:* Understanding of previously taught information is evaluated and reinforced.
- Assist the patient to the supine position. ➥*Rationale:* CO measurements are most accurate in the supine position.

---

*CO-Set may be used in lieu of these items. The CO-Set is a closed system that contains IV tubing with a snap clamp, syringe, and stopcock.

Procedure	for Measurement of Cardiac Output with the Closed or Open Thermodilution Method	
Steps	**Rationale**	**Special Considerations**
1. **HH**		
2. Select the injectate delivery system: open or closed method. **(Level B*)**	Both systems are reliable.[29,34,37]	A closed system may eliminate cost and time expenditures of individual syringe preparation. The closed system has infection control benefits because of reduction of multiple entries into the system.[31]
3. Select cold or room temperature injectate. **(Level B)**	Room temperature injectate may be used for most patients. Research on room temperature versus cold injectate supports the accuracy of either method.[7,9,12,22,38,43] Cold injectate may improve the accuracy of CO measurement for patients with low or high CO.[43]	The acceptable temperature range for cold and room temperature injectate varies by system (manufacturer). Generally, room temperature is 18°C to 25°C, and cold is 0° to 12°C.
4. Select the injectate bolus amount (generally, 10 mL). **(Level B)**	An injectate of 10 mL may be used for most patients.[12,28,33]	Volumes of 5 mL may necessitate additional injections because of greater variability of individual measurements.[28]
5. Connect the CO cable to the PA catheter.	Prepares the system.	
6. Select the computation constant consistent with the type and size of the PA catheter, injectate volume, and injectate temperature. Confirm the injectate delivery system.	The computation constant is a correction factor determined by the catheter manufacturer that corrects for the gain of indicator (heat) that occurs as the injectate (5% dextrose in water [D_5W]) moves through the catheter from the hub of the injectate port to the injection port opening in the RA. The catheter manufacturer provides a table to determine the correct computation constant. The computation constant must be accurate for valid and reliable CO measurements.	Carefully select the correct computation constant for the type and catheter size, injectate volume, and cold or room temperature injectate. Confirm the setting on the CO computer/monitor. Recheck the computation constant before each series of CO measurements.
7. Connect the CO computer to the power source if it is a stand-alone device or turn on the CO computer or module.	Supplies the energy source.	
8. Note the temperature of the injectate (on the computer or monitor screen).	The injectate temperature should be at least 10°C less than the patient's core temperature.[25]	Follow manufacturer's recommendations.
9. Position the patient supine, with the head of the bed elevated no more than 20 degrees. **(Level B)**	Studies of patients in the supine position with the head of bed flat or elevated up to 20 degrees have not shown significant differences in TDCO measurements.[17,20,23,47]	One study supports the accuracy of CCO values with patients with the head of the bed elevated to 45 degrees.[11,16]

*Level B: Well-designed controlled studies with results that consistently support a specific action, intervention, or treatment

Procedure	for Measurement of Cardiac Output with the Closed or Open Thermodilution Method—*Continued*	
Steps	**Rationale**	**Special Considerations**
	Consistency in patient position may increase stability in consecutive CO readings.	The patient's medical condition and level of instability may determine positioning.
		Position should be documented and communicated.
		Consistent positioning when obtaining CO measurements over time decreases measurement variability.
		Cautiously use CO values obtained from lateral positions. The lateral recumbent position increases variability in CO measurements.[10,46]
10. Verify the position of the PA catheter by assessing both the RA and PA waveforms for proper waveform contours.	Proper positioning of the PA catheter ensures that the distal thermistor is located in the pulmonary artery. The distal thermistor sensor calculates the time-temperature data. Excessive coiling of the PA catheter in the RA or right ventricle can result in poor positioning of the distal thermistor in relation to the injectate port.[21]	Improper positioning of the PA catheter tip may result in false values.[14,15,21,26]
11. Observe the patient's cardiac rate and rhythm.	A rapid heart rate or dysrhythmias may decrease CO and lead to variability in CO measurements.	
12. If possible, consider restricting infusions delivered through the introducer or other central lines. **(Level C*)**	TDCO measurements obtained during administration of other infusions can cause variability in CO measurements (by as much as 40% higher).[18,45]	

*Level C: Qualitative studies, descriptive or correlational studies, integrative reviews, systematic reviews, or randomized controlled trials with inconsistent results

Procedure	for Closed-Method of Syringe Preparation and Cardiac Output Determination	
Steps	**Rationale**	**Special Considerations**

Note: Follow Steps 1 to 12 of the Procedure for Measurement of Cardiac Output with the Closed or Open Thermodilution Method.

1. **HH**		
2. **PE**		
3. Obtain the injectate solution of 5% dextrose in water (D$_5$W).	The specific gravity of D$_5$W is a component in the formula used to derive CO with the TDCO method.	
4. Aseptically connect the IV tubing to the injectate solution.	Prepares the system.	
5. Hang the IV injectate solution on an IV pole; prime the tubing.	Eliminates air from the tubing.	
6. Remove the sterile cap from the proximal lumen of the PA catheter.	Prepares for the injectate connection.	

Procedure continues on following page

Procedure	for Closed-Method of Syringe Preparation and Cardiac Output Determination—*Continued*	

Steps	Rationale	Special Considerations
7. Connect the injectate tubing to the proximal lumen of the PA catheter via a three-way Luer-Lok stopcock (see Figs. 67-4 and 67-5).	Connects the injectate solution to the PA catheter.	
8. Connect the injectate syringe to the three-way stopcock (see Figs. 67-4 and 67-5).	The syringe is used for solution injection.	Connect the system so that the CO syringe is in a straight line with the PA catheter to decrease resistance with injection of solution.
9. Connect the inline temperature probe (see Figs. 67-4 and 67-5).	Measures the injectate temperature.	Verify temperature.
10. If using cold injectate, set up the cold injectate system (e.g., CO-Set closed injectate system; see Fig. 67-4).	If using cold injectate, cool the injectate solution to 0°C to 12°C (32°F to 53°F).	Refer to manufacturer recommendations. Cold injectate may be proarrhythmic in some patients.[32,42]
11. Turn the stopcock so that it is open to the injectate solution (closed to the patient) and withdraw 10 mL of the injectate solution into the syringe.	Prepares for injection.	
12. Turn the stopcock so that it is closed to the injectate solution and open to the patient. Support the stopcock with the palm of the nondominant hand.	Minimal handling (less than 30 seconds) of the syringe is recommended to avoid thermal indicator variation that may introduce error into the CO calculation.[5,8,26]	Syringe holders or automatic injector devices are available and can be used to aid in injectate administration.
13. Activate the CO computer, and wait for the "ready" message.	The CO computer or module needs to be ready before injection of solution.	Follow manufacturer guidelines.
14. Before administering the bolus injectate, observe for a steady baseline temperature (e.g., the line before the CO curve begins should be flat without undulations) on the monitor screen (see Figs. 67-2B and 67-3A).	An abnormal baseline may increase variability in CO measurements and introduce error.[1]	Patients with advanced systolic heart failure (low ejection fraction) are more prone to a wavering initial baseline from unstable PA blood temperature. If possible, have the patient lie still and not talk while you are preparing to administer the bolus injection.
15. Observe the patient's respiratory pattern. Prepare to begin administering the injectate at end expiration to decrease variance in CO measurements from the respiratory cycle. (**Level C***)	End expiration is defined as the phase of the respiratory cycle preceding the start of inspiration. Significant variations in transthoracic pressure during respiration can affect CO by altering venous return.[19,35,40,41]	
16. Administer the bolus injectate rapidly and smoothly in 4 seconds or less.	Prolonged injection time may result in false low CO. Rates of 2 to 4 seconds for injection of 5 to 10 mL of injectate yield accurate results.[5,13,39]	A prolonged injection time interferes with time and temperature calculations. One respiratory cycle is generally less than 4 seconds. One ventilation cycle on a ventilator is generally 4 seconds.

*Level C: Qualitative studies, descriptive or correlational studies, integrative reviews, systematic reviews, or randomized controlled trials with inconsistent results

| Procedure | for Closed-Method of Syringe Preparation and Cardiac Output Determination—*Continued* | | |

Steps	Rationale	Special Considerations
17. Assess the CO curve and value on the monitor screen (see Figs. 67-2 and 67-3).	The CO curve must be a normal curve. A normal curve starts at baseline (baseline must be a straight, flat, nonwavering line) with a smooth upstroke and a gradual downstroke. If the CO curve is not normal, the CO measurement obtained from the injection should be discarded. Abnormal contours of the curve may indicate improper catheter position. An abnormal CO curve may represent technical error.	Normal CO is 4 to 8 L/min. Abnormal CO curves may also provide information about the patient's clinical condition, such as tricuspid valve regurgitation.
18. Repeat Steps 11 through 17 (up to three times total for cold injectate and up to five times total for room temperature injectate).	Discard all CO measurements that do not have normal CO curves or have wandering baselines.	Allow 60 seconds between each CO measurement to ensure consistency and accuracy.
19. Determine the CO measurement by calculating the average of three measurements within 10% of a middle (median) value. (**Level E***)	Determines accurate CO value.[44]	
20. Return the proximal stopcock at the RA lumen to the original position.	Continues RA monitoring.	
21. Continue infusions delivered through the introducer or other central lines.	Continues therapy.	
22. Observe the PA and RA waveforms on the monitor.	Continues hemodynamic monitoring.	
23. Discard used supplies in appropriate receptacles.	Removes and safely discards used supplies.	
24. **HH**		
25. Determine the hemodynamic calculations. Compare the values with prior values and determine whether the plan of care requires alterations.	Assesses cardiac performance and hemodynamic status.	

*Level E: Multiple case reports, theory-based evidence from expert opinions, or peer-reviewed professional organizational standards without clinical studies to support recommendations

| Procedure | for Open Method of Syringe Preparation and Cardiac Output Determination | | |

Steps	Rationale	Special Considerations

Note: Follow Steps 1 to 12 of the Procedure for Measurement of Cardiac Output with the Closed or Open Thermodilution Method.

1. **HH**
2. **PE**

| 3. Prepare syringes or obtain manufactured prefilled syringes for CO determination. | Prepares the injectate for CO determination. | Prefilled syringes may decrease variability related to injectate volume. |

Procedure continues on following page

Procedure for Open Method of Syringe Preparation and Cardiac Output Determination—*Continued*

Steps	Rationale	Special Considerations
A. Clean the injectate port of the D$_5$W IV bag with an alcohol wipe. Apply a dispensing port to the bag's injectate port	Reduces surface contamination. A dispensing port negates the use of needles and reduces the incidence of accidental needle sticks.	Not necessary with manufactured prefilled sterile syringes.
B. Aseptically withdraw the injectate solution from the D$_5$W IV bag into three to five 10-mL syringes and cap securely.	Prepares the injectate for CO measurements.	Additional syringes may be necessary because syringes may be inadvertently dropped or contaminated.
C. If not using immediately, label the container or syringes with the date and time they were prepared.	Prefilled syringes at the bedside or in the refrigerator must be labeled (e.g., "for CO injection only").	
4. Cold injectate: Cool the syringes by filling a syringe container with sterile water and ice.	Iced slush is used to cool syringes. Use of water and ice prevents air pockets that can cause variability in the temperature of different injectate syringes.	Not necessary with room temperature syringes. Handling of a cold syringe causes warming and hampers validity of CO measurements.[5,8,26] Cold injectate may be proarrhythmic.[32,42]
5. Remove the nonvented cap from the right atrial lumen stopcock of the PA catheter.	Prepares the stopcock.	
6. Aseptically connect one of the sterile CO injectate syringes onto the right atrial lumen stopcock of the PA catheter.	Reduces the risk of introducing microorganisms into the system.	
7. Turn the stopcock so that it is closed to the flush solution and open between the injectate syringe and the patient. Support the stopcock with the palm of the nondominant hand.	Prepares the system for injectate administration.	
8. Connect the inline temperature probe (see Figs. 67-4 and 67-5).	Measures the injectate temperature.	Verify temperature.
9. Activate the CO computer, and wait for the "ready" message.	The CO computer or module needs to be ready before injection of solution.	Follow manufacturer guidelines.
10. Before administering the bolus injectate, observe for a steady baseline temperature (e.g., the line before the CO curve begins should be flat without undulations) on the monitor screen (see Figs. 67-2, *B* and 67-3, *A*).	An abnormal baseline may increase variability in CO measurements and introduce error.[1]	Patients with advanced systolic heart failure (low ejection fraction) are more prone to a wavering initial baseline from unstable PA blood temperature. If possible, have the patient lie still and not talk while you are preparing to administer the bolus injection.
11. Observe the patient's respiratory pattern. Prepare to begin administering the injectate at end expiration to decrease variance in CO measurements from the respiratory cycle. **(Level C*)**	End expiration is defined as the phase of the respiratory cycle preceding the start of inspiration. Significant variations in transthoracic pressure during respiration can affect CO by altering venous return.[19,35,40,41]	

*Level C: Qualitative studies, descriptive or correlational studies, integrative reviews, systematic reviews, or randomized controlled trials with inconsistent results

Procedure for Open Method of Syringe Preparation and Cardiac Output Determination—*Continued*

Steps	Rationale	Special Considerations
12. Administer the bolus injectate rapidly and smoothly in 4 seconds or less.	Prolonged injection time may result in false low CO. Rates of 2 to 4 seconds for injection of 5 to 10 mL of injectate yield accurate results.[5,13,39]	A prolonged injection time interferes with time and temperature calculations. One respiratory cycle is generally less than 4 seconds. One ventilation cycle on a ventilator is generally 4 seconds.
13. Assess the CO curve and value on the monitor screen (see Figs. 67-2 and 67-3).	The CO curve must be a normal curve. A normal curve starts at baseline (baseline must be a straight, flat, nonwavering line) with a smooth upstroke and a gradual downstroke. If the CO curve is not normal, the CO measurement obtained from the injection should be discarded. Abnormal contours of the curve may indicate improper catheter position. An abnormal CO curve may represent technical error.	Normal CO is 4 to 8 L/min. Abnormal CO curves may also provide information about the patient's clinical condition, such as tricuspid valve regurgitation.
14. Repeat Steps 6 through 13 (up to three times total for cold injectate and up to five times total for room temperature injectate).	Obtains CO measurements. Discard all CO measurements that do not have normal CO curves or have wandering baselines.	Allow 60 seconds between each CO measurement to ensure consistency and accuracy. Asepsis is essential as the stopcock is turned and syringes are exchanged between CO measurements.
15. Determine the CO measurement by calculating the average of three measurements within 10% of a middle (median) value. **(Level E*)**	Determines accurate CO value.[44]	
16. After the last injectate is completed: A. Turn the right atrial lumen stopcock of the PA catheter so that the system is open between the patient and the transducer B. Aseptically remove the last injectate syringe C. Place a new, sterile, nonvented cap on the stopcock port.	Closes the system; maintains the sterility of the system.	
17. Observe the PA and RA waveforms on the monitor.	Continues hemodynamic monitoring.	
18. Discard used supplies in appropriate receptacles.	Removes and safely discards used supplies.	
19. 🅷🅷		
20. Determine hemodynamic calculations. Compare values with prior values and determine whether the plan of care requires alterations.	Assesses cardiac performance and hemodynamic status.	

*Level E: Multiple case reports, theory-based evidence from expert opinions, or peer-reviewed professional organizational standards without clinical studies to support recommendations

Procedure continues on following page

Procedure for Measurement of Cardiac Output with Continuous Cardiac Output Method		
Steps	**Rationale**	**Special Considerations**
1. **HH**		
2. **PE**		
3. Turn on the CO computer or module.	Provides energy.	
4. Connect the CO cable to the PA catheter.	Supplies the energy source.	
5. Observe the right atrial waveform. The proximal lumen opening of the PA catheter should be located in the RA.	A right atrial waveform indicates that the thermal filament is properly placed. The thermal filament should be located in the right ventricle between the infusion port and the distal tip of the catheter. Advancement of the thermal filament into the PA results in erroneous measurements.	The thermal filament should float free in the right ventricle to prevent the loss of indicator (heat) into the cardiac tissue. If the loss of indicator occurs, the CO value is overestimated, giving erroneous readings.
6. Position the patient supine with the head of the bed elevated up to 45 degrees. (**Level C***)	CCO measurements are most accurate in a supine position, but head-of-bed angle can be varied for comfort, between 0 and 45 degrees.[16]	Additional studies are needed to determine the effect of patient body position on CCO measurements. Document body position at the time of hemodynamic data collection.
7. Check the heat signal indicator on the CO computer or module per manufacturer's recommendations.	CCO systems assess the quality of the measured thermal signal. Relationships are in response to thermal noise or signal to noise ratio.	CCO monitors provide messages for troubleshooting signal-to-noise ratio interferences. Refer to manufacturer recommendations. Technologic advances suppress the effects of blood thermal noise.[48]
8. Note that the CCO values reflect an average of the preceding 3 to 6 minutes of data collection.	CCO measurements are averaged over the preceding 3 to 6 minutes and are not individual measurements.	CCO values are updated every 30 to 60 seconds. Continuous data collection reflects phasic changes in the respiratory cycle. CCO measurements are not timed to the respiratory cycle.
9. When documenting CCO values, also document other hemodynamic findings.	Provides data regarding hemodynamic status.	
10. Compare the CCO value with the patient's current clinical status and hemodynamic findings.	CCO is a global assessment parameter and must be appreciated as part of the patient's total hemodynamic profile at a given time.	CCO method eliminates many of the potential user-related and technique-related errors associated with intermittent bolus CO. Research shows clinically acceptable correlation between the TDCO technique and the CCO method in the steady state.[1,6,27,29,30] Future studies are needed to determine efficacy in patients in various phases of acute hemodynamic instability and in specific patient populations. Also, the effects of changes in positioning need to be studied further, especially in patients with structural or functional heart damage.

*Level C: Qualitative studies, descriptive or correlational studies, integrative reviews, systematic reviews, or randomized controlled trials with inconsistent results

Procedure for Measurement of Cardiac Output with Continuous Cardiac Output Method—*Continued*

Steps	Rationale	Special Considerations
11. Note: The CCO catheter system can be used to obtain TDCO. Follow Steps 1 to 12 of the Procedure for Measurement of Cardiac Output with the Closed or Open Thermodilution Method CO and then follow the steps for either the Closed-or Open-Method of Syringe Preparation and Cardiac Output Determination.		
12. Discard used supplies in appropriate receptacles.	Removes and safely discards used supplies.	
13. 🅷🅷		

Expected Outcomes

- Accurate CO measurement are obtained
- Hemodynamic profile and derived parameters are obtained with accuracy, whether through the continuous or intermittent method
- Sterility and patency of the PA catheter is maintained.

Unexpected Outcomes

- Inability to accurately measure CO
- Erroneous readings because of technical, equipment, or operator error
- Contamination of the system
- Occlusion of the proximal PA lumen

Patient Monitoring and Care

Steps	Rationale	Reportable Conditions
		These conditions should be reported if they persist despite nursing interventions.
1. Maintain patency of the PA catheter (see Procedures 73 and 75).	PA catheter patency is essential for accurate monitoring.	• Inability to maintain PA catheter patency
2. Monitor RA and PA waveforms for confirmation of proper catheter position.	Proper placement determines accurate hemodynamic and CO measurement.	• Abnormal RA or PA waveforms or values
3. Maintain the sterility of the PA catheter.	Reduces the risk for catheter-related infections.	• Fever, site redness, drainage, or symptoms consistent with infection
4. Calculate cardiac index, systemic vascular resistance, and other parameters as prescribed or indicated.	Determines cardiac performance and current hemodynamic status.	• Abnormal cardiac index, systemic vascular resistance, or other hemodynamic values
5. Monitor vital signs and respiratory status hourly and as indicated.	Changes in vital signs or respiratory status may indicate hemodynamic compromise.	• Sudden or significant change in the patient's clinical status
6. Include the fluid volume used in the TDCO in the patient's total fluid volume intake.	Additional volume given intermittently should be included in the total intake for accurate fluid volume assessment.	• Signs or symptoms of fluid overload (e.g., respiratory distress, crackles, increased PADP or PAOP, elevated jugular venous pressure, new or worsening S3 gallop, worsening edema)

Procedure continues on following page

Patient Monitoring and Care —*Continued*

Steps	Rationale	Reportable Conditions
7. Assess the patient's response to therapies.	Hemodynamic monitoring may expedite treatment decisions.	• Significant worsening or improvement in CO, volume parameters (PAOP, RAP), and vascular resistance (pulmonary vascular resistance [PVR] and systemic vascular resistance [SVR])
8. If using a closed system delivery set (CO-Set), change the system components (tubing, syringe, stopcocks, and IV solution) every 96 hours with the hemodynamic monitoring system (see Procedure 76).	No recommendations exist that are specific to the closed system delivery set.	

Documentation

Documentation includes the following:
- Patient and family education
- CO, cardiac index, SVR, volume indicators (PAOP and RAP)
- CO curves
- Baseline PA blood temperature
- Continuous or intermittent bolus method
- Volume and temperature of injectate
- Concurrent headrest elevation, vital signs, and hemodynamic measurements
- Titration or administration of medications that affect CO (e.g., dobutamine or milrinone; epinephrine, norepinephrine), vascular resistance (e.g., intravenous nitrates or arterial vasodilator therapy—nitroprusside or nesiritide), and intravascular volume (e.g., intravenous loop or thiazide diuretics)
- Significant medical therapies or nursing interventions that affect CO (e.g., intraaortic balloon pump or ventricular assist device therapies, volume expanders, position changes), vascular resistance, or intravascular volume (e.g., sedation, blood/blood products, headrest elevation, fluid restriction, sodium restriction)
- Unexpected outcomes
- Additional interventions, including psychosocial or emotional/psychiatric interventions that might influence hemodynamic trends

References

CR 1. Albert NM, Spear B, Hammell J: Agreement and clinical utility of two techniques for measuring cardiac output in patients with low cardiac output, *Am J Crit Care* 8: 464-474, 1999.

CR 2. Baillard C, et al: Haemodynamic measurements (continuous cardiac output and systemic vascular resistance) in critically ill patients: transesophageal Doppler versus continuous thermodilution, *Anaesth Intensive Care* 27:33-37, 1999.

CR 3. Balik M, Pachl J, Hendl J: Effect of the degree of tricuspid regurgitation on cardiac output measurements by thermodilution, *Intensive Care Med* 28:1117-1121, 2002.

CR 4. Berthelsen PG, et al: Thermodilution cardiac output: cold vs. room temperature injectate and the importance of measuring the injectate temperature in the right atrium, *Acta Anaesthesiol Scand* 46:1103-1110, 2002.

CR 5. Bilfinger TV, Lin CY, Anagnostopoulos CE: In vitro determination of accuracy of cardiac output measurement by thermal dilution, *J Surg Res* 33:409-414, 1982.

CR 6. Boldt J, et al: Is continuous cardiac output measurement using thermodilution reliable in the critically ill patient? *Crit Care Med* 22:1913-1918, 1994.

CR 7. Bourdillon PDV, Fineberg N: Comparison of iced and room-temperature injectate for thermodilution cardiac output, *Cathet Cardiovasc Diagn* 17:116-120, 1989.

CR 8. Bridges EJ: Hemodynamic monitoring. In Woods SL, et al, editors: *Cardiac nursing,* ed 5, Philadelphia, 2005, JB Lippincott Williams & Wilkins, 478-526.

CR 9. Daily EK, Mersch J: Thermodilution cardiac outputs using room and ice temperature injectate: comparison with the FICK method, *Heart Lung* 16:294-300, 1987.

CR 10. Doering L, Dracup K: Comparisons of cardiac output in supine and lateral positions, *Nurs Res* 37:114-118, 1988.

CR 11. Driscoll A, et al: The effect of patient position on the reproducibility of cardiac output measurements, *Heart Lung* 24:38-44, 1995.

CR 12. Elkayam U, et al: Cardiac output by thermodilution technique: effect of injectate's volume and temperature on accuracy and reproducibility in the critically ill, *Chest* 84:418-422, 1983.

CR 13. Enghof E, Sjogren S: Thermal dilution for measurement of cardiac output in the pulmonary artery catheter in man in relation to choice of indicator volume and injection time, *Ups J Med Sci* 78:33-37, 1973.

14. Frazier SK: Hemodynamic monitoring. In Moser D, Reigel B, editors: *Cardiac nursing: a companion to Braunwald's heart disease,* Philadelphia, 2008, Saunders.

15. Gawlinski A: *Protocols for practice: hemodynamic monitoring series: cardiac output monitoring,* Aliso Viejo, CA, 1998, American Association of Critical-Care Nurses.

16. Giuliano KK, et al: Backrest angle and cardiac output measurement in critically ill patients, *Nurs Research* 52:242-248, 2003.

17. Grap MJ, et al: Use of backrest elevation in critical care: a pilot study, *Am J Crit Care* 8:495-496, 1999.

18. Griffin K, et al: Thermodilution cardiac output measurements during simultaneous volume infusion through the venous infusion port of the pulmonary artery catheter, *J Cardiothorac Vasc Anesth* 11:437-439, 1997.

19. Groeneveld AB, et al: Effect of mechanical ventilatory cycle on thermodilution right ventricular volumes and cardiac output, *J Appl Physiol* 89:89-96, 2000.

20. Grose BL, Wood SL, Laurent DJ: Effect of backrest position on cardiac output measured by the thermodilution method in acutely ill patients, *Heart Lung* 10:661-665, 1981.

21. Kalassian KG, Raffin TA: The technique of thermodilution cardiac output measurements, *J Crit Illness* 11:249-256, 1996.

22. Kiely M, Byers LA, Greenwood R: Thermodilution measurement of cardiac output in patients with low output: room temperature versus iced injectate, *Am J Crit Care* 7:436-438, 1998.

23. Kleven M: Effect of backrest position on thermodilution cardiac output in critically ill patients receiving mechanical ventilation with positive end-expiratory pressure, *Heart Lung* 13:303-304, 1984.

24. Lehmann KG, Platt MS: Improved accuracy and precision of thermodilution cardiac output measurement using a dual thermistor catheter system, *J Am Coll Cardiol* 33:883-891, 1999.

25. Levett JM, Replogle RL: Thermodilution cardiac output: a critical analysis and review of the literature, *J Surg Res* 27:392-404, 1979.

26. Loveys BJ, Woods SL: Current recommendations for thermodilution cardiac output measurement, *Progress Cardiovasc Nurs* 1:24-32, 1986.

27. Marcum J, et al: A comparison of varying injectate volumes in determining thermodilution cardiac output in critically ill postsurgical patients, *Am J Crit Care* 2:262, 1995.

28. McCloy K, Leung S, Beldon J: Effects of injectate volume on thermodilution measurements of cardiac output in patients with low ventricular ejection fraction, *Am J Crit Care* 8:86-92, 1999.

29. Medin DL, et al: Validation of continuous thermodilution cardiac output in critically ill patients with analysis of systematic errors, *J Crit Care* 13:184-189, 1998.

30. Mihaljevic T, et al: Continuous versus bolus thermodilution cardiac output measurement: a comparative study, *Crit Care Med* 23:944-949, 1995.

31. Nelson LD, Martinez OV, Anderson HB: Incidence of microbial colonization in open versus closed delivery systems for thermodilution injectate, *Crit Care Med* 14:291-293, 1986.

32. Nishikawa R, Dohi S: Slowing of heart rate during cardiac output measurement by thermodilution, *Anesthesiology* 57:538-539, 1982.

33. Pearl RG, et al: Effect of injectate volume and temperature on thermodilution cardiac output determination, *Anesth* 64:798-801, 1986.

34. Plachetka JR, et al: Comparison of two closed systems for thermodilution cardiac output, *Crit Care Med* 9:487-489, 1981.

35. Riedinger MS, Shellock FG, Swan HJ: Reading pulmonary artery and pulmonary capillary wedge pressure waveforms with respiratory variations, *Heart Lung* 10:675-678, 1981.

36. Rocca GD, et al: Continuous and intermittent cardiac output measurement: pulmonary artery catheter versus aortic transpulmonary technique, *Br J Anaesth* 88:350-356, 2002.

37. Rodig G, et al: Intraoperative evaluation of a continuous versus intermittent bolus thermodilution technique of cardiac output measurement in cardiac surgical patients, *Eur J Anesthesiol* 15:196-201, 1998.

38. Shellock FG, Riedinger MS: Reproducibility and accuracy of using room-temperature vs ice-temperature injectate for thermodiltion cardiac output determination, *Heart Lung* 12:175-176, 1983.

39. Shellock FG, et al: Thermodilution cardiac output determination in hypothermic postcardiac surgery patients: room vs. ice temperature injectate, *Crit Care Med* 11:668-670, 1983.

40. Snyder JV, Powner DJ: Effects of mechanical ventilation on the measurement of cardiac output by thermodilution, *Crit Care Med* 10:677-682, 1982.

41. Stevens JH, et al: Thermodilution cardiac output measurement:effects of the respiratory cycle on its reproducibility, *JAMA* 253:2440-2442, 1985.

42. Todd MM: Atrial fibrillation induced by right atrial injection of cold fluid during thermodilution cardiac output determination: a case report, *Anesthesiology* 59:253-255, 1983.

43. Wallace DC, Winslow EH: Effects of iced and room-temperature injectate on cardiac output measurements in critically ill patients with low and high cardiac outputs, *Heart Lung* 22:55-63, 1993.

44. Weil MH: Measurement of cardiac output, *Crit Care Med* 5:117-119, 1977.

45. Wetzel RC, Latson TW: Major errors in thermodilution cardiac output measurement during rapid volume infusion, *Anesthesiology* 62:684-687, 1985.

46. Whitman GR, Howaniak DL, Verga TS: Comparison of cardiac output measurements in 20-degree right- and left-lateral recumbent positions, *Heart Lung* 11:256-257, 1982.

47. Wilson AE, et al: Effect of backrest position on hemodynamic and right ventricular measurements in critically ill adults, *Am J Crit Care* 5:264-270, 1996.

48. Woods S, Osguthorpe S: Cardiac output determination, *AACN Clin Issue Crit Care Nurs* 4(1):81-97, 1993.

Additional Readings

Ahrens T: Hemodynamic monitoring, *Crit Care Nurs Clin North Am* 11:19-31, 1999.

Brandsteller RD, et al: Swan-Ganz catheter: misconceptions, pitfalls, and incomplete user knowledge: an identified trilogy in need of correction, *Heart Lung J Acute Crit Care* 27:218-222, 1998.

CR Burchell SA, et al: Evaluation of a continuous cardiac output and mixed venous oxygen saturation catheter in critically ill surgical patients, *Crit Care Med* 25:388-391, 1997.

CR Ditmyer CE, Shively M, Burns CB: Comparison of continuous with intermittent bolus thermodilution cardiac output measurement, *Am J Crit Care* 4: 460-465, 1995.

CR Headley JM: Strategies to optimize the cardiorespiratory status of the critically ill, *AACN Clin Issues Crit Care Nurs* 6:121-134, 1995.

CR Headley J: *Invasive hemodynamic monitoring: physiological principles and clinical application,* Irvine, CA, 2002, Edwards Lifesciences.

CR Hollenberg SM, Hoyt J, Pulmonary artery catheters in cardiovascular disease, *N Horiz* 5:207-213, 1997.

CR Jansen JR, et al: Mean cardiac output by thermodilution with a single controlled injection, *Crit Care Med* 29: 1868-1873, 2001.

CR Sandham JD, et al: A randomized, controlled trial of the use of pulmonary-artery catheters in high-risk surgical patients, *N Engl J Med* 348:5-14, 2003.

CR Taylor RW: Controversies in pulmonary artery catheterization, *N Horiz* 5:1-296, 1997.

Central Venous Catheter Removal

PURPOSE: Central venous catheters are removed when therapy is completed, when the presence of the catheter presents a risk for complications (e.g., the catheter is occluded or malpositioned), or when the patient has a catheter-related infection.

Teresa Preuss, Debra Lynn-McHale Wiegand

PREREQUISITE NURSING KNOWLEDGE

* Knowledge of the normal anatomy and physiology of the vasculature and cardiovascular system is necessary.
* Knowledge of normal coagulation values is needed.
* Principles of aseptic technique should be known.
* Advanced cardiac life support knowledge and skills are necessary.
* Clinical and technical competence in central venous catheter (CVC) removal is necessary.
* Knowledge of the state nurse practice act is important because some states do not allow this intervention to be performed by a registered nurse.
* Knowledge of potential complications associated with the removal of the CVC is needed.
* An air embolism can occur during or after the removal of the catheter as a result of air drawn in along the subcutaneous tract and into the vein. During inspiration, negative intrathoracic pressure is transmitted to the central veins. Any opening external to the body to one of these veins may result in aspiration of air into the central venous system. The pathologic effects depend on the volume and rate of air aspirated. Signs and symptoms include: respiratory distress, agitation, cyanosis, gasp reflex, sucking sound, hypotension, petechiae, cardiac dysrhythmias, and altered mental status.

EQUIPMENT

* Goggles or face shield
* Face mask, sterile glows, nonsterile gloves
* Antiseptic solution (e.g., 2% chlorhexidine-based preparation)
* Sterile scissors
* 4 × 4 gauze pads
* One roll of 2-inch tape
* Two moisture-proof absorbent pads
  Additional equipment to have as needed includes the following:
* Additional dressing supplies (e.g., transparent dressing)
* Sterile specimen container (needed if culture of catheter tip will be obtained)
* Antibiotic ointment
* Suture removal kit
* Emergency equipment

PATIENT AND FAMILY EDUCATION

* Explain the procedure to the patient and family and the reason for catheter removal. ➤➤*Rationale:* This explanation provides information and decreases anxiety.
* Explain the importance of the patient lying still during the catheter removal. ➤➤*Rationale:* This explanation ensures patient cooperation and facilitates safe removal of the catheter.

- Instruct the patient and family to report any signs and symptoms of shortness of breath, bleeding, or discomfort at the site of catheter removal. ➤➤*Rationale:* Identifies patient discomfort and early recognition of complications.

PATIENT ASSESSMENT AND PREPARATION

Patient Assessment

- Assess vital signs and the neurovascular status of the extremity distal to the catheter insertion site. ➤➤*Rationale:* This assessment provides baseline data.
- Assess the patient's current coagulation values. ➤➤*Rationale:* If the patient has abnormal coagulation study results, hemostasis may be difficult to obtain.
- Assess the catheter site for redness, warmth, tenderness, or presence of drainage. ➤➤*Rationale:* Determines if signs or symptoms of infection are present.

Patient Preparation

- In collaboration with the physician, determine when the CVC should be removed. ➤➤*Rationale:* The invasive catheter is removed when it is no longer indicated.

- In collaboration with the physician, determine whether the tip of the catheter will be cultured. ➤➤*Rationale:* This discussion determines additional supplies that may be needed.
- Verify correct patient with two identifiers. ➤➤ *Rationale:* Prior to performing a procedure, the nurse should ensure the correct identification of the patient for the intended intervention.
- Ensure that the patient and family understand preprocedural teaching. Answer questions as they arise, and reinforce information as needed. ➤➤*Rationale:* Understanding of previously taught information is evaluated and reinforced.
- Place the patient in a supine position with the head of the bed in a slight Trendelenburg's position (or flat if Trendelenburg's position is contraindicated or not tolerated by the patient). ➤➤*Rationale:* A normal pressure gradient exists between atmospheric air and the central venous compartment that promotes air entry if the compartment is open. Placing the patient in a head-down position decreases the risk of air being drawn into the venous circulation.
- Start a new peripheral intravenous (IV) line or ensure that an existing peripheral IV line is patent. ➤➤*Rationale:* IV access is established for fluids or medications.

Procedure	**for Central Venous Catheter Removal**		
Steps	**Rationale**	**Special Considerations**
1. **HH**		
2. **PE**		All health care providers in the room should wear a face mask.
3. Transfer or discontinue IV solution.	Prepares the catheter for removal.	
4. Open the sterile scissors or suture removal kit and sterile gauze pads.	Prepares supplies for use.	
5. Place a moisture-proof absorbent pad under the patient's upper torso and another close to the catheter site.	Collects blood and body fluids associated with removal; serves as a receptacle for the contaminated catheter.	
6. Place the patient supine in slight Trendelenburg's position.[1,3-6,9,12] **(Level E*)**	Minimizes the risk for venous air embolus. Cases have been reported of venous air embolus occurring after removal of CVCs while patients were in the Fowler's position.	Place the patient flat if Trendelenburg's position is contraindicated or not tolerated by the patient or a femoral CVC will be removed. If the CVC is in the femoral vein, extend the patient's leg and ensure the groin area is adequately exposed.
7. Have the patient turn his or her head away from the catheter site (if removing an internal jugular or subclavian catheter).	Decreases the risk for contamination.	
8. Remove the catheter dressing and discard.	Prepares for removal.	

*Level E: Multiple case reports, theory-based evidence from expert opinions, or peer-reviewed professional organizational standards without clinical studies to support recommendations

Procedure for Central Venous Catheter Removal—*Continued*

Steps	Rationale	Special Considerations
9. Remove the nonsterile gloves, perform hand hygiene, and apply a pair of sterile gloves.	Decreases the risk for contamination.	
10. Remove the securing device or, if present, cut sutures and gently pull the sutures through the skin.	Allows for removal of the catheter.	Ensure that the entire suture is removed. Retained sutures can form epithelialized tracts that can lead to infection.
11. Ask the patient to take a deep breath in and hold it (if removing an internal jugular or subclavian catheter).[8,10,12,13] **(Level E*)**	Minimizes the risk for venous air embolus.	If the patient is receiving positive pressure ventilation, withdraw the catheter during the inspiratory phase of the respiratory cycle or while delivering a breath via a bag-valve device.
12. Withdraw the catheter, pulling parallel to the skin and using a steady motion.	Minimizes trauma.	Antibiotic ointment may be applied to the exit wound to seal the opening.[4] If resistance is met, do not continue to remove the catheter. Notify the advanced practice nurse or physician immediately.
13. As the catheter exits the site, apply pressure with a gauze pad.	Minimizes the risk for venous air embolus and promotes hemostasis.	The distal end of a multilumen catheter should be removed quickly because the exposed proximal and medial openings could permit the entry of air.
14. Have the patient exhale after the catheter is removed.	Once the catheter is removed the patient can breathe normally.	
15. Lay the catheter on the moisture-proof absorbent pad. Check to be sure that all of the catheter was removed.	Ensures the removal of the entire catheter.	Keep the catheter tip sterile and obtain a culture if prescribed.
16. Continue applying firm direct pressure over the insertion site with the gauze pad until bleeding has stopped.	Ensures hemostasis.	Because CVCs are placed in large veins, hemostasis may take up to 10 minutes to occur. Pressure may be needed for a longer period of time if the patient has been receiving anticoagulant therapy or if coagulation studies are abnormal.
17. Apply a sterile air occlusive dressing over the site.[1,2,4,6,8,9] **(Level E)**	Decreases the risk for infection at the insertion site and minimizes the risk for venous air embolism.	Label the dressing with the date, time, and your initials. The dressing should remain in place for a minimum of 12 hours.[4]
18. Maintain bed rest for at least 30 minutes after catheter removal.[4]	May decrease the risk of a postprocedure venous air embolism.	
19. Dispose of used supplies in appropriate receptacles.	Removes and safely discards used supplies.	
20. 🅷🅷		

*Level E: Multiple case reports, theory-based evidence from expert opinions, or peer-reviewed professional organizational standards without clinical studies to support recommendations

Procedure continues on following page

Expected Outcomes

- The catheter is removed intact
- Hemostasis is achieved at the catheter site

Unexpected Outcomes

- Inability to remove the catheter
- Catheter not removed intact
- Venous air emboli
- Persistent bleeding
- Hematoma
- Pain

Patient Monitoring and Care

Steps	Rationale	Reportable Conditions
		These conditions should be reported if they persist despite nursing interventions.
1. Assess the patient's vital signs, pulse oximetry, and level of consciousness before and after the CVC is removed.	Provides baseline data and data that identify changes in patient condition.	- Abnormal vital signs - Shortness of breath or tachypnea - Cyanosis or decreased oxygen saturation - Changes in mental status
2. If signs and symptoms of venous air embolus are present, immediately place the patient in the left lateral Trendelenburg's position.	Venous air embolus is a potentially life-threatening complication. The left lateral Trendelenburg's position prevents air from passing into the left side of the heart and traveling into the arterial circulation.	- Respiratory distress - Agitation - Cyanosis - Gasp reflex - Sucking sound - Hypotension - Petechiae - Cardiac dysrhythmias - Altered mental status
3. After removal of the CVC, assess the site for signs of bleeding every 15 minutes × 2, every 30 minutes × 2, and then 1 hour later.	Bleeding or a hematoma can develop if there is still bleeding from the vessel.	- Bleeding - Hematoma development
4. Remove the dressing and assess for site closure 24 hours after CVC removal.	Verifies healing and closure of the site.	- Abnormal healing
5. Daily assess the need for the CVC. If long-term use of the CVC is needed, consider changing the CVC every 7 days. **(Level C*)**	The Centers for Disease Control and Prevention (CDC)[7] and research findings[2] recommend that CVCs do not need to be changed more frequently than every 7 days. There are no specific recommendations regarding routine replacement of CVCs that need to be in place for greater than 7 days.[2,7,11] CVCs should be changed over a guidewire when emergently inserted (e.g., trauma resuscitation), the catheter malfunctions, a positive blood culture is obtained after the CVC was inserted, or sepsis develops without an identified source.[2]	- Signs and symptoms of infection at the CVC catheter insertion site - Signs and symptoms of sepsis

*Level C: Qualitative studies, descriptive or correlational studies, integrative reviews, systematic reviews, or randomized controlled trials with inconsistent results

Patient Monitoring and Care —*Continued*

Steps	Rationale	Reportable Conditions
	CVCs should be removed and reinserted at a new site when there is a skin infection at the catheter insertion site (i.e., redness, swelling, or drainage at or around the insertion site) or a positive culture at the insertion site.[2]	
6. Follow institution standard for assessing pain. Administer analgesia as prescribed.	Identifies need for pain interventions.	Continued pain despite pain interventions

Documentation

Documentation should include the following:
- Patient and family education
- Date and time of catheter removal
- Site assessment
- Pain assessment, interventions, and effectiveness

- Application of air occlusive dressing
- Patient tolerance of the procedure
- Unexpected outcomes and interventions

References

CR 1. Ely EW, et al: Venous air embolism from central venous catheterization: a need for increased physician awareness, *Crit Care Med* 27:2113-2117, 1999.

CR 2. Eyer S, et al: Catheter-related sepsis: prospective, randomized study of three methods of long-term catheter maintainence, *Crit Care Med* 18:1073-1079, 1990.

CR 3. Hsiung GR, Swanson PD: Cerebral air embolism after central venous catheter removal, *Neurolgy* 55:1063-1064, 2000.

CR 4. Kim DK, et al: The CVC removal distress syndrome: an unappreciated complication of central venous catheter removal, *Am Surgeon* 64:344-347, 1998.

CR 5. McCarthy PM, et al: Air embolism in single-lung transplant patients after central venous catheter removal, *Chest* 107:1178-1179, 1995.

CR 6. Mennim P, Cormac FC, Taylor JD: Venous air embolism associated with removal of central venous catheter, *BMJ* 305:171-172, 1992.

CR 7. O'Grady NP, et al: Guidelines for the prevention of intravascular catheter-related infections, *Am J Infect Control* 30:476-489, 2002.

8. Oztekin DS, et al: Comparison of complications and procedural activities of pulmonary artery catheter removal by critical care nurses versus medical doctors, *Nurs Crit Care* 13:105-115, 2008.

CR 9. Pronovost PJ, Wu AW, Sexton JB: Acute decompensation after removing a central line: practical approaches to increasing safety in the intensive care unit, *Ann Intern Med* 140:1025-1033, 2004.

CR 10. Rountree WD: Removal of pulmonary artery catheters by registered nurses: a study in safety and complications, *Focus Crit Care* 18:313-318, 1991.

CR 11. Safdar N, Klugar DM, Maki DG: A review of risk factors for catheter-related bloodstream infection caused by percutaneously inserted, noncuffed central venous catheters: implications for preventive strategies, *Medicine* 81:466-472, 2002.

CR 12. Turnage WS, Harper JV: Venous air embolism occurring after removal of a central venous catheter, *Anesth Analg* 72:559-560, 1991.

CR 13. Wadas TM: Pulmonary artery catheter removal, *Crit Care Nurse* 14:62-72, 1994.

Additional Reading

Deceuninck O, DeRoy L, Moruzi S, et al: Massive air embolism after central venous catheter removal, *Circulation* 116:e516-e518, 2007.

Central Venous Catheter Site Care

P U R P O S E : Site care of the central venous catheter allows for assessment and care of the catheter insertion site.

Teresa Preuss, Debra Lynn-McHale Wiegand

PREREQUISITE NURSING KNOWLEDGE

- Understanding of the principles of aseptic technique is needed.
- Knowledge of the signs and symptoms of catheter-related infection and sepsis is necessary.
- Most serious catheter-related infections are associated with central venous catheters (CVCs), especially those that are placed in the intensive care setting.[7]
- Bloodstream infections related to the use of CVCs are an important cause of patient morbidity, mortality, and increased healthcare costs.[2]
- Topical antibiotic ointment or creams are not recommended on the catheter insertion site. The use of antibiotic ointment or cream can potentially promote fungal infections and antimicrobial resistance.[7,8]

EQUIPMENT

- Nonsterile and sterile gloves
- Transparent dressing or sterile 4 × 4 gauze
- Roll of 2-inch tape
- Face mask
- Prepackaged sterile dressing kit (may include some of the above items)
- Antiseptic solution (e.g., 2% chlorhexidine based)
- Chlorhexidine-impregnated sponge
  Additional equipment as needed includes the following:
- Stabilizing device (used with nonsutured central venous catheters)

PATIENT AND FAMILY EDUCATION

- Explain the dressing change procedure. **➤➤***Rationale:* Explanation prepares the patient and decreases patient anxiety.
- Explain the importance of patient positioning during the dressing change. **➤➤***Rationale:* Patient cooperation is increased; the potential for contamination is decreased.

PATIENT ASSESSMENT AND PREPARATION

Patient Assessment

- Assess the patient's arm, shoulder, neck, and chest on the same side as the catheter insertion site for signs of pain, swelling, or tenderness. Assess the patient's leg size and assess for signs of pain, swelling, or tenderness on the same side as the catheter insertion site if the CVC is placed in the femoral vein. **➤➤***Rationale:* Assessment evaluates for thrombophlebitis or venous thrombosis.
- Assess for signs and symptoms of infection. Signs and symptoms may include redness, swelling, and drainage at the catheter site or fever, chills, and positive blood cultures. **➤➤***Rationale:* Infection is a potential complication of any invasive catheter.
- Assess the patient's history for sensitivity to antiseptic solutions. **➤➤***Rationale:* Assessment decreases risk for allergic reactions.

Patient Preparation

- Verify correct patient with two identifiers. ➛*Rationale:* Prior to performing a procedure, the nurse should ensure the correct identification of the patient for the intended intervention.
- Ensure that the patient and family understand preprocedural teaching. Answer questions as they arise, and reinforce information as needed. ➛*Rationale:* Understanding of previously taught information is evaluated and reinforced.
- If the patient is on ventilatory support, assess the patient's need for suctioning before beginning the procedure. Femoral catheter sites need to be inspected for potential contamination with urine or stool. ➛*Rationale:* The risk for catheter site contamination by secretions or excretions is minimized.

Procedure for Central Venous Catheter Site Care

Steps	Rationale	Special Considerations
1. HH		
2. PE		
3. Prepare supplies.	Prepares equipment.	
4. Position the patient so that the CVC site is easily accessible.	Prepares for dressing change.	If the CVC is in the femoral vein, extend the patient's leg and ensure the groin area is adequately exposed while maintaining patient privacy and comfort.
5. Have the patient turn his or her head away from the catheter insertion site (if performing site care on an internal jugular or subclavian catheter).	Decreases the risk for site contamination.	
6. Apply a face mask.	Reduces the transmission of microorganisms.	
7. Remove and discard the central venous catheter dressing.	Exposes the catheter site for inspection and site care.	
8. Inspect the catheter, insertion site, and surrounding skin.	Assesses for signs of infection, catheter dislodgment, leakage, or loose sutures.	
9. Remove and discard gloves in the appropriate receptacle.	Removes and safely discards used supplies.	
10. HH		
11. Apply sterile gloves.	Maintains aseptic and sterile technique.	
12. Cleanse the skin, catheter, and stabilizing device with 2% chlorhexidine-based preparation.[1-3,5,7,8] **(Level A*)**	Reduces the rate of recolonization of skin flora.	Allow the solution to dry.
13. Apply chlorhexidine impregnated sponge to site.[6-8] **(Level D*)**	Reduces the transmission of microorganisms.	Follow institution standard.
14. Apply a sterile air occlusive dressing.	Provides a sterile environment.	Use either a transparent dressing alone or gauze dressing with tape. If the patient is diaphoretic or if the site is bleeding or oozing, a gauze dressing is preferred.[7]
15. Document date and time of dressing change on the external dressing.	Indicates when the dressing was changed.	
16. Discard used supplies in appropriate receptacles.		
17. HH	Removes and safely discards used supplies.	

*Level A: Meta-analysis of quantitative studies or metasynthesis of qualitative studies with results that consistently support a specific action, intervention, or treatment
*Level D: Peer-reviewed professional organizational standards with clinical studies to support recommendations

Procedure continues on following page

Expected Outcomes

- Dressing remains dry, sterile, and intact
- Catheter site remains free from infection
- Catheter remains in place without dislodgment

Unexpected Outcomes

- Catheter-related infection
- Accidental removal or dislodgement of the catheter
- Impaired integrity of the skin under the dressing

Patient Monitoring and Care

Steps	Rationale	Reportable Conditions
		These conditions should be reported if they persist despite nursing interventions.
1. Replace gauze dressings every 2 days and transparent dressings at least every 7 days.[4,7] **(Level D*)** Follow institution standard.	Decreases the risk for infection at the catheter site. The Centers for Disease Control and Prevention (CDC) recommends replacing the dressing when it becomes damp, loosened, or soiled or when inspection of the site is necessary.[7]	
2. Assess for signs and symptoms of infection.	The catheter should be removed if signs of infection are present.	• Signs and symptoms of infection at catheter insertion site • Signs and symptoms of sepsis
3. Follow institution standard for assessing pain. Administer analgesia as prescribed.	Identifies need for pain interventions.	• Continued pain despite pain interventions

Documentation

Documentation should include the following:

- Patient and family education
- Date and time of the procedure
- Assessment of the catheter site
- Type of dressing applied

- Date and time of dressing change and initials or signature of the person changing the dressing (also documented on the dressing)
- Unexpected outcomes
- Additional interventions
- Pain assessment, interventions, and effectiveness

*Level D: Peer-reviewed professional organizational standards with clinical studies to support recommendations

References

1. Balamongkhon B, Thamlikitkul V: Implementation of chlorhexidine gluconate for central venous catheter site care at Siriraj Hospital, Bangkok, Thailand, *Am J Infect Control* 35:585-588, 2007.
CR 2. Chaiyakunapruk N, Veenstra DL, Lipsky BA, et al: Chlorhexidine compared with povidone-iodine solution for vascular catheter-site care: a meta-analysis, *Ann Intern Med* 136:792-807, 2002.
CR 3. Eggimann P, Harbarth S, Constantin M: Impact of a prevention strategy targeted at vascular-access care on incidence of infections acquired in intensive care, *Lancet* 355:1864-1868, 2000.
4. Infusion Nurses Society: Infusion nursing standards of practice, *J Infus Nurs* 29:S1-S92, 2006.
5. Maenthaisong R, Chaiyakunapruk N, Visanu T: Cost-effective analysis of chlorhexidine gluconate compared with povidone-iodine solution for catheter-site care in Siriraj Hospital, Thailand, *J Med Assoc Thai* 89:S94-S101, 2006.
CR 6. Maki DG, Narans LL, Knasinski V, et al: Prospective, randomized, investigator-masked trial of novel chlohexidine-impregnated disk (Biopatch) on central

venous and arterial catheters [abstract], *Infect Control Hosp Epidemiol* 21:96, 2000.
CR 7. O'Grady NP, et al: Guidelines for the prevention of intravascular catheter-related infections, *Am J Infect Control* 30:476-89, 2002.
CR 8. Safdar N, Klugar DM, Maki DG: A review of risk factors for catheter-related bloodstream infection caused by percutaneously inserted, noncuffed central venous catheters: implications for preventive strategies, *Medicine* 81:466-472, 2002.

Additional Readings

Alexander M, Corrigan A, Gorski L, eds: *Infusion Nurses Society Infusion Nursing: An Evidence-Based Approach,* ed 3, 2010, Saunders.
CR Gillies D, et al: Gauze and tape and transparent polyurethane dressings for central venous catheters, Cochrane Database Sys Rev, Chichester, UK, 2003, John Wiley & Sons, Ltd.
Maki DG, Kluger DM, Crnich CJ: The risk of bloodstream infection in adults with different intravascular devices: a system review of 200 published prospective studies, *May Clin Proc* 81:1159-1171, 2006.

Central Venous/Right Atrial Pressure Monitoring

P U R P O S E : Central venous/right atrial pressure monitoring provides information about the patient's intravascular volume status and right ventricular preload. The central venous pressure or the right atrial pressure allows for evaluation of right-sided heart hemodynamics and evaluation of patient response to therapy. Central venous pressure and right atrial pressure are used interchangeably.

Teresa Preuss, Debra Lynn-McHale Wiegand

PREREQUISITE NURSING KNOWLEDGE

- Knowledge of the normal anatomy and physiology of the cardiovascular system is needed.
- Knowledge of the principles of aseptic technique and infection control is necessary.
- Knowledge is needed of the principles of hemodynamic monitoring.
- The central venous pressure (CVP)/right atrial pressure (RAP) represents right-sided heart preload or the volume of blood found in the right ventricle at the end of diastole.
- CVP/RAP influences and is influenced by venous return and cardiac function. Although the CVP/RAP is used as a measure of changes in the right ventricle, the relationship is not linear. Because the right ventricle has the ability to expand and alter its compliance, changes in volume can occur with little change in pressure.
- The CVP/RAP normally ranges from 2 to 8 mm Hg in the adult.
- The central venous catheter is inserted in a central vein with the tip of the catheter placed in the proximal superior vena cava.
- Knowledge is needed of the setup, leveling, and zeroing of the hemodynamic monitoring system (see Procedure 76).
- Understanding of *a*, *c*, and *v* waves is necessary. The *a* wave reflects right atrial contraction. The *c* wave reflects closure of the tricuspid valve. The *v* wave reflects the right atrial filling during ventricular systole. The CVP/RAP measurement is the mean of the *a* wave.
- CVP/RAP values are useful in evaluation of volume status, effect of medication therapy (especially medication that decreases preload), and cardiac function (Table 70-1).
- Monitoring parameters from the femoral catheter is not recommended. The catheter is too distant from the right atrium to produce reliable data.

TABLE 70-1	Central Venous Pressure
Conditions Causing Increased CVP	
Elevated intravascular volume	
Depressed right-sided cardiac function (RV infarct, RV failure)	
Cardiac tamponade	
Constrictive pericarditis	
Pulmonary hypertension	
Chronic left ventricular failure	
Conditions Causing Decreased CVP	
Reduced intravascular volume*	
Decreased mean arterial pressure (MAP)	
Venodilation	

*Although the measured CVP is low, cardiac function may be depressed, normal, or hyperdynamic when there is reduced vascular volume.
RV, Right ventricular.

EQUIPMENT

* Pressure transducer system, including flush solution recommended according to institution standard, a pressure bag or device, pressure tubing with transducer, and flush device (see Procedure 76)
* Pressure module and cable for interface with the monitor
* Dual-channel recorder
* Leveling device (low-intensity laser or carpenter level)
* Nonsterile gloves
* Nonvented caps

Additional equipment to have available as needed includes the following:

* Indelible marker

PATIENT AND FAMILY EDUCATION

* Discuss the purpose of the central venous catheter and monitoring with both the patient and family. ➤➤*Rationale:* This discussion reduces anxiety and includes the patient and family in the plan of care.
* Explain the patient's expected participation during the procedure. ➤➤*Rationale:* The explanation encourages patient assistance.

PATIENT ASSESSMENT AND PREPARATION

Patient Assessment

* Determine hemodynamic, cardiovascular, and peripheral vascular status. ➤➤*Rationale:* This assessment provides baseline data.

* Determine the patient's baseline pulmonary status. If the patient is mechanically ventilated, note the type of support, ventilator mode, and presence or absence of positive end-expiratory pressure (PEEP) or continuous positive airway pressure (CPAP). ➤➤*Rationale:* The presence of mechanical ventilation alters hemodynamic waveforms and pressures.
* Assess for signs and symptoms of fluid volume deficit. Signs and symptoms may include thirst, oliguria, tachycardia, and dry mucous membranes. ➤➤*Rationale:* Assessment data should correlate with a decreased CVP/RAP value.
* Assess for signs and symptoms of fluid volume excess. Signs and symptoms may include dyspnea, abnormal breath sounds (i.e., crackles), S_3 heart sound, peripheral edema, tachycardia, and jugular vein distention. ➤➤*Rationale:* Assessment data should correlate with an increased CVP/RAP value.

Patient Preparation

* Verify correct patient with two identifiers. ➤➤*Rationale:* Prior to performing a procedure, the nurse should ensure the correct identification of the patient for the intended intervention.
* Ensure that the patient and family understand teaching. Answer questions as they arise, and reinforce information as needed. ➤➤*Rationale:* Understanding of previously taught information is evaluated and reinforced.
* Place the patient in the supine position with the head of the bed flat or elevated up to 45 degrees. ➤➤*Rationale:* This positioning prepares the patient for hemodynamic monitoring.

Procedure	for Central Venous/Right Atrial Pressure Monitoring	
Steps	**Rationale**	**Special Considerations**
1. **HH**		
2. **PE**		
3. Position the patient in the supine position with the head of the bed from 0 to 45 degrees. **(Level B*)**	Studies have determined that the CVP/RAP is accurate in this position.[3-5,7,11,13,15,26,27]	CVP/RAP may be accurate for patients in the supine position with the head of the bed elevated up to 60 degrees,[5,15] but additional studies are needed to support this. Only one study[12] supports the accuracy of hemodynamic values for patients in the lateral positions; other studies do not.[3,9,11,19,25] The majority of studies support the accuracy of hemodynamic monitoring for patients in the prone position.[1,2,8,10,14,20,24] Two studies demonstrated that prone positioning caused an increase in hemodynamic values.[21,23]

*Level B: Well-designed, controlled studies with results that consistently support a specific action, intervention, or treatment

Procedure for Central Venous/Right Atrial Pressure Monitoring—*Continued*

Steps	Rationale	Special Considerations
4. Level the air-fluid interface of the monitoring system to the phlebostatic axis (see Procedure 76 and Figs. 76-7 and 76-9).	The phlebostatic axis is at approximately the level of the atria and should be used as the reference point for the air-fluid interface.	Mark the location of the phlebostatic axis if not already identified.
5. Zero the transducer (see Procedure 76).	Allows the monitor to use atmospheric pressure as a reference for zero.	
6. Run a dual-channel strip of the electrocardiogram (ECG) and CVP/RAP waveform (Fig. 70-1).	Right atrial pressures should be determined from the graphic recording so that end expiration can be properly identified.	Some monitors have the capability of "freeze framing" waveforms. A cursor can be used to determine pressure measurements.
7. Measure the CVP/RAP at end expiration.	Measurement is most accurate as the effects of intrathoracic pressure changes are minimized.	
8. With the dual-channel recorded strip, draw a vertical line from the beginning of the P wave of one of the ECG complexes down to the CVP/RAP waveform. Repeat this with the next ECG complex (see Fig. 73-7).	Compares electrical activity with mechanical activity. Usually, three waves are present on the CVP/RAP waveform.	At times, the *c* wave is not present.
9. Align the PR interval with the CVP/RAP waveform (see Fig. 73-7).	The *a* wave correlates with this interval.	
10. Identify the *a* wave (see Fig. 70-1).	The *a* wave is seen approximately 80 to 100 ms after the P wave. The *c* wave follows the *a* wave, and the *v* wave follows the *c* wave.	The *a* wave reflects atrial contraction. The *c* wave reflects closure of the tricuspid valve. The *v* wave reflects passive filling of the right atrium.

Procedure continues on following page

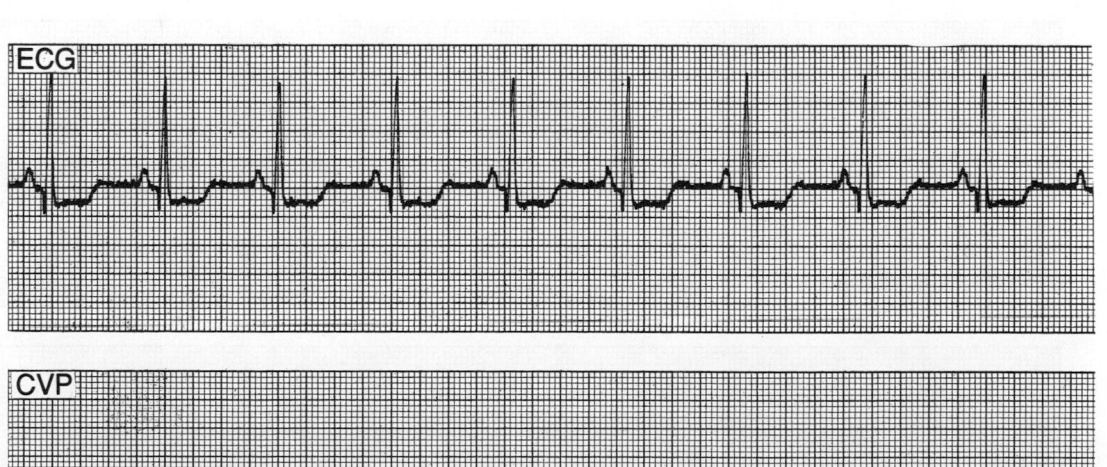

FIGURE 70-1 CVP waveform with *a, c,* and *v* waves present. The *a* wave is usually seen just after the *p* wave of the ECG. The *c* wave appears at the time of the RST junction on the ECG. The *v* wave is seen in the TP interval.

Procedure   for Central Venous/Right Atrial Pressure Monitoring—*Continued*

Steps	Rationale	Special Considerations
11. Identify the scale of the CVP/RAP tracing (see Figs. 70-2 and 73-8).	Aids in determining the pressure measurement.	The RAP scale commonly is set at 20 mm Hg. Scale settings may vary based on monitoring equipment.
12. Measure the mean of the *a* wave to obtain the RAP (Fig. 70-2; see Fig 73-8).	The *a* wave represents atrial contraction and reflects ventricular filling at end diastole.	
13. Discard used supplies in appropriate receptacles.	Removes and safely discards used supplies.	
14. 🅷🅷		

Expected Outcomes

- Accurate CVP/RAP measurements
- Adequate and appropriate waveforms
- CVP/RAP readings that correlate with physical findings
- Evaluation of information obtained to guide therapeutic interventions

Unexpected Outcomes

- Inaccurate readings
- CVP/RAP readings that do not correlate with physical findings
- Infection
- Sepsis
- Occluded catheter

Patient Monitoring and Care

Steps	Rationale	Reportable Conditions
		These conditions should be reported if they persist despite nursing interventions.
1. Recheck leveling whenever the patient position changes.	Ensures an accurate reference point at phlebostatic axis.	

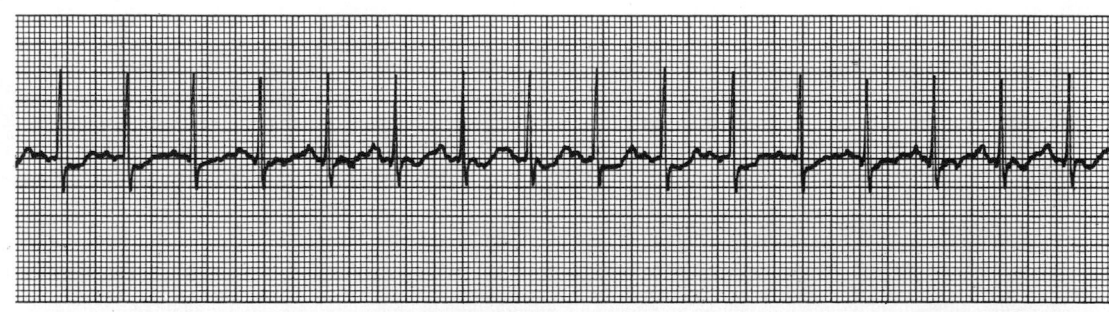

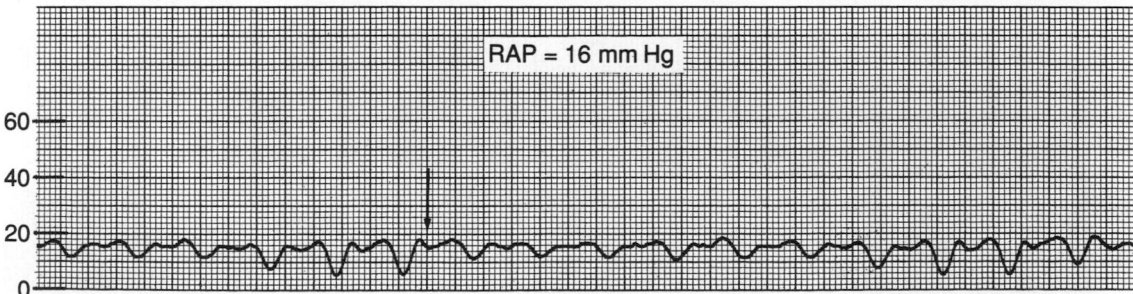

FIGURE 70-2   Reading the RAP from paper printout at end expiration in a spontaneously breathing patient. While observing the patient, identify inspiration. The point just before inspiration is end expiration. *Arrow* indicates the point of end expiration. Reading is taken as a mean value. The RAP value for this patient is 16 mm Hg.

Patient Monitoring and Care —*Continued*

Steps	Rationale	Reportable Conditions
2. Zero the transducer during initial setup or before insertion, if disconnection occurs between the transducer and the monitoring cable, if disconnection occurs between the monitoring cable and the monitor, and when the values obtained do not fit the clinical picture. Follow manufacturer's recommendations regarding routine zeroing of the system.	Ensures accuracy of the hemodynamic monitoring system; minimizes the risk for contamination of the system.	
3. Monitor the pressure transducer system (pressure tubing, transducer, stopcocks, etc) for air and eliminate air from the system.	Air emboli are potentially fatal.	
4. Assess central venous catheter patency every 8 hours and administer thrombolytics as prescribed if the catheter is occluded.[6,22] **(Level B*)**	Ensures catheter patency.	• Occluded catheter
5. Continuously monitor the CVP/RAP waveform and obtain the hemodynamic value hourly and as necessary with changes in patient condition. Follow institution standard.	Provides for continuous waveform analysis and assessment of patient status.	• Abnormal CVP/RAP values or waveforms
6. Change the hemodynamic monitoring system (flush solution, pressure tubing, transducer, and stopcocks) every 96 hours. **(Level B)** The flush solution may need to be changed more frequently if near empty of solution.	The Centers for Disease Control and Prevention (CDC)[17] and research findings[16,18] recommend that the hemodynamic flush system can be used safely for 96 hours. This recommendation is based on research conducted with disposable pressure monitoring systems used for peripheral and central lines.	
7. Perform a dynamic response test (square wave test) at the start of each shift, with a change of the waveform, or when the system is opened to air (see Fig. 62-3).	An optimally damped system provides an accurate waveform.	• Overdamped or underdamped waveforms that cannot be corrected with troubleshooting procedures
8. Maintain the pressure bag or device at 300 mm Hg.	At 300 mm Hg, each flush device delivers approximately 1 to 3 mL/hr to maintain patency of the system.	
9. Obtain a CVP/RAP waveform strip to place on the patient's chart at the start of each shift and whenever there is a change in the waveform or patient condition.	Allows assessment of the waveform and the CVP/RAP measurement.	

Documentation

Documentation should include the following:
- Patient and family education
- CVP/RAP pressures and waveform
- Site assessment
- Occurrence of unexpected outcomes and interventions

*Level B: Well-designed, controlled studies with results that consistently support a specific action, intervention, or treatment

References

CR 1. Blanch L, et al: Short-term effect of prone position in critically ill patients with acute respiratory distress syndrome, *Intensive Care Med* 23:1003-1039, 1997.

CR 2. Brussel T, et al: Mechanical ventilation in the prone position for acute respiratory failure after cardiac surgery, *J Cardiothorac Vasc Anesth* 7:541-546, 1993.

CR 3. Cason CL, et al: Effects of backrest elevation and position on pulmonary artery pressures, *Cardiovasc Nurs* 26:1-5, 1990.

CR 4. Chulay M, Miller T: The effect of backrest elevation on pulmonary artery and pulmonary capillary wedge pressures in patients after cardiac surgery, *Heart Lung* 13:138-140, 1984.

CR 5. Clochesy J, Hinshaw AD, Otto CW: Effects of change of position on pulmonary artery and pulmonary capillary wedge pressure in mechanically ventilated patients, *NITA* 7:223-225, 1984.

CR 6. Deitcher SR, et al: Safety and efficacy of alteplase for restoring function in occluded central venous catheters: results of the cardiovascular thrombolytic to open occluded lines trial, *J Clin Oncol* 20:317-324, 2002.

CR 7. Dobbin K, et al: Pulmonary artery pressure measurement in patients with elevated pressures: effect of backrest elevation and method of measurement, *Am J Crit Care* 1:61-69, 1992.

CR 8. Fridrich P, et al: The effects of long-term prone positioning in patients with trauma-induced adult respiratory distress syndrome, *Anesth Analg* 83:1206-1211, 1996.

CR 9. Groom L, Frisch SR, Elliot M: Reproducibility and accuracy of pulmonary artery pressure measurement in supine and lateral positions, *Heart Lung* 19:147-151, 1990.

CR 10. Jolliet P, Bulpa P, Chevrolet JC: Effects of prone position on gas exchange and hemodynamics in severe acute respiratory distress syndrome, *Crit Care Med* 26:1977-1985, 1998.

CR 11. Keating D, et al: Effect of sidelying positions on pulmonary artery pressures, *Heart Lung* 15:605-610, 1986.

CR 12. Kennedy GT, Bryant A, Crawford MH: The effects of lateral body positioning on measurements of pulmonary artery and pulmonary wedge pressures, *Heart Lung* 13:155-158, 1984.

CR 13. Lambert CW, Cason CL: Backrest elevation and pulmonary artery pressures: research analysis, *Dimens Crit Care Nurs* 9:327-335, 1990.

CR 14. Langer M, et al: The prone position in ARDS patients, *Chest* 94:103-107, 1982.

CR 15. Laulive JL: Pulmonary artery pressures and position changes in the critically ill adult, *Dimens Crit Care Nurs* 1:28-34, 1982.

CR 16. Luskin RL, et al: Extended use of disposable pressure transducers: a bacteriologic evaluation, *JAMA* 255:916-920, 1986.

CR 17. O'Grady NP, et al: Guidelines for the prevention of intravascular catheter-related infections, *Am J Infect Control* 30:476-489, 2002.

CR 18. O'Malley MK, et al: Value of routine pressure monitoring system changes after 72 hours of use, *Crit Care Med* 22:1424-1430, 1994.

CR 19. Osida C: Measurement of pulmonary artery pressures: supine verses side-lying head elevated positions, *Heart Lung* 18:298-299, 1989.

CR 20. Pappert D, et al: Influence of positioning on ventilation-perfusion relationships in severe adult respiratory distress syndrome, *Chest* 106:1511-1516, 1994.

CR 21. Pelosi P, et al: Effects of the prone position on respiratory mechanics and gas exchange during acute lung injury, *Am J Respir Crit Care Med* 157:387-393, 1998.

CR 22. Ponec D, et al: Recombinant tissue plasminogen activator (Alteplase) for restoration of flow in occluded central venous access devices: a double-blind placebo-controlled trial: the cardiovascular thrombolytic to open occluded lines (COOL) efficacy trial, *J Vasc Interv Radiol* 12: 951-955, 2001.

CR 23. Voggenreiter G, et al: Intermittent prone positioning in the treatment of severe and moderate posttraumatic lung injury, *Crit Care Med* 27:2375-2382, 1999.

CR 24. Vollman KM, Bander JJ: Improved oxygenation utilizing a prone positioner in patients with acute respiratory distress syndrome, *Intensive Care Med* 22:1105-1111, 1996.

CR 25. Wild L: Effect of lateral recumbent positions on measurement of pulmonary artery and pulmonary artery wedge pressures in critically ill adults, *Heart Lung* 13:305, 1984.

CR 26. Wilson AE, et al: Effect of backrest position on hemodynamic and right ventricular measurements in critically ill adults, *Am J Crit Care* 5:264-270, 1996.

CR 27. Woods SL, Mansfield LW: Effect of body position upon pulmonary artery and pulmonary capillary wedge pressures in noncritically ill patients, *Heart Lung* 5:83-90, 1976.

Additional Readings

Bridges EJ: Pulmonary artery pressure monitoring: when, how, and what else to use, *AACN Adv Crit Care* 17: 286-305, 2006.

CR Darovic GO: *Hemodynamic monitoring: invasive and noninvasive clinical application,* ed 3, Philadelphia, 2002, Saunders.

CR Keckeisen M: *Protocols for practice: hemodynamic monitoring series: pulmonary artery pressure monitoring,* Aliso Viejo, CA, 1997, American Association of Critical-Care Nurses.

Magder S: Invasive intravascular hemodynamic monitoring: technical issues, *Crit Care Clin* 23:401-414, 2007.

Left Atrial Catheter: Care and Assisting with Removal

P U R P O S E :   The left atrial catheter measures pressure from the left atrium for assessment of left ventricular function after cardiac surgery in the setting of severe left ventricular dysfunction, pulmonary hypertension, presence of circulatory assist devices, or cardiac transplantation.[2] The left atrial catheter provides information about left-sided intracardiac pressure. Hemodynamic information obtained with the left atrial catheter is used to guide therapeutic interventions, including administration of fluids and medications and titration of vasoactive and inotropic medications.

Barbara Leeper

PREREQUISITE NURSING KNOWLEDGE

- Knowledge of the cardiovascular anatomy and physiology is necessary.
- Understanding of basic dysrhythmia recognition and treatment of life-threatening dysrhythmias is needed.
- Advanced cardiac life support knowledge and skills are necessary.
- Understanding is needed of the setup of the hemodynamic monitoring system (see Procedure 76).
- Understanding of hemodynamic monitoring is necessary (see Procedure 73).
- Principles of aseptic technique should be understood.
- The left atrial pressure (LAP) waveform is configured similarly to that of a pulmonary artery occlusion pressure or pulmonary artery wedge pressure waveform (Fig. 71-1).
- Understanding of *a*, *c*, and *v* waves is necessary. The *a* wave reflects left atrial contraction. The *c* wave reflects closure of the mitral valve. The *v* wave reflects passive filling of the left atrium during left ventricular systole.
- The LAP is measured with a polyvinyl catheter placed in the left atrium during cardiac surgery. The left atrial catheter can be inserted via a needle puncture of the right superior pulmonary vein, with subsequent threading into the left atrium, or it can be inserted via direct cannulation

of the left atrium through a needle puncture at the intraatrial groove.[20]
- LAP monitoring may be used in the following situations:
  - ❖ For patients with prosthetic tricuspid or pulmonic valves, in whom pulmonary artery catheters are contraindicated

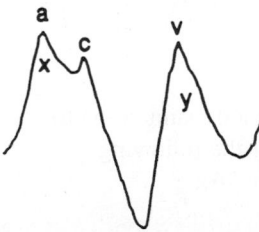

FIGURE 71-1   LAP (left atrial pressure) waveform and its components: *a* wave, the presystolic wave resulting from atrial contraction; *x* descent, the downslope of the *a* wave caused by atrial relaxation; *c* wave, a sharp inflection caused by mitral valve closure; *v* wave, an atrial pressure wave rising to a peak during late ventricular systole caused by filling of the atrium while the mitral valve is closed; *y* descent, the downslope of the *v* wave caused by early diastolic runoff through the mitral valve. Changes in the waveform configuration may indicate valve or myocardial disease. For example, an elevated *a* wave is seen in mitral stenosis and an elevated *v* wave in mitral insufficiency. Both the *a* and the *v* waves are elevated in cardiac tamponade.

❖ For patients with abnormal heart anatomy (e.g., those with a single ventricle or tricuspid atresia)

❖ For patients with high pulmonary artery pressures, which may interfere with the correlation of pulmonary artery diastolic pressure (PADP) with pulmonary artery occlusion pressure (PAOP)

❖ For accurate information when vasoconstriction medications are infused in conjunction with pulmonary vasodilator medications

❖ For patient monitoring after cardiac transplantation

• The normal LAP is 4 to 12 mm Hg.

• One danger with use of this catheter is the potential for air or a blood clot embolus to enter the left atrium and be carried to the brain or other body organs. Close attention to the hemodynamic monitoring system and assessment of the waveform are imperative.

EQUIPMENT

• Left atrial catheter (inserted in the operating room)
• Hemodynamic monitoring system (see Procedure 76).
• Sterile dressing supplies
• Indelible marker
• Nonsterile gloves and mask
• Gown and goggles or face shield

Additional equipment to have available, if needed, includes the following:

• Air filter (institution-specific) between the left atrial (LA) catheter and the pressure transducer tubing
• Suture removal kit or supplies

PATIENT AND FAMILY EDUCATION

• Assess the patient and family understanding of LAP monitoring. ➛*Rationale:* Assessment provides information about patient and family knowledge.

• Discuss the purpose of the catheter. ➛*Rationale:* This discussion informs the patient and family about the catheter and may also decrease anxiety.

• Discuss with the patient and family the location of the catheter and the importance of not touching the catheter or putting tension on the catheter tubing. ➛*Rationale:* This discussion may prevent LA catheter contamination and inadvertent LA catheter removal.

PATIENT ASSESSMENT AND PREPARATION

Patient Assessment

• Assess the patient's hemodynamic, cardiovascular, peripheral vascular, and neurovascular status. ➛*Rationale:* The assessment provides baseline data that can be used to compare with the LAP.

• Assess the patient's current laboratory test results, including coagulation studies. ➛*Rationale:* Assessment identifies laboratory value abnormalities. Baseline coagulation studies are helpful in determining the risk for bleeding.

Patient Preparation

• Verify correct patient with two identifiers. ➛*Rationale:* Prior to performing a procedure, the nurse should ensure the correct identification of the patient for the intended intervention.

• Ensure that the patient and family understand teaching. Answer questions as they arise, and reinforce information as needed. ➛*Rationale:* Understanding of previously taught information is evaluated and reinforced.

• Consider administration of sedation as prescribed. ➛*Rationale:* An agitated or restless patient could accidentally pull out the LA catheter.

Procedure | for Care of the Left Atrial Catheter

Steps	Rationale	Special Considerations
1. **HH**		
2. **PE**		
3. Check the hemodynamic monitoring system for the following (see Procedure 76):	Ensures that the hemodynamic monitoring system is set up appropriately.	The LA hemodynamic monitoring system is set up in the operating room. **Do not use the rapid flush technique to ensure patency; this may introduce air into the catheter or system. The LA catheter should be flushed only if needed by a physician.** Follow institution standard.
A. Flush bag has solution.	Maintains catheter patency.	
B. Pressure in the flush bag is maintained at 300 mm Hg.	At 300 mm Hg, the flush system delivers 1 to 3 mL/hr to maintain patency of the system.	
C. Connections are tight.	Maintains a closed, sterile system.	
D. The entire system is air-free.	Reduces the risk for air embolization.	

Procedure   for Care of the Left Atrial Catheter—*Continued*

Steps	Rationale	Special Considerations
4. Connect the pressure cable from the left atrial transducer to the bedside monitor.	Connects the LA catheter to the bedside monitoring system.	
5. Set the scale on the bedside monitor for LAP monitoring.	Permits waveform analysis.	The scale for LAP is commonly set at 20 mm Hg. Scale settings may vary based on monitoring equipment.
6. Level the left atrial air-fluid interface (zeroing stopcock) to the phlebostatic axis (see Procedure 76).	The phlebostatic axis approximates the level of the atria and should be used as the reference point for patients in the supine position.	The reference point for the atria changes when a patient is in the lateral position (see Procedure 76).
7. Secure the system to the intravenous (IV) pole or patient's chest.	Ensures that the air-fluid interface (zeroing stopcock) is maintained at the level of the phlebostatic axis. If the air-fluid interface is above the phlebostatic axis, the LAP is falsely low. If the air-fluid interface is below the phlebostatic axis, the LAP is falsely high.	The point of the phlebostatic axis should be marked with an indelible marker.
8. Zero the left atrial hemodynamic monitoring system (see Procedure 76).	Zeroing negates the effects of atmospheric pressure.	
9. Position the patient in the supine position with the head of the bed from 0 to 30 degrees. **(Level C*)**	Ensures the accuracy of the LAP.	Studies have determined that right atrial (RA) and pulmonary artery (PA) pressures are accurate with the head of the bed elevated to 45 degrees.[3-7,12,14,15,23,24] A study conducted with LA catheters determined that LA pressures are accurate with the head of the bed elevated to 30 degrees.[21] Refer to Procedure 76 for information on lateral and prone positioning. Research for lateral and prone positioning has been conducted on PA catheters, not LA catheters.
10. Run a dual-channel strip of the electrocardiogram (ECG) and the left atrial waveform.	The LAP should be determined from the graphic strip as the effect of ventilation can be identified.	
11. Measure the LAP at end expiration.	Measurement is most accurate as the effects of pulmonary pressures are minimized.	
12. With the dual-channel recorded strip, draw a vertical line from the beginning of the P wave of one of the ECG complexes down to the LAP waveform. Repeat this with the next ECG complex.	Compares electrical activity with mechanical activity. Three waveforms are present between the two lines drawn.	
13. Align the end of a QRS complex of the ECG strip with the LAP waveform.	Compares electrical activity with mechanical activity.	

*Level C: Qualitative studies, descriptive or correlational studies, integrative reviews, systematic reviews, or randomized controlled trials with inconsistent results

Procedure continues on following page

Procedure   for Care of the Left Atrial Catheter—*Continued*

Steps	Rationale	Special Considerations
14. Identify the *a* wave.	The *a* wave correlates with the end of the P wave of the ECG. The *c* wave correlates with the middle of the QRS complex of the ECG. The *v* wave follows the *c* wave and correlates with the end of the T wave of the ECG.[17]	
15. Measure the mean of the *a* wave to obtain the LAP.	The *a* wave represents left atrial contraction and reflects left ventricular filling at end diastole.	If the patient's positive end-expiratory pressure (PEEP) is more than 10 mL H₂O, adjustments in determining the pressure may be necessary.
16. Set alarms. Upper and lower alarm limits are set on the basis of the patient's current clinical status and the LAP values.	Activates the bedside and central alarm system.	
17. Continuously monitor the waveform for any changes (overdamping, left ventricular waveform, or absence of a waveform) and correlate with changes in physical findings.	Indicates problems with the LA catheter that require troubleshooting.	Overdamping may be caused by a hypovolemic state, air in the system, or a clot in the catheter. The presence of a left ventricular waveform (Fig. 71-2) indicates that the catheter has migrated into the left ventricle. Cardiac arrest, a clotted catheter, a perforated left ventricle, or a problem within the hemodynamic monitoring system may cause an absent waveform. **It is important in all of these situations, *not* to irrigate the catheter.**[20]
18. **Do not use the LA catheter for blood withdrawal, routine administration of medications, or IV therapy. The catheter is for pressure monitoring.**	Each time the left atrial line is entered, there is a significant risk for introducing air emboli or bacteria directly into the heart.[8]	Follow institution standard. In rare circumstances, such as severe pulmonary hypertension, a physician may determine the need for placement of a left atrial catheter and prescribe a vasoactive medication or inotrope to be infused through the catheter.[9,10,11,13] This is not considered to be routine practice and is only performed in special cases. An IV push medication should rarely be administered through a LA catheter and should only be administered by a physician or advanced practice nurse.
19. Discard uses supplies in appropriate receptacles.	Removes and safely discards used supplies.	
20. **HH**		

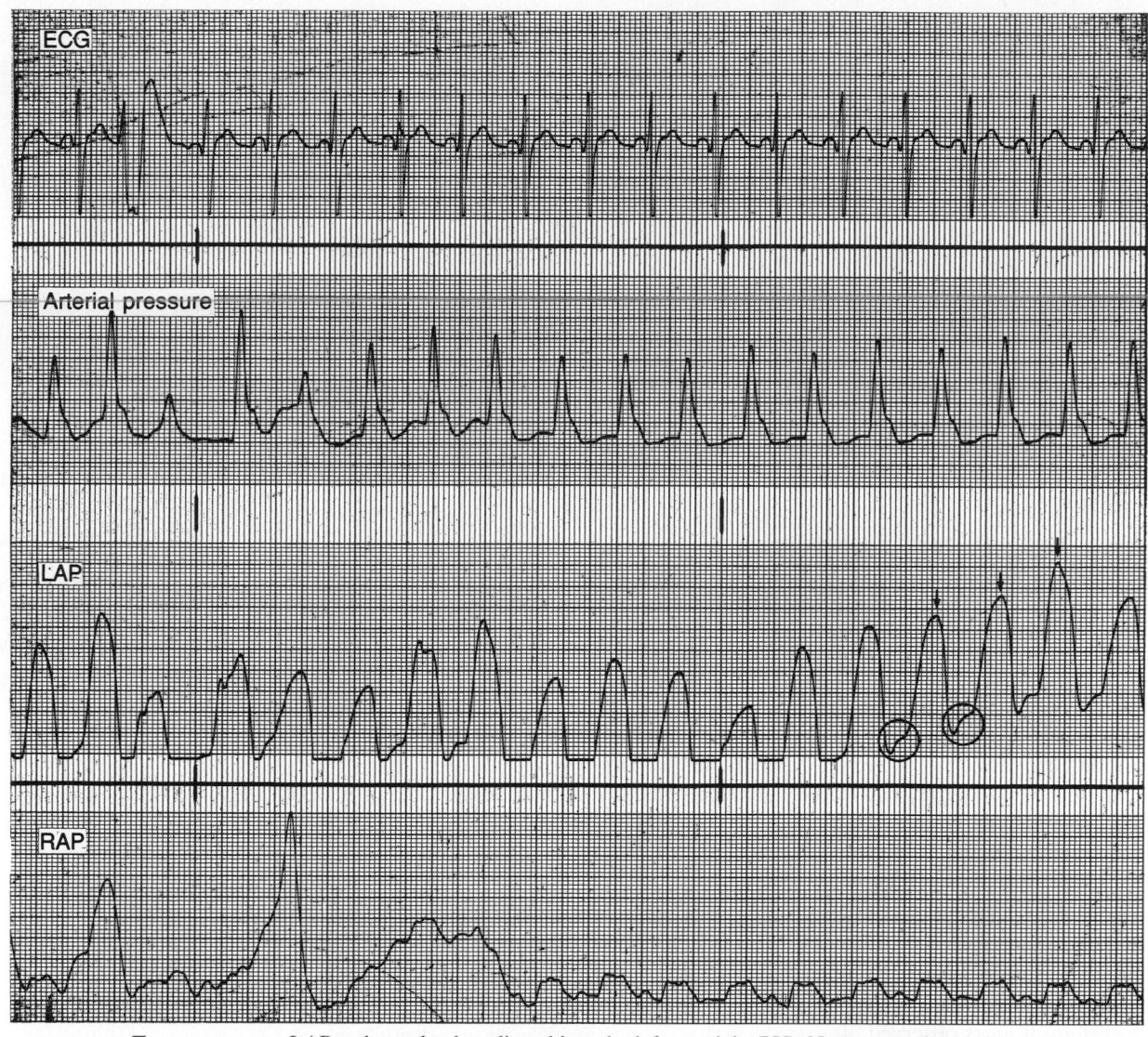

FIGURE 71-2   LAP catheter that has slipped into the left ventricle (LV). Note anacrotic notch on upstroke of LV waveform *(circled)*. Note also that paper was not calibrated in this example. *LAP,* left atrial pressure, *ECG,* electrocardiogram, *RAP,* right atrial pressure.

Procedure   for Assisting with Removal of the Left Atrial Catheter

Steps	Rationale	Special Considerations
1. **HH**		
2. **PE**		
3. Position the patient in the supine position.	Prepares the patient and provides access to the site.	All healthcare providers in the room should wear a face mask.
4. Turn off the LAP alarm.	Monitoring is no longer needed.	
5. Turn the stopcock off to the patient.	Turns off the administration of flush solution and stops hemodynamic monitoring.	
6. Remove the dressing.	Prepares for LA catheter removal.	
7. Clip the sutures if present.	Frees the LA catheter for removal.	
8. Assist the physician or advanced practice nurse as needed with catheter removal and hold firm pressure on the site.	Provides assistance if needed.	

Procedure continues on following page

Procedure   for Assisting with Removal of the Left Atrial Catheter—*Continued*

Steps	Rationale	Special Considerations
9. Apply a sterile occlusive dressing to the site.	Decreases the risk for infection until the insertion site has healed.	
10. Dispose of used supplies in appropriate receptacle.	Removes and safely discards used supplies.	
11. 🄷🄷		

Expected Outcomes

- Normal cerebral, myocardial, and peripheral perfusion
- LAP readings that correlate with physical findings
- Normal LAP value (4 to 12 mm Hg)
- LAP catheter removed when prescribed

Unexpected Outcomes

- Infection
- Hemorrhage at removal site
- Air embolus
- Cardiac tamponade caused by LA line removal.
- Retention, migration, or embolization of the catheter[20]

Patient Monitoring and Care

Steps	Rationale	Reportable Conditions
		These conditions should be reported if they persist despite nursing interventions.
1. Recheck leveling whenever patient position changes.	Ensures accurate reference point for the left atrium.	
2. Continuously monitor the LA waveform and obtain pressure measurements every hour and as needed. Follow institution standard.	Identifies trends in monitoring.	• Abnormal LAP values and waveforms
3. Monitor the LAP hemodynamic monitoring system every 1 to 2 hours for integrity of the system and for presence of air bubbles in the system. If air is observed, it must be removed immediately.	Air emboli are potentially fatal.	• Suspected air emboli • Air in the system that requires assistance with removal
4. Zero the transducer at the time of the patient's admission to the intensive care unit (ICU), if the transducer and the monitoring cable become disconnected, if the monitoring cable and the monitor become disconnected, and when the values obtained do not fit the clinical picture. Follow manufacturer's recommendations.	Ensures the accuracy of the hemodynamic monitoring system.	
5. Change the hemodynamic monitoring system (flush solution, pressure tubing, transducer, and stopcock) every 96 hours. **(Level B*)**	The Centers for Disease Control and Prevention (CDC)[18] and research findings[16,18,19] recommend that the hemodynamic flush system can be used safely for 96 hours. This recommendation is based on research conducted with disposable pressure monitoring systems used for peripheral and central lines. No studies report these data specific to left atrial catheters.	

*Level B: Well-designed, controlled studies with results that consistently support a specific action, intervention, or treatment

Patient Monitoring and Care —*Continued*

Steps	Rationale	Reportable Conditions
6. Replace gauze dressings every 2 days and transparent dressings at least every 7 days.[14,22] **(Level D*)**	Decreases the risk for infection at the catheter site. The CDC[18] has made no recommendations specifically for the frequency of routine LA catheter dressing changes. The CDC[18] recommends replacing dressings when the dressing becomes damp, loosened, or soiled or when inspection of the site is necessary.	
7. Follow institution standard for site care and application of antimicrobial ointment to the LA catheter site.	Routine use of antimicrobial ointment at central venous catheter insertion sites is not recommended because of the potential to promote fungal infections and antimicrobial resistance.[1,18] Specific data are not available related to LA catheter sites.	
8. Obtain LA waveform strips to place on the patient's chart at the start of each shift and whenever a change in the waveform occurs.	The printed waveform allows assessment of the adequacy of the waveform, presence of damping, and respiratory variation.	
9. Before removal of the LA catheter, assess the patient's prothrombin time (PT), partial thromboplastin time (PTT), international normalized ratio (INR), and platelet levels.	Ensures that the patient does not have any difficulty forming a clot at the LA insertion site after its removal. Failure to form a clot can lead to cardiac tamponade. PT, PTT, and INR values should be normal before the catheter is removed. The platelet count should be at least 60,000/mm^3 before the catheter is removed.	• Abnormal coagulation results
10. After removal of the LA catheter, follow these steps: A. Maintain bed rest for 2 hours. B. Monitor vital signs, chest tube drainage, and heart sounds every 15 minutes × 4, every 30 minutes × 2, and then again in 1 hour.	Changes in vital signs and increased bleeding from the chest tube (e.g., greater than 100 mL/hr) suggest that the insertion site did not clot and that the patient is hemorrhaging.	• Tachycardia • Hypotension • Increased chest tube bleeding • Cessation of chest tube bleeding • Narrowing of pulse pressure • Muffled heart sounds
11. Follow institution standard for assessing pain. Administer analgesia as prescribed.	Identifies need for pain interventions.	• Continued pain despite pain interventions

*Level D: Peer-reviewed professional organizational standards with clinical studies to support recommendations

Documentation

Documentation should include the following:
- Patient and family education
- Left atrial pressure waveform recording strip (identify the *a* and *v* waves, inspiration and expiration, and the location where the LAP value was determined)
- Pain assessment, interventions, and effectiveness
- Amount of intake of flush solution
- Assessment of the dressing or catheter insertion site or both
- Unexpected outcomes
- Additional interventions

References

CR 1. Akl BF, Pett SB Jr., Wernly JA et al: Unusual complication of direct left atrial pressure monitoring line, *J Thorac Cardiovasc Surg* 88:1033-1035, 1984.

CR 2. Bojar RM: *Manual of perioperative care in cardiac and thoracic surgery,* ed 4, Malden, MA, 2005, Blackwell Sciences, 229-230.

CR 3. Bridges EJ, Woods SL: Pulmonary artery pressure measurement: state of the art, *Heart Lung* 22:99-111, 1993.

CR 4. Cason CL, et al: Effects of backrest elevation and position on pulmonary artery pressures, *Cardiovasc Nurs* 26:1-5, 1990.

CR 5. Chulay M, Miller T: The effect of backrest elevation on pulmonary artery and pulmonary capillary wedge pressures in patients after cardiac surgery, *Heart Lung* 13:138-40, 1984.

CR 6. Clochesy J, Hinshaw AD, Otto CW: Effects of change of position on pulmonary artery and pulmonary capillary wedge pressure in mechanically ventilated patients, *NITA* 7:223-225, 1984.

CR 7. Dobbin K, et al: Pulmonary artery pressure measurement in patients with elevated pressures: effect of backrest elevation and method of measurement, *Am J Crit Care* 1:61-69, 1992.

CR 8. Ducharme FM, et al: Incidence of infection related to arterial catheterization in children: a prospective study, *Crit Care Med* 16:272-276, 1988.

CR 9. Fullerton DA, St Cyr JA, Albert JD, et al: Hemodynamic advantage of left atrial epinephrine administration after cardiac operations, *Ann Thorac Surg* 56:1263-1266, 1986.

CR 10. Haider W, Zwolfer W, Hiesmayr M, et al: Improved cardiac performance and reduced pulmonary vascular constriction by epinephrine administration via a left atrial catheter in cardiac surgical patients, *J Cardiothorac Vasc Anesth* 7:684-687, 1993.

CR 11. Hochberg MS, Gielschinsky I, Parsonnet V, et al: Pulmonary inactivation of vasopressors following cardiac operations, *Ann Thorac Surg* 41:200-203, 1986.

CR 12. Keating D, et al: Effect of sidelying positions on pulmonary artery pressures, *Heart Lung* 15:605-610, 1986.

CR 13. Kelleher RM, Rose AA, Ordway L: Prostaglandins for control of pulmonary hypertension in the postoperative cardiac surgery patient: nursing implications, *Crit Care Nurs Clin North Am* 3:741-748, 1991.

CR 14. Lambert CW, Cason CL: Backrest elevation and pulmonary artery pressures: research analysis, *Dimens Crit Care Nurs* 9:327-335, 1990.

CR 15. Laulive JL: Pulmonary artery pressures and position changes in the critically ill adult, *Dimens Crit Care Nurs* 1:28-34, 1982.

CR 16. Luskin RL, et al: Extended use of disposable pressure transducers: a bacteriologic evaluation, *JAMA* 255:916-920, 1986.

CR 17. Mark JB: *Atlas of cardiovascular monitoring,* New York, 1998, Churchill Livingstone, 18, 24.

CR 18. O'Grady NP, et al: Guidelines for the prevention of intravascular catheter-related infections, *Am J Infect Control* 30:476-489, 2002.

CR 19. O'Mailley MK, et al: Value of routine pressure monitoring system changes after 72 hours of use, *Crit Care Med* 22:1424-1430, 1994.

CR 20. Recker DH: Procedure for left atrial catheter insertion, *Crit Care Nurse* 5:36-41, 1985.

CR 21. Retailliau MA, McGregor LM, Woods SL: The effect of the backrest position on the measurement of left atrial pressure in patients after cardiac surgery, *Heart Lung* 14:477-483, 1985.

CR 22. Taylor T: Monitoring left atrial pressures in the open-heart surgical patient, *Crit Care Nurse* 6:62-68, 1986.

CR 23. Wilson AE, et al: Effect of backrest position on hemodynamic and right ventricular measurements in critically ill adults, *Am J Crit Care* 5:264-270, 1996.

CR 24. Woods SL, Mansfield LW: Effect of body position upon pulmonary artery and pulmonary capillary wedge pressures in noncritically ill patients, *Heart Lung* 5:83-90, 1976.

Additional Readings

CR Ahrens TS, Taylor LA: *Hemodynamic waveform analysis,* Philadelphia, 1992, Saunders.

CR Gawlinski A: Facts and fallacies of patient positioning and hemodynamic management, *J Cardiovasc Nurs* 12:1-15, 1997.

CR Leitman BS, et al: The left atrial catheter: its uses and complications, *Radiology* 185:611-612, 1992.

CR Rao PS, Sathyanarayana PV: Transseptal insertion of left atrial line: a simple and safe technique, *Ann Thorac Surg* 55:785-786, 1993.

CR Santini F, et al: Routine left atrial catheterization for the postoperative management of cardiac surgical patients: is the risk justified? *Eur J Cardiothoracic Surg* 16:218-221, 1999.

CR Yeo TC, et al: Retained left atrial catheter: an unusual cardiac source of embolism identified by transesophageal echocardiography, *J Am Soc Echocardiogr* 11:66-70, 1998.

AP Pulmonary Artery Catheter Insertion (Perform)

P U R P O S E : Pulmonary artery catheters are used for determination of hemodynamic status in critically ill patients. Pulmonary artery catheters provide information about right-sided and left-sided intra-cardiac pressures and cardiac output. Additional functions available are fiberoptic monitoring of mixed venous oxygen saturation, intracardiac pacing, and assessment of right ventricular volumes and ejection fraction.

Desiree A. Fleck

PREREQUISITE NURSING KNOWLEDGE

- Knowledge of the normal anatomy and physiology of the cardiovascular system is needed.
- Knowledge of the normal anatomy and physiology of the vasculature and adjacent structures of the neck is necessary.
- Knowledge of the principles of sterile technique is essential.
- Clinical and technical competence in central line insertion and suturing is important.
- Clinical and technical competence in pulmonary artery (PA) catheter insertion is essential. Competence in chest radiograph interpretation is needed.
- Basic dysrhythmia recognition and treatment of life-threatening dysrhythmias should be understood.
- Advanced cardiac life support knowledge and skills are needed.
- Understanding of PA pressure monitoring (see Procedure 73) is necessary.
- Hemodynamic information obtained with a PA catheter is routinely used to guide therapeutic interventions, including

administration of fluids and diuretics and titration of vasoactive and inotropic medications.[1-3,10,11]
- Understanding is needed of *a*, *c*, and *v* waves. The *a* wave reflects atrial contraction. The *c* wave reflects closure of the atrioventricular valves. The *v* wave reflects passive filling of the atria during ventricular systole.
- Information can be gathered regarding cardiac output (CO), cardiac index (CI), systemic vascular resistance (SVR), pulmonary vascular resistance (PVR), stroke volume/stroke index (SV/SI), mixed venous oxygenation (Svo_2), right heart pressures (pulmonary artery pressure [PAP] and right atrial pressure [RAP]), and a reflection of left ventricular end-diastolic pressure (LVEDP) and volume (LVEDV). Also, information regarding right ventricular ejection fraction (RVEF) and end-diastolic volume (RVEDV) can be determined with certain catheters.
- CO and Svo_2 can be obtained intermittently or continuously.
- There are several types of PA catheters with different functions (e.g., pacing, mixed venous oxygenation saturation monitoring, continuous CO or right ventricular volume monitoring). Catheter selection is based on patient need.
- The PA catheter contains a proximal lumen port, a distal lumen port, a thermistor lumen port, and a balloon inflation lumen port (see Fig. 73-1). Some catheters also have additional infusion ports that can be used for the infusion of medications and intravenous fluids.

- The distal lumen port is used for monitoring systolic, diastolic, and mean pressures in the PA. The proximal lumen (or injectate) port is used for monitoring the right atrial pressure and injection of the solution used to obtain cardiac outputs. The balloon inflation lumen port is used to obtain the pulmonary artery occlusion pressure (PAOP) or pulmonary artery wedge pressure (PAWP).
- The standard 7.5F PA catheter is 110 cm long and has black markings at 10-cm increments and wide black markings at 50-cm increments to facilitate insertion and positioning (see Fig. 73-1). The catheter should reach the PA after advancing 40 to 55 cm from the internal jugular vein, 35 to 50 cm from the subclavian vein, 60 cm from the femoral vein, 70 cm from the right antecubital fossa, and 80 cm from the left antecubital fossa.
- Central venous access may be obtained in a variety of places (see Procedure 81).
- The right subclavian vein is a more direct route than the left subclavian vein for placement of a PA catheter because the catheter does not cross the midline of the thorax.[1,2,9,13]
- Use of an internal jugular vein minimizes the risk for a pneumothorax. The preferred site for catheter insertion is the right internal jugular vein. The right internal jugular vein is a "straight shot" to the right atrium.[13]
- Knowledge of West's lung zones helps attain proper placement of the PA catheter (Fig. 72-1).

The PA catheter should lie in lung zone 3, below the level of the left atrium in the dependent portion of the lung.[19] In lung zone 3, both arterial and venous pressures exceed alveolar pressure and PAOP reflects vascular pressures rather than alveolar pressures.[19]

- Common indications for insertion of a PA catheter include the following[1,2,7,8,12,14,16]:
  - ❖ Acute coronary syndrome or myocardial infarction (MI) complicated by hemodynamic instability, heart failure, cardiogenic shock, mitral regurgitation, ventral septal rupture, subacute cardiac rupture with tamponade, postinfarction ischemia, papillary muscle rupture, or severe heart failure (e.g., cardiomyopathy, constrictive pericarditis)
  - ❖ Hypotension unresponsive to fluid replacement or with heart failure
  - ❖ Cardiac tamponade, significant dysrhythmias, right ventricular infarct, acute pulmonary embolism, and tricuspid insufficiency
  - ❖ Anesthesia in cardiac surgery with any of the following:
    - ○ Evidence of previous MI
    - ○ Resection of ventricular aneurysm
    - ○ Coronary artery bypass graft (reoperation)
    - ○ Coronary artery bypass graft (left main or complex coronary disease)
    - ○ Complex cardiac surgery (multivalvular surgery)
    - ○ High-risk surgery (e.g., pulmonary hypertension)
  - ❖ General surgery:
    - ○ Vascular procedures (abdominal aneurysm repair, aortobifemoral bypass)
    - ○ Patients at high risk[1,15,17]
    - ○ Hypotensive anesthesia[1]
  - ❖ Cardiac disorders:
    - ○ Unstable angina that necessitates vasodilator therapy

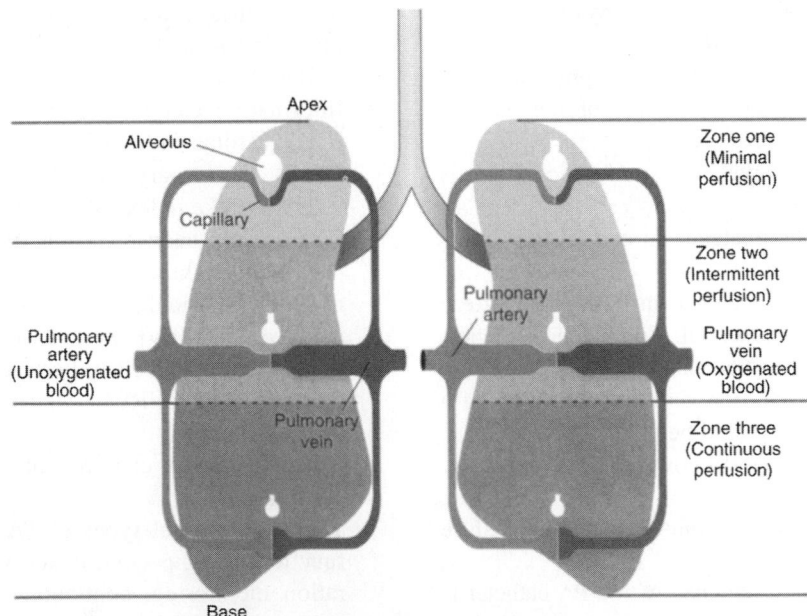

FIGURE 72-1   West's lung zones. Schema of the heart and lungs demonstrating the relationship between the cardiac chambers and the blood vessels and the physiologic zones of the lungs. Zone 1 (PA>Pa>Pv): Absence of blood flow. Zone 2 (Pa>PA>Pv): Intermittent blood flow. Zone 3 (Pa> Pv>PA): Continuous blood flow, resulting in an open channel between the pulmonary artery catheter and the left atrium. *PA,* Pulmonary artery; *Pa,* pressure arterial; *Pv,* pressure venous. *(From Copstead LC, Banasik JL: Pathophysiology: biological and behavioral perspectives, ed 2, Philadelphia, 2000, Saunders.)*

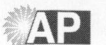

- o Heart failure unresponsive to conventional therapy (cardiomyopathy)[1,2,18]
- o Pulmonary hypertension during acute medication therapy
- o Distinguishing cardiogenic from noncardiogenic pulmonary edema
- o Constrictive pericarditis or cardiac tamponade
- o Evaluation of pulmonary hypertension for a precardiac transplant workup
- ❖ Pulmonary disorders:
  - o Acute respiratory failure with chronic obstructive pulmonary diseases
  - o Cor pulmonale with pneumonia
  - o Optimization of positive end-expiratory pressure (PEEP) and volume therapy in patients with acute respiratory distress syndrome[1]
- ❖ Patients who need intraaortic balloon pump therapy
- ❖ Critically ill pregnant patients (e.g., severe preeclampsia with unresponsive hypertension, pulmonary edema, persistent oliguria)
- ❖ Extensive multisystem infection
- ❖ Severe shock states
- ❖ Drug overdose
- ❖ Major trauma or burn
- ❖ Azotemia
- Relative contraindications to PA catheter insertion include the following:
  - ❖ Preexisting left bundle-branch block
  - ❖ Presence of fever (>101°F [38°C])
  - ❖ Mechanical tricuspid valve
  - ❖ Coagulopathic state
  - ❖ Presence of an endocardial pacemaker
  - ❖ History of heparin-induced thrombocytopenia

EQUIPMENT

- Percutaneous sheath introducer kit and sterile catheter sleeve
- PA catheter (non–heparin-coated catheters and latex-free PA catheters are available)
- Bedside hemodynamic monitoring system with pressure and cardiac output monitoring capability
- Pressure modules and cables for interface with the monitor
- Cardiac output cable with a thermistor/injectate sensor
- Pressure transducer system, including flush solution recommended according to institution standard, a pressure bag or device, pressure tubing with transducers, and flush device (see Procedure 76)
- Dual-channel recorder
- Sterile normal saline intravenous fluid for flushing the introducer and catheter infusion ports
- Antiseptic solution (e.g., 2% chlorhexidine-based preparation)
- Head covering, fluid-shield masks, sterile gowns, sterile gloves, nonsterile gloves, and sterile drapes
- 1% lidocaine without epinephrine
- Sterile basin or cup

- Sterile water or normal saline solution
- Sterile dressing supplies
- Chlorhexidine-impregnated sponge
- Stopcocks (may be included with the pressure tubing systems)
- Nonvented caps or needleless caps
- Leveling device (low-intensity laser or carpenter level)
  Additional equipment to have available as needed includes the following:
- Fluoroscope
- Emergency equipment
- Temporary pacing equipment
- Indelible marker
- Transducer holder and intravenous (IV) pole
- Heparin
- 3-mL syringe

PATIENT AND FAMILY EDUCATION

- Explain the procedure and the reason for the PA catheter insertion. ➥*Rationale:* Explanation decreases patient and family anxiety.
- Explain the need for sterile technique and explain that the patient's face may be covered. ➥*Rationale:* The explanation decreases patient anxiety and elicits cooperation.
- Inform the patient of expected benefits and potential risks. ➥*Rationale:* The patient is given information to make an informed decision.
- Explain the patient's expected participation during the procedure. ➥*Rationale:* Patient assistance is encouraged.

PATIENT ASSESSMENT AND PREPARATION

Patient Assessment

- Determine the patient's medical history of cervical disk disease or difficulty with vascular access. ➥*Rationale:* Baseline data are provided.
- Determine the patient's medical history of pneumothorax or emphysema. ➥*Rationale:* Patients with emphysematous lungs may be at higher risk for puncture and pneumothorax depending on the approach.
- Determine the patient's medical history of anomalous veins. ➥*Rationale:* Patients may have a history of dextrocardia or transposition of the great vessels, which leads to greater difficulty in catheter placement.
- Assess the intended insertion site. ➥*Rationale:* Scar tissue may impede placement of the catheter.
- Assess the patient's cardiac and pulmonary status. ➥*Rationale:* Some patients may not tolerate supine or Trendelenburg's position for extended periods.
- Assess vital signs and pulse oximetry. ➥*Rationale:* Baseline data are provided.
- Assess for electrolyte imbalances (potassium, magnesium, and calcium). ➥*Rationale:* Electrolyte imbalances may increase cardiac irritability.
- Assess the electrocardiogram (ECG) for left bundle-branch block. ➥*Rationale:* Right bundle-branch block has

been associated with PA catheter insertion. Caution should be used because complete heart block may ensue.[9,15]

- Assess for heparin and latex sensitivity or allergy. ➤*Rationale:* PA catheters are heparin-bonded and contain latex. If the patient has a heparin allergy or a history of heparin-induced thrombocytopenia, consider the use of a non–heparin-coated catheter.[15,17] If the patient has a latex allergy, use a latex-free PA catheter.
- Assess for a coagulopathic state and determine whether the patient has recently received anticoagulant or thrombolytic therapy. ➤*Rationale:* These patients are more likely to have complications related to bleeding and may need interventions before insertion of the PA catheter.

Patient Preparation

- Verify correct patient with two identifiers. ➤*Rationale:* Prior to performing a procedure, the nurse should ensure the correct identification of the patient for the intended intervention.
- Ensure that the patient understands preprocedural teaching. Answer questions as they arise, and reinforce information as needed. ➤*Rationale:* Understanding of previously taught information is evaluated and reinforced.

- Obtain informed consent. ➤*Rationale:* Informed consent protects the rights of a patient and makes a competent decision possible for the patient.
- Perform a pre-procedure verification and time out, if nonemergent. ➤*Rationale:* Ensures patient safety.
- Place the patient in the supine position and prepare the area with the antiseptic solution (e.g., 2% chlorhexidine–based preparation).[13,15] ➤*Rationale:* The site access is prepared for PA catheter insertion.
- Prescribe sedation or analgesics as needed. ➤*Rationale:* Sedation and analgesics minimize anxiety and discomfort. Movement of the patient may inhibit insertion of the PA catheter.
- If the patient is obese or muscular and the preferred site is the internal jugular vein or subclavian vein, place a towel posteriorly between the shoulder blades. ➤*Rationale:* This action helps extend the neck and provide better access to the subclavian and internal jugular veins.
- If the brachial vein is used, stabilize the arm on a padded arm board. ➤*Rationale:* Visualization of the brachial vein is aided.
- Drape sterile drapes over the prepared area. ➤*Rationale:* Sterile drapes provide an aseptic work area.

Procedure   for Performing Pulmonary Artery Catheter Insertion

Steps	Rationale	Special Considerations
1. HH		
2. PE		All healthcare providers in the room should have on protective equipment including goggles or face shields and masks.
3. Obtain central venous access with an introducer (see Procedure 81).	The PA catheter is inserted into a central vein.	Fully drape the patient with exposure of only the insertion site.
4. Open the PA catheter kit.	Prepares the equipment.	
5. Estimate the length of the catheter needed by holding the catheter over the insertion site and extending it to the sternal notch.	Helps ensure proper placement. The catheter should reach the PA after advancing 40 to 55 cm from the internal jugular vein, 35 to 55 cm from the subclavian vein, 60 cm from the femoral vein, 70 cm from the right antecubital fossa, and 80 cm from the left antecubital fossa.	Before inserting the catheter, attempt to curl the catheter in the direction it will float.
6. Hand off the ports of the PA catheter to the critical care nurse for connection to the hemodynamic monitoring system (see Procedure 73).	Connects the ports to the flush system; connects the transducer systems to the bedside monitor.	
7. Flush all open lumens.	Removes air from the PA catheter.	
8. Insert the recommended amount of air (1.5 mL) into the balloon and immerse the inflated balloon in sterile water or normal saline solution.	Checks for integrity of the balloon.	If an air leak is present, air bubbles are noted.
9. Ensure that the PA catheter thermistor is connected to the cardiac output monitor or module.	Allows the core or blood temperature to be monitored and is needed for cardiac output measurement.	

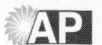

Procedure for Performing Pulmonary Artery Catheter Insertion—*Continued*

Steps	Rationale	Special Considerations
10. If a PA catheter with the ability to monitor mixed venous oxygenation is being inserted, the fiberoptics are calibrated before removal from the package (see Procedure 16). **(Level M*)**	Calibrates the system.	Calibrate the catheter according to manufacturer's guidelines.
11. Ensure that the critical care nurse has leveled and zeroed the hemodynamic monitoring system (see Procedure 76).	Prepares the monitoring system so that PA pressures can be obtained during catheter insertion.	
12. Insert the catheter through the sterile catheter sleeve **(Level B*)**.	Maintains sterility of the PA catheter to allow repositioning of the catheter.[4-6]	
13. While observing the monitor and the markings on the PA catheter (Fig. 72-2), follow these steps: A. Advance the catheter through the introducer to the superior vena cava into the right atrium. B. Inflate the balloon with 1.5 mL of air. C. Advance the catheter through the tricuspid valve, into the right ventricle. D. Continue to advance the catheter from the right ventricle through the pulmonic valve into the PA. E. Advance the catheter to obtain a PAOP. F. Deflate the balloon. G. Observe the PA waveform.	Waveforms and values change while moving from the superior vena cava to the right atrium to the right ventricle to the pulmonary artery and into the wedge position.	When inserting the PA catheter into the subclavian vein, have the patient bring his or her ear to the shoulder on the side of the insertion site. This creates a sharp angle between the jugular and subclavian veins and may help prevent misdirection of the catheter into the internal jugular vein. During insertion, monitor the ECG tracing for dysrhythmias. Run a graphic strip of the insertion waveforms.
14. Ensure proper placement by wedging the PA catheter again, and confirm placement with a paper tracing.	Ensures proper placement and accurate readings.	
15. Extend the sterile catheter sleeve over the catheter and secure in place. **(Level M)**	May maintain catheter sterility for catheter repositioning.[6]	The duration of catheter sterility in the sleeve is unknown.[6]
16. Apply an occlusive, sterile dressing.	Reduces the incidence of infection.	Dressings may be a sterile gauze or a sterile, transparent, semipermeable dressing.[13,15] Follow institution standard for application of a chlorhexidine-impregnated sponge (see Procedure 69).
17. Note the centimeter marking at the introducer site.	Aids in ensuring placement and troubleshooting.	
18. Obtain a chest radiograph.	Confirms catheter placement.	
19. Discard used supplies in appropriate receptacles.	Removes and safely discards used supplies.	
20. **HH**		

*Level B: Well-designed, controlled studies with results that consistently support a specific action, intervention or treatment
*Level M: Manufacturer's recommendations only

Procedure continues on following page

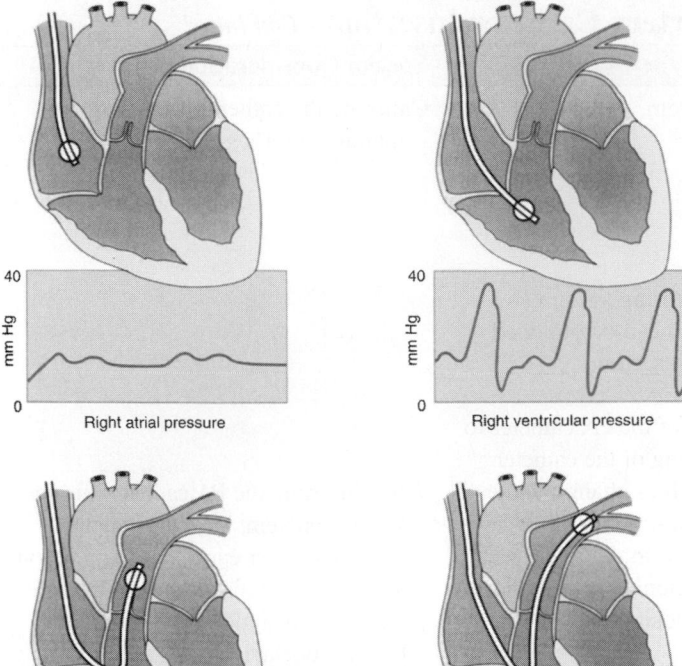

40 mm Hg 0
Right atrial pressure

40 mm Hg 0
Right ventricular pressure

40 mm Hg 0
Pulmonary artery

40 mm Hg 0
Pulmonary artery
occlusive pressure

FIGURE 72-2   Pulmonary artery catheter advancing through the heart with appropriate waveforms. *(Adapted from Bucher L, Melander S: Critical care nursing, Philadelphia, 1999, Saunders.)*

Expected Outcomes

- Accurate placement of the pulmonary artery catheter
- Adequate and appropriate waveforms
- Ability to obtain accurate information about cardiac pressures
- Evaluation of information to guide therapeutic interventions

Unexpected Outcomes

- Pneumothorax or hemothorax
- Infection
- Ventricular dysrhythmias
- Misplacement (e.g., carotid artery, vertebral artery, subclavian artery)
- Valvular damage
- Vessel wall erosion
- Hemorrhage
- Hematoma
- Pericardial or ventricular rupture
- Venous air embolism
- Cardiac tamponade
- Sepsis
- Pulmonary artery infarction
- Pulmonary artery rupture
- Pulmonary artery catheter balloon rupture
- Pulmonary artery catheter knotting
- Heparin-induced thrombocytopenia or thrombosis
- Thromboembolism
- Pain

Patient Monitoring and Care

Steps	Rationale	Reportable Conditions
		These conditions should be reported if they persist despite nursing interventions.
1. Perform systematic cardiovascular, peripheral vascular, and hemodynamic assessments before and immediately after insertion:		
A. Assess level of consciousness.	Assesses for signs of adequate perfusion; air embolism may present with restlessness; patient may present with decreased level of consciousness if the catheter is advanced into the carotid artery.	• Change in level of consciousness
B. Assess vital signs.	Demonstrates response to the procedure and effectiveness of therapies performed.	• Abnormal vital signs
C. Assess postinsertion hemodynamic values: pulmonary artery systolic pressure (PASP), pulmonary artery diastolic pressure (PADP), RAP, PAOP, CO, CI, SVR, and other parameters as needed.	Obtains baseline data and assesses patient status.	• Abnormal hemodynamic pressures or cardiac parameters
2. Assess the central line insertion site for hematoma or hemorrhage.	If coagulopathies are present, a pressure dressing may be needed.	• Bleeding that does not stop • Hematoma
3. Assess heart and lung sounds after PA catheter insertion.	Abnormal heart or lung sounds may indicate cardiac tamponade, pneumothorax, or hemothorax.	• Diminished or muffled heart sounds • Absent or diminished breath sounds unilaterally
4. Assess the results of the chest radiograph.	Ensures adequate placement in lung zone 3 below the level of the left atrium.	• Abnormal chest radiograph results
5. Monitor for signs and symptoms of cardiac tamponade and air embolism.	Identifies complications.	• Signs or symptoms of cardiac tamponade or air embolism
6. Monitor the centimeter marking at the introducer site.	May be helpful in troubleshooting the PA catheter.	• Changes in the external centimeter marking • Abnormal PA waveforms
7. Follow institution standard for assessing pain. Administer analgesia as prescribed.	Identifies need for pain interventions.	• Continued pain despite pain interventions

Documentation

Documentation should include the following:
- Patient and family education
- Completion of informed consent
- Universal Protocol requirements
- Insertion of PA catheter and sheath introducer
- Type and size of catheter placed
- Size of introducer sheath
- PA pressure values on insertion (RAP, right ventricular systolic and diastolic pressures, PASP, PADP, PAOP)
- Graphic strip of insertion
- Insertion site of the PA catheter
- Centimeter mark at the edge of the introducer
- Any difficulties encountered during placement (e.g., ventricular ectopy, new bundle-branch blocks)
- Patient tolerance
- Confirmation of placement (e.g., chest radiograph)
- Initial values after placement of the catheter (PAPs, PAOP, RAP, CO, CI, SVR, PVR, Svo$_2$)
- Occurrence of unexpected outcomes
- Additional interventions
- Pain assessment, interventions, and effectiveness

References

CR 1. American Society of Anesthesiology: Practice guidelines for pulmonary artery catheters, *Anesthesiology* 99:988,1014, 2003.

CR 2. Amin DK, Shah PK, Swan HJC: Deciding when hemodynamic monitoring is appropriate, *J Crit Illn* 8:1053-1061, 1993.

CR 3. Bridges EJ, Woods SL: Pulmonary artery measurement: state of the art, *Heart Lung* 22:99-111, 1993.

CR 4. Burns D, Burns D, Shively M: Critical care nurses' knowledge of pulmonary artery catheters, *Am J Crit Care* 5:49-54, 1996.

CR 5. Cohen Y, et al: The "hands-off" catheter and the prevention of systemic infections associated with pulmonary artery catheter: a prospective study, *Am J Respir Crit Care Med* 157:284-287, 1998.

6. Corcoran TB, Grape S, Duff O, et al: The pulmonary artery catheter sleeve: protective or infective? *Anaesth Intensive Care* 37(2):290-295, 2009.

CR 7. Darovic GO: Pulmonary artery pressure monitoring. In *Hemodynamic monitoring: invasive and noninvasive clinical application*, Philadelphia, 2002, Saunders.

CR 8. Davis D, et al: Impact of formal continuing medical education: do conferences, workshops, rounds and other traditional continuing education activities change physician behavior or health care outcomes? *JAMA* 282:867-874, 1999.

CR 9. Eggimann P, et al: Impact of a prevention strategy targeted at vascular-access care on incidence of infections acquired in intensive care, *Lancet* 355:1864-1868, 2000.

CR 10. Herbert KA, Glancy DL: Indications for Swan-Ganz catheterization, *Heart Dis Stroke* 3:196-200, 1994.

CR 11. Iberti TJ, et al: A multicenter study of physicians' knowledge of the pulmonary artery catheter, *JAMA* 22:2928-2933, 1990.

CR 12. Iberti TJ, et al: Assessment of critical care nurses' knowledge of the pulmonary artery catheter, *Crit Care Med* 22:1674-1678, 1994.

13. Lorente L, Henry C, Martin M., et al: Central venous catheter-related infection in a prospective and observational study of 2,595 catheters, *Crit Care* 9:R631-R635, 2005.

CR 14. Morris AH, Chapman RH: Wedge pressure confirmation by aspiration of pulmonary capillary blood, *Crit Care Med* 13:756-759, 1985.

CR 15. O'Grady NP, et al: Guidelines for the prevention of intravascular catheter-related infections, *Am J Infect Control* 30:476-489, 2002.

CR 16. Pulmonary Artery Consensus Conference Participants: Pulmonary Artery Catheter Consensus Conference: consensus statement, *Crit Care Med* 25:910-925, 1997.

CR 17. Silver D, Kapsch DN, Tsoi EK: Heparin-induced thrombocytopenia, thrombosis, and hemorrhage, *Ann Surg* 198:301-306, 1983.

CR 18. Sandham JD, Hull LD, Brant LF, et al: A randomized, controlled trial of the use of pulmonary-artery catheters in high-risk surgical patients, *N Engl J Med* 348:5-14, 2003.

CR 19. West JB, Dollery CT, Naimark A: Distribution of blood flow in isolated lung: relation to vascular and alveolar pressure, *J Appl Physiol* 19:713-724, 1964.

Additional Readings

Ahrens TS, Taylor LK: *Hemodynamic waveform analysis*, Philadelphia: 1992, Saunders.

American Association of Critical Care Nurses: Evaluation of the effects of heparinized and nonheparinized flush solutions on the patency of arterial pressure monitoring lines: the AACN Thunder Project, *Am J Crit Care* 2:3-15, 1993.

Amin DK, Shah PK, Swan HJC: The Swan-Ganz catheter: techniques for avoiding common errors, *J Crit Illn* 8:1263-1271, 1993.

Amin DK, Shah PK, Swan HJC: The technique of inserting a Swan-Ganz catheter, *J Crit Illn* 8:1147-1156, 1993.

Baxter JK, et al: Effectiveness of right heart catheterization: time for a randomized trial, *JAMA* 277:108, 1997.

Blot F, Chachaty E, Raynard B, et al: Mechanisms and risk factors for infection of pulmonary artery catheters and introducer sheaths in cancer patients admitted to an intensive care unit, *J Hosp Infect* 48(4):289-297, 2001.

Chernow B: Pulmonary artery flotation catheters: a statement by the American College of Chest Physicians and the American Thoracic Society, *Chest* 111:261, 1997.

Connors AF, et al: The effectiveness of right heart catheterization in the initial care of critically ill patients, *JAMA* 276:889-897, 1996.

Daily EK, Schroeder JS: T*echniques in bedside hemodynamic monitoring*, ed 5, St Louis, 1994, Mosby.

Darovic GO: *Hemodynamic monitoring: invasive and noninvasive clinical application*, Philadelphia, 2002, Saunders.

Friesinger GC, Williams SV, ACP/ACC/AHA Task Force on Clinical Privileges in Cardiology: Clinical competence in hemodynamic monitoring, *J Am Coll Cardiol* 15:1460, 1990.

Gardner PE, Bridges EJ: Hemodynamic monitoring. In Woods SL, et al, editors: *Cardiac nursing*, ed 3, Philadelphia, 1995, Lippincott, 424-458.

Ginosar Y, Pizov R, Sprung CL: Arterial and pulmonary artery catheters. *In Critical care medicine*, St Louis, 1995, Mosby.

Hadian M, Pinsky MR: Evidence-based review of the use of the pulmonary artery catheter: impact, data and complications, *Crit Care* 10(Suppl 3):S11-S18, 2006.

Harvey S, et al: Assessment of the clinical effectiveness of pulmonary artery catheters in management of patients in intensive care (PAC-Man): a randomized controlled trial, *Lancet* 366 (9484):472-477, 2005.

Harvey S, et al: Pulmonary artery catheters for adult patients in intensive care, *Cochrane Database Syst Rev* July 19:3, 2006.

Keckeisen M: *Protocols for practice: hemodynamic monitoring series: pulmonary artery pressure monitoring*, Aliso Viejo, CA, 1997, American Association of Critical-Care Nurses.

Leeper B: Monitoring right ventricular volumes: a paradigm shift, *AACN Clin Issues Adv Pract Acute Crit Care* 14:208-219, 2003.

Pinsky MR: Hemodynamic monitoring over the past 10 years, *Crit Care* 10:117-119, 2006.

Pulmonary Artery Catheter Consensus Conference Participants: Pulmonary Artery Catheter Consensus Conference: consensus statement, *Crit Care Med* 25:910-925, 1997.

Rapoprot LJ, Teres D, Steingrub J: Patient characteristics and ICU organizational factors that influencing of frequency of PA catheter, *JAMA* 283:2555, 2000.

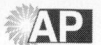

Swan JHC: What role today for hemodynamic monitoring, *J Crit Illn* 8:1043-1050, 1993.

Swan JHC, Ganz W, Forrester JS: Catheterization of the heart in a man with the use of a flow-directed balloon-tipped catheter, *N Engl J Med* 280:447, 1970.

The American Society of Anesthesiologists' Task Force on Pulmonary Artery Catheterization: Practice guidelines for pulmonary catheterization, *Anesthesiology* 78:380-394, 1993.

The National Heart, Lung, and Blood Institute Acute Respiratory Distress Syndrome Clinical Trial Network, Wheeler

AP, et al: Pulmonary artery vs central venous catheter to guide treatment of acute lung injury, *N Engl J Med* 354(21):2213-2224, 2006.

Tuggle D: *Optimizing hemodynamics: strategies for fluid and medication titration in shock*, AACN advanced critical care nursing, Philadelphia, 2009, Elsevier, 1099-1133.

Wiener R, Welch H: Trends in the use of the pulmonary artery catheter in the United States 1993-2004, *JAMA* 298(4): 423-429, 2007.

Pulmonary Artery Catheter Insertion (Assist) and Pressure Monitoring

P U R P O S E : Pulmonary artery catheters are used to determine hemodynamic status in critically ill patients. Pulmonary artery catheters provide information about right-sided and left-sided intracardiac pressures and cardiac output. Additional functions available are fiberoptic monitoring of mixed venous oxygen saturation, intracardiac pacing, and assessment of right ventricular volumes and ejection fraction. Hemodynamic information obtained with a pulmonary artery catheter is used to guide therapeutic intervention, including administration of fluids and diuretics and titration of vasoactive and inotropic medications.

Teresa Preuss, Debra Lynn-McHale Wiegand

PREREQUISITE NURSING KNOWLEDGE

- Knowledge of the normal cardiovascular anatomy and physiology is needed.
- Knowledge of the normal pulmonary anatomy and physiology is necessary.
- Knowledge of principles of aseptic technique is needed.
- Basic dysrhythmia recognition and treatment of life-threatening dysrhythmias should be understood.
- Advanced cardiac life support knowledge and skills are necessary
- Knowledge of the anatomy of the pulmonary artery (PA) catheter (Fig. 73-1) and the location of the PA catheter in the heart and pulmonary artery (Fig. 73-2) is important.
- Knowledge of the setup of the hemodynamic monitoring system (see Procedure 76) is essential.
- Understanding of normal hemodynamic values (see Table 67-1) is needed.
- The pulmonary artery catheter contains a proximal injectate lumen port, a PA distal lumen port, a thermistor connector, and a balloon-inflation valve. Some catheters also have two infusion ports, right atrial (RA) and right

ventricular (RV) lumens, that can be used for infusion of medications and intravenous fluids.
- The PA distal lumen is used to monitor systolic, diastolic, and mean pressures in the pulmonary artery. This lumen also allows for sampling of mixed venous blood. The proximal injectate lumen is used to monitor the right atrial pressure and inject the solution used to obtain cardiac output (CO). The balloon-inflation valve is used to obtain the pulmonary artery occlusion pressure (PAOP).
- PAOP may be referred to as pulmonary artery wedge pressure.
- The PA diastolic pressure and the PAOP are indirect measures of left ventricular end-diastolic pressure (LVEDP). Usually, the PAOP is approximately 1 to 4 mm Hg less than the pulmonary artery diastolic pressure (PADP). Because these two pressures are similar, the PADP is commonly followed, which minimizes the frequency of balloon inflation, thus decreasing the potential of balloon rupture and pulmonary artery trauma.
- Differences between the PADP and the PAOP may exist for patients with pulmonary hypertension, chronic obstructive lung disease, acute respiratory distress syndrome (ARDS), pulmonary embolus, and tachycardia.

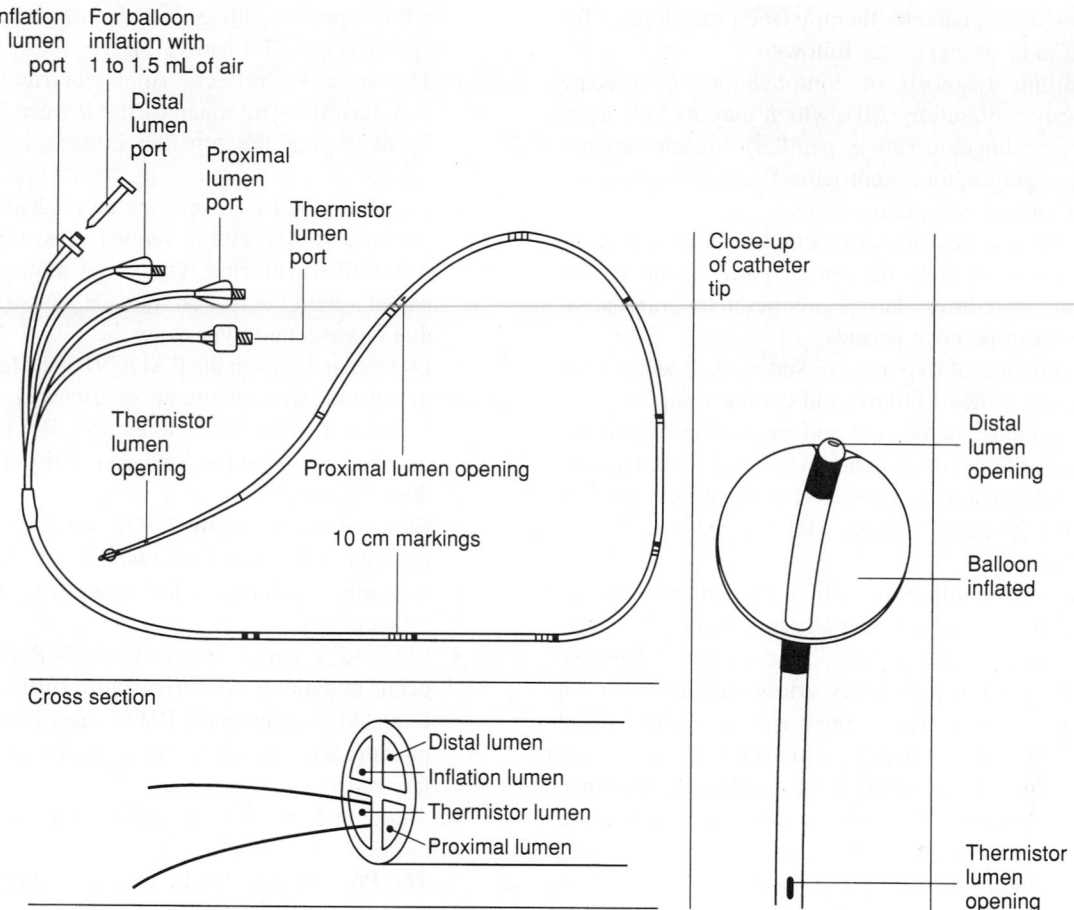

FIGURE 73-1   Anatomy of the pulmonary artery (PA) catheter. The standard no. 7.5 Fr thermodilution PA catheter is 110 cm in length and contains four lumens. It is constructed of radiopaque
polyvinyl chloride. Black markings are on the catheter in 10-cm increments beginning at the distal
end. At the distal end of the catheter is a latex rubber balloon of 1.5-mL capacity, which, when inflated, extends slightly beyond the tip of the catheter without obstructing it. Balloon inflation cush-
ions the tip of the catheter and prevents contact with the right ventricular wall during insertion. The
balloon also acts to float the catheter into position and allows measurement of the pulmonary artery
occlusion pressure. The narrow black bands represent 10-cm lengths, and the wide black bands indicate 50-cm lengths. *(From Visalli F, Evans P: The Swan-Ganz catheter: a program for teaching
safe effective use, Nursing 81[11]:1, 1981.)*

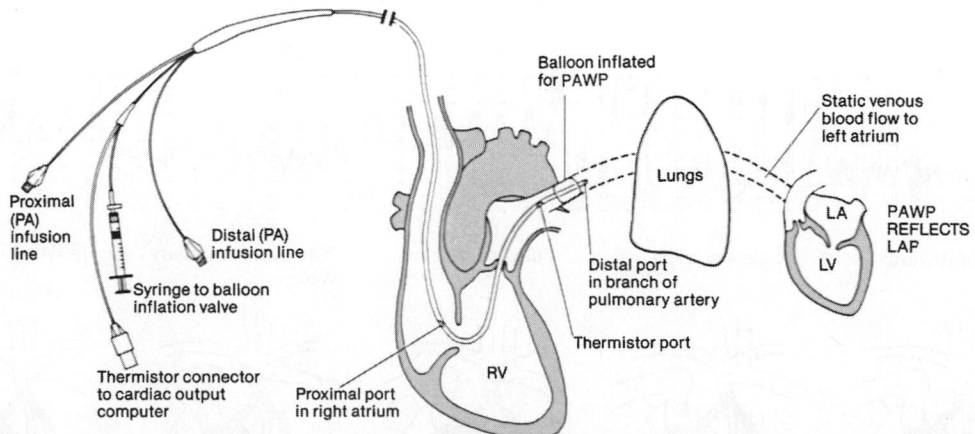

FIGURE 73-2   Pulmonary artery (PA) catheter location within the heart. Pulmonary artery occlusion pressure (PAOP) is an indirect measure of left atrial (LA) and left ventricular (LV) end-diastolic
pressure. Pulmonary artery occlusion pressure (PAOP) is also referred to as pulmonary artery wedge
pressure (PAWP). *(From Kersten LD: Comprehensive respiratory nursing, Philadelphia, 1989,
Saunders.)*

- Indications for PA catheter therapy (see Procedure 72 for additional indications) are as follows:
  - ❖ Aid in the diagnosis of complications after acute myocardial infarction (MI), which may include heart failure, cardiogenic shock, papillary muscle rupture, mitral regurgitation, ventricular septal rupture, or cardiac rupture with tamponade.
  - ❖ Assessment of ventricular function in heart failure.
  - ❖ Management of high-risk cardiac patients undergoing surgical procedures during preoperative, intraoperative, or postoperative periods.
  - ❖ Differentiation of hypotensive states, such as hypovolemia, sepsis, heart failure, and cardiac tamponade.
  - ❖ Hemodynamic monitoring and evaluation of patients with major organ dysfunction who need fluid management and infusion of vasoactive medications, such as patients with burns, trauma, ARDS, or gastrointestinal bleeding.
- Hemodynamic monitoring with a PA catheter has no absolute contraindications, but an assessment of risk versus benefit to the patient should be considered. Relative contraindications to pulmonary artery catheter insertion include presence of fever, presence of a mechanical tricuspid valve, and a coagulopathic state. A patient with left bundle-branch block may have a right bundle-branch block develop during PA catheter insertion, resulting in complete heart block. In these patients, a temporary pacemaker should be readily available.
- Pulmonary artery pressures may be elevated as a result of pulmonary artery hypertension, pulmonary disease, mitral valve disease, left ventricular failure, atrial or ventricular left-to-right shunt, pulmonary emboli, or hypervolemia.
- Pulmonary artery pressures may be decreased due to hypovolemia or vasodilation.
- Waveforms that occur during insertion include RA, RV, PA, and pulmonary artery occlusion (PAO; Fig. 73-3).
  - ❖ The *a* wave reflects atrial contraction, the *c* wave reflects closure of the atrioventricular valve, and the *v* wave reflects passive filling of the atria during ventricular systole (Figs. 73-4 and 73-5).
  - ❖ The *a* wave reflects right ventricular filling at end diastole. The mean of the *a* wave is determined by averaging the top and bottom values of the *a* wave.
  - ❖ Elevated *a* and *v* waves may be evident in right atrial pressure (RAP/central venous pressure [CVP]) and in PAOP waveforms. These elevations may occur in patients with cardiac tamponade, constrictive pericardial disease, and hypervolemia.
  - ❖ Elevated *a* waves in the RAP/CVP waveform may occur in patients with pulmonic or tricuspid stenosis, right ventricular ischemia or infarction, RV failure, pulmonary artery hypertension, and atrioventricular (AV) dissociation.
  - ❖ Elevated *a* waves in the PAOP waveform may occur in patients with mitral stenosis, acute left ventricular ischemia or infarction, left ventricular failure, and AV dissociation.
  - ❖ Elevated v waves in the RAP/CVP waveform may occur in patients with tricuspid insufficiency.
  - ❖ Elevated *v* waves in the PAOP waveform may occur in patients with mitral insufficiency or a ruptured papillary muscle.
- Insertion and placement verification should occur as follows:
  - ❖ The PA catheter may be inserted through the subclavian, internal jugular, femoral, external jugular, or antecubital veins.
  - ❖ The standard 7.5 Fr PA catheter is 110 cm long and has black markings at 10-cm increments and wide black markings at 50-cm increments for facilitation of insertion and positioning (see Fig. 73-1). The catheter should reach the PA after being advanced 40 to 55 cm from the internal jugular vein, 35 to 50 cm from the subclavian vein, 60 cm from the femoral vein, 70 cm from the right antecubital fossa, and 80 cm from the left antecubital fossa.

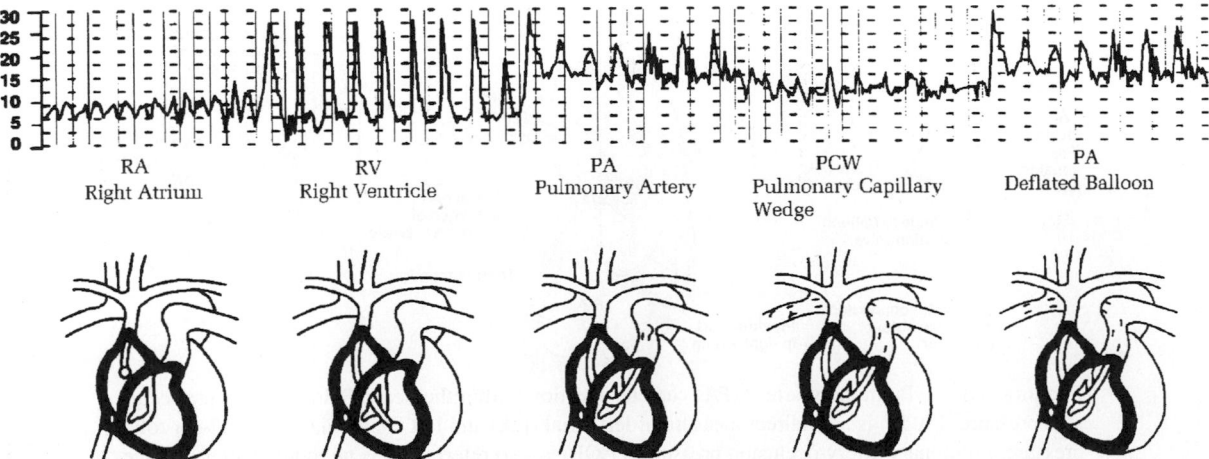

RA	RV	PA	PCW	PA
Right Atrium	Right Ventricle	Pulmonary Artery	Pulmonary Capillary Wedge	Deflated Balloon

FIGURE 73-3 Schematic of waveform progression as a pulmonary artery catheter is inserted through the various cardiac chambers. *(From Abbott Critical Care Systems, Mountain View, CA.)*

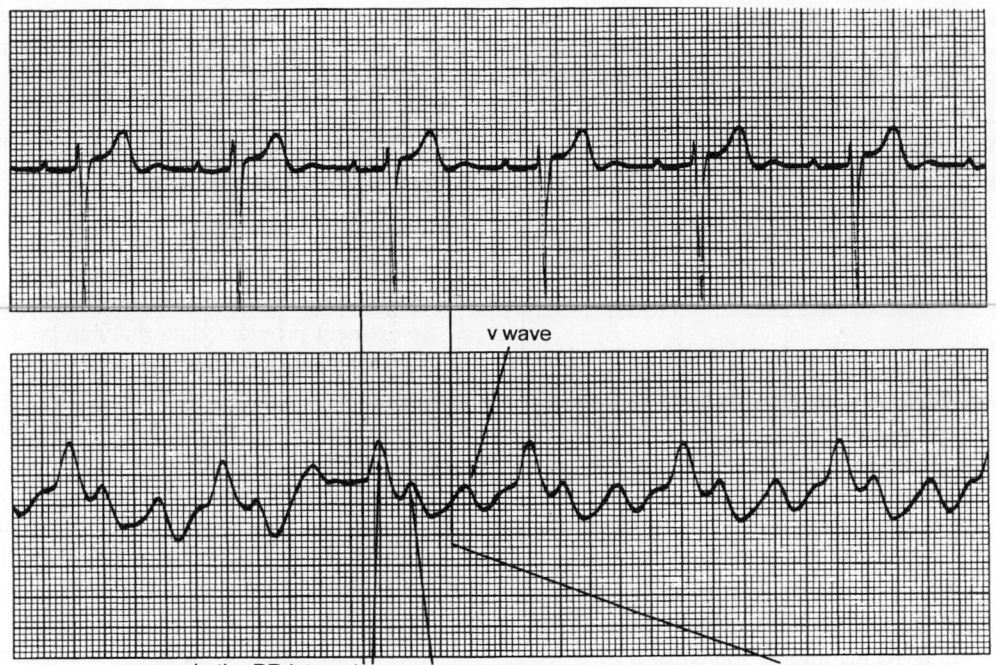

v wave

a wave in the PR interval   c waves at the end of the QRS   v waves after the T wave

FIGURE 73-4   Identification of *a*, *c*, and *v* waves in the waveform for right atrial and central venous pressure (RA/CVP). Atrial waveforms are characterized by three components: *a*, *c*, and *v* waves. The *a* wave reflects atrial contraction, the *c* wave reflects closure of the tricuspid valve, and the *v* wave reflects passive filling of the atria. *(From Ahrens TS, Taylor LK: Hemodynamic waveform analysis, Philadelphia, 1992, Saunders.)*

ECG

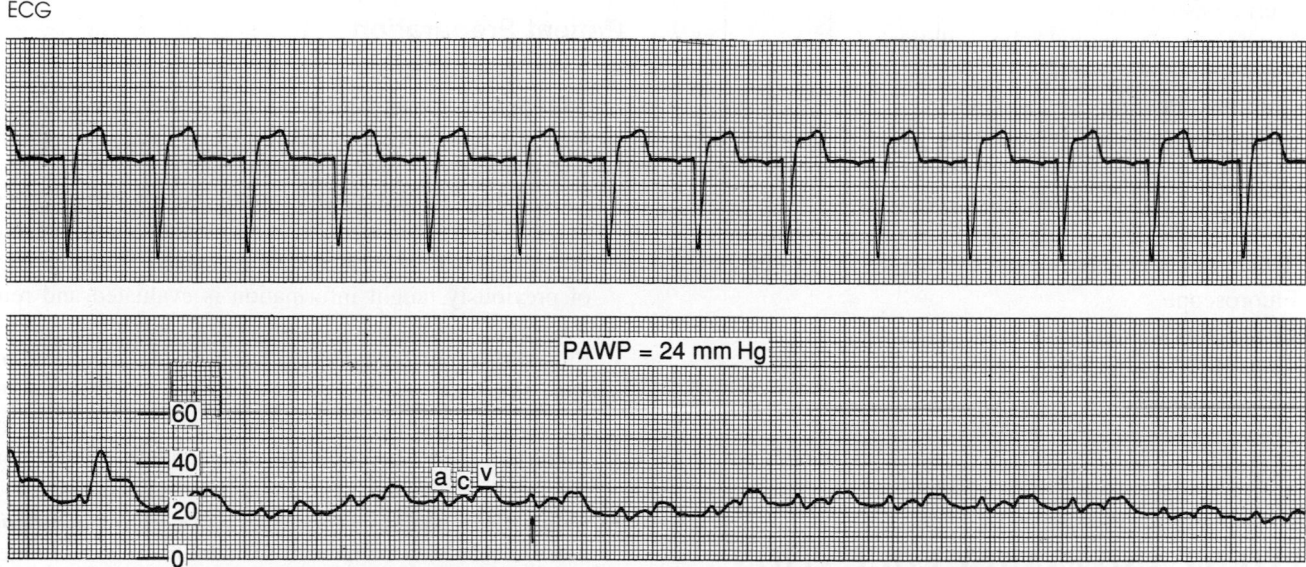

PAWP = 24 mm Hg

FIGURE 73-5   Normal pulmonary artery occlusion pressure (PAOP) waveform. Note the delay in the *a*, *c*, and *v* waves because of the time needed for the mechanical events to show a pressure change. This waveform is from a spontaneously breathing patient. The *arrow* indicates end expiration, where the mean of *a* wave pressure is measured. Pulmonary artery occlusion pressure (PAOP) is also referred to as pulmonary artery wedge pressure (PAWP).

❖ Verification of PA catheter placement is validated with waveform analysis. Correct catheter placement shows a PAO tracing when the balloon is inflated and a PA tracing when the balloon is deflated.

❖ Catheter placement is also verified with chest radiography.

❖ The PA catheter balloon contains latex, which may cause allergic reactions. Latex-free catheters are available.

EQUIPMENT

- PA catheter (non–heparin-coated PA catheters and latex-free PA catheters are available)
- Percutaneous sheath introducer kit and sterile catheter sleeve
- Pressure modules and cables for interface with the monitor
- Cardiac output cable with a thermistor/injectate sensor
- Pressure transducer system, including flush solution recommended according to institution standard, a pressure bag or device, pressure tubing with transducers, and flush device
- Dual-channel recorder
- Sterile normal saline intravenous (IV) solution for flushing of the introducer and catheter infusion ports
- Antiseptic solution (e.g., 2% chlorhexidine-based preparation)
- Head covers, fluid-shield masks, sterile gowns, sterile gloves, nonsterile gloves, and sterile drapes
- 1% lidocaine without epinephrine
- Sterile basin or cup
- Sterile water or normal saline solution
- Sterile dressing supplies
- Chlorhexidine-impregnated sponge
- Stopcocks (may be included in some pressure tubing systems)
- Nonvented caps or needleless caps
- Leveling device (low-intensity laser or carpenter level) Additional equipment as needed includes the following:
- Fluoroscope
- Emergency equipment
- Temporary pacing equipment
- Indelible marker
- Transducer holder and intravenous (IV) pole
- Heparin
- 3-mL syringe

PATIENT AND FAMILY EDUCATION

- Provide the patient and family with information about the PA catheter, reason for the PA catheter, and explanation of the equipment. ➤*Rationale:* The patient and family understand the procedure, why it is needed, and how it will help manage care. Patient and family anxiety may decrease.

- Explain the patient's expected participation during the procedure. ➤*Rationale:* This explanation will encourage patient assistance.

PATIENT ASSESSMENT AND PREPARATION
Patient Assessment

- Determine baseline hemodynamic, cardiovascular, peripheral vascular, and neurovascular status. ➤*Rationale:* Assessment provides data that can be used for comparison with postinsertion assessment data and hemodynamic values.
- Determine the patient's baseline pulmonary status. If the patient is mechanically ventilated, note the type of support, ventilator mode, and presence or absence of positive end-expiratory pressure (PEEP) or continuous positive airway pressure (CPAP). ➤*Rationale:* The presence of mechanical ventilation alters hemodynamic waveforms and pressures.
- Assess the patient's medical history specifically related to problems with venous access sites, cardiac anatomy, and pulmonary anatomy. ➤*Rationale:* Identification of obstructions or disease should be made before the insertion attempt.
- Assess the patient's current laboratory profile, including electrolyte, coagulation, and arterial blood gas results. ➤*Rationale:* Laboratory abnormalities are identified. Baseline coagulation studies are helpful in determination of the risk for bleeding. Electrolyte and arterial blood gas imbalances may increase cardiac irritability.

Patient Preparation

- Verify correct patient with two identifiers. ➤*Rationale:* Prior to performing a procedure, the nurse should ensure the correct identification of the patient for the intended intervention.
- Ensure that the patient and family understand preprocedural teaching. Answer questions as they arise, and reinforce information as needed. ➤*Rationale:* Understanding of previously taught information is evaluated and reinforced.
- Ensure that informed consent has been obtained. ➤*Rationale:* Informed consent protects the rights of the patient and makes a competent decision possible for the patient.
- Perform a pre-procedure verification and time out, if nonemergent. ➤*Rationale:* Ensures patient safety.
- Validate the patency of the peripheral IV line. ➤*Rationale:* Access may be needed for administration of emergency medications or fluids.
- Assist the patient to the supine position. ➤*Rationale:* This position prepares the patient for skin preparation, catheter insertion, and setup of the sterile field.
- Sedate the patient or provide prescribed analgesics as needed. ➤*Rationale:* Movement of the patient may inhibit insertion of the PA catheter.

Procedure	for Assisting with Pulmonary Artery Catheter Insertion and Pressure Monitoring		
Steps	**Rationale**	**Special Considerations**	

Assisting with PA Catheter Insertion

Steps	Rationale	Special Considerations
1. **HH**		
2. Prepare the flush solution (see Procedure 76). Follow institution standard for adding heparin to the IV bag, if heparin is not contraindicated. **(Level B*)**	Heparinized flush solutions are commonly used to minimize thrombi and fibrin deposits on catheters that might lead to thrombosis or bacterial colonization of the catheter.	Although heparin may prevent thrombosis,[23,28] it has been associated with thrombocytopenia and other hematologic complications.[5] Further research is needed regarding use of heparin versus normal saline to maintain PA catheter patency.
3. Prime or flush the entire pressure transducer system (see Procedure 76).	Removes air bubbles. Air bubbles introduced into the patient's circulation can cause air embolism. Air bubbles within the tubing dampen the waveform.	Air is more easily removed from the hemodynamic tubing when the system is not under pressure.
4. Apply and maintain pressure in the pressure bag or device at 300 mm Hg.	Each flush device delivers 1 to 3 mL/hr to maintain patency of the hemodynamic system.	
5. **HH**		
6. **PE**		All health care personnel involved in the procedure needs to apply head coverings, fluid-shield masks, sterile gowns, and gloves.
7. Assist the physician or advanced practice nurse with apply sterile drapes, opening the PA catheter and introducer kits. Assist as needed with fully draping the patient with exposure of only the insertion site.	Aids in maintaining sterility.	
8. When the sheath introducer is in place, connect a normal saline IV solution to the infusion port.	Maintains the patency of the sheath introducer infusion port.	
9. Connect the pressure transducer system to the PA distal and proximal ports of the PA catheter, and flush all lumens.	Removes air from the pulmonary artery catheter.	Flush additional infusion ports before insertion.
10. Connect the pressure cables from the PA distal and proximal injectate transducers to the bedside monitor (see Fig. 76-2).	Connects the pulmonary artery catheter to the bedside monitoring system.	
11. Connect the thermistor connector of the PA catheter to the CO monitor or module (see Fig. 76-3).	Allows the core temperature to be monitored and is needed for CO measurement.	
12. If inserting a PA catheter with the ability to monitor mixed venous oxygenation, the fiberoptics are calibrated before removal from the package (see Procedure 16).	Calibrates the system before insertion.	Follow manufacturer guidelines for catheter calibration.

*Level B: Well-designed, controlled studies with results that consistently support a specific action, intervention, or treatment

Procedure continues on following page

Procedure for Assisting with Pulmonary Artery Catheter Insertion and Pressure Monitoring—*Continued*

Steps	Rationale	Special Considerations
13. Set the scales for each pressure tracing.	Permits waveform analysis.	The scale for the RA/CVP pressure commonly is set at 20 mm Hg, and the PA scale commonly is set at 40 mm Hg. Scale settings may vary based on monitoring equipment. Scales can be adjusted based on patient pressures.
14. Examine the PA catheter for defects in construction and check balloon integrity.	Ensures integrity of the PA catheter.	The inflated balloon can be placed in a container of sterile normal saline solution or water. No air bubbles should be seen. If air bubbles are seen, a defect exists in the balloon integrity.
15. Level the RA (proximal injectate) air-fluid interface (zeroing stopcock) and the PA (distal) air-fluid interface (zeroing stopcock) to the phlebostatic axis (see Figs. 76-7 and 76-9).	The phlebostatic axis approximates the level of the atria and is the reference point for patients in the supine position.	The reference point for the atria changes when a patient is in the lateral position (see Fig. 76-8).
16. Zero the system connected to the PA lumen and to the RA lumen of the PA catheter by turning the stopcock of each system off to the patient, opening it to air, and zeroing the monitoring system (see Procedure 76).	Prepares each monitoring system so that pressures can be obtained during catheter insertion.	
17. The physician or advanced practice nurse places a sterile plastic sleeve over the PA catheter, attaching it to the PA catheter before the catheter is inserted.[20] **(Level B*)**	A sterile sleeve prevents contamination of the PA catheter, allows repositioning of the catheter after the initial insertion, and reduces blood stream infections.[8,20]	Research has not yet determined how long the sleeve remains sterile.
18. As insertion begins, continuously run an electrocardiogram (ECG) and PA distal waveform strip.	Provides documentation of RA, RV, and PA pressures during insertion and dysrhythmia occurrence during insertion.	A dual-channel recorder is preferred because then the ECG and the PA waveform can be simultaneously recorded.
19. After the tip of the PA catheter is in the right atrium, inflate the balloon with no more than 1.25 to 1.5 mL of air and close the gate valve or the stopcock (Fig. 73-6).	The inflated balloon helps to advance the PA catheter through the right side of the heart and into the PA, minimizing the chance of endocardial damage. Closing the gate valve or the stopcock holds air in the balloon during insertion.	The presence of the tip of the catheter in the right atrium is determined by observing the PA distal waveform during insertion (see Fig. 73-3).
20. Observe for RA, RV, PA, and then PAO waveforms (see Fig. 73-3).	Placement in the PA is validated with waveform analysis.	Monitor the ECG tracing as the PA catheter is inserted because ventricular dysrhythmias may result from right ventricular irritability. Right ventricular pressures are obtained only during insertion.

*Level B: Well-designed, controlled studies with results that consistently support a specific action, intervention, or treatment

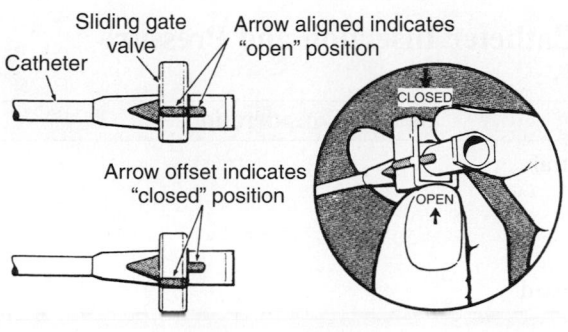

Sliding gate valve

Catheter

Arrow aligned indicates "open" position

CLOSED

Arrow offset indicates "closed" position

OPEN

Gate Valve Operation

FIGURE 73-6 Pulmonary artery catheter gate valve. *Top left:* Gate valve in the open position. *Bottom left:* Gate valve in the closed position. *(From Baxter Edwards Corporation.)*

Procedure	for Assisting with Pulmonary Artery Catheter Insertion and Pressure Monitoring—*Continued*	
Steps	**Rationale**	**Special Considerations**
21. Verify that the PA catheter is in the proper position. When the balloon is deflated, the monitor shows a PA tracing; when the balloon is inflated, the monitor shows a PAO tracing.	When the balloon is inflated, the catheter floats from the pulmonary artery to a smaller arteriole.	The catheter usually reaches the PA after being advanced 40 to 55 cm from the internal jugular vein, 35 to 50 cm from the subclavian vein, 60 cm from the femoral vein, 70 cm from the right antecubital fossa, and 80 cm from the left antecubital fossa. Placement may vary depending on patient size. A chest radiograph is obtained to verify catheter position.
22. After the pulmonary artery catheter is in place, open the balloon inflation gate valve or stopcock and remove the PA syringe.	The gate valve or stopcock is closed during insertion to retain air in the balloon. The air is then released so that continuous monitoring of the PA waveform can be performed.	Air is expelled from the PA syringe, and the empty syringe is reconnected to the end of the balloon inflation valve.
23. Reassess accurate leveling, and secure the system to the patient's chest or arm or to a pole mount.	Ensures that the air-filled interface (zeroing stopcock) is maintained at the level of the phlebostatic axis. If the air-fluid interface is above the phlebostatic axis, PA pressures are falsely low. If the air-fluid interface is below the phlebostatic axis, PA pressures are falsely high.	Leveling ensures accuracy. The point of the phlebostatic axis should be marked with an indelible marker, especially with use of a pole-mount setup.
24. Zero both the RA and PA hemodynamic monitoring systems (see Procedure 76).	Ensures accuracy of the system with the established reference point.	
25. Observe the waveform and perform a dynamic response test (square wave test; see Fig. 62-3).	Results indicate whether the system is correctly damped.	
26. Assist if needed with applying an occlusive, sterile dressing to the insertion site (see Procedure 69).	Reduces the risk for infection.	Follow institution standard for application of a chlorhexidine-impregnated sponge (see Procedure 69).
27. Document the external centimeter marking of the PA catheter at the introducer exit site.	Identifies the length of the PA catheter inserted and allows for evaluation of PA catheter movement.	If the centimeter marking is not visible at the exit site, measure the distance from the introducer exit site to the nearest visible marking.

Procedure continues on following page

Procedure	**for Assisting with Pulmonary Artery Catheter Insertion and Pressure Monitoring**—*Continued*		
Steps	**Rationale**	**Special Considerations**	

Steps	Rationale	Special Considerations
28. Set the alarms. Upper and lower alarm limits are set on the basis of the patient's current clinical status and hemodynamic values.	Activates the bedside and central alarm system.	
29. Discard used supplies in an appropriate receptacle.	Removes and safely discards used supplies.	
30. **HH**		
31. Ensure prescribed chest radiograph is completed.	Verifies catheter placement.	

Obtaining PA Pressure Measurements
RA/CVP

Steps	Rationale	Special Considerations
1. Position the patient in the supine position with the head of the bed from 0 to 45 degrees. **(Level B*)**	Studies have determined that the RA and PA pressures are accurate in this position.[3,6,7,10,17,19,21,32,33]	RA and PA pressures may be accurate for patients in the supine position with the head of the bed elevated up to 60 degrees,[7,21] but additional studies are needed to support this. Only one study[18] supports the accuracy of hemodynamic values for patients in the lateral positions; other studies do not.[3,13,17,25,31] The majority of studies support the accuracy of hemodynamic monitoring for patients in the prone position.[1,2,12,16,20,26,30] Two studies demonstrated that prone positioning caused an increase in hemodynamic values.[27,29]
2. Run a dual-channel strip of the ECG and RA waveform (Fig. 73-7).	RA pressures should be determined from the graphic strip because the effect of ventilation can be identified.	Digital data can be used to determine RA pressure if ventilation does not affect the RA pressure waveform. Some monitors have the capability of "freeze framing" waveforms. A cursor can be used to determine pressure measurements.
3. Measure RA pressure at end expiration.	Measurement is most accurate as the effects of pulmonary pressures are minimized.	

---

*Level B: Well-designed, controlled studies with results that consistently support a specific action, intervention, or treatment

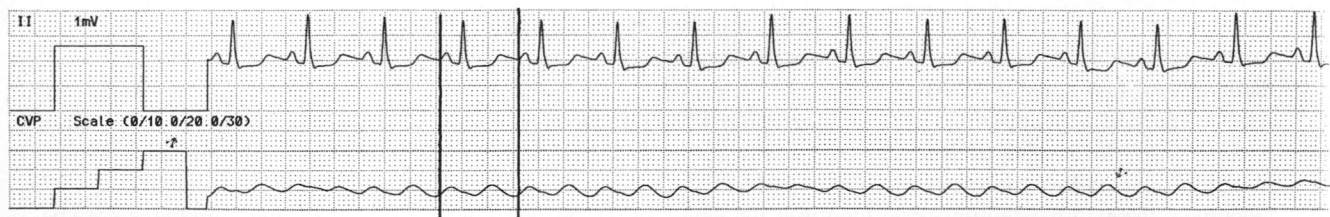

FIGURE 73-7   Note *vertical lines* drawn from the beginning of the P wave of two of the electrocardiogram (ECG) complexes down to the right atrial (RA) waveform. The first positive deflection of the RA waveform is the *a* wave; the second positive deflection is the *v* wave. The *c* wave, which would lie between the *a* wave and the *v* wave, is not evident in this strip.

Procedure	for Assisting with Pulmonary Artery Catheter Insertion and Pressure Monitoring—*Continued*	
Steps	**Rationale**	**Special Considerations**
4. With the dual-channel recorded strip, draw a vertical line from the beginning of the P wave of one of the ECG complexes down to the RA waveform. Repeat this with the next ECG complex (see Fig. 73-7).	Compares electrical activity with mechanical activity. Usually three waves are present on the RA waveform.	At times, the *c* wave is not present.
5. Align the PR interval with the RA waveform.	The *a* wave correlates with this interval.	
6. Identify the *a* wave.	The *a* wave is seen approximately 80 to 100 ms after the P wave. The *c* wave follows the *a* wave, and the *v* wave follows the *c* wave.	The *a* wave reflects atrial contraction. The *c* wave reflects closure of the tricuspid valve. The *v* wave reflects passive filling of the atria.
7. Identify the scale of the RA tracing (Fig. 73-8).	Aids in determination of the pressure measurement.	The RA scale commonly is set at 20 mm Hg. Scale settings may vary based on monitoring equipment.

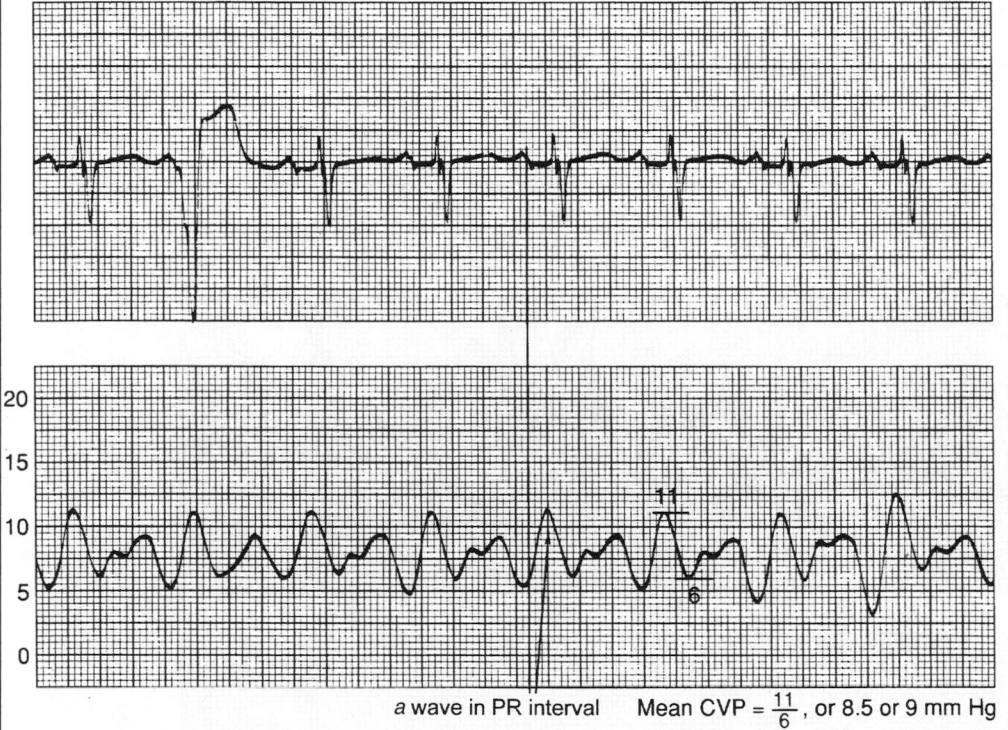

FIGURE 73-8   Obtaining measurements of right atrial and central venous pressures (RA/CVP). Aligning the *a* wave on the RA/CVP waveform with the PR interval on the electrocardiogram facilitates accurate measurement of RA/CVP at end diastole. *(From Ahrens TS, Taylor LK: Hemodynamic waveform analysis, Philadelphia, 1992, Saunders.)*

a wave in PR interval   Mean CVP = $\frac{11}{6}$, or 8.5 or 9 mm Hg

8. Measure the mean of the *a* wave to obtain the RA pressure (RAP; see Fig. 73-8).	The *a* wave represents atrial contraction and reflects right ventricular filling at end diastole.	

Procedure continues on following page

Procedure	for Assisting with Pulmonary Artery Catheter Insertion and Pressure Monitoring—*Continued*	

Steps	Rationale	Special Considerations
PA Systolic and Diastolic Pressures		
1. Position the patient in the supine position with the head of the bed from 0 to 45 degrees. **(Level B*)**	Studies have determined that the RA and PA pressures are accurate in this position.[3,6,7,10,17,19,21,32,33]	RA and PA pressures may be accurate for patients in the supine position with the head of the bed elevated up to 60 degrees,[7,21] but additional studies are needed to support this. Only one study[18] supports the accuracy of hemodynamic values for patients in the lateral positions; other studies[3,13,17,25,31] do not. The majority of the studies[1,2,12,16,20,26,30] support the accuracy of hemodynamic monitoring for patients in the prone position, yet two studies showed that prone positioning caused an increase in hemodynamic values.[27,29]
2. Run a dual-channel strip of the ECG and PA waveform (Fig. 73-9).	PA pressures are determined from the graphic strip because the effect of ventilation can be identified.	Some monitors have the capability of "freeze framing" waveforms. A cursor can be used to determine pressure measurements.
3. Measure the PA pressure at end expiration.	Measurement is most accurate as the effects of pulmonary pressures are minimized.	

*Level B: Well-designed, controlled studies with results that consistently support a specific action, intervention, or treatment

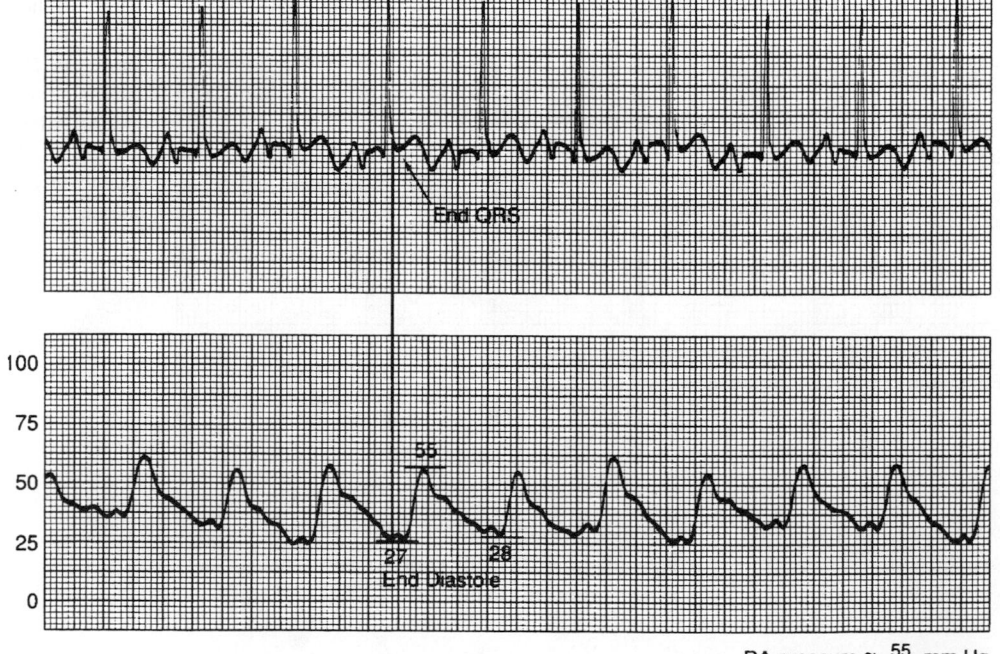

PA pressure ≅ $\frac{55}{28}$ mm Hg

FIGURE 73-9 Obtaining measurements of pressure in the pulmonary artery (PA). For systolic pressure, align the peak of the systolic waveform with the QT interval on the electrocardiogram (ECG). For PA diastolic pressure, use the end of the QRS as a marker to detect the PA diastolic phase. Obtain the reading just before the upstroke of the systolic waveform. *(From Ahrens TS, Taylor LK: Hemodynamic waveform analysis, Philadelphia, 1992, Saunders.)*

Procedure for Assisting with Pulmonary Artery Catheter Insertion and Pressure Monitoring—*Continued*

Steps	Rationale	Special Considerations
4. Identify the QT interval on the ECG strip.	Demonstrates ventricular depolarization.	
5. Align the QT interval with the PA waveform.	Compares electrical activity with mechanical activity.	
6. Identify the scale of the PA tracing.	Aids in determination of the pressure measurement.	The PA scale is commonly set at 40 mm Hg. Scale settings may vary based on monitoring equipment.
7. Measure the PA systolic pressure at the peak of the systolic waveform on the PA waveform (see Fig. 73-9).	Reflects the highest systolic pressure.	
8. Align the end of the QRS complex with the PA waveform (see Fig. 73-9).	The end of the QRS complex correlates with ventricular end-diastolic pressure.	
9. Measure the PA diastolic pressure at the point of the intersection of this line (see Fig. 73-9).	This point occurs just before the upstroke of the systolic pressure.	
PAOP		
1. Position the patient in the supine position with the head of the bed from 0 to 45 degrees. **(Level B*)**	Studies have determined that the RA and PA pressures are accurate in this position.[3,6,7,10,17,19,21,32,33]	RA and PA pressures may be accurate for patients in the supine position with the head of the bed elevated up to 60 degrees,[7,21] but additional studies are needed to support this. Only one study[18] supports the accuracy of hemodynamic values for patients in the lateral positions; other studies[3,13,17,25,31] do not. The majority of the studies[1,2,12,16,20,26,30] support the accuracy of hemodynamic monitoring for patients in the prone position, but two studies demonstrated that prone positioning caused an increase in hemodynamic values.[27,29]
2. Fill the PA syringe with 1.5 mL of air.	More than 1.5 mL of air may rupture the PA balloon and the pulmonary arteriole.	
3. Connect the PA syringe to the gate valve or stopcock of the balloon port of the PA catheter (see Fig. 73-6).	This port is designed for PA balloon air inflation.	
4. Run a dual-channel strip of the ECG and PA waveform.	The PAO pressures are determined from the graphic strip because the effect of ventilation can be identified.	Some monitors have the capability of "freeze framing" waveforms. A cursor can be used to determine pressure measurements.
5. Slowly inflate the balloon with air until the PA waveform changes to a PAO waveform (Fig. 73-10).	A slight resistance is usually felt during inflation of the balloon. Overinflation of the balloon can cause pulmonary arteriole infarction or rupture, resulting in potentially life-threatening hemorrhage.[14]	Only enough air is needed to convert the PA waveform to a PAO waveform. Thus, the entire amount of 1.5 mL of air is not necessarily needed.

*Level B: Well-designed, controlled studies with results that consistently support a specific action, intervention, or treatment

Procedure continues on following page

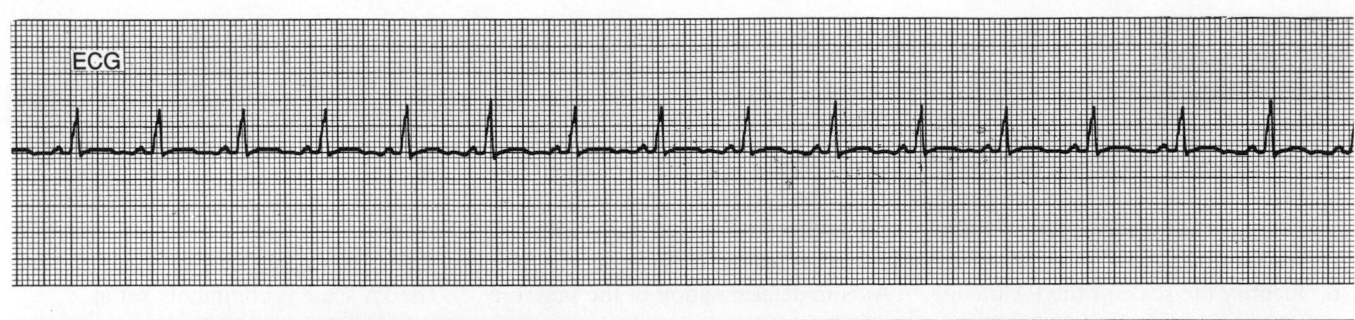

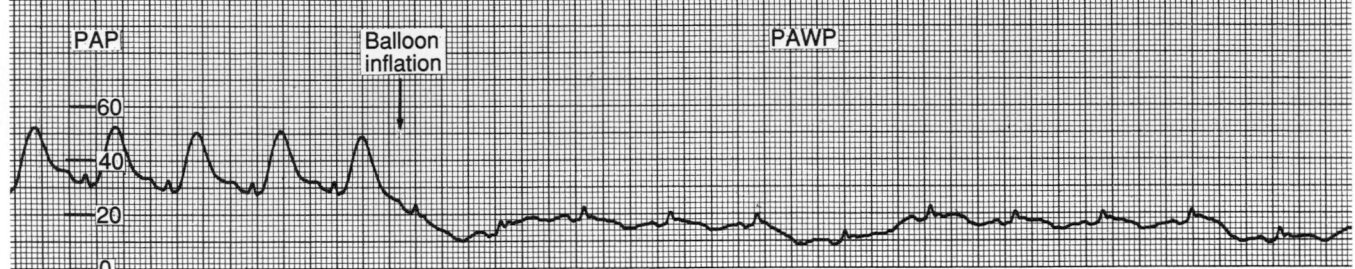

FIGURE 73-10 Change in pulmonary artery pressure (PAP) waveform to pulmonary artery occlusion pressure waveform with balloon inflation. The balloon is inflated while the bedside monitor is observed for change in the waveform. Balloon inflation *(arrow)* in patient with normal pulmonary artery occlusion pressure. Pulmonary artery occlusion pressure (PAOP) is also referred to as pulmonary artery wedge pressure (PAWP).

Procedure	for Assisting with Pulmonary Artery Catheter Insertion and Pressure Monitoring—*Continued*	
Steps	**Rationale**	**Special Considerations**
6. Inflate the PA balloon for no more than 8 to 15 seconds (two to four respiratory cycles).	Prolonged inflation of the balloon can cause pulmonary arteriole infarction and rupture, with potentially life-threatening hemorrhage.[14]	
7. Disconnect the syringe from the balloon-inflation port. **(Level M*)**	Allows air to passively escape from the balloon.	Active withdrawal of air from the balloon can weaken the balloon, pull the balloon structure into the inflation lumen, and possibly cause balloon rupture.
8. Observe the monitor as the PAO waveform changes back to the PA waveform.	Ensures adequate balloon deflation.	
9. Expel air from the syringe.	The syringe should remain empty so that accidental balloon inflation does not occur.	
10. Reconnect the syringe to the end of the balloon-inflation valve.	The syringe that is manufactured for the PA catheter should be connected to the PA catheter so that it is not lost. This syringe can only be filled with 1.5 mL of air, thus serving as a safety feature to minimize the chance of balloon overinflation.	

*Level M: Manufacturer's recommendations only

Procedure for Assisting with Pulmonary Artery Catheter Insertion and Pressure Monitoring—*Continued*

Steps	Rationale	Special Considerations
11. Follow institution standard regarding keeping the gate valve or the stopcock open.	The most important considerations are that the syringe is attached to the balloon-inflation port, the syringe is empty, and the PA distal waveform reflects a pulmonary artery waveform.	
12. With the dual-channel recorded strip, draw a vertical line from the beginning of the P wave of one of the ECG complexes down to the PAO waveform. Repeat this with the next ECG complex.	Compares electrical activity with mechanical activity. Two to three waves are present on the PAO waveform.	The *c* waves commonly are not present on PAO waveforms because of the distance the pressure needs to travel back to the transducer.
13. Align the end of a QRS complex of the ECG strip with the PAO waveform (Fig. 73-11).	Compares electrical activity with mechanical activity.	
14. Identify the *a* wave (see Fig. 73-11).	The *a* wave correlates with the end of the QRS complex. The *c* wave follows the *a* wave, and the *v* wave follows the *c* wave.	If only two waves are present, the first wave is the *a* wave and the second wave is the *v* wave.

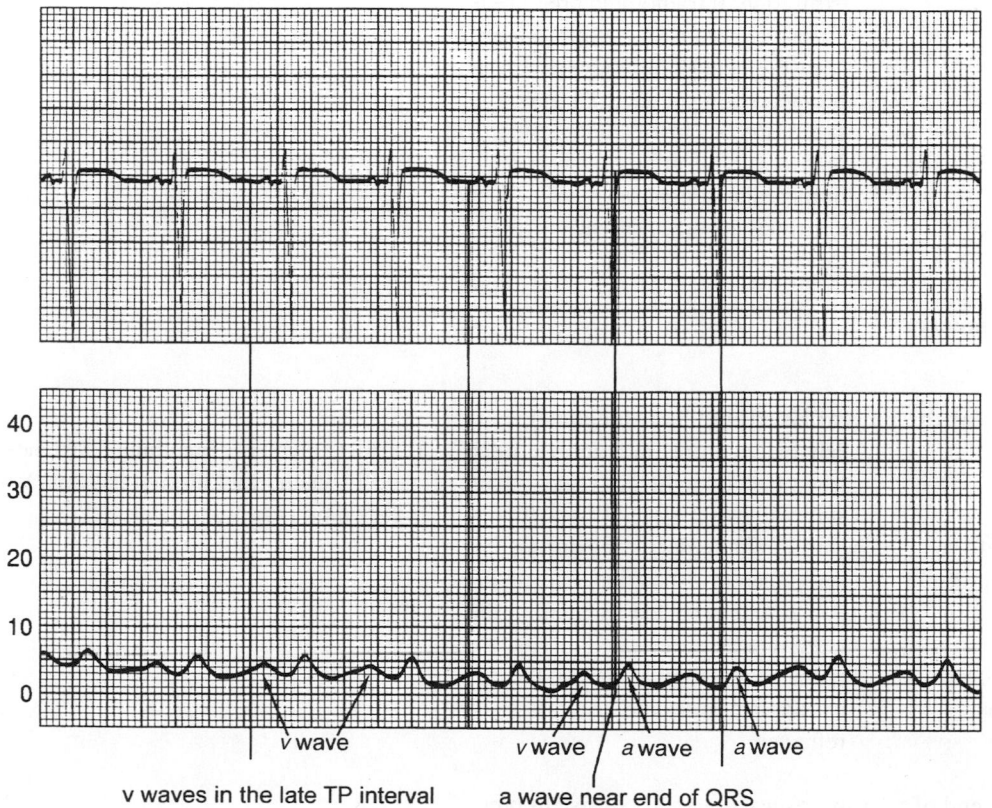

40
30
20
10
0

v wave   *v* wave / *a* wave / *a* wave

v waves in the late TP interval   a wave near end of QRS

FIGURE 73-11   Obtaining measurement of the pulmonary artery occlusion pressure (PAOP). For accurate readings, align the *a* wave from the PAO waveform with the end of the QRS on the electrocardiogram (ECG) at end diastole. Pulmonary artery occlusion pressure (PAOP) is also referred to as pulmonary artery wedge pressure (PAWP). *(From Ahrens TS, Taylor LK: Hemodynamic waveform analysis, Philadelphia, 1992, Saunders.)*

Steps	Rationale	Special Considerations
15. Identify the scale of the PAO tracing.	Aids in determination of pressure measurement.	PA scale commonly is set at 40 mm Hg.
16. Measure the mean of the *a* wave to obtain the PAOP (see Fig. 73-5).	The *a* wave represents atrial contraction and reflects left ventricular filling at end diastole.	If PEEP is being used and the PEEP is more than 10 cm H_2O, adjustments in determination of the pressures may be necessary. Follow institution standard.

Procedure continues on following page

Procedure	**for Assisting with Pulmonary Artery Catheter Insertion and Pressure Monitoring—*Continued***	
Steps	**Rationale**	**Special Considerations**
17. Compare the PADP with the PAOP.	The PAOP is commonly 1 to 4 mm Hg less than the PADP. Significant differences between PADP and PAOP may exist for patients with pulmonary hypertension, chronic obstructive lung disease, ARDS, pulmonary embolus, and tachycardia. PADPs that correlate with PAOPs represent left ventricular filling pressures.	
18. Follow PADP if a close correlation is found between PADP and PAOP.	Ensures accuracy of determination of left ventricular filling pressures.	Minimizes the number of times the PA balloon is inflated.
19. Follow the PAOP if greater than 4 mm Hg of difference is found between PAOP and PADP.	Ensures accuracy of measurements.	

Measurement of Hemodynamic Pressures at End Expiration

1. Measure all hemodynamic pressures at end expiration to ensure accuracy.	Atmospheric and alveolar pressures are approximately equal at end expiration. Intrathoracic pressure is closest to zero at end expiration. Measurement of hemodynamic pressures is most accurate at end expiration because pulmonary pressures have minimal effect on intracardiac pressures.	
2. Determine end expiration by observing the rise and fall of the chest during breathing and use of graphic hemodynamic, respiratory, or continuous airway pressure waveforms.	Determines accuracy of end expiration.	

Determining End Expiration for the Patient Breathing Spontaneously

1. Record a strip of the PA waveform.	A labeled recording aids in determination of accurate hemodynamic pressure values.	In patients who are breathing spontaneously, the normal inspiratory:expiratory ratio is approximately 1:2.
2. Note that the pressure waveform dips down during the inspiratory phase of breathing (Fig. 73-12).	Pleural pressure decreases during spontaneous inspiration, and this decrease is reflected by a fall in the cardiac pressures.	
3. Note that the pressure waveform elevates during the expiratory phase of breathing (see Fig. 73-12).	As pleural pressures equalize, the cardiac pressures are accurately reflected.	
4. Measure the pressure at the end of the expiratory phase (see Fig. 73-12).	Ensures accurate and consistent pressure measurements.	

Determining End Expiration for the Patient Receiving Mechanical Ventilation

1. Record a strip of the PA waveform.	A labeled recording aids in determination of accurate hemodynamic pressure values.	

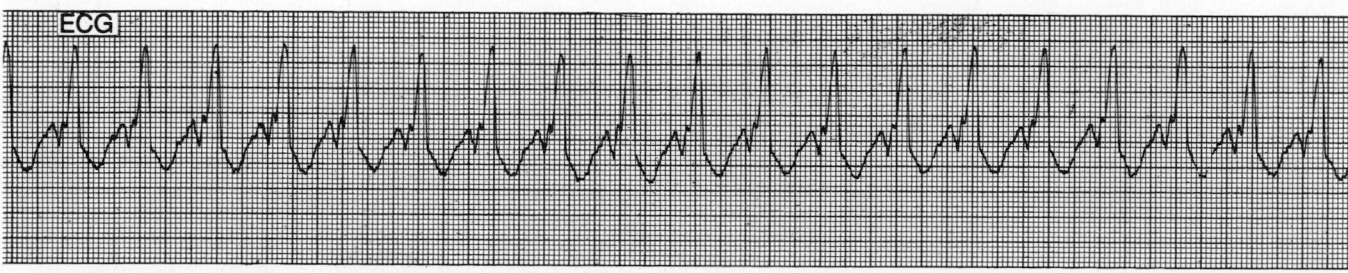

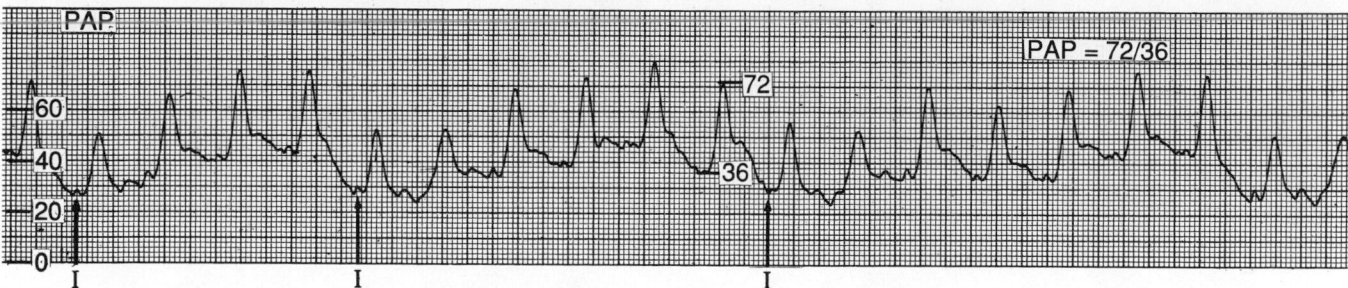

FIGURE 73-12 Respiratory fluctuations of pulmonary artery pressure (PAP) waveform in a spontaneously breathing patient. The location of inspiration *(I)* is marked on the waveform. The points just before inspiration are end expiration, where readings are taken.

Procedure	for Assisting with Pulmonary Artery Catheter Insertion and Pressure Monitoring—*Continued*	
Steps	**Rationale**	**Special Considerations**
2. Note that the pressure waveform elevates as a breath is delivered by the ventilator (Fig. 73-13).	As the ventilator delivers a breath to the lungs, an increase in pleural pressure results. This increase in pleural pressure causes an increase in intracardiac pressures.	
3. Note that the pressure waveform dips down as the breath is exhaled (see Fig. 73-13).	As the mechanical breath is exhaled, pulmonary pressures decrease and intracardiac pressures are accurately and consistently measured.	

Determining End Expiration for the Patient Receiving Intermittent Mandatory Mechanical Ventilation

1. Record a strip of the PA waveform.	A labeled recording aids in determination of accurate hemodynamic pressure monitoring.	
2. If the patient is receiving intermittent mandatory ventilation, measure the pressure during the end expiration.	Ensures accurate determination of pressure values.	
3. Note that the pressure waveform elevates as a breath is delivered by the ventilator (Fig. 73-14).	As the ventilator delivers a breath to the lungs, an increase in pleural pressure results. This increase in pleural pressure causes an increase in intracardiac pressures.	
4. Note that the pressure waveform dips down as the breath is exhaled (see Fig. 73-14).	As the mechanical breath is exhaled, pulmonary pressures decrease and intracardiac pressures are more accurately reflected.	
5. Identify the patient's spontaneous breath (see Fig. 73-14).	This breath may occur just before triggered ventilator breaths.	
6. Determine end expiration.	Ensures accuracy of measurements.	Airway pressure waveforms can be used to facilitate identification of end expiration.

Procedure continues on following page

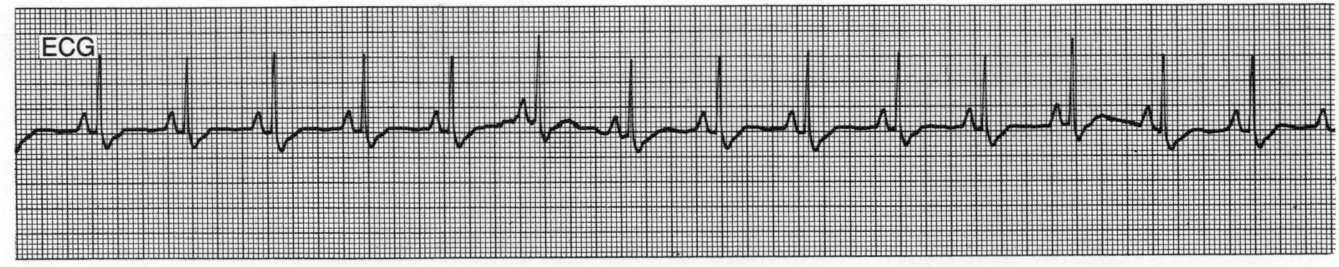

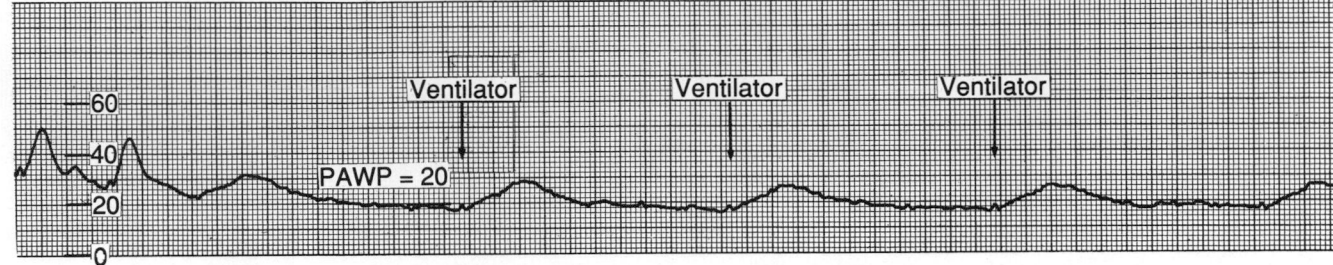

FIGURE 73-13   Patient on mechanical ventilation (on pressure support-type ventilator) who had no spontaneous respiration because of neuromuscular-blocking agent (vecuronium). The point of end expiration is located just before the ventilator artifact. Pulmonary artery occlusion pressure (PAOP) is also referred to as pulmonary artery wedge pressure (PAWP).

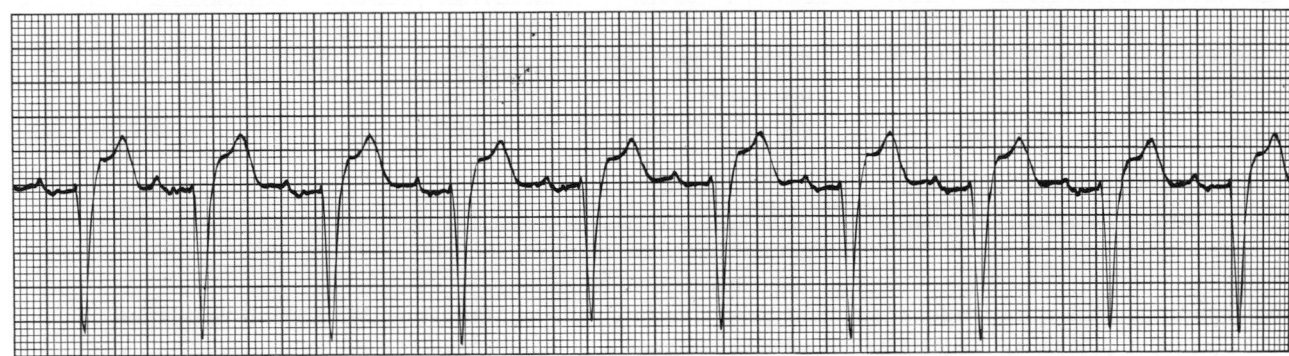

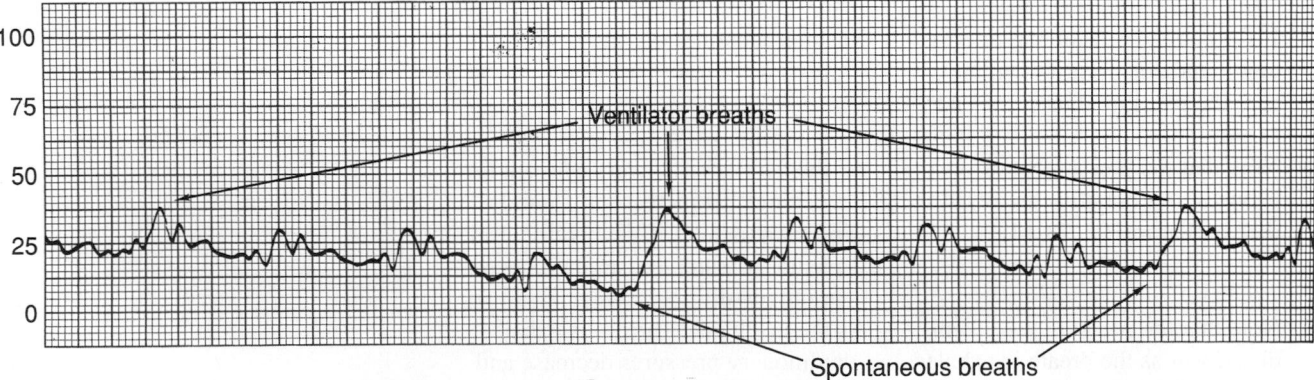

FIGURE 73-14   Intermittent mandatory ventilation (IMV) mode of ventilation and the effect on the pulmonary artery (PA) waveform. *(From Ahrens TS, Taylor LK: Hemodynamic waveform analysis, Philadelphia, 1992, Saunders.)*

Expected Outcomes	Unexpected Outcomes
• Accurate placement of the pulmonary artery catheter • Adequate and appropriate waveforms • Ability to obtain accurate information about cardiac pressures • Evaluation of information obtained to guide therapeutic interventions	• Pneumothorax or hemothorax • Infection • Ventricular dysrhythmias • Heart block • Misplacement (e.g., carotid artery, subclavian artery) • Hemorrhage • Hematoma • Pericardial or ventricular rupture • Venous air embolism • Cardiac tamponade • Sepsis • Pulmonary artery infarction • Pulmonary artery rupture • Pulmonary artery catheter balloon rupture • Pulmonary artery catheter knotting • Pseudoaneurysm formation • Heparin-induced thrombocytopenia • Thrombosis • Valvular damage • Pain

Patient Monitoring and Care

Steps	Rationale	Reportable Conditions
		These conditions should be reported if they persist despite nursing interventions.
1. Recheck leveling whenever patient position changes.	Ensures accurate reference point for the left atrium.	
2. Zero the transducer during initial setup or before insertion if disconnection occurs between the transducer and the monitoring cable, if disconnection occurs between the monitoring cable and the monitor, and when the values obtained do not fit the clinical picture. Follow manufacturer's recommendations for disposable systems.	Ensures accuracy of the hemodynamic monitoring system.	
3. Place sterile nonvented caps on all stopcocks. Replace with new sterile caps whenever the caps are removed.	Stopcocks can be a source of contamination. Stopcocks that are part of the initial setup are commonly vented. Vented caps need to be replaced with nonvented caps to maintain sterility.	
4. Monitor the pressure transducer system (pressure tubing, transducer, stopcocks, etc) for air and eliminate air from the system.	Air emboli are potentially fatal.	• Suspected air emboli

Procedure continues on following page

Patient Monitoring and Care —*Continued*

Steps	Rationale	Reportable Conditions
5. Continuously monitor hemodynamic waveforms and obtain hemodynamic values (pulmonary artery systolic pressure [PASP], PADP, RAP) hourly and as necessary with condition changes. Follow institution standard for obtaining hemodynamic values.	Provides for continuous waveform analysis and assessment of patient status.	• Abnormal hemodynamic waveforms or pressures
6. Obtain CO, cardiac index (CI), and systemic vascular resistance (SVR) and additional parameters immediately after catheter insertion and as necessary per patient condition.	Monitors patient status.	• Abnormal hemodynamic parameters or significant changes in hemodynamic parameters
7. Change the hemodynamic monitoring system (flush solution, pressure tubing, transducers, and stopcocks) every 96 hours. **(Level B*)** The flush solution may need to be changed more frequently if near empty of solution.	The Centers for Disease Control and Prevention (CDC)[23] and research findings[22,24] recommend that the hemodynamic flush system can be used safely for 96 hours. This recommendation is based on research conducted with disposable pressure monitoring systems used for peripheral and central lines.	
8. Perform a dynamic response test (square wave test) at the start of each shift, with a change of the waveform, or when the system is opened to air (see Fig. 62-3).	An optimally damped system provides an accurate waveform.	• Overdamped or underdamped waveforms that cannot be corrected with troubleshooting procedures
9. Label the tubing with the date and time the system was prepared.	Identifies when the system needs to be changed.	
10. Maintain the pressure bag or device at 300 mm Hg.	At 300 mm Hg, each flush device delivers approximately 1 to 3 mL/hr to maintain patency of the system.	
11. Do not fast flush the catheter for longer than 2 seconds.[9]	Pulmonary artery rupture may occur with prolonged flushing of high-pressure fluid.	• Hemoptysis
12. Never flush the PA catheter when the balloon is wedged in the pulmonary artery.	Excessive PA pressure may cause PA damage or rupture.	• Hemoptysis
13. Use aseptic technique when withdrawing from or flushing the PA catheter.	Prevents bacterial contamination of the system.	
14. Clear the system, including stopcocks, of all traces of blood after blood withdrawal.	Blood can become a medium for bacterial growth.[23] Clots also may be flushed into the catheter if all blood is not eliminated.	
15. Maintain sterility and integrity of the plastic sleeve covering the PA catheter.	Any tear in the sleeve breaks the sterile barrier, making catheter repositioning no longer possible.	• Defects in the integrity of the plastic sleeve
16. Blood products and albumin should never be infused through the PA catheter.	Viscous blood may occlude the catheter. The accuracy of the PA monitoring system may be adversely affected.	

*Level B: Well-designed, controlled studies with results that consistently support a specific action, intervention, or treatment

Patient Monitoring and Care —*Continued*

Steps	Rationale	Reportable Conditions
17. IV fluids are never infused via the distal lumen of the PA catheter and are rarely infused via the proximal lumen of the PA catheter.	PA monitoring is not possible, and a life-threatening situation can occur (e.g., undetected wedged PA catheter).	
18. Replace gauze dressings every 2 days and transparent dressings at least every 7 days.[15,23] **(Level D*)**	Decreases the risk for infection at the catheter site. The CDC recommends replacing the dressing when the dressing becomes damp, loosened, or soiled or when inspection of the site is necessary.[23]	• Signs or symptoms of infection
19. Perform central venous catheter site care (see Procedure 69).	Ensures consistency of dressing change and indicates when the next change will occur.	
20. Obtain PA waveform strips to place on the patient's chart at the start of each shift and whenever a change in the waveform occurs.	The printed waveform allows assessment of the adequacy of the waveform, presence of damping, or respiratory variation.	
21. Consider changing PA catheters every 7 days. **(Level B*)**	The CDC[23] and research findings[4,11] recommend that PA catheters do not need to be changed more frequently than every 7 days. There are no specific recommendations regarding routine replacement of PA catheters that need to be in place for greater than 7 days.[11,23] PA catheters should be removed and replaced if they malfunction. PA catheters should be removed and the introducers should be changed over a guidewire, followed by insertion of new PA catheters, when a positive blood culture is obtained after the PA catheter was inserted and sepsis develops without an identified source.[11] PA catheters should be removed and reinserted at a new site when there is a skin infection at the catheter insertion site (i.e., redness, swelling, or drainage at or around the insertion site) or a positive culture at the insertion site.[4,11]	• Signs and symptoms of PA catheter site infection • Signs and symptoms of sepsis
22. Follow institution standard for assessing pain. Administer analgesia as prescribed.	Identifies need for pain interventions.	• Continued pain despite pain interventions

*Level B: Well-designed, controlled studies with results that consistently support a specific action, intervention, or treatment
*Level D: Peer-reviewed professional organizational standards with clinical studies to support recommendations

Procedure continues on following page

Documentation

Documentation should include the following:
- Patient and family education
- Universal Protocol requirements
- Completion of informed consent
- Insertion of the PA catheter
- External centimeter marking of PA catheter noted at exit site
- Patient tolerance of procedure
- Confirmation of PA catheter placement (e.g., waveforms, chest radiograph)
- Date and time of PA catheter site care and dressing change

- Pain assessment, interventions, and effectiveness
- Cardiac rhythm during PA catheter insertion and monitoring
- Site assessment
- PA pressures (RA/CVP, PA systolic, diastolic, mean, and PAOP)
- Waveforms (RA/CVP, pulmonary artery pressure [PAP], PAOP)
- CO/CI and SVR
- Occurrence of unexpected outcomes and interventions

References

CR 1. Blanch L, et al: Short term effects of prone position in critically ill patients with acute respiratory distress syndrome, *Intensive Care Med* 23:1033-1039, 1997.

CR 2. Brussel T, et al: Mechanical ventilation in the prone position for acute respiratory failure after cardiac surgery, *J Cardiothorac Vasc Anesth* 7:541-546, 1993.

CR 3. Cason CL, et al: Effects of backrest elevation and position on pulmonary artery pressures, *Cardiovasc Nurs* 26:1-5, 1990.

CR 4. Chen Y, et al: Comparison between replacement at 4 days and 7 days on the infection rate for pulmonary artery catheters in an intensive care unit, *Crit Care Med* 31:1353-1358, 2003.

CR 5. Chong BH: Heparin-induced thrombocytopenia, *Br J Haematol* 89:431-439, 1995.

CR 6. Chulay M, Miller T: The effect of backrest elevation on pulmonary artery and pulmonary capillary wedge pressures in patients after cardiac surgery, *Heart Lung* 13:138-140, 1984.

CR 7. Clochesy J, Hinshaw AD, Otto CW: Effects of change of position on pulmonary artery and pulmonary capillary wedge pressure in mechanically ventilated patients, *NITA* 7:223-225, 1984.

CR 8. Cohen Y, et al: The "hands-off" catheter in the prevention of systemic infections associated with pulmonary artery catheter: a prospective study, *Am J Respir Crit Care Med* 157:284-287, 1998.

CR 9. Daily EK, Schroeder JS: *Techniques in bedside hemodynamic monitoring,* ed 5, St Louis, 1994. Mosby.

CR 10. Dobbin K, et al: Pulmonary artery pressure measurement in patients with elevated pressures: effect of backrest elevation and method of measurement, *Am J Crit Care* 1:61-69, 1992.

CR 11. Eyer S, et al: Catheter-related sepsis: prospective, randomized study of three methods of long-term catheter maintenance, *Crit Care Med* 18:1073-1079, 1990.

CR 12. Fridrich P, et al: The effects of long-term prone positioning in patients with trauma-induced adult respiratory distress syndrome, *Anesth Analg* 83:1206-1211, 1996.

CR 13. Groom L, Frisch SR, Elliot M: Reproducibility and accuracy of pulmonary artery pressure measurement in supine and lateral positions, *Heart Lung* 19:147-151, 1990.

CR 14. Hannan AT, Brown M, Bigman O: Pulmonary artery catheter induced hemorrhage, *Chest* 85:128-131, 1984.

CR 15. Infusion Nurses Society: Infusion nursing standards of practice, *J Infusion Nurs* 29:S1-S92, 2006.

CR 16. Jolliet P, Bulpa P, Chevrolet JC: Effects of prone position on gas exchange and hemodynamics in severe acute respiratory distress syndrome, *Crit Care Med* 26:1977-1985, 1998.

CR 17. Keating D, et al: Effect of sidelying positions on pulmonary artery pressures, *Heart Lung* 15:605-610, 1986.

CR 18. Kennedy GT, Bryant A, Crawford MH: The effects of lateral body positioning on measurements of pulmonary artery and pulmonary wedge pressures, *Heart Lung* 13:155-158, 1984.

CR 19. Lambert CW, Cason CL: Backrest elevation and pulmonary artery pressures: research analysis, *Dimens Crit Care Nurs* 9:327-335, 1990.

CR 20. Langer M, et al: The prone position in ARDS patients, *Chest* 94:103-107, 1988.

CR 21. Laulive JL: Pulmonary artery pressures and position changes in the critically ill adult, *Dimens Crit Care Nurs* 1:28-34, 1982.

CR 22. Luskin RL, et al: Extended use of disposable pressure transducers: a bacteriologic evaluation, *JAMA* 255:916-920, 1986.

CR 23. O'Grady NP, et al: Guidelines for the prevention of intravascular catheter-related infections, *Am J Infect Control* 30:476-489, 2002.

CR 24. O'Malley MK, et al: Value of routine pressure monitoring system changes after 72 hours of use, *Crit Care Med* 22:1424-1430, 1994.

CR 25. Osika C: Measurement of pulmonary artery pressures: supine verses side-lying head-elevated positions, *Heart Lung* 18:298-299, 1989.

CR 26. Pappert D, et al: Influence of positioning on ventilation-perfusion relationships in severe adult respiratory distress syndrome, *Chest* 106:1511-1516, 1994.

CR 27. Pelosi P, et al: Effects of the prone position on respiratory mechanics and gas exchange during acute lung injury, *Am J Respir Crit Care Med* 157:387-393, 1998.

CR 28. Randolph AG, et al: Benefit of heparin in central venous and pulmonary artery catheters, *Chest* 113:165-171, 1998.

CR 29. Voggenreiter G, et al: Intermittent prone positioning in the treatment of severe and moderate posttraumatic lung injury, *Crit Care Med* 27:2375-2382, 1999.

CR 30. Vollman KM, Bander JJ: Improved oxygenation utilizing a prone positioner in patients with acute respiratory distress syndrome, *Intensive Care Med* 22:1105-1111, 1996.

CR 31. Wild L: Effect of lateral recumbent positions on measurement of pulmonary artery and pulmonary artery wedge pressures in critically ill adults, *Heart Lung* 13:305, 1984.

CR 32. Wilson AE, et al: Effect of backrest position on hemodynamic and right ventricular measurements in critically ill adults, *Am J Crit Care* 5:264-270, 1996.

CR 33. Woods SL, Mansfield LW: Effect of body position upon pulmonary artery and pulmonary capillary wedge pressures in noncritically ill patients, *Heart Lung* 5:83-90, 1976.

Additional Readings

CR Abreu AR, Campos MA, Krieger BP: Pulmonary artery rupture induced by a pulmonary artery catheter: a case report and review of the literature, *J Intensive Care Med* 19: 291-296, 2004.

CR Ahrens TS, Taylor LA: *Hemodynamic waveform analysis,* Philadelphia, 1992, Saunders.

CR American Association of Critical-Care Nurses: *AACN practice alert: pulmonary artery pressure measurement,* 2004, available at www.aacn.org.

CR Anonymous: Pulmonary artery catheter consensus conference: consensus statement, *Crit Care Med* 25:910-925, 1997.

CR Bridges EJ: Pulmonary artery pressure monitoring: when, how, and what else to use, *AACN Adv Crit Care* 17: 286-305, 2006.

CR Daily EK: Hemodynamic waveform analysis, *J Cardiovasc Nurs* 15:6-22,87-88, 2001.

CR Darovic GO: *Hemodynamic monitoring: invasive and noninvasive clinical application,* ed 3, Philadelphia, 2002, Saunders.

CR Houghton D, et al: Routine daily chest radiography in patients with pulmonary artery catheters, *Am J Crit Care* 11: 261-265, 2002.

CR Keckeisen M: *Protocols for practice: hemodynamic monitoring series: pulmonary artery pressure monitoring,* Aliso Viejo, CA, 1997, American Association of Critical-Care Nurses.

CR Liu C, Webb C: From the Food and Drug Administration: pulmonary artery rupture: serious complication associated with pulmonary artery catheters, *Int J Trauma Nurs* 6: 19-26, 2000.

CR Ott K, Johnson K, Ahrens T: New technologies in the assessment of hemodynamic parameters, *J Cardiovasc Nurs* 15:41-55, 2001.

CR Quaal SJ: Improving the accuracy of pulmonary artery catheter measurement, *J Cardiovasc Nurs* 15:71-82, 2001.

CR Quaal SJ: Is it necessary to perform a square wave test routinely to test for accuracy in hemodynamic monitoring? Or is it recommended only if there is a problem? *Crit Care Nurse* 15:92-93, 1995.

Rauen CA, Flynn MB, Bridges E: Evidence-based practice habits: transforming research into bedside practice, *Crit Care Nurse* 29:46-59, 2009.

Rizvi K, et al: Effect of airway pressure display on interobserver agreement in the assessment of vascular pressures in patients with acute lung injury and acute respiratory distress syndrome, *Crit Care Med* 33:98-103, 2005.

Pulmonary Artery Catheter Removal

P U R P O S E :   The pulmonary artery catheter is removed when the patient's condition is improved sufficiently that hemodynamic monitoring is no longer necessary, when there is risk for complications from the presence of the catheter (e.g., dysrhythmias, pseudoaneurysm), or when there is risk for infection associated with the prolonged use of intravascular catheters.

Teresa Preuss, Debra Lynn-McHale Wiegand

PREREQUISITE NURSING KNOWLEDGE

- Knowledge of the normal cardiovascular anatomy and physiology is necessary.
- Knowledge of normal values for intracardiac pressures is important.
- Knowledge of normal coagulation values is needed.
- Knowledge of normal waveform configurations for right atrial pressure (RAP), right ventricular pressure (RVP), pulmonary artery pressure (PAP), and pulmonary artery occlusive pressure (PAOP) is necessary.
- Venous access routes should be known.
- Principles of aseptic technique should be known.
- Advanced cardiac life support knowledge and skills are needed.
- Potential complications associated with removal of the pulmonary artery (PA) catheter should be understood.
- Clinical and technical competence in PA catheter removal is necessary.
- Knowledge of the state nurse practice act is important because some states do not allow this intervention to be performed by a registered nurse.
- Air embolism can occur during the removal of the catheter. Air embolism after the removal of the catheter is a result of air drawn in along the subcutaneous tract and into the vein. During inspiration, negative intrathoracic pressure is transmitted to the central veins. Any opening external to the body to one of these veins may result in aspiration of

air into the central venous system. The pathologic effects depend on the volume and rate of air aspirated.
- Indications for the removal of the PA catheter include the following:
  - ❖ The patient's condition no longer necessitates hemodynamic monitoring.
  - ❖ Complications occur because of the presence of the PA catheter.
  - ❖ The patient shows evidence of a catheter-related infection that may be associated with the PA catheter.
- Contraindications to percutaneous removal of the PA catheter include the following:
  - ❖ The PA catheter is knotted (observed on chest radiograph).
  - ❖ A permanent pacemaker, temporary transvenous pacemaker, or implantable cardioverter defibrillator (ICD) is present (catheter should be removed by an advanced practice nurse or a physician).

EQUIPMENT

- 1.5-mL syringe
- Sterile and nonsterile gloves
- Gown
- Fluid-shield face mask or goggles
- 4 × 4 sterile gauze pads
- Central line dressing kit
- Two moisture-proof absorbent pads
- One roll of 2-inch tape

Additional equipment to have available as needed includes the following:
- Obturator/cap for hemostasis valve
- Additional dressing supplies (e.g., transparent dressing)
- Suture removal kit
- Emergency equipment

PATIENT AND FAMILY EDUCATION

- Explain the procedure and the reason for removal of the catheter. ➤➤*Rationale:* This explanation provides information and decreases anxiety.
- Explain the importance of the patient lying still during the removal of the catheter. ➤➤*Rationale:* The explanation ensures patient cooperation and facilitates safe removal of the catheter.
- Instruct the patient and family to report any shortness of breath, bleeding, or discomfort at the insertion site after removal of the catheter. ➤➤*Rationale:* Identifies patient discomfort and early recognition of complications.

PATIENT ASSESSMENT AND PREPARATION

Patient Assessment

- Assess the electrocardiogram (ECG), vital signs, and neurovascular status of the extremity distal to the catheter insertion site. ➤➤*Rationale:* This assessment serves as baseline data.
- If the introducer will also be removed, assess the current coagulation values of the patient. ➤➤*Rationale:* If the patient has abnormal coagulation study results, hemostasis may be difficult to obtain after the introducer catheter is removed.
- Verify catheter position with waveform analysis or chest radiograph. ➤➤*Rationale:* Accuracy of catheter position is ensured.

- Determine whether the patient has a permanent pacemaker, temporary transvenous pacemaker, or ICD. ➤➤*Rationale:* PA catheter removal by a critical care nurse is contraindicated in the presence of a permanent pacemaker, temporary transvenous pacemaker, or ICD. Entanglement of the PA catheter and the pacemaker electrodes can occur.
- Assess the integrity of the PA catheter. ➤➤*Rationale:* The PA catheter should be removed by an advanced practice nurse or physician if the catheter or introducer is not intact (e.g., visible cracks are noted).
- Assess the catheter site for redness, warmth at the site, tenderness, or presence of drainage. ➤➤*Rationale:* Signs and symptoms of infection are assessed.

Patient Preparation

- In collaboration with the physician, determine when the PA catheter should be removed. ➤➤*Rationale:* The invasive catheter is removed when it is no longer indicated.
- Verify correct patient with two identifiers. ➤➤*Rationale:* Prior to performing a procedure, the nurse should ensure the correct identification of the patient for the intended intervention.
- Ensure that the patient and family understand preprocedural teaching. Answer questions as they arise, and reinforce information as needed. ➤➤*Rationale:* Understanding of previously taught information is evaluated and reinforced.
- Place the patient in a supine position with the head of the bed in a slight Trendelenburg's position (or flat if Trendelenburg's position is contraindicated or not tolerated by the patient). ➤➤*Rationale:* A normal pressure gradient exists between atmospheric air and the central venous compartment that promotes air entry if the compartment is open. The lower the site of entry below the heart, the lower the pressure gradient, thus minimizing the risk of venous air embolism.

Procedure | for Pulmonary Artery Catheter Removal

Steps	Rationale	Special Considerations
1. 🄷🄷		
2. 🄿🄴		All health care providers in the room should wear a face mask.
3. Place a moisture-proof absorbent pad under the patient's upper torso and another under the PA catheter.	Collects blood and body fluids associated with removal; serves as a receptacle for the contaminated catheter.	
4. Place the patient supine in slight Trendelenburg's position.[3,5-7,12] **(Level E*)**	Minimizes the risk for venous air embolus.	Place the patient flat if Trendelenburg's position is contraindicated, not tolerated by the patient, or a femoral PA catheter will be removed. If the PA catheter is in the femoral vein, extend the patient's leg and ensure the groin area is adequately exposed.

*Level E: Multiple case reports, theory-based evidence from expert opinions, or peer-reviewed professional organizational standards without clinical studies to support recommendations

Procedure continues on following page

Procedure for Pulmonary Artery Catheter Removal—*Continued*

Steps	Rationale	Special Considerations
5. Have the patient turn his or her head away from the PA catheter and insertion site.	Decreases the risk for contamination.	
6. Transfer or discontinue intravenous (IV) solution and flush solutions.	Prepares the catheter for removal.	
7. Open supplies.	Prepares for removal.	
8. Remove the syringe from the balloon inflation port, ensure that the gate valve or stopcock is in the open position, and observe the PA waveform (see Fig. 73-6).	Allows air to passively escape from the balloon and ensures adequate balloon deflation.	Myocardial or valvular tissues can be damaged if the PA catheter is removed with the balloon inflated.
9. Turn off all stopcocks to the patient.	Prepares for removal.	
10. Unlock the sheath from the introducer catheter.	Prepares for removal.	
11. Remove the old dressing.	Prepares for removal.	Signs of local or systemic infection may determine the need to send a culture of the catheter tip.
12. Discard nonsterile gloves in appropriate receptacle, perform hand hygiene and apply sterile gloves.	Removes and safely discards used supplies. Reduces the transmission of microorganisms; Standard Precautions.	
13. If present, clip the sutures securing the PA catheter.	Frees the PA catheter for removal.	
14. Ask the patient to take a deep breath in and hold it.[9-13] **(Level E*)**	Minimizes the risk for venous air embolus.	If the patient is receiving positive pressure ventilation, withdraw the catheter during the inspiratory phase of the respiratory cycle or while delivering a breath via a bag-valve device.
15. While stabilizing the introducer catheter, gently withdraw the PA catheter with a constant, steady motion (Fig. 74-1).	Ensures the removal of an intact catheter.	Observe the ECG tracing during removal. Dysrhythmias may occur during removal but are usually self-limiting.[1,9,11] If resistance is met, do not continue to remove the catheter and notify the advanced practice nurse or physician immediately. Resistance may be caused by catheter knotting, kinking, or wedging.
16. Temporarily cover the hemostasis valve with a sterile-gloved finger until the obturator/cap is secured.	The hemostasis valve must be occluded to minimize the risk for air embolus and hemorrhage.	The introducer may remain in place to provide central venous access.
17. Have the patient exhale once the PA catheter is removed.	Once the catheter is removed the patient can breathe normally.	
18. Place the PA catheter on the moisture-proof absorbent pad and check to be sure that the entire catheter was removed.	Allows for assessment of the catheter.	
19. If the introducer remains in place, perform site care and apply a sterile dressing to the site.	Decreases the risk for infection at the insertion site.	
20. If the introducer is to be removed, clip sutures or remove the securing device.	Frees the introducer for removal.	

*Level E: Multiple case reports, theory-based evidence from expert opinions, or peer-reviewed professional organizational standards without clinical studies to support recommendations

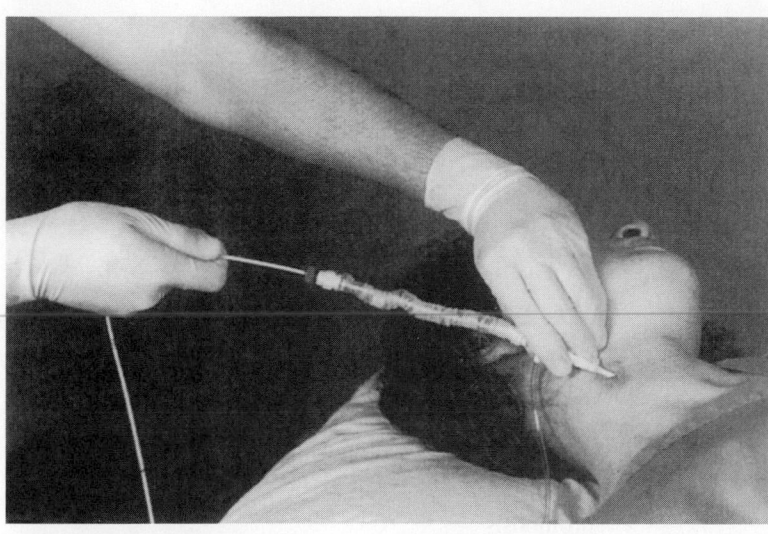

FIGURE 74-1 While stabilizing the introducer, gently withdraw the PA catheter using a constant, steady motion. *(From Wadas TM: Pulmonary artery catheter removal, Crit Care Nurse 14:63, 1994.)*

Procedure | for Pulmonary Artery Catheter Removal—*Continued*

Steps	Rationale	Special Considerations
21. Ask the patient to take a deep breath in and hold it.[9,11-13] **(Level E*)**	Minimizes the risk for venous air embolus. Cases have been reported of venous air embolus occurring after removal of central venous catheters while patients were in the Fowler's position.	If the patient is receiving positive pressure ventilation, withdraw the catheter during the inspiratory phase of the respiratory cycle or while delivering a breath via a bag-valve device. If the introducer is in the femoral vein, extend the patient's leg and ensure the groin area is adequately exposed.
22. Withdraw the introducer, pulling parallel to the skin and using a steady motion.	Minimizes trauma.	Antibiotic ointment may be applied to the exit wound to seal the track opening.[5] If resistance is met, do not continue to remove the introducer. Notify the advanced practice nurse or physician immediately.
23. As the introducer exits the site, apply pressure with a gauze pad.	Minimizes the risk for venous air embolus and promotes hemostasis.	
24. Have the patient exhale once the introducer is removed.	Once the catheter is removed the patient can breathe normally.	
25. Lay the introducer on the moisture-proof absorbent pad. Check to be sure that all of the introducer was removed.	Ensures the removal of the entire introducer.	
26. Continue applying firm, direct pressure over the insertion site with the gauze pad until bleeding has stopped.	Ensures hemostasis.	Because central venous catheters are placed in large veins, 10 minutes may be needed for hemostasis to occur. Pressure may be needed for a longer period of time if the patient has been receiving anticoagulant therapy or if coagulation study results are abnormal.
27. Apply a sterile air occlusive dressing to the insertion site.[3,5,7,9] **(Level E)**	Decreases the risk for infection at the insertion site and minimizes the risk for venous air embolus.	Mark the dressing with the date, time, and your initials. Indicates when the dressing was placed. The dressing should remain in place for a minimum of 12 hours.[5]

*Level E: Multiple case reports, theory-based evidence from expert opinions, or peer-reviewed professional organizational standards without clinical studies to support recommendations

Procedure continues on following page

Procedure　for Pulmonary Artery Catheter Removal—*Continued*

Steps	Rationale	Special Considerations
28. Maintain bed rest for at least 30 minutes after catheter removal.[5]	May decrease the risk of a postprocedure venous air embolism.	
29. Dispose of used supplies in appropriate receptacles.	Removes and safely discards used supplies.	
30. 𝐇𝐇		

Expected Outcomes

- The PA catheter is removed
- The introducer may or may not be removed

Unexpected Outcomes

- Dysrhythmias
- Valvular damage
- PA rupture
- Thrombosis
- Venous air emboli
- Uncontrolled bleeding
- Infection
- Inability to percutaneously remove the PA catheter because of knotting or kinking
- Hematoma
- Pain

Patient Monitoring and Care

Steps	Rationale	Reportable Conditions
		These conditions should be reported if they persist despite nursing interventions.
1. Assess the need for the PA catheter daily. If long-term use of the PA catheter is needed; consider changing the PA catheter every 7 days. **(Level B*)**	The Centers for Disease Control (CDC)[8] and research findings[2,4] and Prevention recommend that PA catheters do not need to be changed more frequently than every 7 days. There are no specific recommendations regarding routine replacement of PA catheters that need to be in place for greater than 7 days.[4,8] The PA catheter should be removed and the introducer should be changed over a guidewire when a positive blood culture is obtained after the PA catheter was inserted and sepsis develops without an identified source.[4] A new PA catheter can then be inserted through the new introducer. PA catheters should be removed and reinserted at a new site when there is a skin infection at the catheter insertion site (i.e., redness, swelling, or drainage at or around the insertion site) or a positive culture at the insertion site.[2,4]	- Signs and symptoms of infection at the PA catheter insertion site - Signs and symptoms of sepsis

*Level B: Well-designed, controlled studies with results that consistently support a specific action, intervention, or treatment

Patient Monitoring and Care —*Continued*

Steps	Rationale	Reportable Conditions
2. Monitor the patient's vital signs, pulse oximetry, and level of consciousness before and after the PA catheter or introducer removal.	Provides baseline data and data that identify changes in patient condition	• Abnormal vital signs • Persistent shortness of breath or tachypnea • Cyanosis or decreased oxygen saturation • Changes in mental status
3. Monitor the patient's cardiac rate and rhythm during PA catheter withdrawal.	Ventricular dysrhythmias may occur as the PA catheter passes through the right ventricle.	• Ventricular dysrhythmias that occur after the PA catheter is removed
4. Monitor for signs and symptoms of venous air embolus, and if present, immediately place the patient in the left lateral Trendelenburg's position.	Venous air embolus is a potentially life-threatening complication. The left lateral Trendelenburg's position prevents air from passing into the left side of the heart and traveling into the arterial circulation.	• Respiratory distress • Agitation • Cyanosis • Gasp reflex • Sucking sound • Hypotension • Petechiae • Cardiac dysrhythmias • Altered mental status
5. After removal of the introducer, assess the site for signs of bleeding every 15 minutes × 2, every 30 minutes × 2, and then 1 hour later.	Bleeding or a hematoma can develop if there is still bleeding from the vessel.	• Abnormal vital signs or signs of bleeding
6. Remove the dressing and assess for site closure 24 hours after introducer removal.	Verifies healing and closure of the site.	• Abnormal healing
7. Follow institution standard for assessing pain. Administer analgesia as prescribed.	Identifies need for pain interventions.	• Continued pain despite pain interventions

Documentation

Documentation should include the following:
• Patient and family education
• Patient assessment before and after removal of the PA catheter
• Patient's response to the procedure
• Pain assessment, interventions, and effectiveness
• Date and time of removal
• Occurrence of unexpected outcomes
• Nursing interventions taken
• Application of an air occlusive dressing
• Site assessment

References

CR 1. Baldwin IC, Heland M: Incidence of cardiac dysrhythmias in patients during pulmonary artery catheter removal after cardiac surgery, *Heart Lung* 29:155-160, 2000.

CR 2. Chen Y, et al: Comparison between replacement at 4 days and 7 days on the infection rate for pulmonary artery catheters in an intensive care unit, *Crit Care Med* 31:1353-1358, 2003.

CR 3. Ely EW, et al: Venous air embolism from central venous catheterization: a need for increased physician awareness, *Crit Care Med* 27:2113-2117, 1999.

CR 4. Eyer S, et al: Catheter-related sepsis: prospective, randomized study of three methods of long-term catheter maintainence, *Crit Care Med* 18:1073-1079, 1990.

CR 5. Kim DK, et al: The CVC removal distress syndrome: an unappreciated complication of central venous catheter removal, *Am Surgeon* 64:344-347, 1998.

CR 6. McCarthy PM, et al: Air embolism in single-lung transplant patients after central venous catheter removal, *Chest* 107:1178-1179, 1995.

CR 7. Mennim P, Cormac FC, Taylor JD: Venous air embolism associated with removal of central venous catheter, *BMJ* 305:171-172, 1992.

CR 8. O'Grady NP, et al: Guidelines for the prevention of intravascular catheter-related infections, *Am J Infect Control* 30:476-489, 2002.

9. Oztekin DS, et al: Comparison of complications and procedural activities of pulmonary artery catheter removal by critical care nurses versus medical doctors, *Nurs Crit Care* 13:105-115, 2008.

CR 10. Peter DA, Saxman C: Preventing air embolism when removing CVCs: an evidence-based approach to changing practice, *Medsurg Nurs* 12:223-229, 2003.

CR 11. Rountree WD: Removal of pulmonary artery catheters by registered nurses: a study in safety and complications, *Focus Crit Care* 18:313-318, 1991.

CR 12. Turnage WS, Harper JV: Venous air embolism occurring after removal of a central venous catheter, *Anesth Analg* 72:559-560, 1991.

CR 13. Wadas TM: Pulmonary artery catheter removal, *Crit Care Nurse* 14:62-72, 1994.

Additional Readings

CR Arnaout S, et al: Rupture of the chordae of the tricuspid valve after knotting of the pulmonary artery catheter, *Chest* 120:1742-1744, 2001.

CR Darovic GO: *Hemodynamic monitoring: invasive and noninvasive clinical application,* ed 3, Philadelphia, 2002, Saunders.

Mirski MA, Lele AV, Fitzsimmons L, et al: Diagnosis and treatment of vascular air embolism, *Anesthesiology* 106:164-177, 2007.

CR Woodrow P: Central venous catheters and central venous pressure, *Nursing Standard* 16:45-52,54, 2002.

Pulmonary Artery Catheter and Pressure Lines, Troubleshooting

P U R P O S E :   Troubleshooting of the pulmonary artery catheter is important to maintain catheter patency, to ensure that data from the pulmonary artery catheter are accurate, and to prevent the development of catheter-related and patient-related complications.

Teresa Preuss, Debra Lynn-McHale Wiegand

PREREQUISITE NURSING KNOWLEDGE

- Knowledge of the cardiovascular anatomy and physiology is needed.
- Knowledge of the pulmonary anatomy and physiology is necessary.
- An understanding of basic dysrhythmia recognition and treatment of life-threatening dysrhythmias is important.
- Advanced cardiac life support knowledge and skills are needed.
- Knowledge of principles of aseptic technique is necessary.
- Understanding of the set-up of the hemodynamic monitoring system (see Procedure 76) is needed.
- Anatomy of the pulmonary artery (PA) catheter (see Fig. 73-1) and the location of the PA catheter in the heart and pulmonary artery (see Fig. 73-2) should be understood.
- Pulmonary artery occlusion pressure may be referred to as pulmonary artery wedge pressure.
- After wedging of the PA catheter, air is passively removed by disconnecting the syringe from the balloon-inflation port. Active withdrawal of air from the balloon is avoided because it can weaken the balloon, pull the balloon structure into the inflation lumen, and possibly cause balloon rupture.
- The pulmonary artery diastolic pressure (PADP) and the pulmonary artery occlusion pressure (PAOP) are indirect measures of left ventricular end-diastolic pressure

(LVEDP). Usually, the PAOP is approximately 1 to 4 mm Hg less than the PADP. Because these two pressures are similar, the PADP is commonly followed, which minimizes the frequency of balloon inflation, thus decreasing the potential of balloon rupture.
- Differences between the PADP and the PAOP may exist for patients with pulmonary hypertension, chronic obstructive lung disease, adult respiratory distress syndrome, pulmonary embolus, and tachycardia.
- Pulmonary artery pressures (PAPs) may be elevated because of pulmonary artery hypertension, pulmonary disease, mitral valve disease, left ventricular failure, atrial or ventricular left-to-right shunt, pulmonary emboli, or hypervolemia.
- PAPs may be decreased because of hypovolemia or vasodilation.
- The waveforms that occur during insertion should be recognized, including right atrial (RA), right ventricular (RV), PA, and pulmonary artery occlusion (PAO; see Fig. 73-3).
- *a* wave reflects atrial contraction. The *c* wave reflects closure of the atrioventricular valves. The *v* wave reflects passive filling of the atria during ventricular systole (see Figs. 73-4 and 73-5).
- Knowledge of normal hemodynamic values (see Table 67-1) is needed.
- Elevated *a* and *v* waves may be evident in RA or central venous pressure (CVP) and in PAO waveforms. These elevations may occur in patients with cardiac tamponade, constrictive pericardial disease, and hypervolemia.

- Elevated *a* waves in the RA or CVP waveform may occur in patients with pulmonic or tricuspid stenosis, right ventricular ischemia or infarction, right ventricular failure, pulmonary artery hypertension, and atrioventricular (AV) dissociation.
- Elevated *a* waves in the PAO waveform may occur in patients with mitral stenosis, acute left ventricular ischemia or infarction, left ventricular failure, and AV dissociation.
- Elevated *v* waves in the RA or CVP waveform may occur in patients with tricuspid insufficiency.
- Elevated *v* waves in the PAO waveform may occur in patients with mitral insufficiency or ruptured papillary muscle.

EQUIPMENT

- Nonsterile gloves
- Syringes (5- or 10-mL)
- Sterile nonvented caps
- Sterile 4 × 4 gauze
- Stopcocks
- Needleless blood sampling access device
- Pressure monitoring cables
- Pressure transducer system, including flush solution recommended according to institution standard, a pressure bag or device, pressure tubing with transducers, and flush device
- Dual-channel recorder
- Leveling device (low-intensity laser or carpenter level)
  Additional equipment to have available as needed includes the following:
- Emergency equipment
- Blood specimen tubes

PATIENT AND FAMILY EDUCATION

- Explain the troubleshooting procedures to the patient and family. ➺*Rationale:* The patient and family are kept informed, and anxiety is reduced.

- Explain the patient's expected participation during the procedure. ➺*Rationale:* This explanation will encourage patient assistance.
- Inform the patient and family of signs and symptoms to report to the critical care nurse, including chest pain, palpitations, new cough, tenderness at the insertion site, and chills. ➺*Rationale:* The patient is encouraged to report signs of discomfort and potential PA catheter complications.

PATIENT ASSESSMENT AND PREPARATION
Patient Assessment

- Monitor PA waveforms continuously. ➺*Rationale:* The PA catheter may migrate forward into a wedged position or may loop around and move back into the right ventricle.
- Assess the configuration of the PA catheter waveforms. ➺*Rationale:* Thrombus formation at the tip of the catheter lumen may be evidenced by an overdamped waveform.
- Assess the patient's hemodynamic and cardiovascular status. ➺*Rationale:* The patient's clinical assessment should correlate with the PA catheter readings.
- Assess the patient and the PA catheter site for signs of infection. ➺*Rationale:* Infection can develop because of the invasive nature of the PA catheter.

Patient Preparation

- Verify correct patient with two identifiers. ➺*Rationale:* Prior to performing a procedure, the nurse should ensure the correct identification of the patient for the intended intervention.
- Ensure that the patient understands preprocedural teaching. Answer questions as they arise, and reinforce information as needed. ➺*Rationale:* Understanding of previously taught information is evaluated and reinforced.
- Determine the patency of the patient's intravenous catheters. ➺*Rationale:* Access may be needed for administration of emergency medication or fluids.

Procedure	for Pulmonary Artery Catheter and Pressure Lines, Troubleshooting	
Steps	**Rationale**	**Special Considerations**
1. **HH**		
2. **PE**	Reduces the transmission of microorganisms; Standard Precautions.	
Troubleshooting an Overwedged Balloon		
1. Identify an overwedged balloon (Fig. 75-1).	Determines the need for troubleshooting.	Overinflation of the balloon can cause pulmonary arteriole infarction or rupture, resulting in life-threatening hemorrhage.
2. Remove the syringe from the gate valve or the stopcock of the PA balloon inflation port.	Passively removes air from the PA balloon.	Ensure that the gate valve or stopcock is in the open position (see Fig. 73-6).

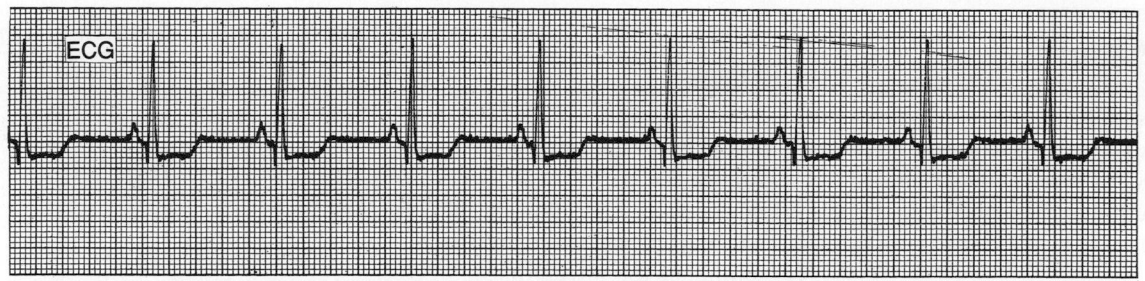

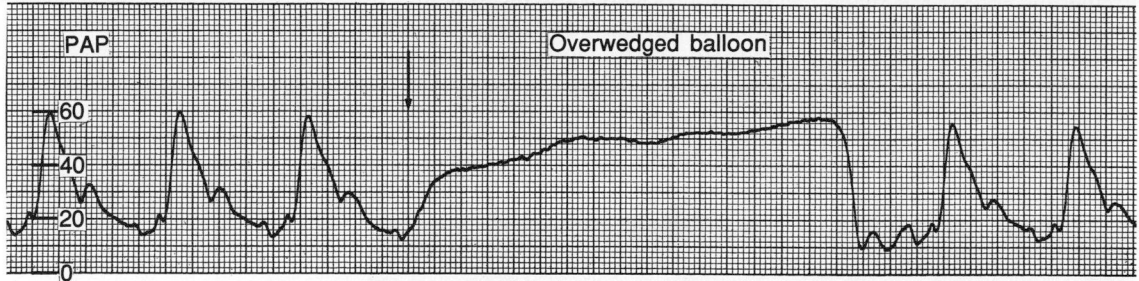

FIGURE 75-1 Balloon inflation *(arrow).* Overwedging of balloon (balloon has been overinflated). The danger of overinflating the balloon is that the pulmonary artery (PA) vessel may rupture from the pressure of the balloon. *ECG,* electrocardiogram; *PAP,* Pulmonary artery pressure.

Procedure	for Pulmonary Artery Catheter and Pressure Lines, Troubleshooting—*Continued*	
Steps	**Rationale**	**Special Considerations**
3. Note the change in the PA waveform from the overinflated waveform to the PA waveform.	As the balloon deflates, the PA waveform returns.	
4. Note and record the external centimeter marking of the PA catheter at the introducer exit site.	Identifies whether the PA catheter has migrated forward from the previously documented measurement.	The advanced practice nurse or the physician may need to reposition the catheter.
5. Note and record the amount of air needed to wedge the PA catheter.	Prevents overwedging of the PA catheter balloon.	
Preventing an Overwedged Balloon		
1. Fill the syringe with 1.5 mL of air.	More than 1.5 mL of air may rupture the PA balloon and the pulmonary arteriole.	
2. Connect the PA syringe to the gate valve or stopcock of the balloon inflation port of the PA catheter.	This port is designed for PA balloon air inflation.	
3. Slowly inflate the balloon with air until the PA waveform changes to a PAO waveform (see Fig. 73-10).	Only enough air is needed to convert the PA waveform to a PAO waveform.	
4. Inflate the PA balloon for no more than 8 to 15 seconds (2 to 4 respiratory cycles).	Avoids prolonged pressure on the pulmonary arteriole.	
5. Disconnect the syringe from the balloon inflation port.	Allows air to passively escape from the balloon.	
6. Observe the monitor as the PAO waveform changes back to the PA waveform.	Ensures adequate balloon deflation.	
7. Expel air from the syringe.	The syringe should remain empty so that accidental balloon inflation does not occur.	
8. Reconnect the empty syringe to the end of the balloon inflation port.	Retains the safety syringe.	

Procedure continues on following page

Procedure   for Pulmonary Artery Catheter and Pressure Lines, Troubleshooting—*Continued*

Steps	Rationale	Special Considerations

Troubleshooting an Absent Waveform

1. Check to see whether there is a kink in the pulmonary artery catheter.

   Kinks may inhibit waveform transmission.

2. Ensure that all connections are tight.

   Loose connections allow air into the system and can overdamp or eliminate the waveform.

3. Ensure that the stopcock is open to the transducer (Fig. 75-2).

   The stopcocks open to the system allow waveform transmission from the vascular system to the monitor; stopcocks closed to transducer prevent waveform transmission to the monitor and oscilloscope.

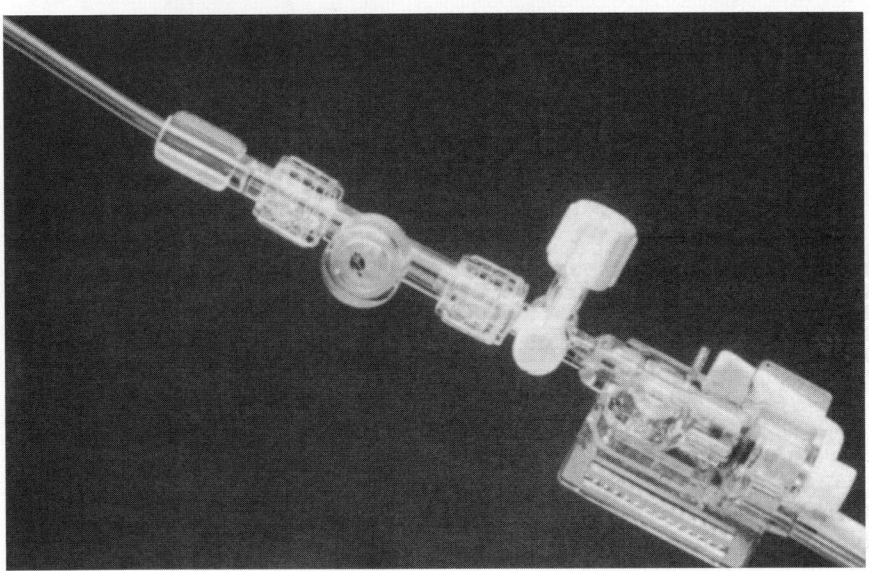

FIGURE 75-2 The stopcock is open to the transducer. *(From Ahrens TS, Taylor LK: Hemodynamic waveform recognition, Philadelphia, 1993, Saunders.)*

4. Check that the cables are in the appropriate pressure modules.

   Necessary for signal transmission.

5. Ensure that the pressure cables are securely plugged into the monitor.

   No waveform is transmitted without proper connection.

6. Ensure that the correct monitor parameters are turned on.

   Necessary for specific parameter monitoring.

7. Ensure the correct scale has been chosen for pressure being monitored (e.g., 40 mm Hg scale is used for PA monitoring).

   A larger scale (e.g., 100 mm Hg) causes the waveform to be smaller and possibly to not be visible on the oscilloscope.

8. Level and zero the monitoring system (see Procedure 76).

   Ensures accurate functioning of the monitoring system.

9. Aspirate through the stopcock that is closest to the catheter to check for blood return (see Fig. 66-2).

   Ensures patency of the PA catheter.

   A clotted catheter has no waveform and no blood return when aspirated.

10. Replace the monitoring cable.

    A faulty cable can result in an absent waveform.

    If the cable is changed, zero the monitoring system.

11. Replace the disposable pressure tubing with transducer.

    A faulty transducer can result in an absent waveform.

    If the disposable pressure tubing with transducer is changed, zero the monitoring system.

12. Notify the advanced practice nurse or the physician if troubleshooting is unsuccessful.

    The catheter needs to be removed or replaced.

Procedure	for Pulmonary Artery Catheter and Pressure Lines, Troubleshooting—*Continued*	
Steps	**Rationale**	**Special Considerations**
Troubleshooting an Overdamped Waveform		
1. Obtain a monitor strip of the over-damped waveform (Fig. 75-3).	The waveform can be compared with the previous waveforms.	
2. Ensure that all connections are tight.	Loose connections allow air into the system and can overdamp the waveform.	

Procedure continues on following page

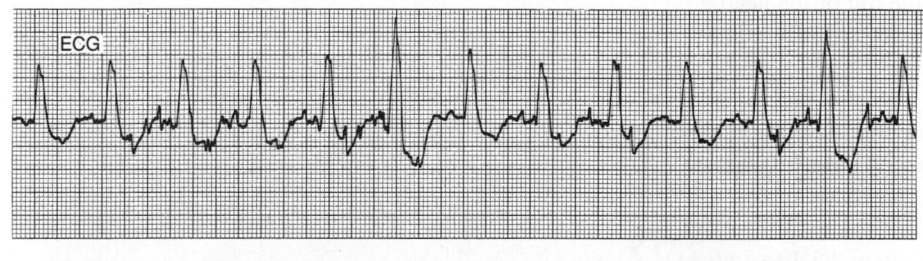

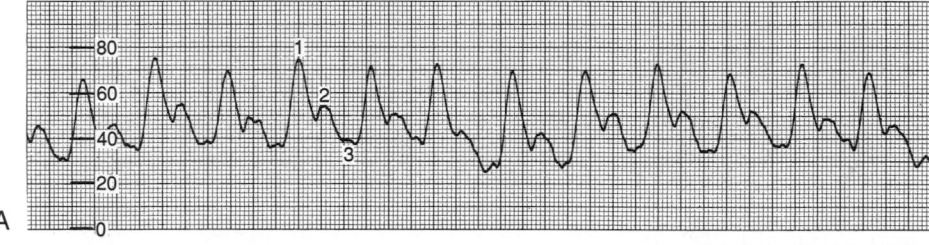

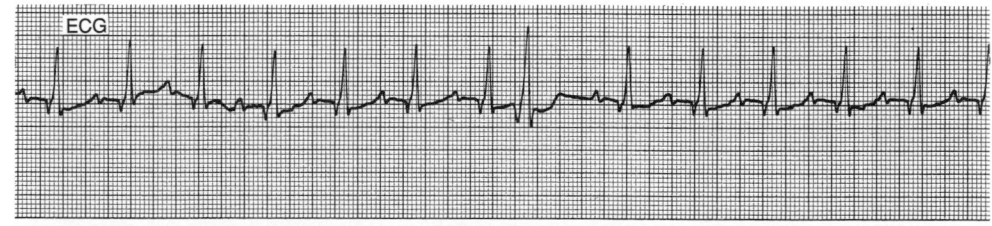

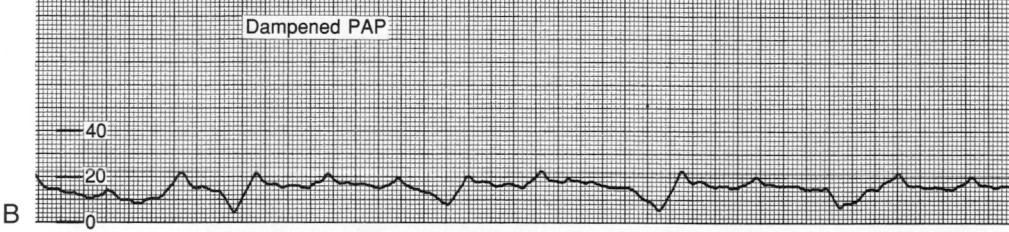

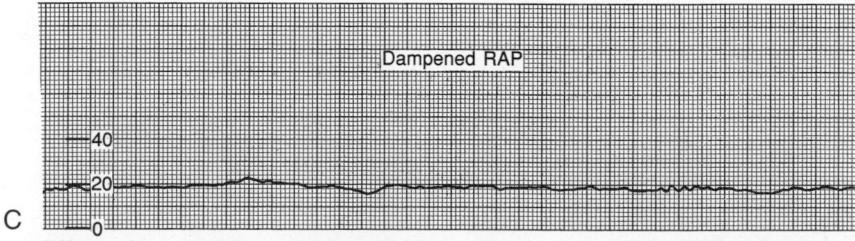

FIGURE 75-3   Effects of overdamping on PAP and RAP waveforms. **A,** Normal waveform with elevated pulmonary artery (PA) pressures *(1,* systole; *2,* dicrotic notch; *3,* diastole). **B,** Overdamped PAP waveform. **C,** Overdamping of RAP waveform. Overdamping of the waveform may result from clots at the catheter tip, catheter against vessel or heart wall, air in lines, stopcock partially closed, or deflated pressure bag. *ECG,* electrocardiogram; *PAP,* Pulmonary artery pressure; *RAP,* right atrial pressure.

Procedure	for Pulmonary Artery Catheter and Pressure Lines, Troubleshooting—*Continued*	
Steps	**Rationale**	**Special Considerations**
3. Ensure that there is fluid in the flush bag and that the pressure on the flush bag or device is delivering 300 mm Hg.	Low counterpressure from the intravenous (IV) flush bag results in an overdamped waveform.	
4. Check all tubing for air bubbles. If air exists within the transducer, follow these steps:	Removes air from the system, prevents the air from entering the patient, and ensures accurate monitoring of waveforms.	Check that the IV flush bag and pressure tubing drip chamber contain fluid.
A. Remove the nonvented cap at the top port of the stopcock or cleanse the top of the needleless cap with an antiseptic solution.		
B. Insert a sterile syringe or a needleless blood sampling access device into the top port of the stopcock or the top of the needleless cap of the stopcock (see Figs. 65-1 and 66-1).		
C. Turn the stopcock off to the patient (see Figs. 64-4, *A* and 65-3).		
D. Fast flush the air from the transducer and system into the syringe or insert a blood specimen tube into the needleless blood sampling access device.		
E. Open the system to the transducer (see Figs. 65-1 and 66-1).		
F. Remove the syringe or the needleless blood sampling access device from the stopcock.		
G. Zero the hemodynamic monitoring system (see Procedure 76).		
H. If not using a needleless cap, place a new sterile nonvented cap on the top port of the stopcock.		
I. Evaluate and then monitor the waveform.		
5. If air exists between the pressure bag and a stopcock, follow these steps:		
A. Remove the nonvented cap at the top port of the stopcock or cleanse the top of the needleless cap with an antiseptic solution.		
B. Insert a sterile syringe or a needleless blood sampling access device into the top port of the stopcock or the top of the needleless cap of the stopcock (see Figs. 65-1 and 66-1).		

Procedure for Pulmonary Artery Catheter and Pressure Lines, Troubleshooting—*Continued*

Steps	Rationale	Special Considerations

C. Turn the stopcock off to the patient (see Figs. 64-4, *A* and 65-3).

D. Fast flush the air from the transducer and system into the syringe or insert a blood specimen tube into the needleless blood sampling access device.

E. Open the system to the transducer (see Figs. 65-1 and 66-1).

F. Remove the syringe or the needleless blood sampling access device from the stopcock.

G. If not using a needleless cap, place a new sterile nonvented cap on the top port of the stopcock.

H. Evaluate and then monitor the waveform.

6. If the air is between the patient and a stopcock (Fig. 75-4), follow these steps:

A. Remove the nonvented cap at the top port of the stopcock or cleanse the top of the needleless cap with an antiseptic solution.

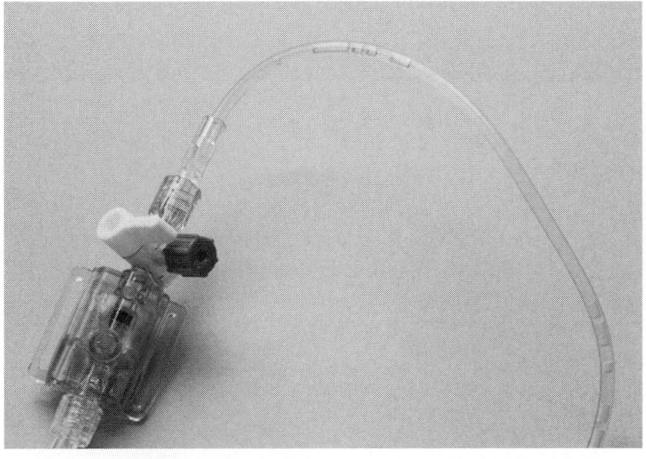

FIGURE 75-4   Air between the patient and stopcock. (*Courtesy Edwards Lifesciences, Irvine, CA.*)

B. Insert a sterile syringe or a needleless blood sampling access device into the top port of the stopcock or the top of the needleless cap of the stopcock (see Figs. 65-1 and 66-1).

C. Turn the stopcock off to the flush solution (see Figs. 65-2, 65-4, and 66-2.

D. Gently pull the air back into the syringe or insert a blood specimen tube into the needleless system.

Procedure continues on following page

Procedure	for Pulmonary Artery Catheter and Pressure Lines, Troubleshooting—*Continued*	
Steps	**Rationale**	**Special Considerations**

E. When all the air is removed, turn the stopcock off to the patient (see Figs. 64-4, *A* and 65-3).

F. Fast flush the blood from the top port of the stopcock. — Clears the tubing of blood.

G. Open the system to the transducer (see Figs. 65-1 and 66-1).

H. Remove the syringe or needleless blood sampling access device from the stopcock.

I. Zero the hemodynamic monitoring system (see Procedure 76).

J. If not using a needleless cap, place a new sterile nonvented cap on the top port of the stopcock.

K. Fast flush the system.

L. Evaluate and then monitor the waveform.

7. Aspirate through the stopcock of the catheter to check for adequate blood return. — Ensures that blood flows easily within the catheter and assesses for the presence of clots.

A. Remove the nonvented cap at the top port of the stopcock or cleanse the top of the needleless cap with an antiseptic solution.

B. Connect a 5- to 10-mL syringe to the stopcock or to the needleless cap.

C. Turn the stopcock off to the flush solution (see Figs. 65-4 and 66-2).

D. Gently aspirate until blood enters the syringe.

E. Turn the stopcock open to the transducer (see Figs. 65-1 and 66-1).

F. Fast flush the blood back into the patient.

G. Turn the stopcock off to the patient (see Figs. 64-4, *A* and 65-3) and fast flush the blood from the top port of the stopcock or the needleless cap into the syringe.

H. Open the stopcock to the transducer (see Figs. 65-1 and 66-1).

I. Remove the syringe from the top port of the stopcock or the needleless cap.

J. Zero the hemodynamic monitoring system (see Procedure 76).

Procedure for Pulmonary Artery Catheter and Pressure Lines, Troubleshooting—*Continued*		
Steps	**Rationale**	**Special Considerations**

Steps	Rationale	Special Considerations
K. If not using a needleless cap, place a new sterile nonvented cap on the top of the stopcock. L. Evaluate and then monitor the waveform.		
8. Check the transducer for the presence of blood. If blood is present, follow these steps:	Ensures accurate monitoring of waveforms.	
A. Remove the nonvented cap at the top port of the stopcock or cleanse the top of the needleless cap with an antiseptic solution.		
B. Turn the stopcock off to the patient (see Fig. 76-4).		
C. Connect a 5- to 10-mL syringe to the stopcock or to the needleless cap or insert a needleless blood sampling access device.		
D. Fast flush the blood from the transducer into the syringe or insert a blood specimen tube into the needleless access device.		
E. Remove the syringe or the needleless access device.		
F. Turn the stopcock open to the transducer (see Fig. 76-5).		
G. Zero the hemodynamic monitoring system (see Procedure 76).		
H. If not using a needleless cap, place a new sterile nonvented cap on the top port of the stopcock.		
I. Evaluate and monitor the waveform.		
9. Perform a dynamic response test (square wave test; see Fig. 62-3).	Overdamped waveforms do not accurately represent pulmonary artery pressure waveforms.	
10. Notify the advanced practice nurse or physician if troubleshooting is unsuccessful.	The catheter needs to be removed or replaced.	

Troubleshooting a Continuously Wedged Waveform

Steps	Rationale	Special Considerations
1. Identify the wedged waveform (see Fig. 73-5).	Confirms the need for troubleshooting.	Continuous monitoring of the PA waveform is necessary to assess for the presence of the PA waveform. PA catheters should be wedged for only 8 to 15 seconds (2 to 4 respiratory cycles) to obtain a PAOP measurement.
2. Remove the PA balloon inflation syringe and ensure that the gate valve or stopcock is open (see Fig. 73-6) and that the balloon is deflated.	Ensures that air is not trapped within the PA balloon.	

Procedure continues on following page

Procedure   for Pulmonary Artery Catheter and Pressure Lines, Troubleshooting—*Continued*

Steps	Rationale	Special Considerations
3. Assist the patient in changing position, or if possible, ask the patient to cough.	May help the catheter float out of the wedge position.	Monitor the PA waveform for a change from a PAO waveform to a PA waveform.
4. If troubleshooting is unsuccessful, notify the advanced practice nurse or physician.	Immediate repositioning of the catheter is necessary because prolonged wedging can lead to PA infarction.	The critical care nurse may withdraw the PA catheter according to institution policy.
5. Never flush a wedged PA catheter.	Flushing the catheter in the wedged position may lead to PA rupture and hemorrhage.	

Troubleshooting a Catheter in the Right Ventricle (RV)

Steps	Rationale	Special Considerations
1. Identify the RV waveform (Fig. 75-5).	The RV waveform resembles the PA waveform. The RV waveform, however, does not have a dicrotic notch. In addition, the diastolic pressure of the RV waveform is lower than the PADP. The normal PADP is 8 to 15 mm Hg; the normal RV diastolic pressure is 0 to 8 mm Hg.	Note the external centimeter marking.
2. Inflate the PA balloon with 1.5 mL of air.	The inflated PA balloon may readily float into position in the PA.	
3. Observe for change in the waveform from RV to PA to PAO (see Fig. 73-3).	Waveform analysis aids in identification of PA catheter position.	The catheter may not advance to the PA or PAO waveforms.
4. Remove the syringe from the PA inflation balloon port.	Air is released passively from the PA balloon.	Air is expelled from the PA syringe, and the empty syringe is reconnected to the end of the balloon inflation valve.
5. Observe the waveform.	The waveform should change from the PAO waveform to a PA waveform.	

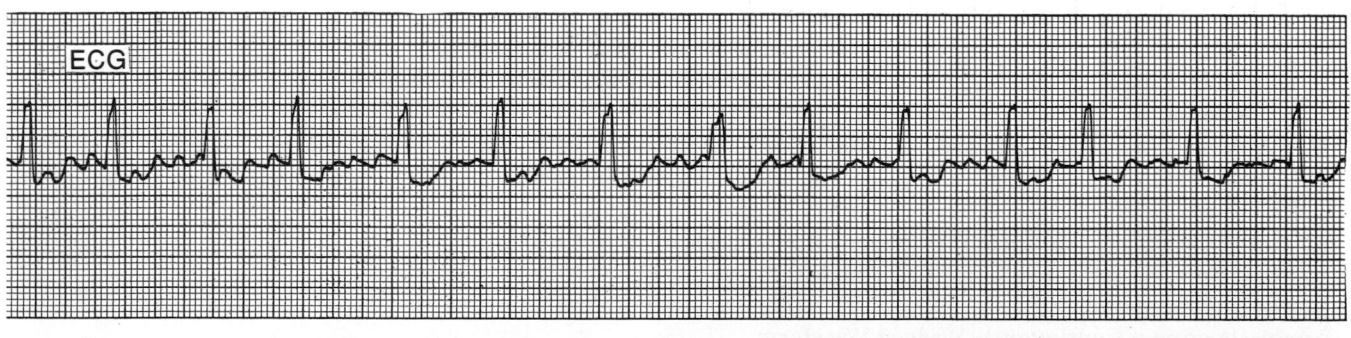

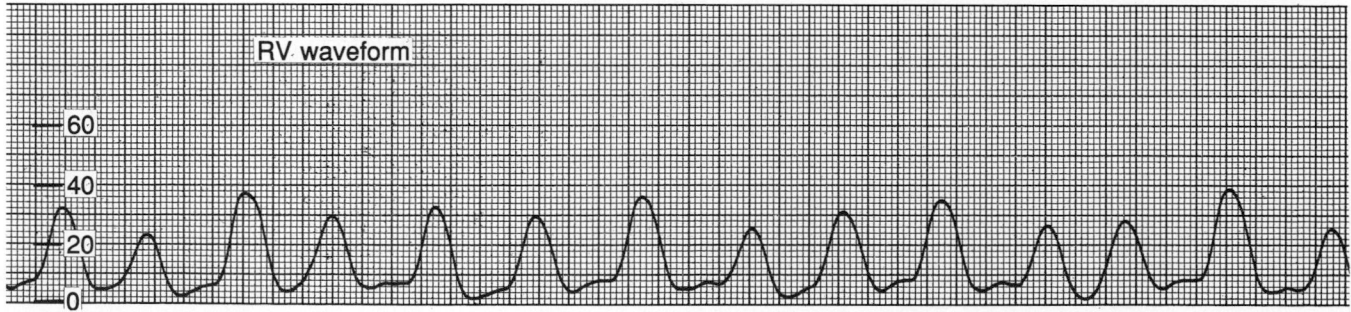

FIGURE 75-5   RVP waveform. This waveform was seen coming from the PA (distal) lumen of a PA catheter. The catheter was coiled in the RV. *ECG,* electrocardiogram; *RV,* right ventricle.

Procedure for Pulmonary Artery Catheter and Pressure Lines, Troubleshooting—*Continued*

Steps	Rationale	Special Considerations
6. If the RV pressure waveform is still present, inflate the PA balloon port with 1.5 mL of air.	An inflated PA balloon cushions the catheter tip and prevents endocardial irritation.	The PA catheter tip may cause ventricular dysrhythmias. If the PA balloon is inflated, the ventricular dysrhythmias may decrease because the inflated balloon may cause less irritation of the endocardium.
7. Assist the patient with a change of position.	The inflated PA catheter may float into the PA after a position change.	
8. Observe for change in waveform from RV to PA to PAO (see Fig. 73-3).	Waveform analysis aids identification of the PA catheter position.	
9. Remove the syringe from the PA balloon port.	Deflates the PA balloon.	
10. If troubleshooting is unsuccessful, notify the advanced practice nurse or physician.	The PA catheter cannot remain in the right ventricle because it may trigger life-threatening ventricular dysrhythmias. Immediate repositioning is necessary.	If ventricular dysrhythmias are present, consider temporarily leaving the balloon inflated until the catheter is repositioned in the PA. If the balloon remains inflated, continuous visual monitoring is necessary in case the catheter floats into the wedge position. The critical care nurse may advance or remove the PA catheter according to institution policy.

Troubleshooting an Inability to Wedge the PA Catheter

Steps	Rationale	Special Considerations
1. Note the external centimeter marking of the PA catheter at the introducer exit site and compare this with the most recent documented marking.	Determines whether the catheter has moved from its previous location. Most PA catheters are in the correct position if the external markings of the catheter are between 45 and 55 cm. The PA catheter tip may not be distal enough in the PA to float into the wedge position.	The advanced practice nurse or physician may need to reposition the catheter.
2. Ensure that the PA balloon is inflated with the maximum 1.5 mL of air.	The full 1.5 mL of air may be necessary to wedge some PA catheters. An insufficient amount of air can prevent wedging.	Repositioning the patient may aid in changing the position of the catheter and may facilitate successful wedging of the PA catheter.
3. Resistance should be felt when inflating the PA balloon.	Resistance is present when the PA balloon is intact.	The balloon may rupture because of overinflation, frequent inflations, or repeated aspiration of air from the balloon rather than allowing it to passively deflate.
4. If no resistance is felt or if blood is aspirated from the balloon lumen, follow these steps:	If the balloon is ruptured, no resistance is felt during an inflation attempt. Blood may also come back through the balloon lumen.	
A. Immediately discontinue balloon inflation attempts.		
B. Remove the syringe.		
C. Close the gate valve or stopcock.		
D. Tape the balloon inflation port closed and label the tape that the balloon should not be used.		

Procedure continues on following page

Procedure	for Pulmonary Artery Catheter and Pressure Lines, Troubleshooting—*Continued*	
Steps	**Rationale**	**Special Considerations**

Steps	Rationale	Special Considerations
5. If the balloon is ruptured or troubleshooting is unsuccessful, notify the advanced practice nurse or physician.	A new PA catheter may be placed, or PADP may be followed if the PADP correlated with the PAOP.	

Troubleshooting Unexpected Changes in PAP

Steps	Rationale	Special Considerations
1. Ensure that the patient is in the supine position with the head of bed from 0 to 45 degrees. **(Level B*)**	Studies have determined that the RA and the PA pressures are accurate in this position.[3-6,10,12,14,22,23,]	RA and PA pressures may be accurate for patients in the supine position with the head of the bed elevated up to 60 degrees,[5,14] but additional studies are needed to support this. Only one study[11] supports the accuracy of hemodynamic values for patients in lateral positions; other studies do not.[3,8,10,16,21] The majority of studies support the accuracy of hemodynamic monitoring for patients in the prone position.[1,2,7,9,13,17,20] Two studies demonstrated that prone positioning caused an increase in hemodynamic values.[18,19]
2. Ensure that the air-fluid interface (zeroing stopcock) is level with phlebostatic axis (see Procedure 76).	Ensures accurate pressure values. If the transducer is higher or lower than the phlebostatic axis, pressures are inaccurate.	
3. Zero the hemodynamic monitoring system (see Procedure 76).	Ensures accuracy of the monitoring system.	
4. Check for air bubbles in the pressure monitoring system and eliminate bubbles if present (see Troubleshooting an Overdamped Waveform section previously in this procedure).	Air overdamps the waveform (see Fig. 75-3), resulting in lower readings.	
5. Obtain hemodynamic parameters and correlate with patient assessment data.	Hemodynamic and assessment data should correlate.	
6. If PAP changes are accurate, titrate fluids or vasoactive agents as prescribed or notify advanced practice nurse or physician.	Hemodynamic data guide therapeutic intervention.	

Troubleshooting Blood Backup into a PA Catheter or Pressure Transducer System

Steps	Rationale	Special Considerations
1. Turn the stopcock off to the patient (see Fig. 76-4).	Prevents blood from going into the transducer.	If blood reaches the transducer, it may have to be replaced.
2. Ensure that all connections are tight and that all stopcocks are closed to air and have nonvented or needleless caps.	Loose connections or open stopcocks cause a decrease in pressure within the fluid-filled system and blood may exert a back pressure into the pressure tubing.	A crack in the system necessitates replacing the entire monitoring system.
3. Ensure that there is fluid in the flush bag and that the pressure on the flush bag or device is delivering 300 mm Hg.	Low pressure from the bag results in blood back-up.	

*Level B: Well-designed, controlled studies with results that consistently support a specific action, intervention, or treatment

Procedure	for Pulmonary Artery Catheter and Pressure Lines, Troubleshooting—*Continued*	
Steps	**Rationale**	**Special Considerations**
4. Once the source of the problem is located and corrected, flush the entire line to remove blood from the system.	Prevents clot formation within the monitoring system. Blood can become a medium for bacterial growth.[15]	
5. Zero the hemodynamic monitoring system (see Procedure 76).	Ensures accuracy of the monitoring system.	
6. Evaluate and monitor the PA waveform.	Ensures presence of the correct waveform and system functioning.	

Troubleshooting When the Patient Develops Hemoptysis or Bloody Secretions from the Endotracheal Tube During PA Catheter Monitoring

1. Notify the physician immediately.	PA perforation with hemorrhage is a potentially lethal complication of a PA catheter.	
2. Maintain patency of the airway.	Prevents hypoxemia and respiratory arrest.	Prepare for intubation if the patient is not already intubated.
3. Remain with the patient for monitoring and reassurance.	Reduces anxiety and fear; provides essential assessment.	
4. Be prepared to follow these steps: 　A. Send blood specimens for coagulation studies and type and cross-match. 　B. Obtain a chest radiograph. 　C. Prepare the patient for the operating room.	Blood loss from the PA can be fatal. Immediate surgical repair of the PA is necessary.	

After all troubleshooting interventions:

1. Removes and safely discards used supplies.
2. 🄷🄷

Expected Outcomes

- Normal pulmonary tissue perfusion
- Absence of PA catheter–related dysrhythmias
- Absence of signs of PA catheter–related infection
- Absence of discomfort associated with PA catheter
- Accurate pulmonary artery waveforms and pressures

Unexpected Outcomes

- PA balloon rupture
- Pulmonary infarction and rupture
- PA catheter–related infection resulting in sepsis
- Discomfort at the PA catheter insertion site
- Ventricular tachycardia unresponsive to antidysrhythmic medications

Patient Monitoring and Care

Steps	**Rationale**	**Reportable Conditions**
		These conditions should be reported if they persist despite nursing interventions.
1. The PA waveforms should be continuously monitored.	Provides assessment of proper placement of the PA catheter and abnormal waveforms such as PAO or RV waveforms.	• Abnormal waveforms (e.g., continued PAO waveform and RV waveforms)

Procedure continues on following page

Patient Monitoring and Care —*Continued*

Steps	Rationale	Reportable Conditions
2. Pressure alarms should be set and remain on at all times.	Alerts the critical care nurse to pressure changes and to disconnections in the pressure monitoring system.	• Abnormal hemodynamic values
3. Evaluate the hemodynamic monitoring system and waveform configurations.	Ensures that the system is intact and functioning appropriately.	• Abnormal waveforms
4. Monitor hemodynamic status (PA, PAO, RA, cardiac output or cardiac index, systemic vascular resistance, etc).	Guides appropriate therapy.	• Abnormal hemodynamic monitoring values
5. Assess the hemodynamic waveforms and pressure values before and after troubleshooting.	Identifies that troubleshooting has been successful.	• Unsuccessful troubleshooting attempts
6. Follow institution standard for assessing pain. Administer analgesia as prescribed.	Identifies need for pain interventions.	• Continued pain despite pain interventions

Documentation

Documentation should include the following:
- Patient and family education
- Troubleshooting intervention and outcome
- Occurrence of unexpected outcomes and interventions
- Pain assessment, interventions, and effectiveness

- Patient tolerance of procedure
- Site assessment
- External centimeter marking of PA catheter noted at exit site

References

1. Blanch L, et al: Short term effects of prone position in critically ill patients with acute respiratory distress syndrome, *Intensive Care Med* 23:1033-1039, 1997.
2. Brussel T, et al: Mechanical ventilation in the prone position for acute respiratory failure after cardiac surgery, *J Cardiothorac Vasc Anesth* 7:541-546, 1993.
3. Cason CL, et al: Effects of backrest elevation and position on pulmonary artery pressures, *Cardiovasc Nurs* 26:1-5, 1990.
4. Chulay M, Miller T: The effect of backrest elevation on pulmonary artery and pulmonary capillary wedge pressures in patients after cardiac surgery, *Heart Lung* 13:138-140, 1984.
5. Clochesy J, Hinshaw AD, Otto CW: Effects of change of position on pulmonary artery and pulmonary capillary wedge pressure in mechanically ventilated patients, *NITA* 7:223-225, 1984.
6. Dobbin K, et al: Pulmonary artery pressure measurement in patients with elevated pressures: effect of backrest elevation and method of measurement, *Am J Crit Care* 1:61-69, 1992.
7. Fridrich P, et al: The effects of long-term prone positioning in patients with trauma-induced adult respiratory distress syndrome, *Anesth Analg* 83:1206-1211, 1996.
8. Groom L, Frisch SR, Elliot M: Reproducibility and accuracy of pulmonary artery pressure measurement in supine and lateral positions, *Heart Lung* 19:147-151, 1990.
9. Jolliet P, Bulpa P, Chevrolet JC: Effects of prone position on gas exchange and hemodynamics in severe acute respiratory distress syndrome, *Crit Care Med* 26:1977, 1998.
10. Keating D, et al: Effect of sidelying positions on pulmonary artery pressures, *Heart Lung* 15:605-610, 1986.
11. Kennedy GT, Bryant A, Crawford MH: The effects of lateral body positioning on measurements of pulmonary artery and pulmonary wedge pressures, *Heart Lung* 13:155-158, 1984.
12. Lambert CW, Cason CL: Backrest elevation and pulmonary artery pressures: research analysis, *Dimens Crit Care Nurs* 9:327-335, 1990.
13. Langer M, et al: The prone position in ARDS patients, *Chest* 94:103-107, 1988.
14. Laulive JL: Pulmonary artery pressures and position changes in the critically ill adult, *Dimens Crit Care Nurs* 1:28-34, 1982.
15. O'Grady NP, et al: Guidelines for the prevention of intravascular catheter-related infections, *Am J Infect Control* 30:476-489, 2002.
16. Osika C: Measurement of pulmonary artery pressures: supine verses side-lying head-elevated positions, *Heart Lung* 18:298-299, 1989.
17. Pappert D, et al: Influence of positioning on ventilation-perfusion relationships in severe adult respiratory distress syndrome, *Chest* 106:1511-1516, 1994.
18. Pelosi P, et al: Effects of the prone position on respiratory mechanics and gas exchange during acute lung injury, *Am J Respir Crit Care Med* 157:387-393, 1998.
19. Voggenreiter G, et al: Intermittent prone positioning in the treatment of severe and moderate posttraumatic lung injury, *Crit Care Med* 27:2375-2382, 1999.

CR 20. Vollman KM, Bander JJ: Improved oxygenation utilizing a prone positioner in patients with acute respiratory distress syndrome, *Intensive Care Med* 22:1105-1111, 1996.

CR 21. Wild L: Effect of lateral recumbent positions on measurement of pulmonary artery and pulmonary artery wedge pressures in critically ill adults, *Heart Lung* 13:305, 1984.

CR 22. Wilson AE, et al: Effect of backrest position on hemodynamic and right ventricular measurements in critically ill adults, *Am J Crit Care* 5:264-270, 1996.

CR 23. Woods SL, Mansfield LW: Effect of body position upon pulmonary artery and pulmonary capillary wedge pressures in noncritically ill patients, *Heart Lung* 5:83-90, 1976.

Additional Readings

Bridges EJ: Pulmonary artery pressure monitoring: when, how, and what else to use, *AACN Adv Crit Care* 17: 286-305, 2006.

CR Darovic GO: *Hemodynamic monitoring: invasive and noninvasive clinical application,* ed 3, Philadelphia, 2002, Saunders.

CR Keckeisen M: *Protocols for practice: hemodynamic monitoring series: pulmonary artery pressure monitoring,* Aliso Viejo, CA, 1997, American Association of Critical-Care Nurses.

Rauen CA, Flynn MB, Bridges E: Evidence-based practice habits: transforming research into bedside practice, *Crit Care Nurse* 29:46-59, 2009.

Single-Pressure and Multiple-Pressure Transducer Systems

P U R P O S E :   Single-pressure and multiple-pressure transducer systems provide a catheter-to-monitor interface so that intravascular and intracardiac pressures can be measured. The transducer detects a biophysical event and converts it to an electronic signal.

Teresa Preuss, Debra Lynn-McHale Wiegand

PREREQUISITE NURSING KNOWLEDGE

- Knowledge of the anatomy and physiology of the cardiovascular system is needed.
- Knowledge of principles of aseptic technique is necessary.
- Fluid-filled pressure monitoring systems used for bedside hemodynamic pressure monitoring are based on the principle that a change in pressure at any point in an unobstructed system results in similar pressure changes at all other points of the system.
- Pressure transducers detect the pressure waveform generated by ventricular ejection and convert that pressure wave into an electrical signal, which is transmitted to the monitoring equipment for representation as a waveform on the oscilloscope.
- Invasive measurement of intravascular (arterial) pressure requires insertion of a catheter into an artery.
- Invasive measurement of intracardiac (right atrial and pulmonary artery) pressures requires insertion of a catheter into the pulmonary artery.
- A single-pressure transducer system is used to measure pressure from a single catheter (e.g., arterial catheter, central venous; Fig. 76-1).
- A double-pressure transducer system is used to measure pressure from two catheters (e.g., arterial and central venous) or two ports (e.g., pulmonary artery and right atrial) from a single catheter (e.g., pulmonary artery catheter; Fig. 76-2).
- A triple-pressure transducer system is commonly used to measure pressures from the arterial and pulmonary artery catheters. With this system, arterial pressures, pulmonary

artery pressures, and right atrial pressures can be obtained (Fig. 76-3).
- For accuracy of the hemodynamic values obtained from any transducer system, leveling and zeroing are essential.

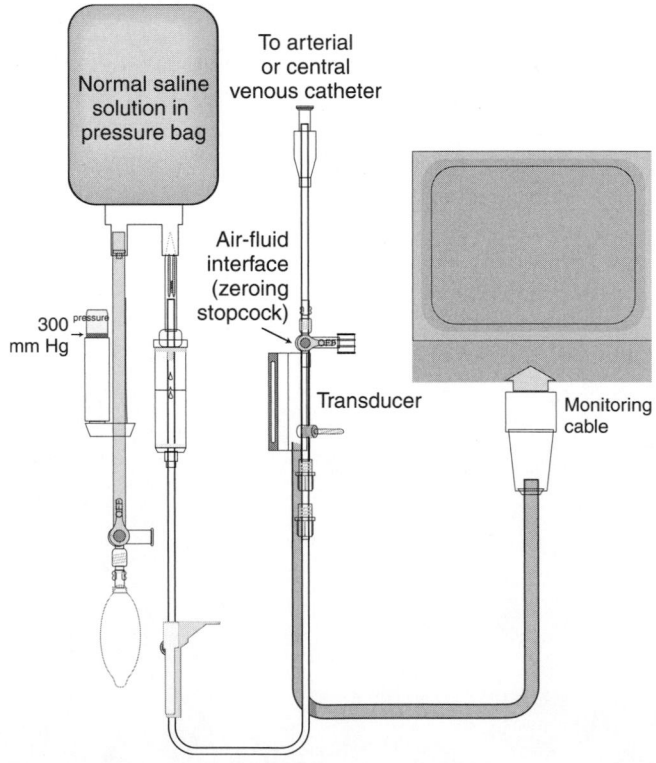

FIGURE 76-1   Single-pressure transducer system. *(Drawing by Paul W. Schiffmacher, Thomas Jefferson University, Philadelphia, PA.)*

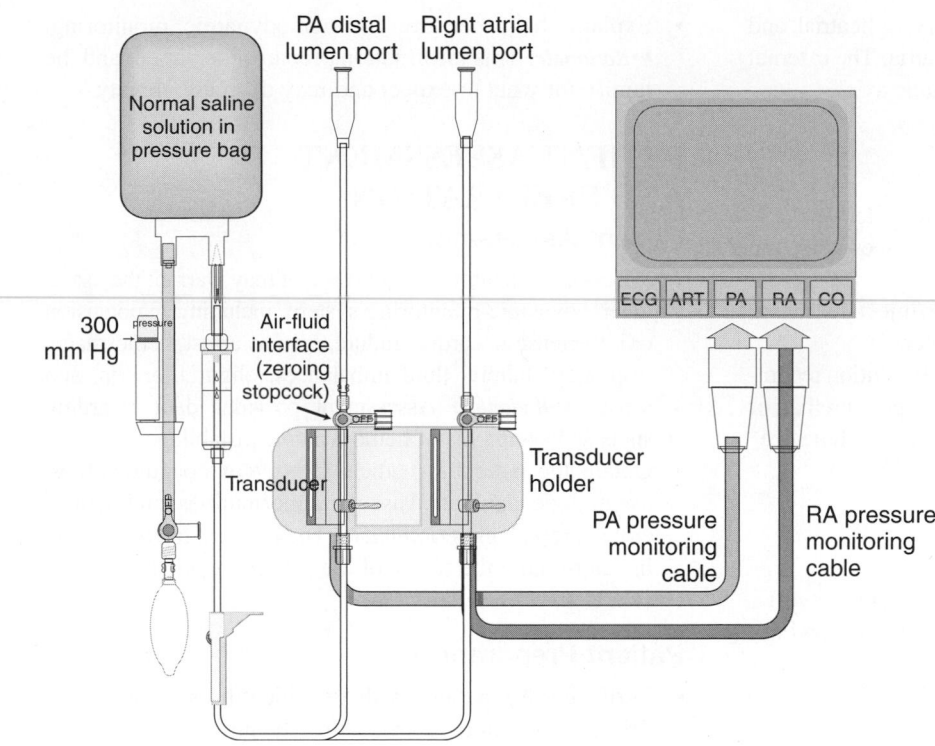

Normal saline
solution in
pressure bag

PA distal
lumen port

Right atrial
lumen port

300
mm Hg

pressure

Air-fluid
interface
(zeroing
stopcock)

Transducer

Transducer
holder

PA pressure
monitoring
cable

RA pressure
monitoring
cable

ECG ART PA RA CO

FIGURE 76-2 Double-pressure transducer system. *ECG,* Electrocardiogram; *ART,*
arterial; *CO,* cardiac output. *(Drawing by
Paul W. Schiffmacher, Thomas Jefferson
University, Philadelphia, PA.)*

Normal saline
solution in
pressure bag

To patient's
arterial
catheter

Balloon
inflation
valve and
syringe

Right
ventricular
infusion
for IV fluid

Pulmonary
artery
catheter

Right
atrial
infusion
for IV fluid

300
mm Hg

pressure

Air-fluid
interface
(zeroing
stopcock)

PA distal
lumen port

Right atrial
lumen port

Transducer

Transducer
holder

Pressure
tubing

ECG ART PA RA CO

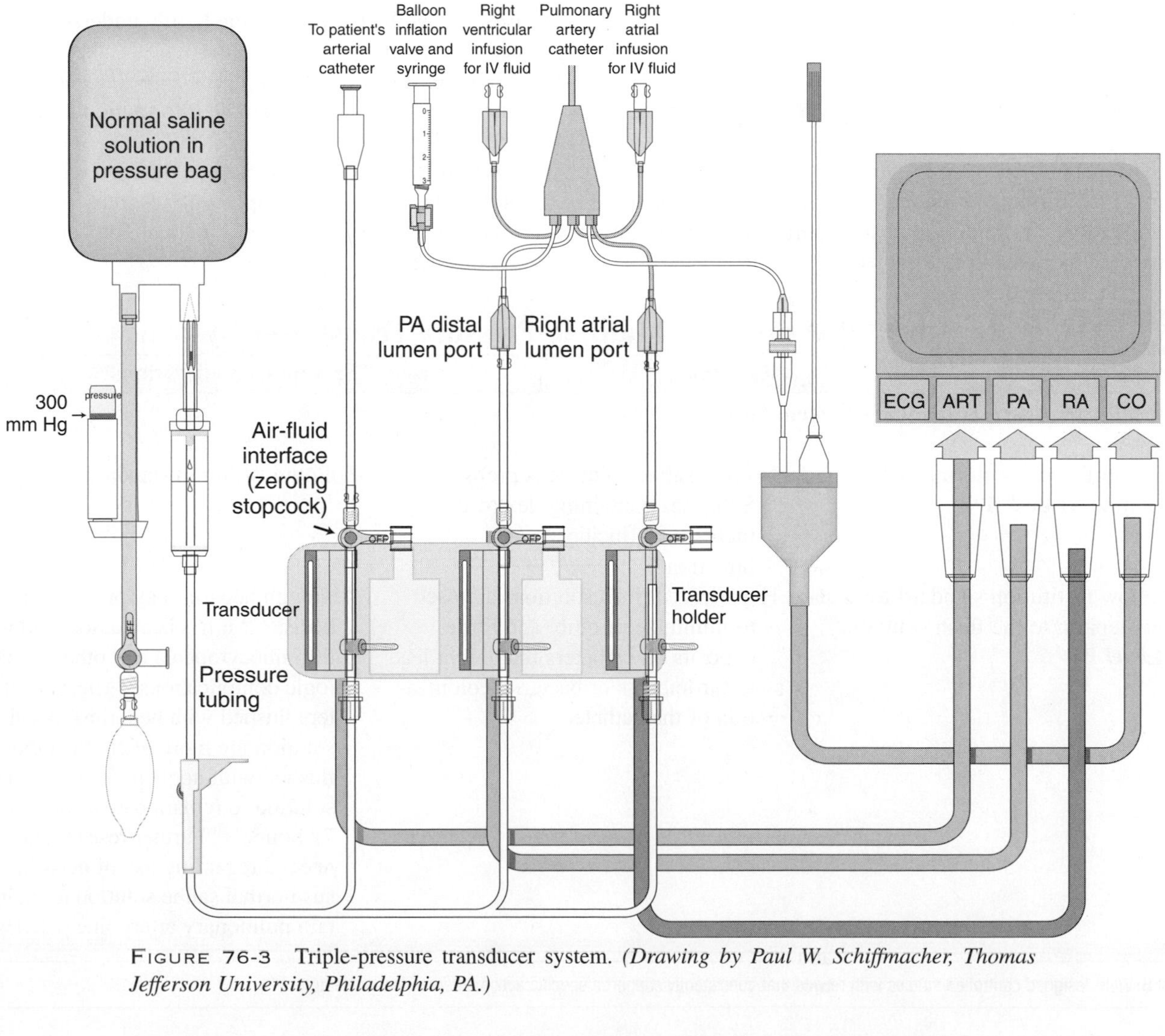

FIGURE 76-3 Triple-pressure transducer system. *(Drawing by Paul W. Schiffmacher, Thomas
Jefferson University, Philadelphia, PA.)*

- All hemodynamic values (pulmonary artery, right atrial, and arterial) are referenced to the level of the atria. The external reference point of the atria is the phlebostatic axis.

EQUIPMENT

- Invasive catheter (e.g., arterial, pulmonary artery)
- Pressure modules and cables for interface with the monitor
- Cardiac output cable with a thermistor/injectate sensor for use with the pulmonary artery catheter
- Pressure transducer system, including flush solution recommended according to institution standard, a pressure bag or device, pressure tubing with transducers, and flush device
- Monitoring system (central and bedside monitor)
- Dual-channel recorder
- Indelible marker
- Nonvented caps
- Leveling device (low-intensity laser or carpenter level)

Additional equipment as needed includes the following:

- Heparin
- 3-mL syringe
- Stopcocks
- 4 × 4 gauze pads or hydrocolloid gel pad
- Tape
- Nonsterile gloves
- Transducer holder and intravenous (IV) pole

PATIENT AND FAMILY EDUCATION

- Assess patient and family understanding of hemodynamic monitoring and the reason for its use. ➤*Rationale:* Clarification or reinforcement of information is an expressed patient and family need.
- Explain the procedure for hemodynamic monitoring. ➤*Rationale:* This information prepares the patient and the family for what to expect and may decrease anxiety.

PATIENT ASSESSMENT AND PREPARATION

Patient Assessment

- Assess the patient for conditions that may warrant the use of a hemodynamic monitoring system, including hypotension or hypertension, cardiac failure, cardiac arrest, hemorrhage, respiratory failure, fluid imbalances, oliguria, anuria, and sepsis. ➤*Rationale:* Assessment provides data regarding signs and symptoms of hemodynamic instability.
- Obtain the patient's medical history of coagulopathies, use of anticoagulants, vascular abnormalities, and peripheral neuropathies. ➤*Rationale:* The medical history assists in determining the safety of the procedure and aids in site selection.

Patient Preparation

- Verify correct patient with two identifiers. ➤*Rationale:* Prior to performing a procedure, the nurse should ensure the correct identification of the patient for the intended intervention.
- Ensure that the patient and the family understand preprocedural teaching. Answer questions as they arise, and reinforce information as needed. ➤*Rationale:* Understanding of previously taught information is evaluated and reinforced.
- Position the patient in the supine position with the head of bed flat or elevated up to 45 degrees. ➤*Rationale:* This positioning prepares the patient for hemodynamic monitoring.

Procedure for Single-Pressure and Multiple-Pressure Transducer Systems

Steps	Rationale	Special Considerations
Disposable Pressure Transducer System Setup		
1. HH		
2. Use an IV bag of normal saline solution. **(Level B*)**	Normal saline solution is preferred. Solutions containing dextrose increase the incidence of infection.[7,25,27,37]	Follow institution standard.
3. Follow institution standard for adding heparin to the flush solution. **(Level B)**	Heparinized flush solutions are used to minimize thrombi and fibrin deposits on catheters that might lead to thrombosis or bacterial colonization of the catheter.	Although heparin may prevent thrombosis,[27,34] it has been associated with thrombocytopenia and other hematologic complications.[9] Arterial catheters flushed with heparinized saline solution are more likely than those flushed with nonheparinized saline solution to remain patent for up to 72 hours.[1,20] Further research is needed regarding use of heparin versus normal saline solution to maintain pulmonary artery line patency.

*Level B: Well-designed controlled studies with results that consistently support a specific action, intervention, or treatment

Procedure for Single-Pressure and Multiple-Pressure Transducer Systems—*Continued*

Steps	Rationale	Special Considerations
4. Label the IV bag, indicating the date and time the solution was hung, the dose of heparin (if used), and your initials.	Identifies the contents of the IV flush bag and identifies when the IV bag needs to be changed.	
5. Open the prepackaged pressure transducer kit with aseptic technique. A. A single-pressure tubing kit can be used for right atrial or arterial monitoring (see Fig. 76-1). B. A double-pressure tubing kit can be used for pulmonary artery and right atrial monitoring (see Fig. 76-2). C. A triple-pressure tubing kit can be used for arterial, pulmonary artery, and right atrial monitoring (see Fig. 76-3).	Provides the correct pressure tubing.	Assemble the pressure transducers, pressure tubing, and stopcocks if not preassembled by the manufacturer. Use the minimal number of stopcocks and tubing length to avoid under-damped waveforms.
6. Tighten all connections.	Prepares the system.	
7. Spike the outlet port of the IV solution with the pressure tubing.	Allows access to the IV flush solution.	Separate flush systems are needed if invasive catheters are inserted at different times.
8. Open the roller clamp and squeeze the drip chambers to fill the chamber half full.	Primes the drip chamber.	Filling the drip chamber at least half-way is important to prevent air bubbles from entering the tubing and allows the nurse to see that the solution is flowing when performing a manual flush of the invasive line.
9. Insert the IV bag into the pressure bag or device on the IV pole. Do not inflate the pressure bag.	Priming the tubing under pressure increases turbulence and may cause air bubbles to enter the tubing.	Air should never be allowed to develop in a hemodynamic system. Micro or macro air emboli can migrate to major organs and present a potentially life-threatening complication.
10. Flush the entire system, including transducer, stopcock, and pressure tubing with the flush solution. A. With the flush device, flush solution from the IV bag through to the tip of the pressure tubing. B. Turn the stopcock off to the patient end of the tubing (Fig. 76-4). C. With the flush device, flush solution from the IV bag through the stopcock. D. Replace the vented cap on the stopcock with a nonvented cap. E. Open the stopcock to the transducer (Fig. 76-5).	Eliminates air from the system.	Vented caps are placed by the manufacturer and permit sterilization of the entire system. These vented caps need to be replaced with sterile nonvented caps to prevent bacteria and air from entering the system.

Procedure continues on following page

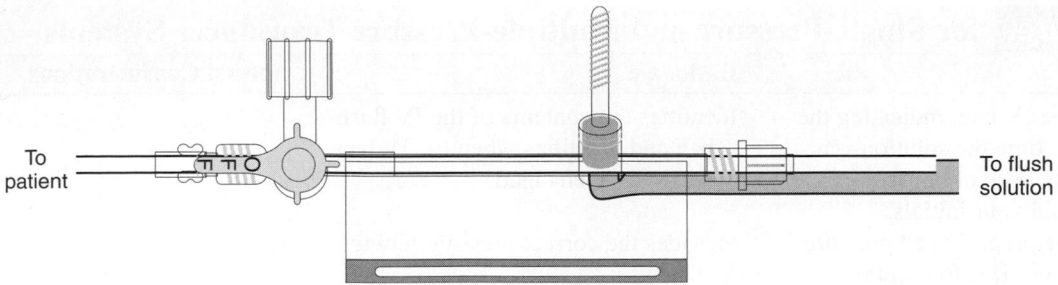

FIGURE 76-4   Stopcock off to the patient. *(Drawing by Paul W. Schiffmacher, Thomas Jefferson University, Philadelphia, PA.)*

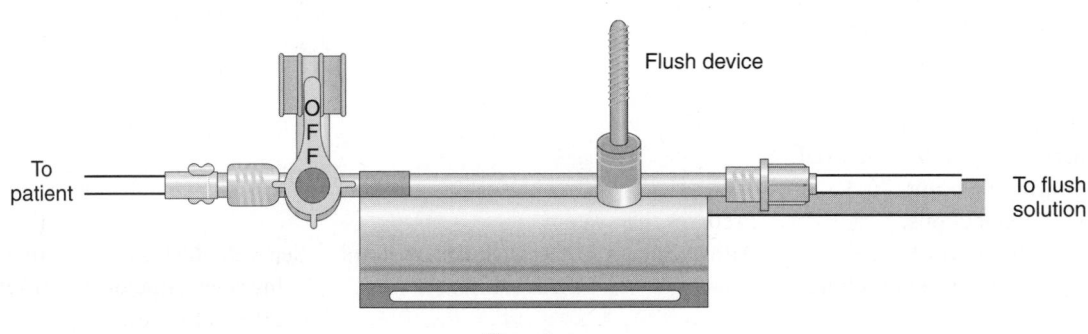

FIGURE 76-5   Stopcock open to the transducer. *(Drawing by Paul W. Schiffmacher, Thomas Jefferson University, Philadelphia, PA.)*

Procedure	**for Single-Pressure and Multiple-Pressure Transducer Systems**—*Continued*	
Steps	**Rationale**	**Special Considerations**
11. With use of a double-pressure or triple-pressure tubing kit, **repeat Step 10** with each of the pressure transducer systems.	Eliminates air from the systems.	
12. Inflate the pressure bag or device to 300 mm Hg.	Inflating the pressure bag to 300 mm Hg allows approximately 1 to 3 mL/hr of flush solution to be delivered through the catheter, thus maintaining catheter patency and minimizing clot formation.	
13. With use of a pole mount, insert the transducer into the pole mount holder (Fig. 76-6).	Secures the transducer.	
14. With sterile technique, connect the end of each transducer tubing to the appropriate catheter port (e.g., pulmonary artery [PA], right atrial [RA], arterial).	Allows for monitoring of pressures.	Prior to assisting with connections protective equipment needs to be applied.
15. 🄷🄷		
16. Label the pressure tubing, indicating the date, time, and your initials.	Identifies when the pressure tubing needs to be changed.	

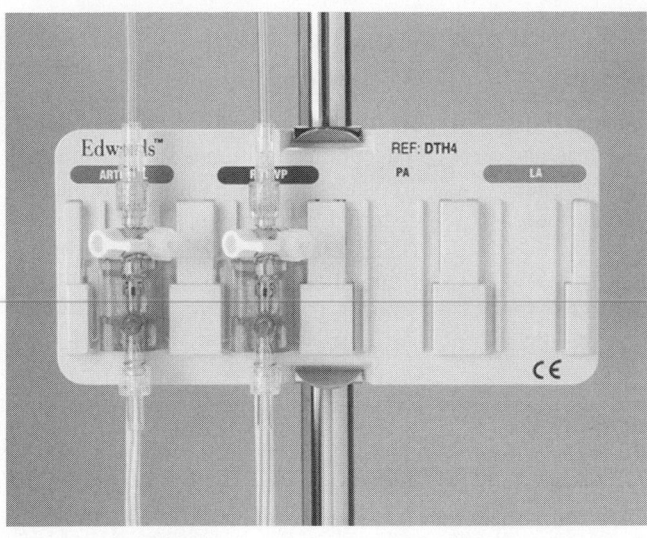

FIGURE 76-6   Transducers in pole mount. *(Courtesy Edwards Lifesciences, Irvine, CA.)*

Procedure	for Single-Pressure and Multiple-Pressure Transducer Systems—*Continued*	
Steps	**Rationale**	**Special Considerations**
Monitor Setup		
1. Turn on the bedside monitor.	Prepares the monitor.	
2. Plug the pressure cables into the appropriate pressure modules in the bedside monitor (see Fig. 76-3).	Necessary for signal transmission to the monitor.	Some monitors are preprogrammed to display the waveform that corresponds to the module for cable insertion (e.g., first position arterial, second position pulmonary artery, third position right atrial).
3. Turn the parameters on (e.g., PA, RA, arterial).	Visualizes the correct waveforms.	
4. Set the appropriate scale for the pressure being measured.	Necessary for visualization of the complete waveform and to obtain accurate readings. Waveforms vary in amplitude depending on the pressure within the system.	The scale for right atrial pressure is commonly set at 20 mm Hg. The scale for pulmonary artery pressure is commonly set at 40 mm Hg. The scale for arterial blood pressure is commonly set at 180 mm Hg. Scales may vary based on monitoring equipment. Scales can be adjusted based on patient pressures.
Leveling the Transducer		
1. 🔲		
2. Position the patient in the supine position with the head of the bed from 0 to 45 degrees. **(Level B*)**	Studies have determined that the RA and the PA pressures are accurate in this position.[8,10-12,16,21,23,41,42]	RA and PA pressures may be accurate for patients in the supine position with the head of the bed elevated up to 60 degrees,[11,23] but additional studies are needed to support this. Only one study[18] supports the accuracy of hemodynamic values for patients in lateral positions; other studies do not.[4,8,14,16,29,36,40] The majority of studies support the accuracy of hemodynamic monitoring for patients in the prone position.[3,6,13,15,22,31,39] Two studies demonstrated that prone positioning caused an increase in hemodynamic values.[33,38]

*Level B: Well-designed controlled studies with results that consistently support a specific action, intervention, or treatment

Procedure continues on following page

Procedure | for Single-Pressure and Multiple-Pressure Transducer Systems—*Continued*

Steps	Rationale	Special Considerations
3. Locate the phlebostatic axis for the supine position (Fig. 76-7).	The phlebostatic axis is at approximately the level of the atria and should be used as the reference point for the air-fluid interface.	The reference point for the left lateral decubitus position is the fourth intercostal space (ICS) at the left parasternal border (Fig. 76-8).[17,30] The reference point for the right lateral decubitus position is the fourth ICS at the midsternum (see Fig. 76-8).[17,30]

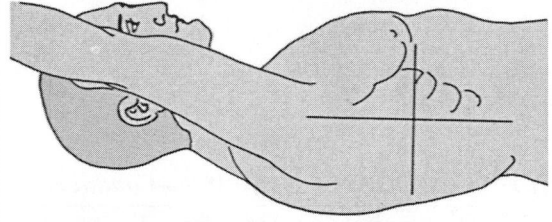

FIGURE 76-7   Phlebostatic axis in the supine position.

A. Identify the fourth ICS on the edge of the sternum.
B. Draw an imaginary line along the fourth ICS laterally, along the chest wall.
C. Draw a second imaginary line from the axilla downward, midway between the anterior and posterior chest walls.
D. The point at which these two lines cross is the level of the phlebostatic axis.
E. Mark the point of the phlebostatic axis with an indelible marker.

4. Use a leveling device (low-intensity laser or carpenter's level) to align the air-fluid interface with the phlebostatic axis.	Ensures that the air-fluid interface is level with the phlebostatic axis. Leveling to the phlebostatic axis reflects accurate central arterial pressure values.	

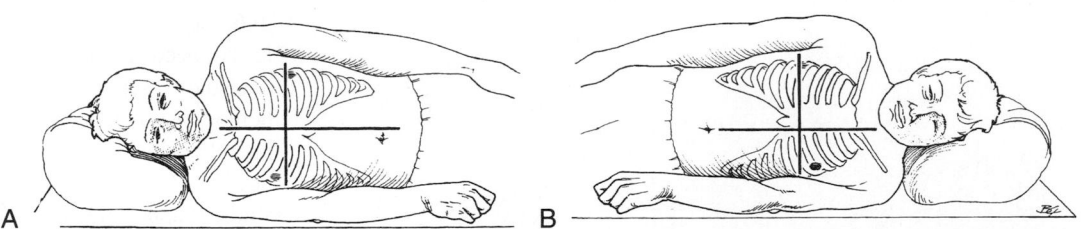

FIGURE 76-8   Reference points for the hemodynamic monitoring system for patients in lateral positions. **A,** For the right lateral position, the reference point is the intersection of the fourth intercostal space and the midsternum. **B,** For the left lateral position, the reference point is the intersection of the fourth intercostal space and the left parasternal border. *(From Keckelsen M: Protocols for practice: hemodynamic monitoring series: pulmonary artery monitoring, Aliso Viejo, CA, 1997, American Association of Critical-Care Nurses.)*

Procedure	for Single-Pressure and Multiple-Pressure Transducer Systems—*Continued*	
Steps	**Rationale**	**Special Considerations**

Pole mount[2,35]:
Low-intensity laser:
  A. Place the low-intensity laser leveling device next to the air-fluid interface (zeroing stopcock).
  B. Point the laser light at the phlebostatic axis.
  C. Move the pole mount holder up or down until the interface is level with the phlebostatic axis.

Carpenter level:
  A. Place one end of the carpenter level next to the air-fluid interface (zeroing stopcock).
  B. Place the other end of the carpenter level at the phlebostatic axis.
  C. Move the pole mount holder up or down until the interface is level with the phlebostatic axis. (Fig. 76-9).

5. With patient mount:
  A. Place the pulmonary artery distal/PA air-fluid interface (zeroing stopcock) at the phlebostatic axis.

          Ensures that the air-fluid interface is level with the phlebostatic axis.
          Leveling to the phlebostatic axis reflects accurate central arterial pressure values.

  B. Place the pulmonary artery proximal (RA) and arterial air-fluid interfaces (zeroing stopcocks) directly next to the pulmonary artery distal/PA air-fluid interface.

          Leveling the arterial interface to the tip of an arterial catheter reflects the transmural pressure of a particular point in the arterial tree (e.g., radial artery) and not central arterial pressure.[5,19,26,32]

  C. Place a 4 × 4 gauze or hydrocolloid gel pad between each of the transducers and the patient's skin.

          May prevent skin breakdown.

  D. Secure each of the systems in place with tape.

6. **HH**

Procedure continues on following page

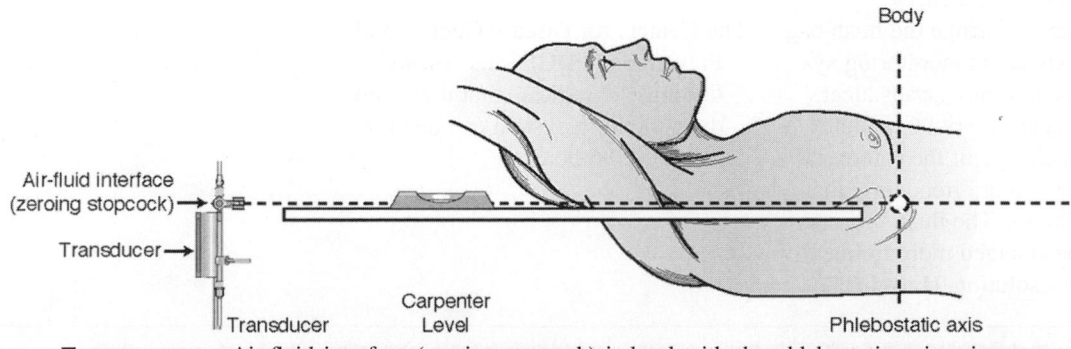

FIGURE 76-9   Air-fluid interface (zeroing stopcock) is level with the phlebostatic axis using a carpenter level. *(Drawing by Paul W. Schiffmacher, Thomas Jefferson University, Philadelphia, PA.)*

Procedure for Single-Pressure and Multiple-Pressure Transducer Systems—*Continued*

Steps	Rationale	Special Considerations
Zeroing the transducer		
1. **HH**		
2. Turn the stopcock off to the patient end of the tubing (see Fig. 76-4).	Prepares the system for the zeroing procedure.	
3. Remove the nonvented cap from the stopcock, opening the stopcock to air.	Allows the monitor to use atmospheric pressure as a reference for zero.	
4. Push and release the zeroing button on the bedside monitor. Observe the digital reading until it displays a value of zero.	The monitor automatically adjusts itself to zero. Zeroing negates the effects of atmospheric pressure.	Some monitors require that the zero be turned and adjusted manually. Some systems also may require calibration. Refer to manufacturer's guidelines for specific information.
5. Place a new, sterile nonvented cap on the stopcock.	Maintains sterility.	
6. Turn the stopcock so that it is open to the transducer (see Fig. 76-5).	Permits pressure monitoring and maintains catheter patency.	
7. Discard used supplies in appropriate receptacles.	Removes and safely discards used supplies.	
8. **HH**		

Expected Outcomes

- The pressure monitoring system is prepared aseptically
- The hemodynamic monitoring system remains intact with secure connections
- The phlebostatic axis is accurately identified
- The air-fluid interface of the transducer is leveled to the phlebostatic axis
- The pressure monitoring system is zeroed

Unexpected Outcomes

- Loose connections within the hemodynamic monitoring system
- Stopcocks left open to air without nonvented caps
- Air bubbles within the system
- Pressure bag inflated to less than 300 mm Hg

Patient Monitoring Care

Steps	Rationale	Reportable Conditions
		These conditions should be reported if they persist despite nursing interventions.
1. Check the IV flush bag every 4 hours and as needed.	Ensures that the IV flush bag contains solution to maintain catheter patency.	
2. Check that the IV flush bag is maintained at 300 mm Hg every 4 hours and as needed.	Maintains catheter patency.	
3. Arterial lines: Change the flush bag and hemodynamic monitoring system (pressure tubing, transducer, and stopcocks) every 96 hours or with each change of the catheter if it is changed more frequently than every 96 hours. The flush bag may need to be changed more frequently if empty of solution. **(Level B*)**	The Centers for Disease Control and Prevention (CDC)[27] and research findings[24,28] indicate that the hemodynamic flush system can be used safely for 96 hours.	

*Level B: Well-designed controlled studies with results that consistently support a specific action, intervention, or treatment

Patient Monitoring and Care —*Continued*

Steps	Rationale	Reportable Conditions
4. Pulmonary artery and central venous lines: Change the flush bag and hemodynamic monitoring system (pressure tubing, transducer, and stopcocks) every 96 hours or with each change of the catheter if it is changed more frequently than every 96 hours. The flush bag may need to be changed more frequently if empty of solution. **(Level B*)**	The CDC[27] and research findings[24,28] indicate that the hemodynamic flush system can be used safely for 96 hours.	
5. Zero the hemodynamic monitoring system during initial setup or before insertion, after insertion, if disconnection occurs between the transducer and the monitoring cable, if disconnection occurs between the monitoring cable and the monitor, and when the values obtained do not fit the clinical picture. Follow manufacturer's recommendations for disposable systems.	Ensures the accuracy of the hemodynamic monitoring system.	
6. Check the hemodynamic monitoring system every 4 hours and as needed.	Ensures that all connections are tightly secured and that there are no cracks in the system. Ensures that the system is closed with nonvented caps on all stopcocks. Ensures that the system is free of air bubbles.	
7. Set the hemodynamic monitoring system alarms.	Provides immediate alarm for high and low pressures.	

Documentation

Documentation should include the following:
- Patient and family education
- Date and time of hemodynamic monitoring system preparation
- Hemodynamic monitoring system leveling and zeroing
- Type of flush solution
- Unexpected outcomes
- Additional nursing interventions

*Level B: Well-designed controlled studies with results that consistently support a specific action, intervention, or treatment

References

CR 1. American Association of Critical-Care Nurses: Evaluation of the effects of heparinized and nonheparinized flush solutions on the patency of arterial pressure monitoring lines: the AACN Thunder Project, *Am J Crit Care* 2:3-15, 1993.

CR 2. Bisnaire D, Robinson L: Accuracy of leveling hemodynamic transducer systems, *CACCN* 10:16-19, 1999.

CR 3. Blanch L, et al: Short term effects of prone position in critically ill patients with acute respiratory distress syndrome, *Intensive Care Med* 23:1033-1039, 1997.

CR 4. Bridges EJ, et al: Effect of 30 degree lateral recumbent position on pulmonary artery and pulmonary artery wedge pressures in critically ill adult cardiac surgery patients, *Am J Crit Care* 9:262-275, 2000.

CR 5. Bridges EJ, et al: Direct arterial vs. oscillometric monitoring of blood pressure: stop comparing and pick one [comment], *Crit Care Nurse* 17:96-97,101-102, 1997.

CR 6. Brussel T, et al: Mechanical ventilation in the prone position for acute respiratory failure after cardiac surgery, *J Cardiothorac Vasc Anesth* 7:541-546, 1993.

CR 7. Buxton AE, et al: Failure of disposable domes to prevent septicemia acquired from contaminated pressure transducers, *Chest* 74:508-513, 1978.

CR 8. Cason CL, et al: Effects of backrest elevation and position on pulmonary artery pressures, *Cardiovasc Nurs* 26:1-5, 1990.

CR 9. Chong BH: Heparin-induced thrombocytopenia, *Br J Haematol* 89:431-439, 1995.

CR 10. Chulay M, Miller T: The effect of backrest elevation on pulmonary artery and pulmonary capillary wedge pressures in patients after cardiac surgery, *Heart Lung* 13:138-140, 1984.

CR 11. Clochesy J, Hinshaw AD, Otto CW: Effects of change of position on pulmonary artery and pulmonary capillary wedge pressure in mechanically ventilated patients, *NITA* 7:223-225, 1984.

CR 12. Dobbin K, et al: Pulmonary artery pressure measurement in patients with elevated pressures: effect of backrest elevation and method of measurement, *Am J Crit Care* 1:61-69, 1992.

CR 13. Fridrich P, et al: The effects of long-term prone positioning in patients with trauma-induced adult respiratory distress syndrome, *Anesth Analg* 83:1206-1211, 1996.

CR 14. Groom L, Frisch SR, Elliot M: Reproducibility and accuracy of pulmonary artery pressure measurement in supine and lateral positions, *Heart Lung* 19:147-151, 1990.

CR 15. Jolliet P, Bulpa P, Chevrolet JC: Effects of prone position on gas exchange and hemodynamics in severe acute respiratory distress syndrome, *Crit Care Med* 26: 1977-1985, 1998.

CR 16. Keating D, et al: Effect of sidelying positions on pulmonary artery pressures, *Heart Lung* 15:605-610, 1986.

CR 17. Keckeisen M: *Protocols for practice: hemodynamic monitoring series: pulmonary artery pressure monitoring,* Aliso Viejo, CA, 1997, American Association of Critical-Care Nurses.

CR 18. Kennedy GT, Bryant A, Crawford MH: The effects of lateral body positioning on measurements of pulmonary artery and pulmonary wedge pressures, *Heart Lung* 13:155-158, 1984.

CR 19. Kirkhoff KT, Rebenson-Piano M: Mean arterial pressure readings: variations with positions and transducer level, *Nurs Res* 33:343-345, 1984.

CR 20. Kulkarni M, et al: Heparinized saline versus normal saline in maintaining patency of the radial artery catheter, *Can J Surg* 37:37-42, 1994.

CR 21. Lambert CW, Cason CL: Backrest elevation and pulmonary artery pressures: research analysis, *Dimens Crit Care Nurs* 9:327-335, 1990.

CR 22. Langer M, et al: The prone position in ARDS patients, *Chest* 94:103-107, 1988.

CR 23. Laulive JL: Pulmonary artery pressures and position changes in the critically ill adult, *Dimens Crit Care Nurs* 1:28-34, 1982.

CR 24. Luskin RL, et al: Extended use of disposable pressure transducers: a bacteriologic evaluation, *JAMA* 255: 916-920, 1986.

CR 25. Maki DG, Martin WT: Nationwide epidemic of septicemia caused by contaminated infusion products: IV: growth of microbial pathogens in fluids for intravenous infusion, *J Infect Dis* 131:267-272, 1975.

CR 26. McGhee BH, Bridges MEJ: Monitoring arterial blood pressure: what you may not know, *Crit Care Nurse* 22:60-79, 2002.

CR 27. O'Grady NP, et al: Guidelines for the prevention of intravascular catheter-related infections, *Am J Infect Control* 30:476-489, 2002.

CR 28. O'Malley MK, et al: Value of routine pressure monitoring system changes after 72 hours of use, *Crit Care Med* 22:1424-1430, 1994.

CR 29. Osika C: Measurement of pulmonary artery pressures: supine verses side-lying head-elevated positions, *Heart Lung* 18:298-299, 1989.

CR 30. Paolella LP, et al: Topographic location of the left atrium by computed tomography: reducing pulmonary artery catheter calibration error, *Crit Care Med* 16:1154-1156, 1988.

CR 31. Pappert D, et al: Influence of positioning on ventilation-perfusion relationships in severe adult respiratory distress syndrome, *Chest* 106:1511-1516, 1994.

CR 32. Pauca AL, et al: Does radial artery pressure accurately reflect aortic pressure? *Chest* 102:1193-1198, 1992.

CR 33. Pelosi P, et al: Effects of the prone position on respiratory mechanics and gas exchange during acute lung injury, *Am J Respir Crit Care Med* 157:387-393, 1998.

CR 34. Randolph AG, et al: Benefit of heparin in central venous and pulmonary artery catheters, *Chest* 113:165-171, 1998.

CR 35. Rice WP, et al: A comparison of hydrostatic leveling methods in invasive pressure monitoring, *Crit Care Nurse* 20:20,22-30, 2000.

CR 36. Ross CJ, Jones R: Comparisons of pulmonary artery pressure measurements in supine and 30 degree lateral positions, *Can J Cardiovasc Nurs* 6:4-8, 1995.

CR 37. Solomon SL, et al: Nosocomial fungemia in neonates associated with intravascular pressure-monitoring devices, *Pediatr Infect Dis* 5:680-685, 1986.

CR 38. Voggenreiter G, et al: Intermittent prone positioning in the treatment of severe and moderate posttraumatic lung injury, *Crit Care Med* 27:2375-2382, 1999.

CR 39. Vollman KM, Bander JJ: Improved oxygenation utilizing a prone positioner in patients with acute respiratory distress syndrome, *Intensive Care Med* 22:1105-1111, 1996.

CR 40. Wild L: Effect of lateral recumbent positions on measurement of pulmonary artery and pulmonary artery wedge pressures in critically ill adults, *Heart Lung* 13:305, 1984.

CR 41. Wilson AE, et al: Effect of backrest position on hemodynamic and right ventricular measurements in critically ill adults, *Am J Crit Care* 5:264-270, 1996.

CR 42. Woods SL, Mansfield LW: Effect of body position upon pulmonary artery and pulmonary capillary wedge pressures in noncritically ill patients, *Heart Lung* 5:83-90, 1976.

Additional Readings

CR Darovic GO: *Hemodynamic monitoring: invasive and noninvasive clinical application,* ed 3, Philadelphia, 2002, Saunders.

CR Imperial-Perez F, McRae M: *Protocols for practice: hemodynamic monitoring series: arterial pressure monitoring,* Aliso Viejo, CA, 1998, American Association of Critical-Care Nurses.

CR Kee LL, et al: Echocardiographic determination of valid zero reference levels in supine and lateral positions, *Am J Crit Care* 2:72-80, 1993.

CR Mermel LA, Maki DG: Epidemic bloodstream infections from hemodynamic pressure monitoring: signs of the times, *Infect Control Hosp Epidemiol* 10:47-53, 1989.

CR Pearson ML: Hospital infection control practices advisory committee: guideline for prevention of intravascular device-related infections, *Infect Control Hosp Epidemiol* 17:438-473, 1996.

CR Quaal SJ, Weir C: Effect of head of bed position on pulmonary artery pressure measurements: a review of the literature, *Online J Knowledge Synthesis Nurs* 2:1-10, 1995.

CR Shih F: Patient positioning and the accuracy of pulmonary artery pressure measurements, *Int J Nurs Studies* 36:497-505, 1999.

CR Vollman KM: What are the practice guidelines for prone positioning of acutely ill patients? Specifically, what are the recommendations related to hemodynamic monitoring and tube feeding? *Crit Care Nurse* 21:84-86, 2001.

Special Cardiac Procedures

AP Arterial and Venous Sheath Removal

P U R P O S E : Arterial and venous sheaths are placed for cardiac catheterizations and interventional procedures. Achieving and maintaining hemostasis after their removal is essential to prevent access site complications.

Rose B. Shaffer

PREREQUISITE NURSING KNOWLEDGE

- Knowledge of the femoral artery and vein anatomy is important.
- The technique for the percutaneous approach to the insertion of the arterial and venous sheaths should be understood.
- Technical and clinical competence in removal of arterial and venous sheaths is needed.
- Knowledge about anticoagulation and antiplatelet therapy used during interventional procedures is essential.
- Understanding of the technology (i.e., activated clotting time [ACT] machine) used to determine the timing of arterial sheath removal and knowledge of the institution's standards regarding removal of arterial sheaths are important.
- The importance of peripheral vascular and neurovascular assessment of the affected extremity (e.g., assessment of the quality and strength of the pulse to be accessed and the pulses distal to the access site, assessment for a bruit) should be understood.
- Knowledge about the variety of hemostasis options available should include the following:
  - Manual compression alone or in combination with non-invasive hemostasis pads (e.g., Syvek Patch, Marine

Polymer Technologies, Inc, Danvers, MA; Clo-Sur P.A.D., Scion Cardio-Vascular, Inc, Miami, FL; D-Stat Dry, Vascular Solutions, Minneapolis, MN).
  - Mechanical compression devices (e.g., CompressAR, Advanced Vascular Dynamics, Portland, OR; FemoStop, Radi Medical Systems, Wilmington, MA; Fig. 77-1).
  - Collagen plug devices (e.g., VasoSeal, Datascope Corp, Montvale, NJ; Angioseal, St Jude Medical, St Paul, MN).

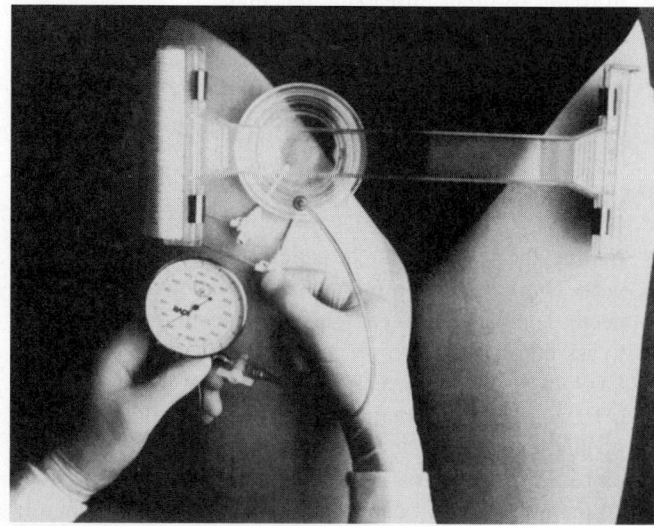

FIGURE 77-1   FemoStop in the correct position. *(From Barbiere C: A new device for control of bleeding after transfemoral catheterization, Crit Care Nurse 15[1]:52, 1995.)*

❖ Percutaneous suture-mediated closure devices (e.g., Perclose, Abbott Vascular Devices, Redwood City, CA; X-Site, Datascope Corp)

❖ Percutaneous staple-mediated closure devices (e.g., Angiolink, Medtronic, Santa Rosa, CA; Starclose, Abbott Vascular Devices).

• Collagen plug devices, percutaneous suture-mediated closure devices, and percutaneous staple-mediated closure devices can be deployed into the artery by the physician at the end of the catheterization or interventional procedure.

• Sheath removal can be associated with many complications, including the following:

❖ External bleeding at the site

❖ Internal bleeding (e.g., localized hematoma or retroperitoneal bleed)

❖ Vascular complications (e.g., pseudoaneurysm, arteriovenous [AV] fistula, dissection, thrombus, or embolus)

❖ Neurovascular complications (sensory or motor changes in the affected extremity)

❖ Vasovagal complications

EQUIPMENT

• Cardiac monitoring system
• Blood pressure monitoring system
• Antiseptic solution (e.g., 2% chlorhexidine-based preparation)
• Nonsterile gloves
• Sterile gloves
• Protective eyewear
• Dressing supplies
• 10-mL syringe
  Additional equipment as needed includes the following:
• Selected hemostasis option (mechanical compression device or noninvasive hemostasis pad)
• Alcohol pads
• Indelible marker
• Selected analgesic and/or sedative as prescribed
• Portable Doppler ultrasound machine
• Suture removal kit
• ACT machine
• Readily available emergency medications (e.g., atropine), additional intravenous fluids, and resuscitation equipment

PATIENT AND FAMILY EDUCATION

• Explain the procedure to the patient and the family. ➤*Rationale:* This explanation provides information and may help decrease anxiety and fear. This also encourages the patient to ask questions and voice concerns about the procedure.

• Explain the importance of bed rest, of not lifting the head off the pillow, of maintaining the head of the bed at no higher than 30 degrees, and of keeping the affected extremity straight for a specified time to maintain hemostasis after the procedure. ➤*Rationale:* The patient is prepared for what to expect after the procedure, and patient cooperation is elicited to decrease the risk for bleeding, hematoma, and other vascular complications.

• Explain that the procedure may produce discomfort and that pressure will be felt at the site until hemostasis is achieved. Encourage the patient to report discomfort, and reassure the patient that analgesia and or sedation will be provided. ➤*Rationale:* Explanation prepares the patient for what to expect and allays fears.

• After sheath removal, instruct the patient to report any warm, wet feeling or pain at the puncture site. Also, instruct the patient to report any sensory or motor changes in the affected extremity. ➤*Rationale:* This aids in the early recognition of complications and identifies the need for additional pain interventions.

PATIENT ASSESSMENT AND PREPARATION

Patient Assessment

• Assess the patient's medical history for bleeding disorders. ➤*Rationale:* Bleeding disorders may increase the risk for bleeding or vascular complications.

• Assess the patient's platelet count, prothrombin time (PT), with international normalized ratio (INR), and partial thromboplastin time (PTT) before sheath removal. ➤*Rationale:* Laboratory results should be within acceptable limits to decrease the risk for bleeding after sheath removal.

• Assess the patient's complete blood count (CBC). ➤*Rationale:* Assessment determines baseline data.

• Assess the patient's ACT before sheath removal. ➤*Rationale:* Results should be within acceptable limits to decrease the risk for bleeding after sheath removal.

• Assess the patient's electrocardiographic (ECG) rhythm and vital signs. ➤*Rationale:* Baseline data are established. Collaborate with the advanced practice nurse or physician if the patient's blood pressure is elevated; elevated blood pressure may need to be treated before sheath removal to achieve and maintain hemostasis.

• Review the documented baseline assessment of the access site before vascular access, including assessment for presence or absence of bruit. ➤*Rationale:* Baseline assessment data are established.

• Assess the extremity distal to the sheath for quality and strength of pulses, color, temperature, sensation, and movement. ➤*Rationale:* Baseline assessment data are established before sheath removal.

• Assess for patency of the intravenous (IV) access and ensure that more than 500 mL of intravenous fluid remains in the IV solution or is readily available. ➤*Rationale:* This assessment allows for emergency medication or fluids to be administered if necessary (e.g., vasovagal reaction).

Patient Preparation

• Verify correct patient with two identifiers. ➤*Rationale:* Prior to performing a procedure, the nurse should ensure the correct identification of the patient for the intended intervention.

• Ensure that the patient and the family understand preprocedural teaching. Answer questions as they arise, and

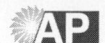

reinforce information as needed. ➤➤*Rationale:* Understanding of previously taught information is evaluated and reinforced.
- Administer analgesia or sedation as prescribed before removal of the sheaths. ➤➤*Rationale:* Pain and anxiety are managed.
- Place the patient with the head of the bed flat. ➤➤*Rationale:* This positioning improves the ability to achieve hemostasis.

- Mark the distal pulses with an indelible marker. ➤➤*Rationale:* Marking facilitates the ability to locate pulses after the procedure.
- If a mechanical device is used to maintain pressure, position the device under the patient. ➤➤*Rationale:* The device is positioned before sheath removal because patient movement must be minimized after sheath removal.

Procedure for Arterial and Venous Sheath Removal

Steps	Rationale	Special Considerations
1. **HH**		
2. **PE**		
3. Place a blood pressure cuff on the patient's arm and obtain the patient's blood pressure.	Establishes a baseline blood pressure before sheath removal.	Monitor the patient's blood pressure every 5 minutes during arterial sheath removal until hemostasis is achieved. If possible, place the blood pressure cuff on the opposite arm of the IV to allow for uninterrupted flow of IV fluids.
4. Place the patient's head of bed flat.	Prepares the patient for the procedure and improves the ability to achieve hemostasis.	
5. Administer analgesia or sedation as prescribed. **(Level B*)**	Analgesia and sedation have been shown to reduce the discomfort associated with sheath removal.[10,20,23]	The routine use of subcutaneous lidocaine infiltrated around the catheter site has not been proven to reduce the discomfort associated with sheath removal.[5,10,20,23]
6. Turn off the arterial catheter alarm.	Monitoring is no longer needed; prevents the alarm from sounding.	
7. Open the suture removal kit if the sheaths are sutured in place.	Prepares for sheath removal.	
8. Remove the arterial and venous sheath dressing.	Prepares for sheath removal.	
9. Clean the arterial and venous sites with an antiseptic solution (e.g., 2% chlorhexidine solution).	Decreases the risk for infection.[14]	Follow institution standard.
10. If using a noninvasive hemostasis pad in conjunction with manual compression, open the pad using sterile technique.	Prepares for sheath removal and ensures sterility.	
11. Attach a 10-mL syringe to the blood sampling port of the stopcock, turn the stopcock off to the flush bag, and gently draw back 5 to 10 mL of blood into the syringe.	Ensures there is no clot in the catheter.	Notify the physician or advanced practice nurse if unable to withdraw blood.
12. Discard the nonsterile gloves in the appropriate receptacle.	Removes and safely discards used supplies.	
13. **HH**		

*Level B: Well-designed controlled studies with results that consistently support a specific action, intervention, or treatment

Procedure continues on following page

Procedure | for Arterial and Venous Sheath Removal—*Continued*

Steps	Rationale	Special Considerations
14. Apply sterile gloves.	Maintains asepsis.	
15. Remove sutures, if present.	Prepares for sheath removal.	Additional stabilizing devices may be used and removed.
16. Palpate the femoral pulse.	Allows for more accurate positioning of the hemostasis option (manual or mechanical).	
17. Determine the method that will be used to achieve hemostasis. (**Level B***)	Both manual and mechanical compression devices are effective in achieving hemostasis and reducing the risk of groin complications.[3,4,8,15,16,22]	Collagen plug devices, percutaneous suture-mediated closure devices, and percutaneous staple-mediated closure devices are deployed into the artery by the physician at the end of the catheterization or interventional procedure. Studies comparing arterial closure devices to either manual or mechanical compression are inconclusive regarding the optimal method of arterial closure.[11,13]
18. Position the hemostasis option (manual or mechanical) 1 to 2 cm above the site where the arterial sheath enters the skin. (If using a noninvasive hemostasis pad in conjunction with manual pressure, **see Step 21.**) With manual pressure, ensure positioning with the arms straight down, directly over the femoral artery.	The arterial puncture site (arteriotomy) is superior and medial to the skin puncture site since the arterial sheath is inserted at a 45-degree angle to the artery. Body weight can then be used to apply firm pressure.	If the patient is obese or has a large abdomen, a second person may be needed to assist with sheath removal.
19. Simultaneously depress the hemostasis option (manual or mechanical) and gently remove the arterial sheath from the femoral artery during exhalation.	Prevents external bleeding. Removing the arterial sheath during the exhalation phase of the respiratory cycle may prevent the patient from "bearing down" during arterial sheath removal.	Never withdraw the sheath if resistance is met. Notify the physician or advanced practice nurse.
20. Continue to apply firm pressure.	Firm pressure is needed to achieve hemostasis.	The distal pulse may decrease during application of full pressure but should not be completely obliterated. If manual compression is being performed, another person is needed to assess distal perfusion.
A. Maintain manual pressure above the arterial puncture site for approximately 20 minutes.		The length of time needed to achieve hemostasis depends on several factors, including the size of sheath used; the type of procedure; the use of bivalirudin, heparin, or antiplatelet medications during the procedure; the ACT level at the time of sheath removal; and the patient's anatomy at the femoral insertion site. Patients who are hypertensive or obese may need a longer application of pressure.

*Level B: Well-designed controlled studies with results that consistently support a specific action, intervention, or treatment

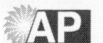

Procedure for Arterial and Venous Sheath Removal—*Continued*

Steps	Rationale	Special Considerations
B. Maintain the mechanical compression device. **(Level M*)**		With use of a mechanical device, set the pressure of the device according to manufacturer recommendation and institution standard. Tissue damage may occur if prolonged pressure is maintained (i.e., longer than 2 to 3 hours).[2] During mechanical compression, monitoring of the arterial puncture site and distal pulses is essential.
21. With use of a noninvasive hemostasis pad in conjunction with manual compression:		Follow manufacturer guidelines.
A. Apply manual pressure 1 to 2 cm proximal to the skin insertion site **(see Step 18)**.		
B. Place the noninvasive hemostasis pad directly over the puncture site before removing the sheath.		
C. Remove the sheath.		
D. Reduce the proximal pressure to allow a small amount of blood from the arterial puncture site to moisten the noninvasive hemostasis pad; then, quickly reapply the proximal manual pressure.	Noninvasive hemostasis pads must be moistened to activate the hemostatic mechanism.	
E. Hold firm manual pressure proximal to the skin insertion site and over the noninvasive hemostasis pad at the puncture site.		
F. Gradually release the proximal pressure after 3 to 4 minutes; however, pressure should be maintained over the puncture site for at least 10 minutes.		The total time of compression depends on the same factors listed for manual compression **(see Step 20 A)**.
G. Place a new sterile gauze over the hemostasis pad and cover with a sterile dressing.	Maintains asepsis.	The noninvasive hemostasis pad is left in place for 24 hours.
22. While achieving hemostasis, assess the circulation of the extremity distal to the site of the arterial sheath removal.	Verifies adequate circulation while hemostasis is achieved.	The pulse may decrease during application of full pressure but should not be completely obliterated. If manual compression is being performed, another person is needed to assess distal perfusion.
23. With use of manual compression or mechanical compression, discontinue pressure once hemostasis is achieved.	Pressure is no longer needed.	With use of a mechanical device, follow manufacturer recommendations, institution standard, or physician prescription regarding the gradual reduction of pressure from the device. Notify the physician or advanced practice nurse if unable to achieve hemostasis.

*Level M: Manufacturer's recommendations only.

Procedure continues on following page

Procedure   for Arterial and Venous Sheath Removal—*Continued*

Steps	Rationale	Special Considerations
24. With use of a venous sheath, remove the venous sheath approximately 5 to 10 minutes after removal of the arterial sheath and maintain manual pressure over both sites for approximately 10 additional minutes or until hemostasis is achieved.[1]	Achieves both arterial and venous hemostasis. The arterial sheath is removed first because pressure needs to be applied to the arterial site longer than the venous site to achieve hemostasis. In addition, the venous line may be used to give additional IV fluids or medications, if needed (e.g., vasovagal reaction).	Follow manufacturer guidelines and institution standard. For example, if the FemoStop device is used, the venous sheath is removed first to reduce the risk of AV fistula formation. Collagen plug devices, percutaneous suture-mediated devices, and percutaneous staple-mediated closure devices are not used for venous punctures. Noninvasive hemostasis pads may be used in conjunction with manual pressure to achieve hemostasis for venous punctures.
25. After hemostasis is achieved, palpate the area around the arterial site.	Determines whether any bleeding has occurred around the arterial site.	If bleeding is noted around the arterial site after hemostasis is achieved, apply manual pressure and notify the physician or advanced practice nurse.
26. Apply a sterile dressing to the arterial or venous sites.	Maintains asepsis.	If a collagen plug device or a percutaneous suture-mediated or staple-mediated closure device is deployed in the arteriotomy immediately after the procedure. Pressure is usually held for at least 10 minutes after the venous sheath is removed.
27. Discard used supplies in appropriate receptacles.		
28. **HH**		

Expected Outcomes

- Arterial and venous sheaths removed with hemostasis achieved
- Adequate peripheral vascular and neurovascular integrity of the extremity distal to the site of sheath removal (positive sensation, movement, capillary refill, color, temperature, pulse)
- No evidence of peripheral vascular or neurovascular complications
- Cardiovascular and hemodynamic stability

Unexpected Outcomes

- Inability to remove the arterial or venous sheaths
- Inability to achieve hemostasis
- Impaired perfusion to the extremity distal to the site of sheath removal
- Impaired motor/sensory status of the extremity distal to the site of sheath removal
- Development of a hematoma or new bruit
- Development of a retroperitoneal bleed
- Development of a pseudoaneurysm or arteriovenous fistula
- Vasovagal response during the removal of the arterial sheath (ensure patent IV, with IV fluids and emergency medications and equipment available)
- Hemodynamic instability
- Angina or shortness of breath
- Decrease in hemoglobin greater than 2 g compared with preprocedure values
- Unrelieved pain

Patient Monitoring and Care

Steps	Rationale	Reportable Conditions
		These conditions should be reported if they persist despite nursing interventions.
1. Assess the peripheral vascular and neurovascular status of the affected extremity after arterial sheath removal: every 15 minutes × 4, every 30 minutes × 2, then every 60 minutes × 4.	A thrombus, embolus, or dissection may precipitate changes in peripheral vascular or neurovascular status, necessitating early intervention.	• Change in strength of pulses in the affected extremity (diminished or absent) • Coldness or coolness of the distal extremity • Paresthesia in the affected extremity • Pallor, cyanosis of the affected extremity • Pain in the affected extremity • Decrease in mobility of the affected extremity
2. Obtain vital signs after removal of the arterial sheath: every 15 minutes × 4, every 30 minutes × 2, then every 60 minutes × 4.	Changes in vital signs may occur because of a vasovagal response or blood loss.	• Abnormal vital signs
3. Assess the puncture site: every 15 minutes × 4, every 30 minutes × 2, then every 60 minutes × 4, including assessment of presence or absence of bruit.	Detects presence of bleeding, hematoma, or bruit.	• Bleeding at arterial or venous sites • Hematoma development • New bruit • Pain at the access site
4. Monitor the ECG during and after sheath removal.	Detects the presence of dysrhythmias. Bradydysrhythmias are common with vasovagal reactions.	• Dysrhythmias
5. After hemostasis is achieved, the patient's head of bed can be elevated up to 30 degrees. (**Level B***)	Minimizes back discomfort and does not increase vascular complications.[6,17]	• Occurrence of bleeding • Hematoma development • Abnormal vital signs • New bruit • Changes in peripheral vascular or neurovascular status • Back pain not relieved with position changes or analgesics

6. Maintain bed rest for 2 to 6 hours after arterial sheath removal when manual or mechanical pressure is used. (**Level B**)
    With collagen plug devices, percutaneous suture-mediated closure devices, percutaneous staple-mediated closure devices, and noninvasive hemostasis pads, the bed rest time is decreased to between 1 and 4 hours, depending on the manufacturer's recommendations; follow institution standard.
    Maintain bed rest for a maximum of 4 hours after venous sheath removal. Follow institution standard.
	Minimizes back discomfort, minimizes complications of bed rest, and does not increase vascular complications.[7,9,12,18,19,21]
	Bed rest times vary depending on the size of sheath used; the type of procedure; the use of bivalirudin, heparin, or antiplatelet medications during the procedure; and institution protocol.
	Patients with venous punctures need less time in bed than with arterial punctures because the incidence of complications is decreased.
		• Occurrence of bleeding
		• Hematoma development
		• Abnormal vital signs
		• New bruit
		• Changes in peripheral vascular or neurovascular status
		• Back pain not relieved with position changes or analgesics

*Level B: Well-designed controlled studies with results that consistently support a specific action, intervention, or treatment

Procedure continues on following page

Patient Monitoring and Care —*Continued*

Steps	Rationale	Reportable Conditions
7. Follow institution standard for assessing pain. Administer analgesia as prescribed.	Identifies need for pain interventions.	• Continued pain despite pain interventions

Documentation

Documentation should include the following:
- Patient and family education
- Date and time of sheath removal
- Site of arterial and venous sheath removal
- Quality of arterial and venous sheaths removed (e.g., intact, cracked)
- Any difficulties with removal
- Patient tolerance of the procedure
- Pain assessment, interventions, and effectiveness
- Any medications administered
- Time hemostasis obtained

- Method of hemostasis
- Site assessment after hemostasis's obtained, including presence or absence of a bruit
- Heart rate and rhythm, blood pressure, and respiratory rate
- Peripheral vascular and neurovascular checks to the affected extremity
- Occurrence of unexpected outcomes
- Nursing interventions
- Evaluation of any nursing intervention

References

1. Baim DS, Simon DI: Percutaneous approach including trans-septal and apical puncture. In Baim DS, editor: *Grossman's cardiac catheterization, angiography, and intervention*, ed 7, Philadelphia, 2006, Lippincott Williams & Wilkins, 79-106.
2. Barbiere CC: A new device for control of bleeding after transfemoral catheterization: the FemoStop system, *Crit Care Nurse* 15:51-53, 1995.
3. Benson LM, et al: Determining best practice: comparison of three methods of femoral sheath removal after cardiac interventional procedures, *Heart Lung J Acute Crit Care* 34:115-121, 2004.
4. Bogart MA: Time to hemostasis: a comparison of manual versus mechanical compression of the femoral artery, *Am J Crit Care* 4:149-156, 1995.
5. Bowden SM, Worrey JA: Assessing patient comfort: Local infiltration of lidocaine during femoral sheath removal, *Am J Crit Care* 4:368-369, 1995.
6. Coyne C, et al: Controlled trial of backrest elevation after coronary angiography, *Am J Crit Care* 3:282-288, 1994.
7. Fowlow B, Price P, Fung T: Ambulation after sheath removal: a comparison of 6 and 8 hours of bedrest after sheath removal in patients following a PTCA procedure, *Heart Lung J Acute Crit Care* 24:28-37, 1995.
8. Jones T, McCutcheon H: Effectiveness of mechanical compression devices in attaining hemostasis after femoral sheath removal, *Am J Crit Care* 11:155-162, 2002.
9. Keeling AW, et al: Reducing time in bed after percutaneous transluminal coronary angioplasty (TIBS III), *Am J Crit Care* 9:185-187, 2000.
10. Kiat Ang C, et al: Effect of local anesthesia and intravenous sedation on pain perception and vasovagal reactions during femoral arterial sheath removal after percutaneous coronary intervention, *Int J Cardiol* 116:321-326, 2005.
11. Koreny M, et al: Arterial puncture closing devices compared with manual compression after cardiac catheterization: systematic review and meta-analysis, *JAMA* 291:350-357, 2004.
12. Logemann T, et al: Two versus six hours of bed rest following left-sided cardiac catheterization and a meta-analysis of early ambulation trials, *Am J Cardiol* 84:486-488, 1999.
13. Nikolsky E, et al: Vascular complications associated with arteriotomy closure devices in patients undergoing percutaneous coronary procedures, *J Am Coll Cardiol* 44:1200-1209, 2004.
14. O'Grady NP, et al: Guidelines for the prevention of intravascular catheter- related infections, Centers for Disease Control and Prevention, *MMWR Recommend Rep* 51(RR-10):1-29, 2002.
15. Rudisill PT, et al: Study of mechanical versus manual-mechanical compression following various interventional cardiology procedures, *J Cardiovasc Nurs* 11:15-21, 1997.
16. Simon A, et al: Manual versus mechanical compression for femoral artery hemostasis after cardiac catheterization, *Am J Crit Care* 7:308-313, 1998.
17. Sulzbach LM, Munro BH, Hirshfeld JW: A randomized clinical trial of the effect of bed position after PTCA, *Am J Crit Care* 4:221-226, 1995.
18. Tagney J, Lackie D: Bed-rest post-femoral arterial sheath removal: what is safe practice? A clinical audit, *Nurs Crit Care* 10:167-173, 2005.
19. Vlasic W, Almond D, Massel D: Reducing bedrest following arterial puncture for coronary interventional procedures-impact on vascular complications: the BAC Trial, *J Invasive Cardiol* 13:788-792, 2001.
20. Wadas TM, Hill J: Is lidocaine infiltration during femoral sheath removal really necessary? *Heart Lung J Acute Crit Care* 27:31-36, 1998.
21. Walker S, et al: Comparison of complications in percutaneous coronary intervention patients mobilized at 3, 4 and 6 hours after femoral arterial sheath removal, *J Cardiovasc Nurs* 23:407-413, 2008.

CR 22. Walker SB, Cleary SR, Higgins M: Comparison of the FemoStop device and manual pressure in reducing groin puncture site complications following coronary angioplasty and coronary stent placement, *Int J Nurs Pract* 7:366-375, 2001.

23. Wensley CJ, et al: Pain relief for the removal of femoral sheath in interventional cardiology patients, *Cochrane Database Syst Rev* 4:Art. No.:CD006043. DOI: 10.1002/14651858. CD006043.pub2, 2008.

Additional Readings

CR Chlan LL, Sabo J, Savik K: Effects of three groin compression methods on patient discomfort, distress, and vascular complications following a precutaneous coronary intervention procedure, *Nurs Res* 54:391-398, 2005.

CR Christensen BV, et al: Vascular complications after angiography with and without the use of sandbags, *Nurs Res* 47:51-53, 1998.

CR Cura FA, et al: Safety of femoral closure devices after percutaneous coronary interventions in the era of glycoprotein IIb/IIIa platelet blockade, *Am J Cardiol* 86:780-782, 2000.

Dressler DK, Dressler KK: Caring for patients with femoral sheaths: after percutaneous coronary intervention, sheath removal and site monitoring are the nurse's responsibility, *AJN* 106:64A-64H, 2006.

Dueling JHH, et al: Closure of the femoral artery after cardiac catheterization: a comparison of Angio-Seal, StarClose, and manual compression, *Cathet Cardiovasc Interv* 71:518-523, 2008.

Dumont CJP, et al: Predictors of vascular complications post diagnostic cardiac catheterization and percutaneous coronary intervention, *Dimens Crit Care Nurs* 25:137-142, 2006.

CR Galli A, Palatnik A: Ask the experts: what is the proper activated clotting time (ACT) at which to remove a femoral sheath after PCI? What are the best "protocols" for sheath removal? *Crit Care Nurse* 25:88-95, 2005.

Juergens CP, et al: Vaso-vagal reactions during femoral arterial sheath removal after percutaneous coronary intervention and impact on cardiac events, *Int J Cardiol* 127:252-254, 2007.

Kim M: Vascular closure devices, *Cardiol Clin* 24:277-286, 2006.

CR Nickolaus MJ, Gilchrist IC, Ettinger SM: The way to the heart is all in the wrist: transradial catheterization and interventions, *AACN Clin Issues* 12:62-71, 2001.

Sabo J, Chlan LL, Savik K: Relationships among patient characteristics, comorbidities, and vascular complications post-percutaneous coronary intervention, *Heart Lung J Acute Crit Care* 37:190-195, 2008.

CR Schickel S, et al: Removal of femoral sheaths by registered nurses: issues and outcomes, *Crit Care Nurse* 16:32-36, 1996.

CR Smith TT, Labriola R: Developing best practice in arterial sheath removal for registered nurses, *J Nurs Care Qual* 16:61-67, 2001.

Pericardial Catheter Management

PURPOSE: An indwelling pericardial catheter allows for the slow and complete evacuation of a pericardial effusion. The catheter also allows for the infusion of medications, such as antibiotics or chemotherapeutic agents, into the pericardial space.

Mary Ellen Kern

PREREQUISITE NURSING KNOWLEDGE

- Knowledge of the anatomy and physiology of the cardiovascular system, the principles of cardiac conduction, electrocardiogram (ECG) lead placement, basic dysrhythmia interpretation, and electrical safety is needed.
- Understanding of sterile technique is essential.
- Advanced cardiac life support knowledge and skills are needed.
- Pericardial effusion is an excessive collection of fluid in the pericardial space.
- The pericardial space normally contains 20 to 50 mL of fluid. Injury to the pericardium causes increased production of pericardial fluid, formation of fibrin, and cellular proliferation.[2,13]
- Pericardial fluid has electrolyte and protein profiles similar to plasma.[13]
- Causes of pericardial effusion are numerous and include infection, malignant neoplasms, autoimmune disorders, kidney failure, heart failure, acute myocardial infarction, trauma, radiation exposure, inflammatory disorders, and myxedema. Pericardial effusion may also be medication-induced, idiopathic, or a complication of invasive procedures.[7,13,14]
- Pericardiocentesis is an effective treatment for pericardial effusion (see Procedures 45 and 46). An indwelling pericardial catheter may be left in place after a pericardiocentesis to drain excess or continued excess production of pericardial fluid.

- The pericardial catheter may be connected to a closed drainage system (Fig. 78-1).
- The pericardial catheter may also be left in place to allow the instillation of certain medications (i.e., nonabsorbable corticosteroid or antineoplastic agents) depending on the patient's underlying disease state.[8,12]

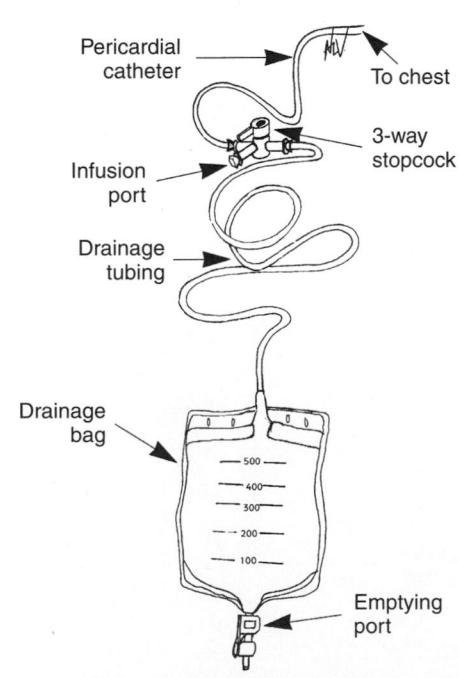

FIGURE 78-1 Indwelling pericardial catheter system. *(From Hammel WJ: Care of patients with an indwelling pericardial catheter, Crit Care Nurse 18[5]:40-45, 1998.)*

- The indwelling pericardial catheter is usually removed within 48 to 72 hours after placement to avoid the risk of infection or iatrogenic pericarditis.[13,14] The indwelling pericardial catheter may be left in place for longer periods of time to promote the resolution of a pericardial effusion or cardiac tamponade.[1] Pericardial catheters are immediately removed if there is an abrupt rise in the white blood cell (WBC) level.[12]
- Pericardial catheters are usually removed when the total amount of drainage has decreased to less than 25 to 30 mL over the preceding 24 hours.[1,13,14]
- Extended catheter drainage is associated with a reduction of the re-occurrence of cardiac tamponade compared with a single pericardiocentesis in patients with pericardial effusion related to malignancy.[2,3]

EQUIPMENT

- Pericardial catheter
- Sterile drapes: small drapes and a full-body drape
- Sterile and nonsterile gloves, gowns, masks, protective eyewear
- Sterile 0.9% normal saline solution for irrigation and sterile basin
- Anticoagulant flush available for dwell as prescribed (i.e., heparin)
- Sterile syringes: 3-, 5-, 30-, or 60-mL Luer-Lok
- Sterile 1000-mL vacuum bottle available for the initial procedure
- Antiseptic solution (e.g., 2% chlorhexidine-based preparation)
- Sterile 4 × 4 gauze
- Sterile transparent occlusive dressing
- Adhesive tape
- Sterile three-way Luer-Lok stopcock with nonvented caps and replacement caps
  Additional equipment as needed includes the following:
- Drainage tubing
- Pericardial drainage bag
- Cytotoxic disposal receptacle (when chemotherapeutic or cytotoxic agents are prescribed and used to avoid aerosolization of the medication once disconnected from the patient)

PATIENT AND FAMILY EDUCATION

- Explain the need for the indwelling pericardial catheter and the reason for its insertion. ➤➤*Rationale:* The explanation decreases patient and family anxiety.
- Explain the need for frequent monitoring while the pericardial catheter remains in place. ➤➤*Rationale:* This information may decrease patient and family anxiety.
- Explain that the catheter may be uncomfortable and may cause some discomfort at the insertion site, possibly with inspiration, and that pain medication will be available to administer at the time of the procedure and

afterward to promote comfort. ➤➤*Rationale:* This explanation prepares and informs the patient of the pain management plan.
- Describe the possible signs and symptoms of cardiac tamponade to the patient and family. ➤➤*Rationale:* Teaching the patient and family will help them to recognize a possible reoccurrence of pericardial effusion.

PATIENT ASSESSMENT AND PREPARATION

Patient Assessment

- Assess the patient's cardiovascular and hemodynamic status: heart rate and rhythm, blood pressure (BP), respiratory rate, heart sounds, peripheral pulses, and if available, pulmonary artery pressures (PAPs), pulmonary artery occlusion pressure (PAOP), right atrial pressure (RAP), cardiac output (CO), cardiac index (CI), and systemic vascular resistance (SVR). ➤➤*Rationale:* The patient's baseline values are established for future comparison.
- Assess the patient for dyspnea, tachypnea, tachycardia, muffled heart sounds, precordial dullness to percussion, or impaired consciousness; hypotension (systolic BP, <100 mm Hg or decreased from patient's baseline); if available, cerebral perfusion pressure (CPP) of less than 70 mm Hg; increased jugular venous pressure/jugular distention; pulsus paradoxus (inspiratory fall in systolic BP sounds) greater than 12 to 15 mm Hg; equalization of RAP, PAOP, and pulmonary artery diastolic pressure; and decreased CO/CI.[14] ➤➤*Rationale:* Signs and symptoms of possible cardiac tamponade are assessed.
- Determine the patient's allergy history (e.g., heparin, antiseptic solutions). ➤➤*Rationale:* This assessment decreases the risk for allergic reactions by avoiding known allergenic products.

Patient Preparation

- Verify correct patient with two identifiers. ➤➤*Rationale:* Prior to performing a procedure, the nurse should ensure the correct identification of the patient for the intended intervention.
- Ensure that the patient and family understand preprocedural teaching. Answer questions as they arise, and reinforce information as needed. ➤➤*Rationale:* Understanding of previously taught information is evaluated and reinforced.
- Ensure that in nonemergent situations, informed consent has been obtained. ➤➤*Rationale:* Informed consent protects the rights of the patient and makes a competent decision possible for the patient.
- Perform a pre-procedure verification and time out, if nonemergent. ➤➤*Rationale:* Ensures patient safety.
- Administer analgesia or anxiolytic as prescribed before pericardial catheter insertion. ➤➤*Rationale:* Comfort is promoted and anxiety is reduced.

Procedure   for Pericardial Catheter Management

Steps	Rationale	Special Considerations
General Management of the Patient with a Pericardial Catheter Without a Drainage System		
1. **HH**		Consider putting a mask on the patient during the actual procedure if the patient is not intubated in a contained system, especially if the patient has methicillin-resistant *Staphylococcus aureus* (MRSA)–positive results on nasal swab or known colonization.
2. **PE**		
3. Assist the physician or advanced practice nurse with the pericardio-centesis (see Procedures 45 and 46) as the pericardial catheter is inserted over a guidewire and is positioned in the pericardial sac.	Provides assistance as needed.	The pericardial catheter may be in-serted in the operating room, in a special procedure environment (e.g., cardiac catheterization labora-tory or interventional laboratory), or at the bedside.
4. Determine that the connections between the pericardial catheter and the stopcock are tight.	Ensures that the integrity of the system is intact.	At the completion of the pericardial tap, the stopcock is turned off to the patient and a sterile nonvented cap is placed on the stopcock port.
5. Observe the drainage of pericar-dial fluid for color, amount, and consistency.	Ensures pericardial catheter patency. The presence of fibrin matrix in the drainage can result in obstruction of the catheter and be problematic for future manual taps.	Pericardial fluid is commonly straw-colored, serous drainage. A two-dimensional (2-D) or Doppler echo-cardiogram is usually performed after the pericardiocentesis to assess for reaccumulation of pericardial fluid.[10]
6. Perform catheter site care:	Prevents infection.	Consider placing a mask on the patient during the procedure if the patient is not intubated.
A. **HH**		
B. **PE**		
C. Remove the dressing and discard it in an appropriate receptacle.	Allows for site assessment and prepares for site care.	
D. Assess the catheter, insertion site, suture, and surrounding skin.	Assess for signs of infection, catheter dislodgment, leakage, or loose sutures.	
E. Remove and discard the non-sterile gloves in an appropriate receptacle.	Maintains aseptic technique.	
F. **HH**		
G. Apply sterile gloves.		
H. Cleanse the skin around the pericardial catheter insertion site using a back-and-forth motion while applying friction for 30 seconds with an antiseptic solution (e.g., 2% chlorhexidine-based solu-tion).[4,5,9] Allow the antiseptic to remain on the insertion site and to air-dry completely. **(Level D*)**	Reduces the rate of recolonization of skin microflora.	

*Level D: Peer-reviewed professional organizational standards with clinical studies to support recommendations

Procedure for Pericardial Catheter Management—*Continued*

Steps	Rationale	Special Considerations
I. Ensure that the catheter and stopcock are securely anchored to the chest.	Reduces the possibility of dislodgment.	
J. Apply a sterile, occlusive dressing over the catheter insertion site. Label the dressing with the date, time, and initials of the person performing the dressing change.	Provides a sterile environment. Identifies the last dressing change.	
K. Discard used supplies in the appropriate receptacles.		
L. **HH**		
7. *If pericardial fluid removal is desired*, aspirate the pericardial fluid every 4 to 6 hours, as prescribed, or as clinically indicated through a three-way stopcock with sterile technique.[1,2,7]	Removes excess pericardial fluid and relieves symptoms of cardiac tamponade; ensures catheter patency.	Follow institution standard regarding personnel permitted to aspirate and flush pericardial catheters (e.g., registered nurse, advanced practice nurse, physician). Consider placing a mask on the patient during the procedure if the patient is not intubated.
A. **HH**		Pericardial fluid samples may be collected for select diagnostic tests (e.g., protein, glucose, hematocrit, white blood cell count, bacterial or fungal culture).
B. **PE**		
C. Remove the nonvented cap from the infusion port (stopcock is turned off to the patient) of the three-way stopcock.	Prepares the equipment.	
D. Clean the infusion port of the three-way stopcock with an alcohol swab for 15 seconds and allow to dry.	Decreases the risk for infection.	
E. Attach a sterile, 60-mL Luer-Lok syringe to the three-way stopcock.	Connects to the port for pericardial fluid removal without the danger of disconnection.	
F. Turn the stopcock open to the syringe and patient.	Permits the removal of pericardial fluid.	
G. Gently aspirate pericardial fluid.	Gentle removal is necessary to avoid pericardial or myocardial injury.	
H. After completion of the fluid withdrawal, turn the stopcock off to the patient.	Stops pericardial drainage.	
I. Disconnect the specimen syringe from the stopcock.	Removes the specimen.	
J. Connect the flush syringe to the stopcock.	Prepares equipment.	
K. Turn the stopcock open to the syringe and patient and gently flush the pericardial catheter with 2 to 5 mL of sterile (0.9%) normal saline solution or heparinized normal saline solution as prescribed.[1]	Clears the pericardial catheter and maintains catheter patency.	Monitor vital signs and the ECG while flushing the pericardial catheter. Follow institution standard for administration of dwell solution.

Procedure continues on following page

Procedure for Pericardial Catheter Management—*Continued*

Steps	Rationale	Special Considerations
L. Turn the stopcock off to the patient and disconnect the flush syringe.	Removes equipment.	
M. Place a new sterile nonvented cap on the stopcock.	Maintains a sterile, closed system. Prevents pneumopericardium.	
N. Measure the amount of drainage.	Needed for assessing and recording output.	
O. Discard the collected drainage and used supplies in the appropriate receptacles.		
P. 🄷🄷		
8. *If the pericardial catheter is blocked or obstructed to flow:*		Follow institution standard regarding personnel permitted to aspirate and flush pericardial catheters (e.g., registered nurse, advanced practice nurse, or physician).
A. Assess whether there is an external mechanical cause of the pericardial catheter blockage and, if present, correct. Consider the following measures: 1. Correct tubing kinks. 2. Remove tubing that may be compressed under the patient. 3. Turn or reposition the patient.	Relieves mechanical obstruction to flow of pericardial fluid.	
B. Assess for loose tubing connection and, if loosened, tighten the connection.	Ensures an intact pericardial drainage system.	
C. Determine whether the stopcock is in the correct position and, if needed, correct the position.	Facilitates pericardial fluid drainage.	
D. If the previous steps do not relieve the catheter blockage, do the following: 1. 🄷🄷 2. 🄿🄴	Attempts to relieve the blockage.	
3. Turn the stopcock off to the patient and remove the cap from the infusion port of the stopcock.	Prepares the equipment.	
4. Clean the infusion port of the stopcock with an alcohol swab for 15 seconds and allow to dry.	Decreases the risk for infection.	
5. Attach the syringe for the flush and turn the stopcock open to the patient.	Prepares the equipment.	
6. Gently flush the pericardial catheter with 2 to 5 mL of heparinized normal saline solution, as prescribed (e.g., 30 units of heparin per mL of 0.9% normal saline) or sterile normal saline if the patient is sensitive to heparin.[1,2]	Attempts to improve pericardial catheter patency. Heparinized saline solution may be used for a dwell if the drainage tends to be serous or fibrous in consistency.[6]	Monitor vital signs and the ECG while flushing the pericardial catheter.

Procedure for **Pericardial Catheter Management**—*Continued*

Steps	Rationale	Special Considerations
7. Gently attempt to aspirate the flush solution.	Allows drainage of the flush solution and pericardial fluid.	Deduct the flush solution from the measurement of pericardial drainage.
8. Determine whether the pericardial catheter is draining and patent.	Assesses the function of the system.	Obtain vital signs and cardiac parameters.
9. If the above measures do not remove the catheter blockage, notify the physician or advanced practice nurse immediately.	Additional interventions are indicated.	
9. *If medications are prescribed for infusion into the pericardium:*		Follow institution standard for personal protective equipment when administering cytotoxic or antineoplastic medications. Follow institution standard regarding personnel permitted to instill medications into the pericardial sac.
A. **HH**		
B. **PE**		
C. Review the prescribed medication, dose, method of delivery, amount, and time for dwell. Assemble the medication, tubing/pump or syringe, and two flush syringes of 0.9% normal saline (2 to 5 mL each).[1,6,8]	Prepares the equipment.	
D. Ensure that the stopcock is off to the patient and remove the cap from the infusion port.	Prepares the equipment.	
E. Clean the infusion port of the stopcock with an alcohol swab for 15 seconds and allow to dry.	Reduces the risk of infection.	
F. Attach a flush syringe and turn the stopcock open to the patient. Establish the patency of the catheter by gentle infusion and withdrawal of 0.9% normal saline.	Ensures catheter patency.	
G. Turn the stopcock off to the patient and disconnect the flush syringe.	Prepares the equipment.	
H. Attach the prescribed medication (either infusion or syringe). With use of a syringe for delivery, gently instill the medication. With use of an infusion, set the medication infusion rate.	Administers the medication.	Infusion of the medication may activate signs and symptoms of cardiac tamponade.[1] Monitor vital signs, patient presentation, and cardiac parameters if available to identify patient distress and decompensation. If the patient has these symptoms, stop the infusion and notify the advanced practice nurse or the physician.

Procedure continues on following page

Procedure	for Pericardial Catheter Management—*Continued*	
Steps	**Rationale**	**Special Considerations**
I. Turn the stopcock off to the patient when the medication delivery is complete.	Stops the medication administration.	
1. Disconnect the syringe or tubing.	Removes the equipment.	
2. Attach a flush syringe of 0.9% normal saline.	Prepares the equipment.	
3. Turn the stopcock open to the patient and gently instill the flush solution.	Ensures that the medication is fully in the pericardium and not in the catheter.	
J. Turn the stopcock off to the patient and apply a sterile, nonvented cap to the infusion port.	Closes the system.	
K. Allow the medication to dwell for the prescribed time.	Allows time for the medication to act.	
L. When the dwell time is completed, remove the infusion port cap and attach a syringe large enough to retrieve the medication plus the pericardial fluid accumulation.	Prepares the equipment.	
M. Gently withdraw the medication and pericardial drainage.	Removes the medication.	Retrieval of the medication should be equivalent to the amount that was instilled, plus the flush solution and additional pericardial fluid that accumulated during the dwell time.
N. Turn the stopcock off to the patient and disconnect the syringe.	Removes the equipment.	
O. Attach a flush syringe of 2 to 5 mL of 0.9% normal saline with heparin if prescribed.[13,14]	Prepares the equipment.	
P. Turn the stopcock open to the patient and instill the 0.9% normal saline flush or heparin flush.	Clears the pericardial catheter.	
Q. Turn the stopcock off to the patient, remove the flush syringe and apply a sterile nonvented cap to the infusion port.	Closes the pericardial catheter system and maintains a closed system.	
R. Discard used supplies in the appropriate receptacles.		Discard any chemotherapeutic agent, tubing, and flush in the designated cytotoxic receptacle.
S. 🅷🅷		

General Management of the Patient with a Pericardial Catheter Closed Drainage System

1. 🅷🅷		
2. 🅿🅴		
3. Assist the physician or the advanced practice nurse with the pericardiocentesis (see Procedures 45 and 46) as the pericardial catheter is inserted over a guidewire and placed in the pericardial sac.	Provides assistance as needed.	The pericardial catheter may be inserted in the operating room, in a special procedure environment (e.g., cardiac catheterization laboratory or interventional laboratory), or at the bedside.
4. Determine that connections between the pericardial catheter, stopcock, tubing, and drainage bag are tight.	Ensures that the integrity of the system is intact.	At the completion of the pericardial tap, a nonvented sterile cap is placed on the stopcock port and the stopcock is turned off to the patient or open to drainage as prescribed.

Procedure for Pericardial Catheter Management—*Continued*

Steps	Rationale	Special Considerations
5. Position the drainage bag lower than the catheter insertion point, and observe the drainage of pericardial fluid for color, amount, and consistency.	Promotes drainage and is preventive for catheter blockage. The presence of fibrin matrix in the drainage can result in obstruction of the catheter.	Pericardial fluid is commonly straw-colored, serous drainage. A 2-D or Doppler echocardiogram is often performed after a pericardiocentesis to assess for reaccumulation of pericardial fluid.[10]
6. Perform catheter site care. A. **HH** B. **PE**	Prevents infection and avoids dislodgment of the catheter.	Observe the site for any evidence of drainage and notify the physician or advanced practice nurse of this finding.
C. Remove the dressing and discard it in an appropriate receptacle.	Allows for site assessment and prepares for site care.	
D. Assess the catheter, insertion site, suture, and surrounding skin.	Assess for signs of infection, catheter dislodgment, leakage, or loose sutures.	
E. Remove and discard the non-sterile gloves in an appropriate receptacle.	Maintains aseptic technique.	
F. **HH**		
G. Apply sterile gloves and establish a sterile field.		
H. Cleanse the skin around the pericardial catheter insertion site using a back-and-forth motion while applying friction for 30 seconds with an antiseptic solution (e.g., 2% chlorhexidine-based solution).[4,5,9] Allow the antiseptic to remain on the insertion site and to air-dry completely. **(Level D*)**	Reduces the rate of recolonization of skin microflora.	
I. Ensure that the catheter and the stopcock are securely anchored to the chest.	Reduces the possibility of dislodgement.	
J. Apply a sterile, occlusive dressing over the catheter insertion site. Label the dressing with the date, time, and initials of the person performing the dressing change.	Provides a sterile environment. Identifies the last dressing change.	
K. Discard used supplies in the appropriate receptacles.		
L. **HH**		
7. *If pericardial fluid removal is desired*, intermittently or continuously drain the pericardial fluid as prescribed by turning the stopcock off to the infusion port and open between the patient and the drainage bag (see Fig. 78-1).	Removes excess pericardial fluid.	Follow institution standard regarding personnel permitted to drain pericardial catheters (e.g., registered nurse, advanced practice nurse, or physician).

*Level D: Peer-reviewed professional organizational standards with clinical studies to support recommendations

Procedure continues on following page

Procedure	**for Pericardial Catheter Management—*Continued***	
Steps	**Rationale**	**Special Considerations**
A. Intermittent drainage: In the case of intermittent drainage, the stopcock is usually off to the patient and opened every 4 to 6 hours to drainage or as clinically indicated with Doppler scan or 2-D echocardiogram and patient presentation until the accumulation of fluid is resolved (follow prescribed regimen).		
B. Continuous drainage: In continuous drainage, the stopcock is open between the patient and the drainage bag and off to the infusion port (follow prescribed regimen).		
C. Empty the pericardial drainage bag at least every 8 hours.	Reduces the possibility of colonization in the bag and the potential reflux of fluid to the patient.	Pericardial fluid samples may be collected for selected diagnostic tests.
1. HH		
2. PE		
3. Turn the stopcock off to the patient.	Decreases the risk for pneumopericardium.	
4. Open the emptying port of the drainage bag and drain the pericardial fluid into a receptacle for measurement and waste disposal.	Allows drainage collection.	
5. Close the port and secure the drainage bag.	Closes and secures the system.	
6. Resume the prescribed drainage mode.	Continues treatment.	
D. After completion of intermittent fluid drainage, temporarily turn the stopcock off to the patient for the flush procedure.		Monitor vital signs and the ECG while flushing the pericardial catheter.
1. Remove the infusion port cap and clean the infusion port with an alcohol swab for 15 seconds and allow to dry.	Prepares the system.	
2. Connect the flush syringe, open the stopcock to the patient, and gently flush the pericardial catheter with 2 to 5 mL of sterile normal saline solution or prescribed solution (e.g., heparinized solution).[1]	Clears the pericardial catheter and maintains catheter patency.	
3. Turn the three-way stopcock off to the patient and disconnect the flush syringe.	Maintains a closed system; prevents pneumopericardium.	
4. Place a new sterile nonvented cap on the infusion port.	Maintains asepsis.	

Procedure for Pericardial Catheter Management—*Continued*

Steps	Rationale	Special Considerations
8. *If the pericardial catheter is blocked or obstructed to flow:*		Follow institution standards regarding personnel permitted to aspirate pericardial catheters (e.g., registered nurse, advanced practice nurse, or physician).
A. Determine whether the drainage system is lower than the insertion point and reposition if needed.	Facilitates drainage.	
B. Assess whether there is an external mechanical cause of pericardial catheter blockage and, if present, correct. Consider the following measures: 1. Correct tubing kinks. 2. Remove tubing that may be compressed under the patient. 3. Turn or reposition the patient.	Relieves a mechanical obstruction to flow of pericardial fluid.	
C. Assess for loose tubing connection, and if loosened, tighten the connection.	Ensures an intact pericardial drainage system.	
D. Determine whether the stopcock is in the correct position, and if needed, correct the position.	Facilitates pericardial fluid collection.	
E. If the previous steps do not relieve the catheter blockage, do the following: 1. 🅷🅷 2. 🅿🅴 3. Remove the cap from the stopcock. 4. Clean the infusion port of the stopcock with an alcohol swab for 15 seconds and allow to dry. 5. Connect the flush syringe, open the stopcock to the patient, and gently flush the pericardial catheter with 2 to 5 mL of sterile normal saline solution or prescribed solution (e.g., heparinized solution).[1] 6. Turn the stopcock off to the infusion port and allow the fluid to passively drain or turn the stopcock off to the drainage bag and gently attempt to aspirate the flush solution through the attached syringe.	Attempts to relieve blockage. Prepares equipment. Decreases the risk for infection. Attempts to improve pericardial catheter patency. Heparinized saline solution may be used if the drainage is serous or fibrous in consistency.[7] Allows drainage of the flush solution and pericardial fluid.	Monitor vital signs and the ECG while flushing the pericardial catheter. Deduct the flush solution from measurement of pericardial drainage. Obtain vital signs and cardiac parameters.

Procedure continues on following page

Procedure | for **Pericardial Catheter Management**—*Continued*

Steps	Rationale	Special Considerations
7. Determine whether the pericardial catheter is draining and patent.	Determines patency of the system.	
8. If the previous measures are ineffective for drainage but the catheter itself is patent, consider changing the tubing and the drainage bag system with the stopcock turned off to the patient at the time of the change.	Prepares the pericardial catheter drainage system.	
9. After the tubing/bag change, assess the patency of the system.	Determines patency.	
10. If the above measures do not remove the catheter blockage, notify the advanced practice nurse or the physician immediately.	Accumulation of fluid in the pericardium without the possibility of drainage may result in tamponade.	
9. *If infusion of medication into the pericardium is desired*:		Follow institution standards regarding personnel permitted to aspirate and flush pericardial catheters (e.g., registered nurse, advanced practice nurse, or physician).
A. **HH**		
B. **PE**		Double-gloving, eyewear or mask, and gown may be indicated for antineoplastic medication administration as may a cytotoxic disposal receptacle for retrieved drainage and flush after instillation.[10]
C. Review the prescribed medication, dose, amount, rate of infusion, and length of dwell time.	Ensures the accuracy of medication administration.	
D. Turn the stopcock off to the patient, remove the infusion port cap, clean the infusion port of the stopcock with an alcohol swab for 15 seconds, and allow to dry.	Decreases the risk for infection.	
E. Connect the medication syringe or IV medication solution to the infusion port of the stopcock. (Patency of the catheter is established by virtue of evident drainage. If there is a question about catheter patency, follow the flush procedure listed in the medication infusion section of Management of the Patient with a Pericardial Catheter Without a Drainage System.)	Prepares the equipment.	

Procedure for Pericardial Catheter Management—*Continued*

Steps	Rationale	Special Considerations
F. Turn the stopcock off to the drainage bag.	Prevents inadvertent instillation of medication into the drainage bag.	
G. Infuse the medication or solution slowly as prescribed.	Provides treatment as prescribed.	Infusion of medication into the pericardial sac may cause iatrogenic cardiac tamponade.
		Assess the patient closely for signs and symptoms of tamponade and chest pain. Stop the infusion if chest pain similar to angina develops or if the patient shows signs of tamponade.[1]
H. If the medication is to dwell in the pericardial space before reestablishment of pericardial drainage:		Discard any chemotherapeutic agent and flush, including antineoplastics, in the designated cytotoxic receptacle.
1. Turn the stopcock off to the patient at the completion of the infusion.		
2. Disconnect the medication syringe or tubing.		
3. Attach a syringe with 2 to 5 mL of 0.9% normal saline flush and turn the stopcock off to the drainage bag.		
4. Gently flush the catheter and turn the stopcock off to the patient for the completion of the dwell time as prescribed.	Ensures that the medication is instilled in the pericardial space and does not lie in the catheter.	
5. Disconnect the syringe and apply a sterile nonvented cap.		
6. After the dwell time is complete, turn the stopcock off to the infusion port and open to drainage.	Allows pericardial drainage to resume.	
7. Measure the amount of the solution infused and the drainage collected.	Ensure that the volume of drainage collected is equal to or greater than the volume of solution instilled.	
8. Resume the prescribed drainage mode: continuous or intermittent. If intermittent, follow the prescription for the drain time after infusion.	The drain time should allow for all of the medication to exit the pericardium.	
a. Once the drain time is completed, clean the infusion port of the stopcock with an alcohol swab for 15 seconds.		

Procedure continues on following page

Procedure for Pericardial Catheter Management—*Continued*

Steps	Rationale	Special Considerations
b. Connect the flush syringe, open the stopcock to the patient, and gently flush the pericardial catheter with 2 to 5 mL of sterile normal saline solution or prescribed solution (e.g., heparinized solution).[1] c. Turn the stopcock off to the patient until the next time the patient is due for intermittent drainage. d. Discard used supplies in appropriate receptacles. e. 🄷🄷		

Expected Outcomes

- Patent pericardial drainage system
- Resolution of pericardial effusion
- Hemodynamic stability
- Patient free of infection
- Patient free of pain and anxiety
- Medications administered as prescribed

Unexpected Outcomes

- Infection
- Pain
- Catheter blockage
- Reaccumulation of pericardial fluid
- Cardiac tamponade and hemodynamic instability
- Dysrhythmias
- Cardiac arrest

Patient Monitoring and Care

Steps	Rationale	Reportable Conditions
		These conditions must be reported if they persist despite nursing interventions.
1. Perform systematic cardiovascular and hemodynamic assessments at least every 60 minutes and as patient status necessitates or as prescribed.	Determines cardiac and hemodynamic status.	- Signs of cardiac tamponade: dyspnea, tachypnea, tachycardia, hypotension, increased jugular venous pressure, pulsus paradoxus, muffled heart sounds, precordial dullness to percussion, and altered level of consciousness; equalization of RAP, pulmonary artery (PA) diastolic, PAOP; CI less than 2.5 L/min/m^2; dysrhythmias
2. Assess the patency of the pericardial catheter: A. Without a closed drainage system, every 4 to 6 hours and as needed and as prescribed. B. With a closed drainage system, every hour and as needed or as prescribed.	Pericardial catheter blockage may predispose the patient to excessive accumulation of pericardial fluid that may lead to cardiac tamponade.	- Inability to obtain pericardial drainage or cessation of pericardial drainage - Signs and symptoms of cardiac tamponade - Evidence of accumulation of pericardial fluid on Doppler or 2-D echocardiography
3. Assess the amount and type of fluid draining from the pericardial catheter.	Monitors the type and amount of pericardial fluid drainage.	- Change in the amount or color of pericardial drainage from the patient's baseline

Patient Monitoring and Care —*Continued*

Steps	Rationale	Reportable Conditions
4. Change the pericardial dressing every 24 hours.	Provides an opportunity to assess for signs and symptoms of infection. Infective pericarditis is associated with high mortality and morbidity rates.[7] The Centers for Disease Control and Prevention (CDC) recommends replacing dressings on intravascular catheters when the dressing becomes damp, loosened, or soiled or when inspection of the site is necessary.[9]	• Elevated WBC levels • Elevated temperature • Signs and symptoms of infection at the insertion site (e.g., pain, erythema, drainage)
5. If in use, change the pericardial tubing and drainage bag every 72 hours.[1]	Reduces the incidence of infection.	
6. Follow institution standard for assessing pain. Administer analgesia as prescribed.	Identifies need for pain interventions. The patient may experience chest pain or pleuritic-type pain while the pericardial catheter is in place.	• Continued pain despite pain interventions
7. Identify parameters that show clinical readiness for removal of the indwelling pericardial catheter.	Facilitates early removal of the pericardial catheter; decreases infection risk.	• Pericardial drainage less than 25 to 30 mL over the previous 24 hours[2] • Hemodynamic stability as evidenced by systolic BP greater than 100 mm Hg, CI greater than 2.5 L/min/m^2, no pulsus paradoxus, no equalization of RAP, PA diastolic pressure, PAOP[1,2] • Absence of pericardial effusion shown on 2-D echocardiography or Doppler echocardiography[2,7]
8. Identify situations in which the pericardial effusion cannot be resolved with use of pericardial drainage via tap or closed system.	Unresolved pericardial effusion can be life-threatening.	• Hemodynamic instability • Continued pericardial effusion

Documentation

Documentation should include the following:
- Patient and family education
- Completion of inform consent
- Universal Protocol requirements
- Patient tolerance of the indwelling pericardial catheter
- Pericardial catheter insertion site assessment
- Dressing, tubing, and drainage bag changes
- Amount of pericardial drainage each shift, including the net volumes when the catheter is flushed or medications are infused
- Volumes of injectate or aspirate

- Characteristics of the pericardial drainage: color, consistency, and any changes
- Hemodynamic status
- Pain assessment, interventions, and effectiveness
- Occurrence of unexpected outcomes/treatments
- Nursing interventions

References

1. Cornily JC, et al: Cardiac tamponade in medical patients: a 10 year follow-up survey, *Cardiology* 111(3):197-201, 2008.
2. Gandhi S, et al: Has the clinical presentation and clinician's index of suspicion of cardiac tamponade changed over the past decade? *Echocardiography* 25(3):237-241, 2008.
CR 3. Hammel WJ: Care of patients with an indwelling pericardial catheter, *Crit Care Nurse* 18:40-45, 1998.
4. Infusion Nurses Society: *Policies and procedures for infusion nursing,* ed 3rd ed., Norwood, MA: 2006, Author.
5. Intravenous Nurses Society: (2006). Infusion nursing standards of practice, *J Infus Nurs* 29(1S):S1-S90, 2006.
6. Johnson KK, Soundarraj D, Patel P: Tenecteplase for malignant pericardial effusion, *Pharmacotherapy* 27(2):303-305, 2007.
7. Kolski BC, et al: Echocardiographic assessment of the accuracy of computed tomography in the diagnosis of hemodynamically significant pericardial effusions, *J Am Soc Echocardiogr* 21(4):377-379, 2007.
8. Maruyama R, et al: Catheter drainage followed by the instillation of bleomycin to manage malignant pericardial effusion in non-small cell lung cancer: a multi-institutional phase II trial, *J Thorac Oncol* 2(1):65-68, 2007.

CR 9. O'Grady NP, et al: Guidelines for the prevention of intravascular catheter-related infections: Centers for Disease Control and Prevention, *MMWR Recommend Rep* 51(RR-10):1-29, 2002.
10. Seferovic PM, et al: Management strategies in pericardial emergencies, *Herz* 31(9):891-900, 2006.
11. Staltari D, et al: Laparoscopic pericardio-peritoneal window: An alternative approach in the treatment of recurrent pericardial effusion, in-hospital evolution and survival, *Surg Laparosc Endosc Percutan Tech* 17(2):116-119, 2007.
12. Swanson N, Mirza I, Wijesinghe N, et al: Primary percutaneous balloon pericardiotomy for malignant pericardial effusion, *Cath Cardiovasc Interv* 71(4):504-507, 2008.
13. Valley VT, et al: *Pericarditis and cardiac tamponade,* available at www.eMedicine.com, updated May 12, 2008.
14. Yarlagadda C: *Cardiac tamponade,* available at www.eMedicine.com, updated May 24, 2008.

Additional Reading

Field JN, editor: *ACLS provider manual,* Dallas, 2006, American Heart Association, 51-58.

Transesophageal Echocardiography (Assist)

P U R P O S E : Transesophageal echocardiography offers an alternative approach for obtaining high-quality images of the heart structure that are not well visualized with a conventional transthoracic approach. A transesophageal echocardiography obtains images of the heart from a transducer inside the esophagus. The esophagus lies immediately behind the heart, and with this technology, clear images of the heart can be obtained.

Linda M. Hoke, Janice Y. Dawson

PREREQUISITE NURSING KNOWLEDGE

- Knowledge of cardiovascular anatomy and physiology is necessary.
- Knowledge of basic dysrhythmia recognition and treatment of life-threatening dysrhythmias is needed.
- Advanced cardiac life support knowledge and skills are necessary.
- A topical anesthetic is used in the oropharyngeal area; thus, the patient's gag reflex may be diminished or absent, putting the patient at risk for aspiration.[12,15]
- It is essential to understand the institution's intravenous (IV) conscious sedation guideline.
- Sedation can put the patient at risk for respiratory depression.[3,5,15]
- A fiberoptic probe with an ultrasound transducer is inserted through the mouth and into the esophagus just behind the heart (Fig. 79-1). The transducer located at the tip of the probe sends high-frequency sound waves toward the heart, which return as echoes. The echoes are converted, by computer, into moving images of the heart. The image is displayed on a screen and can be recorded on videotape or compact disk (CD), printed on paper, or sent electronically to a picture archiving communication system (PACS). This test is used to visualize structures of the heart and aorta that may not be seen with a standard transthoracic echocardiogram (TTE) and to clarify structures, that may be otherwise poorly seen. The test may be performed as an outpatient or inpatient procedure or in the operating room.[3,16,18]

- Various modes of echocardiography are used to examine the heart, blood vessels, valve function, and blood flow. The three techniques are as follows[17]:
  - Motion-mode (M-mode) echocardiography: This is a one-dimensional echocardiogram that visualizes time, depth, and intensity. It looks like a tracing instead of a picture of the heart and is used to measure the exact size of the heart chambers.
  - Two-dimensional (2-D) echocardiography: This shows the actual shape and motion of the different heart structures. These images represent "slices" of the heart in motion.
  - Doppler echocardiography: This assesses the flow of blood through the heart. The signals that represent blood flow are displayed as a series of black-and-white tracings or color images on the screen.
- Transesophageal echocardiography (TEE) imaging is more risky than transthoracic imaging because of the insertion of the probe in the esophagus and the need for IV conscious sedation.[4,16]
- Indications for TEE are as follows:
  - Evaluation of (pre) clot formation in the heart, especially in the atria and appendages, in patients with an atrial dysrhythmia.[3,6,15,18,20]
  - Evaluation of spontaneous echocardiographic contrast or "smoke" presenting as dynamic echoes within the left atrium and appendage, which resembles swirling smoke in 2-D images. It is manifested by erythrocyte and platelet aggregates in regions of low blood flow; it has a significant correlation with previous embolic

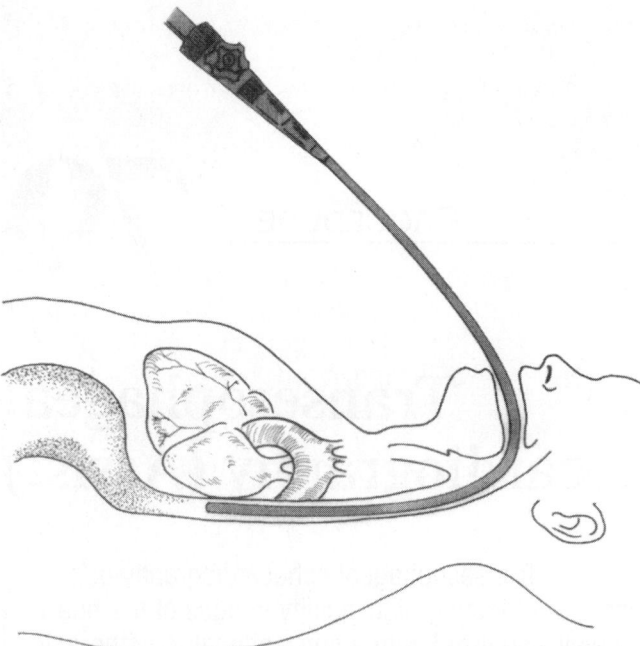

FIGURE 79-1 TEE probe inserted through the mouth and into the esophagus just behind the heart. *(From Brown LM, Brown AS: Transesophageal echocardiography: implications for the critical care nurse, Crit Care Nurs 14:56, 1994.)*

events and may serve as a marker for increased risk for embolism.[3,6,15,18,20]

❖ TEE before cardioversion is advocated in patients in whom early cardioversion would be clinically beneficial. Patients with atrial fibrillation undergoing electrical cardioversion with short-term anticoagulation therapy have lower hemorrhagic complications. Cardioversion may be performed more safely, after only a short period of anticoagulant therapy, in patients without atrial cavity or appendage thrombus. with TEE. Cardioversion is delayed in patients at high risk with thrombus detected by TEE. Conventional treatment has been to give patients undergoing elective cardioversion therapeutic anticoagulation therapy for 3 weeks before and 4 weeks after cardioversion, to decrease the risk for thromboembolism.[11,12,16]

❖ Transient ischemic attack or stroke evaluation to rule out cardiac source of emboli and structure abnormalities (e.g., patent foramen ovale) or other abnormalities not identified before a neurologic event.[3,15,16]

❖ Multiple factors may obstruct the penetration of the ultrasound beams from the transthoracic approach. Poor-quality TTE images can be found in patients with obesity, chronic obstructive lung disease, chest wall deformities, multiple chest trauma, and thick surgical chest dressings.[3,15]

❖ Assessment of native cardiac valve defects, particularly of the mitral valve.[1-3,15]

❖ Assessment of prosthetic cardiac valve function.[3,15,16,18]

❖ Assessment of intracardiac foreign bodies, tumors, or masses.[3,15,16,18]

❖ Assessment of vegetative endocarditis and abscess.[3,8,15,16]

❖ Assessment of congenital heart defects.[3,15,16,18]

❖ The superior sensitivity and specificity of TEE for aortic disease, including aneurysm, dissection, atherosclerosis, mobile plaque, congenital aortic disease, pseudoaneurysm, and traumatic aortic disruption, make it the test of choice in many clinical situations.[3,15,16,18]

❖ Disease in the ascending and transverse aorta often necessitates a TEE for complete evaluation; however, a short portion of the distal ascending aorta and proximal transverse arch is usually not visible. This portion is a blind area because of the carina passing between the aorta and the esophagus.[3,15,16,18]

❖ TEE used in combination with stress test for the evaluation of patients with coronary artery disease. Transesophageal echocardiography–dobutamine stress echocardiography (TEE-DSE) has been reported to be highly accurate for detection of ischemia in patients with suspected coronary artery disease.[19]

❖ Transesophageal atrial pacing stress echocardiography (TAPSE) is an efficient alternative to DSE for the detection of coronary artery disease. The heart rate can be rapidly increased, resulting in myocardial ischemia in regions supplied by stenosed coronary arteries. In contrast to TEE-DSE, termination of pacing results in nearly instantaneous restoration of the patient's intrinsic heart rate.[10]

❖ Intraoperative guide to left ventricular function and intracardiac blood flow and evaluation of cardiac surgical repair.[13]

❖ Assessment of a donor heart for transplant.[18]

❖ Intracardiac shunt evaluation. Right-sided echocardiography saline contrast studies are performed to document an atrial septal defect or a patent foramen ovale and to increase the signal strength of the tricuspid regurgitant jet to allow a more accurate estimate of pulmonary artery pressures.[18] Saline contrast for TEE is an IV injection of microbubbles formed by agitating a saline solution. This saline contrast results in a marked increase in echogenicity of the right-sided cardiac chambers.[22]

❖ Cardiac assessment in the interventional laboratory during percutaneous interventions, such as transcatheter closure for atrial septal defects and ventricular septal defects.[16,18]

❖ Cardiac assessment during interventional procedures, such as balloon mitral valvuoplasty, nonsurgical reduction of the ventricular septum in patients with hypertrophic cardiomyopathy, and transseptal catheterization for placement of a catheter during radiofrequeny ablation of cardiac dysrythmias.[16,18]

❖ Cardiac evaluation of left ventricular assist devices for optimal device performance, evaluation of hypoxemia, correct positioning of the cannula to optimize left ventricular filling, and determination of the patient's ability to be weaned from the mechanical device.[16,18]

❖ Assessment of the critically ill patient as an alternative for the technically limited TTE study.

❖ Assessment of unexplained hypotension, volume status, suspected massive pulmonary embolism, unexplained hypoxemia, and complications of cardiothoracic surgery.[17,18]

- Contraindications to TEE can be divided into absolute and relative.
- Absolute contraindications are[3,12,18]:
  ❖ Tumor of the upper gastrointestinal (GI) tract
  ❖ Esophageal obstruction, stenosis, fistulae, or varices
  ❖ A history of esophageal radiation or unresolved esophageal dilation
  ❖ GI bleeding
  ❖ Gastric volvulus or perforation
  ❖ Perforated viscus
  ❖ Patients who ate within 6 to 8 hours of the study
  ❖ Unwilling patients
  ❖ Inability to obtain intravenous access
- Relative contraindications are[13]:
  ❖ Upper GI surgery
  ❖ Severe thrombocytopenia (platelets 20,000 to 50,000/mm^3)
  ❖ Oropharyngeal distortion
  ❖ Prior esophageal surgery
  ❖ Esophagitis
  ❖ Loose teeth
- Antibiotics are no longer administered before the procedure in patients with a prosthetic valve. Echocardiography does not pose a risk for infection.[23]

EQUIPMENT

- Omniplane transesophageal probe
- Echocardiography machine (compatible with the probe)
- Constant low wall suction with connecting tubing and rigid pharyngeal suction tip catheter
- Protective mask and goggles
- Nonsterile gloves
- Barrier gowns
- Water-soluble lubricant (institution-specific)
- Oxygen with both nasal prongs and mask available
- Topical anesthetic such as 2% or 4% lidocaine solution with an administration device (i.e., mucosal atomization device), 2% viscous lidocaine, or benzocaine spray (institution-specific)
- Premedications for sedation and appropriate reversal agents (as prescribed)
- Alcohol prep pads
- IV insertion kit and IV setup with solution (usually 0.9% normal saline [NS] solution)
- Three-way stopcock and syringes for saline contrast injection (at least two 10-mL syringes with normal saline flush solution)
- Syringes for sedation medications (at least one 5-mL and one 10-mL)
- Tongue depressor
- Emesis basin

- Tonsillar forceps and cotton balls with radiopaque string attached (institution-specific)
- Flashlight (to assess the oropharyngeal area, especially in the case of trauma)
- Disposable bite guard (may use the type with or without a strap to hold it in place)
- Thermometer
- Continuous electrocardiographic (ECG) monitoring
- Continuous oximetric monitoring
- Automatic blood pressure cuff (with manual blood pressure cuff available for backup use)
- Pillow (to support/position neck when the patient lies on the left side during the procedure)
  Additional equipment as needed includes the following:
- Methylene blue, if benzocaine spray is used
- Emergency equipment
- Emergency intubation equipment
- Continuous capnography (institution-specific)[7]

PATIENT AND FAMILY EDUCATION

- Explain the procedure and the indication for therapy and the patient's role in the procedure. ➥*Rationale:* Information about the procedure increases patient cooperation and decreases patient and family anxiety and apprehension.
- Ensure that the patient understands the preparation for the procedure, which includes nothing by mouth (NPO) after midnight, or a minimum of 6 to 8 hours. Before the test, the patient may take daily medications, with a sip of water, as prescribed by the physician.[3,12] ➥*Rationale:* Undigested material in the stomach increases the risk for aspiration. Missing a daily medication dose may not be advisable.
- Explain to the patient that the local anesthetic may make the tongue and throat feel swollen and that he or she may feel unable to swallow. The gag reflex will be inhibited by the local anesthetic and may last approximately 1 hour after administration. The patient may experience gagging or retching during the numbing process and during the initial passage of the probe. ➥*Rationale:* The explanation may assist in decreasing patient anxiety during the procedure.
- Explain that the patient will be sedated to decrease anxiety, to increase comfort, and for ease in passing the probe. ➥*Rationale:* This information may decrease patient and family anxiety.
- Explain that the patient will be monitored closely during and after the procedure. ➥*Rationale:* The explanation assists in decreasing the patient and family anxiety.

PATIENT ASSESSMENT AND PREPARATION
Patient Assessment

- Confirm medications the patient has taken within the last 4 hours. ➥*Rationale:* Recent sedative, analgesic, and vasoactive medications may affect the patient's tolerance

and response to the medications given during the procedure.
- Assess the patient's baseline cardiac rhythm. ➡**Rationale:** The patient's rhythm may have converted if the indication for the procedure was a dysrhythmia. Passage of a large-bore tube may cause vagal stimulation and brady-dysrhythmias.
- Assess the patient's baseline respiratory, hemodynamic, and neurologic assessment before anesthetizing the posterior pharynx and administering any sedative agents. ➡**Rationale:** Baseline assessment data provide information to use as a comparison for further assessment once medications have been administered.
- Assess the patient's baseline vital signs, oxygen saturation, and if applicable, carbon dioxide level. ➡**Rationale:** Close monitoring of vital signs and oxygenation during the procedure and comparison with baseline are essential to assess the patient's tolerance of the procedure.
- Assess the patient's baseline pain characteristic, site, and severity. ➡**Rationale:** Baseline assessment data provide information to use as a comparison during and after the procedure.
- Assess the patient for a history of substance use. ➡**Rationale:** Substance use may affect the patient's tolerance and response to the medications given during the procedure.

Patient Preparation

- Verify correct patient with two identifiers. ➡**Rationale:** Prior to performing a procedure, the nurse should ensure the correct identification of the patient for the intended intervention.
- Ensure that the patient and family understand preprocedural teaching. Answer questions as they arise, and reinforce information as needed. ➡**Rationale:** Understanding of previously taught information is evaluated and reinforced. Patient and family anxiety is decreased.
- Ensure that informed consent has been obtained. ➡**Rationale:** Informed consent is necessary before invasive procedures and the administration of conscious sedation. Informed consent protects the rights of the patient and makes a competent decision possible for the patient; however, in emergency circumstances, time may not allow the form to be signed.

- Perform a pre-procedure verification and time out, if non-emergent. ➡**Rationale:** Ensures patient safety.
- Ensure that the patient has not eaten for at least 6 to 8 hours before the procedure. ➡**Rationale:** Undigested material in the stomach increases the risk for aspiration.
- Instruct the patient to void before the procedure. ➡**Rationale:** Voiding before the procedure minimizes disruption of the examination.
- Initiate or continue ECG monitoring, apply an automatic blood pressure cuff, and initiate oxygen saturation monitoring and if prescribed, capnography. ➡**Rationale:** These measures allow for close cardiovascular and respiratory monitoring during the procedure. Follow institution standard regarding capnography monitoring.
- Ensure the IV access is in place and functional. ➡**Rationale:** IV access is needed to administer premedications and for possible emergency medications.
- Maintain IV infusion during the procedure. ➡**Rationale:** IV infusion maintenance ensures the IV is functioning and available should an emergency situation arise.
- Have the patient remove any dentures or dental prostheses. ➡**Rationale:** Dentures may interfere with the safe passage of the transesophageal probe.
- Set up the suction system with the connecting tubing and a rigid pharyngeal suction tip attached and ready for use. ➡**Rationale:** This setup is necessary for suctioning the patient's oral secretions during the procedure.
- Administer a small amount of supplemental oxygen if prescribed. ➡**Rationale:** Administration of oxygen may maintain adequate patient oxygenation during the procedure.
- Have a sedative (e.g., midazolam, diazepam) or analgesic (e.g., morphine sulfate, fentanyl) available (as prescribed) and administer when requested. Naloxone and flumazenil must be available for narcotic or sedative reversal. ➡**Rationale:** Sedatives and analgesics reduce patient anxiety, promote comfort, facilitate cooperation during the procedure, and decrease myocardial workload.
- Have atropine available at the bedside. ➡**Rationale:** Atropine is necessary if a vagal reaction occurs with the insertion and passage of the transesophageal probe.
- Have the saline contrast agent available if prescribed. ➡**Rationale:** The contrast agent enhances the ability to evaluate cardiac structures and function.

Procedure	for Transesophageal Echocardiography (Assist)	
Steps	**Rationale**	**Special Considerations**
1. **HH**		
2. **PE**		
3. Assist if needed with anesthetizing the posterior pharynx with the topical agent.	Decreases discomfort caused by passage of the probe.	If possible, allow the patient to sit up to increase comfort and decrease anxiety or the feeling of choking.
A. Position the patient in the left lateral position. Use pillows to ensure correct alignment of the spine with the head and body.[3]	This position allows secretions to collect in the dependent areas of the mouth for ease of suctioning and is the position of choice to prevent aspiration in case the patient vomits.	Patients with endotracheal intubation can be examined in the supine position.

Procedure for Transesophageal Echocardiography (Assist)—*Continued*

Steps	Rationale	Special Considerations
B. Reassess vital signs, oxygen saturation, neurologic status, and pain before administration of IV conscious sedation.	Reconfirms any change in patient condition.	
4. Administer IV conscious sedation as prescribed.[3,4,7,12] (**Level E***).	Allows the patient to cooperate in facilitating passage of the probe during the procedure.	Ensure that the appropriate antagonists are readily available. The patient may need additional medication throughout the procedure.
5. Assist the physician as needed with the insertion of the probe.[12,15]		
A. Insert the bite guard.	Prevents the patient from biting the probe or the inserter's fingers. Prevents damage to the teeth and mouth.	Gag and cough reflexes may be compromised by topical anesthetics, and the patient may vomit as the probe is passed, increasing the risk for aspiration.
B. Assist with lubrication of the distal end of the probe as prescribed.	Minimizes mucosal injury and irritation and facilitates the ease of passage of the probe.	
C. Assist the patient to slightly bend his or her head in a forward flex.	Eases insertion of the probe into the esophagus.	
D. Encourage the patient to simulate swallowing while the probe is being passed as directed by the physician.	The swallowing maneuver causes the epiglottis to close the trachea and directs the probe into the esophagus.	
E. Suction the oral secretions as needed to ensure patency of the airway.	Because of the diminished gag reflex and the presence of the probe in the patient's pharynx, swallowing of oral secretions may not be possible.	Manipulation of the probe in the esophagus and stomach may cause stimulation of gastric secretions, which may necessitate additional suctioning.
F. Provide the patient with reassurance and encouragement to keep the bite guard in place, maintain left lateral position, hold still without attempts to speak, and focus on his or her breathing pattern.	Decreases patient anxiety and promotes patient cooperation.	
6. Assist with the administration of the saline contrast agent as prescribed.	Enhances the view of the cardiac structures and function.	
7. Assist with the removal of the probe from the patient, and place the probe in an appropriate receptacle for cleaning.	Reduces the transmission of microorganisms; Standard Precautions.	
8. Discard used supplies in appropriate receptacles.	Removes and safely discards used supplies.	
9. [HH]		
10. Continue constant assessment and monitoring until the effects of IV conscious sedation and topical anesthetic have worn off.	Ensures patient safety.	Keep the patient on the left side with his or her head slightly elevated until the gag, swallow, and cough reflexes are intact.

*Level E: Multiple case reports, theory-based evidence from expert opinions, or peer-reviewed professional organizational standards without clinical studies to support recommendations

Procedure continues on following page

Expected Outcomes

- Clear visualization of cardiac structures and function
- Immediate preliminary diagnosis
- Note: Negative study results are helpful in excluding cardiac sources of compromise[17,18]

Unexpected Outcomes

- Esophageal or gastric perforation
- Vasovagal hypotension from esophageal manipulation
- Substernal chest pain
- Temporary dysphagia
- Aspiration
- Respiratory depression
- Hematoma in the oropharynx
- Hypotension
- Hypertension
- Dysrhythmias
- Laryngospasm
- Bronchospasm
- Change in neurologic status
- Air embolism in patients with right-to-left shunt with use of saline contrast
- Heart failure
- Pain
- Methemoglobinemia

Patient Monitoring and Care

Steps	Rationale	Reportable Conditions
		These conditions should be reported if they persist despite nursing interventions.
1. Assess and monitor cardiovascular, respiratory, and neurologic status at a minimum of 5-minute intervals during and 15-minute intervals after the TEE procedure, until the patient's condition returns to baseline for at least 30 minutes.	Ensures patient safety and identifies potential complications.	Alterations of the following: • Neurologic status • Oxygenation • Carbon dioxide level • Heart rate and rhythm • Blood pressure
2. Maintain IV access.	Ensures IV patency for possible emergency medications.	
3. Assess and monitor the patient's sedation score (follow institution preference for tool) at a minimum of 5-minute intervals during and 15-minute intervals after the TEE procedure until the patient's condition returns to baseline for at least 30 minutes.	Determines the patient's response to IV conscious sedation. Determines if additional sedation is needed.	• Abnormal sedation score
4. Follow the institution standard for assessing pain at a minimum of 5-minute intervals during and 15-minute intervals after the TEE procedure until the patient's condition returns to baseline for at least 30 minutes. Administer analgesia as prescribed.	May indicate a complication of the procedure or identify the need for pain interventions.	• New onset of pain • Continued pain despite pain interventions • Unresolved discomfort not relieved after the probe removal
5. Monitor for signs and symptoms of esophageal perforation.[14]	Identifies complications.	
A. Esophageal perforation in the cervical area.		• Pain at the base of the neck • Dysphagia • Crepitus

Patient Monitoring and Care —*Continued*

Steps	Rationale	Reportable Conditions
B. Thoracic perforation.		• Deep back pain • Dysphagia • Tachycardia
C. Abdominal esophageal perforation.		• Dysphagia in the upper epigastric region that is more retrosternal in nature
D. A severe perforation can include hemothorax or pneumothorax.		• Chest pain • Respiratory distress • Tachypnea • Dyspnea • Hypotension • Tachycardia
6. Monitor for intraprocedure complications or reasons to terminate the TEE early.[7,9,12,21]	Determines the patient's response to the procedure. Identifies complications.	• Patient becomes agitated or unable to cooperate or has a significant change in neurologic status • Dental or oropharyngeal trauma • Hypoxemia • Hypercapnia • New dysrhythmia • New hypotension or hypertension • Perforation or subcutaneous emphysema • GI or other bleeding • Chest pain • Benzocaine-induced methemoglobinemia
7. Assess for the return of normal pharyngeal function. Keep the patient on the left side with his or her head slightly elevated until the gag, swallow, and cough reflexes are intact.	Topical anesthesia decreases the gag, swallow, and cough reflexes, thus increasing the patient's risk of aspiration. The left lateral position is the position of choice to prevent aspiration.	• Prolonged absence of gag, swallow, or cough reflexes
8. Provide clear liquids when prescribed after return of the patient's pharyngeal function. Progress the patient's nutritional intake to solid food as tolerated.	Topical anesthesia decreases the gag reflex and increases the risk for aspiration. Mild throat discomfort is common as the topical anesthetic wears off.	• Nausea • Vomiting • Unusual throat or stomach discomfort • Increase in throat discomfort after 24 hours, possibly indicating a hematoma

Documentation

Documentation should include the following:
- Date and time of procedure
- Initial patient assessment
- Preprocedure and postprocedure patient and family education
- Preprocedure verifications and time-out.
- Completion of informed consent form.
- Vital signs, pulse oximetry, capnography, neurologic status, and pain evaluation immediately before sedation and during and after the procedure
- Medications administered and their effectiveness
- Assessments of gag, swallow, and cough reflexes
- Time of probe insertion and removal
- Characteristics of any secretions obtained when suctioned
- Total intake of IV solutions
- Occurrence of unexpected outcomes

References

1. de Waroux JB, Pouleur AC, Goffinet C, et al: Functional anatomy of aortic regurgitation: accuracy, prediction of surgical repairability, and outcome implications of transesophageal echocardiography, *Circulation* 116: 264-269, 2007.
2. Duran CM: TEE: the 'roadmap' for mitral valve repair, *J Heart Valve Dis* 15:521-523, 2006.

CR 3. Feigenbaum H, Armstrong WF, Thomas R: *Feigenbaum's echocardiography*, Philadelphia, 2004, Lippincott Williams & Wilkins.

CR 4. Ferson D, Thakar D, Swafford J, et al: Use of deep intravenous sedation with propofol and the laryngeal mask airway during transesophageal echocardiography, *J Cardiothoracic Vasc Anesth* 17:443-446, 2003.

CR 5. Fu ES, Downs JB, Schweiger JW, et al: Supplemental oxygen impairs detection of hypoventilation by pulse oximetry, *Chest* 126:1552-1558, 2004.

6. Fuster V, Ryden LE, et al: ACC/AHA/ESC 2006 guidelines for the management of patients with atrial fibrillation: a report of the American College of Cardiology/American Heart Association Task Force on Practice Guidelines and the European Society of Cardiology Committee for Practice Guidelines (Writing Committee to Revise the 2001 Guidelines for the Management of Patients With Atrial Fibrillation): developed in collaboration with the European Heart Rhythm Association and the Heart Rhythm Society, *Circulation* 114(7):e257-354, 2006.

7. Green SM: Research advances in procedural sedation and analgesia, *Ann Emerg Med* 49:31-36, 2007.

CR 8. Harris KM, Li DY, L'Ecuyer P, et al: The prospective role of transesophageal echocardiography in the diagnosis and management of patients with suspected infective endocarditis, *Echocardiography* 20:57-62, 2003.

9. Kane GC, Hoehn SM, Behrenbeck TR, et al: Benzocaine-induced methemoglobinemia based on the Mayo Clinic experience from 28,478 transesophageal echocardiograms: incidence, outcomes, and predisposing factors, *Arch Intern Med* 167:1977-1982, 2007.

10. Kobal SL, Pollick C, Atar S, et al: Stress echocardiography in octogenarians: transesophageal atrial pacing is accurate, safe, and well tolerated, *J Am Soc Echocardiogr* 19:1012-1016, 2006.

11. Maltagliati A, Galli CA, Tamborini G, et al: Usefulness of transoesophageal echocardiography before cardioversion in patients with atrial fibrillation and different anticoagulant regimens, *Heart* 92:933-938, 2006.

12. Marchiondo K: Transesophageal imaging and interventions: nursing implications, *Crit Care Nurse* 27:25-28,30,32, 2007.

13. Marymont J, Murphy GS: Intraoperative monitoring with transesophageal echocardiography: indications, risks, and training, *Anesthesiol Clin* 24:737-753, 2006.

CR 14. Min JK, Spencer KT, Furlong KT, et al: Clinical features of complications from transesophageal echocardiography: a single-center case series of 10,000 consecutive examinations, *J Am Soc Echocardiogr* 18:925-929, 2005.

15. Oh JK, Seward JB, Tajik AJ: *The echo manual*, Philadelphia, 2006, Lippincott Williams & Wilkins.

CR 16. Peterson GE, Brickner ME, Reimold SC: Transesophageal echocardiography: clinical indications and applications, *Circulation* 107:2398-2402, 2003.

CR 17. Rose DD: Transesophageal echocardiography as an alternative for the assessment of the trauma and critical care patient, *AANA J* 71:223-228, 2003.

CR 18. Sengupta PP, Khandheria BK: Transoesophageal echocardiography, *Heart* 91:541-547, 2005.

CR 19. Siddiqui TS, Stoddard MF: Safety of dobutamine stress transesophageal echocardiography in obese patients for evaluation of potential ischemic heart disease, *Echocardiography* 21:603-608, 2004.

CR 20. Singer DE, Albers GW, Dalen JE, et al: Antithrombotic therapy in atrial fibrillation: the Seventh ACCP Conference on Antithrombotic and Thrombolytic Therapy, *Chest* 126(3):429S-456S, 2004.

CR 21. Soto RG, Fu ES, Vila H Jr, et al: Capnography accurately detects apnea during monitored anesthesia care, *Anesth Analg* 99:379-382, 2004.

22. Trevelyan J, Steeds RP: Comparison of transthoracic echocardiography with harmonic imaging with transoesophageal echocardiography for the diagnosis of patent foramen ovale, *Postgrad Med J* 82:613-614, 2006.

23. Wilson W, Taubert KA, Gewitz M, et al, American Heart Association Rheumatic Fever, Endocarditis, and Kawasaki Disease Committee, American Heart Association Council on Cardiovascular Disease in the Young, American Heart Association Council on Clinical Cardiology, American Heart Association Council on Cardiovascular Surgery and Anesthesia, and Quality of Care and Outcomes Research Interdisciplinary Working Group: Prevention of infective endocarditis: guidelines from the American Heart Association: a guideline from the American Heart Association Rheumatic Fever, Endocarditis, and Kawasaki Disease Committee, Council on Cardiovascular Disease in the Young, and the Council on Clinical Cardiology, Council on Cardiovascular Surgery and Anesthesia, and the Quality of Care and Outcomes Research Interdisciplinary Working Group, *Circulation* 116(15):1736-1754, 2007.

Additional Readings

CR Ball M: SGNA position statement. statement on the use of sedation and analgesia in the gastrointestinal endoscopy setting, *Gastroenterol Nurs* 26(5):209-201, 2003.

CR Gilman G, Nelson JM, Murphy AT, et al: The role of the nurse in clinical echocardiography, *J Am Soc Echocardiogr* 18(7):773-777, 2005.

CR Hashimoto S, Nakatani S, Tanimura M, et al: Usefulness of conscious sedation with midazoram during transesophageal echocardiographic examination, *J Cardiol* 44(5):195-200, 2004.

Hoole SP, Falter F: Evaluation of hypoxemic patients with transesophageal echocardiography, *Crit Care Med* 35(8 Suppl):S408-S413, 2007.

Jiminez MA, Polena S, Coplan NL, et al: Methemoglobinemia and transesophageal echo, *Proceed Western Pharmacol Soc* 50:134-135, 2007.

Mart CR, Parrish M, Rosen KL, et al: Safety and efficacy of sedation with propofol for transoesophageal echocardiography in children in an outpatient setting, *Cardiol Young* 16(2):152-156, 2006.

CR Miyake M, Izumi C, Takahashi S, et al: Efficacy of transesophageal echocardiography in patients with cardiac arrest or shock, *J Cardiol* 44(5):189-194, 2004.

Pino RM: The nature of anesthesia and procedural sedation outside of the operating room, *Curr Opin Anaesthesiol* 20(4):347-351, 2007.

Porembka DT: Importance of transesophageal echocardiography in the critically ill and injured patient, *Crit Care Med* 35(8 Suppl):S414-S430, 2007.

Subramaniam B, Talmor D: Echocardiography for management of hypotension in the intensive care unit, *Crit Care Med* 35(8 Suppl):S401-S407, 2007.

AP Arterial Puncture

P U R P O S E :   Arterial puncture is performed to obtain a sample of blood for arterial blood gas analysis.

Linda Bucher, Joel M. Brown II

PREREQUISITE NURSING KNOWLEDGE

- An arterial blood gas (ABG) analysis measures the pH and the partial pressure of oxygen (Pao_2) and carbon dioxide ($Paco_2$). ABG samples are also analyzed for oxygen saturation (Sao_2) and for bicarbonate (HCO_3^-) values. These analyses are done primarily to evaluate a patient's oxygenation status, acid-base balance, and ventilation.[3,5] Additional laboratory tests (e.g., ammonia and lactate levels) can be performed on arterial blood samples.
- Patient indications for ABGs vary and include patients with chronic obstructive pulmonary disease (COPD), acute respiratory distress syndrome (ARDS), and pneumonia. ABG analysis frequently is performed on patients in shock, receiving cardiopulmonary resuscitation (CPR), or experiencing changes in respiratory therapy or status.[3,5]
- Knowledge of principles of aseptic technique is necessary.
- Knowledge is needed of the anatomy and physiology of the vasculature and adjacent structures.
- The brachial artery is a continuation of the axillary artery in the upper extremity. It bifurcates just below the elbow (Fig. 80-1). From the bifurcation, the ulnar artery moves down the forearm on the medial side and the radial artery on the lateral side.[20]
- The preferred artery for arterial puncture is the radial artery. Although this artery is smaller than the ulnar artery, it is more superficial and can be more easily stabilized during the procedure.[6] The use of the brachial artery is a safe and reliable alternative site for arterial puncture.[16]
- At times, the femoral artery is used for arterial puncture. The use of this artery can be technically difficult because of the proximity of the artery to the femoral vein (Fig. 80-2).
- Arterial cannulation is considered for patients who need frequent arterial blood samples, continuous arterial pressure monitoring, or evaluation of vasoactive medication therapy (see Procedures 61 and 62).[5]
- The most common complications associated with arterial puncture include pain, vasospasm, hematoma formation, infection, hemorrhage, and neurovascular compromise.[5,9,16,19]

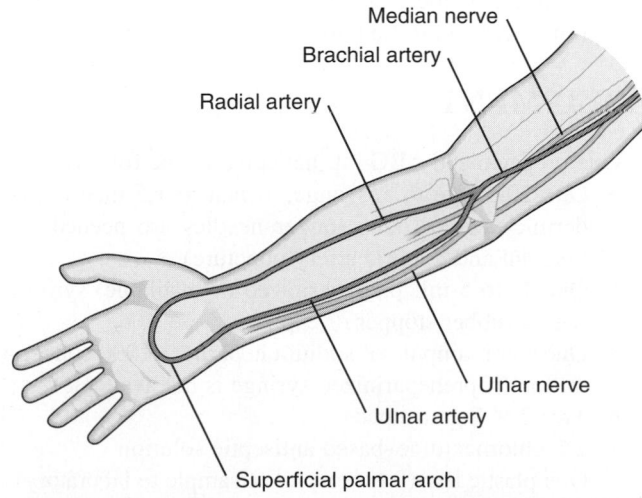

FIGURE 80-1   Anatomic landmarks for locating the radial and brachial arteries.

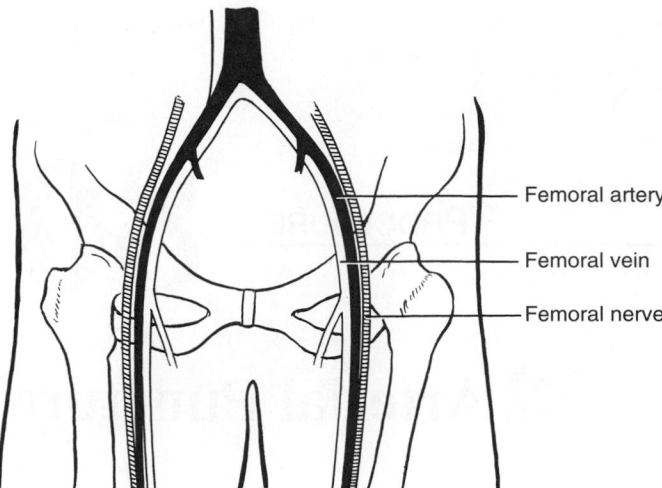

FIGURE 80-2   Anatomic landmarks for locating the femoral artery.

- Site selection proceeds as follows:
  - ❖ Use the radial artery as first choice. The radial artery is small and easily stabilized as it passes over a bony groove located at the wrist (see Fig. 80-1).
  - ❖ Use the brachial artery as second choice, except in the presence of poor pulsation from shock, obesity, or sclerotic vessel (e.g., because of previous cardiac catheterization). The brachial artery is larger than the radial artery. Hemostasis after arterial puncture is enhanced by its proximity to bone if the entry point is approximately 1.5 inches above the antecubital fossa (see Fig. 80-1).
  - ❖ Use the femoral artery in the case of cardiopulmonary arrest or altered perfusion to the upper extremities. The femoral artery is a large superficial artery located in the groin (see Fig. 80-2). It is easily palpated and punctured. Complications related to femoral artery puncture include hemorrhage and hematoma because bleeding can be difficult to control; inadvertent puncture of the femoral vein because of the close proximity of the vein to the artery; infection because aseptic technique in the groin area is difficult to maintain; and limb ischemia if the femoral artery is damaged.

EQUIPMENT

- One prepackaged ABG kit that contains the following:
  - ❖ One 20-gauge to 25-gauge, 1-inch to 1.5-inch hypodermic needle (note: longer needles are needed for brachial and femoral artery puncture)
  - ❖ One 1- to 5-mL preheparinized (if available) syringe with a rubber stopper or cap
  - ❖ One 1-mL ampule of sodium heparin, 1:1000 concentration (if preheparinized syringe is not available)
  - ❖ Two 2 × 2 gauze pads
  - ❖ 2% chlorhexidine–based antiseptic solution
  - ❖ One plastic bag (for transport of sample to laboratory)
  - ❖ One adhesive bandage

- Appropriate laboratory form, specimen label
- One pair of nonsterile examination gloves and eye protection
- 1% lidocaine (without epinephrine), 1-mL, or eutectic mixture of local anesthetics (EMLA) cream
  Additional supplies as needed include the following:
- Small rolled towel (to support the patient's wrist)
- Sterile gloves
- 1-mL syringe with 25-gauge needle (if lidocaine is used)
- Ice

PATIENT AND FAMILY EDUCATION

- Explain the reason for the arterial puncture to the patient and family. ➥*Rationale:* Clarification of information is an expressed patient and family need and helps to diminish anxiety, enhance acceptance, and encourage questions.
- Describe the overall steps of the procedure, including the patient's role in the procedure. ➥*Rationale:* This explanation decreases patient anxiety, enhances cooperation, and provides an opportunity for the patient to voice concerns and prevents accidental movement during the procedure.

PATIENT ASSESSMENT AND PREPARATION

Patient Assessment

- Determine the need for arterial cannulation versus puncture. ➥*Rationale:* Repeated arterial punctures increase patient discomfort and the risk for complications.
- Assess for factors that influence ABG measurements, including anxiety, endotracheal suctioning, nebulizer treatment, change in oxygen therapy/ventilator settings, patient positioning, body temperature, metabolic rate, and respiratory rate. ➥*Rationale:* These conditions or therapies can alter blood gas analysis.
- Assess the patient's current anticoagulation therapy, known blood dyscrasias, and pertinent laboratory values (e.g., platelets, partial thromboplastin time [PTT], prothrombin time [PT], and international normalized ratio [INR]) before the procedure. ➥*Rationale:* Anticoagulation therapy, blood dyscrasias, or alterations in coagulation studies could prolong hemostasis at the puncture site and increase the risk for hematoma formation or hemorrhage.
- Assess the patient's allergy history (e.g., lidocaine, antiseptic solutions, tape). ➥*Rationale:* Assessment decreases the risk for allergic reactions.
- Assess the patient's past surgical history (e.g., use of radial artery for coronary artery bypass surgery, fistulas, or shunts). ➥*Rationale:* Arterial puncture should be avoided in extremities affected by these conditions.
- Ascertain the patient's nondominant hand, if possible. ➥*Rationale:* A complication to the nondominant hand may have fewer consequences.

Patient Preparation

- Verify correct patient with two identifiers. ➥*Rationale:* Prior to performing a procedure, the nurse should ensure the correct identification of the patient for the intended intervention.
- Ensure that the patient and family understand preprocedural teaching. Answer questions as they arise, and reinforce information as needed. ➥*Rationale:* Understanding of previously taught information is evaluated and reinforced.
- Perform a preprocedure verification and time-out, if non-emergent. ➥*Rationale:* Ensures patient safety.
- If the patient is receiving oxygen or mechanical ventilation, check that the current therapy has been underway for at least 20 to 30 minutes before obtaining ABGs.[5,8,11,14,18] ➥*Rationale:* Accurate laboratory results are achieved, which is most important in patients with an abnormal ventilation/perfusion ratio.[14]
- Position the patient appropriately. ➥*Rationale:* Positioning enhances the accessibility to the insertion site and promotes patient comfort.
- Radial artery puncture:
  - ❖ Assist the patient to a semirecumbent position. ➥*Rationale:* A position of comfort decreases anxiety and may facilitate respiratory effort.
  - ❖ Elevate and hyperextend the wrist. A small rolled towel may be placed under the wrist for support.

➥*Rationale:* This action moves the artery closer to the skin surface, making the artery easier to palpate.
  - ❖ Palpate for the presence of a strong radial pulse. ➥*Rationale:* Identification and localization of the pulse increases the chance of a successful arterial puncture.
- Brachial artery puncture:
  - ❖ Assist the patient to a semirecumbent position. ➥*Rationale:* A position of comfort decreases anxiety and may facilitate respiratory effort.
  - ❖ Elevate and hyperextend the patient's arm. A small pillow may be placed under the arm for support. ➥*Rationale:* This action increases accessibility for puncture.
  - ❖ Rotate the patient's arm and palpate for the presence of a strong brachial pulse. ➥*Rationale:* Identification and localization of the pulse increase the chance of a successful arterial puncture.
- Femoral artery puncture:
  - ❖ Assist the patient to a supine, straight-leg position. ➥*Rationale:* This position provides the best position for localizing the femoral artery pulse.
  - ❖ Palpate for the presence of a strong femoral pulse. ➥*Rationale:* Identification and localization of the pulse increase the chance of a successful arterial puncture.

Procedure for Arterial Puncture

Steps	Rationale	Special Considerations
1. **HH**		Ensure that hospital policy permits registered nurses (RNs) to perform radial, brachial, and femoral arterial punctures.
2. If the radial artery is to be used, perform the modified Allen's test before the puncture (Fig. 80-3). **(Level C*)**	The modified Allen's test has been recommended before a radial artery puncture to assess the patency of the ulnar artery and an intact superficial palmar arch.[5,11,14,17]	The modified Allen's test does not always ensure adequate flow through the ulnar artery. A Doppler ultrasound flow indicator can also be used to further verify blood flow.[1,2,14]
A. With the patient's hand held overhead, instruct the patient to open and close the hand several times.	Forces the blood from the hand.	If the patient is unconscious or unable to perform the procedure, clench the fist passively for the patient.
B. With the patient's fist clenched, apply direct pressure on the radial and ulnar arteries.	Obstructs the flow of blood to the hand.	
C. Instruct the patient to lower and open the hand.	Observe for pallor.	Perform passively if the patient is unconscious or unable to assist.

*Level C: Qualitative studies, descriptive or correlational studies, integrative reviews, systematic reviews, or randomized controlled trials with inconsistent results

Procedure continues on following page

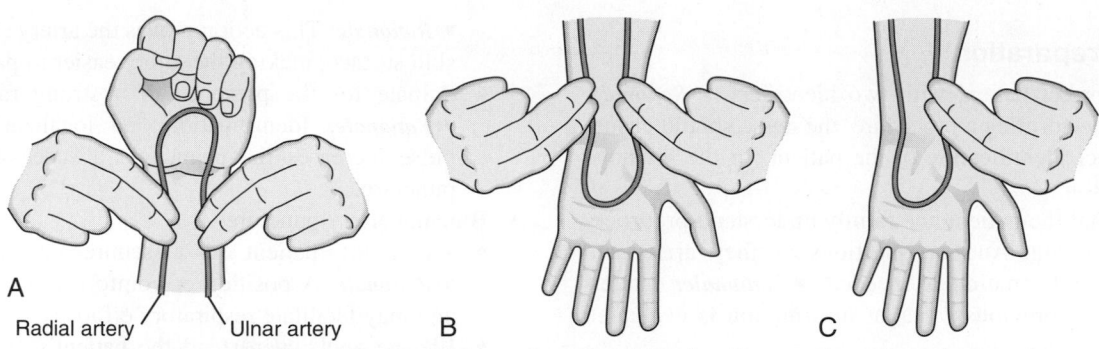

Radial artery   Ulnar artery   **B**   **C**

Figure 80-3   Modified Allen's test. Elevate the patient's hand and instruct the patient to open and close the fist several times. **A,** With the patient's fist clenched, simultaneously occlude the radial and ulnar arteries. **B,** Instruct the patient to lower and open his or her fist. Observe for pallor in the patient's hand. **C,** Release the pressure over the ulnar artery and observe the hand for the return of color. *(From Bucher L, Melander SD: Critical care nursing, Philadelphia, 1999, Saunders.)*

Procedure	**for Arterial Puncture**—*Continued*	
Steps	**Rationale**	**Special Considerations**
D. Release the pressure over the ulnar artery and observe the hand for return of color.[5,11,14]	Return of color within 7 seconds indicates patency of the ulnar artery and an intact superficial palmar arch and is interpreted as a positive Allen's test. If color returns between 8 and 14 seconds, the test is considered equivocal. If it takes 15 or more seconds for color to return, the test is considered a negative test.	If the test is negative or equivocal, the radial artery should not be used and the modified Allen's test should be performed on the opposite hand.
3. If a preheparinized syringe is not available, heparinize the syringe and needle. A. Assemble a 22-gauge needle on the syringe and prime the entire syringe barrel and needle with 1 mL of heparin. Once done, expel the heparin from the syringe.	Prevents specimen coagulation. Excess heparin in the syringe can lower the pH and Pa_{CO_2}.	A small-bore needle is less likely to cause vasospasm of the artery during the procedure.
B. Eliminate any visible air bubbles from the syringe.	Maintains the accuracy of ABG values.	
4. **PE**		
5. Prepare the site with a 2% chlorhexidine–based antiseptic solution.[4] A. Cleanse the site with a back-and-forth motion while applying friction for 30 seconds. B. Allow the antiseptic solution to dry.	Limits the introduction of potentially infectious skin flora into the vessel during the puncture.	
6. Locally anesthetize the puncture site per institution policy. **(Level C*)**	Provides local anesthesia for arterial puncture.	Most patients report pain during arterial puncture.[6,7] Patients have reported reduced pain when a local, intradermal anesthetic agent is used before the arterial puncture.[7,9]

*Level C: Qualitative studies, descriptive or correlational studies, integrative reviews, systematic reviews, or randomized controlled trials with inconsistent results

Procedure for Arterial Puncture—*Continued*

Steps	Rationale	Special Considerations
A. Use a 1-mL syringe with a 25-gauge needle to draw up 0.5 mL of 1% lidocaine without epinephrine.	Minimizes vessel trauma. The absence of epinephrine decreases the risk for peripheral vasoconstriction.	Research exploring the efficacy of lidocaine ointment, amethocaine gel, and EMLA cream as alternatives to intradermal lidocaine for management of the pain associated with arterial puncture has shown mixed results.[10,12,13,15,21] If these alternatives are used, manufacturer's recommendations should be followed.
B. Aspirate before injecting the local anesthetic.	Determines whether a blood vessel has been inadvertently entered.	
C. Inject intradermally and then with full infiltration around the artery puncture site. Use approximately 0.2 to 0.3 mL for an adult.	Decreases the incidence of localized pain with injection of all skin layers.	
7. Perform the percutaneous puncture of the selected artery.		
A. Palpate and stabilize the artery with the index and middle fingers of the nondominant hand.	Increases the likelihood of correctly locating the artery and decreases the chance of vessel rolling.	Use sterile gloves if the site of the artery puncture is palpated after it is antiseptically prepared.
B. With the needle bevel up and the syringe at a 30- to 60-degree angle to the radial or brachial artery, puncture the skin slowly (Figs. 80-4 and 80-5). For a femoral artery puncture, a 60- to 90-degree angle is used (Fig. 80-6).	A slow, gradual thrust promotes entry into the artery without inadvertently passing through the posterior wall.	Enter at an angle that is comfortable for your hand. Certainty of position is more important than angle entry. If too much force is used, the needle may touch the periosteum of the bone and cause considerable pain.
C. Observe the syringe for a flashback of blood.	Pulsation of blood into the syringe verifies that the artery has been punctured.	Flashback occurs more easily with a glass syringe than a plastic syringe. Gentle aspiration may be necessary with a plastic syringe.
D. If the puncture is unsuccessful, withdraw the needle to the skin level, angle slightly toward the artery, and readvance. Do not withdraw the needle.	Prevents the necessity of a second puncture and changes the needle angle to facilitate the location of the artery.	Excessive probing of the artery may cause injury to it, and to the nerve.

Procedure continues on following page

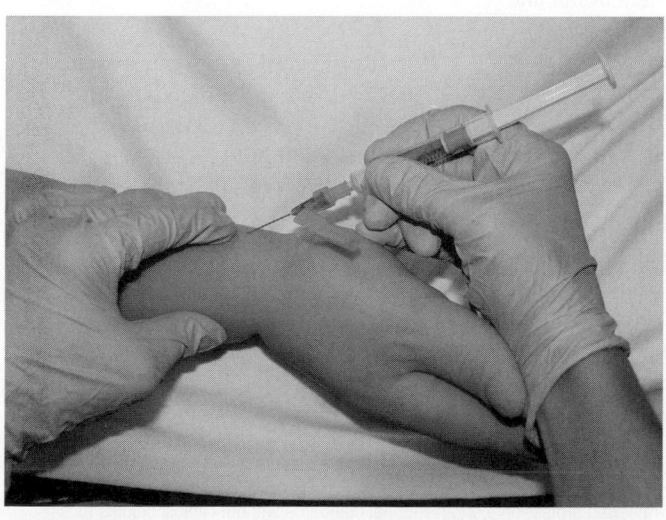

FIGURE 80-4 Radial artery puncture with the syringe at a 30-degree angle to the artery.

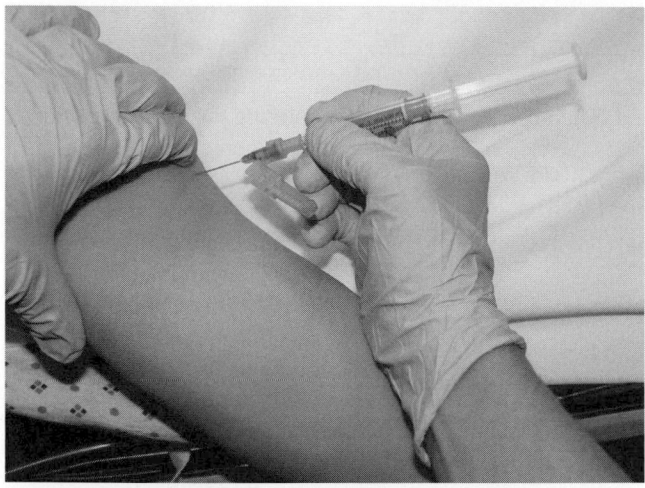

FIGURE 80-5   Brachial artery puncture with the syringe at a 45-degree angle to the artery.

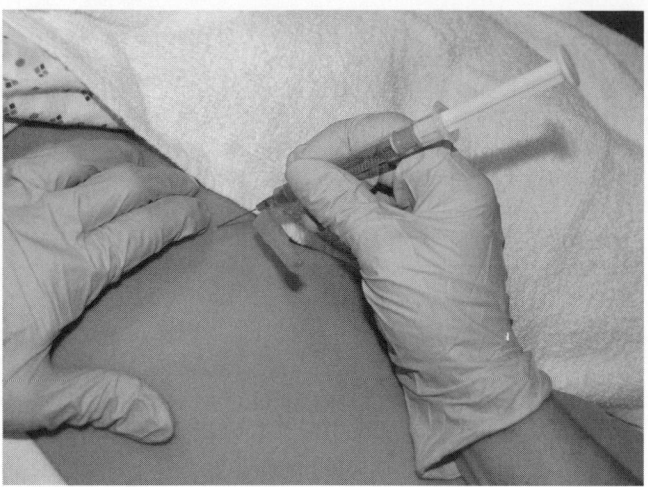

FIGURE 80-6   Femoral artery puncture with the syringe at a 60-degree angle to the artery.

Procedure for Arterial Puncture—*Continued*		
Steps	**Rationale**	**Special Considerations**
8. Obtain 1 mL of blood.	An accurate ABG can be done on as little as 0.2 mL of blood.	Sample volumes may vary with equipment used. Obtain more than 1 mL of blood for rechecking and additional studies, as necessary.
9. Withdraw the needle while stabilizing the barrel of the syringe.	Prevents inadvertent aspiration of air during withdrawal.	Equipment may vary. If a safety guard is available, it should be snapped onto the needle with a one-handed technique by gently pressing the device against a hard surface.
10. Press a gauze pad firmly over the puncture site for at least 5 minutes or until hemostasis is established.[5] Never ask the patient to assist in applying the pressure. Cover the puncture site with an adhesive bandage once hemostasis is achieved.[6]	Hematomas and hemorrhage can occur if pressure is not applied and maintained correctly. Hematomas can cause circulatory impedance and pain and can predispose to infection. The patient's status can be unpredictable, and he or she should not be involved in this aspect of the procedure. If the patient were to fail to apply and maintain pressure correctly, the risk for hematoma and hemorrhage would increase.	If the patient is receiving anticoagulation therapy or has a bleeding dyscrasia, pressure may need to be applied for as long as 15 minutes. Check dependent areas for hematoma or internal bleeding.
11. Check the syringe for air bubbles and express any air bubbles by slowly ejecting some of the blood onto a 2 × 2 gauze pad.	Air bubbles can alter the Pao_2 results.[5,14]	If a safety guard is present, it should be removed and a blood/air filter should be placed on the syringe. Excess air should be evacuated through the blood/air filter.
12. Seal the needle or tip of the syringe immediately with a rubber stopper or cap, respectively. Gently roll the syringe for 30 seconds.	Prevents leakage of blood and air from entering the sample. Mixes blood and heparin, thus preventing clot formation.	
13. Label the specimen and completely immerse the sample into a plastic bag with crushed ice and water.[14] **(Level E*)**	Ice decreases the temperature of the sample to approximately 4°C, which slows oxygen metabolism and may enhance accuracy of the results.	Follow institution policy regarding necessity of the use of ice, a mixture of crushed ice and water, or other coolant for transporting ABG samples.

*Level E: Multiple case reports, theory-based evidence from expert opinions, or peer-reviewed professional organizational standards without clinical studies to support recommendations

Procedure for Arterial Puncture—*Continued*

Steps	Rationale	Special Considerations
14. Complete the laboratory form per institution protocol. Note the percentage of oxygen therapy, respiratory rate, and ventilator settings, if appropriate, and the patient's temperature and time the specimen was drawn.	Helps the laboratory to perform the analysis accurately.	Policies may vary regarding the type of patient information required for laboratory analysis.
15. Expedite the delivery of the sample to the laboratory.	Ideally, the blood gas analysis should be performed within 10 minutes of collection to ensure the accuracy of results.[6,11,14]	
16. Discard used supplies in appropriate receptacles; dispose of needles and other sharp objects in appropriate containers.	Reduces the transmission of microorganisms; Standard Precautions. Safely removes sharp objects.	
17. **HH**		

Expected Outcomes

- The ABG sample is collected correctly such that the accuracy of the results is enhanced
- The puncture site remains free of hematoma, hemorrhage, and infection
- The peripheral vascular and neurovascular systems remain intact (free of complications)
- Alterations in the ABGs are identified and treated accordingly

Unexpected Outcomes

- Pain/severe discomfort during the procedure
- Complications during the puncture or vasospasm
- Complications after the puncture: changes in the color, size, temperature, sensation, or pulse of the extremity used for the arterial puncture; hematoma, hemorrhage, or infection at the puncture site

Patient Monitoring and Care

Steps	Rationale	Reportable Conditions
		These conditions should be reported if they persist despite nursing interventions.
1. Observe the puncture site for signs of hemostasis after the procedure.	Postpuncture bleeding can occur in any patient but is more likely to occur in patients with coagulopathies or patients who are receiving anticoagulation therapy.	• Excessive bleeding • Hematoma • Internal bleeding in dependent areas • Abnormal vital signs
2. Assess the puncture site and involved extremity for signs of postpuncture complications.	Arterial puncture can result in peripheral vascular and neurovascular compromise of the extremity distal to the puncture site.	• Changes in color, size, temperature, sensation, movement, or pulse in the extremity used for arterial puncture
3. Assess the puncture site for signs or symptoms of infection.	Determines necessity for further treatment.	• Erythema, warmth, hardness, tenderness, or pain at the puncture site • Presence of purulent drainage from the puncture site
4. Follow institution standard for assessing pain. Administer analgesia as prescribed.	Identifies need for pain interventions.	• Continued pain despite pain interventions

Procedure continues on following page

Documentation

Documentation should include the following:
- Patient and family education
- Results of the modified Allen's test or Doppler ultrasound scan, if done
- Arterial site used
- Local anesthetic used (if applicable)
- Patient's tolerance of the procedure

- Patient's temperature and amount and type of oxygen therapy
- Pain assessment, interventions, and effectiveness
- Postpuncture site assessment and care
- Sample results
- Unexpected outcomes
- Additional nursing interventions

References

CR 1. Abu-Omar Y, et al: Duplex ultrasonography predicts safety of radial artery harvest in the presence of an abnormal Allen test, *Ann Thorac Surg* 77:116-119, 2004.

2. Barone JE, Madlinger RV: Should an Allen Test be performed before artery cannulation? *J Trauma* 61:468-470, 2006.

3. Carlson KK, editor: *Advanced critical care nursing,* St Louis, 2009, Saunders.

CR 4. Centers for Disease Control and Prevention: Guidelines for the prevention of intravascular catheter-related infections, *MMWR* 51(RR-10):1-31, 2002.

5. Chernecky CC, Berger BJ, editors: *Laboratory tests and diagnostic procedures,* ed 5, St Louis, 2008, Saunders.

CR 6. Flynn JC, editor: *Procedures in phlebotomy,* ed 3, St Louis, 2004, Saunders.

CR 7. Giner J, et al: Pain during arterial puncture, *Chest* 110:1443-1445, 1996.

CR 8. Hess D, et al: The validity of assessing arterial blood gases 10 minutes after an Fio_2 change in mechanically ventilated patients without chronic pulmonary disease, *Respir Care* 30:1037-1041, 1985.

9. Hudson TL, Dukes SF, Reilly K: Use of local anesthesia for arterial punctures, *Am J Crit Care* 15:595-599, 2006.

CR 10. Hussey VM, Poulin MV, Fain JA: Effectiveness of lidocaine hydrochloride on venipuncture sites, *AORN J* 66:472-475, 1997.

11. Intravenous Nurses Society: Infusion nursing standards of practice, *J Infus Nurs* 29(1S):S1-S90, 2006.

CR 12. Joly LM, et al: Topical lidocaine-prilocaine cream (EMLA) versus local infiltration of anesthesia for radial artery cannulation, *Anesth Analg* 87:403-406, 1998.

CR 13. Lander J, et al: Evaluation of a new topical anesthetic agent: a pilot study, *Nurs Res* 45:50-52, 1996.

CR 14. National Committee for Clinical Laboratory Standards: *Procedures for the collection of arterial blood specimens: approved standard H11-A4,* ed 4, Wayne, PA, 2004, National Committee for Clinical Laboratory Standards.

CR 15. Nott M, Peacock J: Relief of injection pain in adults: EMLA cream for 5 minutes before venipuncture, *Anaesthesia* 45:772-774, 1990.

CR 16. Okeson GC, Wulbrecht PH: The safety of brachial artery puncture for arterial blood sampling, *Chest* 14:748-751, 1998.

17. Oettle AC, et al: Evaluation of Allen's test in both arms and arteries of left and right-handed people, *Surg Radiol Anat* 28:3-6, 2006.

CR 18. Sherter CB, et al: Prolonged rate of decay of arterial Po_2 following oxygen breathing in chronic airway obstruction, *Chest* 67:259, 1975.

19. Siegel JD, et al, and the Healthcare Infection Control Practices Advisory Committee: *Guideline for isolation precautions: preventing transmission of infectious agents in healthcare settings,* 2007, retrieved October 10, 2008, from www.cdc.gov/ncidod/dhqp/pdf/guidelines/Isolation2007.pdf.

20. Thibodeau GA, Patton KT: *Anatomy and physiology,* ed 6, St Louis, 2007, Mosby.

CR 21. Tran NQ, Pretto JJ, Worsnop CJ: A randomized controlled trial of the effectiveness of topical amethocaine in reducing pain during arterial puncture, *Chest* 122:1357-1360, 2002.

Additional Reading

Infusion Nurses Society: *Policies and procedures for infusion nurses,* ed 2, Norwood, MA, 2006, Infusion Nurses Society.

81

AP Central Venous Catheter Insertion (Perform)

P U R P O S E : Central venous catheters are inserted for measurement of right atrial pressure and central venous pressure with jugular or subclavian catheter placement. Clinically useful information can be obtained about right ventricular preload, cardiovascular status, and fluid balance in patients who do not need pulmonary artery pressure monitoring. Central venous catheters also are placed for infusion of vasoactive medications, total parenteral nutrition, and hemodialysis access. In addition, central venous catheters are used to administer medication and intravenous products to patients with limited peripheral intravenous access and to provide access for pulmonary artery catheters and transvenous pacemakers.

Desiree A. Fleck

PREREQUISITE NURSING KNOWLEDGE

- Knowledge of the normal anatomy and physiology of the cardiovascular system is needed.
- Clinical and technical competence in central line insertion and suturing is important.
- Knowledge of the principles of sterile technique is essential.
- Knowledge of the anatomy and physiology of the vasculature and adjacent structures of the neck, groin, and arm is needed.
- Competence in chest radiographic interpretation is necessary.
- Advanced cardiac life support knowledge and skills are needed.

AP This procedure should be performed only by physicians, advanced practice nurses, and other healthcare professionals (including critical care nurses) with additional knowledge, skills, and demonstrated competence per professional licensure or institution standard.

- Indications for a central venous catheter (CVC) include the following[4,7]:
  - ❖ Blood loss
  - ❖ Hypotension after major surgery
  - ❖ Right ventricular ischemia or infarction
  - ❖ Hemodialysis access
  - ❖ Administration of total parenteral nutrition
  - ❖ Lack of peripheral venous access
  - ❖ Assessment of hypovolemia or hypervolemia
  - ❖ Monitoring of CVC pressures
  - ❖ Long-term infusions of medications
  - ❖ Placement of pulmonary artery catheters
  - ❖ Transvenous pacemakers
- Placement of a CVC can guide treatment after major surgery and during active bleeding.
- The central venous pressure (CVP) can be helpful in the differentiation of right ventricular failure from left ventricular failure.
- The CVP is commonly elevated during or after right ventricular failure, ischemia, or infarction because of decreased compliance of the right ventricle while the pulmonary artery occlusion pressure is normal.

- The CVP can be helpful in the determination of hypovolemia. The CVP value is low if the patient is hypovolemic. Venodilation also decreases CVP.
- Relative contraindications of CVC insertion include the following[4,7]:
  - ❖ Fever
  - ❖ Coagulopathies
  - ❖ Presence of a permanent pacemaker
  - ❖ Persistent shock
  - ❖ Obstruction of the superior or inferior vena cava, innominate vein, subclavian veins, or internal jugular veins
  - ❖ Respiratory distress
- The CVP provides information regarding right heart filling pressures and right ventricular function and volume.
- The CVP historically was measured with a water manometer system but is now measured with a single-pressure transducer system (see Procedures 70 and 76).
- The CVP waveform is identical to the right atrial pressure (RAP) waveform.
- The normal CVP value is 2 to 6 mm Hg.
- Electrocardiographic (ECG) monitoring is essential in the accurate interpretation of the CVP value.
- Understanding is needed of *a, c,* and *v* waves. The *a* wave reflects right atrial contraction; the *c* wave reflects closure of the tricuspid valve; and the *v* wave reflects right atrial filling during ventricular systole (see Figs. 70-1 and 73-7).
- Dysrhythmias may alter CVP or RAP waveforms.
- The risk for a pneumothorax is minimized with use of an internal jugular vein. The preferred site for catheter insertion is the right internal jugular vein. The right internal jugular vein is a "straight shot" to the right atrium.
- The right or left subclavian veins are also sites for central catheter placement. Placement of a CVC through the right subclavian vein is a shorter and more direct route than the left subclavian vein because it does not cross the midline of the thorax.[4,7]
- Femoral veins may be accessed but have the disadvantages of limiting the patient to bed rest with immobilization of the leg and increasing the patient's risk of infection.
- The presence of a pacemaker may alter the choice of placement of a CVC because of a risk for dislodging pacemaker leads with insertion of a CVC.
- Complications may occur during or after insertion of a central venous catheter (see Table 81-1).

EQUIPMENT

- CVC insertion kit
- CVC of choice (single, dual, or triple lumen) usually supplied with insertion needle, dilator, syringe, and guidewire.
- Large sterile drapes or towels
- 1% lidocaine without epinephrine
- One 25-gauge ⅝-inch needle
- Large package of 4 × 4 gauze sponges
- Suture kit (hemostat, scissors, needle holder)
- 3-0 or 4-0 nylon suture with curved needle

- Three-way stopcock
- Syringes: one 10- to 12-mL syringe; two 3- to 5-mL syringes; two 22-gauge, 1½-inch needles
- Masks, head coverings, goggles (shield and mask combination may be used), sterile gloves, and sterile gowns
- No. 11 scalpel
- Skin protectant pads or swab sticks
- Roll of 2-inch tape
- Dressing supplies
- Waterproof pad
- Chlorhexidine-impregnated sponge
- Antiseptic solution (e.g., 2% chlorhexidine-based preparation)
- Nonsterile gloves
- Normal saline flush syringes or 0.9% sodium chloride vials, 10- to 30-mL

Additional equipment as needed includes the following:
- Hemodynamic monitoring system (see Procedure 76)
- Sutureless catheter securement device
- Intravenous (IV) solution with Luer-Lok administration set for IV infusion
- Luer-Lok extension tubing
- Bedside monitor and oscilloscope with pulse oximetry
- Supplemental oxygen supplies
- Emergency equipment
- Package of alcohol pads or swab sticks
- Package of povidone-iodine pads or swab sticks
- Heparin flushes
- Needleless caps
- Arm board

PATIENT AND FAMILY EDUCATION

- Explain the need for the CVC insertion and assess patient and family understanding. ➥*Rationale:* Clarification and understanding of information decrease patient and family anxiety levels.
- Explain the procedure and the time involved. ➥*Rationale:* Explanation increases patient cooperation and decreases patient and family anxiety levels.
- Explain the need for sterile technique and that the patient's face may be covered. ➥*Rationale:* The explanation decreases patient anxiety and elicits cooperation.
- Explain the benefits and potential risks for the procedure. ➥*Rationale:* Information is offered so that the patient can make an informed decision.

PATIENT ASSESSMENT AND PREPARATION

Patient Assessment
- Determine the patient's medical history of cervical disk disease or difficulty with vascular access. ➥*Rationale:* Baseline data are provided.
- Determine the patient's medical history of pneumothorax or emphysema. ➥*Rationale:* Patients with emphysematous lungs may be at increased risk for puncture and pneumothorax, depending on the approach.

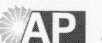

TABLE 81-1	**Complications of Central Venous Catheter Insertion**		
Complication	**Clinical Manifestation**	**Treatment**	**Prevention**

Pneumothorax	Sudden respiratory distress
	Chest pain
	Hypoxia/cyanosis
	Decreased breath sounds
	Resonance to percussion
		Confirmation with chest
		  radiograph
		Symptomatic treatment
		Small pneumothorax:
		  Bed rest
		  O_2
		Pneumothorax > 25%:
		  Chest tube
		  Cardiopulmonary support
			Proper patient preparation
			Sedation as necessary
			Proper patient positioning
			Adequate hydration status
			Technique and angle of the needle/catheter on
			  insertion
			Avoidance of multiple passes with the needle
			Healthcare provider is skilled and experienced in
			  insertion technique

Tension
  pneumothorax
	Most likely to occur in patients
	  on ventilatory support
	Respiratory distress
	Rapid clinical deterioration:
	  Cyanosis
	  Jugular venous distention
	    (may not be present with
	    severe hypovolemia)
	  Hypotension
	  Decreased cardiac output
		Treatment must be rapid and
		  aggressive
		Immediate air aspiration
		  followed by chest tube
		Cardiopulmonary support
			Proper patient preparation
			Sedation as necessary
			Proper patient positioning
			Adequate hydration status
			Reduction of PEEP to ≤5 cm H_2O at the time of
			  venipuncture
			Technique and angle of the needle/catheter on
			  insertion
			Avoidance of multiple passes with the needle
			Healthcare provider is skilled and experienced in
			  insertion technique
			Use of peripherally inserted central venous
			  catheter

Delayed
  pneumothorax
	Slow onset of respiratory
	  symptoms
	Subcutaneous emphysema
	Persistent pleuritic chest or
	  back pain
		Confirmation with chest
		  radiograph
		Chest tube
		Cardiopulmonary support
			Proper patient preparation
			Sedation as necessary
			Proper patient positioning
			Adequate hydration status
			Technique and angle of the needle/catheter on
			  insertion
			Avoidance of multiple passes with the needle
			Healthcare provider is skilled and experienced in
			  insertion technique
			Use of peripherally inserted central venous
			  catheter

Hydrothorax
  hydromedias-
  tinum
	Dyspnea
	Chest pain
	Muffled breath sounds
	High glucose level of chest
	  drainage
	Low-grade fever
		Stop infusion
		Confirmation with chest
		  radiograph; contrast injec-
		  tion may be helpful
		Cardiopulmonary support
			Proper patient preparation
			Sedation as necessary
			Proper patient positioning
			Adequate hydration status
			Technique and angle of the needle/catheter on
			  insertion
			Avoidance of multiple passes with the needle
			Healthcare provider is skilled and experienced in
			  insertion technique
			Use of peripherally inserted central venous
			  catheter
			Placement of catheter tip in lower superior vena
			  cava
			Aspiration of blood before catheter use to confirm
			  vascular placement

Hemothorax	Respiratory distress
	Hypovolemic shock
	Hematoma in the neck with
	  jugular insertions
		Confirmation with chest
		  radiograph
		Chest tube
		Thoracotomy for arterial repair
		  if indicated
			Correction of coagulopathies before insertion
			Adequate hydration status
			Avoidance of multiple passes with the
			  needle
			Evaluation with Doppler scan studies or venogram
			  of suspected thrombosis from prior cannulation
			  before insertion

Continued

TABLE 81-1	**Complications of Central Venous Catheter Insertion—cont'd**		
Complication	**Clinical Manifestation**	**Treatment**	**Prevention**
Arterial puncture/ laceration	Return of bright red blood in the syringe under high pressure Pulsatile blood flow on disconnection of the syringe Arterial waveform/pressures when the catheter is connected to the transducer system Arterial saturation of sample sent for blood gas analysis Deterioration of clinical status: Hemorrhagic shock Respiratory distress Bleeding from catheter site may or may not be observed Deviation of trachea with large hematoma in the neck Hemothorax may be detected on chest radiograph	Application of pressure for 3 to 5 minutes or as needed to promote hemostasis after removal of the needle Elevate head of bed if condition is hemodynamically stable Chest tube as indicated Thoracotomy for arterial repair if indicated	Correction of coagulopathies before insertion Adequate hydration status Avoidance of multiple passes with the needle Evaluation with Doppler scan studies or venogram of suspected thrombosis from prior cannulation before insertion Use of small-gauge needle to first locate the vein
Bleeding/ hematoma; venous or arterial bleeding	Bleeding from insertion site Hematoma formation not likely to be seen with subclavian approach Bleeding may occur internally without visible evidence Tracheal compression Respiratory distress Carotid compression	Application of pressure to the insertion site Thoracotomy for arterial repair Tracheostomy for tracheal deviation from hematoma With the femoral approach, manual pressure slightly above the inadvertent arterial puncture site (see Procedure 77 for femoral sheath removal)	Correction of coagulopathies before insertion Adequate hydration status Avoidance of multiple passes with the needle at venipuncture Use of small-gauge needle to first locate the vein Immediate control of femoral bleeding may prevent large blood loss or hematoma formation
Cardiac dysrhythmias	Cardiac dysrhythmias: Premature atrial complexes Atrial fibrillation or flutter Premature ventricular complexes Supraventricular tachycardia Ventricular tachycardia Sudden cardiovascular collapse	Withdraw the guidewire or catheter from the heart; dysrhythmias should stop if the cause was mechanical in nature Pharmacologic treatment of persistent dysrhythmias	Avoidance of entry into the heart with the guidewire Observation of cardiac monitor; tall, peaked P waves can be identified as the catheter tip enters the right atrium
Air embolism	Symptoms depend on amount of air drawn in, especially with patients who are spontaneously breathing Sudden cardiovascular collapse Tachypnea, apnea, tachycardia Hypotension, cyanosis, anxiety Diffuse pulmonary wheezes "Mill wheel" churning heart murmur Neurologic deficits, paresis, stroke, coma Cardiac arrest	Stop airflow Position patient on left side in Trendelenburg's position Oxygen administration Air aspiration; transthoracic needle or intracardiac catheter Cardiopulmonary support	Adequate hydration status Head-down tilt or Trendelenburg's position during catheter insertion Use of small-bore needle for insertion Application of thumb over needle or catheter hub during disconnection; needle or hub should not be exposed longer than 1 second Advancement of catheter during positive-pressure cycle in patients on ventilatory support Avoidance of nicking of catheter with careful suturing technique Avoidance of catheter exchange from large-bore catheter (pulmonary artery) to smaller catheter Use of Luer-Lok connections Minimal risk with peripherally inserted central venous catheter

TABLE 81-1	Complications of Central Venous Catheter Insertion—cont'd		
Complication	**Clinical Manifestation**	**Treatment**	**Prevention**
Catheter malposition	Pain in ear or neck Swishing sound in ear with infusion Sharp anterior chest pain Pain in ipsilateral shoulder blade Cardiac dysrhythmia Observation on chest radiograph Signs or symptoms may be absent No blood return on aspiration	Ensure that the bevel of the insertion needle is positioned downward (toward feet of patient) before placing guidewire Repositioning of catheter with guidewire or new venipuncture Catheter removal	Proper patient positioning Anthropometric measurement for accurate intravascular catheter length Avoidance of use of force when advancing the catheter Use of a guidewire or blunt-tipped stylet
Catheter embolism	Cardiac dysrhythmias Chest pain Dyspnea Hypotension Tachycardia May be clinically silent	Location of fragment on radiograph Transvenous retrieval of catheter fragment Thoracotomy	Use of "over a guidewire" (Seldinger) insertion technique Extreme caution with use of through-the-needle catheter designs; never withdraw a catheter through the needle Use of guidewire or stylet within a catheter that is inserted through a needle
Cardiac tamponade	Retrosternal or epigastric pain Dyspnea Venous engorgement of face and neck Restlessness, confusion Hypotension, paradoxic pulse Muffled heart sounds Mediastinal widening Pleural effusion Cardiac arrest	Treatment must be rapid and aggressive Discontinuation of infusions through the central line Aspiration through the catheter Emergency pericardiocentesis Emergency thoracotomy	Catheter tip position: Parallel to the walls of the superior vena cava 1 to 2 cm above the junction of the superior vena cava and right atrium Use of soft, flexible catheters Minimal risk with peripherally inserted central venous catheter
Tracheal injury	Subcutaneous emphysema Pneumomediastinum Air trapping between the chest wall and the pleura Respiratory distress with puncture of endotracheal tube cuff	Emergency reintubation (for punctured endotracheal tube cuff) Aspiration of air in mediastinum	Healthcare provider is skilled and experienced in insertion techniques Use of peripherally inserted central venous catheter
Nerve injury	Patient has tingling/numbness in arm or fingers Shooting pain down the arm Paralysis Diaphragmatic paralysis (phrenic nerve injury)	Remove catheter if brachial plexus injury is suspected	Healthcare provider is skilled and experienced in insertion technique Minimal risk with peripherally inserted central venous catheter
Sterile thrombophlebitis	Potential complication of the peripherally inserted central venous catheter Redness, tenderness, swelling along the course of the vein Pain in the upper extremity or shoulder	Application of heat for 48 to 72 hours Removal of catheter	Strict aseptic technique during catheter insertion Adequate skin preparation
Pulmonary embolism	Potential complication of catheter exchange Often clinically silent Chest pain, dyspnea, coughing, tachycardia, anxiety, fever	Spiral chest CT scan Lung perfusion scan Cardiopulmonary support with large pulmonary embolism	Avoidance of catheter exchange in veins with thrombosis

CT, Computed tomography; *PEEP,* positive end-expiratory pressure.

- Determine the patient's medical history of anomalous veins. ➤➤*Rationale:* Patients may have a history of dextro-acardia or transposition of the great vessels, which leads to greater difficulty in catheter placement.
- Assess the intended insertion site. ➤➤*Rationale:* Scar tissue may impede placement of the catheter. Permanent pacemakers or implantable cardioverter defibrillators may preclude placement. Previous surgery and previous placement of a CVC may cause a thrombus to be present.
- Assess the patient's cardiac and pulmonary status. ➤➤*Rationale:* Some patients may not tolerate a supine or Trendelenburg's position for extended periods of time.
- Assess vital signs and pulse oximetry. ➤➤*Rationale:* Baseline data are provided.
- Assess electrolyte levels (e.g., potassium, magnesium, calcium). ➤➤*Rationale:* Electrolyte abnormalities may increase cardiac irritability.
- Assess the patient for heparin sensitivity or allergy. ➤➤*Rationale:* CVCs are heparin-bonded, although non–heparin-bonded catheters are available. If the patient has a heparin allergy or has a history of heparin-induced thrombocytopenia, use a non–heparin-coated catheter.
- Assess for a coagulopathic state and determine whether the patient has recently received anticoagulant or thrombolytic therapy. ➤➤*Rationale:* These patients are more likely to have complications related to bleeding and may need interventions before insertion of the CVC.

Patient Preparation

- Verify correct patient with two identifiers. ➤➤*Rationale:* Prior to performing a procedure, the nurse should ensure the correct identification of the patient for the intended intervention.
- Ensure that the patient and family understand preprocedural teaching. Answer questions as they arise, and reinforce information as needed. ➤➤*Rationale:* Understanding of previously taught information is evaluated and reinforced.
- Obtain informed consent. ➤➤*Rationale:* Informed consent protects the rights of the patient and makes a competent decision possible for the patient; however, in emergency circumstances, time may not allow for this form to be signed.
- Perform a pre-procedure verification and time out, if non-emergent. ➤➤*Rationale:* Ensures patient safety.
- Prescribe sedation or analgesics as needed. ➤➤*Rationale:* The patient may need sedation or analgesics to promote comfort and to ensure adequate cooperation and appropriate placement.
- If the patient is obese or muscular and the preferred site is the internal jugular vein or subclavian vein, place a towel posteriorly between the shoulder blades. ➤➤*Rationale:* This placement helps extend the neck and provide better access to the subclavian and internal jugular veins.

Procedure	**for Performing Central Venous Catheter Insertion**	
Steps	**Rationale**	**Special Considerations**
1. HH		
2. PE		All healthcare providers in the room should have on protective equipment including goggles or face shields and masks.
3. Place a waterproof pad under the patient's back.	Avoids soiling of bed linens.	
4. Remove nonsterile gloves.		
5. HH		
6. Apply sterile gown and gloves.	Minimizes the risk of infection; maintains sterile precautions.	Follow institution standard for maximal sterile barrier precautions.
7. Prepare the site using 2% chlorhexidine-based antiseptic solution.[2, 3, 5] Cleanse the site with a back-and-forth motion while applying friction for 30 seconds (Refer to Figure 82-1). Allow the antiseptic to remain on the insertion site and to air-dry completely before catheter insertion.[2, 3, 5] **(Level D*)**	Limits the introduction of potentially infectious skin flora into the vessel during the puncture.	

*Level D: Peer-reviewed professional organizational standards with clinical studies to support recommendations

Procedure for Performing Central Venous Catheter Insertion—*Continued*

Steps	Rationale	Special Considerations
8. Discard used supplies in appropriate receptacles.		
9. 🅷🅷		
10. Open the CVC insertion kit and drop the remaining sterile items onto the sterile field.	Maintains aseptic technique and prepares the work area.	
11. Apply a new pair of sterile gloves.	Maintains sterility.	
12. Place sterile drapes over the prepped area.	Provides an aseptic work area.	
13. Fully drape the patient with exposure of only the insertion site.	Minimizes the risk of infection; maintains aseptic and sterile precautions.	
14. Determine the anatomy of the access site.	Helps ensure proper placement of the CVC.	
15. Check landmarks again for the intended catheter insertion site.	Ensures proper placement of the catheter.	
16. Estimate the length of the catheter needed. This can be done by holding the catheter from the insertion site to the sternal notch.	Helps ensure proper placement.	

Internal Jugular Vein (Fig. 81-1)

Steps	Rationale	Special Considerations
1. Locate the carotid artery via palpation.	Helps prevent placing the introducer in the carotid artery.	
2. Identify the jugular vein and mark it if necessary.	Identifies the intended insertion site.	
3. Instruct the patient to turn his or her head away from the insertion site.	Helps identify the landmarks.	Someone from the healthcare team may need to assist the patient to turn his or her head.
4. Ensure that the patient is in a 15- to 25-degree Trendelenburg's position.	Helps to decrease the risk for air embolism. Helps engorge the veins for identification of the correct site.	
5. Identify the internal jugular vein from the triangle between the medial aspect of the clavicle, the medial aspect of the sternal head, and the lateral head of the sternocleidomastoid muscle (see Fig. 81-1).	A high entry can be made from a posterior approach, a lateral approach, an anterior approach, or a central approach.	The midanterior approach may be preferred in an obese patient. The posterior approach may present a slightly higher risk.
6. Administer a local anesthetic.	Promotes patient comfort.	
7. Locate the internal jugular vein with a small needle (i.e., 22 gauge) attached to a 3- or 5-mL syringe: A. Aspirate as the needle is advanced until a flush of blood returns. B. Note the angle and depth of the needle C. Remove the needle	Prepares for procedure.	The internal jugular vein is 3 to 4 cm above the medial clavicle and 1 to 2 cm within the lateral border of the sternocleidomastoid muscle.

Procedure continues on following page

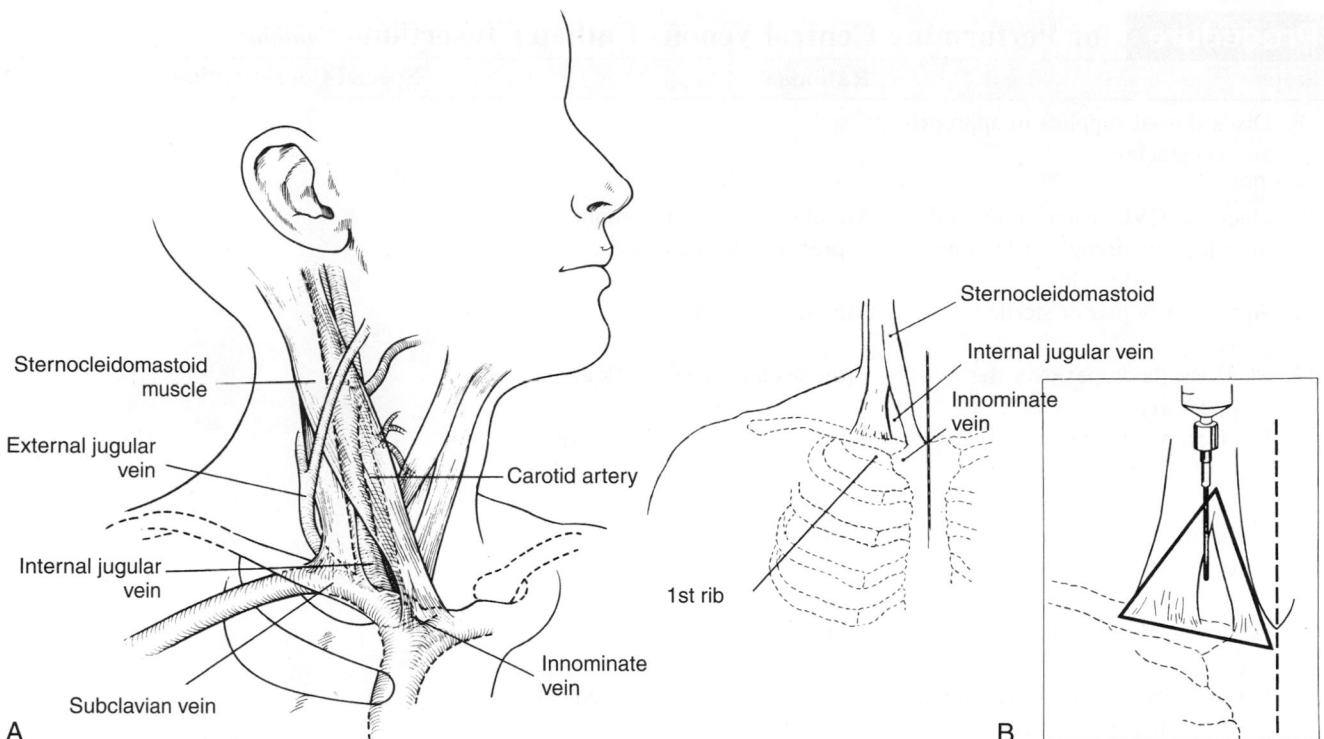

FIGURE 81-1   Anatomy of the jugular vein. **A,** Anatomy of the internal jugular vein showing its lower location within the triangle formed by the sternocleidomastoid muscle and the clavicle. **B,** Triangle drawn over the clavicle and sternal and clavicular portions of the sternocleidomastoid muscle is centered over the internal jugular vein *(inset)*. *(From Dailey EK, Schroeder JS: Techniques in bedside hemodynamic monitoring, St Louis, 1994, Mosby; and Daily PO, Griepp RB, Shumway NE: Percutaneous internal jugular vein cannulation, Arch Surg 101:534-536, 1970. Copyright 1970, American Medical Association.)*

Procedure for Performing Central Venous Catheter Insertion—*Continued*

Steps	Rationale	Special Considerations

8. Administer additional anesthetic:
  A. Attach a 3- or 5-mL syringe with 2 or 3 mL of 1% lidocaine (without epinephrine) to an 18-gauge needle.
  B. Align the needle with the syringe parallel to the medial border of the clavicular head of the sternocleidomastoid muscle.
  C. Aim at a 30-degree angle to the frontal plane over the internal jugular vein, toward the ipsilateral nipple.
  D. Instill the lidocaine.
	Promotes patient comfort during the procedure. Helps to anesthetize below the subcutaneous tissue.	

9. Use Seldinger's technique for placement of the catheter (Fig. 81-2).	This technique is the preferred method of central venous catheter placement; it uses a dilator and guidewire.	
A. Puncture the skin and advance the needle while maintaining slight negative pressure until a free flow of blood is obtained.	Slight negative pressure helps to ensure placement into the vein and decreases the risk for air embolism and pneumothorax.	If a free flow of blood is not obtained, remove and redirect the needle 5 to 10 degrees more laterally.

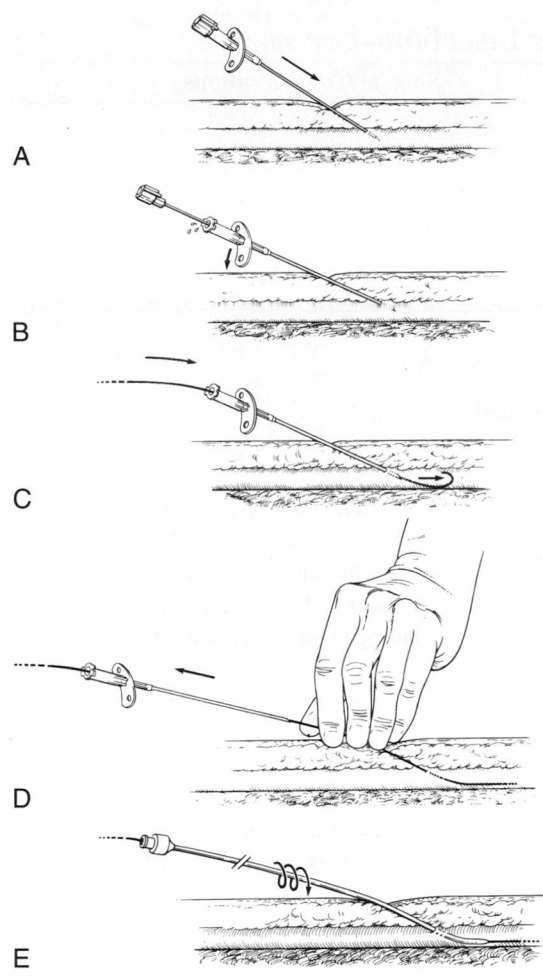

A

B

C

D

E

FIGURE 81-2   Basic procedure for Seldinger's technique. **A,** The vessel is punctured with the needle at a 30- to 40-degree angle. **B,** The stylet is removed, and free blood flow is observed; the angle of the needle is then reduced. **C,** The flexible tip of the guidewire is passed through the needle into the vessel. **D,** The needle is removed over the wire while firm pressure is applied at the site. **E,** The tip of the catheter or sheath is passed over the wire and advanced into the vessel with a rotating motion. *(From Dailey EK, Schroeder JS: Techniques in bedside hemodynamic monitoring, St Louis, 1994, Mosby.)*

Procedure for Performing Central Venous Catheter Insertion—*Continued*

Steps	Rationale	Special Considerations
B. After a free flow of blood is obtained, have the patient hold his or her breath or hum while the syringe is detached and insert the soft-tipped guidewire 10 to 15 cm through the needle.	A free flow of blood indicates the needle is in the vessel. Holding the breath or humming decreases the risk for air embolus.	
C. Remove the needle		
D. Wipe the guidewire with the sterile 4 × 4 gauze	Wiping the guidewire dry eases manipulation.	
E. Instruct the patient to breathe normally		
10. With a no. 11 blade, knife edge up, make a small (2- to 3-mm) stab wound at the insertion site.	Eases the insertion of the dilator through the skin.	
11. Insert the dilator through the skin, over the guidewire, until 10 to 15 cm of wire extends beyond the dilator. Remove the dilator.	The dilator enlarges the vessel and skin opening, easing the insertion of the catheter.	

Procedure continues on following page

Procedure for Performing Central Venous Catheter Insertion—*Continued*

Steps	Rationale	Special Considerations
12. Insert the catheter over the guidewire until 10 to 15 cm of the guidewire extends beyond the catheter. Remove the guidewire. Advance the catheter and note the catheter length at the insertion site.	Helps identify the location.	
13. Aspirate and flush the ports with normal saline solution.	Prevents clotting of the catheter.	
14. Connect to the hemodynamic monitoring system (see Procedure 76) or intravenous fluid.	Necessary for pressure monitoring and maintaining catheter patency.	
15. Suture the catheter in place.	Secures the catheter.	A sutureless catheter-securing device may be used to stabilize the CVC.
16. Apply an occlusive, sterile dressing (see Procedure 69).	Provides a sterile environment.	Follow institution standard for application of a chlorhexidine-impregnated sponge (see Procedure 69).
17. Return the patient to a neutral or head-up position.	Provides comfort.	
18. If monitoring, identify the appropriate waveforms (see Procedure 70).	Ensures accurate monitoring of values.	
19. Assess lung sounds and obtain a chest radiograph.	Confirms placement and assesses for a pneumothorax.	The radiograph needs to be read before administration of total parenteral nutrition or chemotherapeutic agents.
20. Discard used supplies in appropriate receptacles.	Reduces the transmission of microorganisms; Standard Precautions. Safely removes sharp objects.	
21. 🄷🄷		

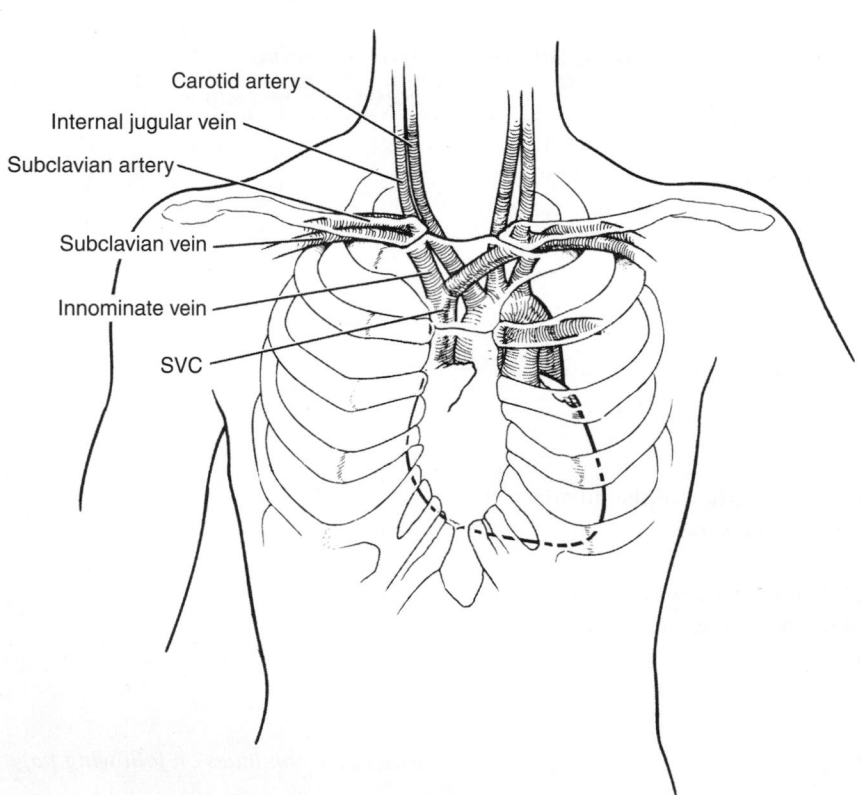

Carotid artery
Internal jugular vein
Subclavian artery
Subclavian vein
Innominate vein
SVC

FIGURE 81-3 Anatomic location of the subclavian vein and surrounding structures. The subclavian vein joins the internal jugular vein to become the innominate vein at about the manubrioclavicular junction. The innominate vein becomes the superior vena cava (SVC) at about the level of the mid manubrium. *(From Dailey EK, Schroeder JS: Techniques in bedside hemodynamic monitoring, St Louis, 1994, Mosby.)*

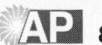

Procedure for Performing Central Venous Catheter Insertion—*Continued*

Steps	Rationale	Special Considerations
Subclavian Vein (Fig. 81-3)		
1. Identify the junction of the middle and medial thirds of the clavicle. The needle insertion should be 1 to 2 cm laterally.	Identifies the landmarks for catheter placement.	Access from the right side is preferred to avoid inadvertent puncture of the thoracic duct.
2. Depress the area 1 to 2 cm beneath the junction with the thumb of the nondominant hand and the index finger 2 cm above the sternal notch.		To avoid the subclavian artery, select a puncture site away from the most lateral course of the vein and do not aim too posteriorly.
3. Instruct the patient to turn his or her head away from the insertion site.	Helps identify the landmarks.	Someone from the health care team may need to assist the patient to turn his or her head.
4. Place the patient in a 15- to 25-degree Trendelenburg's position.	Helps to decrease the risk for air embolism. Helps engorge the veins for identification of the correct site.	
5. Administer a local anesthetic.	Promotes patient comfort.	
6. Locate the subclavian veins with a small needle (i.e., 22 gauge) attached to a 3- or 5-mL syringe:	Prepares for the procedure.	
A. Aspirate as the needle is advanced until a flush of blood returns.		
B. Note the angle and depth of the needle.		
C. Remove the needle.		
7. Use Seldinger's technique for placement of the catheter (Fig. 81-2).	This technique is the preferred method of central venous catheter placement; it uses a dilator and guidewire.	
A. Insert the needle under the clavicle and "walk down" until it slips below the clavicle into the vein while maintaining negative pressure within the syringe until free-flowing blood is returned (Fig. 81-4).	Decreases the risk for pneumothorax. Slight negative pressure helps to ensure placement into the vein and decreases the risk for air embolism and pneumothorax.	Insert at a 45-degree angle to prevent pneumothorax. If it is difficult to depress the needle down, the needle may be bent to form an arc. For the elderly, the subclavian vein may be more inferior. Avoiding a too lateral or too deep needle insertion can reduce the risk for pneumothorax.
B. After a free flow of blood is returned, turn the bevel to the 3 o'clock position. Once in the vein have the patient hold his or her breath or hum, while the syringe is detached and insert the soft-tipped guidewire.	A free flow of blood indicates a vein is entered. Turning the bevel helps the guidewire advance to the correct position. Holding the breath or humming decreases the risk for air embolus.	
C. Remove the needle.		
D. Wipe the guidewire with the sterile 4 × 4 gauze	Wiping the guidewire eases the manipulation of the guidewire.	
E. Instruct the patient to breathe normally.		
8. With a no. 11 blade, knife edge up, make a small (2-mm to 3-mm) stab wound at the insertion site.	Eases the insertion of the dilator through the skin.	

Procedure continues on following page

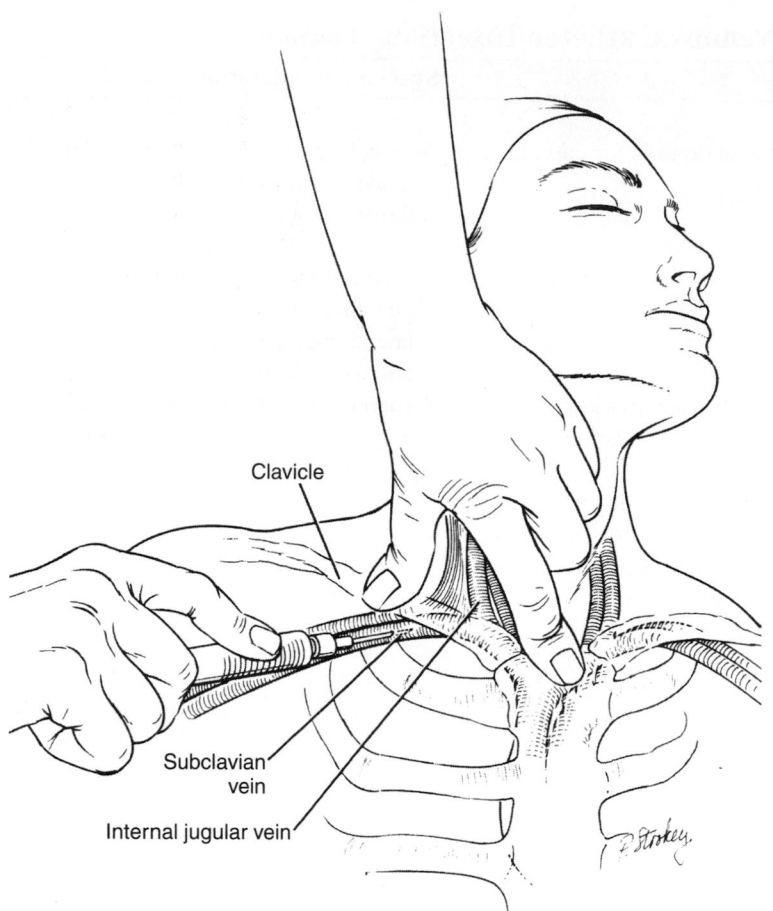

Clavicle

Subclavian
vein

Internal jugular vein

FIGURE 81-4   Puncture of the subclavian vein with the needle inserted beneath the middle third of the clavicle at a 20- to 30-degree angle aiming medially. *(From Dailey EK, Schroeder JS: Techniques in bedside hemodynamic monitoring, St Louis, 1994, Mosby.)*

Procedure for Performing Central Venous Catheter Insertion—*Continued*

Steps	Rationale	Special Considerations
9. Insert the dilator through the skin, over the guidewire, until 10 to 15 cm of guidewire extends beyond the dilator. Remove the dilator.	The dilator enlarges the vessel and skin opening, easing the insertion of the catheter.	
10. Advance the catheter over the guidewire until 10 to 15 cm of the guidewire extends beyond the catheter. Remove the guidewire. Advance the catheter and note the catheter length at the insertion site.	This aids dilation of the subcutaneous tissue to ease insertion and prevents the formation of a false channel.	
11. Aspirate and flush the ports with normal saline solution.	Ensures blood return and maintains catheter patency.	
12. Connect the catheter to the hemodynamic monitoring system (see Procedure 76) or to intravenous fluid.	Necessary for pressure monitoring and catheter patency.	
13. Suture the catheter in place.	Secures the catheter.	A sutureless securing device may be used to stabilize the CVC.
14. Apply an occlusive, sterile dressing to the site.	Decreases the risk for infection.	Follow institution standard for application of a chlorhexidine-impregnated sponge (see Procedure 69).
15. If monitoring, identify appropriate waveforms (see Procedure 70).	Ensures accurate monitoring of values.	

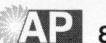

Procedure for Performing Central Venous Catheter Insertion—*Continued*

Steps	Rationale	Special Considerations
16. Assess lung sounds and obtain a chest radiograph.	Confirms placement and assesses for a pneumothorax.	The radiograph must be read before administration of total parenteral nutrition or chemotherapeutic agents.
17. Discard used supplies in appropriate receptacles.	Reduces the transmission of micro-organisms; Standard Precautions. Safely removes sharp objects.	
18. 🅷🅷		
Femoral Vein (see Fig. 80-2)		
1. Identify the anatomy, including the femoral artery (remember NAVEL).	NAVEL is an acronym for remembering the anatomy (Nerve, Artery, Vein, Empty space, Ligament; from lateral to medial).	
2. Administer a local anesthetic.	Anesthetizes the area to provide patient comfort.	

3. Locate the femoral vein with a small needle (i.e., 22 gauge) attached to a 3- or 5-mL syringe:
  A. Aim the needle at a 20- to 30-degree angle.
  B. Aspirate as the needle is advanced until a flush of blood returns.
  C. Note the angle and the depth of the needle.
  D. Remove the needle.
	Anesthetizes the area to provide patient comfort.	

4. Use Seldinger's technique for placement of the catheter (see Fig. 81-2).
  A. Puncture the skin and advance the needle while maintaining slight negative pressure until a free flow of blood is obtained.
  B. After a free flow of blood is obtained, detach the syringe and insert a soft-tipped guidewire through the needle 10 to 15 cm.
  C. Remove the needle.
  D. Wipe the guidewire with a sterile 4 × 4 gauze.
  E. Instruct the patient to breathe normally.
	This technique is the preferred method of CVC placement; it uses a dilator and guidewire.
	
	Negative pressure helps to identify a free flow of blood and ensures proper placement into the vein.
	
	A free flow of blood indicates that the vessel has been accessed.
	Wiping the guidewire eases the manipulation of the guidewire.
		If a free flow of blood is not obtained, remove and redirect the needle 5 to 10 degrees more laterally.

5. With a no. 11 blade, knife edge up, make a small (2-mm to 3-mm) stab wound at the insertion site.	Eases insertion of the introducer through the skin.	
6. Insert the dilator through the skin, over the guidewire until 10 to 15 cm of wire extends beyond the dilator. Remove the dilator.	The dilator dilates the vessel and skin to assist in the ease of the catheter insertion.	

Procedure continues on following page

Procedure   for Performing Central Venous Catheter Insertion—*Continued*

Steps	Rationale	Special Considerations
7. Insert the catheter over the guidewire until 10 to 15 cm of the guide wire extends beyond the catheter. Remove the guidewire. Advance the catheter and note the catheter length at the insertion site.		
8. Suture the catheter in place.	Secures the catheter	A sutureless securing device may be used to stabilize the CVC.
9. Aspirate and flush the ports with normal saline solution.	Ensures blood return and maintains catheter patency.	
10. Connect to the hemodynamic monitoring system (see Procedure 76 or to intravenous fluid.	Necessary for pressure monitoring and catheter patency.	
11. Apply an occlusive, sterile dressing.	Provides a sterile environment.	Follow institution standard for application of a chlorhexidine-impregnated sponge (see Procedure 69).
12. Identify the appropriate waveforms (see Procedure 70).	Ensures the accurate monitoring of values.	
13. Discard used supplies in appropriate receptacles.	Reduces the transmission of microorganisms; Standard Precautions. Safely removes sharp objects.	
14. 🅷🅷		

Median Basilic Vein (Fig. 81-5)

1. Identify the median basilic vein.	Identifies the site for catheter placement.	The basilic vein is deeper and ascends along the ulnar surface of the forearm, joined by the median cubital vein in front of the elbow.

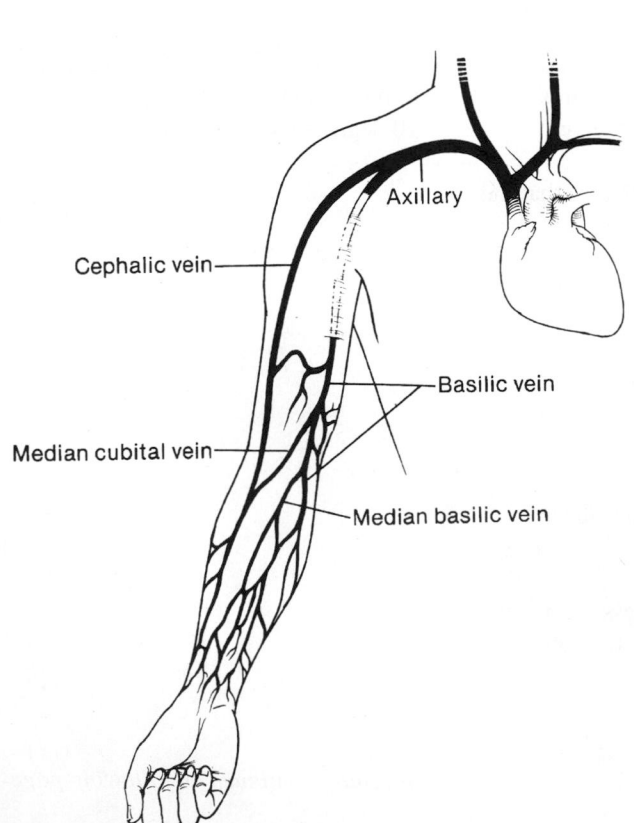

FIGURE 81-5   Anatomy of the veins in the arms. (*From Dailey EK, Schroeder JS: Techniques in bedside hemodynamic monitoring, St Louis, 1994, Mosby.*)

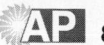

Procedure for Performing Central Venous Catheter Insertion—*Continued*

Steps	Rationale	Special Considerations
2. Further patient preparation includes application of a tourniquet to locate the vein. Abduct the selected arm 30 to 45 degrees and secure it on a flat, padded arm board resting on a flat surface.	Aids preparation and allows for engorgement of the vessel.	
3. Administer a local anesthetic.	Promotes patient comfort.	
4. Use Seldinger's technique for placement of the catheter (see Fig. 81-2).	This technique is the preferred method of central venous catheter placement; it uses a dilator and guidewire.	
A. Apply a venous tourniquet to the upper arm. Maintain traction on the skin distal to the insertion with one hand; puncture the vein with the needle bevel up at a 15- to 20-degree angle.	Allows for better visualization of veins. Helps with insertion and prevents the needle from penetrating too deeply.	Do not attempt to place a central venous catheter in a vein that cannot be seen or palpated.
B. After a free flow of blood is obtained, detach the syringe and insert the soft-tipped guidewire into the vein approximately 2 to 4 cm beyond the tip.	Ensures appropriate placement of the catheter.	If resistance is met, do not force the catheter to advance. Withdraw the catheter 2 to 3 cm, rotate it, and readvance it.
C. Release the tourniquet	Eases manipulation of the guidewire.	
D. Advance the guidewire several centimeters.		
E. Remove the needle		
F. Wipe the guidewire with a sterile 4 × 4 gauze.		
5. Insert the catheter over the guidewire. Remove the guidewire. Note the centimeter marking at the skin.		
6. Suture in place.	Secures the catheter.	A sutureless securing device may be used to stabilize the CVC.
7. Aspirate and flush the ports with normal saline solution.	Maintains catheter patency.	
8. Initiate the intravenous solution.	Maintains catheter patency.	
9. Apply an occlusive, sterile dressing to the insertion site.	Promotes a sterile environment.	Follow institution standard for application of a chlorhexidine-impregnated sponge (see Procedure 69).
10. Immobilize the arm if needed on an arm board.	Ensures that minimal movement of the catheter and sheath occurs.	
11. Discard used supplies in appropriate receptacles.	Reduces the transmission of microorganisms; Standard Precautions. Safely removes sharp objects.	
12. **HH**		

Procedure continues on following page

Expected Outcomes

- Successful placement of the CVC
- If infusing IV solution, the solution infuses without problems
- The *a*, *c*, and *v* waves are identified if hemodynamic monitoring is used
- CVP measurements are obtained

Unexpected Outcomes

- Pain or discomfort during the insertion procedure
- Pneumothorax, tension pneumothorax, hemothorax, or chylothorax
- Nerve injury
- Sterile thrombophlebitis
- Infection
- Cardiac dysrhythmias
- Misplacement (e.g., carotid artery, subclavian artery)
- Inadvertent lymphatic or thoracic duct perforation
- Hemorrhage
- Hematoma
- Venous air embolism
- Pulmonary embolus
- Cardiac tamponade
- Sepsis
- Heparin-induced thrombocytopenia or thrombosis

Patient Monitoring and Care

Steps	Rationale	Reportable Conditions
		These conditions should be reported if they persist despite nursing interventions.
1. Perform cardiovascular, peripheral vascular, and hemodynamic assessments immediately before and after the procedure and as the patient's condition necessitates.	Determines if signs or symptoms of complications are present, for example, an air embolism may present with restlessness and the patient may have decreased level of consciousness if the catheter is advanced into the carotid artery. Changes in CVP may indicate change in volume status. Changes in the CVP waveform may indicate change in right ventricular function or catheter migration.	• Abnormal level of consciousness • Abnormal vital signs • Abnormal waveforms or pressures
2. Assess the insertion site for presence of a hematoma or hemorrhage.	Determines the presence of complications.	• Bleeding that does not stop • Hematoma or expanding hematoma
3. Assess heart and lung sounds before and after the procedure.	Abnormal heart or lung sounds may indicate cardiac tamponade, pneumothorax, chylothorax, or hemothorax.	• Diminished or muffled heart sounds • Absent or diminished breath sounds unilaterally
4. Assess the results of chest radiograph.	Ensures adequate placement and identification of a pneumothorax.	• Abnormal radiograph results
5. Monitor for signs of complications.	May decrease mortality and morbidity if recognized early.	• Signs and symptoms of complications
6. Follow institution standard for assessing pain. Administer analgesia as prescribed.	Identifies need for pain interventions.	• Continued pain despite pain interventions

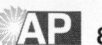
Patient Monitoring and Care —*Continued*

Steps	Rationale	Reportable Conditions
7. Daily assess the need for the CVC. **(Level C*)**	The Centers for Disease Control and Prevention (CDC)[5] and research findings[3] recommend that CVCs do not need to be changed more frequently than every 7 days. No specific recommendations exist regarding routine replacement of CVCs that need to be in place for greater than 7 days.[1,5,6] CVCs should be changed over a guidewire when emergently inserted (e.g., trauma resuscitation), the catheter malfunctions, a positive blood culture is obtained after the CVC was inserted, and sepsis develops without an identified source.[1] CVCs should be removed and reinserted at a new site when there is a skin infection at the catheter insertion site (i.e., redness, swelling, or drainage at or around the insertion site) or a positive culture at the insertion site.[1]	• Signs or symptoms of catheter infection

*Level C: Qualitative studies, descriptive or correlational studies, integrative reviews, systematic reviews, or randomized controlled trials with inconsistent results

Documentation

Documentation should include the following:

- Patient and family education
- Completion of informed consent
- Preprocedure verifications and time-out.
- Insertion of central venous catheter
- Insertion site of central venous catheter
- Vein selected and type and size of catheter placed
- Right atrial pressure and CVP waveform

- Central venous pressure values after insertion
- Centimeter marking at the skin
- Patient response to the procedure
- Pain assessment, interventions, and effectiveness
- Confirmation of placement (e.g., chest radiograph)
- Occurrence of unexpected outcomes
- Additional nursing interventions

References

CR 1. Eyer S, et al: Catheter-related sepsis: prospective, randomized study of three methods of long-term catheter maintainence, *Crit Care Med* 18:1073-1079, 1990.

2. Infusion Nurses Society: *Policies and procedures for infusion nursing* ed 3, Norwood, MA, 2006, AuthorINS.

3. Intravenous Nurses Society: (2006). Infusion nursing standards of practice, *J Infus Nurs* 29(1S): S1-S90, 2006.

CR 4. Kumar A, Darovic GO: Establishment of cardiovascular access. In *Hemodynamic monitoring invasive and noninvasive clinical application*, Philadelphia, 2000, Saunders.

CR 5. O'Grady NP, et al: Guidelines for the prevention of intravascular catheter-related infections, *Am J Infect Control* 30:476-489, 2002.

CR 6. Safdar N, Klugar DM, Maki DG: A review of risk factors for catheter-related bloodstream infection caused by percutaneously inserted, noncuffed central venous catheters: implications for preventive strategies, *Medicine* 81:466-472, 2002.

7. Venus G, Mallory DL: Vascular cannulation. In Civetta J., Taylor, W., & Kirby, R. (eds)., *Critical Care,* ed 5, Philadelphia, 2009, Lippincott, Williams, Wilkins.

Additional Readings

CR Dailey EK, Schroeder JS: *Techniques in bedside hemodynamic monitoring,* ed 5, St Louis, 1994, Mosby.

CR Darovic GO: *Hemodynamic monitoring invasive and noninvasive clinical application*, Philadelphia, 2000, Saunders.

CR Eggimann P, et al: Impact of a prevention strategy targeted at vascular-access care on incidence of infections acquired in intensive care, *Lancet* 355:1864-1868, 2000.

CR Friesinger GC, Williams SV, ACP/AHA Task Force on Clinical Privileges in Cardiology: clinical competence in hemodynamic monitoring, *J Am Coll Cardiol* 15:1460, 1990.

CR Lorente L, Henry C, Martin M, et al: Central venous catheter-related infection in a prospective and observational study of 2,595 catheters, *Crit Care* 9:R631-R635, 2005.

82

Central Venous Catheter Insertion (Assist)

P U R P O S E : Central venous catheters are inserted to measure and obtain right atrial pressure and central venous pressure with jugular or subclavian catheter placement. Clinically useful information can be obtained about right ventricular preload, cardiovascular status, and fluid balance in patients who do not need pulmonary artery pressure monitoring. Central venous catheters also are placed for infusion of vasoactive medications, total parenteral nutrition, hemodialysis access, and the use of pulmonary artery catheters. In addition, central venous catheters are used to administer medication and intravenous products to patients with limited peripheral intravenous access and to provide access for pulmonary artery catheters and transvenous pacemakers.

Desiree A. Fleck

PREREQUISITE NURSING KNOWLEDGE

- Knowledge of the normal anatomy and physiology of the cardiovascular system is needed.
- Knowledge of the anatomy and physiology of the vasculature and adjacent structures of the neck, groin, and arm is necessary.
- Basic dysrhythmia interpretation should be understood.
- Understanding of aseptic technique is necessary. Prevention of infection is a significant concern for patients with indwelling catheters.
- Advanced cardiac life support knowledge and skills are needed.
- Indications for a central venous catheter include the following[4,7]:
  - ❖ Blood loss
  - ❖ Hypotension after major surgery
  - ❖ Right ventricular ischemia or infarction
  - ❖ Hemodialysis access
  - ❖ Administration of total parenteral nutrition or other hyperosmolar solutions
  - ❖ Lack of peripheral venous access
  - ❖ Assessment of hypovolemia or hypervolemia

- ❖ Monitoring of central venous catheter (CVC) pressure
- ❖ Long-term infusion of medications
- ❖ Placement of pulmonary artery catheters
- ❖ Placement of transvenous pacemakers
- Relative contraindications of CVC insertion include the following[4,7]:
  - ❖ Fever
  - ❖ Coagulopathies
  - ❖ Presence of a permanent pacemaker
  - ❖ Persistent shock
  - ❖ Obstruction of the superior or inferior vena cava, innominate vein, subclavian veins, or internal jugular veins
  - ❖ Respiratory distress
- The central venous pressure (CVP) provides information regarding right heart filling pressures and right ventricular function and volume.
- The CVP historically was measured with a water manometer system but now is measured with a single-pressure transducer system (see Procedures 70 and 76).
- The CVP waveform is identical to the right atrial pressure (RAP) waveform.
- The normal CVP value is 2 to 6 mm Hg.

- Electrocardiographic (ECG) monitoring is essential in determination of accurate interpretation of the CVP value.
- Understanding of *a*, *c*, and *v* waves is necessary. The *a* wave reflects right atrial contraction, the *c* wave reflects closure of the tricuspid valve, and the *v* wave reflects right atrial filling during ventricular systole (see Figs. 70-1 and 73-7).
- Dysrhythmias may alter CVP or RAP waveforms.
- The risk for a pneumothorax is minimized with use of an internal jugular vein. The preferred site for catheter insertion is the right internal jugular vein. The right internal jugular vein is a "straight shot" to the right atrium.
- The right and left subclavian veins are also sites for central catheter placement. Placement of a central catheter through the right subclavian vein is a shorter and more direct route than through the left subclavian vein because it does not cross the midline of the thorax.
- Femoral veins may be accessed but have the disadvantage of forcing the patient to be on bed rest with immobilization of that leg and of an increased risk for infection.
- The presence of a pacemaker may alter the choice of placement of a CVC because of a risk for dislodging pacemaker leads with insertion of a CVC.
- Complications may occur during or after insertion of a CVC (see Table 81-1).

EQUIPMENT

- CVC insertion kit
- CVC of choice (single, dual, or triple lumen) usually supplied with insertion needle, dilator, syringe, and guidewire
- Large sterile drapes or towels
- 1% lidocaine without epinephrine
- One 25-gauge, ⅝-inch needle
- Large package of 4 × 4 gauze sponges
- Suture kit (hemostat, scissors, needle holder)
- 3-0 or 4-0 nylon suture with curved needle
- Three-way stopcock
- Syringes: One 10-mL to 12-mL syringe; two 3- to 5-mL syringes; two 22-gauge, 1½-inch needles
- Face masks, head coverings, goggles (shield and mask combination may be used), sterile gloves, and sterile gowns
- No. 11 scalpel
- Skin protectant pads or swab sticks
- Roll of 2-inch tape
- Dressing supplies
- Chlorhexidine-impregnated sponge
- Moisture-proof underpad
- Antiseptic solution (e.g., 2% chlorhexidine–based preparation)
- Nonsterile gloves
- Saline flushes or 0.9% sodium chloride vials, 10 to 30 mL
  Additional equipment as needed includes the following:
- Hemodynamic monitoring system (see Procedure 76)
- Intravenous (IV) solution with Luer-Lok administration set for IV infusion
- Sutureless catheter securement device
- Luer-Lok extension tubing
- Bedside monitor and oscilloscope with pulse oximetry
- Supplemental oxygen supplies
- Emergency equipment
- Package of alcohol pads or swab sticks
- Package of povidone-iodine pads or swab sticks
- Heparin flushes
- Needleless caps
- Arm board

PATIENT AND FAMILY EDUCATION

- Explain the need for the CVC insertion and assess patient and family understanding. ➤*Rationale:* Clarification and understanding of information decrease patient and family anxiety levels.
- Explain the required positioning for the procedure and the importance of the patient not moving during the insertion. ➤*Rationale:* This explanation encourages cooperation and reduces anxiety.
- Explain the need for sterile technique and that the patient's face may be covered. ➤*Rationale:* The explanation decreases patient anxiety and elicits cooperation.

PATIENT ASSESSMENT AND PREPARATION
Patient Assessment

- Assess the patient's vital signs and pulse oximetry. ➤*Rationale:* Baseline data are provided.
- Assess the patient's cardiac and pulmonary status. ➤*Rationale:* Some patients may not tolerate a supine or Trendelenburg's position for extended periods.
- Assess electrolyte levels (e.g., potassium, magnesium, calcium). ➤*Rationale:* Electrolyte abnormalities may increase cardiac irritability.
- Assess the patient's coagulopathic status and determine whether the patient has recently received anticoagulant or thrombolytic therapy. ➤*Rationale:* These patients are more likely to have complications related to bleeding and may need interventions before insertion of the CVC.

Patient Preparation

- Verify correct patient with two identifiers. ➤*Rationale:* Prior to performing a procedure, the nurse should ensure the correct identification of the patient for the intended intervention.
- Ensure that the patient and family understand preprocedural teaching. Answer questions as they arise, and reinforce information as needed. ➤*Rationale:* Understanding of previously taught information is evaluated and reinforced.
- Ensure that informed consent was obtained. ➤*Rationale:* Informed consent protects the rights of the patient and makes a competent decision possible for the patient; however, in emergency circumstances, time may not allow for this form to be signed.
- Perform a pre-procedure verification and time out, if nonemergent. ➤*Rationale:* Ensures patient safety.

- Administer prescribed sedation or analgesics as needed. ➡**Rationale:** The patient may need sedation or analgesia to ensure adequate cooperation and appropriate placement. During the procedure, restlessness and an altered level of consciousness may represent a pneumothorax, hypoxia, or placement in the carotid artery.

- If the patient is obese or muscular and the preferred site is the internal jugular vein or subclavian vein, assist with placing a towel posteriorly between the shoulder blades. ➡**Rationale:** This placement helps extend the neck and provides better access to the subclavian and internal jugular veins.

Procedure	**for Assisting with Central Venous Catheter Insertion**	
Steps	**Rationale**	**Special Considerations**
1. **HH**		
2. Prepare the IV solution or flush solution.	Prepares the infusion system.	
3. Prime the IV tubing or flush the entire pressure transducer system (see Procedure 76).	Removes air bubbles. Air bubbles introduced into the patient's circulation can cause air embolism. Air bubbles with the tubing dampen the waveform.	
4. Apply and maintain pressure in the pressure bag or device at 300 mm Hg.	Each flush device delivers 1 to 3 mL/hr to maintain patency of the hemodynamic system.	
5. Place a moisture-proof pad under under the patient's back.	Avoids soiling of the bed.	
6. **HH**		
7. **PE**		All healthcare providers in the room should have on protective equipment including goggles or face shields and masks.
8. Apply sterile gown and gloves.	Minimizes the risk of infection; maintains sterile precautions.	Follow institution standard for maximal sterile barrier precautions.
9. Assist, if needed, with preparing the site using 2% chlorhexidine-based antiseptic solution.[2,3,5] Cleanse the site with a back-and-forth motion while applying friction for 30 seconds. Allow the antiseptic to remain on the insertion site and to air-dry completely before catheter insertion.[2,3,5]	Limits the introduction of potentially infectious skin flora into the vessel during the puncture.	
(Level D*)		
A. Subclavian insertion: Scrub shoulder to contralateral nipple line and from neck to nipple line (Fig. 82-1, *A*).		
B. Jugular vein insertion: Scrub mid clavicle to opposite border of the sternum and ear to a few inches above the nipple line (Fig. 82-1, *B*).		
C. Femoral vein insertion: Scrub femoral area in a 4- to 6-inch area.		

*Level D: Peer-reviewed professional organizational standards with clinical studies to support recommendations

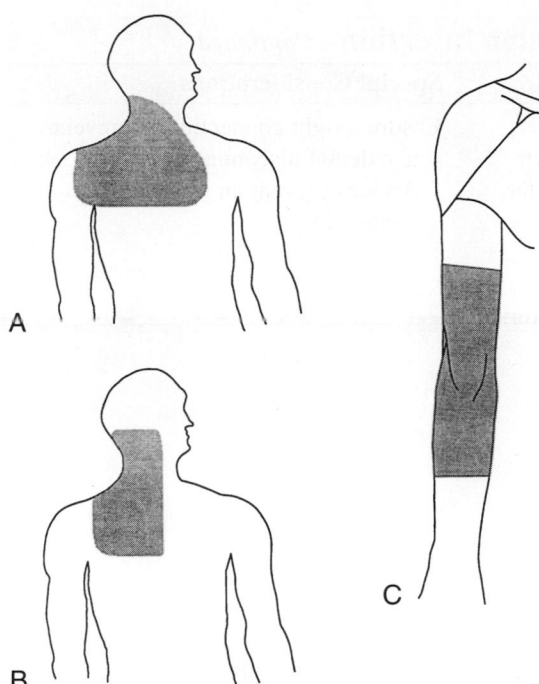

FIGURE 82-1   Area of skin preparation for central venous catheter insertions. **A,** Subclavian insertion: Scrub from shoulder to contralateral nipple line and neck to nipple line. **B,** Jugular insertions: Scrub mid clavicle to opposite border of the sternum and from the ear to a few inches above the nipple. **C,** Peripherally inserted central venous catheters (PICC): Scrub the entire arm. *(Courtesy Suredesign.)*

Procedure for Assisting with Central Venous Catheter Insertion—*Continued*

Steps	Rationale	Special Considerations

10. While the physician or advanced practice nurse completes the skin preparation, ensure patient comfort by explaining what is happening at the time.
   A. Application of the antiseptic solution is cold and wet.
   B. Injection of the local anesthetic may burn or sting as the tissue is infiltrated.
	Reduces anxiety and encourages cooperation.	Continue providing support and comfort throughout the procedure.

11. Assist as needed with applying a full drape to the patient with exposure of only the insertion site.	Minimizies the risk of infection; maintains aseptic and sterile precautions.	
12. Place the bed in a 15- to 25-degree Trendelenburg's position.	Provides venous dilation and increases central venous pressure to reduce the risk for air embolism.	May be contraindicated in certain patients (e.g., those with increased intracranial pressure, elevated venous pressure, respiratory or cardiac compromise).
13. Monitor the heart rate, respiratory rate and rhythm, pulse oximetry, and any patient response to the procedure.	Assessment may indicate occurrence of complications (see Table 81-1) or inadequate pain control.	
14. Observe the cardiac monitor while the guidewire and catheter are advanced, and inform the physician or advanced practice nurse immediately if a dysrhythmia occurs.	Advancement of the guidewire or catheter into the heart may induce cardiac dysrhythmias.	Tall, peaked P waves may be observed as the catheter tip enters the right atrium or if the guidewire has been advanced too far into the right atrium. Dysrhythmias may resolve with withdrawal of the guidewire or catheter. If the dysrhythmia continues, antidysrhythmic medications may be necessary.

Procedure continues on following page

Procedure   for Assisting With Central Venous Catheter Insertion—*Continued*

Steps	Rationale	Special Considerations
15. Once the catheter is placed and blood return is ensured, assist with flushing the lumens with normal saline solution and connecting the IV or hemodynamic monitoring tubing to the catheter.	Maintains aseptic technique. Immediate connection of the IV or monitoring system to the catheter prevents air embolism.	Ensure a tight connection to prevent accidental disconnection. Luer-Lok devices prevent an accidental disconnection.
16. If monitoring: A. Level the CVP air-fluid interface (zeroing stopcock) to the phlebostatic axis (see Procedure 76). B. Zero the system by turning the stopcock off to the patient, opening it to air, and zeroing the monitoring system (see Procedure 76). C. Place a nonvented cap on the top port of the stopcock, turn the stopcock open to the patient, and observe the waveform (Procedure 70). D. Obtain a waveform strip. E. Measure the pressure. F. Set the alarms.	Prepares the hemodynamic monitoring system and assesses the CVP waveform.	
17. Assist as needed with applying a sterile, occlusive dressing (see Procedure 69).	Reduces the risk for infection.	Follow institution standard for application of a chlorhexidine-impregnated sponge (see Procedure 69).
18. Reposition the patient in a comfortable position.	Promotes comfort.	Remove the towel roll, if used.
19. Assist as needed with obtaining a chest radiograph as prescribed.	Ensures that the catheter is placed and determines the presence of complications.	Infusions (especially total parenteral nutrition and chemotherapeutic agents) should not be initiated until catheter placement is confirmed.
20. Discard used supplies in appropriate receptacles.	Reduces the transmission of microorganisms; Standard Precautions. Safely removes sharp objects.	The physician or advanced practice nurse who inserted the catheter should dispose of all sharp objects into the sharps container.
21. ▉▉		

Expected Outcomes

• Successful placement of a CVC
• Infusion of IV solution
• The *a*, *c*, and *v* waves are identified with hemodynamic monitoring
• CVP measurements are obtained

Unexpected Outcomes

• Pain or discomfort during or after the insertion procedure
• Pneumothorax, tension pneumothorax, hemothorax, or chylothorax
• Sterile thrombophlebitis
• Infection
• Cardiac dysrhythmias
• Misplacement of the catheter (e.g., carotid artery, subclavian artery)
• Inadvertent lymphatic or thoracic duct perforation
• Hemorrhage
• Hematoma

Expected Outcomes

Unexpected Outcomes —*Continued*

- Venous air embolism
- Pulmonary embolus
- Cardiac tamponade
- Sepsis
- Heparin-induced thrombocytopenia or thrombosis

Patient Monitoring and Care

Steps	Rationale	Reportable Conditions
		These conditions should be reported if they persist despite nursing interventions.
1. Assess the patient's vital signs, oxygenation saturation, and level of consciousness before the procedure, after the procedure, and as needed during the procedure.	Identifies signs and symptoms of complications and allows for immediate interventions.	• Abnormal vital signs • Abnormal pulse oximetry value • Changes in level of consciousness
2. If the catheter was placed for CVP measurement, assess the waveform.	Ensures that the catheter is in the proper location for monitoring. Allows assessment of *a*, *c*, and *v* waves and measurement of pressure.	• Abrupt and sustained changes in CVP • Abnormal waveform
3. Observe the catheter site for bleeding or hematoma every 15 to 30 minutes for the first 2 hours after insertion.	Postinsertion bleeding may occur in a patient with coagulopathies or arterial punctures, with multiple attempts at vein access, or with the use of through-the-needle introducer designs for insertion.	• Bleeding that does not stop • Hematoma or expanding hematoma
4. Assess heart and lung sounds before and after the procedure.	Abnormal heart or lung sounds may indicate cardiac tamponade, pneumothorax, chylothorax, or hemothorax.	• Diminished or muffled heart sounds • Absent or diminished breath sounds unilaterally
5. Daily assess the need for the CVC. **(Level C*)**	The Centers for Disease Control and Prevention (CDC)[5] and research findings[3] recommend that CVCs do not need to be changed more frequently than every 7 days. No specific recommendations exist regarding routine replacement of CVCs that need to be in place for greater than 7 days.[1,5,6] CVCs should be changed over a guidewire when emergently inserted (e.g., trauma resuscitation), the catheter malfunctions, a positive blood culture is obtained after the CVC was inserted, and sepsis develops without an identified source.[1]	• Signs or symptoms of catheter infection

*Level C: Qualitative studies, descriptive or correlational studies, integrative reviews, systematic reviews, or randomized controlled trials with inconsistent results

Procedure continues on following page

Patient Monitoring and Care —*Continued*

Steps	Rationale	Reportable Conditions
	CVCs should be removed and reinserted at a new site when there is a skin infection at the catheter insertion site (i.e., redness, swelling, or drainage at or around the insertion site) or a positive culture at the insertion site.[1]	
6. Follow institution standard for assessing pain. Administer analgesia as prescribed.	Identifies need for pain interventions.	• Continued pain despite pain interventions

Documentation

Documentation should include the following:

- Patient and family education
- Completion of patient and family education
- Universal Protocol requirements
- Catheter location
- Medications administered
- Date and time of procedure
- Catheter type
- Lumen size
- Right atrial pressure and CVP waveform
- Central venous pressure values after insertion

- Centimeter marking at the skin
- Patient response to the procedure
- Pain assessment, interventions, and effectiveness
- Fluids administered
- Type of dressing applied
- Occurrence of unexpected outcomes
- Additional nursing interventions

References

CR 1. Eyer S, et al: Catheter-related sepsis: prospective, randomized study of three methods of long-term catheter maintenance, *Crit Care Med* 18:1073-1079, 1990.

2. Infusion Nurses Society: *(2006). Policies and procedures for infusion nursing.,* ed 3, Norwood, MA:, 2006, AuthorINS.

CR 3. Intravenous Nurses Society: (2006). Infusion nursing standards of practice, *J Infus Nurs* 29(1S): S1-S90, 2006.

4. Kumar A, Darovic GO: Establishment of cardiovascular access. In Darovic, GO: *Hemodynamic monitoring invasive and noninvasive clinical application,* Philadelphia, 2000, Saunders.

CR 5. O'Grady NP, et al: Guidelines for the prevention of intravascular catheter-related infections, *Am J Infect Control* 30:476-489, 2002.

CR 6. Safdar N, Klugar DM, Maki DG: A review of risk factors for catheter-related bloodstream infection caused by percutaneously inserted, noncuffed central venous catheters: implications for preventive strategies, *Medicine* 81: 466-472, 2002.

7. Venus G, Mallory DL: Vascular cannulation. In Civetta J., Taylor, W., & Kirby, R. (eds)., *Critical Care,* ed 5, Philadelphia, 2009, Lippincott, Williams & Wilkins.

Additional Readings

CR Dailey EK, Schroeder JS: *Techniques in bedside hemodynamic monitoring,* ed 5, St Louis, 1994, Mosby.

CR Darovic GO: *Hemodynamic monitoring invasive and noninvasive clinical application,* Philadelphia, 2000, Saunders.

CR Eggimann P, et al: Impact of a prevention strategy targeted at vascular-access care on incidence of infections acquired in intensive care, *Lancet* 355:1864-1868, 2000.

CR Friesinger GC, Williams SV, ACP/AHA Task Force on Clinical Privileges in Cardiology: Clinical competence in hemodynamic monitoring, *J Am Coll Cardiol* 15:1460, 1990.

CR Lorente L, Henry C, Martin M., et al: Central venous catheter-related infection in a prospective and observational study of 2,595 catheters, *Crit Care* 9:R631-R635, 2005

AP Implantable Venous Access Device: Access, Deaccess, and Care

P U R P O S E :   Implantable venous access devices or ports are used for delivery of medications, parenteral solutions, blood products, and cytotoxic agents and for blood sampling for patients who need long-term venous access.

Anne C. Muller

PREREQUISITE NURSING KNOWLEDGE

- Understanding of the implantable venous access device, including the septum and outer borders, is needed.
- Knowledge of the anatomy of the venous system is necessary.
- Understanding is needed of the principles of medication delivery. Intermittent use necessitates flushing with normal saline solution (NS) after each use and instillation of heparin as prescribed.
- Understanding of the principles of aseptic and sterile technique is necessary.
- The properties of chemotherapeutic or cytotoxic agents and preferred delivery techniques should be understood.
- Understanding of the consequences of infiltration of vesicant substances is needed.
- Implanted venous access devices are surgically placed, totally implanted in a cutaneous pocket (usually in the chest wall), and designed to provide venous access for intermittent or continuous infusions, maintaining a patient's intact body image when not accessed.
- Implanted devices consist of a slim tube or catheter connected to a reservoir, which is covered by a disc 2 to 3 cm

in width (Figs. 83-1 and 83-2). The disc is made of silicone and is referred to as the septum. Provided a noncoring needle is used to access the septum, the septum is capable of resealing when deaccessed. The internal catheter is connected to the patient's venous system and may consist of either silicone or polyurethane.[5,15]

- The implanted venous access device is percutaneously accessed with a noncoring needle.
- The use of a noncoring needle allows for repeated access of the venous device without damage to the silicone core.
- The noncoring needle chosen should be of optimal length, with the most common length for adults 1½ or 1¾ inches. Patients with increased subcutaneous tissue

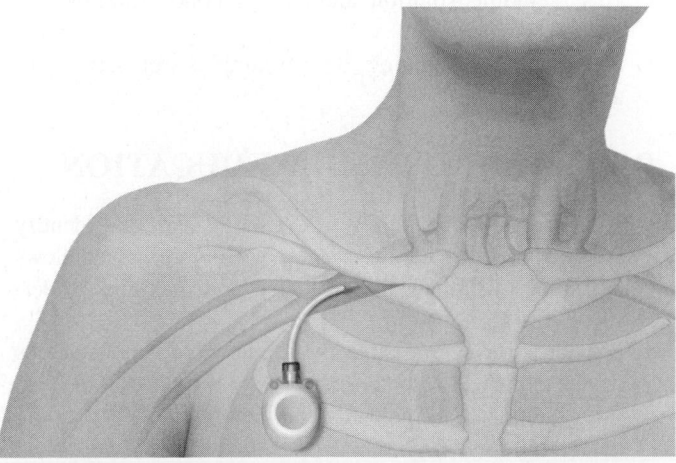

FIGURE 83-1   Port placement. *(Courtesy of Bard Corporation).*

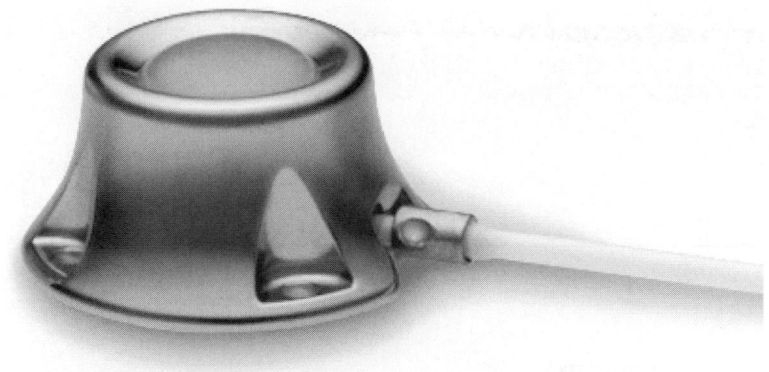

FIGURE 83-2   PORT-A-CATH® reservoir with self-sealing septum and catheter. *(Courtesy of Smiths Medical ASD, Inc., St. Paul, MN.)*

may need a longer needle for access. Too short a needle may cause the flanges to press against the skin surrounding the portal chamber, leading to patient discomfort and possibly resulting in damage to the skin overlying the venous access device. Too long a needle may result in a rocking motion that can cause discomfort, possible migration out of the portal septum, or damage to the integrity of the septum, impairing it for further use.

EQUIPMENT

- Nonsterile gloves
- Sterile gloves
  Noncoring needle, winged with 90-degree angle and extension tubing (available in lengths of ¾, 1, 1¼, 1½, and 1¾ inches)
- Dressing supplies
- Skin antiseptic solution (e.g., 2% chlorhexidine–based solution)
- Two 10-mL syringes
- Luer-Lok vial access device
- Prepierced needleless injection cap
- Single-use 30-mL vial NS
- ½-inch steri-strips
- Heparin flush, 100 units/mL concentration
- Central venous catheter dressing change kit
- Needleless blood sampling access device
  Additional equipment as needed includes the following:
- 10% betadine solution and 70% alcohol solution site preparation swabs
- Supplies for obtaining blood samples for laboratory analysis

PATIENT AND FAMILY EDUCATION

- Assess patient and family readiness to learn and identify factors that affect learning. ➦*Rationale:* Assessment allows the nurse to individualize teaching and maximize understanding.
- Provide information about the implantable venous access device and the methods used for accessing it. ➦*Rationale:* Information assists the patient and family in understanding the procedure and decreases patient and family anxiety.

- Explain the patient's role during the procedure and expected outcomes. ➦*Rationale:* The patient is able to participate in care, and cooperation is encouraged.
- Explain the anticipated sensations during the access procedure. ➦*Rationale:* Explanation allows the patient to alert the healthcare provider to unusual or unexpected sensations during the procedure.
- Explain site care and signs and symptoms of infection and infiltration. ➦*Rationale:* Explanation enables the patient and family to participate in care, and the patient is encouraged to report untoward events to healthcare providers.

PATIENT ASSESSMENT AND PREPARATION

Patient Assessment

- Review the patient's medical history specifically related to problems with device implantation, complications with previous access, and allergies to antiseptic solutions. ➦*Rationale:* Baseline data are provided.
- Obtain the patient's vital signs. ➦*Rationale:* Baseline data are provided.
- Review the patient's current laboratory status, including coagulation results. ➦*Rationale:* Baseline coagulation studies are helpful in determination of the risk for bleeding. If results are abnormal, consult with the primary care provider before accessing the device.[2]

Patient Preparation

- Verify correct patient with two identifiers. ➦*Rationale:* Prior to performing a procedure, the nurse should ensure the correct identification of the patient for the intended intervention.
- Ensure that the patient and family understand preprocedural teaching. Answer questions as they arise, and reinforce information as needed. ➦*Rationale:* Understanding of previously taught information is evaluated and reinforced.
- Assist the patient to a supine position with the head of the bed elevated up to a 30-degree angle. ➦*Rationale:* Positioning prepares the patient and allows optimal access to the implanted venous access device.

Procedure for Implantable Venous Access Device: Access, Deaccess, and Care

Steps	Rationale	Special Considerations
Accessing an Implantable Venous Access Device		
1. HH		Both conventional antiseptic that contains soap and water and waterless alcohol-based gels or foams are considered acceptable by the Centers for Disease Control and Prevention (CDC).[4]
2. PE		
3. Remove the patient's gown away from the venous access device.	Optimizes the viewing area.	
4. Palpate the subcutaneous tissue to determine the borders of the access device.[2,5] Palpate the venous access device borders and locate the septum and the center of the septum. **(Level M*)**	Allows for palpation of the venous access device borders and identification of the septal center.	
5. Assess the site for signs and symptoms of infection (e.g., erythema, induration, pain, or tenderness at the site).	Minimizes the risk of accessing an infected area.	Erythema, swelling, or tenderness may indicate system leakage. A radiograph is recommended if leakage is suspected.[3,5]
6. Discard gloves in the appropriate receptacle.	Removes and safely discards used supplies.	
7. HH		
8. Open the central venous catheter dressing kit with the sterile inner surface of the wrap to create a sterile field.	Maintains asepsis and prepares supplies. Creates a sterile field.	Disinfect the table as needed. Venous access devices have the lowest risk for catheter-related blood system infections, provided that aseptic and sterile techniques are used throughout care delivery.[4]
9. Prepare supplies:	Places equipment within reach during the procedure.	
A. With sterile technique, remove the wrapper from two 10-mL syringes and place them on the sterile field.	Maintains the sterility of the procedure.	
B. Remove the packaging and place the winged or safety noncoring needle with extension tubing, needleless injection cap, needleless blood sampling access device, and steri-strips on the sterile field.	Protects the healthcare provider from potential needle injury. Maintains sterile technique.	
10. Remove the cap from the NS vial and wipe the top of the NS vial with an alcohol wipe and allow to dry.	Reduces microorganisms.	
11. Aseptically connect the needleless blood sampling access device to the vial.	Reduces microorganisms.	

*Level M: Manufacturer's recommendations only

Procedure continues on following page

Procedure   for Implantable Venous Access Device: Access, Deaccess, and Care—*Continued*

Steps	Rationale	Special Considerations
12. Prepare supplies: A. Put a sterile glove on your dominant hand. B. With the sterile hand, pick up a 10-mL syringe. C. With the nonsterile hand, pick up the NS vial with the needleless blood sampling access device attached. D. Use the sterile gloved hand to withdraw 10 mL of NS. E. With the sterile hand, pick up the second 10-mL syringe. F. As above, use the sterile gloved hand to withdraw 10 mL of NS.	Prepares the supplies for procedure.	
13. Apply the remaining sterile glove.	Maintains asepsis.	
14. With sterile technique: A. Attach the needleless injection cap to the extension tubing on the noncoring needle. B. Attach the 10-mL NS syringe to the needleless cap. C. Prime the tubing with NS away from the sterile field.	Prepares the equipment. Removes air from the extension tubing, preventing possible air embolism.	
15. Retain the priming syringe on the needleless cap and return the primed equipment to the sterile field.		
16. Cleanse the implanted venous access device site or port with a 2% chlorhexidine-based antiseptic solution. Cleanse the site using a back-and-forth motion while applying friction for 30 seconds. Allow the antiseptic to remain on the insertion site and to dry completely before catheter insertion.[4,9,10]	Reduces the risk of infection.	
17. Pick up the noncoring needle with the NS syringe attached with the dominant hand and remove the protective cap.		
18. Use the nondominant hand to stabilize the borders of the venous access device.		
19. Triangulate the venous access device between the thumb and first two fingers of the nondominant hand (Fig. 83-3).	Stabilizes the venous access device within the chest wall and prevents slippage. Protects the healthcare provider from a potential needle injury.	

Procedure	for Implantable Venous Access Device: Access, Deaccess, and Care—*Continued*	
Steps	**Rationale**	**Special Considerations**
20. With the dominant hand, firmly grasp the protective cap or wings of the noncoring needle and insert it firmly into the center of the port septum using a 90-degree angle perpendicular to the skin surface (Fig. 83-4).		
21. Advance the needle through the skin and septum until reaching the base of the portal reservoir (Fig. 83-5).		With use of a noncoring safety needle, grasp the vertical fin between the thumb and middle finger and press downward with the index finger.[4,11,13]
22. Note that resistance is felt as the needle reaches the base of the reservoir.		Once the septum is punctured, avoid tilting or rocking the needle, which may cause fluid leakage or damage to the system.[2]
23. Flush the venous access device with 5 mL of NS.	Determines the patency of the venous access device.	Avoid use of syringes with less than a 10-mL volume for flushing or administration of infusate. Smaller syringes exert pressure exceeding 40 psi and may cause catheter rupture or fragmentation with possible embolization.[2,5,13]
24. Observe the skin surrounding the noncoring needle for leakage of fluid or infiltration at the access site.	Assesses for potential access problems.	

Procedure continues on following page

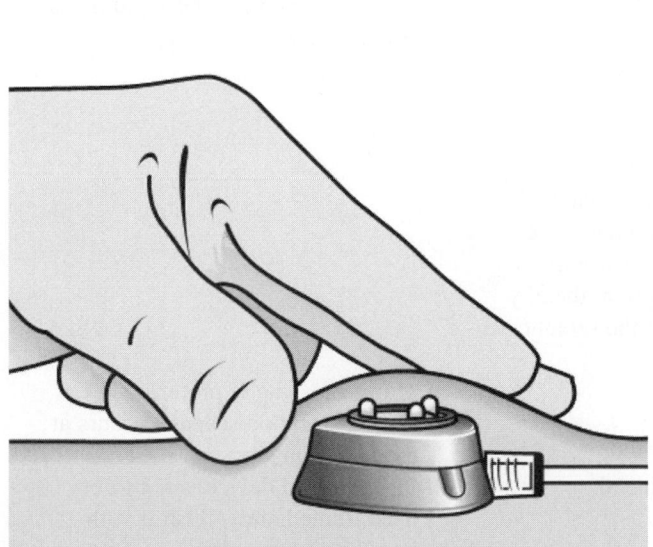

FIGURE 83-3 Triangulating the PowerPort® Implanted Port with the non-dominant hand. *(Courtesy of Bard Corporation.)*

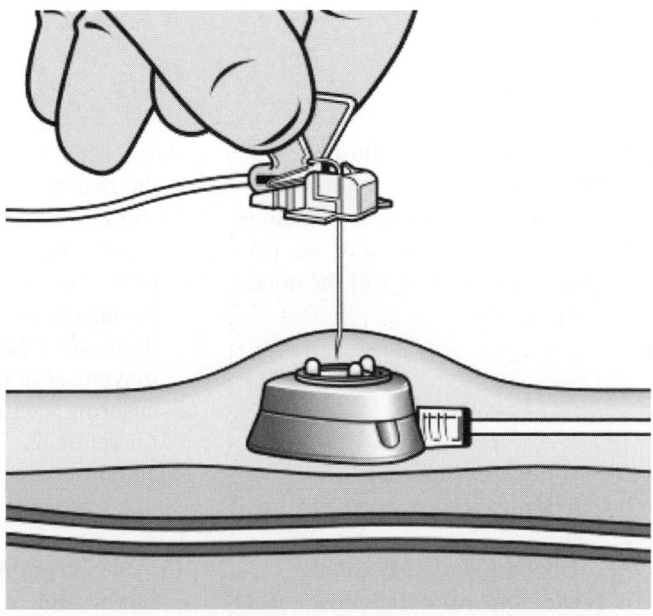

FIGURE 83-4 Needle access of the PowerPort® Implanted Port with a non-coring PowerLoc® Needle. *(Courtesy of Bard Corporation.)*

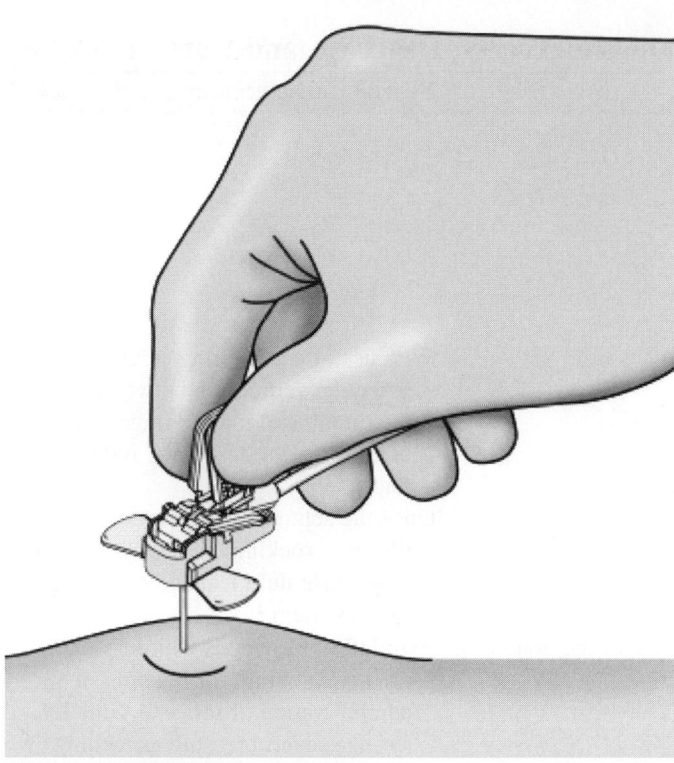

FIGURE 83-5   The non-coring PowerLoc® Needle is inserted until the base of the port reservoir is felt. *(Courtesy of Bard Corporation.)*

Procedure   for Implantable Venous Access Device: Access, Deaccess, and Care—*Continued*

Steps	Rationale	Special Considerations
25. Gently aspirate blood, then flush with the remaining 5 mL of NS.	Verifies placement.	If a blood return is not evident, gently flush with the push-pull method and reposition the patient. If a blood return is still not evident, continue the access procedure and apply a dressing to minimize the risk of infection. Contact the patient's physician. Administer a lytic agent and obtain a radiographic or dye shadow study as prescribed.[5,8,16] Some authorities suggest re-accessing to determine if the septum has been pierced.[13]
26. Position the wings flush with the patient's skin.	Anchoring minimizes discomfort for the patient.	
27. Stabilize the needle by attaching steri-strips in a cross or star pattern over the wings of the noncoring needle.	Stabilizes the needle inserted in the septal core and minimizes rocking of the needle, which can cause damage to the septum and patient discomfort. Minimizes needle movement in the septum, thereby ensuring integrity of the septal core for future use.	
28. Apply a sterile, occlusive dressing.	Maintains asepsis.	A gauze dressing is preferred if oozing or blood seepage occurs at the insertion site.
29. Label the dressing with the date, time of cannulation, needle gauge and length, and your initials.	Provides important clinical information.	If the accessed device is not to be used immediately, flush it with heparin as prescribed.

Procedure for Implantable Venous Access Device: Access, Deaccess, and Care—*Continued*

Steps	Rationale	Special Considerations
30. Initiate continuous or intermittent infusion.	Begins therapy.	
31. Discard used supplies in appropriate receptacles.	Removes and safely discards used supplies.	
32. HH		

Deaccessing an Implantable Venous Access Device

1. HH		
2. PE		
3. Flush the venous access device with 10 mL of NS, followed by heparin as prescribed (e.g., 5 mL of 100 units/mL heparin).[2,12]	Prepares and optimizes catheter patency while not in use.	
4. Loosen the transparent or gauze dressing and steri-strips from the site.	Facilitates removal.	
5. Use the thumb and forefinger of the dominant hand to grasp the dressing and steri-strips along with the winged flanges of the needle.	Prepares for needle removal.	
6. With the nondominant hand, apply gentle stabilizing pressure to the venous access device while removing the needle by pulling straight up and out in a firm, continuous motion.	Minimizes patient discomfort and ensures controlled withdrawal of a sharp object.	With use of a noncoring safety needle, grasp the horizontal flanges securely, pull up, and squeeze the flanges together. The flanges fold together, forcing the needle inside the locked wings and covering the needle. The wings will lock in place.
7. Assess the site for redness or drainage.	Identifies possible complications.	
8. Discard the noncoring needle in a designated container.	Safely removes sharp objects.	
9. Apply a dressing to the site if oozing occurs.	Provides absorption.	
10. Discard supplies in appropriate receptacles.	Removes and safely discards used supplies.	
11. HH		

Obtaining a Blood Specimen from an Implantable Venous Access Device

1. HH		
2. PE		
3. If present, shut off the intravenous (IV) infusion and disconnect the IV tubing from the extension tubing on the noncoring needle.	Maintains asepsis.	
4. Place a sterile cap on the end of the IV tubing.	Maintains asepsis.	
5. Thoroughly cleanse the injection cap with an alcohol wipe and allow it to dry. Do not remove the cap.[7,9,14]	Minimizes infection and healthcare provider exposure to blood and body fluids.[4]	
6. Attach a 10-mL syringe with NS and flush the venous access device.	Clears the catheter of medication or IV fluid.	
7. Attach a new sterile 10-mL syringe or a needleless blood sampling access device.	Prepares supplies.	

Procedure continues on following page

Procedure for Implantable Venous Access Device: Access, Deaccess, and Care—*Continued*

Steps	Rationale	Special Considerations
8. Determine the appropriate discard volume. (**Level E***)	Clears the catheter of solution. The discard volume includes the dead space and the blood diluted by the flush solution. Portal reservoirs average 0.5 mL volume; catheters average 0.6 mL for single-lumen systems.[2] Recommendations are that at least three times the dead space be withdrawn.[7]	Blood for coagulation tests should not be withdrawn through a heparinized catheter if the results will be used to monitor anticoagulant therapy or to determine if a patient has a coagulopathy.[1,13,15] Follow institution standard.
9. Gently aspirate the discard volume into the syringe or engage a blood specimen tube into the needleless blood sampling access device to obtain the discard volume and allow the tube to passively fill.[6,7,14]	Withdraws the discard.	Minimizes needle-stick injury, exposure to blood, and decreases infection risk to the patient by reducing incidence of opening the catheter system.[7,12]
10. Remove the discard syringe or blood specimen tube.	Prepares for blood sampling.	
11. Insert a new syringe into the injection cap or place a new blood specimen tube into the needleless blood sampling access device.	Prepares for removal of the specimen sample.	
12. Slowly and gently aspirate blood or engage the blood specimen tube into the needleless blood sampling access device.	Obtains the blood specimen.	
13. Remove the syringe or the blood specimen tube.	Removes the specimen.	
14. After the blood specimen is obtained, flush the port with 10 mL of NS.	Clears blood from the system.	Flush with an additional 10 to 20 mL of NS if the blood does not clear completely from the extension tubing.[8]
15. Clamp the extension tubing.		
16. Apply a new injection cap with strict aseptic technique.	Reduces infection.	
17. Reconnect the IV and continue the infusion.	Resumes therapy.	If the IV infusion is completed, administer heparin as prescribed.
18. Label the specimen(s) and the laboratory form.	Properly identifies the patient and laboratory tests to be performed.	
19. Discard used supplies in appropriate receptacles.	Removes and safely discards used supplies.	
20. HH		
21. Send the laboratory specimen(s) for analysis.	Expedites determination of laboratory results.	

*Level E: Multiple case reports, theory-based evidence from expert opinions, or peer-reviewed professional organizational standards without clinical studies to support recommendations

Expected Outcomes

- Site without redness, pain, or tenderness
- Venous access device stable
- Venous access device is accessed without difficulty
- Venous access device flushes easily without evidence of resistance or infiltration
- No evidence or leakage at the septal site
- Blood specimens are obtained as prescribed
- Venous access device is deaccessed without difficulty

Unexpected Outcomes

- Port reddened, tender, or painful on palpation
- Implanted device unstable in chest wall with palpation
- Patient describes burning sensation in the subcutaneous tissue with flushing or infusion
- Sluggish or no blood return with aspiration
- Evidence of leakage of flush solution at the septal site
- Patient describes pain at site, chest, ear, or shoulder with flushing
- Signs or symptoms of local or systemic infection
- Swollen neck or arm

Patient Monitoring and Care

Steps	Rationale	Reportable Conditions
		These conditions should be reported if they persist despite nursing interventions.
1. During IV infusions, assess the venous access device for patency and signs of infiltration every 4 hours and as needed.	Determines adequate functioning of the venous access device.	• Signs or symptoms of infiltration at the venous access site
2. Follow institution standard for frequency and type of dressing change.	The dressing should be changed if it becomes damp, loosened, or soiled or when inspection of the site is necessary.[5]	• Signs or symptoms of infection
3. Replace gauze dressings every 2 days and transparent dressings at least every 7 days.[4,9,10] **(Level D*)** Follow institution standard.	Decreases the risk for infection at the catheter site. The Centers for Disease Control (CDC) recommends replacing the dressing when it becomes damp, loosened, or soiled or when inspection of the site is necessary.[4]	
4. Follow institution standard for assessing pain. Administer analgesia as prescribed.	Identifies need for pain interventions.	• Continued pain despite pain interventions
5. Follow-up care for deaccessed device includes reaccessing the device to administer monthly flush with 5 mL of 100 units of heparin as prescribed.[2,11,12,14]	Maintains catheter patency.	
6. Assess for signs and symptoms of infection.	Determines the presence of infection.	• Redness, pain, or drainage at the site; fever, elevated white blood cell count

*Level D: Peer-reviewed professional organizational standards with clinical studies to support recommendations

Documentation

Documentation should include the following:
- Location and cannulation of the device
- Needle length and gauge
- Appearance of blood return
- Access of the site
- De-access of the site

- Specimens obtained and sent for analysis
- Laboratory results
- Pain assessment, interventions, and effectiveness
- Unexpected outcomes
- Additional interventions

References

CR 1. Barton JC, Poon MC: Coagulation testing of Hickman catheter blood in patients with acute leukemia, *Arch Intern Med* 146(11):2165-2169, 1986.

CR 2. Beck SL, et al: *Standards of care for the patient with a venous access device*, Salt Lake City, UT, 1990, American Cancer Society, Utah Division.

3. Camp-Sorrell, D: Accessing and Deaccessing Ports: Where is the evidence?, *Clin Jour of Oncol Nurs*, 13:587-590, 2009.

CR 4. CDC: Guidelines for the prevention of intravascular catheter related bloodstream infection, *MMWR* 5:1-26, 2002.

CR 5. Deltec Incorporated: *Clinician information Port-A-Cath®, Port-A-Cath II and P.A.S. Port systems,* St Paul, MN, 2002, Deltec, Inc, 1-24.

CR 6. Frey AM: Drawing blood from vascular access devices, *J Infusion Nurs* 26:285-293, 2003.

7. Hartkopf L: Implanted Ports, computed tomography, power injectors, and catheter rupture, *Clin J of Oncol Nurs*, 12:809812, 2008.

CR 8. Himberger J, Himberger L: Accuracy of drawing blood through infusing intravenous lines, *Heart Lung* 30:66-73, 2001.

9. Infusion Nurses Society: Infusion nursing standards of practice, *J Infus Nurs* 29:S1-S92, 2006.

10. Infusion Nurses Society: *Policies and procedures for infusion nursing.,* ed 3, Norwood, MA, 2006, Author INS.

11. Johnson K: Power injectable portal systems, *J of Radiol Nurs* 28:27-31, 2009.

CR 12. Mayo DJ, Dimond EP, Framer W, et al: Discard volumes necessary for clinically useful coagulations studies from heparinized Hickman catheters, *Oncol Nurs Forum* 23(4):671-675, 1996.

CR 13. Polovich M, Whitford J, and Olsen M: Oncology Nurses Society: *Chemotherapy and biotherapy guidelines and recommendations for practice*, Pittsburgh, ed 3, 2009, Oncology Nursing Press, Inc.

CR 14. Pinto KM: Accuracy of coagulation values obtained from a heparinized central venous catheter, *Oncol Nurs Forum* 21(3):573-575, 1994.

15. Schummer W, Schummer C, Schelenz C: Case Report: The malfunction of implanted venous access devices, *Brit J of Nurs*, 12(4):210-214, 2009.

CR 16. Yucha C, DeAngelo E: The minimum discard volume, *J Intraven Nurs* 19:141-146, 1996.

Additional Readings

CR Camp-Sorrell D, Mermel L, Kluger D, et al: *The efficacy of chlorhexidine-impregnated sponge (BioPatch) for the prevention of intravascular catheter related infection: a prospective, randomized, controlled multi-center trial*, abstract of the 40th Interscience Conference on Antimicrobial Agents and Chemotherapy 422, 2000.

CR Rosenthal K: Pinpointing intravascular device complications, *Nurs Manage* June:37-42, 2003.

CR Sabel M, Smith J: Principles of chronic venous access: recommendations based on the Roswell Park experience, *Surg Oncol* 6:171-177, 1988.

CR Seemann S, Reinhardt A: Blood sample collection from a peripheral catheter system compared with phlebotomy, *J Intraven Nurs* 23:290-297, 2000.

CR Sterba K: Controversial issues in the care and maintenance of vascular access devices in the long-term/subacute care client, *J Infus Nurs* 24:249-254, 2001.

CR Wu P-y, Yeh Y-C, Huang C-H, et al: Spontaneous migration of a Port-A-Cath catheter into ipsilateral jugular vein in two patients with severe cough, *Ann Vasc Surg* 19:734-736, 2005.

84

Intraosseous Devices

P U R P O S E :   Intraosseous access is indicated when intravenous access cannot be obtained or cannot be obtained in a timely manner (within 90 seconds[10]) and access to venous circulation is needed for the administration of medications or fluids.

Robin Scott, Michael W. Day

PREREQUISITE NURSING KNOWLEDGE

- Intraosseous (IO) access is a safe and reliable access point into the noncollapsible marrow cavity that allows direct access to the venous circulation.

- The Volkmann's canals that are located throughout the bone connect with the medullary canal and the blood vessels of the periosteum (Fig. 84-1). When medications and fluids are introduced into the medullary canal, they flow through the vascular plexi directly into the vascular system.[6]

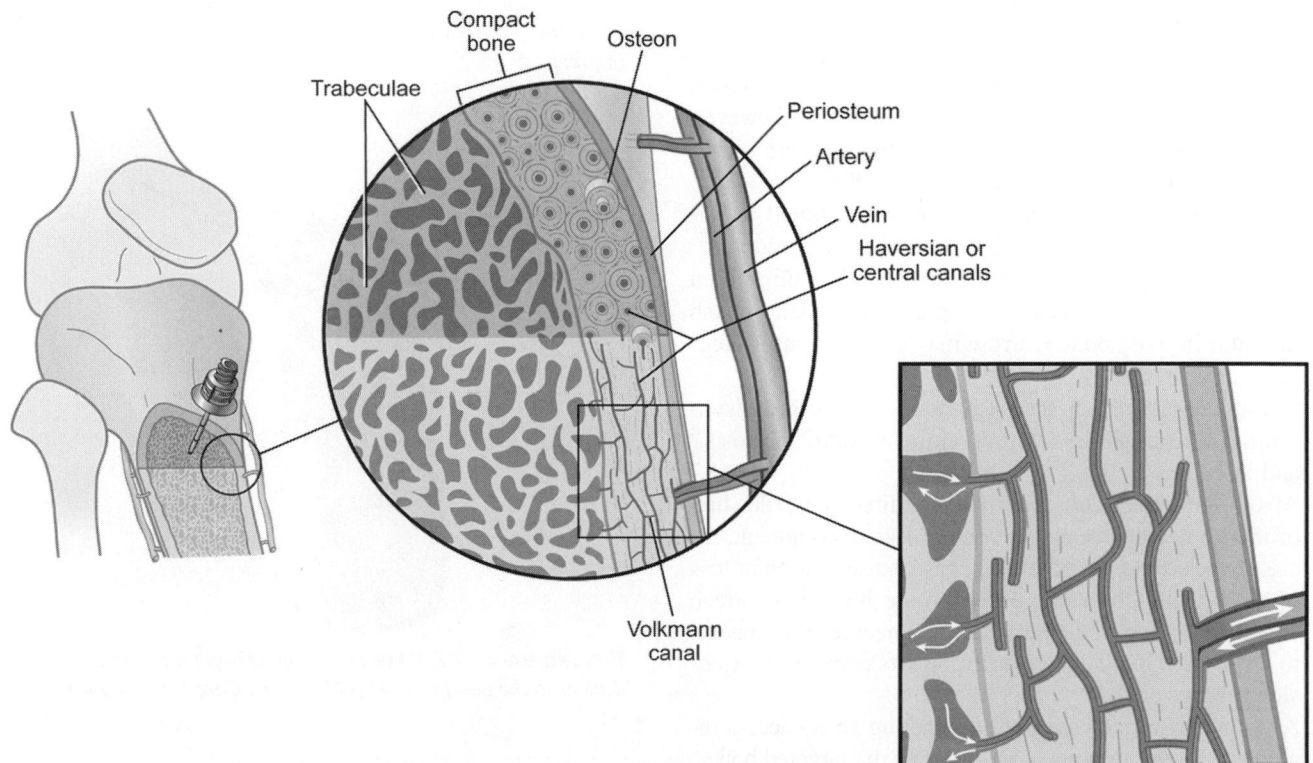

FIGURE 84-1   IO Circulation. *(From Day MW: Intraossesous devices in the adult trauma patient, Crit Care Nurs. In press.)*

- Insertion devices are available for insertion of IO needles.[6] These devices include the bone injection gun (BIG; Waismed, a Persys Medical Co, Houston, TX; Fig. 84-2), the FAST1 adult intraosseous infusion system (Pyng Medical Corp, Vancouver, BC, Canada, Fig. 84-3), and the EZ-IO (Vidacare Corp, Shavano Park, TX; Fig. 84-4). These three devices are approved by the US Food and Drug Administration (FDA) for IO access in adult patients. Two of the devices (BIG, EZ-IO) use a specially designed needle with a stylet or trocar. The third device (FAST1) uses a metal-tipped plastic catheter.

- In adults, the available IO access sites, depending on the specific device and following each manufacturer's guidelines, include:
  - ❖ Tibial plateau: 1 to 2 cm distal to the tibial tuberosity[3,5,8]
  - ❖ Distal tibia: 1 to 2 cm above the medial malleolus[7]
  - ❖ Sternum: 1.5 cm below the sternal notch[5,8]
  - ❖ Greater tubercle of the proximal humerus[8]

- IO blood can be used for many laboratory tests, including typing and screening, electrolyte values, chemistries, blood gas values, drug levels, and hemoglobin levels.[2] However, specimen samples from the marrow have a lower correlation to serum levels after 30 minutes of resuscitation.[3] In addition, drawing of blood from an IO device may not be recommended by specific manufacturers and has the potential of occluding the device.

- The onset of action for medications is similar to that of intravenous (IV) medications.[13] However, administration via the IO route may result in lower serum concentrations versus the IV route for the following medications: ceftriaxone, chloramphenicol, phenytoin, tobramycin, and vancomycin.[5]

- Marrow-toxic medications should not be infused via the IO route.[8]

- All resuscitation medications, isotonic fluids, and blood products may be given via the IO route[2,3,5,14]; however, myonecrosis has been reported with the infusion of hypertonic saline solution via the IO route.[10,12]

- Medications administered via the IO route should be followed by a 5- to 10-mL flush of normal saline solution.[4]

- Fluids running into an IO line should be administered with a pressure bag because the pressure needed to push the fluid into the bone marrow may exceed that of volumetric IV pumps.

- Complications of IO access include compartment syndrome, osteomyelitis, fracture, extravasation,[5] necrosis,[5] and infection.[7]

- A syringe should not be attached directly to the hub of the IO needle because it could cause dislodgment, increase the size of the hole, and cause extravasation or loss of the IO site. To extend access to the IO needle, attach extension tubing to the hub of the IO needle and secure it to the skin.[11] Some device insertion kits come with extension tubing.

- Absolute contraindications to attempting an IO access include previous attempts or fractures of the targeted bone.

- Relative contraindications to IO access include infection at the access site, previous bone surgery at the

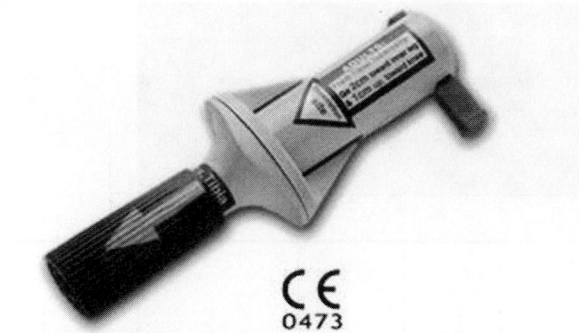

FIGURE 84-2   Bone injection gun (BIG; adult). *(From Day MW: Intraosseous devices in the adult trauma patient, Crit Care Nurs. In press.)*

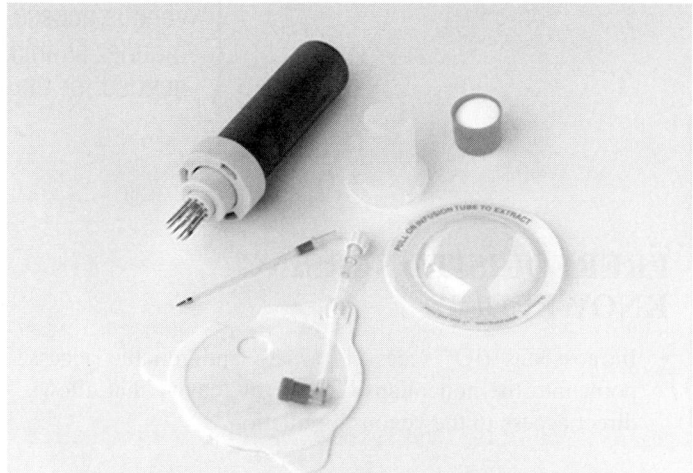

FIGURE 84-3   The FAST1 infusion set. *(From Day MW: Intraosseous devices in the adult trauma patient, Crit Care Nurs. In press.)*

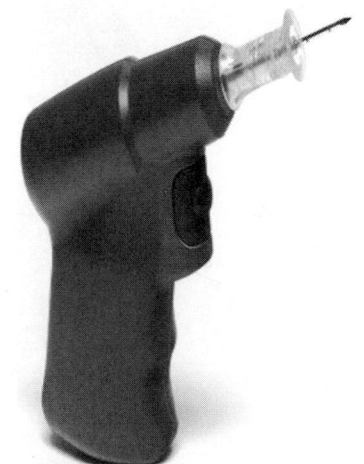

FIGURE 84-4   EZ-IO power driver. *(From Day MW: Intraosseous devices in the adult trauma patient, Crit Care Nurs. In press.)*

insertion site, fractures above the insertion site,[9] and bone disorders, such as osteoporosis and osteogenesis imperfecta.[3] Another relative contraindication to the FAST1 is skin damage at the insertion site, which may preclude the adherence of the target patch used to secure the device.

- IO access in obese patients may be more difficult. The EZ-IO has a needle set specifically designed for the patient with "excessive tissue" at the insertion site.
- IO access is meant to be a temporary venous access; IO lines should be removed as soon as other venous access is obtained or within 24 hours of insertion.

EQUIPMENT

- Nonsterile gloves
- Antiseptic solution (e.g., 2% chlorhexidine-based preparation)
- IO insertion device (follow manufacturer's guidelines for information that may be age or weight based)
- Tape
- IV tubing
- Isotonic crystalloid fluid, as prescribed
- Two 5- to 10-mL syringes
- Prescribed medications
- Pressure bag for IV solution
- Dressing supplies
  Additional equipment as needed includes the following:
- Blood specimen tubes
- 1% lidocaine without epinephrine
- 2% lidocaine without epinephrine
- Sterile 2 × 2 gauze pads
- Large needle forceps

PATIENT AND FAMILY EDUCATION

- Explain to the patient and family the reason for the IO access. ➥*Rationale:* Clarification of information is an expressed patient need and helps to diminish anxiety, enhance acceptance, and encourage questions.

- Describe the major steps of the procedure, including the patient's role in the procedure. ➥*Rationale:* Explanation decreases patient anxiety, enhances cooperation, provides an opportunity for the patient to voice concerns, and prevents accidental contamination of the sterile field and equipment.
- Explain the expected outcomes of the procedure. ➥*Rationale:* Explanation reduces anxiety and clarifies the duration and goals of IO access.

PATIENT ASSESSMENT AND PREPARATION

Patient Assessment

- Assess the patient for fractures or infections at the insertion site, for previous bone surgeries at the site, and for a history of osteoporosis or fractures of the target bone. ➥*Rationale:* An alternate site should be accessed to avoid possible complications associated with the previous conditions.
- Obtain the patient's baseline vital signs and cardiac rhythm. ➥*Rationale:* Baseline data facilitate the identification of clinical problems and identify the urgency of obtaining IO access.
- If possible, determine the patient's allergy history (e.g., lidocaine, antiseptic solutions). ➥*Rationale:* This assessment decreases the risk for allergic reactions by avoiding known allergenic products.

Patient Preparation

- Verify correct patient with two identifiers. ➥*Rationale:* Prior to performing a procedure, the nurse should ensure the correct identification of the patient for the intended intervention.
- Ensure that the patient and family understand preprocedural teaching. Answer questions as they arise, and reinforce information as needed. ➥*Rationale:* Understanding of previously taught information is evaluated and reinforced.
- Perform a pre-procedure verification and time out, if non-emergent. ➥*Rationale:* Ensures patient safety.

Procedure	for Intraosseous Access	
Steps	**Rationale**	**Special Considerations**
1. HH		
2. PE		
3. Assist the patient to a position of comfort for access of the appropriate insertion site.	Prepares the patient for the procedure and allows for optimal visualization.	
4. Palpate the intended insertion site. A. Proximal tibia: 1. Identify the tibial tuberosity. 2. Move 2 cm medially and 1 cm proximally	Guides IO device placement.	

Procedure continues on following page

Procedure | for Intraosseous Access—*Continued*

Steps	Rationale	Special Considerations

B. Distal tibia:
  1. Identify the medial malleolus.
  2. Move two finger widths proximally at the midline of the medial aspect of the leg.
C. Sternum:
  1. Identify the sternal notch.
  2. Move 1.5 cm below the sternal notch.[5,8]
D. Humerus:
  1. Identify the greater tubercle.
  2. Move one finger width lateral from the greater tubercle.		

5. Cleanse the intended site and surrounding area with antiseptic solution (e.g., 2% chlorhexidine-based preparation).[2,4,9,14] **(Level D*)**	Limits the introduction of potentially infectious skin flora into the insertion site.	
6. Stabilize the insertion site with the nondominant hand.[4]	Prevents movement of the limb during insertion.	
7. FAST1 insertion: **(Level M*)** (see Fig. 84-3) A. The FAST1 is inserted into the sternum. B. Identify the sternal notch and apply the target patch. C. With firm pressure, apply the delivery device at a 90-degree angle to the manubrium and push until the device releases the FAST1 device. D. The stabilizer points penetrate the skin, mark the depth of the manubrium, and deliver the FAST1 device into the bone. E. Remove the delivery device. F. The FAST1 device is embedded in the manubrium. G. Connect the tubing that is affixed to the target patch to the FAST1 device.	Inserts the IO device.	Follow manufacturer's guidelines. It is *critical* that the FAST1 be held perpendicular to the sternum and *not* the patient's body. The amount of pressure needed to deliver the FAST1 device may necessitate the use of two hands.
8. BIG insertion (see Fig. 84-2): **(Level M*)** A. The BIG can be inserted into the proximal tibia or the humerus. B. Palpate the appropriate landmarks with the dominant hand, and with the nondominant hand, place the barrel of the BIG on the skin perpendicular to the intended insertion site.	Inserts the IO needle.	The BIG device is color coded. The adult device is blue.

*Level D: Peer-reviewed professional organizational standards with clinical studies to support recommendations
*Level M: Manufacturer's recommendations only

Procedure for Intraosseous Access—*Continued*

Steps	Rationale	Special Considerations
C. With the dominant hand, squeeze and remove the red safety latch. D. Grasp the "shoulders" of the BIG with the fingers of the dominant hand while the palm presses down into the BIG and deploys the needle and trocar. E. Remove the BIG and stabilize the needle. F. Remove the trocar from the needle and secure the needle to the skin by taping the red safety latch around it.		
9. EZ-IO insertion (see Fig. 84-4): **(Level M*)** A. The EZ-IO can be inserted into the proximal tibia, the distal tibia, or the humerus. B. Connect the appropriately sized needle to the power driver (Fig. 84-5). C. Palpate the appropriate landmark. D. Stabilize the limb and advance the needle at a 90-degree angle through the skin until the bone is felt. E. When the 5-mm mark is visible, apply steady, firm pressure and activate the power driver until the needle hub contacts the skin or a sudden decrease in resistance is noted. F. Stabilize the needle and remove the power driver. G. Remove the stylet from the needle by turning it counterclockwise while withdrawing it.	Inserts the IO needle.	Follow manufacturer's guidelines for selection of the size of the needle based on patient weight. If the 5-mm mark is not visible, the needle is withdrawn and a larger size is attached and advanced into the insertion site.

*Level M: Manufacturer's recommendations only

Procedure continues on following page

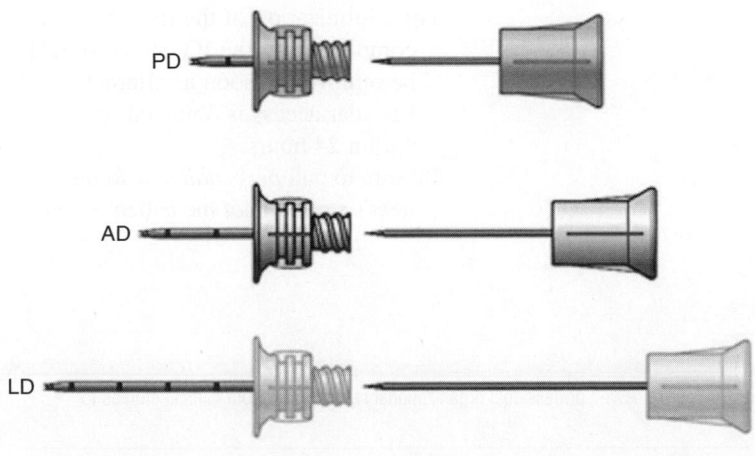

PD

AD

LD

FIGURE 84-5 EZ-IO needle sets. (*From Day MW: Intraossesous devices in the adult trauma patient, Crit Care Nurs. In press.*)

Procedure for Intraosseous Access—*Continued*

Steps	Rationale	Special Considerations
10. Secure the IO catheter or needle as recommended by the manufacturer.	Prevents the needle from moving.	
11. Apply a sterile, occlusive dressing.	Promotes a sterile environment.	

12. Confirm placement by:
  A. Aspirating blood or marrow.[2-4,7,11,14]
  B. Flushing the needle with 10 mL of normal saline solution.[2,3,7,11,14]
	Verifies needle placement in the marrow cavity.	If blood specimens are needed, attach a 5-mL syringe and aspirate bone marrow and blood from the site.[2,3,7,11,14]
		Follow institution standard. Aspiration of marrow may occlude the IO device with bone.[4]
		Lack of marrow aspirate does not indicate improper placement.
		If swelling or infiltration is observed, remove the IO device and attempt IO access in another bone.

13. Securely attach the tubing and tape it to the patient's skin.	Secures the tubing system.	Care should be taken when positioning and transferring the patient to avoid dislodgment of the IO device.
14. Infuse IV fluids with a pressure bag or manual pressure.	IO lines often need pressure to ensure adequate flow.	The pressure limits on infusion pumps may be exceeded by the resistance of fluid flow through an IO.
15. If the patient is alert, infuse lidocaine (without epinephrine) into the IO device as prescribed.[3,9-11] **(Level E*)**	Promotes comfort.	The infusion of fluids and medications can be painful to the conscious patient.
16. Administer prescribed medications via the IO device and follow each medication with a 5- to 10-mL normal saline solution flush as prescribed.[1,4] **(Level E)**	Following medications with a saline solution flush ensures delivery of medication into the marrow cavity and blood vessels.	
17. Discard used supplies in appropriate receptacles.	Removes and safely discards used supplies.	
18. **HH**		

Procedure for Removal of the Intraosseous Access

1. **HH**		
2. **PE**		
3. Replace the IO site within 24 hours or as soon as venous access is obtained.[10,11]	IO access is a temporary access site.	
4. Follow manufacturer's guidelines for removal:	IO device is no longer needed.	Follow manufacturer's guidelines. For minimization of the risk of complications, the IO device should be removed as soon as alternate vascular access is obtained or within 24 hours. Be sure to pull *perpendicular* to the patient's sternum *not* the patient's body.

A. FAST1:
    1. Grasp the IO device.
    2. Pull the IO device up, perpendicular to the manubrium.		

*Level E: Multiple case reports, theory-based evidence from expert opinions, or peer-reviewed professional organizational standards without clinical studies to support recommendations

Procedure for Intraosseous Access—*Continued*

Steps	Rationale	Special Considerations

B. BIG removal:
   1. Grasp the IO device hub with the red safety latch.
   2. Simultaneously rotate and withdraw the IO device.
 C. EZ-IO removal:
   1. Attach a 5 to 10 mL syringe to the hub of the IO device.
   2. Stabilize the limb.
   3. Simultaneously rotate clockwise and pull the IO device out.
   4. If the hub separates from the body of the IO device, grasp the body with large needle forceps and rotate the body and pull out.		

5. Apply an occlusive, sterile dressing to the site.	Promotes a sterile environment.	
6. Discard used supplies in appropriate receptacles.	Reduces the transmission of microorganisms; Standard Precautions. Safely removes sharp objects.	
7. 🄷🄷		

Expected Outcomes

- Access to venous circulation for the administration of medications and fluids
- The IO line remains patent
- The tip of the IO needle lies in the marrow cavity
- The insertion site, catheter, and systemic circulation remain free of infection

Unexpected Outcomes

- Inability to provide medications or fluids
- Infection
- Extravasation
- Complications such as compartment syndrome, fractures, osteomyelitis, and necrosis
- Pain

Patient Monitoring and Care

Steps	Rationale	Reportable Conditions
		These conditions should be reported if they persist despite nursing interventions.
1. Observe the IO insertion site for signs and symptoms of infection.	Identifies complication.	- Edema around the site - Pain, tenderness, or erythema around the site - Drainage from the site - Increased temperature - Elevated white blood cell (WBC) count
2. Observe the IO insertion site for signs and symptoms of extravasation or compartment syndrome.	A misplaced needle or excessive movement of the needle after insertion may lead to a leakage of fluids outside of the marrow cavity and can impair circulation to the extremity.	- Increased circumference of the extremity - Increased pain in the extremity - Change in extremity sensation, temperature, or pulses
3. Follow institution standard for assessing pain. Administer analgesia as prescribed.	Identifies need for pain interventions.	- Continued pain despite pain interventions

Procedure continues on following page

Documentation

Documentation should include the following:

- Patient and family education
- Preprocedure verification and time out.
- Site of insertion
- Number of IO insertion attempts
- Sites of previous IO insertion attempts
- Brand of the IO device inserted and if appropriate, manufacturer's needle description
- Confirmation of IO needle placement
- Date and time of insertion

- Type and amount of anesthetic used
- Assessment of insertion site
- Method of securing the IO needle in place
- Problems encountered during or after the procedure
- Pain assessment, interventions, and effectiveness
- Vital signs and cardiac rhythm
- Date and time the IO device is removed
- Assessment of site after the IO device is removed

References

1. American Heart Association: Access for medication, part 3: intraosseous access. In *Advanced cardiac life support provider manual, student CD*, 2006, AHA.
2. Bailey P: *Intraosseous cannulation, UpToDate database*, 2008, retrieved July 15, 2009. from www.uptodate.com/online/content/topic.do?topicKey=ped_proc/4947&view=print#, Waltham, MA.
3. Blumberg SM, Gorn M, Crain EF: Intraosseous infusion: a review of methods and novel devices, *Pediatr Emerg Care* 24:50-59, 2008.
4. Bosomworth NJ: The occasional intraosseous infusion, *Can J Rural Med* 13:80-83, 2008.
5. Buck ML, Wiggins BS, Sesler JM: Intraosseous drug administration in children and adults during cardiopulmonary resuscitation, *Ann Pharmacother* 41:1679-1686, 2007.
6. Day MW: Intraosseous devices in the adult trauma patient, *Crit Care Nurs*. In press.
CR 7. Gluckman W, Forti RJ: *Intraosseous cannulation, emedicine*, 2003, retrieved June 29, 2009, from http://emedicine.medscape.com/article/908610-overview.
8. Holleran RS: Procedure 67 intraosseous access. In Proehl J, editor: *Emergency nursing procedures*, ed 4, St Louis, 2009, Elsevier.
9. Infusion Nurses Society: *The role of the registered nurse in the insertion of intraosseous (IO) access devices, INS Position Statement*, 2009, INS, Norwood, MA.
10. Langley DM, Moran M: Intraosseous needles: not just for kids anymore, *J Emerg Nurs* 34:318-319, 2007.
11. MacKinnon KA: Intraosseous vascular use at Signature Healthcare Brockton Hospital Department of Emergency Services, *J Emerg Nurs*. In press, 2009.
12. Ong MEH, Chan YH, Oh JJ, et al: An observational, prospective study comparing tibial and humeral intraosseous access using the EZ-IO, *Am J Emerg Med* 27:8-15, 2009.
13. Von Hoff DD, Kuhn JG, Burris HA, et al: Does intraosseous equal intravenous? A pharmacokinetic study, *Am J Emerg Med* 26:31-38, 2008.
CR 14. Vreede E, Bulatovic A, Rosseel P, et al: *Article 10 intraosseous infusion, update in anesthesia, 12*, 2000, retrieved June 29, 2009, from www.nda.ox.ac.uk/wfsa/html/u12/u1210_01.htm.

Additional Readings

Brenner T, Bernhard M, Helm M, et al: Comparison of two intraosseous infusion systems for adult emergency medical use, *Resuscitation* 78:314-319, 2008.
CR Gunal I, Kose N, Gurer D: Compartment syndrome after intraosseous infusion: an experimental study in dogs, *J Pediatr Surg* 31(11):1491-1493, 1996.
CR Rosetti VA, Thompson BM, Miller J, et al: Intraosseous infusion: an alternative route of pediatric intravascular access, *Ann Emerg Med* 14:885-888, 1985.

PROCEDURE **85**

AP Peripherally Inserted Central Catheter

P U R P O S E : Peripherally inserted central catheters are used to deliver central venous therapy for up to 1 year and to provide venous access for patients who need multiple venipunctures. Peripherally inserted central catheters are used for administration of long-term antibiotic therapy, chemotherapy, total parenteral nutrition, analgesia, blood products, intermittent inotropic (e.g., dobutamine) therapy, power injections, and fluids. The length and type of therapy should determine the type of central venous access device selected.

Linda Bucher, Linda V. Sanderson

PREREQUISITE NURSING KNOWLEDGE

- Successful completion of specialized education in peripherally inserted central catheter (PICC) insertion and demonstrated competency are necessary.[5,6] In addition, opportunities to demonstrate clinical competency on a regular basis (e.g., yearly) may be needed.
- Clinical and technical competence is needed in suturing PICC lines in place (if permitted by registered nurse [RN] in state of practice).
- Sterile technique should be understood.
- Knowledge is necessary of the anatomy and physiology of the vasculature and adjacent structures in the upper extremity, neck, and chest.
- Ideally, the patient receiving a PICC should have a peripheral vein that can accommodate a 14- or 16-gauge introducer needle. If necessary, a 22-G microintroducer can be used to dilate a vein to accommodate an introducer sheath. The smallest device in the largest vein allows for maximal hemodilution of the infusate and minimizes the risk of phlebitis and thrombosis.[2]

- The basilic and cephalic antecubital fossa veins are the preferred veins for cannulation with a PICC (Fig. 85-1). The basilic vein is the larger of the two veins and is the vein of choice for insertion of a PICC. The cephalic vein has been associated with an increased risk of thrombosis and is the vein of choice for patients who need crutches. Patient preference for arm selection (e.g., nondominant hand, lifestyle, activity restrictions, ability to care for the catheter) should be considered with selection of the insertion site.[2] Once inserted, the PICC is advanced to the superior vena cava.[5,6]
- Patient indications for the insertion of a PICC are not limited to inpatient therapies. A PICC is used increasingly for patients receiving intravenous (IV) therapy in the home setting for chronic heart failure, cancer treatment, chronic pain management, nutritional support, and fluid replacement (e.g., hyperemesis gravidarum).
- PICCs may be preferred over percutaneously inserted central venous catheters for patients with trauma of the chest (e.g., burns) or certain pulmonary disorders (e.g., chronic obstructive pulmonary disease, cystic fibrosis).[7] PICCs eliminate the risks associated with insertion of percutaneously inserted central venous catheters in the neck or chest (e.g., pneumothorax).[2]
- PICCs are contraindicated in patients with sclerotic veins and a history of renal disease and in extremities affected by mastectomy, arteriovenous graft, fistula, or radial artery surgery.

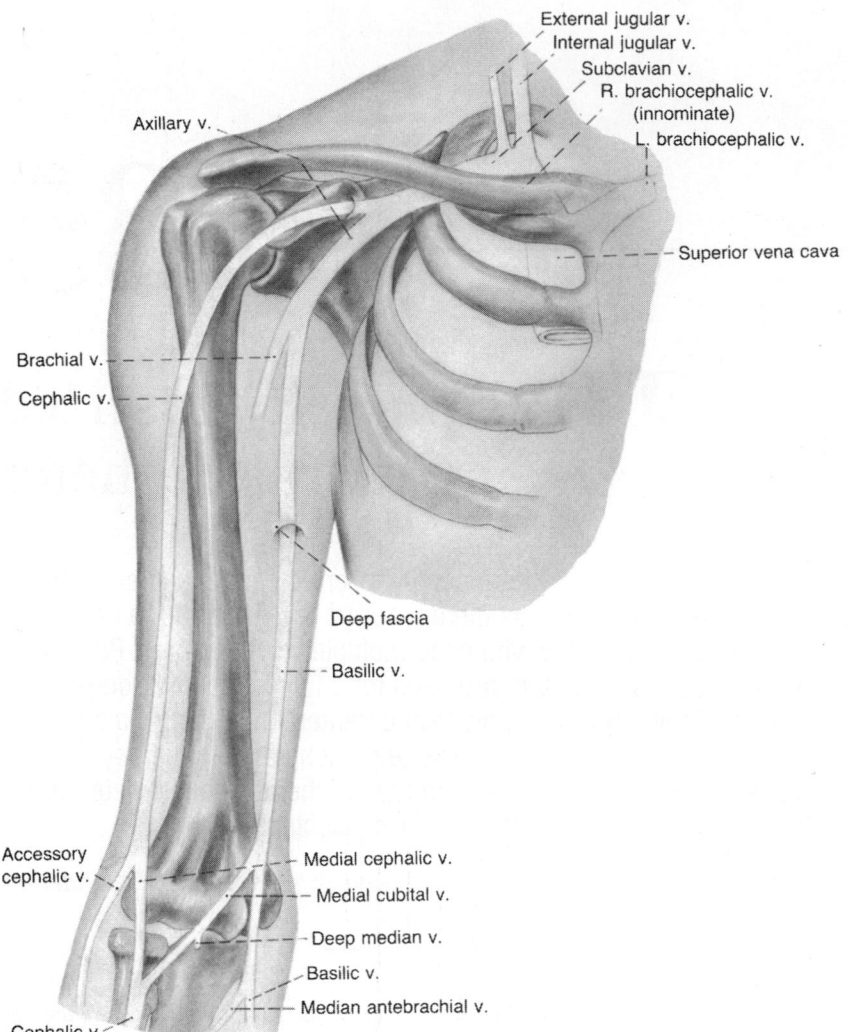

External jugular v.
Internal jugular v.
Subclavian v.
R. brachiocephalic v.
(innominate)
L. brachiocephalic v.

Axillary v.

Superior vena cava

Brachial v.
Cephalic v.

Deep fascia

Basilic v.

Accessory
cephalic v.

Medial cephalic v.

Medial cubital v.

Deep median v.

Basilic v.

Median antebrachial v.

Cephalic v.

FIGURE 85-1　Location of the veins of the right shoulder and upper arm. *(From Jacob SW, Francone CA: Elements of anatomy and physiology, ed 2, Philadelphia, 1989, Saunders.)*

- IV therapy via the PICC poses fewer and less severe complications (including infections) compared with percutaneously inserted central venous catheters. The most common complications associated with the PICC are phlebitis and catheter occlusion.[1,7]
- A variety of PICCs are available for use. PICCs are flexible catheters that are made of silicone or polyurethane. Catheter diameters range from 23 gauge to 16 gauge, and catheter length ranges from 40 cm (16 inches) to 60 cm (24 inches). For adults, 18- or 20-gauge catheters that are 60 cm in length are the standard. PICCs are available as single-lumen, double-lumen, and triple-lumen catheters, with and without valves. Some PICCs are designed to handle power injections (e.g., contrast media for computed tomographic [CT] scans).
- A PICC can be inserted with or without the use of a guidewire. When a guidewire is used, venous access is achieved with a small gauge (20- or 22-gauge) peripheral IV catheter. Once the IV catheter is inserted, the stylet is removed and the guidewire is threaded through the IV catheter. The IV catheter is then removed, and the dilator/introducer is inserted over the guidewire. The dilator and guidewire are removed, leaving the introducer in the

vein to allow for passage of the PICC into the vein. Once the PICC is in place, the introducer is removed. This approach is referred to as the modified Seldinger method.[2] Care must be taken with the use of a guidewire. Although advancement of the introducer is enhanced by the firmness provided by the guidewire, the guidewire can inadvertently traumatize the vessel.[7]
- A PICC can also be inserted through a cannula. This insertion involves a venipuncture with a short peripheral IV catheter. The stylet is removed, and the PICC is threaded into the vein. The short peripheral IV catheter is removed by pulling it over the end of the PICC.[2]
- Ultrasound scan technology is available to assist with vein assessment and PICC insertion (Fig. 85-2). Successful completion of specialized education is needed.
- A variety of safety-engineered introducers are available and should be used to reduce the risk for blood exposure and needle-stick injury.[5,6,9]
- Verification of the PICC tip placement requires a chest radiograph after insertion.[2,5,6,11]
- PICCs can be placed at the patient's bedside, in interventional radiology, or in specialized rooms dedicated for PICC insertion.

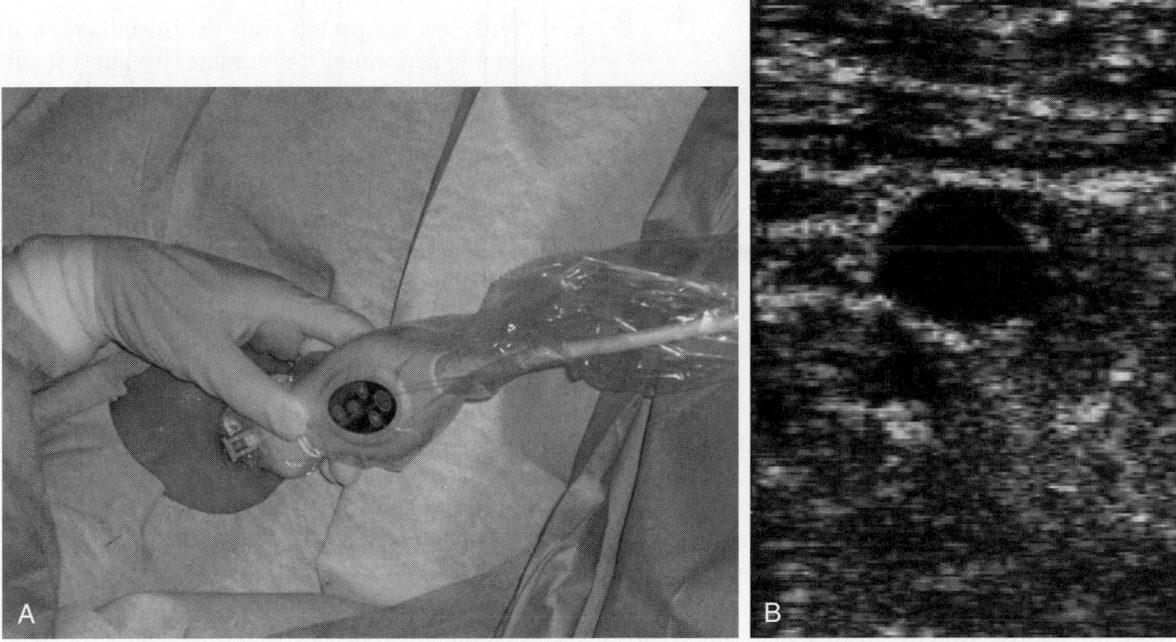

FIGURE 85-2 Use of ultrasound scan technology to assist with vein location. **A,** Ultrasound scan probe is positioned over the insertion site. **B,** Depiction of ultrasound scan–assisted catheter insertion. *(Courtesy of Bard Access Systems, Salt Lake City.)*

EQUIPMENT

- Catheter insertion kit
- PICC catheter of choice
- Single-use tourniquet or blood pressure cuff
- Sterile and nonsterile measuring tape
- Waterproof underpad/linen saver
- Sterile gown
- Head cover
- Mask
- Goggles
- Two pairs of nonpowdered sterile gloves
- Sterile drapes and towels, including one fenestrated drape
- Antiseptic solution (e.g., 2% chlorhexidine-based preparation)
- 10-mL vial of heparin (concentration and use per institution policy)
- 30-mL vial of normal saline (NS) solution
- Luer-Lok injection port (cap) with short extension tubing
- One to three 10-mL, 20-gauge, 1-inch needle syringes (blunt needles recommended), depending on the number of lumens
- Sterile 4 × 4 gauze pads or sponges
- 1% lidocaine without epinephrine, or 1 to 2 mL of eutectic mixture of local anesthetics (EMLA) cream (optional)
- Sterile 2 × 2 gauze pads or sponges
- Sterile, transparent, semipermeable dressing

Additional equipment as needed includes the following:
- One 1-mL, 25-gauge, 5/8-inch needle syringe (if intradermal lidocaine is used)
- One 3-0 or 4-0 nylon suture on a small, curved cutting needle (if suturing is used)
- Alternative catheter securement device (e.g., sterile wound closure strips; if suturing is not used)

PATIENT AND FAMILY EDUCATION

- Explain the reason for the PICC, the benefits and risks associated with the catheter, and the alternatives to PICC placement. ➻*Rationale:* Clarification of information is an expressed patient need and helps to diminish anxiety, enhance acceptance, and encourage questions.
- Describe the major steps of the procedure, including the patient's role in the procedure. ➻*Rationale:* Explanation decreases patient anxiety, enhances cooperation, provides an opportunity for the patient to voice concerns, and prevents accidental contamination of the sterile field and equipment.
- Instruct the patient and family to refuse injections, venipunctures, and blood pressure measurements on the arm with the PICC. ➻*Rationale:* The risk for catheter-related complications and catheter damage is minimized.
- Provide appropriate patient and family discharge education regarding the care and maintenance of the PICC. ➻*Rationale:* Education reduces the risk for catheter-related complications from lack of knowledge and skills needed to care for the PICC after discharge.

PATIENT ASSESSMENT AND PREPARATION

Patient Assessment

- Assess the patient's medical history for mastectomy, fistula, shunt, or radial artery surgery. ➺*Rationale:* PICC insertion should be avoided in extremities affected by these conditions to preserve veins for future needs and because the risk for complications is increased.
- Obtain the patient's baseline vital signs and cardiac rhythm. ➺*Rationale:* Cardiac dysrhythmias can occur if the catheter is advanced into the heart. Baseline data facilitate the identification of clinical problems and the efficacy of interventions.
- Assess the vasculature of the antecubital space of both arms, focusing on the basilic and cephalic veins (see Fig. 85-1). A tourniquet or blood pressure cuff should be applied on the mid–upper arm for vein assessment and then removed. ➺*Rationale:* Proper vein selection increases the success of insertion and decreases the incidence of postinsertion complications.
- Determine the patient's allergy history (e.g., lidocaine, heparin, EMLA cream, antiseptic solutions, tape, latex). ➺*Rationale:* Assessment decreases the risk for allergic reactions with avoidance of known allergenic products.

Patient Preparation

- Verify correct patient with two identifiers. ➺*Rationale:* Prior to performing a procedure, the nurse should ensure the correct identification of the patient for the intended intervention.
- Ensure that the patient and family understand preprocedural teaching. Answer questions as they arise, and reinforce information as needed. ➺*Rationale:* Understanding of previously taught information is evaluated and reinforced.
- Ensure that informed consent has been obtained. ➺*Rationale:* Informed consent protects the rights of the patient and allows the patient to make a competent decision.
- Perform a pre-procedure verification and time out, if non-emergent.➺*Rationale:* Ensures patient safety.
- Assist the patient to a semi-Fowler or dorsal recumbent position, depending on the patient's clinical condition and level of comfort. ➺*Rationale:* The upright position allows gravity to assist in directing the catheter downward when the catheter is advanced into the innominate vein and superior vena cava. It also may help avoid inadvertent placement of the catheter into the jugular vein.
- Position the selected arm at 45 degrees of extension from the body for anthropometric measurement. For catheter placement in the superior vena cava, use the nonsterile measuring tape to measure the distance from the selected insertion site to the shoulder (Fig. 85-3, *A*) and from the shoulder to the sternal notch (Fig. 85-3, *B*). Add 3 inches (7.5 cm; or the measured distance from the sternal notch to the third intercostal space) to this number for catheter placement in the superior vena cava. ➺*Rationale:* Extension of the extremity allows for displacement of the catheter with arm movement. Accurate measurement

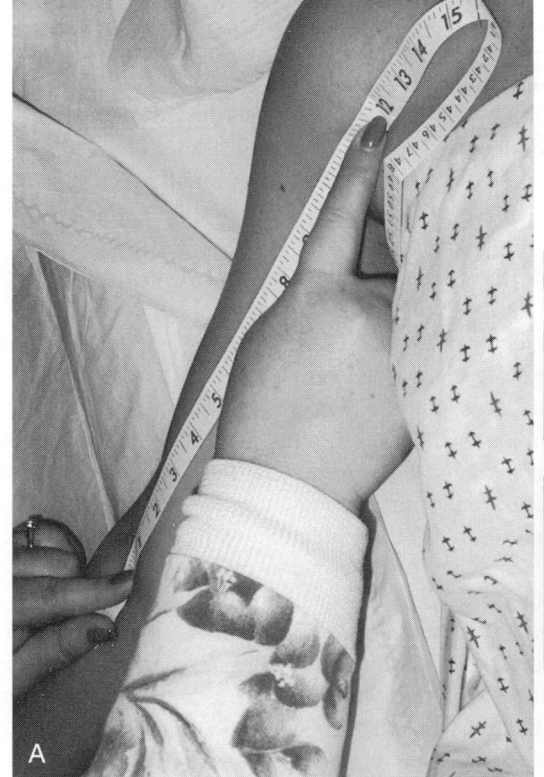

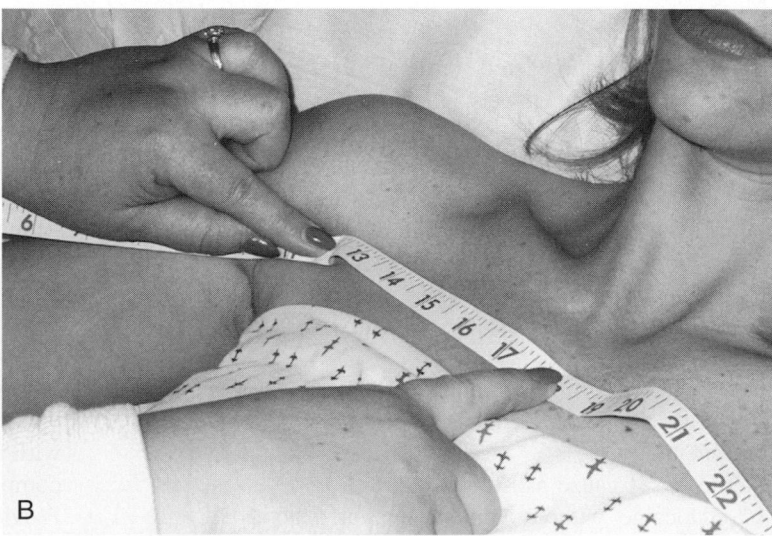

FIGURE 85-3 Measurement of the catheter length for placement in the superior vena cava. **A,** First, measure the distance from the selected insertion site to the shoulder. **B,** Continue measuring from the shoulder to the sternal notch and add 3 inches (7.5 cm) to this number.

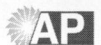

ensures proper tip position in the superior vena cava and determines the length of the catheter to be inserted.

- Measure the mid–upper arm circumference of the selected extremity. ➤*Rationale:* Measurement provides a baseline for evaluation of suspected thrombosis. Increases of greater than 2 cm over baseline are supportive of venous occlusion.
- Stabilize the position of the arm with a towel or pillow. ➤*Rationale:* Stabilization increases patient comfort, secures the work area, and facilitates access to the selected vein.

- Instruct the patient on proper head positioning. The head is positioned to the contralateral side (away from the insertion site) throughout the procedure, except when the catheter is advanced from the axillary vein to the superior vena cava. At this point, the patient is instructed to position his or her head toward the ipsilateral side (toward the insertion site) with the chin dropped to the shoulder. ➤*Rationale:* Proper positioning limits the risk for the catheter being inadvertently directed into the jugular vein.

Procedure for Peripherally Inserted Central Catheter

Steps	Rationale	Special Considerations
1. **HH**		
2. **PE**		
3. Place a waterproof pad under the selected arm.	Avoids soiling of bed linens.	
4. Wash the insertion area with soap and water.	Prepares insertion site.	
5. Discard used supplies and remove gloves.	Removes and safely discards used supplies.	
6. **HH**		
7. With the measuring tape, perform the preinsertion anatomic measurements (see Fig. 85-3). Make a note of the required catheter length.	Catheters are provided at various lengths.	
8. Position the tourniquet high on the upper extremity, near the axilla, but do not constrict venous blood flow at this time.	Placement high on the extremity avoids contamination of the sterile field.	A blood pressure cuff may be used in place of a tourniquet.
9. Open the PICC insertion tray and drop the remaining sterile items onto the sterile field.	Maintains aseptic technique; prepares the work area, including procurement of all necessary equipment; avoids interruption of the procedure and contamination of the work area.	
10. **HH**		
11. Apply sterile gown and sterile gloves.	PICC insertion is a sterile procedure.	Personnel protective equipment (e.g., head cover, mask, goggles) is needed as well as sterile equipment. Blood splashing may occur with the use of guidewires, stylets, and breakaway or peel-away introducers.
12. Prepare the catheter according to manufacturer's recommendations.	Each manufacturer recommends a specific preparation protocol for each type of catheter.	
13. Fill the 10-mL syringe with NS. Add the injection port (cap) to the short extension tubing and prime it with NS. Leave the syringe attached.	Prepares the system.	If inserting a double-lumen or triple-lumen catheter, prime the additional lumen of the catheter with NS.

Procedure continues on following page

Procedure for Peripherally Inserted Central Catheter—*Continued*

Steps	Rationale	Special Considerations
14. Prepare the site with a 2% chlorhexidine-based antiseptic solution.[1,5,6] Cleanse the site with a back-and-forth motion while applying friction for 30 seconds. Allow the antiseptic to remain on the insertion site and to air-dry completely before catheter insertion.[1,5,6] **(Level D*)**	Limits the introduction of potentially infectious skin flora into the vessel during the puncture.	
15. Discard gloves in the appropriate receptacle.	Removes and safely discards used supplies.	
16. 🖐		
17. Apply the tourniquet (or blood pressure cuff) snugly, approximately 6 inches (15 cm) above the antecubital fossa.	Provides vasodilation of the vein for venipuncture.	Constriction should effectively cause venous distention without arterial occlusion. A blood pressure cuff may be used and may be more effective, especially if the patient is obese. After the cuff is inflated, palpate the radial artery to assess for arterial blood flow.
18. Apply a new pair of sterile gloves.	PICC insertion is a sterile procedure.	
19. Instruct the patient to lift his or her arm; place a sterile drape underneath and the fenestrated drape over the prepared area, leaving the venipuncture site exposed. Place a sterile 4 × 4 gauze pad over the tourniquet.	Maintains the sterile field and facilitates aseptic technique.	Use of ultrasound scan technology may be used to assist with catheter insertion (see Fig. 85-2).
20. Instruct the patient to turn his or her head away from the insertion site.	Prevents contamination of the field by organisms from the patient's respiratory tract.	
21. Inject a skin weal of approximately 0.5 mL of 1% lidocaine without epinephrine at or adjacent to the venipuncture site. **(Level B*)**	Provides local anesthesia for venipuncture with large-gauge needles and introducers. Local anesthesia should be administered with insertion of a PICC.[3-6,8,10]	Patients report less pain when a local anesthetic agent is used before venipuncture.[3,4] Lidocaine may produce stinging, burning, obliteration of the vein, or venospasm. The use of EMLA (a topical anesthetic cream) before venipuncture has been researched.[3,8,10] If it is used, manufacturer's recommendations should be followed.
22. Perform the venipuncture according to catheter design and manufacturer's instructions.	Catheters vary according to design and introducing techniques.	

*Level B: Well-designed, controlled studies with results that consistently support a specific action, intervention, or treatment
*Level D: Peer-reviewed professional organizational standards with clinical studies to support recommendations

Procedure | for Peripherally Inserted Central Catheter—*Continued*

Steps	Rationale	Special Considerations
23. Perform the modified Seldinger technique (Fig. 85-4):		
A. Insert a peripheral IV and observe for blood return in the flashback chamber (see Fig. 85-4, *1*).		Place a finger over the orifice of the catheter to limit blood loss and risk for air embolism (see Fig. 85-4, *2*).
B. Remove the stylet and advance the guidewire 2 to 4 inches (5 to 10 cm) through the IV catheter (see Fig. 85-4, *2*).[7]		If no blood return is found, the procedure should be terminated and an alternate access site selected.
C. Remove the IV catheter and insert the dilator/introducer over the guidewire (see Fig. 85-4, *4*).	Use of a guidewire enhances the advancement of the dilator/introducer.	A small skin nick may be performed at the venipuncture site to facilitate the advancement of the dilator/introducer (see Fig. 85-4, *3*). If a scalpel is not provided in the PICC insertion kit, a no. 11 blade should be used.
D. Gently advance the dilator/introducer until the tip is well within the vein (see Fig. 85-4, *5*).		
E. Remove the dilator and guidewire, leaving the introducer in place (see Fig. 85-4, *6*).[7]		Place a finger over the orifice of the introducer to limit blood loss and the risk for air embolism (see Fig. 85-4, *6*).
F. Insert the catheter approximately 6 to 8 inches (15 to 20 cm).	Establishes venous access.	Sterile forceps may be used to insert the catheter into the introducer and advance the catheter into the vein (see Fig. 85-4, *7*).
24. Release the tourniquet with sterile technique (e.g., with a sterile 4 × 4 gauze pad).	Continued vasodilation may not be necessary for catheter advancement.	If a blood pressure cuff is used, it may remain inflated throughout the advancement of the catheter. Leaving the tourniquet in place (or the blood pressure cuff inflated) may facilitate catheter advancement if vascular insufficiency is evident.
25. Instruct the patient to turn his or her head toward the cannulated arm and to drop his or her chin to the chest.	Changes the angle of the jugular vein and decreases the potential for malpositioning of the catheter in the jugular vein.	
26. Advance the remainder of the catheter until approximately 4 inches (10 cm) remain. Observe the heart rate and rhythm.	Cardiac dysrhythmias may occur if the catheter is advanced into the heart.	Never advance the catheter if resistance is felt. Excessive pushing could lead to perforation of the vein or myocardium.
27. Instruct the patient to return his or her head to the contralateral side (away from the insertion site).	Prevents contamination of the field by organisms from the patient's respiratory tract.	
28. Pull the introducer out of the vein and away from the insertion site and remove (see Fig. 85-4, *8* and *9*).	The introducer sheath is not needed once the catheter is in place.	Methods of removing the introducer vary according to the manufacturer.

Procedure continues on following page

Modified Seldinger Technique

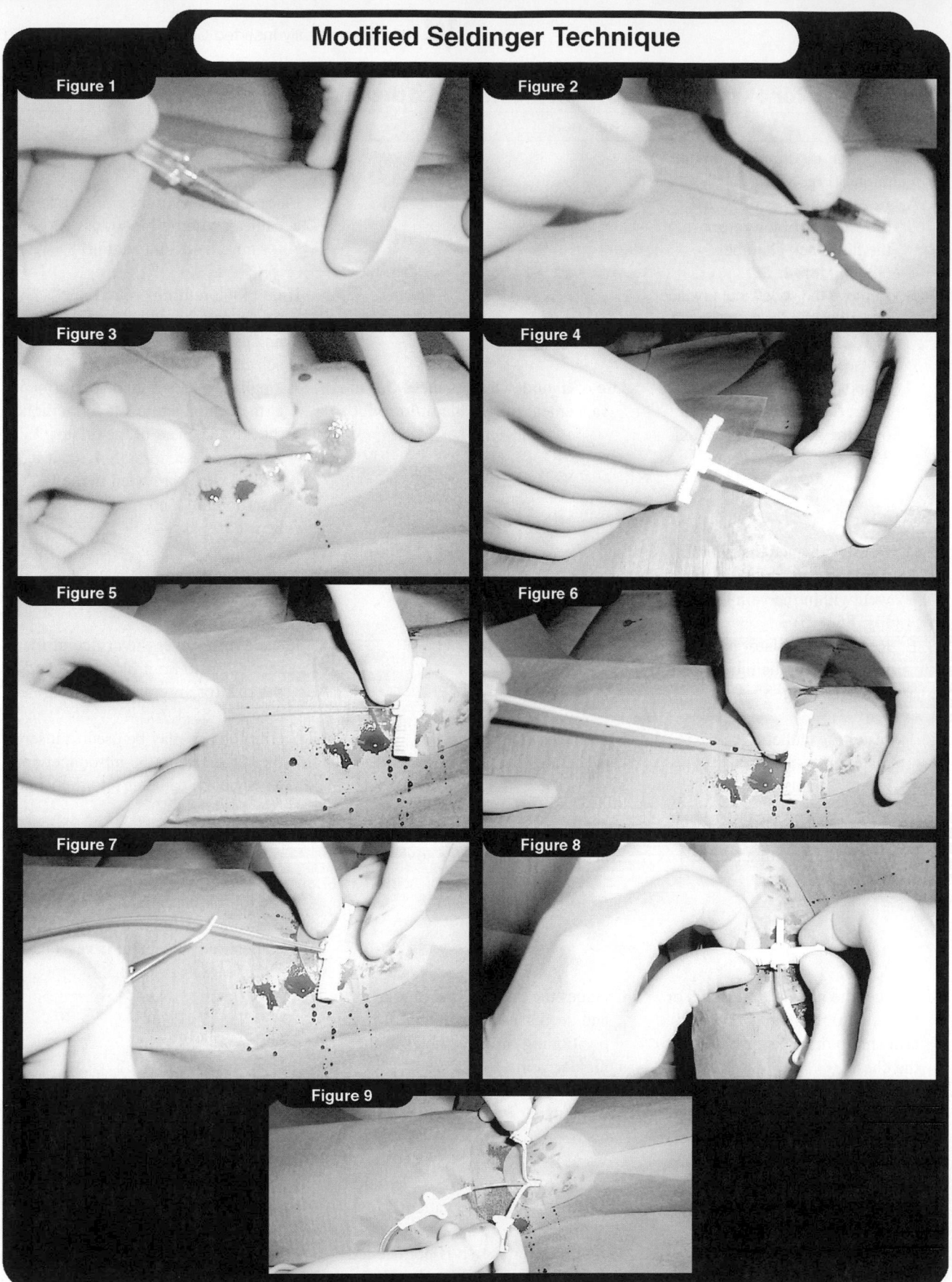

FIGURE 85-4   Modified Seldinger technique. **1,** Insertion of the peripheral intravenous catheter. **2,** Advancement of the guidewire through the catheter. **3,** Small skin nick to facilitate the advancement of the dilator/introducer. **4,** Insertion of the dilator/introducer over the guidewire. **5,** Advancement of the dilator/introducer. **6,** Removal of the dilator and guidewire. **7,** Insertion of the catheter using sterile forceps. **8,** Removal of the introducer. **9,** Introducer peeled apart and removed. *(Courtesy Bard Access Systems, Salt Lake City, UT.)*

Procedure for Peripherally Inserted Central Catheter—*Continued*

Steps	Rationale	Special Considerations
29. Measure the length of the catheter remaining outside the skin and reposition, if necessary, to the predetermined length. Approximately 1 inch (2.5 cm) of the catheter should remain externally.	Ensures proper catheter tip position.	
30. Attach the primed extension tubing (with injection port) to the catheter; aspirate for evidence of blood, and flush with NS with use of a push/pause technique.	Use of extension tubing provides easier access to the catheter and reduces local trauma at the insertion site. Aspiration affirms patency of the catheter. The push/pause technique during flushing optimizes catheter long-term patency.[5,6]	
31. Inject the recommended amount and concentration of heparin as prescribed into the catheter, clamp the extension tubing, and remove the syringe. Repeat the procedure with use of a double-lumen or triple-lumen catheter.	Maintains catheter patency and prevents backflow of blood in the catheter.	Recommendations vary regarding the use, amount, and concentration of heparin to maintain catheter patency.[2,11] Contraindicated in persons with known allergies to heparin. Institution standards should be followed.
32. Secure the catheter at the insertion site by suturing or by applying an alternate catheter securement device (Fig. 85-5).	Prevents inward or outward migration of the catheter.	A nylon suture is recommended. Follow institution standard.
33. Cover the insertion site with a sterile, 2 × 2 gauze pad. Cover the site with a sterile, transparent, semipermeable dressing.[7]	Decreases catheter-related infections.	A 2 × 2 gauze can be folded and placed immediately below the insertion site to act as a "wick" for any drainage in the first 24 hours. It is not needed after the first dressing change, thus will be in place for only 24 hours.
34. Discard used supplies in appropriate receptacles.	Reduces the transmission of microorganisms; Standard Precautions. Safely removes sharp objects.	
35. **HH**		
36. Prepare the patient for a chest radiograph.	Confirms placement of the catheter tip and detects any complications.	Some PICCs require contrast media for good visualization. Infusions should not be initiated until the catheter tip placement is confirmed.

Expected Outcomes

- The PICC tip is positioned in the superior vena cava
- The PICC remains patent
- The insertion site and upper extremity remain free of phlebitis and thrombophlebitis
- The insertion site, catheter, and systemic circulation remain free of infection

Unexpected Outcomes

- Pain or severe discomfort during the procedure
- Complications on insertion, such as cardiac dysrhythmias, pericardial tamponade, air embolism, catheter embolism, arterial puncture, and nerve (brachial plexus) injury
- Complications after insertion, such as phlebitis, thrombophlebitis, catheter occlusion, infection (e.g., insertion site, catheter, systemic), and infiltration

Procedure continues on following page

Patient Monitoring and Care

Steps	Rationale	Reportable Conditions
		These conditions should be reported if they persist despite nursing interventions.
1. Observe the patient for signs or symptoms of cardiac dysrhythmias and pericardial tamponade during the procedure. If cardiac dysrhythmias occur, pull the catheter back and reassess the patient.	Cardiac dysrhythmias may occur if the catheter is advanced into the heart. Pericardial tamponade may occur if the catheter penetrates the atrium.	• Cardiac dysrhythmias • Hemodynamic instability (changes in vital signs, level of consciousness, peripheral pulses, narrow pulse pressure, jugular venous distention)
2. Assess the patient and obtain the chest radiographic report confirming proper catheter tip placement before initiating any intravenous solutions.	Ensures accurate catheter tip placement and aids in identification of potentially life-threatening complications.	• Abnormal chest radiographic report • Change in lung sounds • Chest pain • Respiratory distress
3. Observe the dressing and insertion site every 30 minutes for the first 4 hours after insertion.	Postinsertion bleeding may occur in patients with coagulopathies or with arterial punctures, multiple attempts at venipuncture, or use of the through-the-needle introducer design for insertion.	• Excessive bleeding, hematoma • Abnormal vital signs

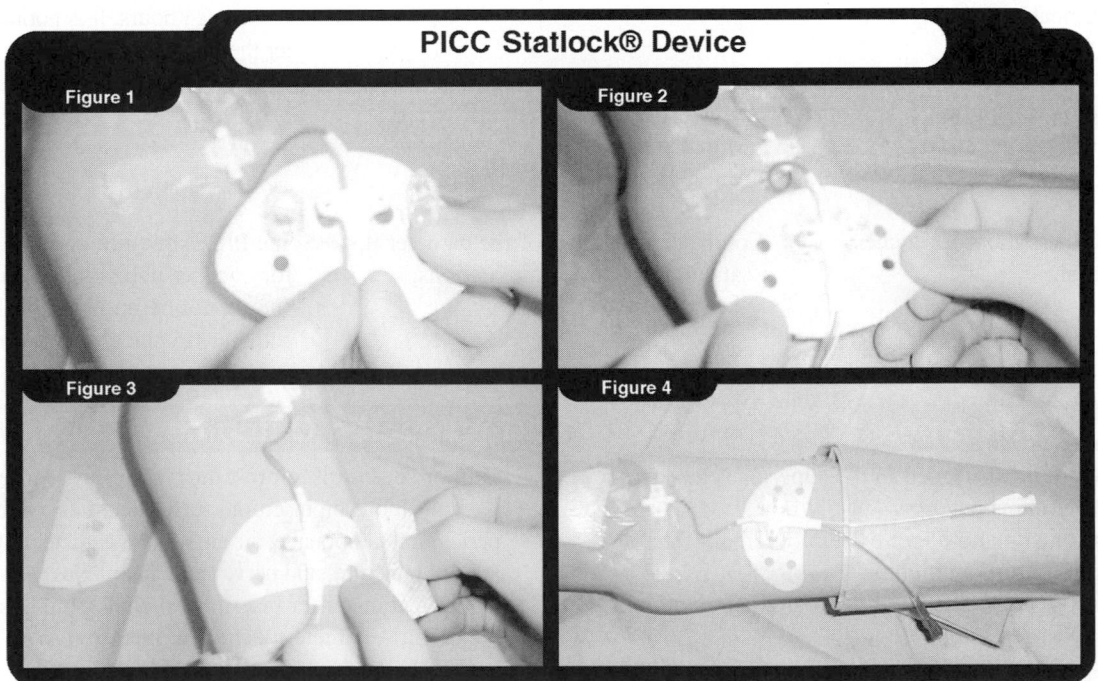

FIGURE 85-5   PICC Statlock device. **1,** Insertion of the wings of the PICC onto the device. **2,** Placement of the device on the forearm. **3,** Application of the sterile, transparent, semipermeable dressing over the device. **4,** Device properly secured. *(Courtesy Bard Access Systems, Salt Lake City UT.)*

Patient Monitoring and Care —*Continued*

Steps	Rationale	Reportable Conditions
4. Assess the insertion site and upper extremity every shift for signs and symptoms of phlebitis, thrombophlebitis, or infiltration.	Mechanical phlebitis is the most common complication within the first 72 hours after insertion. Thrombophlebitis may occur within 0 to 10 days of catheter insertion.	• Pain along the vein • Edema at the puncture site • Erythema • Ipsilateral swelling of the arm, neck, or face • Venous occlusion (changes in arm circumference greater than 2 cm from baseline) • Infiltration (infusion continues in spite of restriction to venous blood flow by tourniquet)
5. Assess the catheter for venous blood return and patency before initiating infusions. Connect a 10-mL syringe filled with 10 mL of NS to the extension tubing. Release the clamp and aspirate slowly to verify blood return. Flush with 10 mL of NS (with a push/pause technique) and then administer the infusion.	Verifies position of the catheter in the vascular space and patency before initiation of infusions.	• Catheter occlusion (failure to obtain blood return on aspiration or resistance to irrigation)
6. Assess the catheter for dislodgment or migration by measuring the length of the external catheter.	The catheter may no longer be properly positioned if the length of the external catheter is longer or shorter than the length measured at the time of insertion.	• Change in external catheter length • Catheter occlusion • Cardiac dysrhythmias • Pain or burning during infusions • Palpation of the catheter in the internal jugular vein • Palpation of a coiled catheter • Infiltration
7. The initial dressing should be left in place for 24 hours. After this, assess the insertion site and upper forearm while performing a sterile dressing change. Transparent, semipermeable dressings should be changed at least weekly.[1] Sterile gauze dressings should be changed every 48 hours.[5,6] Dressings should be changed if they become damp, loosened, or visibly soiled.[1]	Policies may vary regarding the type of dressing and frequency of dressing changes after the initial dressing change.	• Redness, warmth, hardness, tenderness or pain, or swelling at the insertion site • Presence of purulent drainage from the insertion site • Local rash or pustules
8. Monitor the insertion site and patient for signs and symptoms of local or systemic infection.	The incidence of infection related to the catheter may result from failure to maintain asepsis during insertion, failure to comply with dressing change protocols, immunosuppression, frequent access to the catheter, and long-term use of a single IV access site.	• Redness, warmth, hardness, tenderness or pain, or swelling at the insertion site • Presence of purulent drainage from the insertion site • Local rash or pustules • Fever, chills, or elevated white blood cell count • Nausea and vomiting

Procedure continues on following page

Patient Monitoring and Care —*Continued*

Steps	Rationale	Reportable Conditions
9. Avoid measuring blood pressure, performing venipunctures, or administering injections in the extremity with a PICC. Follow institution standard regarding placing a sign at the patient bedside regarding avoiding use of the extremity with the PICC.	Minimizes the risk for catheter-related complications and catheter damage.	
10. Follow institution standard for assessing pain. Administer analgesia as prescribed.	Identifies need for pain interventions.	• Continued pain despite pain interventions

Documentation

Documentation should include the following:

- Patient and family education
- Completion of informed consent
- Preprocedure verification and time-out
- Known allergies
- Mid–upper arm circumference
- Date and time of the procedure
- Catheter type, size, and length, including the length of catheter remaining outside the insertion site
- Type and amount of local anesthetic (if used)
- The location of the PICC insertion site and the vein accessed
- The method of securing catheter (suture, Steri-Strips)
- Confirmation of the catheter tip placement
- Problems encountered during or after the procedure or nursing interventions
- Patient tolerance of the procedure
- Pain assessment, interventions, and effectiveness
- Vital signs and cardiac rhythm
- Assessment of the insertion site

References

CR 1. Centers for Disease Control and Prevention: Guidelines for the prevention of intravascular catheter-related infections, *MMWR* 51(RR-10):2-29, 2002.

CR 2. Eddins J: Central venous access. In Phillips L, editor: *Manual of I.V. therapeutics,* ed 4, Philadelphia, 2005, F.A. Davis.

CR 3. Fetzer SJ: Reducing venipuncture and intravenous insertion pain with eutectic mixture of local anesthetic: a meta-analysis, *Nurs Res* 51:119-124, 2002.

CR 4. Hussey VM, Poulin MV, Fain JA: Effectiveness of lidocaine hydrochloride on venipuncture sites, *AORN J* 66:472-475, 1997.

5. Infusion Nurses Society: *Policies and procedures for infusion nursing,* ed 3, Norwood, MA, 2006, INS.

6. Intravenous Nurses Society: Infusion nursing standards of practice, *J Infus Nurs* 29(1S):S1-S90, 2006.

CR 7. Josephson DL: *Intravenous infusion therapy for nurses,* ed 2, Clifton Park, NY, 2004, Thomson Delmar Learning.

CR 8. Lander J, et al: Evaluation of a new topical anesthetic agent: a pilot study, *Nurs Res* 45:50-52, 1996.

CR 9. National Committee on Safer Needle Devices: *Using safer needle devices: the time is now,* Washington, DC, 1997, National Committee on Safer Needle Devices.

CR 10. Nott M, Peacock J: Relief of injection pain in adults: EMLA cream for 5 minutes before venipuncture, *Anaesthesia* 45:772-774, 1990.

CR 11. Oncology Nursing Society (ONS): *Access device guidelines: recommendations for nursing practice and education,* ed 2, Pittsburgh, 2004, ONS.

Additional Readings

Alexander M, Corrigan A, Gorski L, Hankins J, Perucca R. editors. Infusion Nurses Society: *Infusion Nursing: An evidence-based approach,* ed 3, 2010, Saunders.

CR Potter PA, Perry AG, editors: *Basic nursing: a critical thinking approach,* ed 5, St Louis, 2003, Mosby.

Weinstein SM: *Plumer's principles and practice of intravenous therapy,* ed 8, Philadelphia, 2006, Lippincott Williams & Wilkins.

Unit III
Neurologic
System

SECTION TWELVE

Neurologic Monitoring

PROCEDURE

86

Bispectral Index Monitoring

P U R P O S E : The bispectral index is a processed electro-encephalogram-based parameter used in critically ill adults for assessment of level of consciousness and response to sedative, hypnotic, and anesthetic agents.[1-4,10,13,16] The bispectral index also may indicate an arousal response to painful stimulation.[2] Information derived from bispectral index monitoring may be used to guide sedative, hypnotic, and analgesic therapy.[2,4,10,16]

Richard B. Arbour

PREREQUISITE NURSING KNOWLEDGE

- Understanding of cerebral physiology is needed.
- Sedative, hypnotic, anesthetic, and analgesic agents produce clinical effects as a result of binding, in a dose-related manner, with specific receptors in the brain modulating cerebral physiology.[24,34]
- Understanding of the interrelationship between the electrical activity of the brain and cerebral metabolism is necessary.
- Electroencephalogram (EEG) tracings are obtained and recorded through the application of scalp electrodes and detect electrical activity in the brain.[33]

- Examination of EEG waveforms provides a complement to central nervous system (CNS) evaluation obtained through clinical neurologic assessment.
- On its basic level, EEG activity requires multiple energy-using steps, which need to occur in succession. These steps include electrical impulse discharge at the thalamus and impulse conduction to the cerebral cortex with associated presynaptic release of neurotransmitters.
- Any clinical state or therapy that affects cerebral metabolism may also affect the EEG.[12,18,22,30]
- See Table 86-1 for terminology associated with bispectral index (BIS) technology.
- The close relationship between BIS and EEG activity should be understood.[25,33,35,36]

TABLE 86-1	Bispectral Index Monitoring Terminology
Bispectral Index (BIS)	Processed EEG that assesses level of consciousness and response to sedative, hypnotic, and analgesic therapy.
Digital Signal Converter (DSC)	Amplifies, filters, and digitizes the patient's EEG signals.
Electroencephalogram (EEG)	Measures electrical activity of the brain.
Electromyelograph (EMG)	Measures the presence of muscle activity or detects high frequency artifact from patient care devices.
Signal Quality Index (SQI)	A measure of the signal quality for the EEG channel source and is calculated based on impedance to electronic signal, electrode contact artifact and other variables.
Suppression Ratio (SR)	Percentage of EEG suppression (isoelectric EEG) over the past 63 seconds of collected data.

- When BIS monitoring is initiated, a sensor is placed across the patient's forehead per manufacturer recommendations to detect one channel of EEG activity (Fig. 86-1).
- EEG activity is then subjected to multiple processing steps.

❖ The EEG signal is filtered and digitized within the amplifier head box (digital signal converter [DSC])[2-4] (Fig. 86-4, *A*) or BISx[5-7] near the patient's head (Fig. 86-2, *A* and 86-3, *A*).
❖ Artifacts (low-frequency and high-frequency) are eliminated.

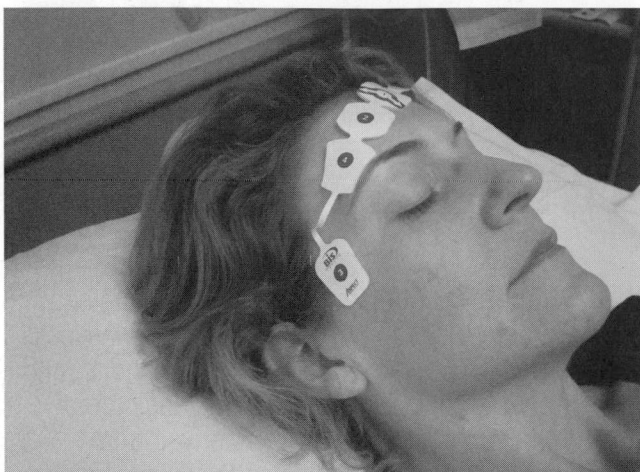

FIGURE 86-1   BIS sensor in place illustrating anatomic landmarks for optimal sensor placement. BIS Extend sensor in place. Sensor may be placed on right or left side.

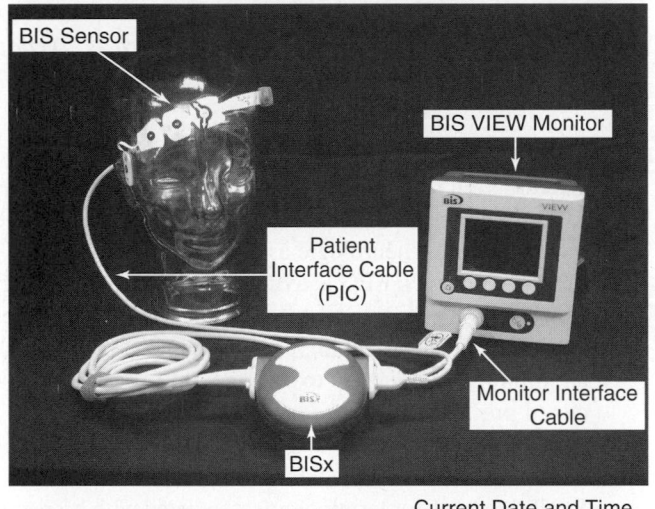

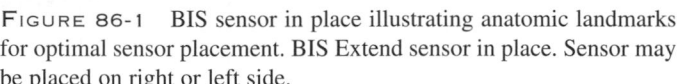

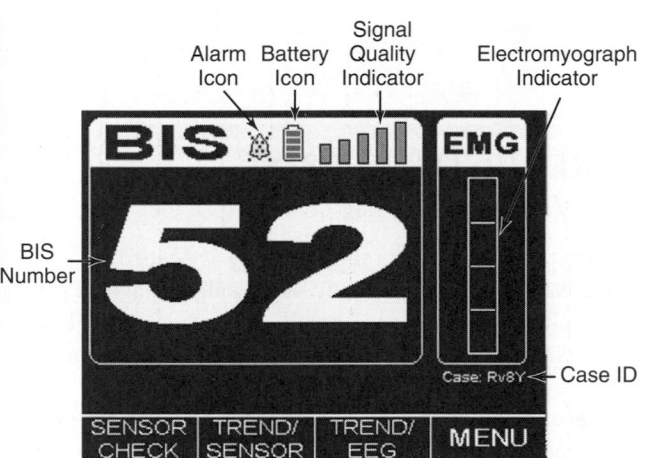

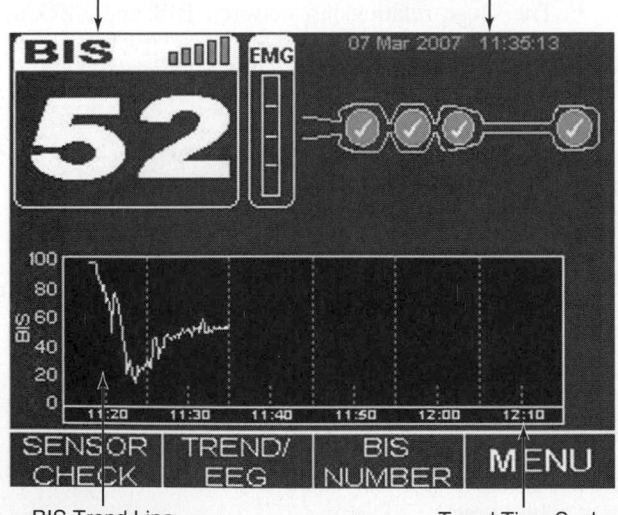

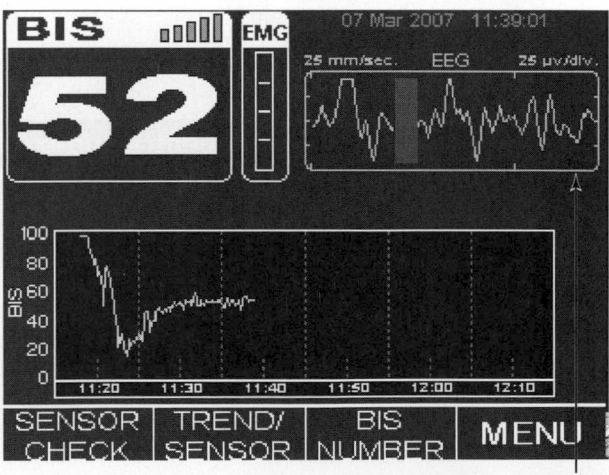

FIGURE 86-2   BIS VIEW monitoring system, including location of menu and power control keys, BISx, BIS index/trend, EMG, EEG, and sensor status displays. (*Courtesy Aspect Medical Systems, Norwood, MA.*)

❖ Multiple processing steps are applied for calculation of a specific EEG state (frequency and amplitude) associated with the level of sedation, arousal, or anesthesia.

❖ The level of EEG suppression and near suppression is determined.

❖ The EEG features are combined to form the BIS, a single value that correlates with the level of consciousness and the specific EEG state.[3,10,33,36]

❖ The BIS value is a single number based on the previous 10 to 30 seconds of EEG data (depending on the smoothing rate setting on the monitoring system) and is updated frequently; thus, changes in BIS value may lag behind clinical changes.[5,6]

❖ The BIS monitor provides a single channel of an EEG tracing from the right or left frontal-temporal montage electrode placement (BIS A2000™, BIS VISTA™, BIS VIEW™; Fig. 86-4B).[3-6]

• The BIS monitor may also provide bilateral EEG data acquisition from right and left frontal-temporal electrode placement (BIS VISTA bilateral monitoring system).[7]

• Understanding of factors that affect cerebral metabolism and EEG activity is needed.

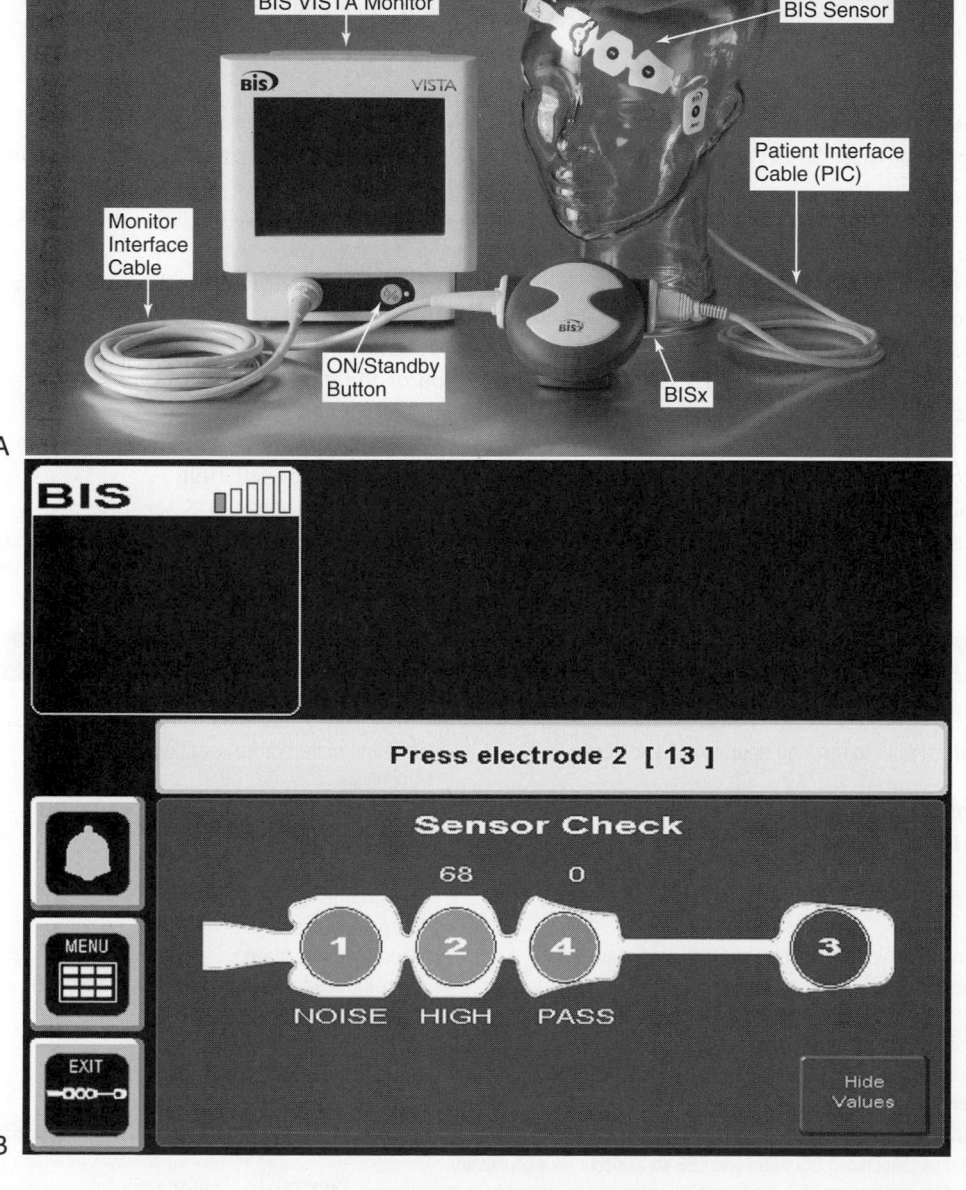

FIGURE 86-3 BIS VISTA monitoring system illustrating display, BISx, and location of menu and power control keys. *(Courtesy Aspect Medical Systems, Norwood, MA.)*

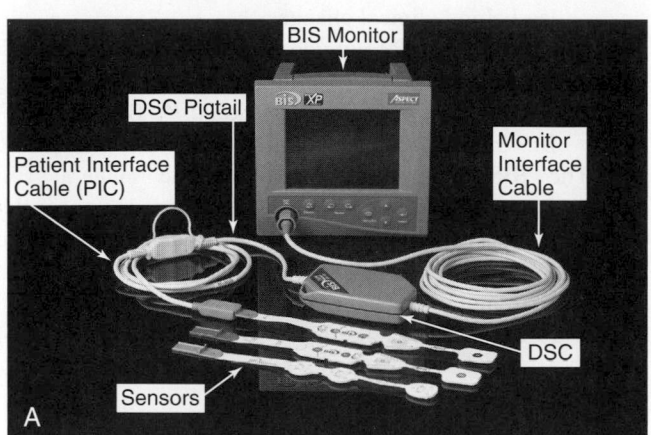

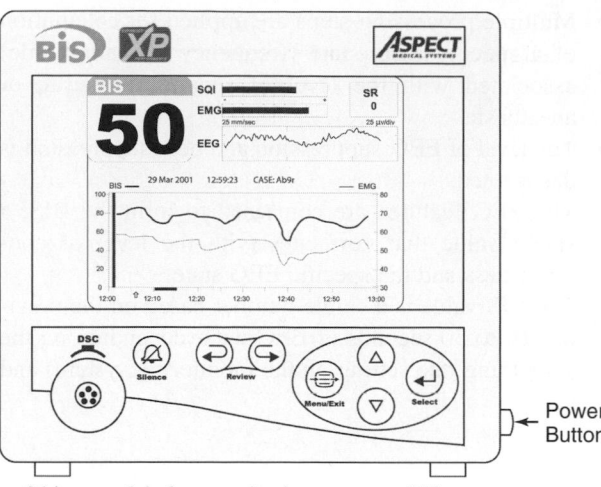

FIGURE 86-4   Equipment and accessories for use of bispectral index monitoring system: BIS monitor, patient cable, patient interface cable, digital signal converter, and available sensors (Extend sensor, Quatro sensor, and pediatric sensors shown). BIS Extend sensor automatically defaults to a 30-second smoothing rate, which may be preferable when patients are lightly sedated and minimal changes in drug delivery or patient stimulation exist, conditions that may apply to an intensive care setting. The BIS Quatro sensor automatically defaults to a 15-second smoothing rate and may be preferable when rapid changes in hypnotic level are anticipated or when maximal sensitivity in assessment of arousal response is desired, which may be helpful in an operating room setting. (*Courtesy Aspect Medical Systems, Norwood, MA.*)

- ❖ Sedation (dose-related): Related to the modulation of the EEG state and level of consciousness from medication administration.[1-3,34]
- ❖ Analgesic agents (dose-related): Related to attenuation of the arousal response or sedation as a side effect of opioid analgesia in higher doses.[1,2,16,34]
- ❖ Anesthetic agents (dose-related).[25,36,37]
- ❖ Cerebral injury or hypoperfusion (hemodynamic stability, global neurologic injury, severe hypoxemia): Related to direct alterations in cerebral metabolic stability.[9,18,26,29]
- • Potential indications for BIS monitoring include:
  - ❖ Use of neuromuscular blockade: BIS monitoring may help in identification of patients at risk for awareness, recall, and pain during paralysis.[2,23,39,40]

- ❖ Use of BIS values to guide sedation and analgesia.[2]
- ❖ Titration of sedation or analgesia in patients receiving controlled ventilation.[5,7,15,23]
- ❖ Avoidance of extremes of undersedation and oversedation.[1,37]
- ❖ Titration of medications for medication-induced coma.[10,32,35]
- ❖ Procedural sedation.[16]
- ❖ Determination of the dosage of sedation or analgesia during end-of-life care.[12,20]
- • Table 86-2 provides BIS values and correlation with clinical endpoints and level of sedation.
- • See Fig. 86-1 for placement of the BIS sensor.
- • Knowledge of factors that affect the BIS value is necessary.

TABLE 86-2	BIS Values, Corresponding Level of Sedation, and EEG State[3,13,17,20]	
BIS Value	**Corresponding Level of Sedation**	**Descriptors**
100	Awake state; patient able to respond appropriately to verbal stimulation	Baseline state before sedation Anxiolysis
80	Patient able to respond to loud verbal, limited tactile stimulation, such as mild prodding/shaking	High-frequency EEG activity (Beta augmentation) Moderate sedation
60	Low probability of explicit recall; patient unresponsive to verbal stimulation	Low-frequency EEG activity Deep sedation
40	Patient unresponsive to verbal stimulation, less responsive to physical stimulation	Deep hypnotic state Drug-induced coma; burst-suppression EEG pattern
20	Minimal responsiveness	
0	No responsiveness mediated by brain function; spinal reflexes may be present	Isoelectric or completely suppressed EEG

Note: Levels of sedation and responsiveness, and corresponding BIS value and EEG state, occur on a continuum.
(Adapted from Arbour R: Continuous nervous system monitoring: EEG, the bispectral index and neuromuscular transmission, AACN Clin Iss 14(2):192, 2003.)

❖ Sedation: Decrease in BIS value.[11,14,15,21]

❖ Analgesia: Decrease in BIS value from attenuation of cerebral arousal or sedation occurring as a side effect of high-dose opioid analgesia.[1,2]

❖ Neuromuscular blocking agents: Decrease in BIS value related to attenuation of high-frequency muscle activity across the patient's forehead.[8,17,23,40]

❖ Painful (noxious) stimulation: If analgesia is inadequate, arousal response may be produced within the cerebral cortex.[1,2,19]

❖ Sleep: BIS range is lower (20 to 70) during deep sleep, and BIS range is higher (75 to 92) during rapid eye movement (REM) sleep.[21]

❖ Hypothermia: Decrease in BIS value.[3,22,27]

❖ Cerebral ischemia: Decrease in BIS value.[21,26,28,38]

❖ Neurologic injury: Decrease in BIS value[3,8,16] depending on location of injury and degree to which overall cerebral metabolism is affected.[1,3,18]

❖ Encephalopathic states: Severe anoxic or ischemic encephalopathy (decrease in BIS value).[1,3]

❖ Electromyographic (EMG) activity (high-frequency activity from muscle activity across forehead)[3,6] may cause increase in BIS value independent of hypnotic state.[8,17,19,40]

❖ High-frequency electrical artifact from patient care equipment, such as pacemaker, or muscle activity, such as rapid head or eye movement (increase in BIS value).

• Knowledge is needed of BIS display screen, monitor controls, and information array available on BIS monitor (Figs. 86-2, 86-3 and 86-4).

• Knowledge of data obtained from BIS monitoring is necessary.

❖ The BIS value is a single number on a linear (0 to 100) scale that reflects the level of sedation or cerebral arousal. BIS values correspond with specific clinical endpoints, indicating arousal and consciousness. A BIS value at or near 100 typically corresponds with an awake state. A BIS value at or near 0 corresponds with an isoelectric or near-isoelectric EEG reading and a deeply comatose patient.[12,19,25,33]

❖ The suppression ratio (SR) represents the percentage of suppressed EEG over the last 63 seconds of collected data within the EEG data sample. This parameter may be elevated in patients receiving high-dose propofol or barbiturates. The SR may also be elevated in a patient with severe cerebral injury, such as encephalopathy or catastrophic brain trauma. An SR of 15 indicates that the EEG signal was isoelectric over an interval of 15% of the previous 63 seconds of collected data.[3,4,10,25]

❖ The EMG displays the power (in decibels) within the range of 70 to 110 Hz (cycles per second). This frequency range includes electrical activity from muscle artifact and patient care devices.[3,4,10,25]

• Interpretation of BIS value:

❖ BIS is interpreted over time, in response to stimulation and within the context of whether therapeutic endpoints and overall goals of therapy are met.[1,2,4,25]

❖ Decisions to increase or decrease titration of sedative or analgesic therapy should be based on clinical assessment and judgment, goals of therapy, and the BIS value.[1,2,25]

❖ Relying on the BIS alone for sedation and analgesia management is not recommended.[1,3]

❖ Movement such as in response to painful stimulation may occur with low BIS values.

❖ BIS values should be interpreted with caution in patients with brain injury or disease and in those receiving psychoactive medications.

❖ BIS monitoring is not intended for regional cerebral ischemia monitoring. With use of BIS in the presence of known CNS injury, a baseline BIS value is recommended before administration of sedative, analgesic, or anesthetic agents.[4,25]

❖ Elevation in BIS value may result from:
  ○ Sources of noxious stimuli (arousal response and potential increase in EMG activity).[17]
  ○ Decrease in level of neuromuscular blockade (affecting EMG activity).[1-3,38,40]
  ○ Interruption in sedative therapy, development of tolerance.
  ○ Interruption in analgesic therapy, development of tolerance.
  ○ REM sleep.
  ○ Seizure activity (potentially).
  ○ Shivering (particularly in combination with EMG activity).
  ○ Environmental noise: Cerebral arousal from excessive auditory stimulation.

❖ Decrease in BIS value may result from:
  ○ Attenuation of arousal response or EMG activity after opioid administration.[1,2,4,25]
  ○ Administration of a neuromuscular blocking agent.[2,3,39,40]
  ○ Attenuation of EMG activity.[3,8,25]
  ○ Excessive sedative dose.[1-3]
  ○ Excessive analgesic dosing.
  ○ Hypothermia (patient cooling).[3,22,27]
  ○ Progression to deeper stages of sleep.
  ○ Hemodynamic instability.[21,26,28,31]
  ○ Cerebral hypoperfusion.[9,21,28]
  ○ Onset or evolution of neurologic injury.[3,26,30,38]

• Knowledge of sedative and analgesic therapy is needed.

• Specific medication therapies (e.g., opioids, benzodiazepines, propofol) should be known.[13,32,34,35]

• Indications and contraindications of specific medication classes should be understood.

• Goals of care should be known.

• Clinical assessment for establishing goals and end points of therapy is necessary.[2,3,24,25]

• Knowledge of medication effects on BIS value is needed.

❖ Opioids: May decrease in a dose-related manner (with the side effect of sedation at higher doses) and decrease BIS value related to attenuation of the arousal response from pain.[2,3,15,25]

❖ Benzodiazepines: Decrease BIS value in a dose-related manner.

❖ Propofol: Decrease in BIS value in dose-related manner.

- Single-agent therapy with ketamine may not result in a dose-related decrease in BIS value.[25] Ketamine results in increased cerebral blood flow and activation of EEG, specifically in higher frequencies.[13] Higher EEG frequencies are associated with lighter levels of sedation.[1,3] The BIS value may remain elevated in the presence of deeper sedation, as determined with clinical assessment.[25]
- Knowledge of neuromuscular blockade and monitoring issues is necessary.
  - Differentiation between monitoring level of sedation and cortical arousal and monitoring level of neuromuscular blockade.
  - Monitoring level of sedation and cortical arousal is a phenomenon mediated by the CNS and is evaluated with clinical assessment of level of consciousness and arousal and with a processed EEG parameter such as the BIS. Medication effects evaluated include CNS depressants, such as propofol, barbiturates, benzodiazepines, and opioids at higher doses.
  - Monitoring level of neuromuscular blockade is a phenomenon mediated by the peripheral nervous system (PNS) and measures the effects of neuromuscular blocking agents at producing varying degrees of skeletal muscle relaxation. The degree of neuromuscular blockade is evaluated two ways. First is clinical assessment of ventilator synchrony, resolution of life-threatening agitation, and the degree to which clinical goals and end points are met. Second is peripheral nerve stimulation and assessment of the evoked response. Peripheral nerve stimulation is commonly performed at the ulnar nerve in the wrist. After nerve localization and electrode placement, an electrical stimulus is applied and the localized response of the target muscle is assessed (see Procedure 38).
  - Risk of awareness and pain during paralysis should be understood.
  - Clinical goals for aggressive sedation and analgesia during paralysis should be known.
  - Knowledge of monitoring parameters is needed.
  - Hemodynamic changes (marginal value and affected by multiple factors) should be understood.
  - Diaphoresis (affected by multiple factors) should be understood.
  - Knowledge of EEG-based monitoring (BIS) is necessary.
- Initial monitoring and setup of the sensor and equipment includes:
  - Signal quality index (SQI) is displayed on the monitor screen. The SQI bar that extends to the right side of the SQI bar graph display indicates optimal (100%) EEG signal quality. The BIS value on the numeric region of the monitor display is shown as a solid number. SQI less than 50% (SQI less than middle range of display) is indicated by a BIS value shown as an outlined number. If SQI is inadequate for calculation of a BIS value, no data are displayed.[3,4,25]

EQUIPMENT

- BIS monitor
- Digital signal converter
- Patient interface cable
- BIS sensor
- Detachable power cord
- Alcohol pads
- Gauze pads
- Nonsterile gloves
  Additional equipment includes the following:
- Soap and water
- Emergency equipment

PATIENT AND FAMILY EDUCATION

- Assess factors that affect the patient (if still awake) and family readiness to learn. ➤➤*Rationale:* Teaching is individualized to specific patient and family needs.
- Explain the purpose of BIS monitoring, including content regarding specific information obtained, how it may be used, and an explanation of the equipment. ➤➤*Rationale:* The patient (if still awake) and family may experience less anxiety and have increased understanding of the patient equipment at the bedside.
- Explain to the patient (if appropriate) and family what will happen with the initiation of BIS monitoring (skin preparation, placement of electrodes, moderate pressure for electrode contact). ➤➤*Rationale:* The explanation prepares the patient and family for events associated with initiation of BIS monitoring and also provides an opportunity to reinforce preprocedural teaching and assess level of understanding.
- Although rare, some patients may have mild skin irritation develop in the area in contact with the sensor. This irritation typically resolves within 1 hour after sensor removal. ➤➤*Rationale:* The patient and family are prepared for the possible minor issue with sensor application and the possible need for removal or repositioning of the sensor.
- Explain that BIS monitoring and electrode placement pose no risk to the patient beyond that of mild skin irritation (in rare instances) and that the patient experiences no discomfort as part of monitoring procedure. ➤➤*Rationale:* Anxiety may be decreased.

PATIENT ASSESSMENT AND PREPARATION
Patient Assessment

- Assess the patient's level of sedation, responsiveness, and arousal. ➤➤*Rationale:* Baseline data are provided.
- In collaboration with other healthcare providers, establish overall goals and endpoints of sedative and analgesic therapy. ➤➤*Rationale:* A coordinated plan is established with integration of the BIS data into decision making regarding sedation and analgesia.

- Assess the skin at the intended sites for sensor placement. ➻*Rationale:* Provides baseline information regarding the patient's skin.
- Assess the patient's neurologic status. ➻*Rationale:* Baseline data are provided. BIS values may be decreased with significant neurologic injury, which needs to be determined before initiation of BIS monitoring. If possible, obtain a baseline BIS value before initiating therapy with sedative, analgesic, or anesthetic agents.

Patient Preparation

- Verify correct patient with two identifiers. ➻*Rationale:* Prior to performing a procedure, the nurse should ensure the correct identification of the patient for the intended intervention.
- Determine anatomic landmarks for the BIS sensor placement. ➻*Rationale:* Landmarks provide for accurate placement of the sensor.

Procedure	for Bispectral Index Monitoring	
Steps	**Rationale**	**Special Considerations**
1. Connect the power cord to the monitor and plug it into the electrical wall outlet.	Prepares the equipment.	Equipment may vary because a stand-alone monitor may be used or a module may be used that is incorporated into the bedside monitoring system.
2. With use of the BIS A2000 system, connect the digital signal converter (DSC) and the patient interface cable to the monitor (see Fig. 86-4, *A*). With use of the BIS VIEW or BIS VISTA systems, connect the BISx and related cable to the monitor (see Fig. 86-2,*A* and and 86-3, *A*).[4-7]	Prepares the equipment.	
3. Turn on the monitor and observe as a system check is run. **(Level M*)**	The system initiates a self test to ensure that the equipment and connections are operating effectively.	If a hardware problem exists, such as DSC failure, a message appears on the display, indicating the need for hardware part replacement or service. If a problem exists, an error message appears. Refer to the operator manual.[4]
4. **HH**		
5. **PE**		
6. Cleanse the intended sensor area with alcohol pads and dry with gauze. **(Level M*)**	A thorough skin preparation removes debris and oily residue from the skin and facilitates optimal electrical contact for EEG data acquisition.[4-7]	Mild soap and water is an acceptable alternative. Ensure that the skin is dry before applying the sensors.

*Level M: Manufacturer's recommendations only

Procedure continues on following page

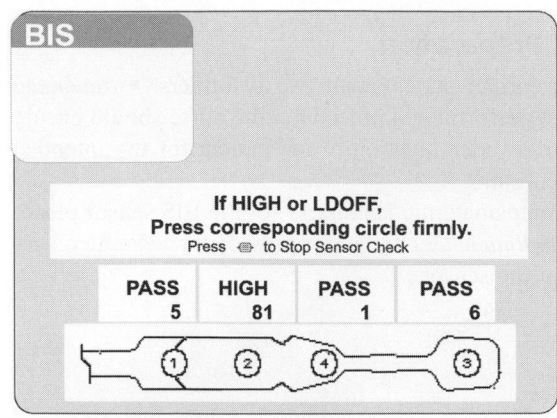

If HIGH or LDOFF,
Press corresponding circle firmly.
Press ⊕ to Stop Sensor Check

PASS	HIGH	PASS	PASS
5	81	1	6

FIGURE 86-5   BIS sensor check at start of monitoring.[4] Circle 1 is positioned at center of forehead approximately 2 inches (5 cm) above nose. Circle 4 is placed directly above and parallel to the eyebrow. Circle 3 is placed on the temple area between the hairline and the outer canthus of the eye. Circle 2 is placed between circles 1 and 4 on the patient's forehead. *(Courtesy Aspect Medical Systems, Norwood, MA.)*

Procedure | for Bispectral Index Monitoring—*Continued*

Steps	Rationale	Special Considerations
7. Attach the BIS sensor to the patient's forehead (Fig. 86-1; see Fig. 86-5). A. Position circle 1 electrode at the center of the forehead, approximately 2 inches above the patient's nose. B. Position circle 4 electrode directly above and parallel to the eyebrow. C. Position circle 3 electrode on the temple area between the hairline and the outer canthus of the eye. D. Position circle 2 electrode between the first and fourth sensors on the patient's forehead. E. Press the edges of the sensors to ensure adhesion and seal in the conductive gel. F. Press each of the electrodes with continuous direct pressure for 5 seconds to ensure optimal skin contact. G. With use of the BIS VISTA bilateral monitoring systems, refer to operator's manual. **(Level M*)**	Ensures consistency of the anatomic location for sensor placement and optimizes the electrical contact between the monitoring system and the skin for facilitation of EEG data acquisition. EEG data acquisition begins shortly after optimal connection is established between the patient and the monitoring system.	The conductive parts of the electrodes, sensor, or connectors should not contact other conductive parts of the monitoring system. The patient interface cable should be carefully placed and secured. Data acquisition begins when impedances are acceptable. Electrodes that show high impedance are highlighted on the sensor check display seen at start-up. For electrodes identified as having high impedance, repeat pressing of electrodes to optimize electrical contact. If significant artifact is present, the DSC should be moved away from sources of external electrical or mechanical artifact. Sources of artifact include fluid or forced-air warming systems, ventricular assist devices, high-frequency ventilation, suction, pacemakers, and oscillating mattresses.[25,40-42] Sensor check is initiated automatically. In the event of an error message, such as high impedance or sensor removal, repreparation and replacement of the sensor may be necessary.[4-7]
8. Insert the sensor tab into the patient interface cable until it is engaged.	Connects the BIS sensor and the patient interface cable.	

*Level M: Manufacturer's recommendations only

Procedure for Bispectral Index Monitoring—*Continued*

Steps	Rationale	Special Considerations
9. Secure the digital signal converter to an accessible location near the patient's head (e.g., patient's pillow or sheet), avoiding close proximity to sources of mechanical or electrical interference.	The digital signal converter amplifies, filters, and digitizes the patient's EEG signals. It is located close to the patient's head to minimize the vulnerability of the EEG signal to interference from other electronic equipment or patient care devices.[4-7]	
10. Access the setup menu by pressing "MENU/EXIT" on the monitor to select the specific monitor settings, including BIS smoothing rate, event markers, and display type (Fig. 86-6). This also provides access to the advanced setup menu. The up and down keys may be used to scroll through options. Choice of setting is made by pressing "SELECT."[4-6] **(Level M)**	Settings such as display type and BIS smoothing rate (in seconds) may be chosen.	A 10- or 15-second smoothing rate provides increased sensitivity and expedited feedback to altered hypnotic or arousal states.[5,6] A 30-second smoothing rate generates a smoother trend with less variability, is less sensitive to artifact, and is often chosen for long-term monitoring.[5,6] Ten-second, fifteen-second, and thirty-second smoothing rate options are available.[5-8]
11. As noted previously, access the advanced setup menu by initially pressing "MENU/EXIT" and then highlighting "Advanced Setup" by using the up or down arrows. Press select when "Advanced Setup" is highlighted (Fig. 86-7).	Used to select secondary parameters displayed with BIS trend, such as EMG activity, SR, and SQI, and to alter settings that may be changed less frequently. SQI of 100% indicates an optimal EEG signal. SR is the percentage of suppressed (isoelectric) EEG over the previous 63 seconds within the EEG data sample.[5,10,25,35]	If BIS is used to monitor a patient's sedation level during neuromuscular blockade, selection of EMG as a secondary parameter may provide early information regarding "lightening" of the blockade (EMG activity may increase). If used during deep sedation for controlled ventilation, EMG may indicate a pain/arousal response and indicate the need for analgesia.[3] Increased EMG activity may also indicate a lighter state of sedation or increased muscle activity.[3,25,39,40] If BIS is used to monitor a patient in a drug-induced coma, SR may be monitored as a secondary parameter for continuous evaluation of the degree of EEG suppression.[10,35]
12. Select additional settings as needed, including: A. Intervals for collection of data in the BIS log. B. "Advanced Setup" as outlined earlier to change the alarm limits and the display type.	The settings, such as the interval for recording of the BIS log values, log displays, alarm limits, and alternative displays such as EEG density spectral array, may be changed based on clinical or other needs for data collection.	The density spectral array display shows changes and trends in the power spectrum of the EEG over time. The BIS log display shows BIS numeric values averaged over the previous minute and can be displayed at varying intervals such as 1, 5, 15, or 60 minutes.[4] Up to 400 hours of data can be stored in the BIS A2000.[6] Approximately 1200 hours of data may be stored in the BISx for later retrieval and review.[5,6] The EEG display provides a single channel of raw EEG from a frontal montage.[4-6]

Procedure continues on following page

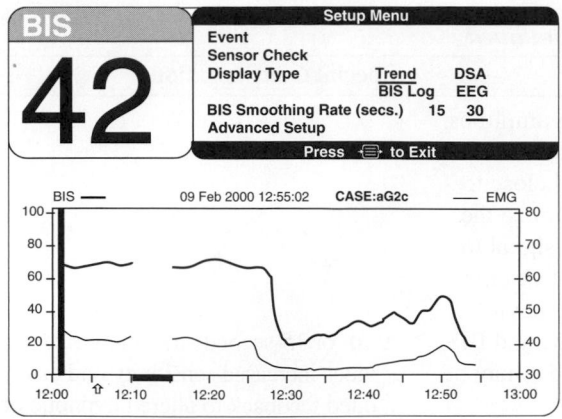

FIGURE 86-6 Setup menu for selection of monitor settings optimal to specific patient needs.[4] Display of specific monitoring parameters such as BIS trend and smoothing rate may be adjusted on this display. *(Courtesy Aspect Medical Systems, Norwood, MA.)*

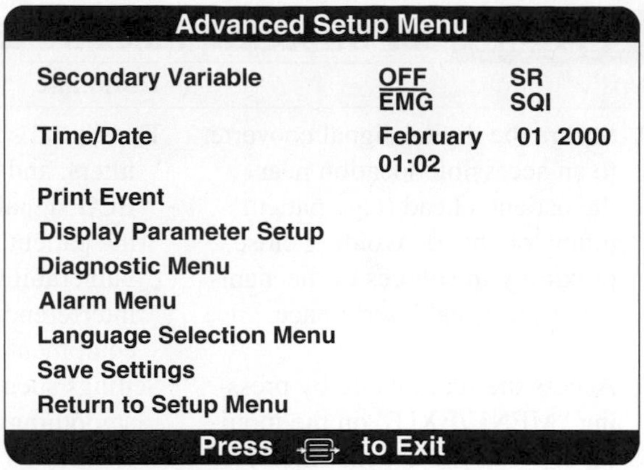

FIGURE 86-7 Advanced setup menu enabling the operator to select secondary monitoring parameters to be displayed with BIS trend and other, less frequently changed settings. Secondary parameters that may be selected include electromyography (EMG), suppression ratio (SR), and signal quality index (SQI).[4] *(Courtesy Aspect Medical Systems, Norwood, MA.)*

Procedure for Bispectral Index Monitoring—*Continued*

Steps	Rationale	Special Considerations
13. When the monitor settings have been adjusted to a specific patient, BIS data collection can begin.	BIS data collection can proceed after all preparatory steps and monitor settings are completed appropriately. This ensures optimal electrical contact between the patient and the monitoring system and optimal electrical safety. In addition, confirmation of display settings and secondary parameters at the outset of monitoring effectively tailors the monitor display and data acquisition to the specific patient.	
14. Observe the monitor display for: A. High impedance alarm (it is highlighted on the sensor check display at start-up): If displayed, press each electrode again to optimize electrical contact. Remove the sensor, cleanse the skin, and place a new sensor if necessary. B. Lead off alarm (it is displayed as "LDOFF"): If present, check whether the sensor has loosened. Remove the sensor, cleanse the skin, and apply another sensor. C. Artifact: If artifact is present, move the digital signal converter away from sources of external electrical or mechanical artifact.	Data acquisition begins when impedances are acceptable. Artifact may result from use of fluid or forced-air warming systems, ventricular assist devices, high-frequency ventilation, suction, pacemakers, and oscillating mattresses.[25,40-42]	A sensor check is initiated automatically during the system start up (see Fig. 86-5).

Procedure | for Bispectral Index Monitoring—*Continued*

Steps	Rationale	Special Considerations
15. For a patient receiving neuromuscular blockade, sedation, or analgesia therapy, the medication should be titrated for a BIS value between 45 and 60. **(Level C*)**	A BIS value less than 60 is associated with a low probability of explicit recall. A patient with a BIS value less than 45 is approaching a deep hypnotic state.[2,3,25,35]	If the BIS value exceeds 60 in a patient receiving neuromuscular blockade in association with stimulation such as airway suctioning or chest physiotherapy, additional analgesics are indicated. If the BIS value decreases to less than 40 to 45, downward titration of sedative therapy may be indicated. In addition, the patient should be evaluated for additional clinical changes such as hypotension, hypothermia, or cerebral ischemia, which may cause a decrease in the BIS value.[27,28,30,38]
16. For a patient receiving deep sedation for controlled ventilation, correlate the goal for the BIS value with specific clinical endpoints of therapy.	Correlation of the BIS value with clinical goals of therapy identifies patients who may be progressing to deeper levels of sedation and those who may be at risk for impending breakthrough agitation.[29]	With increased agitation and a BIS value less than 60, movement may be related to pain or reflex responses to noxious stimulation. Additional analgesia should be considered.
17. Discard used supplies in an appropriate receptacle.	Removes and safely discards used supplies.	
18. ▦		

*Level C: Qualitative studies, descriptive or correlational studies, integrative reviews, systematic reviews, or randomized controlled trials with inconsistent results

Expected Outcomes

- Optimal placement of the BIS sensor consistent with anatomic landmarks and manufacturer recommendations
- Skin remaining intact in the area of the BIS sensor placement
- Data acquisition and display after monitor setup and completion of self-test
- SQI of more than 50, indicating optimal EEG data acquisition
- Clear EEG waveform visible on the monitor display
- BIS decrease in response to sedative administration in dose-related manner
- BIS decrease after analgesia administration
- BIS value increase after significant noxious stimulation
- BIS values equal between right and left frontal-temporal montage EEG sensor placement
- BIS data effective in providing feedback on the state of the brain in response to sedative, analgesic, or hypnotic administration that can be used to direct therapy

Unexpected Outcomes

- Skin irritation in the area of the BIS sensor placement
- SQI significantly less than 50, indicating suboptimal EEG signal acquisition
- A sudden decrease in the BIS value independent of changes in sedative or analgesic therapy (may indicate hemodynamic compromise, cerebral ischemia, or the onset or progression of significant neurologic injury)
- A sudden rise in the BIS independent of stimulation, increased EMG activity, or an outward change in the patient's condition (may indicate seizure activity)
- BIS completely unresponsive to noxious stimulation such as endotracheal suctioning or invasive procedures
- BIS values significantly unequal between the right and left frontal-temporal montage sensor placement (may indicate unilateral cerebral injury or ischemia)
- BIS values that do not correlate with clinical assessment of sedation level and respond inconsistently to administration of sedative, hypnotic, or analgesic agents

Procedure continues on following page

Patient Monitoring and Care

Steps	Rationale	Reportable Conditions
		These conditions should be reported if they persist despite nursing interventions.
1. Follow institutional standard for assessing pain. Administer analgesia as prescribed.	Identifies need for pain interventions.	• Continued pain despite pain interventions
2. Assess the skin condition in the area of the sensor placement.	Ensures that the skin is intact.	• Altered skin integrity or irritation after sensor placement
3. Maintain the digital signal converter (DSC or BISx) in close proximity to the patient's head.	Decreases the vulnerability of the EEG signals to electrical interference from other sources.	
4. Monitor the BIS values and secondary parameters, including SQI, EMG, and SR, as determined by goals of care, clinical status, and response to interventions. For example, during rapid administration of sedative or analgesic agents before the anticipated use of neuromuscular blockade therapy, it may be appropriate to monitor and record the BIS value multiple times per hour. As therapy is stabilized, BIS can be monitored hourly.	Identifies trends in BIS and secondary parameters. Decrease in SQI to less than 50% may indicate suboptimal EEG data acquisition.	• Increase in EMG activity without a change in medication therapy (may indicate increased arousal response [pain] or lightening of neuromuscular blockade and result in increase in BIS independent of hypnotic state or decreasing level of sedation or analgesia) • Significant difference in BIS value between right and left frontal montage EEG (may indicate unilateral cerebral injury) • BIS value absolutely invariant to significant noxious stimulation (may indicate significant cerebral injury) • Increased suppression ratio (may indicate onset or evolution of cerebral injury, hemodynamic compromise, ischemia, or excessively deep hypnotic state[3])
5. Identify goals or end points of therapy at the beginning of BIS monitoring.	Patient outcomes are improved with an organized, research-based approach to care.[1-3,10]	• Not progressing toward achievement of goals or end point of therapy
6. Observe BIS values at least hourly and in response to titration of medication therapy.	Determines changes in BIS values in response to medication therapy and interventions. Also provides the ability to use "event marker" to closely correlate changes in BIS and secondary parameters for later review.	• Abnormal BIS values or trends: BIS value not decreasing in response to upward titration of sedative or hypnotic therapy; BIS value not increasing after downward titration of sedative or hypnotic therapy
7. Change the BIS sensor at least every 24 hours or more frequently as needed (e.g., diaphoresis, loose electrodes).	Maintains optimal electrical contact between the patient and the monitoring system.	

Patient Monitoring and Care —*Continued*

Steps	Rationale	Reportable Conditions
8. Observe the EEG channel at least every 2 hours and as determined by the patient's clinical state and therapeutic interventions.	The EEG amplitude and frequency change based on the patient's clinical state, evolving injury, and medication therapy.[3,10,33,34] The EEG also (under normal conditions) changes in response to varying levels and types of stimulation.[10,11,14,20] In most conditions, electrocardiographic (ECG) artifact is not visible in an EEG waveform.[3] ECG artifact visible in the EEG channel may indicate significant EEG suppression.[3]	• A decrease in EEG frequency or amplitude (e.g., if this occurs with a decrease in the BIS value, may indicate neurologic injury) • A significant decrease in the BIS value that is inconsistent with the medication therapy may indicate critical pathology and warrant further evaluation with neuroimaging diagnostic EEG or clinical examination
9. Observe the BIS value in response to stimulation.	The BIS value should, in most patients, rise in response to stimulation. The EEG, on which the BIS is based, normally responds to external stimulation. An EEG unresponsive to stimulation may indicate significant neurologic injury and possibly poor prognosis.[1,3,33,36]	• Significant ECG artifact in the EEG channel • A BIS value that is unresponsive to noxious stimulation • A significant difference in BIS values or suppression ratio (SR) between the right and left frontal-temporal montage (may indicate unilateral cerebral injury)

Documentation

Documentation should include the following:
- Goals and end points of sedative or analgesic therapy
- Family education regarding BIS monitoring
- Clinical assessment (if appropriate) of level of sedation
- BIS value at start of monitoring and with changes or titration of therapy
- BIS value recording on flow sheet at least hourly and more frequently as indicated (Fig. 86-8)
- Pain assessment, interventions, and evaluation of interventions
- Occurrence of skin irritation at the site of the BIS sensor placement with action taken
- Unexpected outcomes and interventions
- Sudden changes in BIS value (increase or decrease) independent of obvious clinical changes or alterations of medication therapy

- Suppression ratio (SR) (as appropriate) for BIS use in medication-induced coma
- SQI and EMG activity (as appropriate)
- Documentation of left versus right frontal montage (location of the BIS sensor on the right or the left side)
- BIS value before and after noxious stimulation and the difference between these two values
- Change in the BIS value in response to noxious or painful stimulation
- For case reviews to track, BIS values or trends and response to stimulation or therapeutic interventions over time; printout/strip of BIS trend data can be obtained if printer is available (Fig. 86-9)

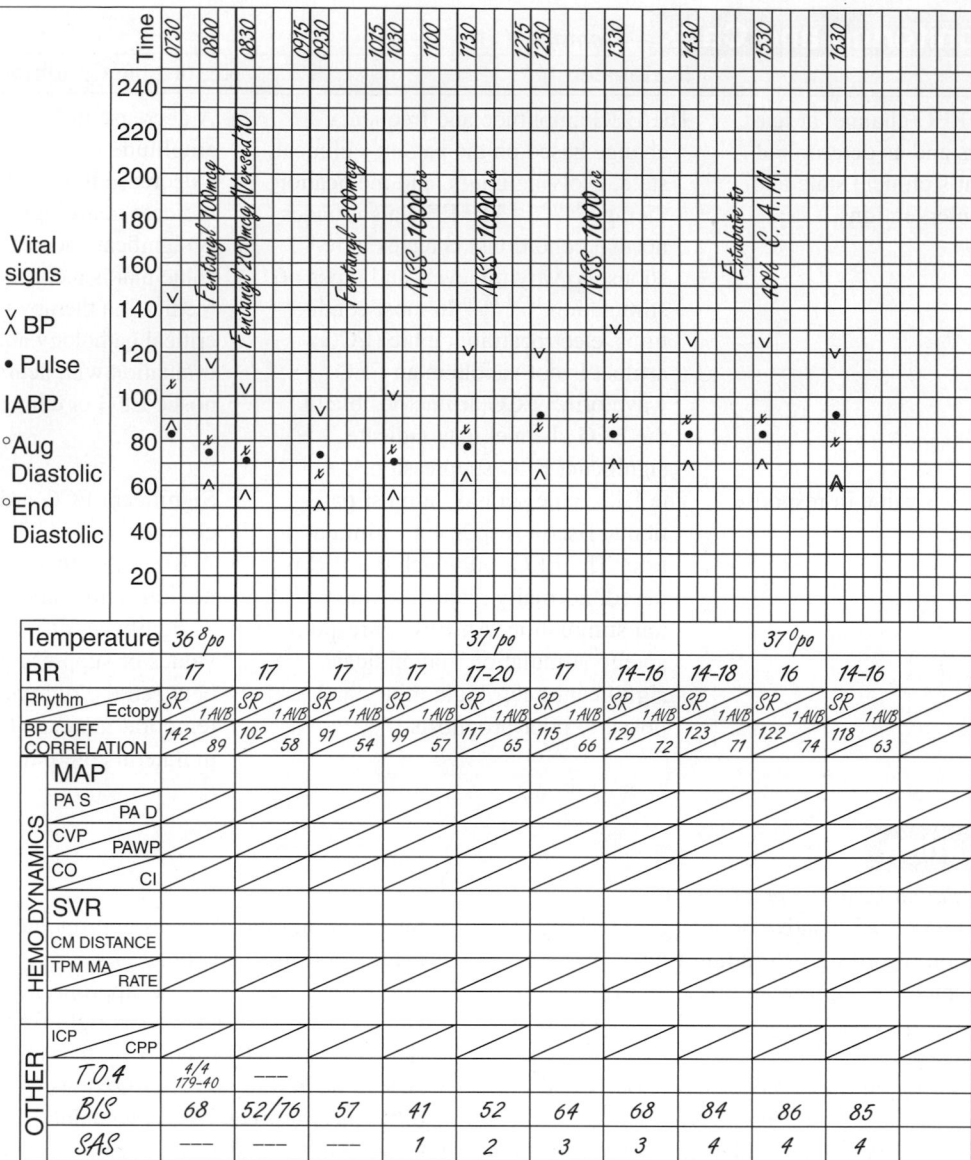

Time	0730	0800	0830	0915 0930	1015 1030	1100	1130	1215 1230	1330	1430	1530	1630			
Temperature	36 8po				37 1po					37 0po					
RR	17	17	17	17	17-20	17	14-16	14-18	16	14-16					
Rhythm / Ectopy	SR / 1AVB	SR / 1AVB	SR / 1AVB	SR / 1AVB	SR / 1AVB	SR / 1AVB	SR / 1AVB	SR / 1AVB	SR / 1AVB	SR / 1AVB					
BP CUFF CORRELATION	142 / 89	102 / 58	91 / 54	99 / 57	117 / 65	115 / 66	129 / 72	123 / 71	122 / 74	118 / 63					
T.O.4	4/4 179-40	----													
BIS	68	52/76	57	41	52	64	68	84	86	85					
SAS	----	----	----	1	2	3	3	4	4	4					

FIGURE 86-8 Documentation of BIS values over time and after medication administration in critically ill patient. At 7:30 AM, the patient was still receiving neuromuscular blockade with a BIS value of 68. Additional sedation/analgesia was administered (fentanyl and midazolam), with resulting BIS decline to 52. After stimulation, BIS value elevated to 76, necessitating supplemental dosing with analgesics (fentanyl). BIS value remained at less than 60, and neuromuscular blockade was discontinued. The upward trend in the BIS value tracked recovery of consciousness to baseline mental status. (*Courtesy Aspect Medical Systems, Norwood, MA.*)

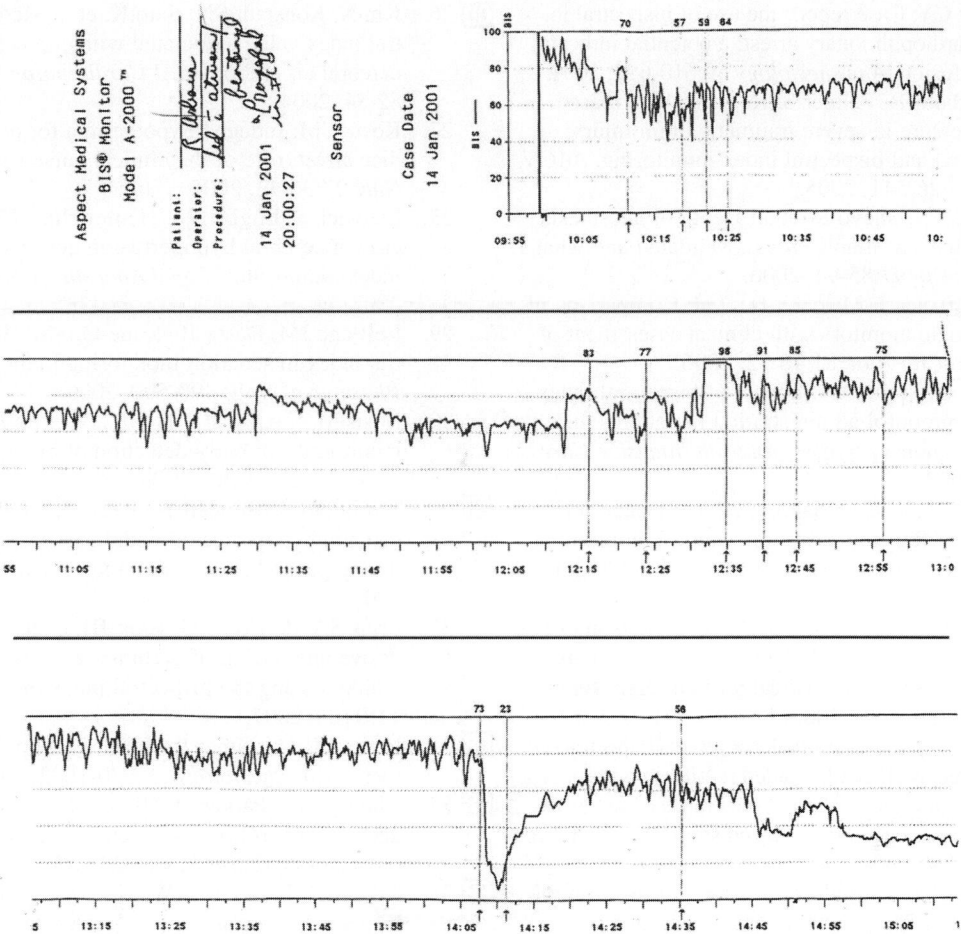

FIGURE 86-9 An illustration of BIS trend recording of sedation/analgesia management in critically ill patient. BIS monitoring was initiated at approximately 10:00 AM. Sedation was managed initially with fentanyl and lorazepam. Decline in BIS from between 90 and 97 to between 55 and 65 occurred over 25 to 30 minutes in response to therapy. Decline in BIS value matched clinical assessment of increased level of sedation. The patient had periods of breakthrough agitation and ventilator dyssynchrony beginning at 12:15 PM. Agitation was refractory to current therapy despite upward titration of sedation and analgesia. The sedation management was changed to propofol at approximately 14:05 PM. The precipitous drop in BIS value indicated increased sedation. Propofol was titrated back in a controlled, incremental manner. Sedation was more closely and optimally managed with application of BIS monitoring and avoiding, in a controlled manner, extremes of excessive sedation and inadequate sedation/risk of agitation and ventilator dyssynchrony. This tracing has been used in electronic format beginning in June 2003 for educational purposes on behalf of Aspect Medical Systems. *(Courtesy Aspect Medical Systems, Norwood, MA.)*

References

1. Arbour R: Impact of bispectral index monitoring on sedation and outcomes in critically ill patients: a case series, *Crit Care Nurs Clin North Am* 18:227-241, 2006.

CR 2. Arbour R: Using bispectral index monitoring to detect potential breakthrough awareness and limit duration of neuromuscular blockade: case report and discussion, *Am J Crit Care* 13:66-73, 2004.

CR 3. Arbour R: Continuous nervous system monitoring, EEG, the bispectral index and neuromuscular transmission, *AACN Clin Issues* 14:185-207, 2003.

4. Aspect Medical Systems: *A-2000™ Bispectral Index™ (BIS) monitoring system operating manual,* Norwood, MA, 2006, Aspect Medical Systems, Inc.

5. Aspect Medical Systems: *BIS VIEW™ monitoring system operating manual,* Norwood, MA, 2007, Aspect Medical Systems, Inc.

6. Aspect Medical Systems: *BIS VISTA monitoring system operating manual,* Norwood, MA, 2008, Aspect Medical Systems, Inc.

7. Aspect Medical Systems: *BIS VISTA monitoring system bilateral monitoring addendum operating manual,* Norwood, MA, 2008, Aspect Medical Systems Inc.

CR 8. Aspect Medical Systems: *Overview: the effects of electromyography (EMG) and other high-frequency signals on the bispectral index (BIS),* Norwood, MA, 2000, Aspect Medical Systems, Inc.

CR 9. Azim N, Wang CY: Case report: the use of bispectral index during a cardiopulmonary arrest: a potential indicator of cerebral perfusion, *Anesthesiology* 59:610-612, 2004.

CR 10. Bader MK, Arbour R, Palmer S: Refractory increased intracranial pressure in severe traumatic brain injury: barbiturate coma and bispectral index monitoring, *AACN Clin Issues* 16:526-541, 2005.

11. Brunh J, Myles PS, Sneyd R, et al: Depth of anesthesia monitoring: what's available, what's validated and what's next? *Br J Anaesth* 97:85-94, 2006.

12. Chisholm CJ, Zurica J, Mironov D, et al: Comparison of electrophysiologic monitors with clinical assessment of sedation, *Mayo Clin Proc* 81:46-52, 2006.

13. Chiu CL, Ong G, Majid AA: Impact of bispectral index monitoring on propofol administration in patients undergoing cardiopulmonary bypass, *Anaesth Intensive Care* 35:342-347, 2007.

14. Consales G, Chelazzi C, Rinaldi S, et al: Bispectral index compared to Ramsay score for sedation monitoring in intensive care units, *Minerva Anestesiol* 72:329-336, 2006.

CR 15. Courtman SP, Wardurgh A, Petros AJ: Comparison of the bispectral index monitor with the Comfort score in assessing level of sedation of critically ill children, *Intens Care Med* 29:2239-2246, 2003.

16. Dahaba AA, Lischnig U, Kronthaler R, et al: Bispectral-index-guided versus clinically guided remifentanyl/propofol analgesia/sedation during interventional radiological procedures: an observer-blinded randomized study, *Anesth Analg* 103:378-384, 2006.

CR 17. Dahaba AA: Different conditions that could result in the bispectral index indicating an incorrect hypnotic state, *Anesth Analg* 101:765-773, 2005.

CR 18. Escudero D, Otero J, Muniz G, et al: The bispectral index scale: its use in the detection of brain death, *Transplant Proc* 37:3661-3663, 2005.

CR 19. Fraser GL, Riker RR: Bispectral index monitoring in the intensive care unit provides more signal than noise, *Pharmacotherapy* 25(5 Pt 2):19S-27S, 2005.

CR 20. Gambrell M: Using the BIS monitor in palliative care: a case study, *J Neurosci Nurs* 37:140-143, 2005.

21. Hashimoto H, Nakamura H, Hirota K: Marked reduction in bispectral index with severe bradycardia without hypotension in a diabetic patient undergoing ophthalmic surgery, *J Anesth* 22:300-303, 2008.

22. Honan D, Doherty D, Frizelle H: A comparison of the effects on bispectral index of mild vs. moderate hypothermia during cardiopulmonary bypass, *Eur J Anaesthesiol* 23:385-390, 2006.

23. Inoue S, Kawaguchi M, Sasaoka N, et al: Effects of neuromuscular block on systemic and cerebral hemodynamics and bispectral index during moderate or deep sedation in critically ill patients, *Intens Care Med* 32:391-397, 2006.

CR 24. Jacobi J Fraser GL, Coursin DB, et al: Clinical practice guidelines for the sustained use of sedatives and analgesics in the critically ill adult, *Crit Care Med* 30:119-141, 2002.

CR 25. Kelly SD: *Monitoring level of consciousness during anesthesia and sedation: a clinician's guide to the bispectral index: Aspect Medical Systems,* 2003, retrieved June 4, 2004, from http://www.aspectmedical.com/resources/handbook/default.mspx.

CR 26. Kin N, Konstadt SN, Sato K, et al: Reduction of bispectral index value associated with clinically significant cerebral air embolism, *J Cardiothorac Vasc Anesth* 18: 82-84, 2004.

27. Kosik TM: Induced hypothermia for patients with cardiac arrest: role of the clinical nurse specialist, *Crit Care Nurs* 27:36-42, 2007.

28. Lauwick S, English M, Hemmerling TM: An unusual case of cerebral hypoperfusion detected by bispectral index monitoring, *Can J Anaesth* 54:680-681, 2007.

29. LeBlanc JM, Dasta JF, Kane-Gill SL: Role of the bispectral index in sedation monitoring in the ICU, *Ann Pharmacother* 40:490-500, 2006.

30. Misis M, Raxach JG, Molto HP, et al: Bispectral index monitoring for early detection of brain death, *Transplant Proc* 40:1279-1281, 2008.

CR 31. Morimoto Y, Monden Y, Ohtake K, et al: The detection of cerebral hypoperfusion with bispectral index monitoring during general anesthesia, *Anesth Analg* 100:158-161, 2005.

32. Prins SA, de Hoog M, Blok JH, et al: Continuous noninvasive monitoring of barbiturate coma in critically ill children using the bispectral index monitor, *Crit Care* 11:R108, 2007.

CR 33. Rampil IJ: A primer for EEG signal processing in anesthesia, *Anesthesiology* 89:980-1002, 1998.

CR 34. Rhoney DH, Parker D: Use of sedative and analgesic agents in neurotrauma patients: effects on cerebral physiology, *Neurol Res* 23:237-259, 2001.

CR 35. Riker RR, Fraser GL, Wilkins ML: Comparing the bispectral index and suppression ratio with burst suppression of the electroencephalogram during pentobarbital infusions in adult intensive care patients, *Pharmacotherapy* 23: 1087-1093, 2003.

CR 36. Rosow C, Manberg PJ: Bispectral index monitoring, *Anesth Clin North Am* 19:946-966, 2001.

37. Sackey PV, Radell PJ, Granath F, et al: Bispectral index as a predictor of sedation depth during isoflurane or midazolam sedation in ICU patients, *Anaesth Intens Care* 35:348-356, 2007.

CR 38. Sen I, Puri GD, Bapuraj JR: Early detection of cerebral vasospasm during a neurointerventional procedure using the BIS, *Anaesth Intens Care* 33:691-692, 2005.

CR 39. Tobias JD, Grindstaff R: Bispectral index monitoring during the administration of neuromuscular blocking agents in a pediatric intensive care unit patient, *J Intens Care Med* 20:233-237, 2005.

CR 40. Vivien B, Di Maria S, Quattera A, et al: Overestimation of bispectral index in sedated intensive care unit patients revealed by administration of muscle relaxant, *Anesthesiology* 99:9-17, 2003.

41. Vretzakis G, Draguomanis C, Argiriadou H, et al: Inaccuracy of BIS values produced by the cardiopulmonary bypass machine during operative repair of an aortic dissection, *J Cardiothorac Vasc Anesth* 20:68-70, 2006.

42. Zanner R, Schneider G, Kochs EF: Falsely increased bispectral index values caused by the use of a forced-air-warming device, *Eur J Anaesthesiol* 23:618-619, 2006.

Additional Readings

Arbour R: Electroencephalograph-derived monitoring, In Littlejohns LR, Bader MK, editors: *AACN-AANN protocols for practice: monitoring technologies in critically ill patients,* Sudbury, MA, 2009, Jones and Bartlett, 175-197

CR Claassen J, Mayer SA, Kowalski RG, et al: Detection of electrographic seizures with continuous EEG monitoring in critically ill patients, *Neurology* 62:1743-1748, 2004.

CR Deogaonkar A, Gupta R, DeGeorgia M, et al: Bispectral index monitoring correlates with sedation scales in brain-injured patients, *Crit Care Med* 32:2403-2406, 2004.

CR March K, Wellwood J, Arbour R: Technology. In Bader MK, Littlejohns LR, editors: *AANN core curriculum for neuroscience nursing,* St Louis, 2004, Saunders, 199-204.

CR Markand ON: Pearls, perils and pitfalls in the use of the electroencephalogram, *Semin Neurol* 23:7-46, 2003.

CR Nasraway SA: The bispectral index: expanded performance for everyday use in the intensive care unit? *Crit Care Med* 33:685-687, 2005.

Parker BM: Anesthetics and anesthesia techniques: impacts on perioperative management and postoperative outcomes, *Clev Clin J Med* 73(Suppl 1):S13-S17, 2006.

CR Tonner PH, Wei C, Bein B, et al: Comparison of two bispectral index algorithms in monitoring sedation in postoperative intensive care patients, *Crit Care Med* 33:580-584, 2005.

CR Watson BD, Kane-Gill SL: Sedation assessment in critically ill adults: 2001-2004 update, *Ann Pharmacother* 38:1898-1906, 2004.

CR Welsby IJ, Ryan M, Booth JV, et al: The bispectral index in the diagnosis of perioperative stroke: a case report and discussion, *Anesth Analg* 96:435-437, 2003.

Brain Tissue Oxygen Monitoring: Insertion (Assist), Care, and Troubleshooting

P U R P O S E : Brain tissue oxygen monitoring is performed in the patient with severe brain injury for measurement and continuous monitoring of regional brain tissue oxygenation. Monitoring of brain tissue oxygen provides important information relative to the delivery of oxygen to cerebral tissue of the injured brain.

Eileen Maloney-Wilensky, Stephanie A. Bloom, Michael F. Stiefel

PREREQUISITE NURSING KNOWLEDGE

- Incorporated as an adjunct monitor of trends in concert with concurrent neurologic multimodality monitoring parameters (intracranial pressure [ICP], cerebral perfusion pressure [CPP], systemic jugular venous oxygen [$SjvO_2$]), brain tissue oxygen saturation (also abbreviated as $PbtO_2$, $PbrO_2$, $PtiO_2$, tiO_2) monitoring reflects the oxygenation of cerebral tissue local to the sensor placement.[4,22,30]
- In institutions where $SjvO_2$ is used as a monitoring parameter, the difference between $SjvO_2$ measurements and $PbtO_2$ values must be noted. $SjvO_2$ is a measure of the oxygen contained in the blood draining from the cerebral venous sinuses into the jugular bulb (a measure of global brain oxygenation), whereas $PbtO_2$ measures regional (local to the catheter placement in the cerebral white matter) brain tissue oxygenation.[22,24,26]
- Understanding of neuroanatomy and physiology, specifically intracranial dynamics, is needed.
- Knowledge of sterile and aseptic technique is necessary.
- Currently, only one brain tissue oxygen monitoring system is available.[24]
- A brain tissue oxygen probe may be inserted through an intracranial bolt or tunneled.[2,30]
- $PbtO_2$ monitoring provides information that reflects brain tissue oxygen levels associated with cerebral oxygen demand and systemic oxygen delivery.

- $PbtO_2$ values are relative within an individual. Establishing and following the patient's cerebral oxygen trends provides the healthcare providers with information that will aid in the assessment and treatment of cerebral hypoxia.
- Indications for $PbtO_2$ monitoring include patients at risk for secondary injury from cerebral edema. Conditions most likely to cause cerebral edema include severe traumatic brain injury, aneurysmal and traumatic subarachnoid hemorrhage, brain tumor, stroke, and any condition that increases ICP.
- Contraindications for $PbtO_2$ monitoring include patients with a coagulopathy, those receiving anticoagulation therapy, and those with an insertion site infection.
- $PbtO_2$ probes are safe with a 1.5-T magnetic resonance imaging (MRI) system as long as the fiberoptic ICP catheter is not in place.[11]
- $PbtO_2$ probes are safe with computed tomography (CT).
- Cerebral oxygen data are accurate and reliable when the $PbtO_2$ probe is located in the deep white matter of the brain, the location where oxygen availability is most stable.
- Parameters such as ICP and brain tissue temperature can be measured immediately at the time of probe placement.
- Monitoring of $PbtO_2$ values may be delayed as long as 2 hours as time is needed for the brain tissue to settle after the microtrauma caused by probe placement.[5-7,12,28]

- The normal range for brain tissue oxygen values is between 20 and 35 mm Hg.[12,13,17,18,24] Treatment goals usually aim to keep the $Pbto_2$ equal to or greater than 20 mm Hg.[30]
- A $Pbto_2$ of less than 15 mm Hg is a critical threshold associated with a greater chance of functional disability and mortality related to cerebral ischemia.[1,3,12,25]
- A $Pbto_2$ of less than 10 mm Hg is directly associated with severe disability, poor outcome at discharge, and death.[1,3,28]
- A $Pbto_2$ of less than 5 mm Hg is indicative of cerebral cell death and an approximately 90% mortality rate.[1,3,14,23,25]
- Brain tissue oxygen values can be used to manage potential cerebral hypoxia. Clinical interventions can be aimed at increasing oxygen delivery or decreasing cerebral oxygen demand.
- Decreases in $Pbto_2$ values occur when cerebral blood flow or cerebral oxygen delivery is inadequate or states of increased metabolic demands exist, indicating the potential for secondary brain injury.
- Increases in $Pbto_2$ values denote decreased oxygen uptake by cerebral cells that may be caused by states of increased oxygen delivery or decreased oxygen utilization.

- Table 87-1 outlines treatment options for patients with a decrease or increase in $Pbto_2$ values.
- $Pbto_2$ probe placement: The physician placing the probe device determines the catheter placement location after review of the CT scan and after consideration of the most appropriate monitoring area based on diagnosis and pathology, avoiding areas of infarct or hematoma.[4,17] Placement of the probe may be ipsilateral or contralateral to the pathology.[26]
  - ❖ The probe may be placed in the nondominant hemisphere (e.g., right frontal region) to minimize risk of injury from catheter insertion.[6,12,29] The right hemisphere is a safer location for probe placement than the left hemisphere because speech function is located in the left hemisphere in most individuals.
  - ❖ Placement may be near a lesion when the clinical goal is to monitor oxygen availability to damaged but salvageable tissue.
  - ❖ If a patient has a subarachnoid hemorrhage, the probe may be placed in the area of the brain expected to develop vasospasm. Placement is determined by the distribution of subarachnoid blood on CT scan and by aneurysm location.[16,21]

TABLE 87-1 **Management of Increased or Decreased $Pbto_2$ Values**

Decreased $Pbto_2$ Values

Increased oxygen demand	Increased ICP	Treat the increased ICP with diuretics, CSF drainage, sedation (e.g., barbiturates, propofol), craniotomy.
	Pain	Administer analgesics.
	Shivering	Rewarm, if needed, or administer agents to stop shivering (e.g., demerol, thorazine, paralytic agents).
	Agitation	Administer sedation agents.
	Seizures	Administer benzodiazepines and adjunct anticonvulsant agents.
	Fever	Treat the underlying cause of the fever, initiate a cooling device, if needed, and administer antipyretic agents.
Decreased oxygen delivery	Hypotension	Administer isotonic fluids (normal saline or hypertonic saline solution) or vasopressors.
	Hypovolemia	Administer isotonic fluids (normal saline or hypertonic saline solution), blood replacement.
	Anemia	Administer blood replacement products.
	Hypoxia	Increase Fio_2, PEEP, interventions to mobilize pulmonary secretions and maximize pulmonary function.

Increased $Pbto_2$ values

Increased oxygen delivery	Hyperdynamic (elevated ICP)	Consider sedation agents, temperature management, and/or positioning to treat elevated ICP
Decreased oxygen demand	Hypothermia	Rewarm to achieve normothermia or mild hypothermia as prescribed for management of cerebral metabolism.
	Sedatives Anesthesia Neuromuscular blockade agents	Decrease sedation, anesthesia, or paralysis as prescribed.

PEEP, Positive end-expiratory pressure.

❖ Manufacturer's recommended guidelines for probe device removal manufacturer's guidelines or replacement is 5 to 7 continuous days per device. Drift may affect accuracy after 5 days.[9] Practice may vary based on institutional guidelines.

EQUIPMENT

- Sterile gowns, sterile drapes, sterile gloves, nonsterile gloves, caps, goggles, and face masks
- Shave preparation kit
- Antiseptic solution
- Pbto$_2$ monitor (Fig. 87-1) or module
- Connecting cables
- Cranial access tray
- Pbto$_2$ probe
- Scalpel
- Dressing supplies, including 4 × 4 gauze and tape
- Sterile dry gauze; may be placed at the insertion site

Additional equipment to have available as needed includes the following:

- An intravenous (IV) arm board may be used to stabilize the monitor probe and cable
- Intracranial bolt system

- Extra transparent and soft cloth adhesive dressing or any appropriate dry, sterile occlusive dressing
- A compatible fiberoptic ICP catheter may be inserted through the intracranial bolt system as well and will require a separate monitor to measure ICP

PATIENT AND FAMILY EDUCATION

- Assess patient or family understanding of the purpose of Pbto$_2$ monitoring. Most patients who need brain tissue oxygen monitoring are in an altered level of consciousness with a score of 8 or less on the Glasgow Coma Scale; education is directed toward the family.[3] ➥*Rationale:* Understanding may reduce anxiety and stress, stimulates requests for clarification or additional information, and increases awareness of the goals, duration, and expectations of the monitoring system.
- Explain the insertion process, patient monitoring, and care involving the Pbto$_2$ monitoring system. ➥*Rationale:* Explanation may alleviate anxiety and stress and stimulates requests for clarification or additional information.
- Explain the expected outcomes of the Pbto$_2$ system. ➥*Rationale:* Explanation may decrease patient and family anxiety and stress by increasing awareness of Pbto$_2$ monitoring duration and therapy goals.

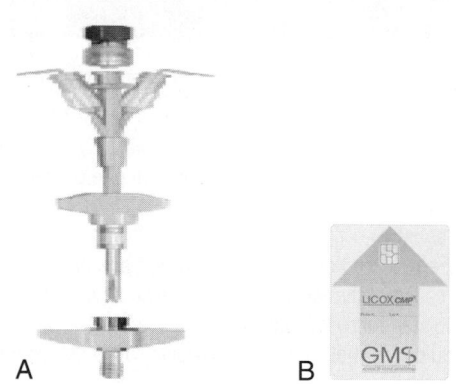

A   B

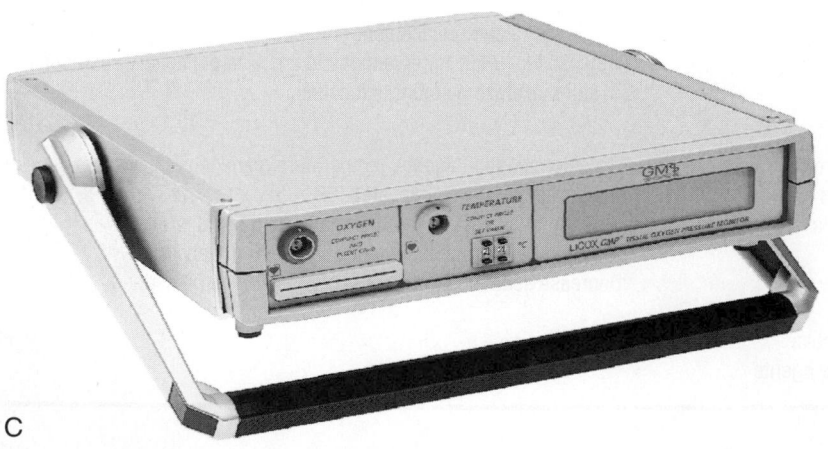

C

FIGURE 87-1   **A,** Model IM3 triple-lumen introducer. **B,** Smart card where calibration data for the oxygen probe is electronically stored. **C,** Licox CMP monitor, AC 3.1. *(Courtesy Integra Neurosciences, Plainsboro, NJ.)*

PATIENT ASSESSMENT AND PREPARATION

Patient Assessment

- Assess the patient's neurologic status. ➤*Rationale:* Performing a baseline neurologic assessment enables the nurse to identify changes that may occur as a result of the $Pbto_2$ probe insertion.
- Assess the patient for signs or symptoms of local infection at the intended insertion location. ➤*Rationale:* Evidence of local infection is a contraindication to brain tissue oxygen catheter placement.
- Obtain and review coagulation laboratory results (e.g., complete blood count, platelet count, prothrombin time, partial thromboplastin time, bleeding time, and international normalized ratio). ➤*Rationale:* Assessment identifies the patient's risk for bleeding.

Patient Preparation

- Verify correct patient with two identifiers. ➤*Rationale:* Prior to performing a procedure, the nurse should ensure the correct identification of the patient for the intended intervention.
- Ensure that the patient and family understand the procedure teaching. Answer questions as they arise, and reinforce information as needed. Most patients who need brain tissue oxygen monitoring are in an altered level of consciousness with a Glasgow Coma Scale score of eight or less. ➤*Rationale:* Information previously taught is evaluated and reinforced.
- Ensure that informed consent has been obtained. ➤*Rationale:* Informed consent protects the rights of the patient and makes a competent decision possible for the patient; however, in emergency circumstances, time may not allow for the consent form to be signed.
- Perform a pre-procedure verification and time out, if non-emergent. ➤*Rationale:* Ensures patient safety.
- Administer sedation or analgesia as prescribed before beginning the insertion procedure. ➤*Rationale:* Sedation or analgesia facilitates the insertion process.
- Assist the patient to the semi-Fowler's position with the head in the neutral position and the head of bed elevated 30 to 45 degrees. ➤*Rationale:* Patients who are candidates for brain tissue oxygen monitoring may have increased ICP. Elevating the head of the bed and placing the head in the neutral position act to decrease intracranial pressure by enhancing jugular venous outflow and provides for optimal insertion accessibility.

Procedure for Brain Tissue Oxygen Monitoring: Insertion (Assist), Care, and Troubleshooting

Steps	Rationale	Special Considerations
1. 🔲		
2. Plug the $Pbto_2$ monitor power cord into an AC wall outlet.	Provides the power source.	
3. Attach the cables (e.g., oxygen cable, temperature cable) to the $Pbto_2$ monitor.	Prepares the equipment.	Refer to manufacturer's guidelines as needed. Monitors and cables may be color-coded.
4. 🔲		
5. Apply goggles or masks with face shields, caps, gowns, and sterile gloves.	Prepares for sterile procedure.	
6. Assist as needed with site preparation (e.g., shave preparation and cleansing with antiseptic solution).	Prepares for sterile procedure.	Antiseptic solution choice should be determined by institutional policy. Use of povidone-iodine versus chlorhexidine is controversial. The antiseptic solution should be allowed to dry before initial incision.[8] Studies suggest chlorhexidine is neurotoxic.[8]
7. Assist as needed in draping the head, neck, and chest of the patient.	Prepares a sterile environment for the insertion process.	
8. Assist as needed with opening of the sterile trays and probes.	Facilitates efficiency of the insertion process.	
9. Turn on the $Pbto_2$ monitor.	Prepares the monitor.	

Procedure continues on following page

Procedure	for Brain Tissue Oxygen Monitoring: Insertion (Assist), Care, and Troubleshooting—*Continued*		
Steps	**Rationale**	**Special Considerations**	
10. Insert the calibration card for calibration of the monitor unique to each Pbto$_2$ probe.[9,10,14,16,19] **(Level M*)**	The Licox monitor (Integra NeuroSciences, Plainsboro, NJ) requires insertion of a calibration card referred to as the "smart card," which has numbers on it that match those on the oxygen probe that is being inserted. This card is placed into a card slot located on the front of the monitor. The calibration card can only be used with the probe that has the same numbers on it (and is included in the same packaging; see Fig. 87-1, *B*).[9,10,14,16,19]	If the calibration card is lost, another corresponding Pbto$_2$ probe and "smart card" must be used.	
11. Assist as needed with insertion of an intracranial bolt (see Procedure 88).	May be inserted before Pbto$_2$ probe insertion.		
12. Assist as needed with insertion of the oxygen probe and temperature probe.	Facilitates the insertion process.	The oxygen probe and temperature probe may be separate (triple-lumen bolt system) or may be combined (double-lumen bolt system). The additional lumen is for the ICP probe.	
13. Connect the oxygen and temperature probes to the monitor cables.	Prepares for monitoring.		
14. Observe the temperature and Pbto$_2$ values.[6,7,27,28]	Initiates monitoring. The temperature values should be accurate; however, time is needed for the brain tissue to settle after the microtrauma caused by catheter placement.		
15. If possible, use a cable to transfer the values from the Pbto$_2$ monitor to the bedside monitor. Set the upper and lower alarm limits.	Allows integration of the monitoring systems. The currently available brain tissue oxygen monitoring system does not have an alarm system. Integrating the monitoring system with the bedside monitor allows: (1) a larger display of the numeric values; and (2) audible upper and lower alarm limits.[10]	Refer to monitor guidelines for specific information.	
16. After the system has been placed, apply a sterile occlusive dressing at the insertion point.	Prevents contamination of the insertion site by microorganisms and protects the site.	A dressing (formed with dry sterile gauze) provides a base to secure the device to an arm board or other securing method.	
17. Secure the Pbto$_2$ monitor cables with two points of tension to avoid tension on the Pbto$_2$ and ICP probes. A. Anchor the cables at the patient's head and at the shoulder.	The monitoring cables need to be secured so that no tension or disruption of the device occurs at the insertion site.		

*Level M: Manufacturer's recommendations only

Procedure	**for Brain Tissue Oxygen Monitoring: Insertion (Assist), Care, and Troubleshooting**—*Continued*	
Steps	**Rationale**	**Special Considerations**
B. Secure the cables so that they do not get entangled in the side rails and do not touch the floor.	Supports the entire mechanism.	One method to secure the monitor cables is: A. Place an IV arm board or stability anchor to a conical gauze dressing where the device and cables can be secured. B. Anchor the cables from the patient's head to the shoulder in place with a transparent or soft cloth adhesive dressing (Fig. 87-2). The first tension point is directly on the patient's head where the dressing is anchored to the skin at the point of insertion. The second tension point is at the patient's shoulder. C. Place rolled towels under the secured system.

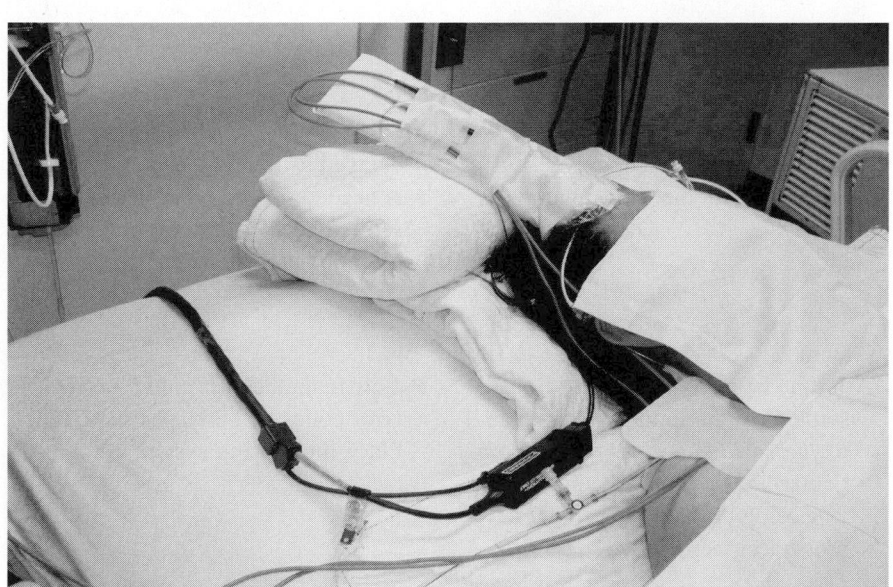

FIGURE 87-2 Demonstration of securing the IM3 hyphenate triple-lumen system (oxygen probe, temperature probe, and ICP catheter). *(Courtesy University of Pennsylvania: Brain oxygen monitor clinical practice guidelines.)*

C. Allow enough slack to accommodate for patient movement and turning.	Prevents gravity drag and tension on the cables and the device.	
18. Discard used supplies in appropriate receptacles.	Removes and safely discards used supplies. Safely removes sharp objects.	

19. **HH**

Brain Tissue Oxygenation Monitor Set-up with the Bedside Monitor

1. Connect the brain oxygen monitor to the bedside monitor with the attached cable.	Allows integration of the monitoring systems.	Refer to monitor guidelines for specific information.

Procedure continues on following page

Procedure	for Brain Tissue Oxygen Monitoring: Insertion (Assist), Care, and Troubleshooting—*Continued*		
Steps	**Rationale**	**Special Considerations**	
2. Select a pressure module and label the parameter. A waveform need not be displayed, only a numeric display.	Prepares the equipment.	Each bedside monitor may have its own unique labels for parameters that are being added (e.g., brain oxygen).	
3. Manually adjust the temperature on the front of the monitor to the established number of degrees Celsius determined by the institution. **(Level M*)**	Prepares the equipment.	Follow institutional guidelines. If a separate brain temperature probe or combined brain tissue oxygen and brain temperature probe is not in use, the temperature on the front of the monitor must be adjusted manually every hour to equal the patient's core temperature for accurate determination of the $Pbto_2$.[10]	
4. Disconnect the blue and green cables from the brain oxygen monitor.	Prepares the equipment.		
5. Select the designated pressure module and zero the bedside monitor.	Prepares the equipment.		
6. Plug the blue and green cables back into the front of the brain oxygen monitor.[10]	Allows integration of the monitoring systems.		
7. Note the difference between the brain oxygen monitor reading and the bedside monitor reading.	Confirms that data on the brain oxygen monitor accurately correlate with the bedside monitor.		
8. Readings should be within 1 mm Hg when the blue and green cables are connected to the Licox system at the head of the patient and after the brain tissue has had time to settle (20 to 120 minutes) after Licox insertion.[5-7,12,28] **(Level C*)**	Confirms that data on the brain oxygen monitor accurately correlate with the bedside monitor.	Monitoring of $Pbto_2$ values may be delayed as long as 2 hours as time is needed for the brain tissue to settle after the microtrauma caused by probe placement.[5-7,12,28]	

Troubleshooting the $Pbto_2$ Monitoring System

1. Perform an oxygen challenge test as prescribed.
  A. Place the ventilator fraction of inspired oxygen (Fio_2) setting on 100% for 2 to 5 minutes.
  B. Observe the monitor as an accurate probe will show an increase in $Pbto_2$. **(Level C)**
	After the brain tissue has had time to settle from the initial insertion, an oxygen challenge is performed particularly if the $Pbto_2$ reading is unexpectedly low or a question of probe accuracy exists.	Follow manufacturer guidelines for error codes that are specific to the $Pbto_2$ monitoring system.	

C. If no response to the increased Fio_2 is seen, inform the physician because a head CT scan may be prescribed to confirm correct probe placement.[15,16,28] **(Level C)**	Head CT scan may be obtained after insertion to check catheter placement. Follow hospital-specific guidelines.		
2. Note whether an electrical disturbance has occurred.	Strong electromagnetic disturbances can result in $Pbto_2$ measurement errors. Errors can continue for a few seconds after the disturbance.	These disturbances may occur when a high-frequency scalpel or cautery is used or during cardioversion.	

*Level C: Qualitative studies, descriptive or correlational studies, integrative reviews, systematic reviews, or randomized controlled trials with inconsistent results
*Level M: Manufacturer's recommendations only

Procedure	for Brain Tissue Oxygen Monitoring: Insertion (Assist), Care, and Troubleshooting—*Continued*	
Steps	**Rationale**	**Special Considerations**
3. Note whether a cable is damaged; if so, replace the cable.	If the probe cable or the extension cable is damaged, measured values can be incorrect or the measurement can be interrupted.	
4. Avoid changes in the temperature of the temperature probe connector:	The temperature measurement may be inaccurate if the connector of the temperature probe is subjected to significant changes in temperature or if the temperature of the connector is beyond the defined range of 18° to 30° C.[10]	
A. Avoid holding the temperature probe connector.	If the probe connector is held with a warm hand, the temperature measurement may be inaccurate until it is released.	
B. Protect the temperature probe connector from direct sunlight or warming devices.[1] **(Level M*)**	Warming of the connector can cause inaccurate temperature readings.[10]	

Removal of the Brain Tissue Oxygen Monitoring System

1. HH		
2. PE		
3. Position the patient in a semi-Fowler's position.	Prepares for removal.	
4. Turn off the Pbto$_2$ monitor.	Facilitates the removal process.	
5. Assist as needed with removal of the dressing.	Prepares for removal.	
6. Assist as needed with removal of the monitoring probes.	Facilitates the removal process.	
7. Apply an occlusive sterile dressing to the site.	Reduces the risk for infection.	Assess for bleeding, cerebrospinal fluid (CSF) leak, and signs and symptoms of infection.
8. Discard used supplies in appropriate receptacles.	Removes and safely discards used supplies.	
9. HH		

Expected Outcomes

- Pbto$_2$ probe placed in the correct position; monitoring able to begin after brain tissue has had time to settle (20 minutes to 2 hours)
- Pbto$_2$ value between 20 and 35 mm Hg, or as prescribed, as an acceptable value for the individual patient
- Accurate and reliable Pbto$_2$ monitoring
- Early detection of cerebral hypoxia
- Immediate intervention and management of compromised cerebral oxygenation hypoxia

Unexpected Outcomes

- Brain tissue oxygen reading low, with no response to oxygen challenge
- Infection
- Hematoma from placement

*Level M: Manufacturer's recommendations only

Procedure continues on following page

Patient Monitoring and Care

Steps	Rationale	Reportable Conditions
		These conditions should be reported if they persist despite nursing interventions.
1. Assess the patient's baseline neurologic status, vital signs, and ICP every 15 minutes and more frequently if necessary during and immediately after the procedure.	Provides assessment of patient status before and during the procedure.	• Changes in neurologic status • Changes in vital signs • Changes in ICP and CPP

2. Perform an oxygen challenge test as prescribed.
  A. Place the ventilator Fio_2 setting on 100% for 2 to 5 minutes.
  B. An accurate probe shows an increase in $Pbto_2$.[9,10,17,29]
  (Level C*)
	After the brain tissue has had time to settle from the initial insertion, perform an oxygen challenge, particularly if the $Pbto_2$ reading is unexpectedly low or a question exists of probe accuracy, reliability, or validity.	• Lack of variation response to oxygen challenge

3. Obtain the patient's temperature every 1 to 2 hours or as prescribed.	Provides a comparison of cerebral and body temperatures. Although the temperature measurements do not correlate exactly, a parallel trend should be seen.	• Abnormal temperatures
4. Maintain the $Pbto_2$ value between 20 and 35 mm Hg or as prescribed.[6,13,18,25-29] **(Level C)**	Represents normal values.	• Elevated $Pbto_2$ values • Decreased $Pbto_2$ values
5. Follow institution standard for assessing pain. Administer analgesia as prescribed.	Identifies need for pain interventions.	Continued pain despite pain interventions

*Level C: Qualitative studies, descriptive or correlational studies, integrative reviews, systematic reviews, or randomized controlled trials with inconsistent results

Documentation

Documentation should include the following:
- Patient and family education
- Preprocedure verifications and time out
- Completion of informed consent
- Insertion of the $Pbto_2$ probe
- Patient tolerance of the procedure
- Site assessment
- Neurologic assessments

- Hourly values, including $Pbto_2$, brain tissue temperature, and other hemodynamic (e.g., vital signs, cardiac parameters: cardiac output [CO], cardiac index [CI], systemic vascular resistance [SVR]), and neurologic multimodality monitoring in use (e.g., ICP, CPP, $Sjvo_2$).
- Occurrence of unexpected outcomes and interventions
- Pain assessment, interventions, and effectiveness

References

CR 1. Bardt TF, et al: Monitoring of brain tissue Po_2 in traumatic brain injury: effect of cerebral hypoxia on outcome, *Acta Neurochir (Wien)* 71(Suppl):153-156, 1998.

2. Bhatia A, Gupta AK: Neuromonitoring in the intensive care unit: II: cerebral oxygenation monitoring and microdialysis, *Intens Care Med* 33:1322-1328, 2007.

3. Bratton SL, et al: Guidelines for the management of severe traumatic brain injury: X: brain oxygen monitoring and thresholds, *J Neurotrauma* 24:S65-S70, 2007.

CR 4. De Georgia MA, Deogaonkar A: Multimodal monitoring in the neurological intensive care unit, *Neurologist* 11: 45-54, 2005.

CR 5. Dings J, Meixenberger J, Roosen K: Brain tissue PO_2 monitoring: catheter stability and complications, *Neurol Res* 19:241-245, 1997.

CR 6. Dings J, et al: Clinical experience with 118 brain tissue oxygen partial pressure catheter probes, *Neurosurgery* 43:1082-1095, 1998.

CR 7. Haitsma IK, Maas AIR: Advanced monitoring in the intensive care unit: brain tissue oxygen tension, *Curr Opin Crit Care* 8:115-120, 2002.

8. Hebl JR: The importance and implications of aseptic techniques during regional anesthesia, *Reg Anesth Pain Med* 31:311-323, 2006.

9. Integra NeuroSciences: *LICOX®IMC complete neuro-monitoring directions for use. model IP2.P* complete brain IMC-PROBE KIT,* Plainsboro, NJ, 2004, Integra NeuroSciences.

10. Integra NeuroSciences: *LICOX CMP brain oxygen monitoring system operations manual,* Plainsboro, NJ, 2004, Integra Neurosciences.

11. Integra NeuroSciences: *MRI safety of the Licox IT2 complete brain tunneling probe kit, including the model CC1.P1 oxygen and temperature probe and model VK5.2 parenteral probe guide at 1.5 Tesla,* Plainsboro, NJ, 2006, Integra Neurosciences.

12. Lang EW, et al: Direct cerebral oxygenation monitoring: a systematic review of recent publications, *Neurosurg Rev* 30:99-106, 2007.

CR 13. Maas AIR, et al: Monitoring cerebral oxygenation: experimental studies and preliminary clinical results of continuous monitoring of cerebrospinal fluid and brain tissue oxygen tension, *Acta Neurochir* 59(Suppl):50-57, 1993.

14. Mazzeo AT, Bullock R: Monitoring brain tissue oximetry: will it change management of critically ill neurologic patients? *J Neurol Sci* 261:1-9, 2007.

CR 15. Meixensberger J, et al: Brain tissue oxygen guided treatment supplementing ICP/CPP therapy after traumatic brain injury, *J Neurol Neurosurg Psychiatry* 74:760-764, 2003.

CR 16. Meixensberger J, et al: Monitoring of brain tissue oxygenation following severe subarachnoid hemorrhage, *Neurol Res* 25:445-450, 2003.

CR 17. Mulvey JM, et al: Multimodality monitoring in severe traumatic brain injury: the role of brain tissue oxygenation monitoring, *Neurocrit Care* 1:391-402, 2004.

CR 18. Sarrafzadeh AS, et al: Cerebral oxygenation in contusioned vs. nonlesioned brain tissue: monitoring of $PtiO_2$ with Licox and Paratrend, *Acta Neurochir (Wien)* 71(Suppl):186-189, 1998.

19. Stewart C, et al: The new licox combined brain tissue oxygen and brain temperature monitor: assessment of in vitro accuracy and clinical experience in severe traumatic brain injury, *Neurosurgery* 63:1159-1165, 2008.

CR 20. Stiefel MF, et al: Cerebral oxygenation following decompressive hemicraniectomy for the treatment of refractory intracranial hypertension, *J Neurosurg* 101(2):241-247, 2004.

CR 21. Stiefel MF: The effect of nimodipine of cerebral oxygenation following subarachnoid hemorrhage, *J Neurosurg* 101(4):594-599, 2004.

CR 22. Stiefel MF, et al: Multi-modality monitoring in the management of refractory intracranial hypertension: a case report, *J Trauma* 59(3):757-761, 2005.

CR 23. Stiefel MF, et al: Reduced mortality rate in patients with severe traumatic brain injury treated with brain tissue oxygen monitoring, *J Neurosurg* 103(5):805-811, 2005.

24. Tisdall MM, Smith M: Mulimodal monitoring in traumatic brain injury: current status and future directions, *Br J Anaesth* 99:61-67, 2007.

CR 25. Valadka AB, et al: Relationship of brain tissue Po2 to outcome after severe head injury, *Crit Care Med* 26:1576-1581, 1998.

CR 26. Valadka AB, et al: Brain tissue Po2: correlation with cerebral blood flow, *Acta Neurochirurgica* 81(Suppl):299-301, 2002.

CR 27. van den Brink WA, et al: Monitoring brain oxygen tension in severe head injury: the Rotterdam experience, *Acta Neurochir* 71(Suppl):190-194, 1998.

CR 28. van den Brink WA, et al: Brain oxygen tension in severe head injury, *Neurosurgery* 46:868-878, 2000.

CR 29. van Santbrink H, et al: Continuous monitoring of partial pressure of brain tissue oxygen in patients with severe head injury, *Neurosurgery* 38:21-31, 1996.

30. Wartenberg KE, Schmidt JM, Mayer SA: Multimodality monitoring in neurocritical care, *Crit Care Clin* 23:507-538, 2007.

Additional Readings

CR Bader MK, Littlejohns LR, March K: Brain tissue oxygen monitoring II: implications for critical care teams and case study, *Crit Care Nurse* 23:29-38, 40-42, 44, 2003.

Blissitt PA: Brain oxygen monitoring. In Bader MK, Littlejohns LR, editors: *AACN AANN protocols for practice: monitoring technologies in critically ill neuroscience patients,* Boston, 2009, Jones and Bartlett, 103-144.

CR Gracias VH, et al: Cerebral cortical oxygenation: a pilot study, *J Trauma Injury Infect Crit Care* 56(3):469-474 2004.

CR Maloney Wilensky E, et al: Brain tissue oxygen practice guidelines using the LICOX CMP monitoring system, *J Neurosci Nurs* 37(5):278-288, 2005.

CR Littlejohns LR, Bader MK: Guidelines for the management of severe head injury: clinical application and changes in practice, *Crit Care Nurse* 21:48-65, 2001.

CR Littlejohns LR, Bader MK, March K: Brain tissue oxygen monitoring in severe brain injury: I: research and usefulness in critical care, *Crit Care Nurse* 23:17-25, 2003.

CR Patterson J, et al: Successful outcome in severe traumatic brain injury: a case study, *J Neurosci Nurs* 37(5):236-242, 2005.

CR Smith MJ, et al: Packed red blood cell transfusion increases local cerebral oxygenation, *Crit Care Med* 33:1104-1108, 2005.

Stiefel MF, et al: Conventional neurocritical care does not ensure cerebral oxygenation after traumatic brain injury, *J Neurosurg* 105:568-575, 2006.

Intracranial Bolt and Fiberoptic Catheter Insertion (Assist), Intracranial Pressure Monitoring, Care, Troubleshooting, and Removal

P U R P O S E : The fiberoptic catheter is a device utilized for continuous measurement of intracranial pressure (ICP). The fiberoptic catheter is placed in the brain parenchyma and reflects pressure exerted by the intracranial contents, brain tissue, blood, and cerebrospinal fluid (CSF), within the skull. The fiberoptic catheter is inserted through a bolt. Unlike a ventricular catheter, which is attached to an external transducer and drainage system, the fiberoptic catheter does not allow for CSF drainage.

Tess Slazinski

PREREQUISITE NURSING KNOWLEDGE

- A fundamental understanding of neuroanatomy and physiology is needed.
- Knowledge of aseptic and sterile technique is necessary.
- Proper equipment assembly and setup specific to the fiberoptic intracranial pressure monitoring device must be understood.
- Intracranial pressure (ICP) is the pressure exerted by the intracranial contents, brain tissue, blood and cerebrospinal fluid (CSF). Increased intracranial pressure occurs when the intracranial volume exceeds the brain's ability to compensate for increased volume.[13]
- Normal ICP ranges from 0 to 15 mm Hg; sustained ICPs of greater than 20 mm Hg are generally considered neurologic emergencies.[3,10]
- ICP is measured via a catheter inserted into the brain parenchyma. The catheter is inserted through an intracranial bolt (Fig. 88-1).

- The normal ICP waveform has three or four peaks with P_1 of greater amplitude than P_2 and P_3. P_1 is thought to reflect arterial pressure; P_2 and P_3 and P_4 (when present) have been described as choroid plexus or venous in origin (Fig. 88-2).[13] The amplitude of P_2 may exceed P_1 with increased ICP or decreased intracranial compliance (Fig. 88-3).
- ICP waveform trends include *a*, *b*, and *c* waves. The *a* waves, also referred to as plateau waves, are associated with ICP values of 50 to 100 mm Hg and last 5 to 20 minutes. The a waves (Fig. 88-4) are associated with abrupt neurologic deterioration and herniation. The *b* waves (Fig 88-5), with ICP values of 20 to 50 mm Hg and lasting 30 seconds to 2 minutes, may become *a* waves. The *c* waves (Fig. 88-6) may coincide with ICPs as high as 20 mm Hg but are short lasting and without clinical significance.[1]
- Cerebral perfusion pressure (CPP) is the pressure at which the brain is perfused. CPP is calculated by subtracting the ICP from the mean arterial pressure (MAP). Normal

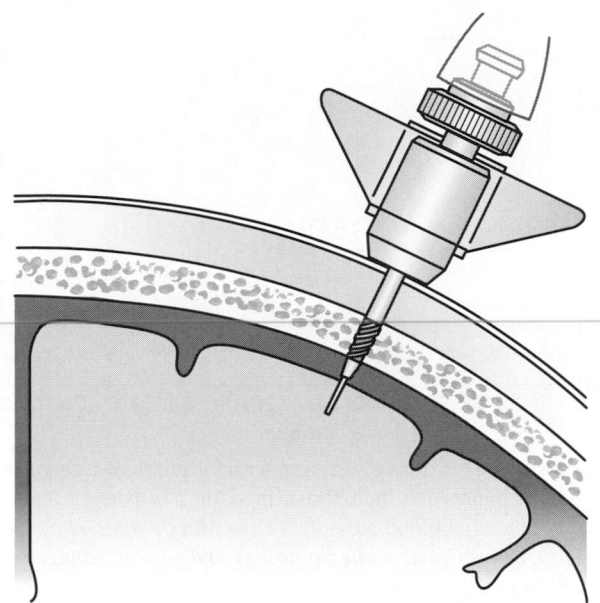

FIGURE 88-1   Intracranial bolt inserted into the parenchyma. *(From Littlejohns L, Bader MK: AACN-AANN protocols for practice: monitoring technologies in critically ill neuroscience patients, Sudbury, MA, 2009, Jones and Bartlett, 35.)*

CPP is thought to be approximately 80 mm Hg.[11] In severe traumatic brain injury, the CPP for adults should range between 50 and 70 mm Hg.[2] Patients with other neurologic injuries may require individualized CPP parameters reflective of the neuropathology and brain perfusion needs. Research continues regarding the relationship between cerebral blood flow and CPP.

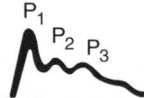

FIGURE 88-2   Components of the intracranial pressure waveform: P_1, P_2 and P_3.

- ICP and CPP must be considered together in management of the patient. Cerebral autoregulation is the intrinsic ability of the cerebral vessels to constrict and dilate as needed to maintain adequate cerebral perfusion. Cerebral autoregulation is impaired with brain injury and the cerebral blood flow becomes passively dependent on the systemic blood pressure. The cerebral blood vessels are no longer able to react to maintain CPP in response to a change in blood pressure.[3]
- Sustained ICP elevations of 20 mm Hg or greater necessitate immediate reporting and intervention. ICP waveform changes that indicate loss of cerebral compliance or cerebral autoregulation should be reported immediately.[8,10,13]
- ICP monitoring is indicated for the following:
  - ❖ Traumatic brain injury with a Glasgow Coma Scale score of less than or equal to 8 and abnormal computed tomography (CT) scan results or normal CT scan results with two of the following: hypotension; greater than 40 years of age; and motor posturing[2]
  - ❖ Intracranial hemorrhage[13]
  - ❖ Subarachnoid hemorrhage[13]
  - ❖ Hydrocephalus[13]
  - ❖ Fulminant hepatic failure with encephalopathy[13]
  - ❖ Ischemic stroke with massive edema[13]
  - ❖ Meningitis[13]
  - ❖ Cysts[13]
- Contraindications for ICP monitoring include infection and coagulopathies.
- Concerns with accuracy of ICP monitoring values primarily relate to displacement, misplacement, or breakage of the catheter and drift (especially after 5 days).[11,13]
- Management of the patient with increased ICP and decreased CPP is a multi-tiered approach that includes positioning, maintaining normothermia, administration of pharmacologic agents, and surgical procedures.[6,9]

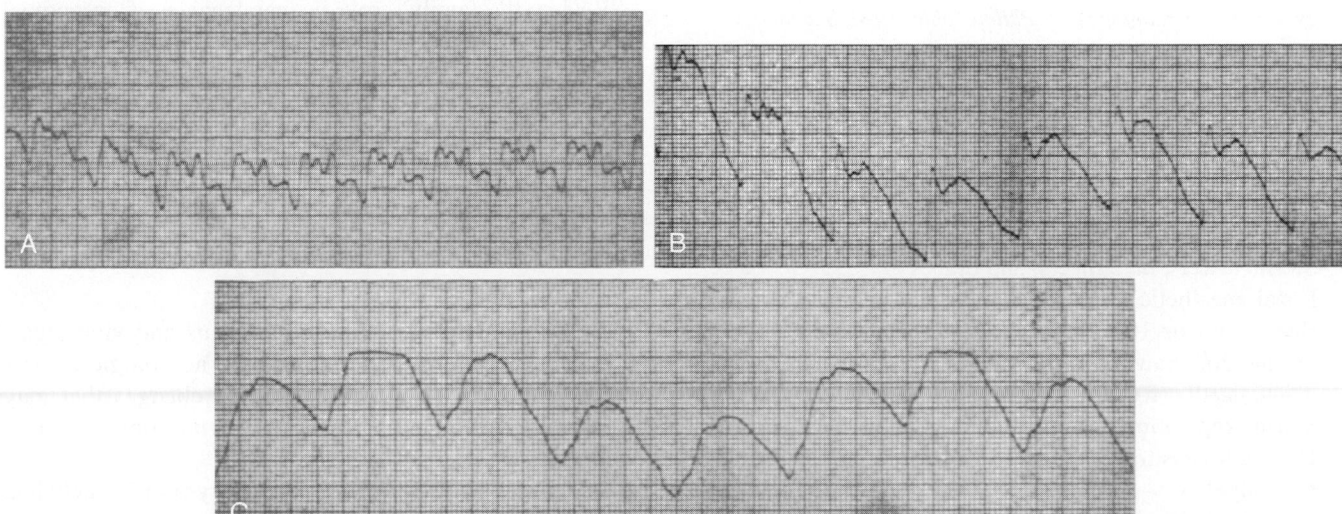

FIGURE 88-3   Example of intracranial pressure waveforms with P_2 elevation indicating decreased cerebral compliance.

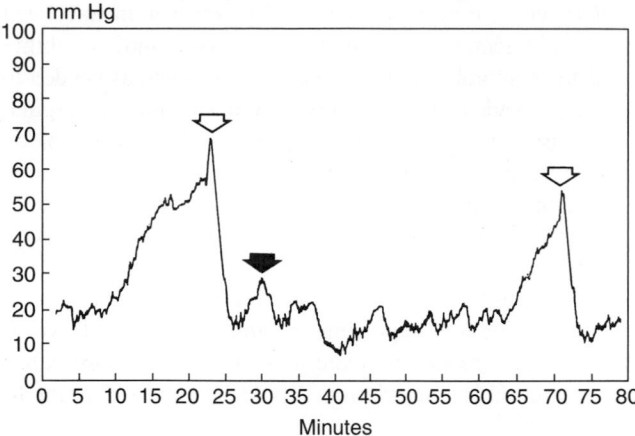

FIGURE 88-4   *a* or plateau waves. *Open arrows* indicate plateau elevations in intracranial pressure. Note that when intracranial pressure falls, it does not return to baseline preceding the first wave *(closed arrow). (From Marshall SB, et al: Neuroscience critical care: pathophysiology and patient management, Philadelphia, 1990, Saunders.)*

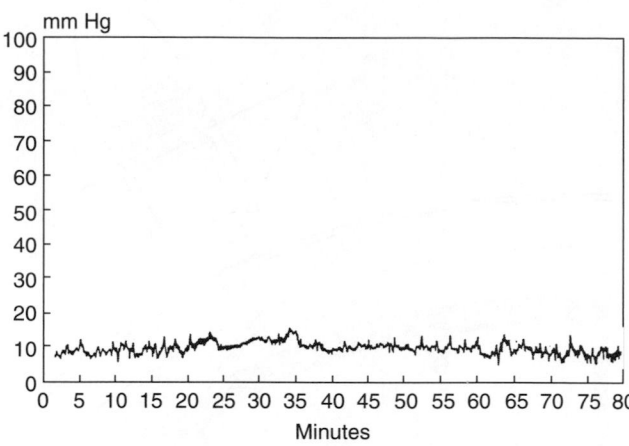

FIGURE 88-6   *c* waves. The intracranial pressure changes are much less impressive than those in *a* or *b* waves and reflect changes in arterial blood pressure. *(From Marshall SB, et al: Neuroscience critical care: pathophysiology and patient management, Philadelphia, 1990, Saunders.)*

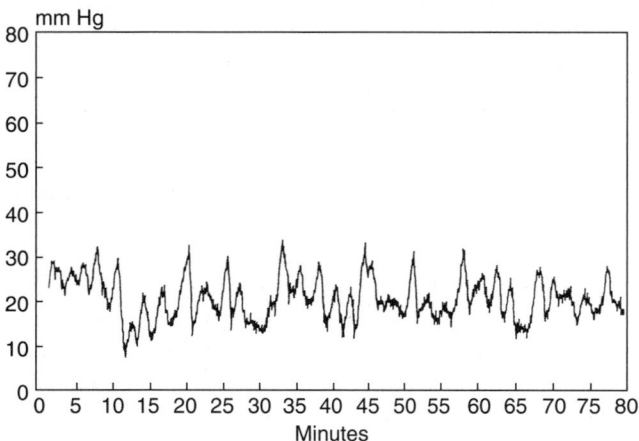

FIGURE 88-5   Elevations in intracranial pressure represent *b* waves. The intracranial pressure rise is steep and rapid but to heights less than those observed with *a* waves and much briefer. *(From Marshall SB, et al: Neuroscience critical care: pathophysiology and patient management, Philadelphia, 1990, Saunders.)*

EQUIPMENT

- Antiseptic solution
- Sterile gloves, surgical caps, masks, goggles or face shields, and sterile surgical gowns
- Sterile towels, half-sheets, and drapes
- Local anesthetic (lidocaine 1% or 2% without epinephrine), 5-ml or 10-mL Luer-Lok syringe with 18-gauge needle (for drawing up lidocaine), and 23-gauge or 25-gauge needle (for administration of lidocaine)
- Shave preparation kit
- Cranial access tray
  - ❖ Scalpel
  - ❖ Scalpel retractor
  - ❖ Forceps
  - ❖ Needles/needle holders

- Monitoring equipment
  - ❖ Pressure box (bedside monitor)
  - ❖ Pressure cable
  - ❖ Stand-alone monitor (for interpretation of fiberoptic data)
  - ❖ Preamp fiberoptic catheter connector cable
  - ❖ Monitoring cable to connect to bedside monitor
- Sterile dressing supplies

PATIENT AND FAMILY EDUCATION

- Assess patient and family understanding of fiberoptic catheters. ➥*Rationale:* Explanations to patient and family specific needs may allay fears.
- Explain the fiberoptic catheter insertion procedure. Review normal parameters and patient care after insertion. Review the family's role in maintenance of an optimal ICP with limitation of patient stimulation. ➥*Rationale:* Explanation of expected interventions may allay patient and family anxieties, encourage questions, and promote therapeutic family interaction.

PATIENT ASSESSMENT AND PREPARATION
Patient Assessment

- Assess the patient's neurologic status and vital signs. ➥*Rationale:* Performing a baseline neurologic assessment enables the nurse to identify changes that may occur during or as a result of the fiberoptic catheter placement.
- Assess the patient's current laboratory profile, including complete blood count (CBC) or platelet count, prothrombin time (PT), international normalized ratio (INR), and partial thromboplastin time (PTT). ➥*Rationale:* Baseline

coagulation study results determine the risk for bleeding during intracranial bolt and catheter insertion.

- Assess for allergies. **➤➤Rationale:** Assessment minimizes the risk of allergic reaction.

Patient Preparation

- Verify correct patient with two identifiers. **➤➤Rationale:** Prior to performing a procedure, the nurse should ensure the correct identification of the patient for the intended intervention.
- Perform a pre-procedure verification and time out, if nonemergent. **➤➤Rationale:** Ensures patient safety.
- Ensure that informed consent has been obtained. **➤➤Rationale:** Informed consent protects the rights of the

patient and makes a competent decision possible for the patient; however, in emergency circumstances, time may not allow for the consent form to be signed.

- Administer preprocedural analgesia or sedation as prescribed. **➤➤Rationale:** The patient needs to remain still during fiberoptic catheter insertion. In an emergency situation, the patient may already be receiving continuous analgesia and sedation.
- Assist the patient to a supine position with the head of the bed at 30 to 45 degrees and the neck in a midline, neutral position. **➤➤Rationale:** This position provides access for fiberoptic catheter insertion and enhances jugular venous outflow, contributing to possible reduction in intracranial pressure.

Procedure for Intracranial Bolt and Fiberoptic Catheter Insertion (Assist), Intracranial Pressure Monitoring, Care, Troubleshooting, and Removal

Steps	Rationale	Special Considerations
1. 🅷🅷		
2. Apply goggles or masks with face shields, caps, gowns, and sterile gloves.	Prepares for sterile procedure.	
3. Assist as needed with identifying the optimal area for placement of the catheter.	Facilitates catheter placement. Catheters placed adjacent to the intracranial pathology are more likely to identify increased ICP earlier.[13,16-18]	
4. Assist as needed with shaving and cleansing the insertion site with an antiseptic solution.	Reduces transmission of microorganisms and minimizes the risk of infection.	The choice of povidone-iodine or chlorhexidine as an antiseptic agent is controversial. Both should be allowed to dry completely. Studies suggest chlorhexidine is neurotoxic.[5,15]
5. Assist as needed with covering the patient's head and upper thorax with sterile half-sheet and drape.	Protects the insertion site from contamination.	
6. Preparation of the fiberoptic system: A. Ensure that the preamp cable connects from the catheter to the stand-alone monitor. B. Follow manufacturer's instructions for zeroing the catheter before insertion (**Level M***).	The catheter is zeroed before insertion and never rezeroed.[13]	
7. Assist as needed with insertion of the intracranial bolt and fiberoptic catheter.	Facilitates the insertion process.	
8. Apply a sterile occlusive dressing.	Reduces the transmission of microorganisms.	
9. Secure the catheter and preamp cable to the patient in such a way to prevent accidental removal.	Lessens the likelihood of dislodgment and breakage of the catheter.	
10. After fiberoptic catheter placement follow the manufacturer's instructions for the "Cal/Step" interface (**Level M**).	Ensures accurate fiberoptic data at the bedside monitor and allows printing of ICP tracing.	

*Level M: Manufacturer's recommendations only

Procedure continues on following page

Procedure for Intracranial Bolt and Fiberoptic Catheter Insertion (Assist), Intracranial Pressure Monitoring, Care, Troubleshooting, and Removal—*Continued*

Steps	Rationale	Special Considerations
11. Set the appropriate ICP scale for the measured pressure.	Necessary for visualization of the complete ICP waveform and to obtain readings.	
12. Set the monitor alarms.	Goals for ICP management are individualized for each patient based on pathology.	
13. Discard used supplies in an appropriate receptacle.	Removes and safely discards used supplies; safely removes sharp objects.	
14. HH		

Troubleshooting

Steps	Rationale	Special Considerations
1. Assess the integrity of the fiberoptic device. Note the location and presence of any markers on the fiberoptic catheter system that identify location (depth of the catheter).	Occlusion or dislocation may require manipulation or replacement.	Intracranial device manipulation is not a nursing responsibility in most institutions. Notify the physician or advanced practice nurse if the device is occluded or dislocated.
2. Observe for messages or numeric values that indicate a broken catheter.	Breakage requires replacement.	
3. Correct the ICP monitoring device malfunction.	Fiberoptic catheters may become damaged or dislodged, requiring catheter replacement.	Follow manufacturer's instructions and troubleshooting manuals for identifying and correcting common problems.
4. Change the monitoring system, if needed.	Replaces a malfunctioning system.	

Fiberoptic Catheter Removal

Steps	Rationale	Special considerations
1. HH		
2. Ensure healthcare providers who are assisting with catheter removal apply sterile gloves and mask with face shield or goggles.	Minimizes the risk of infection; maintains aseptic and sterile precautions.	
3. Assist with the removal of the fiberoptic catheter.	Facilitates the removal process.	
4. Apply an antiseptic solution and sterile occlusive dressing after the device is removed.	Minimizes contamination by microorganisms.	Observe for any CSF drainage or blood from insertion site.
5. Discard used supplies in an appropriate receptacle.	Removes and safely discards used supplies.	
6. HH		

Expected Outcomes

- Accurate and reliable ICP monitoring, CPP calculation, and assessment of cerebral compliance [7,10]
- Maintenance of ICP within range of 0 to15 mm Hg or as prescribed [7,10,13]
- Early detection of elevated ICP trends [7,10,13]
- Management of increased ICP and decreased CPP [7,10,13]
- Protection of cerebral perfusion with maintenance of CPP within prescribed parameters [7,10]

Unexpected Outcomes

- CSF infection [12,14]
- CSF leakage [13]
- Dislodgment of the fiberoptic catheter [13]
- Dislodgment of the bolt [13]
- Pneumocephalus (rare) [13]
- Cerebral hemorrhage (rare) [2,13]
- Sequelae of sustained increased intracranial pressure and decreased cerebral perfusion pressure: cerebral infarction, herniation, and brain death [6,7,11]

Patient Monitoring and Care

Steps	Rationale	Reportable Conditions
		These conditions should be reported if they persist despite nursing interventions.
1. Assess the patient's neurologic status and vital signs during the procedure.	Evaluates the patient's response to the procedure.	• Changes in neurologic status • Abnormal vital signs
2. Note the ICP waveform and numeric values during the insertion procedure.	Provides baseline data.	• P_2 of greater amplitude than P_1
3. Assess the patient's neurologic status hourly or more often as indicated. [13]	Provides clinical confirmation of and correlation with the monitored ICP data.	• Changes in neurological status
4. Assess the ICP hourly.	Determines the neurologic status.	• Increased ICP • ICP waveform abnormalities • Immediately report sustained ICP elevations of 20 mm Hg or greater [13]
5. Calculate the CPP hourly (or more often as indicated).	A CPP of 50-70 mm Hg should be maintained for adult patients with traumatic brain injury. CPP parameters should be individualized to meet patient perfusion needs.	• Changes in CPP • CPP less than the lowest prescribed parameter may put the patient at risk for cerebral ischemia [2,4]
6. Set the bedside alarm limits based on the parameter goals.	ICP limit is usually set to alarm when ICP is greater than 20 mm Hg; however, this needs to be individualized for each patient.	• Abnormal ICP • Abnormal waveforms
7. Assess the catheter system hourly.	Ensures accuracy and safety of monitoring.	
8. Change the insertion site dressing as needed or based on institution standard.	Practices for head dressing changes and site care vary considerably.	• Significant drainage on ICP insertion site dressing or head dressing • Signs and symptoms of infection
9. Provide a safe environment, preventing inadvertent dislodgment of the fiberoptic catheter through appropriate catheter positioning, sedation, and analgesia as needed and as prescribed.	Catheter dislodgment results in the inability to effectively monitor ICP and may require reinsertion.	• Dislodged device • Abnormal ICP • Abnormal ICP waveform
10. Follow institution standard for assessing pain. Administer analgesia as prescribed.	Identifies need for pain interventions.	• Continued pain despite pain interventions.

Procedure continues on following page

Documentation [10,13]

Documentation should include the following:
- Insertion time and patient response to procedure
- Completion of informed consent
- Preprocedure verifications and time out
- Initial and hourly ICP[10,13]
- Initial and hourly CPP calculation[10,13]
- Insertion site assessment
- Patient and family education

- Initial ICP tracing (include ICP waveform morphology) and any changes in waveform[10,13]
- Nursing interventions used to treat ICP or CPP deviations and expected or unexpected outcomes[10,13]
- Pain assessment, interventions, and effectiveness

References

1. Bershad EM, Humphreis WE, Suarez JI: Intracranial hypertension, *Semin Neurol* 28:690-702, 2008.
2. Bratton SL, Chesnut RM, Ghajar J, et al: Guidelines for the management of severe traumatic brain injury: a joint project of the Brain Trauma Foundation, American Association of Neurological Surgeons (AANS), Congress of Neurological Surgeons (CNS), AANS/CNS Joint Section on Neurotrauma and Critical Care, *J Neurotrauma* 24(Suppl 1):S1-S106, 2007.
3. [CR] Davis JW, Davis IC, Bennink LD, et al: Placement of intracranial pressure monitors: are "normal" coagulation parameters necessary? *J Trauma* 57:1173-1177, 2004.
4. Fan J-Y, Kirkness C, Vicini P, et al: Intracranial pressure waveform morphology and intracranial adaptive capacity, *Am J Crit Care* 17:545-554, 2008.
5. Hebl JR: The importance and implications of aseptic techniques during regional anesthesia, *Reg Anesth Pain Med* 31:311-323, 2006.
6. Hickey JV, Olson DM: Intracranial hypertension: theory and management of increased intracranial pressure. In Hickey JV, editor: *The clinical practice of neurological and neurosurgical nursing*, ed 6, Philadelphia, 2009, Lippincott Williams & Wilkins, 270-307.
7. [CR] Josephson L: Management of increased intracranial pressure, *Dimens Crit Care Nurs* 23:194-207, 2004.
8. [CR] Kirkness CJ, Mitchell PH, Burr RL, et al: Intracranial pressure waveform analysis: clinical and research implications, *J Neurosci Nurs* 32:271-277, 2000.
9. [CR] March K: Application of technology in the treatment of traumatic brain injury, *Crit Care Nurs Q* 23:26-37, 2000.
10. [CR] March K: Intracranial pressure monitoring and assessing intracranial compliance in brain injury, *Crit Care Nurs Clin North Am* 12:429-436, 2002.
11. [CR] March K: Technology. In Bader MK, Littlejohns LR, editors: *AANN core curriculum for neuroscience nursing*, ed 4, St Louis, 2004, Saunders, 199-202.
12. [CR] March K: Intracranial pressure monitoring: why monitor? *AACN Clin Issues* 16:456-475, 2005.
13. March K, Madden L: Intracranial pressure management. In Littlejohns LR, Bader MK, editors: *AACN-AANN protocols for practice: monitoring technologies in critically ill neuroscience patients*, Sudbury, MA, 2009, Jones and Bartlett, 35-69.
14. [CR] O'Grady NP, Alexander M, Dellinger EP, et al: Guidelines for the prevention of intravascular catheter-related infections, *Am J Infect Control* 30:476-489, 2002.
15. Reynolds F: Neurologic infection after neuraxial anesthesia, *Anesthesiol Clin* 26:23-52, 2008.
16. [CR] Sahuqillo J, Poca M, Arribas M, et al: Interhemispheric supratentorial intracranial pressure gradients in head-injured patients: are they clinically important? *J Neurosurg* 90:16-26, 1999.
17. [CR] Slavin KV, Misra M: Infratentorial intracranial pressure monitoring in the neurosurgical intensive care unit, *Neurol Res* 25:880-884, 2003.
18. [CR] Wolfla CE, Luerssen TG, Bowman RM, et al: Brain tissue pressure gradients created by expanding frontal epidural mass lesion, *J Neurosurg* 84:642-647, 1996.

Additional Reading

[CR] Zhong J, Dujovny M, Park HK, et al: Advances in ICP monitoring techniques, *Neurol Res* 25:339-350, 2003.

Combination Intraventricular/ Fiberoptic Catheter Insertion (Assist), Monitoring, Nursing Care, Troubleshooting, and Removal

P U R P O S E : The combination intraventricular/fiberoptic catheter combines the capability of external ventricular drainage of cerebrospinal fluid with monitoring of intracranial pressure. This hybrid device can be used to monitor intracranial pressure intermittently or continuously and to drain cerebrospinal fluid intermittently or continuously.[16]

Tess Slazinski

PREREQUISITE NURSING KNOWLEDGE

- A fundamental understanding of neuroanatomy and physiology is needed.
- Knowledge of aseptic and sterile technique is necessary.
- Proper equipment assembly and setup specific to fiberoptic intracranial pressure monitoring device should be understood.
- Intracranial pressure (ICP) is the pressure exerted by the intracranial contents, brain tissue, blood, and cerebrospinal fluid (CSF) within the cranium. Increased ICP occurs when the intracranial volume exceeds the brain's ability to compensate for increased volume.[16,18] Increased ICP contributes to secondary neuronal injury.
- The ventricular catheter with external strain gauge transducer is considered the gold standard for ICP monitoring.[3,4] The external ventricular drain (EVD) is considered the most accurate and reliable method of monitoring ICP and ICP waveform and allows for CSF drainage.[3] However, the fluid-filled system of the external ventricular catheter has the greatest infection rate[1,2] and hemorrhage rate and requires repeated zeroing and leveling with the anatomic reference point for the foramen of Monro.[3]

- The parenchymal fiberoptic catheter provides quality ICP monitoring but cannot be rezeroed once inserted, cannot be used for CSF drainage, and is subject to drift, particularly after 5 days.[3,14]
- The combination catheter has some of the advantages and disadvantages of both the ventricular catheter with an external strain gauge transducer and the fiberoptic transducer tipped catheter. The combination catheter can only be zeroed before insertion. However, because the transducer is in the tip of the fiberoptic catheter, there is no external strain gauge transducer and therefore no repetitive zeroing and leveling of a transducer with the anatomic reference point for the foramen of Monro. In addition, the combination catheter allows for CSF drainage but still requires attention to the level of the reference point of the drip chamber to the anatomic reference point for the foramen of Monro and setting of the pressure level at the top of the graduated burette (drip chamber) to prevent underdrainage or overdrainage of CSF.[12]
- The anatomic reference point for the foramen of Monro is the external auditory canal.[11]
- Normal ICP ranges from 0 to 15 mm Hg; sustained ICPs of greater than 20 mm Hg are generally considered neurologic emergencies.[17]

- The normal ICP waveform has three or four peaks, with P_1 being of greater amplitude than P_2 and P_2 of greater amplitude than P_3. P_1 is thought to reflect arterial pressure; P_2, P_3, and P_4 (if present) have been described as choroid plexus or venous in origin (see Fig. 88-2).[18] The amplitude of P_2 may exceed P_1 with increased ICP or decreased intracranial compliance (see Fig. 88-3).
- ICP waveform trends include a, b, and c waves. The a waves, also referred to as plateau waves, are associated with ICP values of 50 to 100 mm Hg and last 5 to 20 minutes. The a waves (see Fig. 88-4) are associated with abrupt neurologic deterioration and herniation. The b waves (see Fig. 88-5) with ICP values of 20 to 50 mm Hg, lasting 30 seconds to 2 minutes, may become a waves. The c waves (see Fig. 88-6) may coincide with ICPs as high as 20 mm Hg but are short lasting and without clinical significance.[3,10,18]
- Cerebral perfusion pressure (CPP) is a derived mathematic calculation that indirectly reflects the adequacy of cerebral blood flow. The CPP is calculated by subtracting the ICP from the mean arterial pressure (MAP); thus CPP = MAP − ICP. The normal CPP range for adults is approximately 60 to 100 mm Hg, or a mean of 80 mm Hg. The optimal CPP for a given patient and clinical condition is not entirely known. ICP and CPP should be managed concomitantly. According to the Brain Trauma Foundation Guides, an acceptable CPP for an adult with a severe traumatic brain injury (Glasgow Coma Scale [GCS] score of equal to or less than 8) lies between 50 and 70 mm Hg.[4] Patients with aneurysmal subarachnoid hemorrhage vasospasm may need higher CPPs to maintain adequate perfusion through vasospastic cerebral blood vessels. Patients with strokes, aneurysmal subarachnoid hemorrhage, or other neurologic injuries may require higher or individualized CPP parameters reflective of the neuropathology and brain perfusion needs. Research continues regarding the relationship between cerebral blood flow and CPP.
- ICP and CPP must be considered together in management of the patient.
- Cerebral autoregulation is the intrinsic ability of the cerebral vessels to constrict and dilate as needed to maintain adequate cerebral perfusion. Cerebral autoregulation is impaired with brain injury, and the cerebral blood flow becomes passively dependent on the systemic blood flow. The cerebral blood vessels are no longer able to react to maintain CPP in response to a change in blood pressure.
- Sustained ICP elevations of 20 mm Hg or greater necessitate immediate reporting and intervention. ICP waveform changes that indicate loss of cerebral compliance or cerebral autoregulation should be reported immediately.[11,16]
- ICP monitoring is indicated for the following:
  - Traumatic brain injury with a GCS score less than 8 and abnormal computed tomographic (CT) scan or normal CT scan with two of the following: hypotension, age more than 40 years, and posturing[4]
  - Intracranial hemorrhage[18]
  - Aneurysmal subarachnoid hemorrhage[18]
  - Hydrocephalus[18]
  - Fulminant hepatic failure with encephalopathy[18]
  - Ischemic stroke with massive edema[18]
  - Meningitis[18]
  - Cysts[18]
- CSF drainage is indicated for the following[12]:
  - Acute hydrocephalus[12]
  - Subarachnoid hemorrhage[12]
  - Intracerebral hemorrhage[12]
  - Traumatic brain injury[12]
  - Postoperative craniotomy[12]
  - Meningitis[12]
- Consequences of CSF underdrainage include headache, neurologic deterioration, hydrocephalus, increased intracranial pressure, secondary neuronal injury, herniation, and death.
- Consequences of CSF overdrainage include headache, subdural hematoma, pnemocephalus, ventricular collapse, herniation, and death.
- A contraindication for ICP monitoring is coagulopathies.
- Issues regarding accuracy primarily relate to displacement, misplacement, or breakage of the fiberoptic catheter and drift (especially after 5 days).[3,16]
- Management of the patient with increased ICP and decreased CPP is a multi-tiered approach that includes nursing interventions (e.g., positioning, maintaining normothermia) and the administration of pharmacologic agents and surgical procedures.[4,10,16]

EQUIPMENT

- Antiseptic solution
- Sterile gloves, surgical caps, masks, goggles or face shields, and sterile surgical gowns
- Sterile towels, half-sheets, and drapes
- Local anesthetic (lidocaine 1% or 2% without epinephrine), 5- or 10-mL Luer-Lok syringe with 18-gauge needle (for drawing up of lidocaine), and 23-gauge or 25-gauge needle (for administration of lidocaine)
- Shave preparation kit
- Cranial access tray
  - Scalpel
  - Scalp retractor
  - Forceps
  - Needles/needle holders
  - Intraventricular/fiberoptic catheter
  - Calibration screwdriver (single-use)
- Monitoring equipment
  - Pressure module (bedside monitor)
  - Pressure cable
  - Stand-alone monitor (for interpretation of fiberoptic data)
  - Preamp cable connector cable
  - Monitoring cable to connect to bedside monitor
- External ventricular drainage system
- Sterile dressing supplies

PATIENT AND FAMILY EDUCATION

- Assess patient and family understanding of the purpose of the intraventricular and fiberoptic catheter. ➤*Rationale:* Explaining the purpose of the procedure may decrease patient and family anxiety.
- Explain the intraventricular and fiberoptic catheter insertion procedure. Review normal parameters and patient care after insertion. Review the family's role in maintenance of an optimal ICP with limitation of patient stimulation. ➤*Rationale:* Explanation of expected interventions may allay patient and family anxieties, encourage questions, and promote therapeutic family interaction.

PATIENT ASSESSMENT AND PREPARATION

Patient Assessment

- Assess the patient's neurologic status. ➤*Rationale:* A baseline neurologic assessment enables the nurse to identify changes that may occur during or as a result of the intraventricular/fiberoptic catheter placement.
- Assess the patient's current laboratory profile, including complete blood count (CBC), platelet count, prothrombin time (PT), international normalized ratio (INR), and partial thromboplastin time (PTT). ➤*Rationale:* Baseline coagulation studies determine the risk for bleeding during intraventricular catheter insertion.

- Assess for allergies. ➤*Rationale:* Insertion of the intraventricular fiberoptic catheter may necessitate local anesthetic, an antiseptic to clean the site, and analgesia and sedation. Assessment minimizes the risk of allergic reaction.

Patient Preparation

- Verify correct patient with two identifiers. ➤*Rationale:* Prior to performing a procedure, the nurse should ensure the correct identification of the patient for the intended intervention.
- Ensure that informed consent has been obtained. ➤*Rationale:* Informed consent protects the rights of the patient and makes a competent decision possible for the patient; however, in emergency circumstances, time may not allow for the consent form to be signed.
- Perform a pre-procedure verification and time out, if nonemergent. ➤*Rationale:* Ensures patient safety.
- Administer preprocedural analgesia or sedation as prescribed. ➤*Rationale:* The patient needs to remain still during catheter insertion. In an emergency situation, the patient may already be receiving continuous analgesia and sedation.
- Assist the patient to a supine position with the head of the bed at 30 to 45 degrees and the neck in a midline, neutral position. ➤*Rationale:* This position provides access for intraventricular/fiberoptic catheter insertion and enhances jugular venous outflow, contributing to possible reduction in intracranial pressure.

Procedure	for Combination Intraventricular/Fiberoptic Catheter Insertion (Assist), Monitoring, Nursing Care, Troubleshooting, and Removal	
Steps	**Rationale**	**Special Considerations**
1. **HH**		
2. Attach the external drainage system to an intravenous (IV) pole.	Preparation of the external ventricular drainage system allows for stability when priming the tubing.	External ventricular drainage systems are either pole mount or panel systems. Both systems require attachment to an IV pole for stability.
3. Ensure that all pressure tubing connections on the ventricular drainage system are tightened.	Ensures integrity and sterility of the closed system.	
4. Prime the external ventricular drainage system before patient attachment. Use preservative-free normal saline solution to prevent neuronal damage.[9] (See Figs. 92-1 and 92-2.)	Air needs to be removed from the pressure tubing.	This system does *not* require an external strain gauge flushless transducer because the fiberoptic portion of this catheter is measuring ICP. Use of a syringe filled with sterile, preservative-free normal saline solution to prime the external ventricular drainage system tubing rather than a bag of flush solution lessens the risk of flush solution being administered through the ventricular catheter into the brain.
5. Apply goggles or masks with face shields, caps, gowns, and sterile gloves.	Ensures aseptic and sterile technique.	

Procedure continues on following page

Procedure	for Combination Intraventricular/Fiberoptic Catheter Insertion (Assist), Monitoring, Nursing Care, Troubleshooting, and Removal—*Continued*		

Steps	Rationale	Special Considerations
6. Assist as needed with identifying the optimal area for placement of the catheter. **(Level C*)**	Facilitates catheter placement.	A ventricular catheter is most commonly placed in the nondominant, anterior horn portion of the lateral ventricle.[2]
7. Assist as needed with shaving and cleansing the insertion site with an antiseptic solution.	Reduces the microorganisms and minimizes the risk of infection.	The choice of povidone iodine or chlorhexidine as an antiseptic agent is controversial. Both should be allowed to dry completely. Studies suggest chlorhexidine is neurotoxic.[8,20]
8. Assist as needed with covering the patient's head and upper thorax with sterile drapes.	Protects the insertion site from contamination.[4,15,16]	
9. Fiberoptic system: A. Ensure that the preamp cable connects the catheter to the stand-alone monitor. B. Follow manufacturer's instructions for zeroing the catheter before insertion.	Prepares the system. The catheter is zeroed before insertion and never rezeroed.[17,18]	
10. Assist with the insertion of the intraventricular/fiberoptic catheter.	Facilitates the insertion process.	
11. After intraventricular/fiberoptic catheter placement: A. Follow the manufacturer's instructions for the "Cal/Step" interface. B. Attach the external ventricular drainage device to the proper Y-port. (Refer to Procedure 92.) C. Place the zero reference at the appropriate external anatomic landmark.[12,18] of the external ventricular drainage device. **(Level B*)** (Refer to Fig. 92-2.)	Ensures accurate fiberoptic data at the bedside monitor and allows printing of ICP tracing. The anatmoic reference point for the foramen of Monro is the external auditory canal.[11,17]	Ensure proper CSF drainage amount to prevent ventricular collapse and possible herniation.[9,11]
12. Increase or decrease the height of the graduated burette to the prescribed pressure level.[12]	Ensures proper CSF drainage.	When adjusting the height of the pressure level, the stopcock should be "off" to the patient.
13. The physician will prescribe the desired ICP parameter. (See Procedure 92.)	If the physician prescribes the ICP to be maintained at less than 15 mm Hg, drainage of CSF will be initiated if the patient's ICP is greater than 15 mm Hg.	
14. Monitor the ICP and CPP as prescribed.	Assesses ICP waveform and values and CPP value.	
15. Set the appropriate ICP scale for the measured pressure.	Necessary for visualization of the complete ICP waveform.	

*Level B: Well-designed controlled studies with results that consistently support a specific action, intervention, or treatment
*Level C: Qualitative studies, descriptive or correlational studies, integrative reviews, systematic reviews, or randomized controlled trials with inconsistent results

Procedure for Combination Intraventricular/Fiberoptic Catheter Insertion (Assist), Monitoring, Nursing Care, Troubleshooting, and Removal—*Continued*

Steps	Rationale	Special Considerations
16. Set the monitor alarms.	Goals for ICP management are individualized for each patient based on pathology.	
17. Discard used supplies in appropriate receptacles.	Removes and safely discards used supplies; safely removes sharp objects.	
18. **HH**		

Troubleshooting

Steps	Rationale	Special Considerations
1. Assess the integrity of the intraventricular/fiberoptic device.	Brain tissue or blood may occlude any of the various intracranial devices, resulting in a dampened waveform. Occlusion may necessitate manipulation or replacement.	Intracranial device manipulation is not a nursing responsibility in most institutions. Notify the physician or advanced practice nurse for assistance as needed.
2. Correct the ICP monitoring device malfunction.	Fiberoptic catheters may become damaged or dislodged, requiring catheter replacement.	Follow manufacturer's instructions and troubleshooting manuals for identifying and correcting common problems.
3. Change the monitoring system, if needed.	Ensures a functional system.	

Combination Intraventricular/Fiberoptic Catheter Removal

Steps	Rationale	Special considerations
1. **HH**		
2. Ensure healthcare providers who are assisting with catheter removal don sterile gloves and mask with face shield or goggles.		
3. Assist with the removal of the intraventricular/fiberoptic catheter.	Facilitates the removal process.	Culture the tip of the intraventricular catheter as prescribed.
4. Apply a sterile occlusive dressing after the device is removed.	Minimizes contamination by microorganisms.	
5. Dispose of used supplies and the device in the appropriate receptacle.	Removes and safely discards used supplies; safely removes sharp objects.	
6. **HH**		

Expected Outcomes

- Accurate and reliable ICP monitoring, CPP calculation, and assessment of cerebral compliance[12,18]
- Maintenance of ICP within range of 0 to 15 mm Hg or as prescribed[12,18]
- Early detection of elevated ICP trends[12,18]
- Management of increased ICP and decreased CPP[12,18]
- Protection of cerebral perfusion with maintenance of CPP within prescribed parameters[12,18]

Unexpected Outcomes

- CSF infection[5,14,19]
- CSF leakage
- Dislodging of the interventricular/fiberoptic catheter[15]
- Dislodging of the fiberoptic bolt[15]
- Pneumocephalus[12]
- Cerebral hemorrhage (rare)[12]
- Sequelae of sustained increased ICP and decreased CPP: cerebral infarction, herniation, and brain death[16,18]

Procedure continues on following page

Patient Monitoring and Care

Steps	Rationale	Reportable Conditions
		These conditions should be reported if they persist despite nursing interventions.
1. Assess the patient's neurologic status and vital signs during the procedure.	Evaluates the patient's response to the procedure.	• Changes in neurologic status • Abnormal vital signs
2. Note the ICP waveform and numeric values during the insertion procedure.	Provides baseline data.	• P_2 of greater amplitude than P_1
3. Assess the patient's neurologic status hourly or more often as indicated.	Provides clinical confirmation of and correlation with the monitored ICP data.	• Changes in neurologic status • Changes in vital signs
4. Assess the ICP hourly.	Determines the neurologic status.	• Increased ICP • ICP waveform abnormalities • Immediately report sustained ICP elevations of 20 mm Hg or greater
5. Calculate the CPP hourly (or more often as indicated).	A CPP of 50-70 mm Hg should be maintained for adult patients with traumatic brain injury.[4] CPP parameters should be individualized to meet patient perfusion needs.	• Changes in CPP • CPP less than the lowest prescribed parameter may put the patient at risk for cerebral ischemia[4]
6. Set the bedside alarm limits based on the parameter goals.	ICP limit is usually set to alarm when the ICP is greater than 20 mm Hg; however, this needs to be individualized for each patient.	• Abnormal ICP
7. Assess the catheter system hourly.	Ensures accuracy and safety of monitoring	• Frank blood or clots in the CSF drainage bag may indicate intracranial bleeding • Absence of CSF drainage may indicate an occluded catheter, dislodged catheter, cerebral swelling, or overdrained ventricles • Excessive drainage may lead to infarction and herniation
8. Change the insertion site dressing per institution policy.	Practices for head dressing changes and site care vary considerably.	• Significant drainage on ICP insertion site dressing or head dressing • Signs and symptoms of infection
9. Provide a safe environment, preventing inadvertent dislodgement of the intraventricular/fiberoptic catheter through appropriate catheter positioning, sedation, and analgesia as needed.	Inadvertent dislodgement of the catheter must be avoided because it can result in pneumoencephalopathy or excessive CSF drainage.	• Dislodged device • Abnormal ICP • Abnormal ICP waveform
10. Follow institution standard for assessing pain. Administer analgesia as prescribed.	Identifies need for pain interventions.	• Continued pain despite pain interventions
11. Change the CSF drainage collection device per institutional policy.	Practices for CSF drainage collection device vary considerably.	• Inadvertent disconnection
12. Elevate the patient's head of bed to 30 degrees or as prescribed.	May decrease ICP.	• Elevated ICP

Documentation

Documentation should include the following:
- Completion of informed consent
- Preprocedure verifications and time out
- Insertion time and patient response to procedure
- Initial and hourly ICP reading
- Initial and hourly CPP calculation
- CSF color and clarity
- Insertion site assessment
- Patient and family education

- Initial ICP tracing (include ICP waveform morphology) and any changes in waveform
- Nursing interventions used to treat ICP or CPP deviations and expected or unexpected outcomes
- Hourly amount of CSF drainage
- Pain assessment, interventions, and effectiveness

References

CR 1. Arabi Y, Memish ZA, Balkhy HH, et al: Ventriculostomy-associated infections: incidence and risk factors, *Am J Infect Control* 33:137-143, 2005.

CR 2. Arbour R: Intracranial hypertension: monitoring and nursing assessment, *Crit Care Nurs* 24:19-32, 2004.

3. Bershad EM, Humphreis WE, Suarez JI: Intracranial hypertension, *Semin Neurol* 28:690-702, 2008.

4. Bratton SL, Chesnut RM, Ghajar J, et al: Guidelines for the management of severe traumatic brain injury: a joint project of the Brain Trauma Foundation, American Association of Neurological Surgeons (AANS), Congress of Neurological Surgeons (CNS), AANS/CNS Joint Section on Neurotrauma and Critical Care, *J Neurotrauma* 24(Suppl 1):S1-S106, 2007.

5. Lo CH, Spelman D, Bailey M, et al: External ventricular drain infections are dependent of drain duration: an argument against elective revision, *J Neurosurg* 106:378-383, 2007.

CR 6. Davis JW, Davis IC, Bennink LO, et al: Placement of intracranial pressure monitors: are "normal" coagulation parameters necessary? *J Trauma* 57:1173-1176, 2004.

7. Fan JY, Kirkness C, Vicini P, et al: Intracranial pressure waveform morphology and intracranial adaptive capacity, *Am J Crit Care* 17:545-554, 2008.

8. Hebl JR: The importance and implications of aseptic techniques during regional anesthesia, *Reg Anesth Pain Med* 31:311-323, 2006.

CR 9. Hetherington NJ, Dooley MJ: Potential for patient harm from intrathecal administration of preserved solutions, *Med J Aust* 173:141-143, 2000.

10. Hickey JV, Olson DM: Intracranial hypertension: theory and management of increased intracranial pressure. In Hickey JV, editor: *The clinical practice of neurological and neurosurgical nursing*, ed 6, Philadelphia, 2009, Lippincott Williams & Wilkins, 270-307.

CR 11. Kirkness CJ, Mitchell PH, Burr RL, et al: Intracranial pressure waveform analysis: clinical and research implications, *J Neurosci Nurs* 32:271-277, 2000.

12. Leeper B, Lovasik D: Cerebrospinal drainage systems: external ventricular and lumbar drains. In Littlejohns LR, Bader MK, editors: *AACN-AACN protocols for practice: monitoring technologies in critically ill neuroscience patients*, Sudbury, MA, 2009, Jones and Bartlett, 71-82.

CR 13. Littlejohns LR, Trimble B: Our policy on external ventricular drainage systems includes the procedure for priming the system. Does it really have to be primed?, *Crit Care Nurse* 25:57-59, 2005.

CR 14. Lozier AP, Sciacea RR, Romagnoli MF, et al: Ventriculostomy-related infections: a critical review of the literature, *Neurosurgery* 51:170-181, 2002.

CR 15. March K: Application of technology in the treatment of traumatic brain injury, *Crit Care Nurs Q* 23:26-37, 2000.

CR 16. March K: Intracranial pressure monitoring and assessing intracranial compliance in brain injury, *Crit Care Nurs Clin North Am* 12:429-436, 2000.

CR 17. March K: Technology. In Bader MK, Littlejohns LR, editors: *Core curriculum for neuroscience nursing*, ed 4, Chicago, American Association of Neuroscience Nurses, St Louis, 2004, Saunders, 199-226.

18. March K, Madden L: Intracranial pressure management. In Littlejohns LR, Bader MK, editors: *AACN-AANN protocols for practice: monitoring technologies in critically ill neuroscience patients*, Sudbury, MA, 2009, Jones and Bartlett, 35-69.

CR 19. O'Grady NP, et al: Guidelines for the prevention of intravascular catheter-related infections, *Am J Infect Control* 30:476-489, 2002.

20. Reynolds F: Neurologic infections after neuraxial anesthesia, *Anesthesiol Clin* 26:23-52, 2008.

CR 21. Wilkinson HA, et al: Erroneous measurement of intracranial pressure caused by simultaneous ventricular drainage: a hydrodynamic model study, *Neurosurgery* 24:348-354, 1989.

CR 22. Woodward S, Addison C, Shah S, et al: Benchmarking best practice for external ventricular drainage, *Br J Nurs* 11:47-53, 2002.

Jugular Venous Oxygen Saturation Monitoring: Insertion (Assist), Patient Care, Troubleshooting, and Removal

P U R P O S E :   Jugular venous oxygen saturation (Sjvo$_2$) catheters detect the oxygen saturation of hemoglobin in the blood after cerebral perfusion. The direct and derived parameters obtained from jugular venous oxygen saturation catheters reflect global cerebral oxygenation. Inclusion of jugular venous oxygen saturation data in the clinical management of the patient may prevent the secondary brain injury that occurs as a result of an imbalance between cerebral oxygen delivery and cerebral oxygen demand.[2,43]

Tess Slazinski

PREREQUISITE NURSING KNOWLEDGE

- Fundamental understanding of neuroanatomy and physiology is needed.
- Knowledge of aseptic and sterile technique is necessary.
- The secondary brain injury that occurs as a result of an imbalance in oxygen supply and demand is accompanied by increased intracranial pressure (ICP), potential or actual compromise in cerebral perfusion, or other alterations that lead to cerebral ischemia.[4,29,32]
- Cerebral ischemia results in poor outcomes in critically ill patients.[2,3,5,8,19,35,36]
- Normal jugular venous oxygen saturation (Sjvo$_2$) values range from 55% to 70%.[7,13,33,35,38,40] Sjvo$_2$ values less than 45% to 50% indicate relative cerebral ischemia, especially with frequent desaturations.[7,9,10,12,13,18,25,39]
- Sjvo$_2$ values greater than 70% may demonstrate hyperemia.[8,21,23,26,28,31,32,40] Hyperemia occurs as the result of an increase in cerebral blood flow or hyperdilation of distal cerebrovascular resistance beds and is frequently accompanied by increases in ICP.[20]

- Sjvo$_2$ monitoring is recommended in patients at risk for global cerebral hypoxia, including those with acute severe traumatic brain injury (Glasgow Coma Scale [GCS] score equal to or less than 8)[6,19,26,36,38]; aneurysmal subarachnoid hemorrhage, including vasospasm[9,24]; intraoperative monitoring during craniotomy for tumor, abscess, aneurysm, arteriovenous malformation, spontaneous intracerebral hemorrhage,[24] and carotid endarterectomy for carotid stenosis; intraoperative monitoring during cardiac surgery, especially hypothermic cardiopulmonary bypass and rewarming; patients successfully resuscitated; ICP and cerebral perfusion pressure (CPP) management; controlled hyperventilation for increased ICP; and barbiturate coma for refractory increased ICP.[4]
- Contraindications for Sjvo$_2$ monitoring include coagulopathies, cervical spine injury, local neck trauma, and impaired cerebral venous drainage.[4]
- The Sjvo$_2$ catheter is placed retrograde in the dominant internal jugular vein (usually the right internal jugular vein).[11,14-17,23,33]
- The Sjvo$_2$ catheter tip is positioned at the location of the jugular bulb of the internal jugular vein.[20,23] This is at the mastoid process, approximately at the C1-C2 interspace

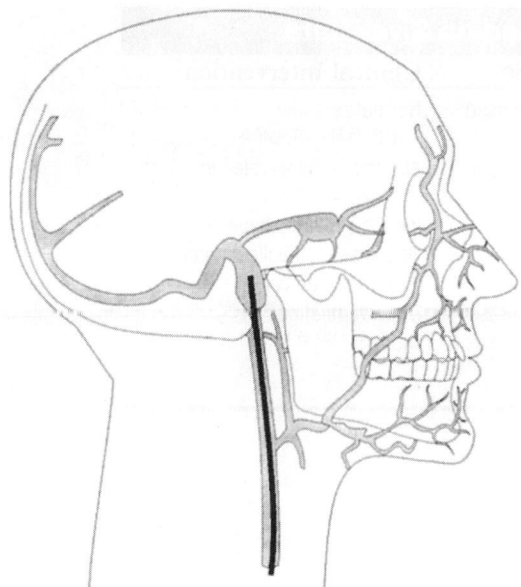

FIGURE 90-1 Placement of the jugular bulb venous catheter. *(From Kidd KC, Criddle L: Using jugular venous catheters in patients with traumatic brain injury, Crit Care Nurse 21:16-22, 2001.)*

(Fig. 90-1).[1] Ultrasound scan devices may be used to locate the jugular bulb to ease bedside placement.

- A decrease in $Sjvo_2$ (55%) may be due to increased demand as a result of pain, hyperthermia, shivering, agitation, or seizures. It may also be due to decreased delivery as a result of hyperventilation (hypocarbia), decreased cardiac output, hypotension, hypovolemia, anemia, hypoxia, and sepsis.[4]
- An increase in $Sjvo_2$ (70%) may be due to decreased demand as the result of hypothermia, anesthesia, paralytics, and sepsis. It may also be due to increased delivery.[4]
- Derived $Sjvo_2$ parameters include arteriovenous jugular oxygen content difference ($Avjdo_2$), the cerebral extraction of oxygen (CEo_2), and the cerebral metabolic rate of oxygen consumption ($CMRo_2$).
  - ❖ $Avjdo_2$ reflects the relationship between cerebral blood flow (CBF) and $CMRo_2$.[27,28,35,41,42]
    - ○ Normal range: 4.0 to 8.0 mL/dL
    - ○ Calculation requires data obtained from both systemic arterial and jugular venous blood gas analysis
  - ❖ CEo_2 reflects the influence of cerebral blood volume change (CBV) and its effect on CBF and $CMRo_2$. Blood volume flow is not equal to blood volume.[27,35,41,45]
    - ○ Normal range: 24% − 42%
    - ○ Equation: $Sao_2 − Sjvo_2$
  - ❖ $CMRo_2$ is the energy needed for cellular function.[35,41] This parameter includes knowledge of the cerebral blood flow and $Avjdo_2$ and is less frequently calculated in the clinical setting. Normal $CMRO_2$ is 3.2 mL/100 g/min.

- The technology used for continuous $Sjvo_2$ monitoring is oximetry, which is based on the unique light absorption spectrum of oxyhemoglobin.[40] Oximetry requires calibration, either in vivo, within the patient's jugular vein, or in vitro, calibration before insertion, outside the body. Formulas and normal ranges for $Sjvo_2$ catheter data and calculations are included in Tables 90-1 and 90-2. Clinical interventions based on $Sjvo_2$ data are shown in Table 90-3.

EQUIPMENT

- Antiseptic solution (e.g., 2% chorhexidine-based preparation)
- Surgical caps, gowns, goggles, sterile gloves, and gowns
- Sterile towels, half-sheets, and drapes
- Local anesthetic (lidocaine 1% or 2% without epinephrine)
- 5- or 10-mL Luer-Lok syringe with an 18-gauge needle (for drawing up of the lidocaine) and a 23-gauge needle (for administration of the lidocaine)
- Introducer set and sheath.
  In addition, the following are needed (if they are not included in the kit):
  - ❖ Sterile needle driver
  - ❖ Sutures
  - ❖ 5 Fr percutaneous transvenous introducer catheter
  - ❖ 4 Fr fiberoptic oximetric $Sjvo_2$ catheter

TABLE 90-1	Formulas for Calculations Using $Sjvo_2$ Data
Calculations	**Formula**
$Avjdo_2$ (mL/dL)	Cao_2 (mL/dL) − $Cjvo_2$ (mL/dL)
CEo_2 (%)	Sao_2 (%) − $Sjvo_2$ (%)

$Avjdo_2$, Arteriovenous jugular oxygen content difference; *Sao_2*, oxygen saturation in arterial blood; *$Sjvo_2$*, jugular venous oxygen saturation; *CEo_2*, cerebral extraction of oxygen; *CBF*, cerebral blood flow"

TABLE 90-2	Normal Ranges for $Sjvo_2$ Data and Calculations
$Sjvo_2$ Data	**Normal Ranges**
$Sjvo_2$	55% − 70%
$Avjdo_2$	4.0 to 8.0 mL/dL
CEo_2	24% − 42%

$Avjdo_2$, arteriovenous jugular oxygen content difference; *$Sjvo_2$*, jugular venous oxygen saturation; *CEo_2*, cerebral extraction of oxygen.

TABLE 90-3	Clinical Interventions Based on $SjvO_2$ Data			
$SjvO_2$	$AvjDO_2$	CEO_2	Clinical Intervention	
Decreased (cerebral blood flow and cerebral oxygen delivery do not meet cerebral metabolic demand)	Increased	Increased	Normalize a low CO_2[19,24,29,31,40,44] Administer hypervolemic therapy[18,29,31] Induce systemic hypertension[31] Decrease metabolic demand[18,22] (barbiturate coma)	
Increased (cerebral blood flow and cerebral oxygen delivery exceed cerebral metabolic demand)	Decreased	Decreased	Hyperventilation[21,24,29,31,32] Diuresis[19,24,29]	

- Optical module and connecting fiberoptic cable
- Oximetric monitor (typically a stand-alone monitor or module)
- Pressure bag setup
  - ❖ 500 mL 0.9% sodium chloride
  - ❖ Pressure tubing
  - ❖ Pressure bag
  - ❖ A pressure waveform is not generated from these catheters; therefore, display of a bedside waveform is not necessary. The system provides 3 mL of fluid an hour to prevent clotting of the catheter.
- Pressure module and cable to interface the oximetric monitor to the bedside monitor
- Sterile occlusive central venous catheter dressing

PATIENT AND FAMILY EDUCATION

- Assess patient and family understanding of $SjvO_2$ catheter monitoring and its purpose. ➤*Rationale:* Knowledge of expectations may allay patient and family fears and anxiety.
- Explain the procedure for insertion, patient monitoring, and patient clinical interventions for the $SjvO_2$ catheter. ➤*Rationale:* Clarification and repeated explanations may reinforce understanding and decrease anxiety.

PATIENT ASSESSMENT AND PREPARATION

Patient Assessment

- Assess the patient's neurologic status and vital signs. ➤*Rationale:* A baseline neurologic examination provides information necessary for recognition of changes during and after catheter insertion.

- Assess the patient for evidence of a local infection or local neck trauma. Verify that the patient does not have a cervical spine injury. ➤*Rationale:* These conditions are contraindications for $SjvO_2$ catheter placement.[38]
- Review current laboratory values such as complete blood count (CBC), prothombin time (PT) partial thromboplastin time (PTT), and international normalized ratio (INR). ➤*Rationale:* Abnormal coagulation study results may be a contraindication for $SjvO_2$ catheter placement.[38]
- Assess for allergies. ➤*Rationale:* Insertion of the $SjvO_2$ catheter may necessitate local anesthetic, an antiseptic to clean the site, and analgesia and sedation. Assessment minimizes the risk of allergic reaction.

Patient Preparation

- Verify correct patient with two identifiers. ➤*Rationale:* Prior to performing a procedure, the nurse should ensure the correct identification of the patient for the intended intervention.
- Perform a pre-procedure verification and time out, if nonemergent. ➤*Rationale:* Ensures patient safety.
- Ensure that informed consent is obtained. ➤*Rationale:* Informed consent protects the rights of the patient and makes competent decision making possible for the patient; however, in emergency circumstances, time may not allow for the consent form to be signed.
- Administer preprocedural analgesia or sedation as prescribed. ➤*Rationale:* Patients need to remain still during $SjvO_2$ catheter insertion. Usually patients are unconscious and may be receiving continuous intravenous analgesia and sedative medications.

Procedure	for Assisting with SjvO₂ Catheter Insertion

Steps	Rationale	Special Considerations
1. [HH]		
2. [PE]		
3. Turn on the oximetric processor (stand-alone monitor). Follow the manufacturer's instructions to perform an in vitro calibration before catheter insertion, if required. **(Level M*)**	Prepares equipment.	Oximetric monitors (depending on the brand) require a 15- to 20-minute warm-up time.
4. With aseptic technique, assemble and prime the tubing system, removing all air bubbles.	Prepares and eliminates air from the monitoring system.	Once the tubing is flushed, apply a pressure bag or device at 300 mm Hg.
5. Position the patient supine with the neck in the neutral position and the head elevated 30 to 45 degrees.	Head elevation provides accessibility for SjvO₂ catheter insertion and augments jugular venous outflow.	
6. Assess the patient's baseline ICP and CPP in this position.	Provides baseline data.	
7. Turn the patient's head away from the selected side for SjvO₂ insertion. Assess the patient's ICP.	Lateral head positioning before the insertion procedure demonstrates the patient's ability to tolerate the procedure. Venous return may be compromised by lateral head positioning.	
8. Assist if needed with preparing the selected insertion site with the antiseptic solution (e.g., 2% chlorhexidine–based preparation).	Reduces the microorganisms and minimizes the risk of infection.	
9. Ensure that healthcare providers put on caps, masks, goggles or face shields, sterile gloves and gowns.	Provides a sterile environment.	
10. If needed, assist with applying the sterile drapes across the patient's upper thorax and neck.	Protects the insertion site from contamination.	Ultrasound may be used to locate the jugular bulb. A sterile plastic drape/sheath is used over the ultrasound scan device to maintain aseptic technique.
11. Assist as needed with opening the percutaneous introducer tray, sheath, and SjvO₂ fiberoptic catheter packaging with aseptic technique.	Facilitates the efficiency of insertion and avoids contamination by microorganisms.	
12. Attach the fluid-filled pressure tubing with pressure bag to the fiberoptic catheter.	Inflating the pressure bag to 300 mm Hg allows approximately 1 to 3 mL/h of flush solution to be delivered through the catheter, thus maintaining catheter patency and minimizing clot formation.	
13. Monitor the patient throughout the insertion procedure: vital signs, ICP, CPP, neurologic status, and pain.	Ensures patient comfort, safety, and success of the insertion attempt.	Lateral head positioning during SjvO₂ catheter insertion may cause increased ICP.
14. Apply an occlusive sterile dressing to the insertion site.	Reduces the risk of infection.	

*Level M: Manufacturer's recommendations only

Procedure continues on following page

Procedure for Assisting with Sjvo₂ Catheter Insertion—*Continued*

Steps	Rationale	Special Considerations

15. Attach the catheter to the oximetry monitor.
  A. If calibrated in vitro, note the $Sjvo_2$ value and signal quality intensity (SQI).
  B. If not calibrated in vitro, perform an in vivo calibration.
  C. Set the oximetry monitor alarms.
	Prepares the system for $Sjvo_2$ monitoring and activates the alarm system.	Obtain an arterial sample and send both the jugular venous and arterial sample to the lab for oximetry determination.

16. If the introducer has a side port, turn the stopcock off to the patient, place a sterile injection cap on the end, and label "Do not infuse."	Side port is not to be used for administration of any intravenous medication.	Some institutions infuse a solution at 10 mL/hr through the introducer in addition to the pressure bag through the catheter. Follow institution standard.
17. Ensure that skull or cervical radiographs are completed after the procedure as prescribed.	The correct position of the tip of the $Sjvo_2$ catheter is at the C1-C2 interspace.[4]	
18. Discard used supplies in an appropriate receptacle.	Removes and safely discards used supplies; safely removes sharp objects.	
19. 🅷🅷		

Procedure for Troubleshooting Sjvo₂ Catheter

Steps	Rationale	Special Considerations
Problem 1: High SQI		
1. Identify the SQI.	Fiberoptic technology provides continuous monitoring of $Sjvo_2$ with analysis of reflected light signals. An SQI of 1 or 2 is usually preferred. High SQI of 4 indicates vessel wall artifact. A high SQI may result in inaccurate values. An SQI of 4 requires intervention (e.g., repositioning the patient's head or the catheter).	
2. Attempt to restore the normal light intensity by adjusting or slightly turning the patient's head to restore a neutral neck alignment.	Vessel wall artifact often happens during turning or positioning the patient; repositioning may correct it.	The physician may need to reposition the catheter.[11,13]
Problem 2: Low Sjvo₂ Values Related to Occlusion		
1. Check the fiberoptic catheter for occlusion.	Low $Sjvo_2$ may indicate clinical deterioration or catheter occlusion.[37]	
2. Cleanse the access port closest to the insertion site and attach a sterile Luer-Lok syringe.	Minimizes the risk of infection.	

Procedure for Troubleshooting Sjvo₂ Catheter—*Continued*

Steps	Rationale	Special Considerations
3. Draw back slowly on the syringe until blood returns freely and a normal light intensity displays.	Ensures optimal light intensity.	
4. If unable to aspirate blood, notify physician.	Catheter may need replacing.	
Problem 3: Sampling and Calibration Errors		
1. Identify the sampling or calibration error.	Slow aspiration of the jugular venous blood sample avoids contamination of the sample with extracerebral venous (facial vein) blood.[29,30]	
2. For in vivo calibration, withdraw a waste sample (1-2 mL) slowly from the jugular venous catheter and discard. Draw the sample from the port of the transducer stopcock.	Slow aspiration of blood is needed.	Obtain an arterial sample and send both the jugular venous and arterial sample to the lab for oximetry determination.
Problem 4: Coiling of the Sjvo₂ Catheter		
1. Identify rhythmic fluctuations in Sjvo₂ trends.	Coiling of the Sjvo₂ catheter within the internal jugular vein may cause rhythmic fluctuations in Sjvo₂ trends that are unrelated to changes in ICP, cerebral perfusion pressure, and systemic blood pressure.[8]	
2. A radiograph may be needed to determine if the catheter is coiled in the internal jugular vein.	Light intensity may remain within an acceptable range even in the presence of coiling of the Sjvo₂ catheter.	
3. If coiling is confirmed, the physician may replace the catheter.		
Problem 5: Sjvo₂ Desaturation		
1. Identify Sjvo₂ desaturation.	Sjvo₂ desaturations are emergent events that necessitate immediate interventions for restoration or enhancement of cerebral blood flow and cerebral oxygen.[8,10,12,13,38]	
2. Confirm the Sjvo₂ data by obtaining a jugular venous blood gas sample for laboratory analysis.	Monitored desaturation should be confirmed with laboratory analysis to rule out monitor malfunction.[11,13]	
3. Perform an in vivo calibration.	Ensures the accuracy of the equipment	

Procedure for Removal of Sjvo₂ Catheter

Steps	Rational	Special Considerations
1. **HH**		
2. **PE**		
3. Inactivate the bedside alarm system.	Monitoring is no longer needed.	
4. Turn the stopcocks on the flush system to the "off" position and assist with catheter removal.	Facilitates the removal process. Observe integrity of catheter.	Follow institution guidelines regarding who can remove the Sjvo₂ catheter.
5. Apply a sterile occlusive dressing after the device is removed.	Reduces the contamination by microorganisms.	

Procedure continues on following page

Procedure   for Troubleshooting Sjvo$_2$ Catheter—*Continued*

Steps	Rationale	Special Considerations
6. After catheter removal observe for signs of bleeding from the insertion site.	Identifies complications.	
7. Dispose of the used supplies and the catheter in the appropriate container.	Removes and safely discards used supplies.	
8. 🅷🅷		

Expected Outcomes

- Accurate and reliable Sjvo$_2$ catheter readings
- Optimization of the balance between cerebral perfusion, cerebral oxygenation, and cerebral metabolic demand
- Early detection and management of compromised cerebral perfusion and impaired cerebral oxygenation

Unexpected Outcomes[4]

- Carotid artery puncture[4,23]
- Excessive bleeding[4]
- Impaired cerebral venous drainage[4]
- Internal jugular venous thrombosis[4,38]
- Infection[4,38]
- Pneumothorax (rare)[4,38]
- Injury to stellate ganglion, phrenic nerve, or cervical ganglion (rare)[4,38]

Patient Monitoring and Care

Steps	Rationale	Reportable Conditions
		These conditions should be reported if they persist despite nursing interventions.
1. Assess the patient's neurologic status, vital signs, and ICP and CPP immediately after Sjvo$_2$ catheter insertion.	Determines the patient's response to the procedure.	- Changes in neurologic status, vital signs, and ICP
2. Assess the Sjvo$_2$ value hourly or more frequently as needed.	Monitors trends in the patient's Sjvo$_2$ values.	
3. Assess the ICP hourly and more frequently if needed.	Sustained ICP elevations greater than 20 mm Hg indicate the potential onset of intracranial hypertension.	- Changes in ICP
4. Calculate Avjdo$_2$ and CEo$_2$ as prescribed.	CEo$_2$ is derived from continuously monitored data. Avjdo$_2$ requires arterial blood gas and jugular venous blood gas analysis.[35]	- Changes in CEo$_2$ and Avjdo$_2$ (see Table 90-3 for possible management strategies)
5. Obtain a jugular venous sample with an ABG syringe and perform an in vivo calibration as recommended by the manufacturer. In vivo calibrations are commonly performed every 24 hours, with Sjvo$_2$ desaturations, and whenever the Sjvo$_2$ value is in question[4] **(Level M*)**	Calibrates the equipment and confirms the accuracy of the data.	

*Level M: Manufacturer's recommendations only

Patient Monitoring and Care —*Continued*

Steps	Rationale	Reportable Conditions
6. After obtaining blood sample, flush the tubing slowly (with a syringe) or with short intermittent pulsed flushes with the pressure tubing flush device, observing ICP during flush.	These catheters are *not* to undergo sustained, high-pressure flushes. Sustained high-pressure flushes may result in increased ICP. Stop flushing if increases in ICP occur.	
7. Assess the integrity of the $Sjvo_2$ catheter hourly or more often as indicated.	Frequent inspection ensures accuracy and safety of the monitoring system.	
8. Change the occlusive dressing per institution policy for central venous lines.	The Centers for Disease Control and Prevention (CDC) recommends replacing dressings when they become damp, loose, or soiled or when inspection of the site is necessary.[35]	• Signs and symptoms of infection
9. Change the intravenous flush solution and tubing for the $Sjvo_2$ catheter per institution policy.	No specific recommendations exist for $Sjvo_2$ tubing changes; however, the CDC recommends that the hemodynamic flush system for the pulmonary artery catheter monitoring can be safely used for 96 hours.[35]	
10. Follow institution standard for assessing pain. Administer analgesia as prescribed.	Identifies need for pain interventions.	• Continued pain despite pain interventions

Documentation

Documentation should include the following:

- Date and time of $Sjvo_2$ catheter insertion, difficulties or abnormalities experienced during insertion
- Completion of informed consent
- Preprocedure verifications and time out
- The depth (in centimeters) of catheter insertion
- Initial ICP reading and CPP
- ICP reading and CPP during and after insertion
- Initial $Sjvo_2$ reading
- Initial $AvjDo_2$ and CEo_2 calculations

- Hourly recording of ICP data
- Hourly recording of $Sjvo_2$, $AvjDo_2$, and CEo_2 data
- Significant changes in $Sjvo_2$, $AvjDo_2$, and CEo_2 and clinical management of those changes
- $Sjvo_2$ dressing and insertion site assessment
- Expected and unexpected outcomes and interventions
- Pain assessment, interventions, and effectiveness

References

CR 1. Bankier AA, et al: Position of jugular oxygen saturation catheter in patients with head trauma: assessment by use of plain films, *Am J Roentgenol* 164:437-441, 1995.

CR 2. Bayir H, et al: Promising strategies to minimize secondary brain injury after head trauma, *Crit Care Med* 31(Suppl):S112-S117, 2003.

CR 3. Bhutra S, et al: Jugular venous oxygen saturation monitoring in comatose neurosurgical patients, *JACP* 15(2):143-147, 1999.

4. Blissitt PA: Brain oxygen monitoring. In Littlejohns LR, Bader MK, editors: *AACN-AANN protocols for practice: monitoring technologies in critically ill neuroscience patients,* Sudbury, MA, 2009, Jones and Bartlett, 103-144.

CR 5. Bouma GJ, et al: Cerebral circulation and metabolism after severe traumatic brain injury: the elusive role of ischemia, *J Neurosurg* 75:685-683, 1991.

6. Bratton SL, Chesnut RM, Ghajar J, et al: Brain oxygen monitoring and thresholds: guidelines for the management of severe traumatic brain injury: A joint project of the Brain Trauma Foundation, American Association of Neurological Surgeons (AANS), Congress of Neurological Surgeons (CNS), AANS/CNS Joint Section on Neurotrauma and Critical Care, *J Neurotrauma* 24(Suppl 1):S65-S70, 2007.

CR 7. Chan MT: Re-defining the ischemic threshold for jugular venous oxygen saturation: a microdialysis study in patient with severe head injury, *Acta Neurochir* 95(Suppl):63-66, 2005.

CR 8. Chieregato A, et al: Detection of early ischemia in severe head injury by means of arteriovenous lactate differences and jugular bulb oxygen saturation: relationship with CPP, severity indexes and outcome: preliminary analysis, *Acta Neurochirurgica* 81(Suppl):289-293, 2002.

CR 9. Citerio G, et al: Jugular saturation (SjVO2) monitoring in subarachnoid hemorrhage (SAH), *Acta Neurochirugica* 71(Suppl):316-319, 1998.

CR 10. Cormio MA, et al: Elevated jugular venous oxygen saturation after severe head injury, *J Neurosurg* 90:9-15, 1999.

CR 11. Dearden NM, Midgley S: Technical considerations in continuous jugular venous oxygen saturation measurement, *Acta Neurochirurgica* 59(Suppl):91-97, 1993.

CR 12. Fandino J, et al: Cerebral oxygenation and systemic trauma related factors determining neurological outcome after brain injury, *J Clin Neurosci* 7:226-233, 2000.

CR 13. Feldman Z, Robertson CS: Monitoring of cerebral hemodynamics with jugular bulb catheters, *Crit Care Clin* 13:51-77, 1997.

CR 14. Ferris EB, et al: The validity of the internal jugular venous blood in studies of cerebral metabolism and blood flow in man, *Am J Physiol* 147:517-521, 1946.

CR 15. Gibbs EL, et al: The cross section areas of the vessels that form the torcular and the manner in which flow is distributed to the right and left lateral sinus, *Anat Rec* 59:419-426, 1934.

CR 16. Gibbs EL, et al: Arterial and cerebral venous blood: arterial-venous differences in man, *J Biol Chem* 144:325-332, 1942.

CR 17. Gibbs FA, et al: Cerebral blood flow preceding and accompanying epileptic seizures in man, *Arch Neurol Psychiatry* (Chicago) 32:257-272, 1934.

CR 18. Gopinath SP: Jugular venous desaturation and outcome after head injury, *J Neurol Neurosurg Psychiatry* 57:717-723, 1994.

CR 19. Graham D, et al: Brain damage in fatal non-missile head injuries with high intracranial pressure, *J Clin Pathol* 41:34-37, 1988.

CR 20. Gupta AK, et al: Measuring brain tissue oxygenation compared with jugular venous oxygenation after traumatic brain injury, *Anesth Analg* 88:549-553, 1999.

CR 21. Imberti R, et al: Cerebral tissue PO2 and SjVO2 changes during moderate hyperventilation in patients with severe traumatic brain injury, *J Neurosurg* 96:91-102, 2002.

22. Iwata M, Kawaguchi M, Inoue S, et al: Effects of increasing concentrations of propofol on jugular venous bulb oxygen saturation in neurosurgical patients under normothermic and mildly hypothermic conditions, *Anesthesiology* 104:33-38, 2006.

CR 23. Jakobsen M, Enevoldsen E: Retrograde catheterization of the right internal jugular vein for serial measurements of cerebral venous oxygen content, *J Cereb Blood Flow Metab* 9:717-720, 1989.

CR 24. Keller E, et al: Jugular venous oxygen saturation thresholds in trauma patients may not extrapolate to ischemic stroke patients: lessons from a preliminary study, *J Neurosurg Anesthesiol* 14:130-136, 2002.

CR 25. Kidd KC, Criddle L: Using jugular venous catheters in patients with traumatic brain injury, *Crit Care Nurse* 21(6):16, 18-22, 2001.

CR 26. Kiening KL, et al: Monitoring of cerebral oxygenation in patients with severe head injuries: brain tissue PO2 versus jugular vein oxygen saturation, *J Neurosurg* 85:751-757, 1996.

CR 27. Komiyama M, et al: Marked regional heterogeneity in venous oxygen saturation in severe head injury studied by superselective intracranial venous sampling, *Neurosurgery* 45(6):1469-1472, 1999.

CR 28. LeRoux PD: Cerebral arteriovenous oxygen difference: a predictor of cerebral infarction and outcome in patients with severe head injury, *J Neurosurg* 87:1-8, 1997.

CR 29. Lubbers DW, et al: Heterogeneity and stability of local PO2 distribution within the brain tissue, *Adv Exp Med Biol* 345:567-574, 1994.

CR 30. March K: Retrograde jugular catheter: monitoring SjO2, *J Neurosci Nurs* 26(1):48-51, 1994.

CR 31. Matta BF, Lam AM: The rate of blood withdrawal affects the accuracy of jugular venous bulb saturation measurements, *Anesthesiology* 86:806-808, 1997.

CR 32. Matta BF, et al: The influence of arterial oxygenation on cerebral venous oxygen saturation during hyperventilation, *Can J Anaesth* 41:1041-1046, 1994.

CR 33. McLeod AD, et al: Measuring cerebral oxygenation during normobaric hyperoxia: a comparison of tissue microprobes, near-infrared spectroscopy, and jugular venous oximetry in head injury, *Anesth Analg* 97:851-856, 2003.

CR 34. Metz C, et al: Monitoring of cerebral oxygen metabolism in the jugular bulb: reliability of unilateral measurements in severe head injury, *J Cereb Blood Flow Metab* 18:332-343, 1998.

CR 35. O'Grady NP, et al: Guidelines for the prevention of intravascular catheter-related infections, *Am J Infect Control* 30:476-489, 2002.

CR 36. Robertson CS, et al: Prevention of secondary ischemic insults after severe head injury, *Crit Care Med* 27:2086-2095, 1999.

CR 37. Robertson CS, et al: Cerebral blood flow, arteriovenous oxygen difference, and outcome in head injured patients, *J Neurol Neurosurg Psychiatry* 55:594-603, 1992.

CR 38. Ross DT, et al: Selective loss of neurons from the thalamic reticular nucleus following severe head injury, *J Neurotrauma* 10:151-165, 1993.

CR 39. Rossi S, et al: Brain oxygen tension, oxygen supply, and consumption during arterial hyperoxia in a model of progressive cerebral ischemia, *J Neurotrauma* 18:163-174, 2001.

CR 40. Schell RM, Cole DJ: Cerebral monitoring: jugular venous oximetry, *Anesth Analg* 90:559-566, 2000.

CR 41. Sheinberg M, et al: Continuous monitoring of jugular venous oxygen saturation in head injured patients, *J Neurosurg* 76:212-271, 1992.

CR 42. Sikes PJ, Segal J: Jugular bulb oxygen saturation monitoring for evaluating cerebral ischemia, *Crit Care Nurs Q* 17(1):9-20, 1994.

CR 43. Stocchetti N, et al: Cerebral venous oxygen saturation studied with bilateral samples in internal jugular veins, *Neurosurgery* 34:38-43, 1994.

CR 44. Stocchetti N, et al: Arterio-jugular difference of oxygen content and outcome after head injury, *Anesth Analg* 99:230-234, 2004.

CR 45. Struchen MA, et al: The relation between acute physiological variables and outcomes on the Glasgow Outcomes Scale and Disability Rating Scale following severe traumatic brain injury, *J Neurotrauma* 18:115-125, 2001.

CR 46. van Santbrink H, et al: Continuous monitoring of partial pressure of brain tissue oxygen in patients with severe head injury, *Neurosurgery* 38:21-31, 1996.

CR 47. White H, Baker A: Continuous jugular venous oximetry in the neurointensive care unit: a brief review, *Can J Anaesth* 49:623-629, 2002.

Additional Readings

CR DeGeorgia MA, Deogaonkar A: Multimodal monitoring in the neurological intensive care unit, *Neurologist* 11:45-54, 2005.

CR Kawano Y, Kawaguchi M, Inoue S, et al: Jugular bulb oxygen saturation under propofol or sevoflurane/nitrous oxide anesthesia during deliberate mild hypothermia in neurosurgical patients, *J Neurosurg Anesthesiol* 16:6-10, 2004.

CR March K: Technology. In Bader MK, Littlejohns LR, editors: *Core curriculum for neuroscience nursing*, ed 4, Chicago, American Association of Neuroscience Nurses, St Louis, 2004, Saunders, 199-226.

CR Smythe PR, Samra SK: Monitors of cerebral oxygenation, *Anesthesiol Clin North Am* 20:293-313, 2002.

Wartenberg KE, Schmidt JM, Mayer SA: Multimodality monitoring in neurocritical care, *Crit Care Clin* 23: 507-538, 2007.

CR Yoshitani K, Kawaguchi M, Iwata M, et al: Comparison of changes in jugular venous bulb oxygen saturation and cerebral oxygen saturation during variations of haemoglobin concentration under propofol and sevoflurane anaesthesia, *Br J Anaesth* 94:341-346, 2005.

Lumbar Subarachnoid Catheter Insertion (Assist) for Cerebrospinal Fluid Drainage and Pressure Monitoring

P U R P O S E :   Patients with a variety of central nervous system conditions and thoracoabdominal aneurysms may benefit from monitoring of intraspinal pressure and maintenance of therapeutic levels of cerebrospinal fluid drainage. Lumbar subarachnoid catheters are used for cerebrospinal fluid pressure monitoring and drainage.[23,40]

Mary Beth Flynn Makic, Debra Lynn-McHale Wiegand

PREREQUISITE NURSING KNOWLEDGE

- Knowledge of the anatomy and physiology of the vertebral column, spinal meninges, spinal cord, nerve roots, and cerebrospinal fluid (CSF) circulation and intracranial and intraspinal dynamics is needed.
- Knowledge of aseptic technique is necessary.
- Normal intraspinal pressure in the adult is 0 to 20 cm H_2O (0 to 15 mm Hg or 50 to 150 mm H_2O) and usually corresponds with intracranial pressure.[24] Intraspinal pressure may be influenced by a number of factors. Further research is needed to ascertain therapeutic levels after various surgical interventions.[21]
- Lumbar subarachnoid catheters, also referred to as lumbar drains or intrathecal catheters, require lumbar puncture (LP) for insertion.[16] Lumbar subarachnoid catheters permit monitoring of CSF pressure. CSF pressure may be monitored intermittently or continuously, and CSF drainage may be performed intermittently or continuously.[23,40]
- Lumbar subarachnoid catheters may be used in the prevention or management of spontaneous, traumatic, or surgical CSF fistulas to allow any tears in the dura mater to heal.[37,41-44] The catheter reduces moisture and pressure at the tear and may be placed before, during, or after surgery.[4,8,11,37,41]
- Lumbar subarachnoid catheters may be used in the diagnostic workup and management of normal pressure hydrocephalus instead of serial lumbar punctures.[12,27,28]
- Lumbar subarachnoid catheters may be used in the perioperative management of intraspinal pressure during and after thoracoabdominal aortic aneurysmal repair to provide adequate room in the intraspinal space to accommodate spinal cord edema and to improve impaired spinal cord perfusion related to spinal cord edema.
- Lumbar subarachnoid catheters may be used instead of or with an external ventricular drain to decrease intracranial pressure and remove blood from the subarachnoid space, which may lessen aneurysmal subarachnoid hemorrhage vasospasm.[13,16,22,26,36] When ventricular and lumbar drainage are used simultaneously, the ventricular drainage output should exceed the lumbar drainage output to lessen the risk of herniation.[12,16,22,38]
- Lumbar subarachnoid catheters may be use in the management of communicating hydrocephalus related to intraventricular, intracerebral hemorrhage.[18,19]
- Complications related to the use of lumbar subarachnoid catheters include infection, headache, nerve root irritation, retained fragments of broken catheters, paraplegia, and neu-

rologic deterioration related to overdrainage, including subdural hematomas, pneumocephalus, and herniation.[1,30,31,33]

- Lumbar subarachnoid catheters have been used, with extreme caution, in the management of patients with meningitis.[26]
- Lumbar subarachnoid catheter drainage is contraindicated with midline mass effect. A computed tomographic (CT) scan before lumbar subarachnoid catheter insertion to confirm discernible basal cisterns and absence of a mass lesion may lessen the risk of herniation.[1,16,21,22]
- A variety of products are available for lumbar subarachnoid catheter drainage systems, making it essential to follow the manufacturer's guidelines for management of the patient[23] to include the type of pressure measurement unit used for patient monitoring (e.g. monitoring pressures in units mm Hg, cm H_2O).

EQUIPMENT

- Antiseptic solution
- Caps, masks with face shields, sterile gowns, and sterile gloves
- Sterile towels, half-sheets, and drapes
- Local anesthetic (lidocaine 1% or 2% without epinephrine)
- 5- or 10-mL Luer-Lok syringe with 18-gauge needle for drawing of lidocaine and 23-gauge needle for administration of lidocaine
- Sutures (2-0 nylon, 3-0 silk)
- Forceps
- Sterile scissors
- Sterile needle holder
- Preservative-free sterile normal saline solution (vial, bag, or prefilled syringe)
- Lumbar catheter tray
- Lumbar puncture tray
- Sterile occlusive dressing
- Tape (1- and 2-inch rolls)
- External transducer with three-way stopcock
- Pressure cable
- External CSF drainage system
- Nonvented sterile caps
  Additional supplies as needed include the following:
- Leveling device
- Rolled towels or small pillows to support the patient during positioning

PATIENT AND FAMILY EDUCATION

- Assess the patient and family understanding of the lumbar subarachnoid catheter system. ➥*Rationale:* Any necessary clarification may limit anxiety for the patient and family.

- Explain insertion, patient monitoring, and care involving the lumbar subarachnoid catheter. ➥*Rationale:* Knowledge of expectations can minimize anxiety and encourage questions regarding goals, duration, and expected outcomes of the lumbar subarachnoid catheter.

PATIENT ASSESSMENT AND PREPARATION

Patient Assessment

- Assess the patient's neurologic status, including level of consciousness, cranial nerves, sensory and motor function in the upper and lower extremities, vital signs, and bowel and bladder function. ➥*Rationale:* Baseline data are provided.
- Assess the patient's current laboratory profile, including complete blood count (CBC), with platelets, partial thromboplastin time (PTT), prothrombin time (PT), and international normalized ratio (INR). ➥*Rationale:* Baseline coagulation study results determine the risk for bleeding during and after lumbar subarachnoid catheter insertion.[16,26,36]
- Assess the patient's medication profile. ➥*Rationale:* Recent anticoagulants or antiplatelet agents may increase the risk of bleeding during and after lumbar subarachnoid catheter insertion.
- Assess known allergies. ➥*Rationale:* Usual medications used during the procedure may be contraindicated by allergy.

Patient Preparation

- Verify correct patient with two identifiers. ➥*Rationale:* Prior to performing a procedure, the nurse should ensure the correct identification of the patient for the intended intervention.
- Ensure that informed consent is obtained. ➥*Rationale:* Informed consent protects the rights of the patient and makes competent decision-making possible for the patient; however, in emergency circumstances, time may not allow for the consent form to be signed.
- Administer preprocedural analgesia or sedation as prescribed. ➥*Rationale:* The patient must be correctly positioned and immobile during lumbar subarachnoid catheter insertion and monitoring and therefore may need sedation or analgesia to tolerate the procedure.
- Administer preprocedural antibiotics as prescribed. ➥*Rationale:* Prophylactic intravenous antibiotics may reduce the risk of infection.
- Perform a pre-procedure verification and time out, if non-emergent. ➥*Rationale:* Ensures patient safety.

Procedure for Lumbar Subarachnoid Catheter Insertion (Assist)

Steps	Rationale	Special Considerations
1. **HH**		
2. **PE**		
3. If pressure monitoring is prescribed, assemble a fluid-filled transducer with stopcock and nonvented cap. Using sterile technique, flush the transducer with preservative-free sterile normal saline solution. **(Level E*)**	Facilitates monitoring after catheter insertion. Preservative in normal saline solution may cause cortical necrosis.[15]	Do not attach a pressurized intravenous (IV) fluid bag to the transducer.
4. Using sterile technique, assemble and flush the sterile CSF drainage system compatible with the lumbar subarachnoid catheter device with preservative-free sterile normal saline solution. **(Level E)**	Prepares the equipment.	Allowing the CSF to flush the system after insertion of the catheter may allow air in the fluid-filled system, resulting in a damped waveform, inaccurate intraspinal pressure values, and decreased drainage. Priming the drainage system with preservative-free sterile normal saline solution, not CSF, is recommended.[25] Follow institutional standard.
5. Attach the fluid-filled transducer to the CSF drainage system.	Prepares the equipment.	The transducer may be attached to the CSF drainage system before either is primed, and the transducer may be flushed at the same time the CSF drainage system is primed.
6. Connect the fluid-filled transducer to the pressure cable and bedside monitor.	Facilitates insertion and immediate lumbar subarachnoid CSF pressure monitoring on insertion.	Ensure that the waveform chosen for CSF monitoring is read on the "mean" setting.
7. Set the reference line of the drip chamber at the level of the transducer, which is typically at zero reference (Figs. 91-1 and 91-2).	Prepares the CSF drainage system for use.	
8. Level the transducer and the zero reference to the anatomic reference point of the patient as prescribed or as per institutional standard (see Fig. 91-1). **(Level E)**	Ensures accurate readings on which to base therapy.	The anatomic reference point will be determined by the physician and may be the external auditory meatus, shoulder height, or the level of catheter insertion.[23]
9. To zero the system prior to attaching to the patient, turn the stopcock off to the patient port, remove the nonvented cap on the stopcock, and zero the monitoring system at the anatomic reference point. Replace the sterile nonvented cap. Follow manufacturer's directions. **(Level M*)**	Allows the monitor to use atmospheric pressure as a reference for zero.	The membrane at the top of the drip chamber may allow zeroing without opening the fluid-coupled system to air.
10. Position the reference level of the drip chamber as prescribed.	The relationship of the reference level of the drip chamber to the anatomic reference point alters the rate of CSF drainage.	
11. Assist the patient to a lateral decubitus position with neck, hips, and knees flexed (knees to chest; see Fig. 95-1 and 96-1).[6,34]	The intervertebral space widens in this position, facilitating the entry of the spinal needle into the subarachnoid space.	All health care providers involved in the procedure need to apply goggles or masks with face shields, caps, sterile gowns, and sterile gloves.

*Level E: Multiple case reports, theory-based evidence from expert opinions, or peer-reviewed professional organizational standards without clinical studies to support recommendations
*Level M: Manufacturer's recommendations only

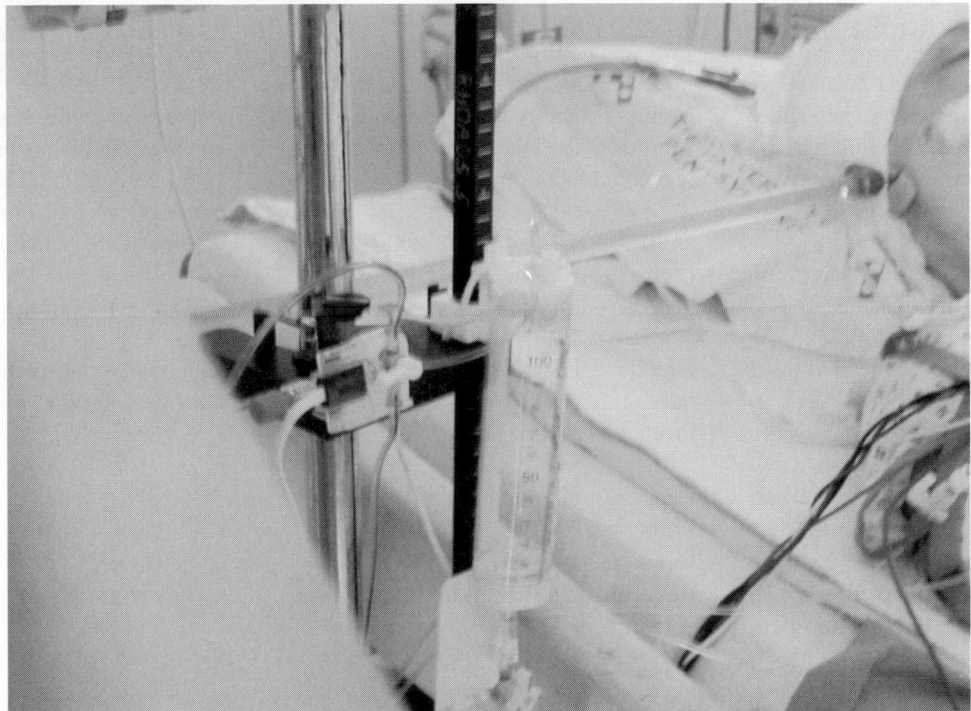

FIGURE 91-1   Drip chamber at the level of the transducer and the external auditory meatus.

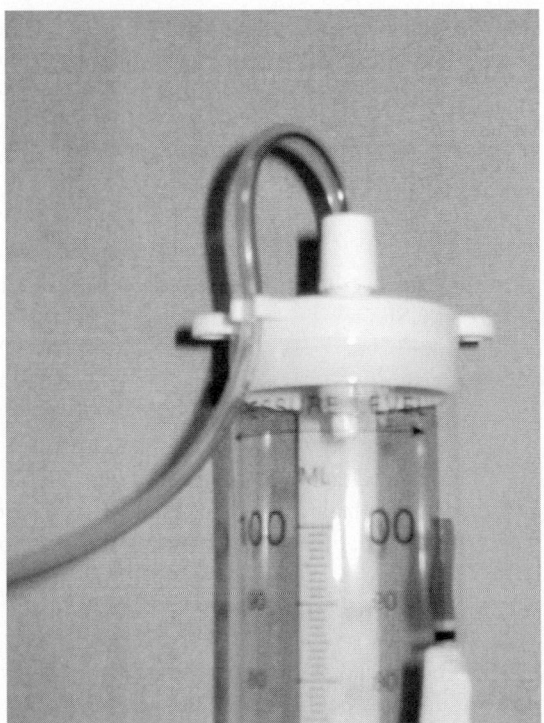

FIGURE 91-2   Top of the drip chamber with reference line.

Procedure for Lumbar Subarachnoid Catheter Insertion (Assist)—*Continued*

Steps	Rationale	Special Considerations
12. Assist the physician or advanced practice nurse as needed with cleansing the intended insertion site with the antiseptic solution.[8,12,26,29] **(Level C*)**	Minimizes the risk for infection and protects the insertion site from recontamination.	The choice of povidone-iodine or chlorhexidine as an antiseptic agent is controversial. Both should be allowed to dry completely. Studies suggest chlorhexidine is neurotoxic.[14,29,32]
13. Assist as needed with draping the patient with sterile sheets and opening sterile trays.	Prepares for catheter insertion.	
14. Provide supplies as needed during catheter insertion.	Facilitates insertion.	Surgeons may insert the catheter during surgery.
15. Note the opening CSF pressure (initial), color, and clarity.	Provides baseline data.	
16. Assist with the application of an occlusive sterile dressing to the catheter insertion site.	Reduces contamination of the insertion site by microorganisms.	
17. Secure the catheter with tape, with care taken not to alter the catheter position.	Reduces the potential for catheter dislodgment.	
18. Attach the CSF drainage system to the lumbar drain.		
19. If the intraspinal pressure is to be monitored, turn the stopcock off to the patient and zero the transducer.	Ensures accurate data on which to base therapy.	
20. If intraspinal pressure is to be monitored, observe the waveform morphology, obtain a strip of the waveform, and measure the CSF pressure.	Provides initial baseline data. Confirms correct placement of the catheter.	Lumbar subarachnoid CSF pressure waveform data are similar to traditional intracranial pressure (ICP) waveform data. Research supports maintenance of an intraspinal pressure of less than 15 mm Hg after thoracic abdominal aortic resection.[2,7,9,21]
21. Position the head of the bed as prescribed. Reassess the level of the transducer, zero reference, and level line of drip chamber. Relevel and rezero as needed. Observe the rate of drainage.	Prevents overdrainage or underdrainage of CSF.	Follow institution standard. Hourly drainage amount is generally 10 to 20 mL/hr.[30]
22. Turn the stopcock to continuously monitor with intermittent drainage or to intermittently monitor with continuous drainage. Set alarm limits. Follow institution standard.	The stopcock must be turned off to the drain to obtain an accurate intraspinal pressure.	Set alarms if continuously monitoring to minimize underdrainage or overdrainage.[8]
23 Discard used supplies in an appropriate receptacle.	Removes and safely discards used supplies; safely removes sharp objects.	
24. **HH**		

*Level C: Qualitative studies, descriptive or correlational studies, integrative reviews, systematic reviews, or randomized controlled trials with inconsistent results

Procedure	for Troubleshooting Lumbar Subarachnoid Catheter Insertion (Assist)		
Steps	**Rationale**	**Special Considerations**	

1. **HH**			
2. If the CSF waveform is damped:	Damping of the waveform can indicate catheter occlusion or risk for catheter displacement.	Catheter occlusion may result from precipitate in the CSF.	
A. Assess the integrity of the lumbar subarachnoid catheter device and correct problems if possible.	Loose connections may cause damped waveforms and increase the risk for infection.		
B. Assess the monitoring system for disconnections and reconnect the system if needed.	Loose cables and connecting devices may contribute to mechanical failure.[23,40]		
C. Assess the level of the transducer, the zero reference point, and the reference line on the drip chamber for the correct position and readjust the position and rezero if needed. (see Figs. 91-1 and 91-2).	The membrane at the top of the drip chamber may allow zeroing without opening the fluid-coupled system to air. However, one-way valves in the drainage system may affect calibration.[20] Also, if the membrane becomes wet, it may no longer permit accurate readings and the drip chamber must be changed.	Changing the drip chamber involves changing the entire CSF drainage system. Responsibility for changing the CSF drainage system varies among institutions and may not be a nursing responsibility in most institutions. Notify the physician or advanced practice nurse for assistance as needed.	
3 Assess for the sudden absence of the pressure waveform or significant changes in pressure measurements without an apparent clinical cause. A. Ensure connections are tight. B. Ensure leveling is correct. C. Rezero the system.	Ensures accurate measurement of CSF pressure.[23,40]	Notify the physician or advanced practice nurse if unable to identify a reversible cause. The CSF drainage system or the catheter may need to be replaced because of catheter dislodgment or blockage.	
4. Assess the flow of CSF through the drainage system by briefly lowering the drip chamber.	Avoids increases in CSF pressure caused by equipment malfunction.[23,41]	Flushing or changing the system may be necessary. Follow institution standard as to who is responsible for flushing the system.	
5. **HH**			

Procedure	for Removal of a Lumbar Subarachnoid Catheter (Assist)		
Steps	**Rationale**	**Special Considerations**	

1. **HH**			
2. **PE**			
3. Assist the physician or advanced practice nurse as needed with removal of the catheter.	Facilitates catheter removal.	Culture the catheter tip as prescribed.	
4. Apply a sterile occlusive dressing.	Reduces the risk of contamination by microorganisms.		
5. Discard used supplies in an appropriate receptacle.	Removes and safely discards used supplies; safely removes sharp objects.		
6. **HH**			
7. Continue to assess the patient's neurologic status and dressing after removal of the catheter for CSF leak.	Removal of the catheter may result in neurologic deterioration related to increased CSF pressure. An overt CSF leak may indicate increased CSF pressure.[1,5]		

Procedure continues on following page

Expected Outcomes

- Accurate and reliable CSF pressure monitoring
- CSF pressure within range of 0 to 15 mm Hg[23] (0 to 20 cm H$_2$O)
- Early detection and management of elevated CSF pressure through CSF drainage[1,26]
- Resolution of any CSF leak[11,37,40,43]
- Resolution of symptoms associated with normal pressure hydrocephalus[4,27,28]
- Prevention of spinal cord damage or reversal of late-onset symptoms associated with thoracoabdominal aneurysm repair[2,7,9,21]

Unexpected Outcomes

- CSF leak or symptoms associated with excessive drainage[9,10,17,21]
- CSF infection[12,33]
- Dislodgment or occlusion of the lumbar subarachnoid catheter[30]
- Tension pneumocephalus[15,30]
- Motor function deficits along the myotome distribution of thoracic or lumbar spinal cord[2,7,9,21]
- Catheter site pain
- Sensory dysfunction involving dermatome distribution of thoracic or lumbar spinal cord[2,7,9,21]
- Bladder or bowel dysfunction[2,7,9,21]
- Decreased level of consciousness in association with herniation[1,5]
- Headache
- Subdural hematoma

Patient Monitoring and Care

Steps	Rationale	Reportable Conditions
		These conditions should be reported if they persist despite nursing interventions.
1. Monitor the patient's neurologic status and vital signs.	Neurologic status changes may result from irritation of spinal nerves associated with subarachnoid catheter placement,[3,21,23,40] spinal cord damage related to thoracoabdominal aneurysm repair,[3,5,21,23,40] subdural hematoma formation, herniation, or tension pneumocranium resulting from overdrainage of CSF.[1,16,22,30]	• Change in level of consciousness • Change in cranial nerve function • Change in sensation of upper and lower extremities • Change in motor function of upper and lower extremities • Changes in bowel and bladder function • Changes in vital signs
2. Follow institution standard for assessing pain. Administer analgesia as prescribed.	Identifies need for pain interventions.	• Continued pain despite pain interventions
3. Assess the lumbar subarachnoid CSF waveform and pressure and the color, clarity, and amount of CSF drainage every hour or as prescribed.	Ensures accurate measurement of CSF pressure and monitoring.[23,40]	• Changes in CSF pressure • Changes in CSF drainage • Changes in the CSF waveform morphology
4. Maintain CSF pressure and drainage as prescribed.	In the management of intraspinal pressure after abdominal aortic aneurysm (AAA) repair, a CSF pressure of less than 15 mm Hg is recommended.[2,21]	• Abnormal CSF pressure
5. Assess the integrity of the lumbar subarachnoid catheter system at least hourly.	Determines accurate functioning of the system.	• Loose connections or other openings in the catheter system
6. Zero the monitoring system with insertion, disconnection, or position changes; when the values do not fit the clinical picture; and according to institution standard.	Ensures accuracy of the monitored data.	

Patient Monitoring and Care —*Continued*

Steps	Rationale	Reportable Conditions
7. Assess the insertion site and change the dressing when loose or soiled. Follow institution standard for dressing changes.	Reduces the risk of infection.	• Signs or symptoms of infection • Significant drainage at the catheter insertion site

8. Continue ongoing assessment of neurologic status hourly, as prescribed, or per institution standard:
  A. Level of consciousness
  B. Cranial nerves
  C. Sensation
  D. Motor function of lower extremities
  E. Bowel and bladder function
  F. Comfort level (including headache)
	Changes in neurologic status or comfort level may indicate dislodgment of the lumbar subarachnoid catheter, spinal cord damage related to thoracoabdominal aneurysm repair, or poorly managed CSF drainage.[23,40]	• Change in level of consciousness
		• Change in cranial nerve function
		• Change in sensation of upper and lower extremities
		• Change in motor function of upper and lower extremities
		• Changes in bowel and bladder function
		• Headache

9. Monitor patient mobility as prescribed to avoid overdrainage or underdrainage.[8,16]	Patients may be permitted to sit or ambulate with specific guidelines for placement or clamping of the drainage system.	• Overdrainage or underdrainage with mobility restrictions
10. Prevent dislodgment of the catheter through ongoing patient education. Ensure that the catheter and drainage system are secured. Provide sedation and analgesia as prescribed.	Catheter dislodgment may result in excessive drainage of CSF.	• Dislodged catheter
11. Change the CSF pressure monitoring and drainage systems according to institution standard.	Reduces the risk of infection.	
12. Obtain or assist with obtaining CSF specimens as prescribed by accessing the sampling port on the CSF drainage system with strict aseptic technique. Follow institution standard.	Currently, insufficient data exist to guide or support decisions on the necessary frequency of routine CSF sampling from lumbar subarachnoid catheters.[26,30]	• Elevated white blood cell (WBC) count • Elevated protein • Decreased glucose in CSF fluid • Gram stain • Culture and sensitivity • CSF cytokines (interleukin [IL]–6) may predict bacterial infection earlier than elevated WBC, elevated protein, and decreased glucose[39]
13. Administer antibiotics as prescribed.	Currently, insufficient data are available to guide or support routine prophylactic antibiotic therapy.[8,12,30]	
14. If overdrainage is suspected, clamp the drain, lower head of the bed,[5,12,16,22,38] and assess neurologic status. (**Level E***)	The patient may be at increased risk of herniation with overdrainage.	• Change in neurologic status and vital signs

*Level E: Multiple case reports, theory-based evidence from expert opinions, or peer-reviewed professional organizational standards without clinical studies to support recommendations

Procedure continues on following page

Documentation

Documentation should include the following:
- Completion of informed consent
- Pre-procedure verifications and time out
- Insertion site assessment
- Insertion of the lumbar subarachnoid catheter, including opening CSF pressure, any difficulties or abnormalities, and patient tolerance
- CSF description (e.g., clarity, color, characteristics)
- Hourly measurement of CSF pressure and amount of drainage

- Waveform tracing at insertion and with continuous monitoring according to institution standard
- Description of expected or unexpected outcomes
- Nursing interventions used to treat elevated CSF pressure and expected or unexpected outcomes
- Pain assessment, interventions, and effectiveness

References

1. Abadal-Centellas JM, et al: Neurologic outcome of post-traumatic refractory intracranial hypertension treated with external lumbar drainage, *J Trauma* 62: 282-286, 2007.
2. Bajwa A, et al: Paraplegia following elective endovascular repair of abdominal aortic aneurysm: reversal with cerebrospinal fluid drainage, *Eur J Vasc Endovasc Surg* 35:46-48, 2007.
3. **CR** Bhama JK, Lin PH, Voloyiannis T, et al: Delayed neurologic deficit after endovascular abdominal aortic aneurysm repair, *J Vasc Surg* 37:690-692, 2003.
4. Bien AG, et al: Utilization of preoperative cerebrospinal fluid drain in skull base surgery, *Skull Base* 17:133-139, 2007.
5. **CR** Bloch J, Regli L: Brain stem and cerebellar dysfunction after lumbar spinal fluid drainage: case report, *J Neurol Neurosurg Psychiatry* 74:992-994, 2003.
6. **CR** Boon JM, Abrahams PH, Meiring JH, et al: Lumbar puncture: anatomical review of a clinical skill, *Clin Anat* 177:544-553, 2004.
7. **CR** Cina CS, et al: Cerebrospinal fluid drainage to prevent paraplegia during thoracic and thoracoabdominal aortic aneurysm surgery: a systematic review and meta-analysis, *J Vasc Surg* 40:36-44, 2004.
8. Dalgic A, et al: An effective and less invasive treatment of post-traumatic cerebrospinal fluid fistula: closed lumbar drainage system, *Minim Invas Neurosurg* 51:154-157, 2008.
9. **CR** Fleck TM, et al: Improved outcome in thoracoabdominal aortic aneurysm repair: the role of cerebrospinal fluid drainage, *Neurocrit Care* 2:11-16, 2005.
10. Fountas KN, et al: Review of the literature regarding the relationship of rebleeding and external ventricular drainage in patients with subarachnoid hemorrhage of aneurysmal origin, *Neurosurg Rev* 29:14-18, 2006.
11. Friedman RA, et al: Management of cerebrospinal fluid leaks after acoustic tumor removal, *Neurosurgery* 61(Suppl):35-39, 2007.
12. Greenberg BM, Williams MA: Infectious complications of temporary spinal catheter insertion for diagnosis of adult hydrocephalus and idiopathic intracranial hypertension, *Neurosurgery* 62:431-435, 2008.
13. Hanggi, D, et al: The effect of lumboventricular lavage and simultaneous low-frequency head-motion therapy after severe subarachnoid hemorrhage: results of a single center prospective phase II trial, *J Neurosurg* 108:1192-1199, 2008.
14. Hebl JR: The importance and implications of aseptic techniques during regional anesthesia, *Regional Anesth Pain Med* 31:311-323, 2006.
15. **CR** Hetherington NJ, Dooley MJ: Potential for patient harm from intrathecal administration of preserved solutions, *Med J Aust* 173:141-143, 2000.
16. Hoekema D, Schmidt RH, Ross I: Lumbar drainage for subarachnoid hemorrhage: technical considerations and safety analysis, *Neurocrit Care* 7:3-9, 2007.
17. **CR** Houle PJ, et al: Pump-regulated lumbar subarachnoid drainage, *Neurosurgery* 46:929-932, 2000.
18. Huttner HB, Schwab S, Bardutzky J: Lumbar drainage for communicating hydrocephalus after ICH with ventricular hemorrhage, *Neurocrit Care* 5:193-196, 2006.
19. Huttner HB, et al: Intracerebral hemorrhage with severe ventricular involvement: lumbar drainage for communicating hydrocephalus, *Stroke* 38:183-187, 2007.
20. Integra: *Accudrain external CSF drainage systems: reference insert-8400,* Plainsboro NJ, 2008, Integra.
21. **CR** Khan SN, Stansby GP: Cerebrospinal fluid drainage for thoracic and thoracoabdominal aortic aneurysm surgery, *Cochrane Database Syst Rev* 4:Art. No: CD003635, 2003.
22. **CR** Klimo P, et al: Marked reduction of cerebral vasospasm with lumbar drainage of cerebrospinal fluid after subarachnoid hemorrhage, *J Neurosurg* 100:215-224, 2004.
23. Leeper B, Lovasik D: Cerebrospinal drainage systems: external ventricular and lumbar drains. In Littlejohns LR, Bader MK, editors: *Monitoring technologies in critically ill neuroscience patients,* Boston, 2009, Jones and Bartlett, 71-101.
24. Lenfeldt N, Koskinen OD, Bergenheim AT, et al: CSF pressure assessed by lumbar puncture agrees with intracranial pressure, *Neurology* 68:155-158, 2007.
25. **CR** Littlejohns LR, Trimble B: Ask the experts: our policy on external ventricular drainage systems includes the procedure for priming the system: does it really have to be primed? *Crit Care Nurse* 25:57-59, 2005.
26. Manosuthi W, et al: Temporary external lumbar drainage for reducing elevated intracranial pressure in HIV-infected patients with cryptoccocal meningitis, *Int J STD AIDS* 19:268-271, 2008.
27. **CR** Marmarou A, et al: The value of supplemental prognostic tests for the preoperative assessment of idiopathic normal-pressure hydrocephalus, *Neurosurgery* 57 (Suppl 2-17):S2-28, 2005.

CR 28. McGirt MJ, et al: Diagnosis, treatment, and analysis of long-term outcomes in idiopathic normal-pressure hydrocephalus, *Neurosurgery* 57:699-705, 2005.

29. Milstone AM, Passaretti CL Perl TM: Chlorhexidine: expanding the armamentarium for infection control and prevention, *Clin Infect Dis* 46:274-281, 2008.

CR 30. Moza K, et al: Indications for cerebrospinal fluid drainage and avoidance of complications, *Otolaryngol Clin North Am* 38:577-582, 2005.

31. Olivar H, et al: Subarachnoid lumbar drains: a case series of fractured catheters and a near miss, *Can J Anaesth* 54:829-834, 2007.

32. Reynolds F: Neurological infections after neuraxial anesthesia, *Anesthesiol Clin* 26:23-52, 2008.

33. Roca B, Pesudo JV, Gonzalez-Darder JM: Meningitis caused by *Enterococcus gallinarum* after lumbar drainage of cerebrospinal fluid, *Eur J Int Med* 17:298-299, 2006.

CR 34. Roos KL: Lumbar puncture, *Semin Neurol* 23:105-114, 2003.

35. Ropper AH, Samuels MA: Special techniques for neurologic diagnosis. In Ropper AH, Samuels MA, editors: *Adams and Victor's principles of neurology,* ed 9, 2009. Text available at www.accessmedicine.com.offcampus. lib.washington.edu/content.aspx?aID=3630099.

CR 36. Ruijs AC, et al: The risk of rebleeding after external lumbar drainage in patients with untreated ruptured cerebral aneurysms, *Acta Neurochir (Wien)* 147:1157-1162, 2005.

37. Sade B, Mohr G, Frenkiel S: Management of intra-operative cerebrospinal fluid leak in transnasal transsphenoidal pituitary microsurgery: use of post-operative lumbar drain and sellar reconstruction without fat packing, *Acta Neurochi (Wien)* 148:13-19, 2006.

CR 38. Samadani U, et al: Intracranial hypotension after intraoperative lumbar cerebrospinal fluid drainage, *Neurosurgery* 52:148-152, 2003.

39. Schade RP, et al: Lack of value of routine analysis of cerebrospinal fluid for prediction and diagnosis of external drainage-related bacterial meningitis, *J Neurosurg* 104:101-108, 2006.

40. Schlosser RJ, et al: Spontaneous cerebrospinal fluid leaks: a variant of benign intracranial hypertension, *Ann Otol Rhinol Laryngol* 115:495-500, 2006.

41. Thompson H, Avanecean D: *Care of the patient with the lumbar drain,* ed 2, Glenview, IL, 2007, American Association of Neuroscience Nurses. Text available at www.aann.org/pubs/guidelines.html.

CR 42. Van Aken MO, et al: Cerebrospinal fluid leakage during transsphenoidal surgery: postoperative external lumbar drainage reduces the risk for meningitis, *Pituitary* 7:89-93, 2004.

43. Viswanathan A, et al: Use of lumbar drainage of cerebrospinal fluid for brain relaxation in occipital lobe approaches in children: technical note, *Surg Neurol* 71: 681-684, 2009.

44. Yilmazlar S, et al: Cerebrospinal fluid leakage complicating skull base fractures: analysis of 81 cases, *Neurosurg Rev* 29:64-71, 2006.

Additional Readings

CR March K, Wellwood, J, Arbour, R: Technology. In Bader MK, Littlejohns LR, editors: *AANN core curriculum for neuroscience nursing,* St Louis, 2004, Saunders, 199-204.

Greenberg, MS: *Handbook of Neurosurgery*, ed 6, New York, NY, Thiem, 2006.

Intraventricular Catheter with External Transducer for Cerebrospinal Fluid Drainage and Intracranial Pressure Monitoring

P U R P O S E :   An intraventricular catheter with an external transducer is used to monitor intracranial pressure and, in the presence of pathology, to alleviate increased intracranial pressure by draining cerebrospinal fluid (CSF) from the ventricular system.

D. Nathan Preuss

PREREQUISITE NURSING KNOWLEDGE

- Knowledge of neuroanatomy and physiology is needed.
- Understanding is needed regarding the assembly and maintenance of the intraventricular catheter with an external transducer and drainage system, care of the insertion site, and drainage techniques.
- Principles of aseptic technique should be understood. Of all the intracranial pressure monitoring devices, external ventricular drains (EVDs) have the greatest risk of infection.[3,6]
- The normal range for intracranial pressure (ICP) is 0 to 15 mm Hg.[3,25,28] This measurement reflects the pressure exerted by the intracranial contents within the skull, including brain, blood, and cerebrospinal fluid.[25]
- Cerebral perfusion pressure (CPP) is a derived mathematic calculation that indirectly reflects the adequacy of cerebral blood flow. The CPP is calculated by subtracting the ICP from the mean arterial pressure (MAP); thus, CPP = MAP − ICP. [3,27] The normal CPP range for adults is approximately 60 to 100 mm Hg[21] or a mean of 80 mm Hg.[19,28] The optimal CPP for a given patient and clinical condition is not entirely known. ICP and CPP should be managed concomitantly. According to the Brain Trauma Foundation Guidelines, an acceptable CPP for an adult with a severe traumatic brain injury (Glasgow Coma Scale [GCS] score of equal to or less than 8) lies between 50 and 70 mm Hg.[6] Patients with aneurysmal subarachnoid hemorrhage vasospasm may need higher CPPs to maintain adequate perfusion through vasospastic cerebral blood vessels.[2] Patients with other neurologic injuries require individualized CPP parameters reflective of the neuropathology and brain perfusion needs.

- Elevations in ICP result when one or more intracranial components—blood, cerebrospinal fluid (CSF), or brain tissue—increase without an accompanying decrease in one or two of the other intracranial components. This is known as the Monro-Kellie doctrine or hypothesis.[3,19]
- Clinical conditions that frequently result in increased intracranial pressure include traumatic brain injury, subarachnoid hemorrhage,[2] intraparenchymal hemorrhage,[8] brain tumor, meningitis, and hydrocephalus.[3,26] An EVD may be indicated in the management of intracranial pressure in each of these conditions.[21]
- Fiberoptic catheters and the microsensors that are placed during surgery in the surgical site or through a bolt in the skull are also used to monitor the ICP. They may be placed in the epidural, subdural, subarachnoid, ventricular, and intraparenchymal spaces.[27,28] These catheters are sentinels for increased ICP but are not designed for

treatment of increased ICP with CSF drainage.[27,28] In contrast, when the ventricular catheter is inserted and transduced at the level of the foramen of Monro, approximately at the level of the external auditory canal, it produces a value and a waveform that reflects the ICP. The EVD is considered the most accurate ICP monitor.[3,6]

- CSF is formed within the lateral ventricles of the cerebral hemispheres by the choroid plexus. From the lateral ventricles, fluid drains into the foramen of Monro, the intraventricular foramina, into the third ventricle adjacent to the thalamus. Although most of the CSF is made in the choroid plexus of the lateral ventricles, the third ventricle contributes some CSF, which then passes through the aqueduct of Sylvius into the fourth ventricle at the pons and medulla. The choroid plexus in the roof of the fourth ventricle contributes an additional small amount of CSF. The fluid then enters into the subarachnoid space, with the major portion of the fluid moving through the foramen of Magendie, where it is dispersed around the spinal cord and through the foramen of Luschka, where it flows around the brain. CSF is absorbed by the arachnoid villi, also known as arachnoid granulations, where it drains into the venous system to be returned to the heart.[5,7]

- CSF is a clear colorless liquid of low specific gravity with no red blood cells and only 0 to 5 white blood cells (WBCs). Approximately 150 mL of CSF circulates within the CSF pathways in the brain and spinal subarachnoid space. CSF is secreted at the rate of 0.35 mL/min or approximately 20 mL/hr.[5]

- ICP waveform morphology reflects transmission of arterial and venous pressure through the CSF and brain parenchyma. The normal ICP waveform has three or four peaks, with P_1 being of greater amplitude than P_2, and P_2 of greater amplitude than P_3. P_1 is thought to reflect arterial pressure; P_2, P_3, and P_4 (when present) have been described as choroid plexus or venous in origin (see Fig. 88-2).[3,27] The amplitude of P_2 may exceed P_1 with increased ICP or decreased intracranial compliance (see Fig. 88-3).

- ICP waveform trends include *a*, *b*, and *c* waves. The *a* waves, also referred to as plateau waves, are associated with ICP values of 50 to 100 mm Hg and last 5 to 20 minutes. The *a* waves are associated with abrupt neurologic deterioration and herniation (Fig. 88-4). The *b* waves (Fig. 88-5), with ICP values of 20 to 50 mm Hg, last 30 seconds to 2 minutes and may become *a* waves. The *c* waves (Fig. 88-6) may coincide with ICPs as high as 20 mm Hg but are short lasting and without clinical significance (see Fig. 88-6).[3]

- Some external ventricular drainage systems may also provide simultaneous drainage and trending of the intracranial pressure.

- Management of acute brain injury is aimed at decreasing secondary brain injury from increased intracranial pressure, decreased cerebral perfusion pressure,

impaired autoregulation, hypotension, hypoxemia, cerebral ischemia, hypercarbia, hyperthermia, hypoglycemia, hyperglycemia, or abnormalities in cerebral blood flow. Interventions should include a decrease in environmental stimuli, elevation of the head of the bed, alignment of the head and neck in a straight position to promote venous drainage, the avoidance of constrictive devices about the neck that might impede arterial flow to the brain and venous drainage from the brain, and attaining and maintaining normothermia without shivering.[3,25]

- In addition to CSF drainage, management of increased ICP frequently requires the use of certain pharmacologic agents to lessen intracranial pressure, including sedation and analgesia, osmotic diuretics, hypertonic saline, neuromuscular blockade, and barbiturates. In the case of barbiturate coma, continuous electroencephalographic (EEG) monitoring for burst suppression is necessary to achieve the desired decrease in cerebral oxygen consumption and electrical stimuli.[13] Additional strategies include decompressive craniectomy and hemispherectomy.[3,12,27,32]

- Underdrainage of CSF may result in sustained increased intracranial pressure and herniation.[21,24,27,28]

- Overdrainage of CSF may result in headache, subdural hematoma, pneumocephalus, and herniation.[21,24,27,28]

EQUIPMENT

- Cranial access tray with drill
- Ventricular catheter
- Pressure monitor tubing kit, including pressure tubing, transducer, a three-way stopcock, or a flushless transducer with stopcock
- Nonvented sterile caps
- External drainage system, including tubing, collection chamber, and drainage bag
- Preservative-free normal saline solution
- Pressure monitoring cable and module
- Sterile syringes
- Shave preparation kit
- Sterile towels, drapes
- Antiseptic solution
- Local anesthetic (lidocaine 1% or 2% without epinephrine)
- Sutures or staples
- Sterile dressing
- Tape
- Laboratory forms and specimen labels (for CSF specimens)
- Sterile CSF specimen tubes (for collection of CSF)
- Caps, masks, sterile drapes, gloves, and gowns
- Suction
- Cautery as required by institutional standard (for bedside insertion)
- Leveling device (e.g. carpenter, laser, or line level)
- IV pole

PATIENT AND FAMILY EDUCATION

- This procedure may be performed at the bedside or in an operating room. The patient may need to be sedated, paralyzed, and intubated. ➤**Rationale:** Patient cooperation during cranial access is of utmost importance. In the presence of an intact neurologic examination, the patient may not need intubation. However, the patient and family should be aware that the patient may need to be intubated to maintain a patent airway, ensure adequate oxygenation, and maintain a normal ICP and an adequate CPP.

- Assess the patient and the family for understanding of ICP pressure monitoring. ➤**Rationale:** Knowledge and information may lessen anxiety.

- Explain the waveforms on the bedside monitor and how this pressure is continually observed for signs of increased ICP. In the case of increased ICP, the drain is opened to drain CSF continuously or intermittently to alleviate the pressure. ➤**Rationale:** This explanation presents to the patient and family a more realistic expectation of the events to come.

PATIENT ASSESSMENT AND PREPARATION

Patient Assessment

- Obtain a baseline assessment to include level of consciousness, mental status, motor and sensation, cranial nerves, and vital signs. ➤**Rationale:** This assessment provides baseline data.

- Obtain the patient's medical and surgical history to include use of aspirin, anticoagulants, prior craniotomies, the presence of aneurysm clips, embolic materials, permanent balloon occlusions, detachable coils, or a ventriculoperitoneal shunt. Obtain laboratory results to assess coagulation status as needed. ➤**Rationale:** The information obtained determines and guides future treatment based on the neurologic examination results and evidence from radiology and angiography.

- Assess for allergies. ➤**Rationale:** Insertion of an external ventricular catheter requires the use of an antiseptic to cleanse the site, local anesthetic, and possibly systemic analgesic and sedation. External ventricular catheters may be impregnated with antibiotics (e.g., clindamycin, rifampin, and minocycline), or systemic antibiotics may be given periprocedurally or prophylactically.[6,21,26]

Patient Preparation

- Verify correct patient with two identifiers. ➤**Rationale:** Prior to performing a procedure, the nurse should ensure the correct identification of the patient for the intended intervention.

- Ensure that the patient and family understand preprocedural teaching. Answer questions as they arise, and reinforce information as needed. ➤**Rationale:** Understanding of previously taught information is evaluated and reinforced.

- Ensure that informed consent has been obtained. ➤**Rationale:** Informed consent protects the rights of the patient and makes a competent decision possible for the patient. However, in emergency circumstances, time may not allow for the consent form to be signed.

- Initiate intravenous (IV) access or assess the patency of the IV. ➤**Rationale:** Readily available IV access is necessary if the patient needs to be sedated or paralyzed or needs other medications.

- Perform a pre-procedure verification and time out, if nonemergent. ➤**Rationale:** Ensures patient safety.

Procedure	**for Pressure Monitoring and Drainage**	
Steps	**Rationale**	**Special Considerations**
External Ventricular Drainage (EVD) System Assembly		
1. 🔲		
2. Open the outer package of the sterile supplies. Apply sterile gloves, gown, and mask with eye shield.	Ensures sterile technique.	
3. With aseptic technique, flush through the pressure tubing and drainage system with preservative-free saline solution, turning the stopcocks as needed to prime the entire system. Remove the syringe and replace with a sterile non-vented cap.	Prepares the drainage system for use; flushes air from the system. If air is left in the tubing, it may alter the numeric value or prevent the flow of CSF.[10,22] Preservative in normal saline may cause cortical necrosis.[16]	Use of a syringe filled with sterile, preservative-free normal saline solution to prime the external ventricular drainage system tubing rather than a bag of flush solution lessens the risk of flush solution being administered through the ventricular catheter into the brain. In addition, the use of a flushless transducer at the zero reference on the drainage system eliminates lengthy tubing that may dampen the waveform (Fig. 92-1).

Procedure | for Pressure Monitoring and Drainage—*Continued*

Steps	Rationale	Special Considerations
4. Connect the end of the EVD drainage system tubing to the distal stopcock of the pressure monitor tubing (Fig. 92-2) if not already included in the drainage system. Tighten all the connections.	Ensures that the system is secure and is a sterile closed system.	
5. Close the clamp or stopcock between the drip chamber and the external ventricular drainage collection bag (see Fig. 92-2).	Ensures the ability to measure hourly drainage in the drip chamber.	
6. Replace all vented caps with nonvented caps.	Vented caps are used by the manufacturer to permit sterilization of the entire system. These caps need to be replaced with sterile nonvented caps to prevent bacteria and air from entering the system.	
7. After flushing the pressure monitor tubing and the external ventricular drainage system tubing, turn the distal stopcock off to the distal tip of the pressure monitor tubing.	The stopcock in this position readies the entire system for connection to the ventriculostomy catheter.	Prevents the backflow of fluid into the drip chamber.
8. Position the reference level of the drip chamber as prescribed.	The relationship of the reference level of the drip chamber to the anatomic reference point alters the rate of CSF drainage.	The reference level of the drip chamber may need to be adjusted after insertion of the ventricular catheter and the initial ICP is obtained.
9. Discard used supplies.	Removes and safely discards used supplies.	
10. **HH**		

Assisting with Insertion of an Intraventricular Catheter

1. **HH**		
2. Apply nonsterile gloves, gowns, and masks with eye shields. After opening outer packaging, apply sterile gloves to handle sterile supplies.	Reduces transmission of microorganisms and body secretions; Standard Precautions.	
3. Ensure the patient is in position for ventricular catheter placement.	Facilitates the insertion of the catheter.	The usual position is supine, with the head of bed elevated. Administer sedation and analgesia as prescribed.
4. Assist as needed with the antiseptic preparation of the insertion site.	Reduces the transmission of microorganisms into the ventricles.	The choice of povidone iodine or chlorhexidine as an antiseptic agent is controversial. Both should be allowed to dry completely. Studies suggest chlorhexidine is neurotoxic.[15] Observe for initiation of CSF drainage, and obtain an opening ICP.
5. Connect the monitoring system to the distal tip of the catheter after it is inserted.		
6. Assist as needed with application of a sterile, occlusive dressing. Secure the catheter to minimize manipulation and the risk of inadvertent removal.[25]	Reduces the risk of infection.	

Procedure continues on following page

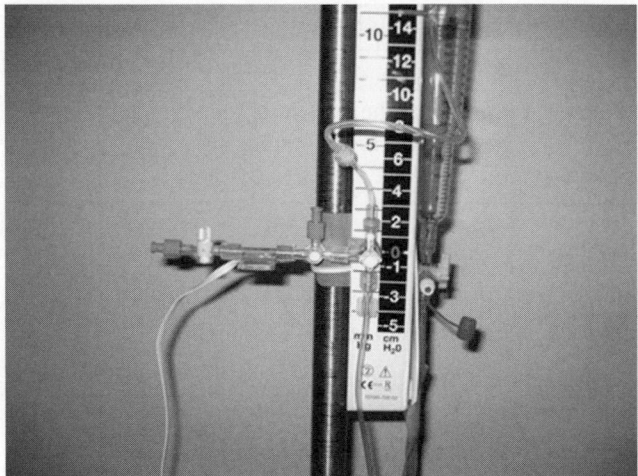

FIGURE 92-1   External ventricular drainage system with flushless transducer at zero reference level. *(Courtesy of Integra Lifesciences Corporation, Plainsboro, NJ.)*

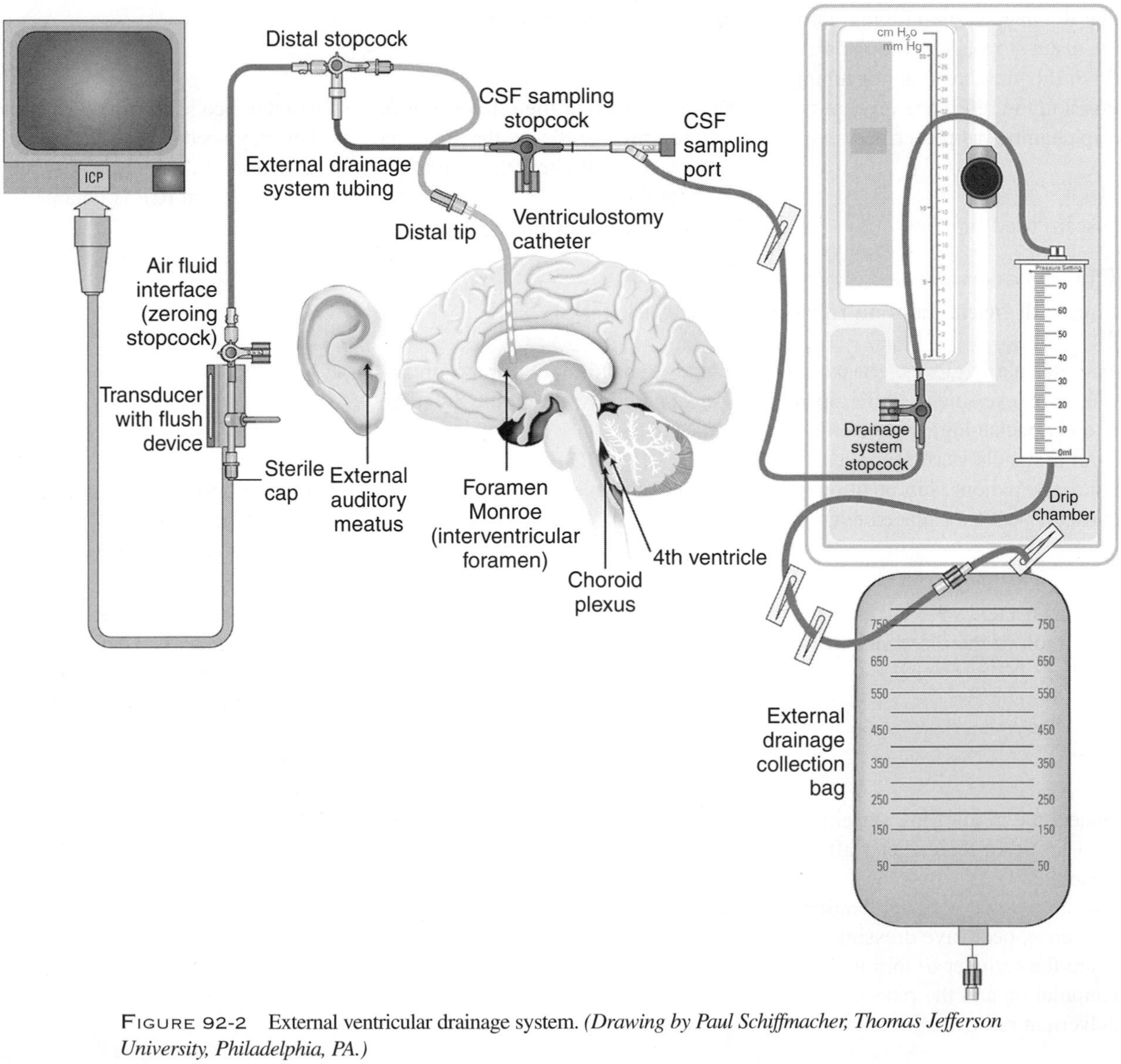

Distal stopcock

CSF sampling stopcock

CSF sampling port

External drainage system tubing

Distal tip

Ventriculostomy catheter

Air fluid interface (zeroing stopcock)

Transducer with flush device

Sterile cap

External auditory meatus

Foramen Monroe (interventricular foramen)

Choroid plexus

4th ventricle

Drainage system stopcock

Drip chamber

External drainage collection bag

FIGURE 92-2   External ventricular drainage system. *(Drawing by Paul Schiffmacher, Thomas Jefferson University, Philadelphia, PA.)*

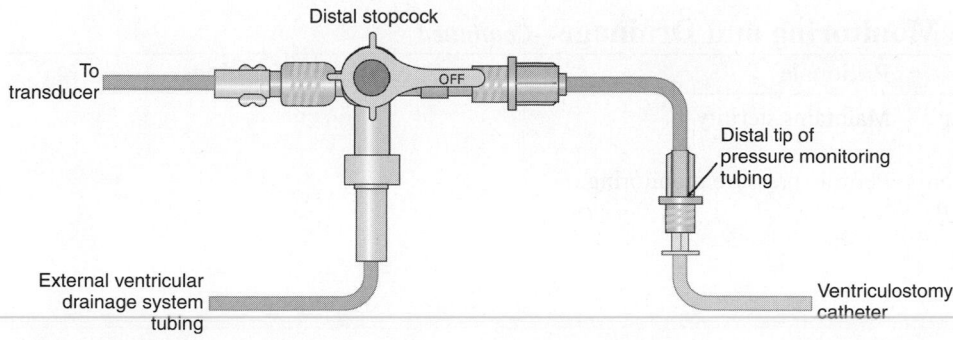

FIGURE 92-3 Distal stopcock turned off to the distal tip of the pressure monitor tubing. *(Drawing by Paul Schiffmacher, Thomas Jefferson University, Philadelphia, PA.)*

Procedure | for Pressure Monitoring and Drainage—*Continued*

Steps	Rationale	Special Considerations
Connecting the EVD Transducer with Bedside Monitor		
1. Turn on the bedside monitor.	Prepares the monitor.	
2. Plug a pressure cable into the appropriate pressure module or port in the bedside monitor (see Fig. 92-2).	The signal is transmitted to the bedside monitor so that it may be transmitted to the oscilloscope for display.	
3. Attach the pressure cable to the transducer connection on the pressure tubing.	Prepares the equipment.	
4. Turn on the ICP parameter.	Visualizes correct waveform.	
5. Set the appropriate scale for the measured pressure.[26,28]	It is necessary to visualize the complete waveform and to obtain corresponding numerical values. Waveforms vary in amplitude, depending on the pressure within the system.	The normal ICP for an adult is within the range of 0 to 15 mm Hg.[9,13]
6. Set the monitor alarm limits for ICP and CPP.	Goals for ICP management are individualized for each patient based on etiology, pathophysiology, and management strategies.	
Leveling the Transducer		
1. HH		
2. Position the patient in the supine position with the head of the bed elevated as prescribed by the physician.[25,27,29] **(Level E*)**	Prepares the patient.	The head of the bed is usually placed at 30 degrees to aid in increasing venous return.[13,26]
3. Place the air-fluid interface (zeroing stopcock) at the level of the external auditory meatus (see Fig. 92-2).[4,29] **Level B*)**	The external auditory meatus approximates the level of the foramen of Monro (intraventricular foramen).[4,9]	Some institutions use the tragus or a line drawn from the outer canthus of the eye.[4,21] Follow institutional policy.
4. HH		
Zeroing the Transducer		
1. HH		Follow institutional standard.
2. PE		
3. Turn the transducer stopcock off to the patient.	Prepares the system for the zeroing procedure.	
4. Remove the nonvented cap from the stopcock, opening the stopcock to air.	Allows the monitor to use atmospheric pressure as a reference for zero.	
5. Push and release the zeroing button on the bedside monitor. Observe the digital reading until it displays a value of zero.	The monitor automatically adjusts itself to zero. Zeroing negates the effects of atmospheric pressure.	Some monitors require that the zero be turned and adjusted manually.

*Level B: Well-designed controlled studies with results that consistently support a specific action, intervention, or treatment
*Level E: Multiple case reports, theory-based evidence from expert opinions, or peer-reviewed professional organizational standards without clinical studies to support recommendations

Procedure continues on following page

Procedure   **for Pressure Monitoring and Drainage—***Continued*

Steps	Rationale	Special Considerations
6. Place a new, sterile nonvented cap on the stopcock.	Maintains sterility.	
7. Turn the stopcock so that it is open to the transducer. Observe the ICP waveform and the corresponding numerical value.	Permits pressure monitoring.	
8. 🄷🄷		
Monitoring Intracranial Pressure		
1. Position the head of the bed as prescribed.	Allows for accurate and consistent monitoring of the ICP.	Ensure that the EVD system is at the prescribed level for ICP measurement (e.g., level with external auditory meatus).
2. Turn the distal stopcock off to the external ventricular drainage system (Fig. 92-4).[21]	Decreases artifact from simultaneous drainage. Allows for accurate monitoring of the ICP.	
3. Record the ICP value and waveform per institutional standard.	Provides a value for ongoing assessment. Allows analysis of the ICP waveform.	The normal ICP waveform has at least three distinct pressure oscillations or peaks. These are referred to as P_1, P_2, and P_3 (see Fig. 88-2).[17,18,24]
4. Monitor ICP and CPP as prescribed.	Assesses ICP waveform and values and CPP value.	If continuous drainage is prescribed, the risk of overdrainage is increased. If the drainage system allows, turn the stopcock to simultaneously drain and to trend the ICP. Set alarms. To obtain an accurate ICP, the stopcock must be turned off to the drain with the catheter open to the transducer only and the waveform and numeric value of the ICP given time to stabilize. The waveform and numeric value of the ICP should correspond.
		Deviations in ICP and CPP may require immediate intervention and should be reported to the physician or advanced practice nurse. If an EVD is in the monitoring position (and off to CSF drainage), special care must be paid to the bedside neurologic examination with regard to the potential for deterioration. The catheter may become obstructed with clot, tissue, or protein. Note any changes in CSF flow. Notify the physician or advanced practice nurse who may need to irrigate the catheter to reestablish patency. Other maneuvers may include turning or stimulating a cough. Some institutional policies allow the critical care nurse to irrigate the catheter with a limited amount of preservative-free saline solution. Follow institutional standard.

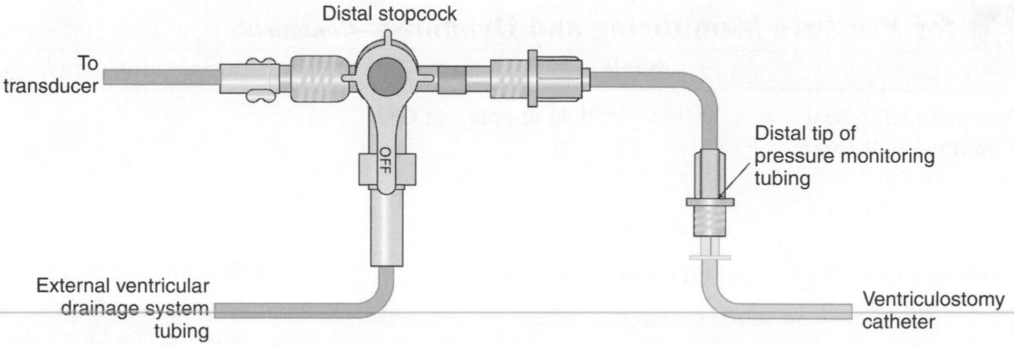

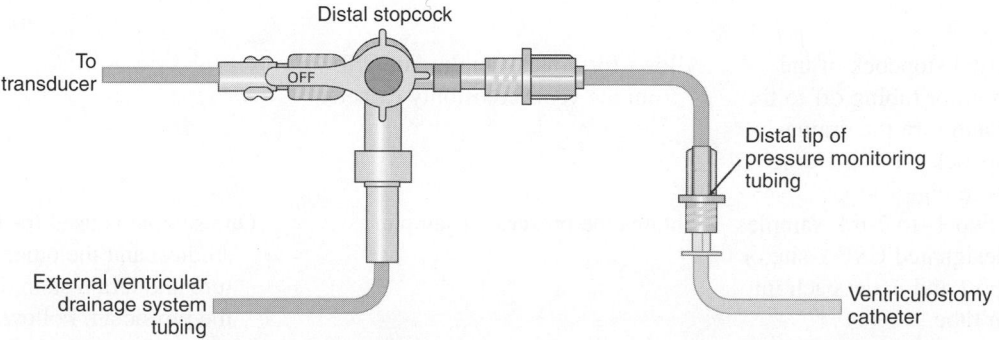

FIGURE 92-4 Distal stopcock turned off to the external drainage system tubing. *(Drawing by Paul Schiffmacher, Thomas Jefferson University, Philadelphia, PA.)*

Procedure | for Pressure Monitoring and Drainage—*Continued*

Steps	Rationale	Special Considerations
Draining CSF from the EVD		
1. The physician will prescribe the desired ICP parameter.	If the physician prescribes the ICP to be maintained at less than 15 mm Hg, drainage of CSF will be initiated if the patient's ICP is greater than 15 mm Hg.	
2. 🅷🅷		
3. To drain the CSF, turn the distal stopcock of the pressure monitoring tubing off to the transducer (Fig. 92-5).[21] **(Level E*)**	Allows the flow of CSF from the ventricles.	Never leave a draining EVD unattended. Excessive drainage may cause overdrainage and a possible collapse of the ventricles, resulting in tearing of the bridging veins of the brain causing a subdural hematoma.
4. Allow 2-5 ml of CSF to enter the drip chamber (see Fig. 92-5).	Prevents overdrainage of CSF.	Never leave a draining EVD unattended.
5. When drainage is completed, turn the distal stopcock off to the external ventricular drainage system (see Fig. 92-4) and note the amount drained and the ICP value.	Check the ICP value to determine whether the parameter is met.	If the patient's CSF is being continuously drained, note and record the amount of drainage every hour. In general, no more than 20 mL, the amount of CSF produced in 1 hour,[5] should be drained each hour.

*Level E: Multiple case reports, theory-based evidence from expert opinions, or peer-reviewed professional organizational standards without clinical studies to support recommendations

Procedure continues on following page

FIGURE 92-5 Distal stopcock turned off to the transducer. *(Drawing by Paul Schiffmacher, Thomas Jefferson University, Philadelphia, PA.)*

Procedure for Pressure Monitoring and Drainage—*Continued*

Steps	Rationale	Special Considerations
6. If the goal was not met, repeat steps 3 to 5 until the ICP parameter is met. 7. 🔲	Allows gradual draining of CSF.	
CSF Sampling		
1. Obtain a physician's order for a CSF sample, including the frequency.	Prepares for the test.	CSF sampling may include glucose, cell count, protein, culture and sensitivity, and Gram stain. If a comparison of serum glucose and CSF glucose is prescribed, a serum glucose sample should be obtained at the same time as the CSF sampling. Normal CSF glucose is two thirds of blood glucose.[5,7]
2. Obtain the supplies for sampling: sterile 3-mL syringes, sterile CSF tubes, antiseptic solution, sterile gloves, mask with face shield, laboratory forms, and specimen labels. 3. 🔲	Prepares the equipment.	
4. Apply sterile gloves and mask with face shield.	Reduces the transmission of microorganisms and body fluids; Standard Precautions.	
5. Cleanse the CSF sampling port with an antiseptic solution (Fig. 92-6). Allow solution to dry.	Reduces the transmission of microorganisms into the ventricles.	Studies suggest chlorhexidine is neurotoxic.[15]

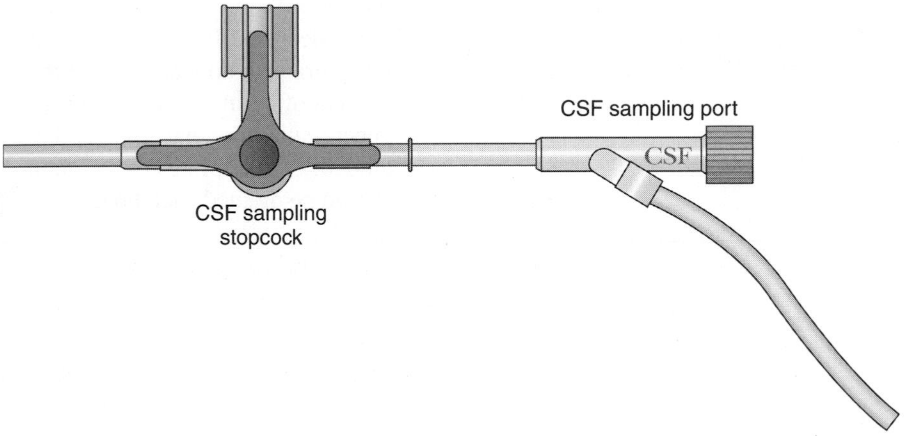

FIGURE 92-6 CSF sampling port. (*Drawing by Paul Schiffmacher, Thomas Jefferson University, Philadelphia, PA.*)

6. Turn the distal stopcock of the pressure monitor tubing off to the transducer and turn the drainage system stopcock off to the drop chamber. (see Fig. 92-5).	Allows for direct sampling of CSF from the ventriculostomy catheter.	
7. Withdraw two 1- to 2-mL samples from the designated CSF Y-site or sampling port and inject each into a specimen tube.	Obtains the prescribed sample.	One sample is used for laboratory studies, and the other is used for culture and Gram stain, if prescribed by the physician. Follow institutional standard regarding obtaining a discard sample (e.g., 1 mL).

Procedure | for Pressure Monitoring and Drainage—*Continued*

Steps	Rationale	Special Considerations
8. Turn the distal stopcock to resume monitoring or open to drainage as prescribed.	Continues monitoring and drainage as prescribed.	
9. Label the CSF specimen tubes and send to the laboratory for analysis.	Prepares the specimen for analysis.	
10. Discard used supplies.	Removes and safely discards used supplies.	
11. ▦		

Expected Outcomes

- Aseptic drainage system[20,24,26]
- Air-fluid interface of the transducer is leveled at the foramen of Monro for accurate ICP and CPP monitoring[21,25,27]
- The monitoring system is zeroed
- Drainage chamber at prescribed level
- Intermittent or continuous drainage as prescribed
- Accurate and reliable monitoring of ICP and CPP[21,25,27]
- Continuous flow of CSF when drainage is initiated; appropriate amount of CSF drainage[21,25,27]
- Immediate management of increased ICP and decreased CPP[21,25,27]
- Improvement or stabilization of neurologic function[21,27,29]

Unexpected Outcomes

- Loose connections within the external ventricular drainage system
- Stopcocks left open to air without nonvented caps
- Air bubbles within the system[22]
- CSF infection[1,11,30]
- CSF leak
- Lack of CSF flow[7]
- Dislodgment or occlusion of the EVD
- Headache from overdrainage[23,29,30]
- Pneumocephalus from overdrainage
- Rebleed from subarachnoid hemorrhage[14,20]
- Subdural hematoma from overdrainage[26]
- EVD-related hemorrhage[26]
- Herniation from underdrainage or overdrainage

Patient Monitoring and Care

Steps	Rationale	Reportable Conditions
		These conditions should be reported if they persist despite nursing interventions.
1. Monitor each of the following parameters continuously or intermittently as prescribed: ICP, CPP, and CSF drainage, amount, color, and clarity.	Assesses neurologic status.	• Any gradual or sudden increase in the ICP, with or without accompanying neurologic changes • Lack of drainage in the presence of significantly increased ICP requires immediate reporting to the physician; this may indicate an occlusion of the catheter[20,26] • Lack of drainage in the presence of significantly increased ICP may also indicate occlusion of the drainage system from persistent contact of CSF catheter with the ventricular wall[9] • Persistent large volumes of the CSF totaling more than 200 mL each day may indicate the need for a CSF shunt[8]

Procedure continues on following page

Patient Monitoring and Care —*Continued*

Steps	Rationale	Reportable Conditions
2. Zero the external ventricular drainage system during the initial setup or before insertion, then after insertion and again if connections between the transducer and the monitoring cable become dislodged, if connections between the monitoring cable and the monitor become dislodged, and when the values do not fit the clinical picture.	Ensures the accuracy of the monitoring process.	
3. When changing the patient's position, maintain the reference level of the EVD at the external auditory meatus.	Minimizes the risk for underdrainage, overdrainage, or erroneous ICP values.	• Increase or decrease in CSF drainage • The inability to obtain CSF drainage • Changes in ICP or neurologic assessment
4. Maintain the reference level of the drip chamber as prescribed.	The relationship of the reference for CSF Drainage and ICP monitoring level of the drip chamber to the anatomic reference point alters the rate of CSF drainage.	• Underdrainage • Overdrainage
5. Check the system every hour and as needed.	Ensures that all connections are tightly secured and that no cracks occur in the system. Ensures that the system is closed with nonvented caps on all stopcocks. Ensures that the system is free of air bubbles.[22]	
6. Set the alarm parameters relative to the ICP and CPP goals established by the physician.	Provides immediate alarm for high pressures (and an immediate alarm for low pressures associated with inadvertent overdrainage).	• Changes in ICP or neurologic assessment
7. All drainage should be measured and recorded as part of the intake and output.	Assesses CSF drainage. Amount, color, and character should be noted.[25]	• Increase or decrease in CSF drainage; change in CSF color, presence of blood or blood-tinged CSF
8. If continuous drainage is used, record and monitor the output every 1 to 2 hours. Maintain the reference point at the foramen of Monro.	Assesses CSF drainage.	• Increase or decrease in CSF drainage; underdrainage or overdrainage
9. Change the dressing at the insertion site daily or as prescribed with aseptic technique. Change bag and drainage system as needed by institutional standard.	Maintains sterility and provides an opportunity for site assessment	• Signs or symptoms of infection • Loosened sutures
10. Follow institutional standard for assessing pain. Administer analgesia as prescribed.	Identifies need for pain interventions.	• Continued pain despite pain interventions

Documentation

Documentation should include the following:
- Initial opening ICP and CPP
- Analysis of waveform[18,25,27,28]
- Description of CSF to include amount, clarity and color
- Insertion site assessment

- Hourly to every 2 hours output or amount drained intermittently[21, 28]
- Hourly ICP and CPP[21,28]
- Neurologic assessment[21,28]
- Site care and change of drainage system or bag
- Pain assessment, interventions, and evaluation

References

CR 1. Arabi Y, Memish ZA, Balkhy HH, et al: Ventriculostomy-associated infections: incidence and risk factors, *Am J Infect Control* 33:137-143, 2005.

2. Bederson JB, Connolly ES, Batjer HH, et al: Guidelines for the management of aneurysmal subarachnoid hemorrhage: a statement for healthcare professionals from a special writing group of the Stroke Council, American Heart Association, *Stroke* 40:994-1025, 2009.

3. Bershad EM, Humphreis WE, Suraz JI: Intracranial hypertension, *Semin Neurol* 28:690-702, 2008.

CR 4. Bisnaire D, Robinson L: Accuracy of levelling intraventricular collection drainage systems, *J Neurosci Nurs* 29:261-268, 1997.

CR 5. Blumenfeld H: *Ventricles and cerebrospinal fluid in neuroanatomy through clinical cases,* Sunderland, MA, 2002, Sinauer Associates, 128-133.

6. Bratton SL, Chesnut RM, Ghajar J, et al: Guidelines for the management of severe traumatic brain injury: a join project of the Brain Trauma Foundation, American Association of Neurological Surgeons (AANS), Congress of Neurological Surgeons (CNS), AANS/CNS Joint Section on Neurotrauma and Critical Care, *J Neurotrauma* 24(Suppl 1):S1-S106, 2007.

7. Brodbelt A, Stoodley M: CSF pathways: a review, *Br J Neurosurg* 21:510-520, 2007.

8. Broderick J, Connolly S, Feldman E, et al: Guidelines for the early management of spontaneous intracerebral hemorrhage in adults: guidelines from the American Heart Association/American Stroke Association Stroke Council, High Blood Pressure Research Council, and the Quality of Care Outcomes in Research Interdisciplinary Working Groups, *Stroke* 38:2001-2023, 2007.

CR 9. Czosnyka M, Pickard JD: Monitoring and interpretation of intracranial pressure, *J Neurol Neurosurg Psychiatry* 75:813-821, 2004.

CR 10. Czosnyka M, Czosnyka ZA, Richards HK, et al: Hydrodynamic properties of extraventricular drainage systems, *Neurosurgery* 52:619-623, 2003.

11. Dasic D, Hanna SJ, Bojanic S, et al: External ventricular drain infection: the effect of a strict protocol on infection rates and a review of the literature, *Br J Neurosurg* 20:296-300, 2006.

CR 12. Dennis LJ, Mayer SA: Diagnosis and management of increased intracranial pressure, *Neurol India* 49 (Suppl 1):S37-S50, 2001.

CR 13. Dunn LT: Raised intracranial pressure, *J Neurol Neurosurg Psychiatry* 73(Suppl I):i23-i27, 2002.

14. Fountas KN, Kapsalaki EZ, Machinis T, et al: Review of the literature regarding the relationship of rebleeding and external ventricular drainage in patients with subarachnoid hemorrhage of aneurysmal origin, *Neurosurg Rev* 29:14-18, 2006.

15. Hebl JR: The importance and implications of aseptic techniques during regional anesth, *Reg Anesth Pain Med* 31:311-323, 2006.

CR 16. Hetherington NJ, Dooley MJ: Potential for patient harm from intrathecal administration of preserved solutions, *Med J Aust* 173: 141-143, 2000.

CR 17. Kinirons B, Mimoz O, Lafendi L, et al: Chlorhexidine versus povidone iodine in preventing colonization of continuous epidural catheters in children, *Anesthesiology* 94:239-244, 2001.

CR 18. Kirkness CJ, Mitchell PH, Burr RL, et al: Intracranial pressure waveform analysis: clinical and research implications, *J Neurosci Nurs* 32:271-277, 2000.

CR 19. Kirkness CJ, March K: Intracranial pressure management. In Bader MK, Littlejohns LR, editors: *AANN core curriculum for neuroscience nursing*, St Louis, 2004, Saunders, 249-267.

20. Komotar R, Zacharia BE, Mocco J, et al: Controversies in the surgical treatment of ruptured intracranial aneurysms: the first annual J. Lawrence Pool Memorial Research Symposium-Controversies in the management of cerebral aneurysms, *Neurosurgery* 62:396-407, 2008.

21. Leeper B, Lovasik D: Cerebrospinal drainage systems: external ventricular and lumbar drains. Littlejohns LR, Bader MK, editors: *AACN-AANN protocols for practice: monitoring technologies in critically ill patients*, Sudbury, MA, 2009, Jones and Bartlett, 71-82.

CR 22. Littlejohns LR, Trimble B: Ask the experts: our policy on external ventricular drainage systems includes the procedure for priming the system. Does it really have to be primed? *Crit Care Nurse* 25:57-59, 2005.

CR 23. Lozier AP, Sciacca RR, Romagnoli MF, et al: Ventriculostomy-related infections: a critical review of the literature, *Neurosurgery* 51:170-182, 2002.

24. Maniker A, Vaynman AY, Karimi RJ, et al: Hemorrhagic complications of external ventricular drainage, *Neurosurgery* 59(ONS Suppl 4):ONS419-424, 2006.

CR 25. March K: Intracranial pressure monitoring and assessing intracranial compliance in brain injury, *Crit Care Nurs Clin North Am* 12:429-436, 2000.

CR 26. March K: Intracranial pressure monitoring: why monitor? *AACN Clin Issues* 16:456-475, 2005.

27. March K, Madden L: Intracranial pressure management. In Littlejohns LR, Bader MK, editors: *AACN-AANN protocols for practice: monitoring technologies in critically ill patients*, Sudbury, MA, 2009, Jones and Bartlett, 35-69.

CR 28. March K, Wellwood, J, Arbour, R: Technology. In Bader MK, Littlejohns LR, editors: *AANN core curriculum for neuroscience nursing*, St Louis, 2004, Saunders, 199-204.

CR 29. Ng I, Lim J, Wong HB: Effects of head posture on cerebral hemodynamics: its influences on intracranial pressure, cerebral perfusion pressure, and cerebral oxygenation, *Neurosurgery* 54:593-598, 2004.

CR 30. O'Grady NP, Alexander M, Dellinger P, et al: Guidelines for the prevention of intravascular catheter-related infections, *Am J Infect Control* 30:476-489, 2002.

31. Reynolds F: Neurologic infections after neuraxial anesthesia, *Anesthesiol Clin* 26:23-52, 2008.

CR 32. Vincent JL, Berre J: Primer on medical management of severe brain injury, *Crit Care Med* 33:1392-1399, 2005.

Additional Reading

CR Dunham CM, Ransom KJ, Flowers LL, et al: Cerebral hypoxia in severely brain-injured patients is associated with admission Glasgow Coma Scale score, computed tomographic severity, cerebral perfusion pressure, and survival, *J Trauma* 56:482-489, 2004.

AP Transcranial Doppler Monitoring

P U R P O S E :   Transcranial Doppler scan measures blood flow velocities in the major branches of the circle of Willis through an intact skull. This measurement supports the grading of vasospasm severity, localization of intracranial stenoses or occlusions, detection of cerebral emboli, monitoring of hemodynamic changes with impaired intracranial perfusion, and assessment of the impact of therapeutic interventions on intracranial hemodynamics.[7-9,18,24]

Anne W. Alexandrov

PREREQUISITE NURSING KNOWLEDGE

- Knowledge of neuroanatomy and physiology is needed.
- Clinical and technical competence related to transcranial Doppler (TCD) ultrasound scan is necessary.
- Noninvasive assessment of the intracranial vasculature is indicated for patients with a subarachnoid hemorrhage, ischemic stroke, sickle cell disease, cerebral emboli, impaired vasomotor reactivity, cerebral circulatory arrest, and other neurovascular disorders.[15,21]
- Successful ultrasound penetration through the skull is possible through intracranial windows, which either lack bone (burr holes, flaps) or consist of thinner bone structure compared with the overall cranial bone thickness. Four windows are available for insonation: temporal, orbital, foraminal, and submandibular (Fig. 93-1).[1-4]
- The transtemporal window allows insonation of the middle cerebral artery (MCA), the anterior cerebral artery (ACA), the posterior cerebral artery (PCA), and the anterior and posterior communicating arteries (AComA and PComA).[1-4]

- The transorbital window allows insonation of the ophthalmic artery (OA) and the internal carotid artery (ICA) siphon.[1-4]
- The transforaminal window allows insonation of the vertebral arteries (VAs) and the basilar artery (BA).[1-4]
- The submandibular window allows insonation of the ICA as it enters the skull.[1-4] TCD scan locates both the depth

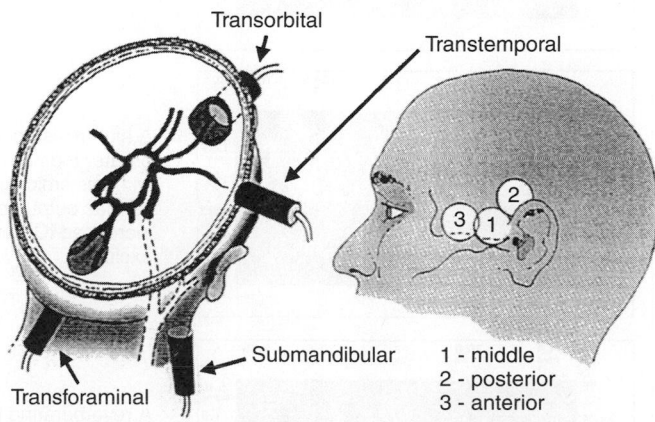

FIGURE 93-1   Four windows of transcranial Doppler insonation *(left image, clockwise):* orbital, temporal, submandibular, and foraminal. The temporal window has three aspects *(right image):* 1, middle; 2, posterior; 3, anterior. *(From Alexandrow AV: Transcranial Doppler ultrasonography, Houston, 1998, University of Texas Medical School.)*

and direction of arterial blood flow relative to the transducer position and the ultrasonic beam direction. Flow moving toward the transducer is displayed as a waveform with a positive velocity spectrum, whereas flow moving away from the transducer is displayed as a waveform with a negative velocity spectrum.[1-4,12,16]

- The TCD scan measures cerebral blood flow velocities that should not be equated to cerebral blood flow (CBF) volume. TCD is an indirect reflection of CBF.[4,15,21]

- The examination should begin with maximal power and gate settings (e.g., power, 100%; gate, 10 to 15 mm) to expedite identification of the temporal window and various arterial segments. Once a good temporal window is established, the power may be reduced to adhere to the U.S. Food and Drug Administration (FDA) principles of (1) "as low as reasonably achievable" (ALARA) and (2) minimization of overall time of patient exposure to ultrasound scan. Transorbital examination should always be performed with minimal power (e.g., 10%) to avoid potential side effects from the heating of orbital structures.[1-4]

- The highest velocity signals for each arterial segment studied, and any abnormal or unusual waveforms, should be measured and stored in the system's computer.[3]

- Criteria for normal insonation depths, flow direction, and mean flow velocities are used for appropriate identification of arteries and diagnosis of abnormalities (Fig. 93-2 and Table 93-1).[2,15,18,21]

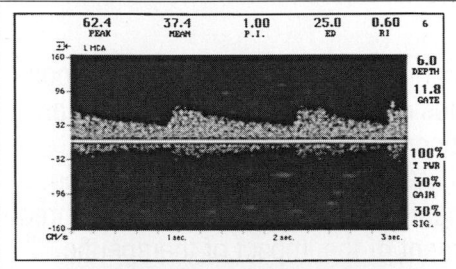

A normal waveform with sharp systolic flow acceleration, stepwise diastolic deceleration, and pulsatility index (PI) range of 0.6 – 1.1.

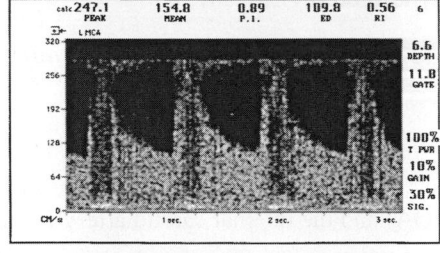

A focal significant MFV increase, with moderate vasospasm (MCA MFV range 120-200 cm/sec, MCA/ICA MFV ratio 3-6). Severe MCA spasm produces MFV greater than 200 cm/sec and ratio greater than 6.

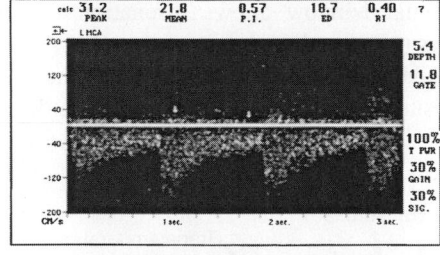

A blunted waveform indicates near occlusion with flow diversion to a branching vessel. Differential diagnosis includes the presence of a proximal ICA obstruction.

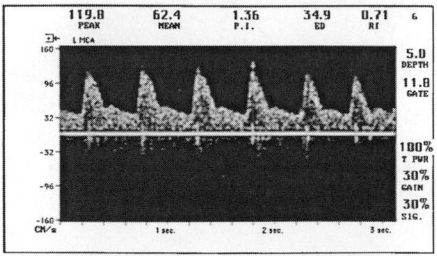

A high resistance waveform with PI greater than or equal to 1.2 can be found with systemic hypertension, increased cardiac output, distal vasospasm or increased ICP after other reasons are excluded.

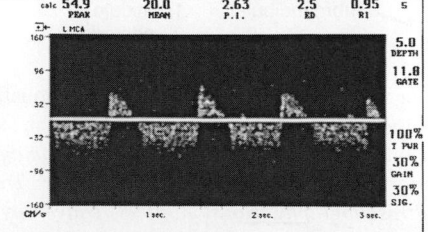

A reverberating flow waveform shows diastolic flow reversal due to ICP equal or exceeding CPP. If found in both MCA and BA, this waveform indicates cerebral circulatory arrest.

FIGURE 93-2 Typical MCA waveforms. Vertical scale is in centimeters per second; horizontal scale is in seconds. Direction of flow: (+), toward the probe; (−), away from the probe. Velocity and pulsatility values (*left to right*): peak systolic, mean, pulsatility index (PI), end-diastolic (ED), resistance index (RI). Depth indicates depth of insonation in centimeters. Gate is the diameter of sample volume in millimeters. Power and gain settings are given in percentages.

TABLE 93-1	Depth, Direction, and Mean Flow Velocities for Circle of Willis Arteries*		
Artery	Depth (mm)	Flow Direction†	MFV for Adults
M1 MCA	45-65	Toward	32-82 cm/sec
A1 ACA	62-75	Away	18-82 cm/sec
ICA siphon	60-64	Bidirectional	20-77 cm/sec
OA	50-62	Toward	Variable
PCA	60-68	Bidirectional	16-58 cm/sec
BA	80-100	Away	12-66 cm/sec
VA	45-80	Away	12-66 cm/sec

*Depth and MFV ranges may vary slightly between reference studies.
†Toward the probe indicates a positive (+) waveform; away from the probe indicates a negative (−) waveform.
M1 MCA, First segment of the middle cerebral artery; *A1 ACA*, first segment of the anterior cerebral artery; *ICA*, internal carotid artery; *OA*, ophthalmic artery; *PCA*, posterior cerebral artery; *BA*, basilar artery; *VA*, vertebral artery.
(Adapted with permission from Alexandrov AV: Transcranial Doppler sonography: principles, examination technique and normal values, Vasc Ultrasound Today 10:141-160, 1998.)

- Criteria for determination of a normal examination are listed in Table 93-2.[2,15,18,21]
- Criteria supporting differential diagnosis are listed in Table 93-3.[2,15,18,21]
- Hemispheric index (HI, also known as the Lindegaard ratio) helps to differentiate vasospasm severity and hyperdynamic blood flow changes (HI = mean flow velocity [MFV] ipsilateral MCA/MFV ipsilateral ICA). Normal values are less than 3.[11,15,18,21]
- The diameter of the vasospastic artery in aneurysmal subarachnoid hemorrhage is inversely related to the mean flow velocity. MCA vasospasm may be further classified as mild, moderate, severe, or critical.[1,12,18,21] Severity of cerebral vasospasm is assessed by MFV value (cm/s) or MCA/ICA ratio[10]:
  - Mild vasospasm has an MFV value of less than 120 or an MCA/ICA ratio of less than 3.
  - Moderate vasospasm has an MFV value from 120 to 150 or an MCA/ICA ratio from 3 to 5.
  - Severe vasospasm has an MFV value from 151 to 200 or an MCA/ICA ratio greater than 6.
  - Critical vasospasm has an MFV value greater than 200 or an MCA/ICA ratio greater than 6.
- Pulsatility of flow refers to vessel resistance and is measured with the pulsatility index (PI); normal range for PI is 0.6 to 1.1.[2,4,15,21] PI (Gosling-King) = [velocity (peak systole) − velocity (end diastole)] ÷ velocity (mean).[4,15,21]
- Hyperventilation increases the PI and decreases mean flow velocity.[4,15,21]
- Hypercapnia decreases PI and increases mean flow velocity.[4,15,21]
- Anatomic variations in the circle of Willis are common (Fig. 93-3).[2,4,15,21] Inability to find an artery with the TCD scan should not be interpreted as arterial occlusion in the absence of other abnormal flow findings (e.g., secondary signs such as high resistance and flow diversion).[4,15,21]
- Clinical conditions, neurologic findings, and the effects of medications (dehydration or increased blood viscosity, hypertension or hypotension) should correlate with examination findings.[2,4,15,21]
- Although subjective, differentiation of Doppler sounds assists with identification of arterial segments and altered flow patterns.[2,4]
- Proximal extracranial, focal intracranial, and distal circulatory conditions are determinants of waveform patterns.[2,4] Waveform classification in patients with ischemic strokes is standardized with use of the Thrombolysis in Brain Ischemia (TIBI) grading scale (Fig. 93-4 and Table 93-4).[9] The TIBI grading system was prospectively validated against angiography; it has excellent reproducibility with greater

TABLE 93-2	Criteria for Normal TCD Scan Findings

1. Optimal windows of insonation, permitting identification of all proximal arterial segments.
2. Direction of flow and depths consistent with criteria in Table 93-1.
3. Side-to-side difference between flow velocities in homologous arteries is less than or equal to 30%.
4. Presence of a normal velocity ratio: MCA greater than or equal to ACA greater than or equal to ICA siphon greater than or equal to PCA greater than or equal to BA greater than or equal to VA.
5. Positive end-diastolic flow velocity of 20% to 50% of the peak systolic velocity values.
6. Low-resistance flow pattern, with PI between 0.6 and 1.1 in all intracranial arteries when Paco$_2$ between 35 and 45 mm Hg.
7. High-resistance flow pattern with PI greater than or equal to 1.2 in the OA only.
8. High-resistance flow patterns with PI greater than or equal to 1.2 in all arteries during hyperventilation or elevated blood pressure.

(Reprinted with permission from Alexandrov AV: Transcranial Doppler sonography: principles, examination technique and normal values, Vasc Ultrasound Today 10:141-160, 1988.)

TABLE 93-3	**Differential Diagnosis**	
Problem	**Findings**	**Differential Diagnosis**
Arterial stenosis	Focal MFV increase above normal values, turbulence, bruits Flow diversion to adjacent arteries Flow alteration distal to site of stenosis (deceleration, low PIs)	Primary arterial stenosis Compensatory flow increase Adjacent artery occlusion Hyperemia
Arterial near occlusion	Blunted waveform Focal decrease in MFV Slow systolic acceleration Slow flow deceleration Flow diversion to adjacent arteries	Near occlusion at the site of insonation Arterial occlusion proximal to insonation site Incorrect vessel identification
Arterial occlusion	No detectable flow Good unilateral window of insonation High-resistance flow proximal to occlusion Flow diversion to adjacent arteries	Primary arterial occlusion Incorrect vessel identification Mass effect

Arterial vasospasm*	Proximal vasospasm:
	    Focal or diffuse elevation of MFV without parallel FV
	       increase in feeding extracranial arteries; HI greater
	       than 3
	Distal vasospasm:
	    Focal increase in flow pulsatility (PI greater than or
	       equal to 1.2), indicating increased resistance distal to
	       site of insonation
	    Increase in MFV in the involved and adjacent arteries
	       may not be present
		Vasospasm
		Hyperemia
		Vasospasm with hyperemia
		Altered cerebral autoregulation
		Increased intracranial pressure

Increased intracranial pressure	Decreased EDV or absent end-diastolic flow
	Rapid flow deceleration
	PI greater than or equal to 1.2
	Note that these findings may be present in patients with
	    increased cardiac output or elevated blood pressure and
	    in elderly individuals
		The presence of PI greater than or equal to 1.2 and
		    positive end-diastolic flow in all arteries may be
		    caused by the following:
		Hyperventilation
		Hypertension
		Increased ICP
		Unilateral PI greater than or equal to 1.2 may be
		    caused by the following:
		Compartmental ICP increase
		Stenoses distal to the site of insonation
		PI greater than or equal to 2.0 associated with absent
		    end-diastolic flow is caused by extreme elevations
		    in ICP and possible cerebral circulatory arrest

Cerebral circulatory arrest	Reversed end-diastolic flow or reverberating flow pattern or
	Minimal systolic flow acceleration with no end-diastolic
	    flow or
	Absent flow signals in all intracranial arterial systems
		Possible or probable circulatory arrest; measure both
		    MCA and BA for 30 minutes; then reassess (tran-
		    sient arrest may occur during transient ICP increase
		    or low blood pressure values)

*Vasospasm criteria have been well established for the proximal MCA.[9,14,15] Fewer criteria and validation studies are available for the posterior circulation vessel and the anterior cerebral artery.[2,14,15] Institutions may set other ranges for possible vasospasm in these vessels.

BA, Basilar artery; *EDV,* end-diastolic velocity; *FV,* flow velocity; *HI,* hemispheric index; *ICP,* intracranial pressure; *MCA,* middle cerebral artery; *MFV,* mean flow velocity; *PI,* pulsatility index.

than 90% agreement in waveform interpretation among expert TCD scan users.[7,8,22] The TIBI system was implemented in a multicenter randomized clinical trial of ultrasound scan–enhanced thrombolysis for acute ischemic stroke to demonstrate superior recanalization rates when systemic tissue plasminogen activator (TPA) therapy was monitored with TCD scan compared with TPA given without ultrasound scan.[5,7-9,18]

• New technology using power motion Doppler (PMD or M-mode) scan can be used to facilitate window and vessel identification and guide spectral Doppler sampling and may reduce the time and effort necessary to learn TCD scanning (see Fig. 93-5).[14,17,19,20,23]

EQUIPMENT

• A pulse-wave TCD scan system
• A 2-MHz probe (single or bilateral)
• Acoustic transmission gel
• Nonsterile gloves
• Tissues or washcloth
• Headphones (optional)

Additional equipment, as needed, includes the following:

• Smaller monitoring transducer with removable handles
• Head frame for monitoring transducer fixation
• Sterile plastic drape

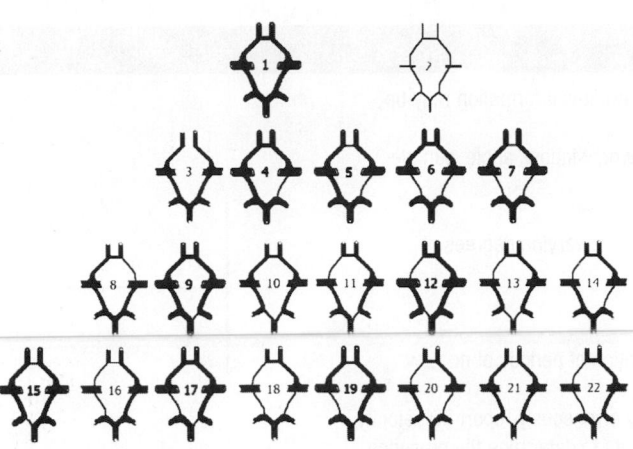

FIGURE 93-3 Variants of the circle of Willis. *(Redrawn from Eftekhar B, Dadmehr M, Ansari S, et al: Are the distributions of variations of circle of Willis different in different populations? Results of an anatomical study and review of literature, BMC Neurol 6:22, 2006.)*

PATIENT AND FAMILY EDUCATION

- Explain the purpose of the diagnostic test and the procedure for testing. ➤*Rationale:* Explanation may decrease patient and family anxiety.
- Explain the need for the patient to remain still and quiet during the procedure. ➤*Rationale:* This explanation may facilitate patient cooperation and completion of the examination.
- Explain that the procedure does not cause any discomfort to the patient. ➤*Rationale:* This explanation may decrease patient and family anxiety.

PATIENT ASSESSMENT AND PREPARATION

Patient Assessment

- Review patient history. ➤*Rationale:* The TCD scan may be used to assist with the diagnosis and management of a number of intracranial arterial conditions, including vasospasm, hyperemia, stenosis, occlusion, intracranial hypertension, cerebral circulatory arrest, cerebral embolization, and vasomotor testing.
- Obtain the patient's blood pressure via arterial line or cuff. ➤*Rationale:* The arterial blood pressure may contribute to the flow velocity and waveform pattern.
- Assess the patient's heart rate and rhythm. ➤*Rationale:* Cardiac dysrhythmias may contribute to the flow velocity and waveform pattern.
- Assess preload or hydration state. ➤*Rationale:* Dehydration may decrease flow velocity because of an increase in blood viscosity and decreased preload pressures.
- Assess for hyperventilation or hypercapnia. ➤*Rationale:* The carbon dioxide level may promote vasoconstriction (hyperventilation) or vasodilation (hypercapnia).
- Assess for pharmacologic agents that may affect velocity findings (e.g., vasodilators, vasopressors). ➤*Rationale:* Vasoconstriction and vasodilation may affect flow velocity.

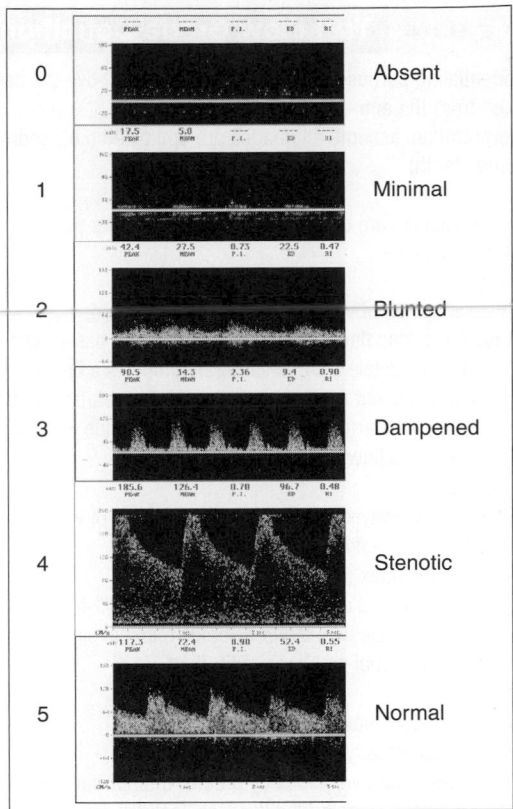

FIGURE 93-4 Thrombolysis in Brain Ischemia (TIBI) grading scale. *(Copyright Health Outcomes Institute, Fountain Hills, AZ)*

- Assess for other factors that may affect velocity findings (e.g., age, hematocrit [Hct], hemoglobin [Hgb], metabolic demand). ➤*Rationale:* Velocities decrease with age; anemia and increased metabolic demand increase velocities.
- Measure intracranial pressure (ICP) and determine cerebral perfusion pressure (CPP) and other intracranial dynamics available (e.g., arterial oxygen saturation, jugular venous oxygen saturation, and brain tissue oxygenation). ➤*Rationale:* These factors may influence the pulsatility of flow and end-diastolic velocities.
- Assess the patient's neurologic status. ➤*Rationale:* Provides baseline data.

Patient Preparation

- Verify correct patient with two identifiers. ➤*Rationale:* Prior to performing a procedure, the nurse should ensure the correct identification of the patient for the intended intervention.
- Ensure that the patient understands preprocedural teaching. Answer questions as they arise, and reinforce information as needed. ➤*Rationale:* Understanding of previously taught information is evaluated and reinforced.
- Assist the patient with positioning. The supine position is best for insonation via the transtemporal, transorbital, or submandibular windows. If the patient is alert with a hemodynamically and neurologically stable condition, assist the patient to a sitting position for insonation through the transforaminal window. If the patient is

TABLE 93-4 | TIBI Flow Grade Definitions

For credentialing purposes, interpret flow signals above the baseline. Supporting flow information may be
gained from the entire image.

For interpretation, assume all images are optimized (i.e., appropriate gain, power, window, angle, sample
volume, depth).

0. Absent.

Absent flow signals are defined by the lack of regular pulsatile flow signals despite varying degrees of
background noise.

1. Minimal.

A: Systolic spikes of variable velocity and duration.

B: Absent diastolic flow during all cardiac cycles based on a visual interpretation of periods of no flow
during end diastole (ED). Reverberating flow is a type of minimal flow.

Caution: Despite absent ED flow with visual interpretation, TCD equipment may erroneously report ED velocity
figures from noise artifacts. Do not rely on machine ED velocity measurements to determine the presence
or absence of ED flow.

2. Blunted.

A: Flattened or delayed systolic flow acceleration of variable duration compared with control.

B: Positive ED velocity.

C: A pulsatility index (PI) less than 1.2.

Caution: Flow velocities are usually greater than 20% lower than those in the comparison side.

Caution: With low velocities, blunted versus minimal signals may be hard to differentiate. Blunted is distinguished by the visual presence of ED flow.

3. Dampened.

A: Normal systolic flow acceleration.

B: Positive ED velocity.

C: Decreased mean velocities by greater than or equal to 30% compared with control (calculate if close).

Caution: With subtle velocity/PI difference, look for dampened waveforms to have a more pulsatile shape.

Caution: Dampened versus blunted signals can be differentiated by dampened signals having a clear peak
systolic complex (initially sharp systolic upstroke without flattening).

Caution: Dampened versus normal signals can be distinguished by dampened having a more abrupt
downslope of late systole and early diastole and other signs of obstruction (i.e., flow diversion; flow velocity
ACA greater than MCA, where flow velocities below the baseline are greater than those above the baseline).

4. Stenotic.

A: Mean flow velocities of greater than or equal to 80 cm/s *and* velocity difference of greater than or equal
to 30% compared with the control side (calculate if close); if velocity difference is less than 30%, look
for additional signs of stenosis, such as turbulence, spectral narrowing.

or

B: If both affected and comparison sides have MFV less than 80 cm/s as a result of low ED velocities,
mean flow velocities greater than or equal to 30% compared with the control side (calculate if close)
and signs of turbulence.

5. Normal.

A: Less than 30% mean velocity difference compared with control (calculate if close).

B: Similar waveform shapes compared with control.

Caution: Hypertensive individuals may have symmetric, high-resistance signals with PI greater than or equal
to 1.2 and low ED velocities.

Caution: Normal versus blunted signals can be differentiated by normal waveforms having initial sharp
systolic upstrokes even if the rest of the waveform shows slow deceleration (note slower
heart rate).

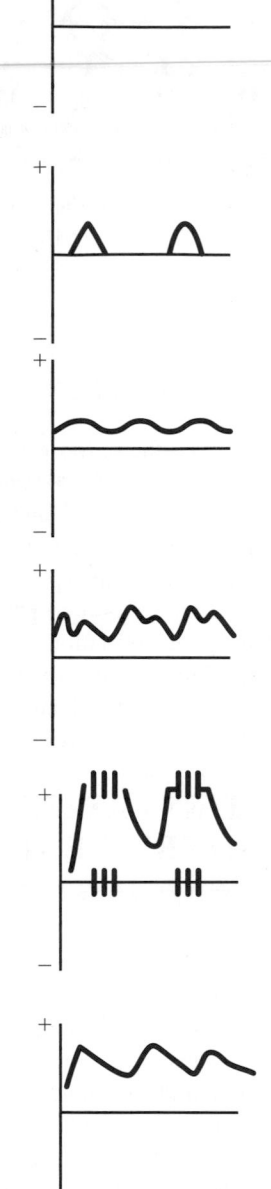

(© 2000 Health Outcomes Institute, Inc. Table 93-3.)

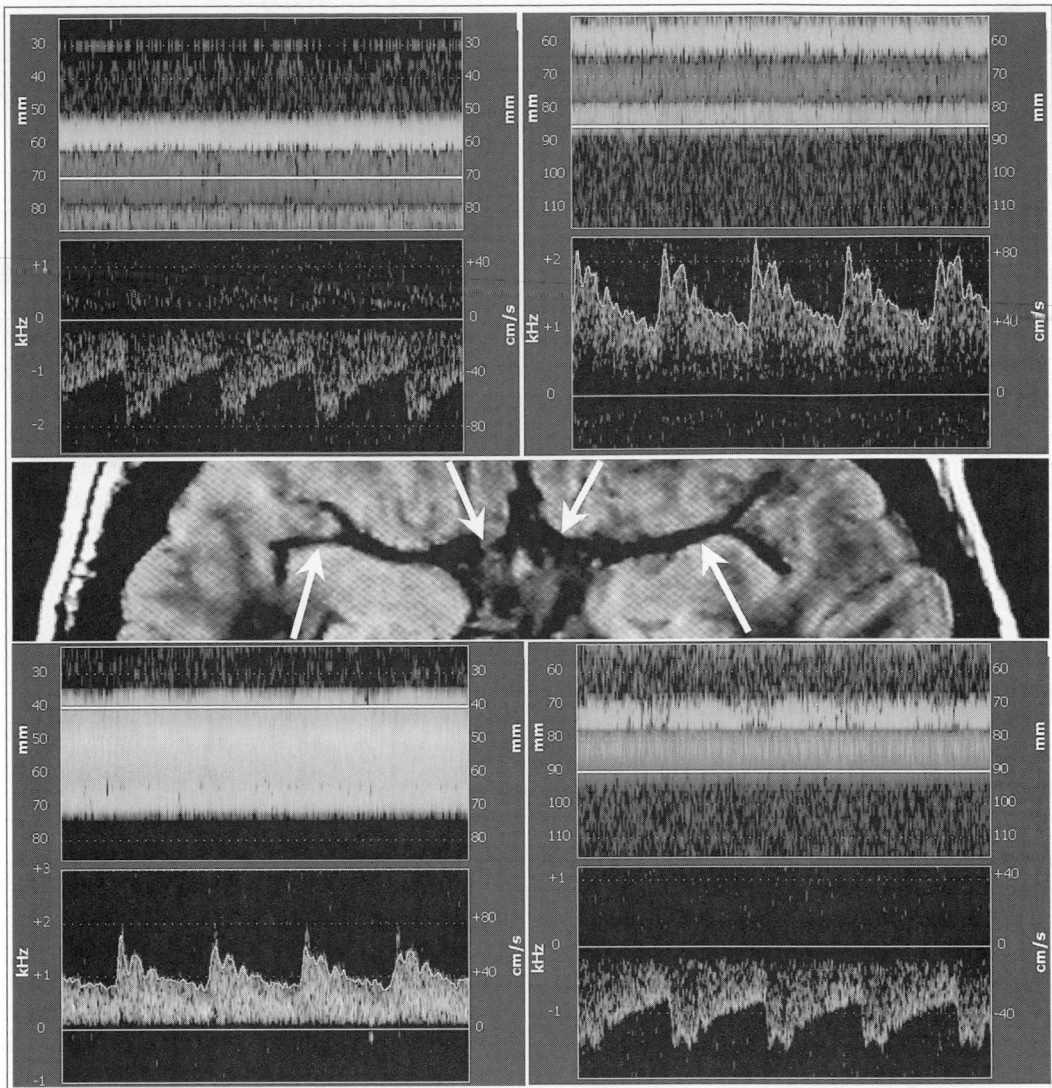

FIGURE 93-5 Power motion Doppler (M-mode). Top frame of each Doppler waveform identifies flow moving toward the probe (above the baseline) and flow moving away from the probe (below); depth is used to denote vessel insonated. *(Copyright Futura/Blackwell Sciences.)*

unable to sit for transforaminal insonation, assist the patient to turn his or her head laterally; if this is not feasible, examine the patient supine with a smaller transducer with a removable handle or a monitoring probe. ➤*Rationale:* The transtemporal, transorbital, and submandibular windows are accessible with the patient in the supine position, whereas the transforaminal window requires a sitting position for proper probe angulation (see Fig. 93-1).

- Ask the patient to close his or her eyes for insonation via the transorbital window. ➤*Rationale:* The probe is placed lightly, without pressure, on the eyelid and angled slightly medially to detect OA and ICA siphon flow signals.
- If necessary, ask the patient to hold his or her breath during insonation via the submandibular window. ➤*Rationale:* Breathing may produce audible and visual artifacts, obstructing assessment of the waveform.

Procedure for Transcranial Doppler Monitoring

Steps	Rationale	Special Considerations
1. **HH**		
2. **PE**		
Transtemporal Insonation		
1. Set the depth at 50 to 56 mm. **(Level E*)**	Depth of 50 to 56 mm allows insonation of the M_1 MCA.[13,15-17]	
2. Set the power to maximum or 100%.	Optimizes the ability to identify the arterial waveforms.	
3. Apply gel to the probe or skin, place the probe above the zygomatic arch, and aim slightly upward and anterior to the contralateral ear (see Fig. 93-1). **(Level E)**	Accesses the transtemporal window.[1,13,15,16]	No temporal window or suboptimal window can be found in 5% to 15% of the population.[4,15,18,21] A sterile plastic drape over the probe and gel may be used to reduce the transmission of microorganisms on a scalp wound or incision.
4. Find a flow signal directed toward the probe that meets MCA flow criteria (see Table 93-1).		
5. Follow the signal until it disappears by holding the probe in a constant position and changing the depth to shallow 40- to 45-mm and deeper 65- to 70-mm settings.	Verifies MCA identification; limits operator error.	
6. Find the ICA bifurcation at 65 mm and obtain both MCA and ACA signals. **(Level E)**	ICA bifurcation is visualized at a depth of 65 mm; a bidirectional MCA/ACA waveform is noted.[4,6,13,16]	
7. Follow the ACA signal to a depth of 70 to 75 mm. **(Level E)**	ACA insonation begins at a depth of 70 to 75 mm.[13,15,16,21]	The contralateral ACA may be insonated at a depth of more than 75 mm in the case of a unilateral suboptimal transtemporal window.
8. Return to the bifurcation and reset the depth to 62 mm while slowly rotating the probe posteriorly by 10 to 30 degrees to find the PCA.	The PCA is commonly detected at depths of 60 to 64 mm.	
9. Find the P_1 PCA signal directed toward the probe and the P_2 PCA signal directed away from the probe.		
10. Record and print findings, including at least waveforms, mean flow velocities, and PIs for all arteries insonated.		Activation of the "envelope" function may be necessary. The envelope is a continuous trace of maximal velocities during the cardiac cycle. If optimized to closely follow the maximal velocities without artifacts, the envelope provides automated calculations of MFV and flow pulsatility that are updated dependent on the display sweep speed.

*Level E: Multiple case reports, theory-based evidence from expert opinions, or peer-reviewed professional organizational standards without clinical studies to support recommendations

Procedure for Transcranial Doppler Monitoring—*Continued*

Steps	Rationale	Special Considerations
Transorbital Insonation		
1. Decrease the power to the minimum or 10%.	Limits eye exposure to ultrasound scan.	
2. Set the depth at 52 mm. **(Level E*)**	Aids in locating the ophthalmic artery (OA).[7,13,16,21]	
3. Place the transducer gently over the eyelid without applying pressure, and turn the transducer slightly medially.	Aligns the ultrasound beam with the OA stem.	
4. Determine flow pulsatility and direction in the distal ophthalmic artery.	PI is equal to or greater than 1.2 because OA is an anastomosis with a high-resistance arterial system (extracranial carotid branches).	
5. Confirm findings at 55 to 60 mm.[4,6,15,21]	Follow the OA course to the ICA siphon.	
6. Reset the depth to 60 to 64 mm and find the ICA siphon flow signals.	The ICA siphon can have bidirectional low-resistance flow signals.	
7. Record and print findings, including peak systolic, end-diastolic, and mean flow velocities, and PI for both the ICA and OA.	Document flow velocity and pulsatility in the ICA siphon and flow direction and pulsatility in the OA (results of Doppler scan spectral analysis for final report).	
Transforaminal Insonation		
1. Use maximal or 100% power.		
2. Set the depth at 75 mm. **(Level E)**	The VA/proximal BA junction is insonated at 75 mm.[5,13,16,21]	
3. Place the probe at midline, 1 inch below the skull edge; aim toward the bridge of the nose.	Allows ultrasound beam penetration through the foramen magnum.	
4. Identify flow directed away from the probe.	Vertebrobasilar arteries normally carry flow from the neck toward the brain (e.g., away from the probe).	
5. Increase the depth to 80 mm, then 90 and 100 mm, to follow the BA from proximal to distal segments.	The proximal BA is insonated at 80 mm, the mid BA is insonated at 90 mm, and the distal BA is insonated at 95 to 100 mm or more.	
6. Confirm findings while slowly decreasing the depth of insonation.	A tortuous BA may be difficult to insonate; operator errors are common.	
7. Set the depth at 60 mm and reposition the probe laterally, aiming at the eye.	Switch from the basilar to the terminal vertebral artery.	
8. Find the VA flow directed away from the probe and follow it at 40 to 60 mm and 60 to 80 mm; repeat examination on the opposite side **(Level E).**	The intracranial portions of the right and left VA are insonated at depths between 40 and 80 mm.[6,13,16,21]	
9. Record and print findings, including peak systolic, end-diastolic, and mean flow velocities, and PI for both the BA and bilateral VA.	Assess flow velocity, pulsatility, and direction in the vertebrobasilar arteries.	

*Level E: Multiple case reports, theory-based evidence from expert opinions, or peer-reviewed professional organizational standards without clinical studies to support recommendations

Procedure continues on following page

Procedure for Transcranial Doppler Monitoring—*Continued*

Steps	Rationale	Special Considerations
Submandibular Insonation		
1. Set the depth at 50 to 60 mm, place the probe laterally under the jaw, and aim upward and medially.	Locate the distal ICA before its entrance to the skull.	Calculate the hemispheric index (HI; Lindegaard ratio): HI = MFV MCA/MFV ICA. Normal values are less than 3. HI is used to differentiate between the first segment of the MCA (M1 MCA) vasospasm after subarachnoid hemorrhage and hyperemia, or a hyperdynamic state.[11,12,15,21]
2. Find a low-resistance flow directed away from the probe that meets ICA criteria (see Table 93-1).	A high-resistance flow pattern is consistent with the external carotid artery, not the ICA.	
3. Repeat the examination on the opposite side.	Assess the contralateral ICA to complete a bilateral spectral Doppler scan study.	
4. Record and print findings, including at least waveforms, mean flow velocities, and PIs for both the right and left ICAs.	Assess flow velocity to calculate the hemispheric index, or the so-called Lindegaard ratio.	
5. Clean the gel from the patient's head.	Promotes comfort.	
6. Discard used supplies in an appropriate receptacle.	Removes and safely discards used supplies.	
7. **HH**		
8. Clean probe according to institutional policy.	Reduces the transmission of microorganisms and body secretions; Standard Precautions.	

Expected Outcomes

- Determination of normal or pathologic flow conditions (notify the physician of pathologic flow findings or inability to obtain flow velocities)
- Recommendation, as needed, for definitive angiographic examination and treatment
- Recognition of technical limitations, including operator skill

Unexpected Outcomes

- Inability to insonate via temporal window in 2% of patients after subarachnoid hemorrhage, aneurysm, or surgical obliteration or edema and in up to 15% to 20% of other adult patients with intact skulls[4,15,18]
- Underestimation of highest detectable velocity because of operator skill

Patient Monitoring and Care

Steps	Rationale	Reportable Conditions
		These conditions should be reported if they persist despite nursing interventions.
1. Monitor respiratory and cardiovascular status during procedure:	Velocity is affected by systemic hemodynamics and the vasomotor response of the resistance vessels in the brain (e.g., arterioles). TCD scan is not associated with the development of changes in the respiratory or cardiovascular status; instead, it is influenced by these changes, should they occur.	• Changes in vital signs • Changes in cardiac rhythm • Changes in respiratory status

Patient Monitoring and Care —*Continued*

Steps	Rationale	Reportable Conditions

A. Partial pressure of carbon dioxide in the arterial blood ($Paco_2$).
   B. Vital signs including mean arterial pressure.
   C. Cardiac rhythm.
   D. Vasoactive medications if used during the procedure.		

2. When conducting the examination with a head frame, loosen the probe fixation after 1 hour and assess the skin. Minimize contact with skin incisions as much as possible.	Tight fixation with a head frame may be necessary to achieve better sound transmission and a constant angle of insonation.	• Skin breakdown • Unrelieved discomfort
3. When monitoring for brain embolization, note the timing of events associated with emboli detection (e.g., placement or removal of aortic cross clamp during cardiac surgery with cardiopulmonary bypass).	Continuous monitoring with TCD scan has shown an association between specific operative events during cardiac surgery with cardiopulmonary bypass and the detection of brain emboli on TCD.	• Events that may affect emboli detection
4. Follow institutional standard for assessing pain. Administer analgesia as prescribed.	Identifies need for pain interventions.	• Continued pain despite pain interventions

Documentation

Documentation should include the following:

- Patient and family education
- Patient name, age, gender, and medical record number (should be included on every page of the written report including waveforms and interpretation)
- Clinical diagnosis (indication for testing)
- Significant, clinically detectable neurologic findings
- Arterial blood pressure, $Paco_2$, cardiac output, ICP (when feasible), and other intracranial dynamics during examination

- Preload as measured by pulmonary artery occlusion pressure (PAOP) and central venous pressure (CVP) to confirm hydration status
- Pain assessment, interventions, and effectiveness
- Flow velocity spectra (waveforms), MFV, and PI in the arteries insonated
- Hard copies of arterial waveforms
- Presence of suboptimal windows indicated in the report
- Interpretation
- Unexpected outcomes
- Additional interventions

References

CR 1. Aaslid R, Markwalder TM, Nornes H: Noninvasive transcranial Doppler ultrasound recording of flow velocity in basal cerebral arteries, *J Neurosurg* 57:769-774, 1982.

CR 2. Alexandrov AV: Transcranial Doppler sonography: principles, examination technique and normal values, *Vasc Ultrasound Today* 10:141-160, 1998.

CR 3. Alexandrov AV, Demchuk AM, Burgin WS: Insonation method and diagnostic flow signatures for transcranial power motion (M-mode) Doppler, *J Neuroimaging* 12:236-244, 2002.

CR 4. Alexandrov AV: *Cerebrovascular ultrasound in stroke prevention and treatment,* Oxford, 2004, Blackwell-Futura Publishing.

CR 5. Alexandrov AV, et al: Ultrasound-enhanced systemic thrombolysis for acute ischemic stroke, *N Engl J Med*, 351:2170-2178, 2004.

6. Alexandrov AV, et al: Practice standards for transcranial Doppler (TCD) ultrasound: part I: test performance, *J Neuroimaging* 17:11-18, 2007.

CR 7. Burgin WS, et al: Transcranial Doppler criteria for recanalization after thrombolysis for middle cerebral artery stroke, *Stroke* 31:1128-1132, 2000.

CR 8. Burgin WS, et al: Validity and reliability of the thrombolysis in brain infarction (TIBI) flow grades, *Stroke* 32:324-325, 2001.

CR 9. Demchuk AM, et al: Thrombolysis in brain ischemia (TIBI) Doppler flow grades predict clinical severity, early recovery, and mortality in patients treated with intravenous tissue plasminogen activator, *Stroke* 32:89-93, 2001.

10. Kassah MY, Majid A, Farooq FU, et al: Transcranial Doppler: an introduction for the primary care physician, *J Am Board Fam Med* 20:65-71, 2007.

CR 11. Lindegaard KF, et al: Cerebral vasospasm diagnosis by means of angiography and blood velocity measurements, *Acta Neurochir (Wien)* 100:12-24, 1989.

CR 12. Lindegaard KF: The role of transcranial Doppler in the management of patients with subarachnoid haemorrhage: a review, *Acta Neurochir* 72(Suppl):59-71, 1999.

CR 13. Lupetin AR, et al: Transcranial Doppler sonography: part 1: principles, technique, and normal appearances, *Radiographics* 15:179-191, 1995.

CR 14. McCartney JP, Thomas-Lukes KM, Gomez CR: *Handbook of transcranial Doppler,* New York, 1997, Springer.

CR 15. Moehring MA, Spencer MP: Power M-mode Doppler (PMD) for observing cerebral blood flow and tracking emboli, *Ultrasound Med Biol* 28:49-57, 2002.

CR 16. Moppet IK, Mahajan RP: Transcranial Doppler ultransonography in anaesthesia and intensive care, *Br J Anaesth* 93:710-724, 2004.

CR 17. Ringelstein EB, et al: Transcranial Doppler sonography: anatomical landmarks and normal velocity values, *Ultrasound Med Biol* 16:745-761, 1990.

18. Saqqur M, et al: Derivation of power M-Mode transcranial Doppler criteria for angiographic proven MCA occlusion, *J Neuroimaging* 16:323-328, 2006.

CR 19. Sloan MA: Transcranial Doppler monitoring of vasospasm after subarachnoid hemorrhage. In Tegeler CH, Baikian VL, Gomez CR, editors: *Neurosonology,* St Louis, 1996, Mosby, 156-171.

CR 20. Sloan MA, et al: Assessment: transcranial Doppler ultrasonography: report of the Therapeutics and Technology Assessment Subcommittee of the American Academy of Neurology, *Neurology* 62:1468-1481, 2004.

CR 21. Tegeler CH, Babikian VL, Gomez CR: *Neurosonology,* St Louis, 1996, Mosby.

22. Tsivgoulis G, et al: Validation of transcranial Doppler with computed tomography angiography in acute cerebral ischemia, *Stroke* 38:1245-1249, 2007.

23. Tsivgoulis G, et al: Applications and advantages of power motion-mode Doppler in acute posterior circulation cerebral ischemia, *Stroke* 39:1197-1204, 2008.

24. White H, Venkatesh B: Applications of transcranial Doppler in the ICU: a review, *Intensive Care Med* 32(7): 981-994, 2006.

Additional Readings

Kirkness C: Cerebral blood flow monitoring. In Littlejohns LR, Bader MK, editors: *AACN-AANN Protocols for Practice: monitoring technologies in critically ill neuroscience patients,* Boston, 2009, Jones and Bartlett, 145-174.

External and Intravascular Warming/Cooling Devices

PURPOSE: An external surface or hydrogel pad temperature management device may be used to increase or decrease the body temperature. An intravascular warming and cooling device may be inserted to increase and decrease the body temperature. External surface cooling devices or intravascular cooling catheters are also used as a therapeutic treatment modality to reduce the body temperature after acute injury (such as cardiac arrest) to decrease cellular metabolism.[19]

Nicole L. Kupchik

PREREQUISITE NURSING KNOWLEDGE

- The hypothalamus is the primary thermoregulatory center for the body; it maintains normothermia through internal regulation of heat production or heat loss. Sensory thermoreceptors are located in the skin and subcutaneous tissue. Superficial or shell-zone temperature information is transmitted by thermoreceptors to the posterior hypothalamus through the spinal cord. Thermoreceptors in the brain, heart, and other deep organs transmit the core-zone temperature. Effective temperature regulation depends on the ability of the posterior hypothalamus to receive and integrate the signals received from the core and shell zones.[9,12,22]
- Knowledge of terms associated with temperature is needed (Table 94-1).
- The hypothalamus regulates temperature in the range of approximately 36.4° to 37.3°C (97.5° to 99.4°F). By initiating physiologic responses to changes above or below this range, the hypothalamus coordinates heat loss or gain. Vasoconstriction and vasodilation control the distribution and flow of blood to the organs, viscera, and skin surface; thus, the amount of heat loss to the environment is influenced by vasomotor activity. In response to heat loss, shivering and vasoconstriction occur, muscles tense and the extremities are drawn closer to the body, and the person conserves heat. In response to heat gain,

sweating and vasodilation occur, muscles relax, and heat is lost through evaporative cooling and to the environment.[12]
- Heat flows from a higher temperature to a lower temperature until the gradient between the two temperatures diminishes. Mechanisms of heat loss include conduction, convection, radiation, and evaporation.[5,9,12,22]
  - ❖ Conduction occurs when heat is lost by direct transfer from one surface to a second adjacent surface of a lower temperature.[5,9,12,22]
  - ❖ Convection occurs when heat is lost by transfer from a surface to the surrounding air.[5,9,12,22]
  - ❖ Radiation occurs when heat (thermal energy) is transferred through air or space between separated surfaces without direct contact.[9,12,22]
  - ❖ Evaporation occurs when heat loss accompanies water loss from the skin to the surrounding air.[9,12,22]
- Alteration in thermoregulation can result from a primary central nervous system injury or disease (e.g., subarachnoid hemorrhage, traumatic brain injury, spinal cord injury, or neoplasm) and metabolic conditions (e.g., diabetes mellitus; toxic levels of ethanol alcohol or other drugs, such as barbiturates and phenothiazines).
- Body temperature is the measurement of the presence or absence of heat. Body heat is generated, conserved, redistributed, or dissipated during all physiologic processes. Factors such as age, circadian rhythm, and hormones influence body temperature.

TABLE 94-1	**Terms Associated with Temperature**
Term	**Definition**
Normothermia/Euthermia	Optimal range of body temperature associated with health.
Hypothermia	Subnormal core body temperature equal to or below 35°C.[21]
Induced hypothermia	Intentional reduction of body temperature to slow metabolic processes. This may be accomplished by surface means (transfer of heat from the skin to the cooling device) or central means (circulatory heat exchange in a cardiopulmonary bypass machine or cooling catheter)
Fever	Response to a pyrogen; the hypothalamus either resets its range higher, maintaining thermoregulation, or a change occurs in the sensitivity of the hypothalamus neuron activity to warmth and coldness.[4]
Hyperthermia	Dysfunction of thermoregulation caused by an injury to the hypothalamus or by a person's heat loss mechanisms being overwhelmed by high environmental heat.

- Body temperature may be measured with a variety of thermometers and at several body sites. Electronic or digital thermometers are used to obtain rectal, oral, and axillary temperatures. Thermistors within catheters or probes measure rectal, nasopharyngeal, esophageal, bladder, brain, and pulmonary artery temperatures. Infrared thermometers measure tympanic membrane and temporal artery temperatures. Choose the method of temperature monitoring that best meets the patient's clinical condition. The most accurate temperature monitoring methods are intravascular (e.g., pulmonary artery catheter), esophageal, and bladder, followed by rectal, oral, and tympanic membrane methods.[9,13,21]
- Variations in temperatures normally occur in the body (Table 94-2).
- Site choice for temperature monitoring is based on the clinical data needed; the patient's condition, safety, and comfort; environmental factors (e.g., room temperature); the indication for a catheter or a probe (e.g., pulmonary artery catheter); and the availability of equipment.
- An esophageal temperature probe can be inserted down the esophageal tract. Accurate placement of the temperature probe is necessary to obtain results similar to monitoring the temperature from the pulmonary artery.
- A consistent temperature site must be monitored during the application of warming or cooling therapy.

- Shivering is an involuntary shaking of the body generated to maintain thermal homeostasis. Shivering causes rhythmic tremors that result in skeletal muscle contraction and is a normal physiologic mechanism to generate heat production.[4,11]
- Early detection of shivering can be accomplished by palpating the mandible and feeling a humming vibration. Electrocardiographic (ECG) artifact from skeletal muscle is seen on the bedside monitor. If not detected early, shivering can progress from visible twitching of the head or neck to visible twitching of the pectorals or trunk, and then to generalized shaking of the entire body and teeth chattering.
- Shivering may be visible on the Bispectral Index Monitor (BIS) in the form of an increase in EMG activity (see Procedure 86).
- Shivering increases the metabolic rate, carbon dioxide (CO_2) production, oxygen consumption (by 40% to 100%),[22] and myocardial work. If cardiopulmonary compensation does not occur to meet these demands, anaerobic metabolism occurs, resulting in acidosis.[11,17,22]
- Shivering is counterproductive to strategies intended to lower temperature.
- At a body temperature below 35°C, the basal metabolic rate can no longer supply sufficient body heat and an exogenous source of heat is needed.
- Table 94-3 outlines techniques to increase heat gain.
- Hypothermia may be categorized as mild (32° to 35°C), moderate (28° to 31.9°C), severe (<28°C), or profound (<16.9°C).[3] In severe to profound hypothermia, attempts

TABLE 94-2	**Normal Variations in Body Temperature Based on a Rectal Temperature of 37°C**
Type of Temperature Measurement	**Degrees Lower Than Rectal Temperature**
Oral	0.3° to 0.5°C[8]
Esophageal	0.2°C[8]
Pulmonary artery	0.2° to 0.3°C[8]
Tympanic membrane	0.05° to 0.25°C[8]
Bladder	0.1° to 0.2°C[8]
Axillary	0.6° to 0.8°C [8]
Brain	0.3° to 2°C higher than rectal[17]
Temporal artery	>0.5° to <1.0°C different than pulmonary artery catheter[9,12]

TABLE 94-3	**Techniques to Increase Heat Gain**
Mechanism of Heat Transfer	**Techniques to Increase Heat Gain**
Radiation	Warming lights, warm environment, room temperature, blankets
Conduction	Warm blankets, circulating water blanket, continuous arteriovenous rewarming, cardiopulmonary bypass
Convection	Thermal fans, circulating air blanket
Evaporation	Head and body covers; warm, humidified oxygen

at defibrillation are usually unsuccessful until the core temperature is above 28°C. The American Heart Association recommends only one attempt at defibrillation and then active rewarming should occur before reattempts at defibrillation.[1]

- Hypothermia may be caused by an increase in heat loss, a decrease in heat production, an alteration in thermoregulation, and a variety of clinical conditions.
- An increase in heat loss may occur from the following:
  - ❖ Accidental (e.g., cold water drowning)
  - ❖ Environmental exposure
  - ❖ Induced vasodilation caused by high levels of ethanol alcohol, barbiturates, phenothiazines, or general anesthesia
  - ❖ Central nervous system dysfunction (e.g., spinal cord injury)
  - ❖ Dermal dysfunction (e.g., burns)
  - ❖ Iatrogenic conditions (e.g., administration of cold intravenous fluids, hemodialysis, cardiopulmonary bypass)
  - ❖ Trauma
- A decrease in heat production is associated with the following:
  - ❖ Endocrine conditions (e.g., hypothyroidism)
  - ❖ Malnutrition
  - ❖ Diabetic ketoacidosis
  - ❖ Neuromuscular insufficiency (e.g., resulting from a pharmacologic paralysis caused by a neuromuscular blocking agent or anesthetic agents)
- Clinical conditions associated with hypothermia are sepsis, hepatic coma, prolonged cardiac arrest, and systemic inflammatory response syndrome (SIRS).
- Severe hypothermia may mimic death; resuscitative efforts should be initiated despite the absence of vital signs.
- Rewarming for cardiac arrest survivors who have undergone therapeutic hypothermia should not occur faster than 0.25° to 0.50°C per hour.[20] Rapid rewarming can cause rewarming acidosis, electrolyte shifts, shivering, hypovolemic shock, temperature afterdrop, and temperature overshoot.[9,16]
- Afterdrop is a decrease in core temperature after rewarming is discontinued.
- Overshoot occurs when the thermoregulator mechanisms rebound or overcompensate.
- Termination of active external rewarming at 36° to 36.5°C may prevent temperature overshoot.
- Rewarming acidosis results from the increase in CO_2 production associated with the temperature increase and from the return of accumulated acids in the peripheral circulation to the heart.
- Rewarming shock occurs when hypothermic vasoconstriction masks hypovolemia. If the patient's circulating volume is insufficient during rewarming vasodilation, sudden decreases in blood pressure, systemic vascular resistance (SVR), and preload occur. In cases of severe to profound hypothermia, peripheral rewarming with external devices should be used with extreme caution. Core methods of rewarming should be considered.
- Hyperthermia occurs when the thermoregulator system of the body absorbs or produces more heat than it is able to release.

- Malignant hyperthermia is a rare, hereditary condition of the skeletal muscle that occurs on exposure to a triggering agent or agents.[2,15] The triggering agents most commonly associated with malignant hyperthermia are anesthetic agents, particularly inhalation anesthetics and succinylcholine. Malignant hyperthermia involves instability of the muscle cell membrane, which causes a sudden increase in myoplasmic calcium and skeletal muscle contractures.
- The earliest indication of malignant hyperthermia is an increase in end-tidal carbon dioxide ($PetCO_2$) of 5 mm Hg more than the patient's baseline. If the $PetCO_2$ is not being monitored, the earliest sign is tachycardia, which occurs within 30 minutes of anesthesia induction. Tachycardia is followed by ventricular ectopy, which may progress to ventricular tachycardia and ventricular fibrillation. Muscle rigidity usually begins in the extremities, chest, or jaws.[2,15]
- A cooling device is used to treat malignant hyperthermia after administration of the triggering agent is stopped and a muscle relaxant (e.g., dantrolene sodium) is given. The muscle relaxant blocks the release of calcium from the sarcoplasmic reticulum without affecting calcium uptake.[15]
- Heat stroke occurs when the outdoor temperature and humidity are excessive and heat is transferred to the body. Increased humidity prevents the body from cooling by evaporation. Other signs of heat stroke include hypotension, tachycardia, tachypnea, mental status changes from confusion to coma, and possibly seizures. The skin is hot and dry, and sweating may occur. The rectal temperature is greater than 40.0° to 41.1°C (104°F to 106°F). Initial interventions include support of airway, breathing, and circulation. Rapid cooling of the patient is the main treatment priority, with a goal of reducing the temperature to 38.3° to 38.9°C (101° to 102°F) within 1 hour.
- Fever occurs in response to a pyrogen and is defined as a temperature more than 38°C.[21] During fever, the hypothalamus retains its function, and shivering and diaphoresis occur to gain or lose body heat. Fever may be an adaptive response and may be considered beneficial in the absence of neurologic disease processes. However, a febrile state increases the heart rate and metabolic rate and may be detrimental to a critically ill patient. The decision to reduce a fever needs to be based on the patient's physical and hemodynamic stability during the fever.[7,21]
- Some external warming or cooling devices transfer warmth or coolness to the patient via conduction. Warmed or cooled fluids circulate through coils or channels in a thermal blanket or pad that is commonly placed under the patient.
- Additional warming and cooling systems are available. Hydrogel pads or external wraps can be placed on the patient's skin in the trunk and upper leg regions. These external systems are controlled through a feedback loop system with a core temperature (e.g., a bladder probe, an esophageal probe) that is attached to a central console

and automatically regulates temperature according to programmed temperature target points. The feedback of patient temperature is compared to the set target temperature and the circulating water temperature is adjusted to ensure the target temperature is maintained.

- Other external devices transfer warmth to the patient via convection. A device used for warming blows warm air through microperforations on the underside of a blanket that is placed over the patient. The air is directed through the blanket onto the patient's skin.[3,12]

- Intravascular cooling and warming devices currently in use include central venous catheters with temperature-controlled saline solution balloons or distal metallic heat transfer elements that cool the blood as it flows by the catheter. The saline solution is not in direct contact with the systemic circulation. These devices may be inserted in the subclavian, internal jugular, or femoral vein.[24] They are attached to a console with an automatic temperature control device that adjusts the pressure, temperature, and flow rate of the circulating saline solution based on the patient's continuously monitored temperature (e.g., rectal, bladder, esophageal) and the set-points established by the healthcare provider).[22]

- Specific information about controls, alarms, troubleshooting, and safety features is available from each manufacturer and must be understood by the nurse before using the equipment.

EQUIPMENT

- Warming or cooling device
- Sheet or bath blanket
- Nonsterile gloves
- Temperature probe, cable, and module to monitor the patient's temperature (varies based on the type of site and thermometer selected and available)
- Pads or blankets needed by the equipment which is going to be used
- Cardiac monitoring (see Procedure 57)

Additional equipment to have available as needed includes the following:

- Hemodynamic monitoring (see Procedure 76)
- Distilled water
- Intravascular cooling/warming central venous catheter
- Console, including cable for monitoring temperature
- Central line insertion tray
- Antiseptic (e.g., chlorhexidine)
- Sterile towels, drapes
- Masks with eye shields, sterile gloves, and sterile gowns
- Occlusive dressing
- Normal saline solution
- Water-soluble lubricant

PATIENT AND FAMILY EDUCATION

- Explain the reason for the use of a warming or cooling device and standard of care, including monitoring of the temperature, expected length of therapy, comfort measures,

and parameters for discontinuation of the device. ➤➤*Rationale:* Explanation encourages the patient and family to ask questions and verbalize concerns about the procedure.

- Assess the patient's and family's understanding of the warming or cooling therapy. ➤➤*Rationale:* Clarification and reinforcement of information are needed during times of stress and anxiety.

- Encourage the patient to notify the nurse of any discomfort. If the patient is unable to verbalize discomfort, look for signs and symptoms of discomfort such as grimacing, changes in heart rate, diaphoresis, etc. ➤➤*Rationale:* Identification of discomfort facilitates early intervention and promotes comfort.

PATIENT ASSESSMENT AND PREPARATION
Patient Assessment

- Assess risk factors, medical history, the cause of the patient's underlying condition, and the type and the length of temperature exposure. ➤➤*Rationale:* Assessment assists in anticipating, recognizing, and responding to the patient's responses and potential side effects to therapy.

- Assess the patient's medication therapy. ➤➤*Rationale:* Medications such as vasopressors and vasodilators may affect heat transfer, increase the potential for skin injury, and contribute to an adverse hemodynamic response.

- Obtain a core temperature (e.g., pulmonary artery, esophageal, bladder). ➤➤*Rationale:* Assessment determines baseline temperature and determines when a warming or cooling device is needed.

- Obtain vital signs and hemodynamic values (if using pulmonary artery monitoring). ➤➤*Rationale:* Assessment determines baseline cardiovascular data. Initially, cold temperatures activate the sympathetic nervous system, resulting in tachycardia, vasoconstriction, and shivering. Rewarming may result in vasodilation and hypotension. Heart failure may occur with malignant hyperthermia and heat stroke.

- Monitor the patient's cardiac rhythm. ➤➤*Rationale:* Monitoring determines the baseline cardiac rhythm. Hypothermia has a negative chronotropic effect on myocardial pacemaker tissue, which may lead to bradycardia. Hypothermia may cause repolarization abnormalities and is susceptible to atrial and ventricular fibrillation.[3] Tachycardia and ventricular dysrhythmias may occur if the patient is hyperthermic.[3,6,22]

- Assess the patient's electrolyte, glucose, arterial blood gas, and coagulation study results. ➤➤*Rationale:* Alterations in temperature balance may result in acid-base imbalance, coagulopathy, electrolyte imbalance, glycemic imbalance, and hypoxemia.[3,6,22,23] Close monitoring of metabolic parameters with careful consideration of replacement during cooling and warming therapy is necessary.[22,23]

- Assess the patient's level of consciousness and neurologic function. ➤➤*Rationale:* Assessment determines baseline neurologic status. A change in mental status, level of consciousness, or impaired neurologic function may occur because of an undesirable high or low temperature or from the condition causing the alteration in temperature. Fatigue, muscle incoordination, poor judgment, weakness, hallucinations, lethargy, and stupor may occur with hypothermia. Seizures may occur with hyperthermia.

- Assess the patient's ventilatory function. ⟶*Rationale:* Hypoventilation, suppression of cough, and mucociliary reflexes associated with hypothermia may lead to hypoxemia, atelectasis, and pneumonia. Hypothermia shifts the oxygenation dissociation curve to the left, and less oxygen is released from oxyhemoglobin to the tissues. Because of peripheral vasoconstriction, digit-based pulse oximetry is often unreliable. Hyperthermia shifts the oxygenation dissociation curve to the right, and oxygen is readily released from oxyhemoglobin.[3,6,22]
- Assess the patient's bowel sounds, abdomen, and gastrointestinal function. ⟶*Rationale:* Assessment determines baseline status. Patients with hypothermia may develop an ileus because of decreased intestinal motility. Vomiting and diarrhea may occur with hyperthermia.
- Assess the patient's skin integrity. ⟶*Rationale:* Assessment provides baseline data. An externally applied warming or cooling device can cause or exacerbate skin injury. Preexisting conditions such as diabetes and peripheral vascular disease increase the patient's risk for skin injury.

Patient Preparation

- Ensure that the patient and family understand preprocedural education. Answer questions as they arise, and reinforce information as needed. ⟶*Rationale:* Understanding of previously taught information is evaluated and reinforced.
- Verify correct patient with two identifiers. ⟶*Rationale:* Prior to performing a procedure, the nurse should ensure the correct identification of the patient for the intended intervention.
- If a warm air device will be used, remove the patient's gown and top sheet. ⟶*Rationale:* The warm air device works via convection and should be in direct contact with the patient's skin for optimal results.
- If the patient is unintentionally hypothermic, cover the patient's head with a blanket or towel or an aluminum cap. ⟶*Rationale:* This action minimizes additional heat loss.
- Ensure that informed consent has been obtained for insertion of intravascular catheters. ⟶*Rationale:* Informed consent protects the rights of the patient and makes a competent decision possible for the patient; however, in emergency circumstances, time may not allow for the consent form to be signed.
- Perform a pre-procedure verification and time out with placement of intravascular catheters, if non-emergent. ⟶*Rationale:* Ensures patient safety.

Procedure for External Warming/Cooling Devices

Steps	Rationale	Special Considerations
Procedure for Obtaining Core Temperatures		
1. **HH**		
2. **PE**		
3. Pulmonary Artery		
A. Connect the cardiac output temperature cable from the bedside monitor to the pulmonary artery catheter.	Measures the temperature of the blood in the pulmonary artery	
B. Observe the temperature display on the bedside monitor.	Provides a temperature value.	
4. Bladder		
A. Connect the bladder temperature cable from the bedside monitor to the bladder probe.	Measures the temperature of the urine in the patient's bladder.	Accuracy of bladder temperatures is influenced by urine volume. Validate the patient's urine output during low urine output conditions.
B. Observe the temperature display on the bedside monitor.	Provides a temperature value.	

Procedure continues on following page

Procedure **for External Warming/Cooling Devices**—*Continued*		
Steps	**Rationale**	**Special Considerations**
5. Esophageal		
A. Assess that the patient does not have any contraindications for placement of an esophageal temperature probe for temperature monitoring.	Ensures that the esophageal temperature probe is inserted safely.	Follow institution policy regarding whether nurses are able to insert esophageal temperature probes. Contraindications for placement of the esophageal temperature probe include: patients with known esophageal strictures or have a history of esophageal cancer, esophageal perforation, and end stage liver disease and varicies.[23]
B. Measure from the opening of the patient's mouth to the earlobe and from the earlobe to the upper part of the sternum for accurate probe placement. Mark the measurement on the tube. Lubricate the tip of the catheter with water-soluble lubricant.	Correct measurement for probe placement is necessary for accurate core temperature monitoring. Eases insertion of the probe.	
C. Insert the esophageal temperature probe into the oral cavity and advance.	Initiates the procedure.	If resistance is met, withdraw the probe and gently advance again; this may indicate tracheal intubation of the probe. Never force the probe.
D. Continue to advance the catheter until the placement marked on the probe reaches the patient's lips.	Positions the probe.	If the patient exhibits signs of respiratory distress, such as coughing or gasping, immediately withdraw the temperature probe.
E. Secure the esophageal temperature sensor to the patient.	Reduces the risk of inadvertent displacement.	
F. Connect the cable from the esophageal probe to the bedside monitor.	Measures the esophageal temperature.	
G. Observe the temperature display on the bedside monitor.	Provides a temperature value.	
H. Placement may be verified with radiograph.	Most catheters have a radiopaque tip visible on radiograph.	
6. Discard used supplies in appropriate receptacle.	Safely discards supplies.	
7. **HH**		

Initiation of a Warming or Cooling Device

Steps	Rationale	Special Considerations
1. **HH**		
2. **PE**		
3. Plug the device into a grounded outlet.	Establishes a power source	
4. Obtain a method for continuously monitoring the patient's core temperature.[12] (**Level E***)	Continuous core temperature monitoring is necessary with use of warming or cooling devices.[12]	Some warming or cooling devices have an adapter for connecting a temperature probe from the patient directly to the device.

Use of Traditional Warming or Cooling Fluid Device

Steps	Rationale	Special Considerations
1. Place a sheet or bath blanket between the patient and the circulating fluid blanket (**Level M***).	Protects the skin.	Avoid applying additional sheets or blankets because efficient heating or cooling occurs with maximal contact between the thermal pad and the patient's skin.

*Level E: Multiple case reports, theory-based evidence from expert opinions, or peer-reviewed professional organizational standards without clinical studies to support recommendations
*Level M: Manufacturer's recommendations only

Procedure	for External Warming/Cooling Devices—*Continued*	
Steps	**Rationale**	**Special Considerations**
2. Fill the reservoir in the unit with distilled water to the indicated full level.	The reservoir must contain enough water for the machine to function properly.	
3. Attach the hoses to the circulating fluid blanket.	Allows the flow of warmed or cooled water to the blanket.	
A. Check that the clamps are closed before connecting the hoses from the device to the blanket.	Prevents water leakage.	
B. After connecting the hoses, ensure that all of the connections are tight before unclamping the hoses.		
C. Check for kinks in the hoses.		
4. Press the start switch on.	Activates the device.	
5. Set the controls.		Follow the institution standard regarding the use of manual or automatic modes.
A. Manual control.		
1. Press the manual control switch on.		
2. Choose the set point for the temperature of the circulating fluid based on prescribed patient body temperature and manufacturer's directions.	The device maintains the circulating fluid in the blanket at the temperature set point.	The patient's temperature must be continuously monitored.[16]
3. Turn the warming or cooling device off when the desired temperature is reached.	The temperature goal is achieved.	Closely monitor the patient's temperature for fluctuation.
B. Automatic control.		
1. Connect the patient temperature probe to the unit before pressing a control mode switch.	Prevents triggering of the temperature probe alarm.	Most warming or cooling devices sound an alarm if the probe relays a low temperature; this may be indicative of probe dislodgment.
2. Select the automatic mode and the set-point based on prescribed patient body temperature and manufacturer's directions.	In the automatic mode, the unit warms or cools the circulating fluid in the blanket based on the set-point (desired temperature) for the patient. A temperature probe connected to the unit monitors the patient's temperature.	The unit operates only if the patient's temperature probe is connected to the unit. Lights on the display panel indicate whether the unit is heating or cooling at any given time.
3. Obtain the patient's temperature from the readout on the display unit.	Indicates the patient's temperature.	
4. Verify the patient's temperature with another source and compare it with the readout on the device's display unit.	Ensures the warming or cooling device's temperature probe is functioning and correlates with the patient's temperature obtained with another method.	
5. The warming or cooling device automatically shuts itself off when the desired patient temperature is reached.	The temperature goal is achieved.	Continue to monitor the patient's temperature by pressing on the monitor only switch.

Procedure continues on following page

Procedure for External Warming/Cooling Devices—*Continued*

Steps	Rationale	Special Considerations
Warming or Cooling Fluid Devices that Use Hydrogel Pads or External Wraps		

1. Apply the adhesive hydrogel pads or the external wraps to the
  A. Upper torso
  B. Over each upper thigh
  C. Additional pads can be placed as needed.
	The pads or the wraps should cover approximately 40% of the patient.	Pads and wraps should be placed over clean, dry, intact skin.

2. Connect the hoses from the pads or wraps to the warming or cooling fluid device.	Prepares the system.	
3. Set the patient's target temperature as prescribed.	Sets the desired temperature.	
4. Activate the automatic mode.	The system will automatically adjust to achieve the target temperature.	
5. Set the minimum and maximum water temperature as prescribed.	Prepares the system.	
6. Set the time to target to the maximum.	Prepares the system.	
7. Follow physician or advance practice nurse prescriptions and follow manufacturer recommendations for warming/cooling device maintenance.	Ensure safe patient monitoring.	
Use of a Warm Air Device		
1. Remove the patient's gown, sheet, and blankets. Then, place the circulating air blanket on top of the patient.	Prepares the equipment.	
2. Place a bath blanket or sheet over the circulating air blanket.	Aids in keeping the air blanket in place.	Maintains privacy.
3. Connect the air blanket to the hose attached to the device.	The blanket inflates as air flows from the hose into it.	A warm air device can increase a patient's temperature 2° to 3°C per hour.[7]
4. Turn the device on and select the temperature of the air that will flow through the blanket.	The device warms the patient by directing warm airstreams directly onto the patient's skin.	The patient's temperature must be continuously monitored.
After the warming or cooling system is initiating:		
1. Discard used supplies in an appropriate receptacle.	Removes and safely discards used supplies.	
2. **HH**		
3. Continuously monitor the patient's temperature, the system, and the patient's response.		Continue to assess the patient's electrolyte, glucose, arterial blood gas, and coagulation study results.[23]

Procedure for Intravascular Warming/Cooling Devices

Steps	Rationale	Special Considerations
1. **HH**		
2. Assist the physician or advanced practice nurse with insertion of the intravascular catheter (see Procedure 81).		The health care provider performing the procedure and those assisting with the procedure should be in sterile attire. All health care providers in the room during the procedure should have on a mask.
3. Connect the tubing from the warming or cooling fluid device to the intravascular catheter.	Prepares the system.	
4. Set the patient's target temperature as prescribed.	Sets the desired temperature.	
5. Activate the warming or cooling system.	Initiates the system.	
6. If intravascular catheter device includes lumens for intravenous fluid administration, maintain patency with intravenous (IV) fluids or saline solution flush as ordered.	Provides venous access for intravenous fluids and medication administration.	
7. Follow physician or advance practice nurse prescriptions for desired patient temperature therapy and monitoring parameters.	Ensure safe patient monitoring.	Follow manufacturer recommendations for warming/cooling device maintenance.
8. Ensure that a post-insertion chest x-ray is obtained if the catheter was placed in the subclavian or internal jugular vein.	Confirms placement.	
9. Discard used supplies in an appropriate receptacle.	Removes and safely discards used supplies; safely removes sharp objects.	
10. **HH**		
11. Continuously monitor the patient's temperature, the system, and the patient's response.		Continue to assess the patient's electrolyte, glucose, arterial blood gas, and coagulation study results.[23]

Expected Outcomes

- External warming or cooling device applied
- Desirable core body temperature achieved

Unexpected Outcomes

- Inability to achieve desired core body temperature
- Hemodynamic instability
- Cardiac dysrhythmias
- Acid-base, electrolyte, glucose, and coagulation imbalance
- Intolerable discomfort
- Shivering
- Skin injury

Procedure continues on following page

Patient Monitoring and Care

Steps	Rationale	Reportable Conditions
		These conditions should be reported if they persist despite nursing interventions.
1. Perform a physical assessment of all systems every 1 to 2 hours.	Alterations in temperature affect every system. The condition that caused the change in temperature may worsen or be refractory to treatment.	• Significant changes in assessment
2. Continuously monitor the patient's temperature.[12] **(Level E*)**	Assesses the patient's response to warming or cooling. Some institutions require two methods of monitoring the patient's temperature when cooling or warming. At least one should have audible alarms for temperatures above and below the desired limit. Follow institution policy.	• Continued hypothermia or hyperthermia (temperature outside of prescribed target temperature)
3. Measure the patient's blood pressure as frequently as indicated by the patient's condition and according to institution standard.	Vasodilation occurs with rewarming, and vasoconstriction may occur with cooling.	• Hypotension or hypertension
4. Palpate the patient's mandible for humming vibration and observe for shivering.	Aids in the early detection and prompt treatment of shivering.	• Shivering • Decreased mixed venous oxygenation saturation • Continued shivering despite prescribed medications
5. Examine the patient's skin condition hourly. Follow manufacturer's recommendations for assessing the patient's skin under hydrogel pads and external wraps (e.g., at least every 4 hours).	Detects signs or symptoms of skin irritation so that the temperature of the device can be adjusted or padding can be placed between the skin and the device.	• Signs or symptoms of skin irritation or injury
6. Continuously monitor the patient's cardiac rate and rhythm.	Detects cardiac dysrhythmias associated with warming or cooling therapy.	• Cardiac dysrhythmias
7. Obtain arterial blood gas results as prescribed and as indicated. Continuously monitor the patient's oxygen saturation and end-tidal carbon dioxide as prescribed.	Detects hypoxemia and acid-base imbalances.	• Decreased oxygen saturation • Abnormal arterial blood gas results
8. Assess for venous thromboembolism (VTE) in vessels that contain intravascular cooling/warming devices.[24] **(Level C*)**	Intravascular cooling devices have been associated with increased risk of VTE.[23]	• VTE or pulmonary emboli
9. Follow the institution standard for assessing pain. Administer analgesia as prescribed.[12]	Identifies need for pain interventions.	• Continued pain despite pain interventions

*Level C: Qualitative studies, descriptive or correlational studies, integrative reviews, systematic reviews, or randomized controlled trials with inconsistent results
*Level E: Multiple case reports, theory-based evidence from expert opinions, or peer-reviewed professional organizational standards without clinical studies to support recommendations

Documentation

Documentation should include the following:
- Patient and family education
- Patient's temperature and site(s) of temperature assessment
- Vital signs, cardiac rhythm, and hemodynamic status
- Physical assessment findings
- Skin assessment
- Postinsertion chest radiograph (intravascular devices placed in the subclavian or internal jugular veins)
- Acid-base, electrolyte, glucose, and coagulation assessment and interventions

- Type of warming or cooling device used
- Mode of cooling or warming device (automatic or manual), patient's set-point or water temperature (as required by institution standard)
- Time external warming or cooling initiated and terminated
- Pain assessment, interventions, and effectiveness of interventions
- Shiver assessment, interventions, and effectiveness of interventions
- Unexpected outcomes
- Additional interventions

References

CR 1. American Heart Association: 2005 Guidelines for cardiopulmonary resuscitation and emergency cardiovascular care, *Circulaton* 112(Suppl 24):IV:1-203, 2005.

2. Anderson-Pompa K, Foster A, Parker L, et al: Genetics and susceptibility to malignant hyperthermia, *Crit Care Nurse* 28:32-36, 2008.

3. Aslam AF, Aslam AK, Vasavada BC, et al: Hypothermia: evaluation, electrocardiographic manifestations and management, *Am J Med* 119:297-301, 2006.

4. Biddle C: The neurobiology of the human febrile response, *AANA J* 74:145-150, 2006.

CR 5. Creechan T, Vollman K, Kravutske ME: Cooling by convection vs cooling by conduction for treatment of fever in critically ill adults, *Am J Crit Care* 10:52-59, 2001.

CR 6. Gentilello L, Moujaes S: Treatment of hypothermia in trauma victims: thermodynamic considerations, *J Intensive Care Med* 10:5-14, 1995.

CR 7. Goheen MSL, Ducharme MB, Kenny GP, et al. Efficacy of forced-air and inhalation rewarming by using a human model for severe hypothermia. *J Appl Physiol,* 83, 1635-1640, 1997.

CR 8. Henker R, Shaver J: Understanding the febrile state according to an individual adaptation framework, *AACN Clin Issues Crit Care Nurs* 2:186-193, 1994.

CR 9. Holtzclaw B: Monitoring body temperature, *AACN Clin Issues Crit Care Nurs* 4:44-55, 1993.

10. Hooper VD, Andrews JO: Accuracy of noninvasive core temperature measurement in acutely ill adults: the state of the science, *Biol Res Nurs* 8:24-34, 2006.

CR 11. Iampietro P, Vaughn JA, Goldman RF, et al: Heat production from shivering, *J Appl Physiol* 15:632-634, 1960.

12. Keresztes PA, Brick K: Therapeutic hypothermia after cardiac arrest, *Dimens Crit Care Nurs* 25:71-76, 2006.

13. Lawson L, Bridges EJ, Ballou I, et al: Accuracy and precision of noninvasive temperature measurement in adult intensive care patients, *Am J Crit Care* 16:485-496, 2007.

CR 14. Lefrant JY, Muller L, de La Coussaye JE, et al: Temperature measurement in intensive care patients: comparison of urinary bladder, oesophageal, rectal, axillary, and inguinal methods versus pulmonary artery core method, *Intensive Care Med* 29:414-418, 2003.

15. Litman RS, Flood CD, Kaplan RF et al: Postoperative malignant hyperthermia: an analysis of cases from the North American Malignant Hyperthermia Registry, *Anesthesiology* 109:825-829, 2008.

CR 16. Loke AY, Chan HC, Chan TM: Comparing the effectiveness of two types of cooling blankets for febrile patients, *Nurs Crit Care* 10:247-254, 2005.

17. Mahmood MA, Zweifler RM: Progress in shivering control, *J Neurol Sci* 261:47-54, 2007.

CR 18. McIlvoy L: Comparison of brain temperature to core temperature: a review of the literature, *J Neurosci Nurs* 36:23-31, 2004.

19. Moore K: Hypothermia in trauma, *J Trauma Nurs* 15:62-64, 2008.

20. Neumar RW, Nolan JP, Adrie C, et al: Post cardiac arrest syndrome: epidemiology, pathophysiology, treatment, and prognostication: a consensus statement from the International Liaison Committee on Resuscitation, *Circulation* 118:2452-2483, 2008.

21. O'Grady NP, Barie PS, Bartlett JG, et al: Guidelines for evaluation of new fever in critically ill adults patients: 2008 update from the American College of Critical Care Medicine and the Infectious Diseases Society of America, *Crit Care Med* 36:1330-1349, 2008.

CR 22. Polderman KH: Application of therapeutic hypothermia in the ICU: opportunities and pitfalls of a promising treatment modality: part 2: practical aspects and side effects, *Intensive Care Med* 30:757-769, 2004.

23. Polderman, K. H., & Ingeborg, H. (2009). Therapeutic hypothermia and controlled normothermia in the intensive care unit: Practical considerations, side effects, and cooling methods. *Critical Care Medicine,* 37, 1101-1119

24. Simosa HF, Petersen DJ, Agarwal SK, et al: Increased risk of deep venous thrombosis with endovascular cooling in patients with traumatic brain injury, *Am Surg* 73:461-464, 2007.

25. Zoll Medical Corporation (2009). Intravascular Temperature Management: Products/Catheter Family, 2009. Text available from: http://www.alsius.com/products/catheters.html.

95

⚜AP Lumbar Puncture (Perform)

P U R P O S E : A lumbar puncture is performed for access to the subarachnoid space to obtain a cerebrospinal fluid sample, measure cerebrospinal fluid pressure, drain cerebrospinal fluid, infuse medications or contrast agents, or place a cerebrospinal fluid drainage catheter.[1-3,7]

Susan Chioffi

PREREQUISITE NURSING KNOWLEDGE

- Knowledge of the anatomy and physiology of the vertebral column, spinal meninges, and cerebrospinal fluid (CSF) circulation, including the location of the lumbar cistern, is needed.
- Technical and clinical competence in performing lumbar punctures (LPs) is necessary.
- Knowledge of sterile technique is needed.
- The presence of meningeal irritation caused by either infectious meningitis or subarachnoid hemorrhage may promote discomfort when the patient is placed in the flexed, lateral decubitus position for the LP.[3-5,17]
- Computed tomography (CT) scan or magnetic resonance imaging (MRI) supersedes the routine use of LP for many diagnoses.[5,7,18,28]
- Indications for LP include the following[4,5,18,28]:
  - ❖ Suspected central nervous system (CNS) infection
  - ❖ Clinical examination results suggestive of subarachnoid hemorrhage accompanied by negative CT scan findings
  - ❖ Suspected Guillain-Barré syndrome
  - ❖ Suspected multiple sclerosis
  - ❖ Intrathecal administration of medications

- ❖ Imaging procedures that require infusion of contrast agents
- ❖ Measurement of CSF pressure
- ❖ CSF drainage in hydrocephalus, pseudotumor cerebri, or CSF fistula
- Contraindications for LP include the following[3,18,28,29]:
  - ❖ Increased intracranial pressure with mass effect
  - ❖ Superficial skin infection localized to the site of entry
  - ❖ Bleeding diathesis (relative contraindication)
  - ❖ Platelet count less than 50,000/mm³
  - ❖ International normalized ratio (INR) greater than 1.5
  - ❖ Anticoagulation therapy (e.g., heparin, warfarin)
- Normal CSF values include the following[18,20,23,28]:
  - ❖ Opening pressure, 0 to 15 mm Hg
  - ❖ White blood cell count, less than 5/mm
  - ❖ Glucose, 60% to 70% of serum blood glucose
  - ❖ Protein, 15 to 45 mg/dL
  - ❖ Clear colorless appearance
  - ❖ Negative culture results
- Recommended CSF tests include the following[18,20,23,28]
  - ❖ Tube #1: Biochemistry:
    - ○ Glucose
    - ○ Protein
    - ○ Protein electrophoresis (if clinically indicated)
  - ❖ Tube #2: Bacteriology:
    - ○ Gram stain
    - ○ Bacterial culture
    - ○ Fungal culture (if clinically indicated); requires larger volume

---

⚜**AP** This procedure should be performed only by physicians, advanced practice nurses, and other healthcare professionals (including critical care nurses) with additional knowledge, skills, and demonstrated competence per professional licensure or institutional standard.

- ○ Tuberculosis culture (if clinically indicated); requires larger volume
- ❖ Tube #3: Hematology:
  - ○ Cell count
  - ○ Differential
- ❖ Tube #4: Optional studies as indicated:
  - ○ Venereal disease research laboratory (VDRL) test
  - ○ Oligoclonal bands
  - ○ Myelin protein
  - ○ Cytology

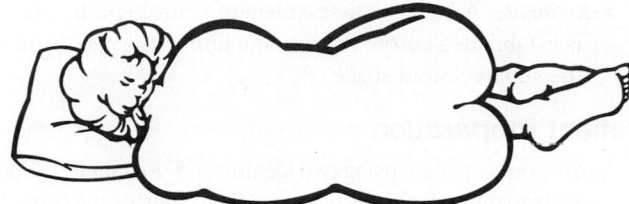

FIGURE 95-1 The lateral decubitus position appropriate for lumbar puncture. The patient flexes the neck, hips, and knees, and the knees are drawn up tightly to the chest. This increases the intraspinous space for facilitation of needle insertion.

EQUIPMENT

- Sterile gloves, caps, masks with eye shields or goggles, and sterile gowns
- Sterile drapes
- Sterile gauze pads
- Antiseptic solution
- Fenestrated drape
- Manometer with three-way stopcock
- Lidocaine, 1% to 2% (without epinephrine)
- 3- to 5-mL syringe
- 20-, 22-, and 25-gauge needles
- 18-, 20-, or 22-gauge spinal needles
- Four numbered capped test tubes
- Adhesive strip or sterile dressing supplies
- Specimen labels
- Laboratory forms
- Glucometer/phlebotomy equipment for serum or whole blood glucose
  Many supplies are available in a lumbar tray.
  Additional equipment, as needed, includes the following:
- Rolled towels or small pillows to support the patient during positioning

PATIENT AND FAMILY EDUCATION

- Explain the purpose of the LP procedure to the patient and family. ➡*Rationale:* Explanation may decrease patient and family anxiety.
- Explain the need for the patient to remain still and quiet in a lateral decubitus position with the neck, knees, and hips flexed (knees to chest); the axis of the hips vertical; the back close to the edge of the bed; the head of the bed flat; and no more than one pillow under the head (Figs. 95-1 and 96-1). If the lumbar puncture is not successful in this position, or the patient cannot tolerate this position, explain that the patient may also be positioned leaning over a bedside table or stand.[5,19,21,23] ➡*Rationale:* Patient cooperation during the examination is elicited; the intervertebral space widens in these positions, facilitating entry of the spinal needle into the subarachnoid space.[2,3,5,6]
- Explain that the procedure may produce some discomfort and that local anesthesia is injected to minimize pain. Also, explain that the patient may receive some mild analgesic and anxiolytic agents as prescribed and needed. ➡*Rationale:* The patient and family are prepared for what to expect.

- Explain that the patient may find it helpful to lie flat for 1 to 4 hours after the LP. ➡*Rationale:* A flat position may promote dural closure; the position was previously thought to reduce the possibility of postprocedural headache, but studies suggest it is not helpful in the prevention of a headache after the procedure.[1,5,12]

PATIENT ASSESSMENT AND PREPARATION
Patient Assessment

- Note any pertinent patient history. ➡*Rationale:* An LP is performed to assist with the diagnosis and management of a number of neurologic disease processes (see previous indications for LP).
- Obtain a baseline neurologic assessment, including assessment for increased intracranial pressure (ICP), before performing the LP. ➡*Rationale:* Increased ICP during the LP may place the patient at risk for a downward shift in intracranial contents (brain herniation) when the pressure is suddenly released from the lumbar subarachnoid space.[3,18,23,28]
- Assess for coagulopathies, active treatment with heparin or warfarin, local skin infections in close proximity to the site, or pertinent medication allergies. ➡*Rationale:* This assessment identifies potential risks for bleeding, infection, and allergic reactions.[2-5]
- Assess the patient's ability to cooperate with the procedure. ➡*Rationale:* Sudden, uncontrolled movement may result in needle displacement with associated injury or need for reinsertion.
- Identify through history and clinical examination vertebral column deformities or tissue scarring that may interfere with the ability to successfully carry out the procedure. ➡*Rationale:* Scoliosis, lumbar surgery with fusion, and repeated LP procedures may interfere with successful cannulation of the subarachnoid space.[3,21]
- Assess for signs and symptoms of meningeal irritation, which include the following:
  - ❖ Nuchal rigidity
  - ❖ Photophobia
  - ❖ Brudzinski's or Kernig's sign
  - ❖ Fever
  - ❖ Headache
  - ❖ Nausea or vomiting
  - ❖ Nystagmus

➤➤*Rationale:* A baseline assessment of neurologic function is established before the introduction of the needle into the subarachnoid space.

Patient Preparation

- Verify correct patient using two identifiers. ➤➤*Rationale:* Prior to performing a procedure, the nurse should ensure the correct identification of the patient for the intended intervention.
- Ensure that the patient and family understand preprocedural teaching. Answer questions as they arise, and reinforce information as needed. ➤➤*Rationale:* Understanding of previously taught information is evaluated and reinforced.
- Obtain informed consent. ➤➤*Rationale:* Informed consent protects the rights of the patient and makes competent decision-making possible for the patient; however, in emergency circumstances, time may not allow for the consent form to be signed.
- Perform a pre-procedure verification and time out, if non-emergent. ➤➤*Rationale:* Ensures patient safety.
- Obtain the patient's history of allergic reactions. ➤➤*Rationale:* History can rule out an allergy to lidocaine, the antiseptic solution, and the analgesia or sedation.
- Prescribe an analgesic medication and/or an anxiolytic medication. ➤➤*Rationale:* These medications may be needed to promote comfort and to decrease anxiety so that positioning can be achieved during the procedure.

Procedure for Lumbar Puncture (Perform)		
Steps	**Rationale**	**Special Considerations**
1. 🔲HH		
2. 🔲PE		
3. Position or assist the critical care nurse with positioning the patient in the lateral recumbent position near the side of the bed with neck, hips, and knees flexed (knees to chest), head of bed flat, and no more than one small pillow under the head (see Figs. 95-1 and 96-1). Ask the critical care nurse to assist the patient in attaining and maintaining the position. The critical care nurse should place an arm behind the patient's head and then the other arm around the knees.	The intervertebral space widens in this position, facilitating the entry of the spinal needle into the subarachnoid space.	If the lumbar puncture is not successful in this position, or the patient cannot tolerate this position, the patient may also be positioned leaning over a bedside table or stand.[3,19,21,23] Also consider performing the LP with fluoroscopy if the patient is morbidly obese or has vertebral column deformities.
4. With the patient in the lateral decubitus position for examination, identify the intervertebral spaces of L3-L4, L4-L5, and L5-S1; the L3-L4 intervertebral space is level with the top of the iliac crests (Fig. 95-2).[3,18] (**Level E***)	The LP is performed below the level of the conus medullaris, which ends at the L1-L2 in the adult. The most common site used for an LP is the L4-L5 interspace, but the L3-L4 or the L5-S1 interspace may be used when cannulation of the L4-L5 interspace is not possible.[4,5,18,27]	An imaginary vertical line is drawn in the midline through the spinous processes between the two iliac crests. A second line is imagined horizontally at the top of the iliac crests and across the spinous processes by the healthcare provider. These lines should intersect the L3-L4 area, and the puncture can be performed at the L3-L4, L4-L5, or L5-S1 interspace.[3,4]
5. 🔲HH		
6. Apply sterile gowns and gloves.	Minimizes the risk of infection; maintains sterile precautions.	

*Level E: Multiple case reports, theory-based evidence from expert opinions, or peer-reviewed professional organizational standards without clinical studies to support recommendations

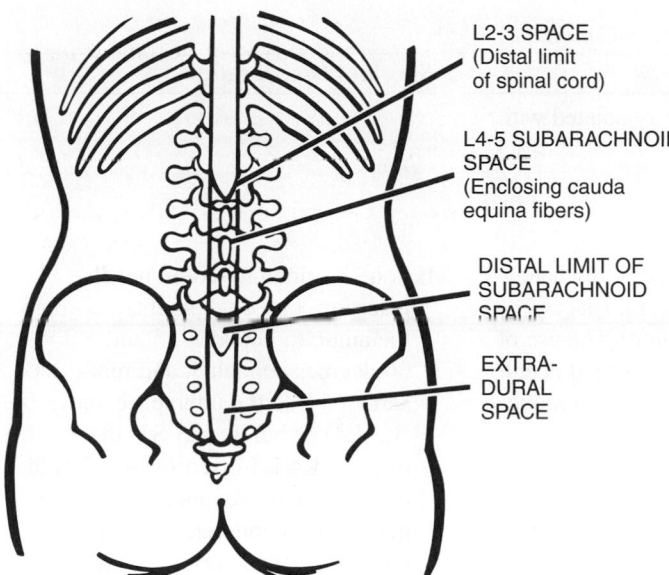

L2-3 SPACE
(Distal limit
of spinal cord)

L4-5 SUBARACHNOID
SPACE
(Enclosing cauda
equina fibers)

DISTAL LIMIT OF
SUBARACHNOID
SPACE

EXTRA-
DURAL
SPACE

FIGURE 95-2 The body of the spinal cord ends at L2-L3. The region below, L4-L5, encloses the cauda equina (a bundle of lumbar and sacral nerve roots) within the subarachnoid space. It is this area that is appropriate for lumbar puncture.

Procedure for Lumbar Puncture (Perform)—*Continued*

Steps	Rationale	Special Considerations
7. Set up a sterile field on the bedside stand. A. Preassemble the manometer, attaching the three-way stopcock; set to the side. B. Open the test tubes and place them in order of use in the tray slots. C. Draw approximately 3 mL of 1% lidocaine with a 20-gauge needle. Change to a 25-gauge needle for a superficial injection; change to a 22-gauge, 1.5-inch needle for a deeper injection.[3,5,7,28]	Prepares equipment for use in the procedure.	Have the critical care nurse or assistant prepare the numbered labels for the test tubes; ensure that the tubes are labeled in the order in which they are filled to facilitate laboratory differentiation of a traumatic tap versus a subarachnoid hemorrhage.[3,20]
8. Cleanse the skin over the L4-L5 puncture site, including one intervertebral space above and below the site with the antiseptic solution.[10,11,16,17] **(Level C*)**	Reduces transmission of microorganisms and minimizes the risk of infection.	The choice of povidone-iodine or chlorhexidine as an antiseptic agent is controversial. Both should be allowed to dry completely. Studies suggest chlorhexidine is neurotoxic.[10,17]
9. Drape the patient with exposure of the insertion site.	Minimizes the risk of infection; maintains sterile precautions.	

*Level C: Qualitative studies, descriptive or correlational studies, integrative reviews, systematic reviews, or randomized controlled trials with inconsistent results

Procedure continues on following page

Procedure for Lumbar Puncture (Perform)—*Continued*

Steps	Rationale	Special Considerations
10. Administer a local anesthetic with a 25-gauge needle, raising a wheal in the skin. Inject a small amount into the posterior spinous region with a 22-gauge needle.[5,28]	Reduces discomfort associated with needle insertion.	
11. Insert a 22-, 20-, or 18-gauge spinal needle bevel up[8] through the skin into the intervertebral space of L4-L5, with the needle at an angle of 15 degrees cephalad, aiming toward the umbilicus and level with the sagittal mid-plane of the body.[3,18] (**Level E***)	Facilitates the passage of the needle between intervertebral spaces toward the dura mater. The use of a smaller atraumatic spinal needle has been associated with a reduced incidence rate of postlumbar puncture headache.[8,9,13,14,29]	If bone is encountered on needle insertion, pull back slightly, correct the angle to between 15 and 40 degrees cephalad, and reinsert.[4,5,28] Use the interspace above (L3-L4) or below (L5-S1) the original L4-L5 insertion site should difficulty with advancement of the needle be encountered despite correction of the insertion angle.[3,4] Variations in the anatomic configuration of the vertebral column, a history of vertebral column surgery, or repeat LPs may necessitate needle insertion at a different level.[3]
12. Once the needle has been advanced approximately 3 to 4 cm, withdraw the stylet and check the hub for CSF. If CSF is not present, replace the stylet and advance slightly. Once CSF is draining, advance the needle another 1 to 2 mm.[3,18] (**Level E**)	In most adults, a 3- to 4-cm insertion depth is sufficient to enter the subarachnoid space.	A "popping" sensation is often associated with penetration of the dura mater.[3,5,18]
13. Attach the stopcock of the manometer to the needle. Have the patient straighten his or her legs and relax his or her position. Measure the opening pressure, and note the color of the fluid in the manometer.[3,18] (**Level E**)	Flexing the legs or straining to maintain a position may artificially elevate the CSF pressure .[3,7,18] Opening pressure or normal CSF pressure measurements taken at the lumbar area range from 0 to 20 cm H_2O (0 to 15 mm Hg or 50 to 150 mm H_2O).	If the patient was sitting on the side of the bed leaning over the bedside table for the lumbar puncture, have the patient lie down on his or her side for the CSF pressure measurement.[4]
14. Consider performing the Queckenstedt test. A. Ask the critical care nurse to simultaneously compress the jugular veins for 10 seconds, if not contraindicated and within institutional policy for the critical care nurse to perform. B. Watch for a change in subarachnoid CSF pressure on the manometer.[5,17]	The Queckenstedt test is used if an obstruction in the spinal subarachnoid space is suspected. A normal response indicates that the pathway between the skull and the lumbar needle is patent. This maneuver is contraindicated in patients with known or suspected elevated intracranial pressure; a sudden release of CSF pressure distally can result in herniation.[5,18]	Normal findings reflect a sharp increase in spinal subarachnoid CSF pressure on compression of the jugular veins; on release, pressure returns to precompression levels. A lack of change in CSF pressure indicates an obstruction of CSF flow. The Queckenstedt test is contraindicated in patients with increased ICP.[5,18]

*Level E: Multiple case reports, theory-based evidence from expert opinions, or peer-reviewed professional organizational standards without clinical studies to support recommendations

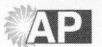

Procedure for Lumbar Puncture (Perform)—*Continued*

Steps	Rationale	Special Considerations

15. Obtain laboratory samples:
  A. Position the first test tube over the stopcock port.
  B. Turn the stopcock and drain CSF from the manometer into the first test tube.
  C. Continue filling test tubes from the hub of the spinal needle; a minimum of 1 to 2 mL CSF should be collected in each of the first three test tubes. The second and fourth test tubes may require up to 8 mL CSF depending on the tests ordered (e.g., fungal or tuberculosis testing).[4,5]
  D. Return the stopcock to the off position and discard the manometer.
	By draining CSF from the manometer into the test tubes, the CSF volume withdrawn is minimized.[3,5] Allows for progressive clearing of CSF blood in the case of a traumatic tap.[4,5,23,28]	In subarachnoid hemorrhage, CSF with the same consistency of blood is drained in all four test tubes. In the case of a traumatic tap, progressive clearing of bloody CSF occurs as drainage continues. Also, the supernatant of centrifuged CSF should be clear if the tap was traumatic and xanthochromic if blood has been present for several hours and has undergone hemolysis.[4,5,23,28]

16. Cover the opening of the needle with a sterile gloved finger. Replace the stylet and withdraw the needle.[1,3,7] **(Level E*)**	Covering the opening of the needle with a sterile gloved finger reduces the contamination by microorganisms. Replacing the stylet before withdrawing the needle prevents unnecessary CSF loss and facilitates needle withdrawal without traction on the spinal nerve roots. Reinsertion of the stylet before withdrawal of the spinal needle has also been associated with a reduced incidence rate of postlumbar puncture headache.[6,8,13,29]	Minimizes postprocedural headache.[1-3] If a lumbar subarachnoid catheter is inserted, refer to Procedure 91.
17. Apply an occlusive sterile dressing to the puncture site.	Decreases the incidence of infection.	
18. Place the patient in a supine or prone position immediately after the procedure.[1,5] **(Level E)**	In the supine position, the patient's weight acts as site pressure. In the prone position, the increased abdominal pressure transmits pressure to the site.[26] Some healthcare providers advocate placing the patient in a supine or prone position for 1 to 4 hours.[1,5]	Whether either the prone or supine position facilitates closure of the dura mater after the LP remains unclear. Neither the supine nor prone position has been shown to prevent postdural puncture headache.[1-3,6,25,26]
19. Label and send specimens to the laboratory. If there is no same-day serum glucose measurement, consider obtaining a serum glucose sample.	Obtains CSF analysis and assists with the differential diagnosis.[5,18,23,28]	Hyperglycemia or hypoglycemia affects CSF glucose values and can interfere with interpretation of results.[5,18,23,28]
20. Discard used supplies in an appropriate receptacle.	Removes and safely discards used supplies; safely removes sharp objects.	
21. ⧉		

*Level E: Multiple case reports, theory-based evidence from expert opinions, or peer-reviewed professional organizational standards without clinical studies to support recommendations with inconsistent results

Procedure continues on following page

Expected Outcomes

- Determination of the characteristics of the CSF that supports establishment of the diagnosis
- Recommendation for definitive treatment that promotes restoration of health or optimal functional status
- Postprocedure headache may occur in up to 70% of patients undergoing LP and is usually self-limiting[8,9,13,18]; the incidence of headache may be reduced with the use of smaller-gauge spinal needles and reinsertion of the stylet before the needle is withdrawn[3,6,13,14,18,29]
- No change in neurologic status after the procedure

Unexpected Outcomes

- In cases of a supratentorial mass or severely elevated intracranial pressure, a shift in intracranial contents (brain herniation) may be promoted by the sudden decrease in pressure incurred with LP[3,4,18,23]
- Injury of the periosteum or spinal ligaments may produce local back pain[5,28]
- Infectious meningitis may result from improper technique that produces contamination[4,5,17,18]
- Traumatic taps may result from inadvertent puncture of the spinal venous plexuses; usually this is a self-limiting process, but it may result in a hematoma in patients with bleeding disorders[3-5,28]
- Transient lower extremity pain may occur from irritation of a spinal nerve[5,28]
- Persistent CSF leak from the puncture site is associated with nonclosure of the dura[3,12]
- Inability to obtain a CSF specimen because of healthcare provider skill level, patient intolerance of the procedure, pathologic blockage of CSF flow, or aberrant anatomy[3]
- Persistent headache despite interventions[3,12-14]

Patient Monitoring and Care

Steps	Rationale	Reportable Conditions
		These conditions should be reported if they persist despite nursing interventions.
1. Monitor the patient's neurologic status, including the development of a change in level of consciousness, pupil size and reactivity, new onset of pain, motor weakness, or numbness in the lower extremities, and the patient's procedural tolerance, throughout and after the procedure.	Changes in neurologic status may be related to sudden intracranial decompression with brain herniation or local irritation of a spinal nerve by the needle or hematoma formation at the puncture site.[2-4,19]	• Deterioration in neurologic status • Transient lower extremity motor or sensory changes associated with spinal nerve irritation or hematoma formation
2. Monitor for postprocedural headache.	Headache occurs in up to 70% of patients after an LP.[8,9,26,28]	• Intractable postprocedural headache
3. Monitor for drainage from the puncture site.	Persistent drainage may indicate an unresolved CSF leak.[1,18,26]	• Drainage from the LP site • Dural tear that necessitates a patch or closure
4. Monitor the patient's neurological status at a minimum of every 4 hours for 24 hours after the LP.	Lower extremity motor or sensory changes may indicate a hematoma at the puncture site.[18]	• Spinal hematoma that necessitates emergent surgical evacuation
5. Monitor the effectiveness of measures taken to prevent or treat postprocedural headache.[13]	Determines level of comfort.	• Unrelieved headache
6. Follow institution standard for assessing pain. Consider administration of mild analgesic agent and encourage patient to remain supine or prone until headache improves.	Additional treatment measures may be necessary to manage postprocedural headache. Although recent studies do not support either the prone or supine position to prevent post dural puncture headache, lying in one of these positions may relieve the headache once it develops.[1,6,8,12,29]	• Intractable postprocedural headache • Dural tear that necessitates patch[9,11,24,27] or closure[26]

Documentation

Documentation should include the following:

- Patient and family education
- Completion of informed consent
- Preprocedure verifications and time-out
- Performance of the procedure, significant findings, CSF appearance, and opening pressure
- Amount of CSF removed
- Patient tolerance of the procedure

- Change in neurologic status associated with the procedure
- CSF specimens obtained
- Pain assessment, interventions, and effectiveness
- Unexpected outcomes
- Additional interventions

References

1. Ahmed SV, Jayawarna C, Jude E: Post-lumbar puncture headache: diagnosis and management, *Postgrad Med J* 82:713-716, 2006.
2. **CR** Armon C, Evans RW: Addendum to assessment: prevention of post-lumbar puncture headaches: report of the Therapeutics and Technology Assessment Subcommittee of the American Academy of Neurology, *Neurology* 65:510-512, 2005.
3. **CR** Boon JM, Abrahams PH, Meiring JH, et al: Lumbar puncture: anatomical review of a clinical skill, *Clin Anat* 17:544-553, 2004.
4. Ellenby MS, Tegtmeyer K, Lai S, et al: Lumbar puncture, *N Engl J Med* 355:e12, 2006.
5. **CR** Euerle B: Spinal puncture and cerebrospinal fluid examination. In Roberts JR, Hedges JR, Chanmugam AS, editors: *Clinical procedures in emergency medicine,* ed 4, St Louis, 2003, Elsevier, 1197-1222.
6. **CR** Evans RW, Armon C, Frohman EM, et al: Assessment: prevention of post-lumbar puncture headaches: report of the Therapeutics and Technology Assessment Subcommittee of the American Academy of Neurology, *Neurology* 55:909-914, 2000.
7. Farley A, McLafferty FA: Lumbar puncture, *Nurs Stand* 22:46-48, 2008.
8. Frank RL: Lumbar puncture and post-dural puncture headaches: implications for the emergency physician, *J Emerg Med* 35:149-157, 2008.
9. Gaiser R: Postdural puncture headache, *Curr Opin Anaesthesiol* 19:249-253, 2006.
10. Hebl JR: The importance and implications of aseptic techniques during regional anesthesia, *Reg Anesth Pain Med* 31:311-323, 2006.
11. **CR** Kinirons B, Mimoz O, Lafendi L, et al: Chlorhexidine versus povidone iodine in preventing colonization of continuous epidural catheters in children, *Anesthesiology* 94:239-244, 2001.
12. **CR** Levine DN, Rapalino O: The pathophysiology of lumbar puncture headache, *J Neurol Sci* 192:1-8, 2001.
13. Lowery S, Oliver A: Incidence of postdural puncture headache and backache following diagnostic/therapeutic lumbar puncture using a 22G cutting spinal needle, and after introduction of a 25G pencil point spinal needle, *Paediatr Anaesth* 18:230-234, 2008.
14. **CR** Luostarinen L, Heinonen T, Luostarinen M, et al: Diagnostic lumbar puncture: comparative study between 22-gauge pencil point and sharp bevel needle, *J Headache Pain* 6:400-404, 2005.
15. **CR** Manthous CA, DeGirolamo A, Haddad C, et al: Informed consent for medical procedures: local and national practices, *Chest* 124:1978-1984, 2003.
16. Milstone AM, Passaretti CL, Perl TM: Chlorhexidine: expanding the armamentarium for infection control and prevention, *Clin Infect Dis* 46:274-281, 2008.
17. Reynolds F: Neurological infections after neuraxial anesthesia, *Anesthesiol Clin* 26:23-52, 2008.
18. **CR** Roos KL: Lumbar puncture, *Semin Neurol* 23:105-114, 2003.
19. Ropper AH, Samuel MA: Special techniques for neurological diagnosis. In Ropper AH, Samuels MA, editors: *Adams and Victor's principles of neurology,* ed 9, New York, 2009, McGraw-Hill. Text available at www.access-medicine.com.offcampus.lib.washington.edu/content.aspx?aID=3630099.
20. **CR** Seehusen DA, Reeves MM, Fomin DA: Cerebrospinal fluid analysis, *Am Fam Physician* 68:1103-1108, 2003.
21. Shah KH, McGillicuddy D, Spear J, et al: Predicting difficult and traumatic lumbar punctures, *Am J Emerg Med* 25:608-611, 2007.
22. Stiffler KA, Jwayyed S, Wilber ST, et al: The use of ultrasound to identify pertinent landmarks for lumbar puncture, *Am J Emerg Med* 25:331-334, 2007.
23. Straus SE, Thorpe KE, Holroyd-Leduc J: How do I perform a lumbar puncture and analyze the results to diagnose bacterial meningitis, *JAMA* 296:2012-2022, 2006.
24. **CR** Sudlow CL, Warlow CC: Epidural blood patching for preventing and treating post-dural puncture headache, *Cochrane Database Syst Rev* 2:CD001791, 2002.
25. **CR** Sudlow CL, Warlow CC: Posture and fluids for preventing post-dural puncture headache, *Cochrane Database Syst Rev* 2:CD001790, 2002.
26. **CR** Turnbull DK, Shepherd DB: Post-dural puncture headache: pathogenesis, prevention, and treatment, *Br J Anaesth* 91:718-729, 2003.
27. van Kooten F, Oedit R, Bakker SL, et al: Epidural blood patch in post dural puncture headache: a randomised, observer-blind, controlled clinical trial, *J Neurol Neurosurg Psychiatry* 79:553-558, 2008.
28. Weaver JP: Cerebrospinal fluid aspiration. In Irwin RS, Rippe JM, editors: *Irwin and Rippe's intensive care medicine,* ed 6, Philadelphia, 2008, Lippincott Williams & Wilkins, 151-158.
29. Williams J, Lye DCB, Umapathi T: Diagnostic lumbar puncture: minimizing complications, *Intern Med J* 38:587-591, 2008.

Additional Readings

Allen SH: How to perform lumbar puncture with the patient in a seated position, *Br J Hosp Med* 67:M46-M47, 2006.

McQuillan KA: The neurologic system. In Alspach JA, editor: *Core curriculum for critical care nursing,* ed 6, Philadelphia, 2006, Saunders, 381-524.

Wilson RK, Williams MA: Normal pressure hydrocephalus, *Clin Geriatr Med* 22:935-951, 2006.

Ziai WC, Lewin JJ: Update in the diagnosis and management of central nervous system infections, *Neurol Clin* 26:427-468, 2008.

Lumbar Puncture (Assist)

PURPOSE: A lumbar puncture is performed for access to the subarachnoid space to obtain a cerebrospinal fluid sample, measure cerebrospinal fluid pressure, drain cerebrospinal fluid, infuse medications or contrast agents, or place a cerebrospinal fluid drainage catheter.[1-3,7]

Susan Chioffi

PREREQUISITE NURSING KNOWLEDGE

- Knowledge of neuroanatomy and physiology is needed.
- A lumbar puncture (LP) at L3-L4 or L4-L5 in an adult is usually performed to obtain a cerebrospinal fluid (CSF) sample.[18]
- Indications for lumbar puncture are as follows:
  - Cerebrospinal fluid analysis may be indicated in the differential diagnosis of subarachnoid hemorrhage, central nervous system (CNS) infection, CNS autoimmune processes, and some malignant diseases.[4,5,18,28]
  - Therapeutically, a lumbar puncture may be used to treat hydrocephalus, cerebrospinal fluid fistulas, and pseudotumor cerebri; to deliver medications or contrast material into the subarachnoid space; or to access the subarachnoid space for placement of a lumbar subarachnoid drain.[4,5,18,28]
- Contraindications for lumbar punctures are as follows[5,18,28,29]:
  - Lumbar punctures are contraindicated if the patient has a known or suspected intracranial mass or elevated intracranial pressure (ICP), noncommunicating hydrocephalus, or infection in the region to be used for lumbar puncture or is coagulopathic or therapeutically anticoagulated. If CSF analysis is necessary, the patient may need pretreatment with fresh frozen plasma, platelets, cryoprecipitate, or the specific factor needed to correct a hematologic abnormality.[5,18,28,29]
  - Lumbar punctures are cautioned against in patients suspected of aneurysmal subarachnoid hemorrhage and in patients with complete spinal blocks. In such cases, a lumbar puncture may be performed if the computed tomographic (CT) scan of the patient's head does not indicate signs of increased ICP, such as significant cerebral swelling, hematoma, intracranial tissue shifts, or herniation.[5,18,28,29]
  - Brain herniation may occur after punctures in the presence of an intracranial mass lesion or increased ICP.[3,18]
- The preferred positioning for a lumbar puncture is lateral decubitus with the neck, hips, and knees flexed (knees to chest); the axis of the hips vertical; the back close to the edge of the bed; head of the bed flat; and no more than a small pillow under the head (see Figs. 95-1 and 96-1).[19] If the lumbar puncture is not successful in this position, or if the patient cannot tolerate this position, the patient may also be positioned sitting on the side of the bed, leaning over a bedside table or stand.[19,21,23,29] This procedure may also be performed with fluoroscopy for patients with marked obesity or spinal deformities. Optimal positioning is necessary to avoid the risk for a "dry tap" or an unsuccessful puncture attempt. Repeated attempts at puncture increase the risk for infection and patient discomfort.[3,18]
- Proper positioning for a lumbar puncture widens the interspinous process space and facilitates the passage of the needle.[2,3,5,6]

EQUIPMENT

- Sterile gloves, caps, masks with eye shield, and sterile gowns
- Sterile drapes
- Sterile gauze pads
- Antiseptic solution
- Fenestrated drape
- Manometer with a three-way stopcock

- Lidocaine, 1% to 2% (without epinephrine)
- 3- to 5-mL syringe
- 18-, 20-, 22-, and 25-gauge needles
- 18-, 20-, or 22-gauge spinal needles
- Four consecutively numbered, capped test tubes
- Adhesive strip or sterile dressing supplies
- Specimen labels
- Laboratory forms
- Glucometer/phlebotomy supplies for concurrent testing of serum or whole blood glucose
  Additional equipment, as needed, includes the following:
- Alcohol pads or swab sticks
- Two over-bed tables (one for sterile field; one to position patient, if necessary)
- Rolled towels or small pillows to support the patient during positioning

PATIENT AND FAMILY EDUCATION

- Explain the purpose of the procedure to the patient and family. ➥*Rationale:* Understanding of the procedure is reinforced, and anxiety may be decreased.
- Explain positioning requirements for the lumbar puncture. ➥*Rationale:* Cooperation with positioning requirements facilitates the procedure.
- Explain that the procedure may cause some mild discomfort; the patient will receive local anesthesia and may also receive some mild analgesia and an anxiolytic. ➥*Rationale:* This prepares the patient for what to expect.

PATIENT ASSESSMENT AND PREPARATION

Patient Assessment

- Obtain vital signs. ➥*Rationale:* Baseline values for the patient are established.
- Perform a neurologic assessment, including level of consciousness, pupil size and reactivity, and motor and sensory function. ➥*Rationale:* Baseline neurologic function is established before the insertion of a needle into the proximity of sensitive neurologic tissue.
- Assess for signs and symptoms of increased ICP. ➥*Rationale:* Increased ICP during the LP may place the patient at risk for a downward shift in intracranial contents

(brain herniation) when the pressure is suddenly released from the lumbar subarachnoid space.
- Assess the patient's current laboratory profile, including complete blood cell count, platelets, prothrombin time, partial thromboplastin time, bleeding time, and international normalized ratio. ➥*Rationale:* Baseline values are established, and any coagulopathies that necessitate intervention before the cisternal or lumbar puncture are identified.
- Assess for signs and symptoms of meningeal irritation, including the following:
  - ❖ Nuchal rigidity
  - ❖ Photophobia
  - ❖ Brudzinski's sign (flexion of the knee in response to flexion of the neck)
  - ❖ Kernig's sign (pain in the hamstrings on extension of the knee with the hip at 90-degree flexion)
  - ❖ Fever
  - ❖ Headache
  - ❖ Nausea or vomiting
  - ❖ Nystagmus
- ➥*Rationale:* Baseline neurologic function is established before introduction of a needle into the subarachnoid space.
- Assess for allergies to local anesthetic, antiseptic, and any analgesic or sedative medications. ➥*Rationale:* Risk of allergic reaction is decreased.[2-5]

Patient Preparation

- Verify correct patient with two identifiers. ➥*Rationale:* Prior to performing a procedure, the nurse should ensure the correct identification of the patient for the intended intervention.
- Ensure that the patient and family understand preprocedural teaching. Answer questions as they arise, and reinforce information as needed. ➥*Rationale:* Understanding of previously taught information is evaluated and reinforced.
- Ensure that informed consent is obtained. ➥*Rationale:* Informed consent protects the rights of the patient and makes competent decision making possible for the patient; however, in emergency circumstances, time may not allow for the consent form to be signed.
- Perform a pre-procedure verification and time out, if nonemergent. ➥*Rationale:* Ensures patient safety.

Procedure for Lumbar Puncture (Assist)

Steps	Rationale	Special Considerations
1. 𝐇𝐇		
2. Ensure that the patient is in the proper lateral decubitus position, near the side of the bed with the neck, hips, and knees flexed (knees to chest). The head of the bed should be flat, and no more than one small pillow should be under the head (Fig 95-1 and 96-1). If difficulty is encountered, an alternative position is to have the patient sit on the edge of the bed, leaning over the bed table .[3,19,29]	The intervertebral space widens in this position, facilitating the entry of the spinal needle into the subarachnoid space.	For lumbar punctures, to help the patient maintain this position, an arm can be placed behind the patient's head and then the other arm around the knees. If difficulty is encountered, an alternative position is to have the patient sit on the edge of the bed, leaning over the bed table (Fig. 96-1).[3,19,29]
3. Administer analgesia and/or anxylotic medications as prescribed.	May be needed to facilitate positioning of the patient and to relieve anxiety.	
4. Apply goggles or masks with face shields, caps, sterile gowns, and sterile gloves.	Minimizes the risk of infection; maintains aseptic and sterile precautions.	
5. Assist as needed with skin preparation with antiseptic solution. (**Level C***)	Reduces microorganisms and helps prevent infection.	The use of povidone-iodine versus chlorhexidine as an antiseptic solution before lumbar puncture is controversial. Chlorhexidine may be neurotoxic. Allowing the site to air dry increases effectiveness of antiseptic solution and minimizes contact with nervous system tissue.[10,11,16,17]
6. Assist as needed with application of sterile drapes.	Decreases the risk for contamination and provides a sterile field for the procedure.	
7. Assist if needed in identifying the appropriate anatomic site for puncture.	The lumbar puncture in an adult is performed below the level of L3 to prevent damage to the spinal cord (the body of the spinal cord ends at L2-L3).	An imaginary line is drawn vertically between the iliac crests, and a second line is imagined horizontally at the top of the spinous processes. These lines should intersect the L3-L4 area, and the puncture can be performed here or one level below at the L4-L5 interspace.[3,4]

*Level C: Qualitative studies, descriptive or correlational studies, integrative reviews, systematic reviews, or randomized controlled trials with inconsistent results

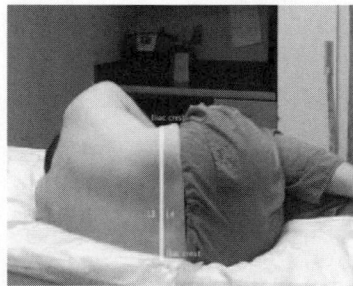

Figure 96-1   Proper positioning of the patient for a lumbar puncture. *(From Ellenby MS, Tegtmeyer K, Lai S, et al: Lumbar puncture: New Engl J Med 355:e12, 2006. Copyright © 2006, Massachusetts Medical Society. All rights reserved.)*

Procedure for Lumbar Puncture (Assist)—*Continued*

Steps	Rationale	Special Considerations
8. Assist with the preparation of local anesthesia as needed. Hold medication vials as needed for removal of local anesthetic to assist the physician or advanced practice nurse in maintaining sterile technique.	Prevents or decreases the pain from the needle insertion.	
9. Once the needle is in place, instruct the patient to relax and breathe normally and to avoid holding his or her breath. Assist the patient to straighten his or her legs when indicated by the physician or advanced practice nurse.[3,7,18] **(Level E*)**	Increased muscle tension or intrathoracic pressure may falsely elevate CSF pressure.[3,7,18]	Patients undergoing lumbar puncture may also straighten their legs because leg flexion can increase intrathoracic pressure.[3,7,18]
10. With aseptic technique, assist with holding the manometer in place when it is attached to the spinal needle via a three-way stopcock.	Secures the position of the manometer.	
11. Assist with obtaining the CSF pressure measurement.	Opening pressure or normal CSF pressure measurements taken at the lumbar area range from 0 to 20 cm H_2O (0 to 15 mm Hg or 50 to 150 mm H_2O). The opening pressure in a traumatic tap is within normal limits, compared with the opening pressure in patients with subarachnoid hemorrhage and meningitis.	The meniscus should show minimal fluctuation related to pulse and respiration.
12. Assist as needed in performing the Queckenstedt test, if not contraindicated or prohibited by institutional policy, by simultaneously compressing the jugular veins for 10 seconds while observing for a change in subarachnoid CSF pressure on the manometer.[5,18] Follow institution policy regarding who may perform the Queckenstedt test.	The Queckenstedt test is used if an obstruction in the spinal subarachnoid space is suspected. A normal response indicates that the pathway between the skull and the lumbar needle is patent. This maneuver is contraindicated in patients with known or suspected elevated intracranial pressure; a sudden release of CSF pressure distally can result in herniation.[5,18]	Normally, a rapid increase in CSF pressure occurs with resultant decrease when compression is released. If a complete or partial spinal block exists, the level does not rise, or it rises slowly, and remains elevated when the jugular veins are released. No increase in CSF pressure may be caused by improper needle placement.[5,18]
13. Assist with the collection of CSF specimens as needed: A. Assist in stabilizing the manometer with one hand. B. Assist with the handoff of each tube as needed (if not placed upright and in order in lumbar puncture tray). Tighten cap of each tube.	Obtains needed CSF specimens.	

*Level E: Multiple case reports, theory-based evidence from expert opinions, or peer-reviewed professional organizational standards without clinical studies to support recommendations

Procedure continues on following page

Procedure | for Lumbar Puncture (Assist)—*Continued*

Steps	Rationale	Special Considerations
14. Label each tube in order of collection with the type of specimen, patient name, and the order in which the specimen was collected (i.e., "# 1 of 3").	Differentiates between subarachnoid hemorrhage and traumatic tap by evaluating each numbered specimen.[4,5,23,28]	Red blood cell (RBC) dissipation through consecutive samples is indicative of a traumatic tap; consistent RBC presence is indicative of a subarachnoid hemorrhage. Also, the supernatant of centrifuged CSF should be clear if the tap was traumatic and xanthrochromic if blood has been present for several hours and has undergone hemolysis.[4,5,23,28]
15. Obtain a serum or whole blood glucose value from the patient as prescribed.	Allows for comparison of the serum glucose value and the CSF glucose concentration. A normal CSF glucose value is approximately two thirds of the blood glucose value.[19,20]	Hyperglycemia increases CSF glucose concentration, and hypoglycemia decreases CSF glucose concentration. Either may interfere with the interpretation of the CSF results.[4,5,18,23,28]
16. Assist the patient to a supine or prone position.[1,5] **(Level E*)**	In the supine position, the patient's weight acts as site pressure. In the prone position, the increased abdominal pressure transmits pressure to the site.[26] Some clinicians advocate placing the patient in a supine or prone position for 1 to 4 hours.[8,9,12,14]	Whether either the prone or supine position facilitates closure of the dura mater after the LP remains unclear. Neither the supine or prone position has been shown to prevent postdural puncture headache.[3,6,25,26]
17. Observe the puncture site, dressing, and linen for CSF leakage or bleeding. Reinforce the dressing as needed.	May indicate continued CSF loss after the procedure. Drainage after lumbar puncture from the insertion site should be minimal.	
18. Discard used supplies in an appropriate receptacle.	Removes and safely discards used supplies; safely removes sharp objects.	
19. 🅷🅷		
20. Send the specimens to the laboratory.	Ensures the specimens are sent for laboratory analysis.	

Expected Outcomes

- Lumbar puncture completed
- CSF samples and results obtained
- Patient's vital signs and level of consciousness stable before, during, and after the procedure
- No change or deterioration in neurologic exam
- Puncture site clean and dry
- No headache, neck stiffness, local pain at puncture site, leg spasms, or elevated temperature related to the procedure

Unexpected Outcomes

- Significant change in vital signs (respiratory changes, bradycardia, and increased systolic blood pressure)
- Change or deterioration in neurologic status (signs of brain herniation, which may include a decrease in the level of consciousness, pupil changes, and motor or sensory impairment)[3-5,18,23]
- Inability to void spontaneously (if able to before procedure)
- Abnormal CSF results
- CSF not obtained or inability to complete procedure
- Prolonged headache, stiff neck, photophobia and an acute increase in temperature related to the procedure[4,5,17,18]
- Excessive drainage at the puncture site[13,14]

*Level E: Multiple case reports, theory-based evidence from expert opinions, or peer-reviewed professional organizational standards without clinical studies to support recommendations

Expected Outcomes	Unexpected Outcomes —*Continued*
	• Persistent headache or low back pain despite interventions
	• New and persistent symptoms of pain, numbness, tingling, weakness, or paralysis in the lower extremities[3-5,28]
	• Spinal or paraspinal abscess
	• Hematoma formation[3-5,28]
	• Implantation of epidermal tumors[4]
	• Vasovagal syncope
	• Seizure
	• Pneumocephalus

Patient Monitoring and Care

Steps	Rationale	Reportable Conditions
		These changes should be reported if they persist despite nursing interventions.
1. Monitor the patient's neurologic, respiratory, and cardiovascular status during the procedure.	Pain or abnormal sensation radiating down one or both legs may result from spinal nerve irritation, which may necessitate a change in patient or needle position. Respiratory depression or an altered level of consciousness may result from brain herniation[2-4,19] or analgesia and sedation.	• Respiratory depression • Changes in level of consciousness • Pupil changes • Motor or sensory changes • Change in vital signs • Bowel or bladder dysfunction
2. Assess vital signs and perform systematic neurologic assessments every 15 minutes for the first hour, every 30 minutes twice, then every hour for the next 4 hours, and at a minimum of every 4 hours for the following 24 hours after the procedure.	A change in vital signs or neurologic assessment could indicate brain herniation, acute hematoma formation at the insertion site, injury to a spinal nerve, or infection.[3,4,18,19]	• Change in vital signs • Changes in level of consciousness • Pupil changes • Motor or sensory changes
3. Monitor the needle puncture site.	Identifies complications at the site.	• Persistent bleeding at the site • Drainage of clear serous fluid
4. Monitor the patient for headache or back or leg pain or discomfort. Follow the institutional standard for assessing pain. Administer analgesia as prescribed.	Identifies traumatic complications of needle placement. Identifies need for management of discomfort.	• Severe, persistent back or leg pain not evident before the procedure • Inability to manage pain • Persistent headache despite interventions[24]
5. Instruct the patient to remain supine or prone in bed for 1 to 4 hours or for the length of time prescribed.[9,12-14] **(Level E*)**	In the supine position, the patient's weight acts as site pressure. In the prone position, the increased abdominal pressure transmits pressure to the site.[26] Some healthcare providers advocate placing the patient in a supine or prone position for 1 to 4 hours.[5,6,25,26]	• Unrelieved headache
6. Ensure adequate oral or intravenous fluid intake.[5,24-26]	May facilitate repletion of CSF.	• Intravascular fluid overload or deficit

*Level E: Multiple case reports, theory-based evidence from expert opinions, or peer-reviewed professional organizational standards without clinical studies to support recommendations

Procedure continues on following page

Documentation

Documentation should include the following:
- Patient and family education
- Completion of informed consent
- Preprocedure verifications and time out
- Date and time of procedure
- Opening pressure
- Status of puncture site
- Specimens sent to the laboratory for analysis

- Amount and character of CSF collected
- CSF laboratory results
- Patient's baseline vital signs and neurologic assessment and tolerance of procedure
- Pain assessment, interventions, and effectiveness
- Any unexpected outcomes
- Additional interventions

References

1. Ahmed SV, Jayawarna C, Jude E: Post-lumbar puncture headache: diagnosis and management, *Postgrad Med J* 82:713-716, 2006.
CR 2. Armon C, Evans RW: Addendum to assessment: prevention of post-lumbar puncture headaches: report of the Therapeutics and Technology Assessment Subcommittee of the American Academy of Neurology, *Neurology* 65:510-512, 2005.
CR 3. Boon JM, Abrahams PH, Meiring JH, et al: Lumbar puncture: anatomical review of a clinical skill, *Clin Anat* 17:544-553, 2004.
4. Ellenby MS, Tegtmeyer K, Lai S, et al: Lumbar puncture, *N Engl J Med* 355:e12, 2006.
CR 5. Euerle B: Spinal puncture and cerebrospinal fluid examination. In Roberts JR, Hedges JR, Chanmugam AS, editors: *Clinical procedures in emergency medicine*, ed 4, St Louis, 2003, Elsevier, 1197-1222.
CR 6. Evans RW, Armon C, Frohman EM, et al: Assessment: prevention of post-lumbar puncture headaches: report of the Therapeutics and Technology Assessment Subcommittee of the American Academy of Neurology, *Neurology* 55:909-914, 2000.
7. Farley A, McLafferty E: Lumbar puncture, *Nurs Stand* 22:46-48, 2008.
8. Frank RL: Lumbar puncture and post-dural puncture headaches: implications for the emergency physician, *J Emerg Med* 35:149-157, 2008.
9. Gaiser R: Postdural puncture headache, *Curr Opin Anaesthesiol* 19:249-253, 2006.
10. Hebl JR: The importance and implications of aseptic techniques during regional anesthesia, *Reg Anesth Pain Med* 31:311-323, 2006.
CR 11. Kinirons B, Mimoz O, Lafendi L, et al: Chlorhexidine versus povidone iodine in preventing colonization of continuous epidural catheters in children, *Anesthesiology* 94:239-244, 2001.
CR 12. Levine DN, Rapalino O: The pathophysiology of lumbar puncture headache, *J Neurol Sci* 192:1-8, 2001.
13. Lowery S, Oliver A: Incidence of postdural puncture headache and backache following diagnostic/therapeutic lumbar puncture using a 22G cutting spinal needle, and after introduction of a 25G pencil point spinal needle, *Paediatr Anaesth* 18:230-234, 2008.
CR 14. Luostarinen L, Heinonen T, Luostarinen M, et al: Diagnostic lumbar puncture: comparative study between 22-gauge pencil point and sharp bevel needle, *J Headache Pain* 6:400-404, 2005.

CR 15. Manthous CA, DeGirolamo A, Haddad C, et al: Informed consent for medical procedures: local and national practices, *Chest* 124:1978-1984, 2003.
16. Milstone AM, Passaretti CL, Perl TM: Chlorhexidine: expanding the armamentarium for infection control and prevention, *Clin Infec Dis* 46:274-281, 2008.
17. Reynolds F: Neurological infections after neuraxial anesthesia, *Anesthesiol Clin* 26:23-52, 2008.
CR 18. Roos KL: Lumbar puncture, *Semin Neurol* 23:105-114, 2003.
19. Ropper AH, Samuel MA: Special techniques for neurological diagnosis. In *Adams and Victor's principles of neurology*, ed 9, New York, 2009, McGraw-Hill.
CR 20. Seehusen DA, Reeves MM, Fomin DA: Cerebrospinal fluid analysis. *Am Fam Physician* 68:1103-1108, 2003.
21. Shah KH, McGillicuddy D, Spear J, et al: Predicting difficult and traumatic lumbar punctures, *Am J Emerg Med* 25:608-611, 2007.
22. Stiffler KA, Jwayyed S, Wilber ST, et al: The use of ultrasound to identify pertinent landmarks for lumbar puncture, *Am J Emerg Med* 25:331-334, 2007.
23. Straus SE, Thorpe KE, Holroyd-Leduc J: How do I perform a a lumbar puncture and analyze the results to diagnose bacterial meningitis, *JAMA* 296:2012-2022, 2006.
CR 24. Sudlow CL, Warlow CC: Epidural blood patching for preventing and treating post-dural puncture headache, *Cochrane Database Syst Rev* 2:CD001791, 2002.
CR 25. Sudlow CL, Warlow CC: Posture and fluids for preventing post-dural puncture headache, *Cochrane Database Syst Rev* 2:CD001790, 2002.
CR 26. Turnbull DK, Shepherd DB: Post-dural puncture headache: pathogenesis, prevention, and treatment, *Br J Anaesth* 91:718-729, 2003.
27. van Kooten F, Oedit R, Bakker SL, et al: Epidural blood patch in post dural puncture headache: a randomised, observer-blind, controlled clinical trial, *J Neurol Neurosurg Psychiatry* 79:553-558, 2008.
28. Weaver JP: Cerebrospinal fluid aspiration. In Irwin RS, Rippe JM, editors: *Irwin and Rippe's intensive care medicine*, ed 6, Philadelphia, 2008, Lippincott Williams & Wilkins, 151-158.
29. Williams J, Lye DCB, Umapathi T: Diagnostic lumbar puncture: minimizing complications, *Intern Med J* 38:587-591, 2008.

Additional Readings

Allen SH: How to perform lumbar puncture with the patient in a seated position, *Br J Hosp Med* 67:M46-M47, 2006.

McQuillan KA: The neurologic system. In Alspach JA, editor: *Core curriculum for critical care nursing*, ed 6, Philadelphia, 2006, Saunders, 381-524.

Wilson RK, Williams MA: Normal pressure hydrocephalus, *Clin Geriatr Med* 22:935-951, 2006.

Ziai WC, Lewin JJ: Update in the diagnosis and management of central nervous system infections, *Neurol Clin* 26: 427-468, 2008.

Cervical Tongs or Halo Ring: Application for Use in Cervical Traction (Assist)

P U R P O S E :   Cervical tongs or a halo ring are inserted into the skull so that weighted traction can be applied to the cervical spine. Cervical traction decompresses the spinal cord and immobilizes and realigns the cervical spine. Realignment and immobilization of the cervical spine decrease the risk of secondary spinal cord injury. Spinal realignment and immobilization allow spinal fractures and supportive structures to heal properly.

Mary Hanson

PREREQUISITE NURSING KNOWLEDGE

- Knowledge of neuroanatomy and physiology is necessary.
- The nurse needs to be knowledgeable about the anatomy and physiology of the spinal column, the special anatomy of the cervical vertebrae, the spinal cord, the cervical spinal nerves, and their areas of peripheral innervation. In addition, it is important that the nurse understands the pathophysiology and manifestations of spinal cord trauma, including ascending edema, spinal shock and related impairment of respiratory function, vasomotor tone, and autonomic nervous system function.
- It is essential that the nurse understands the pathophysiology of spinal cord injury, including the concepts of primary versus secondary spinal cord injury and spinal shock.
- The nurse needs to be knowledgeable about the signs and symptoms of new spinal cord injury or extension of injury, for example, impairment or increased impairment of motor function and sensation, respiratory function, and autonomic nervous system function resulting in loss of vasomotor tone.
- The nurse should be able to state appropriate interventions that may be necessary if new or increased spinal cord injury occurs.

- A number of treatment options are available to manage cervical injuries. The specific treatment for a particular patient depends on the type of injury, the level of injury (e.g., C2 as compared with C6), the specific classification of the injury, and patient characteristics.
- Cervical spine traction is provided to realign, immobilize, and stabilize the cervical spine when it has become unstable as a result of a cervical spine fracture or dislocation caused by trauma or disease, degenerative processes of the cervical vertebrae, or spinal surgery (Fig. 97-1).[3,4] After initial medical stabilization of the patient and assessment and documentation of neurologic function, cervical skeletal traction with the tongs or halo ring can be applied to realign the cervical spine. Tongs or a halo ring may be used with cervical traction to reduce dislocation before the patient undergoes surgery. Occasionally, an unstable cervical spinal injury may necessitate long-term cervical traction for a period of weeks to attain realignment and immobilization to stabilize the spine. The definitive method used to treat cervical fractures depends on the injury classification and physician or institution preference.
- Tongs consist of a body with one pin attached at each end (Fig. 97-2). Tong pins are applied to the outer table of the skull on both sides of the skull. Cervical tongs are available in a variety of types, such as Crutchfield, Gardner-Wells, and Vinke tongs.

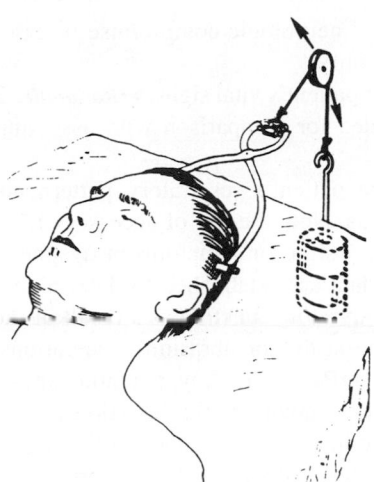

FIGURE 97-1 Continuous traction provided by weight applied to a cervical external fixation device via a rope and pulley system. *(From McRae R: Practical fracture treatment, ed 2, Edinburgh, 1989, Churchill Livingstone.)*

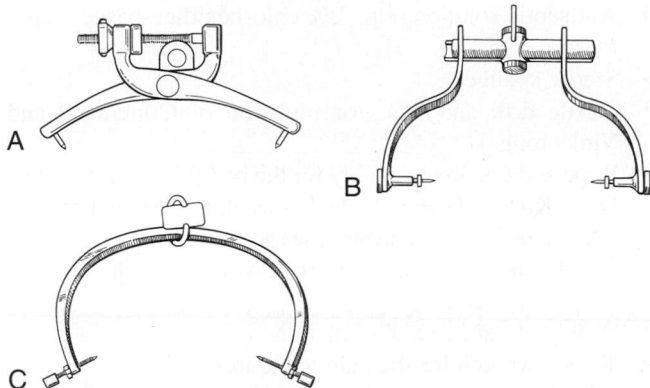

FIGURE 97-2 All three types of cervical tongs consist of a stainless steel body and a pin with a sharp tip attached to each end. **A,** Crutchfield tongs are placed about 5 inches apart in line with the long axis of the cervical spine. **B,** Vinke tongs are placed on the parietal bones, near the widest transverse diameter of the skull. **C,** Gardner-Wells tongs are inserted slightly above the patient's ears.

- The shape, features, insertion site, and placement vary slightly, but the purpose, principles, and care are the same. Physician preference is an important deciding factor in choosing the specific device to be used.[2,11]
- The insertion of Crutchfield and Vinke tongs necessitates an incision to expose the skull. Two holes are made in the outer table of the skull with a twist drill, and the pins are inserted and tightened until there is a firm fit.[2,11]
- Gardner-Wells tongs are inserted by placing the razor-sharp pin edges to the prepared areas of the scalp and tightening the screws until the spring-loaded mechanism indicates that the correct pressure has been achieved. To decrease the possibility of tong displacement, all types of pins are well seated into the outer table of the skull and angled inward.[2,6,11]
- Tongs are made of stainless steel or a graphite body with titanium pins. The graphite body with titanium pins is compatible with magnetic resonance imaging (MRI).
- Traction can be applied with the use of a rope and pulley system or a cable and alignment bracket. Weights are added gradually and followed with radiographic imaging. The physician uses serial radiographs of the cervical spine to assist in determining the optimal amount of traction (measured in pounds) needed to reduce a fracture and provide optimal alignment. Excessive traction may result in stretching of the spinal cord and subsequent damage.[2-4] The addition of traction is managed by the physician.
- Cervical traction also may be applied with a halo ring device. This is a stainless steel or graphite ring that is attached to the skull by four stabilizing pins (two anterior and two posterolateral; Fig. 97-3). Skull pins can be made of stainless steel, titanium, or ceramic material.[1,2,5,7] Pins are threaded through holes in the ring, screwed into the outer table of the skull, and locked into place. Traction can be applied to the ring device with the use of a rope and pulley system or a cable and bracket align-

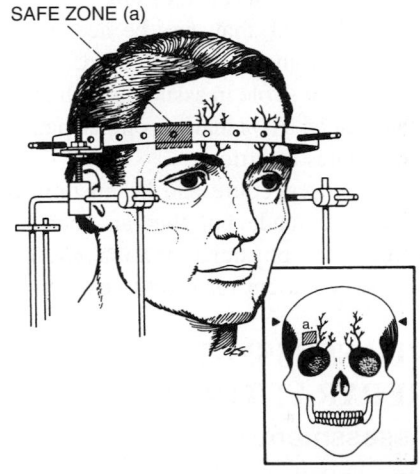

FIGURE 97-3 Placement of halo pins and ring. The anterior pins are placed anterolaterally 1 cm above the orbital ridge. This "safe zone" avoids the temporalis muscle laterally and an orbital nerve plexus and frontal sinus medially. *(From Batte M, et al: The halo skeletal fixator: principles of applications and maintenance, Clin Orthop 239:14, 1989.)*

ment system. Weights are added gradually. After alignment of the cervical spine is achieved, the spine can be immobilized by attaching the ring to a body vest or a custom molded body jacket. The patient then is able to move while the head and neck remain immobile.

EQUIPMENT

- Tongs or halo ring
- Insertion tray, including either the specific type of tongs to be used or the halo ring with insertion pins
- Local anesthetic: lidocaine, 1% to 2% (with or without epinephrine, depending on physician preference)
- Needles (18- and 23-gauge)
- Sterile and nonsterile gloves
- Gowns, masks, and eye shields

- Antiseptic solution (e.g., 2% chlorhexidine-based preparation)
- Sterile sponges
- Sterile drill and bits (for insertion of Crutchfield and Vinke tongs)
- Rope and traction assembly for the bed (If a KCI RotoRest Delta Kinetic Therapy™ bed is used, a cable and bracket alignment system is needed; see Procedure 100.)
- S and C hooks (to attach to the distal end of the rope for weight application)
- Weights to attach to the traction
- Torque wrench for the halo apparatus
  Additional equipment, as needed, includes the following:
- Hair clippers
- Emergency equipment

PATIENT AND FAMILY EDUCATION

- Explain the procedure and the reason for cervical traction. Clarify or reinforce information as needed by the patient or family. Discuss use of any special equipment, such as a special bed, that may be needed. →*Rationale:* Patient and family anxiety is decreased.
- Explain the patient's role in assisting with insertion of the tongs. →*Rationale:* Explanation elicits patient cooperation and facilitates insertion.
- Explain that the procedure can be uncomfortable when the incisions are made but that an anesthetic will be administered by the physician. →*Rationale:* This information prepares the patient for what to expect.

PATIENT ASSESSMENT AND PREPARATION

Patient Assessment

- Conduct a complete neurologic assessment that includes evaluation of cranial nerve function, motor strength of major muscles, sensation (assessment of light touch, pain, and proprioception, noting highest dermatome level), and deep tendon reflexes (biceps, triceps, patella, and Achilles) and superficial reflexes (abdominal and anal wink). →*Rationale:* Baseline data are provided for comparison of postinsertion assessments to determine the presence of neurologic compromise or extension of spinal cord injury.
- Assess the patient's vital signs. →*Rationale:* Baseline data are provided for comparison with assessments after insertion.
- Assess the patient's respiratory pattern and auscultate lung sounds. Note the use of accessory respiratory muscles and any signs or symptoms of dyspnea. →*Rationale:* Baseline data are established to determine any compromise to respiratory function as a result of the procedure.
- Inspect the scalp for abrasions, lacerations, or sites of infection. →*Rationale:* Any potential sites of infection that may contraindicate the insertion of a cervical fixation device into the infected area are identified.
- Assess the level of pain or discomfort and anxiety. →*Rationale:* Assessment establishes data for decision making regarding the need for analgesia or anxiolytics for comfort and cooperation during the insertion procedure.
- Assess for any allergies to an antiseptic agent, local anesthetic or analgesia and anxiolytics. →*Rationale:* Review of medication allergies before administration of a new medication decreases the chances of an allergic reaction.

Patient Preparation

- Ensure that the patient and family understand preprocedural teaching. Answer questions as they arise, and reinforce information as needed. →*Rationale:* Understanding of previously taught information is evaluated and reinforced.
- Verify correct patient with two identifiers. →*Rationale:* Prior to performing a procedure, the nurse should ensure the correct identification of the patient for the intended intervention.
- Ensure that informed consent has been obtained. →*Rationale:* Informed consent protects the rights of the patient and makes a competent decision possible for the patient.
- Perform a pre-procedure verification and time out, if nonemergent. →*Rationale:* Ensures patient safety.
- Ensure that the head of the bed is flat and that the patient's head is in a neutral position by whatever approved means (e.g., hard/rigid collar) have been instituted. →*Rationale:* This measure prevents mobilization of neck, which may increase the risk of injury or extension of spinal cord injury.

Procedure	for Assisting with Application of Tongs or Halo Ring for Cervical Traction	
Steps	**Rationale**	**Special Considerations**
1. Obtain a bed with an orthopedic traction frame, weights, and rope and pulley system attached to the bed or, if prescribed, obtain a KCI RotoRest Delta Kinetic Therapy™ bed with the wire and bracket alignment device.	Traction must be ready to reduce the potential for movement of the head and neck.	May require assistance from other departments; therefore, plan ahead to coordinate.

Procedure	for Assisting with Application of Tongs or Halo Ring for Cervical Traction—*Continued*	

Steps	Rationale	Special Considerations
2. **HH**		
3. **PE**		
4. Assist the physician with tong or halo ring insertion:	Facilitates the procedure.	Because of the high risk for extension of cervical injury, this procedure usually is performed by a neurosurgeon, who can respond rapidly if neurologic deterioration becomes evident.
A. Assist as needed with preparation of the pin sites (clipping a small area of scalp hair if indicated and cleansing with antiseptic solution).	Clipping the hair may prevent it from being trapped when the pins are inserted. Cleansing decreases skin surface bacteria.	
B. Assist if needed with draping the patient, leaving insertion sites exposed.	Aids in maintaining sterility.	
C. Assist as needed with local anesthesia administration.	Decreases patient discomfort during pin insertion.	
D. **HH**		All healthcare personnel involved in the procedure need to apply personal protective and sterile attire (e.g., fluid shield masks, eye shields, gowns, and sterile gloves).
E. Stabilize the patient's head and neck during the procedure.	Maintains alignment of the cervical spine and provides support to the injured areas.	Cervical stabilization can be maintained with the use of a rigid collar or other devices that prevent head rotation and neck flexion or extension. A soft collar is not considered a stabilizing device. The head and shoulder packs of the KCI RotoRest Delta Kinetic Therapy™ bed provide some cervical stability but should not be used as the primary means of stabilizing cervical spine fractures before, during, or after tong or halo insertion. Utmost care must be taken to prevent head and neck flexion or extension. Be prepared for the possibility of respiratory insufficiency, respiratory arrest, hypotension, or cardiac arrest.
F. Carefully follow institution policies regarding manual cervical spine immobilization.	Institutional policies may provide strict guidelines for nursing role in manual cervical spine immobilization during traction placement.	
5. Monitor the patient for changes in respiratory function, neurologic deterioration, and pain.	Identifies evidence of untoward effects or complications related to the procedure. Identifies need for analgesia.	In addition to untoward effects, the patient may need additional reassurance, support, sedation, and analgesia.
6. Follow hospital policy for pin site care (see Procedure 99).	Maintains asepsis.	
7. Assist with application and connection to traction as needed (see Procedure 100).		
A. Maintain the patient's head in a neutral position.	Ensures accurate and safe use of the traction.	

Procedure continues on following page

Procedure for Assisting with Application of Tongs or Halo Ring for Cervical Traction—*Continued*

Steps	Rationale	Special Considerations
B. Assist if needed with the application of prescribed weights.	Provides assistance.	
C. Ensure that weights are unobstructed and hanging freely.[2,8-11] (**Level E***)	Ensures safe use of equipment and maintains principles of traction.	
8. Discard used supplies in an appropriate receptacle.	Removes and safely discards used supplies.	
9. 🅷🅷		

Expected Outcomes

- Tong or halo ring device inserted
- Head and neck immobilized to allow for alignment, stabilization, and healing of fractures
- Prescribed amount of weight applied to tongs or halo
- Traction weights unobstructed and hanging freely
- Improved or stable neurologic function (motor and sensory)
- Patient discomfort minimized

Unexpected Outcomes

- Slippage of tongs or halo pins
- Extension or deterioration of neurologic deficits or spinal cord injury
- Respiratory compromise or arrest
- Hypotensive episode
- Pain
- Bleeding at pin site

Patient Monitoring and Care

Steps	Rationale	Reportable Conditions
		These conditions should be reported if they persist despite nursing interventions.
1. Assess neurological status every 5 minutes during the procedure, including assessment of level of consciousness, movement in arms and legs, sensation, mastication, and eyelid closure.[2,5,7] (**Level E***)	Facilitates early recognition of neurologic deterioration. Bitemporal tongs may interfere with mastication and eyelid closure.[2,5,7]	- Any deterioration or extension of baseline neurologic function (e.g., loss of more dermatomal sensation; decrease in motor strength)
2. Assess respiratory function (respiratory rate, pulse oximetry, lung sounds) before, during, and after the procedure.	Early identification of hypoxia or respiratory distress from neurologic deterioration or other potential complications such as aspiration or oversedation. Decrease in peripheral oxygen saturation may be an early indicator of respiratory compromise.	- Changes in respiratory function (e.g., decrease in oxygen saturation [Sao_2], increase or decrease in respiratory rate, abnormal lung sounds)
3. Provide emotional support and reassurance to the patient during the procedure.	Decreases anxiety and facilitates patient cooperation.	- Unrelieved anxiety
4. Monitor pin sites for hemostasis immediately after the procedure, every 15 minutes × four, every 30 minutes × two, and hourly, or as indicated by institution policy.	The scalp is vascular, and continued bleeding may occur at the pin sites that requires assessment and cleansing.[5,6]	- Evidence of bleeding

*Level E: Multiple case reports, theory-based evidence from expert opinions, or peer-reviewed professional organizational standards without clinical studies to support recommendations

Patient Monitoring and Care —*Continued*

Steps	Rationale	Reportable Conditions
5. Check the security of the traction, bed frame, and bed.	The traction frame is attached to the bed and must be secure.	• Break in the integrity of the traction equipment or the bed frame
6. Maintain the patient's head flat on the bed and ensure that the bed is flat. The head of the bed frame may be on shock blocks or placed in reverse Trendelenburg's position to provide countertraction.[8,9]	The head must be flat on the bed to maintain a neutral position. Countertraction is often provided to prevent the patient from being pulled toward the top of the bed.	• Neck or head twisted or out of neutral alignment
7. If the knot on the traction rope nears the pulley or the wire band nears the bracket, several healthcare providers may slowly pull the patient down in bed. The patient should *never* be pulled up in the bed or traction will be released. Do *not* remove the weights to move the patient toward the foot of the bed.[8-11] **(Level E*)**	The knot of the traction rope must not be resting against the pulley for effective traction. The cover over the wire and bracket alignment device must not be against the alignment screw (head of the bed) for effective traction.	• Evidence of loss of effective traction
8. If cervical traction is lost for whatever reason (e.g., the loop in traction rope holding the weights slips or the pins dislodge), maintain manual cervical spine immobilization, place the patient in a hard/rigid cervical collar, and notify the physician. Elicit the patient's cooperation to minimize extraneous movement.	Immediate intervention is needed to immobilize the patient's head and neck.	• Neurologic or respiratory deterioration • Evidence of loss of effective traction
9. Prepare the patient for a bedside confirmatory radiograph of the cervical spine immediately after insertion and application of weights and as prescribed by the physician.	A radiograph is taken to verify alignment of the cervical spine.	• Abnormal radiographic results
10. If additional weights are added or removed by the physician in an attempt to realign the cervical spine, increase the frequency of neurologic checks. Expect more frequent cervical radiographs or MRI to verify alignment.[2,3]	Monitors for possible risk for secondary spinal cord injury.	• Neurologic or respiratory deterioration
11. Follow institution standard for assessing pain. Administer analgesia as prescribed.	Identifies need for pain interventions.	• Continued pain despite pain interventions

*Level E: Multiple case reports, theory-based evidence from expert opinions, or peer-reviewed professional organizational standards without clinical studies to support recommendations

Procedure continues on following page

Documentation

Documentation should include the following:
- Patient and family education
- Completion of informed consent
- Pre-procedure verifications and time out
- Type of cervical traction applied
- Date and time traction applied
- Local anesthetic used
- Sedation and analgesia used
- Amount of weight applied to the traction
- Weights hanging freely
- Pins secure
- Appearance of pin insertion site and care

- Ongoing comprehensive assessment data and action taken for abnormal response
- Verification of proper functioning and security of traction equipment
- Occurrence of unexpected outcomes
- Patient response to care
- Additional interventions
- Pain assessment, interventions, and effectiveness

References

1. Bono CM: The halo fixator, *J Am Acad Orthop Surg* 15:728-737, 2007.
2. Canale ST, Beaty JH: Cervical spine injuries. In Canale ST, Beaty JH, editors: *Campbell's operative orthopaedics* [electronic resource], ed 11, Philadelphia, 2008, Mosby, 1776-1777.
CR 3. Congress of Neurological Surgeons: Initial closed reduction of cervical spine fracture-dislocation injuries, *Neurosurgery* 50(Suppl 3):S44-S50, 2002.
CR 4. Congress of Neurological Surgeons: Treatment of subaxial cervical spine injuries, *Neurosurgery* 50(Suppl 3):S156-S165, 2002.
CR 5. Hayes VM, Silber JS, Siddiqu FN, et al: Complications of halo fixation of the cervical spine, *Am J Orthop* 34: 271-276, 2005.
6. Hickey JV: Vertebral and spinal cord injuries. In Hickey JV, editor: *The clinical practice of neurological and neurosurgical nursing,* ed 6, Philadelphia, 2009, Wolters Kluwer Health/Lippincott Williams & Wilkins, 410-453.
CR 7. Kang M, Vives MJ, Vaccaro AR: The halo vest: principles of application and management of complications, *J Spinal Cord Med* 26:186-192, 2003.
CR 8. Osmond T: Principles of traction, *Aust Nurs J* 6(Suppl): 1-4, 1999.
CR 9. Styrcula L: Traction basics: part I, *Orthop Nurs* 13(2): 71-74 1994.
CR 10. Styrcula L: Traction basics: part II, *Orthop Nurs* 13(3): 55-59, 1994.
CR 11. Styrcula L: Traction basics: part III, *Orthop Nurs* 13(4): 34-44, 1994.

Additional Readings

CR Davis A: Sensory and motor disorders. In Kinney MR, et al, editors: *AACN clinical reference for critical care nursing*, ed 4, St Louis, 1998, Mosby, 711.
CR Jerome Cervical Spine System: *Application instructions for Jerome Halo Traction Systems,* Morristown, NJ, 2003, Jerome Cervical Spine System.
CR Lee TT, Green BA: Advances in the management of acute spinal cord injury, *Orthop Clin North Am* 33:311-315, 2002.
CR Maher AB, Salmond SW, Pellino TA: *Orthopedic nursing,* ed 3, Philadelphia, 2002, Saunders, 296.
CR McCloskey JC, Bulechek GM, editors: *Iowa Intervention Project: nursing interventions classification (NIC),* ed 3, St Louis, 2000, Mosby.
CR Mollabashy A: Immobilization techniques in cervical spine injury: cervical orthoses, skeletal traction, and halo devices, *Top Emerg Med* 19:3, 1997.

Halo Ring and Vest Care

P U R P O S E : A halo ring attached to a halo vest (commonly referred to as a halo) is designed to immobilize and stabilize the cervical spine. A halo ring and vest may be used alone or in conjunction with surgery for the patient with an unstable cervical spine, as a result of spinal fracture or dislocation; degenerative processes, such as C1-C2 changes from rheumatoid arthritis; or spinal surgery. With the use of the halo ring and vest, vertebral column movement is prevented and subsequent risk of the injury to the spinal cord is reduced.[2] The halo ring and vest may be used as a primary definitive treatment to stabilize the cervical spine, before surgery to reduce spine deformity, or after surgery as an adjunct to interval cervical fixation. This procedure focuses on the management of the patient who needs immobilization with a halo ring and vest.

Mary Hanson

PREREQUISITE NURSING KNOWLEDGE

- Knowledge of neuroanatomy and physiology is necessary.
- The nurse needs to be knowledgeable about the anatomy and physiology of the spinal column, the special anatomy of the cervical vertebrae, the spinal cord, and the cervical spinal nerves and their areas of peripheral innervation. In addition, the nurse must understand the pathophysiology and manifestations of spinal cord trauma, including spinal shock, ascending edema, and related impairment of respiratory function, vasomotor tone, and autonomic nervous system function.
- The nurse must be knowledgeable about the signs and symptoms of new injury or extension of spinal cord injury and the needed interventions.
- Immobilization assists in maintenance of vertebral alignment. In the case of an unstable vertebral column, it also reduces the risk for new injury to the spinal cord.
- A number of treatment options are available to manage cervical injuries. The specific treatment for a particular patient depends on the type of injury, the level of injury (e.g., C2 as compared with C6), the specific classification of the injury, and patient characteristics.

- A halo ring device is a graphite ring attached to the skull with four stabilizing pins (two anterior and two posterolateral; see Fig. 97-3). The pins are threaded through holes in the ring, screwed into the outer table of the skull, and locked into place.
- Direct traction may be applied to the halo ring device with a rope and pulley or cable and bracket alignment system and weights (see Procedures 97 and 100). Patients with a halo ring, pins, and traction applied with weights are cared for similarly to patients in cervical traction with tongs (see Procedures 97 and 100).
- When alignment of the cervical spine is achieved, long-term immobilization of the spine can be achieved by attaching the ring to a body vest or a custom molded body jacket, which allows for mobility of the patient (Fig. 98-1).[2,3]
- With the halo ring and pins in place, traction can be discontinued and a halo vest and struts added for long-term immobilization of the cervical neck (see Fig. 98-1). The advantage of this approach is that the patient can sit upright, mobilize out of bed, and ambulate, if able, while the cervical spine remains stable.
- The nurse must be familiar with the components of the halo-vest device, including the halo ring and pins,

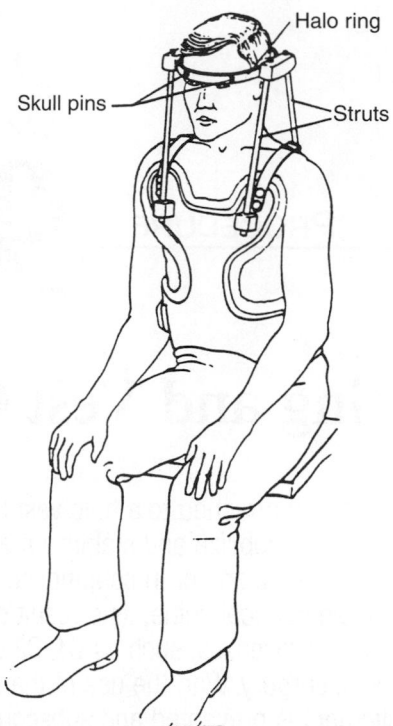

Skull pins — Halo ring — Struts

FIGURE 98-1 Halo-vest apparatus. Supportive struts and ring are attached to a plastic vest, applying cervical traction while allowing for patient mobility. *(From Coalbert MF, Kincaide SL: Halo immobilization device. In Kincaide SL, Lohrman J, editors: Critical care nursing procedures, Philadelphia, 1990, BC Decker, 286.)*

anterior and posterior posts, vest screws, front and back panels of the vest, and shoulder and side buckles.

- Basic cardiac life support knowledge and skills are essential.
- It is important that the nurse knows how to access the patient's anterior chest to administer cardiopulmonary resuscitation (CPR) if cardiac arrest occurs. Refer to information from the manufacturer of the halo vest for specific information on emergency access to the chest. Some vests have a hinged closure; the vest can be lifted up at the hinge to allow quick access to the chest. Other vests are not hinged and require a wrench. The wrench must be available at all times and, depending on institution policy, may be maintained on the front of the vest for instant access to the chest. If the patient needs defibrillation, avoid touching the bars of the traction with the defibrillator.
- The halo-vest side panels may be opened only when the patient is flat and supine.[2,5,8] Unbuckling of the halo vest may result in loss of spine alignment and neurologic compromise.[8] Follow manufacturer's recommendations and institution policies for opening the vest.
- Because the halo vest limits movement of the head, patients must be taught to scan the environment for objects in their path that could lead to falls.
- The halo vest changes the center of gravity and limits movement, thus requiring adaptations for performing activities of daily living (ADLs).[8]

EQUIPMENT

- Halo device (in place)
- Soap and a basin of warm water
- Washcloth and towel
- Alcohol
- Nonsterile gloves
- Flashlight
    Additional equipment to have as needed include the following:
- Sheepskin liner
- Emergency wrench

PATIENT AND FAMILY EDUCATION

- Explain that the reason for the halo ring and vest device is to maintain cervical immobilization. **➤➤Rationale:** Patient and family anxiety is decreased.
- Describe turning, positioning, and skin care procedures before performing them. **➤➤Rationale:** Patient and family anxiety is decreased.
- If the patient is ambulatory, explain modifications in meeting basic needs such as bathing, toileting, eating, dressing, ambulation precautions, and safety needs. **➤➤Rationale:** Self-care skills and awareness of special safety precautions are developed.
- For patients who will be discharged home wearing a halo-vest device, begin a comprehensive teaching program with the patient and family. **➤➤Rationale:** The patient and family are prepared for care in the home environment.
- Explain to the patient and family that the patient cannot be turned with the struts (posts) of the halo-vest device. **➤➤Rationale:** The patient and family are prepared for care in the home environment.
- Explain that precautions must be used when the ambulatory patient with a halo-vest device gets in and out of a car and walks up and down stairs. **➤➤Rationale:** The patient cannot move the head in the halo-vest device to look down.
- Explain that driving, riding a motorcycle or bicycle, and operating machinery are unsafe with a halo-vest device. **➤➤Rationale:** Patients recognize that they cannot turn their head.
- Explain that the pins of the halo transmit vibration and cold sensation to the patient's skull. **➤➤Rationale:** The patient and family are alerted to possible sensations during ADLs.
- Explain that if the pins or screws become loose, the patient should contact the physician immediately. Inform the patient and family not to adjust the pins or screws. **➤➤Rationale:** The patient and family are prepared for care in the home and can identify when emergency care may be needed.
- Explain that if the patient has any decline in neurologic function (i.e., decreased or abnormal sensory function; decline in motor ability; or increase in pain), the physician should be contacted immediately. **➤➤Rationale:** Decline in neurologic function may indicate extension of spinal cord injury and the need for immediate interventions.

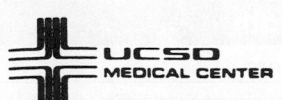

**SPINAL CORD INJURY
ASSESSMENT**

KEY

Sensory: Motor: (Indicate best response)
  S - sharp   0 - none
  D - dull   1 - trace
  H - hyperesthesia   2 - not greater than gravity
  O - absent   3 - greater than gravity
                   4 - slight weakness
                   5 - normal

Source _____ Date _____

Patient Identification

	TIME		06		07		08		09		10		11		12		13		14		15	
			R	L	R	L	R	L	R	L	R	L	R	L	R	L	R	L	R	L	R	L
MOTOR	Shoulder Abduct	C5																				
	Elbow Flexion	C5-C6																				
	Elbow Extension	C7																				
	Wrist Dorsiflexion	C6-7																				
	Thumb-Index Pinch	C7																				
	Hand Grasp	C8																				
	Hip Flexion	L2-3-4																				
	Knee Flexion	L5-S1																				
	Knee Extension	L2-4																				
	Foot Dorsiflex	L5																				
	Foot Plantarflex	S1																				
SENSORY	Cervical	5																				
		6																				
		7																				
		8																				
	Thoracic	1																				
		2																				
		4																				
		5																				
		12																				
	Lumbar	1																				
		2																				
		3																				
		4																				
		5																				
	Sacral	1																				
		2																				
		3, 4, 5																				
	Position	Big Toe																				
	+ −	Index Finger																				
	Deep Pain Big Toe																					
	Initials of Examiner																					

FIGURE 98-2 Sample of flow sheet documentation form for motor and sensory testing. *(From University of California–San Diego Medical Center.)*

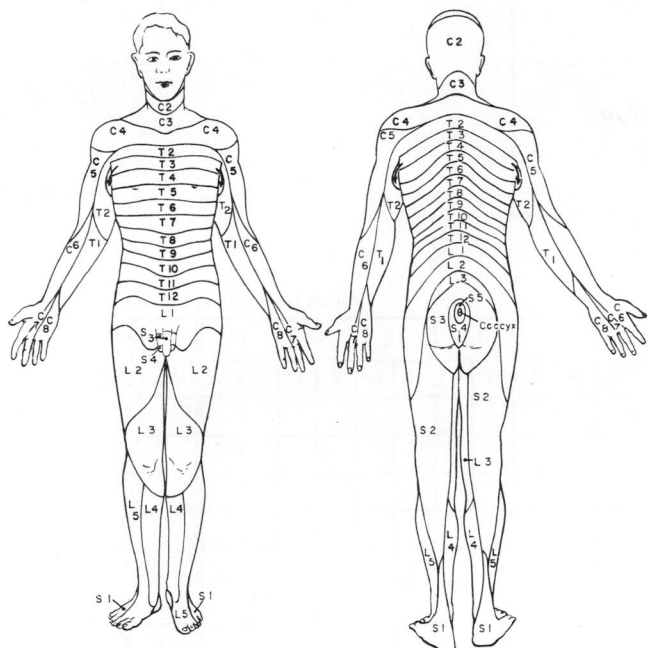

FIGURE 98-3   Sensory dermatomes: guidelines for sensory testing. *(From Barr ML, Kiernan JA: The human nervous system: an anatomical viewpoint, ed 5, Philadelphia, 1988, JB Lippincott, 81.)*

TABLE 98-1	Assessment of Muscle Strength
Motor Score	**Indicators**
5	Normal muscle strength; can maintain high degree of function against maximal resistance.
4	The muscle can go through its normal range of motion, but it can be overcome by increased resistance.
3	The muscle can go through its normal range of motion against gravity only; it cannot tolerate external resistance.
2	The muscle contracts weakly; it does not have sufficient strength to overcome gravity.
1	Visible or palpable muscle contractions may be seen or felt, but no movement is found in the limb.
0	Complete paralysis; no evidence of motor function.

(Adapted from Hickey J: The clinical practice of neurological and neurosurgical nursing, ed 4, Philadelphia, 1997, JB Lippincott.)

PATIENT ASSESSMENT AND PREPARATION

Patient Assessment

- Perform a complete neurologic assessment, including muscle strength and sensation[1] (Figs. 98-2 and 98-3; Table 98-1) before and after halo ring and vest placement and at intervals as prescribed or as designated by institutional protocols thereafter. ➤➤*Rationale:* Baseline data are provided.
- Obtain vital signs before halo ring and vest placement. ➤➤*Rationale:* Baseline data are provided.
- Assess for difficulty swallowing and risk for aspiration.[4,11] ➤➤*Rationale:* Assessment identifies a patient at high risk and the need to modify oral intake.
- Assess the skin at the edges of the vest and where the vest may overlap for redness or abrasion, especially over bony prominences.[8,11] ➤➤*Rationale:* Skin irritation related to the halo-vest device is identified.
- Check the fit of the vest for tightness or looseness. ➤➤*Rationale:* The need for change or modification of the vest is identified. Patient weight loss may contribute to vest looseness.

- Check the halo vest for loose straps or screws, dirt, odor, or evidence of the need to repair the vest. ➤➤*Rationale:* The vest may need to be repaired or the sheepskin liner changed.

Patient Preparation

- Ensure that the patient and family understand preprocedural teaching. Answer questions as they arise, and reinforce information as needed. ➤➤*Rationale:* Understanding of previously taught information is evaluated and reinforced.
- Verify correct patient with two identifiers. ➤➤*Rationale:* Prior to performing a procedure, the nurse should ensure the correct identification of the patient for the intended intervention.
- Assist patients as they lie supine in a neutral position with proper body alignment for the purpose of halo vest application, liner change, and routine skin care. ➤➤*Rationale:* Patients are kept safe and accessible for inspection.
- Observe the sides and back of the vest and adjacent skin with the patient standing, if possible. ➤➤*Rationale:* Observation provides an opportunity to inspect all areas in which the skin and vest come in contact.

Procedure | for Halo Ring and Vest Care

Steps	Rationale	Special Considerations
1. **HH**		
2. **PE**		
3. If unbuckling is prescribed for vest care, position the patient flat in bed on his or her side; then unbuckle one side of the halo vest while maintaining cervical spinal alignment.[2,8] (**Level E***)	Gains access to the underlying skin.	Review the manufacturer's recommendations with regard to vest care. Follow institution policy with regard to vest care.
4. Assess the patient's skin. Use a flashlight while pressing the liner toward the vest to facilitate assessment of the skin.	Determines skin integrity.[8,11]	Insensate patients may be more vulnerable to skin breakdown. The halo vest should fit snugly but not cause skin breakdown or discomfort over pressure areas. The fit of the halo and the sheepskin liner is checked daily. The sheepskin should be smooth and without wrinkles and extend to the edges of the vest to protect the skin from abrasions. The sternum, ribs, scapulae, and clavicle areas are especially at high risk for skin breakdown.
5. Bathe the skin with soap and water. Alcohol may also be used. Minimize moisture to avoid wetting the liner of the vest. If unbuckling the vest is not recommended by manufacturer or institutional policy, pass a damp thin towel between the skin and sheepskin, reaching all skin surfaces.[8]	Cleanses the skin. Alcohol does not leave a film like soap and water; it also leaves a cool, clean feeling to the skin.	Dry the skin thoroughly and avoid excessive lotion or powder; these agents tend to mat the sheepskin liner.
6. Auscultate lung sounds.	Identifies adventitious breath sounds.	Lung sounds may be decreased at the bases in patients with poor diaphragm and intercostal muscle function.[1]
7. Perform anterior and posterior chest physiotherapy, if indicated.	May enhance secretion maintenance and facilitate airway clearance.	A slight decrease in vital capacity related to vest placement may be seen.[11]
8. Rebuckle the vest.[7,8] (**Level E**)	Maintains cervical immobilization.	Ensure that the buckle is secured for proper fit.
9. Turn the patient to the opposite side, keep the head of the bed flat, and **repeat Steps 3 to 8.**[1,2,8,11] (**Level E**)	Facilitates assessment of the opposite side of the patient's body.	

*Level E: Multiple case reports, theory-based evidence from expert opinions, or peer-reviewed professional organizational standards without clinical studies to support recommendations

Procedure continues on following page

Procedure for Halo Ring and Vest Care—*Continued*		
Steps	**Rationale**	**Special Considerations**
10. If unbuckling is prescribed, change or assist with changing the anterior sheepskin liner as needed:	Provides comfort and cleanliness and protects the skin.	Follow institution standard for liner change. The anterior portion of the sheepskin liner may require frequent changes because of secretions or drainage from a tracheostomy or from spills during eating.[8] Protect the sheepskin liner during meals and use towels and plastic when washing the hair to minimize the need to change the liner.[8] Follow manufacturer's recommendations and institutional policy regarding washing, reusing, or discarding the liner.
A. Place the patient supine with the head of the bed flat.	Provides support and alignment	
B. Unbuckle one side strap on the vest while maintaining cervical spine alignment and immobilization.	Provides access to the sheepskin.	
C. Roll the soiled liner on the unbuckled portion of the anterior vest to the center of the vest to facilitate removal of the sheepskin.	Simplifies the liner change.	
D. Match half the clean liner to the corresponding portion of the anterior vest and roll the remainder to the center of the vest.		
E. Buckle the side strap of the vest.	Maintains cervical immobilization.	
F. Unbuckle the other side strap and remove the remainder of the soiled liner.		
G. Unroll the clean liner and match to the corresponding Velcro strips on the vest.		
H. Buckle the side strap.		
11. Change or assist with changing the posterior sheepskin liner as needed:	Promotes comfort and protects the skin.	Follow institution standard for liner change.
A. Position the patient with the head of the bed flat and the patient turned to the side-lying position. Alternately, the patient can be turned prone with a pillow under the chest and a pillow under the head if the patient's respiratory status tolerates this position.	Provides support and protects the skin.	

Procedure	**for Halo Ring and Vest Care**—*Continued*	
Steps	**Rationale**	**Special Considerations**
B. Unbuckle one side strap of the halo vest while maintaining cervical spine alignment and immobilization.	Provides support and alignment.	
C. Roll the soiled liner on the unbuckled portion of the posterior vest to the center of the vest to facilitate removal of sheepskin.	Simplifies the liner change.	
D. Match half the clean liner to the corresponding portion of the posterior vest and roll the remainder to the center of the vest.	Provides comfort and protects the skin.	
E. Buckle the side strap of the vest.	Maintain cervical immobilization.	
F. Roll the patient to the opposite side.	Maintains cervical spine alignment.	
G. Unbuckle the side strap on the vest while maintaining cervical spine alignment and immobilization. Remove the remainder of the soiled liner.	Accesses the opposite side of the liner.	
H. Unroll the clean liner and match to the corresponding Velcro strips on the vest.	Secures the liner in place.	
I. Buckle the side strap.	Maintains cervical immobilization.	
12. Discard used supplies in an appropriate receptacle.	Removes and safely discards used supplies.	
13. **HH**		

Expected Outcomes

- Cervical alignment is maintained
- The underlying skin remains intact and free of irritation
- The vest is functional, fits well, and is clean and odorless
- The pin sites are clean
- Mobility and sensation are maintained if the patient is neurologically intact
- The patient's safety is maintained

Unexpected Outcomes

- Loose pins[4,6]
- Pin site infection, osteomyelitis, or intracranial abscess[4,6,10]
- Poor fit (too loose or too tight) of halo vest or body jacket
- Skin breakdown or irritation under or around the vest[4,6]
- Persistent spinal instability and loss of vertebral alignment[4,6]
- New or worsened injury to the spinal cord caused by spine mobility[4,6]
- New or additional loss of neurologic function
- Orthostatic hypotension
- Respiratory distress
- Injury from fall during ambulation with a halo vest

Procedure continues on following page

Patient Monitoring and Care

Steps	Rationale	Reportable Conditions
		These conditions should be reported if they persist despite nursing interventions.
1. Assess motor and sensory function immediately after application of the halo vest and every 2 to 4 hours per institution standard.	Determines neurological status.	• Any deterioration from baseline neurologic function (e.g., loss of more dermatomal sensation; decrease in motor strength)
2. Monitor for dyspnea, hypoxia, or decreasing tidal volumes (monitor pulse oximetry and measure tidal volumes).	Assesses for hypoxia or respiratory distress from extension of neurologic dysfunction or compromised respiratory function from vest constriction. A decrease in peripheral oxygen saturation or a decrease in tidal volume may be early indicators of respiratory compromise.[2,11]	• Decreased oxygen saturation • Decreased tidal volumes from baseline • Dyspnea
3. Follow institution standard for assessing pain. Administer analgesia as prescribed.	Identifies need for pain interventions.	• Continued pain despite pain interventions
4. Monitor for dysphagia.	Dysphagia is a possible side effect of cervical immobilization with a halo vest and can be associated with altered nutritional status and aspiration.[3,4,6,11]	• Dysphagia
5. Check the fit of the vest, especially if the patient has lost or gained a significant amount of weight.[2,8]	The vest may be too big if significant weight loss occurs or too small if improperly fitted originally or if the patient gains weight.	• Inability to securely fit the vest
6. At least once each shift, observe the skin at the edges of the vest and where the vest may overlap. Replace the vest liner if it is wet or soiled.[2,8]	Promotes comfort and skin integrity.	• Skin irritation noted; the liner is wet or dirty and needs replacement • Call the physician to replace the liner per institution standard.
7. Wash exposed skin with warm water and soap; rinse well and dry. Be careful not to wet the liner.	Maintains cleanliness of the skin and protects the liner.	• Any assistance needed with the liner replacement
8. Provide pin care (see Procedure 99).[7,9,10] **(Level C*)**	Monitors pin sites and prevents infection.	• Evidence of infection
9. Check the integrity of the halo, pins, struts, and vest.[8]	Provides for safe use of equipment and appropriate therapy.	• Any break in the integrity of the equipment
10. Move the patient and the halo vest as a unit to avoid pressure that may dislodge the pins. Never use the anterior or posterior struts (posts) that attach the halo to the vest for moving a patient.[9]	Prevents dislodgment of pins and injury.	• Evidence of dislodgment of pins or the halo
11. Support the patient with pillows when positioning the patient in the proper body alignment.	Provides comfort and prevents dislodgment of the halo-vest device. A pillow behind the patient's head decreases the patient's sensation of being suspended.	• Evidence of dislodgment of the pins or halo

Patient Monitoring and Care —*Continued*

Steps	Rationale	Reportable Conditions
12. Discuss possible changes in body image related to the halo-vest device; provide emotional support.[9]	A dramatic change in body image occurs with the wearing of the halo-vest device and needs to be acknowledged.	• Maladaptation to altered body image
13. Discuss safety in ambulation and fall prevention (e.g., scanning with eyes to compensate for inability to move head; walking more slowly).[9]	Because of the immobilization of the head and neck, the patient is at risk for falls. Consider recommendation of a physical therapy consult.	• Patient fall
14. Follow manufacturer's recommendations and institution policies for obtaining immediate access to the chest in event of an emergency. (Some devices have an anterior vest with a bendable CPR hinge, and some require a wrench for vest removal in emergencies. Keep the wrench readily available at all times.)	Supports basic safety procedures.	• Hemodynamic instability necessitating opening the vest

*Level C: Qualitative studies, descriptive or correlational studies, integrative reviews, systematic reviews, or randomized controlled trials with inconsistent results

Documentation

Documentation should include the following:

- Patient and family education
- Date, time, and name of the physician applying halo vest
- Skin and pin assessment
- Integrity of the vest
- Neurologic (motor/sensory assessment) and pulmonary assessment (tidal volume, pulse oximetry)
- Liner changes
- Date and time of chest physiotherapy performed
- Occurrence of unexpected outcomes
- Patient response to care
- Additional interventions
- Pain assessment, interventions, and effectiveness

References

1. Blissitt PA: Spinal cord injury. In Carlson KK, editor: *Advanced critical care nursing,* Philadelphia, 2009, Saunders, 637-680.
2. Bono CM: The halo fixator, *J Am Acad Orthop Surg* 15:728-737, 2007.
3. Canale ST, Beaty JH: Cervical spine injuries. In Canale ST, Beaty, JH, editors: *Campbell's operative orthopaedics,* ed 11, Philadelphia, 2008, Mosby, 1776-1777.
CR 4. Hayes VM, Silber JS, Siddiqi FN, et al: Complications of halo fixation of the cervical spine, *Am J Orthop* 34:271-276, 2005.
CR 5. Jerome Medical: *Application instructions for Jerome halo traction systems,* Moorestown, NJ, 2003, Jerome Medical.
CR 6. Kang M, Vives MJ, Vaccaro AR: The halo vest: principles of application and management of complications, *J Spinal Cord Med* 26:186-192, 2003.
7. Lethaby A, Temple J, Santy J: Pin site care for preventing infections associated with external bone fixators and pins, *Cochrane Database Syst Rev* 4:CD004551, 2008.
CR 8. Patchen SJ, Timyan L, Atherton S: *Your life in a halo made easier,* Miami and Moorestown, NJ, 2002, University of Miami School of Medicine and Jerome Medical.
CR 9. Patterson MM: Multicenter pin care study, *Orthop Nurs* 24:349-360, 2005.
10. Saeed MU, Dacuycuy MA, Kennedy DJ: Halo pin insertion-associated brain abscess: case report and review of the literature, *Spine* 32:E271-E274, 2007.
11. Taitsman LA, Altman DT, Hecht AC, et al: Complications of cervical halo-vest orthoses in elderly patients, *Orthopedics* 31:446, 2008.

Additional Readings

CR Bernardo LM: Evidence-based practice for pin site care in injured children, *Orthop Nurs* 20:29-34, 2001.
CR McKenzie LL: In search of a standard for pin site care, *Orthop Nurs* 18:73-78, 1999.

Pin Site Care: Cervical Tongs and Halo Pins

P U R P O S E :   Tong and halo pin site care is provided to cleanse and remove exudate from pin sites in an effort to minimize the risk of infection. In addition, pin site care allows assessment of the pin sites for signs and symptoms of infection and pin loosening or displacement.

Mary Hanson

PREREQUISITE NURSING KNOWLEDGE

- The nurse needs to be knowledgeable about the anatomy and physiology of the spinal column, the special anatomy of the cervical vertebrae, the spinal cord, the cervical spinal nerves, and their areas of peripheral innervation. In addition, the nurse must understand the pathophysiology and manifestations of spinal cord injury, including the concepts of primary and secondary spinal cord injury and spinal shock.
- The nurse needs to be knowledgeable of the signs and symptoms of new spinal cord injury or extension of recent spinal cord injury, including impairment of motor and sensory function, respiratory function, and autonomic nervous system function that results in loss of vasomotor tone.
- The nurse needs to be knowledgeable of treatment options available to manage cervical injuries, including cervical spine traction with tongs or a halo ring. Tongs consist of a body with one pin attached at each end (see Fig. 97-2). Tong pins are applied to the outer table of the cranium on both sides of the skull.[3] A halo ring device is also used for management of cervical injuries. This device is a graphite ring that is attached to the skull with four stabilizing pins (two anterior and two posterolateral; see Fig. 98-1). The pins are threaded through holes in the ring, screwed into the outer table of the skull, and locked into place. This device can be attached to traction or vest struts/posts.[2]
- Once inserted, the cervical device (tongs or halo ring) requires special care of the skin at the pin insertion sites (pin site care) to prevent and monitor for infection. Because the pins are inserted through the skin and into the bone, local infections can develop and proliferate and may result in cranial osteomyelitis. Loosening of the pins may also occur.[3-6]
- Various cleansing agents for pin site care have been used, including, but not limited to, 2% chlorhexidene solution, hydrogen peroxide, sterile normal saline solution, antibacterial soap and water, alcohol, and povidone-iodine. None have been found superior.[5,7-10]
- Generally, pin sites do not require a dressing unless excessive drainage occurs at the site.
- Pin sites should be inspected for infection, although the frequency of this inspection has not been clearly identified. Definitive guidelines for the frequency of pin site care, cleansing agents, removal of crust, and the application of dressings have not been established and depend on institutional policies.[7,8]

EQUIPMENT

- Approximately eight cotton-tipped applicators
- Nonsterile gloves
- Cleansing or antiseptic solution
- Sterile container for cleansing solution
- Rinsing solution (as needed)
- Second sterile container for rinsing solution (as needed)
  Additional equipment, to have available as needed, includes the following:
- Hair clippers
- Dressing supplies
- Light source to assist with visualization of posterior pin sites

PATIENT AND FAMILY EDUCATION

- Explain the procedure and the reason for pin care. ➤*Rationale:* Patient and family anxiety may be decreased.
- Explain the patient's role in assisting with the procedure. ➤*Rationale:* Explanation elicits patient cooperation and facilitates the procedure.
- Teach the family if they will perform pin site care for the patient after discharge. ➤*Rationale:* Education elicits family cooperation and comfort in performing the procedure.
- Teach the family to notify the physician if the pins are loose. Teach the family not to adjust the pins. ➤*Rationale:* Safe and appropriate action is elicited.

PATIENT ASSESSMENT AND PREPARATION

Patient Assessment

- Assess the patient's scalp for signs and symptoms of skin irritation; carefully inspect the pin sites for signs and symptoms of infection (e.g., redness, edema, or purulent drainage). ➤*Rationale:* Assessment identifies skin breakdown, irritation, or pin-site infection.
- Assess the patient's pain and anxiety levels. ➤*Rationale:* Interventions may be needed before the procedure to promote patient comfort and decrease anxiety.

Patient Preparation

- Ensure that the patient and family understand preprocedural teaching. Answer questions as they arise, and reinforce information as needed. ➤*Rationale:* Understanding of previously taught information is evaluated and reinforced.
- Verify correct patient with two identifiers. ➤*Rationale:* Prior to performing a procedure, the nurse should ensure the correct identification of the patient for the intended intervention.
- Assist the patient to a supine position. The patient in a halo vest may be sitting up in a position of comfort. ➤*Rationale:* Access to the pins is facilitated for care.

Procedure for Pin Site Care: Cervical Tong and Halo Pins		
Steps	**Rationale**	**Special Considerations**
1. **HH**		
2. **PE**		
3. Prepare the cleansing or antiseptic solution as defined by institution policy in a sterile container. **(Level C*)**	Prepares the cleansing or antiseptic solution for pin care. No cleansing agent has been determined to be superior.[5,7-10]	Solutions may be kept in a covered sterile container for 24 hours. Label with the name of the solution and the date and time the solution was prepared.
4. If needed (after soap or peroxide) place a small amount of rinsing solution (e.g., water or sterile normal saline in a second sterile container.)	Prepares the solution for rinsing off the cleansing solution. No rinsing agent has been determined to be superior.[5,7-10]	This step is not needed if an antiseptic solution is used.
5. Cleanse the area around each pin insertion site with a cotton-tipped swab saturated with cleansing solution. Clean in a single sweeping motion, and then discard the swab. Gently repeat as needed with a new swab each time. Use separate swabs for each site to decrease the chance of cross contamination.[1]	Removes drainage, prevents excessive exudates, and cleanses the area.	Serous drainage may be present the first 2 to 3 days after insertion.
6. If needed, rinse the site with cotton-tipped swabs with the rinsing solution specified by institutional policy.	Removes the cleansing solution and any further exudate.	This step is not needed if an antiseptic solution is used. Apply a dry dressing if excessive drainage is present, and notify the physician.
7. Apply a dry dressing if excessive drainage exists, and notify the physician. **(Level C)**	No particular dressing type or the presence of a dressing has been determined to lessen infection.[6,7]	
8. Discard used supplies in an appropriate receptacle.	Removes and safely discards used supplies.	
9. **HH**		

*Level C: Qualitative studies, descriptive or correlational studies, integrative reviews, systematic reviews, or randomized controlled trials with inconsistent results

Procedure continues on following page

Expected Outcomes

- Pin or tong sites remain intact
- Pin or tong sites remain free of infection

Unexpected Outcomes

- Infection at pin or tong sites, which may be local or may extend into bone (causing osteomyelitis), through the skull (causing intracranial abscess), or into the bloodstream (causing systemic infection)[4,6,9]
- Loose pins[4,6,9]
- Skin irritation, injury, or scarring[4,6,9]
- Bleeding at the pin site[4,6,9]
- Pain at the pin site[4,6,9]
- Loss of cervical spine immobilization related to loose pins[4,6,9]

Patient Monitoring and Care

Steps	Rationale	Reportable Conditions
		These conditions should be reported if they persist despite nursing interventions.
1. Administer pin care as directed by institution policy. Although evidence-based recommendations about the frequency of site care remain unclear, generally care is performed at least every 8 hours and may be reduced to twice a day or daily after drainage subsides.	Keeps pin sites clean and provides an opportunity for assessment of pin sites.	• Evidence of infection
2. Examine each pin site for evidence of bleeding, swelling, drainage, redness, or pin loosening.[2,4,7,9]	Determines the presence of infection or slippage of pins.	• Evidence of bleeding, infection, or abnormal or excessive drainage; pin dislodgment[2,4,7,9]
3. Obtain a sample of drainage if signs and symptoms of infection are present.[4]	Identifies the presence of infectious organisms for further treatment.	• Culture results from exudate; signs and symptoms of infection
4. Monitor for discomfort at the pin sites.	Determines evidence of possible infection or slippage of pin.[4,5]	• Continued discomfort or signs of infection
5. Discuss possible changes in body image related to placement of tongs or a halo ring; provide emotional support.	Acknowledges a change in body image that occurs when external traction or immobilization devices are applied.	• Maladaptation to body image
6. Follow institution standard for assessing pain. Administer analgesia as prescribed.	Identifies need for pain interventions.	• Continued pain despite pain interventions

Documentation

Documentation should include the following:

- Patient and family education
- Condition of skin on scalp
- Condition of skin at pin or tong sites
- Evidence of redness or edema and amount and character of drainage at the pin sites
- Loose pins
- Body temperature
- Neurologic assessment of sensation and motor function
- Occurrence of unexpected outcomes
- Patient response to care
- Additional interventions
- Pin site care performed
- Pain assessment, interventions, and effectiveness

References

1. Bell A, Leader M, Lloyd H: Care of pin sites, *Nurs Stand* 22:44-48, 2008.
2. Bono CM: The halo fixator, *J Am Acad Orthop Surg* 15:728-737, 2007.
3. Canale ST, Beaty JH: Cervical spine injuries. In Canale ST, Beaty JH, editors: *Campbell's operative orthopaedics,* ed 11, Philadelphia, 2008, Mosby, 1776-1777.
CR 4. Hayes VM, Silber JS, Siddiqi FN, et al: Complications of halo fixation of the cervical spine, *Am J Orthop* 34: 271-276, 2005.
5. Holmes SB, Brown SJ: Skeletal pin site care: National Association of Orthopaedic Nurses guidelines for orthopaedic nursing. *Orthop Nurs* 24, 99-107, 2005.
CR 6. Kang M, Vives MJ, Vaccaro AR: The halo vest: principles of application and management of complications, *J Spinal Cord Med* 26:186-192, 2003.
7. Lethaby A, Temple J, Santy J: Pin site care for preventing infections associated with external bone fixators and pins, *Cochrane Database Syst Rev* 4:CD004551, 2008.
CR 8. Patterson MM: Multicenter pin care study, *Orthop Nurs* 24:349-360, 2005.
9. Saeed MU, Dacuycuy MA, Kennedy DJ: Halo pin insertion-associated brain abscess: case report and review of the literature, *Spine* 32:E271-E274, 2007.
10. Wu SC, Crews RT, Zelen C, et al: Use of chlorhexidine-impregnated patch at pin site to reduce local morbidity: the ChiPPS pilot trial, *Int Wound J* 5:416-422, 2008.

Additional Readings

CR Bernardo LM: Evidence-based practice for pin site care in injured children, *Orthop Nurs* 20:29-34, 2001.
CR Davis P, Lee-Smith J, Booth J, et al: Pin site management: towards a consensus: part 2, *J Orthop Nurs* 5:125-130, 2001.
CR Lee-Smith J, Santy J, Davis P, et al: Pin site management: towards a consensus: part 1, *J Orthop Nurs* 5:37-42, 2001.
CR McKenzie LL: In search of a standard for pin site care, *Orthop Nurs* 18:73-78, 1999.

PROCEDURE 100

Cervical Traction Maintenance

PURPOSE: Once cervical traction has been established, the nurse cares for the patient who is immobilized on complete bed rest. Traction must be maintained on a continuous basis until realignment and stabilization with surgical management or orthoses is attained or healing is completed.

Mary Hanson

PREREQUISITE NURSING KNOWLEDGE

- Knowledge of neuroanatomy and physiology is necessary.
- The nurse needs to be knowledgeable about the anatomy and physiology of the spinal column, the special anatomy of the cervical vertebrae, the spinal cord, the cervical spinal nerves, and their areas of innervation. In addition, the nurse must understand the pathophysiology and manifestations of spinal cord trauma, including spinal shock, ascending edema, and related impairment of respiratory function, decreased vasomotor tone, and autonomic nervous system dysfunction.[1,2,10]
- The nurse needs to be knowledgeable about the signs and symptoms of new spinal cord injury or extension of injury and the needed interventions.
- After the cervical tongs are inserted, traction is applied by adding weights to a rope and pulley or cable and bracket alignment device attached to the tongs (see Fig. 97-1). Additional weight may be added gradually, followed with radiographic imaging. The physician uses serial radiographs of the cervical spine to assist in determining the optimal amount of traction (measured in pounds) needed to reduce a fracture and provide optimal alignment. Excessive traction may cause stretching of and damage to the spinal cord; the addition of weight to the traction is managed by the physician.[3,9]
- Once the traction is in place, the patient is maintained on strict bed rest. For facilitation of turning, the patient may be placed on a special bed or turning frame (Fig. 100-1).
- The principles of skeletal traction are the foundation of management of any patient in cervical traction. One must follow such key points as (1) never raising the traction weights, (2) never disconnecting the traction, (3) never allowing the traction weights to rest on the floor, and (4) never allowing other objects to compromise freely hanging weights.

EQUIPMENT

- Cervical traction system in place, including rope and pulley system or cable and bracket alignment device and weights for the Rotating Kinetic Treatment Table (Rotokinetic) (Fig. 100-1) or RotoRest™ Delta Kinetic™ Therapy Bed (Fig 123-1).
- Pillows

Additional equipment, as needed, may include the following:
- Positioning devices
- Specialty bed (e.g., Stryker frame)

PATIENT AND FAMILY EDUCATION

- Explain the procedure and the reason for the traction. ➤➤***Rationale:*** Patient and family anxiety may be decreased.
- Explain the patient's role in maintaining the traction. ➤➤***Rationale:*** Patient cooperation is elicited.
- Explain how the patient's basic needs will be met during the confinement to bed and the maintenance of traction. ➤➤***Rationale:*** The patient and family are reassured that the patient will be cared for and his or her needs met.

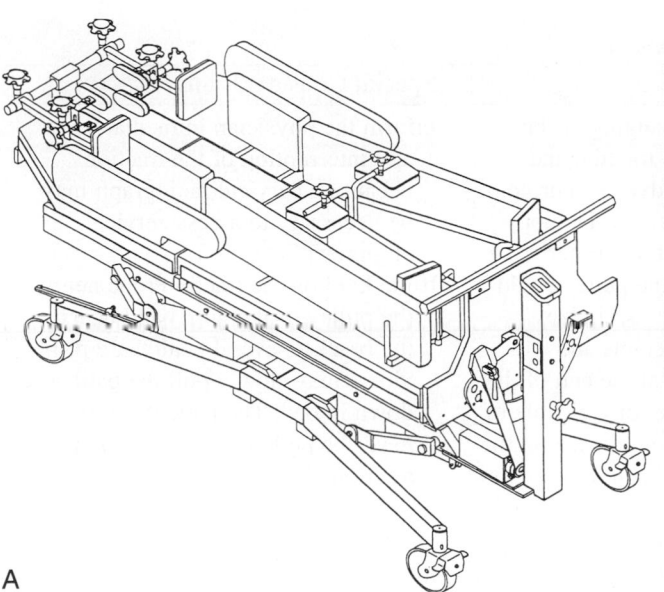
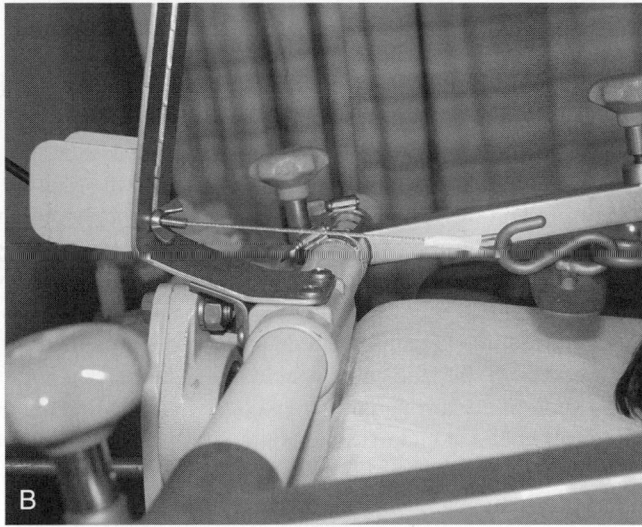

FIGURE 100-1 **A,** The Rotating Kinetic Treatment Table (Kinetic Concepts Inc, San Antonio, TX). The patient is positioned and balanced on the table. The motor mechanism allows the patient to be rotated side to side, thereby displacing weight and assisting to relieve pressure areas. Cervical traction may be applied via a tension system at the head of the bed. Kinetic therapy can also facilitate pulmonary care of the patient, allowing easy access to the thoracic area for physiotherapy and coughing. *(Courtesy Kinetic Concepts Incorporated, San Antonio, TX.)* **B,** Closer view of the tension system for cervical traction.

PATIENT ASSESSMENT AND PREPARATION

Patient Assessment

- Conduct a complete neurologic assessment that includes motor strength of the major muscles, sensory function (assess light touch, pain, and proprioception. Note the highest dermatome level with impaired sensation.) Assess deep tendon reflexes (biceps, triceps, patellar, and Achilles), superficial reflexes, and cranial nerves. **➤➤*Rationale:*** Baseline data are established for determination of any change in neurologic function.
- Assess the patient's comfort. **➤➤*Rationale:*** Spinal injuries are often painful. Changes in pain in the head or neck or at the pin sites may suggest misalignment, pin site infection, or slippage of traction.

Patient Preparation

- Ensure that the patient and family understand preprocedural teaching. Answer questions as they arise, and reinforce information as needed. **➤➤*Rationale:*** Understanding of previously taught information is evaluated and reinforced.
- Verify correct patient with two identifiers. **➤➤*Rationale:*** Prior to performing a procedure, the nurse should ensure the correct identification of the patient for the intended intervention.
- Ensure that body alignment is maintained and that the patient is positioned in the middle of the bed. **➤➤*Rationale:*** Positioning facilitates comfort and even distribution of the traction.
- Check the orthopedic traction frame, rope knot, and pulley or cable and bracket alignment device for secure attachment and function. **➤➤*Rationale:*** Ineffective traction or loss of traction may result in loss of realignment and stabilization of the vertebral column, resulting in spinal cord injury.
- Check the ropes and weights to be sure that they are hanging freely. Check the cable and alignment bracket device for patients treated on a kinetic therapy bed. **➤➤*Rationale:*** Assessment maintains function and prevents slippage of the orthopedic equipment.

Procedure	for Traction Maintenance	
Steps	**Rationale**	**Special Considerations**
1. **HH**		
2. **PE**		
3. Ensure that the orthopedic frame and traction equipment are intact.	Promotes patient safety.	

Procedure continues on following page

Procedure   for Traction Maintenance—*Continued*

Steps	Rationale	Special Considerations
4. Maintain the weights so that they hang freely at all times.[1,4,6,8] **(Level E*)**	Obstruction to free hanging of the weights eliminates traction and could precipitate adverse neurologic responses in the patient. Do not raise the traction at any time.[4,6,8]	Inform the physician immediately of any interruption of the traction because a cervical radiograph may be necessary to assess cervical alignment.
5. Ensure that the rope is able to slide freely through the pulley and that the knot in the rope is not resting on the pulley. If using the cable and bracket alignment device, ensure that the cable is able to slide freely through the bracket (ensure band at end of cable is not resting on bracket).[4,6,8] **(Level E)**	The knot resting on the pulley could interfere with the prescriptive adequacy of the weights and traction. The band at the end of the cable on the bracket of the cable of the bracket alignment device on the kinetic therapy bed could interfere with the prescriptive adequacy of the weights and traction.[4,6,8]	If the knot on the traction rope nears the pulley or the wire band nears the bracket several healthcare providers may slowly pull the patient down in bed. The patient should *never* be pulled up in the bed or traction will be released.
6. Maintain the patient in a straight line (centered on the bed), in a neutral position and aligned with the pulley and rope or cable and bracket alignment device.	Alignment ensures optimal traction that is balanced (does not pull on one side of the body more than on the other side) and prevents traction slippage and pain.	Reposition as necessary; ensure adequate help to prevent extension of a cervical injury.
7. Follow physician prescription regarding turning. When turning manually, logroll with at least three healthcare providers. Follow institution policy for maintaining cervical spinal alignment during repositioning. When turning automatically with kinetic therapy, increase the angle gradually while assessing how the patient responds to turning.	Maintains alignment.	Begin turning only when prescribed by the physician. Turning or moving the patient in a neutral position with a triple logrolling technique requires coordination of turning and preplanning.
8. Use pillows and special positioning devices to maintain the patient in body alignment.	Prevents misalignment and possible extension of a cervical injury.	Do not use pillows under the patient's head; maintain the patient flat on the bed; use pillows to support alignment and maintenance of a neutral position.
9. Discard used supplies in an appropriate receptacle.	Removes and safely discards used supplies.	
10. **HH**		

Expected Outcomes

- The orthopedic traction frame and all traction equipment are secure and functional
- Proper body alignment of the patient is maintained
- The patient is comfortable and safe
- The patient's neurologic function is stable or improved
- The patient tolerates turning

Unexpected Outcomes

- Slippage of tongs, pins, or external fixation device
- Interruption of continuous traction
- Extension or deterioration of neurologic deficits or spinal cord injury
- Pain

*Level E: Multiple case reports, theory-based evidence from expert opinions, or peer-reviewed professional organizational standards without clinical studies to support recommendations

Patient Monitoring and Care

Steps	Rationale	Reportable Conditions
1. Perform a neurologic assessment after cervical traction is initiated and then a minimum of every 2-4 hours, as prescribed or according to institution standard.	Determines neurologic status.	• Any deterioration or extension of baseline neurologic function (e.g., loss of more dermatomal sensation; decrease in motor strength) • Bitemporal tongs may also interfere with eyelid close and mastication[9]
2. Obtain vital signs after cervical traction is initiated and then at minimum every 2-4 hours, as prescribed or according to institution standard.	Determines cardiovascular stability.	• Changes in vital signs
3. Assess respiratory status after cervical traction is initiated and then at minimum every 2-4 hours, as prescribed or according to institution standard (Table 100-1).	Provides early identification of atelectasis, pneumonia, respiratory distress, or extension of neurologic deterioration.	• Abnormal lung sounds • Abnormal respiratory rate or pattern of breathing • Decreased oxygen saturation • Decreased ventilation parameters (e.g., tidal volume, vital capacity) • Increased sputum • Yellow-green sputum • Elevated temperature • Use of accessory muscles
4. Assess cardiac status after cervical traction is initiated and then at minimum every 2-4 hours, as prescribed or according to institution standard (see Table 100-1).	Provides early identification of cardiac dysrhythmias or decompensation.	• Dysrhythmias • Abnormal heart sounds • Hemodynamic instability
5. Perform peripheral vascular assessment after cervical traction is initiated and then at minimum every 2-4 hours, as prescribed or according to institution standard. Consider deep venous thromboembolism (VTE) prophylaxis (e.g., anticoagulation therapy and sequential compression devices).[2,10]	Provides early identification of peripheral vascular insufficiency and DVT.	• Peripheral vascular changes • Signs of DVT
6. Perform gastrointestinal assessment after cervical traction is initiated and then at minimum every 2-4 hours, as prescribed or according to institution standard; consider gastric prophylaxis.[2,10]	Provides early identification of paralytic ileus and gastric distention; prevention of gastric hemorrhage.	• Abdominal distention, nausea, vomiting, decreased bowel sounds, constipation
7. Perform genitourinary assessment after cervical traction is initiated and then at minimum every 2-4 hours, as prescribed or according to institution standard.[2,10]	Provides early identification of urinary tract infection (UTI) and neurogenic bladder.	• Low or high output, distended bladder, signs and symptoms of UTI
8. Perform skin assessment after cervical traction is initiated and then at minimum every 2-4 hours, as prescribed or according to institution standard (see Table 100-1 and 100-2).[2,10]	Provides early recognition of skin breakdown.	• Evidence of skin breakdown

Procedure continues on following page

TABLE 100-1 Acute Physiologic Responses to Immobility and Spinal Cord Injury

Body System	Physiologic Response to Immobility	Physiologic Response to Spinal Cord Injury	Assessment Parameters
Integumentary	Pressure → ischemia → integumentary disruption	Protective motor and sensory functions lost or impaired below the level of the lesion	Inspect bony prominences. Identify preexisting skin disruptions. Assess specific pressure areas related to traction devices and positioning.
Pulmonary	Decreased chest expansion Secretions pool CO_2 retention → respiratory acidosis	Lost or impaired neuromuscular stimulus to the diaphragm, internal and external intercostals, abdominal muscles, and accessory muscles	Observe the thorax for symmetric chest expansion. Identify breathing patterns. Auscultate breath sounds. Respiratory parameters (NIF/FVC). Supplemental O_2 ABG/pulse oximetry. Identify associated pulmonary injury.
Cardiovascular	Increased cardiac workload Thrombus formation Orthostasis	Decreased vasomotor tone Loss of sympathetic response Poor venous return Poikilothermia Spinal shock → autonomic dysreflexia	Monitor vital signs, rhythm interpretation, and hemodynamic parameters. Monitor body/skin temperature. Organ perfusion assessment: level of consciousness and urine output.
Musculoskeletal	Muscle atrophy Joint immobility → Contractures	Loss/impairment of voluntary motor function Flaccid → spastic paralysis	Identify level of lesion. Serial motor/sensory examinations. Assess joint mobility (flaccidity/spasticity). Confirm that the traction and weights are applied correctly.
Neurologic	Increased vasovagal response, bradycardia, hypotension	Neurogenic shock Spinal shock	After spinal shock, assess for autonomic dysreflexia.
Gastrointestinal	Paralytic ileus	Neurogenic bowel	Monitor for absent to hypoactive bowel sounds, inability to tolerate enteral nutrition.
Genitourinary	Bladder atony	Neurogenic bladder Areflexic to eventually reflex voiding	Monitor urine output. Assess for bladder distension.

NIF, Negative inspiratory force; *FVC*, forced vital capacity; *ABG*, arterial blood gas.

Patient Monitoring and Care —*Continued*

Steps	Rationale	Reportable Conditions
9. Perform musculoskeletal assessment every 8 hours (see Table 100-1).[2,10]	Provides early recognition of musculoskeletal contractures.	• Increased spasticity or malpositioning of an extremity
10. Perform nutritional assessment at least once a day.[1,2]	Determines nutritional status.	• Decreased intake, poor skin turgor, intolerance of nutrition
11. Assess anxiety level, pain, and coping.[1,2]	Provides early recognition of anxiety, depression, agitation, and pain.	• Anxiety, depression, agitation, pain, or other untoward responses
12. Perform pin care (frequency may be directed by institutional policy; see Procedure 99). **(Level C*)**	Monitors skin and assesses for infection. No consensus exists regarding pin site care, including cleaning agent, method, or frequency.[5,7,8]	• Evidence of infection
13. Reposition and turn, maintaining neutral body alignment.[1,2] Follow institution standard.	Maintains skin integrity. Prevents complications of immobility.	• Impaired skin integrity

*Level C: Qualitative studies, descriptive or correlational studies, integrative reviews, systematic reviews, or randomized controlled trials with inconsistent results

TABLE 100-2	High-Risk Focus Area Skin Assessment Guide

High-Risk Skin Areas

Devices/ Positions	Forehead	Occiput	Chin	Ear	Clavicle	Scapula	Shoulder	Upper Arm	Elbow	Forearm	Wrist	Thumb Webbing	Axilla	Sternum	Ribs	Iliac Crest: anterior	Iliac Crest: posterior	Sacrum	Groin	Trochanter	Thigh	Knee	Calf	Ankle	Heel	Toe	Pin Sites
Halo-vest device	✓				✓	✓	✓							✓	✓												✓
High-top sneakers																								✓	✓	✓	
Resting arm splints									✓	✓	✓	✓															
Resting foot splints																							✓	✓	✓	✓	
Rotating kinetic table		✓		✓	✓	✓			✓				✓			✓	✓	✓						✓	✓		
Stryker frame: prone	✓		✓											✓						✓					✓		
Stryker frame: supine		✓				✓			✓									✓	✓						✓		
Tenodesis splints										✓	✓	✓															
Tongs: Gardner-Wells		✓																									✓
Crutch-field		✓																									✓
Vinke		✓																									✓

Patient Monitoring and Care —*Continued*		
Steps	**Rationale**	**Reportable Conditions**
14. Perform respiratory management (e.g., mechanical ventilation, supplemental oxygen, deep breathing, suctioning, incentive spirometer, quad coughing, chest physical therapy, bronchoscopy, tracheostomy).[2,10]	Supports respiratory function and oxygenation of all body organs.	• Decreased or increased respirations • Abnormal lung sounds • Decreased oxygen saturation
15. Initiate bladder and bowel programs.[2,10]	Supports adequate emptying of bladder and pattern of bowel activity.	• Bladder distension • Constipation • Decrease in or absence of bowel signs
16. Perform range of motion every two hours and apply splints and other positioners.[1,2]	Maintains intact motor function.	• Evidence of contractures, deformities, functional loss
17. Offer emotional support and other diversional therapy.[1,2]	Supports patient and family through the continuum of care and keeps them actively involved.	

Procedure continues on following page

Patient Monitoring and Care —*Continued*

Steps	Rationale	Reportable Conditions
18. Consult support services as needed.[1,2]	Support services can provide items such as prism glasses to help the patient see, read, and increase visual field.	
19. Follow institution standard for assessing pain. Administer analgesia as prescribed.	Identifies need for pain interventions.	Continued pain despite pain interventions

Documentation

Documentation should include the following:
- Patient and family education
- Ongoing comprehensive assessment data and action taken for abnormal data
- Verification of proper functioning and security of traction equipment (e.g., weights hanging freely, traction rope knot not against pulley, band at end of cable and bracket alignment device not resting on bracket)

- Occurrence of unexpected outcomes
- Patient response to care
- Additional interventions
- Pain assessment, interventions, and effectiveness

References

1. Blissitt PA: Spinal cord injury. In Carlson KK, editor: *Advanced critical care nursing*, Philadelphia, 2009, Saunders/Elsevier, 637-680.
2. Consortium for Spinal Cord Medicine: Early acute management in adults with spinal cord injury: a clinical practice guideline for health-care professionals, Washington, DC, 2008, Paralyzed Veteran's Association.
3. Gupta MC, Benson DR, Keenen TL: Initial evaluation and emergency treatment of the spine-injured patient. In Browner BD, Green NE, Jupiter JB, et al, editors: *Skeletal trauma*, ed 4, Philadelphia, 2008. Saunders, 794-798.
CR 4. Harvey CV: Challenges of traction in critical care: a case study, *Crit Care Nurs Q* 21:1-13, 1998,
5. Lethaby A, Temple J, Santy J: Pin site care for preventing infections associated with external bone fixators and pins, *Cochrane Database of Syst Rev* 4:CD004551, 2008.
CR 6. Osmond T: Clinical update: principles of traction, *Aust Nurs J* 6:S1-S4, 1999.
CR 7. Patterson MM: Multicenter pin care study, *Orthop Nurs* 24:349-360, 2005.
CR 8. Styrcula L: Traction basics: part I, *Orthop Nurs* 13:71-74, 1994.
9. Wood G: Cervical spine injuries. In Canale ST, Beaty JH, editors: *Campbell's operative orthopaedics*, ed 11, St Louis, 2008, Mosby, 1761-1810.
10. Wuermser LA, Ho CH, Chiodo AE, et al: Spinal cord injury medicine: 2: acute care management of traumatic and nontraumatic injury, *Arch Phy Med Rehabil* 88: S55-S61, 2007.

Additional Reading

Hickey JV: Vertebral and spinal cord injuries. In Hickey JV, editor: *The clinical practice of neurological and neurosurgical nursing,* ed 6, Philadelphia, 2009, Wolters Kluwer Health/Lippincott Williams & Wilkins, 410-453.
Sponseller PD, Takenaga RK, Newton P, et al: The use of traction in the treatment of severe spinal deformity, *Spine* 33:2305-2309, 2008.

Epidural Catheters: Assisting with Insertion and Pain Management

P U R P O S E :   Epidural catheters are used to provide regional anesthesia and analgesia by delivering medications directly into the epidural space surrounding the spinal cord. Medications injected into the epidural space are capable of providing dose-related site-specific anesthesia and analgesia. Epidural catheters can be used effectively for short-term (e.g., acute, obstetric, postoperative, trauma) or long-term (e.g., chronic, advanced cancer) pain management.[7,20]

Sarah-Jane Lawless

PREREQUISITE NURSING KNOWLEDGE

- State boards of nursing may have detailed guidelines involving epidural analgesia. Each institution that provides this therapy also has policies and guidelines pertaining to epidural therapy. It is important that the nurse is aware of state guidelines and institution policies.
- The nurse must have an understanding of the principles of aseptic technique.[13,22,23,27]
- The epidural catheter placement and the continuing pain management of the patient should be under the supervision of an anesthesiologist, nurse anesthetist, or acute pain service to ensure positive patient outcomes.[2,12]
- The spinal cord and brain are covered by three membranes, collectively called the meninges. The outer layer is the dura mater. The middle layer is the arachnoid mater, which lies just below the dura mater and, with the dura, forms the dural sac. The innermost layer is the pia mater, which adheres to the surface of the spinal cord and the brain. The cerebrospinal fluid (CSF) circulates in the subarachnoid space, which is also called the intrathecal space.[29]
- The epidural space lies between the dura mater and the bone and ligaments of the spinal canal (Fig. 101-1).

- The epidural space (potential space) contains fat, large blood vessels, connective tissue, and spinal nerve roots.
- Analgesia via an epidural catheter may be given with a continuous, intermittent, or patient-controlled epidural analgesia (PCEA) pump system.[17,29]
- A variety of medication options are available, including local anesthetics, opiates, mixtures of local anesthetics and opiates, α_2-adrenergic agonists (e.g., clonidine), and other agents.[13,17] All medications should be preservative-free for epidural administration.[4,7,12,13]
- The pharmacology of agents given for epidural analgesia, including side effects and duration of action, must be understood.[22]
- Knowledge of the signs and symptoms of profound motor and sensory blockade or overmedication is essential. Intravenous (IV) access, IV volume loading, and immediate availability of an opioid antagonist and vasopressors are necessary.[4,12,22]
- According to the American Pain Society (APS), the most common reason for unrelieved pain in hospitals is the failure of staff to routinely and adequately assess pain and pain relief. Many patients silently tolerate unrelieved pain if not specifically asked about it.[1]
- The Agency for Health Care Policy and Research (AHCPR) urges healthcare professionals to accept the

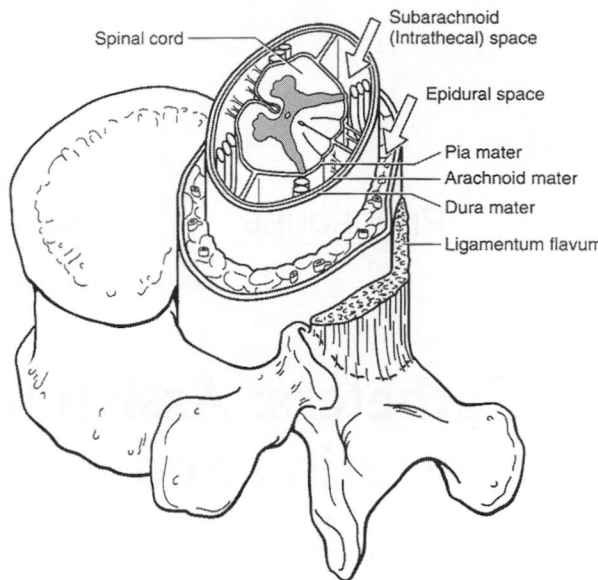

Spinal cord — Subarachnoid (Intrathecal) space

Epidural space

Pia mater
Arachnoid mater
Dura mater

Ligamentum flavum

FIGURE 101-1   Spinal anatomy. The spinal cord is a continuous structure that extends from the foramen magnum to approximately the first or second lumbar vertebral interspace. *(From McCaffery M, Pasero C: Pain: clinical manual, St Louis, 1999, Mosby.)*

patient's self-report as "the single most reliable indicator of the existence and intensity" of pain. Behavioral observations are unreliable indicators of pain levels.[1]

- Pain is an unpleasant sensory and emotional experience associated with actual or potential tissue damage.[1,7]
- No matter how successfully or deftly conducted, surgical operations produce tissue trauma. Trauma caused by surgery or injury initiates a series of biochemical events that release numerous endogenous chemicals, which potentiate mediators of inflammation and pain.[16]
- Pain is just one response to the trauma of surgery. In addition to pain, the substances released from injured tissue evoke stress hormone responses in the patient. Such responses promote pain transmission, breakdown of body tissues, increased metabolic rate, blood clotting, water retention, and impaired immune function and trigger a fight-or-flight alarm reaction with autonomic nervous system stimulation features (e.g., rapid pulse).[1,4,13]
- The psychologic effects of pain include depression, anxiety, and other negative emotions.[1,6,7]
- The patient may attempt to "splint" the injured site, resulting in shallow breathing and cough suppression followed by retained pulmonary secretions and pneumonia.[12,13] Unrelieved pain also may delay the return of normal gastric emptying and cause development of an ileus, impairment of bowel function, and reductions in respiratory tidal volumes, all of which may predispose patients in pain to infection after surgery.[7,8,19,30]
- Epidural analgesia provides a number of well-documented advantages in the postoperative period, including attenuation of the surgical/trauma stress response, excellent analgesia, earlier extubation, less sedation, decreased incidence of pulmonary complications, earlier return of bowel function, decreased deep venous thrombosis,

earlier ambulation, earlier discharge from high-acuity units,[12,14,20,30] and possibly shorter hospital stays.[20,32]

EQUIPMENT

- One epidural catheter kit or the following supplies:
  - ❖ One 25-gauge, ⅝-inch (0.5 × 16 mm) injection needle
  - ❖ One 23-gauge, 1¼-inch (0.6 × 30 mm) injection needle
  - ❖ One 18-gauge, 1½-inch (1.2 × 40 mm) injection needle
  - ❖ One 5-mL Luer-Lok syringe
  - ❖ One 20-mL Luer-Lok syringe
  - ❖ One Luer-Lok loss-of-resistance syringe
  - ❖ One 18-gauge, 3¼-inch (1.3 × 80 mm) epidural needle (pink)
  - ❖ One 0.45 × 0.85 inch epidural catheter
- One introducer stabilizing catheter guide
- One screw-cap Luer-Lok catheter
- One screw-cap Luer-Lok catheter connector
- One 0.2 × m epidural flat filter
- Topical skin antiseptic, as prescribed (e.g., 2% chlorhexidine non–alcohol-based preparation)
- Sterile towels
- Sterile forceps
- Sterile gauze 4 × 4 pads
- Sterile gloves, face masks with eye shields, sterile gowns
- 20 mL normal saline solution
- 5 to 10 mL local anesthetic as prescribed (e.g., 1% lidocaine; local infiltration)
- 5 mL local anesthetic as prescribed to establish the block
- Test dose (e.g., 3 mL 2% lidocaine with epinephrine, 1:200,000)
- Gauze or transparent dressing to cover the epidural catheter entry site
- Tape to secure the epidural catheter to the patient's back and over the patient's shoulder
- Labels stating "Epidural only" and "Not for intravenous injection"
- Pump for administering analgesia (e.g., volumetric pump, dedicated for epidural use with rate and volume limited, which has the ability to be locked to prevent tampering and preferably is a color-coded [e.g., yellow] or patient-controlled epidural analgesia pump)
- Dedicated epidural portless administration set
- Specific observation chart for patient monitoring of the epidural infusion
- Prescribed medication analgesics and local anesthetic medications
- Equipment for monitoring blood pressure, heart rate, and pulse oximetry
  Additional equipment, as needed, includes the following:
- Ice or alcohol swabs for demonstrating level of block
- Capnography equipment desired
- Emergency medications
- Bag-valve-mask device and oxygen
- Intubation equipment

PATIENT AND FAMILY EDUCATION

- Explain the reason and purpose of the epidural catheter. If available, supply easy-to-read written information. ➤*Rationale:* This information prepares the patient and family for what to expect.
- Explain to the patient and family that the insertion procedure can be uncomfortable but that a local anesthetic will be used to facilitate comfort. ➤*Rationale:* Explanation promotes patient cooperation and comfort, facilitates insertion, and decreases anxiety and fear.
- During insertion and therapy, instruct the patient to immediately report adverse side effects, such as ringing in the ears, a metallic taste in the mouth, or numbness or tingling around the mouth, because these are signs indicative of local anesthetic toxicity.[12,29,32] ➤*Rationale:* Immediate reporting identifies side effects and impending serious complications.
- During insertion and therapy, instruct the patient to report changes in pain management (e.g., suboptimal analgesia), numbness of extremities, loss of motor function of lower extremities, acute onset of back pain, loss of bladder and bowel function, itching, and nausea and vomiting.[4,12,13,17] ➤*Rationale:* Education regarding adverse side effects allows for more rapid assessment and management of potential complications.
- If the epidural infusion is patient-controlled, ensure that patient and family understand that only the patient is to activate the medication release. ➤*Rationale:* The patient should remain alert enough to administer his or her own dose. A safeguard to oversedation is that a patient cannot administer additional medication doses if sedated.

PATIENT ASSESSMENT AND PREPARATION

Patient Assessment

- Assess the patient for local infection and generalized sepsis. ➤*Rationale:* Assessment decreases the risk for epidural infection (e.g., epidural abscess).[30] Septicemia and bacteremia are contraindications for epidural catheter placement.[4,8,23,27]
- Assess the patient's concurrent anticoagulation therapy. ➤*Rationale:* Heparin (unfractionated) or heparinoids (e.g. low-molecular-weight heparin) administered concurrently during epidural catheter placement increases the risk for epidural hematoma and paralysis. Care must be taken with insertion and removal of the epidural catheter when patients have received anticoagulation therapy. Anticoagulant and fibrinolytic medications may increase the risk for epidural hematoma and spinal cord damage and paralysis. If used, anticoagulants must be withheld before insertion and removal of the epidural catheter.[21,25,26] Removal of the epidural catheter should be directed by the physician. According to Kleinman and Mikhail,[12] aspirin or nonsteroidal antiinflammatory medications (NSAIDs) by themselves do not pose an increased risk for epidural hematoma, assuming the patient's coagulation profile is within normal limits. Therefore, aspirin or NSAIDs may be administered while the epidural catheter is in place.[12] However, epidural hematomas have been associated with the concurrent administration of the NSAIDs, ketorolac, and anticoagulants.[5,21] Assessment of sensory and motor function must be regularly performed during epidural analgesia for all patients.
- Obtain the patient's vital signs. ➤*Rationale:* Baseline data are provided.
- Assess the patient's pain. ➤*Rationale:* Baseline data are provided.
- Review the patient's medication allergies. ➤*Rationale:* This information may decrease the possibility of an allergic reaction.

Patient Preparation

- Ensure that the patient and family understand preprocedural teaching. Answer questions as they arise, and reinforce information as needed. ➤*Rationale:* Understanding of previously taught information is evaluated and reinforced.
- Verify correct patient with two identifiers. ➤*Rationale:* Prior to performing a procedure, the nurse should ensure the correct identification of the patient for the intended intervention.
- Ensure that informed consent has been obtained. ➤*Rationale:* Informed consent protects the rights of the patient and makes a competent decision possible for the patient.
- Perform a pre-procedure verification and time out, if nonemergent. ➤*Rationale:* Ensures patient safety.
- Wash the patient's back with soap and water and open the gown in the back. ➤*Rationale:* This action cleanses the skin and allows easy access to the patient's back.
- Consider nothing by mouth (NPO), especially if sedation or general anesthesia is to be used. ➤*Rationale:* NPO status decreases the risk for vomiting and aspiration.
- Establish IV access, or ensure the patency of IV lines, and administer IV fluids as prescribed before epidural catheter insertion. ➤*Rationale:* IV access ensures that medications can be given quickly if needed. The administration of IV fluids may decrease hypotension that may occur during epidural infusions.[4,12]
- Reassure the patient. ➤*Rationale:* Anxiety and fears may be reduced.

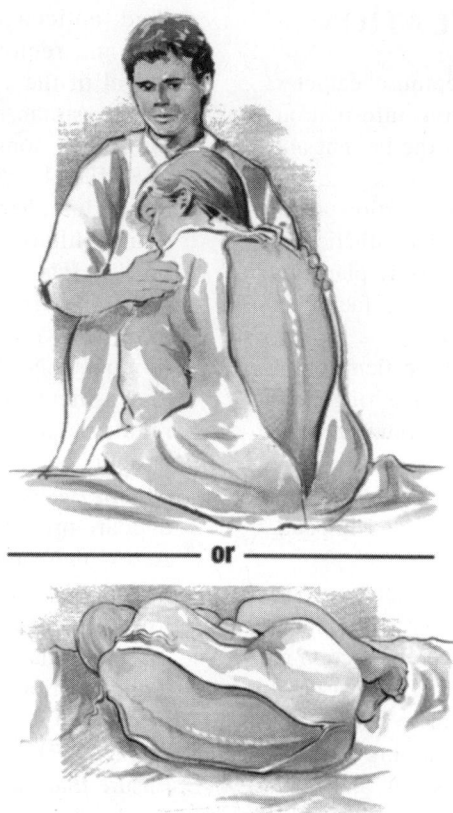

FIGURE 101-2   Patient positioning for placement of epidural catheter. *(Courtesy Astra Pharmaceuticals, London.)*

Procedure	for Pain Management: Epidural Catheters (Assisting with Insertion and Initiating Continuous Infusion)	
Steps	**Rationale**	**Special Considerations**
1. **HH**		
2. **PE**		Health care providers should apply personal protective gear (e.g., face masks with eye shields) and sterile attire (e.g., sterile gowns, sterile gloves).
3. Obtain the prescribed epidural medication infusion from the pharmacy. **(Level B*)**	The medication should be prepared with aseptic technique by the pharmacy with laminar flow or prepared commercially to decrease the risk for an epidural infection.[23,27,28]	All epidural solutions are preservative-free to avoid neuronal injury.[29]
4. Connect the epidural tubing to the prepared epidural medication infusion and prime the tubing.	Removes air from the infusion system.	
5. Ensure that the patient is in position for catheter placement. Assist with holding the patient in position (lateral decubitus knee-to-chest position or leaning over bedside table) and consider preprocedure analgesia or sedation, if necessary (see Fig. 101-2).	Facilitates ease of insertion of the epidural catheter. Both positions open up the interspinous spaces, aiding in epidural catheter insertion (Fig. 101-2).	Movement of the back may inhibit placement of the catheter.

*Level B: Well-designed controlled studies with results that consistently support a specific action, intervention, or treatment

Procedure	for Pain Management: Epidural Catheters (Assisting with Insertion and Initiating Continuous Infusion)—*Continued*		
Steps	**Rationale**	**Special Considerations**
6. Assist as needed with the antiseptic preparation of the intended insertion site. **(Level C*)**	Reduces the transmission of microorganisms into the epidural space.	The choice of povidone-iodine or chlorhexidine as an antiseptic agent for neurological procedures is controversial. Both should be allowed to dry completely. Studies suggest chlorhexidine is neurotoxic.[10,21]
7. Assist if needed with draping the patient with exposure of the insertion site.	Aids in maintaining sterility.	
8. Assist the physician or advanced practice nurse as needed with the epidural catheter placement.	Facilitates catheter insertion.	
9. After the epidural catheter is inserted, assist as needed with application of a sterile, occlusive dressing.	Reduces the incidence of infection.	Use of a transparent dressing allows for ongoing assessment of the insertion site for infection, leakage, or dislodgment.
10. Secure the epidural filter to the patient's shoulder with gauze padding.	Avoids disconnection between the epidural catheter and filter. Gauze padding prevents discomfort and skin pressure from the filter.	
11. The physician or advanced practice nurse administers a bolus dose of medication. **(Level D*)**	Facilitates a therapeutic level of analgesia and confirms correct catheter position.[9]	If a local anesthetic is used for the bolus, monitor the blood pressure frequently, with assessment for possible hypotension. Some analgesia medications (e.g., morphine) may take up to 1 hour to be effective.[12,13,29]
12. Connect the prescribed medication infusion system.	Prepares the infusion system.	
13. Initiate therapy:		
A. Place the system in the epidural pump or PCEA pump and set the rate and volume to be infused.	No other solution or medication (e.g., antibiotic or total parenteral nutrition) should be given through the epidural catheter.[32]	Responses to epidural analgesia vary individually, and epidural analgesia is tailored according to individual responses.
B. Attach an "Epidural only" label to the epidural tubing; tape over the ports, or preferably, use a portless system.[4,32] **(Level E*)**	Inadvertent intravenous administration of some epidural solutions can cause serious adverse reactions, including hypotension and cardiovascular collapse.[11,28]	
C. Do not use a burette.		
D. Lock the key pad on the epidural or PCEA pump.	This is an important safety feature.	
14. Assess the effectiveness of the analgesia. Follow institution standard for assessing pain.	Identifies the need for additional pain medication and interventions.	

*Level C: Qualitative studies, descriptive or correlational studies, integrative reviews, systematic reviews, or randomized controlled trials with inconsistent results
*Level D: Peer-reviewed professional organizational standards with clinical studies to support recommendations
*Level E: Multiple case reports, theory-based evidence from expert opinions, or peer-reviewed professional organizational standards without clinical studies to support recommendations

Procedure continues on following page

Procedure	**for Pain Management: Epidural Catheters (Assisting with Insertion and Initiating Continuous Infusion)**—*Continued*	
Steps	**Rationale**	**Special Considerations**
A. Determine the pain score.	Excellent pain scores should be reported at rest, and very little pain should be experienced with deep breathing, coughing, and movement.	
B. Assess the level of the epidural block with ice or an alcohol swab.[6]	The ideal epidural block should be just above and just below the surgical incision or the trauma site (see the dermatomes described in Fig. 101-3).	
15. Discard used supplies in an appropriate receptacle.	Removes and safely discards used supplies.	
16. **HH**		

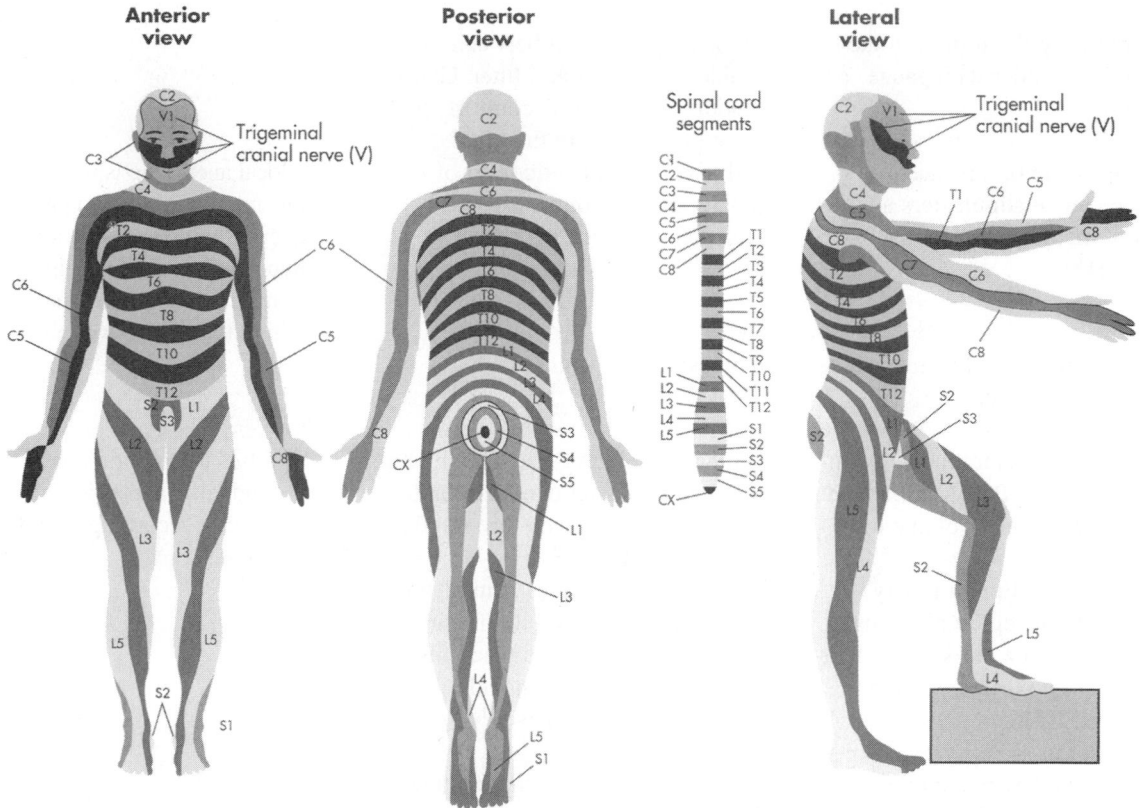

Anterior view   **Posterior view**   **Lateral view**

Figure 101-3   Dermatomes. Segmental dermatome distribution of spinal nerves to the front, back, and side of the body. Dermatomes are specific skin surface areas innervated by a single spinal nerve or group of spinal nerves. Dermatome assessment is done to determine the level of spinal anesthesia for surgical procedures and postoperative analgesia when epidural local anesthetics are used. *C,* Cervical segments; *T,* thoracic segments; *L,* lumber segments; *S,* sacral segments; *CX,* coccygeal segment. *(From McCaffery M, Pasero C: Pain: clinical manual, St Louis, 1999, Mosby.)*

Procedure	for Epidural Catheter (Bolus Dose Administration) Without a Continuous Infusion

Steps	Rationale	Special Considerations
1. **HH**		
2. **PE**		Use mask with face shield.[27]
3. Boldly label the epidural catheter used for intermittent bolus dosing (suggest color coding).[4,32] **(Level E*)**	Reduces the risk for administration of medication into intravenous lines.	
4. Verify correct patient with two identifiers. Verify the correct medication with the five rights of medication administration.	Prior to performing a procedure, the nurse should ensure the correct identification of the patient for the intended intervention and ensure that the correct medication is being administered.	
5. Inform the patient of the procedure.	Prepares the patient for the quick relief of pain.	
6. Prepare the bolus dose as prescribed.	Use only preservative-free dilutant to decrease the risk of neuronal injury.[4,12]	Do not use multidose vials because they increase the risk for contamination and the risk for an epidural infection.[4,13]
7. Prepare and cleanse the epidural port with an antiseptic agent. **(Level C*)**	Do not use an alcohol-based preparation. Use aqueous chlorhexidine or povidone-iodine.	Preparations with alcohol are neurotoxic to the epidural space. The choice of povidone-iodine or chlorhexidine as an antiseptic agent is controversial. Both should be allowed to dry completely. Studies suggest chlorhexidine is neurotoxic.[10,24]
8. Use aseptic technique to administer the epidural bolus:	Administers medication.	Follow state and institution guidelines as to who is able to provide bolus doses.
A. Connect an empty syringe to the catheter port.	Prepares for injection.	
B. Aspirate the epidural catheter, limited by the amount allowed by institution policy. If blood is aspirated, do not reinject the aspirate. Do not inject the medication. Notify the physician. If clear fluid is obtained, it may be CSF. Do not reinject the aspirate. Do not inject the medication. Notify the physician.[6,9,19,29] **(Level D*)**	If blood is obtained, the epidural catheter may have migrated into an epidural vessel. An amount of only 1 to 2 mL of blood may be inconclusive because any blood from an epidural vein may have mixed with blood from the trauma of inserting the catheter. If more than 3 mL is aspirated, the catheter is most likely in an epidural vein.[29] If 5 mL or more of CSF is obtained, the catheter may have migrated into the subarachnoid space.[29]	Administration of epidural medications into the epidural vein or into the subarachnoid space may result in increased sedation, respiratory depression, hypotension, and bradycardia.
C. Connect the syringe with the bolus medication to the catheter port.	Prepares for injection.	

*Level C: Qualitative studies, descriptive or correlational studies, integrative reviews, systematic reviews, or randomized controlled trials with inconsistent results
*Level D: Peer-reviewed professional organizational standards with clinical studies to support recommendations
*Level E: Multiple case reports, theory-based evidence from expert opinions, or peer-reviewed professional organizational standards without clinical studies to support recommendations

Procedure continues on following page

Procedure for Epidural Catheter (Bolus Dose Administration) Without a Continuous Infusion—*Continued*

Steps	Rationale	Special Considerations
D. Administer the medication slowly. Note: If excessive pressure occurs, assess for kinks in the catheter or reposition the patient.	Some resistance will be felt because the diameter of the epidural space is small and the epidural filter is in place.	Excessive pressure may be more pronounced if the epidural catheter is placed at the lumbar dermatome as opposed to the thoracic dermatome. If resistance continues to impair administration of a bolus dose, contact the physician.
9. Assess the effectiveness of the medication. Follow institution standard for assessing pain.	Identifies need for pain interventions. Pain should be relieved or decreased.	Report continued pain despite pain interventions.
10. Monitor vital signs. (**Level D***)	An epidural bolus may cause hypotension, bradycardia, respiratory depression, or increased sedation.[11,28]	Report untoward decreases in blood pressure, heart rate, respirations, oxygen saturation, and sedation.
11. Remove and safely discard used supplies.		
12. HH		

*Level D: Peer-reviewed professional organizational standards with clinical studies to support recommendations

Procedure for Assisting with Removal of the Epidural Catheter

Steps	Rationale	Special Considerations
1. HH	Facilitates the removal procedure.	
2. PE		Health care providers should apply personal protective gear (e.g., face masks with eye shields) and sterile gloves.
3. Assist the physician or advanced practice nurse as needed with removal of the catheter.	Facilitates catheter removal.	
4. Apply a sterile occlusive dressing.	Reduces contamination by microorganisms.	
5. Discard used supplies in an appropriate receptacle.	Removes and safely discards used supplies.	
6. Assess neurologic status, pain, and insertion site after removal of epidural catheter.	Motor or sensory loss in the extremities may be an early warning sign of an epidural abscess or hematoma or may indicate an excessive dose of a local anesthetic.[26,27] An epidural hematoma is a rare but serious complication; if undetected, it may result in permanent paralysis.[13,15,22,31]	Assess for a change in sensory or motor function in extremities, sudden onset of back pain with increasing motor weakness, and loss in bladder and bowel function.
A. Monitor sensory and motor status of lower extremities and ability to void up to 24 hours after removal of the catheter (see Fig. 101-3).[3,8,13,15]		
B. Monitor insertion site for drainage or infection.		
C. Continue to assess pain.		
7. HH		

Expected Outcomes

- The epidural catheter is inserted into the epidural space
- Pain is minimized or relieved
- The patient experiences little or no sedation
- The patient experiences little or no numbness and no motor loss in the limbs
- Hemodynamically stable
- No respiratory problems

Unexpected Outcomes

- Inability to insert the epidural catheter
- Suboptimal pain relief[12]
- Oversedation or drowsiness[11,28]
- Respiratory depression or hypoxia[11,28]
- Hypotension[13,19,29]
- Motor blockade of limbs; lower extremity weakness[12,19,29]
- Sensory loss in the limbs[12,19,29]
- Patchy block (e.g., uneven pain relief)[12]
- Unilateral block (e.g., pain relief on one side of the body only)[12]
- Nausea and vomiting[8,13,17,28]
- Pruritus[2,8,13,17,28]
- Urinary retention[2,8,13,15,28]
- Accidental dural puncture into the subarachnoid space[12,32]
- Dural puncture headache[12,32]
- Epidural catheter tip migration into a vessel or adjacent structure[12]
- Redness or signs of skin breakdown at pressure area sites (e.g., sacrum, heels) from decreased sensation
- High epidural block[13]
- Total spinal blockade[12]
- Occlusion of epidural catheter[12]
- Accidental epidural catheter dislodgment[12]
- Leakage from the epidural catheter insertion site[12,32]
- Cracked epidural filter
- Local anesthetic toxicity[12]
- Anaphylaxis[13]
- Epidural hematoma[8,25,26,28]
- Epidural abscess[8,25,27,28]
- Local erythema or drainage at insertion site[31]
- Nerve or spinal cord injury[12]
- Accidental connection of the epidural solution to the intravenous fluids[32]
- Accidental connection of intravenous fluids to the epidural catheter.
- Local anesthetic toxicity[12,13]
- Cardiopulmonary arrest[12]

Patient Monitoring and Care

Steps	Rationale	Reportable Conditions
		These conditions should be reported if they persist despite nursing interventions.
1. Assess the patient's level of pain with use of a pain scale[9,13,29] every 1 to 2 hours, or more frequently if needed, during the first 12 to 24 hours of therapy. Record the patient's subjective level of pain, with use of the institution's standard pain assessment tool. **(Level D*)**	Describes patient response to pain therapy. A low pain score is expected both at rest and during movement. Analgesic goal is safe, steady pain control at a low level that is acceptable to the patient.	- Moderate to severe pain scores

*Level D: Peer-reviewed professional organizational standards with clinical studies to support recommendations

Procedure continues on following page

Patient Monitoring and Care —*Continued*

Steps	Rationale	Reportable Conditions
2. Assess the patient's level of sedation[9,13,29] with use of the institution's standard assessment scale **(Level D*)**	Sedation precedes opioid-related respiratory depression. A sudden change in sedation scale may indicate that the epidural catheter has migrated into an epidural blood vessel or the intrathecal space.[11]	• Increasing sedation and drowsiness or sudden change in sedation scale
3. Assess respiratory rate the first 20 minutes after administration of the epidural medication, then every 1 to 2 hours and as needed (prn).[11,13,28] **(Level D)**	Provides data for diagnosis of respiratory depression.	• Increasing respiratory depression or sudden change in respiratory rate combined with increasing somnolence
4. Assess heart rate[13,28] every 1 to 2 hours and prn.	Tachycardia may indicate a condition such as shock. Bradycardia may indicate opioid overmedication and sympathetic blockade by the local anesthetic.[12,19]	• Change in heart rate • Abnormal heart rate • Abnormal cardiac rhythm

5. Assess blood pressure every 1 to 2 hours and prn. If hypotension occurs:
    A. Turn off the epidural infusion; notify the physician, advanced practice nurse, pain relief service.
    B. Place the patient in a supine, flat position.
    C. Administer IV fluids as prescribed or according to protocol.
    D. Administer vasopressor medications as prescribed.[13,28]
    E. Use caution when raising patient from lying to sitting or sitting to standing positions.[30]
	Epidural solutions that contain a local anesthetic may cause peripheral and venous dilation, providing a "sympathectomy."[13] The hypotensive effect of a local anesthetic is most common when a patient's fluid status is decreased. Epidural analgesia may not be the sole cause of hypotension but may reveal hypovolemia.	• Hypotension

6. Monitor the infusion rate hourly. Ensure that the control panel is locked if using the volumetric infuser or ensure that the PCEA program is locked in via key or code access.	Ensures that the medication is administered safely.	
7. Monitor oxygen saturation and end-tidal carbon dioxide if prescribed every 1 to 2 hours or continuously as per institution policy.[11,13] **(Level D)**	Assesses oxygenation.	• Oxygen saturation less than 93% or a decreasing trend in oxygenation
8. Obtain the patient's temperature[11,13] every 4 hours; assess more often if febrile. **(Level D)**	Fever may signify an epidural space infection or systemic infection that is a potential risk when an epidural catheter is in place.[13,17,27,31]	• Temperature greater than 101.3°F (38.5°C)
9. Assess the epidural catheter site according to institution standard.[13,31]	Identifies site complications and infection. An epidural abscess is a rare but serious complication. Patient recovery without neurologic injury depends largely on early recognition.[13,17,27,31]	• Redness • Tenderness or increasing diffuse back pain • Pain or paresthesia during epidural injection induration • Swelling or presence of exudate

*Level D: Peer-reviewed professional organizational standards with clinical studies to support recommendations

Patient Monitoring and Care —*Continued*

Steps	Rationale	Reportable Conditions
10. Monitor ability to void and ability to completely empty bladder.[2,8,13] **(Level D*)**	Provides data regarding urinary retention and possible early signs of epidural abscess or epidural hematoma.[8,13,26,27,31]	• Urinary retention • Change in bladder function • Lack of urination for greater than 6 to 8 hours
11. Monitor sensory or motor loss (e.g., leg numbness or inability to bend knees) at least every 4 hours and prn (see Fig. 101-3).[3,8,13,15] **(Level D)**	Motor or sensory loss in the extremities may be an early warning sign of an epidural abscess or hematoma or may indicate an excessive dose of a local anesthetic.[26,27] An epidural hematoma is a rare but serious complication; if undetected, it may result in permanent paralysis.[13,15,17,31]	• Change in sensory or motor function in extremities • Sudden onset of back pain with decreasing motor weakness • Loss in bladder and bowel function (e.g., incontinence)
12. Assess for ringing in the ears, tingling around lips, or a metallic taste.[4,12,13] **(Level D)**	If a local anesthetic is used in the epidural solution, ringing in the ears, tingling around the lips, or a metallic taste may indicate impending local anesthetic toxicity.[4,12,13]	• Ringing in the ears, tingling around the lips, or a metallic taste
13. Monitor and check skin integrity of sacrum and heels every 2 hours and as needed. Change patient's position as needed.	If a local anesthetic is used in the epidural solution, check for pressure points and decubitus ulceration (patient may have sensory loss in lower limbs).[12,19,29]	• Increasing redness or blistering of the skin on the sacrum or heels
14. Change the epidural catheter insertion site dressing as prescribed or if soiled, wet, or loose.	Provides an opportunity to cleanse the area around the catheter and to assess for signs and symptoms of infection that may indicate early signs of an epidural abscess.[13,27]	• Swelling • Site pain • Redness • Leakage of epidural solution or drainage
15. Assess for the presence of nausea or vomiting.[8]	Antiemetics may need to be administered; the medication may need adjustment (e.g., opiates may need to be decreased or removed if nausea and vomiting are not well controlled).	• Unrelieved nausea and vomiting
16. Assess for the presence of pruritus.[2,8] **(Level D)**	Epidural opiates may cause itching. Medications such as antihistamines (may cause sedation) or other low-dose opioid antagonists may be necessary to relieve pruritus. Small doses of naloxone (e.g., 0.04 mg) are effective for pruritus without reversing the analgesia.[12,19] Diphenhydramine or hydroxyzine can also be effective for itching but may cause sedation.[12,19]	• Itching • Redness • Rashes
17. Label the epidural pump and tubing[32] and consider placing the epidural pump on one side of the patient's bed and all other pumps on the other side of the bed.	May aid in minimizing the risk for mistaking the epidural infusion for an IV infusion system. Cardiopulmonary arrest and seizures may occur if the epidural solution is infused intravenously.[12]	• Infusion of IV fluid into the epidural space • Infusion of epidural solution into the IV

*Level D: Peer-reviewed professional organizational standards with clinical studies to support recommendations

Procedure continues on following page

Documentation

Documentation should include the following:
- Patient and family education
- Completion of informed consent
- Pre-procedure verifications and time out
- Any difficulties in insertion
- Type of dressing used
- Confirmation of epidural catheter placement (e.g., decrease in blood pressure, demonstrable block to ice; see Fig. 101-3)
- Site assessment
- Preintervention and serial pain assessment, including levels of motor and sensory blockade (documented on an appropriate flow chart at regular intervals; see Fig. 101-3) and effectiveness of interventions[29]
- Sedation score assessment

- Vital signs and oxygen saturation[11]
- Epidural analgesic medication and medication concentration being infused and infusion rate per hour
- Bolus dose administration and patient response after bolus dose, including effectiveness of pain relief
- Occurrence of unexpected outcomes or side effects
- Nursing interventions taken
- Pump settings when programmed for PCEA
- Medication concentrations, continuous infusion rate, bolus dose, lockout interval, limit for 1 or more hours according to institutional standard
- Pain assessment, interventions, and effectiveness.

References

CR 1. Agency for Health Care Policy and Research, Acute Pain Management Guideline Panel: *Clinical practice guidelines: acute pain management: operative or medical procedures and trauma, AHCPR pub. 92-0032,* Rockville, MD, 1992, Public Health Service, US Department of Health and Human Services.

CR 2. Ashburn MA, Caplan RA, Carr DB, et al: Practice guidelines for acute pain management in the perioperative setting: an updated report by the American Society of Anesthesiologists Task Force on Acute Pain Management, *Anesthesiology* 100:1573-1581, 2004.

3. Bedforth NM, Aitkenhead AR, Hardman JG: Haematoma and abscesses after epidural analgesia an updated report by the American Society of Anesthesiologists Task Force on Acute Pain Management, *Br J Anesth* 101:291-293, 2008.

CR 4. Burkard J, Olson RL, Vacchiano CA: Regional anesthesia. In Nagelhout JJ, Zaglaniczny KL, editors: *Nurse anesthesia,* ed 3, St Louis, 2004, Elsevier Saunders, 977-1030.

CR 5. Chan L, Bailin MT: Spinal epidural hematoma following central neuraxial blockade and subcutaneous enoxaparin: a case report, *J Clin Anesth* 16:382-385, 2004.

6. Dunwoody CJ, Krenzischek DA, Pasero C, et al: Assessment, physiological monitoring, and consequences of inadequately treated acute pain, *J Perianesth Nurs* 23(Suppl 1):S15-S27, 2008.

CR 7. Faut-Callahan M, Hand WR: Pain management. In Nagelhout JJ, Zaglaniczny KL, editors: *Nurse anesthesia,* ed 3, St Louis, 2004, Elsevier Saunders, 1157-1182.

8. Gendall KA, Kennedy RR, Watson AJ, et al: The effect of epidural analgesia on postoperative outcome after gastrointestinal surgery, *Colorectal Dis* 9:584-598, 2007.

CR 9. Gordon DB, Dahl JH, Miaskowski C, et al: American Pain Society recommendations for improving the quality of acute and cancer pain management, *Arch Intern Med* 165:1574-1580, 2005.

CR 10. Hebl JR: The importance and implications of aseptic techniques during regional anesthesia, *Reg Anesth Pain Med* 31:311-323, 2003.

11. Horlocker TT, Burton AW, Connis RT, et al: Practice guidelines for the prevention, detection, and management of respiratory depression associated with neuroaxial opioid administration, *Anesthesiology* 110:218-230, 2009.

12. Kleinman W, Mikhail MS: Spinal, epidural and caudal blocks. In Morgan GE, Mikhail MS, Murray MJ, editors: *Clinical anesthesiology,* ed 4, New York, 2006, McGraw-Hill, 289-323.

CR 13. Mahlmeister L: Nursing responsibilities in preventing, preparing for, and managing epidural emergencies, *J Perinat Neonatal Nurs* 17:19-32, 2003.

14. Marret E, Remy C, Bonnet F: Postoperative pain forum group: meta-analysis of epidural local analgesia versus parenteral opioid analgesia after colorectal surgery, *Br J Surg* 94:665-673, 2007.

15. Meikle J, Bird S, Nightingale JJ, et al: Detection and management of epidural haematomas related to anesthesia in the UK: a national survey of current practice, *Br J Anaesth* 101:400-404, 2008.

16. Mertin S, Sawatzky JA, Diehl-Jones WL, et al: Roadblock to recovery: the surgical stress response, *Dynamics* 18:14-20, 2007.

17. Miaskowski C, Bair M, Chou R, et al: *Principles of analgesic use in the treatment of acute and cancer pain,* ed 6, Glenview, IL, 2008, American Pain Society.

18. Milstone AM, Passaretti CL, Perl TM: Chlorhexidine: expanding the armamentarium for infection control and prevention, *Clin Infect Dis* 46:274-281, 2008.

19. Morgan GE, Mikhail MS, Murray MJ: Pain management. In Morgan GE, Mikhail MS, Murray MJ, editors: *Clinical anesthesiology,* ed 4, New York, 2006, McGraw-Hill Company, 359-412.

CR 20. Pasero C: Improving postoperative outcomes with epidural analgesia, *J Perianesth Nurs* 20:51-55, 2005.

21. Pasero C, McCaffery M: Orthopaedic postoperative pain management, *J Perianesth Nurs* 22:160-172, 2007.

22. Pasero C, Eksterowicz N, Primeau M, et al: The registered nurse's role in the management of analgesia by catheter techniques, *J Perianesth Nurs* 23:53-56, 2008.

23. Ranasinghe JS, Lee AJ, Birnbach DJ: Infection associated with central venous or epidural catheters: how to reduce it, *Curr Opin Anaesthesiol* 21:386-390, 2008.

24. Reynolds F: Neurologic infections after neuroaxial anesthesia, *Anesthesiol Clin* 26:23-52, 2008.

CR 25. Rowlingson JC, Hanson PB: Neuraxial anesthesia and low-molecular-weight heparin prophylaxis in major orthopedic surgery in the wake of the latest American Society of Regional Anesthesia guidelines, *Anesth Analg* 100:1482-1488, 2005.

26. Ruppen W, Derry S, McQuay HJ, et al: Incidence of epidural haematoma and neurological injury in cardiovascular patients with epidural analgesia/anaesthesia: systematic review and meta analysis, *BMC Anesthesiol* 6(10): 2006, accessed September 1, 2009, from www.biomedcentral.com/1471 2253 6 10.

27. Ruppen W, Derry S, McQuay HJ, et al: Infection rates associated with epidural indwelling catheters for seven days or longer: systematic review and meta-analysis, *BMC Palliat Care* (6)3: 2007, accessed September 1, 2009, from www.biomedcentral.com/1472-684X/6/3.

28. Schulz-Stubner S: The critically ill patient and regional anesthesia, *Curr Opin Anaesthesiol* 19:538-544, 2006.

29. St. Marie B: Pain management. In Weinstein SM, editor: Plumer's principles and practice of intravenous therapy, ed 8, Philadelphia, 2007, Lippincott Williams & Wilkins, 576-607.

30. Tenenbein PK, Debrouwere R, Maguire D, et al: Thoracic epidural analgesia improves pulmonary function in patients undergoing cardiac surgery, *Can J Anaesth* 55:344-350, 2008.

31. Wedel DJ, Horlocker TT: Regional anesthesia in the febrile or infected patient, *Reg Anesth Pain Med* 31: 324 333, 2006.

32. Weetman C, Allison W: Use of epidural analgesia in post-operative pain management, *Nurs Stand* 20:54-64, 2006.

Additional Readings

CR Ballantyne JC, McKenna JM, Ryder E: Epidural analgesia-experience of 5628 patients in a large teaching hospital derived through audit, *Acute Pain* 4:89-97, 2003.

Patient-Controlled Analgesia

P U R P O S E : Intravenous patient-controlled analgesia empowers patients to manage their pain by allowing them to administer smaller analgesic doses more frequently. Nurses are responsible for ensuring appropriate patient selection, maintaining the intravenous delivery system, and ensuring that patients are able to safely meet their own needs for pain management through frequent assessment and patient education.

Lorie Ann Meek

PREREQUISITE NURSING KNOWLEDGE

- Pain is an unpleasant sensory and emotional experience that arises from actual or potential tissue damage or is described in terms of such damage.[1] According to the National Institutes of Health, more Americans are affected by pain than by diabetes, heart disease, and cancer combined.[28]
- The most common reason for unrelieved pain in hospitals is the failure of staff to routinely and adequately assess pain and pain relief.[1]
- Additional perceived barriers to adequate pain management are poor pain assessment, patient reluctance to report pain and take analgesics, and physician reluctance to prescribe opioids.[1] Tables 102-1 and 102-2 list guidelines for dosing and considerations for selection of opioids.
- Unrelieved postoperative pain may result in clinical and psychologic changes, an increase in morbidity and mortality, an increase in costs, and a decrease in quality of life. Negative clinical outcomes related to ineffective pain management for patients after surgery include deep vein thrombosis, pulmonary embolism, coronary ischemia, myocardial infarction, pneumonia, poor wound healing, impairment of the immune system, insomnia, and negative emotions.[25] Unrelieved pain may delay recovery and prolong hospital stays.[1,3]
- The Agency for Healthcare Research and Quality (AHRQ) urges healthcare professionals to accept the patient's self-report as "the single most reliable indicator of the existence and intensity" of pain.[1]

- Studies and meta-analyses have shown an increase in patient satisfaction with pain management and an improvement in pain control.[5,18,23,34,38] Intravenous (IV) patient-controlled analgesia (PCA) may be used for both acute and chronic pain.[26]
- Intravenous PCA can be an effective method of pain relief for pediatric and adult patients.[14,18,34,38] Table 102-1 lists dosing guidelines.
- Intravenous PCA can be administered as a continuous (basal) infusion along with patient-initiated boluses or as intermittent patient-initiated boluses exclusively.
- Patient assessment at frequent, regular intervals (at least every 4 hours) should include an evaluation of the patient's vital signs, sedation level with a valid and reliable scale, pain level with a valid and reliable scale, and common opioid side effects, such as pruritus, nausea,[9,12] constipation, and urinary retention.[13] Table 102-2 lists side effects associated with PCA opioids. Patients need more frequent assessments during the first 24 hours after initiation of IV PCA and during the night.[10,11,14,19] Systematic evaluation of agitation and pain can lead to a reduction in pain levels and agitation.[9]
- PCA pump settings should be confirmed at regular intervals.[10,11,19] See Box 102-1 for common terms used when administering patient-controlled analgesia. Adverse events during IV PCA may include respiratory depression and hypoxemia. Opioid antagonists should be readily available.
- Adjunctive medications can be used to improve pain management[7,14,15,27,39] or to improve opioid side effects.[7,15,23,24]

TABLE 102-1	Guidelines for Patient-Controlled Intravenous Opioid Administration for Opioid-Naive Adults and Children with Acute Pain

Adults > 50 kg

Drug*	Usual Starting Dose After Loading	Usual Dose Range	Typical Starting Lockout (min)	Usual Lockout Range (min)
Morphine (1.0 mg/mL)	1.0 mg	0.5-2.5 mg	6	5-10
Hydromorphone (0.2 mg/mL)	0.2 mg	0.05-0.4 mg	6	5-10
Fentanyl (50 mcg/mL)	20 mcg	10-50 mcg	6	5-8

*Typical concentrations are listed in parentheses.

Children < 50 kg

Drug	Usual Starting Dose After Loading	Usual Dose Range	Usual Starting Lockout (doses/h)	Usual Lockout Range (min)	Usual Basal Rate
Morphine (1.0 mg/mL)	0.02 mg/kg/dose	0.01-0.03 mg/kg	5	6-8	0.0-0.03 mg/kg/hr
Hydromorphone (0.2 mg/mL)	0.003-0.004 mg/kg/dose	0.003-0.005 mg/kg	5	6-10	0.00-0.004 mg/kg/hr
Fentanyl (50 mcg/mL)	0.5-1.0 mcg/kg/dose	0.5-1.0 mcg/kg/dose	5	6-8	0.0-0.5 mcg/kg/hr

(Miaskowski C, Blair M, Chou R, et al: Principles of analgesic use in the treatment of acute pain and cancer pain, ed 6, Glenview, IL, 2008, American Pain Society, 42).

- The Joint Commission does not support PCA by proxy (someone other than the patient pushing the PCA button) on the recommendation of the Institute of Safe Medication Practices (ISMP). According to ISMP, patients have experienced oversedation, increased respiratory depression, and death from PCA by proxy.[11,19,21]
- PCA by authorized user (typically nurse or designated family member of patient) is a potential alternative to PCA by proxy. Healthcare institutions that use PCA by authorized user need to have the following in place before this practice is initiated.[2,11,19,21,22,37,41]
  - ❖ Policies that guide the practice, including the patient population
  - ❖ Definition of PCA by an authorized user
  - ❖ Education plan for the authorized user
  - ❖ Documentation of the authorized user and education given
- Patients with an increased risk for complications during IV PCA use include those with:
  - ❖ Age more than 65 years (greater incidence of desaturation)[29]
  - ❖ Morbid obesity (greater incidence of desaturation)[8,29,36]
  - ❖ Sleep apnea or asthma[8,11,20,36]
  - ❖ Concurrent medications that potentiate opiates (e.g., sedation)[11,19]
  - ❖ Impaired organ function[25]
- Careful patient selection is imperative for effective pain management. Patients who may be poor candidates for PCA include the following:
  - ❖ Anyone with cognitive abilities that prohibit understanding and following directions for IV PCA (e.g., infants, young children, patients with a decreased

level of consciousness or with developmental disabilities)[11,19]
  - ❖ Anyone without the physical ability to push the PCA button that controls the dose administration[11,19]
  - ❖ Anyone with a psychologic reason that prohibits using the PCA button for pain management (e.g., psychologic disability, refusal to operate the PCA administration button)[11,19]
- Patients can have as effective or better pain control with epidural analgesia than with IV PCA after various surgical procedures.[6,16,32,33,40]
- A number of medication errors have been reported with IV PCA. Factors associated with errors include improper patient selection, inadequate monitoring, inadequate patient education, medication product mix-ups, programming errors, PCA by proxy, inadequate medical and nursing staff education, prescription errors, and PCA pump design flaws.[11,17,19]
- PCA is available in various routes, including IV, epidural (patient-controlled epidural analgesia [PCEA]; see Procedure 101), subcutaneous, peripheral nerve catheter (see Procedure 103), oral, intranasal, and transdermal.[14,15,25,26,31] The focus of this procedure is IV PCA.

EQUIPMENT

- PCA pump
- PCA tubing with antisiphon valve (may also include a plunger for insertion into PCA medication syringe barrel)
- IV pump
- IV tubing

	Side			Cautions/
Opioid	Effects	Advantages	Disadvantages	Contraindications
Morphine	Nausea Sedation Pruritus Reduced peristalsis Respiratory depression	Vast clinical experience Less experience than other opioids	Slow onset: ~15 min Histamine release Active metabolite (M6G) accumulates in renal patients and causes excessive sedation and other side effects	Allergy (use fentanyl) Renal dysfunction Hepatic dysfunction Asthma (histamine release)
Hydromorphone (Dilaudid)	Nausea Sedation Pruritus Reduced peristalsis Respiratory depression	Faster onset than morphine Less sedation No active metabolites	More expensive than morphine Less clinical experience than morphine Higher potential for abuse	Allergy (use fentanyl) High doses can result in excitation with impaired renal dysfunction
Fentanyl (Sublimaze)	Nausea Sedation Pruritus Reduced peristalsis Respiratory depression	Rapid onset No active metabolites Less constipation compared with morphine	More expensive than morphine Less clinical experience than morphine Short duration of action	Allergy Rapid administration of drug can result in "Stiff Chest" making ventilation difficult

TABLE 102-2   Patient Controlled Analgesia: Considerations in Opioid Selection

(Institute for Safe Medication Practices: Patient-controlled analgesia: making it safer for patients, Horsham, PA, 2006, Institute for Safe Medication Practices.)

BOX 102-1   Key Terms for Patient-Controlled Analgesia[13,25,26,35]

Basal rate: The amount of analgesic administered continuously.

Break-through dose: A bolus dose administered by the nurse, similar to a loading dose when pain is inadequately managed with the current PCA settings.

Cumulative dose limit: The predetermined maximum drug amount that can be delivered over either 1 or more (usually 4) hours.

Demand or PCA dose: The amount of drug administered each time the patient activates the pump.

Loading dose: A bolus dose given before initiation of PCA therapy, usually higher than the dose administered when the patient activates the pump.

Lockout interval: Predetermined period during which the patient cannot initiate doses.

- Prescribed medication (may be in a syringe, bag, or cassette)
- Alcohol wipes
- Non-sterile gloves
- ECG and blood pressure monitoring equipment
- Pulse oximetry equipment
- Normal saline solution or other compatible IV fluid Additional equipment as needed includes:
- Emergency medications, including naloxone
- Bag-valve-mask device and oxygen
- End-title carbon dioxide monitoring equipment

PATIENT AND FAMILY EDUCATION

- Review an appropriate pain rating scale with the patient. The healthcare provider and patient need to establish a mutually agreeable pain level goal. ➤*Rationale:* Review ensures that the patient understands the pain rating scale and enables the nurse to obtain a baseline assessment.

Establishing a pain level goal allows the healthcare provider to know an acceptable goal for pain management.

- Review the principles of PCA use with the patient and family members.[31] If a basal rate has been prescribed, inform the patient that pain medication will be infusing at all times. Explain that if the pain is not relieved with the steady dose, extra medicine can be delivered. Be sure the patient understands what the lockout interval is. If the patient's pain needs are not met, the dosage can and will be changed to meet those needs. ➤*Rationale:* This review may reduce anxiety and preconceptions about PCA use.
- Intravenous PCA is designed for the patient to administer the pain medication. In most circumstances, the patient should be the only one to deliver the demand dose. The ISMP and The Joint Commission do not support PCA by proxy because of adverse events, such as oversedation, respiratory depression, cardiopulmonary arrest, and deaths that have occurred with PCA by proxy.[11,19,20,21] ➤*Rationale:* The patient should remain alert enough to administer his or her own dose. A safeguard to oversedation is that a patient cannot administer additional medication doses if sedated.
- Instruct the patient and family members to report common side effects, such as oversedation, pruritus, nausea or vomiting, constipation, or urinary retention. ➤*Rationale:* Side effects are identified by the patient and family.

PATIENT ASSESSMENT AND PREPARATION

Patient Assessment

- Assess the patient's ability to properly use IV PCA as a method for pain management. ➤*Rationale:* The patient will not achieve adequate pain management if unable to use the PCA.

- Assess the patient's pain and document the intensity, location, and characteristics.[2,3,27] ➤*Rationale:* A baseline assessment permits an accurate evaluation of the efficacy of the PCA.
- Assess the patient's level of consciousness with use of a sedation scale.[28,41] ➤*Rationale:* Sedation generally precedes respiratory depression; a patient who is less alert should be closely monitored if PCA is prescribed.
- Review the patient's medication allergies. ➤*Rationale:* Review of medication allergies before administration of a new medication decreases the chances of an allergic reaction.

Patient Preparation

- Verify correct patient with two identifiers. ➤*Rationale:* Prior to performing a procedure, the nurse should ensure the correct identification of the patient for the intended intervention.
- Ensure that the patient understands the teaching. Answer questions as they arise, and reinforce information as needed.[31] ➤*Rationale:* Understanding of previously taught information is evaluated and reinforced.
- Obtain IV access or ensure patency of the IV. ➤*Rationale:* Analgesia is delivered intravenously.

Procedure | for Initiating Intravenous Patient-Controlled Analgesia

Steps	Rationale	Special Considerations
1. Review the prescription for the PCA, including the medication, concentration, basal rate, loading dose, demand PCA dose, lockout interval, cumulative dose limit (over 1 or more hours), and basal rate as prescribed.[11,19,30,35]	Ensures correct PCA prescription is administered to patient.	Ensure coverage for common side effects, such as pruritus, constipation, or nausea. Follow institution standard. A medication such as naloxone may be prescribed on an as needed basis. Ensure patient is physically, psychologically, and cognitively able to use the PCA for pain management. The use of a basal rate is controversial and may result in oversedation in patients who are opioid naive.[4,26,31]
2. Check for medication allergies or sensitivities. Check for medications that may potentiate the opioid and for adverse effects of the opioid.[11,20] **(Level E)**	Prevents allergic or adverse reactions.	
3. 🄷🄷		
4. Attach the antisiphon valve of the tubing to the medication syringe.	Prepares the equipment.	Many PCA pumps use syringe delivery of the medication. Other PCA pumps use bags and cassettes rather than syringe delivery.
5. Purge the PCA tubing of air.	Removes air from the system. If the tubing is primed to the lowest Y-site, to avoid unintentional bolusing with the first dose, the remainder of the PCA tubing needs to be primed with the IV fluid to prevent an air bolus before connecting to the patient.	If the injector is the plunger of the syringe, attach the antisiphon valve on the tubing to the syringe and manually purge. The PCA may offer the option of purging via the PCA pump before it is attached to the patient.
6. Insert the syringe into the PCA pump by first placing the bottom of the syringe in the lower flanges of the cradle and then place the top portion of the syringe in place.	Prepares the PCA system.	Place the syringe barrel into the pump within the area provided by the upper and lower flanges of the cradle.

*Level E: Multiple case reports, theory-based evidence from expert opinions, or peer-reviewed professional organizational standards without clinical studies to support recommendations

Procedure   for Initiating Intravenous Patient-Controlled Analgesia—*Continued*

Steps	Rationale	Special Considerations
7. Position the medication syringe so that the name and concentration of the drug and the volume markings are visible.	Ensures ready identification of the medication.	
8. Secure the syringe in the cradle.	Ensures proper positioning of the syringe.	
9. Occlude the PCA tubing with the slide clamp.	Contains the medication until the infusion begins.	
10. Insert the IV tubing of the continuous IV solution into the IV pump.	Prepares the infusion pump.	
11. Connect the IV tubing of the continuous IV solution to the lowest Y-site on the PCA medication tubing and ensure the tubing from Y-site to the end of the PCA medication tubing is purged with the IV fluid.	Prepares the system and prevents an air bolus.	
12. Program the PCA pump with the medication name and concentration, the loading dose (as prescribed), PCA dose, lockout interval, cumulative dose limit (over 1 or more hours), and basal rate (as prescribed).	Prepares the system.	
13. Independently verify the patient's identification, medication and medication concentration, PCA pump settings, and tubing[11,17,19] with another health care provider **(Level E*)**	Adverse events can occur as a result of programming errors.	Independent verification of patient identification, medication and concentration, PCA pump settings, and the line attachment before use and before pump refill or programming change may lessen the risk of programming error.[11,17,19]
14. **HH**		
15. **PE**		
16. Program the compatible IV solution at a rate to provide not less than the minimal acceptable rate for a continuous IV solution per institution standard.	Ensures the delivery of the prescribed medication. Highly concentrated medications, such as hydromorphone, may be administered in bolus doses of less than 1 mL, which do not reach the patient quickly through most IV tubing without a continuous IV infusion. Some PCA pumps do not use continuous IV solution; however, the PCA tubing is much smaller.	The medication's basal rate combined with any other IV fluids should total the prescribed hourly IV rate. If the PCA is programmed for bolus dosing only, set the IV solution on no less than the minimal rate for the maintenance IV.
17. Cleanse the IV catheter cap with alcohol and connect the PCA tubing directly to the patient's IV line. Release the slide clamp from the PCA tubing. Initiate continuous IV delivery and PCA therapy.	Connects the PCA to the IV access of patient.	Verify patent IV access before connecting or infusing medication. Extension tubing may result in errors in drug delivery and should not be used.
18. Label the PCA pump and the IV infusion pump.	Ensures quick and clear identification of IV fluids and PCA medications.	

*Level E: Multiple case reports, theory-based evidence from expert opinions, or peer-reviewed professional organizational standards without clinical studies to support recommendations

Procedure | for Initiating Intravenous Patient-Controlled Analgesia—*Continued*

Steps	Rationale	Special Considerations
19. Label the IV tubing and the PCA tubing.	Ensures identification of IV fluids and PCA medications infusing via each IV tubing.	
20. Secure the PCA tubing at two points of tension.	Prevents accidental removal of the IV.	
21. Discard used supplies in an appropriate receptacle.	Removes and safely discards used supplies.	
22. 🅷🅷		

Expected Outcomes

- Pain is minimized or relieved (at an acceptable level for the patient)
- No unmanaged side effects
- Continuous IV access

Unexpected Outcomes

- Extravasation
- Oversedation or respiratory depression
- Loss of IV access and interruption of medication delivery
- Pain not relieved

Patient Monitoring and Care

Steps	Rationale	Reportable Conditions
		These conditions should be reported if they persist despite nursing interventions.
1. Ensure that the medication is infusing properly through the IV.	New infusions may precipitate extravasation; an IV catheter may become dislodged through patient movement.	- Extravasation
2. Assess the patient's pain and level of sedation[9] according to institution policy.	Monitors effectiveness of therapy; identifies need for adjustment. Institutional assessment policies should take into account the expected duration and peak of the medication in use.	- Pain is unrelieved - Altered level of consciousness
3. Monitor the patient's vital signs, including heart rate, blood pressure, respirations, oxygen saturation [Sao_2], and end-tidal CO_2 (as prescribed), according to institution standard.[4,30]	Determines the presence of potential complications	- Change in respiratory status or other vital signs (e.g., respiratory rate, oxygenation via pulse oximetry, end-tidal CO_2)
4. Verify all PCA prescriptions changes and pump changes with another clinician (verify independently).[11,17,19] **(Level E*)**	Decreases the risk of a medication error or programming error.	- Medication dosage and/or programming errors
5. Ensure patient comprehension of PCA use and analgesic goal. Reinforce patient education.[31]	Comprehension can be assessed with patient report and with review of the PCA history for frequency of attempts.	- Patient unable to use PCA - Inability to achieve analgesia goal
6. Assess for the presence of side effects, such as nausea,[12] pruritus, urinary retention,[13] or constipation.	Many side effects from opioid use can be relieved. Side effects can often be managed if pain control is adequate.	- Nausea - Pruritus - Constipation - Urinary retention

*Level E: Multiple case reports, theory-based evidence from expert opinions, or peer-reviewed professional organizational standards without clinical studies to support recommendations

Procedure continues on following page

Patient Monitoring and Care —*Continued*

Steps	Rationale	Reportable Conditions
7. Ensure patient continues to be appropriate candidate for IV PCA.	Pain management may be ineffective and patient may be at higher risk for adverse events if patient not an appropriate candidate.	• Patient cognitively, psychologically, or physically unable to manage IV PCA

Documentation

Documentation should include the following:

- Medication, concentration, basal rate, loading dose, any breakthrough dosing, demand dose, lockout interval, and cumulative dose (verified by another registered nurse after initiation of treatment and with all changes thereafter)[11,17,19,35]
- Pain assessment, interventions, and effectiveness of PCA and other adjunctive pain management
- Patient's baseline and follow-up pain scores with a valid and reliable scale
- Patient's baseline and follow-up sedation scores with a valid and reliable scale

- Total dose of medication administered, per institution standards
- Time the PCA pump was cleared, per institution policy
- Patient teaching and any reinforcement needed
- Side effects of opioids
- Unexpected outcomes
- Vital signs, oxygen saturation, and if used, end-tidal carbon dioxide level
- Appearance and patency of the IV site
- Additional interventions

References

CR 1. Agency for Health Care Policy and Research, Acute Pain Management Guideline Panel: *Clinical practice guidelines: acute pain management: operative or medical procedure and trauma, AHCPR pub. 92-0032*, Rockville, MD, 1992, Agency for Health Care Policy and Research, Public Health Service, US Department of Health and Human Services.

CR 2. Anghelescu DL, Burgoyne LL, Oakes LL, et al: The safety of patient-controlled analgesia by proxy in pediatric oncology patients, *Anesth Analg* 101:1623-1627, 2005.

CR 3. Apfelbaum JL, Chen C, Mehta SS, et al: Postoperative pain experience: results from a national survey suggest postoperative pain continues to be undermanaged, *Anesth Analg* 97:534-540, 2003.

CR 4. Ashburn MA, Caplan RA, Carr DB, et al: Practice guidelines for acute pain management in the perioperative setting: an updated report by the American Society of Anesthesiologists Task Force on Acute Pain Management, *Anesthesiology* 100:1573-1581, 2004.

CR 5. Ballantyne JC, Carr DB, Chalmers TC, et al: Postoperative patient-controlled analgesia: a meta-analysis of initial randomized control trials, *J Clin Anesth* 5:182-193, 1993.

6. Bauer C, Hentz JG, Ducrocq X, et al: Lung function after lobectomy: a randomized, double-blinded trial comparing thoracic epidural ropivacaine/sufentanil and intravenous morphine for patient-controlled analgesia, *Anesth Analg* 105:238-244, 2007.

7. Capdevila X, Dadure C, Bringuier S, et al: Effect of patient-controlled perineural analgesia on rehabilitation and pain after ambulatory orthopedic surgery: a multicenter randomized trial, *Anesthesiology* 105:566-573, 2006.

CR 8. Cashman JN, Dolin SJ: Respiratory and haemodynamic effects of acute postoperative pain management: evidence from published data, *Br J Anesth* 93:212-223, 2004.

9. Chanques G, Jaber S, Barbotte E, et al: Impact of systematic evaluation of pain and agitation in an intensive care unit, *Crit Care Med* 34:1691-1699, 2006.

CR 10. Cohen MR, Smetzer J: Patient-controlled analgesia safety issues, *J Pain Palliat Care Pharmacother* 19:45-50, 2005.

11. Cohen MR, Weber RJ, Moss J: *Patient-controlled analgesia: making it safer for patients*, Horsham, PA, 2006, Institute for Safe Medication Practices. Text available at: http://www.ismp.org/profdevelopment/PCAMonograph.pdf.

CR 12. Culebras X, Corpataux J, Gaggero G, et al: The antiemetic efficacy of droperidol added to morphine patient-controlled analgesia: a randomized controlled multicenter dose-finding study, *Anesth Analg* 97:816-821, 2003.

13. Gallo S, DuRand J, Pshon N: A study of naloxone effect on urinary retention in the patient receiving morphine patient-controlled analgesia, *Orthop Nurs* 27:111-115, 2008.

CR 14. Grass JA: Patient-controlled analgesia, *Anesth Analg* 101:S44-S61, 2005.

15. Grond S, Hall J, Spacek A, et al: Iontophoretic transdermal system using fentanyl compared with patient-controlled intravenous analgesia using morphine for postoperative pain management, *Br J Anaesth* 98(6):806-815, 2007.

16. Gupta A, Fant F, Axelsson K, et al: Postoperative analgesia after radical retropubic prostatectomy: a double-blind comparison between low thoracic epidural and patient-controlled intravenous analgesia, *Anesthesiology* 105:784-793, 2006.

17. Hicks RW, Sikirica V, Nelson W, et al: Medication errors involving patient-controlled analgesia, *Am J Health Syst Pharm* 65:429-440, 2008.

18. Hudcova J, McNicol ED, Quah CS, et al: Patient controlled opioid analgesia versus conventional opioid analgesia for postoperative pain, *Cochrane Database Syst Rev* 4:CD003348, 2006.

CR 19. Institute for Safe Medication Practices: *Safety issues with patient-controlled analgesia: part 1: how errors occur,* Horsham, PA, 2003, Institute for Safe Medication Practices, accessed September 28, 2009, from www.ismp.org/newsletters/acute care/articles/20030710.asp.

CR 20. Institute for Safe Medication Practices: *Safety issues with patient-controlled analgesia: part II: how to prevent errors,* Horsham, PA, 2003, Institute for Safe Medication Practices, accessed September 28, 2009, from www.ismp.org/newsletters/acute care/articles/20030724.asp.

CR 21. Joint Commission on Accreditation of Healthcare Organizations: *Sentinel event alert: patient controlled analgesia by proxy,* Oakbrook Terrace, IL, 2004, Joint Commission on Accreditation of Healthcare Organizations, from www.jointcommission.org/sentinelevents/sentineleventalert/sea_33.htm.

22. Krane EJ: Patient-controlled analgesia: proxy-controlled analgesia? *Anesth Analg* 107:15-17, 2008.

CR 23. Lee Y, Lai HY, Lin PC et al: A dose ranging study of dexamethasone for preventing patient-controlled analgesia-related nausea and vomiting: a comparison of droperidol with saline, *Anesth Analg* 98:1066-1071, 2004.

CR 24. Maxwell LG, Kaufmann SC, Bitzer S, et al: The effects of a small-dose naloxone infusion on opioid-induced side effects and analgesia in children and adolescents treated with intravenous patient-controlled analgesia: a double-blind, prospective, randomized, controlled study, *Anesth Analg* 100:953-958, 2005.

CR 25. Miaskowski C: Patient-controlled modalities for acute postoperative pain management, *J Perianesth Nurs* 20:255-267, 2005.

26. Miaskowski C, Bair M, Chou R, et al: *Principles of analgesic use in the treatment of acute pain and cancer pain,* Glenview, IL, 2008, American Pain Society.

27. Michelet P, Guervilly C, Hélaine A, et al: Adding ketamine to morphine for patient-controlled analgesia after thoracic surgery: influence on morphine consumption, respiratory function, and nocturnal desaturation, *Br J Anaesth* 99:396-403, 2007.

28. National Institutes of Health: *Pain management: fact sheet,* Bethesda, MD, 2007, National Institutes of Health.

29. Overdyk FJ, Carter R, Maddox RR, et al: Continuous oximetry/capnometry monitoring reveals frequent desaturation and bradypnea during patient-controlled analgesia, *Anesth Analg* 105:412-418, 2007.

CR 30. Pasero C, McCaffery M: Safe use of a continuous infusion with IV PCA, *J Perianesth Nurs* 19:42-45, 2004.

31. Pasero C, McCaffery M: Orthopaedic postoperative pain management, *J Perianesth Nurs* 22:160-172, 2007.

32. Roussier M, Mahul P, Pascal J, et al: Patient-controlled cervical epidural fentanyl compared with patient-controlled i.v. fentanyl for pain after pharyngolaryngeal surgery, *Br J Anaesth* 96:492-496, 2006.

33. Schenk MR, Putzier M, Kugler B, et al: Postoperative analgesia after major spine surgery: patient-controlled epidural analgesia versus patient-controlled intravenous analgesia, *Anesth Analg* 103:1311-1317, 2006.

34. Schiessl C, Gravou C, Zernikow B, et al: Use of patient-controlled analgesia for pain control in dying children, *Support Care Cancer* 16:531-536, 2008.

35. St. Marie B: Pain management. In Weinstein SM, editor: *Plumer's principles and practice of intravenous therapy,* ed 8, Philadelphia, 2006, Lippincott Williams & Wilkins, 576-607.

CR 36. Stone JG, Cozine KA, Wald A: Nocturnal oxygenation during patient-controlled analgesia, *Anesth Analg* 89:104-110, 1999.

37. Voepel-Lewis T, Marinkovic A, Kostrzewa A, et al: The prevalence of and risk factors for adverse events in children receiving patient-controlled analgesia by proxy or patient-controlled analgesia after surgery, *Anesth Analg* 107:70-75, 2008.

CR 38. Walder B, Schafer M, Henzi I, Tramèr MR: Efficacy and safety of patient-controlled opioid analgesia for acute postoperative pain: a quantitative systematic review, *Acta Anaesth Scand* 45:795-804, 2001.

39. Webb AR, Skinner BS, Leong S, et al: The addition of a small-dose ketamine infusion to tramadol for postoperative analgesia: a double-blinded, placebo-controlled, randomized trial after abdominal surgery, *Anesth Analg* 104:912-917, 2007.

CR 40. Werawatganon T, Charuluxanun S: Patient controlled intravenous opioid analgesia versus continuous epidural analgesia for pain after intra-abdominal surgery, *Cochrane Database Syst Rev* 1:CD004088, 2005.

41. Wuhrman E, Cooney MF, Dunwoody CJ, et al: Authorized and unauthorized ("PCA by proxy") dosing of analgesic infusion pumps: position statement with clinical practice recommendations, *Pain Manag Nurs* 8:4-11, 2006.

Additional Readings

Helfand M, Freeman M: Assessment and management of acute pain in adult medical inpatients: a systematic review, *Pain Med* 10:1183-1199, 2009.

Hicks RW, Heath WM, Sikirica V, et al: Medication errors involving patient-controlled analgesia, *Jt Comm J Qual Patient Saf* 43:734-742, 2008.

Kim HS, Czuczman GJ, Nicholson WK, et al: Pain levels within 24 hours after UFE: a comparison of morphine and fentanyl patient-controlled analgesia, *Cardiovas Interv Radiol* 31:1100-1107, 2008.

Leung JM, Sands LP, Paul S, et al: Does postoperative delirium limit the use of patient-controlled analgesia in older surgical patients, *Anesthesiology* 111:625-631, 2009.

Schein JR, Hicks RW, Nelson WW, et al: Patient-controlled analgesia-related errors in the postoperative period: causes and prevention, *Drug Safety* 32:549-559, 2009.

Weitz JW, Witkowski TA, Viscusi ER: new and emerging analgesics and analgesic technologies for acute pain management, *Curr Opin Anaesthesiol* 22:608-617, 2009.

Peripheral Nerve Blocks: Assisting with Insertion and Pain Management

PURPOSE: Peripheral nerve blocks are administered as single local anesthetic injections or continuously through a catheter placed into a precise anatomic area to provide site-specific (e.g., femoral, brachial plexus, axillary, intrapleural, extrapleural, paravertebral, tibial, sciatic, and lumbar plexus) prolonged anesthesia or analgesia for postoperative and trauma pain management.[7,33,34] The use of peripheral nerve blocks requires skilled and knowledgeable health care providers.[7,33,34] Catheter placement and the continuing treatment of the patient should be under the direct supervision of an anesthesiologist, nurse anesthetist, or the acute pain service.[22,33]

Sarah-Jane Lawless

PREREQUISITE NURSING KNOWLEDGE

- State boards of nursing may have detailed guidelines involving peripheral nerve blockade. Each institution that provides this therapy also has policies and guidelines pertaining to peripheral nerve blockade. It is important that the nurse is aware of state guidelines and institution policies.
- The nurse must have an understanding of the principles of aseptic technique.[7,10,16,21,35] Peripheral nerve blocks are used as part of a preemptive and multimodal analgesic technique to provide safe and effective postoperative pain management with minimal side effects.[8,10,12,15,19]
- An understanding of the physiology of pain is essential. Pain is defined as an unpleasant sensory and emotional experience associated with actual or potential tissue damage or is described in terms of such damage.[1,7,30]
- Tissue trauma caused by surgery or injury initiates a series of biochemical events that release numerous endogenous chemicals that promote pain transmission, damage to body tissues, alterations in blood clotting, impaired immune function, and autonomic nervous system stimulation.[1] The pathophysiologic effects of pain, such as delayed gastric emptying, development of ileus, and reductions in respiratory tidal volumes, may all predispose patients in pain to postoperative secondary infection.[1,7]

- No matter how successful or how deftly conducted, surgical operations produce tissue trauma and release potent mediators of inflammation and pain.[23] Pain is just one response to trauma or surgery. Substances released from injured tissue evoke stress hormone responses in the patient. Such responses promote breakdown of body tissue; increase metabolic rate, blood clotting, and water retention; impair immune function; and trigger a fight-or-flight alarm reaction with autonomic features (e.g., rapid pulse) and negative emotions.[1,7]

- The patient in pain may attempt to "splint" the injured site, resulting in shallow breathing and cough suppression, followed by retained pulmonary secretions and pneumonia.[3,9,11,16] Unrelieved pain also may delay the return of normal gastric and bowel function in the patient after surgery.[3,5]

- The basis for the efficacy and utility of peripheral nerve blockade in patients with acute pain is the interruption of nociceptive input at its source and through nociceptive transmissions in the peripheral nerve.[7,21] In addition to blocking nociceptors in the incision, a continuous infusion may attenuate pain-mediating substances, such as histamine, bradykinin, and prostaglandins.[23]

- Peripheral nerve blocks with local anesthetics can be used to treat acute pain regionally in a number of ways. These vary from wound infiltration to continuous peripheral nerve blockade with the use of catheters that provide many hours or days of optimal analgesia after surgery or trauma.[12,13,16]

- Peripheral nerve blocks provide well-documented advantages in the postoperative period, including blunting of the surgical/trauma stress response, excellent analgesia, earlier extubation, less sedation, decreased incidence of pulmonary complications, reduction in blood loss, earlier return of bowel function, decreased deep venous thrombosis, earlier ambulation, earlier discharge from high-acuity units, and possibly shorter hospital stays.[7,21,29]

- Peripheral nerve blocks in the outpatient setting have facilitated early patient ambulation and discharge by decreasing side effects, such as drowsiness, nausea, and vomiting.[3,9,11,15] In addition, unlike general anesthesia, peripheral nerve blocks do not alter the level of consciousness. By preserving the patient's level of consciousness, the patient's protective airway reflexes (e.g., cough and gag) are maintained and the need for airway manipulation and intubation is negated. Furthermore, with the use of peripheral nerve blockade, the complications of general anesthesia are avoided.[3] Continuous peripheral nerve blockade improves postoperative analgesia, patient satisfaction, and rehabilitation compared with intravenous opioids for upper and lower extremity procedures.[9,11,15,24,28]

- The anatomic position of the specific catheter is clearly defined and documented after insertion (e.g., femoral, axillary [Figs. 103-1 and 103-2], brachial plexus [Fig. 103-3], intrapleural, extrapleural, paravertebral, tibial, sciatic, and lumbar plexus).[4,29] Radiologic confirmation[5] of the catheter position may be necessary to avoid suboptimal outcomes (e.g., pneumothorax). Catheters may be placed by the surgeon, anesthesiologist, or certified nurse anesthetist (CRNA) under direct vision, via ultrasound scan–guided techniques or with the use of a peripheral nerve stimulator, either adjacent to or directly into the nerve sheath (e.g., sciatic or tibial nerve during surgery for lower limb amputation).[13,16,19-21,26,28] Catheters may also be placed after surgery (e.g., intercostals, intrapleural, axillary, brachial plexus, femoral, and paravertebral; Table 103-1).

- A three-in-one peripheral nerve block can be used for analgesia after proximal lower limb orthopedic surgery. A three-in-one peripheral nerve block provides analgesia to block three nerves, including the lateral femoral cutaneous, femoral, and obturator nerves.[24] This block is as effective as epidural analgesia, with fewer side effects than epidural analgesia (e.g., urinary retention, nausea, and risk for epidural hemorrhage in patients with anticoagulation).[5,6,13,18,24] Some forms of plexus analgesia (e.g., brachial plexus analgesia) in the postoperative setting may serve two purposes: pain relief and sympathetic blockade, the latter of which increases blood flow and may improve outcomes in some cases (i.e., digit reimplantation).[4,13,21,31]

- Analgesia via a catheter may be administered as a continuous infusion with the use of a volumetric pump system, a patient-controlled regional infusion system, or a

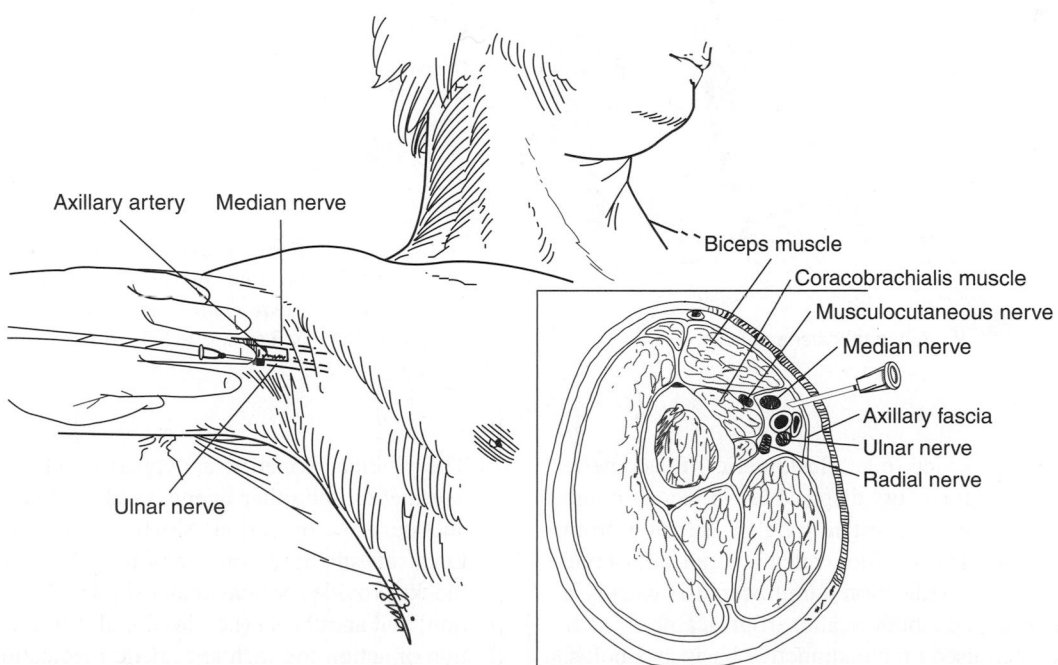

FIGURE 103-1 Location for needle insertion for an axillary block. (*From Sinatra RS: Acute pain: mechanisms & management, St Louis, 1992, Mosby.*)

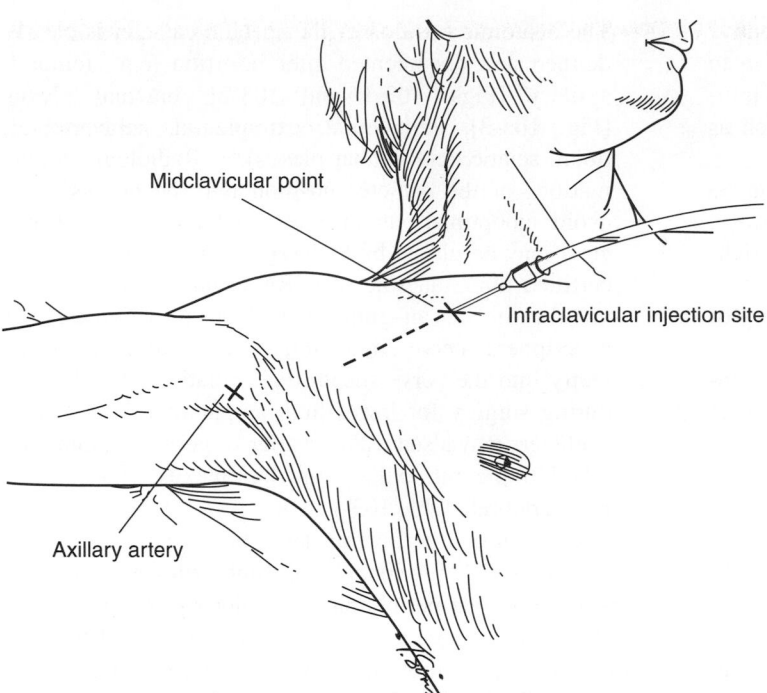

Midclavicular point

Infraclavicular injection site

Axillary artery

FIGURE 103-2   Needle insertion for an axillary block. *(From Sinatra RS: Acute pain: mechanisms & management, St Louis, 1992, Mosby.)*

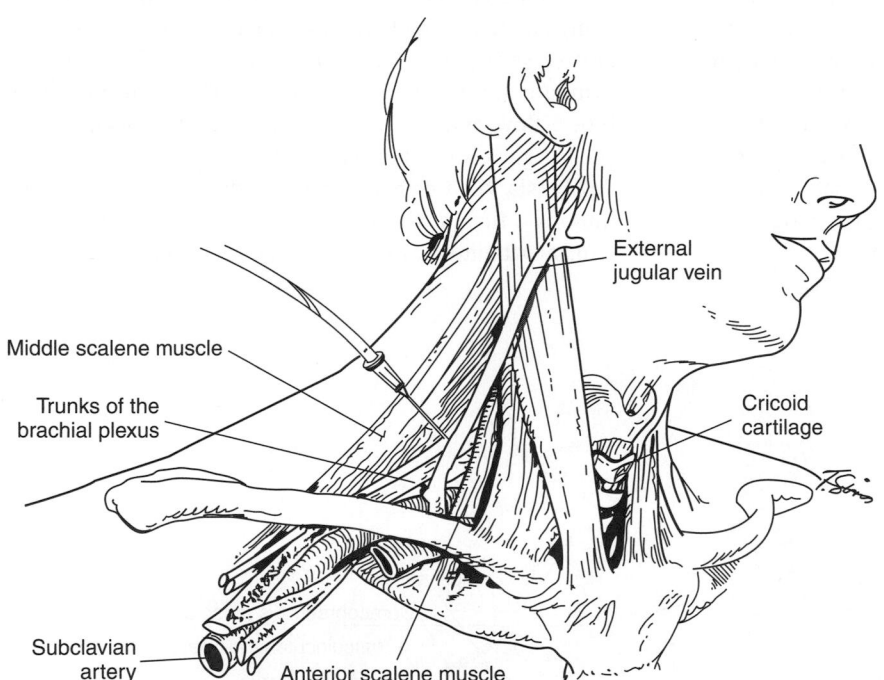

External jugular vein

Middle scalene muscle

Trunks of the brachial plexus

Cricoid cartilage

Subclavian artery

Anterior scalene muscle

FIGURE 103-3   Landmarks for interscalene brachial plexus block. *(From Sinatra RS: Acute pain: mechanisms & management, St Louis, 1992, Mosby.)*

disposable pump device (e.g., elastomeric). Elastomeric pumps are one type of disposable infusion pump designed to provide a constant rate of infusion from a filled reservoir. The infusion rates are not adjustable (Fig. 103-4.)[19,27,31] Medication administered is usually a local anesthetic (e.g., bupivacaine, ropivacaine). Other agents have been used on an adjunctive basis as a bolus, including opioids, clonidine, epinephrine,[13,14] and neostigmine.[15]

- The pharmacokinetics and pharmacodynamics of local anesthetics and other agents used, including side effects and duration of action, should be clearly understood. Local anesthetic medications used for peripheral nerve blocks provide surgical analgesia (i.e., loss of pain sensation) and anesthesia (i.e., loss of all sensation). The duration of action for each anesthetic medication depends on several factors, including the volume injected, concentration of the medication, site of injection, and absorption.

TABLE 103-1	Single-Shot and Continuous Peripheral Nerve Blocks in the Critically Ill	
Block	**Indications**	**Practical Problems**
Interscalene	Shoulder/arm pain (e.g., shoulder dislocation/ fractures, humeral fracture)	Horner's syndrome may obscure neurologic assessment Block of ipsilateral phrenic nerve Close proximity to tracheostomy and jugular vein line sites
Cervical paravertebral (continuous catheter only)	Shoulder/elbow/wrist pain (e.g., shoulder fractures, humeral fracture, elbow fractures, wrist fractures)	Horner's syndrome may obscure neurologic assessment Block of ipsilateral phrenic nerve Patient positioning
Infraclavicular	Arm/hand pain (e.g., elbow fractures, wrist fractures)	Pneumothorax risk Steep angle for catheter placement Interference with subclavian lines
Axillary	Arm/hand pain (e.g., elbow fractures, wrist fractures)	Arm positioning Catheter maintenance
Paravertebral	Unilateral chest or abdominal pain restricted to few dermatomes (e.g., rib fractures)	Patient positioning Stimulation success sometimes hard to visualize
Combination of femoral and sciatic block	Unilateral leg pain (e.g., femoral neck fracture [femoral], tibial and ankle fractures [sciatic])*	Patient positioning Interference of femoral nerve catheters with femoral lines

*Caution: Compartment syndrome.
(Modified from Schulz-Stubner S: The critically ill patient and regional anesthesia, Curr Opin Anaesthesiol 19:538-544, 2006.)

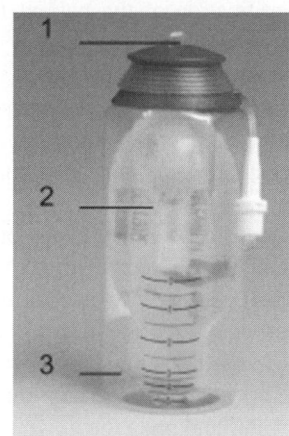

FIGURE 103-4 An elastomeric infusion pump. Parts include: 1, filling port; 2, elastomeric balloon (drug-containing reservoir); and 3, outer protective shell. *(Originally published in Skryabina E, Dunn TS: Disposable infusion pumps, Am J Health Syst Pharm 63:1260-1268, 2006.)* © 2006, American Society of Health-System Pharmacists, Inc. All rights reserved. Reprinted with permission (R1002).

The addition of a vasoconstrictor, such as epinephrine, constricts blood vessels and reduces vascular uptake, which further prolongs the duration of action of the local anesthetic.[13,14] Epinephrine should not be used in peripheral nerve blocks in areas with end arteries, such as ear lobes, the nose, digits, and the penis.[35] Vasoconstrictor medications may cause spasm of blood vessels, resulting in necrosis.[7] Knowledge of signs and symptoms of profound motor and sensory blockade, or overmedication, is essential.[4,7,8,14]

- Sensory and motor blockade may be acceptable or desirable, depending on the physician's goals and preference. The loss of sensation at the site is often the primary goal of blocks, and although motor loss is often acceptable, it is not desirable.[3]
- According to the American Pain Society, the most common reason for unrelieved pain in hospitals is failure of health care providers to routinely and adequately assess pain and pain relief.[2] Many patients silently tolerate unrelieved pain if not specifically asked about it.[1,2,14] Patient self report is considered the best indicator of pain.[2,30] Behavioral observations are unreliable indicators of pain levels.[1,2]
- Contraindications to peripheral nerve blockade include a history of coagulopathy, preexisting neuropathies, anatomic or pathologic deviations at the injection site, and systemic disease or infection.[4-6,8,18,20,35]

EQUIPMENT

- One peripheral nerve catheter kit
- Infusion set for continuous plexus anesthesia with or without an adaptor for a nerve stimulator
- Topical skin antiseptic, as prescribed (e.g., 2% chlorhexidine-based preparation or povidone-iodine)
- Sterile towels
- Sterile forceps
- Sterile gauze 4 × 4 pads
- Sterile gloves, fluid shield face masks, sterile gowns
- 20 mL normal saline solution
- 5 to 10 mL local anesthetic as prescribed (1% lidocaine) for local infiltration
- Local anesthetic as prescribed (to establish the block)
- Occlusive dressing supplies to cover the catheter entry site
- Gauze and tape to secure the catheter to the patient's body
- Labels stating "Local anesthetic only" and "Not for intravenous injection"
- Pump for administration of analgesia (e.g., volumetric pump, dedicated for peripheral nerve block infusion

with rate and volume limited, and preferably a different color from the epidural and intravenous infusion pumps; patient-controlled analgesic pump or a portable infusion device such as an elastomeric [PCA]) pump
- Specific observation chart for patient monitoring of the peripheral nerve block infusion
- Prescribed analgesics and local anesthetics
- Equipment for monitoring blood pressure, heart rate, and pulse oximetry
  Additional equipment, as needed, includes the following:
- Ice or alcohol swabs for demonstrating sensory block
- Emergency medications
- Bag-valve-mask device and oxygen
- Equipment for end-tidal carbon dioxide monitoring
- Intubation equipment
- Peripheral nerve stimulator

PATIENT AND FAMILY EDUCATION

- Explain the reason and purpose of the catheter. If available, supply easy-to-read patient information. ➤➤*Rationale:* The patient and the family know what to expect; anxiety may be reduced.
- Explain to the patient and family that the procedure can be uncomfortable but that a local anesthetic will be used to facilitate comfort. ➤➤*Rationale:* Explanation elicits patient's cooperation and comfort and facilitates insertion; anxiety and fear may be decreased.
- During therapy, instruct the patient to report side effects or changes in pain management (e.g., suboptimal analgesia, profound numbness of extremities [beyond the goal of therapy], lightheadedness, metallic taste, circumoral numbness, dizziness, blurred vision, tinnitus, loss of hearing and seizures).[4,7,14,21] ➤➤*Rationale:* Reporting of pain aids patient's comfort level and identifies side effects.
- Teach the patient to protect the affected extremity from injury and trauma (e.g., burns).[3,4,21] ➤➤*Rationale:* Patient safety is increased, and the limb is protected from injury and trauma.
- If a PCA pump is used, educate the patient and family on its use. Reinforce the education throughout PCA therapy. (see Procedure 102) ➤➤*Rationale:* Prepares the patient and family for effectively using the PCA system.

PATIENT ASSESSMENT AND PREPARATION
Patient Assessment

- Observe the patient for local infection or generalized sepsis. ➤➤*Rationale:* Decreases the risk for infection at the site of catheter insertion. Septicemia and bacteremia are contraindications for peripheral nerve block catheter placement or continuation of therapy.[8,10]

- Assess the patient's concurrent anticoagulant and fibrinolytic therapy.[5,6,35] ➤➤*Rationale:* Heparin (unfractionated and low–molecular-weight heparin) and heparinoids and fibrinolytic agents administered concurrently increase the risk for vessel trauma (e.g., hematoma). Care must be taken with insertion and removal of the peripheral nerve block catheter when patients are on anticoagulant and fibrinolytic therapy.[7] Special institutional guidelines must be observed.[3-6,16,23] Insertion and removal of the peripheral nerve catheter should be directed by the physician.[4-6,18]
- Obtain the patient's vital signs. ➤➤*Rationale:* Provides baseline data.
- Assess the patient's pain. ➤➤*Rationale:* Provides baseline data.
- Review the patient's medication allergies. ➤➤*Rationale:* Review of medication allergies before administration of a new medication decreases allergic reactions.

Patient Preparation

- Verify correct patient with two identifiers. ➤➤*Rationale:* Prior to performing a procedure, the nurse should ensure the correct identification of the patient for the intended intervention.
- Ensure that the patient and family understand the planned procedure. Answer questions as they arise, and reinforce information as needed. ➤➤*Rationale:* Understanding of previously taught information is evaluated and reinforced.
- Ensure that informed consent has been obtained. ➤➤*Rationale:* Informed consent protects the rights of the patient and makes a competent decision possible for the patient.
- Perform a pre-procedure verification and time out, if nonemergent. ➤➤*Rationale:* Ensures patient safety.
- Wash the specific anatomic area of the patient's body with soap and water and open the gown to expose the site for injection while maintaining the patient's privacy and dignity. ➤➤*Rationale:* This action cleanses the skin and allows easy access to the specific anatomic area of the patient's body.
- Consider nothing by mouth (NPO), especially if sedation or general anesthesia is to be used. ➤➤*Rationale:* The risk for vomiting and aspiration is decreased.
- Establish intravenous (IV) access or ensure the patency of IV lines. ➤➤*Rationale:* The need to treat hypotension or respiratory depression may occur.
- Position the patient as appropriate, according to which anatomic area of the body is to be blocked. ➤➤*Rationale:* Prepares the patient for the procedure.
- Reassure the patient. ➤➤*Rationale:* Anxiety and fears may be reduced.

Procedure for Peripheral Nerve Blocks

Steps	Rationale	Special Considerations
1. [HH]		
2. Obtain the prescribed peripheral nerve block medication.	The medication should be prepared with aseptic technique by the pharmacy with laminar flow or prepared commercially	All peripheral nerve block solutions are preservative-free to avoid neuronal injury.
3. Connect the correct tubing to the prepared infusion and prime the tubing.	Removes air from the infusion system.	
4. [PE]		
5. Ensure that the patient is in position for catheter placement.	Facilitates ease of insertion of the peripheral nerve block catheter.	Assist with holding the patient in position or consider sedation, if necessary.
6. Assist as needed with the antiseptic preparation of the intended insertion site. **(Level C*)**	Reduces the transmission of microorganisms into the nerve sheath or plexus space.[10,21]	The choice of povidone-iodine or chlorhexidine as an antiseptic agent for neurological procedures is controversial. Both should be allowed to dry completely. Chlorhexidine may be neurotoxic.[17]
7. Assist if needed with draping the patient with exposure of the insertion site.	Aids in maintaining sterility.	
8. Assist the physician or advance practice nurse as needed with the catheter placement and manipulation of the controls on the peripheral nerve stimulator.[3,21] **(Level C)**	Facilitates catheter insertion. Use of a peripheral nerve stimulator assists with identification of the nerve.[21,25]	
9. After the peripheral nerve catheter is inserted, assist as needed with the application of sterile, occlusive dressing.	Reduces the incidence of infection.[10,21]	
10. Secure the filter to the patient's body with a gauze padding and tape.	Avoids disconnection between the peripheral nerve catheter and the filter. The gauze padding prevents discomfort and skin pressure from the filter.	
11. The physician or advance practice nurse will administer a bolus dose of medication.	Facilitates a therapeutic level of analgesia and ensures correct catheter placement.[35]	An initial test dose of local anesthetic agent with epinephrine may be administered, then a bolus dose. Monitor vital signs and assess the patient's pain. Emergency medications and equipment must be available.[6,23]

*Level C: Qualitative studies, descriptive or correlational studies, integrative reviews, systematic reviews, or randomized controlled trials with inconsistent results

Procedure continues on following page

Procedure | for **Peripheral Nerve Blocks**—*Continued*

Steps	Rationale	Special Considerations
12. Connect the prescribed medication infusion system.	Prepares the infusion system.	
13. Initiate therapy:		
A. Place the system in a volumetric pump or PCA pump and set the rate and volume to be infused.	Prepares the infusion system.	Responses to peripheral nerve block analgesia vary individually, and analgesia is tailored according to individual responses. Note: Peripheral nerve catheters may also be attached to a portable disposable infusion device (e.g., elastomeric pump),[13,19,27,32] which may not have an adjustable rate or volume.[27,32]
B. Attach a Local anesthetic only—Not for intravenous injection label to the tubing and tape over the ports or use a portless system.[4] **(Level C*)**	Do not give any other solution or medication via this catheter. Inadvertent administration of some IV medications into the peripheral nerve block catheter may cause nerve or tissue damage. Inadvertent administration of local anesthetic intravenously can cause hypotension and cardiovascular collapse or arrest.[14,19,21]	
C. Do not use a burette. D. Lock the key pad on the volumetric or PCA pump.		
14. Assess the quality of the analgesia.		
A. Determine the patient's pain based on a consistent and reliable pain assessment tool according to institution policy.[30]	The amount of pain experienced by the patient should be no more than the amount of what is acceptable to the patient.[1,7]	
B. Assist as needed with testing the level of the epidural block with ice or an alcohol swab.	The ideal peripheral nerve block should be just above and just below the surgical incision or the trauma site (see the dermatomes described in Fig. 101-3.)[7,21]	
15. Discard used supplies in an appropriate receptacle.	Removes and safely discards used supplies.	
16. **HH**		

*Level C: Qualitative studies, descriptive or correlational studies, integrative reviews, systematic reviews, or randomized controlled trials with inconsistent results

Expected Outcomes

- Regional analgesic catheter inserted; accurate catheter placement confirmed with use of ultrasound scan, nerve stimulator, or radiologic imaging means when appropriate[4,5,15,20,26,28]
- Pain minimized or relieved[3,28,29]
- No patient sedation or respiratory depression[4,14,35]
- Reduced need for parenteral opioids, thereby also reducing opioid side effects[15,21]
- Reduction in neuropathic pain states, especially after limb amputation[12]
- Temporary numbness and loss of motor control[21]

Unexpected Outcomes

- Inability to insert the catheter
- Untimely or erroneous medication administration[4,7]
- Suboptimal analgesia
- Adverse medication reactions not recognized
- Altered skin integrity from decreased sensory and motor loss[5,7,13,33,34]
- Accidental dislodgment of the catheter delivery system
- Leakage from the catheter insertion site
- Cracked filter on the delivery system
- Inadvertent injection into a blood vessel[3,4,35]
- Ipsilateral Horner's syndrome and hoarseness[4,35]
- Nerve or vessel trauma[3,4,35]
- Hemorrhage or hematoma[5]
- Respiratory distress related to phrenic nerve paralysis or pneumothorax or medication effect[3,15,21,29]
- Sepsis[10]
- Anaphylaxis[4,14]
- Permanent neurologic injuries and damage[4,35]
- Systemic toxicity from local anesthetics (e.g., tachycardia, hypotension, metallic taste, blurred vision, circumoral numbness, tinnitus, decreased hearing, dizziness, confusion progressing to seizures)[4,14,21]

Patient Monitoring and Care

Steps	Rationale	Reportable Conditions
1. Assess the patient's level of pain with a valid and reliable pain scale. Follow institution standard for assessing pain. Administer analgesia as prescribed. Continue to assess frequently, especially during the first 12 to 24 hours of therapy.[7,21,30]	Identifies need for pain interventions. Describes patient's response to pain therapy. A low pain score is expected. Rating pain in this objective manner helps determine appropriate treatment measures.	• Continued pain despite pain interventions
2. Assess the patient's vital signs, oxygenation and ventilatory status, and level of sedation with a valid and reliable sedation scale.[30] Monitoring the patient every 15 minutes has been recommended in the immediate period after initiation of therapy.[21]	Hypotension and sedation may reflect intravenous infusion, systemic toxicity, or the residual effects of sedation administered for catheter placement.[19,21]	Change in respiratory status or other vital signs (e.g., respiratory rate, oxygenation via pulse oximetry, blood pressure) Altered level of consciousness
3. Assess the levels of motor and sensory blockade (see Fig. 101-3).[3,7,21]	Ensures effectiveness of analgesia and maintenance of the block at the correct level.	• Signs and symptoms of overmedication

Procedure continues on following page

Patient Monitoring and Care —*Continued*

Steps	Rationale	Reportable Conditions
4. Monitor the infusion rate according to institution policy. Ensure that the control panel is locked if using a volumetric infuser or ensure that the PCA program is locked via a key or code access. Disposable infusion devices (e.g., elastomeric pump) have been shown to be less accurate than a volumetric pump.[27,32]	Ensures that medication is administered safely and securely. Note: If unable to visualize the volume remaining on a portable infusion device, weighing the device before initiating of therapy and during therapy (with a gram scale) may provide information regarding medication delivered.[27]	
5. Monitor oxygen saturation and capnography (as prescribed) continuously, especially if parenteral opioids are administered (e.g., via IV PCA).[7]	Assesses oxygenation.	• Oxygen saturation less than 93% or decreasing trend in oxygenation
6. Assess temperature regularly; assess more frequently if febrile.	Increasing hyperpyrexia could signify infection.[10]	• Temperature greater than 101.3°F (38.5°C)
7. Assess the catheter site every 4 to 8 hours and as needed.	Identifies site complications.	• A change in the integrity of the peripheral nerve block insertion site (e.g., redness, tenderness, or swelling or the presence of exudate on the dressing)
8. Observe for signs and symptoms of peripheral nerve migration into a blood vessel.	The catheter is no longer in the correct position.	• Unexpected change in sedation scale • Drowsiness • Dizziness • Blurred vision • Slurred speech • Poor balance • Circumoral numbness • Hypotension • Cardiovascular collapse[3,4,14,35]
9. Monitor sensory or motor loss according to the defined goal of therapy. **(Level C*)**	Motor or sensory loss may result from the local anesthetic infusion. Note: With peripheral nerve blockade, sensory loss is usually acceptable and often desirable. Motor loss is not desirable but often acceptable.[3,4,15,21,35]	• Unexpected change in sensory or motor function beyond defined goal of therapy • Interference with respiration or excessive spread of local anesthetic beyond defined area of recommendation[4,7,14,21]
10. Assess for systemic toxicity from the local anesthetic administered through the catheter: metallic taste, blurred vision, circumoral numbness, tinnitus, decreased hearing, dizziness, confusion progressing to seizures.[14,21]	Local anesthetic is used in the solution, and symptoms indicative of systemic toxicity from the agent used to induce anesthesia may occur.	• Metallic taste • Blurred vision • Circumoral numbness • Tinnitus • Decreased hearing • Dizziness • Confusion progressing to seizures[14,21]

*Level C: Qualitative studies, descriptive or correlational studies, integrative reviews, systematic reviews, or randomized controlled trials with inconsistent results

Patient Monitoring and Care —*Continued*

Steps	Rationale	Reportable Conditions
11. Monitor and check the skin integrity of the pressure points relating to the location of the peripheral nerve block (e.g., elbow, sacrum, and heels). Change patient's position as needed. Provide protective positioning.[3,21]	If a local anesthetic is used in the solution, check for decubitus ulceration (patient may have sensory loss in areas adjacent to the area of the peripheral nerve block).[3,21]	• Increasing redness or blistering of the skin on pressure points
12. Change the peripheral nerve block catheter insertion site dressing as prescribed or if soiled, wet, or loose.[6] Note: Usually the dressing is left intact for the duration of therapy unless wet or loose.[5]	Provides an opportunity to cleanse the area around the catheter and to assess for signs and symptoms of infection.[10,21]	• Signs of site infection (e.g., swelling, pain, redness, or presence of drainage) • Leakage of the peripheral nerve block solution
13. Label the peripheral nerve block pump and consider placing the pump on one side of the patient's bed and all other pumps on the other side of the bed.[5]	Aids in minimizing the risk for mistaking the local anesthetic infusion for an IV infusion system.[6]	

Documentation

Documentation should include the following:
• Patient and family education
• Patient tolerance of procedure
• Completion of informed consent
• Completion of a pre-procedure verification and time out
• Catheter location
• Type of dressing used
• Confirmation of peripheral nerve block catheter placement (e.g., radiologic confirmation, stimulating peripheral nerve catheter, ultrasound scan)
• Site assessment
• Assessment of pain and levels of motor and sensory blockade documented on an appropriate flow chart (see Fig. 101-3).

• If PCA is used, document medication concentration, PCA bolus dose, continuous infusion, lockout interval, hourly limits, and total dosage
• Regional analgesic medication and the medication conentration being infused and infusion rate; remaining volume of medication in a disposable infusion device
• Bolus dose administration (if appropriate) and patient response after a bolus dose, including quality of pain relief
• Vital signs and oxygenation saturation.
• Occurrence of unexpected outcomes
• Nursing interventions taken
• Date and time of discontinuation of treatment
• Pain assessment, interventions, and effectiveness

References

CR 1. Agency for Health Care Policy and Research, Acute Pain Management Guideline Panel: *Clinical practice guidelines: acute pain management: operative or medical procedures and trauma,* AHCPR pub. 92-0032, Rockville, MD, 1992, Public Health Service, US Department of Health and Human Services.

2. American Pain Society: *Principles of analgesic use in the treatment of acute and cancer pain,* ed 6, Glenview, IL, 2008, American Pain Society.

CR 3. Barnes S, Russell S: Interscalene blocks in the ambulatory setting, *J Perianesth Nurs* 19:352-354, 2004.

CR 4. Bergman BD, Hebl JR, Kent J, et al: Neurologic complications of 405 consecutive continuous axillary catheters, *Anesth Analg* 96:247-252, 2003.

5. Bickler P, Brandes J, Lee M, et al: Bleeding complications from femoral and sciatic nerve catheters in patients receiving low molecular weight heparin, *Anesth Analg* 103:1036-1037, 2006.

6. Buckenmaier CC, Bleckner LL: Continuous peripheral nerve blocks and anticoagulation, *Br J Anaesth* 101: 139-140, 2008.

7. Burkard J, Vacchiano CA: Regional anesthesia. In Nagelhout JJ, Plaus K, editors: *Nurse anesthesia,* ed 4, St Louis, 2009, Elsevier Saunders, 977-1030.

CR 8. Capdevila X, Pirat P, Bringuler S, et al: Continuous peripheral nerve blocks in hospital wards after orthopedic surgery: a multicenter prospective analysis of the quality of postoperative analgesia and complications in 1,416 patients, *Anesthesiology* 103:1035-1045, 2005.

9. Capdevila X, Dadure C, Bringuier S, et al: Effect of patient-controlled perineural analgesia on rehabilitation and pain after ambulatory orthopedic surgery: a multicenter randomized trial, *Anesthesiology* 105:566-573, 2006.

10. Capdevila X, Jaber S, Pesonen P, et al: Acute neck cellulitis and mediastinitis complicating a continuous interscalene block, *Anesth Analg* 107:1419-1421, 2008.

11. Capdevila X, Ponrouch M, Choquet O: Continuous peripheral nerve blocks in clinical practice, *Curr Opin Anaesthesiol* 21:619-623, 2008.

CR 12. Chelly JE, Ben-David B, Williams BA, et al: Anesthesia and postoperative analgesia: outcomes following orthopedic surgery, *Orthopedics* 26(8 Suppl):S865-S871, 2003.

CR 13. Couture DJ, Cuniff HM, Mave JP, et al: The addition of clonidine to bupivacaine in combined femoral-sciatic nerve block for anterior cruciate ligament reconstruction, *AANA J* 72:273-278, 2004.

CR 14. Cox B, Durieux ME, Marcus MA: Toxicity of local anesthetics, *Best Pract Res Clin Anaesthesiol* 17: 111-136, 2003.

CR 15. Grossi PA, Allegri MB: Continuous peripheral nerve blocks: state of the art, *Curr Opin Anaesthesiol* 18: 522-526, 2005.

16. Hadzic A, Sala-Blanch X, Xu D: Ultrasound guidance may reduce but not eliminate complications of peripheral nerve blocks, *Anesthesiology* 108:557-558, 2008.

17. Hebl JR: The importance and implications of aseptic techniques during regional anesthesia, *Reg Anesth Pain Med* 31:311-323, 2006.

CR 18. Horlocker TT, Wedel DJ, Benzon H, et al: Regional anesthesia in the anticoagulated patient: defining the risks, *Reg Anesth Pain Med* 28:172-197, 2003.

CR 19. Kamming D, Chung F, Williams D, et al: Pain management in ambulatory surgery, *J Perianesth Nurs* 19: 174-182, 2004.

CR 20. Marhofer P, Greher M, Kapral S: Ultrasound guidance in regional anaesthesia, *Br J Anaesth* 94: 7-17, 2005.

21. McCamant KL: Peripheral nerve blocks: understanding the nurse's role, *J Perianesth Nurs* 21:16-24, 2006.

CR 22. McDonnell A, Nicholl J, Read SM: Acute pain teams and the management of postoperative pain: a systematic review and meta-analysis, *J Adv Nurs* 41:261-273, 2003.

23. Mertin S, Sawatzky JA, Diehl-Jones WL, et al: Roadblock to recovery: the surgical stress response, *Dynamics* 18:14-20, 2007.

CR 24. Morau D, Lopez S, Biboulet P, et al: Comparison of continuous 3-in-1 and fascia iliaca compartment blocks for postoperative analgesia: feasibility, catheter migration, distribution of sensory block, and analgesic efficacy, *Reg Anesth Pain Med* 28:309-314, 2003.

25. Pasero C, Eksterowicz N, Primeau M, et al: Registered nurse management and monitoring of analgesia by catheter techniques: position statement, *Pain Manag Nurs* 8:48-54, 2007.

CR 26. Pham-Dang C, Kick O, Collet T, et al: Continuous peripheral nerve blocks with stimulating catheters, *Reg Anesth Pain Med* 28:83-88, 2003.

27. Remerand F, Vuitton AS, Palud M, et al: Elastomeric pump reliability in postoperative regional anesthesia: a survey of 430 consecutive devices, *Anesth Analg* 107:2079-2084, 2008.

CR 28. Salinas FV: Location, location, location: continuous peripheral nerve blocks and stimulating catheters, *Reg Anesth Pain Med* 28:79-82, 2003.

29. Schulz-Stubner S: The critically ill patient and regional anesthesia, *Curr Opin Anaesthesiol* 19:538-544, 2006.

30. Sessler CN, Grap MJ, Ramsay MA: Evaluating and monitoring analgesia and sedation in the intensive care unit, *Crit Care* 12(Suppl 3):S2, 2008, available at http://ccforum.com/content/12/S3/S3, accessed October 15, 2009.

CR 31. Shinaman RC, Mackey S: Continuous peripheral nerve blocks, *Curr Pain Headache Rep* 9:24-29, 2005.

32. Skryabina E, Dunn TS: Disposable infusion pumps, *Am J Health Syst Pharm* 63:1260-1268, 2006.

33. Tsui BCH, Rosenquist RW: Peripheral nerve blockade. In Barash PG, Cullen BF, Stoelting RK, et al, editors: *Clinical anesthesia*, ed 6, Philadelphia, 2009, Lippincott Williams & Wilkins, 955-1002.

34. Wedel DJ, Horlocker TT: Nerve blocks. In Miller RD, Eriksson LI, Fleisher LA, et al, editors: *Miller's anesthesia*, ed 7, London, 2009, Churchill Livingstone, 1639-1674.

35. Wiegel M, Gottschaldt U, Hennebach R, et al: Complications and adverse effects associated with continuous peripheral nerve blocks in orthopedic patients, *Anesth Analg* 104:1578-1582, 2007.

Additional Readings

Mulroy MF, Bernards CM, McDonald SB, et al: *A practical approach to regional anesthesia,* ed 4, Philadelphia, 2008, Lippincott Williams & Wilkins.

Richman JM, Liu SS, Courpas G, et al: Does continuous peripheral nerve block provide superior pain control to opioids? A meta-analysis, *Anesth Analg* 102:248-257, 2006.

Turjanica MA: Postoperative continuous peripheral nerve blockade in the lower extremity total joint arthroplasty population, *Medsurg Nurs* 16:151-154, 2007.

Unit IV
Gastrointestinal
System

SECTION SIXTEEN
**Special
Gastrointestinal
Procedures**

PROCEDURE **104**

Esophagogastric Tamponade Tube

P U R P O S E : Esophagogastric tamponade therapy is used to provide temporary control of bleeding from gastric or esophageal varices.[2]

Kathy Bunzli

PREREQUISITE NURSING KNOWLEDGE

- Tamponade therapy exerts direct pressure against the varices with the use of a gastric or esophageal balloon and may be used for cases that are unresponsive to medical therapy or that are too hemodynamically unstable for endoscopy or sclerotherapy.[1,3]
- Esophagogastric tamponade tubes are used to control bleeding from either gastric or esophageal varices. The suction lumens allow the evacuation of accumulated blood from the stomach or esophagus. The suction lumens also allow for the intermittent instillation of saline solution to assist in the evacuation of blood or clots.
- Three types of tubes are available for esophagogastric tamponade therapy. The two most common are the Sengstaken-Blakemore (C.R. BARD, Inc., Covington, Georgia) tube (Fig. 104-1) has a gastric and esophageal balloon and a gastric suction lumen. The four-lumen Minnesota tube (Fig. 104-2) has gastric and esophageal balloons and separate gastric and esophageal suction lumens. The third, the Linton or Linton-Nachlas tube, (Mallinckrodt Inc. Tyco Health Care Group, Hampshire, UK) has a gastric balloon and separate gastric and esophageal suction lumens and is used only for treatment of bleeding gastric varices. The Minnesota tube is considered the preferred tube for esophagogastric tamponade therapy because it allows for suction above and below the balloons. ·
- Esophagogastric tamponade tubes may be introduced via either the nasogastric or the orogastric route. The tubes are then advanced through the oropharynx and esophagus and into the stomach.
- Contraindications include esophageal strictures or recent esophageal surgery, congestive heart failure, respiratory failure, hiatal hernia, and cardiac dysrhythmias.[3] Because of the risk for aspiration, the patient may need endotracheal intubation for airway protection.
- Sedation should be considered, but dosing should be individualized on the basis of the likelihood of liver injury with its concomitant alteration in the metabolism of medications. The plan for sedation is individualized with the goal of achieving patient comfort through a safe use of medications if needed.
- Head of bed (HOB) should be at least 30 to 45 degrees at all times to reduce risk of aspiration.[6]

EQUIPMENT

- Tamponade tube (Sengstaken-Blakemore, Minnesota, or Linton-Nachlas)
- Irrigation kit (or catheter-tip, 60-mL syringe and basin)
- Nasogastric (NG) tubes (one for Sengstaken-Blakemore tube)
- Normal saline (NS) solution for irrigation
- NS solution, 500 mL (provides weight for traction on the tube)
- Water-soluble lubricant
- Topical anesthetic agent
- Sphygmomanometer or pressure gauge
- Four rubber-shod clamps
- Adhesive tape
- Two suction setups and tubing

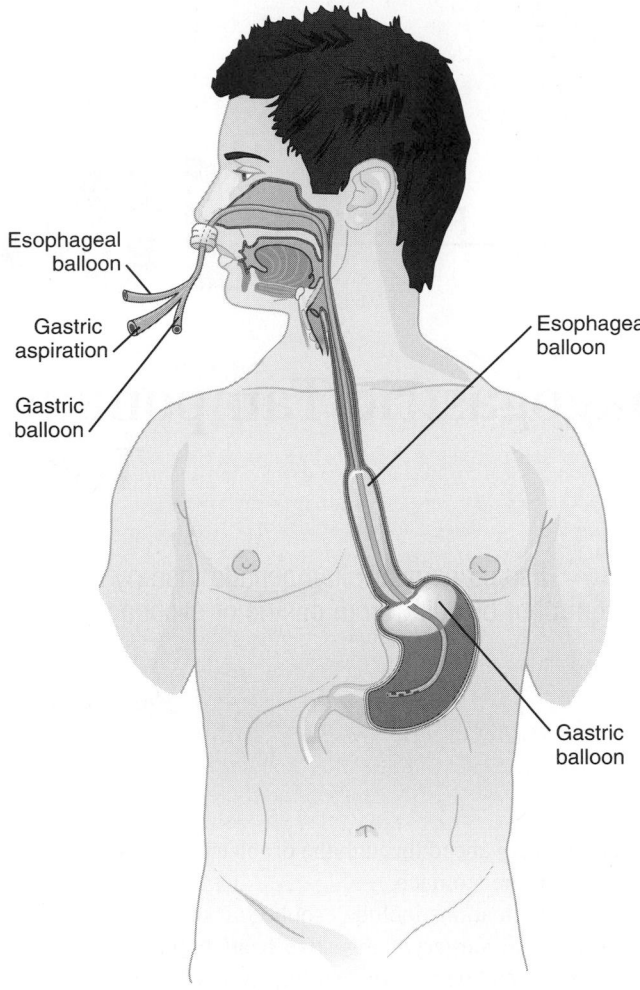

Esophageal balloon

Gastric aspiration

Gastric balloon

Esophageal balloon

Gastric balloon

FIGURE 104-1   Sengstaken-Blakemore tube in place with both the esophageal and gastric balloons inflated. *(From Carlson KK, editor: AACN: advanced critical care nursing, Philadelphia, 2009, Saunders, 751.)*

- Endotracheal suction equipment
- Cardiac monitor
- Emergency medications, including atropine
- Emergency equipment, including transcutaneous pacemaker and intubation equipment
- Scissors, to be kept at bedside
  Additional equipment (to have available based on patient need) includes the following:
- Rubber cube sponge (used for nasal tamponade tube placement)
- Balanced suspension traction apparatus with 1 pound of weights, 500 mL of NS solution (Fig. 104-3), or football helmet with face mask (Figs. 104-4)
- Lopez enteral valve (Fig. 104-5)[7] (ICU, Medical, San Clemente, CA), a three-way stopcock used to attach a 60-mL catheter-tip syringe and the handheld manometer to the Minnesota tube

PATIENT AND FAMILY EDUCATION

- Explain the procedure and reason for the tube insertion. ➧*Rationale:* Patient anxiety may be decreased.
- Explain the patient's role in assisting with the passage of the tube and maintenance of tamponade traction. ➧*Rationale:* Patient cooperation is elicited during the insertion and tamponade therapy.
- Explain that the procedure can be uncomfortable because the gag reflex may be stimulated, causing the patient to be nauseated or to vomit. ➧*Rationale:* Patient cooperation is elicited during the insertion.

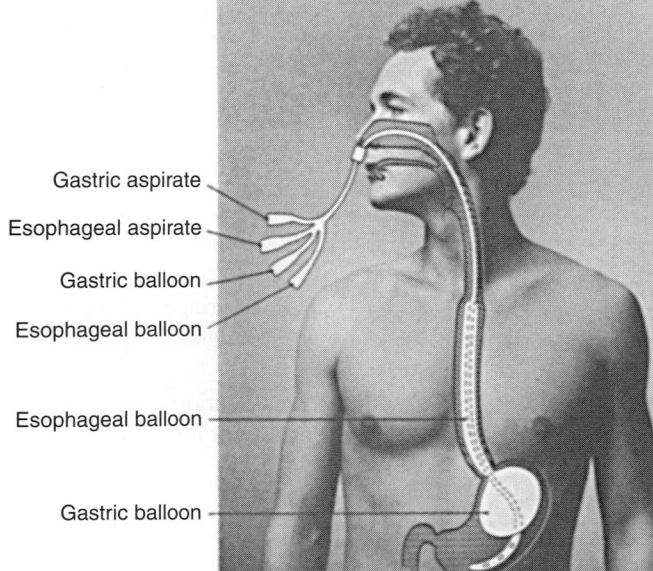

Gastric aspirate

Esophageal aspirate

Gastric balloon

Esophageal balloon

Esophageal balloon

Gastric balloon

FIGURE 104-2   Minnesota four-lumen tube. *(From Swearingen PL: Photo atlas of nursing procedures, Reading, MA, 1991, Addison-Wesley.)*

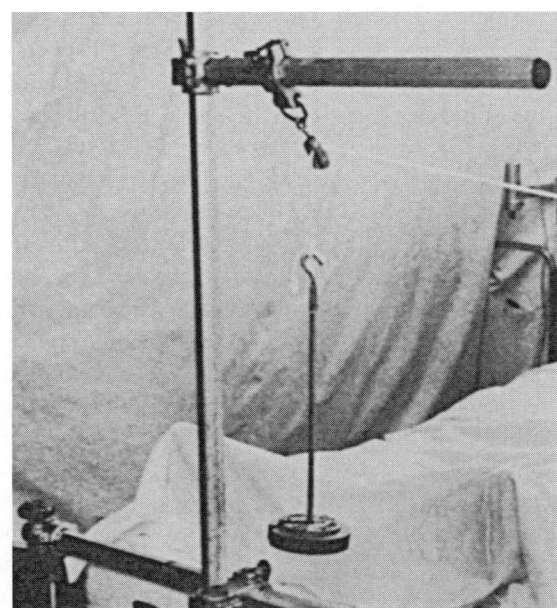

FIGURE 104-3   Balanced suspension traction securing tamponade tube and placement. *(From DeGroot KD, Damato M: Critical care skills, Norwalk, CT, 1987, Appleton & Lange.)*

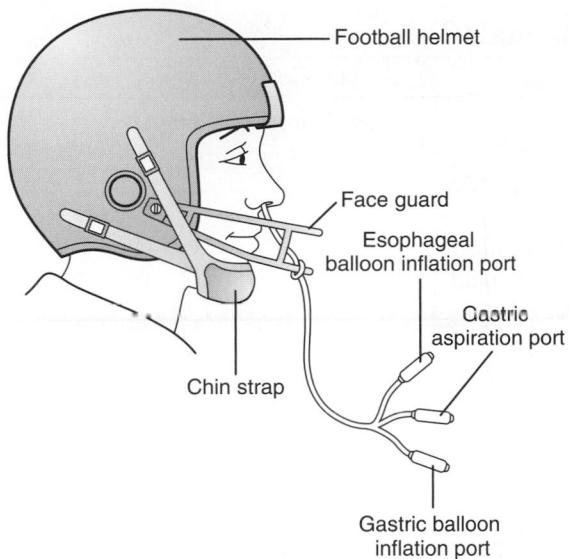

FIGURE 104-4 Tamponade tube secured in position with helmet.

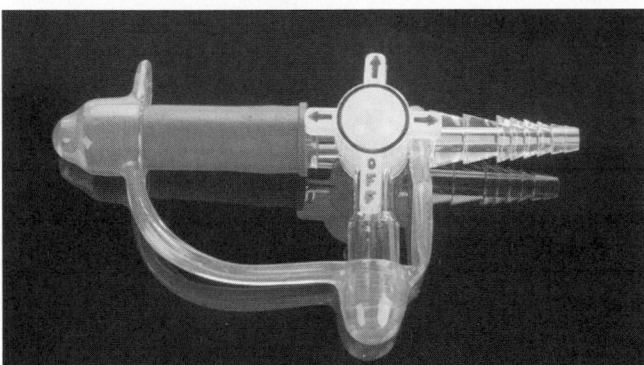

FIGURE 104-5 Lopez valve. *(Courtesy of ICU Medical, Inc. San Clemente, CA.)*

PATIENT ASSESSMENT AND PREPARATION

Patient Assessment

- Assess signs and symptoms of major blood loss:
  ❖ Tachycardia
  ❖ Tachypnea
  ❖ Hypotension
  ❖ Decreased urine output
  ❖ Decreased filling pressures (pulmonary artery pressure, pulmonary capillary wedge pressure and central venous pressure)
  ❖ Decreased platelet counts
  ❖ Decreased hematocrit and hemoglobin values
  ❖ Change in level of consciousness (LOC)

➤*Rationale:* Esophageal or gastric varices can cause significant blood loss.
- Assess the baseline cardiac rhythm. ➤*Rationale:* Passage of a large-bore tube into the esophagus may cause vagal stimulation and bradycardia.
- Assess the baseline respiratory status (i.e., rate, depth, pattern, and characteristics of secretions). ➤*Rationale:* Use of topical anesthetic agents in the nares or oropharynx may alter the gag or cough reflex, increasing the risk for aspiration. Passage of a large-bore tube may impair the airway. Large amounts of blood in the stomach predispose a patient to vomiting and potential aspiration.
- Assess the patient's ability to protect the airway. ➤*Rationale:* Multiple factors can influence the patient's ability to protect the airway, including presence of vomiting and depressed mental status.
- Assess the mental status. ➤*Rationale:* Patients with altered mental status should be intubated and mechanically ventilated prophylactically to prevent airway complications.
- If anticipating a nasal esophageal tube placement:
  ❖ Absolute contraindications include a history of transphenoidal hypophysectomy. ➤*Rationale:* This type of surgical procedure may predispose placement of the tube into the cranial vault.
  ❖ Assess for medical history of nasal deformity, surgery, trauma, epistaxis, or coagulopathy. ➤*Rationale:* The risk for complications and bleeding with nasal insertion is increased.
  ❖ Evaluate patency of nares. Occlude one naris at a time, and ask the patient to breathe through the nose. Select the naris with the best airflow. ➤*Rationale:* Choosing the most patent naris eases insertion and may improve patient tolerance of the tube.
  ❖ The nasal route is not recommended in patients with coagulopathy. ➤*Rationale:* The risk for bleeding and complications is increased.

Patient Preparation

- Ensure that the patient and family understand preprocedural teachings. Answer questions as they arise, and reinforce information as needed. ➤*Rationale:* Understanding of previously taught information is evaluated and reinforced.
- Measure the tube from the bridge of the nose to the earlobe to the tip of the xiphoid process. Mark the length of tube to be inserted. ➤*Rationale:* Estimating the length of tube to be inserted helps place the distal tip in the stomach.
- If the patient is alert, place the patient in high Fowler's or semi-Fowler's position. If the patient is unconscious or obtunded, place the patient head down in the left lateral position. ➤*Rationale:* Positioning facilitates the passage of the tube into the stomach and reduces the risk for aspiration.

Procedure | for Inserting Esophagogastric Tamponade Tube

Steps	Rationale	Special Considerations
1. **HH**		Check for latex allergy.
2. **PE**		
3. Attach the gastric balloon port to the sphygmomanometer or pressure gauge (Fig. 104-6).	Measuring the pressure of the gastric balloon as it is inflated immediately on insertion may prevent its inflation in the esophagus, which could cause esophageal rupture.	
4. Test the tamponade tube balloon integrity:	Ensures integrity of esophageal balloon.[1]	
A. If applicable, inflate the esophageal balloon with the volume indicated in the package insert. **(Level M*)**		
B. Inflate the gastric balloon with 100, 200, 300, 400, and 500 mL of air, noting the pressure reading at each stage of inflation. **(Level M)**	Knowing the pressure required at each stage of inflation may prevent inadvertent perforation of the esophagus after insertion.[1]	
C. Hold the air-filled balloon under water to test for air leaks. **(Level M)**	Ensures integrity of balloon.[1]	
D. Actively and completely deflate the balloon and clamp. **(Level M)**	Deflated balloon eases insertion.[1]	
5. Insert a nasogastric tube into the stomach, drain contents, and then remove tube.	Emptying the stomach of blood/gastric contents decreases the risk for aspiration and minimizes occlusion of the tube with blood clots.	
6. Lubricate balloons and distal 15 cm of tube with water-soluble lubricant. **(Level E*)**	Minimizes mucosal injury and irritation during insertion; facilitates insertion.[1]	Use only water-soluble lubricant. Oil-based lubricants, such as petroleum jelly, may cause respiratory complications if inadvertently aspirated. Oil-based lubricants may also damage the latex in the tube and may cause the balloon to rupture.[1]

*Level E: Multiple case reports, theory-based evidence from expert opinions, or peer-reviewed professional organizational standards without clinical studies to support recommendations

*Level M: Manufacturer's recommendations only

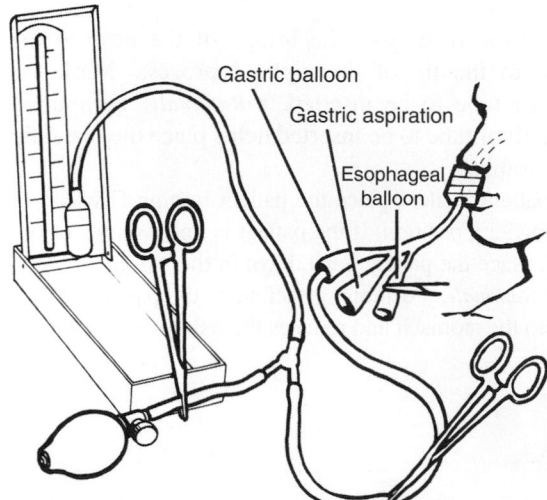

Gastric balloon
Gastric aspiration
Esophageal balloon

FIGURE 104-6 Inflation of esophageal balloon. *(Courtesy of Davol, Inc. Warwick, RI)*

Procedure for Inserting Esophagogastric Tamponade Tube—*Continued*

Steps	Rationale	Special Considerations
7. Apply the topical anesthetic agent to the posterior oropharynx as prescribed by the physician or advanced practice nurse (apply to nostril if nasally inserted). **(Level D*)**	Decreases discomfort caused by insertion.[1]	*Caution:* Gag and cough reflexes may be compromised by topical anesthetic, increasing the risk for aspiration. Keep emergency intubation equipment easily available.
8. Assist practitioner with insertion of the tamponade tube into mouth or selected nostril. The tube is advanced into stomach to at least the 50-cm mark on the tube or 10 cm beyond the estimated length needed to reach the stomach. (Fig. 104-7) **(Level E*)**	Ensures placement of entire gastric balloon in stomach.[1]	Heart rate may decrease as a result of vagal stimulation. Should symptomatic bradycardia occur, atropine may be administered or transcutaneous pacing initiated as prescribed (or per institutional protocol).
9. Lavage stomach via gastric suction port with NS solution until clear of large blood clots. **(Level E)**	Ensures patency and prevents clots from blocking the tube.[5,8]	
10. Connect gastric suction port to intermittent suction at 60 to 120 mm Hg. **(Level E)**	Provides for evacuation of gastric contents and for assessment of continued bleeding.[3,5,8]	
11. Connect esophageal suction port to intermittent suction at 120 to 200 mm Hg (Minnesota tube only). **(Level D)**	Provides for evacuation of secretions and for assessment of continued bleeding.[1,3]	

---

*Level D: Peer-reviewed professional organizational standards with clinical studies to support recommendations

*Level E: Multiple case reports, theory-based evidence from expert opinions, or peer-reviewed professional organizational standards without clinical studies to support recommendations

---

Procedure continues on following page

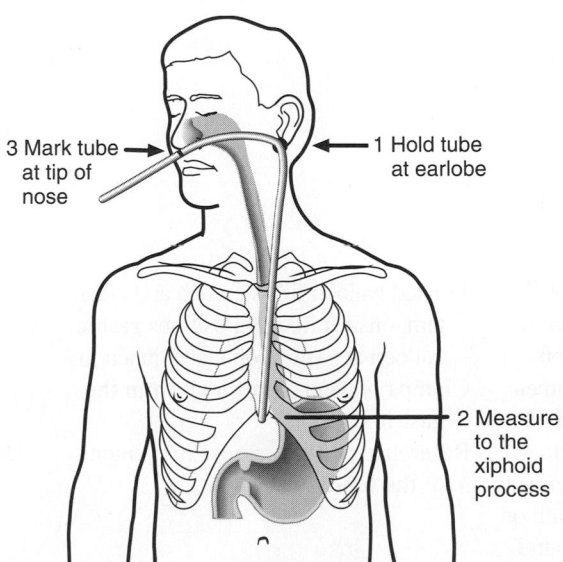

3 Mark tube at tip of nose

1 Hold tube at earlobe

2 Measure to the xiphoid process

FIGURE 104-7 Measuring nasogastric tube. *(From Luckmann J: Saunders manual of nursing care, Philadelphia, 1997, Saunders, 1262.)*

Procedure for Inserting Esophagogastric Tamponade Tube—*Continued*

Steps	Rationale	Special Considerations
12. Tube placement must be confirmed:		
A. Aspirate drainage from gastric suction port. **(Level M*)**	Prevents gastric balloon from being inflated in the esophagus, causing rupture.[1]	The ability to simply aspirate fluid from the tube is often interpreted as confirmation of gastric intubation. Caution is needed because several reports have shown that fluid can also be aspirated after endotracheal intubation. The gold standard to confirm placement is an abdominal or chest radiograph to ensure proper placement of tamponade tube.[1,4,7]
B. The physician or other advanced practitioner slowly inflates the gastric balloon with increments of 100 mL of air, up to a total 500 mL, observing the pressure on the sphygmomanometer or pressure gauge at each increment. (If the pressure exceeds preinflation pressure for a particular volume by more than 15 mm Hg, all of the air is withdrawn and the tube is advanced an additional 10 cm.) **(Level E*)**	A pressure difference of more than 15 mm Hg indicates that the gastric balloon is in the esophagus.[3,5,8]	pH testing of gastric secretions may also be used to assess placement. Auscultation to confirm gastric tube placement by placing a stethoscope over the stomach and instilling 20 to 50 mL of air via syringe is no longer accepted practice. Numerous reports are found in the literature of tubes improperly placed but believed in the correct location with the auscultation method of assessment.
C. On full inflation of the gastric balloon, clamp the gastric balloon lumen with a rubber-shod clamp. An abdominal radiograph is obtained.	Outline of gastric balloon can be visualized on radiograph. Ensures placement of entire gastric balloon with the stomach.[3,8]	The gastric balloon inflation process may be simplified with the use of a Lopez enteral valve, (Fig. 104-5) which can be connected to one side of the gastric balloon. The catheter-tip syringe goes into the large port, and the manometer in another, and the tapered end of the valve goes into the Minnesota tube. This alternative may eliminate the need to repeatedly clamp and unclamp the tubing while measuring the volume of air injected through the 60-mL catheter-tip syringe.
13. On radiographic confirmation of placement, the tube is withdrawn until slight resistance is met. Double-clamp the gastric balloon lumen with rubber-shod clamp. **(Level M*)**	Inflated balloon fills stomach and creates tamponade effect.[3,8] Positions gastric balloon at gastroesophageal junction. Clamps prevent an air leak from the gastric balloon.[1,3,8]	
14. Use permanent marker or tape to mark the tamponade tube placement at the opening at either the mouth or nose. Place the tape marker around tube as it exits the mouth or nose.	Reference point to assess movement of the tube.	Document the marking and assess the tube for possible migration based on marking.

*Level E: Multiple case reports, theory-based evidence from expert opinions, or peer-reviewed professional organizational standards without clinical studies to support recommendations
*Level M: Manufacturer's recommendations only

Procedure for Inserting Esophagogastric Tamponade Tube—*Continued*

Steps	Rationale	Special Considerations
15. The practitioner performing the tube insertion performs or prescribes inflation of the esophageal balloon if bleeding is not controlled with gastric tamponade. A. Clamp the tube and disconnect the sphygmomanometer or pressure gauge from the gastric balloon port and attach it to the esophageal balloon port. **(Level M*)**	Produces direct pressure on esophageal vessels.[1,3,4]	Maintain esophageal balloon pressures as prescribed or per institution protocol.
B. Gradually inflate the esophageal balloon to 25 to 45 mm Hg. **(Level M)**	Higher pressures may cause esophageal necrosis.[1]	Patient may have chest pain with inflation. Monitor electrocardiographic (ECG) changes during placement, removal, or inflation of the balloon.
C. Double-clamp the esophageal balloon port with rubber-shod clamps. **(Level M)**	Prevents air leaks from esophageal balloon.[1]	
16. If bleeding has not stopped, gentle traction is applied to the tube. **(Level M)** A. Apply gentle traction (1) Use 1 pound of weight attached to tube with balance suspension traction (see Fig. 104-3). (2) For alternative traction, use a 500 mL of NS solution bag. Attach bag to tube with balance system (see Figs. 104-3.)	Fixes position of gastric balloon and exerts pressure on varices.[1,5,8]	
B. Tape tube to sponge cube at naris, if tube is passed nasally. **or**	Prevents excessive pressure on nares.	
C. Apply football helmet to the patient's head and tape tube to chin or faceguard (see Fig. 104-4).		Pad the inside of helmet to ensure a snug fit and to prevent pressure ulcer formation on the occipital region of the head.
17. Place the head of the bed at 30 to 45 degrees. **(Level D*)**	Promotes comfort, minimizes aspiration, and may prevent ventilator-associated pneumonia (if patient is intubated).[4]	
18. Sengstaken-Blakemore tube only: A. Insert an NG tube to just above the esophageal balloon. **(Level D)**	Reduces secretions and accumulated blood.[1,5,8]	If the gastric tube migrates upward, it may result in complete blockage of airway.
B. Use permanent marker or tape to mark the tamponade tube placement at the opening of either the mouth or nose.	Reference point to assess migration of tube.	

*Level D: Peer-reviewed professional organizational standards with clinical studies to support recommendations
*Level M: Manufacturer's recommendations only

Procedure continues on following page

Procedure | for Inserting Esophagogastric Tamponade Tube—*Continued*

Steps	Rationale	Special Considerations
C. Connect to intermittent suction 120 to 200 mm Hg. **(Level D)**	Reduces secretions and accumulated blood.[1,8]	
D. The position of the Sengstaken-Blakemore tube should be checked and documented every hour.		
19. Gastric balloon inflated:		
A. The gastric inflated balloon should be kept at the minimal pressure required to control bleeding (approximately 25 mm Hg for at least 48 hours) and deflated for 12 to 24 hours to assess for any new bleeding. **(Level M*)**	Underinflation can lead to tube displacement into the esophagus. Overinflation can lead to mucosal and submucosal ischemia.[1]	
B. The Sengstaken-Blakemore tube should remain in place for a short period of time. **(Level E*)**	Minimizes the opportunity for mucosal trauma.[2]	
20. Changes with inflation or deflation of the tamponade tube should be performed or prescribed by a physician or advanced practitioner:		
A. Connect sphygmomanometer to the esophageal balloon port.	The esophageal balloon is inflated if the bleeding continues after the inflation of the gastric balloon. Do not inflate the esophageal balloon first.	
B. With use of the second access port, gradually inflate the esophageal balloon to 25 to 45 mm Hg.	High pressures can lead to mucosal and submucosal ischemia.	Higher pressures may cause pain with inflation. Monitor ECG for changes during placement, inflation, or removal of the esophageal balloon.
C. Double-clamp the esophageal balloon port with rubber-shod clamps. **(Level M)**	Prevent esophageal trauma.	
D. The physician or advanced practitioner must deflate the esophageal balloon to make any changes to the tube's position. **(Level D*)**	Ensures adequate balloon inflation for tamponade. Prevents mucosal ischemia, necrosis, and injury,[1,3,8] Prevents air leaks from the esophageal balloon.[1]	
Discontinuing Tamponade Therapy		
21. Discontinue tamponade therapy in stages. **(Level E)**	Provides for gradual reduction in tamponade to assess cessation of bleeding.[1,8]	
A. Deflate the esophageal balloon (if inflation was needed to control bleeding) by unclamping the esophageal balloon port and aspirating with an irrigation syringe to actively deflate the balloon.		Never deflate gastric balloon while esophageal balloon remains inflated. A deflated gastric balloon may allow an inflated esophageal balloon to migrate in the airway. If the airway becomes obstructed, immediately cut both balloon ports to deflate the balloons and remove the tube immediately.

*Level D: Peer-reviewed professional organizational standards with clinical studies to support recommendations

*Level E: Multiple case reports, theory-based evidence from expert opinions, or peer-reviewed professional organizational standards without clinical studies to support recommendations

*Level M: Manufacturer's recommendations only

Procedure for Inserting Esophagogastric Tamponade Tube—*Continued*

Steps	Rationale	Special Considerations
B. Observe for the recurrence of bleeding over 24 hours. If bleeding recurs, reinflate the esophageal balloon as directed by the physician or advanced practitioner or assist with this step of the procedure.	Bleeding may recur with the release of pressure on the esophageal varices.[1,8]	
C. If no further bleeding is noted, the gastric balloon is deflated by unclamping the gastric balloon port and aspirating with an irrigation syringe to actively deflate the balloon (this step is ordered or performed by a physician or advanced practitioner).		
D. Observe for the recurrence of bleeding over 24 hours. If bleeding recurs, reinflate the gastric balloon or assist with this step of the procedure as needed based on institutional practice.	Bleeding may recur with the release of pressure on esophageal varices.	
E. If bleeding has not recurred in 24 hours, assist with the removal of the tube by cutting the balloon lumens with scissors and slowly withdrawing the tube. (**Level E***)	Ensures complete balloon deflation before removal.[1,8]	
22. Dispose of equipment and soiled material in appropriate receptacle.	Standard Precautions.	
23. **HH**		

Expected Outcomes

- Cessation of variceal bleeding
- Gastric decompression and evacuation

Unexpected Outcomes

- Inappropriate placement of tamponade tube
- Gastric or esophageal necrosis
- Esophageal rupture
- Airway obstruction
- Cardiac dysrhythmias (during insertion or removal)
- Aspiration of gastric or oropharyngeal contents
- Erosion of mucosa around nares

Patient Monitoring and Care

Steps	Rationale	Reportable Conditions
		These conditions should be reported if they persist despite nursing interventions.
1. Maintain tamponade therapy as needed: maximum of 24 to 36 hours for esophageal balloon; 48 to 72 hours for gastric balloon. (**Level D***)	Longer inflation time may cause necrosis or ulceration.[1]	• Continued bleeding

*Level D: Peer-reviewed professional organizational standards with clinical studies to support recommendations
*Level E: Multiple case reports, theory-based evidence from expert opinions, or peer-reviewed professional organizational standards without clinical studies to support recommendations

Procedure continues on following page

Patient Monitoring and Care —*Continued*

Steps	Rationale	Reportable Conditions

2. Provide care to nares every 2 hours when tube is inserted nasally.
  A. Remove dried blood or secretions from the nasal orifice and proximal nares.
  B. Apply lubricating ointment or lotion to keep the mucosa moist.
	Prevents drying and ulcerations of the mucosa.	• Breakdown of tissue around the nares

3. Provide oral care every 2 hours.	Prevents drying and ulcerations of the mucosa and is also a strategy to thwart the development of ventilator-assisted pneumonia (VAP).	• Mouth, tongue, or lip ulcerations
4. Provide frequent oral suctioning. (**Level E***)	Esophageal balloon prevents swallowing of secretions and saliva.[4,5]	• Bloody oral secretions
5. Monitor the esophageal balloon pressure hourly. Maintain esophageal balloon pressures at 25 to 45 mm Hg (pressures vary with respirations and may intermittently reach 70 mm Hg). (**Level E**)	Prevents excessive pressure on esophageal tissues.[1,5] Sudden loss of pressure may indicate rupture of balloon or esophagus.	• Continued esophageal bleeding • Sudden loss of balloon pressure
6. Decrease the esophageal balloon pressure by 5 mm Hg every 3 hours (as per physician order or assist the physician or other advanced practitioner in this step of the procedure) until pressure is 25 mm Hg, without evidence of bleeding. (**Level E**)	Use of the lowest possible pressure to create tamponade effect reduces the possibility of necrosis.[1,5]	• Continued esophageal bleeding
7. Assist with the complete deflation of the esophageal balloon for 30 minutes every 8 hours or perform this step as prescribed by physician or other advanced practitioner per institutional protocol. (**Level E**)	Intermittent relief of the pressure may prevent necrosis of esophageal tissue.[1]	• Continued esophageal bleeding
8. Evaluate for recurrence of variceal bleeding.	Bleeding may occur despite tamponade therapy.	• Continued bleeding
9. Monitor for airway patency and respiratory status.	Presence or movement of a large-bore tube may impair the upper airway.	• Tachypnea • Stridor • Cough • High-pressure alarms on mechanical ventilator
10. Keep scissors at the bedside to immediately deflate the balloons. (**Level E**)	Inadvertent deflation of the gastric balloon may result in blockage of the airway by the esophageal balloon.[1]	
11. Obtain an abdominal radiograph every 24 hours or sooner if there is any indication of displacement of the tamponade tube. (**Level E**)	Inadvertent deflation of the gastric balloon may cause blockage of the airway by the esophageal balloon.[1,3,5,8]	

*Level E: Multiple case reports, theory-based evidence from expert opinions, or peer-reviewed professional organizational standards without clinical studies to support recommendations

Patient Monitoring and Care —*Continued*

Steps	Rationale	Reportable Conditions
12. Monitor the gastric output. Irrigate the gastric suction port with 50 mL of NS solution every 30 minutes, or as needed, to keep the lumen patent. **(Level E)**	Blood clots may occlude the gastric lumen.[1]	• Continued gastric bleeding • Change in characteristics of output (color, quantity)
13. Monitor the esophageal output. Irrigate the esophageal suction port (or NG with Sengstaken-Blakemore) with 5 to 10 mL of NS solution every 2 to 4 hours, or as needed, to maintain patency. **(Level M*)**	Blood clots may occlude the esophageal suction lumen (or NG tube).[1]	• Continued esophageal bleeding • Change in characteristics of drainage (color, quantity)

Documentation

Documentation should include the following:

- Patient and family education
- Date and time of the insertion
- Name of the provider inserting tube
- Tube type
- Any difficulties with the insertion
- Patient tolerance of the tube insertion, including pressures with specific balloon volumes
- Confirmation of placement with an abdominal radiograph
- Type and maintenance of the traction device
- Amount and type of suction applied to the various lumens
- Esophageal and gastric balloon pressures as applicable
- Periodic deflation of the esophageal balloon
- Appearance and volume of gastric and esophageal drainage, if present
- Nasal or oral care
- Tube site assessments (nasal or oral)
- Unexpected outcomes
- Deflation sequence of the esophageal and gastric balloons
- Medications administered during the tube insertion (if applicable)

*Level E: Multiple case reports, theory-based evidence from expert opinions, or peer-reviewed professional organizational standards without clinical studies to support recommendations
*Level M: Manufacturer's recommendations only

References

1. Bard Medical: Bard Medical Division, 8195 Industrial Boulevard, Covington, GA 30014 *Instructions for passing Minnesota four lumen esophagogastic tamponade tube for the control of bleeding from esophageal varicies,* 2006.
2. Christensen T, Christensen M: The implementation for guideline of care for patients with Sengstaken-Blakemore tube in situ in a general intensive care unit using transitional change theory, *Intensive Crit Care Nurs* 23:234-242, 2007.
3. Day M: Gastrointestinal bleeding. In Carlson K, editor: *Advanced critical care nursing,* St Louis, 2009, Saunders, 748-751.
4. Hilinski A, Stark ML: Memory aide to reduce the incidence of ventilator-associated pneumonia, *Crit Care Nurse* 26(5): 80-81, 2006.
5. Isaacs KL: *Balloon tamponade: handbook of gastroenterologic procedures,* ed 4, 2005, Philadelphia, Lippincott Williams & Wilkins, 119-120, retrieved August 17, 2009, from www.findarticles.com/p/articles/mi.
6. Mallinckrodt Inc. Tyco Health Care Group, 154 fareham road gosport, hampshire, UK, po 13 oas *Linton-Nachlas tube,* retrieved April 19, 2009, from www.gpnotebook.co.uk/simplepage.cfm.
7. Martin RK, Hassanein T: Liver dysfunction and failure. In Carlson KK, editor: *Advanced critical care nursing,* Philadelphia, 2009, Saunders/Elsevier, 759-764.
8. Treger R, Graham TP, Dea SK: *Sengstaken-Blakemore tube: treatment & medication,* 2008, retrieved April1, 2009, from http//emedicine.medscape.com/article/81020-treatment.

Additional Reading

Garcia-Tsao G: Portal hypertension, *Curr Opin Gastroenterol* 22(3):254-262, 2006.

Gastric Lavage in Hemorrhage and Overdose

P U R P O S E :　With suspected gastric hemorrhage, gastric lavage can be used for the initial assessment of upper gastrointestinal bleeding to potentially identify the severity of bleeding and clear the stomach of blood and clots. Gastric lavage may improve visualization of the gastric fundus in preparation for endoscopy or endoscopic treatments. In overdose, gastric lavage can be used to evacuate drugs or toxins within 1 hour of ingestion, potentially minimizing the consequences of systemic absorption of drugs or toxins.

Ann G. Will

PREREQUISITE NURSING KNOWLEDGE

- Gastric lavage is not recommended as a routine procedure in the management of hemorrhage and overdose. Current evidence (Level D*) shows limited improvement in patient outcomes after lavage, and the procedure may contribute to additional complications, including gastric or esophageal perforation, aspiration, laryngospasm, dysrhythmias, hypothermia, fluid and electrolyte abnormalities, and hypoxia.[2,3,5,7-10] The risk-benefit ratio of gastric lavage should be considered before the procedure is performed.
- The use of gastric lavage has been found to be of potential benefit in some cases of hemorrhage and overdose. Specific indications for the use of gastric lavage include:
  - ❖ Gastrointestinal (GI) hemorrhage: The patient who has had GI hemorrhage may present with signs and symptoms of volume loss and a decrease in oxygen-carrying capacity. These symptoms include tachypnea, tachycardia, hypotension, orthostatic changes, decreased hemodynamic filling pressures, decreased urine output, pallor, cold and clammy skin, confusion, anxiety, and somnolence. The patient may also show signs of hematemesis, maroon or tarry stools, or hematochezia.

Gastric lavage in GI hemorrhage may be helpful in clearing the stomach of blood and clots to facilitate evaluation of the source of bleeding and to improve visualization of the gastric fundus in preparation for endoscopic treatment.[5,10] The presence of bright red blood in the aspirate could be an indicator for the need for urgent enodoscopy.[5]

- ❖ Overdose: The American Academy of Clinical Toxicology and European Association of Poisons Centres and Clinical Toxicologists do not recommend the use of gastric lavage in the routine management of poisoned patients because of the limited evidence of improved patient outcomes and potential risks of the procedure.[3,9] However, in specific poisoning cases, gastric lavage could be of some benefit (Level D*). Indications include if lavage is initiated in symptomatic patients within 1 hour (60 minutes) of ingestion of a potentially life-threatening amount of highly toxic substance, if the substance slows GI motility, or if the substance is a sustained-release medication.[3,7-9] Gastric lavage is contraindicated in the use of overdose if the patient has consumed strong corrosives or hydrocarbons (e.g., gasoline, strong acids, or alkali) and if the pills or pill fragments are known to be larger than the opening of the orogastric (OG) tube.[6,9] The administration of activated charcoal (AC) has been used in combination with gastric lavage for specific toxins; however, its use must be approached

---

*Level D: Peer-reviewed professional organizational standards with clinical studies to support recommendations

cautiously because the combination of therapies may result in an increased risk for aspiration.[7,8] It should be noted that the end point of gastric lavage is not clearly defined if particulate cannot be clearly observed; however, the amount of lavage fluid instilled should approximate the amount of fluid returned.[7-9] Gastric lavage after overdose or toxin ingestion has variable efficacy. The amount of toxin or drug recovered depends on variables such as time from ingestion, whether liquid or pills were ingested, specific agent ingested, and size of lavage tube used. Even if lavage is performed close to the time of ingestion, not all the ingested toxin will be recovered and treatment related to effects of the overdose will still be necessary.[6-9]

- Nonintubated patients who need gastric lavage must be alert and have adequate pharyngeal and laryngeal reflexes. If the patient has a limited gag reflex or is unable to protect the airway, the patient should be intubated before gastric lavage is performed.[6,9,11] All patients undergoing gastric lavage should be positioned in the left lateral decubitus position to assist with passage of the gastric tube.[7-9]
- Passage of the lavage tube may cause vagal stimulation and precipitate bradydysrhythmias.
- Patients with esophageal varices, coagulopathy, a recent history of upper GI tract surgery, or an underlying pathology should be carefully evaluated for the risk/benefit ratio before gastric lavage is performed.[6,9]

EQUIPMENT

- Adult lavage tube, external diameter 12 to 13.3 mm[9]
  - ❖ No. 36 to 40 Fr gastric tube or
  - ❖ No. 30 English gastric tube
- 60-mL irrigating syringe
- Water-soluble lubricant
- Lavage fluid (warm normal saline solution or tap water)
- Measurable container for lavage fluid
- Disposable basin or suction canister for aspirate
- Suction source and connecting tubing
- Rigid pharyngeal suction-tip (Yankauer) catheter
- Endotracheal suction equipment
- Tape for securing nasogastric (NG) or OG tube
- Stethoscope
- Cardiac monitor
- Pulse oximeter
- Automatic blood pressure cuff
- Nonsterile gloves
- Eye and face protection
- Barrier gowns

  Additional equipment, to have available based on patient need, includes the following:
- Specimen container for aspirate (for overdose)
- Absorptive agent for instillation (for overdose, if prescribed)
- Emergency intubation and cardiac equipment
- Bite block or oral airway (if patient needs intubation for procedure)
- Emergency medications

PATIENT AND FAMILY EDUCATION

- Explain the indications and procedure for gastric lavage. ➤*Rationale:* Patient and family anxiety may be decreased.
- Evaluate the patient and family understanding of the risks and benefits of gastric lavage. ➤*Rationale:* The patient and family may be unaware of the risks and benefits of the procedure.
- Explain the patient's role in assisting with passage of the tube and lavage of the stomach. ➤*Rationale:* The patient's cooperation during the procedure is elicited.
- Explain the purpose of the cardiac monitor, automatic blood pressure cuff, and pulse oximeter. ➤*Rationale:* Patient and family anxiety may be decreased.
- Assess the need for family presence during the procedure. ➤*Rationale:* Patient and family anxiety may be decreased and patient cooperation during the procedure could potentially be improved.
- Evaluate patient and family need for information on prevention of accidental ingestion of drugs or toxic agents. ➤*Rationale:* The patient and family may be unaware or uninformed that the agent or drug is potentially toxic.
- Evaluate patient and family need for information on emergency treatment for accidental ingestion of drug or toxic agents. ➤*Rationale:* Emergency first aid measures may be helpful with some ingestions to decrease potential toxicity or systemic absorption.

PATIENT ASSESSMENT AND PREPARATION
Patient Assessment

- Perform baseline cardiovascular and neurologic assessments and assess hemodynamic status, cardiac rhythm, and vital signs. ➤*Rationale:* Passage of the lavage tube may cause changes in heart rate, blood pressure, or vagal stimulation, which can precipitate bradydysrhythmias or other electrocardiographic (ECG) changes, including ST elevation.[9] In the overdose case, toxic levels of certain classes of drugs can also cause ECG changes.[3]
- Perform baseline respiratory assessment and pulse oximetry. ➤*Rationale:* Gastric lavage has been shown to cause changes in oxygen saturation, leading to hypoxia. Patients who are unable to protect the airway should be intubated before gastric lavage.
- Signs and symptoms of major blood loss are as follows:
  - ❖ Tachycardia
  - ❖ Tachypnea
  - ❖ Decreased urine output
  - ❖ Hypotension
  - ❖ Decreased hemodynamic filling pressures
  - ❖ Pallor, cold and clammy skin
  - ❖ Changes in mental status or somnolence
  - ❖ Hematemesis
  - ❖ Maroon or tarry stools
  - ❖ Hematochezia

➤*Rationale:* Esophageal or gastric varices can cause significant blood loss. The clinical presentation is dependent on amount of blood lost.

- Evaluate the patient for a history of esophageal varices, recent GI surgery, coagulopathy, or underlying pathology. ➤*Rationale:* Varices, recent surgery, coagulopathies, or other contraindications may predispose the patient to complications during lavage tube insertion.
- Obtain baseline coagulation studies, hematocrit and hemoglobin values, basic metabolic panel, renal and liver function tests, and blood type. ➤*Rationale:* Baseline information is provided so that treatment can be determined and progress can be more accurately monitored.
- Serum toxicology screen, urinalysis, urine toxicology screen, and anion gap (overdose case) are other laboratory tests that also may be monitored. ➤*Rationale:* Baseline information for diagnosis is provided so that intervention can be made appropriately and patient progress can be more accurately monitored.[3]
- Obtain arterial blood gas (ABG) values. ➤*Rationale:* Overdose victims with hypoventilation and patients with GI hemorrhage with significant blood loss or comorbid disease are at risk for hypoxia, hypercapnea, and acid-base disorders.
- Assess adequacy of gag reflex. ➤*Rationale:* Lack of an adequate gag reflex indicates the need for endotracheal intubation before lavage begins.[6,9,11]
- Assess the type of drugs or toxic substances ingested, quantity ingested, and time since ingestion. Use of common toxidromes (classifications of the signs and symptoms that develop with poisoning) can help to identify unknown ingested substances (for the overdose case).[3] ➤*Rationale:* Certain substances may require neutralization before tube evacuation is attempted. A poison control center should be contacted if the practitioner is unsure that lavage is indicated. Side effects can be anticipated if the drugs or toxins that were swallowed and the quantity are known.

- Perform careful skin assessment (overdose case). ➤*Rationale:* Assessment may give evidence regarding toxin ingested because various drugs can cause cutaneous changes. Changes to look for include diaphoresis, bullae, acneiform rash, flushed appearance, and cyanosis.
- Assess any odors present (overdose case). ➤*Rationale:* Some toxins have a distinctive odor, which can aid in identification of substance ingested.
- Perform a 12-lead ECG and continuous cardiac monitoring. ➤*Rationale:* In an overdose case, the drug or toxin ingested may be cardiotoxic. For the patient with a GI hemorrhage, comorbid disease states may increase risk for tissue hypoxia and ischemia.

Patient Preparation

- Ensure that the patient understands preprocedural teachings. Answer questions as they arise, and reinforce information as needed. ➤*Rationale:* Understanding of previously taught information is evaluated and reinforced.
- Place the patient on a cardiac monitor, automatic blood pressure cuff, and pulse oximeter. Set up oropharyngeal suction. ➤*Rationale:* This action allows for close cardiovascular and respiratory system monitoring during the procedure and ensures suction is available for the procedure.
- Establish and maintain intravenous (IV) access. For the patient with GI hemorrhage, place a minimum of two large-bore IVs or provide central access. ➤*Rationale:* IV access is necessary for emergency IV medication administration and volume resuscitation in the case of GI hemorrhage.[5]
- Position patient in left lateral decubitus position.[7,8] ➤*Rationale:* This position facilitates passage of the tube into the stomach. The left lateral position is the position of choice to prevent aspiration if the patient should vomit.
- Apply oxygen via nasal prongs or mask as needed. Continue to evaluate the patient for possible need of airway intubation. ➤*Rationale:* Supplemental oxygen may optimize the patient's oxygen saturation.

Procedure	for Gastric Lavage in Hemorrhage and Overdose	
Steps	**Rationale**	**Special Considerations**
1. **HH**		
2. **PE**		
3. Coat the distal end of the lavage tube with water-soluble lubricant.	Minimizes mucosal injury and irritation during insertion of the tube.	
4. Place the bed in a semi-Fowler's position with the head of the bed up 10 to 20 degrees, a slight reverse Trendelenburg's position. Place the patient in the left lateral decubitus position.	The left lateral decubitus position maximizes access to the stomach and minimizes pyloric emptying. The slight reverse Trendelenburg's position also decreases movement of stomach contents into the duodenum and possibly helps minimize risk of aspiration during procedure.	Ensure adequate ventilation and oxygenation while the patient is positioned for gastric lavage.

Procedure	**for Gastric Lavage in Hemorrhage and Overdose**—*Continued*	
Steps	**Rationale**	**Special Considerations**
5. Prepare suction, lavage fluids, tape, and emergency equipment.	Preprocedure setup facilitates smooth technique, minimizes complications, and prepares for emergency situations.	If the patient does not have an intact gag reflex, endotracheal intubation should be done before the procedure.[6,9,11]
6. Insert a large OG or NG tube.[5-9] **(Level D*)**	A large-bore OG tube (number 36 to 40 Fr for adults) is preferred for the evacuation of blood, clots, undigested pills, or pill fragments. A smaller bore tube may become occluded with solid material.	For overdose situations, an OG tube should be placed that is large enough to capture the pill particulate.[6-9] A smaller bore nasogastric tube may be used if liquid poisons were ingested.[6-8] Do not cut the end of the tube to create a larger opening because rough edges on the tube can injure the mucosal lining of the GI tract.[6]
A. Measure the distance from the bridge of the patient's nose to the ear and then from the earlobe to the tip of the xiphoid process (see Fig. 11-2). Mark this distance on the tube.		
B. Insert an oral airway (see Procedure 11) or bite block if necessary.		Remove patient dentures.
C. Position the tube toward the posterior pharynx over the tongue.	Prevents patient from biting on the lavage tube or harming the practitioner during insertion of the lavage tube.	
D. Pass the tube slowly into the stomach, encouraging the patient to attempt to swallow as the tube is advanced. Continue to advance the tube until the mark previously placed on the tube is reached.	Rapid passage of the tube may lead to perforation or stimulate vomiting, leading to an increased risk of aspiration.	Asking the patient to flex the head forward may facilitate advancement of the tube. Heart rate may decrease as a result of vagal stimulation. Have atropine ready for use as necessary. Have oropharyngeal suction available.
7. Aspirate with a 60-mL syringe for return of stomach contents, and obtain radiographic confirmation of placement.[1] **(Level D)**	The position of the lavage tube must be confirmed to be in the stomach because of the risk for endotracheal placement of the lavage tube and subsequent pulmonary complications. Radiographic confirmation of lavage tube placement is currently the only definitive way to confirm tube placement; however, aspiration of stomach contents is suggestive of gastric placement.[1]	Ask the patient to phonate to ensure that the tube has not improperly been placed in the trachea.[7,8]
8. After placement is confirmed, secure the tube with tape, and aspirate gastric contents through the lavage tube with a 60-mL syringe.	Manual aspiration withdraws gastric contents and toxic agents or blood and clots out of the stomach.	In cases of overdose, save the aspirate in a specimen container and send to the laboratory for analysis if necessary.

*Level D: Peer-reviewed professional organizational standards with clinical studies to support recommendations

Procedure continues on following page

Procedure for Gastric Lavage in Hemorrhage and Overdose—*Continued*

Steps	Rationale	Special Considerations
9. Perform intermittent lavage (with either room-temperature normal saline solution or tap water).[5-9] **(Level D*)**	In overdose cases, lavage aids in removing toxic substances from the stomach before absorption. In GI hemorrhage, lavage aids in clearing the stomach of blood and clots to help identify the severity of bleeding and improve visualization of the gastric fundus in preparation for endoscopic evaluation or treatment.	
A. Slowly instill lavage fluid into the lavage tube with a 60-mL irrigating syringe (for adults, use 200 to 300 mL of fluid).[6-8] **(Level D)**	Small amounts of lavage fluid are used to limit fluid from entering the duodenum during lavage.[9]	Lavage fluid should be slightly warmed or at room temperature to prevent hypothermia in children, the elderly, or individuals receiving large amounts of lavage fluids.
B. Aspirate gastric contents through the lavage tube with an irrigating syringe.	Evacuates stomach contents, blood, clots, or ingested toxic agents.	The amount of lavage fluid returned should approximate the amount instilled.
or		
C. Connect lavage tube to low intermittent suction.	Low levels of suction (<60 mm Hg) should be used to prevent suction-induced mucosal damage to the GI tract.	
D. For patients with GI hemorrhage, continue intermittent lavage until the aspirate is clear of blood and clots.[5,10] **(Level D)**	Gastric lavage may help to identify the severity of bleeding and clear the stomach of blood and clots to improve visualization for endoscopic evaluation and treatment.[5,10] The presence of bright red blood can be an indicator of the need for urgent endoscopic treatment.[5]	The presence of coffee ground aspirate may indicate a resolving or previous GI bleed. Note that the absence of blood or coffee ground aspirate does not rule out the presence of current or past bleeding.[5]
E. In the overdose case, continue intermittent lavage until the aspirate is clear of the toxic substance or particulate matter.[7-9] Once lavage is complete, activated charcoal can be instilled through the tube if indicated. **(Level E*)**	Gastric lavage may help to remove life-threatening levels of ingested toxic substances from symptomatic patients if performed within 1 hour of ingestion.[3,7-9] Activated charcoal is used for absorption of the residual substance ingested (unable to be removed with lavage). If the patient is alert and has an intact gag reflex, activated charcoal can be swallowed.	Note that the end point of gastric lavage is not clearly defined if particulate cannot be clearly observed and that the lack of poor lavage return does not rule out significant ingestion of the toxic substance.[7-9]
10. Remove the OG or NG tube.	The OG or NG tube should be for single use only.[9]	
A. Clamp lavage tube with rubber-shod clamp.	Prevents leakage of contents remaining within lumen and possible aspiration of contents during removal.	
B. Pull lavage tube out slowly and steadily.	Minimizes risk for vomiting or complications.	If the lavage tube does not remove easily, discontinue removal and evaluate for causes of obstruction.
11. Dispose of equipment in appropriate receptacle.	Standard Precautions.	

*Level D: Peer-reviewed professional organizational standards with clinical studies to support recommendations

*Level E: Multiple case reports, theory-based evidence from expert opinions, or peer-reviewed professional organizational standards without clinical studies to support recommendations

Procedure | for Gastric Lavage in Hemorrhage and Overdose—*Continued*

Steps	Rationale	Special Considerations
12. Remove barrier gown, face and eye protection, and gloves. Perform proper hand-washing technique.	Reduces transmission of microorganisms.	
13. Document procedure in patient record.		

Expected Outcomes

- Evacuation of blood and clots from the stomach
- Prevention of blood aspiration
- Improved visualization of the gastric fundus for endoscopy
- Identification of the severity of GI hemorrhage
- Prevention or minimization of systemic complications from the absorption of drugs or toxic agents
- Minimization of mucosal damage by toxic agents

Unexpected Outcomes

- Endotracheal intubation rather than gastric intubation with lavage tube
- Esophageal or gastric perforation
- Trauma to the nose, throat, or esophagus
- Epistaxis if NG route is used for lavage
- Hypothermia in the elderly patient
- Bradydysrhythmias or ECG changes
- Pulmonary aspiration of gastric contents
- Movement of gastric contents into the duodenum, potentially increasing the amount of toxin absorbed
- Fluid and electrolyte imbalance
- Laryngospasm
- Hypoxia or hypercapnia
- Intubation as a result of hypoxia, aspiration, or other respiratory compromise
- Prolonged absence of the gag reflex

Patient Monitoring and Care

Steps	Rationale	Reportable Conditions
		These conditions should be reported if they persist despite nursing interventions.
1. Monitor vital signs every 15 minutes throughout the procedure and every hour after lavage for at least 4 hours or longer, depending on patient condition.	Continued blood loss or side effects of drugs or toxins ingested may cause changes in vital signs. Cold lavage fluid may cause hypothermia in the elderly patient. Complications from the procedure may not present during or immediately after the procedure.	• Increase in heart rate 10 to 20 beats or more above baseline • Decrease in systolic blood pressure 20 to 30 mm Hg or more below baseline • Respiratory rate lower than 8 or higher than 24 breaths per minute or rate changes greater than 20% of baseline normal • Temperature lower than 97.5°F (36.5°C) or higher than 101°F (38°C)
2. Monitor the neurologic status continuously throughout the procedure and after lavage.	Side effects from toxic agents ingested or significant blood loss may lead to a decrease in level of consciousness.	• Decreasing level of consciousness • Loss of gag reflex
3. Monitor respiratory status continuously throughout procedure and after lavage: 　A. Pulse oximetry 　B. Respiratory rate 　C. Work of breathing 　D. Oxygen requirements	Aspiration is a potential complication because of a change in level of consciousness, loss of gag reflex, or vomiting.	• Decrease in oximetry below baseline or 90% • Increase in respiratory rate above baseline • Symptoms of shortness of breath • Increasing oxygen requirements

Procedure continues on following page

Patient Monitoring and Care —*Continued*

Steps	Rationale	Reportable Conditions
4. Monitor cardiac status continuously throughout the procedure and after the lavage: A. Heart rate B. Heart rhythm C. ECG intervals D. Signs and symptoms of decreased cardiac output	Bradydysrhythmias may be caused by passage of the lavage tube or an increase in heart rate may indicate continued blood loss. Toxic effect of drugs ingested may also cause ECG changes, including prolongation of the PR, QRS, and QT intervals.	• Heart rate less than 60 beats per minute or greater than 100 beats per minute with or without a decrease in blood pressure below baseline • Chest pain, diaphoresis, change in level of consciousness, and shortness of breath • Change in ECG rhythm or length of PR, QRS, and QT intervals from baseline
5. Assess for normal pharyngeal function. After lavage, keep the patient in the left lateral position with slight head elevation until normal gag reflex returns.	The left lateral position is the position of choice to prevent aspiration should the patient not be able to control secretions or emesis.	• Prolonged absence of gag reflex
6. For the patient with GI hemorrhage:		• Bright red emesis or bleeding from the lavage tube or NG tube • Decrease in hemoglobin or hematocrit below baseline • Decrease in systolic blood pressure 20 to 30 mm Hg or more below baseline • Increase in pulse 10 to 20 beats per minute or more above baseline • Urine output less than 0.5 to 1 mL/kg/hr • Increasing confusion or decreasing level of consciousness • Continued bleeding • Changes in pulmonary status • Increase in blood pressure 20 to 30 mm Hg or more above baseline with initiation of vasoactive medications
A. Measure blood volume loss.	Aids in assessment of fluid balance and volume resuscitation requirements.	
B. Monitor for recurrence of bleeding, color, and consistency of gastric drainage, serial hemoglobin and hematocrit, postural vital signs, urine output, and change in level of consciousness.	Bleeding may recur despite interventions.	
C. Administer crystalloid IV fluids for volume resuscitation. Switch to the administration of packed red blood cells and fresh frozen plasma (FFP) or platelets when available for volume replacement and reversal of coagulopathies.	Replaces volume, prevents hemorrhagic shock, and improves oxygen-carrying capacity. Goal hemoglobin level should be 8 g/dL.[4]	

Patient Monitoring and Care —*Continued*

Steps	Rationale	Reportable Conditions
D. Administer proton pump inhibitors (PPIs) as prescribed by physician or advanced practice nurse. Initiation of a PPI should not occur before endoscopic evaluation.[12]	PPIs inhibit the proton pump in the parietal cells of the stomach, suppressing gastric acid secretion.	
E. Administer vasoactive medications such as vasopressin or octreotide as prescribed by physician or advanced practice nurse when a diagnosis of GI hemorrhage is suspected.[4]	Vasoactive medications such as vasopressin and octreotide provide specific vasoconstriction to the GI tract, thereby reducing blood flow to that area.	
F. Prepare the patient for possible endoscopy.	Endoscopic evaluation is the gold standard in the diagnosis and treatment of GI hemorrhage and should occur within 24 hours of initial presentation.[4,12]	
7. For the patient with drug overdose:		• Patient reporting intent to harm self • Patient reporting that ingestion was a suicide attempt • Deviation of test results outside normal limits
A. Evaluate the patient's need for follow-up psychiatric support for suicide ideation.	The drug or toxin ingestion may be a result of suicidal ideations.	
B. Institute suicide precautions until the patient has been cleared by psychiatric services. Precautions include removal of objects from the patient's room that could be used by the patient to inflict self-harm.		
C. In the hours and days after ingestion, repeat laboratory tests, including electrolytes, glucose, blood urea nitrogen and creatinine, liver function, and drug or toxin levels.	Laboratory tests ordered depend on the drug or toxins ingested. Lavage may cause electrolyte abnormalities. Liver function tests may be necessary if the drug is toxic to the liver. Drug or toxin level tests validate the clearance of the drug or toxin from the patient's system.	

Documentation

Documentation should include the following:

- Patient and family education
- History of ingestion of drug or toxin or upper GI bleeding
- Date, time, and reason for lavage
- Type and size of lavage tube inserted
- Patient tolerance of tube placement and lavage procedure
- Verification of lavage tube placement (method used)
- Type and amount of lavage fluid used
- Unexpected outcomes
- Nursing interventions
- Amount and characteristics of aspirate
- Assessment of gastric drainage after lavage
- Name and dose of medications given after the lavage
- Aspirated specimen sent to laboratory for analysis
- Referral to psychiatry if suicide is suspected
- Occurrence of rebleed in the patient with GI hemorrhage
- Blood products given during volume resuscitation

References

CR 1. American Association of Critical-Care Nurses: *AACN practice alert: verification of feeding tube placement,* 2005, retrieved April 26, 2009 from www.aacn.org/WD/Practice/ Docs/PracticeAlerts/Verification_of_Feeding_Tube_Placement_05-2005.pdf.

2. Caravati EM, Erdman AR, Scharman EJ, et al: Long-acting anticoagulant rodenticide poisoning: an evidence-based consensus guideline for out-of hospital management, *Clin Toxicol* 45(1):1-22, 2007.

3. Criddle LM: An overview of pediatric poisonings, *AACN Adv Crit Care* 18(2):109-118, 2007.

4. Garcia-Tsao G, Sanyal AJ, Grace ND, et al: Practice guidelines: prevention and management of gatroesophageal varices and variceal hemorrhage in cirrhosis, *Am J Gastroenterol* 102(9):2086-2102, 2007.

5. Gralnek IM, Barkun AN, Bardou M: Management of acute bleeding from a peptic ulcer, *N Engl J Med* 359(9):928-937, 2008.

6. Greene S, Harris C, Singer J: Gastrointestinal decontamination of the poisoned patient, *Pediatr Emerg Care* 24(3):176-189, 2008.

CR 7. Heard K: Gastrointestinal decontamination, *Med Clin North Am* 89(6):1067-1078, 2005.

8. Heard K: The changing indications of gastrointestinal decontamination in poisonings, *Clin Lab Med* 26(1):1-12, 2006.

CR 9. Kulig K: Position paper: gastric lavage: American Academy of Clinical Toxicology; European Association of Poisons Centres and Clinical Toxicologists, *J Toxicol Clin Toxicol* 42(7):933-943, 2004.

CR 10. Lee SD, Kearney DJ: A randomized controlled trial of gastric lavage prior to endoscopy for acute upper gastrointestinal bleeding, *J Clin Gastroenterol* 38(10): 861-865, 2004.

11. Madden M: Responding to pediatric poisoning, *Nursing* August:52-55, 2008.

12. Palmer K, Nairn M: Management of acute gastrointestinal blood loss: summary of SIGN guidelines, *BMJ* 337(a1832):928-933, 2008.

Additional Readings

Li Y, Tse ML, Gawarammana I, et al: Systematic review of controlled clinical trials of gastric lavage in acute organophosphorus pesticide poisoning, *Clin Toxicol* 47(3):179-192, 2009.

Larkin GL, Claassen C: Trends in emergency department use of gastric lavage for poisoning events in the United States, 1993-2003, *Clin Toxicol* 45(2):164-168, 2007.

Scottish Intercollegiate Guidelines Network: *Management of acute upper and lower gastrointestinal bleeding: a national clinical guideline,* 2008, retrieved April, 26, 2009 from www.sign.ac.uk/guidelines/fulltext/105/index.html.

Intraabdominal Pressure Monitoring

P U R P O S E : Intraabdominal hypertension and abdominal compartment syndrome occur when the abdominal contents expand in excess of the capacity of the abdominal cavity, compromising abdominal organ perfusion and resulting in organ dysfunction or failure and associated mortality.[3,5,9,13,14,17,20,23,25]

John J. Gallagher

PREREQUISITE NURSING KNOWLEDGE

- Understanding of gastrointestinal anatomy and physiology is necessary.
- Knowledge of aseptic technique is essential.
- Intraabdominal hypertension (IAH) and abdominal compartment syndrome (ACS) occur when the abdominal contents expand in excess of the capacity of the abdominal cavity, compromising abdominal organ perfusion and resulting in organ dysfunction or failure and associated mortality.[3,5,9,13,14,17,20,23,25]
- Four major categories of risk are associated with the development of IAH and ACS (Table 106-1).[3,17] They include:
  - Diminished abdominal wall compliance
  - Increased intestinal intraluminal contents
  - Increased peritoneal cavity contents
  - Capillary leakage into the bowel wall and mesentery/ fluid resuscitation
- IAH is defined as a sustained or repeated pathologic elevation of intraabdominal pressure (IAP) to more than or equal to 12 mm Hg.[3,17]
- IAH is graded by severity[3,17]:
  - Grade I: IAP, 12 to 15 mm Hg
  - Grade II: IAP, 16 to 20 mm Hg
  - Grade III: IAP, 21 to 25 mm Hg
  - Grade IV: IAP, >25 mm Hg
- ACS is defined as IAP more than or equal to 20 mm Hg that is associated with new organ dysfunction or failure.[1,3,17,20,21,25] ACS is categorized into three types[3,12,17]:

- Primary ACS: Associated with injury or disease of the abdominopelvic region.
- Secondary ACS: Associated with disease outside the abdominopelvic region (sepsis, burns, fluid resuscitation).
- Recurrent ACS: ACS that redevelops after previous medical or surgical treatment of primary or secondary ACS.
- Both IAH and ACS may compromise perfusion to the visceral organs represented by the parameter: abdominal perfusion pressure (APP).[3,6-8,17] APP is derived as:

$$APP = \text{mean arterial pressure (MAP)} - IAP \text{ or bladder pressure}$$
or
$$APP = MAP - IAP$$

- APP should be maintained at more than 50 to 60 mm Hg to maintain adequate perfusion to the abdominal organs and reduce the chance of organ dysfunction.[3,6,7,17]
- Measurement of bladder pressure via an indwelling urinary bladder catheter is considered the reference standard for the measurement of IAP and may be performed with equipment readily available in the critical care environment (Fig. 106-1).[2,3,8,15,17,22] Commercially prepared kits designed for measurement of IAP are also available and may provide advantages in efficiency, standardization of measurement technique, and data reproducibility. Instructions for specific setup and operation of commercially prepared devices are provided by the manufacturer. Note that regardless of the device used, a standardized procedure for measurement should

TABLE 106-1	**Patients at Risk for Development of Intraabdominal Hypertension and Abdominal Compartment Syndrome[3,17] (Levels C, D, E*)**

Reduced Abdominal Wall Compliance

- Acute respiratory failure with elevated intrathoracic pressure
- Abdominal surgery with primary fascial or tight closure
- Major trauma or burns
- Prone positioning
- HOB > 30 degrees
- Central obesity/high body mass index (BMI)

Increased Intestinal Intraluminal Contents

- Gastroparesis
- Ileus
- Colonic pseudoobstruction

Increased Peritoneal Cavity Contents

- Hemoperitoneum/pneumoperitoneum
- Ascites

Capillary Leak/Fluid Resuscitation

- Acidosis (pH, <7.2)
- Hypotension
- Hypothermia (core temperature, <33°C)
- Massive transfusion (>10 units/24 hr)
- Coagulopathy
- Platelets <55,000/mm^3
- Prothrombin time (PT) >15 seconds
- Partial thromboplastin time (PTT) >2 times normal
- International standardized ratio (INR) >1.5
- Massive fluid resuscitation (5 L/24 hr)
- Pancreatitis
- Oliguria
- Sepsis
- Major burns or trauma

Damage control laparotomy

---

*Level C: Qualitative studies, descriptive or correlational studies, integrative reviews, systematic reviews, or randomized controlled trials with inconsistent results

*Level D: Peer-reviewed, professional organizational standards with clinical studies to support recommendations

*Level E: Multiple case reports, theory-based evidence from expert opinions, or peer-reviewed professional organizational standards without clinical studies to support recommendations

be used to prevent measurement variability between practitioners.[12,15,22]

- The bladder acts as a passive reservoir and accurately reflects IAP when intravesicular volumes of 25 mL or less are used. Larger volumes previously suggested (50 to 100 mL) are not necessary and may in fact overdistend the bladder, falsely elevating measured bladder pressure (IAP).[3,11,18]
- Normal IAP is 0 mm Hg and may even be subatmospheric. In patients who are critically ill, it may rise to 5 to 7 mm Hg.[3,17]
- IAP should be measured with the patient in the supine position. The transducer should be leveled or zeroed at the iliac crest in the midaxillary line (Fig. 106-2).[2,3,17,24]
- IAP should be measured at end expiration. Wait an appropriate time (10 to 60 seconds) after saline solution instillation to allow for equilibration of the monitor to a steady state pressure reading.[3,17]

- IAP should be expressed in millimeters of mercury (mm Hg; 1 mm Hg = 1.36 cm H_2O).[3,17]
- Serial monitoring of bladder pressures is useful in detection of the onset of IAH and the progression to the more severe condition of ACS. Recommendations are that measurements be repeated every 2 to 4 hours in patients with IAP more than or equal to 12 mm Hg so a trend may be established and increases in pressure are detected.[3,17]
- Bladder pressure measurement may be contraindicated in certain conditions, such as bladder trauma, bladder surgery, and neurogenic bladder. Risks and benefits of measurement should be discussed with the physician before the procedure is performed in these patients.
- In patients who do not have a urinary catheter in place, the risks and benefits of catheter placement for the purpose of bladder pressure measurement should be considered.

Bladder Pressure Monitoring Setup

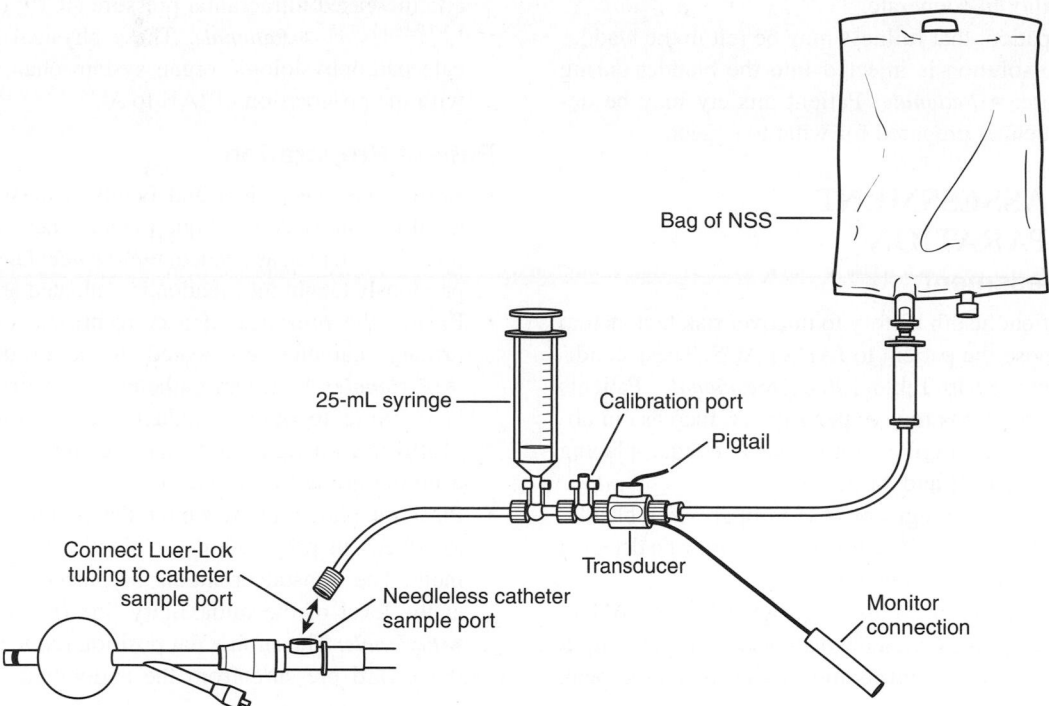

Bag of NSS

25-mL syringe

Calibration port

Pigtail

Connect Luer-Lok tubing to catheter sample port

Needleless catheter sample port

Transducer

Monitor connection

FIGURE 106-1   Bladder pressure monitoring setup. *(Illustration by John J. Gallagher.)*

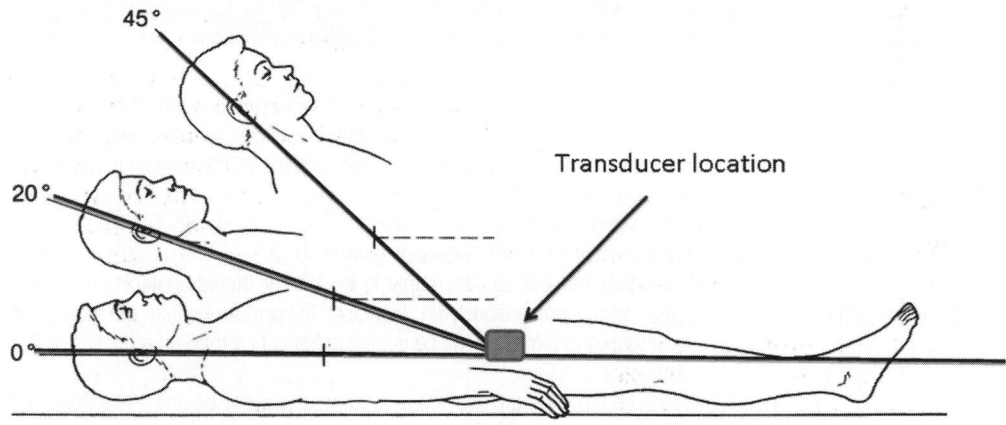

45°

20°

0°

Transducer location

The correct transducer position at the iliac crest in the mid-axillary line in the supine position and with head of bed elevation.

FIGURE 106-2   Correct position of the transducer for bladder pressure measurement. *(Illustration by John J. Gallagher.)*

EQUIPMENT

- Nonsterile gloves
- Cardiac monitor and pressure cable for interface with the monitor
- 500- or 1000-mL intravenous (IV) bag of normal saline (NS) solution
- Pressure transducer system, including pressure tubing with flush device, transducer, and two stopcocks
- 25-mL Luer-Lok syringe
- Clamp
- Chlorhexidine swab sticks

Note: Commercial bladder pressure monitoring system may be substituted for the previous list.

PATIENT AND FAMILY EDUCATION

- Explain the procedure of bladder pressure measurement and its purpose to the patient and family. ➤➤*Rationale:* Patient and family anxiety may be decreased. Understanding of how the procedure is performed may promote the patient's ability to cooperate.

- Inform the patient that fullness may be felt in the bladder when saline solution is injected into the bladder during the procedure. ➤➤*Rationale:* Patient anxiety may be decreased. Patient is prepared for what to expect.

PATIENT ASSESSMENT AND PREPARATION

Patient Assessment

- Obtain a patient health history to uncover risk factors that may predispose the patient to IAH or ACS. These conditions are outlined in Table 106-1. ➤➤*Rationale:* Patients with these conditions may experience an increase in abdominal cavity fluid collection or tissue edema, placing them at risk for IAH and ACS.[3,17]
- Assess the patient for signs of IAH through serial bladder pressure measurement.[3,17] Rationale: IAH may be detected early through IAP measurement.
- Assess the patient for signs of progression of IAH to ACS. These findings include decreased cardiac output and blood pressure, oliguria and anuria, increased peak inspiratory pressures (PIPs), hypercarbia and hypoxia, and increased intracranial pressure (ICP); (Table 106-2).[1-5,7,9,13,16,17,25,] ➤➤*Rationale:* These physical findings indicate pathophysiologic organ system changes associated with the progression of IAH to ACS.[3,5-7,9,13,16,17,25]

Patient Preparation

- Ensure that the patient and family understand preprocedural teachings. Answer questions as they arise, and reinforce information as needed. ➤➤*Rationale:* Understanding of previously taught information is evaluated and reinforced.
- Ensure the presence of a conventional (single-lumen) urinary catheter connected to a drainage system. ➤➤*Rationale:* A urinary catheter with a drainage system is required to obtain bladder pressure measurements. Multilumen irrigation urinary catheters also may be used but are not required.
- Place the patient in the supine flat position (if this can be tolerated) in preparation for bladder pressure measurement. The transducer should be placed at the iliac crest at the level of the midaxillary line (see Fig. 106-2).[3,17] ➤➤*Rationale:* The supine flat position reduces the effect of downward pressure from the abdominal organs on the

TABLE 106-2	Physiologic Changes Associated with Intraabdominal Hypertension and Abdominal Compartment Syndrome[3,5-7,9,13,16,17,25] (Levels C, D, E*)
Organ System	**Rationale**
Cardiovascular ↑ CVP, PAP, PCWP, SVR ↓ CO (more pronounced with hypovolemia) ↓ Venous return from lower extremities (risk for DVT)	Increased abdominal pressure prevents venous return (preload reduction) and impedes arterial outflow (increase in afterload). Transmitted backpressure from the abdominal cavity falsely elevates CVP, PAP, PCWP, PVR, and SVR. CVP and PCWP may be corrected for the influence of increased IAP as follows[5]: CVP corrected = CVP measured − IAP/2 PCWP corrected = PCWP measured − IAP/2
Renal ↑ Renal blood flow → ↓GFR → ↓urine output	Increased IAP reduces cardiac output to the kidney, thereby reducing perfusion pressure to the glomerulus. Simultaneously IAP increases the pressure within the renal parenchyma, leading to reduction in filtration. The combination leads to a marked reduction in GFR and urine production.
Pulmonary ↑ Intrathoracic pressures ↑ Peak inspiratory pressures ↓ Tidal volume → hypercarbia + ↓Pao$_2$ ↓ Compliance	Increased IAP causes an increase in intrathoracic pressure and limits diaphragm excursion, resulting in hypoventilation and hypoxia.
Neurologic ↑ICP ↓CPP	Increased IAP impedes venous outflow from the brain, increasing cerebral venous congestion.
Gastrointestinal/hepatic effect ↓Celiac and portal blood flow ↓Lactate clearance ↓Mucosal blood flow → ↓ pHi	Increased IAP reduces perfusion to the abdominal organs. Capillary blood flow becomes obstructed as the IAP rises. When the IAP achieves and surpasses the venous capillary pressure, capillary blood flow is reduced or ceases. Transfer of oxygen/nutrients stops leading to anaerobic metabolism.

*Level C: Qualitative studies, descriptive or correlational studies, integrative reviews, systematic reviews, or randomized controlled trials with inconsistent results
*Level D: Peer-reviewed, professional organizational standards with clinical studies to support recommendations
*Level E: Multiple case reports, theory-based evidence from expert opinions, or peer-reviewed professional organizational standards without clinical studies to support recommendations

CO, Cardiac output; *CPP,* cerebral perfusion pressure; *CVP,* central venous pressure; *DVT,* deep venous thrombosis, *GFR,* glomerular filtration rate; *IAP,* intraabdominal pressure; *ICP,* intracranial pressure; *Pao$_2$,* partial pressure of arterial oxygen; *PAP,* pulmonary artery pressure; *PCWP,* pulmonary capillary wedge pressure; *pHi,* intramucosal pH; *PVR,* pulmonary vascular resistance; *SVR,* systemic vascular resistance.

bladder, reducing the chance that IAP is falsely elevated. Patients who cannot tolerate the supine position (head injury, respiratory compromise) may have measurements taken with the head of the bed (HOB) elevated.[3,17] If the patient must remain with the HOB elevated, the transducer must be placed at the level of the bladder (iliac crest; see Fig. 106-2).

- Documentation should reflect the degree of reverse Trendelenburg's or HOB elevation when measurements are not obtained in the supine position.[2,3,17,24] ➧*Rationale:*

IAP results can be evaluated in light of the patient's position at the time of measurement. Note that the phlebostatic axis should not be used to level the transducer for bladder pressure measurement.

- Verify correct patient with two identifiers. ➧*Rationale:* Prior to performing a procedure, the nurse should ensure the correct identification of the patient for the intended intervention.
- Perform a pre-procedure verification and time out, if non-emergent. ➧*Rationale:* Ensures patient safety.

Procedure for Intraabdominal Pressure Monitoring[2,3,10,11,15,17,22,24] (see Fig. 106-1)

Steps	Rationale	Special Considerations
1. **HH**		
2. **PE**		
3. Assemble the entire pressure transducer system as shown (see Fig. 106-1) and flush the system with normal saline (NS) solution.	Ensures that all air is out of the system.	
4. Attach the 25- or 30-mL syringe to the distal stopcock (see Fig. 106-1).	The syringe is used to fill the bladder with saline solution from the IV bag.	
5. Connect the system to the pressure module of the monitoring system with the transducer cable. Select a 30–mm Hg scale.	Connects the system for monitoring. The 30–mm Hg scale is sufficient to measure most IAP ranges.	
6. With the patient in the supine position and the HOB flat, level the fluid interface (zeroing stopcock) to the iliac crest at the level of the midaxillary line.[3,17] **(Level D*)** If the patient must remain with the HOB elevated, the transducer must be placed at the level of the bladder (iliac crest; see Fig. 106-2). Note: The phlebostatic axis should not be used to level the transducer for bladder pressure measurement.	The supine position limits the effect of the abdominal cavity contents on the bladder that may falsely elevate bladder pressure measurements. Approximates the level of the bladder and should be used as the reference point.	Marking the position ensures consistent use of the same reference point. The transducer may be secured to an IV pole beside the patient and leveled in the standard fashion or it may be placed on the patient at the level described. If the patient is unable to be placed in the supine position, the degree of HOB elevation should be noted on the medical record along with the bladder pressure to allow future measurements to be done in the same position so they may be compared with one another accurately.
7. Zero the IAP monitoring system.	Negates the effect of atmospheric pressure. Ensures accuracy of the system with the established reference point.	
8. Clamp the bladder drainage system just distal to the catheter and drainage bag connection on the drainage bag tubing.	Prevents drainage of saline solution out of the bladder during bladder filling.	

*Level D: Peer-reviewed professional organizational standards with clinical studies to support recommendations

Procedure continues on following page

Procedure	**for Intraabdominal Pressure Monitoring**[2,3,10,11,15,17,22,24]—*Continued*	
Steps	**Rationale**	**Special Considerations**
9. Cleanse the sampling port on the urinary drainage system with a chlorhexidine swab and aseptically attach the end of the pressure tubing to the sampling port.	Cleansing the sampling port reduces the incidence of nosocomial urinary tract infection (UTI) from system contamination.	
10. Turn the stopcock attached to the syringe off to the patient and open to the fluid bag and syringe. Activate the fast-flush mechanism (pigtail) while pulling back on the syringe plunger to fill the syringe to 25 mL.[3,11,17,18] **(Level C*)**		
11. Turn the stopcock off to the fluid bag and open to the syringe and patient. Inject the 25 mL of saline solution into the bladder.[3,11,17,18] **(Level C)**	The fluid-filled bladder accurately reflects IAP. Use of a volume of 25 mL prevents overdistention of the bladder and false elevation of the bladder pressure.	
12. Expel any air seen between the clamp and the urinary catheter by opening the clamp and allowing the saline solution to flow back past the clamp; then reclamp.[19,22] **(Level E*)**	Air in the system may dampen the pressure reading.	
13. Measure the IAP at end expiration with the graphic scale on the monitor display and numeric display of the mean pressure (Fig. 106-3).[3,17] **(Level D*)**	Measurement at end expiration is most accurate when the effects of pulmonary pressures are minimized.	The numeric mean IAP pressure displayed on the monitor may be used in most circumstances. The numeric reading is a mean pressure value, reflecting the average of both inspiratory and expiratory IAP. Consider reading the IAP from the monitor graphic scale or a printed strip if noticeable excursions are found in the waveform with ventilation.
14. Once a reading has been obtained, unclamp the urinary drainage system. The pressure monitoring system may be left connected or disconnected and capped to maintain sterility of the system. Note: The urinary drainage system should be left unclamped between readings.	Unclamping the drainage system discontinues pressure measurement and resumes the normal urinary drainage function of the catheter system. Note: If the monitoring system is maintained connected to the urinary catheter, repeated reentry into the catheter tubing is avoided.	Monitoring requires clamping the drainage system and filling the bladder to obtain a reading. Minimizing entry into the urinary drainage system may reduce the chance of UTI. Specific data to support this practice in IAP measurement do not exist.
15. Record the bladder pressure on the patient flow sheet and remember to subtract the 25 mL of instilled saline solution from the hourly urine output.	The volume of instilled normal saline solution falsely elevates the calculation of hourly urine output if it is not subtracted.	

*Level C: Qualitative studies, descriptive or correlational studies, integrative reviews, systematic reviews, or randomized controlled trials with inconsistent results
*Level D: Peer-reviewed professional organizational standards with clinical studies to support recommendations
*Level E: Multiple case reports, theory-based evidence from expert opinions, or peer-reviewed professional organizational standards without clinical studies to support recommendations

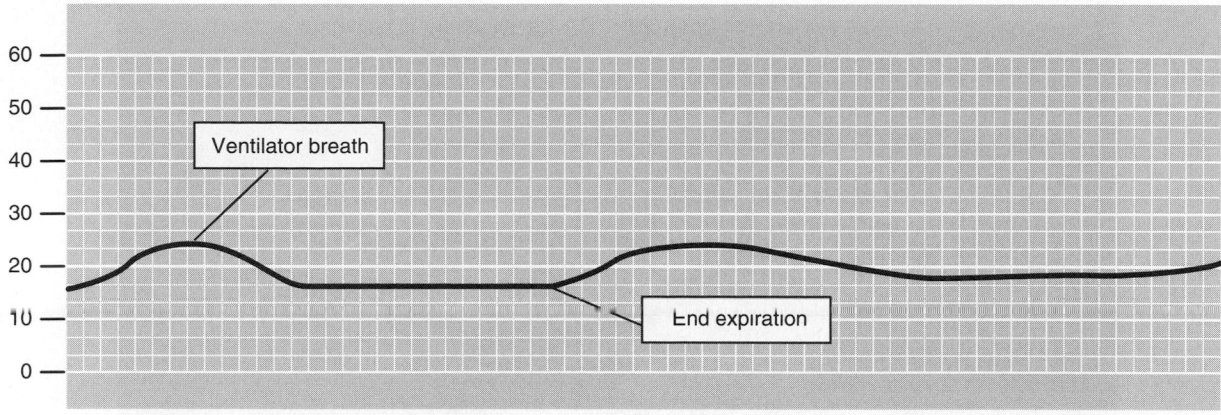

FIGURE 106-3   IAP waveform. The IAP read at end expiration is 16 mm Hg in this patient on mechanical ventilation.

Procedure	for Intraabdominal Pressure Monitoring[2,3,10,11,15,17,22,24]—*Continued*	
Steps	Rationale	Special Considerations
16. Report IAP readings as per institutional protocol, especially if they are trending upward or if they are associated with other assessment findings that indicate the development of IAH and ACS. 17. Discard used supplies, remove gloves and discard in appropriate receptacle. 18. **HH**	Early detection of elevated IAP and implementation of interventions to reduce IAP are essential to reduce the morbidity and mortality associated with IAH and ACS.	

Procedure	for Intraabdominal Pressure Monitoring with the Wolfe Tory Medical AbViser (Wolfe Tory Medical, Salt Lake City, Utah) Bladder Pressure Monitoring System with AutoValve (Fig. 106-4)	
Steps	Rationale	Special Considerations
Note: Please refer to manufacturer's instructions provided with the device for assembly and use (www.wolfetory.com). 1. **HH** 2. **PE** 3. After opening the AbViser package, insert the spike into the bag of sterile saline solution (Fig. 106-5, *Step 1*). 4. Prime the system with saline solution by aspirating and compressing the syringe to remove all air from the tubing. Continue this process until saline solution runs through the AutoValve at the distal end of the system (see Fig. 106-5, *Step 2*).	Removes all air from the system to establish a fluid column for accurate pressure measurement.	

Procedure continues on following page

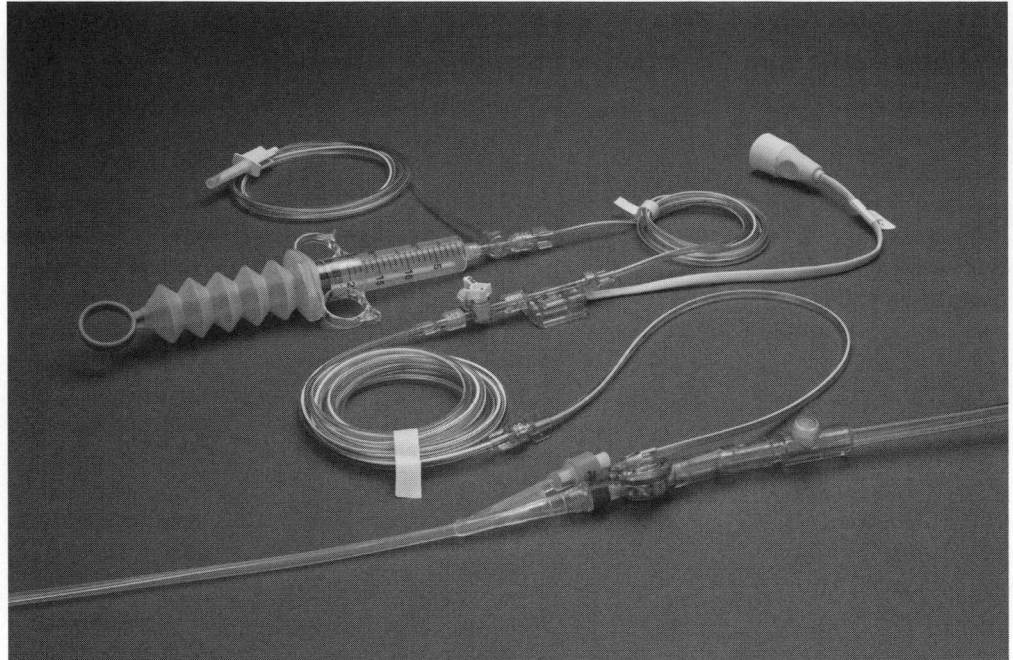

FIGURE 106-4   Commercially prepared bladder pressure measurement system (AbViser). *(Courtesy of Wolfe Tory Medical, Salt Lake City, UT.)*

Procedure	for Intraabdominal Pressure Monitoring with the Wolfe Tory Medical AbViser (Wolfe Tory Medical, Salt Lake City, Utah) Bladder Pressure Monitoring System with AutoValve—*Continued*

Steps	Rationale	Special Considerations
5. Place a sterile drape under the urinary catheter/drain bag connection and prepare the connection with antiseptic solution (see Fig. 106-5, *Step 3*).	Reduces the chance of bacterial contamination of the urinary drainage system.	
6. With aseptic technique, detach the urinary catheter from the drainage bag (see Fig. 106-5, *Step 3*).	Reduces the chance of bacterial contamination of the urinary drainage system.	
7. Pick up the AutoValve and tear the perforation on the protective bag, exposing the barbed end of the AutoValve. Slide the urinary catheter over the barbed end of the AutoValve. Connect the other end of the AutoValve to the urinary drainage bag connection. Ensure the connections are dry and wrap the tape strip included with the kit around the catheter/ AutoValve connection (see Fig. 106-5, *Step 3*).	Reduces the risk of contamination; secures the connection to reduce the chance of system component separation.	
8. Hang the syringe in a convenient spot with the S-hook included with the kit.		

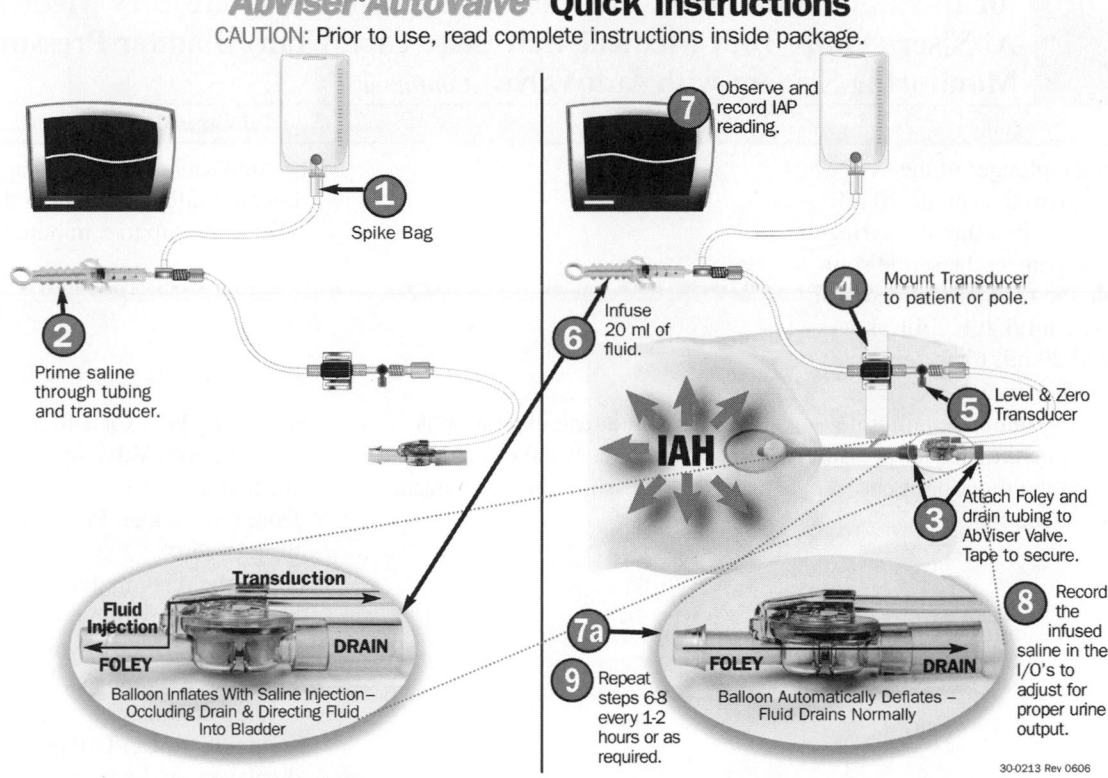

AbViser·AutoValve™ **Quick Instructions**
CAUTION: Prior to use, read complete instructions inside package.

1 — Spike Bag

2 — Prime saline through tubing and transducer.

Transduction
Fluid Injection
FOLEY   DRAIN
Balloon Inflates With Saline Injection–
Occluding Drain & Directing Fluid
Into Bladder

7 — Observe and record IAP reading.

6 — Infuse 20 ml of fluid.

4 — Mount Transducer to patient or pole.

5 — Level & Zero Transducer

3 — Attach Foley and drain tubing to AbViser Valve. Tape to secure.

IAH

8 — Record the infused saline in the I/O's to adjust for proper urine output.

7a

FOLEY   DRAIN
Balloon Automatically Deflates –
Fluid Drains Normally

9 — Repeat steps 6-8 every 1-2 hours or as required.

30-0213 Rev 0606

FIGURE 106-5   AbViser® Bladder Pressure Monitoring System. *(Courtesy of Wolfe Tory Medical, Salt Lake City, UT.)*

Procedure	**for Intraabdominal Pressure Monitoring with the Wolfe Tory Medical AbViser (Wolfe Tory Medical, Salt Lake City, Utah) Bladder Pressure Monitoring System with AutoValve—***Continued*	
Steps	**Rationale**	**Special Considerations**
9. Attach the pressure transducer to the patient or pole mount at the level of the iliac crest in the midaxillary line (see Fig. 106-5, *Step 4).*	Approximates the level of the bladder and should be used as the reference point.	Marking the position may ensure consistent use of the same reference point. The transducer may be secured to an IV pole beside the patient and leveled in the standard fashion, or it may be secured to the patient at the level described.
10. Connect the AbViser system to the monitor with the pressure transducer cable. Select a 30–mm Hg scale on the monitor	Connects to the system for monitoring. The 30–mm Hg scale is sufficient to measure most IAP ranges.	
11. Zero the pressure transducer at the level of the iliac crest (see Fig. 106-2) in the midaxillary line (see Fig. 106-5, *Step 5).*	Negates the effect of atmospheric pressure. Ensures accuracy of the system with the established reference point.	
12. After zeroing the transducer, ensure that the stopcock is open to the patient and transducer.		
13. Place the patient in the supine position	Limits the effect of the abdominal cavity contents on the bladder that may falsely elevate bladder pressure measurements.	If the patient is unable to be placed in the supine position, the degree of HOB elevation should be noted on the medical record along with the bladder pressure measurement.

Procedure continues on following page

Procedure	for Intraabdominal Pressure Monitoring with the Wolfe Tory Medical AbViser (Wolfe Tory Medical, Salt Lake City, Utah) Bladder Pressure Monitoring System with AutoValve—*Continued*

Steps	Rationale	Special Considerations
14. Retract the plunger of the syringe on the system to aspirate 20 mL of saline solution into the syringe and briskly inject the saline solution into the bladder (for pediatric patients, 1 mL/kg + 2 mL, not to exceed 20 mL total; see Fig. 106-5, *Step 6*).		The AutoValve closes to retain the injected saline solution in the bladder for up to 3 minutes.
15. Allow the system to equilibrate and then note the bladder pressure reading on the monitor at end expiration (see Fig. 106-5, *Step 7*).	Measurement at end expiration is most accurate, as the effects of pulmonary pressures are minimized.	The reading lasts for 1 to 3 minutes until the AutoValve opens, allowing for drainage of the saline solution from the bladder. Pressure should drop to zero. Note: If the reading does not go to zero, fluid may remain in the drainage tubing. Drain any remaining fluid into the drainage bag and the reading should go to zero. The numeric mean IAP pressure displayed on the monitor may be used in most circumstances. The numeric reading is a mean pressure value, reflecting the average of both inspiratory and expiratory IAP. Consider reading the IAP from the monitor graphic scale or a printed strip if noticeable excursions are found in the waveform with ventilation.
16. Confirm that the AutoValve has opened and that urine is draining normally (see Fig. 106-5, *Step 7, A*).		The valve remains open until the next volume of fluid is infused.
17. Discard used supplies, remove gloves and discard in appropriate receptacle.		
18. 🄷🄷		
19. Record the bladder pressure on the patient flow sheet and remember to subtract the 20 mL of instilled saline solution from the hourly urine output (see Fig. 106-5, *Step 8*).	The volume of instilled normal saline solution falsely elevates the hourly urine output calculation if it is not subtracted.	
20. Repeat measurement every 2 hours or as clinically indicated (see Fig. 106-5, *Step 9*).	Measurements should be trended to detect the onset of IAH.	

Procedure	for Intraabdominal Pressure Monitoring with the Holtech Abdo-Pressure System, Charlottenlund, Denmark	
Steps	**Rationale**	**Special Considerations**

Note: Intended for patients who are at least 20 pounds. Please refer to manufacturer's instructions provided with the device for assembly and use (www.holtech-medical.com).

1. 🔲HH
2. 🔲PE
3. Open the Abdo-Pressure pouch and close the tube clamp.
4. Place the urine collection device under the patient's bladder and tape the drainage tube to the bedsheet. Carefully disinfect the catheter connection before disconnecting.
5. Insert the Abdo-Pressure between catheter and drainage device. Perform aseptically.

		This step is key in preventing contamination of the urinary drainage system.

6. Prime the Abdo-Pressure with 20 mL of sterile saline solution through its needle-free injection/sampling port.

	Removes air from the system.	Prime only once, at initial setup, or subsequently, to remove any air from the manometer tube. The manometer tube should always be fluid filled.
		Note: In patients who are anuric, re-priming at each pressure determination is not necessary. The fluid returned to the bladder from the manometer tube provides an adequate volume for a reliable pressure determination.
		Carefully disinfect the needle-free port before urine sampling.

7. Place the "0 mm Hg" mark of the manometer tube at the midaxillary line at the iliac crest and elevate the filter vertically above the patient (Fig. 106-6).

	Approximates the level of the bladder and should be used as the reference point for accurate measurement.	

8. Open the clamp and read the bladder pressure (end-expiration value) when the fluid meniscus has stabilized (see Fig. 106-6).

	Allows for equilibration of the fluid column to accurately represent bladder pressure.	Slow descent (>20 to 30 seconds) of the meniscus during a bladder pressure determination suggests a blocked or kinked urinary catheter.

9. Close the clamp and place the Abdo-Pressure in its drainage position (Fig. 106-7).

	Allows normal flow through the urinary drainage system.	Avoid a U-bend of the large urimeter drainage tube (which will impede urine drainage).
		Never empty the manometer tube into the urine drainage device during use.
		The Abdo-Pressure tube should be fluid filled during drainage. Only reprime with sterile saline solution to remove any air or bladder debris in the manometer tube.

10. Discard used supplies; remove gloves and discard in appropriate receptacle.
11. 🔲HH

Procedure continues on following page

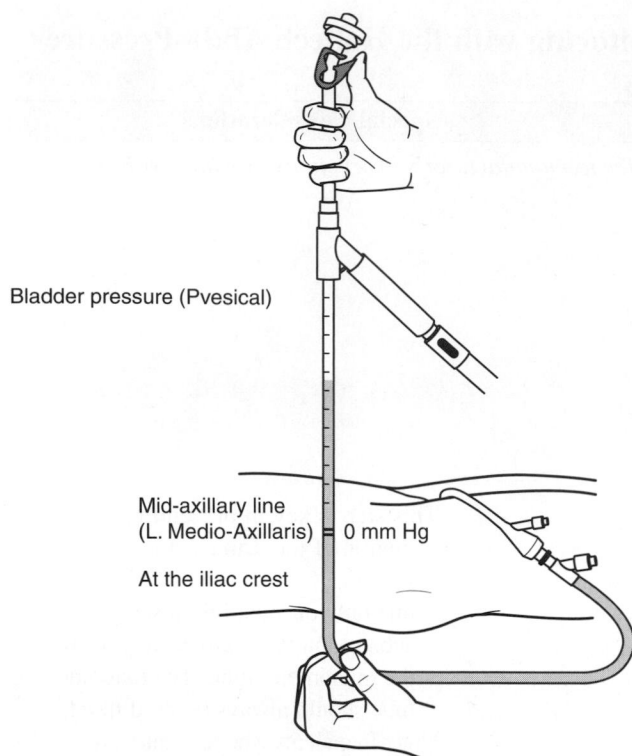

Bladder pressure (Pvesical)

Mid-axillary line
(L. Medio-Axillaris) = 0 mm Hg

At the iliac crest

FIGURE 106-6   Commercially prepared Abdo-Pressure bladder pressure monitoring system. *(Redrawn with permission from Holtech Medical.)*

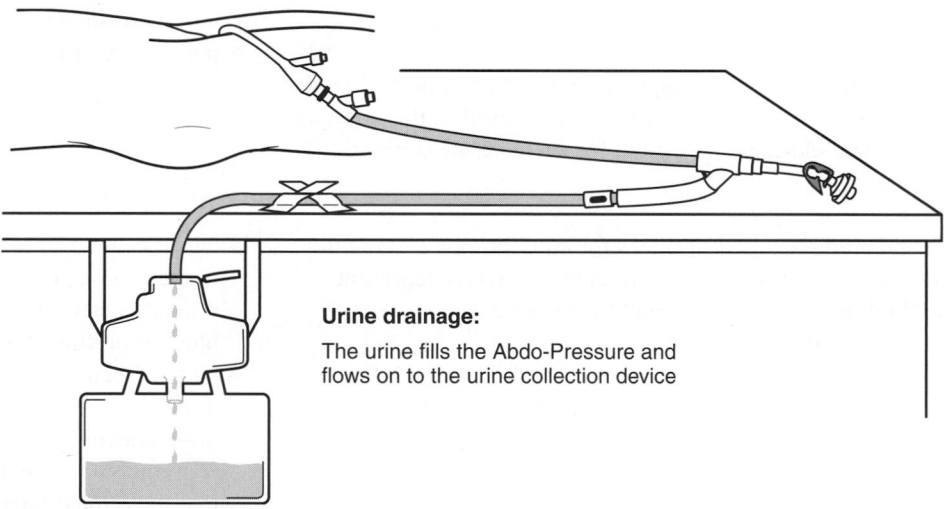

Urine drainage:

The urine fills the Abdo-Pressure and flows on to the urine collection device

FIGURE 106-7   The urine fills the Abdo-Pressure and flows on to the urine collection device. *(Redrawn with permission from Holtech Medical.)*

Procedure	for Intraabdominal Pressure Monitoring with the Holtech Abdo-Pressure System, Charlottenlund, Denmark—*Continued*	
Steps	**Rationale**	**Special Considerations**
12. Replace the Abdo-Pressure whenever the Foley catheter or the urine collection device is replaced. Note: Never use the Abdo-Pressure for more than 7 days.		

Expected Outcomes

- Intraabdominal pressure (IAP) monitoring achieved
- Compartment pressure within normal limits
- Elevated compartment pressure detected and therapeutic intervention initiated

Unexpected Outcomes

- Inability to monitor IAP
- Inaccurate pressure readings obtained
- Development of a nosocomial UTI from urinary drainage system manipulation
- Patient discomfort

Patient Monitoring and Care[1,3,5,7-9,12,13,17,20,21,23,25]

Steps	Rationale	Reportable Conditions
		These conditions should be reported if they persist despite nursing interventions.
1. Monitor IAP every 2 to 4 hours or more frequently, depending on clinical need.[3,17] **(Level D*)**	Serial measurements detect a trended increase in IAPs, reflecting development of IAH or ACS.	- IAP >12 mm Hg - APP <60 mm Hg
2. Assess the patient for signs of increasing IAP, including: A. Decrease in blood pressure and cardiac output. B. Oliguria or anuria. C. Increase in peak inspiratory pressures. D. Hypoxia and hypercarbia. E. Elevated ICP.[3,5,9,13,16,17] **(Levels C*, D, E*)**	Patients may have symptoms develop slowly over time. The symptoms may mimic other clinical conditions, such as acute respiratory distress syndrome (ARDS), acute renal failure, congestive heart failure, and intracranial hypertension.	- Decrease in blood pressure and cardiac output - Oliguria or anuria - Increase in peak inspiratory pressures - Hypoxia and hypercarbia - Elevated ICP
3. Monitor for signs and symptoms of UTI.[19,22] **(Level E)**	Frequent breaks in the integrity of the urinary drainage system may contribute to the development of UTI.	- Temperature elevation - Elevated white blood cell count - Increased urine sediment or cloudiness of urine

*Level C: Qualitative studies, descriptive or correlational studies, integrative reviews, systematic reviews, or randomized controlled trials with inconsistent results
*Level D: Peer-reviewed professional organizational standards with clinical studies to support recommendations
*Level E: Multiple case reports, theory-based evidence from expert opinions, or peer-reviewed professional organizational standards without clinical studies to support recommendations

Procedure continues on following page

Documentation

Documentation should include the following:
- Patient and family education
- Assessment findings before obtaining IAPs
- Intraabdominal (bladder) pressure value
- APP value
- Postprocedure assessment
- Changes in the patient's assessment that indicate onset of IAH or ACS

- The amount of fluid instilled into the bladder to be subtracted from the hourly urine output
- Unexpected outcomes
- Additional interventions
- Reportable conditions

References

CR 1. Balogh Z, et al: Secondary abdominal compartment syndrome is an elusive early complication of traumatic shock resuscitation, *Am J Surg* 184:538-543, 2002.
2. Cheatham ML, et al: The impact on body position on intra-abdominal pressure measurement: a multicenter analysis, *Crit Care Med* 37:2187-2190, 2009.
3. Cheatham ML, et al: Results from the International Conference of Experts on Intra-abdominal Hypertension and Abdominal Compartment Syndrome: II: recommendations, *Intensive Care Med* 33(6):951-962, 2007.
4. Cheatham ML, Safcsak K: Is the evolving management of IAH/ACS improving survival? *Acta Clinica Belgica* 62(Suppl 1):268-Abstract 061, 2007.
5. Cheatham ML, Malbrain MLNG: Cardiovascular implications of abdominal compartment syndrome, *Acta Clinica Belgica* 62(Suppl 1):98-112, 2007.
6. Cheatham ML, Malbrain MLNG: Abdominal perfusion pressure. In Cheatham ML, Malbrain MLNG, Sugrue M, editors: *Abdominal compartment syndrome,* Georgetown, TX, 2006, Landes Biomedical, 69-81.
CR 7. Cheatham ML, et al: Abdominal perfusion pressure: a superior parameter in the assessment of intraabdominal hypertension, *J Trauma* 56:237-242, 2000.
CR 8. Cheatham ML, Safcak K: Intraabdominal pressure: a revised method for measurement, *J Am Coll Surg* 186:594-595, 1998.
CR 9. Cullen D, et al: Cardiovascular, pulmonary, and renal effects of massively increased intraabdominal pressure in critically ill patients, *Crit Care Med* 17:118-122, 1989.
CR 10. De Potter TJ, Dits H, Malbrain MLNG: Intra- and interobserver variability during in vitro validation of two novel methods for intra-abdominal pressure monitoring, *Intensive Care Med* 31(5):747-751, 2005.
11. De Waele JJ, et al: Saline volume in transvesical intra-abdominal pressure measurement: enough is enough, *Intensive Care Med* 32(3):455-459, 2006.
CR 12. Gracias VH, et al: Abdominal compartment syndrome in the open abdomen, *Arch Surg* 137:1298-1300, 2002.
CR 13. Kashtan J, et al: Hemodynamic effects of increased intraabdominal pressure, *J Surg Res* 30:249-255, 1981.
14. Kimball EJ, et al: Clinical awareness of intra-abdominal hypertension and abdominal compartment syndrome in 2007, *Acta Clinica Belgica* 62(Suppl 1):66-73, 2007.
15. Kimball EJ, et al: Reproducibility of bladder pressure measurements in critically ill patients, *Intensive Care Med* 33(7): 1195-98 (2007).
CR 16. Kron I, Harman K, Nolan SP: The measurement of intraabdominal pressure as a criterion for abdominal re-exploration, *Ann Surg* 199:28-30, 1984.
17. Malbrain MLNG, Delaet I, Cheatham ML: Consensus conference definitions and recommendations on intraabdominal hypertension (IAH) and the abdominal compartment syndrome (ACS): the long road to the final publications: how did we get there? *Acta Clinica Belgica* 62(Suppl 1):44-59, 2007.
18. Malbrain MLNG, Deeren D: Effect of bladder volume on measuring intravesical pressure: a prospective cohort study, *Crit Care Forum* 10(4):1-6, 2006.
19. Malbrain MLNG, Jones F: Intra-abdominal pressure measurement techniques. In Ivatury RR, Cheatham ML, Malbrain M, et al, editors: *Abdominal compartment syndrome,* Georgetown, TX, 2006, Landis Bioscience.
CR 20. Malbrain MLNG, et al: Incidence and prognosis of intraabdominal hypertension in a mixed population of critically ill patients: a multiple-center epidemiological study, *Crit Care Med* 33(2):315-322, 2005.
CR 21. Malbrain MLNG, et al: Prevalence of intra-abdominal hypertension in critically ill patients: a multicentre epidemiological study, *Intensive Care Med* 30(5):822-829, 2004.
CR 22. Malbrain MLNG: Different techniques to measure intra-abdominal pressure (IAP): time for a critical re-appraisal, *Intensive Care Med* 30(3):357-371, 2004.
CR 23. Malbrain MLNG: Abdominal perfusion pressure as a prognostic marker in intraabdominal hypertension. In Vincent JL, editor: *Yearbook of intensive care and emergency medicine,* Berlin, Heidelberg, New York, 2002, Springer, 792-814.
24. Vasquez DG, Berg-Copas GM, Wetta-Hall R: Influence of semi-recumbent position on intra-abdominal pressure as measured by bladder pressure, *J Surg Res* 139(2):280-285, 2007.
25. Wolfe TR, Kimball EJ, McLean B: The interrelationship of severe sepsis, sepsis resuscitation and the abdominal compartment syndrome, *Int J Intensive Care* Spring: 87-91, 2008.

Additional Readings

Ivatury RR, Cheatham ML, Malbrain M, et al, editors: *Abdominal compartment syndrome*, Georgetown, TX, 2006, Landis Bioscience.
World Society of the Abdominal Compartment Syndrome: *World Society of the Abdominal Compartment Syndrome* (website). www.wsacs.org. Accessed June 10, 2009.
Abdominal Compartment Syndrome: *Abdominal Compartment Syndrome.org* (website). Sponsored by Wolfe Tory Medical. www.abdominalcompartmentsyndrome.org. Accessed June 10, 2009.
Intra-abdominal Pressure Monitoring: *Holtech Medical* (website). www.holtech-medical.com. Accessed June 10, 2009.
Wolfe Tory Medical, Inc.: *Wolfe Tory Medical* (website). www.wolfetory.com. Accessed June 10, 2009.

![AP] Paracentesis (Perform)

PURPOSE: Abdominal paracentesis is performed to remove fluid from the peritoneal cavity for diagnostic or therapeutic purposes.

Eleanor Fitzpatrick

PREREQUISITE NURSING KNOWLEDGE

- Knowledge of anatomy and physiology of the abdomen is important to avoid unexpected outcomes.
- Intestines and bladder lie immediately beneath the abdominal surface.
- Large volumes of ascitic fluid tend to float the air-filled bowel toward the midline, where it may be easily perforated during the procedure.
- The cecum is relatively fixed and is much less mobile than the sigmoid colon; therefore, bowel perforations are more frequent in the right lower quadrant than in the left.
- Peritoneal fluid is normally straw-colored, serous fluid secreted by the cells of the peritoneum. Grossly bloody fluid in the abdomen is abnormal.
- The peritoneal fluid collected is used to evaluate and diagnose the cause of ascites, acute abdominal conditions such as peritonitis or pancreatitis, and blunt or penetrating trauma to the abdomen.
- Therapeutic paracentesis is used to reduce intraabdominal and diaphragmatic pressures to relieve dyspnea and respiratory compromise and prevent hernia formation and diaphragmatic rupture.[12,15,16,19] These complications are seen in those patients with tense, refractory ascites with failed medical interventions such as sodium restriction and diuresis.[5,15,19]
- Ascitic fluid is produced as a result of a variety of conditions.[10] These conditions may include interference in venous return because of heart failure, constrictive pericarditis, or tricuspid valve insufficiency; obstruction of flow in the vena cava or portal vein; disturbance in electrolyte balance, such as sodium retention; depletion of plasma proteins because of nephrotic syndrome or starvation; lymphoma, leukemia, or neoplasms that involve the liver or mediastinum; ovarian malignant disease; chronic pancreatitis; and cirrhosis of the liver.
- Analysis of the ascitic fluid can determine the cause of ascites. A serum-to-ascites albumin gradient should be calculated by subtracting the ascitic fluid albumin level from the serum albumin value. This calculation differentiates portal hypertensive from nonportal hypertensive ascites.[5,7,9,10,14,19]
- Paracentesis is contraindicated in patients with an acute abdomen, who need immediate surgery. Coagulopathies and thrombocytopenia are considered relative contraindications. Coagulopathy should preclude paracentesis only in the case of clinically evident fibrinolysis or clinically evident disseminated intravascular coagulation.[12,16]
- Caution should be used when paracentesis is performed in patients with severe bowel distention, previous abdominal surgery (especially pelvic surgery), pregnancy (use open technique after first trimester), distended bladder that cannot be emptied with a Foley catheter, or obvious infection at intended site of insertion (cellulitis or abscess).
- The insertion site should be midline one third the distance from the umbilicus to the symphysis, or 2 to 3 cm below the umbilicus (Fig. 107-1). An alternate position is a point one third the distance from the umbilicus to the anterior iliac crest (left side preferred).[5,19]
- Ultrasound scan can be used before paracentesis to locate fluid and during the procedure to guide insertion of catheter. The ultrasound scan may be performed by the

---

![AP] This procedure should be performed only by physicians, advanced practice nurses, and other healthcare professionals (including critical care nurses) with additional knowledge, skills, and demonstrated competence per professional licensure or institutional standard.

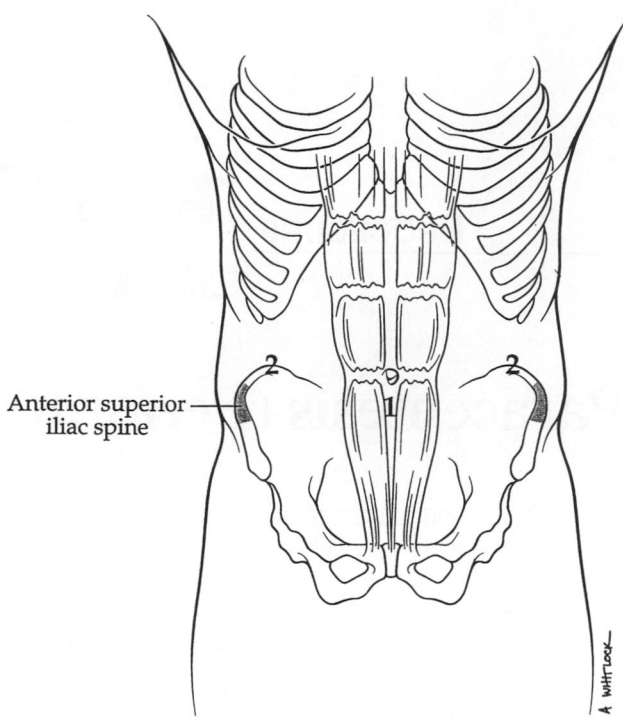

FIGURE 107-1 Preferred sites for paracentesis: *1,* Primary site is infraumbilical in midline through linea alba. *2,* Preferred alternate (lateral rectus) site is in either lower quadrant, approximately 4 to 5 cm cephalad and medial to the anterior superior iliac spine. *(From Roberts JR, Hedges JR: Clinical procedures in emergency medicine, ed 4, Philadelphia, 2004, Saunders.)*

(Label in figure: Anterior superior iliac spine)

practitioner performing the procedure or by other personnel trained to conduct the study. Ultrasound scan–guided paracentesis has a higher success rate when compared with the procedure performed with physical examination as the lone assessment tool.[8] Endoscopic transgastric ultrasound scan has also been used in the diagnosis of malignant ascites.[12]

- A semipermanent catheter or a shunt may be an option for patients with rapidly reaccumulating ascites.[13,15,16]
- When large-volume paracentesis (>5 L) is performed in patients with cirrhosis and other disorders, the infusion of albumin, 6 to 8 g/L of fluid removed, may prevent the onset of circulatory compromise associated with massive fluid shifting.[1,3,6,7,18]

EQUIPMENT

- Commercially prepared kit or the following:
  - Personal protective equipment, including sterile gloves, mask, goggles, and gown
  - Skin-cleansing solution (povidone-iodine or chlorhexidine preparation)
  - Sterile marking pen
  - Sterile towels or sterile drape
  - Local anesthetic for injection: 1% or 2% lidocaine with epinephrine
  - 5- or 10-mL syringe with 21- or 25-gauge needle for anesthetic

- Trocar with stylet, needle (16-, 18- or 20-gauge), or angiocatheter, depending on abdominal wall thickness
- 25- or 27-gauge 1½-inch needle
- 20- or 22-gauge spinal needles
- 20-mL syringe for diagnostic tap
- 50-mL syringe if using stopcock technique
- Four sterile tubes for specimens
- Scalpel and no. 11 knife blade
- Three-way stopcock
- Sterile 1-L collection bottles with connecting tubing
- Nylon skin suture material on cutting needle (4-0 or 5-0) and needle holder
- Mayo scissors and straight scissors
- Four to six sterile 4 × 4 gauze pads
- Sterile gauze dressing with tape or adhesive strip
- Stoma bag
- Soft wrist restraints

PATIENT AND FAMILY EDUCATION

- Explain the indications, procedure, and risks to the patient and family. ➤*Rationale:* Explanation may decrease patient anxiety and encourages patient and family cooperation and understanding of the procedure.
- Explain the patient's role in assisting with the procedure and postprocedure care. ➤*Rationale:* Patient cooperation during and after the procedure is elicited.
- Explain the signs and symptoms to report, such as fever, abdominal pain, decreased urine output, bleeding, and leakage of fluid from surgical wound site. ➤*Rationale:* Unexpected outcomes may not manifest themselves for a period of time after the procedure.

PATIENT ASSESSMENT AND PREPARATION

Patient Assessment

- Obtain the medical history and perform a review of systems for abdominal injury, major gastrointestinal pathology, liver disease, and portal hypertension. ➤*Rationale:* Certain conditions of the gastrointestinal tract may be diagnosed and treated with paracentesis. Contraindications to paracentesis may be identified.
- Identify the presence of any allergies to medication or other substances. ➤*Rationale:* Patients may have allergies to skin preparations or anesthetics used before the invasive procedure is performed. Identification assists the practitioner in choosing the most appropriate skin preparation and anesthetic.
- Assess respiratory status (i.e., rate, depth, excursion, gas exchange, and use of accessory muscles). ➤*Rationale:* Paracentesis may be indicated to decrease work of breathing.
- Obtain baseline vital signs, including heart rate, blood pressure, and pulse oximetry. ➤*Rationale:* Hypotension and dysrhythmias may occur with rapid changes in intraabdominal pressure.

- Obtain baseline pain assessment. ➥*Rationale:* Changes in level of pain during or after the procedure may be an indicator of complications.
- Obtain baseline fluid and electrolyte status. ➥*Rationale:* Removal of peritoneal fluid may cause compartment shifting of intravascular volume, electrolytes, and proteins, leading to a decreased circulating volume.
- Assess bowel or bladder distention. ➥*Rationale:* Distension increases the risk for bowel or bladder perforation during the procedure.
- Assess abdominal girth. ➥*Rationale:* Information on changes in fluid accumulation within the peritoneal cavity is provided.
- Obtain coagulation study results (i.e., prothrombin time [PT], partial thromboplastin time [PTT], and platelets). ➥*Rationale:* Abnormal clotting may increase the risk for bleeding during and after the procedure. Therapy may be necessary to correct clotting abnormalities before the procedure.[2]

Patient Preparation

- Ensure that the patient understands preprocedural teachings. Answer questions as they arise, and reinforce information as needed. ➥*Rationale:* Understanding of previously taught information is evaluated and reinforced.
- Obtain a written informed consent form. ➥*Rationale:* Paracentesis is an invasive procedure that requires a signed informed consent form.

- Decompress the bladder either by having the patient void or by inserting a Foley catheter. ➥*Rationale:* A distended bladder increases the risk for bladder perforation during the procedure.
- Obtain plain and upright radiographs of the abdomen before the procedure is performed. ➥*Rationale:* Air is introduced during the procedure and may confuse the diagnosis later.
- Perform a pre-procedure verification and time out, if non-emergent. ➥*Rationale:* Ensures patient safety.
- Verify correct patient with two identifiers. ➥*Rationale:* Prior to performing a procedure, the nurse should ensure the correct identification of the patient for the intended intervention.
- Check that all relevant documents and studies are available before the procedure is started. ➥*Rationale:* This measure ensures that the correct patient receives the correct procedure.
- Place the patient in the supine position (may tilt to side of collection slightly for improved fluid positioning). ➥*Rationale:* Fluid accumulates in the dependent areas.
- Examine abdomen for areas of shifting dullness. Find landmarks and mark appropriately. ➥*Rationale:* Shifting dullness indicates fluid.
- If the patient has altered mental status, soft wrist restraints may be needed. ➥*Rationale:* The patient must not move his or her hands into the sterile field once it has been established.

Procedure | for Performing Paracentesis

Steps	Rationale	Special Considerations
1. HH		
2. PE		
3. Prepare equipment and sterile field. Label all medications, medication containers (e.g., syringes, medicine cups, basins), and other solutions that are to be used during the procedure.	Provides a sterile field to decrease risk for infection; Universal Protocol.	Maintain aseptic technique.
4. Cleanse insertion site with povidone-iodine solution or chlorhexidine product.[4,11] **(Level C*)**	Reduces risk for infection.	Allergies should be identified before a skin preparation product is chosen. Use sterile technique.
5. With the patient in the supine position, determine the site for trocar insertion. Site should be midline one third the distance from the umbilicus to the symphysis (2 to 3 cm below the umbilicus; see Fig. 107-1).	Determines correct site for trocar placement. Alternate position is a point one third the distance from the umbilicus to the anterior iliac crest (left side preferred).	Avoid the rectus muscle because of increased risk for hemorrhage from epigastric vessels; surgical scars because of increased risk for perforation caused by adhesion of bowel to the wall of the peritoneum; and upper quadrants because of the possibility of undetected hepatomegaly.[5]
6. Apply sterile gloves and sterile gown.	Reduces transmission of micro-organisms and body secretions.	
7. Apply sterile drapes to outline the area to be tapped.	Provide sterile field to decrease risk for infection.	

*Level C: Qualitative studies, descriptive or correlational studies, integrative reviews, systematic reviews, or randomized controlled trials with inconsistent results

Procedure continues on following page

Procedure for Performing Paracentesis—*Continued*

Steps	Rationale	Special Considerations
8. Inject the area with local anesthetic (lidocaine with epinephrine preferred). Initially infiltrate the skin and subcutaneous tissues; then direct needle perpendicular to the skin and infiltrate the peritoneum.	Local anesthesia minimizes pain and discomfort. Epinephrine helps eliminate unwanted abdominal wall bleeding and false-positive results.	Maximum dose of lidocaine is 30 mL of 1% or 15 mL of 2%. Assess for anesthesia of area. Resistance is felt as the needle perforates the peritoneum.
9. With the no. 11 blade and scalpel holder, create a skin incision large enough to allow threading a 3- to 5-mm catheter.	Promotes easier insertion of the catheter	If lavage is necessary, the opening is large enough to thread the lavage catheter.
10. Insert an 18-gauge needle attached to a 20- or 50-mL syringe through the anesthetized tract into the peritoneum. Apply slight suction to the syringe as it is advanced. Grasp the needle close to the skin as it is advanced.	Provides access to peritoneal fluid for evacuation. Slight suction is applied to indicate when the peritoneum is entered and if a blood vessel is entered. Grasping the needle as it is advanced prevents accidental thrusting into the abdomen and possible viscus perforation.	Inserted through a small stab wound at midline below umbilicus. A small pop is felt as the needle advances through the anterior and posterior muscle fascia and enters the peritoneum.
11. Once in the cavity, direct the needle at a 60-degree angle toward the center of the pelvic hollow. When fluid returns, fill the syringe (Fig. 107-2).	Collection of fluid for laboratory studies to provide information about the patient's status.	Usually, diagnostic tests are ordered dependent on the patient's status and reason for paracentesis.[5] Tests may include the following: tube 1: lactate dehydrogenase (LDH), glucose, albumin; tube 2: protein, specific gravity; tube 3: cell count and differential; tube 4: save until further notice. If indicated, Gram stain, acid-fast bacillus (AFB) stain, bacterial and fungal cultures, amylase, and trigliceride tests may be performed.[2,5,7,8] Also, send a specimen for cytology if malignancy is suspected.
12. Attach syringes or stopcock and tubing and gently aspirate or siphon fluid via gravity or vacuum into collection device. Drains may be left in and allowed to drain for 6 to 12 hours.[17-19] **(Level E*)**	Initiates therapy.	Monitor amount of fluid removed. Removal of large amount of fluid (> 5 L) may cause hypotension.[8,13,18] If large amounts are removed or hypotension is seen, consider intravenous (IV) albumin to maintain intravascular volume.[8,13,18] **(Level E)** No evidence shows that leaving the drain in for 24 to 48 hours or more is safer or more effective.

*Level E: Multiple case reports, theory-based evidence from expert opinions, or peer-reviewed professional organizational standards without clinical studies to support recommendations

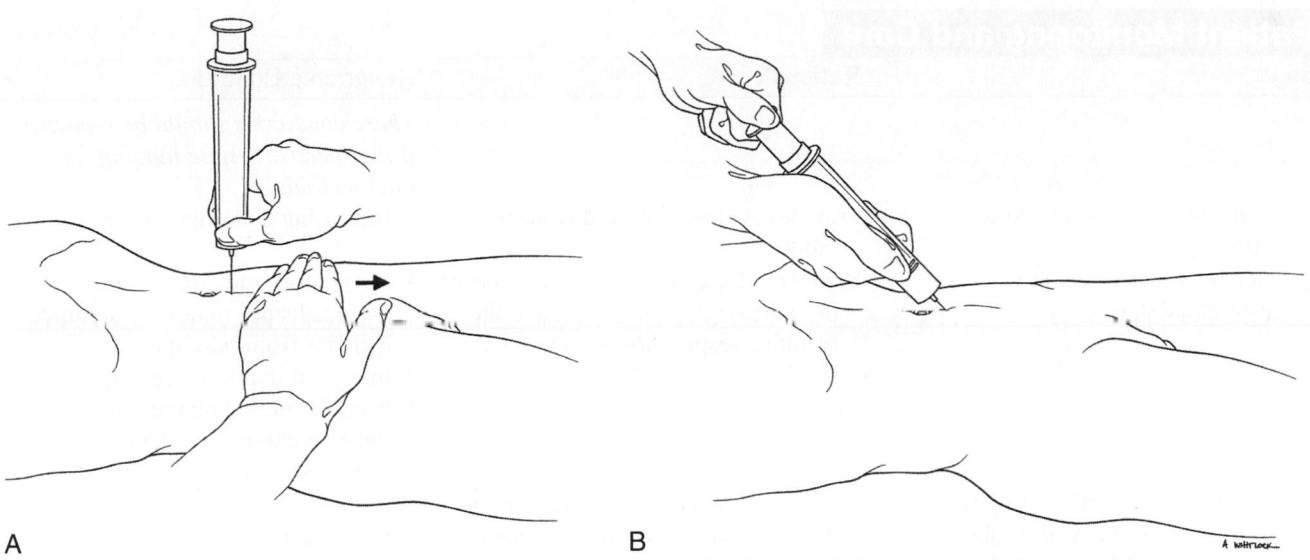

A   B

FIGURE 107-2 **A,** Z-track method of paracentesis. The skin is pulled approximately 2 cm caudal in relation to the deep abdominal wall by the non–needle-bearing hand while the paracentesis needle is slowly being inserted directly perpendicular to the skin. **B,** After the peritoneum is penetrated and fluid return obtained, the skin is released. Note that the needle is angulated caudally. *(From Roberts JR, Hedges JR: Clinical procedures in emergency medicine, ed 4, Philadelphia, 2004, Saunders.)*

Procedure | for Performing Paracentesis—*Continued*

Steps	Rationale	Special Considerations
13. After the fluid is removed, gently remove the catheter and apply pressure to the wound. If the wound is still leaking fluid after 5 minutes of direct pressure, suture the puncture site with a mattress suture (see Procedure 124) and apply a pressure dressing. If significant leakage is found, apply a stoma bag over the site until drainage becomes minimal.	Keeps insertion site clean and dry. Reduces risk for infection.	
14. Apply a sterile dressing to wound site.	Provides a barrier to infection and collects fluid that may leak from wound site.	
15. Dispose of used equipment and soiled material in appropriate receptacle.	Standard Precautions.	
16. **HH**		

Expected Outcomes

- Evacuation of peritoneal fluid for laboratory analysis
- Decompression of peritoneal cavity
- Relief of respiratory compromise
- Relief of abdominal discomfort

Unexpected Outcomes

- Perforation of bowel, bladder, or stomach
- Lacerations of major vessels (mesenteric, iliac, aorta)
- Abdominal wall hematomas
- Laceration of catheter and loss in peritoneal cavity
- Incisional hernias
- Local or systemic infection
- Hypovolemia, hypotension, shock
- Bleeding from insertion site
- Ascitic fluid leak from insertion site
- Peritonitis

Procedure continues on following page

Patient Monitoring and Care

Steps	Rationale	Reportable Conditions
		These conditions should be reported if they persist despite nursing interventions.
1. Evaluate changes in abdominal girth.	Provides evidence of fluid reaccumulation.	• Increasing abdominal girth
2. Monitor for changes in the respiratory status.	Removal of ascitic fluid should relieve pressure on the diaphragm and the resulting respiratory distress.	• Respiratory rate greater than 24 breaths per minute or significant increase from baseline • Increased depth of breathing • Irregular breathing pattern • Pulse oximetry less than 92%, or significant decrease from baseline
3. Monitor for potential complications, including bowel or bladder perforation, bleeding, and intravascular volume loss.	Paracentesis interrupts the integrity of the skin and underlying peritoneum.	• Hematuria • Hypotension • Tachycardia
4. Monitor vital signs, temperature, and insertion site for drainage or evidence of infection.	Rapid changes in intraabdominal pressure may affect heart rate and blood pressure. Infection is a complication of paracentesis.	• Hypotension • Dysrhythmias • Increased temperature • Purulent drainage from insertion site • Redness, swelling at insertion site • Abnormal laboratory results (e.g., increased white blood cell [WBC] count)
5. Monitor intake and output.	Provides data for evaluation of fluid balance status.	• Inappropriate fluid balance or changes from baseline fluid status
6. Monitor abdominal pain and level of weakness.	Patients often feel weak and have abdominal discomfort for a few hours after the procedure follow institution standard for assessing pain. Identifies need for pain interventions.	• Continued pain despite pain interventions, if performed
7. Evaluate laboratory data when returned.	Provides for evaluation of condition and aids in diagnosis.	• Red blood cell (RBC) count greater than 100,000/mm^3 • Amylase value greater than 2.5 times normal • Alkaline phosphatase value greater than 5.5 mg/dL • WBC count greater than 100/mm^3 • Positive culture results[7,9]

Documentation

Documentation should include the following:
- Patient and family education
- Date and time of procedure
- Patient tolerance of procedure
- Assessment of insertion site after procedure
- Amount and characteristics of fluid removed
- Specimens sent for laboratory analysis
- Postprocedure vital signs, respiratory status
- Postprocedure comfort/pain level
- Abdominal girth
- Unexpected outcomes
- Nursing interventions

References

1. Arora G, Keeffe EB: Management of chronic liver failure until liver transplantation, *Med Clin North Am* 92(4):839-860, 2008.
2. Dib N, Oberti F, Cales P: Current management of the complications of portal hypertension: variceal bleeding and ascites, *Can Med Assoc J* 174(10):1433-1443, 2006.
3. Dong MH, Saab S: Complications of cirrhosis, *Disease-A-Month* 54(7):445-456, 2008.
4. Edmiston CE, Seabrook GR, Johnson CP, et al: Comparative of a new and innovative 2% chlorhexidine gluconate-impregnated cloth with 4% chlorhexidine gluconate as topical antiseptic for preparation of the skin prior to surgery, *Am J Infect Control* 35(2):89-96, 2007.
5. Ferri FF: Paracentesis. In Ferri F, editor: *Practical guide to the care of the medical patient*, ed 7, Philadelphia, 2007, Mosby/Elsevier.
6. **CR** Gines P, Arroyo V, Quintero E, et al: Comparison of paracentesis and diuretics in the treatment of cirrhotics with tense ascites-results of a randomized study, *Gastroenterology* 93(2):234-241, 1987.
7. Grewal P, Martin P: Pretransplant management of the cirrhotic patient, *Clin Liver Dis* 11(2):431-439, 2007.
8. Han MK, Hyzy R: Advances in critical care management of hepatic failure and insufficiency, *Crit Care Med* 34(9 Suppl):S225-S231, 2006.
9. Hauser SC, editor: *Mayo Clinic gastroenterology and hepatology board review*, ed 2, Rochester, MN, 2006, Mayo Clinic Scientific Press.
10. Heidelbaugh JJ, Sherbondy M: Cirrhosis and chronic liver failure: part II: complications and treatment, *Am Fam Physician* 74(5):767-776, 2006.
11. **CR** Hibbard JS: Analyses comparing the antimicrobial activity of current antiseptic agents: a review, *J Infusion Nurs* 28(3):194-207, 2005.
12. Kaushik N, Khalid A, Brody D, et al: EUS-guided paracentesis for the diagnosis and management of malignant ascites, *Gastrointest Endosc* 64(6):908-913, 2006.
13. McGibbon A, Chen G, Peltekian K, et al: An evidence-based manual for abdominal paracentesis, *Dig Dis Sci* 52(12):3307-3315, 2007.
14. **CR** Pare P, Talbot J, Hoefs JC: Serum-ascites albumin concentration gradient: a physiologic approach to the differential diagnosis of ascites, *Gastroenterology* 85(2):240-244, 1983.
15. Rodes J, editor: *Textbook of hepatology: from basic science to clinical practice*, ed 3, Malden, MA, 2007, Blackwell Publishing Ltd.
16. Rosenberg SM: Palliation of malignant ascites, *Gastroenterol Clin* 35(1):189-199, 2006.
17. Saab S, Nieto JM, Lewis SK, et al: TIPS versus paracentesis for cirrhotic patients with refractory ascites, *Cochrane Database Syst Rev* 3: 2008.
18. Sanchez W, Talwalkar JA: Palliative care for patients with end-stage liver disease ineligible for liver transplantation, *Gastroenterol Clin* 35(1):201-219, 2006.
19. Schiff ER, Sorrell MF, Maddrey WC: *Schiff's diseases of the liver*, ed 10, Philadelphia, 2007, Lippincott Williams & Wilkins.

Additional Readings

Garcia-Tsao G: Portal hypertension, *Curr Opin Gastroenterol* 22(3):254-262, 2006.
Hou W & Sanyal A.J: Ascites: Diagnosis and management, *Med Clin North Am*, 93(4), 801-817, 2009.
Minor MA, Grace ND: Pharmacologic therapy of portal hypertension, *Clin Liver Dis* 10(3):563-581, 2006.
Thomsen TW, Shaffer RW, White B, et al: Videos in clinical medicine: paracentesis, *N Engl J Med* 355(19):e21, 2007.

PROCEDURE **108**

Paracentesis (Assist)

P U R P O S E :   Abdominal paracentesis is performed to remove fluid from the peritoneal cavity for diagnostic or therapeutic purposes.

Eleanor Fitzpatrick

PREREQUISITE NURSING KNOWLEDGE

- Knowledge of anatomy and physiology of the abdomen is important to avoid unexpected outcomes.
- Intestines and bladder lie immediately beneath the abdominal surface.
- Large volumes of ascitic fluid tend to float the air-filled bowel toward the midline, where it may be easily perforated during the procedure.
- The cecum is relatively fixed and is much less mobile than the sigmoid colon; therefore, bowel perforations are more frequent in the right lower quadrant than in the left.
- Peritoneal fluid is normally straw-colored, serous fluid secreted by the cells of the peritoneum. Grossly bloody fluid in the abdomen is abnormal.
- The peritoneal fluid collected is used to evaluate and diagnose the cause of ascites, acute abdominal conditions such as peritonitis or pancreatitis, and blunt or penetrating trauma to the abdomen.
- Therapeutic paracentesis is used to reduce intraabdominal and diaphragmatic pressures to relieve dyspnea and respiratory compromise and to prevent hernia formation and diaphragmatic rupture.[12,15,16,19] These complications are seen in those patients with tense, refractory ascites with failed medical interventions, such as sodium restriction and diuresis.[5,15,19]
- Ascitic fluid is produced as a result of a variety of conditions.[10] These conditions may include interference in venous return because of heart failure, constrictive pericarditis, or tricuspid valve insufficiency; obstruction of flow in the vena cava or portal vein; disturbance in electrolyte balance, such as sodium retention; depletion of plasma proteins because of nephrotic syndrome or starvation; lymphoma, leukemia, or neoplasms that involve the liver or mediastinum; ovarian malignant disease; chronic pancreatitis; or cirrhosis of the liver.

- Analysis of the ascitic fluid can determine the cause of ascites. A serum-to-ascites albumin gradient should be calculated by subtracting the ascitic fluid albumin level from the serum albumin. This calculation differentiates portal hypertensive from nonportal hypertensive ascites.[5,7,9,10,14,19]
- Paracentesis is contraindicated in patients with an acute abdomen, who need immediate surgery. Coagulopathies and thrombocytopenia are considered relative contraindications. Coagulopathy should preclude paracentesis only in the case of clinically evident fibrinolysis or clinically evident disseminated intravascular coagulation.[12,16]
- Caution should be used when paracentesis is performed in patients with severe bowel distention, previous abdominal surgery (especially pelvic surgery), pregnancy (use open technique after first trimester), distended bladder that cannot be emptied with a Foley catheter, or obvious infection at intended site of insertion (cellulitis or abscess).
- The insertion site should be midline one third the distance from the umbilicus to the symphysis (2 to 3 cm below the umbilicus; see Fig. 107-1). An alternate position is a point one third the distance from the umbilicus to the anterior iliac crest (left side preferred).[5,19]
- Ultrasound scan can be used before paracentesis to locate fluid and during the procedure to guide insertion of catheter. Ultrasound scan–guided paracentesis has a higher success rate when compared with procedures performed with the physical examination as the lone assessment tool.[8]

- Endoscopic transgastric ultrasound scan has also been used in the diagnosis of malignant ascites.[12]
- A semipermanent catheter or a shunt may be an option for patients with rapidly reaccumulating ascites.[13,15,16]
- When large-volume paracentesis (>5 L) is performed in patients with cirrhosis and other disorders, the infusion of albumin, 6 to 8 g/L of fluid removed, may prevent the onset of circulatory compromise associated with massive fluid shifting.[1,3,6,7,18]

EQUIPMENT

- Commercially prepared kit or the following:
  - ❖ Personal protective equipment, including sterile gloves, mask, goggles, and gown
  - ❖ Skin-cleansing solution (povidone-iodine or chlorhexidine preparation)
  - ❖ Sterile marking pen
  - ❖ Sterile towels or sterile drape
  - ❖ Local anesthetic for injection: 1% or 2% lidocaine with epinephrine
  - ❖ 5- or 10-mL syringe with 21- or 25-gauge needle for anesthetic
  - ❖ Trocar with stylet, needle (16-, 18-, or 20-gauge), or angiocatheter, depending on abdominal wall thickness
  - ❖ 25- or 27-gauge 1½-inch needle
  - ❖ 20- or 22-gauge spinal needles
  - ❖ 20-mL syringe for diagnostic tap
  - ❖ 50-mL syringe if using stopcock technique
  - ❖ Four sterile tubes for specimens
  - ❖ Scalpel and no. 11 knife blade
  - ❖ Three-way stopcock
  - ❖ Sterile 1-L collection bottles with connecting tubing
  - ❖ Nylon skin suture material on cutting needle (4-0 or 5-0) and needle holder
  - ❖ Mayo scissors and straight scissors
  - ❖ Four to six sterile 4 × 4 gauze pads
  - ❖ Sterile gauze dressing with tape or adhesive strip
  - ❖ Stoma bag
  - ❖ Soft wrist restraints

PATIENT AND FAMILY EDUCATION

- Explain the indications, procedure, and risks to the patient and family. ➤➤*Rationale:* Explanation may decrease patient anxiety and encourages patient and family cooperation and understanding of the procedure.
- Explain the patient's role in assisting with the procedure and postprocedure care. ➤➤*Rationale:* Patient cooperation during and after the procedure is elicited.
- Explain the signs and symptoms to report, such as fever, abdominal pain, decreased urine output, bleeding, and leakage of fluid from surgical wound site. ➤➤*Rationale:* Unexpected outcomes may not manifest themselves for a period of time after the procedure.

PATIENT ASSESSMENT AND PREPARATION

Patient Assessment

- Obtain the medical history and a review of systems for abdominal injury, major gastrointestinal pathology, liver disease, and portal hypertension. ➤➤*Rationale:* Certain conditions of the gastrointestinal tract may be diagnosed and treated with paracentesis. Contraindications to paracentesis may be identified.
- Identify the presence of any allergies to medication or other substances. ➤➤*Rationale:* Patients may have allergies to skin preparations or anesthetics used before the invasive procedure is performed. Identification assists the practitioner in choosing the most appropriate skin preparation and anesthetic.
- Assess respiratory status (i.e., rate, depth, excursion, gas exchange, and use of accessory muscles). ➤➤*Rationale:* Paracentesis may be indicated to decrease the work of breathing.
- Obtain baseline vital signs, including heart rate, blood pressure, and pulse oximetry. ➤➤*Rationale:* Hypotension and dysrhythmias may occur with rapid changes in the intraabdominal pressure.
- Obtain a baseline pain assessment. ➤➤*Rationale:* Changes in the level of pain during or after the procedure may be an indicator of complications.
- Obtain baseline fluid and electrolyte status. ➤➤*Rationale:* Removal of peritoneal fluid may cause compartment shifting of intravascular volume, electrolytes, and proteins, leading to a decreased circulating volume.
- Assess bowel or bladder distention. ➤➤*Rationale:* Distension increases the risk for bowel or bladder perforation during the procedure.
- Assess abdominal girth. ➤➤*Rationale:* Information on changes in fluid accumulation within the peritoneal cavity is provided.
- Obtain coagulation study results (i.e., prothrombin time [PT], partial thromboplastin time [PTT], and platelets). ➤➤*Rationale:* Abnormal clotting may increase the risk for bleeding during and after the procedure. Therapy may be necessary to correct clotting abnormalities before the procedure.[2]

Patient Preparation

- Ensure that the patient understands preprocedural teachings. Answer questions as they arise, and reinforce information as needed. ➤➤*Rationale:* Understanding of previously taught information is evaluated and reinforced.
- Ensure that a written informed consent form has been obtained by the practitioner performing the procedure. The assisting practitioner may be a witness to the signing of the consent if needed. ➤➤*Rationale:* Paracentesis is an invasive procedure and requires a signed informed consent form.
- Decompress the bladder either by having the patient void or by inserting a Foley catheter. ➤➤*Rationale:* A distended bladder increases the risk for bladder perforation during the procedure.

- The physician or advanced practice nurse orders plain and upright radiographs of the abdomen before the procedure is performed. ➤➤*Rationale:* Air is introduced during the procedure and may confuse the diagnosis later.
- Perform a pre-procedure verification and time out with the physician or advanced practice nurse, if non-emergent. ➤➤*Rationale:* Ensures patient safety.
- Check that all relevant documents and studies are available before the procedure is started. ➤➤*Rationale:* This measure ensures that the correct patient receives the correct procedure.

- Place the patient in the supine position (may tilt to side of collection slightly for improved fluid positioning). ➤➤*Rationale:* Fluid accumulates in the dependent areas.
- The physician or advanced practice nurse will examine the abdomen for areas of shifting dullness, find landmarks, and mark appropriately. ➤➤*Rationale:* Shifting dullness indicates fluid.
- If the patient has altered mental status, soft wrist restraints may be needed. ➤➤*Rationale:* The patient must not move his or her hands into the sterile field once it has been established.

Procedure for Assisting with Paracentesis

Steps	Rationale	Special Considerations
1. **HH**		
2. **PE**		
3. Assist in preparing the equipment and sterile field. Label all medications, medication containers (e.g., syringes, medicine cups, basins), and other solutions that are to be used during the procedure.	Provides a sterile field to decrease risk for infection. Universal Protocol.	Maintain aseptic technique.
4. Assist physician or nurse practitioner to cleanse insertion site with povidone-iodine solution or chlorhexidine preparation.[4,11] **(Level C*)**	Reduces risk for infection.	Allergies should be identified before a skin preparation product is chosen. Use sterile technique.
5. Assist the physician or advanced practice nurse with the application of sterile gloves, gown, and mask as well as sterile drapes to outline the area to be tapped.	Provides sterile field to decrease risk for infection.	
6. Assist physician or advanced practice nurse to draw up local anesthetic (lidocaine with epinephrine preferred).	Local anesthesia minimizes pain and discomfort. Epinephrine helps eliminate unwanted abdominal wall bleeding and false-positive results.	Maximum dose of lidocaine is 30 mL of 1% or 15 mL of 2%. Assess for anesthesia of area.
7. Assist in collection of peritoneal fluid for laboratory analysis.	Collection of fluid for laboratory studies to provide information about the patient's status.	Usually diagnostic tests are ordered depending on patient's status and reason for paracentesis.[5] These tests may include the following: tube 1: lactate dehydrogenase (LDH), glucose, albumin; tube 2: protein, specific gravity; tube 3: cell count and differential; tube 4: save until further notice. If indicated, Gram stain, acid-fast bacillus (AFB) stain, bacterial and fungal cultures, amylase, and triglyceride tests may be ordered.[2,5,7,8] Also, collect a specimen for cytology if malignancy is suspected.

*Level C: Qualitative studies, descriptive or correlational studies, integrative reviews, systematic reviews, or randomized controlled trials with inconsistent results

Procedure for Assisting with Paracentesis—*Continued*

Steps	Rationale	Special Considerations
8. Assist the physician or advanced practice nurse in attaching syringes or stopcock and tubing and aspirating or siphoning fluid via gravity or vacuum into collection device. Drains may be left in and allowed to drain for 6 to 12 hours.[17,18,19] **(Level E*)**	Initiates therapy.	Monitor amount of fluid removed. Removal of large amount of fluid (> 5 L) may cause hypotension.[8,13,18] If large amounts are removed or hypotension seen, intravenous (IV) albumin to maintain intravascular volume may be considered.[8,13] No evidence shows that leaving the drain in for 24 to 48 hours or more is safer or more effective.
9. After the fluid and catheter are removed, apply pressure to the wound. If the wound is still leaking fluid after 5 minutes of direct pressure, the physician or advanced practice nurse may suture the puncture site (see Procedure 124) and apply a pressure dressing. If significant leakage is found, apply a stoma bag over the site until drainage becomes minimal.	Keeps the insertion site clean. Reduces the risk for infection.	Inspect catheter to ensure it is intact.
10. Apply a sterile dressing to wound site.	Provides a barrier to infection and collects fluid that may leak from wound site.	
11. Dispose of used equipment and soiled material in appropriate receptacle.	Standard Precautions.	
12. **HH**		

Expected Outcomes

- Evacuation of peritoneal fluid for laboratory analysis
- Decompression of peritoneal cavity
- Relief of respiratory compromise
- Relief of abdominal discomfort

Unexpected Outcomes

- Perforation of bowel, bladder, or stomach
- Lacerations of major vessels (mesenteric, iliac, aorta)
- Abdominal wall hematomas
- Laceration of catheter and loss in peritoneal cavity
- Incisional hernias
- Local or systemic infection
- Hypovolemia, hypotension, shock
- Bleeding from insertion site
- Ascitic fluid leak from insertion site
- Peritonitis

Patient Monitoring and Care

Steps	Rationale	Reportable Conditions
		These conditions should be reported if they persist despite nursing interventions.
1. Evaluate changes in abdominal girth.	Provides evidence of fluid reaccumulation.	- Increasing abdominal girth

*Level E: Multiple case reports, theory-based evidence from expert opinions, or peer-reviewed professional organizational standards without clinical studies to support recommendations

Procedure continues on following page

Patient Monitoring and Care —*Continued*

Steps	Rationale	Reportable Conditions
2. Monitor for changes in the respiratory status.	Removal of ascitic fluid should relieve pressure on the diaphragm and the resulting respiratory distress.	• Respiratory rate greater than 24 breaths per minute or significant increase from baseline • Increased depth of breathing • Irregular breathing pattern • Pulse oximetry less than 92%, or significant decrease from baseline
3. Monitor for potential complications, including bowel or bladder perforation, bleeding, and intravascular volume loss.	Paracentesis interrupts the integrity of the skin and underlying peritoneum.	• Hematuria • Hypotension • Tachycardia
4. Monitor vital signs, temperature, and insertion site for drainage or evidence of infection.	Rapid changes in intraabdominal pressure may affect heart rate and blood pressure. Infection is a complication of paracentesis.	• Hypotension • Dysrhythmias • Increased temperature • Purulent drainage from insertion site • Redness, swelling at insertion site • Abnormal laboratory results (increased white blood cell [WBC] count)
5. Monitor intake and output.	Provides data for evaluation of the fluid balance status.	• Inappropriate fluid balance or changes from baseline fluid status
6. Monitor abdominal pain and level of weakness. Follow institutional standards for assessing pain.	Patients often feel weak and have abdominal discomfort for a few hours after the procedure. Identifies need for pain interventions.	• Continued pain despite pain interventions, if performed
7. Evaluate the laboratory data when returned.	Provides for evaluation of the condition and aids in diagnosis.	• Red blood cell (RBC) count greater than 100,000/mm^3 • Amylase value greater than 2.5 times normal • Alkaline phosphatase value greater than 5.5 mg/dL • WBC count greater than 100/mm^3 • Positive culture results[7,9]

Documentation

Documentation should include the following:

- Patient and family education
- The date and time of the procedure
- Patient tolerance of the procedure
- Assessment of the insertion site after the procedure
- The amount and characteristics of fluid removed

- Specimens sent for laboratory analysis
- Postprocedure vital signs, respiratory status
- Postprocedure comfort/pain level
- Abdominal girth
- Unexpected outcomes
- Nursing interventions

References

1. Arora G, Keeffe EB: Management of chronic liver failure until liver transplantation, *Med Clin North Am* 92(4):839-860, 2008.
2. Dib N, Oberti F, Cales P: Current management of the complications of portal hypertension: variceal bleeding and ascites, *Can Med Assoc J* 174(10):1433-1443, 2006.
3. Dong MH, Saab S: Complications of cirrhosis, *Disease-A-Month* 54(7):445-456, 2008.
4. Edmiston CE, Seabrook GR, Johnson CP, et al: Comparative of a new and innovative 2% chlorhexidine gluconate-impregnated cloth with 4% chlorhexidine gluconate as topical antiseptic for preparation of the skin prior to surgery, *Am J Infect Control* 35(2):89-96, 2007.
5. Ferri FF: Paracentesis. In Ferri F, editor: *Practical guide to the care of the medical patient*, ed 7, Philadelphia, 2007, Mosby/Elsevier.

CR 6. Gines P, Arroyo V, Quintero E, et al: Comparison of paracentesis and diuretics in the treatment of cirrhotics with tense ascites-results of a randomized study, *Gastroenterology* 93(2):234-241, 1987.

7. Grewal P, Martin P: Pretransplant management of the cirrhotic patient, *Clin Liver Dis* 11(2):431-439, 2006.

8. Han MK, Hyzy R: Advances in critical care management of hepatic failure and insufficiency, *Crit Care Med* 34(9 Suppl):S225-S231, 2006.

9. Hauser SC, editor: *Mayo Clinic gastroenterology and hepatology board review,* ed 2, Rochester, MN, 2006, Mayo Clinic Scientific Press.

10. Heidelbaugh JJ, Sherbondy M: Cirrhosis and chronic liver failure: part II: complications and treatment, *Am Fam Physician* 74(5):767-776, 2006.

CR 11. Hibbard JS: Analyses comparing the antimicrobial activity of current antiseptic agents: a review, *J Infusion Nurs* 28(3):194-207, 2005.

12. Kaushik N, Khalid A, Brody D, editor: EUS-guided paracentesis for the diagnosis and management of malignant ascites, *Gastrointest Endosc* 64(6):908-913, 2006.

13. McGibbon A, Chen G, Peltekian K, et al: An evidence-based manual for abdominal paracentesis, *Dig Dis Sci* 52(12):3307-3315, 2007.

CR 14. Pare P, Talbot J, Hoefs JC: Serum-ascites albumin concentration gradient: a physiologic approach to the differential diagnosis of ascites, *Gastroenterology* 85(2):240-244 , 1983.

15. Rodes J, editor: *Textbook of hepatology: from basic science to clinical practice,* ed 3, Malden, MA, 2007, Blackwell Publishing Ltd.

16. Rosenberg SM: Palliation of malignant ascites, *Gastroenterol Clin* 35(1):189-199, 2006.

17. Saab S, Nieto JM, Lewis SK, et al: TIPS versus paracentesis for cirrhotic patients with refractory ascites, *Cochrane Database Syst Rev* 3: 2008.

18. Sanchez W, Talwalkar JA: Palliative care for patients with end-stage liver disease ineligible for liver transplantation, *Gastroenterol Clin* 35(1):201-219, 2006.

19. Schiff ER, Sorrell MF, Maddrey WC: *Schiff's diseases of the liver,* ed 10, Philadelphia, 2007, Lippincott Williams & Wilkins.

Additional Readings

Garcia-Tsao G: Portal hypertension, *Curr Opin Gastroenterol* 22(3):254-262, 2006.

Hou W, Sanyal AJ: Ascites: diagnosis and management, *Med Clin of North Amer*, *93(4), 801-817,* 2009.

Minor MA, Grace ND: Pharmacologic therapy of portal hypertension, *Clin Liver Dis* 10(3):563-581, 2006.

Thomsen TW, Shaffer RW, White B, et al, editors: Videos in clinical medicine: paracentesis, *N Engl J Med* 355(19): e21, 2007.

AP Peritoneal Lavage (Perform)

PURPOSE: Percutaneous peritoneal lavage is performed for both therapeutic and diagnostic purposes.

Jenny Bosley

PREREQUISITE NURSING KNOWLEDGE

- Knowledge of the anatomy and physiology of the abdomen is important to avoid unexpected outcomes.
- The intestines and the bladder lie immediately beneath the abdominal surface. In children, the bladder is an abdominal organ. In adults, a full bladder is raised out of the pelvis.
- The cecum is relatively fixed and is much less mobile than the sigmoid colon; therefore, bowel perforations are more frequent in the right lower quadrant than in the left.
- A distended stomach can extend to the anterior abdominal wall.
- Peritoneal fluid is normally straw-colored, serous fluid secreted by the cells of the peritoneum. Grossly bloody fluid, a red blood cell (RBC) count of greater than 100,000/mm^3,[2,5,9] or the presence of bacteria or bile in the return fluid in the abdomen is abnormal. A white blood cell (WBC) count greater than 500,000/mm and the presence of bile or amylase in the lavage fluid are parameters, in addition to the RBC count, that can lead to operative intervention.[2,5,9]
- Diagnostic peritoneal lavage is a highly sensitive tool for diagnosis of visceral injuries in the abdominal cavity.[1,5,8]
- Diagnostic peritoneal lavage is used after blunt abdominal trauma or in trauma patients who have head injuries, are unconscious, or have preexisting paraplegia to determine the presence of the following[2]:
  - ❖ Hemoperitoneum (blood in lavage returns)
  - ❖ Organ injury (intestinal enzymes or microorganisms in lavage returns)
- Therapeutic lavage is used to:
  - ❖ Irrigate and cleanse purulent exudate in patients with peritonitis or intraabdominal abscess
  - ❖ Warm the abdominal cavity in patients with hypothermia
  - ❖ Remove unwanted or toxic chemicals through peritoneal dialysis
  - ❖ Obtain cytology specimens in patients with cancer
- For trauma patients with stab wounds and gunshot wounds to the lower chest or anterior abdomen, diagnostic peritoneal lavage is controversial; most trauma centers operate on patients with gunshot wound injuries to the lower chest or anterior abdomen.[1]
- Diagnostic peritoneal lavage can be used as a tool in patients with hypotension of uncertain etiology in the presence of trauma.[6]
- Diagnostic peritoneal lavage is not necessary if abdominal surgery is already indicated.[7,9]
- Because it is an invasive procedure, diagnostic peritoneal lavage does have a small risk of visceral injury (0.6%).[5]
- Diagnostic peritoneal lavage is 95% sensitive and 99% specific for intraperitoneal blood; however, it cannot exclude retroperitoneal hemorrhage, disruption of the diaphragm, or hollow viscus perforation.[5,7]
- Computed tomography (CT) scan frequently is used in trauma patients with hemodynamically stable conditions as the diagnostic procedure of choice.[5] Also, abdominal ultrasound scan and focused abdominal sonography in trauma (FAST) have been increasingly used to screen blunt abdominal trauma cases for hemoperitoneum.[9]

- In patients with hemodynamically unstable conditions, diagnostic peritoneal lavage (DPL) may be preferred because of its high sensitivity.[1,2,5,9] DPL is quick, inexpensive, safe, and highly sensitive to the presence of blood in the peritoneal cavity.[5] Patients with hemodynamically unstable conditions may also go directly to the operating room (OR) for laparotomy.
- Complementary CT scan and DPL decreases nontherapeutic laparotomy rates and allows nonoperative management of those patients with solid-organ injury.[9]
- Peritoneal lavage is absolutely contraindicated in an acute abdomen that needs immediate surgery as indicated by free air on radiography or penetrating abdominal trauma.
- Relative contraindications for DPL include the following[5,6]:
  - Thrombocytopenia
  - Coagulopathy[7]
  - Morbid obesity[7]
  - Severe bowel distention
  - Advanced cirrhosis[7]
  - Previous abdominal surgery, especially pelvic surgery
  - Distended bladder that cannot be emptied with a Foley catheter
  - Obvious infection at intended site of insertion (cellulitis or abscess)
  - Pregnancy of greater than 12 weeks' gestation[7]
- Use caution when performing DPL in patients with suspected pelvic fractures (may use a supraumbilical site) because of false-positive results[7]; if DPL is performed in pregnant patients of more than 12 weeks' gestation, use an open technique, superior to the uterus.[7]
- Insertion site should be midline, one third the distance from the umbilicus to the symphysis, or 2 to 3 cm below the umbilicus (see Fig. 107-1). An alternate position is a point one third the distance from the umbilicus to the anterior iliac crest (left side preferred).
- Ultrasound scan can be used before peritoneal lavage to locate fluid and during the procedure to guide insertion of the catheter.[9]

EQUIPMENT

- Commercially prepared kit or the following:
  - Personal protective equipment, including sterile gloves, mask, goggles, and gown
  - Skin cleansing solution (chlorhexidine or povidone-iodine)
  - Sterile marking pen
  - Sterile towels or sterile drape
  - Razor to shave area, if necessary
  - Local anesthetic for injection: 1% or 2% lidocaine with epinephrine
  - 5- or 10-mL syringe with 25- or 27-gauge needle for anesthetic
  - Scalpel and no. 11 knife blade
  - Trocar with stylet; needle (16-, 18-, or 20-gauge) or angiocatheter; depending on abdominal wall thickness may use guidewire with floppy tip and 9 to 18 Fr peritoneal lavage catheter
  - 20-mL syringe for diagnostic tap

- Sterile intravenous (IV) tubing (without valves) with appropriate sterile connectors for lavage catheter and IV bags
- Sterile tubes for specimens
- Warmed Ringer's lactate (RL), normal saline (NS), or antibiotic solution for infusion into abdomen
- Three-way stopcock for therapeutic lavage
- Nylon skin suture material on cutting needle (4-0 or 5-0) and needle holder
- Four to six sterile 4 × 4 gauze pads
- Sterile gauze dressing with tape or adhesive strip
- Soft wrist restraints
- Pressure bag

PATIENT AND FAMILY EDUCATION

- Explain the indications, the procedure, and the risks to the patient and family. →*Rationale:* Explanation may decrease patient anxiety and may encourage patient and family cooperation and understanding of procedure.
- Explain the patient's role in assisting with the procedure and postprocedure care. →*Rationale:* Patient cooperation during and after the procedure is elicited.
- Explain the signs and symptoms to report, such as fever, abdominal pain, decreased urine output, bleeding, and leakage of fluid from wound site. →*Rationale:* Unexpected outcomes may not manifest themselves for a period of time after the procedure.

PATIENT ASSESSMENT AND PREPARATION
Patient Assessment

- Obtain the medical history and a review of systems to identify abdominal injury, peritonitis, intraabdominal abscess, or pregnancy. →*Rationale:* Certain conditions of the gastrointestinal tract may be diagnosed and treated with peritoneal lavage. Contraindications to peritoneal lavage may be identified.[6]
- Identify the presence of any allergies to medication or other substances. →*Rationale:* Patients may have allergies to skin preparations or anesthetics used before the invasive procedure is performed. This identification assists the practitioner in choosing the most appropriate skin preparation and anesthetic.
- Assess for bowel or bladder distention. →*Rationale:* Distention increases the risk for bowel or bladder perforation during the procedure.[7]
- Coagulation studies (i.e., prothrombin time [PT], partial thromboplastin time [PTT], and platelets). →*Rationale:* Abnormal clotting studies may increase the risk for bleeding during and after the procedure. Therapy may be necessary to correct clotting abnormalities before the procedure is performed.
- Obtain plain radiographs of the abdomen and upright abdominal films if possible (before the procedure). →*Rationale:* Air is introduced during the procedure and may confound the diagnosis later.[7]

- Obtain baseline vital signs and pain assessment according to institutional standard. ➤➤*Rationale:* Practitioner can identify intraprocedure or postprocedure changes that may be indicative of complications.

Patient Preparation

- Ensure that the patient understands preprocedural teachings. Answer questions as they arise, and reinforce information as needed. ➤➤*Rationale:* Understanding of previously taught information is evaluated and reinforced.
- Obtain signed informed consent from the patient or decision maker, if possible. In a trauma situation or unresponsive patient, this may be implied consent. ➤➤*Rationale:* Peritoneal lavage is an invasive procedure that requires a signed consent form.
- Have patient void or insert a urinary drainage catheter. ➤➤*Rationale:* A distended bladder increases the risk for bladder perforation during the procedure.[7]
- Insert a nasogastric tube unless contraindicated (e.g., in significant facial trauma) and attach to low intermittent suction. ➤➤*Rationale:* A distended stomach increases the risk for perforation during the procedure.[6]
- Perform a pre-procedure verification and time out, if nonemergent. ➤➤*Rationale:* Ensures patient safety.

- Verify correct patient with two identifiers. ➤➤*Rationale:* Prior to performing a procedure, the physician or advanced practice nurse should ensure the correct identification of the patient for the intended intervention.
- Check that all relevant documents and studies are available before starting the procedure. ➤➤*Rationale:* This measure ensures that the correct patient receives the correct procedure.
- Place the patient in the supine position (may tilt to side of collection slightly for improved fluid positioning). ➤➤*Rationale:* Fluid accumulates in the dependent areas.
- Examine abdomen for landmarks and mark appropriately. Shave area, if necessary. ➤➤*Rationale:* Correct placement of catheter for peritoneal lavage minimizes complications.
- For the patient with pain or agitation who is unable to cooperate with the procedure, consider analgesia or sedation. If sedation is needed for the procedure, institution-specific moderate sedation monitoring should be performed. ➤➤*Rationale:* Analgesia and sedation provide for patient comfort and safety during procedure.
- If the patient has altered mental status, soft wrist restraints may be needed. ➤➤*Rationale:* The patient must not move his or her hands into the sterile field once it has been established.

Procedure   for Performing Peritoneal Lavage

Steps	Rationale	Special Considerations
1. **HH**		
2. **PE**		
3. Label all medications, medication containers (e.g., syringes, medicine cups, basins), or other solutions that are to be used during the procedure.	Provides additional safety for the patient undergoing the procedure.	
4. Prepare the equipment and sterile field and apply sterile gown and gloves.	Facilitates easy access to needed equipment.	Maintain aseptic technique.
5. Set up lavage equipment. A. Attach the IV tubing to lavage fluid and clear tubing of air. B. Attach the IV tubing to one port of the three-way stopcock and attach the drainage collector to the second port of the three-way stopcock. **or** C. Use IV tubing with a roller clamp and use the lavage fluid bag as the drainage bag.	Provides a closed system for instillation and drainage of lavage fluid.	
6. Cleanse the insertion site with povidone-iodine solution or chlorhexidine preparation.	Reduces risk for infection.	Allergies should be identified before a skin preparation product is selected. Use sterile technique.

Procedure for Performing Peritoneal Lavage—*Continued*

Steps	Rationale	Special Considerations
7. Apply sterile drapes to outline the insertion site. Site should be in the midline about one third the distance from the umbilicus to the symphysis (usually 2 to 3 cm below the umbilicus; see Fig. 107-1). An alternate position is a point about one third the distance from the umbilicus to the anterior iliac crest (left side preferred).	Minimizes the risk of infection. Maintains aseptic and sterile precautions.	Avoid the rectus muscle because of increased risk for hemorrhage from epigastric vessels; avoid surgical scars because of increased risk for perforation caused by adhesion of bowel to the wall of the peritoneum; avoid the upper quadrants because of the possibility of undetected hepatomegaly.[2,3] (**Level D***)
8. Inject the area with local anesthetic (lidocaine with epinephrine preferred). Initially direct the needle perpendicular to the skin and infiltrate the peritoneum with anesthetic.	Local anesthesia minimizes pain and discomfort. Epinephrine helps eliminate unwanted abdominal wall bleeding and false-positive results.	Maximum dose of lidocaine is 30 mL of 1% or 15 mL of 2%. Assess for anesthesia of area. Resistance is felt as the needle perforates the peritoneum.
9. With the no. 11 blade scalpel, create a vertical skin incision large enough to allow threading of a 3-mm to 5-mm lavage catheter. Spread the subcutaneous tissue and incise the fascia to expose the peritoneum. Nick the peritoneal membrane to pass the catheter.	To create an opening large enough to thread the lavage catheter.	When the subcutaneous tissue is nicked with the scalpel, a tough, gritty sensation is felt.
10. Insert an 18-gauge needle attached to a 20- or 50-mL syringe perpendicular through the anesthetized tract into the peritoneum. Apply slight suction to the syringe as it is advanced. Grasp the needle close to the skin as it is advanced (see Fig. 107-2).	Provides access to the peritoneal space. Slight suction is applied to indicate when the peritoneum is entered or if a blood vessel is entered. Grasping the needle as it is advanced prevents accidental thrusting into the abdomen and possible viscus perforation.	The needle is inserted through a small incision at midline below umbilicus. A small pop is felt as the needle advances through the anterior and posterior muscle fascia and enters the peritoneum.
11. Once in the cavity, direct the needle at a 60-degree angle toward the center of the pelvic hollow. If fluid returns, fill the syringe.	Collection of fluid for laboratory studies.	A free return of 10 mL of blood is a strong positive finding for a hemoperitoneum.[4] If blood is returned, remove the needle and prepare for immediate surgical intervention.
12. If the tap is dry, perform the lavage technique.	Accurately assesses for hemoperitoneum.	
13. Introduce the guidewire through the 18-guage needle.	Provides an access for insertion of the peritoneal lavage catheter.	The wire should insert easily. If any resistance is felt, advance or redirect the needle until the wire feeds easily. Difficulty in advancing the catheter may indicate the stylet is not in the peritoneal cavity or that there may be adhesions.
14. Insert about half of the wire into the pelvis and remove the needle. Hold on to the guidewire continuously.	Letting go of the guidewire could allow the wire to inadvertently migrate into peritoneum.	

*Level D: Peer-reviewed professional organizational standards with clinical studies to support recommendations

Procedure continues on following page

Procedure for Performing Peritoneal Lavage—*Continued*

Steps	Rationale	Special Considerations
15. Slide the peritoneal lavage catheter over the wire with gently twisting motions (Fig. 109-1).	A twisting motion minimizes visceral perforation and displaces the abdominal contents.	Always keep a firm hold on the wire to prevent it from slipping into the peritoneal cavity.

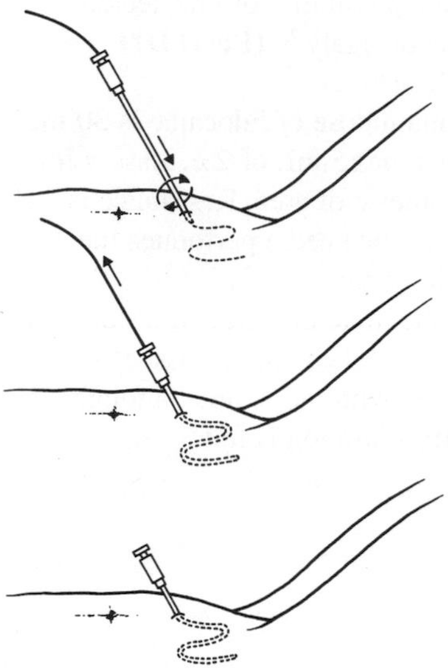

FIGURE 109-1   The plastic catheter is placed over the guidewire and inserted into the peritoneal cavity by means of a twisting motion at the skin level. After the catheter has been advanced, the guidewire is removed. *(From Pfenninger JL, Fowler GC, editors: Pfenninger and Fowler's procedures for primary care, ed 2, St Louis, 2003, Mosby.)*

Steps	Rationale	Special Considerations
16. Remove the wire after the catheter is in the peritoneal cavity.		Aspiration may be attempted. If it is dry, proceed to lavage.
17. Attach the lavage catheter to the remaining port of the stopcock and tubing to withdraw the peritoneal fluid.	Fluid may be gently aspirated, siphoned via gravity, or collected into a vacuum device.	Retain the first 100 mL of fluid for laboratory analysis. **Refer to Step 26** for specific laboratory tests.[1,9] **(Level B*)**
18. Instill the lavage fluid: A. If a drainage collector is used, turn the stopcock off to the drainage collector. B. Open clamp on the IV tubing. C. Instill 700 to 1000 mL of warmed RL or NS solution or antibacterial fluid.	Directs lavage fluid into the peritoneal space.	Infuse over 10 to 15 minutes. This may be done with a pressure bag to decrease time.
19. Rotate the patient side to side (if not contraindicated).	Facilitates sampling of fluid that may accumulate in pockets on either side. Mixes the solution with any free material in abdominal cavity.	

*Level B: Well-designed controlled studies with results that consistently support a specific action, intervention, or treatment

Procedure for Performing Peritoneal Lavage—*Continued*

Steps	Rationale	Special Considerations

20. Drain the lavage fluid:
  A. If the drainage collector is used, turn the stopcock off to the IV tubing.
  B. If the drainage collector is not used, lower the IV bag to a level below the patient.
  C. Allow the fluid to drain into the drainage collector or lowered IV bag.
	Directs lavage fluid from the peritoneal space to the drainage collector.	In therapeutic lavage, consider the dwell time of the fluid before drainage (usually 5 to 10 minutes). When draining fluid, be careful that no tension is put on the tubing.

21. Rotate the patient side to side (if not contraindicated).	Facilitates the drainage of fluid that may accumulate in pockets on either side.	Lavage fluid may be absorbed into the intravascular space, creating a potential fluid volume excess. Twisting the catheter may free the catheter from adhering to peritoneum and facilitate drainage of fluid.
22. **Repeat Steps 18 to 21** as needed.	Continued lavage may be needed to cleanse the peritoneal space.	
23. If the lavage is positive for blood, prepare the patient for immediate surgery. Leave the incision open and cover with a sterile, NS solution–soaked dressing.	Immediate repair of the bleeding site is needed.	
24. After the fluid is removed, gently remove the catheter and apply pressure to the wound. Suture the puncture site with a mattress suture with 4-0 nylon (see Procedure 124) and apply a dressing.	Keeps the insertion site clean. Reduces the risk for infection. Provides a barrier to infection and collects the fluid that may leak from the wound site.	Inspect the catheter to ensure it is intact.
25. Prepare and send the fluid specimens for laboratory analysis.	Provides information about patient status.	Have the first 100 mL of fluid analyzed for RBCs, WBCs, bilirubin, amylase, lipase, alkaline phosphate, and culture and sensitivity.[9] **(Level B*)**
26. Dispose of equipment and soiled material in appropriate receptacle.	Standard Precautions.	
27. Remove all personal protective equipment, discard supplies, and perform hand hygiene.	Reduces transmission of microorganisms.	

Expected Outcomes

- Lavage fluid returns obtained for diagnostic evaluation
- Peritoneum cleansed of purulent exudate and microorganisms
- Stable vital signs, rise in temperature in the patient with hypothermia
- No increase in pain level
- No adverse effects

Unexpected Outcomes

- Perforation of bowel, bladder, or stomach
- Lacerations of major vessels (mesenteric, iliac, aorta)
- Laceration of catheter or guidewire with loss in peritoneal cavity
- Local or systemic infection
- Hypovolemia, hypotension
- Bleeding from insertion site
- Inadequate drainage of lavage fluid
- Respiratory compromise

*Level B: Well-designed controlled studies with results that consistently support a specific action, intervention, or treatment

Procedure continues on following page

Patient Monitoring and Care

Steps	Rationale	Reportable Conditions
		These conditions should be reported if they persist despite nursing interventions.
1. Monitor for changes in respiratory status (i.e., rate, depth, and pattern).	Retained lavage fluid puts pressure on diaphragm and intraabdominal organs, causing breathing difficulty.	• Respiratory rate significantly (>20%) increased from baseline • Increased depth of breathing • Irregular breathing pattern • Pulse oximetry less than 92%, or significant decrease from baseline
2. Monitor for potential complications, including bowel or bladder perforation, bleeding, and intravascular volume loss. Assess presence and level of abdominal pain.	Peritoneal lavage interrupts the integrity of the skin and underlying peritoneum. Pain is an indicator of many of the potential complications and identifies the need for management of discomfort.	• Acute abdominal pain, distention, rigidity, and guarding • Continued pain despite pain interventions • Decreased bowel sounds • Fever, chills • Blood in urine • Hypotension • Tachycardia
3. Monitor vital signs for evidence of infection.	Infection is a complication of peritoneal lavage.	• Increased temperature • Labile blood pressure
4. Monitor insertion site for drainage or evidence of infection.	Infection is a complication of peritoneal lavage.	• Purulent drainage from insertion site • Redness, swelling at insertion site
5. Monitor intake and output.	Provides data for evaluation of fluid balance status.	• Urine output less than 30 mL/hr • Symptoms of excess volume losses caused by significant drainage of fluid or blood from catheter • Signs of overzealous fluid resuscitation in the face of trauma (hypertension, edema, rising peak inspiratory pressures in the intubated and ventilated patient, falling pulse oximetry [Spo_2] levels)
6. Evaluate laboratory data when returned.	Provides for an evaluation of the condition and aids in diagnosis.	• RBC count greater than 100,000/mm³ • Amylase value greater than 2.5 times normal • Alkaline phosphate value greater than 5.5 mg/dL • Positive bilirubin • Vegetable matter present • WBC count greater than 500,000/mm • Positive culture results

Documentation

Documentation should include the following:
- Patient and family education
- Date and time of the procedure
- Patient tolerance of the procedure
- Assessment of the insertion site after the procedure
- Type and amount of the fluid instilled and the dwell time
- True drainage (total drainage minus lavage fluid input)
- Medications administered
- Amount and characteristics of the fluid removed
- Specimens sent for laboratory analysis
- Vital signs and respiratory status before and after procedure
- Assessment of pain level according to institutional standards and any acute changes
- Unexpected outcomes
- Nursing interventions

References

CR 1. Brakenridge SC, et al: Detection of intra-abdominal injury using diagnostic peritoneal lavage after shotgun wound to the abdomen, *J Trauma* 54:329-331, 2003.

2. Crandall M, West MA: Evaluation of the abdomen in the critically ill patient: opening the black box, *Curr Opin Crit Care* 12:333-339, 2006.

3. Ferri FF: Paracentesis. In Ferri FF, editor: *Practical guide to the care of the medical patient,* ed 7, Philadelphia, 2007, Mosby/Elsevier.

4. Griffin XL, Pullinger R. Are diagnostic peritoneal lavage or focused abdominal sonography for trauma safe screening interventions for hemodynamically stable patients after blunt abdominal trauma? A review of the literature, *J Trauma* 62:779-784, 2007.

5. Jansen JO, Yule SR, Loudon MA: Investigation of blunt abdominal trauma, *BMJ* 336:938-942, 2008.

CR 6. Marx JA: Peritoneal procedures. In Roberts JR, Hedges JR, editors: *Clinical procedures in emergency medicine,* ed 4, Philadelphia, 2004, Saunders, 733-749.

CR 7. Proehl J, editor. Diagnostic peritoneal lavage. *Emergency nursing procedures,* ed 4, St Louis, 2008, Elsevier.

CR 8. Sato T, Hirose Y, Saito H, et al: Diagnostic peritoneal lavage for diagnosing blunt hollow visceral injury: the accuracy of two different criteria and their combination, *Surg Today* 35:935-939, 2005.

9. Thacker LK, Parks J, Thal ER: Diagnostic peritoneal lavage: is 100,000 RBC's a valid figure for penetrating abdominal trauma? *J Trauma Injury Infect Crit Care* 62:853-857, 2007.

Additional Readings

CR Bode PJ, van Vugt AB: Ultrasound in the diagnosis of injury, *Injury* 27:379-383, 1996.

CR Brown MA, et al: Blunt abdominal trauma: screening US in 2,693 patients, *Radiology* 218:352-358, 2001.

CR Goletti O, et al: The role of ultrasonography in blunt abdominal trauma: results in 250 consecutive cases, *J Trauma* 36:178-181, 1994.

CR Gonzalez RP, et al: Complementary roles of diagnostic peritoneal lavage and computed tomography in the evaluation of blunt abdominal trauma, *J Trauma* 51:1128-1134, 2001.

CR Liu A, Kaufmann C, Ritchie R: A computer-based simulator for diagnostic peritoneal lavage, *Stud Health Technol Inform* 81:278-285, 2001.

CR Marx JA, et al: Limitations of computed tomography in the evaluation of acute abdominal trauma: a prospective comparison with diagnostic peritoneal lavage, *J Trauma* 25:933-937, 1985.

CR Maxwell-Armstrong C, et al: Diagnostic peritoneal lavage analysis: should trauma guidelines be revised? *Emerg Med J* 19:524-525, 2002.

CR Root HD, et al: Diagnostic peritoneal lavage, *Surgery* 57:633-637, 1965.

Peritoneal Lavage (Assist)

PURPOSE: Percutaneous peritoneal lavage is performed for both therapeutic and diagnostic purposes.

Jenny Bosley

PREREQUISITE NURSING KNOWLEDGE

- Knowledge of the anatomy and physiology of the abdomen is needed.
- The Intestines and the bladder lie immediately beneath the abdominal surface. In children, the bladder is an abdominal organ. In adults, a full bladder is raised out of the pelvis.
- The cecum is relatively fixed and is much less mobile than the sigmoid colon; therefore, bowel perforations are more frequent in the right lower quadrant than in the left.
- A distended stomach can extend to the anterior abdominal wall.
- Peritoneal fluid is normally straw-colored, serous fluid secreted by the cells of the peritoneum.
- Grossly bloody fluid, a red blood cell (RBC) count of greater than 100,000/mm[3],[2,5,9] and the presence of bacteria or bile in the return fluid in the abdomen are abnormal. A white blood cell (WBC) count greater than 500,000/mm and the presence of bile or amylase in the lavage fluid are parameters, in addition to the RBC count, that can lead to operative intervention.[2,5,9]
- Diagnostic peritoneal lavage is a highly sensitive tool for diagnosis of visceral injuries in the abdominal cavity.[1,5,8]
- Diagnostic peritoneal lavage is used after blunt abdominal trauma or in trauma patients with head injuries, those who are unconscious, or those with pre-existing paraplegia to determine the presence of the following[2]:
  - ❖ Hemoperitoneum (blood in lavage returns)
  - ❖ Organ injury (intestinal enzymes or microorganisms in lavage returns)

- Therapeutic lavage is used to:
  - ❖ Irrigate and cleanse purulent exudate in patients with peritonitis or intraabdominal abscess
  - ❖ Warm the abdominal cavity in patients with hypothermia
  - ❖ Remove unwanted or toxic chemicals through peritoneal dialysis
  - ❖ Obtain cytology specimens in patients with cancer
- For trauma patients with stab wounds and gunshot wounds to the lower chest or anterior abdomen, diagnostic peritoneal lavage is controversial; most trauma centers operate on patients with gunshot wound injuries to the lower chest or anterior abdomen.[1]
- Diagnostic peritoneal lavage can be used as a tool in patients with hypotension of uncertain etiology, in the presence of trauma.[6]
- Diagnostic peritoneal lavage is not needed if abdominal surgery is already indicated.[7,9]
- Because it is an invasive procedure, diagnostic peritoneal lavage does have a small risk of visceral injury (0.6%).[5]
- Diagnostic peritoneal lavage is 95% sensitive and 99% specific for intraperitoneal blood; however, it cannot exclude retroperitoneal hemorrhage, disruption of the diaphragm, or hollow viscus perforation.[5,7]
- Computed tomographic (CT) scan frequently is used in hemodynamically stable trauma cases as the diagnostic procedure of choice.[5] Also, abdominal ultrasound scan and focused abdominal sonography in trauma (FAST) have been increasingly used to screen blunt abdominal trauma cases for hemoperitoneum.[9]
- In patients with hemodynamically unstable conditions, diagnostic peritoneal lavage (DPL) may be preferred by some practitioners because of its high sensitivity.[1,2,5,9] DPL is quick, inexpensive, safe, and highly sensitive to the presence of blood in the peritoneal

cavity.[5] Hemodynamically unstable cases may also go directly to the operating room for laparotomy.

- Complementary CT and DPL decreases nontherapeutic laparotomy rates and allows nonoperative management of those patients with solid-organ injury.[9]
- Peritoneal lavage is absolutely contraindicated in an acute abdomen that needs immediate surgery as indicated by free air on radiograph or penetrating abdominal trauma.
- Relative contraindications for DPL include the following[5,6]:
  - ❖ Thrombocytopenia
  - ❖ Coagulopathy[7]
  - ❖ Morbid obesity[7]
  - ❖ Severe bowel distension
  - ❖ Advanced cirrhosis[7]
  - ❖ Previous abdominal surgery, especially pelvic surgery
  - ❖ Distended bladder that cannot be emptied with a Foley catheter
  - ❖ Obvious infection at intended site of insertion (cellulitis or abscess)
  - ❖ Pregnancy of greater than 12 weeks' gestation[7]
- Practitioners should use caution when performing DPL in patients with suspected pelvic fractures (a supraumbilical site may be used) because of false-positive results[7]; if performed in pregnant patients of more than 12 weeks' gestation, an open technique, superior to the uterus, is used.[7]
- The practitioner who performs peritoneal lavage should choose an insertion site midline, one third the distance from the umbilicus to the symphysis, or 2 to 3 cm below the umbilicus (see Fig. 107-1). An alternate position is a point one third the distance from the umbilicus to the anterior iliac crest (left side preferred).
- The physician or advanced practice nurse can use ultrasound scan before peritoneal lavage to locate fluid and during the procedure to guide insertion of the catheter.[9]

EQUIPMENT

- Commercially prepared kit or the following:
  - ❖ Personal protective equipment, including sterile gloves, mask, goggles, and gown
  - ❖ Skin cleansing solution (chlorhexidine or povidone iodine)
  - ❖ Sterile marking pen
  - ❖ Sterile towels or sterile drape
  - ❖ Razor to shave area, if necessary
  - ❖ Local anesthetic for injection: 1% or 2% lidocaine with epinephrine
  - ❖ 5- or 10-mL syringe with 25- or 27-gauge needle for anesthetic
  - ❖ Scalpel and no. 11 knife blade
  - ❖ Trocar with stylet; needle (16-, 18-, or 20-gauge) or angiocatheter; depending on abdominal wall thickness may use guidewire with floppy tip and 9 to 18 Fr peritoneal lavage catheter
  - ❖ 20-mL syringe for diagnostic tap
  - ❖ Sterile intravenous (IV) tubing (without valves) with appropriate sterile connectors for lavage catheter and IV bags

- ❖ Sterile tubes for specimens
- ❖ Warmed Ringer's lactate (RL), normal saline (NS), or antibiotic solution for infusion into abdomen
- ❖ Three-way stopcock for therapeutic lavage
- ❖ Nylon skin suture material on cutting needle (4-0 or 5-0) and needle holder
- ❖ Four to six sterile 4 × 4 gauze pads
- ❖ Sterile gauze dressing with tape or adhesive strip
- ❖ Soft wrist restraints
- ❖ Pressure bag

PATIENT AND FAMILY EDUCATION

- Reinforce the indications, the procedure, and the risks to the patient and family. ➜*Rationale:* Patient anxiety may be decreased, and patient and family cooperation and understanding of procedure are encouraged.
- Explain the patient's role in assisting with the procedure and postprocedure care. ➜*Rationale:* Patient cooperation during and after the procedure is elicited.
- Explain the signs and symptoms to report, such as fever, abdominal pain, decreased urine output, bleeding, and leakage of fluid from wound site. ➜*Rationale:* Unexpected outcomes may not manifest themselves for a period of time after the procedure.

PATIENT ASSESSMENT AND PREPARATION
Patient Assessment

- Obtain the medical history and perform a review of systems to identify abdominal injury, peritonitis, intraabdominal abscess, or pregnancy. ➜*Rationale:* Certain conditions of the gastrointestinal tract may be diagnosed and treated with peritoneal lavage. Contraindications to peritoneal lavage may be identified.[6]
- Identify the presence of any allergies to medication or other substances. ➜*Rationale:* Patients may have allergies to skin preparations or anesthetics used before the invasive procedure is performed. Identification assists the practitioner in choosing the most appropriate skin preparation and anesthetic.
- Assess for bowel or bladder distention. ➜*Rationale:* Distension increases the risk for bowel or bladder perforation during the procedure.[7]
- Assess coagulation study results (i.e., prothrombin time [PT], partial thromboplastin time [PTT], and platelets). ➜*Rationale:* Abnormal clotting study results may increase the risk for bleeding during and after the procedure. Therapy may be necessary to correct clotting abnormalities before the procedure is performed.
- Plain and upright radiographs of the abdomen should be ordered by the physician or advanced practice nurse, and upright abdominal films if possible (before the procedure). ➜*Rationale:* Air is introduced during the procedure and may confound the diagnosis later.[7]
- Obtain baseline vital signs and pain assessment according to institutional standard. ➜*Rationale:* The practitioner can identify intraprocedure or postprocedure changes that may be indicative of complications.

Patient Preparation

- Ensure that the patient understands preprocedural teachings. Answer questions as they arise, and reinforce information as needed. ➤➤*Rationale:* Understanding of previously taught information is evaluated and reinforced.

- Ensure that a written informed consent form has been obtained by the practitioner performing the procedure (if possible). The healthcare provider who is assisting may be a witness to the signing of the consent if needed. In a trauma situation or with an unresponsive patient, this consent may be implied. ➤➤*Rationale:* Peritoneal lavage is an invasive procedure that requires a signed consent form.

- Have the patient void or insert a urinary drainage catheter. ➤➤*Rationale:* A distended bladder increases the risk for bladder perforation during the procedure.[7]

- Insert a nasogastric tube unless contraindicated (e.g., in significant facial trauma) and attach to low intermittent suction. ➤➤*Rationale:* A distended stomach increases the risk for perforation during the procedure.[6]

- Perform a pre-procedure verification and time out, if nonemergent. ➤➤*Rationale:* Ensures patient safety.

- Verify correct patient with two identifiers. ➤➤*Rationale:* Prior to performing a procedure, the physician or advanced practice nurse and the healthcare provider assisting in the procedure should ensure the correct identification of the patient for the intended intervention.

- Check that all relevant documents and studies are available before starting the procedure. ➤➤*Rationale:* This measure ensures that the correct patient receives the correct procedure.

- Place the patient in the supine position (may tilt to side of collection slightly for improved fluid positioning). ➤➤*Rationale:* Fluid accumulates in the dependent areas.

- The physician or advanced practice nurse examines the abdomen for landmarks and marks appropriately. ➤➤*Rationale:* Correct placement of the catheter for peritoneal lavage minimizes complications.

- For the patient with pain or agitation who is unable to cooperate with the procedure, consider analgesia or sedation. If sedation is needed for the procedure, institution-specific moderate sedation monitoring should be performed. ➤➤*Rationale:* Analgesia or sedation provides for patient comfort and safety during the procedure.

- If the patient has altered mental status, soft wrist restraints may be needed. ➤➤*Rationale:* The patient must not move his or her hands into the sterile field once it has been established.

Procedure for Assisting with Peritoneal Lavage

Steps	Rationale	Special Considerations
1. **HH**		
2. **PE**		Include protective goggles.
3. Assist the physician, advanced practice nurse, or other healthcare provider performing the procedure with applying personal protective and sterile equipment (e.g. head cover, mask, eye protection, sterile gown).	Minimizes the risk of infection. Maintains aseptic and sterile precautions.	
4. Label all medications, medication containers (e.g., syringes, medicine cups, basins), or other solutions that are to be used during the procedure.	Provides additional safety for the patient undergoing the procedure.	
5. Assist in preparing the equipment and sterile field and apply sterile gloves.	Facilitates easy access to needed equipment.	Maintain aseptic technique.
6. Assist in setting up the lavage equipment. A. Assist with attaching the IV tubing to the lavage fluid and clear tubing of air.	Provides closed system for instillation and drainage of lavage fluid.	

Procedure for Assisting with Peritoneal Lavage—*Continued*		
Steps	**Rationale**	**Special Considerations**
B. Assist with attaching the IV tubing to one port of the three-way stopcock and drainage collector to second port of the three-way stopcock.		
or		
C. Use IV tubing with a roller clamp and use the lavage fluid bag as the drainage bag.		
7. Assist the physician or advanced practice nurse to cleanse insertion site with povidone-iodine solution or chlorhexidine preparation.	Minimizes risk for infection.	Allergies should be identified before a skin preparation product is selected. Use sterile technique.
8. Assist with the placement of sterile drapes to expose the insertion site. Site should be in the midline about one third the distance from the umbilicus to the symphysis (usually 2 to 3 cm below the umbilicus; see Fig. 107-1). Alternate position is a point about one third the distance from the umbilicus to the anterior iliac crest (left side preferred).	Minimizes the risk of infection. maintains aseptic and sterile precautions.	The rectus muscle should be avoided by the practitioner because of increased risk for hemorrhage from epigastric vessels; surgical scars should be avoided because of increased risk for perforation caused by adhesion of bowel to the wall of the peritoneum; the upper quadrants should be avoided because of the possibility of undetected hepatomegaly.[2,3] **(Level D*)**
9. Assist the practitioner with injecting the area with local anesthetic (lidocaine with epinephrine preferred). Initially, the needle should be directed perpendicular to the skin and the peritoneum infiltrated with anesthetic.	Local anesthesia minimizes pain and discomfort. Epinephrine helps eliminate unwanted abdominal wall bleeding and false-positive results.	Maximum dose of lidocaine is 30 mL of 1% or 15 mL of 2%. The physician or advanced practice nurse assesses for anesthesia of area.
10. With the no. 11 blade scalpel, the practitioner creates a vertical skin incision large enough to allow threading of a 3- to 5-mm lavage catheter. The subcutaneous tissue is spread and the fascia incised to expose the peritoneum. The peritoneal membrane is nicked to pass the catheter.	Creates an opening large enough to thread the lavage catheter.	
11. The practitioner inserts an 18-gauge needle attached to a 20- or 50-mL syringe perpendicular through the anesthetized tract into the peritoneum. The practitioner applies slight suction to the syringe as it is advanced and grasps the needle close to the skin as it is advanced (see Fig. 107-2).	Provides access to the peritoneal space. Slight suction is applied to indicate when the peritoneum is entered or if a blood vessel is entered. The needle is grasped as it is advanced to prevent accidental thrusting into the abdomen and possible viscus perforation.	Inserted through small incision at midline below umbilicus.

*Level D: Peer-reviewed professional organizational standards with clinical studies to support recommendations

Procedure continues on following page

Procedure for Assisting with Peritoneal Lavage—*Continued*

Steps	Rationale	Special Considerations
12. Once in the cavity, the needle is directed at a 60-degree angle toward the center of the pelvic hollow. If fluid returns, the syringe can be filled.	Collection of fluid for laboratory studies.	A free return of 10 mL of blood is a strong positive finding for a hemo-peritoneum.[4] If blood is returned, the needle should be removed and the nurse should prepare the patient for immediate surgical intervention.
13. If the tap is dry, the lavage technique is performed.	Accurately assesses for hemoperitoneum.	
14. Assist with guidewire insertion, introduced through the 18-gauge needle.	Provides access for insertion of the peritoneal lavage catheter.	The wire should insert easily. Diffi-culty in advancing the catheter may indicate the stylet is not in the peritoneal cavity or that adhesions are present.
15. About half of the wire is inserted into the pelvis, and the needle is removed. The physician or advanced practice nurse holds on to the guidewire continuously.	Letting go of the guidewire could allow the wire to inadvertently migrate into peritoneum.	
16. The peritoneal lavage catheter is slid over the wire, with gently twisting motions (see Fig. 109-1).	Twisting motion minimizes visceral perforation and displaces abdominal contents.	The practitioner should always keep a firm hold on the wire to prevent it from slipping into the peritoneal cavity.
17. The wire is removed after the catheter is in the peritoneal cavity.		Aspiration may be attempted. If it is dry, lavage can be performed.
18. Assist with attaching the lavage catheter to remaining port of stop-cock and tubing to withdraw perito-neal fluid.	Fluid may be gently aspirated, siphoned via gravity, or collected into a vacuum device.	Retain first 100 mL of fluid for labo-ratory analysis. **Refer to Step 26** for specific laboratory tests.[1,9] **(Level B*)**
19. Lavage fluid is instilled: A. If a drainage collector is used, turn the stopcock off to the drainage collector. B. Open the clamp on IV tubing. C. Instill 700 to 1000 mL of warmed RL or NS solution or antibacterial fluid.	Directs lavage fluid into peritoneal space.	Infuse over 10 to 15 minutes. This may be done with a pressure bag to decrease time.
20. Rotate the patient side to side (if not contraindicated).	Facilitates sampling of fluid that may accumulate in pockets on either side. Mixes the solution with any free material in the abdominal cavity.	
21. Drain lavage fluid: A. If a drainage collector is used, turn the stopcock off to the IV tubing. B. If a drainage collector is not used, lower the IV bag to a level below the patient. C. Allow fluid to drain into the drainage collector or lowered IV bag.	Directs the lavage fluid from the peritoneal space to the drainage collector.	In therapeutic lavage, consider dwell time of fluid before drainage (usually 5 to 10 minutes). When draining fluid, be careful that there is no tension on the tubing.

*Level B: Well-designed controlled studies with results that consistently support a specific action, intervention, or treatment

Procedure | for Assisting with Peritoneal Lavage—*Continued*

Steps	Rationale	Special Considerations
22. Rotate the patient side to side (if not contraindicated).	Facilitates drainage of fluid that may accumulate in pockets on either side.	Lavage fluid may be absorbed into the intravascular space, creating a potential fluid volume excess. Twisting of the catheter may free the catheter from adhering to peritoneum and facilitate drainage of fluid.
23. **Repeat Steps 19 to 22** as needed.	Continued lavage may be needed to cleanse the peritoneal space.	
24. If the lavage is positive for blood, prepare the patient for immediate surgery. Leave the incision open and cover with a sterile NS solution–soaked dressing.	Immediate repair of the bleeding site is needed.	
25. After the fluid is removed, the catheter is gently removed by the physician or advanced practice nurse and pressure is applied to the wound. The puncture site is sutured and a dry dressing is applied.	Keeps the insertion site clean. Reduces the risk for infection. Provides a barrier to infection and collects fluid that may leak from wound site.	The catheter should be inspected on removal to ensure it is intact.
26. Prepare and send the fluid specimens for laboratory analysis.	Provides information about patient status.	Have the first 100 mL of fluid analyzed for RBCs, WBCs, bilirubin, amylase, lipase, alkaline phosphate, and culture and sensitivity.[9] **(Level B*)**
27. Dispose of equipment and soiled material in appropriate receptacle.	Standard Precautions.	
28. Remove all personal protective equipment, discard supplies, and perform hand hygiene.	Reduces transmission of microorganisms.	

Expected Outcomes

- Lavage fluid returns obtained for diagnostic evaluation
- Peritoneum cleansed of purulent exudate and microorganisms
- Stable vital signs, rise in temperature in the patient with hypothermia
- No increase in pain level
- No adverse effects

Unexpected Outcomes

- Perforation of bowel, bladder, or stomach
- Lacerations of major vessels (mesenteric, iliac, aorta)
- Laceration of catheter or guidewire with loss in peritoneal cavity
- Local or systemic infection
- Hypovolemia, hypotension
- Bleeding from insertion site
- Inadequate drainage of lavage fluid
- Respiratory compromise

*Level B: Well-designed controlled studies with results that consistently support a specific action, intervention, or treatment

Procedure continues on following page

Patient Monitoring and Care

Steps	Rationale	Reportable Conditions
		These conditions should be reported if they persist despite nursing interventions.
1. Monitor for changes in respiratory status (i.e., rate, depth, and pattern).	Retained lavage fluid puts pressure on diaphragm and intraabdominal organs, causing difficulty in breathing.	• Respiratory rate significantly (>20%) increased from baseline • Increased depth of breathing • Irregular breathing pattern • Pulse oximetry less than 92%, or significant decrease from baseline
2. Monitor for potential complications, including bowel or bladder perforation, bleeding, and intravascular volume loss. Assess presence and level of abdominal pain.	Peritoneal lavage interrupts the integrity of the skin and underlying peritoneum. Pain is an indicator of many of the potential complications and identifies a need for management of discomfort.	• Acute abdominal pain, distention, rigidity, and guarding • Continued pain despite pain interventions • Decreased bowel sounds • Fever, chills • Blood in urine • Hypotension • Tachycardia
3. Monitor vital signs for evidence of infection.	Infection is a complication of peritoneal lavage.	• Increased temperature • Labile blood pressure
4. Monitor insertion site for drainage or evidence of infection.	Infection is a complication of peritoneal lavage.	• Purulent drainage from insertion site • Redness, swelling at insertion site
5. Monitor intake and output.	Provides data for evaluation of fluid balance status.	• Urine output less than 30 mL/hr • Symptoms of excess volume losses caused by significant drainage of fluid or blood from catheter • Signs of overzealous fluid resuscitation in the face of trauma (hypertension, edema, rising peak inspiratory pressures in the intubated and ventilated patient, falling pulse oximetry [Spo_2] levels)
6. Evaluate laboratory data when returned.	Provides for an evaluation of the condition and aids in diagnosis.	• RBCs greater than 100,000/mm^3 • Amylase value greater than 2.5 times normal • Alkaline phosphate value greater than 5.5 mg/dL • Positive bilirubin results • Vegetable matter present • WBCs greater than 500,000/mm • Positive culture results

Documentation

Documentation should include the following:

- Patient and family education
- Date and time of the procedure
- Patient tolerance of the procedure
- Assessment of the insertion site after the procedure
- Type and amount of fluid instilled and the dwell time
- True drainage (total drainage minus lavage fluid input)
- Medications administered

- Amount and characteristics of the fluid removed
- Specimens sent for laboratory analysis
- Preprocedure and postprocedure vital signs, respiratory status
- Assessment of pain level according to institutional standards and any acute changes
- Unexpected outcomes
- Nursing interventions

References

CR 1. Brakenridge SC, et al: Detection of intra-abdominal injury using diagnostic peritoneal lavage after shotgun wound to the abdomen, *J Trauma* 54:329-331, 2003.

2. Crandall M, West MA: Evaluation of the abdomen in the critically ill patient: opening the black box, *Curr Opin Crit Care* 12:333-339, 2006.

3. Ferri FF: Paracentesis. In Ferri, editor: *Practical guide to the care of the medical patient*, ed 7, Philadelphia, 2007, Mosby/Elsevier.

4. Griffin XL, Pullinger R: Are diagnostic peritoneal lavage or focused abdominal sonography for trauma safe screening interventions for hemodynamically stable patients after blunt abdominal trauma? A review of the literature, *J Trauma* 62:779-784, 2007.

5. Jansen JO, Yule SR, Loudon MA: Investigation of blunt abdominal trauma, *BMJ* 336:938-942, 2008.

CR 6. Marx JA: Peritoneal procedures. In Roberts JR, Hedges JR, editors: *Clinical procedures in emergency medicine*, ed 4, Philadelphia, 2004, Saunders, 733-749.

CR 7. Proehl J, editor. Diagnostic peritoneal lavage. In *Emergency nursing procedures*, ed 4, St Louis, 2008, Elsevier.

CR 8. Sato T, Hirose Y, Saito H, et al: Diagnostic peritoneal lavage for diagnosing blunt hollow visceral injury: the accuracy of two different criteria and their combination, *Surg Today* 35:935-939, 2005.

9. Thacker LK, Parks J, Thal ER: Diagnostic peritoneal lavage: is 100,000 RBC's a valid figure for penetrating abdominal trauma? *J Trauma Injury Infect Crit Care* 62:853-857, 2007.

Additional Readings

CR Bode PJ, van Vugt AB: Ultrasound in the diagnosis of injury, *Injury* 27:379-383, 1996.

CR Brown MA, et al: Blunt abdominal trauma: screening US in 2,693 patients, *Radiology* 218:352-358, 2001.

CR Goletti O, et al: The role of ultrasonography in blunt abdominal trauma: results in 250 consecutive cases, *J Trauma* 36:178-181, 1994.

CR Gonzalez RP, et al: Complementary roles of diagnostic peritoneal lavage and computed tomography in the evaluation of blunt abdominal trauma, *J Trauma* 51:1128-1134, 2001.

CR Liu A, Kaufmann C, Ritchie R: A computer-based simulator for diagnostic peritoneal lavage, *Stud Health Technol Inform* 81:278-285, 2001.

CR Marx JA, et al: Limitations of computed tomography in the evaluation of acute abdominal trauma: a prospective comparison with diagnostic peritoneal lavage, *J Trauma* 25:933-937, 1985.

CR Maxwell-Armstrong C, et al: Diagnostic peritoneal lavage analysis: should trauma guidelines be revised? *Emerg Med J* 19:524-525, 2002.

CR Root HD, et al: Diagnostic peritoneal lavage, *Surgery* 57:633-637, 1965.

Endoscopic Therapy

P U R P O S E :   Endoscopic therapy is performed to control or prevent bleeding from esophageal or gastric varices, gastric or duodenal ulcer sites, or other selected causes of upper gastrointestinal bleeding.

Eleanor Fitzpatrick

PREREQUISITE NURSING KNOWLEDGE

- Upper gastrointestinal (GI) hemorrhage is a relatively common, potentially life-threatening emergency that requires rapid assessment and resuscitation.[11] Esophagogastroduodenoscopy (EGD) is the diagnostic and therapeutic modality for nonvariceal and variceal upper GI bleeding.[2,3,12] Endoscopic therapy reduces the rate of rebleeding, blood transfusion requirements, and the need for surgery.[2,3]

- Endoscopic therapies are the interventions of choice for many upper and lower GI bleeding lesions. Upper endoscopic therapies include injection therapy, ablative therapy, such as heater probe, and mechanical therapy, such as endoclips or endoscopic banding.[2]

- For all upper endoscopic interventions, a fiberoptic endoscope is passed through the esophagus and into the stomach and duodenum to identify the site of bleeding. The nurse assisting the endoscopist prepares all of the equipment potentially needed during the procedure. Once the site of bleeding is found, any of the endoscopic techniques identified previously may be used.

- Endoscopic variceal ligation (EVL) is the preferred endoscopic method for control of acute esophageal bleeding and for prevention of rebleeding, unless excess bleeding prevents effective band placement and ligation.[11] Endoscopic sclerotherapy (EST), which involves injection of a sclerosant into or adjacent to a varix, may be used. EST has largely been replaced by the use of EVL, which is a type of mechanical therapy.[1,4,9,12]

- For gastric varices, a promising intervention is gastric variceal occlusion (GVO) with tissue adhesives such as

N-butyl-cyanoacrylate. Studies are ongoing, but tissue adhesives are not yet approved for use in the United States.[9,12]

- Injection therapy is used for hemostasis for bleeding from peptic ulcer disease, Mallory-Weiss tears, and other lesions and for postprocedure related bleeding.[11] Epinephrine is the injection agent of choice for these maladies in the United States.[2]

- The several proposed mechanisms of action of the various sclerosing agents include vasoconstriction, esophageal or vascular smooth muscle spasm, compression of the bleeding vessel by submucosal edema or by the volume of sclerosing agent used (tamponade effect), and actual coagulation of the vessel. Ultimately, vessel thrombosis occurs.

- A variety of sclerosing agents are available (Table 111-1). The physician or advanced practice nurse who performs the endoscopy prescribes the agents to be used.

- Endoscopic therapy can combine a number of interventions to promote hemostasis, including esophageal band ligation, injection therapy, laser therapy, thermal coagulation, and transjugular intrahepatic portosystemic shunt (TIPS), a radiologic intervention.[2,11,12]

- Ablative therapies, such as the use of a heater probe or bipolar electrocoagulation, are other endoscopic techniques for the management of bleeding from peptic ulcer disease and other nonvariceal causes of upper GI bleeding. These therapies are effective as they result in coagulation of a bleeding vessel.[2,8]

- Passage of the large-bore therapeutic endoscope may stimulate the vagal response in the patient and precipitate bradydysrhythmias.

TABLE 111-1	**Sclerosing Agents**
Sclerosants Used for Bleeding Varices[4]	**Sclerosants Used for Other Causes of Upper GI Bleeding[2]**
Sodium morrhuate (5%)	Epinephrine (1:10,000 to 1:20,000)
Ethanolamine oleate (5%)	Ethyl alcohol (volumes greater than 1 to 2 mL can lead to tissue damage)
Sodium tetradecyl sulfate	Thrombin
Ethanolamine acetate	Polidocanol
Polidocanol (0.5% to 1%)	Sodium tetradecyl sulfate
Ethanol (can cause ulceration)	

- As a result of the sedation and topical anesthetic used, the patient's gag reflex may be diminished or absent, putting the patient at risk for aspiration.
- Sedation can put the patient at risk for respiratory depression. A moderate sedation protocol is recommended for use to guide monitoring of the patient. This protocol should include the use of recommended monitoring and emergency equipment.

EQUIPMENT

- Therapeutic large-caliber endoscope (rigid or flexible; however, the flexible scope is the usual type used for upper endoscopy)
- Endoscopic injector needle (23- to 26-gauge, 2- to 5-mm needle; as ordered by physician)
- Three 10-mL syringes filled with sclerosing agent, as prescribed by physician
- Additional therapeutic equipment should be available for management of nonvariceal upper GI bleeding (i.e., laser or thermal equipment, endoloops or endoclips)
- Esophageal bands should be available for management of known or suspected variceal upper GI bleeding
- Suction setup with connecting tubing
- Rigid pharyngeal suction-tip (Yankauer) catheter
- Safety goggles for each healthcare provider and the patient
- Nonsterile gloves
- Barrier gowns
- Nonsterile 4-inch gauze or washcloth
- Water-soluble lubricant
- Topical anesthesia
- Premedications (as prescribed by physician)
- Two 30- to 60-mL syringes
- Normal saline (NS) solution or tap water for irrigation
- Oral airway or bite block
- Cardiac monitor
- Pulse oximeter
- Automatic blood pressure cuff
- Emergency intubation equipment
  Additional equipment, to have available as needed, includes the following:
- Nasogastric (NG) tube, Minnesota tube, or Sengstaken-Blakemore tube for esophagogastric tamponade (see Procedure 104)

PATIENT AND FAMILY EDUCATION

- Explain the procedure and indication for endoscopic therapy and the patient's role in the procedure. ➤➤*Rationale:* Patient and family anxiety may be decreased.
- Explain that the patient will be sedated for comfort and for ease in passing the endoscope. ➤➤*Rationale:* Patient and family anxiety may be decreased.
- Explain that the patient will be monitored closely during and after the procedure. ➤➤*Rationale:* Patient and family anxiety may be decreased.

PATIENT ASSESSMENT AND PREPARATION
Patient Assessment

- Assess for a history of upper GI bleeding, and the source of this bleeding, and baseline hematocrit and hemoglobin levels. ➤➤*Rationale:* This assessment is used as a basis for assessment of bleeding or continued bleeding after endoscopic therapy.
- Assess baseline cardiac rhythm. ➤➤*Rationale:* Passage of a large-bore tube may cause vagal stimulation and bradydysrhythmias.
- Obtain baseline coagulation study results (i.e., prothrombin time [PT], partial thromboplastin time [PTT], platelet count). ➤➤*Rationale:* Abnormal coagulation values increase the potential for bleeding after endoscopic therapy.
- Review respiratory, hemodynamic, and neurologic assessment before the administration of any sedative agents. ➤➤*Rationale:* Baseline assessment data provide information to use as a comparison for further evaluation once medications have been administered.
- Obtain baseline vital signs and pulse oximeter reading. ➤➤*Rationale:* Close monitoring of vital signs and pulse oximetry during the procedure and comparison with baseline values are essential to assess patient's tolerance of the procedure.
- Assess sedation score (Aldrete score, Ramsay scale, or the Richmond Agitation/Sedation Score are commonly used) based on blood pressure, pulse, oxygen saturation, level of consciousness, and respiratory status. ➤➤*Rationale:* Use of a scoring system standardizes assessment of the patient's tolerance of moderate sedation.

Patient Preparation

- Verify correct patient with two identifiers. ➻*Rationale:* Prior to performing a procedure, the nurse should ensure the correct identification of the patient for the intended intervention.
- Ensure that the patient understands preprocedural teachings. Answer questions as they arise, and reinforce information as needed. ➻*Rationale:* Understanding of previously taught information is evaluated and reinforced.
- Ensure that informed consent has been obtained. ➻*Rationale:* Informed consent protects the rights of the patient and makes a competent decision possible for the patient.
- Check that all relevant documents and studies are available before starting the procedure. ➻*Rationale:* This measure ensures that the correct patient receives the correct procedure.
- Place the patient on a cardiac monitor and apply a pulse oximeter and automatic blood pressure cuff. ➻*Rationale:* This allows for close cardiovascular and respiratory monitoring during the procedure.
- Ensure venous access is in place. ➻*Rationale:* Venous access is needed for premedications and emergency medications.

- Ensure that the patient has been on nothing-by-mouth (NPO) status for at least 4 hours before the procedure. ➻*Rationale:* Undigested material in the stomach increases the risk for aspiration and decreases visualization of the GI tract.
- Have sedatives (common sedatives used include midazolam, diazepam, meperidine, and fentanyl) available (as prescribed) and administer when requested. Naloxone and flumazenil should be available for narcotic or sedative reversal. ➻*Rationale:* Sedation decreases patient anxiety and facilitates cooperation during the procedure.
- Set up the suction with connecting tubing and rigid pharyngeal suction tip attached and a catheter ready. ➻*Rationale:* This set up is necessary for suctioning the patient's oral secretions during the procedure.
- Have atropine available at the bedside. ➻*Rationale:* Atropine is necessary if a vagal reaction occurs with the insertion and passage of the endoscope.
- Remove the patient's dentures. ➻*Rationale:* Dentures interfere with safe passage of the endoscope.
- Protect the patient's eyes with goggles or a waterproof covering. ➻*Rationale:* Protection is provided against accidental exposure to blood or the sclerosing agents. Sclerosing agents are eye irritants.

Procedure	**for Assisting with Endoscopic Therapy**	
Steps	**Rationale**	**Special Considerations**
1. HH		
2. PE		
3. VP		
4. Position patient in the left lateral position. **(Level E*)**	The left lateral position allows predictable views of the stomach as the scope is advanced. This position allows secretions to collect in the dependent areas of the mouth for ease of suctioning and is the position of choice to prevent aspiration should the patient vomit.	
5. Perform or assist the physician with gastric lavage (see Procedure 105).	Large amounts of blood or clots in the stomach or esophagus can impair visualization of varices and increase the risk for aspiration during the procedure.	
6. Administer premedications as ordered.	Allows patient cooperation during the endoscopy and facilitates the passage of the endoscope.	

*Level E: Multiple case reports, theory-based evidence from expert opinions, or peer-reviewed professional organizational standards without clinical studies to support recommendations

Procedure | for Assisting with Endoscopic Therapy—*Continued*

Steps	Rationale	Special Considerations
7. Assist physician or advanced practice nurse with insertion of the endoscope.		Gag and cough reflexes may be compromised by topical anesthetics, and the patient may vomit as the endoscope is passed, increasing the risk for aspiration. Have emergency intubation equipment available. Monitor heart rate, rhythm, and respiratory status during the endoscopy.
A. Anesthetize the posterior pharynx with a topical agent as requested.	Decreases the discomfort caused by passage of the endoscope.	
B. Insert an oral airway (see Procedure 11) or bite block.	Prevents the patient from biting the endoscope or the inserter's fingers.	
C. Lubricate 20 to 30 cm of the distal end of endoscope with water-soluble lubricant. (Many physicians and advanced practice nurses prefer to lubricate the scope themselves.)	Minimizes mucosal injury and irritation and facilitates ease of passage of the endoscope.	
D. Encourage the patient to simulate swallowing while the tube is passed.	Swallowing maneuver causes the epiglottis to close the trachea and directs endoscope into esophagus.	
E. Suction oral pharynx as needed.	Because of the diminished gag reflex and the presence of the endoscope in the patient's pharynx, oral secretions may not be able to be swallowed. Blood from the GI tract may be vomited and could be aspirated because of the diminished gag reflex.	
8. The physician or advanced practice nurse performing the EGD may request that the nurse prepare equipment for thermal or laser coagulation of a bleeding site.	This technique is frequently used to control bleeding from many upper gastrointestinal sites.	
9. Inject irrigant via the endoscope as requested.	Cleanses area to increase visualization of the tissue.	
10. If a bleeding site is to be sclerosed, manipulate the sclerosing needle as requested (Fig. 111-1). Inject sclerosant if requested.	Ensures that the sclerosing needle is in proper position for injection and does not injure tissue during movement of endoscope.	The needle must be retracted before manipulation of endoscope.
11. Endoscopic bands or endoclips may also be requested by the physician or advanced practice nurse performing the intervention (Fig. 111-2).	In EVL, or banding, a rubber band is deployed from the endoscope and contracts around a lesion that has been raised with endoscopic suction into a specially fitted, transparent endoscopic cap (Fig. 111-2).[2]	

Procedure continues on following page

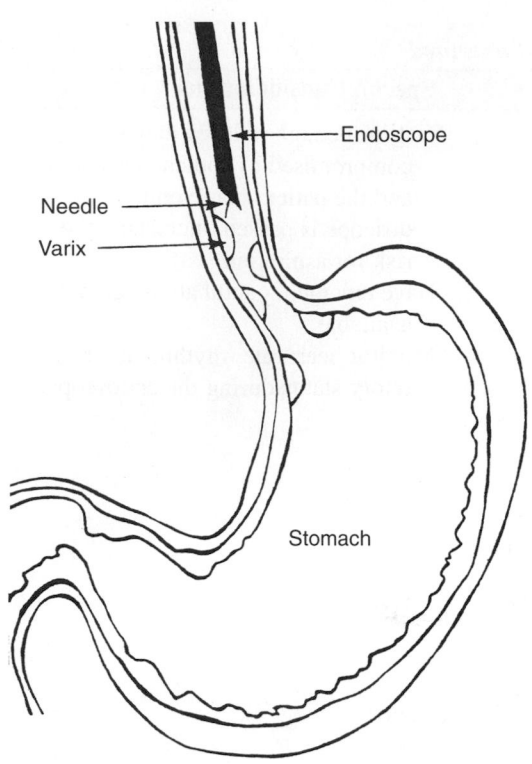

FIGURE 111-1 Injection of sclerosing agent into engorged varix. *(From Pierce JD, Wilkerson E, Griffiths SA: Acute esophageal bleeding and endoscopic injection therapy, Crit Care Nurse 10:67-72, 1990.)*

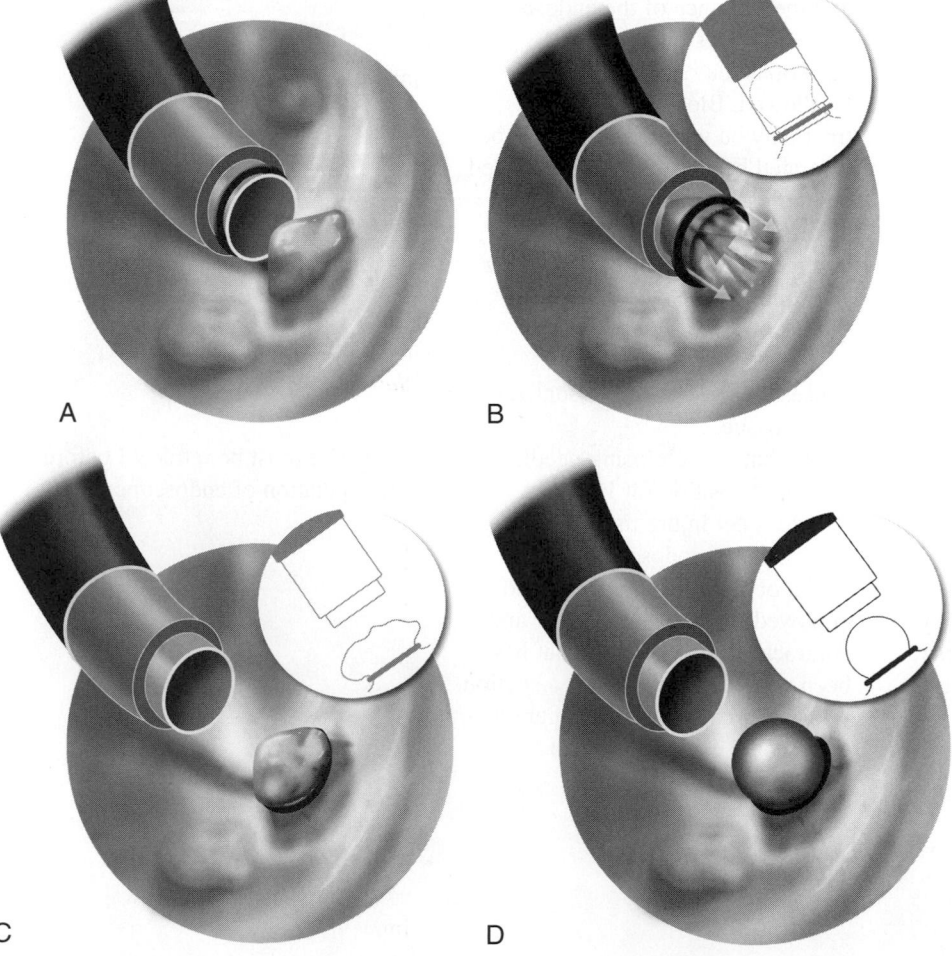

FIGURE 111-2 Endoscopic variceal ligation (EVL). **A,** Endoscope placement over varix. **B,** The varix is drawn into the distal portion of the endoscope. **C,** A rubber band is dropped over the varix. **D,** The rubber band contracts around the varix, causing it to sclerose and eventually slough. *(Drawings by Paul Schiffmacher, Medical Illustrator, Medical Media Services at Thomas Jefferson University Hospital, Philadelphia.)*

Procedure for Assisting with Endoscopic Therapy—*Continued*

Steps	Rationale	Special Considerations
12. Insert NG tube or esophagogastric tamponade tube (see Procedure 104) after removal of endoscope, as requested.	NG tube provides assessment of continued or recurrent bleeding. Esophagogastric tamponade tube may be used to apply pressure to oozing varices.	Suction applied to a NG tube can cause mucosal damage or disrupt fragile varices and initiate bleeding. A chest radiograph may be performed to rule out aspiration or esophageal perforation.
13. Dispose of equipment and discard used supplies in appropriate receptacles. The endoscope should be returned to the GI laboratory for proper disinfection.	Removes and safely discards used supplies, reduces the transmission of microorganisms; Standard Precautions. Safely removes sharp objects.	
14. **HH**	Reduces transmission of micro-organisms; Standard Precautions.	

Expected Outcomes

- Hemostasis at site of GI bleeding without recurrent bleeding or prevention of bleeding from esophageal varices
- Stabilization of hematocrit and hemoglobin values

Unexpected Outcomes

- Continued or recurrent bleeding from ligated (banded) or injected varices
- Continued or recurrent bleeding from ulcer site treated with injection, ablative, or mechanical therapy
- Esophageal, gastric, or duodenal sloughing or ulceration
- Esophageal, gastric, or duodenal perforation
- Substernal chest pain
- Fever
- Temporary dysphagia
- Allergic response to sclerosing agent
- Aspiration pneumonia
- Pleural effusion
- Atelectasis
- Bacteremia/sepsis

Patient Monitoring and Care

Steps	Rationale	Reportable Conditions
		These conditions should be reported if they persist despite nursing interventions.
1. Monitor cardiovascular, respiratory, and neurologic status every 5 to 15 minutes during and after endoscopy until patient condition returns to preprocedure status, then every 30 minutes to 1 hour for 2 to 4 hours. Includes: A. Level of consciousness B. Vital signs C. Oximetry D. Electrocardiogram	Changes in vital signs, heart rhythm, and oximetry may indicate complications related to the procedure.	• Altered level of consciousness from baseline • Oximetry reading below baseline • Pulse above or below baseline • Fever greater than 101°F • Decrease in blood pressure 20 to 30 mm Hg below baseline
2. Follow institutional standard for assessing pain.	May indicate continued bleeding or reaction to sclerosant. Identifies need for pain interventions.	• Same pain status as before procedure • New onset of chest pain • Continued pain despite pain interventions

Procedure continues on following page

Patient Monitoring and Care —*Continued*

Steps	Rationale	Reportable Conditions
3. Monitor output from NG tube or any vomitus.	Signs of continued or recurrent bleeding.	• Bright red vomitus or NG drainage
4. Monitor serial hematocrit and hemoglobin results as prescribed.	Continued fall in the hematocrit and hemoglobin value indicates continued or recurrent bleeding.	• Decreasing hematocrit and hemoglobin value below baseline
5. Monitor postural vital signs once the patient is able to be out of bed.	Postural changes indicate volume loss.	• Decrease in blood pressure 20 to 30 mm Hg below baseline • Increase in pulse 10 to 20 beats per minute above baseline
6. Assess for return of normal pharyngeal function. Keep patient on left side with slight head elevation until gag, swallow, and cough reflexes are intact. Remain with patient until reflexes return.	Some endoscopic therapies can cause transient dysphagia. Topical anesthesia decreases the gag reflex and increases the risk for aspiration. The left lateral position is the position of choice to prevent aspiration should the patient not be able to control secretions or vomit.	• Prolonged absence of gag, swallow, or cough reflex
7. Provide clear liquids when prescribed after return of pharyngeal function. Diet should be progressed slowly to solid food.	Food may act as an irritant to the sclerosed ulcer or variceal sites	• Nausea • Vomiting of bright red blood
8. Administer antacids, histamine (H$_2$) blockers, sulcralfate, proton pump inhibitors, somatostatin, or octreotide as ordered.[5,7,10,13] **(Level A*)**	Antacids neutralize gastric acid. Histamine blockers decrease gastric acid secretion. Sulcralfate reacts with gastric acid, forming a paste that adheres to ulcer sites. Proton pump inhibitors inhibit the proton pump in the parietal cells of the stomach, suppressing gastric acid secretion. Somatostatin and octreotide (synthetic somatostatin) lower portal pressure with splanchnic vasoconstriction.[3,6,9]	
9. Continue patient and family education.		
A. Explain signs and symptoms to report (fever, chest pain, difficulty swallowing, vomiting bright red blood, difficulty breathing).	Unexpected outcomes can occur within hours or may be delayed days or weeks after endoscopic therapy.	
B. Explain diet progression.	Decreases risk for aspiration of liquid or food before patient is ready for swallowing.	
C. Explain medication therapy.	Knowledge and understanding about the medication regimen promotes safe, effective medication use.	

*Level A: Meta-analysis of quantitative studies or metasynthesis of qualitative studies with results that consistently support a specific action, intervention, or treatment

Documentation

Documentation should include the following:

- Completion of informed consent
- Preprocedure verifications and time out
- Date and time of procedure
- Initial patient assessment
- Preprocedure and postprocedure patient and family education
- Baseline vital signs
- Baseline pulse oximetry
- Premedications administered
- Gastric lavage (if performed) and patient's tolerance
- Vital signs and pulse oximetry during endoscopic therapy
- Type of intervention: injection, ablative or mechanical; sclerosing agents administered and amount; number of bands or clips placed; and location if applicable

- Time of insertion of NG or tamponade tube (if inserted) and patient's tolerance, characteristics of any drainage from NG tube, radiographic documentation of placement of NG or tamponade tube, and initial pressure applied
- Postendoscopic therapy vital signs and pulse oximetry
- Position of patient after procedure
- Assessment of gag, swallow, and cough reflexes
- Postprocedure medications administered
- Unexpected outcomes
- Nursing interventions
- Sedation score
- Pain assessment, interventions, and effectiveness

References

1. Abraldes JG, Bosch J: The treatment of acute variceal bleeding, *Clin Gastroenterol* 41(Suppl):S312-S317, 2007.
2. Cappell MS, Friedel D: Acute nonvariceal upper gastrointestinal bleeding: endoscopic diagnosis and therapy, *Med Clin North Am* 92(3):511-550, 2008.
3. Cappell MS, Friedel D: Initial management of acute upper gastrointestinal bleeding: from initial evaluation up to gastrointestinal endoscopy, *Med Clin North Am* 92(3):491-509, 2008.
4. Dib N, Oberti F, Cales P: Current management of the complications of portal hypertension: variceal bleeding. *Can Med Assoc J*, 174(10), 1433-1443, 2006.
CR 5. Di Mario F, Battaglia G, Leandro G, et al: Short-term treatment of gastric ulcer: a meta analytical evaluation of blind trials, *Dig Dis Sci* 41(6):1108-1131, 1996.
6. Ferri FF: Paracentesis. In Ferri F, editor: *Practical guide to the care of the medical patient,* ed 7, Philadelphia, 2007, Mosby/Elsevier.
CR 7. Gisbert JP, Gonzalez L, Calvet X, et al: Proton pump inhibitors versus H2 antagonists: a meta analysis of their efficacy in treating bleeding peptic ulcer, *Aliment Pharm Ther* 15(7):917-926, 2001.
8. Hauser SC, editor: *Mayo Clinic Gastroenterology and Hepatology Board review,* ed 2, Rochester, MN, 2006, Mayo Clinic Scientific Press.
9. Longacre AV, Garcia-Tsao G: A commonsense approach to esophageal varices, *Clin Liver Dis* 10(3):613-625, 2006.
CR 10. Messori A, Trippoli S, Vaiani M, et al: Bleeding and pneumonia in intensive care patients given ranitidine and sulcralfate in the prevention of stress ulcer: a meta analysis of randomized controlled trials, *BMJ* 321(7):1103-1106, 2003.
11. Tariq SH, Mekhjian G: Gastrointestinal bleeding in older adults, *Clin Geriatr Med* 23(4):769-784, 2007.
12. Toubia N, Sanyal AJ: Portal hypertension and variceal hemorrhage, *Med Clin North Am* 92(3):551-574, 2008.
CR 13. Tryba M: Prophylaxis of stress ulcer bleeding: a meta analysis, *J Clin Gastroenterol* 13(Suppl 2):S44-S55, 1991.

Additional Readings

DiMaio CJ: Nonvariceal upper gastrointestinal bleeding, *Gastrointest Endosc Clin North Am* 17(2):253-272, 2007.

Heidelbaugh JJ, Sherbondy M: Cirrhosis and chronic liver failure: part II, complications and treatment, *Am Fam Physician* 74(5):767-776, 2006.

Khan S, Tudur Smith C, Williamson P, et al: Portosystemic shunts versus endoscopic therapy for variceal rebleeding in patients with cirrhosis, *Cochrane Database Syst Rev* 3: 2008.

CR Leung JW, Chung SC: Endoscopic injection of adrenaline in bleeding peptic ulcers, *Gastrointest Endosc* 33(2):73-75, 1987.

Lim CH, Vani D, Shah SG, et al: The outcome of suspected upper gastrointestinal bleeding with 24-hour access to upper gastrointestinal endoscopy: a prospective cohort study, *Endoscopy* 38(6):581-585, 2006.

Marmo R, Rotondano G, Piscopo R, et al: Dual therapy versus monotherapy in the endoscopic treatment of high-risk bleeding ulcers: a meta-analysis of controlled trials, *Am J Gastroenterol* 102(2):279-289, 2007.

Shibli AB, Tachauer A, Smruti R: Outpatient management of cirrhosis, *South Med J* 99(6):559-561, 2006.

Siersema PD: Therapeutic esophageal interventions for dysphagia and bleeding, *Curr Opin Gastroenterol* 22(4):442-447, 2006.

Talwalkar JA: Cost effectiveness of treating esophageal varices, *Clin Liver Dis* 10(3):679-689, 2006.

Zaman A: Portal hypertension-related bleeding: management of difficult cases, *Clin Liver Dis* 10(3):353-370, 2006.

Continuous Renal Replacement Therapies

P U R P O S E :   Continuous renal replacement therapies are used in the critical care unit setting for volume regulation, acid-base control, electrolyte regulation, drug intoxications, management of azotemia, and immune modulation. These methods are most often used in critically ill patients whose hemodynamic status does not tolerate the rapid fluid and electrolyte shifts associated with hemodialysis or who need continuous removal or regulation of solutes and intravascular volume.

Sonia M. Astle

PREREQUISITE NURSING KNOWLEDGE

- Continuous renal replacement therapy (CRRT) is an extracorporeal blood purification therapy intended to substitute for impaired renal function over an extended period of time for, or attempted for, 24 hours per day.
- CRRT can be accomplished through a variety of methods, with either arteriovenous access or venovenous access. The venovenous access is used almost exclusively because of its less invasive nature.[10,18] The following methods of CRRT are included as listed (details outlined in Table 112-1):
  - ❖ Slow continuous ultrafiltration (SCUF)
  - ❖ Continuous venovenous hemofiltration (CVVH)
  - ❖ Continuous venovenous hemodialysis (CVVHD)
  - ❖ Continuous venovenous hemodiafiltration (CV-VHDF)[2-4,11]
- Basic knowledge is required of the principles of diffusion, ultrafiltration (UF), osmosis, oncotic pressure, and hydrostatic pressure and how they pertain to fluid and solute management during dialysis.
  - ❖ *Diffusion:* The passive movement of solutes through a semipermeable membrane from an area of higher to lower concentration until equilibrium is reached.

- ❖ *Convective transport:* The rapid movement of fluid across a semipermeable membrane from an area of high pressure to an area of low pressure with transport of solutes. When water moves across a membrane along a pressure gradient, some solutes are carried along with the water and do not require a solute concentration gradient (also called solute drag). Convective transport is most effective for the removal of middle-molecular-weight and large-molecular-weight solutes.
- ❖ *UF:* The bulk movement of solute and solvent through a semipermeable membrane in response to a pressure difference across the membrane. This movement is usually achieved with positive pressure in the blood compartment in the hemofilter and negative pressure in the dialysate compartment. Blood and dialysate run countercurrent. The size of the solute molecules as compared with the size of molecules that can move through the semipermeable membrane determines the degree of UF.
- ❖ *Osmosis:* The passive movement of solvent through a semipermeable membrane from an area of higher to lower concentration.
- ❖ *Oncotic pressure:* The pressure exerted by plasma proteins that favor intravascular fluid retention and movement of fluid from the extravascular to the intravascular space.

TABLE 112-1	**Continuous Renal Replacement Therapies**				
Ultrafiltration Mode of Therapies	Principles Involved	Access	Indications	Advantages	Complications/ Disadvantages
SCUF (slow, continuous ultrafiltration)	Ultrafiltration	Venovenous	Patient with diuretic-resistant, volume-overloaded, hemodynamically unstable condition who cannot tolerate rapid fluid shifts	Continuous, gradual treatment (fewer high and low extremes) Precise fluid control can be done in patient with low mean arterial pressure	Anticoagulation, bleeding Hypotension Hypothermia Access complications (bleeding, clotting, infection) Requires strict monitoring of fluid and electrolyte replacement to avoid deficits or overload Air embolism Critical care setting only Recommended 1:1 nurse/patient ratio Poor control of azotemia; dialysis may be needed Minimal solute clearance Poor emergent treatment of hyperkalemia/acidosis Requires training of critical care nurses in use of pump
CVVH (continuous venovenous hemofiltration)	Ultrafiltration Convection Solute removal	Venovenous	Patient with volume-overloaded, hemodynamically unstable condition with azotemia or uremia	Precise fluid control can be done in patient with low mean arterial pressure Ease of initiation	Anticoagulation, bleeding Hypotension Hypothermia Access complications (bleeding, clotting, infection) Requires strict monitoring of fluid and electrolyte replacement to avoid deficits or overload Air embolism Critical care setting only Recommended 1:1 nurse/patient ratio Waste product removal not as efficient as CVVHDF Requires training of critical care nurses in use of pump
CVVHD (continuous venovenous hemodialysis)	Ultrafiltration Diffusion Solute removal	Venovenous	Patient with volume-overloaded, hemodynamically unstable condition with azotemia or uremia	Precise fluid control can be done in patient with low mean arterial pressure Ease of initiation	Same as CVVH Hyperglycemia Hypernatremia Hypophosphatemia
CVVHDF (continuous venovenous hemodiafiltration)	Ultrafiltration Convection Diffusion Solute removal	Venovenous	Patient with volume-overloaded, hemodynamically unstable condition with azotemia or uremia, catabolic acute renal failure, electrolyte imbalances/metabolic acidosis	Precise fluid control can be done in patient with low mean arterial pressure Better solute clearance than CVVH/ CVVHD Ease of initiation	Same as CVVH Hyperglycemia Hypernatremia Hypophosphatemia

Adapted from Giuliano K, Pysznik E: Renal replacement therapy in critical care: implementation of a unit-based CVVH program, Crit Care Nurse 18:40-45, 1998.

❖ *Hydrostatic pressure:* The force exerted by arterial blood pressure that favors the movement of fluid from the intravascular to the extravascular space.

❖ *Absorption:* The process by which drug molecules pass through membranes and fluid barriers and into body fluids.

❖ *Adsorption:* The adhesion of molecules (solutes) to the surface of the hemofilter, charcoal, or resin.

• CRRT uses an artificial kidney (i.e., hemofilter, dialyzer) with a semipermeable membrane to create two separate compartments: the blood compartment and the dialysis solution compartment. The semipermeable membrane allows the movement of small molecules (e.g., electrolytes) and middle-size molecules (creatinine, vasoactive substances) from the patient's blood into the dialysis solution but is impermeable to larger molecules (red blood cells, plasma proteins).

• Each dialyzer has four ports: two end ports for blood (in one end and out the other) and two side ports for dialysis solution ultrafiltrate (in one end and out the other). In most cases, the blood and dialysate are run through the dialyzer in opposite or countercurrent directions.

• With hollow-fiber dialyzers, the blood flows through the center of hollow fibers, and the dialysis solution (dialysate) flows around the outside of the hollow fibers. The advantages of hollow-fiber filters include a low priming volume, low resistance to flow, and high amount of surface area. The major disadvantage is the potential for clotting as a result of the small fiber size.

• All dialyzers have UF coefficients; thus, the dialyzer selected varies in different clinical situations.[1-5] The higher the UF coefficient, the more rapid the fluid removal. UF coefficients are determined with in vivo measurements done by each dialyzer manufacturer.

• Clearance refers to the ability of the dialyzer to remove metabolic waste products or drugs from the patient's blood. The blood flow rate, the dialysate flow rate, and the solute concentration affect clearance. Clearance occurs by the processes of diffusion, convection, and UF.

• The dialysate (when used during CRRT) is composed of water, a buffer (i.e., lactate or bicarbonate), and various electrolytes. Most solutions also contain glucose. The buffer helps neutralize acids that are generated as a result of normal cellular metabolism and that usually are excreted by the kidney. The concentration of electrolytes is usually the normal plasma concentration, which helps to create a concentration gradient for removal of excess electrolytes. The glucose aids in increasing the oncotic pressure in the dialysate (thus aiding in fluid removal) and in caloric replacement. Although glucose comes in various concentrations, it is usually used in normal plasma concentrations to prevent hyperglycemia.

• Heparin or citrate is often used during CRRT to prevent clotting of the circuit during treatment. Saline solution flushes can be used alone or with other anticoagulants to maintain circuit patency.[3-7,9]

• An anticoagulant is used to maintain vascular access patency when CRRT is not in use.[3,10]

• If the patient is taking angiotensin-converting enzyme (ACE) inhibitors, contact with certain filters or membranes in the CRRT system can cause an anaphylactic reaction and severe hypotension as a result of increased levels of bradykinin, a potent vasodilator. ACE inhibitors are recommended to be withheld for 48 to 72 hours before treatment, if possible.

• Continuous venovenous renal replacement therapy is achieved with a pumped system.

• The patient's volume status and serum electrolyte levels are changed gradually so that patients have fewer problems than they do with hemodialysis. Specifics of these therapies are outlined in Table 112-1.[1,2,4,7,13-15,17]

• SCUF (Fig. 112-1) is a nonpumped system, CVVH (Fig. 112-2), CVVHD (Fig. 112-3), and CVVHDF (Fig. 112-4)

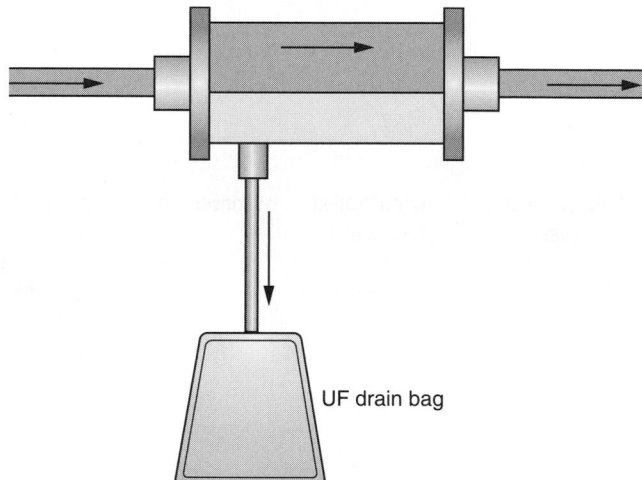

FIGURE 112-1 Slow continuous ultrafiltration (SCUF). Fluid removal, no fluid replacement. *(Copyright Rhonda K. Martin. All rights reserved. Used with permission.)*

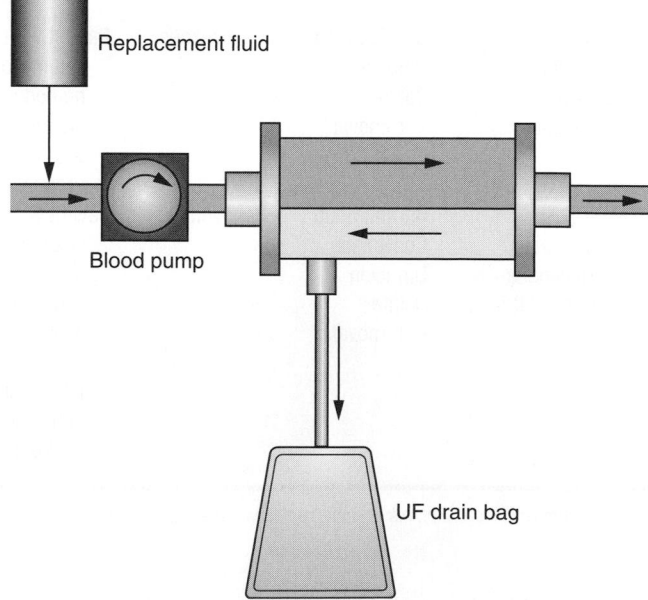

FIGURE 112-2 Continuous venovenous hemofiltration (CVVH). Fluid removal and fluid replacement. *(Copyright Rhonda K. Martin. All rights reserved. Used with permission.)*

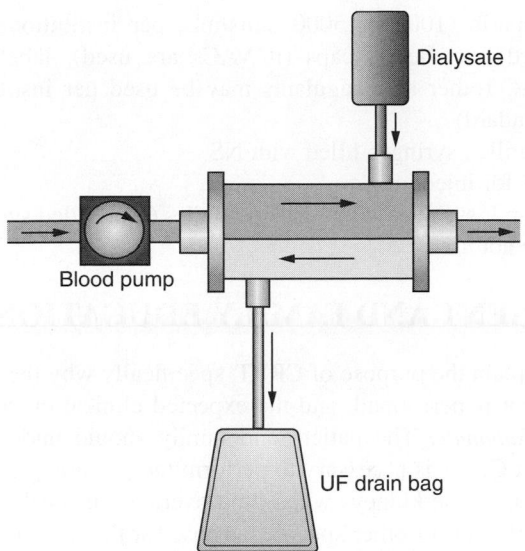

FIGURE 112-3   Continuous venovenous hemodialysis (CVVHD). Fluid and solute removal with dialysate. *(Copyright Rhonda K. Martin. All rights reserved. Used with permission.)*

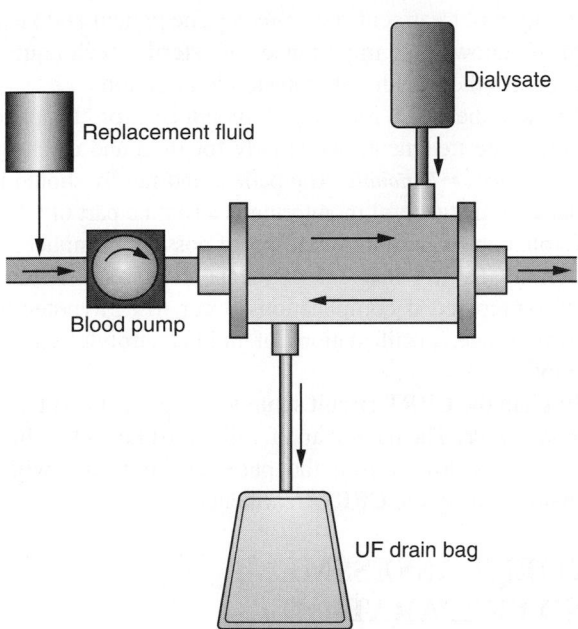

FIGURE 112-4   Continuous venovenous hemodiafiltration (CVVHDF). Fluid replacement with dialysate. *(Copyright Rhonda K. Martin. All rights reserved. Used with permission.)*

use pumped systems. These therapies are used to remove both plasma water and solutes and require venous access, most commonly provided with a double-lumen vascular access catheter (VAC). External arteriovenous (AV) hemodialysis shunts or surgically created AV hemodialysis anastomoses have been used in the past for CRRT; however, because of increased incidence rates of vascular injury, bleeding, and infection, they are *not* recommended for CRRT access.[1,10] Common sites for the VAC are the internal jugular, subclavian, and femoral veins. The internal jugular approach is the preferred access. Cannulation

of the subclavian vein may cause stenosis and prevent placement of upper extremity grafts or fistulas if long-term dialysis is necessary.[3,10] Femoral cannulation is associated with increased infection.[3,10,16,19,20]

- A blood pump provides the pressure that drives the system; the blood circuit consists of blood lines, a blood pump, and various monitoring devices. The blood lines carry the blood to and from the patient. The blood pump controls the speed of the blood through the circuit. The monitoring devices include arterial and venous pressure monitors and an air detection monitor to prevent air that may have entered the circuit from being returned to the patient. Anticoagulant, dialysate, and replacement fluids can also be added to the system.
  - ❖ Integrated pump systems have separate pumps for blood, dialysate, ultrafiltrate/effluent, and replacement fluids (Fig. 112-5). The pumps are controlled by a computerized control module. Blood flow rate, dialysate flow rate, anticoagulation rate, and fluid removal rates are entered by the nurse per medical guidelines. Dialysate, ultrafiltrate/effluent, and replacement fluids are measured by weight or volumetric scales on the unit. The module calculates and adjusts pump speeds to achieve the selected fluid goal. The module also records and displays treatment data.
- SCUF (see Fig. 112-1) is used primarily to remove plasma water. A hemofilter with a large surface area, high sieving coefficient, and low resistance is used to facilitate slow continuous fluid removal.

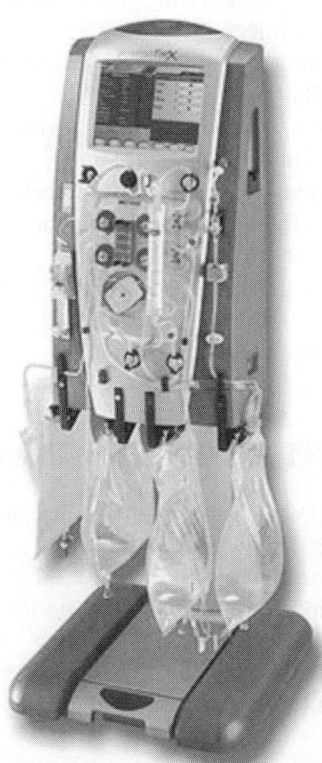

FIGURE 112-5   Gambro Prismaflex CRRT machine. *(Courtesy Gambro USA, Lakewood, Colo.)*

- CVVH (see Fig. 112-2) removes fluids and solutes via convection. Replacement solution is part of the setup; the replacement solution creates a solute drag effect.
- CVVHD (see Fig. 112-3) is used to remove solutes primarily via diffusion. Dialysate solution is part of the setup; flow of the dialysate is countercurrent to the blood flow.
- CVVHDF (see Fig. 112-4) removes fluids and solutes via diffusion and convection. Dialysate runs countercurrent to the blood flow. Intravenous or blood circuit replacement fluid is used continuously based on the amount of UF removed each hour and net fluid goals for the patient.
- Other extended renal replacement therapy techniques or "hybrid" techniques (sustained low-efficiency dialysis [SLED], extended daily dialysis [EDD]) generally use standard hemodialysis equipment with reduced blood flow and dialysate rates to gradually remove plasma water and solutes. They are used from 4 to 12 hours a day.

EQUIPMENT (FOR INITIATION)

- Dedicated vascular access
- Hemofilter/pump system with blood lines
- Replacement fluid, as ordered
- Dialysate fluid, as ordered
- Fluid shield, face masks, or goggles
- Sterile and nonsterile gloves
- Fluid warmer
- Two 10-mL prefilled syringes with normal saline (NS) solution
- Two 5-mL and 10-mL syringes and blunt-tip needles (to draw up NS for injection)
- NS for injection (if prefilled NS syringes are not used)
- Sterile NS solution, 3L
- Dressing supplies (alcohol wipes, sterile barrier, gauze pads, transparent dressing, tape)
- Povidone-iodine, hypochlorite, or chlorhexidine bactericidal solution (follow institution standard)
- Sterile container
- Heparin, 1000 units/mL, or citrate (for priming follow institution standard)
- Hemostats (extra clamps if needed)
- Drainage bag

EQUIPMENT (FOR TERMINATION)

- Intravenous (IV) accessory spike to connect NS bag to arterial tubing
- Hemostats (extra clamps if needed)
- Dressing supplies (alcohol wipes, sterile barrier, gauze pads, transparent dressing, tape)
- Povidone-iodine, hypochlorite, or chlorhexidine bactericidal solution (follow institution standard)
- NS, 1000 mL
- Sterile container
- Sterile and nonsterile gloves
- Fluid shield, face mask, or goggles

- Heparin (1000 or 5000 units/mL, per institution standard), needleless caps (if VACs are used), labels for VAC (other anticoagulants may be used per institution standard)
- Prefilled syringes filled with NS
- NS for injection
- 10-mL syringes and blunt-tip needles (if prefilled syringes are not used)

PATIENT AND FAMILY EDUCATION

- Explain the purpose of CRRT, specifically why the treatment is performed, and the expected clinical outcomes. ➤*Rationale:* The patient and family should understand that CRRT is necessary to perform the physiologic functions of the kidneys when fluid overload or renal failure is present (or other specific purpose for the therapy).
- Explain the procedure, including risks, anticipated length of treatment, and patient positioning, and review any questions the patient may have. ➤*Rationale:* Explanation provides information and may decrease patient anxiety.
- Explain the need for careful sterile technique for the duration of treatment. ➤*Rationale:* The patient and family must know the importance of sterile technique to decrease the likelihood of systemic infection.
- Explain the need for careful monitoring of the patient during the treatment, particularly for fluid and electrolyte imbalance. ➤*Rationale:* The patient and family should understand that careful monitoring is a routine part of CRRT.
- Explain the signs and symptoms of possible complications during CRRT. ➤*Rationale:* Patients and family should be fully prepared if complications occur (e.g., hypotension, hemorrhage, manifestations of fluid/electrolyte/acid-base imbalance).
- Explain the CRRT circuit setup to the patient and family. ➤*Rationale:* The patient and family must know that blood will be removed from the patient's body and will be visible during the CRRT treatment.

PATIENT ASSESSMENT AND PREPARATION
Patient Assessment

- Assess baseline vital signs, including hemodynamic parameters, weight, laboratory values (blood urea nitrogen (BUN), creatinine, electrolytes, hemoglobin, hematocrit), and neurologic status. ➤*Rationale:* Patients in renal failure often have altered baseline assessment results, both in physical assessment and in laboratory values. Knowledge of this information before treatments are started is helpful so that interventions, including net fluid balance and dialysate fluid, can be individualized. Alterations during treatment are common because of the rapid removal of fluid and solutes.
- Assess the insertion site for signs and symptoms of infection. ➤*Rationale:* Insertion sites provide a portal of entry for infection, which may result in septicemia if unrecognized or untreated. If the insertion site appears to be

infected, further interventions (e.g., site change, culture, antibiotic treatment) may be necessary.

- Assess patency of VAC and the ability to easily aspirate blood from both ports. →*Rationale:* Adequate blood flow is necessary during a treatment to facilitate optimal fluid and solute removal. Patent catheter ports are necessary for adequate blood flow.
- Assess adequate circulation to the distal parts of the access limb. →*Rationale:* The placement of vascular access may compromise circulation.

Patient Preparation

- Verify correct patient with two identifiers. →*Rationale:* Prior to performing a procedure, the nurse should ensure the correct identification of the patient for the intended intervention.
- When CRRT is initiated, ensure that informed consent has been obtained. →*Rationale:* Informed consent pro-

tects the rights of the patient and makes a competent decision possible for the patient.
- Ensure that patient understands preprocedural teachings. Answer questions as they arise, and reinforce information as needed. →*Rationale:* Understanding of previously taught information is evaluated and reinforced.
- Position the patient in a comfortable position (that also facilitates optimal blood flow through the vascular access). →*Rationale:* The patient and family must understand that movement during the procedure may affect the blood flow through the system and that a comfortable position before the initiation of therapy is important. They should also understand that different access sites may require different patient positions to facilitate optimal blood flow. Choose a position that allows for setup of the sterile field. The nurse who sets up the sterile field and initiates therapy must be able to easily reach all the necessary supplies.

Procedure	for Initiation and Termination of Continuous Renal Replacement Therapy

Steps	Rationale	Special Considerations
Systems (SCUF, CVVH, CVVHD, CVVHDF)		
1. HH		
2. PE		
3. Verify orders, which should include the following: A. Modality B. Vascular access C. Type of hemofilter/dialyzer D. Anticoagulant type, concentration, infusion rate, monitoring parameters E. Replacement fluid and rate (if used) F. Hourly ultrafiltration rate G. Hourly net fluid goal H. Dialysate solution and rate (if used) I. Blood pressure/vital sign parameters J. Laboratory testing **(Level C*)**	Familiarizes nurse with the individualized patient treatment and reduces the possibility of error.[3,4]	Ensure patient weight and laboratory values are recorded before initiation of therapy.

*Level C: Qualitative studies, descriptive or correlational studies, integrative reviews, systematic reviews, or randomized controlled trials with inconsistent results

Procedure continues on following page

Procedure for Initiation and Termination of Continuous Renal Replacement Therapy—*Continued*

Steps	Rationale	Special Considerations
4. Turn on the system. Set up system according to manufacturer's instructions, attach any prescribed solutions, and prepare anticoagulant infusion (if ordered), replacement fluid, dialysate, and flush infusion (if ordered).	Correct system setup is imperative for safety and optimal functioning. Use of anticoagulants prolongs the function of the hemofilter.[3,4]	Pump must be plugged into a generator outlet because some pumps do not have battery power. Heparin, if ordered, is usually administered on a prefilter port; citrate is usually administered at the arterial port of the VAC.
For integrated pump units (Prismaflex, Diapact, NxStage, Aquarius), follow manufacturer's instructions and prompts from the control screen.	Ensures correct system setup.	Replacement solutions are administered through the arterial or venous infusion port as ordered (usually arterial) with blood tubing. Connect 1 L NS to arterial infusion port (for flushing system). Dialysate solution (if CVVHD/CVVHDF is used) is connected to the outlet port of the hemofilter near the venous end with blood tubing.

Automated setup instructions include:
  Select therapy/modality
  Calibration (if indicated)
  Load set
  Priming
  Anticoagulant
  Dialysate/replacement fluid rates
  Blood flow rate
  Fluid removal rate
After priming per manufacturer instructions, **go to Step 5.**
		Each integrated pump is loaded and primed with various methods, ranging from assembly and priming of all components to "one-touch" circuit loading and priming. Some unit's air detectors are activated after the machine is primed.

5. With the protective caps on, place the arterial and venous blood lines on the patient's bed near the VAC.	Leave the priming bag, collection bag, and protective caps in place to preserve sterility of the system until the blood lines are attached to the VAC.	Some systems have a collection bag for the priming solution, which stays attached to the venous blood line until it is attached to the VAC.
6. Remove gloves and discard in appropriate receptacle.	Reduces transmission of microorganisms; Standard Precautions.	
7. HH		
8. PE		
9. Prepare sterile field with sterile barrier under the VAC.	Prepares material and maintains aseptic technique.	
10. Place 4 × 4 gauze pads onto the sterile field. Open sterile container, syringes, blunt-tip needles, and NS (or prefilled NS syringes) and place on sterile field.	Prepares material and maintains aseptic technique.	
11. Add bactericidal solution to sterile container. (**Level D***)	Prepares solution used to cleanse VAC ports. Povidone-iodine, hypochlorite, and chlorhexidine solutions are acceptable bactericidal agents.[3,10,19]	
12. HH		
13. Apply sterile gloves.	Maintains aseptic technique.	
14. Attach blunt-tip needles to two 10-mL syringes; with help of assistant, fill NS or use prefilled syringes per institutional standard.	Prepares syringe for VAC flushing.	With Quinton catheters, 20 to 30 mL per lumen flush for hemocaths and permacaths is recommended.[1]

*Level D: Peer-reviewed professional organizational standards with clinical studies to support recommendations

Procedure	for Initiation and Termination of Continuous Renal Replacement Therapy—*Continued*		

Steps	Rationale	Special Considerations
15. Saturate four of the 4 × 4 pads in bactericidal solution. Using two of the soaked pads perform a 1-minute scrub of the arterial and venous ports of the VAC.	Prevents introduction of infection.	Be sure to remove any crust or drainage.
16. Using the other two soaked pads wrap one pad each around arterial and venous ports and leave in place for 3 to 5 minutes.	Reduces transmission of micro organisms.[3,9,15,19]	
17. After 3 to 5 minutes, remove the bactericidal-soaked 4 × 4 pad and discard in appropriate receptacle.	Safely discards used supplies.	
18. Ensure clamps are closed on the arterial and venous ports of the VAC; then remove cap from arterial port of the VAC and discard.	Provides access to arterial side of the VAC; Standard Precautions.	Be sure clamp is closed before removing arterial port cap.
19. Attach an empty 5-mL syringe to the arterial port, open the clamp, and gently aspirate 5 mL of blood and anticoagulant. Close the clamp, remove syringe, and discard in appropriate receptacle. **(Level D*)**	Verifies patency of arterial port. Note any resistance, which could mean a clotted or kinked port. Prevents bolus of anticoagulant to the patient and decreases transmission of microorganisms.[3,10]	Never forward-flush an indwelling port until first aspirating. This prevents dislodgment/embolism of clots and prevents a bolus of anticoagulant to the patient. Observe for clots. A clotted or kinked port decreases blood flow and reduces efficacy of the treatment.
20. **Repeat Steps 18 and 19** on the venous port.	Provides access to venous side of catheter; Standard Precautions.	
21. Attach 10-mL syringe with NS flush solution to arterial port. Open clamp and flush; then close clamp.	Prevents clotting of blood until dialysis is initiated.	Note any resistance on flushing.
22. **Repeat Step 21** on venous port.		
23. Disconnect protective cap or priming bag from arterial blood line, attach to arterial port of the VAC, and secure the connection.	Loose connections introduce air into the circuit.	
24. Disconnect the protective cap from the venous blood tubing, attach to the venous port of the VAC, and secure the connection.	Loose connections introduce air into the circuit.	
25. Open the clamps on the arterial and venous blood lines.	Opens the circuit in preparation of starting the blood pump.	Perform final check for air in the blood circuit.
26. Turn on the blood pump and gradually turn the blood flow rate to the ordered rate.	Prevents hypotension from rapid blood and fluid shifts.	Observe for blood leaks, air in the system, and pressure alarms. Assess the patient's vital signs, which should remain within 20% of baseline parameters.
27. Start the replacement fluid solution, if ordered.	Fluid loss without replacement may cause hypotension.	Fluids may be warmed to prevent hypothermia per institution standard.[9,12]
28. Start dialysate infusion, if ordered.	Starts hemodialysis or hemodiafiltration.	
29. Check that all alarms are on and parameters are set.	Ensures safe delivery of therapy.	

*Level D: Peer-reviewed professional organizational standards with clinical studies to support recommendations

Procedure continues on following page

| Procedure | for Initiation and Termination of Continuous Renal Replacement Therapy—*Continued* | | |

Steps	Rationale	Special Considerations
30. Note blood pump flow rate, arterial and venous monitor pressures, transmembrane filter pressure, amount and color of UF, and vital signs on initiation and hourly or per institutional standard.	Ensures safe delivery of therapy.	Increased arterial monitor pressure indicates problems with the vascular access or blood inflow. Increased venous monitor pressure indicates clotting of the hemofilter or system.
31. Dispose of used materials in the appropriate receptacle.	Safely discards used supplies.	
32. **HH**		
33. Prepare a fluid balance flow sheet and calculate the net fluid gain/ loss prescribed each hour.	Accurate calculations of hourly fluid balance prevent hypervolemia and hypovolemia and ensure that clinical goals are being met.	Hourly fluid balance is usually calculated by subtracting the total output (including UF) from the total intake.

Flushing

1. **HH**		
2. **PE**		
3. Connect NS with flushed tubing to the arterial port.	Prepares port for flushing.	
4. Clamp the arterial side of the circuit (proximal to the arterial infusion port).	Prevents any more blood from entering the circuit via the arterial port during flushing.	**Note:** Be sure that NS flush is running freely to prevent rupture or back filtration. Hemostasis and clot formation in the arterial limb of the tubing are a possibility if the flushing procedure is prolonged.
5. Open the NS flush while the pump continues to run. Note the amount infused.	Flushing allows the nurse to assess the patency of the system.[4]	Flushing contributes to the patient's IV intake; the volume of fluid should be documented. When the circuit is flushed of blood, clots may be observed. Flushing does not dissolve existing clots.
6. If no clots are observed, turn off the NS and unclamp the arterial circuit to allow hemofiltration to continue.	Continues therapy	If numerous clots are observed, the hemofilter may need to be replaced.
7. Discard used equipment in appropriate receptacle.	Safely discards used supplies.	
8. **HH**		

Termination

1. **HH**		
2. **PE**		
3. Turn off all infusions into the circuit.	Prepares for termination of therapy.	
4. With IV accessory spike, attach NS flush solution to arterial infusion port.	Prepares for flushing blood from tubing.	

Procedure	for Initiation and Termination of Continuous Renal Replacement Therapy—*Continued*		

Steps	Rationale	Special Considerations
5. Continue terminating, depending on type of pump. Press the "End Treatment" option and follow instructions.	Follow instructions on the pump for termination. The blood should be flushed through the circuit to prevent unnecessary blood loss.	If clots are identified beyond the venous bubble trap, stop the pump; do not return blood to patient. Blood from the arterial port of the VAC is not returned to the patient because of the possibility of clot formation, and the machine does not detect clots in that location.
6. Once hemofilter and venous line are flushed, stop the pump.	Blood is cleared from tubing.	
7. When the entire circuit is clear of blood, turn off the pump and clamp off both the arterial and venous access ports and the arterial and venous circuit lines.	Prevents air from entering access ports and fluid leaking from circuit lines.	
8. If the VAC is to be discontinued, remove it now per institution standard.	CRRT therapy may no longer be needed.	If the VAC is not discontinued, instill both ports with anticoagulant per institution standard.
9. Record the amount of NS infused.	Ensures accurate fluid balance.	The flush solution is fluid given to the patient and must be recorded as intake.
10. If VAC is not to be removed, prepare sterile field. Open and place sterile barrier under the VAC.	Prepares material and maintains aseptic technique.	
11. Place 4 × 4 gauze pads onto the sterile field. Open sterile container, syringes, blunt-tip needles, and NS (or prefilled NS syringes) and place on sterile field.	Prepares material and maintains aseptic technique.	
12. Add bactericidal solution to sterile container. **(Level D*)**	Prepares solution used to cleanse VAC ports. Povidone-iodine, hypochlorite and chlorhexidine solutions are acceptable bactericidal agents.[3,10,19]	
13. Remove gloves and discard in appropriate receptacle.	Safely discards used supplies.	
14. 🅷🅷		
15. 🅿🅴		
16. Attach blunt-tip needles to two 10-mL syringes; with help of assistant, fill syringes with NS or use prefilled syringes per institutional standard.	Prepares syringe for VAC flushing.	With Quinton catheters, 20 to 30 mL per lumen flush for hemocaths and permacaths is recommended.[1]
17. Saturate four of the 4 × 4 pads in bactericidal solution. Using two of the soaked pads perform a 1-minute scrub of the arterial and venous ports of the VAC.	Prevents introduction of infection.	Be sure to remove any crust or drainage.

*Level D: Peer-reviewed professional organizational standards with clinical studies to support recommendations

Procedure continues on following page

Procedure for Initiation and Termination of Continuous Renal Replacement Therapy—*Continued*

Steps	Rationale	Special Considerations
18. Using the other two soaked pads, wrap one pad each around the arterial and venous ports and leave in place for 3 to 5 minutes.	Reduces transmission of microorganisms.[3,9,15,19]	
19. After 3 to 5 minutes, remove the bactericidal-soaked 4 × 4 pad and discard in appropriate receptacle.	Safely discards used supplies.	
20. Be sure clamps are closed on the arterial and venous ports of the VAC, then disconnect the arterial blood line from the arterial vascular access.	Opens system under sterile conditions for system termination.	Be sure port clamp is closed before removing arterial line.
21. **Repeat Step 20** on the venous system line.		
22. Attach 10-mL syringe with NS to arterial port. Open clamp and flush, then close clamp.	Prevents clotting of blood until anticoagulant is instilled.	
23. **Repeat Step 22** on venous port.		
24. Instill anticoagulant into each access port according to institution standard. Use only the volume listed on the vascular access.	Maintains patency of accesses.	Use only the amount listed on the access to avoid instilling anticoagulant into the patient. Label each port with date, time, anticoagulant used, and nurse's initials.
25. Clamp and cap the arterial and venous ports with sterile needleless caps; tape securely.	Maintains sterility of VAC.	
26. Change vascular access dressings according to institution standard.	Prevents infection.	
27. Dispose of used equipment in the appropriate receptacle.	Safely discards used supplies.	
28. [HH]		
Emergency Termination		
1. Clamp arterial and venous vascular access ports and circuit lines.	Stops treatment.	Emergency termination is used to emergently move the patient or for serious complications, including blood leak, hemofilter rupture, clotting, circuit disconnection, and dialyzer/circuit reaction.
2. [HH]		
3. Apply mask and sterile gloves.	Maintains aseptic technique.	
4. Disconnect circuit bloodlines from the VAC ports.	Disconnects patient from CRRT machine.	Blood in the circuit is lost during emergency termination.
5. Flush VAC with NS, instill with anticoagulant per institution standard, and apply sterile caps to VAC ports.	Maintains VAC patency.	
6. Stop all infusions related to CRRT treatment.	Prevents fluid and electrolyte imbalances.	
7. Dispose of used equipment in appropriate receptacles.	Safely discards used supplies.	
8. [HH]		

Expected Outcomes

- VAC accessed without complications
- Blood easily aspirated from the access site
- Accumulated fluid and waste products removed
- Acid-base balance restored
- BUN and creatinine values restored to baseline levels
- Electrolyte levels within baseline values
- Hemodynamic stability and maintenance of optimal intravascular volume
- Nutritional status maintained

Unexpected Outcomes

- Clotting/decreased patency of the access sites
- Crack in the VAC or end caps
- Bleeding from insertion site or access site
- Signs and symptoms of infection at the insertion or access site
- Dislodgment of the VAC
- Decreased circulation in the extremity with the vascular access
- Hematoma formation at the access site
- Physiologic complications (dysrhythmias, chest pain, fluid or electrolyte imbalance, complications related to anticoagulation, air embolism, hypotension, seizures, nausea and vomiting, headaches, muscle cramping, dyspnea)
- Introduction of pathogens into the circuit
- Technical problems with the blood pump (blood leak, air leak, clotting, disconnection of circuit, hemolysis, hemofilter rupture)
- Hypothermia
- Malnutrition

Patient Monitoring and Care

Steps	Rationale	Reportable Conditions
		These conditions should be reported if they persist despite interventions.
1. Obtain and record predialysis and daily weight.	Predialysis weight is an important factor in deciding how much UF is needed during treatment. It also helps to guide ongoing treatment.[3]	• Abnormal increase or decrease in weight
2. Perform ongoing assessments, including the following: A. Vital signs B. Jugular vein distention C. Presence of edema D. Intake and output E. Neurologic assessment F. Pulmonary assessment	Provides information in response to treatment.[1,4,7,9] Monitors for complications.	• Hypotension • Hypertension • Tachycardia/bradycardia • Tachypnea/bradypnea • Fever • Hypothermia • Jugular vein distention • Crackles • Edema • Change in level of consciousness, dizziness • Change in cardiac rhythm
3. Monitor the circulation to the extremity where the VAC is located.	To assess for any decrease in perfusion distal to the VAC site.[3,4]	• Diminished capillary refill • Diminished or absent peripheral pulses, pain • Pale, mottled, or cyanotic • Cool to touch • Diminished or absent movement or sensation.

Procedure continues on following page

Patient Monitoring and Care —*Continued*

Steps	Rationale	Reportable Conditions
4. Monitor electrolytes, glucose, and albumin during treatment as per institutional standard.	Must be monitored because of continued fluid and electrolyte shifts during treatment. Amino acids are also lost through the hemofilter.	• Hyperkalemia or hypokalemia • Hypernatremia or hyponatremia • Hypercalcemia or hypocalcemia • Hyperglycemia or hypoglycemia • Hypermagnesemia or hypomagnesemia • Hyperphosphatemia or hypophosphatemia • Hypoalbuminemia
5. Administer medications to correct electrolyte abnormalities as ordered during treatment. **(Level D*)**	Patients with renal failure are predisposed to many electrolyte abnormalities. During CRRT, medications or electrolyte replacements may be given as ordered for individual patients.[3,4] Renal diet with adjusted protein, potassium, phosphorous, carbohydrate, and fluid intake that takes into account the patient's current catabolic state, renal function, adequacy of dialysis, and removal of amino acids via dialysis is required.[3,4,8]	• Hyperkalemia or hypokalemia • Hypernatremia or hyponatremia • Hypercalcemia or hypocalcemia • Hyperglycemia or hypoglycemia • Hypermagnesemia or hypomagnesemia • Hyperphosphatemia or hypophosphatemia • Hypoalbuminemia • Unexpected change in weight (loss or gain)
6. Monitor the CRRT circuit (e.g., occlusions; kinks in UF, blood, or vascular access lines; hemofilter). **(Level D)**	Disconnections or introduction of air into the circuit are always possible during treatment. Bleeding or exsanguination can also occur.[3,4,7,10] Clotting of the circuit is a potential complication. If hemofilter becomes clotted, the extracorporeal blood volume should be returned to the patient quickly. Blood leaks from the dialyzer into the dialysate may occur and necessitate termination of treatment. In the event of a filter leak, do *not* return circuit blood to the patient. Venous or arterial pressures that are out of range may indicate dialyzer or access malfunction.	• Disconnections, cracks, or leaks • Excessive clotting • Blood leaks/hemofilter rupture • Malfunction of dialyzer or access
7. Monitor UF for rate, clarity, and air bubbles. **(Level D)**	A decrease in UF production can occur from clotting of the dialyzer.[3,4,7,10] Pink or blood-tinged UF is indicative of filter leak or rupture.	• Decrease in UF production • Change in color or characteristics of UF • Air in UF • Suspicion of clotting in the circuit
8. Administer anticoagulant as ordered.	Heparin or citrate is often used to prevent clotting of the circuit.[3,4] Heparin/citrate dose varies according to patient condition and laboratory values.	

*Level D: Peer-reviewed professional organizational standards with clinical studies to support recommendations

Patient Monitoring and Care —*Continued*

Steps	Rationale	Reportable Conditions
9. Monitor anticoagulation as per institutional standard.	Because heparin or citrate commonly is used to prevent system clotting, coagulation studies should be routinely monitored.	• Abnormal coagulation study results
10. Monitor the vascular access. **(Level D*)**	Bleeding can occur from either the venous or arterial access site. Clotting of the access can occur.[3,4,7,10,19]	• Decrease in access function or patency
11. Monitor condition of access site.	Bleeding or infection can occur as access site complications.[3,4,16,20]	• Bleeding • Site redness or edema • Warmth • Purulent drainage • Pain or tenderness • Fever
12. Initiate and monitor rate of replacement fluids.	Prevents hypotension. Replacement fluids are dependent on patient's baseline assessment.	
13. Monitor the patient for complications associated with CRRT treatment.	Several complications are possible with CRRT.[3,4,6,7,9,11]	• Muscle cramps • Dialysis disequilibrium (headache, nausea and vomiting, hypertension, decreased sensorium, seizures, coma) • Air embolism • Dialyzer reaction (hypotension, pruritus, back pain, angioedema, anaphylaxis) • Hypoxemia • Hypothermia
14. Monitor the blood pump for proper functioning.	Any type of equipment is subject to malfunctioning. The nurse operating the blood pump must be competent with its operation, understand troubleshooting methods, and know when to take the pump out of service.	• Problems with the blood pump
15. Follow institution standard for assessing pain. Administer analgesia as prescribed.	Identifies need for pain interventions.	• Continued pain despite pain interventions

Documentation

Documentation should include the following:
- Patient and family education
- Date and time of treatment initiation, mode of therapy, filter change
- Condition of vascular access regarding patency, quality of blood flow, ease of access procedure
- Date and time of VAC insertion and dressing change
- Condition of insertion site and any signs or symptoms of infection
- Blood flow rate and arterial and venous monitoring pressures
- Type and content of dialysis and replacement fluids
- Anticoagulation type and dose
- Completion of informed consent.
- Vital signs/hemodynamic parameters
- Status of pulse distal to vascular access site
- Hourly fluid balance calculation
- Patient's response to CRRT and daily progress toward treatment goals
- Unexpected outcomes
- Nursing interventions
- Daily weight
- Laboratory assessment data
- Pain assessment, interventions, and effectiveness.

*Level D: Peer-reviewed professional organizational standards with clinical studies to support recommendations

References

CR 1. Bellomo R, Ronco C, Mehta R: Nomenclature for continuous renal replacement therapies, *Am J Kidney Dis* 28:S2-S7, 1996.

2. Bouman CS: High-volume hemofiltration as adjunctive therapy for sepsis and systemic inflammatory response syndrome: background, definition and a descriptive analysis of animal and human studies, *Adv Sepsis* 6:74-57, 2007.

3. Craig M: Slow extended daily dialysis (SLEDD) and continuous renal replacement therapies (CRRT). In Counts C, editor: *Core curriculum for nephrology nursing*, ed 5, Pitman, NJ, 2008, American Nephrology Nurses' Association, 132-229.

4. Dirkes S, Hodge K: Continuous renal replacement therapy in the adult intensive care unit: history and current trends, *Crit Care Nurse* 27:61-81, 2007.

5. Fiore GB, Ronco C: Principles and practice of internal hemodiafiltration, *Contrib Nephrol* 158:177-184, 2007.

6. Gibney N, et al: Volume management by renal replacement therapy in acute kidney injury, *Int J Artif Organs* 31:145-155, 2008.

CR 7. Giuliano K, Pysznik E: Renal replacement therapy in critical care: implementation of a unit-based CVVH program, *Crit Care Nurse* 18:40-45, 1998.

8. Goldstein-Fuchs J: Nutrition and chronic kidney disease. In Molzahn A, Butera E, editors: *Contemporary nephrology nursing: principles and practice*, ed 2, Pitman, NJ, 2006, American Nephrology Nurses' Association, 371-391.

CR 9. Jones S: Heat loss and continuous renal replacement therapy, *AACN Clin Issues* 15:223-230, 2004.

10. National Kidney Foundation (NKF): KDOQI clinical practice guidelines for vascular access: update 2006, *Am J Kidney Dis* 48:S176-S307, 2006.

11. Ricci Z, Ronco C: Dose and efficiency of renal replacement therapy: continuous replacement therapy versus intermittent hemodialysis versus extended daily dialysis, *Crit Care Med* 36:S229-S237, 2008.

CR 12. Rickard C, et al: Preventing hypothermia during continuous veno-venous haemodiafiltration: a randomized controlled study, *J Adv Nurs* 47:393-400, 2004.

13. Ronco C, et al: Potential interventions in sepsis-related acute kidney injury, *Clin J Am Soc Nephrol* 3:531-544, 2008.

14. Ronco C, et al: Outcome comparisons of intermittent and continuous therapy in acute kidney injury: what do they mean? *Int J Artif Organs* 31:213-220, 2008.

15. Pannu N, et al: Renal replacement therapy in patients with acute renal failure, *JAMA* 299:793-805, 2008.

16. Pronovost P, et al: An intervention to decrease catheter-related blood stream infections in the ICU, *N Engl J Med* 355:2725-2734, 2006.

17. Tolwani AJ, et al: Standard versus high-dose CVVHDF for ICU-related acute renal failure, *J Am Soc Nephrol* 19:1233-1238, 2008.

18. Uchino S, et al: Continuous renal replacement therapy: a worldwide practice survey, *Intensive Care Med* 33:1563-1570, 2007.

19. White RB: Vascular access for hemodialysis. In Molzahn A, Butera E, editors: *Contemporary nephrology nursing: principles and practice*, ed 2, Pitman, NJ, 2006, American Nephrology Nurses' Association, 559-578.

CR 20. Young E, et al: Incidence and influencing factors associated with exit site infections in temporary catheters for hemodialysis and apheresis, *Nephrol Nurs J* 32:41-50, 2005.

Additional Readings

Clark WR, et al: Recent clinical advances in the management of critically ill patients with acute renal failure, *Blood Purification* 24:487-498, 2006.

Oudemans-van Straaten HM, et al: Anticoagulation strategies in continuous renal replacement therapy: can the choice be evidence based? *Intensive Care Med* 32:188-202, 2006.

Palsson R, et al: Choice of replacement solution and anticoagulation in continuous venovenous hemofiltration, *Clin Nephrol* 65:34-42, 2006.

Hemodialysis

P U R P O S E :   Hemodialysis is performed for volume regulation, acid-base control, electrolyte regulation, management of azotemia, and the treatment of drug intoxications.

Sonia M. Astle

PREREQUISITE NURSING KNOWLEDGE

- Hemodialysis (Fig. 113-1) may be needed for the onset of acute renal failure, for maintenance therapy for patients with chronic renal failure, or for patients with acute drug intoxication.[9]
- Requirements for ensuring adequate therapy include: 1, an appropriate prescription; 2, a high level of nursing expertise; 3, an efficiently operating hemodialysis machine; 4, satisfactory access; 5, an informed patient; and 6, ongoing data review.[11]
- Knowledge of the principles of diffusion, ultrafiltration (UF), osmosis, oncotic pressure, and hydrostatic pressure as they pertain to fluid and solute management during dialysis is neccessary.[2,4,5]
  - *Diffusion* is the passive movement of solutes through a semipermeable membrane from an area of higher to lower concentration until equilibrium is reached.
  - *Ultrafiltration* is the bulk movement of solute and solvent through a semipermeable membrane with a pressure movement. This movement is usually achieved with positive pressure in the blood compartment of the hemofilter and negative pressure in the dialysate compartment. Blood and dialysate run countercurrent to each other (in opposite directions). The size of the solute molecules as compared with the size of molecules that can move through the semipermeable membrane determines the degree of UF.
  - *Osmosis* is the passive movement of solvent through a semipermeable membrane from an area of higher to lower concentration.
  - *Oncotic pressure* is the pressure exerted by plasma proteins that favors intravascular fluid retention and movement of fluid from the extravascular to the intravascular space.
  - *Hydrostatic pressure* is the force exerted by arterial blood pressure that favors the movement of fluid from the intravascular to the extravascular space.
  - *Absorption* is the process by which drug molecules pass through membranes and fluid barriers and into body fluids.
  - *Adsorption* is the adhesion of molecules (solutes) to the surface to the hemofilter, charcoal, or resin.
  - *Convective transport* is the rapid movement of fluid across a semipermeable membrane from an area of high pressure to an area of low pressure with transport of solutes. When water moves across a membrane along a pressure gradient, some solutes are carried along with the water and do not require a solute concentration gradient (also called solute drag). Convective transport is most effective for the removal of middle-molecular-weight and large-molecular-weight solutes.
- Vascular access is needed to perform hemodialysis and can be provided with a double-lumen vascular access catheter (VAC), an external arteriovenous (AV) shunt, or a surgically created AV anastomosis (e.g., fistula or graft). Common sites for the VAC include the internal jugular or subclavian vein. Common sites for the external shunt include the forearm (radial artery to cephalic vein) or the leg (posterior tibial artery to long saphenous vein). The AV fistula or graft is used for long-term dialysis management.
- The subclavian vein is not recommended for temporary access because of the increased incidence of vascular stenosis, which makes the vein of the ipsilateral arm unsuitable for chronic dialysis if needed. The internal jugular or leg veins are more commonly used.

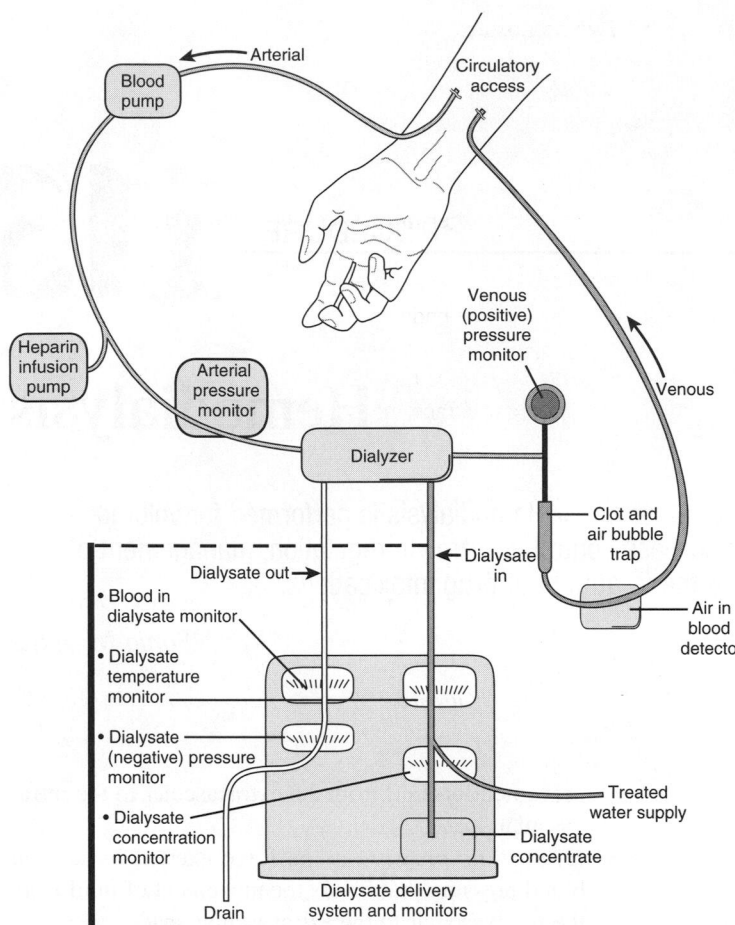

Figure 113-1   Components of a typical hemodialysis system. *(From Thompson JM, et al, editors: Mosby's manual of clinical nursing, St Louis, 1989, Mosby.)*

- Hemodialysis uses an artificial kidney (hemofilter, dialyzer) with a semipermeable membrane to create two separate compartments: the blood compartment and the dialysis solution (dialysate) compartment. The semipermeable membrane allows the movement of small molecules (e.g., electrolytes, urea, drugs) and middle-weight molecules (creatinine) from the patient's blood into the dialysate but is impermeable to larger molecules (blood cells, plasma proteins).

- Each dialyzer has four ports: two end ports for blood (in one end and out the other) and two side ports for dialysis solution (also in one end and out the other). In most cases, the blood and dialysate are run through the dialyzer in opposite or countercurrent directions.

- The hollow-fiber dialyzer is the most commonly used dialyzer. With this dialyzer, the blood flows through the center of hollow fibers and the dialysate flows around the outside of the hollow fibers. The advantages of hollow-fiber filters include a low priming volume, low resistance to flow, and high amount of surface area. The major disadvantage is the potential for clotting because of the small fiber size.

- Parallel-plate dialyzers are designed as sheets of membrane over supporting structures. Blood and dialysate pass through alternate spaces of the dialyzer. The major disadvantages of this type of filter are the increase in allergic dialyzer reactions and lower filter surface area.

- All dialyzers have UF coefficients; thus, the dialyzer selected varies in different clinical situations. The higher the UF coefficient, the more rapid the fluid removal. UF coefficients are determined with in vivo measurements done by each dialyzer manufacturer.

- Clearance refers to the ability of the dialyzer to remove metabolic waste products from the patient's blood. The blood flow rate, the dialysate flow rate, and the solute concentration affect clearance. Clearance occurs by the processes of diffusion, convection, and UF.[2-4,8-10]

- The blood circuit consists of blood lines, a blood pump, and various monitoring devices. The blood lines carry the blood to and from the patient. The blood pump controls the speed of the blood through the circuit. The monitoring devices include arterial and venous pressure monitors and an air detection monitor to prevent air entering the circuit from being returned to the patient.

- The dialysate is composed of water, a buffer (e.g., acetate or bicarbonate), and various electrolytes. Most solutions also contain glucose. The buffer helps neutralize acids that are generated as a result of normal cellular metabolism and usually are excreted by the kidney. The concentration of electrolytes is usual normal plasma concentrations, which help to create a concentration gradient for removal of excess electrolytes. The glucose, available in various concentrations, promotes the removal of plasma water.

- Heparin is usually used during dialysis to prevent clotting of the circuit. In patients with coagulopathies, normal saline solution flushes can be used to keep the blood circuit patent.[5] Heparin should be avoided in patients with a history of heparin-induced thrombocytopenia (HIT).[2,10]

- Because large volumes of water are used during treatments to generate the dialysate, the water must be purified before patient use to prevent patient exposure to potentially harmful substances present in the water supply (e.g., calcium carbonate, sodium chloride, and iron).

- Other extended renal replacement therapy techniques or "hybrid" techniques (sustained low-efficiency dialysis [SLED], extended daily dialysis [EDD]) generally use standard hemodialysis equipment and techniques with reduced blood flow and dialysate rates to gradually remove plasma water and solutes in the critically ill patient. They are used from 4 to 12 hours a day.[8]

- The adequacy of dialysis and assessment of the patient's residual renal function should be evaluated on a periodic basis. Adequacy of dialysis can be measured with urea kinetic modeling (Kt/V) or urea clearance.[2,4,14,15] Residual renal functioning can be monitored with urine creatinine clearance.[14,15] Collaboration with the nephrology team is necessary to monitor these parameters.[2,4,5]

EQUIPMENT

- Fluid shield face masks or goggles
- Sterile and nonsterile gloves
- Sterile gowns
- Sharps container
- Sterile normal saline (NS) solution, 3 L
- Two 10-mL syringes with blunt-tip cannulas
- Two 3-mL syringes
- Dressing supplies (sterile barrier, 4 × 4 gauze pads, transparent dressing, tape)
- Povidone-iodine, hypochlorite, or chlorhexidine bactericidal solution (follow institution standard)
- Heparin (1000 units/mL; for both priming and infusion, as ordered)
- Sterile bowl for soaking of 4 × 4 pads with bactericidal solution
- Antiseptic solution
- Hemostats
- Replacement fluid, as ordered
- Dialysate fluid, as ordered
- Alcohol wipes

Additional equipment for graft cannulation includes the following:

- Two 10-mL syringes with blunt-tip cannulas
- NS solution for injection
- Two fistula needles
- Chlorhexidine swabs
- 1% lidocaine and two tuberculin syringes with 25-gauge needles
- Two hemostats

Additional equipment for initiation of hemodialysis includes the following:

- Dialysis machine, tubing, dialyzer, and dialysate solution/water treatment setup

- Two hemostats
- One 30-mL syringe

Additional equipment, to have available depending on patient need, includes the following:

- One tourniquet (AV fistula only)
- Loading dose of heparin (if ordered)
- Equipment for termination of hemodialysis includes the following:
    - ❖ Four hemostats
    - ❖ 2 × 2 gauze pads
    - ❖ NS solution, 1000 mL
    - ❖ Four bandages, tape
    - ❖ Fluid shield face masks or goggles
    - ❖ Nonsterile gloves

PATIENT AND FAMILY EDUCATION

- Explain the procedure and review any questions the patient may have. ➥*Rationale:* Explanation provides information and may decrease patient anxiety.

- Explain the need for sterile technique for the duration of treatment. ➥*Rationale:* Explanation decreases the chance of systemic infection because pathogens can be transported throughout the entire body via the circulation.

- Explain the purpose of hemodialysis. ➥*Rationale:* Hemodialysis is necessary to perform the physiologic functions of the kidneys when renal failure is present.

- Explain the need for careful monitoring of the patient during the treatment for fluid and electrolyte imbalance. ➥*Rationale:* Dialysis treatment puts the patient at risk for imbalance because of the rapid movement of fluid and electrolytes from the patient during treatment.

- Explain the importance of input from the patient on how he or she is feeling during the treatment. ➥*Rationale:* Hypotension is a common occurrence during treatment; the patient may experience light-headedness or dizziness if hypotension is present. Patient knowledge of this possibility should help decrease anxiety.

- Explain the hemodialysis circuit setup to the patient. ➥*Rationale:* The patient and family must be aware that blood will be removed from the patient's body and will be visible during the hemodialysis treatment.

PATIENT ASSESSMENT AND PREPARATION

Patient Assessment

- Assess baseline vital signs, weight, neurologic status, physical assessment of all body systems, and fluid and electrolyte status. ➥*Rationale:* Patients in renal failure often have altered baseline assessments, both in physical assessment and in the laboratory values. Having this information before treatments are started is helpful so that interventions, including the dialysate, can be individualized. Alterations during treatment are common because of the rapid removal of fluid and solutes.

- Assess graft, fistula, or VAC site for signs or symptoms of infection. ➥*Rationale:* Because dialysis access sites are used frequently, infection is always a potential risk. Dialysis access sites should only be used for dialysis, and not for other intravenous access needs, except in an emergency situation. Insertion sites provide a portal of entry for infection, which may result in septicemia if unrecognized or untreated. If the insertion site appears to be infected, further interventions (e.g., site change, culture, and antibiotic treatment) may be necessary.

- Assess VAC patency and the ability to easily aspirate blood from both ports. ➟*Rationale:* Adequate blood flow is necessary during a treatment to facilitate optimal fluid and solute removal. Patent VAC ports are necessary for adequate blood flow.
- With AV fistula use, assess the site for presence of bruit, erythema, swelling, and quality of blood flow. ➟*Rationale:* Physical assessment of the fistula can indicate patency of the graft and the possible presence of infection.
- Assess the circulation to the distal parts of the access limb. ➟*Rationale:* The placement of a vascular access may compromise circulation.

Patient Preparation

- Verify correct patient with two identifiers. ➟*Rationale:* Prior to performing a procedure, the nurse should ensure the correct identification of the patient for the intended intervention.
- Ensure the patient understands preprocedural teachings. Answer questions as they arise, and reinforce information as needed. ➟*Rationale:* Understanding of previously taught information is evaluated and reinforced.
- Position the patient in a comfortable position (that also facilitates optimal blood flow through the access site and allows for the setup of a sterile field). ➟*Rationale:* Facilitation of patient comfort helps to minimize the amount of patient movement during treatment, which can change the amount of blood flow through the access site. Different access sites may require different patient positions to facilitate optimal blood flow.
- With AV fistula use, ask the patient whether he or she wants lidocaine used on the access site before the fistula is accessed. ➟*Rationale:* Patient comfort is promoted, and anxiety may be reduced.

Procedure for Hemodialysis

Steps	Rationale	Special Considerations
Cannulation of AV Fistula or Graft		
1. **HH**		
2. **PE**		
3. Wash access site for 1 full minute with antiseptic solution and a 4 × 4 gauze pad; rinse off with water.	Reduces the transmission of microorganisms.	
4. Place arm on an aseptic barrier.	Maintains aseptic technique.	
5. Starting at the site for insertion and moving out in concentric circles for 2 to 3 inches, wash access area with bactericidal swabs or soaked 2 × 2 gauze pad. (**Level B***)	Povidone-iodine, hypochlorite, or chlorhexidine bactericidal solution reduces the transmission of microorganisms. Allow all to air dry. Chlorhexidine has a rapid and prolonged antimicrobial effect; apply solution with back-and-forth friction scrub for 30 seconds.[2] Povidone-iodine solution serves as a bactericidal agent and requires a 2- to 3-minute scrub for bacteriostatic effect.[1,2,13,16-18] Hypochlorite has a rapid and prolonged antimicrobial effect.[4]	Skin asepsis is crucial; however, the most effective method for skin cleansing has not yet been established.
6. With two 10-mL syringes with blunt-tip cannulas, draw up prescribed flush solution in each syringe.	Prepares syringes for flushing fistula/graft.	Use an amount of heparinized saline solution that is consistent with institution standard. In some cases, only saline solution is used. Activated clotting times (ACTs) provide information regarding the patient's anticoagulation status.
7. Attach flush to fistula needle tubing and prime through fistula needles.	Prevents clotting of blood in fistula needles.	

*Level B: Well-designed controlled studies with results that consistently support a specific action, intervention, or treatment

Procedure for Hemodialysis—*Continued*

Steps	Rationale	Special Considerations
8. Clamp tubing.	Prevents loss of heparinized solution and backflow of blood.	
9. Apply tourniquet to upper portion of access limb (AV fistula cannulation).	Facilitates site determination for cannulation.	
10. Select site to be used. **(Level D*)**	Decreases recirculation of dialyzed blood.	Arterial site should be at least 3 inches from arterial anastomosis Venous needle must be in the direction of venous flow and, if possible, 3 inches or more from the arterial needle.[1,2,13,17]
11. Grasp butterfly wings or hub of fistula needle between thumb and index finger of dominant hand with needle tip bevel up.	Provides secure grasp of needle on cannulation.	Before insertion of fistula needle, lidocaine may be injected intradermally to make a small wheal, per patient preference.[2]
12. Remove needle guard.	Exposes fistula needle.	
13. Hold skin taut with nondominant hand.	Prevents rolling of vessel.	
14. With dominant hand, insert needle at a 45-degree angle to the skin (if lidocaine was used, use same puncture site for needle).		
A. AV fistula: Advance bevel up to hub of the needle.	Accesses arterial vascular system.	
B. AV graft: As soon as tip is through the graft, rotate needle 180 degrees and advance needle to hub, with bevel down. **(Level D)**	Accesses arterial vascular system. Bevel-down position prevents shearing of graft.[5,13]	Prevents shearing of graft material.
15. Remove tourniquet before infusing NS or heparin solution (AV fistula).	Prevents clotting.	
16. Unclamp needle and tubing clamp and aspirate blood.	Verifies correct placement and patency of access.	
17. Infuse flush solution; reclamp tubing.	Prevents clotting and backflow of blood.	
18. Secure needle with adhesive tape over insertion site.	Maintains angle of needle so that it floats freely in the vessel/graft.	
19. **Repeat Steps 11 to 18** for insertion of second needle.	Cannulation of venous site.	Hemodialysis can now be initiated.
20. Discard used equipment in appropriate receptacle.	Safely discards used supplies.	
21. 🅷🅷		
Accessing a VAC		
1. 🅷🅷		
2. 🅿🅴		
3. Prepare sterile field with sterile barriers, 2 × 2 pads, 4 × 4 pads, and transparent dressing.	Prepares material and maintains aseptic technique.	
4. Open sterile needles and syringes. Place on sterile field.	Readies equipment and maintains aseptic technique to prevent transmission of microorganisms.	

*Level D: Peer-reviewed professional organizational standards with clinical studies to support recommendations

Procedure continues on following page

Procedure | for Hemodialysis—*Continued*

Steps	Rationale	Special Considerations
5. Attach blunt-tip adaptors to 10-mL syringes; prepare flush solution according to institutional standard.	Prepares syringe for VAC flushing.	Refer to manufacturer's recommendations for amount of flush to be used.
6. Remove dressing from exit site, with care taken not to contaminate or dislodge cannula.	Allows access to exit site.	Inspect for signs and symptoms of exit-site infection: drainage, crusting, swelling, redness, exudate, or symptoms of pain at the site.
7. Discard soiled dressing and gloves in appropriate receptacle.	Safely discards used supplies.	
8. **HH**		
9. Apply sterile gloves.	Maintains aseptic technique.	
10. Place sterile barrier beneath VAC.	Sets up sterile field.	Do not touch VAC with gloves. Should gloves accidentally touch the VAC, a glove change is necessary to maintain aseptic technique.
11. Saturate four of the 4 × 4 pads in bactericidal solution. Using one of the soaked pads, perform a 1-minute scrub of the arterial port of the VAC. (**Level D***)	Povidone-iodine, chlorhexidine, and hypochlorite preparations are the only currently approved bactericidal agents.[1,2,7,13]	Be sure to remove any crust or drainage.
12. Wrap one bactericidal-soaked 4 × 4 pad around arterial port and leave in place for approximately 3 to 5 minutes.	Reduces transmission of microorganisms.	
13. After 3 to 5 minutes, remove soaked 4 × 4 pad and discard in appropriate receptacle.	Safely discards used supplies.	
14. Remove cap from arterial port of VAC and discard in appropriate receptacle.	Provides access to arterial port of VAC; Safely discards used supplies.	Be sure slide clamp is closed before removing arterial cap.
15. Attach an empty 3-mL syringe to the arterial port, open the slide clamp, and gently aspirate 3 mL of blood. Close the slide clamp, remove syringe, and discard in appropriate receptacle.	Removes indwelling heparin from the VAC port and assesses patency.	If difficulty is found in aspirating blood, notify physician or advanced practice nurse. If serum laboratory work is required, attach another empty syringe to the arterial port and aspirate required amount of blood.
16. **Repeat Steps 10 to 14** on the venous port.	Verifies patency of venous port; decreases transmission of microorganisms.	Observe for clots.
17. Attach flush syringe to arterial port, open slide clamp, and gently aspirate 2 to 3 mL of blood; slowly flush port; then close slide clamp.	Positive pressure prevents backup of blood into the port after flushing.	Syringe should be left attached to VAC port until replaced with dialyzer tubing connector.
18. **Repeat Step 16** on venous port.	Prevents clotting of blood until dialysis is initiated.	Syringe should be left attached to VAC port until replaced with dialyzer tubing connector.
19. Soak two 2 × 2 pads in bactericidal solution and cleanse connection site.	Minimizes the risk of infection.	

*Level D: Peer-reviewed professional organizational standards with clinical studies to support recommendations

Procedure for Hemodialysis—*Continued*

Steps	Rationale	Special Considerations
20. Remove flush syringe from arterial port. Attach arterial line from dialysis tubing securely to the arterial port of the VAC with a Luer-Lok connector. Place the venous line from the dialysis machine in the container for priming fluid discard. Leave the recirculating adaptor on the line.	Connects the patient to the dialysis machine.	
21. Tape connections securely.	Reduces the possibility of accidental disconnection of the lines.	Follow institution standard.
22. Open the clamps on the arterial port of the VAC and dialysis tubing, and turn on blood pump at a slow rate (50 to 100 mL/min).	Primes the dialysis line with blood.	
23. When the venous drip chamber located on the hemodialysis machine is pink, turn off the blood pump; clamp the venous line. Remove flush syringe from the venous port and securely attach the port to the venous tubing with a Luer-Lok connector.	Indicates blood has circulated through dialyzer to the venous line.	The venous port should be left in clamped position.
24. Secure connections.	Reduces the possibility of accidental disconnection of lines.	
25. Discard used equipment in appropriate receptacle.	Safely discards used supplies.	
26. **HH**		
27. Proceed to the initiation of hemodialysis.	Continues treatment.	
Disconnecting From the VAC		
1. **HH**		
2. **PE**		
3. Open syringes, caps, needles, and 4 × 4 gauze pads; place on sterile field.	Maintains aseptic technique.	
4. Fill two syringes with desired amount of heparin, depending on type of VAC used. Fill two 10-mL syringes with NS solution.	Heparin is used to maintain patency of access.[2]	Follow institutional standard regarding use of heparin.
5. Place sterile barrier under VAC ports.	Sets up a sterile field.	
6. Wrap both VAC ports with bactericidal-soaked 4 × 4 pads and scrub for 1 minute. **(Level D*)**	Reduces transmission of microorganisms. Maintains asepsis.	Povidone-iodine, chlorhexidine, and hypochlorite preparations are the only currently approved bactericidal agents.[1,2,7,13]
7. Remove nonsterile gloves, discard in appropriate receptacle.	Safely discards used supplies.	
8. **HH**		
9. Apply sterile gloves.	Maintains aseptic technique.	
10. Clamp arterial and venous ports.	Prevents blood loss from catheter.	

*Level D: Peer-reviewed professional organizational standards with clinical studies to support recommendations

Procedure continues on following page

Procedure for Hemodialysis—*Continued*		
Steps	**Rationale**	**Special Considerations**
11. Using the same bactericidal-soaked 4 × 4 pad to handle the dialysis tubing, disconnect arterial line from the arterial port of the VAC.		
12. Attach a 3- or 5-mL syringe with heparin to the arterial access and unclamp slide clamp; inject pre-scribed amount of heparin.	Maintains catheter patency by preventing clotting of blood.	Heparin dosage varies depending on type of catheter used and institution standard. In some cases, the catheter may be flushed with NS solution only. Use only the amount of hepa-rin listed on the catheter to avoid instilling anticoagulant into the patient. Label each catheter port with date, time, anticoagulant used, and nurse's initials.[2]
13. Clamp, disconnect syringe, and cap the arterial port.	Prevents loss of blood.	
14. **Repeat Steps 9 to 12** on venous port.	Maintains patency by preventing clotting of blood.	
15. Apply povidone-iodine ointment to the VAC insertion site at each dressing change.	Lowers incidence of catheter-related infections.	Follow institutional standard regarding use of ointment.
16. Apply dressing to VAC site at each hemodialysis treatment or when the dressing becomes damp, loosened, or soiled. **(Level B*)**	Prevents contamination of VAC exit site.[1,2,13,16-18]	Dressing should be maintained and changed at least weekly.
17. Discard used equipment in appropriate receptacle.	Safely discards used supplies.	
18. 🅷🅷		
Initiation and Termination of Hemodialysis		

1. Verify orders, which should include:
  A. Vascular access
  B. Hours of treatment
  C. Type of hemofilter/dialyzer
  D. Blood flow rate
  E. Anticoagulant type, concentra-tion, infusion rate, monitoring parameters
  F. Ultrafiltration goal
  G. Dialysate solution and rate (if used)
  H. Blood pressure and vital sign parameters
  I. Laboratory testing
(Level D*)
	Familiarizes nurse with the individual-ized patient treatment and reduces the possibility of error.[2,5,13]	Ensure patient weight and laboratory values are recorded before initiation of therapy.

2. Set up dialysis machine according to manufacturer's instructions.	Ensures safe and proper assembly and allows for testing of all patient alarms and the proper functioning of the machine before the VAC/graft/fistula is accessed.	
3. 🅷🅷		

*Level B: Well-designed controlled studies with results that consistently support a specific action, intervention, or treatment
*Level D: Peer-reviewed professional organizational standards with clinical studies to support recommendations

Procedure for Hemodialysis—Continued

Steps	Rationale	Special Considerations
4. **PE**		
5. Access VAC, graft, or fistula.	Allows access to site.	
6. If patient has a graft or fistula, wash access arm for 1 full minute with antiseptic solution and a sterile 4 × 4 gauze pad. Place arm on sterile barrier.	Reduces transmission of microorganisms and establishes a sterile field.	
7. Connect arterial access to arterial blood line with a Luer-Lok connector.	Provides a circuit between the patient and the dialyzer.	
8. Place the venous dialyzer tubing line into the retaining clamps of the fluid receptacle on the side of the dialysis machine.	Prevents contamination of venous tubing.	Be careful not to immerse the end of the venous line below the fluid level.
9. Tape arterial cannula connections securely.	Prevents potential catheter disconnection.	
10. Remove clamp from arterial line.	Permits flow of blood.	
11. Adjust blood pump to 50 to 100 mL/min until blood reaches the venous drip chamber.	Slow rate prevents symptoms of rapid blood loss and allows for assessment of blood flow from the arterial line.	Heparin loading dose, if ordered, may be given via bolus in arterial line.
12. Turn off blood pump.	Prevents blood loss from dialyzer and cannula.	
13. Clamp the end of the venous tubing below the drip chamber with a bulldog clamp.	Prevents introduction of air.	
14. Remove venous line tubing from fluid container, remove the recirculation adaptor, and connect to the venous access cannula with a Luer-Lok connector.	Completes pathway circuit for return of blood from the dialyzer to the patient.	
15. Tape venous connections securely.	Prevents potential catheter disconnection.	
16. Remove clamp from venous tubing.	Permits flow of blood.	
17. Turn on blood pump and adjust blood flow rate.	Initiates flow of blood from patient to the dialyzer.	
18. Immediately turn on foam detector switch from bypass to alarm position.	Sets the foam detector alarm monitor to "on."	The air/foam monitor detects minute air leaks.
19. Adjust the blood level in the arterial and venous drip chambers to three quarters full.	Prevents accumulation of air in tubing and dialyzer.	
20. Turn dialyzer over so that arterial (red) port is at the top.	Establishes countercurrent flow.	
21. If patient is receiving systemic heparinization, set parameters on heparin infusion pump as prescribed.	Provides anticoagulation.	
22. Secure cannula connections.	Additional precaution against accidental disconnection.	
23. Slowly increase blood pump speed to prescribed rate while continuing to assess patient (level of consciousness, symptoms of chest pain, dysrhythmias, and changes in hemodynamic variables).	Prevents complications of rapid removal of blood.	If any question exists as to how well the patient will tolerate hemodialysis, the pump speed should be started at 100 mL/min and gradually increased to goal.

Procedure continues on following page

Procedure for Hemodialysis—*Continued*

Steps	Rationale	Special Considerations
24. Set arterial and venous alarm parameters.	Sets the safety alarm system.	
25. Observe the patient's transmembrane pressure (TMP) display.	Removes desired UF.	To calculate TMP, the following formula may be used: Weight to be removed $\times$ 500 mL $-$ KUF = TMP With *KUF* the coefficient of ultrafiltration of the dialyzer. Each type/size of dialyzer has a different KUF, which can be obtained from the package insert.
26. Set TMP or negative pressure and alarms.	Allows for UF.	Most machines automatically adjust based on treatment time and volume removal goal.
27. Discard used equipment in appropriate receptacle.	Safely discards used supplies.	
28. 🅷🅷		
29. Continuously monitor patient status and machine function throughout treatment.	Prevents complications and minimizes effects of fluid and electrolyte shifts.	Patient assessment should include vital signs and symptoms related to fluid and electrolyte shifts (e.g., cramping, hypotension, nausea, vomiting). Monitor the machine for blood flow rate, arterial and venous pressure readings, dialysate pressure, TMP, and blood circuit for clotting or air.

Termination

Steps	Rationale	Special Considerations
1. 🅷🅷		
2. 🅿🅴		
3. Set the arterial, venous, and dialysate pressure alarms to the maximum low/high limits.	Prevents machine from alarming when terminating dialysis as pressures drop.	
4. Turn off TMP or negative pressure.	Removes negative pressure, thereby stopping UF.	
5. Turn off the heparin infusion pump.	Discontinues heparinization before the end of dialysis, thus allowing clotting times to return to normal shortly after treatment.	May be done 30 minutes to 1 hour before termination of treatment, depending on institutional standard.
6. Decrease the blood pump flow rate.	Reduces blood flow.	
7. Check the amount of NS solution left in the circuit for adequate blood return; hang a new bag if necessary.	Minimizes the danger of air embolism on return of blood to patient.	NS solution (100 to 300 mL) is used to return blood to patient.
8. Maintain the blood level in the arterial and venous drip chambers at three quarters full.	Prevents air in tubing and dialyzer.	
9. Turn off the blood pump.	Stops blood flow.	
10. Unclamp the NS solution flush line on the arterial side of the blood circuit. Allow flush to infuse until lines are pink-tinged.	Clears the line of blood.	

Procedure for Hemodialysis—*Continued*

Steps	Rationale	Special Considerations
11. Clamp the arterial tubing between patient and blood pump and on the vascular access.	Prevents loss of blood if the tubing becomes separated.	
12. Place a sterile 4 × 4 under the vascular access. Disconnect the arterial dialysis tubing from the arterial vascular access	Prevents contamination.	
13. Turn on blood pump and simultaneously unclamp the patient end connector of the arterial tubing.	Promotes slow return of blood in tubing back to patient.	
14. Clear the blood tubing and dialyzer with saline solution until rinse-back is achieved.	Promotes rinse-back of blood to patient.	Satisfactory rinse-back is achieved when venous chamber has pink-tinged fluid.
15. Turn off blood pump.	Terminates flow of blood.	
16. Clamp venous access.	Prevents backflow of blood.	
17. When using a VAC, instill and dwell the catheter ports with prescribed anticoagulant.	Prevents clotting of catheter ports.	Follow manufacturers recommendation for amount of anticoagulant to be instilled in each port of the VAC. Follow institution standard for use of anticoagulant. .
18. AV fistula/AV graft: When fistula needles are used, remove both cannulas from patient's access site, one at a time. With a sterile 2 × 2 gauze pad, apply moderate pressure to access site until bleeding has stopped.	Discontinues vascular access. Promotes hemostasis at access sites.	
19. Dress access site with sterile 2 × 2 gauze pad and bandages.	Provides protective barrier.	
20. Sanitize single-patient machine according to established procedure.	Reduces transmission of microorganisms and readies it for future use.	
21. Dispose of used equipment in appropriate receptacle.	Safely discards used supplies.	
22. **HH**		

Expected Outcomes

- Catheter/fistula/graft accessed with no complications
- Blood easily aspirated from the access site
- Pulsating blood flow in the dialysis tubing set
- Accumulated waste products removed
- Acid-base balance restored
- Blood urea nitrogen (BUN) and creatinine values restored to baseline levels
- Electrolyte values restored to baseline levels
- Accumulated fluid removed; dry weight restored
- Nutritional status maintained

Unexpected Outcomes

- Clotting or decreased patency of the AV fistula or catheter lumens
- Poor blood flow
- Bleeding from the insertion site or access site
- Signs or symptoms of infection at the insertion or access site
- Dislodgment of the catheter
- Decreased circulation in the vascular access limb
- Hematoma formation at the accessed site
- Physiologic complications (dysrhythmias, chest pain, fluid-electrolyte imbalance, hypotension, seizures, nausea and vomiting, headaches, muscle cramping, dyspnea)
- Technical problems with the dialysis machine

Procedure continues on following page

Patient Monitoring and Care

Steps	Rationale	Reportable Conditions
		These conditions should be reported if they persist despite nursing interventions.
1. Perform and record a predialysis weight and daily weights. **(Level D*)**	Predialysis weight is an important factor in deciding how much UF is needed during treatment. It also helps to guide ongoing treatment.[2,4-6]	• Abnormal increase or decrease in weight
2. Perform ongoing assessments, including the following: A. Vital signs B. Jugular vein distention C. Presence of edema D. Intake and output E. Neurologic assessment F. Pulmonary assessment **(Level D)**	Provides information in response to treatment.[2,4-6] Monitors for complications.	• Hypotension • Hypertension • Tachycardia/bradycardia • Tachypnea/bradypnea • Fever • Hypothermia • Jugular vein distention • Crackles • Edema • Change in level of consciousness, dizziness • Change in cardiac rhythm
3. Monitor the circulation to the extremity where the graft/fistula is located. A. Capillary refill B. Pulses distal to access C. Color/temperature of extremity D. Sensation **(Level D)**	To assess for any decrease in perfusion distal to the graft site.[1,2,10,13]	• Diminished capillary refill • Diminished or absent peripheral pulses • Pale, mottled, or cyanotic extremity • Cool to touch • Diminished or absent movement • Pain
4. Monitor electrolytes and glucose during treatment as per institutional standard.	Must be monitored because of continued fluid and electrolyte shifts during treatment.	• Hyperkalemia or hypokalemia • Hypernatremia or hyponatremia • Hypercalcemia or hypocalcemia • Hyperglycemia or hypoglycemia • Hyperphosphatemia or hypophosphatemia
5. Administer medications to correct electrolyte abnormalities as ordered during treatment.	Patients with renal failure are predisposed to many electrolyte abnormalities. During dialysis, several medications/electrolyte replacements may be given, as ordered for individual patients.[1,16]	
6. Monitor the dialysis circuit (e.g., occlusions, kinks, or leaks; blood or clots in vascular access lines). **(Level D)**	Disconnections or introduction of air into the circuit are always possible during treatment. Bleeding or exsanguination also can occur.[1,2,4-6] Clotting of the circuit is a potential complication. If hemofilter becomes excessively clotted, the extracorporeal blood volume should be returned to the patient quickly. Blood leaks from dialyzer into the dialysate may occur and necessitate termination of treatment. Venous or arterial pressures, which are out of range, may indicate dialyzer or access malfunction.	• Disconnections, cracks, or leaks • Bleeding • Excessive clotting • Blood leaks/hemofilter rupture • Malfunction of dialyzer or access

*Level D: Peer-reviewed professional organizational standards with clinical studies to support recommendations

Patient Monitoring and Care —*Continued*

Steps	Rationale	Reportable Conditions
7. Monitor UF for rate, clarity, and air bubbles. **(Level D*)**	A decrease in UF production can occur from clotting of the dialyzer.[2,13] Pink or blood-tinged UF is indicative of filter leak or rupture.	• Decrease in UF production • Change in color or characteristic of UF • Air in UF
8. Administer heparin as ordered. **(Level D)**	Heparin is often used to prevent clotting of the circuit.[2,10,13] Heparin dose varies according to patient condition and laboratory values.	• Suspicion of clotting in the circuit
9. Monitor anticoagulation as per institutional standard.	Because heparin is commonly used to prevent system clotting, coagulation studies should be routinely monitored.	• Abnormal coagulation studies

10. Monitor the patency of vascular access.
  A. Gently palpate along entire length of graft or over access for a thrill (feeling of vibration or purring under fingers).
  B. Auscultate for the presence of bruit (sounds like rushing water). **(Level D)**
	Bleeding can occur from either the venous or arterial catheter or AV fistula. Clotting of the access can occur.[1,2,12]
	Absence of a bruit does not confirm occlusion. Use Doppler scan if unable to hear a bruit with a stethoscope.
		• Decrease in access function or patency
		• Absence of bruit or thrill

11. Monitor the patient for complications associated with dialysis treatment. **(Level B*)**	Several complications are possible with dialysis.[1,2,4,12,13,16,18]	• Muscle cramps • Dialysis disequilibrium (headache, nausea/vomiting, hypertension, decreased sensorium, convulsions, coma) • Air embolism • Dialyzer reaction (hypotension, pruritus, back pain, angioedema, anaphylaxis) • Hypoxemia • Abnormal laboratory values

12. Administer medications to correct metabolic abnormalities as ordered.	Patients with renal failure are predisposed to many metabolic abnormalities. Common medications administered to patients with renal failure include the following[2,7,16]:
	  A. Vitamin D and calcium carbonate to increase the serum calcium level and prevent or treat bone disease.
	  B. Erythropoietin and iron to treat anemia.
	  C. Deferoxamine mesylate to remove excessive iron.
	  D. Phosphate binders to treat hyperphosphatemia.	

*Level B: Well-designed controlled studies with results that consistently support a specific action, intervention, or treatment
*Level D: Peer-reviewed professional organizational standards with clinical studies to support recommendations

Procedure continues on following page

Patient Monitoring and Care —*Continued*

Steps	Rationale	Reportable Conditions
	E. Renal diet may also be prescribed, with adjusted protein, potassium, phosphorus, carbohydrate, and fluid intake that takes into account the patient's current catabolic state, residual renal function, adequacy of dialysis, and removal of amino acids with dialysis.[2,7]	
13. Place a sign above patient's bed indicating which limb has the vascular access (AV graft or fistula).	Blood pressures and blood draws should not be done on the access arm.	
14. Follow institution standard for assessing pain. Administer analgesia as prescribed.	Identifies need for pain interventions.	• Continued pain despite pain interventions

Documentation

Documentation should include the following:
- Patient and family education
- Date and time of treatment initiation
- Condition of catheter or AV fistula regarding patency, quality of blood flow, ease of access procedure
- Condition of insertion site and any signs or symptoms of infection
- Presence of bruit if an AV fistula is used
- Needle gauge size used for cannulation
- Type of machine used for dialysis
- Pain assessment, interventions, and effectiveness.

- Arterial and venous pressures during treatment
- Pump speed
- Length of dialysis treatment
- Vital signs throughout the treatments
- Unexpected outcomes
- Any medications/intravenous (IV) fluids given during treatment
- Nursing interventions
- Predialysis and postdialysis weight
- Laboratory assessment data

References

CR 1. Allon M: Dialysis catheter-related bacteremia: treatment and prophylaxis, *Am J Kidney Dis* 44:779-791, 2004.

2. Amato RL, et al: Hemodialysis. In Counts CS, editor: *Core curriculum for nephrology nursing,* ed 5, Pitman, NJ, 2008, American Nephrology Nurses Association, 657-681.

3. Bouman CS: High-volume hemofiltration as adjunctive therapy for sepsis and systemic inflammatory response syndrome: background, definition and a descriptive analysis of animal and human studies, *Adv Sepsis* 6:74-77, 2007.

CR 4. Burrows-Hudson S, Prowant B: *Nephrology nursing standards of practice and guidelines for care,* Pitman, NJ, 2005, American Nephrology Nurses Association.

5. Challinor P: Hemodialysis. In Thomas N, editor: *Renal nursing,* ed 3, Edinburg, 2008, Ballierre Tindall, 181-222.

CR 6. Dinwiddie LC: Managing catheter dysfunction for better patient outcomes: a team approach, *Nephrol Nurs J* 31:653-660, 2004.

7. Goldstein-Fuchs J: Nutrition and chronic kidney disease. In Molzahn A, Butera E, editors: *Contemporary nephrology nursing: principles and practice,* ed 2, Pitman, NJ, 2006, American Nephrology Nurses' Association, 371-391.

CR 8. Golper T: Hybrid renal replacement therapies in critically ill patients: sepses, kidney and multiple organ dysfunction, *Contrib Nephrol* 114:278-283, 2004.

CR 9. Kellum JA, et al: The 3rd International Consensus Conference of the Acute Dialysis Quality Initiative (ADQI), *Int J Artif Organs* 28:441-444, 2005.

CR 10. Kraus MA: Renal replacement therapy, part 1: indications and modalities, In Molitoris BA, editor: *Critical care nephrology,* London, 2005, Remedica, 151-156.

11. Latham CE: Hemodialysis technology. In Molzahn A, Butera E, editors: *Contemporary nephrology nursing: principles and practice,* ed 2, Pitman, NJ, 2006, American Nephrology Nurses' Association, 548.

12. MacRae JM, et al: The cardiovascular effects of arteriovenous fistulas in chronic kidney disease: a cause for concern? *Semin Dialysis* 19:349-352, 2006.

13. National Kidney Foundation (NKF): KDOQI clinical practice guidelines for vascular access: update 2006, *Am J Kidney Dis* 48:S176-S307, 2006.

CR 14. Palevsky PM, et al: Design of the VA/NIH Acute Renal Failure Trial Network (AN) Study: intensive versus conventional renal support in acute renal failure, *Clin Trials* 2:423-435, 2005.

15. Palevsky PM, et al: Intensity of renal support in critically ill patients with acute kidney injury, *N Engl J Med* 359: 7-20, 2008.

16. Robins DC: Hemodialysis: prevention and management of treatment complications. In Molzahn A, Butera E, editors: *Contemporary nephrology nursing: principles and practice,* ed 2, Pitman, NJ, 2006, American Nephrology Nurses' Association, 581-623.

17. White RB: Vascular access for hemodialysis. In Molzahn A, Butera E, editors: *Contemporary nephrology nursing: principles and practice,* ed 2, Pitman, NJ, 2006, American Nephrology Nurses' Association, 559-578.

[CR] 18. Young EJ, et al: Incidence and influencing factors associated with exit site infections in temporary catheters for hemodialysis and apheresis, *Nephrol Nurs J* 32:41-50, 2005.

Additional Readings

Ball L: The buttonhole technique for arteriovenous fistula cannulation, *Nephrol Nurs J* 33:299-304, 2006.

Bellomo R, et al: Acute renal failure: definition, outcome measures, animal models, fluid therapy and information technology needs: the Second International Consensus Conference of the Acute Dialysis Quality Initiative (ADQI) Group, *Crit Care* 8:R204-R212, 2004.

[CR] Burrowes JD, Van Houten G: Herbs and dietary supplement use in patients with stage 5 chronic kidney disease, *Nephrol Nurs J* 33:85-88, 2006.

Fry AC, Farrington K: Management of acute renal failure, *Postgrad Med J* 82:106-116, 2006.

Desai AA et al: Identifying best practices in dialysis care: results of cognitive interviews and a national survey of dialysis providers, *Clin J Am Soc Nephrol* 3:1066-1076, 2008.

Denhaerynck K, et al: Prevalence and consequences of nonadherence to hemodialysis regimens, *Am J Crit Care* 16:222-235, 2007.

[CR] Gomez N: Practice issues in nephrology nursing: focus on issues from ANNA's special interest groups: National Symposium Special Interest Group presentations, *Nephrol Nurs J/J Am Nephrol Nurs Assoc* 30:333-341, 2003.

Liangos O: Epidemiology and outcomes of acute renal failure in hospitalized patients: a national survey, *Clin J Am Soc Nephrol* 1:43-51, 2006.

[CR] Metta R, et al: Spectrum of acute renal failure in the intensive care unit: the PICARD experience, *Kidney Int* 66: 1613-1621, 2004.

Ostermann M, et al: Acute kidney injury in the intensive care unit according to RIFLE, *Crit Care Med* 35:1837-1843, 2007.

Overberger P, et al: Management of renal replacement therapy in acute kidney injury: a survey of practitioner prescribing practices, *Clin J Am Soc Nephrol* 2:623-630, 2007.

Pupim LB, et al: Nutrition and metabolism in kidney disease, *Semin Nephrol* 26:134-157, 2006.

Rauf AA, et al: Intermittent hemodialysis versus continuous renal replacement therapy for acute renal failure: I: the intensive care unit: an observational outcomes analysis, *J Intensive Care Med* 23:195-203, 2008.

[CR] Uchino S, et al: Acute renal failure in critically ill patients: a multinational, multicenter study, *JAMA* 294:813-818, 2005.

Peritoneal Dialysis

PURPOSE: Peritoneal dialysis is used for the removal of fluid and toxins, the regulation of electrolytes, and the management of azotemia.

Sonia M. Astle

PREREQUISITE NURSING KNOWLEDGE

- Peritoneal dialysis (PD) works on the principles of diffusion and osmosis; thus, a basic knowledge of these concepts is necessary.
  - *Diffusion* is the passive movement of solutes through a semipermeable membrane from an area of higher concentration to one of lower concentration. When this concept is applied to peritoneal dialysis, diffusion occurs because the patient's blood contains waste products (solute), which give it a higher osmolarity (concentration) than the dialysate. So, waste products in the blood diffuse across the semipermeable membrane into the dialysate solution.
  - *Osmosis* is the passive movement of solvent through a semipermeable membrane from an area of lower concentration to one of higher concentration. The dextrose added to the dialysate gives it a higher osmotic gradient than that of the patient's blood. So, excess water in the blood is pulled into the dialysate via osmosis.
- PD uses the peritoneal membrane as the semipermeable membrane for both fluid and solutes.[4,10,14]
- Sterile dialysis fluid (dialysate) is infused into the peritoneal cavity of the abdomen through a flexible catheter (Fig. 114-1).
- A small-framed adult can usually tolerate 2 to 2.5 L of dialysate, whereas a large-framed adult may be able to tolerate up to 3 L in the abdominal cavity. The larger the volume of dialysate, the more effective the removal of blood urea nitrogen (BUN) and creatinine[6,9,11]; however, peritoneal clearance may be improved with more frequent exchange rather than an increase in the

exchange volume.[5] The most limiting factor of the volume of dialysate is that it may cause direct pressure on the diaphragm and cause a compromise of respiratory excursion.[4,14,15] The PD dialysate contains higher concentrations of glucose than normal serum levels. These higher concentrations aid in the removal of water via osmosis and small-to-middle-weight molecules (urea, creatinine) via diffusion. Several concentrations of glucose are available in commercially prepared dialysate solutions. The higher the concentration of glucose in the dialysate, the greater the amount of fluid removal. Icodextrin, a relatively new alternative to glucose solutions, may be used as the osmotic agent. This glucose polymer is metabolized to maltose and is not readily absorbed.[6,8,12,13]

- PD involves repeated fluid exchanges or cycles. Each cycle has three phases: instillation, dwell, and drain.
  - During the instillation phase, the dialysate is infused via gravity into the patient's peritoneal cavity through a peritoneal catheter.[1,2,12]
  - During the dwell phase, the dialysate remains in the patient's peritoneal cavity, allowing osmosis and diffusion to occur. Dwell time varies based on the patient's clinical need.
  - During the drain phase, the dialysate and excess extracellular fluid, wastes, and electrolytes are drained via gravity from the peritoneal cavity via the catheter.
- PD can be performed either manually with a dialysis administration set with a drainage bag or with a cycler machine (Fig. 114-2). With a cycler machine, multiple exchanges are programmed into the machine and run automatically. Cycler machines are infrequently found in the hospital setting but are often used by outpatients for evening and night exchanges.

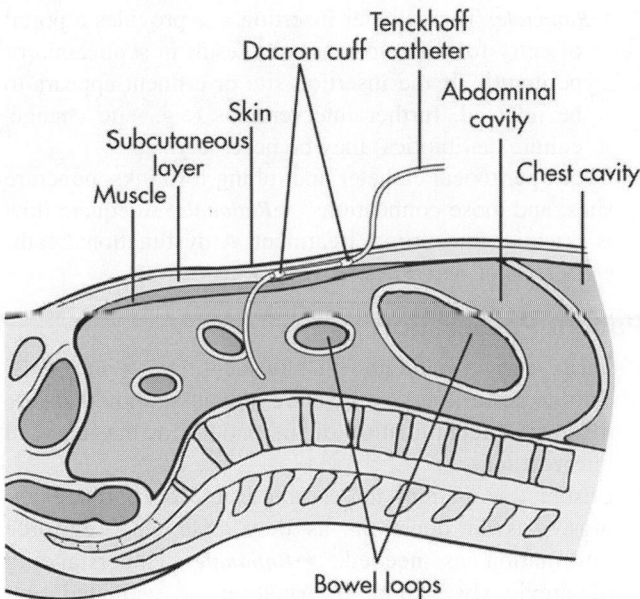

FIGURE 114-1 Tenckhoff catheter used in peritoneal dialysis. *(From Lewis SM et al (2007). Medical-surgical nursing: Assessment and management of clinical problems, ed 7, Mosby.)*

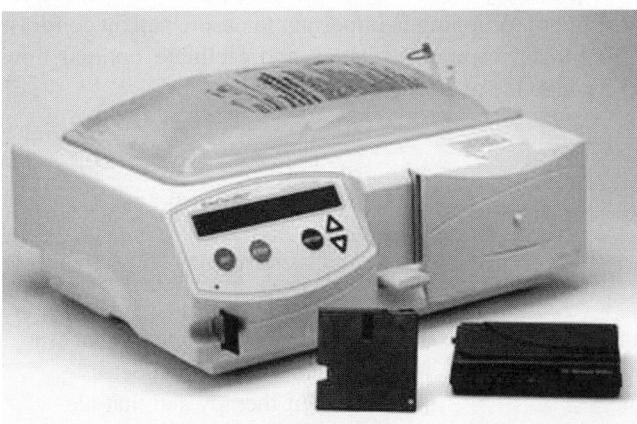

FIGURE 114-2 Baxter HomeChoice Pro PD Cycler. *(Courtesy Baxter International, Inc, Deerfield, IL.)*

- PD catheters can become clogged with the build-up of fibrin. Heparin is sometimes added to the dialysate or used as a separate flush to prevent occlusion.[1,4,9,14,15]
- PD dialysate should be warmed to the appropriate temperature in a commercial warmer. *Never* warm the solution in a standard microwave oven, which heats unevenly and does not regulate the fluid temperature.[14,15]
- After each cycle of PD, assess the patient's vital signs, fluid balance, and any signs of infection and communicate abnormal findings to the physician.
- The adequacy of dialysis and assessment of the patient's residual renal function should be evaluated on a periodic basis. Adequacy of dialysis can be measured with urea kinetic modeling (Kt/V) or urea clearance.[6,11] Residual renal functioning can be monitored with urine creatinine clearance. Collaboration with the nephrology team is necessary to monitor these parameters.

EQUIPMENT

- Masks
- Goggles or fluid shield face masks
- Sterile and nonsterile gloves
- Sterile 4 × 4 gauze pads
- Sterile containers
- Povidone-iodine, chlorhexidine, or hypochlorite solutions
- Tape
- Sterile barriers
- Plastic hemostats
  Additional equipment, to have available depending on patient need, includes the following:
- Equipment for culture
- Equipment for cell count/hematocrit
  Additional equipment for initiation of PD includes the following:
- PD administration set with drainage bag
- Warmed dialysate solution
- Cycler with tubing (if being used)
  Additional equipment for termination of PD includes the following:
- Sterile catheter caps
- Labels for catheter

PATIENT AND FAMILY EDUCATION

- Explain the purpose of PD. ➤*Rationale:* PD is necessary to perform the physiologic functions of the kidneys when renal failure is present. PD uses the lining inside the abdomen, called the peritoneal cavity, as a filter to clean the blood and remove excess fluid.
- Explain the procedure and review any questions. ➤*Rationale:* Explanation provides information and may decrease patient anxiety.
- Explain the need for careful sterile technique when the abdominal catheter is accessed. ➤*Rationale:* Sterile technique is used to decrease the chance of peritoneal infection because pathogens can be introduced into the abdominal cavity via the catheter.
- Explain the three phases of PD. ➤*Rationale:* Because each phase is different, the patient must be informed of all three phases and the purposes, interventions, and possible complications of each.
- Explain the potential for feelings of fullness and possibly shortness of breath during the dwell phase. ➤*Rationale:* The pressure of the dialysate fluid on the diaphragm may cause the patient to have these feelings, which are normal for the dwell phase.

PATIENT ASSESSMENT AND PREPARATION

Patient Assessment

- Obtain baseline vital signs, respiratory status, abdominal assessment, blood glucose level, and pertinent laboratory results (potassium, sodium, calcium, phosphorus, magnesium, renal function tests, complete blood count). ➤*Rationale:*

Patients in renal failure often have altered baseline assessments, according to both physical assessment and laboratory values. The availability of this information before treatments are started is helpful so that interventions, including the type and amount of dialysate fluid, can be individualized.

- Assess volume status, as indicated by the following:
  - ❖ Skin turgor
  - ❖ Mucous membranes
  - ❖ Edema
  - ❖ Breath sounds
  - ❖ Weight
  - ❖ Intake and output
  - ➤➤*Rationale:* PD is often initiated for the control of hypervolemia.[9] Knowledge of a patient's pretreatment volume status is essential to allow for the individualization of treatment goals and interventions.
- Assess PD catheter and abdominal exit site for signs and symptoms of infection, leakage or drainage, or signs and symptoms of peritonitis[3,6-9,15]:
  - ❖ Cloudy or bloody dialysate solution
  - ❖ Leakage at the catheter site
  - ❖ Subcutaneous fluid in abdomen, groin, or upper thighs
  - ❖ Abdominal pain
  - ❖ Fever
  - ❖ Chills
  - ❖ Rebound tenderness

➤➤*Rationale:* The catheter insertion site provides a portal of entry for infection that can result in septicemia or peritonitis. If the insertion site or effluent appears to be infected, further interventions (e.g., site change, culture, antibiotics) may be necessary.

- Check peritoneal catheter and tubing for kinks, puncture sites, and loose connections. ➤➤*Rationale:* Adequate flow is essential for optimal treatment. A dysfunctional catheter can alter outcomes.

Patient Preparation

- Verify correct patient with two identifiers. ➤➤*Rationale:* Prior to performing a procedure, the nurse should ensure the correct identification of the patient for the intended intervention.
- Ensure that patient understands preprocedural teachings. Answer questions as they arise, and reinforce information as needed. ➤➤*Rationale:* Understanding of previously taught information is evaluated and reinforced.
- Assist the patient in applying a mask. ➤➤*Rationale:* The risk for airborne and nasal pathogens is decreased.
- Reposition patient to a comfortable position. ➤➤*Rationale:* Proper positioning is important to ensure patient comfort, optimize respiratory status, and facilitate optimal flow through the abdominal catheter.

Procedure   for Peritoneal Dialysis

Steps	Rationale	Special Considerations
PD Initiation and Discontinuation		
1. Verify PD orders, which should include: A. Manual or automated delivery system B. Dialysis solution type, volume, dextrose/icodextrin and calcium concentrations, and additional medications C. Fill volume/time, dwell time, drain volume/time D. Vital sign parameters E. Laboratory testing	Familiarizes nurse with the individualized patient treatment and reduces the possibility of error.	Ensure that patient weight and laboratory values are recorded before initiation of therapy and that the patient is wearing a mask and is properly positioned.
2. **HH**		
3. **PE**		
4. Remove dialysate bag from protective pouch; check for expiration date, clarity, and leaks.	Assesses for contamination of dialysate.	Consider obtaining and recording bag weight to accurately assess intake and output.
5. Connect dialysate bag to PD administration set; prime tubing with dialysate; clamp tubing.	Fills tubing with dialysate; decreases chance of introducing air into the abdominal cavity.	Signs of air instillation into the peritoneum include referred shoulder and back pain.
6. Prepare sterile field. Open sterile container package or sterile 4 × 4 gauze packs.		

Procedure   for Peritoneal Dialysis—*Continued*

Steps	Rationale	Special Considerations
7. Pour povidone-iodine, hypochlorite, or chlorhexidine bactericidal solution (follow institution standard) into sterile container or onto sterile 4 × 4 gauze pads.	Maintains aseptic technique.	
8. Remove dressing covering catheter connector site and discard.	Allows visualization of catheter connector site.	Note odor or drainage on the old dressing.
9. Remove nonsterile gloves.		
10. **HH**		
11. Apply sterile gloves.	Maintains aseptic technique.	
12. Saturate four of the 4 × 4 pads in bactericidal solution. Using one of the soaked pads, perform a 1-minute scrub of the catheter-cap connection.	Reduces transmission of microorganisms.	Be sure to remove any crust or drainage.
13. Wrap one bactericidal-soaked 4 × 4 gauze pad around catheter-cap connection; leave in place for approximately 3 to 5 minutes.	Reduces transmission of microorganisms.	
14. After 3 to 5 minutes, remove 4 × 4 gauze pad; discard in appropriate receptacle.	Safely discards used supplies.	
15. With the nondominant hand, pick up the PD catheter with a sterile 4 × 4 gauze pad; remove cap.	Maintains aseptic technique.	
16. Connect catheter to dialysate administration set.	Ensure a tight connection.	

Instillation Cycle

Steps	Rationale	Special Considerations
17. Clamp the tubing to the drainage bag and unclamp any clamps between the dialysate and the patient.	Provides open access between catheter and PD tubing, allowing inflow of dialysate.	
18. Set flow rate as prescribed.		Time for inflow depends on the height of the dialysate bag, position of patient, and the patency of the catheter.
19. When inflow is complete, clamp the dialysate tubing and the patient's catheter. Disconnect the PD administration tubing and empty dialysate bag from the patient's catheter per manufacturer's instructions.	Clamping prevents backflow. Dwell cycle is now beginning.	
20. Remove gloves; discard soiled equipment in appropriate receptacle.	Safely discards used supplies.	
21. **HH**		

Dwell Cycle

Steps	Rationale	Special Considerations
22. Begin dwell cycle.	Allow for exchange across the peritoneal membrane of fluid, toxins, and electrolytes.	Dwell time is determined by the number of cycles needed in a 24-hour period. If a cycler is used, the cycles are preprogrammed.

Procedure continues on following page

Procedure | for Peritoneal Dialysis—*Continued*

Steps	Rationale	Special Considerations
Drain Cycle		
23. **HH**		
24. Clamp the tubing from the dialysate to the catheter.	Prevents backflow.	If a cycler is used, follow manufacturer's instructions for system setup.
25. Place the drainage bag below midabdominal area. Unclamp the drainage bag and the catheter to permit drainage from peritoneal cavity into the drainage bag.	Enhances gravity.	Allow 15 to 20 minutes for outflow; observe and record characteristics (cloudy, bloody, clear, yellow) and amount of outflow. Reposition patient if flow stops or is sluggish. Notify physician or advanced practice nurse (APN) if drainage is cloudy or bloody.
26. Monitor vital signs as prescribed during outflow.	Assess for hypotension, tachycardia related to hypovolemia, and sudden release of intraabdominal pressure.	Notify physician or APN if patient becomes hypotensive or tachycardic or has abdominal pain.
27. Clamp the catheter when effluent is completely drained.	Decreases leakage and contamination.	Obtain and record bag weight to accurately assess intake and output.
28. Begin the next instillation phase per physician's order.		
Discontinuation of PD		
29. **HH**		
30. **PE**		
31. Observe outflow of last PD cycle.	Turning the patient from side to side ensures that patient's abdomen is empty of dialysate.	
32. Clamp both the catheter and the PD tubing.	Prevents leakage and contamination.	
33. Prepare sterile field. Open sterile container, sterile catheter cap, and 4 × 4 sterile gauze packages.	Maintains aseptic technique.	
34. Pour bactericidal solution into a sterile container with sterile catheter cap.	Prevents contamination; some institutions do not use a bactericidal soak for new caps but instead simply attach a new sterile cap.	Follow institutional standards.
35. Remove and discard nonsterile gloves.	Safely discards used supplies.	
36. **HH**		
37. Apply sterile gloves.	Maintains aseptic technique.	
38. Place new sterile catheter cap on sterile field.		
39. With sterile 4 × 4 gauze pads, disconnect the catheter from the PD tubing.		
40. Carefully connect the sterile cap to catheter.	Maintains aseptic technique.	
41. Securely tape catheter to abdomen.	Prevents accidental dislodgment.	
42. Apply dressing.		Dressing should be applied and changed per institution standard.
43. Remove gloves and discard soiled materials in appropriate receptacle.	Safely discards used supplies.	
44. **HH**		
Catheter Exit Site Care		
1. **HH**		
2. **PE**		

Procedure for Peritoneal Dialysis—*Continued*

Steps	Rationale	Special Considerations
3. Prepare sterile field. Open sterile 4 × 4 gauze pads and sterile container.	Maintains aseptic technique.	
4. Pour bactericidal solution into sterile container.	Reduces transmission of microorganisms.	
5. Remove and discard old dressing into appropriate receptacle.	Allows for visualization of catheter site.	Be careful not to tug or dislodge the catheter. Note any odor or drainage on old dressing.
6. Inspect catheter exit site and surrounding area for leakage, infection, or trauma.	Provides assessment for complications.	Note any pain, warmth, crusting, bleeding, tenderness, redness, or swelling that may indicate infection.
7. Gently palpate subcutaneous catheter segments and cuff.	Check for pain, erythema, edema, or accumulated drainage.	Obtain culture if drainage is present and notify physician or APN if the listed signs or symptoms are present.
8. Remove nonsterile gloves.		
9. **HH**		
10. Apply sterile gloves.	Maintains aseptic technique.	
11. Use a sterile 4 × 4 gauze pad to hold the catheter off the skin.	Helps prevent contamination of catheter by skin flora.	
12. Use povidone-iodine, hypochlorite, or chlorhexidine–soaked 4 × 4 gauze pads to cleanse catheter and exit site; allow them to air dry. **(Level D*)**	Acts as a bactericidal agent.	When cleansing skin, begin at exit site and move outward in concentric circles. Keep cleansing solutions out of the catheter sinus track.[4]
13. Apply a new catheter site dressing with sterile gauze or a transparent occlusive dressing. **(Level D)**	Gauze wicks drainage away from the site.	Transparent occlusive dressings are not recommended in the first 2 weeks after catheter placement because they allow pooling of secretions in the sinus track.[4]
14. Remove gloves and discard soiled supplies in appropriate receptacle.	Safely discards used supplies.	
15. **HH**		

Expected Outcomes

- Catheter and exit site maintained without complications
- Instillation and drainage of dialysate without problems
- Respiratory status not compromised during treatment
- BUN and creatinine values restored to baseline levels
- Electrolyte values restored to baseline levels
- Glucose control maintained
- Accumulated fluid removed
- Nutritional status maintained
- Peritoneum and abdomen intact

Unexpected Outcomes

- Drainage/leakage from the exit site
- Poor dialysate flow during instillation or drainage
- Signs and symptoms of peritonitis
- Inability to drain the total amount of instilled dialysate
- Signs or symptoms of infection at the insertion or access site
- Dislodgment of the abdominal catheter
- Tubing disconnection
- Physiologic complications during treatment
- Introduction of pathogens into the abdominal catheter
- Diaphragmatic impingement
- Viscous perforation by PD catheter
- Malnutrition
- Protein or blood loss from peritonitis

*Level D: Peer-reviewed professional organizational standards with clinical studies to support recommendations

Procedure continues on following page

Patient Monitoring and Care

Steps	Rationale	Reportable Conditions
		These conditions should be reported if they persist despite nursing interventions.
1. Perform and record a predialysis and daily weight. **(Level D*)**	Predialysis weight is an important factor in deciding how much PD is needed during treatment. It also helps to guide ongoing treatment and nutritional status.[1-4,14,15]	• Abnormal increase or decrease in weight

2. Perform baseline and ongoing assessments, including the following: **(Level D)**
  A. Vital signs
  B. Jugular vein distention
  C. Presence or absence of edema
  D. Skin turgor
  E. Mucus membranes
  F. Intake and output
  G. Pulmonary assessment, including expiratory tidal volume and peak inspiratory pressures on the ventilated patient
  H. Abdominal assessment
	Important to establish a baseline before initiation of treatment.[4,14,15] Monitors for complications.	• Hypotension
		• Hypertension
		• Fever
		• Hypothermia
		• Jugular vein distention
		• Dry mucous membranes
		• Shortness of breath
		• Crackles
		• Edema
		• Abdominal distention or tenderness
		• Rebound tenderness
		• Decreased tidal volume
		• Increased peak inspiratory pressures

3. Monitor BUN, creatinine, and electrolyte levels during treatment at a frequency determined by institutional standard.	Fluids and electrolyte levels shift during treatment.[4]	• Hyperglycemia • BUN or creatinine levels abnormal for patient • Hyperkalemia or hypokalemia • Hypernatremia or hyponatremia • Hypercalcemia or hypocalcemia

4. Administer medications to correct metabolic abnormalities as ordered. **(Level D)**	Patients with renal failure are predisposed to many metabolic abnormalities. Common medications administered to patients with renal failure include the following:[4,14,15]
	  Vitamin D and calcium carbonate prealbumin to increase the serum calcium level and prevent or treat bone disease.
	  Erythropoietin and iron to treat anemia.
	  Deferoxamine mesylate to remove excessive iron.
	  Stool softeners because constipation can impair drainage of PD fluid.
	  Phosphate binders to treat hyperphosphatemia.
	  Renal diet may also be prescribed, with adjusted protein, phosphorus, carbohydrate, and fluid intake that takes into account the patient's current catabolic state, residual renal function, adequacy of dialysis, and removal of amino acids by dialysis.[4,14,15]
		• Hypercalcemia or hypocalcemia
		• Abnormal hemoglobin or hematocrit values
		• Hyperphosphatemia or hypophosphatemia
		• Decreased albumin or prealbumin levels

*Level D: Peer-reviewed professional organizational standards with clinical studies to support recommendations

Patient Monitoring and Care —*Continued*

Steps	Rationale	Reportable Conditions
5. Monitor serum glucose at the beginning of the treatment and at frequencies throughout the treatment according to institutional standard.	The glucose in the dialysate solution predisposes patients to hyperglycemia, especially patients with diabetes.[1,9] Administer insulin as ordered to maintain glucose control.	• Hyperglycemia or hypoglycemia
6. Monitor the integrity of the PD setup. **(Level D*)**	Disconnections in the setup provide a portal of entry for pathogen that can lead to peritonitis.[1,4,7,9,13]	• Fever • Tachycardia • Cloudy or bloody dialysate
7. Monitor for signs and symptoms of infection at catheter exit site.	Identifies need for intervention.	• Site redness or edema • Warmth • Bleeding • Purulent drainage • Pain or tenderness • Fever
8. Monitor the ease with which the dialysate is both instilled and drained through the abdominal catheter.	Patients may need repositioning to facilitate flow through the abdominal catheter. Catheters may also become kinked or occluded. Fibrin clots can obstruct outflow; heparin may be added to the dialysate solution. Rapid infusion can cause abdominal pain.	• Inability to instill or drain fluid through the abdominal catheter
9. Follow institution standard for assessing pain. Administer analgesia as prescribed.	Identifies need for pain interventions.	• Continued pain despite pain interventions

Documentation

Documentation should include the following:
- Patient and family education
- Date and time of treatment initiation
- Treatment/exchange number
- Condition of abdominal catheter and exit site at time of treatment
- Date and time of dressing application
- Patient weight before and after treatment
- Pain assessment, interventions, and effectiveness

- Intake and output
- Length and parameters of treatment
- Dialysate solution used
- Vital signs/hemodynamic parameters throughout the treatment
- Unexpected outcomes
- Nursing interventions
- Laboratory assessment data

*Level D: Peer-reviewed professional organizational standards with clinical studies to support recommendations

References

CR 1. Ash SR: Chronic peritoneal dialysis catheters: procedures for placement, maintenance and removal, *Semin Nephrol* 22:221-236, 2002.

2. Ash SR: Chronic peritoneal dialysis catheters: challenges and design solutions, *Int J Artif Organs* 29:85-94, 2006.

CR 3. Bernardini J, et al: Randomized, double-blind trial of antibiotic exit site cream for prevention of exit site infection in peritoneal dialysis patients, *J Am Soc Nephrol* 16:539-545, 2005.

CR 4. Burrows-Hudson S, Prowant B: *Nephrology nursing standards of practice and guidelines for care,* Pitman, NJ, 2005, American Nephrology Nurses' Association.

CR 5. Churchill DN: Impact of peritoneal dialysis dose guidelines on clinical outcomes, *Perit Dial Int* 25:S95-S98, 2005.

6. Crabtree JH: Rescue and salvage procedures for mechanical and infectious complications of peritoneal dialysis, *Int J Artif Organs* 29:67-84, 2006.

7. Diaz-Buxo JA: Complications of peritoneal catheters: early and late, *Int J Artificial Organs* 29:50-58, 2006.

8. Goffin E: Aseptic peritonitis and icodextrin, *Perit Dial Int* 26:314-316, 2006.

9. Luongo M, Biel L: Peritoneal dialysis in the acute care setting. In Counts C, editor: *Core curriculum for nephrology nursing,* ed 5, Pitman, NJ, 2008, American Nephrology Nurses' Association, 215-230.

10. McIntyre CS: Update on peritoneal dialysis solutions, *Kidney Int* 71:486-490, 2007.

11. National Kidney Foundation (NKF): KDOQI clinical practice guidelines for vascular access: update 2006, *Am J Kidney Dis* 48:S176-S307, 2006.

12. Negoi D, et al: Current trends in the use of peritoneal dialysis catheters, *Adv Perit Dial* 22:147-152, 2006.

13. Piraino B: Peritoneal Dialysis infections recommendations [review], *Contrib Nephrol* 150:181-186, 2006.

14. Prowant BF, et al: Peritoneal dialysis. In Counts CS, editor: *Core curriculum for nephrology nursing,* ed 5, Pitman, NJ, 2008, American Nephrology Nurses' Association, 657-681.

15. Wild J: Peritoneal dialysis. In Thomas N, editor: *Renal nursing,* ed 3, Edinburg, 2008, Ballierre Tindall, 223-275.

Additional Readings

Chin AI, Yeun JY: Encapsulating peritoneal sclerosis: an unpredictable and devastating complication of peritoneal dialysis, *Am J Kidney Dis* 47:697-712, 2006.

CR Crabtree JH, et al: Optimal peritoneal dialysis catheter type and exit site location: an anthropometric analysis, *ASAIO J* 51:743-747, 2005.

CR Erixon M, et al: Take care in how you store your PD fluids: actual temperature determines the balance between reactive and non-reactive GDPs, *Perit Dial Int* 25: 583-590, 2005.

Scanziani R, et al: Imaging work-up for peritoneal access care and peritoneal dialysis complications, *Int J Artif Organs* 29:142-152, 2006.

Unit VI
Hematologic System

SECTION EIGHTEEN

Fluid Management

PROCEDURE

115

Use of a Massive Infusion Device and a Pressure Infusor Bag

P U R P O S E :   A massive transfusion is defined as 10 or more units of blood within the first 24 hours of admission.[3,13] Rapid infusers are used to warm and quickly infuse multiple units of blood and intravenous fluids into patients with hemodynamically unstable conditions. Patients with severe trauma, gastrointestinal hemorrhage, postoperative hemorrhage, and intravascular losses, as occur in septic shock and burns, may need the rapid administration of large volumes of blood products and intravenous fluids to restore and maintain intravascular volumes. A pressure infusor bag is used to administer a large amount of intravenous fluid or blood products to a patient with life-threatening hemorrhage within a prescribed period of time.

D. Nathan Preuss

PREREQUISITE NURSING KNOWLEDGE

- Knowledge of aseptic technique and principles of fluid resuscitation and blood transfusions is essential.
- A unit of fresh whole blood contains approximately 500 mL of warm blood with a hematocrit of 38% to 50%, a platelet count of 150,000 to 400,000, essentially full coagulation function, and 1500 mg of fibrinogen.[1] The combination of one unit of packed red blood cells (PRBCs), one unit of platelets, one unit of fresh frozen plasma (FFP), and a 10 pack of cryoprecipitate provides 660 mL of fluid with a hematocrit of 29%, a platelet count of 87,000, coagulation activity approximating 65%, and 750 mg of fibrinigen.[1]
- Events from the battlefields of Afghanistan and Iraq have shown the need to rethink current practices regarding massive transfusion (MT). The Joint Theater Trauma Registry has refocused attention to rapid correction of trauma-induced coagulopathy, permissive hypotension, the early correction of hypothermia and acidosis, and the increased use of component blood transfusion therapy.[1,13]

Damage control resuscitation emphasizes treatment of the lethal triad of hypothermia, acidosis, and coagulopathy with surgical techniques.[1,9] The use of MT occurs in 3% to 5% of all civilian trauma and 8% to 10% of all military trauma.[3,10,15]

- Hemorrhage is a major cause of death in the first hours after trauma.[11,15]
- Current strategies suggest an MT protocol with predefined blood protocols, permissive hypotension, minimizing of crystalloid products, and MT protocol of 1:1 FFP:PRBC during the first 24 hours for patients who are hypocoagulable with traumatic injuries.[4,6,9] Aggressive use of FFP and platelets drastically reduces 24-hour mortality rates and early coagulopathy in patients with trauma.[5]
- Previously, the goal of shock resuscitation has been to support blood pressure, urine output, and reverse metabolic changes associated with ischemia and blood loss. Current civilian and combat strategies seek to immediately identify coagulopathy and simultaneously treat hypothermia and acidosis (which can impair thrombin generation rates) and achieve hemostasis to then

volume load with blood components in ratios of 1:1 FFP:PRBC.[9]

- Use of a rapid infusion device, such as the one described in this procedure (Fig. 115-1), can warm and infuse fluids at rates from 75 to 30,000 mL/hr (Level 1, Inc, Rockland, MA). The tubing is made of soft plastic that expands to allow rapid infusion of fluids under pressure. Some rapid infusers include automated pressure chambers to compress intravenous (IV) bags. They allow for fast and easy bag changes and can accommodate both 1-L IV bags and 500-mL blood product bags. Pressure is maintained at a constant 300 mm Hg and is turned on and off via a simple toggle switch at the top of each pressure chamber. Older infusers simply have an IV pole from which to hang fluids, and separate pressure infusor bags must be used.

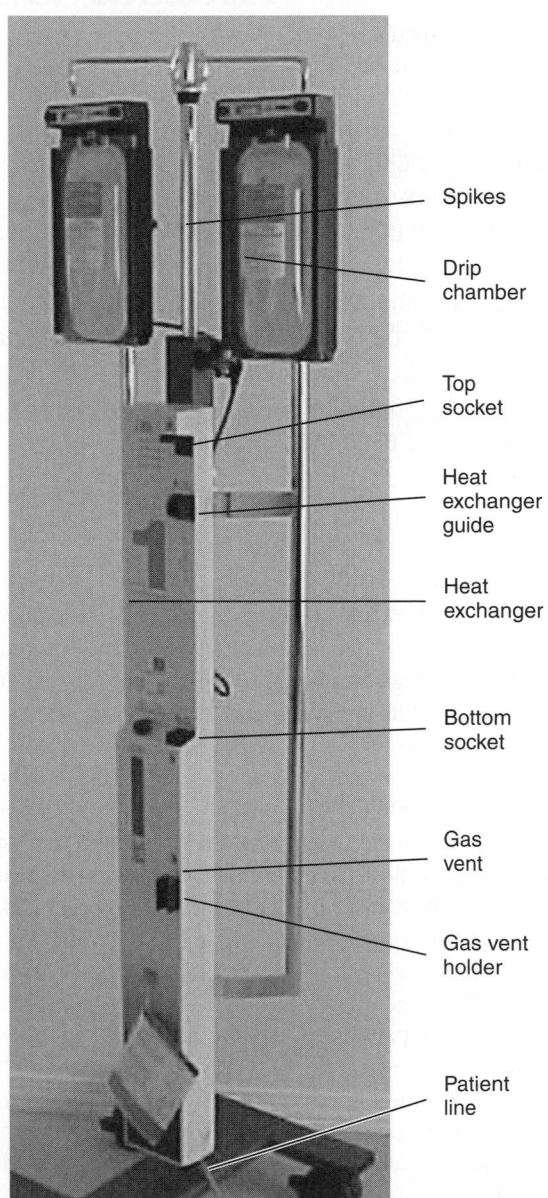

FIGURE 115-1   Level 1 rapid infuser. (*Courtesy Level 1, Inc, Rockland, Mass.*)

- IV catheters for aggressive fluid resuscitation should have a large bore and short diameter to facilitate the rapid infusion of large volumes of IV fluids and blood products. Usually, multiple IVs are used, including peripheral and central sites. Venous access may also be obtained surgically via a venous cut-down of the basilic or saphenous veins when peripheral access cannot be obtained.[12]

- Both crystalloid and colloid IV solutions are used for resuscitating patients who are hypovolemic with hemodynamically unstable conditions. Crystalloids directly increase the intravascular volume. Colloids expand plasma volume by pulling interstitial fluid back into the vascular space via osmosis. Numerous crystalloid and colloid preparations are available in isotonic, hypotonic, and hypertonic preparations. Crystalloids most commonly used in aggressive fluid resuscitation are 0.9% normal saline (NS) and lactated Ringer's (LR) solutions.

- The use of colloids such as albumin, dextran, and hetastarch allows the effective restoration of intravascular volume with smaller amounts of fluid; however, these colloids coat red blood cells (RBCs) and platelets, which may result in type and cross-match difficulties and clotting problems. Even slight overresuscitation with colloids increases the risk for fluid overload and pulmonary edema.[12,14]

- Blood and blood products are natural colloids used to replace lost blood and restore coagulation factors. In the patient with significant ongoing hemorrhage, infusion of blood and clotting factors is critical to restoring intravascular volume. Type O-negative blood is the universal donor for all patients and can be given in extreme emergencies before the completion of typing and cross-matching. PRBCs and whole blood are used to replace oxygen-carrying components; FFP, platelets, and cryoprecipitate are used to replace essential clotting factors.[2]

- When large volumes of IV fluids are being infused into patients, the fluids must be warmed to prevent hypothermia. (Although institutions vary in what constitutes large volumes, a good rule of thumb is to institute fluid rewarming measures when more than 2 L of fluid are required in less than 1 hour.)

- Hypothermia is a common consequence of aggressive fluid resuscitation and has serious physiologic consequences. It is correlated with mortality when the patient's body temperature decreases below 34°C[17] and significantly prolongs coagulation times at or below 35°C.[7] Moderate hypothermia (32° to 34°C) reduces coagulation factor activity approximately 10% for each degree Celsius decrease in temperature while markedly affecting platelet function.[8] Measures to prevent and treat hypothermia include solar blankets, heated blankets, body bags, warmed blood products and fluids, continuous arteriovenous rewarming, and cardiopulmonary bypass, used in extreme cases of hypothermia (see Procedure 94).[1]

- Patients who have received multiple transfusions and aggressive fluid resuscitation are at risk for multiple

Image labels:
Spikes
Drip chamber
Top socket
Heat exchanger guide
Heat exchanger
Bottom socket
Gas vent
Gas vent holder
Patient line

complications as a result of shock and from the fluids and blood products themselves. These sequelae may include fluid overload, adult respiratory distress syndrome, acute tubular necrosis, hypothermia, hypokalemia, hypocalcemia, hemolytic and allergic reactions, and air embolism.[14]

EQUIPMENT

- Rapid infuser (see Fig. 115-1)
- Disposable fluid administration sets (Fig. 115-2)
- Replaceable filter with gas vent (Fig. 115-3)
- Blood administration set
- Pressure infusor bag
- IV pole
- IV fluids or blood products as prescribed
- Sterile or distilled water for warmer
- Nonsterile gloves
- Fluid shield face mask or goggles
- Antiseptic solution
  Additional equipment to have available as needed:
- Emergency equipment

PATIENT AND FAMILY EDUCATION

- Explain the need for rapid infusion of fluids, the purpose of warming fluids, and how the equipment operates. ➤*Rationale:* Patient and family anxiety about unfamiliar equipment at the bedside is decreased.

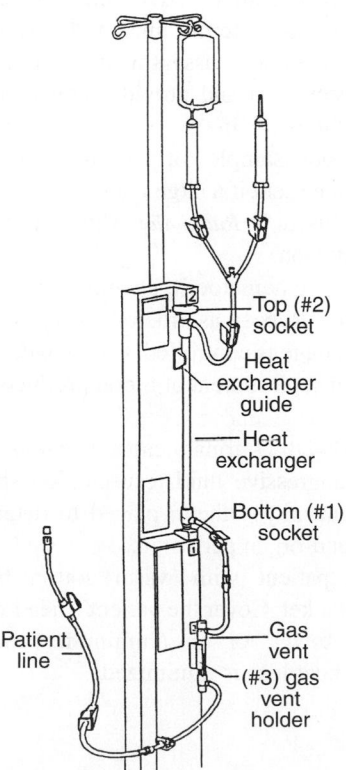

FIGURE 115-2 Placement of tubing in Level 1 rapid infuser. (*Courtesy Level 1, Inc, Rockland, MA.*)

- Explain that prevention of hypothermia is among the top priorities in the resuscitation of the patient. ➤*Rationale:* The patient and family can understand the plan of care.

PATIENT ASSESSMENT AND PREPARATION

Patient Assessment

- Assess blood pressure, heart rate, respiratory rate, peripheral pulses, and level of consciousness. ➤*Rationale:* Assessment is necessary to determine the severity of the patient's volume depletion and shock.
- Assess temperature using a bladder probe or pulmonary artery catheter. ➤*Rationale:* Assessment is necessary to assess for the development of hypothermia while large volumes of fluids are infused. Core temperatures most accurately reflect true body temperature.
- Assess patient history, including precipitating events, surgical and medical interventions thus far, and history of cardiac problems. ➤*Rationale:* Potential or actual need for massive fluid resuscitation and risk for fluid overload are identified.
- Assess hemodynamic parameters, including baseline central venous pressure (CVP) and, if available, pulmonary artery pressure (PAP), pulmonary capillary wedge pressure (PCWP), cardiac output (CO) and cardiac index (CI), systemic vascular resistance (SVR), and mixed venous oxygen saturation (Svo_2). Assessment of right ventricular ejection fraction, oxygen delivery and consumption, and oxygen extraction ratio should also be included if the technology is available. ➤*Rationale:* Baseline information is provided about patient's preload, afterload, and cardiac contractility.
- Assess laboratory values to include arterial blood gas, serum electrolyte, serum lactate, base deficit, hemoglobin, hematocrit, and coagulation studies. ➤*Rationale:* Baseline oxygenation, presence of metabolic acidosis, severity of ongoing hemorrhage, and severity of coagulopathy are measured so that the need for intervention and the effectiveness of interventions can be determined.
- Assess patency of multiple large-bore IV sites. ➤*Rationale:* Multiple sites are often necessary to infuse enough fluids and blood products to support the patient's vital signs. Extra sites in addition to those used for rapid infusion should be kept patent in case one of the other sites becomes nonfunctional or is accidentally pulled out.

Patient Preparation

- Verify correct patient with two identifiers. ➤*Rationale:* Prior to performing a procedure, the nurse should ensure the correct identification of the patient for the intended intervention.
- Ensure that informed consent has been obtained. ➤*Rationale:* Informed consent protects the rights of the patient and makes a competent decision possible for the patient.

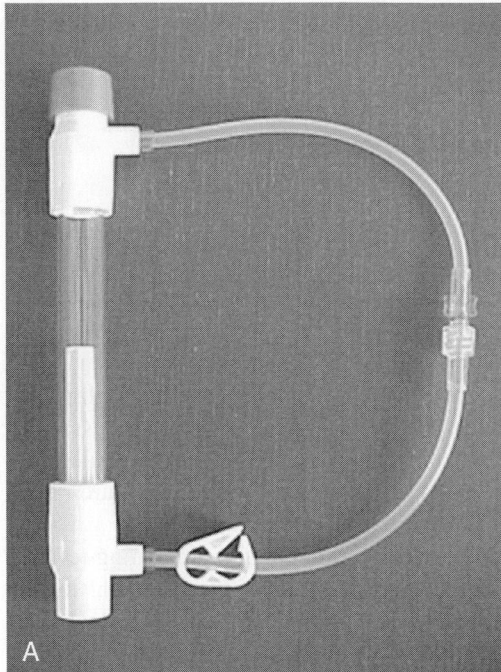
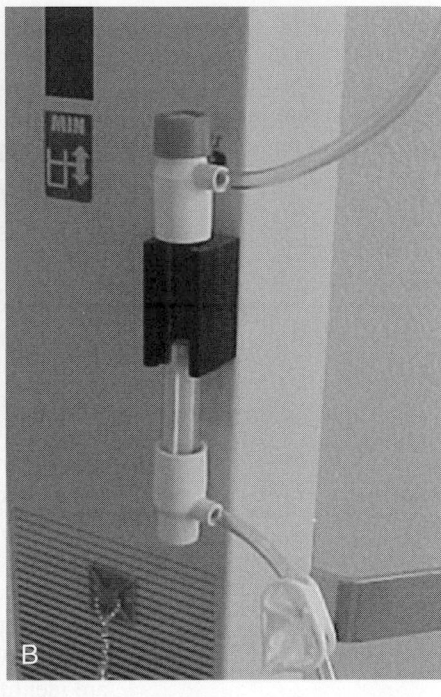

A

B

FIGURE 115-3 **A,** Rapid infuser filter showing male/female connecting ends on the right. **B,** Insertion of the filter in the Level 1 rapid infuser with the clamp open. *(Courtesy Level 1, Inc, Rockland, MA.)*

- Ensure that the patient and family understand the need and purpose for rapid infusion. Answer questions as they arise, and reinforce information as needed. ➤*Rationale:* Understanding of previously taught information is evaluated and reinforced.
- Place additional peripheral IV sites. ➤*Rationale:* Aggressive fluid resuscitation requires additional IV access besides the one site being used with the rapid infuser. Backup IV sites can be used if other sites infiltrate or become pulled out; extra sites may also be used to infuse medications, such as vasopressors, that should be kept separate from rapid infusion lines. Ideal sites for large IV catheter access are the antecubital fossae, saphenous veins, and the veins of the forearm and upper arm.
- Assist the physician or advanced practice nurse with placement of central venous access or pulmonary artery catheter or both. ➤*Rationale:* This placement allows for the assessment of volume status before and after infusion of fluids and blood products. It also allows for assessment of core temperature with pulmonary artery catheter thermistor and provides central venous access in the event vasoactive medications are needed.
- Place an automatic blood pressure monitor on the patient's arm that is not being infused with the rapid infusion device. Set it to check blood pressure every

5 minutes. ➤*Rationale:* Assessment of patient's hemodynamics and response to fluid replacement is provided. This is used temporarily until an arterial line can be placed by the physician or advanced practice nurse.
- Assist the physician or advanced practice nurse with placement of an arterial line. ➤*Rationale:* Placement allows for continuous assessment of the blood pressure during resuscitation and provides convenient access for blood sampling.
- Obtain a blood sample for type and cross-match. Two tubes should be sent if a large volume of blood is expected to be transfused. ➤*Rationale:* This action prepares for blood transfusion.
- Obtain baseline hematocrit, chemistry panel, and coagulation studies. Repeat, as ordered, every 15 to 60 minutes until hemorrhage is controlled. ➤*Rationale:* These studies guide proper replacement of blood products and essential electrolytes.
- Place an indwelling urinary catheter. ➤*Rationale:* Patients who need aggressive fluid resuscitation should have an indwelling urinary catheter placed to determine volume status and end-organ perfusion.
- Cover the patient with warm cotton blankets or a warm-air blanket. Cover the patient's head with a warmed blanket, a towel, or an aluminum cap. ➤*Rationale:* Additional heat loss is minimized.

Procedure for Use of Massive Infusion Device

Steps	Rationale	Special Considerations
1. [HH]		
2. [PE]		
3. Verify order for infusion of IV fluids and blood products.	Determines products and amounts to be infused.	The order from the physician or advanced practice nurse should include volume and type of additional IV fluids and blood products, laboratory work, and rapid infuser.
		Follow institution standard for performing pre-transfusion blood verification with another qualified health care provider.
4. Verify order for use of a fluid warmer. (**Level C***)	Warming fluids helps to prevent hypothermia.[1,7]	The order from the physician or advanced practice nurse should include rationale for use of a fluid warmer.
5. Turn on device.	Allows system to warm before moving fluid through the warming chamber.	Follow manufacturer's guidelines for set-up of each device.
6. Open Y-set fluid administration package provided by the manufacturer. Close all clamps.	Prevents accidental spillage of blood or fluid. Prevents flow of fluid through circuit before machine is warmed.	
7. Spike fluid or blood with both sides of the Y-set.	Allows for smooth transition from an empty bag to the next bag.	
8. Hang fluid bags on small hooks inside the rapid infuser pressure chambers, leaving the chamber doors open (see Fig. 115-1) or place fluid bags in separate pressure infusor bags.	Clearing the tubing of air is easier if the tubing is primed while the bags are still unpressurized.	Autotransfusion bags do not fit into the pressure chambers. Caution needs to be maintained so that air is not pushed through the tubing and into the patient causing an air embolism. Follow institution standard regarding removal of air from infusion bags.
9. Push the bottom end of the heat exchanger rod firmly into the bottom socket and snap the heat exchanger into the guide (see Fig. 115-2).	The bottom of the heat exchanger must be firmly placed or it will not fit into the top socket.	Being too gentle results in improper placement of the tubing and the warmer will not run.
10. Slide the top socket up and place the top end of the exchanger into the placement tract.	Locks the warming chamber into place at both the top and the bottom sockets.	
11. Slide the top heat exchanger socket down over the heat exchanger tube until the pole latch clicks into place.	Secures heat exchanger.	
12. Snap the gas vent filter into the holder on the lower portion of the pole assembly with the orange end up (see Fig. 115-3).	Filters air and blood clots from tubing.	Only fits into the machine one way because the tubing is not long enough to be placed incorrectly.
13. Squeeze drip chambers so that they are half full.	Minimizes entrapment of bubbles in the tubing. Allows visualization of the drip chamber so that drip rate can be assessed.	

*Level C: Qualitative studies, descriptive or correlational studies, integrative reviews, systematic reviews, or randomized controlled trials with inconsistent results

Procedure continues on following page

Procedure for Use of Massive Infusion Device—*Continued*		
Steps	**Rationale**	**Special Considerations**
14. Open the clamp on one side of the Y-set.	Make sure that only one side of the Y-tubing is open during priming; otherwise, fluid is pumped from one bag to the other and not through the tubing.	
15. Remove the male Luer-Lok cap at the end of the IV tubing; open the clamps.	Does not prime unless the end cap has been removed.	
16. Remove the filter from its holder and invert it. Prime the tubing; close the roller clamp. Turn the filter back over and replace it in its holder.	Prevents entrapment of large amounts of air.	
17. Tap the filter or air eliminator against the cabinet several times. Monitor fluid line for bubbles during use.	Releases any residual trapped air.	Never administer fluids if air bubbles are found between the filter chamber and the patient connection. Run IV fluid into the trash container to rid tubing of any residual air. When no more bubbles are observed leaving the gas vent filter, all the air has been vented from the filter or air eliminator.
18. Open the roller clamp partially and slowly infuse fluid.	Infusing slowly allows for assessment of any air bubbles. The air filter eliminates bubbles in the tubing.	If unable to clear line of air and more than $\frac{1}{4}$ inch of air is present at the top of the filter, replace the filter.
19. Replace male Luer-Lok cap at the end of the tubing; close the clamps.	Maintains asepsis of tubing.	
20. Close the pressure chamber doors and latch.	Positions fluid bags for pressurization when the machines are turned on and the pressure switch is activated.	Be certain that the latch is secure before the chamber is pressurized.
21. Perform all function and alarm checks as per manufacturer instructions.	Validates proper equipment function.	
22. Wait for the temperature readout to reach the operating temperature of 41°C.	Prevents hypothermia by ensuring the chamber is warm before fluids are run through it and into the patient.	
23. Flip the toggle switch at the top of the pressure chamber to "on/+" or inflate the separate pressure bags.	Pressurizes the chambers.	The pressure automatically inflates to 300 mm Hg. Fluids infuse via gravity flow without being pressurized; however, high flow rates cannot be achieved unless the pressure bags are inflated.
24. Cleanse the injection site with antiseptic solution.[2,16] (**Level B***)	Reduces the risk for infection.	Follow institutional standard. Chlorhexidine and povidone-iodine solutions may be more effective than alcohol in reducing external microbial contamination.[2]
25. Connect the distal end of the tubing to the patient's IV.	Prepares for infusion.	
26. Open the roller clamp to infuse the fluid.	Fluids or blood products now infuse under pressure.	It is best to infuse one side at a time, especially when blood products are infusing, to prevent mixing of fluids and blood products. The pressure system is designed to leave a small volume remaining to prevent air emboli.

*Level B: Well-designed controlled studies with results that consistently support a specific action, intervention, or treatment

Procedure   for Use of Massive Infusion Device—*Continued*

Steps	Rationale	Special Considerations
27. Set the rate by gradually opening the clamp.	Fluids given via rapid infusers are administered as boluses over short periods; roller clamps are usually left wide open until the bolus is complete.	If a slower bolus is desired, adjust the roller clamp to decrease the flow of fluid.
Changing the Bags		
1. Close the top clamp on the side of the Y-connector with the empty fluid bag.	Prevents air from entering the tubing.	Follow manufacturer's guidelines for changing infusion bags for each device.
2. Open the clamp on the side of the Y-connector with the full fluid bag; infuse the fluid.	Keeping one side of the Y-connector spiked with fluid ready to infuse is helpful when patients have severely unstable conditions and need immediate boluses of fluid.	
3. Turn the "on/+" switch above the pressure chamber to the "off" position and remove the empty bag.	Releases pressure from the pressure chamber.	
4. Replace the empty fluid bag with a full one.	The next bag of IV fluid must be ready to infuse to avoid delays in infusion in case the patient's blood pressure falls precipitously.	
5. Close the pressure chamber door and latch; flip the control switch above the pressure chamber to "on/+."	Repressurizes chamber.	
Replacing the Filter or Air Eliminator		
1. Close the clamps on the disposable fluid administration set just proximal to the filter and between the filter and the patient connection.	The filter should be replaced after 3 hours of use, after 4 units of blood, or if fluid rate slows because of clotting.	Follow manufacturer's guidelines for replacing the filter or air eliminator for each device.
2. Remove the old filter or air eliminator from the holder and place the new filter or air eliminator in the holder.	Keep the old filter or air eliminator connected to the disposable fluid administration set until ready to change to new one. Minimizes potential for contaminating exposed tubing ends.	
3. Disconnect the old filter or air eliminator at the upper Luer-Lok and connect the tubing to the new filter.	Prepares for placement of new equipment.	
4. Disconnect the patient line Luer-Lok from the old filter or air eliminator and connect to the new one.	Prepares for placement of new equipment.	
5. Open the clamp just proximal to the filter or air eliminator to restart fluid. Invert the filter until completely filled with fluid, then turn back to proper position and replace in holder. Open the clamp between the filter and the patient connection.	Infusion of fluid resumes.	

Procedure continues on following page

Procedure	for Use of Massive Infusion Device—*Continued*		
Steps	**Rationale**	**Special Considerations**	
6. Remove the filter or air eliminator from the holder and tap until all bubbles are eliminated; reinsert. Check patient line for bubbles before opening the roller clamp.	Facilitates removal of bubbles.	If air bubbles are present, disconnect the tubing from the patient and infuse into the trash container until the line is clear of air. Reconnect to the patient and resume the infusion. If alarm sounds after setup, check to ensure filter is properly snapped into place.	
Troubleshooting Alarms			
1. If the alarm sounds and the disposable light is illuminated, check to be sure the disposable tubing set is properly placed in the machine.	The system will not run if the disposable tubing is not completely set into the machine.	The tubing set can become inadvertently dislodged. Follow manufacturer's guidelines for troubleshooting alarms for each device.	
2. If the alarm sounds and the water level light is illuminated, check the water level in the chamber and replace as needed with sterile or distilled water.	The system will not run if the water level is too low.		
3. If the system alarms "overtemp," turn the machine off and use a different rapid infuser.	Fluids inadequately warmed cause hypothermia. Fluids overly warmed cause hemolysis of red blood cells.	Notify biomedical engineering of the problem.	
Transporting a Patient with a Rapid Infuser			
1. Turn the rapid infuser off.	If the infuser is still on when the administration set is removed from its holder, water will spurt out of the warming chamber and aluminum tube.	Follow manufacturer's guidelines for each device to transport a patient with a rapid infuser.	
2. Remove the disposable administration set from its holder on the infuser and place it in the bed alongside the patient or hang it on the transport IV pole.	The rapid infusers described here do not operate on a battery. Fluids infuse via gravity, or separate pressure infusor bags can be used.	Fluids run briskly via gravity drainage. If pressure is still necessary to infuse fluids, separate pressure infusor bags need to be used as long as the machine is not plugged in. Interventions to minimize heat loss must be in place while the infuser is not plugged in. Aluminum head covering, warmed cotton blankets, and warm-air blankets help prevent heat loss. Removing the administration set from the machine and transporting the patient separately from the infuser is less awkward and minimizes the risk for pulling out the IV lines during transport.	
3. Plug the infuser into an electric outlet once you reach the intended destination.	Establishes power source.		
4. Return administration set into the infuser. Turn the machine on. Return fluid bags to pressure chambers.	The infuser is now ready to repressurize the chambers and warm the fluid. Any bubbles are eliminated by the filter.	If bubbles are not removed and more than ¼ inch of air is at the top of the filter, the filter must be replaced.	
5. Discard used supplies in the appropriate receptacle.	Safely discards used supplies.		
6. **HH**			

Procedure for Pressure Infusor Bag Use

Steps	Rationale	Special Considerations
1. **HH**		
2. **PE**		
3. Obtain and set up IV fluid or blood component system.	The infusion system should be assembled before inserting the IV fluid or blood product into the pressure infusor bag.	If administering blood products, follow institution standard for performing pre-transfusion blood verification with another qualified health care provider.
4. Cleanse the injection site with antiseptic solution.[2,16] **(Level B*)**	Reduces the risk for infection.	Follow institutional standard. Chlorhexidine and povidone-iodine solutions may be more effective than alcohol in reducing external microbial contamination.[2]
5. If administering a blood component, piggyback the blood tubing into the 0.9% NS solution or connect directly into the IV line.	Allows transfusion to proceed.	Follow institutional standard for use of 0.9% NS solution as primary IV fluid line. Fresh frozen plasma and platelets should be given directly into the IV line. Do not piggyback them.
6. Open the roller clamp on the tubing.	Allows infusion to proceed.	Rate of infusion is dependent on the amount of pressure applied to the unit, not the position of the roller clamp.
7. Place the unit of blood or IV fluid through the mesh or plastic cover of the deflated pressure infusor bag so the entire bag to be infused remains within the mesh or plastic panel.	Allows pressure to be evenly applied.	Do not allow the top of the bag to be infused appear above the mesh or plastic covering because this interferes with flow.
8. Secure the bag to be infused in place with Velcro strap or hang on hook in the pressure infusor bag. Hang the infusor bag on the IV pole.	Prevents bag to be infused from slipping out of the bag when hung from the IV pole.	A standard sphygmomanometer cuff should never be used to administer large-volume transfusions because it does not exert uniform pressure on all parts of the component container.
9. Inflate the pressure infusor bag to achieve the desired rate of flow.	Pressure of infusor bag is used to adjust flow, not the position of the roller clamp.	The pressure should not exceed 300 mm Hg to avoid damaging red blood cells, rupturing the IV or blood bag, dislodging the IV catheter, or injuring the vein. The patient may have discomfort in an extremity if a peripheral catheter is used; if appropriate, decrease the pressure to maintain patient comfort.
10. When infusion is complete, deflate the pressure infusor bag.	Slows infusion.	
11. If infusing blood, close the roller clamp to the blood component and flush the primary infusion tubing with 0.9% NS solution if used as primary IV line.	Allows the patient to receive blood sequestered in the tubing.	

*Level B: Well-designed controlled studies with results that consistently support a specific action, intervention, or treatment

Procedure continues on following page

Procedure for Pressure Infusor Bag Use—*Continued*

Steps	Rationale	Special Considerations
12. When the infusion is complete, don nonsterile gloves and disconnect the IV fluid, NS solution or blood tubing from the IV line.	Completes infusion; Standard Precautions.	
13. Discard used supplies in appropriate receptacle.	Safely discards used supplies.	Blood container and administration set should be handled as hazardous waste.
14. ⊞		

Expected Outcomes

- Patient's blood pressure and heart rate return to baseline
- Patient's core temperature remains above 36.0°C
- CVP, PAP, PCWP, CO, CI, and SVR reflect return of euvolemia and hemodynamic stability
- IV sites remain patent
- Rapid flow of blood components
- Urine output at least 0.5 mL/kg/hr

Unexpected Outcomes

- Blood pressure remains below baseline despite multiple liters of fluid and blood products
- Core temperature falls below 36.0°C so that more aggressive rewarming interventions become necessary
- Hypothermia-induced coagulopathy develops as temperature falls below 35°C
- Inability to restore normal intravascular status occurs, as seen by CVP less than 6, PCWP less than 6, CO less than 4 L/min, CI less than 2 L/min/m², or SVR greater than 1500 dynes/sec
- Infiltration of IV secites occurs
- Clotting of rapid infuser filter occurs
- Anuria or oliguria with urinary output less than 0.5 mL/kg/hr occurs
- Patient discomfort

Patient Monitoring and Care

Steps	Rationale	Reportable Conditions
		These conditions should be reported if they persist despite nursing interventions.
1. Monitor the patient's vital signs every 5 to 15 minutes as indicated. As the patient's condition becomes more stable, assessment of vital signs may be done less frequently (every 15 to 30 minutes until the blood pressure remains stable for more than 2 hours).	Determines severity of shock, responsiveness to fluids and blood products, and the need for additional fluids.	• Systolic blood pressure below 90 mm Hg despite fluid administration • Abnormal vital signs

Patient Monitoring and Care —*Continued*

Steps	Rationale	Reportable Conditions
2. Assess the patient's core temperature every 15 to 30 minutes. **(Level C*)**	Patients who are in severe shock have impaired thermogenesis. This, in combination with the infusion of inadequately warmed fluids, leads to hypothermia. Hypothermia-induced coagulopathies begin at a core temperature of 35°C and exacerbate any hemorrhage already occurring. Also, severe physiologic complications from hypothermia, such as cardiovascular instability, electrolyte changes, urine concentration problems, and shifts in the oxygen-hemoglobin dissociation curve, affect the patient's ability to respond to physiologic stress. Prevention of hypothermia is a critical goal for patients undergoing massive fluid resuscitation.[1,7]	• Worsening hypothermia or unrelieved hypothermia
3. Assess the integrity of IV sites every 15 minutes.	IV sites under pressure are at higher risk for infiltration. Also, lines can be inadvertently pulled out during radiographic filming, turning, and other aspects of patient care during a massive resuscitation. Multiple IV sites are recommended to be available at all times in the event an IV infiltrates or is pulled out.	Infiltrated IV sites
4. Assess hemodynamic parameters every 15 to 30 minutes.	Determines intravascular volume status and responsiveness to interventions. Patients may still be inadequately resuscitated even though vital signs, urine output, and hemodynamic parameters have returned to normal. A complete clinical picture (including laboratory tests in conjunction with vital signs, urine output, and hemodynamic parameters) is the best way to determine whether a patient has been adequately resuscitated.[12]	• Abnormal trends in hemodynamic monitoring
5. Assess urine output every 30 to 60 minutes.	Urine output is an assessment of end-organ perfusion. If little or no urine is produced, it is assumed that the kidneys are not being perfused and, therefore, other major viscera are also probably not being adequately perfused. Trauma to the urinary tract may interfere with accurate assessment of urine output because clots may block urine drainage and laceration to ureters may result in extravasation of urine into the peritoneum.	• Urine output less than 0.5 mL/kg/hr

*Level C: Qualitative studies, descriptive or correlational studies, integrative reviews, systematic reviews, or randomized controlled trials with inconsistent results

Procedure continues on following page

Patient Monitoring and Care —*Continued*

Steps	Rationale	Reportable Conditions
6. Draw hemoglobin, hematocrit, and coagulation studies as prescribed. These are usually measured every 30 to 60 minutes or after transfusion of blood and blood components.	Determines presence of ongoing blood loss and coagulopathy.[7]	• Abnormal hemoglobin, hematocrit, and coagulation results
7. Draw arterial blood gases and lactic acid as prescribed and indicated.	Determines persistence of metabolic acidosis and identifies need for additional interventions to improve perfusion to major organs.[12]	• Abnormal laboratory results
8. Draw electrolytes as prescribed.	Patients undergoing large-volume resuscitation are at risk for hypokalemia, hypomagnesemia, hypocalcemia, and hypophosphatemia.	• Abnormal laboratory results
9. Monitor the patient for signs and symptoms of a transfusion reaction. If a transfusion reaction is suspected, stop the transfusion.	Blood component replacement therapy constitutes the infusion of a foreign substance into the recipient.	• Signs and symptoms of a transfusion reaction.
10. Follow institution standard for assessing pain. Administer analgesia as prescribed.	Identifies need for pain interventions.	• Continued pain despite pain interventions

Documentation

Documentation should include the following:

- Patient and family education
- Completion of informed consent
- Rationale for use of the rapid infuser
- Blood pressure, heart rate, respiratory rate, lung sounds, and peripheral pulses throughout the resuscitation
- The patient's core temperature while the rapid infusers are used
- Hemodynamic parameters, including CVP, PAP, PCWP, CO, CI, and SVR
- Urine output, estimated blood loss, other measured output
- Laboratory results, including arterial blood gases, hematocrit, hemoglobin, electrolytes, and lactic acid
- Appearance of IV sites
- IV insertions
- Total IV fluids and blood products in intake and output record
- Unexpected outcomes
- Additional interventions
- Pain assessment, interventions, and effectiveness

References

1. Beekley AC: Damage control resuscitation: a sensible approach to the exsanguinating patient, *Crit Care Med* 36:S267-S274, 2008.
2. Casey AL, et al: A randomized, prospective clinical trial to assess the potential infection risk associated with the PosiFlow needleless connector, *J Hosp Infection* 54:288-293, 2003.
3. Como JJ, et al: Blood transfusion rates in the care of acute trauma, *Transfusion* 44:809-813, 2004.
4. Cotton BA, et al: Predefined massive transfusion protocols are associated with a reduction in organ failure and postinjury complications, *J Trauma* 66:41-49, 2009.
5. Dente CJ, et al: Improvements in early mortality and coagulopathy are sustained better in patients with blunt trauma after institution of a massive transfusion protocol in a civilian level 1 trauma center, *J Trauma* 66:1616-1624, 2009.
6. Duchesne JC, et al: Review of current blood transfusions strategies in a mature level 1 trauma center: were we wrong for the last 60 years? *J Trauma* 65:272-277, 2008.
7. Gubler KD, et al: The impact of hypothermia on dilutional coagulopathy, *J Trauma* 36:847-851, 1994.
8. Hess JR, Lawson JH: The coagulopathy of trauma versus disseminated intravascular coagulation, *J Trauma* 60: S12-S19, 2006.
9. Holcomb JB, et al: Damage control resuscitation: directly addressing the early coagulopathy of trauma, *J Trauma* 62:307-310, 2007.
10. Holcomb JB: Damage control resuscitation, *J Trauma* 62:S36-S37, 2007.
11. Kauvar DS, Lefering R, Wade CE: Impact of hemorrhage on trauma outcome: an overview of epidemiology, clinical presentations, and therapeutic considerations, *J Trauma* 60:S3-S11, 2006.

CR 12. Koran Z, Newberry L: Vascular access and fluid replacement. In Emergency Nurses Association, Newberry L, editors: *Sheehy's emergency nursing*, ed 5, St Louis, 2003, Mosby, 147.

13. McLaughlin DF, et al: A predictive model for massive transfusion in combat casualty patients, *J Trauma* 64:S57-S63, 2008.

CR 14. McQuillan KA: Initial management of traumatic shock. In McQuillan KA, et al:, editors *Trauma nursing: from resuscitation through rehabilitation*, ed 3, Philadelphia, 2002, Saunders, 151.

15. Nunez TC, et al: Early prediction of massive transfusion in trauma: simple as ABC (assessment of blood consumption)? *J Trauma* 66:346-352, 2009.

CR 16. O'Grady NP, et al: Guidelines for the prevention of intravascular catheter-related infections, *Am J Infect Control* 30(8):476-489, 2002.

17. Shaz BH, et al: Transfusion management of trauma patients, *Anesth Analg* 108:1760-1768, 2009.

Additional Readings

CR American Association of Blood Banks: *Primer of blood administration,* revised 12/02, Bethesda, MD, 2002, The Association.

Snyder CW, et al: The relationship of blood product ration to mortality: survival benefit or survival bias? *J Trauma* 66:358-364, 2009.

CR Stammers AH, et al: Utilization of rapid-infusor devices for massive transfusion, *Perfusion* 20:65-69, 2005.

Special Hematologic Procedures

Apheresis and Therapeutic Plasma Exchange (Assist)

P U R P O S E :   Apheresis techniques are used to remove cells, plasma, and other substances from blood. These procedures are used as adjunctive treatments in many diseases, especially in antibody-mediated conditions that produce autoantibodies.

Sonia M. Astle

PREREQUISITE NURSING KNOWLEDGE

* Therapeutic apheresis (i.e., hemapheresis) is a technique for selective removal of cells, plasma, and substances from the patient's circulation to promote clinical improvement. The different apheresis techniques vary according to the component of the blood removed or replaced or the substance removed.
  * *Plasma exchange* is the process of replacing the plasma removed with an equal amount of either plasma or fluid (most commonly a combination of 5% albumin and normal saline solution).
  * *Cytapheresis* is the selective removal of the cellular components of blood. Blood is withdrawn from the patient and a specific cellular component is retained (i.e., white blood cell); the remainder of other cells and plasma is returned to the donor or patient.
  * *Leukocytapheresis* is the removal of white blood cells from the blood; the remaining blood is returned to the patient. It is most commonly used as a therapeutic method for blast cell reduction in leukemias (leukocytosis).
  * *Erythrocytapheresis* is the process of removing erythrocytes (red blood cells) from whole blood.
  * *Thrombocytapheresis* is the selective removal of platelets (thrombocytes).
  * *Plasma adsorption/perfusion* is the removal of plasma with a hollow fiber filter. Blood is returned to the patient, and the plasma is pumped over an adsorptive column that removes certain proteins or pathogens. The treated plasma is then returned to the patient.

* *Lymphoplasmaphersis* is the separation and removal of lymphocytes and plasma from the withdrawn blood, with the remainder of the blood retransfused into the donor.
* *Immunoadsorption* is the removal of an antigen in the blood by a specific antibody lining the surface of a filter or cartridge.
* *Photopheresis* uses apheresis techniques to remove and return blood to the patient. Photosensitizing drugs are given to the patient, and white blood cells are removed and exposed to an ultraviolet light, then returned to the patient. Photopheresis induces cellular changes that have been shown to be effective in certain diseases such as cutaneous T-cell, graft-versus-host disease, post–bone marrow transplant, and solid organ transplant rejection. Apheresis techniques are also used for the procurement of peripheral stem cells for bone marrow transplantation.
* During plasma exchange procedures, the plasma removed must be replaced; the most common replacement fluids are albumin, fresh frozen plasma (FFP), thawed plasma (derived from thawed FFP and maintained at low temperatures for use within 1 to 5 days), and normal saline.[1] Because clotting factors are transiently reduced by plasma exchange, FFP can also be used as a fluid replacement in patients when bleeding is an issue.
* Plasma volume is an estimate of the patient's total volume based on gender, height, weight, and hematocrit value. Exchange volume is the ratio of the patient's plasma volume to be removed and replaced; this is usually 1:1 or 1.5:1 of the patient's estimated plasma volume.[4]

- In plasma exchange, an average of 3 to 5 L of plasma is removed and replaced.[4]
- Treatments can be done with two different machines.[4]
  - *Centrifugal apheresis machine:* Separates plasma and other blood components with use of a centrifuge (Fig. 116-1).
  - *Filtration:* A hollow-fiber cell separator, permeable to plasma proteins, is used to remove the patient's plasma via an apheresis machine or continuous renal replacement machines adapted for pheresis (Fig. 116-2).
- Treatment length and frequency vary according to the disease being treated, rate of production of the substance being removed, and the patient's response to treatment. Acute conditions, such as thrombotic thrombocytopenia purpura or graft-versus-host disease, usually require daily treatments for 5 to 7 days.[6,7] Other conditions usually require plasma exchanges two or three times weekly for up to 6 weeks.[2,5-7] The total amount of plasma to be exchanged is used as a guide for treatment. A single treatment, referred to as a plasma exchange, usually takes 2 to 3 hours with a centrifugal machine and 2 to 6 hours with filtration methods.[4]
- Apheresis procedures are performed by healthcare professionals such as registered nurses or blood bank personnel, with special knowledge and skills in apheresis. These procedures are commonly performed both in critical care units and on an outpatient basis, depending on the type of disease being treated and on the patient's condition.
- The most commonly used apheresis systems use two large-bore peripheral venous catheters, a double-lumen vascular access catheter (VAC), or a dialysis graft or fistula to access the vascular system. Peripherally inserted central venous catheters or implantable venous access ports do not provide for adequate blood flow and are not acceptable for use.[4]
- The system should be primed with an anticoagulant (e.g., heparin or citrate) to prevent clotting. If citrate is used, the patient must be monitored closely for hypocalcemia.

Citrate works as an anticoagulant by binding calcium (Ca^{++}), therefore decreasing the amount of Ca^{++} available for normal clotting.[4]

- Plasma exchange is used to treat antibody-mediated disorders because the pathogenic antibodies are contained in the plasma. Removal of these antibodies through plasma exchange reduces the number of circulating antibodies, temporarily decreasing the patient's symptoms.
- Conditions treated by plasma exchange may include the following[2,5-7]:
  - Myasthenia gravis
  - Guillain-Barré syndrome
  - Various hematologic disorders
  - Nephrologic disorders
  - Rhematologic disorders
  - Poisoning
  - Drug overdose/drug toxicity
  - Acute liver failure
  - Solid organ transplantation for ABO incompatibility and rejection
  - Cytokine-mediated injury, such as sepsis, burns, and multisystem organ dysfunction syndrome (MODS); experimental use
- Current indication categories for therapeutic apheresis, as endorsed by the American Association of Blood Banks (AABB) and the American Society for Apheresis (ASFA), are listed in Table 116-1.
- If the patient is taking angiotensin-converting enzyme (ACE) inhibitors, contact with certain filters or membranes in the apheresis system can cause an anaphylactic reaction and severe hypotension as a result of increased levels of

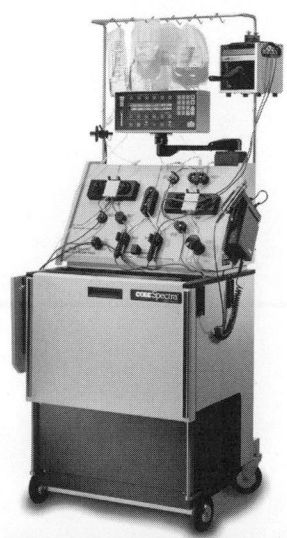

FIGURE 116-1   COBE Spectra Apheresis System. (© *Caridian-BCT, Inc. 2010. Used with permission.*)

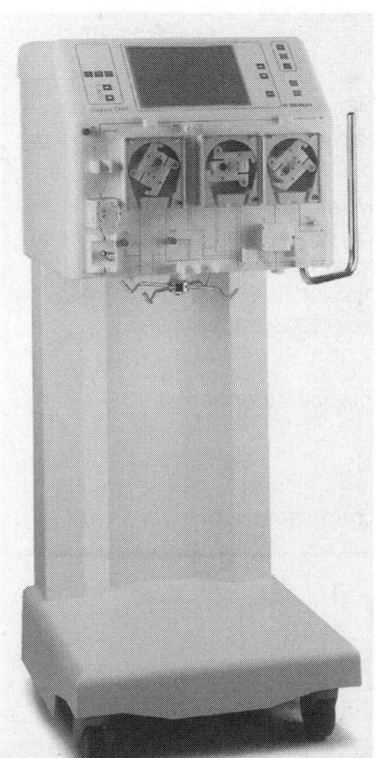

FIGURE 116-2   The B. Braun Diapact CRRT system can also be used for therapeutic plasma exchange and plasma adsorption/perfusion. (*Photo courtesy B. Braun Medical, Inc.*)

TABLE 116-1	Indication Categories for Therapeutic Apheresis	
Disease	**Procedure**	**Indication Category***
Autoimmune		
Catastrophic antiphospholipid syndrome	Plasma exchange	III
Cryoglobulinemia	Plasma exchange	I
Pemphigus vulgaris	Plasma exchange	III
	Extracorporeal photopheresis	III
Systemic lupus erythematosus		
Manifestations other than nephritis	Plasma exchange	III
Hematologic		
ABO-incompatible hematopoietic progenitor cell transplantation	Plasma exchange	II
Autoimmune hemolytic anemia: warm autoimmune hemolytic anemia: cold agglutinin disease	Plasma exchange	III
Babesiosis		
Severe	Erythrocytaphesis	II
Coagulation factor inhibitors	Immunoadsorption	III
	Plasma exchange	III
Cutaneous T-cell lymphoma; mycosis fungoides		
Erythrodermic	Extracorporeal photopheresis	I
Nonerythrodermic	Extracorporeal photopheresis	IV
Erythrocytosis; polycythemia vera		
Symptomatic	Erythrocyapheresis	II
Graft-versus-host disease		
Skin	Extracorporeal photopheresis	II
Nonskin	Extracorporeal photopheresis	III
Hyperleukocytosis		
Leukostasis	Leukocytapheresis	I
Prophylaxis	Leukocytapheresis	III
Hyperviscosity in monoclonal gammopathies	Plasma exchange	I
Idiopathic thrombocytopenic purpura		
Refractory	Immunoadsorption	II
Refractoy or nonrefractory	Plasma exchange	IV
Malaria		
Severe	Erythrocytapheresis	II
Myeloma and acute renal failure	Plasma exchange	III
Posttransfusion purpura	Plasma exchange	III
Red cell alloimmunization in pregnancy	Plasma exchange	II
Sickle cell disease		
Life-threatening and organ-threatening	Erythrocytapheresis	I
Stroke prophylaxis	Erythrocytapheresis	II
Prevention of iron overload	Erythrocytapheresis	II
Thrombotic thrombocytopenic purpura	Plasma exchange	I
Metabolic		
Familial hypercholesterolemia		
Homozygotes	Selective removal	I
Heterozygotes	Selective removal	II
	Plasma exchange	II
Hypertriglyceridemic pancreatitis	Plasma exchange	III

TABLE 116-1	Indication Categories for Therapeutic Apheresis—cont'd	

Disease	Procedure	Indication Category*
Overdose and poisoning		
Mushroom poisoning	Plasma exchange	II
Other compounds	Plasma exchange	III
Phytanic acid storage disease (Refsum's disease)	Plasma exchange	II
Sepsis	Plasma exchange	III
Thyrotoxicosis	Plasma exchange	III
Miscellaneous		
Dilated cardiomyopathy	Immunoadsorption	P
Inflammatory bowel disease	Adoptive cytapheresis	P
Macular degeneration, age-related	Membrane differential filtration	P
Neurologic		
Acute disseminated encephalomyelitis	Plasma exchange	III
Acute inflammatory demyelinating polyneuropathy (Guillain-Barré syndrome)	Plasma exchange	I
Chronic inflammatory demyelinating polyradiculoneuropathy	Plasma exchange	I
Lambert-Eaton myasthenic syndrome	Plasma exchange	II
Multiple sclerosis		
Acute central nervous system (CNS) inflammatory demyelinating disease	Plasma exchange	II
Devic's syndrome	Plasma exchange	III
Chronic progressive	Plasma exchange	III
Myasthenia gravis	Plasma exchange	I
Paraproteinemic polyneuropathies		
Immunoglobulin (IgG)/IgA	Plasma exchange	I
IgM	Plasma exchange	II
Multiple myeloma	Plasma exchange	III
IgG/IgA/IgM	Immunoadsorption	III
Pediatric autoimmune neuropsychiatric disorders associated with streptococcal infections (PANDAS); Sydenham's chorea		
Severe PANDAS	Plasma exchange	I
Severe Sydenham's chorea (SC)	Plasma exchange	I
Rasmussen's encephalitis	Plasma exchange	II
Stiff-person syndrome	Plasma exchange	III
Renal		
Antineutrophil cytoplasmic antibodies (ANCA)–associated rapidly progressive glomerulonephritis (Wegener's granulomatosis)	Plasma exchange	II
Antiglomerular basement membrane disease (Goodpasture's syndrome)	Plasma exchange	I
Focal segmental glomerulosclerosis		
Primary	Plasma exchange	III
Secondary	Plasma exchange	III
Hemolytic uremic syndrome; thrombotic microangiopathy; transplant-associated microangiopathy		
Idiopathic hemolytic uremic syndrome (HUS)	Plasma exchange	III
Other	Plasma exchange	III
Transplant-associated microangiopathy	Plasma exchange	III
Diarrhea-associated pediatric	Plasma exchange	IV
Rapidly progressive glomerulonephritis	Plasma exchange	III
Renal transplantation: antibody-mediated rejection; human leukocyte-associated (HLA) desensitization		
Antibody-mediated rejection	Plasma exchange	II
HLA desensitization	Plasma exchange	II

Continued

TABLE 116-1	Indication Categories for Therapeutic Apheresis—cont'd	
Disease	**Procedure**	**Indication Category***
Rheumatic		
Rheumatoid arthritis, refractory	Immunoadsorption	II
Scleroderma (progressive systemic sclerosis)	Plasma exchange	III
	Extracorporeal photopheresis	IV
Transplantation		
ABO-incompatible solid organ transplantation		
Kidney	Plasma exchange	II
Heart (infants)	Plasma exchange	II
Liver	Plasma exchange	III
Heart transplant rejection		
Prophylaxis	Extracorporeal photopheresis	I
Treatment	Extracorporeal photopheresis	II
	Plasma exchange	III
Lung transplant	Extracorporeal photopheresis	III

*Indication categories as established by the American Medical Association:
I, Standard therapy, acceptable but not mandatory. *II*, Available evidence tends to favor efficacy; conventional therapy usually tried first. *III*, Inadequately tested at this time. *IV*, No demonstrated value in controlled trials. *P*, Pending, includes diseases that can be treated with therapeutic apheresis using devices that are not available in the United States or do not have US Food and Drug Administration (FDA) clearance (ASAF category).
From Szczepiorkowski ZM, Shaz BH, Bandarenko N, et al: The new approach to assignment of ASFA categories: introduction to the fourth special issue: clinical applications of therapeutic apheresis, J Clin Apheresis 22:96-105, 2007.

bradykinin, a potent vasodilator. ACE inhibitors are recommended to be withheld for 48 to 72 hours before treatment.
- Invasive procedures should be delayed until after the treatment, unless FFP is used as a replacement fluid.
- Potential complications of apheresis techniques include the following:
  - Bleeding
  - Thrombocytopenia
  - Red blood cell (RBC) lysis/hemolysis
  - Air embolism
  - Blood leak
  - Circuit clotting
  - Hypovolemia
  - Hypotension
  - Hypothermia
  - Vascular access complications
  - Fever/chills
  - Shock
  - Anaphylaxis
  - Allergic reactions
  - Transfusion reactions
  - Electrolyte imbalances
  - Dysrhythmias
  - Citrate toxicity
  - Infection

EQUIPMENT

- Blood cell separator machine
- Blood cell separator tubing set
- Replacement fluids
- Hemostats
- Appropriate laboratory specimen tubes
- Vascular access dressings and flushes
- Nonsterile gloves
- Fluid shield face masks or goggles
- Caps

PATIENT AND FAMILY EDUCATION

- Explain the procedure, including risks, length of treatment, and patient positioning, and answer any questions the patient may have. ➤➤*Rationale:* Explanation provides information and may decrease patient anxiety.
- Explain the purpose of the apheresis procedure, why this treatment is being performed, and the expected clinical outcomes. ➤➤*Rationale:* Plasmapheresis is used to treat antibody-mediated disorders.
- Explain the need for careful sterile technique for the duration of treatment. ➤➤*Rationale:* Sterile technique is important to decrease the chance of systemic infection because pathogens can be transported throughout the entire body via the circulation.
- Explain the need for careful monitoring of the patient for complications. ➤➤*Rationale:* Hypocalcemia, hypotension, bleeding, and hypothermia are all potential complications of apheresis.
- Explain the importance of the patient informing the nurse how he or she is feeling during the treatment. ➤➤*Rationale:* Patient symptoms can be important signs of complications related to the procedure. Examples include lightheadedness as a sign of hypotension and numbness and tingling as a sign of hypocalcemia.
- Explain the importance of preventing bleeding complications: pressure dressings at vascular sites, avoiding shaving, and care of access catheter. ➤➤*Rationale:* Alterations in blood composition and anticoagulation can put the patient at risk for bleeding.

- Explain the apheresis circuit setup to the patient and family. ➤➤*Rationale:* Blood will be removed from the patient's body and will be visible during the plasmapheresis treatment.

PATIENT ASSESSMENT AND PREPARATION

Patient Assessment

- Obtain baseline vital signs, body system assessment, hemodynamic parameters (if appropriate), weight, and pretreatment fluid balance. ➤➤*Rationale:* Total body assessment should be based specifically on the patient's diagnosis and reason for treatment. Pretreatment assessment provides a baseline for comparison once the treatment is started, allowing for appropriate modification of intervention as needed. Changes in weight during and after treatment are an indicator of fluid balance.
- Review medications and ensure that the patient has not taken an ACE inhibitor within 48 hours. ➤➤*Rationale:* Contact with certain fibers or membranes in the apheresis system can cause an anaphylactic reaction and severe hypotension.
- Assess pretreatment laboratory values. ➤➤*Rationale:* Baseline values are needed of the complete blood count (CBC) with differential, platelet count, and electrolytes before these are altered by treatment. Coagulation parameters are particularly important: fibrinogen, prothrombin time (PT), activated clotting time (ACT), and partial thromboplastin time (PTT), if heparin is used; and ACT and ionized Ca^{++}, if citrate is used. Serum sodium and serum bicarbonate levels/pH also should be evaluated in patients when citrate is used as the anticoagulant. Disease-specific tests should also be obtained pretreatment as needed.
- Obtain vascular access. ➤➤*Rationale:* A properly functioning vascular access is necessary to perform plasmapheresis.

Patient Preparation

- Verify correct patient with two identifiers. ➤➤*Rationale:* Prior to performing a procedure, the nurse should ensure the correct identification of the patient for the intended intervention.
- Ensure that informed consent has been obtained. ➤➤*Rationale:* Informed consent protects the rights of the patient and makes a competent decision possible for the patient.
- Ensure that patient understands preprocedural teachings. Answer questions as they arise, and reinforce information as needed. ➤➤*Rationale:* Understanding of previously taught information is evaluated and reinforced.
- Assist the patient to a position of comfort that also facilitates optimal blood flow through the vascular access. ➤➤*Rationale:* Facilitating patient comfort helps to minimize the amount of patient movement during treatment. Movement can change the blood flow through the access site. Different access sites may require different patient positions to facilitate optimal blood flow.

Procedure for Assisting with Apheresis/Plasmapheresis		
Steps	**Rationale**	**Special Considerations**
1. Verify apheresis orders.	Familiarizes nurse with the individualized patient treatment and reduces the possibility of error.	
2. Review the following with the apheresis nurse: A. Exchange volume B. Anticoagulant C. Replacement fluids D. Baseline patient assessment, including 　(1) Vital signs 　(2) Jugular vein distention 　(3) Presence of edema 　(4) Intake and output 　(5) Neurologic assessment 　(6) Pulmonary assessment 　(7) Renal assessment 　(8) Parameters/treatment for heart rate and blood pressure 　(9) Laboratory monitoring 　(10) Procedure for emergency resuscitation	Sets joint goals and actions to provide for patient safety and optimize the patient's outcome.[4]	

Procedure continue on following page

Procedure for Assisting with Apheresis/Plasmapheresis—*Continued*

Steps	Rationale	Special Considerations
3. Gather supplies for vascular access.	Prepares for the procedure.	The process of vascular access depends on whether the site is central or peripheral.
4. Assist in gathering the supplies for apheresis procedure.	Prepares for the procedure.	Obtaining and sending laboratory specimens may be part of the apheresis setup as the vascular system is accessed.
5. Ensure that appropriate replacement fluid is available. Warm replacement fluids.	Maintains correct electrolyte balance; avoids hypothermia.[4]	Replacement fluids should be slightly warmed before infusion unless contraindicated (e.g., blood products should be maintained at a specific temperature before infusion to maintain viability of the product). Never use a microwave to warm fluids. Some patients also may need an increase in the ambient room temperature or ventilator cascade and warming blankets to avoid hypothermia. Most apheresis systems have inline blood warmers.
6. Infuse fluid boluses as needed before initiation.	Maintains hemodynamic stability.	
7. **HH**		
8. **PE**		
9. Assist with setup and priming of the apheresis circuit as needed.	Ensures safe and proper assembly and complete removal of air from the circuit.	
10. After setup, discard used supplies in the appropriate receptacle.	Safely discards used supplies.	
11. **HH**		
12. Tape and secure all connections.	Prevents inadvertent disconnection of the system.	

Expected Outcomes

- Therapeutic goals achieved
- Optimal fluid balance is maintained
- Laboratory values are maintained within expected range
- Properly functioning access site
- Patient remains pain free or has pain controlled to an acceptable goal

Unexpected Outcomes

- Complications related to the treatment (e.g., hypotension, hypocalcemia, hypothermia, hypokalemia, hypernatremia, metabolic alkalosis, air embolism, blood leak, bleeding, and infection)
- Poor blood flow through the vascular access
- Bleeding from the access site
- Dislodgment of the access catheter
- Hematoma formation at the access site
- Technical problems with apheresis circuit
- Hemolysis

Patient Monitoring and Care

Steps	Rationale	Reportable Conditions
		These conditions should be reported if they persist despite nursing interventions.
1. Monitor the patient during and after the apheresis treatment: A. Vital signs B. Hemodynamic parameters C. Jugular vein distention D. Presence of edema E. Intake and output F. Neurologic assessment G. Pulmonary assessment H. Renal assessment I. Apheresis circuit J. Laboratory values as ordered (if plasma is removed, include prothrombin time/international normalized ratio [INR], fibrinogen, platelet count) **(Level C*)**	Patients can experience complications, such as hypotension, hypothermia, blood leak, air embolism, transfusion reactions, hypocalcemia, RBC hemolysis, thrombocytopenia, citrate toxicity, and bleeding, that may need intervention.[1,3-5]	• Hypotension • Hypertension • Tachycardia/bradycardia • Tachypnea/bradypnea • Fever • Hypothermia • Jugular vein distention • Crackles • Edema • Change in level of consciousness • Dizziness • Change in cardiac rhythm • Blood leak • Hemolysis • Thrombocytopenia • Dysrhythmias • Coagulopathies • Allergic reaction • Transfusion reaction
2. Monitor serum ionized Ca^{++}, magnesium, serum sodium, and serum bicarbonate levels/pH (if citrate is used as an anticoagulant).	Citrate binds with Ca^{++} and can cause hypocalcemia. It also metabolizes to sodium and bicarbonate, which may cause hypernatremia, metabolic alkalosis, and citrate toxicity.[4]	• Hypocalcemia • Hypernatremia • Metabolic alkalosis • Increased anion gap
3. Monitor ACT/PTT (if heparin is used as an anticoagulant).	These values primarily reflect the activity of the intrinsic clotting pathway.	• Prolonged ACT/PTT
4. Administer replacement fluid as needed.	Replacement fluids are important during the treatment to maintain adequate intravascular volume.	• Hypotension • Tachycardia • Decreased central venous and pulmonary artery pressures • Decreased urine output
5. Hold medication administration.	Many medications are withheld during treatment, including vasopressors and pain medications, especially those that are protein-bound.[8] Some medications, such as antihypertensive agents, anticholinergic agents, and Ca^{++} supplements, may be withheld during treatment.[4] Analgesics and antipyretics may be indicated during a treatment, although these medications may mask the symptoms of transfusion reaction.[8]	
6. Monitor the access and dressing sites after the termination of the apheresis procedure. **(Level C)**	Bleeding or signs or symptoms of infection can be complications of the vascular access.[9]	• Bleeding • Redness, tenderness, pain, or warmth at the access insertion site • Generalized bleeding or fever

*Level C: Qualitative studies, descriptive or correlational studies, integrative reviews, systematic reviews, or randomized controlled trials with inconsistent results

Procedure continues on following page

Patient Monitoring and Care —*Continued*

Steps	Rationale	Reportable Conditions
7. Appropriately label VACs that contain indwelling anticoagulant.	Prevents the infusion of anticoagulant into the patient.	• Bleeding • Bruising • Oozing • Dysrhythmias

8. Receive report from the apheresis nurse, including:
  A. Amount and type of fluids removed
  B. Amount and type of fluids given
  C. Exchange volume and fluid balance
  D. Patient reactions during treatment
  E. Medications given during treatment
	For proper patient evaluation and documentation.	

9. Follow institutional standard for assessing pain. Administer analgesia as prescribed.	Identifies need for pain interventions.	• Continued pain despite pain interventions

Documentation

Documentation should include the following:
• Patient and family education
• Completion of informed consent
• Date and time of treatment initiation
• Condition of vascular access
• Intake/output/fluid balance
• Vital signs throughout the apheresis treatment
• Daily weight

• Patient's response to apheresis and daily progress toward treatment goals
• Unexpected outcomes
• Nursing interventions
• Laboratory assessment data
• Pain assessment, interventions, and effectiveness.

References

1. Garner Sf, et al: Apheresis donors and platelet function: inherent platelet responsiveness influences platelet quality, *Transfusion* 48:673-680, 2008.
2. McLeod BC: Evidence based therapeutic apheresis in autoimmune and other haemolytic anemias, *Curr Opin Hematol* 14:647-654, 2007.
3. Rahman T, Harper L: Plasmapheresis in nephrology: an update, *Curr Opin Nephrol Hypertens* 15:603-609, 2006.
4. Rohe RM, et al: Therapeutic plasma exchange. In Counts C, editor: *Core curriculum for nephrology nursing,* ed 5, Pitman, NJ, 2008, American Nephrology Nurses' Association, 277-308.
5. Roth SH: Role of apheresis in rheumatoid arthritis, *Drugs* 66:1903-1908, 2006.
6. Szczepiorkowski ZM, et al: The new approach to assignment of ASFA categories: introduction to the fourth special issue: clinical applications of therapeutic apheresis, *J Clin Apher* 22:96-105, 2007.
7. Szczepiorkowski ZM, et al: Guidelines on the use of therapeutic apheresis in clinical practice: evidence-based approach from the Apheresis Applications Committee of the American Society for Apheresis, *J Clin Apheresis* 22:106-175, 2007.
8. Tobian AA, et al: Transfusion premedications: a growing practice not based on evidence, *Transfusion* 47:1089-1096, 2007.
CR 9. Young EJ, et al: Incidence and influencing factors associated with exit site infections in temporary catheters for hemodialysis and apheresis, *Nephrol Nurs J* 32:41-50, 2005.

Additional Readings

Heddle NM, et al: Comparing the efficacy and safety of apheresis and whole blood-derived platelet transfusions: a systematic review, *Transfusion* 48:1447-1458, 2008.
George JN: Evaluation and management of patients with thrombotic thrombocytopenic purpura, *J Intensive Care Med* 22:82-91, 2007.
Greenberg BM: Idiopathic transverse myelitis: corticosteroids, plasma exchange, or cyclophosphamide, *Neurology* 68:1614-1617, 2007.
Thompson GR, et al: Recommendations for the use of LDL apheresis, *Atherosclerosis* 198:247-255, 2008.
Van de Watering L: The intention-to-treat principle in clinical trails and meta-analyses of leukoreduced blood transfusions in surgical patients, *Transfusion* 47:573-581, 2007.

AP Bone Marrow Biopsy and Aspiration (Perform)

P U R P O S E : The acquisition of a bone marrow aspirate from the core of the bone is used in the diagnosis of hematopoietic disorders. It is also used to follow the effectiveness of treatment in patients undergoing conventional chemotherapy, to assess response in the post autologous blood and marrow transplant period as well as treatment response and engraftment in the post allogeneic stem cell transplant. The preferred site for a bone marrow aspirate and biopsy is the posterior iliac crest.[1] The sternum may be used in aspiration of marrow; however, a core biopsy cannot be obtained from the sternum because of the risk of damage to underlying internal organs, most significantly the heart.[6,8]

Eileen C. Finnegan

PREREQUISITE NURSING KNOWLEDGE

- A thorough understanding is needed of the anatomy and physiology of the posterior and anterior iliac crest and the sternum.
- Clinical and technical competence in performing a bone marrow aspirate and biopsy is necessary.
- Essential knowledge of sterile technique is needed.
- An understanding is needed of institutional policies and procedures for administration of intravenous (IV) pharmacologic agents, including conscious sedation (if indicated) and intradermal and epicortical local anesthesia (lidocaine in most cases; procaine may be used in cases of lidocaine allergy) and procedural care of the patient receiving conscious sedation (if used).
- Knowledge is needed of information to be gained from a bone marrow aspirate sample (i.e., identification of normal and abnormal hematopoietic elements, identification of malignant clones with flow cytometry, identification of chromosomal abnormalities that occur in hematologic malignant diseases, identification of molecular diagnostic studies that show gene rearrangements and translocations, and the performance of chimerism studies in patients after allogeneic transplant).
- A bone marrow biopsy is used for morphologic analysis of hematopoietic cells and for assessment of the architecture of the bone marrow that may be abnormal in certain disease states.
- Indications for bone marrow aspiration and biopsy include the following:
  - To diagnosis a hematologic abnormality
  - To monitor a hematologic disease state after initial diagnosis or therapy
  - To diagnose bone marrow involvement before stem cell collection and for staging of various malignant states
  - To assess the status of disease after autologous bone marrow or hematopoietic stem cell transplant
  - To assess chimerism disease status and immune reconstitution after an allogeneic bone marrow or hematopoietic stem cell transplant
  - To evaluate immunodeficiency syndromes or to confirm an infectious disease process in the marrow

- Contraindications to bone marrow biopsy and aspirate are the presence of hemophilia, severe disseminated intravascular coagulopathy, or other related severe bleeding disorders. Thrombocytopenia alone is not a contraindication to bone marrow examination.[3,5] The use of anticoagulant medications may pose serious bleeding risk; therefore, coagulation studies should be obtained in these patients. The decision on whether anticoagulation can be safely withheld prior to and restarted after the procedure is patient dependent.

EQUIPMENT

- Bone marrow aspiration and biopsy kit, which includes the following:
  - ❖ Povidone-iodine or chlorhexidine-alcohol antiseptic preparation
  - ❖ Sterile fenestrated drape (2)
  - ❖ 1 vial lidocaine (1% or 2%; 5-10mLs)
  - ❖ 5 or 10-mL syringe for drawing up lidocaine
  - ❖ Filter needle (if lidocaine drawn from glass vial)
  - ❖ Needles of appropriate lengths to anesthetize both skin and periosteum
  - ❖ Sterile 4 × 4 and 2 x 2 gauze pads
  - ❖ Small scalpel blade
  - ❖ Illinois needle (for bone marrow aspirate)
  - ❖ Jamshidi bone biopsy needle (for core biopsy)
  - ❖ 20-mL syringe for bone marrow aspirate
  - ❖ Blunt tip needles
  - ❖ Multiple 10-ml syringes with slip tips or adaptor for leur lock
  - ❖ Adhesive bandage
- Sterile gloves
- Sterile gowns
- Fluid shield face mask or goggles
- Required tubes for specimen processing: two edetate disodium (EDTA; lavender top) and two sodium heparin (green top) tubes (follow institution standard)
- Glass slides and cover plate
- 2½- to 6-inch spinal needle (may be required for anesthetizing periosteum in the obese patient)
- Extra-long Jamshidi needle (may be needed to acquire core specimen in obese patient)
- Container for bone core biopsy specimen, including appropriate fixative (10% formalin or 2 ×2 cotton gauze soaked with sterile saline solution to keep specimen from drying out)
- 1 vial of 100 units/mL heparin (follow institution standard)
- 1 Additional vial of lidocaine (1% or 2%; 20 mL)

Additional equipment for patients receiving conscious sedation:

- Pulse oximeter
- Automated blood pressure monitor
- Oxygen
- Suction
- Ambu bag
- IV pharmacologic agents for sedation (i.e., midazolam, 2 to 4 mg; fentanyl, 25 to 50 mcg; lorazepam, 1 to 2 mg)

- IV opiate and benzodiazepine antagonist agents (i.e., naloxone and flumazenil)
- Emergency equipment

PATIENT AND FAMILY EDUCATION

- Assess patient and family understanding of the bone marrow aspiration and biopsy procedure and the reason for it. ➥*Rationale:* Clarification of the procedure and reinforcement of information are expressed patient and family needs in times of stress and anxiety.
- Inform the patient and family (if permitted by patient) that the results will be shared with them as soon as they are available. ➥*Rationale:* The patient and family are usually anxious about the results.
- Explain the actual procedure to the patient and family. ➥*Rationale:* The patient and family are prepared for what to expect; anxiety may be decreased.
- Review safety requirements for patients who will receive pharmacologic agents for sedation (i.e., must have transportation and escort home and may not drive until the following day). ➥*Rationale:* This review ensures patient safety and healthcare provider's accountability for patients receiving sedation.
- Encourage the patient to verbalize any pain experienced during the procedure. ➥*Rationale:* Additional lidocaine, pain medication, or sedation medication can be administered. Poor relaxation can cause the large gluteal muscles to spasm, making the procedure more difficult for all involved.
- Instruct patient and family to keep pressure dressing clean, dry, and in place for 24 hours after the procedure. ➥*Rationale:* Proper dressing care reduces chance of bleeding and minimizes chance of infection at the site.
- Advise patient and family that a wrapped ice bag applied to the site over clothing may add comfort. The ice should never be applied directly to the skin. ➥*Rationale:* Ice reduces swelling, decreases chance of hematoma, and adds comfort.
- Avoid applying heat to the procedure site. ➥*Rationale:* Heat could exacerbate bleeding.
- Advise against non-steroidal anti-inflammatory drugs or aspirin for 24 hours after biopsy. ➥*Rationale:* This measure reduces the chance of bleeding or hematoma at site.
- Advise use of acetaminophen for pain relief, if not contraindicated. ➥*Rationale:* Acetaminophen relieves pain and does not promote bleeding.

PATIENT ASSESSMENT AND PREPARATION
Patient Assessment

- Assess patient's home medications, including over-the-counter medications that can increase clotting time. ➥*Rationale:* Assessment can decrease risk of bleeding and hematoma.
- Assess the need for antianxiety or analgesic medication or conscious sedation. ➥*Rationale:* If the patient is

very anxious before the procedure or has had severe pain with previous bone marrow procedures, small doses of analgesia or sedation promote patient comfort. Tense muscles can create a technically difficult procedure and add to pain and anxiety.

- Assess coagulation studies in patients who are taking anticoagulant medications. **➟Rationale:** Patients at risk for bleeding complications are identified.

- Assess the ability of the patient to lie on his or her stomach or side, with the head of the bed at no greater than a 25-degree elevation. **➟Rationale:** Access to and control of the posterior iliac crest is best obtained with the patient lying flat, or with the head of the bed only slightly raised, in a side-lying or prone position.

- Assess vital signs and oxygenation status. **➟Rationale:** Baseline data are provided. Assessment ensures that the blood pressure and oxygenation status can be maintained if the patient is placed on his or her side or prone.

- Assess the posterior iliac crest with palpation. In select cases, the anterior iliac crest may be used as a result of positioning limitations or excessive tissue surrounding the posterior iliac crest. However, an increased risk of injury to the surrounding nerves and blood vessels makes this procedure more complicated. The sternum is used for aspiration only in very select cases because of potential fatal complications with this procedure. It should be performed with cardiac monitoring by a physician. **➟Rationale:** Assessment identifies the most suitable area for obtaining optimal samples with a minimum of risk of discomfort and danger to the patient.

- Assess for recent bone marrow aspiration and biopsy sites. **➟Rationale:** The patient may have a painful experience if an additional biopsy is performed at a site that has not yet healed from a previous procedure. Penetration of scar tissue from previous bone marrow biopsy sites may also be difficult.

Patient Preparation

- Ensure that the patient and family understand pre- and postprocedural teachings and discharge instructions. Answer questions as they arise, and reinforce information as needed. **➟Rationale:** Understanding of previously taught information is evaluated and reinforced. The patient and family understand postprocedure care.

- Verify correct patient with two identifiers. **➟Rationale:** Prior to performing a procedure, the nurse should ensure the correct identification of the patient for the intended intervention.

- Obtain informed consent for bone marrow aspiration and biopsy and, if indicated, conscious sedation. **➟Rationale:** Informed consent protects the rights of the patient and makes a competent decision possible for the patient.

- Perform a pre-procedure verification and time out, if nonemergent. **➟Rationale:** Ensures patient safety.

- Prescribe analgesia or sedation, if needed. **➟Rationale:** Patient may need analgesia or sedation to ensure adequate cooperation and minimize discomfort during the procedure.

- Follow institution standard for a patient receiving conscious sedation. **➟Rationale:** Preparation ensures that appropriate emergency equipment and medical staff are available.

- Obtain IV access for patients receiving sedation. **➟Rationale:** A secure patent IV line is necessary for administration of IV pharmacologic agents and, if necessary, emergency antagonist agents.

- Obtain a complete blood count and differential via venipuncture. **➟Rationale:** Many pathologists prefer to review a peripheral blood sample in conjunction with the marrow to make a complete and accurate diagnostic evaluation.

- Confirm availability of personnel who will assist with the procedure. If the procedure is to be performed without assistance, prepare all equipment and walk through the procedure for concise and accurate specimen acquisition. **➟Rationale:** Slide preparation, specimen processing, and additional supplies require an appropriately trained assistant for the procedure if available.

- Assist the patient to an appropriate position depending on the patient's comfort and the practitioner's preference. **➟Rationale:** Positioning ensures good visualization and control of the posterior iliac crest.

- Ensure site markings have been made where appropriate. Site may be marked with sterile marking pen. **➟Rationale:** Procedure site is identified.

Procedure	for Performing Bone Marrow Biopsy and Aspiration	
Steps	**Rationale**	**Special Considerations**
Bone Marrow Aspiration		
1. **HH**		
2. **PE**		Apply mask.
3. Open the bone marrow procedure tray; add any additional supplies in a manner that preserves sterility.	Maintains sterility of the procedure.	An extra overbed works well as a procedure table. Clean before and after each use.
4. **HH**		
5. Apply sterile gown and gloves.	Maintains sterility of the procedure.	

Procedure continues on following page

Procedure for Performing Bone Marrow Biopsy and Aspiration—*Continued*

Steps	Rationale	Special Considerations
6. Prepare all necessary syringes, including lidocaine syringe and those requiring anticoagulant.	Ensures adequate preparation for the procedure and reduces distraction once the procedure is started.	
7. Prepare the intended site with the antiseptic swabs and place sterile drape.	Minimizes risk for infection.	
8. With a 25- to 30-gauge needle, inject the skin with lidocaine, creating a wheal.[6]	A small-gauge needle lessens the discomfort associated with administration of local anesthesia.	
9. With a 21-gauge 1½-inch needle (or spinal needle if necessary), infiltrate the periosteum with lidocaine in a "peppering" fashion. Stabilization of the site of aspiration with stretching the skin with the thumb and forefinger of the opposite hand is helpful.	If the periosteum is not numb, the patient will have extreme discomfort. Also, assessing the area of the posterior iliac crest in an obese patient is often difficult. Use of the spinal needle helps the practitioner locate an appropriate site.	If additional lidocaine is needed, ask the assistant to invert the extra vial. If the 1½-inch needle does not reach the bone, use the 3½-inch spinal needle to reach it. The spinal needle can also be used to assess the geography of the posterior iliac crest and allows the practitioner to assess the depth of the bone. It is helpful to anesthetize an area of about a quarter to half dollar size so that adjustments can be made in needle placement.
10. Make an incision above the biopsy site with a small scalpel. Advance the aspirate needle through the incision (while continuing to stretch the skin) to the periosteum with firm pressure and slight rotation; penetrate the cortex. A slight sensation of "giving" is often noticed as the marrow cavity or medulla is reached.	Slight rotation of the needle allows for smooth entry into the marrow cavity.	If the patient experiences excessive pain, it is recommended that the needle be placed in another section of bone or additional lidocaine be applied to the outer surface of the bone.
11. Remove the stylet, attach the 20-mL syringe primed with EDTA, and aspirate 3- to 5-mL of marrow. Immediately hand this syringe to the assistant or place a drop onto a glass slide and verify presence of spicules in the sample if an assistant is not available.	The syringe is inverted to mix the EDTA and marrow specimen. The first aspirate sample is used to make the slides and to place in the lavender-top EDTA tubes for clot sections or polymerase chain reaction (PCR) studies.	A volume of spicules is most often found toward the end of the syringe; therefore, place marrow in lavender-top tubes first after spicules have been identified.
12. If aspirate is not obtained or is aparticulate, replace the stylet, reposition the needle, and attempt to aspirate again. With each pull, rotate the needle slightly.[6] **(Level C*)**	If marrow cannot be obtained after three attempts, another needle may be needed because of blunting.	At times, it is difficult to obtain a bone marrow aspirate. Difficulty can occur if a patient is aplastic or if the marrow space is packed by disease. This is known as a "dry tap." In these cases, the practitioner should try to obtain a good core biopsy specimen for pathology analysis. The touch preparation in this case becomes a crucial step in providing the pathologist with material suitable for morphologic examination.[6]

*Level C: Qualitative studies, descriptive or correlational studies, integrative reviews, systematic reviews, or randomized controlled trials with inconsistent results

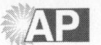

Procedure	for Performing Bone Marrow Biopsy and Aspiration—*Continued*	
Steps	**Rationale**	**Special Considerations**
13. Obtain additional samples as needed in the 10-mL syringe containing heparin. Place in the green-top sodium heparin tubes (with the help of the assistant if available).	Heparinized aspirate is used for flow cytometry, chromosome analysis, and chimerism studies.	Invert syringe to mix heparin and marrow. Follow institution standard for use of heparinized and non-heparinized tubes for obtaining samples.
14. Have the assistant invert all of the tubes several times.	Aspirate samples can clot quickly if not thoroughly mixed with anticoagulant.	
15. Replace stylet, recap needle and remove the aspiration needle from the site with a gentle pulling motion. Apply firm pressure with sterile gauze. If obtaining a bone biopsy, **proceed to Step 1 (next section).**	Ensures adequate hemostasis and reduces chance of infection.	Replacing the stylet decreases discomfort with removal of the aspirate needle.
16. If a bone marrow biopsy is not being obtained, hold pressure for 5 minutes or until bleeding has stopped. Apply pressure dressing.	Ensures adequate hemostasis and reduces chance of infection.	
17. If a biopsy is not being obtained, discard used supplies in appropriate receptacle.	Safely discards used supplies.	
18. **HH**		

Bone Marrow Biopsy

1. Make a 5-mm skin incision, pass the Jamshidi needle through the incision, and advance the needle until the periosteum is reached.	Allows smooth entry of the marrow needle into the skin.	Some sections of bone are extremely hard, making placement of the Jamshidi needle difficult. If hard bone is encountered, another section of bone should be used. If a section of bone is extremely soft, it is often difficult to obtain an adequate biopsy, and another section of bone should be chosen. Be sure all of periosteum is anesthetized.
2. Rotate the needle slightly until it is firmly seated in the bone.	Requires constant smooth pressure.	
3. Remove the stylet, replace the cap on the needle, and advance the needle approximately 1 to 2 cm with a slight rotating motion.	Removing the stylet allows the core section of bone to fill the needle. Replacing the cap provides suction to keep the specimen in the needle.	
4. Verify the length of the biopsy sample, with the stylet used as a guide.	Gently insert the stylet so as not to push the core back or damage it.	Optimal length of biopsy sample should be between 1.5 and 2.0 cm.
5. Before removal, the Jamshidi needle should be rotated 360 degrees in each direction three to five times. Place the cap back on the hub, and gently back the needle out of the bone, skin, and muscle, while applying firm gentle pressure.	Giving the Jamshidi needle a few 360-degree turns and creating a vacuum by placing the cap over the top of the needle during removal increases the likelihood that the bone core will be retained within the needle.	If no cap is available for the needle, place thumb over needle to create vacuum.

Procedure continues on following page

Procedure for Performing Bone Marrow Biopsy and Aspiration—*Continued*

Steps	Rationale	Special Considerations
6. Apply firm pressure to the site for 5 minutes or until bleeding has stopped; apply the adhesive pressure dressing. Assist patient to supine position and place small rolled towel directly under site to apply additional direct pressure.	Reduces chance of bleeding at the site. Prevents infection.	May apply wrapped ice pack over clothes directly to site to reduce swelling, create hemostasis, and decrease pain.
7. If available, attach a guide to the distal end of the biopsy needle. With the blunt obturator supplied, remove the core sample by passing the obturator through the guide and pushing the sample out through the needle hub (large end).	Removing the core sample this way prevents damage to the bone by not forcing it through the narrower "drill" end of the needle.	
8. With the help of the assistant (if available) place the bone core sample on a glass slide. With an additional glass slide, gently touch the slide against the length of the biopsy sample to make 3 to 4 imprints. Place core sample in specimen container with appropriate solution for processing (i.e., 10% formalin or sterile 2 × 2 gauze soaked with sterile saline solution).	A touch preparation can be useful for a complete pathology analysis.	Core specimen should be kept moist to prevent decay before processing.
9. Ensure specimens are sent to appropriate laboratory for analysis.	Specimens require staining and decalcification for studies.	
10. Discard used supplies in appropriate receptacle.	Safely discards used supplies.	
11. [HH]		

Expected Outcomes

- Adequate bone marrow aspirate and core biopsy specimens obtained
- Spicules in the aspirate (unless the patient is aplastic); aspirate not clotted
- Minimal bleeding and discomfort (patient may feel a dull ache for a few days after the procedure)

Unexpected Outcomes

- Difficulty obtaining a bone marrow aspirate
- Excessive pain
- Inability to perform procedure because of patient fear or intolerance
- Hematoma
- Retroperitoneal bleed
- Local infection

Patient Monitoring and Care

Steps	Rationale	Reportable Conditions
		These conditions should be reported if they persist despite nursing interventions.
1. Follow institutional standard for assessing pain. Administer analgesia as prescribed. **(Level B*)**	Identifies need for pain interventions. Promotes patient comfort.[2,4,7]	- Continued pain despite pain interventions

*Level B: Well-designed controlled studies with results that consistently support a specific action, intervention, or treatment

Patient Monitoring and Care —*Continued*

Steps	Rationale	Reportable Conditions
2. Assess vital signs, oxygenation, level of consciousness, and electrocardiogram rhythm during the procedure and until patient is completely recovered from sedation medications.	Monitors patient response to positioning, the procedure, and medications.	• Changes in vital signs, decreases in oxygen saturation (Sao_2), changes in cardiac rhythm, or level of consciousness
3. Assess the site after the procedure.	Monitors for signs and symptoms of complications.	• Bleeding, hematoma, and infection

Documentation

Documentation should include the following:
- Patient and family education
- Completion of informed consent
- Procedure verification and time-out
- Date and time of the procedure
- Indication for the procedure
- Preparation for the procedure
- Any complications that occurred

- Any medications used
- Specimens obtained
- Additional interventions
- For patients receiving conscious sedation, documentation that institution-approved discharge criteria has been met
- Pain assessment, interventions, and effectiveness

References

CR 1. Bain BJ: Bone marrow aspiration, *J Clin Pathol* 54: 657-663, 2001.

CR 2. Burkle CM, et al: Morbidity and mortality of deep sedation in outpatient bone marrow biopsy, *Am J Hematol* 77:250-256, 2004.

CR 3. Ellis LD, Jensen WN, Westerman MP: Needle biopsy of bone and marrow; an experience with 1,445 biopsies, *Arch Intern Med* 114:213-221, 1964.

4. Gudgin EJ, Besser MW, Craig JIO: Entonox as a sedative for bone marrow aspiration and biopsy, *Int J Lab Hematol* 30:65-67, 2008.

CR 5. Hyun BH, Gulati GL, Ashton JK: Bone marrow examination: techniques and interpretation, *Hematol Oncol Clin North Am* 2:513-523, 1988.

CR 6. Riley RS, et al: A pathologist's perspective on bone marrow aspiration and biopsy: 1: performing a bone marrow examination, *J Clin Lab Anal* 18:70-90, 2004.

CR 7. Vanhelleputte P, et al: Pain during bone marrow aspiration: prevalence and prevention, *J Pain Symptom Manage* 26: 860-866, 2003.

CR 8. Van Marum RJ, Te Velde L: Cardiac tamponade following sternal puncture in two patients, *Netherlands J Med* 59: 39-40, 2001.

Additional Readings

CR Aboul-Nasr R, et al: Comparison of touch imprints with aspirate smears for evaluating bone marrow specimens, *Am J Clin Pathol* (6)III:753-758, 1999.

CR Bain BJ: Bone marrow trephine biopsy, *J Clin Pathol* 54:737-742, 2001.

CR Huyn BH, Stevenson AJ, Hanua CA: Fundamentals of bone marrow examination, *Hematol Oncol Clin North Am* 8:651-663, 1994.

CR Lawson S, et al: Trained nurses can obtain satisfactory bone marrow aspirates and trephine biopsies, *J Clin Pathol* 52:154-156, 1999.

CR Lin EM: *Advanced practice in oncology nursing: case studies and review,* Philadelphia, 2001, Saunders.

CR Litwack K: *Core curriculum for perianesthesia nursing,* ed 4, Philadelphia, 1999, Saunders.

CR Quinn DMD, Schick L: *Perianesthesia nursing core curriculum: preoperative, phase 1 and phase II PACU nursing,* Philadelphia, 2004, Saunders.

CR Ryan DH, *Cohen HJ: Bone marrow aspiration and morphology, hematology basic principles and practice,* ed 3, New York, 2000, Churchill Livingstone.

CR Trewhitt KG: Bone marrow aspirate and biopsy collection and interpretation, *Oncol Nurs Forum* 28:1409-1415, 2001.

Bone Marrow Biopsy and Aspiration (Assist)

PURPOSE: Bone marrow aspiration and biopsy are used for diagnosis and classification of various hematopoietic diseases, identification of metastatic disease, monitoring of clinical response to treatment, and assessment of engraftment after bone marrow or stem cell transplantation.

Eileen C. Finnegan

PREREQUISITE NURSING KNOWLEDGE

- A thorough understanding is needed of the anatomy and physiology of the posterior and anterior iliac crest and the sternum. The preferred site for a bone marrow aspirate and biopsy is the posterior iliac crest.[1] The sternum may be used to aspirate marrow; however, a core biopsy cannot be obtained from the sternum because of risk of damage to underlying organs, most significantly the heart.[6,8]
- Clinical and technical competence in assisting with a bone marrow aspirate and biopsy is necessary.
- Clinical and technical competence in preparing slides and caring for a core biopsy is needed.
- Knowledge of sterile technique is necessary.
- Understanding is needed of institutional policies and procedures for administration of and monitoring of intravenous (IV) and oral pharmacologic agents, including conscious sedation (if indicated).
- Procedural care of the patient receiving IV conscious sedation or oral antianxiolytics or pain medication should be understood.
- Bone marrow aspirate is used in identification of normal and abnormal hematopoietic elements. The aspirate is also used to identify malignant clones with flow cytometry, to identify chromosomal abnormalities that occur in hematologic malignant disease, to perform molecular diagnostic studies of gene rearrangements and translocations, and to

perform chimerism studies in patients after allogeniec transplant.
- The bone marrow biopsy is used for morphologic analysis of hematopoietic cells and for assessment of the architecture of the bone marrow that may be abnormal in certain disease states.
- Indications for bone marrow aspiration and biopsy include the following:
  - ❖ To diagnosis a hematologic abnormality
  - ❖ To monitor a hematologic disease state after initial diagnosis or therapy
  - ❖ To diagnose bone marrow involvement before stem cell collection and for staging of various malignant states
  - ❖ To assess the status of disease after autologous bone marrow or hematopoietic stem cell transplant
  - ❖ To assess chimerism disease status and immune reconstitution after an allogeneic bone marrow or hematopoietic stem cell transplant
  - ❖ To evaluate immunodeficiency syndromes or to confirm an infectious disease process in the marrow
- Contraindications to bone marrow biopsy and aspirate are the presence of hemophilia, severe disseminated intravascular coagulopathy, or other related severe bleeding disorders. Thrombocytopenia alone is not a contraindication to bone marrow examination.[3,5] The use of anticoagulant medications may pose serious bleeding risk; therefore, coagulation studies should be obtained in these patients. The decision on whether anticoagulation can be

safely withheld prior to and restarted after the procedure is patient dependent.

EQUIPMENT

- Bone marrow aspiration and biopsy kit, which includes the following:
  - ❖ Povidone-iodine or chlorhexidine-alcohol antiseptic preparation
  - ❖ Sterile fenestrated drape (2)
  - ❖ 1 vial of lidocaine (1% or 2%; 5-10 mL)
  - ❖ 5 or 10-mL syringe for drawing up lidocaine
  - ❖ Needles of appropriate lengths to anesthetize both skin and periosteum
  - ❖ Sterile 4 × 4 and 2 × 2 gauze pads
  - ❖ Small scalpel blade
  - ❖ Bone marrow aspirate needle (Illinois needle)
  - ❖ Jamshidi bone biopsy needle (regular or extra long)
  - ❖ 20-mL syringe for bone marrow aspirate
  - ❖ 10-mL syringes for marrow aspiration
  - ❖ Edetate disodium (EDTA) sterile solution (15 mg/mL; 2 mL total)
  - ❖ Blunt needles for drawing up EDTA, heparin, saline solution
  - ❖ Adhesive bandage
- Sterile gloves
- Filtered needle (if lidocaine drawn from glass vial)
- Fluid shield face mask or goggles
- Specimen bags and labels
- Required tubes for specimen processing: two EDTA (lavender top) and two sodium heparin (green top) tubes (follow institution standard)
- Glass slides and cover plate
- 2½- to 6-inch spinal needle (may be required for anesthetizing periosteum in the obese patient)
- Container for bone biopsy specimen including appropriate fixative (10% formalin or sterile saline solution–soaked sterile gauze)
- 1 additional vial of lidocaine (1% or 2%)
- 1 vial of 100 unit/mL heparin (follow institution standard)

Additional equipment for patients receiving conscious sedation:
- Pulse oximeter
- Automated blood pressure monitor
- Oxygen
- Suction
- Ambu bag
- IV pharmacologic agents (i.e., midazolam, 2 to 4 mg; fentanyl, 25 to 50 mcg; lorazepam, 1 to 2 mg)
- IV opiate and benzodiazepine antagonist agents (i.e., naloxone and flumazenil)
- Emergency equipment

PATIENT AND FAMILY EDUCATION

- Assess patient and family understanding of the bone marrow aspiration and biopsy procedure and the reason for it. ➻*Rationale:* Clarification of the procedure and reinforce-

ment of information may reduce patient and family anxiety and stress.
- Inform the patient and family (if permitted by patient) that the results will be shared with them as soon as they are available. ➻*Rationale:* The patient and family are usually anxious about the results.
- Explain the actual procedure to the patient and family. ➻*Rationale:* The patient and family are prepared for what to expect. Anxiety is decreased. The patient is involved in care.
- Review safety requirements for patients who will receive pharmacologic agents for sedation (i.e., must have transportation and escort home and may not drive until the following day). ➻*Rationale:* Review ensures patient safety and healthcare provider's accountability for patients receiving sedation.
- Encourage the patient to verbalize any pain experienced during the procedure. ➻*Rationale:* Additional lidocaine, pain medication, or sedation medication can be administered. Patient becomes a participant in care.
- Instruct patient and family to keep pressure dressing clean, dry, and in place for 24 hours after the procedure. Ask patient or family to assess for bruising or hematoma. Advise the use of ice pack to site to reduce pain and hematoma. ➻*Rationale:* Proper dressing care reduces chance of bleeding and minimizes chance of infection at the site.
- Avoid applying heat to the procedure site. ➻*Rationale:* Heat could exacerbate bleeding.
- Advise against non-steroidal anti-inflammatory drugs or aspirin for 24 hours after biopsy. ➻*Rationale:* This measure reduces the chance of bleeding or hematoma at site.
- Advise use of acetaminophen for pain relief, if not contraindicated. ➻*Rationale:* Acetaminophen relieves pain and does not promote bleeding.

PATIENT ASSESSMENT AND PREPARATION

Patient Assessment

- Assess patient's home medications, including over-the-counter medications that can increase clotting time. ➻*Rationale:* Assessment decreases risk of bleeding and hematoma.
- Assess the need for antianxiety or analgesic medication or conscious sedation. ➻*Rationale:* If the patient is very anxious before the procedure or has had severe pain with previous bone marrow procedures, small doses of analgesia or sedation promote patient comfort. Relaxation of surrounding muscles makes procedure easier on patient and provider.
- Assess coagulation studies in patients who are taking anticoagulant medications. ➻*Rationale:* Patients at risk for bleeding complications are identified.
- Assess the ability of the patient to lie on his or her stomach or side, with the head of the bed at no greater than a 25-degree elevation. ➻*Rationale:* Access to and control of the posterior iliac crest is best obtained with the patient

lying flat, or with the head of the bed only slightly raised, in a side-lying or prone position.

- Assess vital signs and oxygenation status. **➙Rationale:** Baseline data are provided. Assessment ensures that the blood pressure and oxygenation status can be maintained if the patient is placed on his or her side or prone.
- Assess for recent bone marrow aspiration and biopsy sites. **➙Rationale:** The patient may have a painful experience if an additional biopsy is performed at a site that has not yet healed from a previous procedure. Penetration of scar tissue from areas of previous biopsies also may be difficult.

Patient Preparation

- Ensure that the patient and family understand pre- and postprocedural teachings and discharge instructions. Answer questions as they arise, and reinforce information as needed. **➙Rationale:** Understanding of previously taught information is evaluated and reinforced. The patient and family understand postprocedure care. The patient is made a participant in care.
- Verify correct patient with two identifiers. **➙Rationale:** Prior to performing a procedure, the nurse should ensure the correct identification of the patient for the intended intervention.
- Obtain informed consent for bone marrow aspiration and biopsy and, if indicated, conscious sedation. **➙Rationale:**

Informed consent protects the rights of the patient and makes a competent decision possible for the patient.

- Perform a pre-procedure verification and time out, if non-emergent. **➙Rationale:** Ensures patient safety.
- Administer analgesia or sedation as prescribed. **➙Rationale:** Patient may need analgesia or sedation to ensure adequate cooperation and minimize discomfort during the procedure.
- Follow institution standard for a patient receiving conscious sedation. **➙Rationale:** Preparation ensures that appropriate emergency equipment and medical staff are available.
- Obtain IV access for patients receiving sedation. **➙Rationale:** A secure patent IV line is necessary for administration of IV pharmacologic agents and, if necessary, emergency antagonist agents.
- Obtain a complete blood count and differential via venipuncture. **➙Rationale:** Many pathologists prefer to review a peripheral blood sample in conjunction with the marrow to make a complete and accurate diagnostic evaluation.
- Confirm availability of personnel who will assist with the procedure. **➙Rationale:** Slide preparation, specimen processing, and obtaining additional supplies require an appropriately trained assistant for the procedure.
- Assist the patient to an appropriate position depending on the patient's comfort and the practitioner's preference. **➙Rationale:** Positioning ensures good visualization and control of the posterior iliac crest.

Procedure | for Assisting with Bone Marrow Biopsy and Aspiration

Steps	Rationale	Special Considerations
1. 🄷🄷		
2. Ensure that the patient is positioned properly.	Prepares patient for the procedure.[6]	With an outpatient setting, ensure patient safety on examination table.
3. Assist the physician or advanced practice nurse with opening and assembling necessary supplies.	Prepares supplies. Maintains sterile technique.	
4. 🄷🄷		
5. Assist healthcare provider performing the procedure with applying personal protective and sterile equipment. (sterile gown, sterile gloves, mask, goggles)	Maintains sterile technique.	Gowns may be required in some settings, such as the blood and marrow transplant unit.
6. Assist with or draw up 2 mL of EDTA into one of sterile syringes (10 or 20-mL) depending on number of specimens needed.	Ensures adequate slide preparation because EDTA is used to preserve spicules.	EDTA tubes usually have a lavender top.
7. Assist with or draw up 200 mg of heparin into one of syringes (10-mL or 20-mL) depending on number if specimens needed.	Heparinized aspirate is used for flow cytometry, chromosome analysis, and chimerism studies.	Heparinized tubes usually have a green top. Follow institution standard for use of heparinized and non-heparinized tubes for obtaining samples.
8. Follow institutional standard for administration of prescribed IV pharmacologic agents, including conscious sedation. **(Level B*)**	Promotes patient comfort and reduces anxiety.[2,4,7]	Ensure emergency equipment available and functional. Make others aware procedure is occurring in case assistance is needed.

*Level B: Well-designed controlled studies with results that consistently support a specific action, intervention, or treatment

Procedure   for Assisting with Bone Marrow Biopsy and Aspiration—*Continued*

Steps	Rationale	Special Considerations

9. Assist with processing the aspirate obtained in the nonheparinized (EDTA) syringe first.
  A. The aspirate in the 20-mL nonheparinized (EDTA) syringe should be placed in lavender-top tubes and used for slide preparation, clot analysis, and polymerase chain reaction (PCR) studies.
  B. The aspirate in the heparinized syringes should be placed into green-top sodium heparin tubes.
	Nonheparinized (EDTA) bone marrow aspirate can clot if it is not placed in the appropriate tubes soon after it is obtained.	If no spicules are visible in the aspirate syringe, there will be no hematopoietic elements for morphologic analysis. It may be necessary to attempt aspiration after repositioning the aspirate needle to an alternate site, or the patient may have an "empty marrow." If no blood can be aspirated at all, the procedure may be documented as a "dry tap."

10. Assist as needed with performing touch preparation with the bone biopsy core sample, and place sample in 10% formalin fixative or sterile saline solution–soaked sterile gauze in container.	A touch preparation can be useful for a complete pathology analysis, especially if the aspirate is aparticulate or a "dry tap."[6]	
11. Assist with holding pressure for 5 minutes or until bleeding has stopped. Apply pressure dressing.	Ensures adequate hemostasis and reduces chance of infection.	Have patient lie on back with small towel role or covered ice pack under biopsy site to reduce risk of bleeding, hematoma, and pain.
12. Follow institutional postprocedural recovery plan for patients who have received conscious sedation.	Ensures recovery parameters have been met.	
13. Label and send samples for laboratory analysis.	Ensures accuracy of results and timeliness of laboratory analyses.	Ensure that paperwork for specimens is correctly completed to avoid delays in processing.
14. Discard used supplies in appropriate receptacle.	Safely discards used supplies.	
15. 🅷🅷		

Expected Outcomes

- Adequate bone marrow aspirate and core biopsy specimens obtained
- Minimal bleeding and discomfort (patient may feel a dull ache for a few days after the procedure)
- Spicules in the aspirate (unless the patient is aplastic); aspirate not clotted

Unexpected Outcomes

- Inability to obtain specimens
- Excessive pain
- Hematoma
- Retroperitoneal bleed
- Local infection

Patient Monitoring and Care

Steps	Rationale	Reportable Conditions
		These conditions should be reported if they persist despite nursing interventions.
1. Follow institutional standard for assessing pain. Administer analgesia as prescribed. **(Level B*)**	Identifies need for pain interventions. Promotes patient comfort.[2,4,7]	- Continued pain despite pain interventions

*Level B: Well-designed controlled studies with results that consistently support a specific action, intervention, or treatment

Procedure continues on following page

Patient Monitoring and Care —*Continued*

Steps	Rationale	Reportable Conditions
2. Monitor vital signs, level of consciousness, oxygenation, and electrocardiogram rhythm during the procedure and until patient is completely recovered from sedation medications.	Determines the patient response to positioning and the procedure.	• Changes in vital signs or level of consciousness • Decreased oxygen saturation (Sao_2) • Cardiac dysrhythmias
3. Assess the site after the procedure.	Monitors for signs and symptoms of complications.	• Bleeding • Hematoma • Infection

Documentation

Documentation should include the following:

- Patient and family education
- Completion of informed consent
- Procedure verification and time-out
- Indication for the procedure
- Date and time of the procedure
- Practitioner performing the procedure
- Person assisting with procedure
- Any complications that occurred

- Any medications used
- Specimens obtained
- Additional interventions
- For patients receiving conscious sedation, documentation that institution-approved discharge criteria has been met
- Pain assessment, interventions, and effectiveness

References

CR 1. Bain BJ: Bone marrow aspiration, *J Clin Pathol* 54: 657-663, 2001.

CR 2. Burkle CM, et al: Morbidity and mortality of deep sadation in outpatient bone marrow biopsy, *Am J Hematol* 77:250-256, 2004.

CR 3. Ellis LD, Jensen WN, Westerman MP: Needle biopsy of bone and marrow: an experience with 1,445 biopsies, *Arch Intern Med* 114:213-221, 1964.

4. Gudgin EJ, Besser MW, Craig JIO: Entonox as a sedative for bone marrow aspiration and biopsy, *Int J Lab Hematol* 30:65-67, 2008.

CR 5. Hyun BH, Gulati GL, Ashton JK: Bone marrow examination: techniques and interpretation, *Hematol Oncol Clin North Am* 2:513-523, 1988.

CR 6. Riley RS, et al: A pathologist's perspective on bone marrow aspiration and biopsy: 1: performing a bone marrow examination, *J Clin Lab Anal* 18:70-90, 2004.

CR 7. Vanhelleputte P, et al: Pain during bone marrow aspiration: prevalence and prevention, *J Pain Symptom Manage* 26:860-866, 2003.

CR 8. Van Marum RJ, Te Velde L: Cardiac tamponade following sternal puncture in two patients, *Netherlands J Med* 59:39-40, 2001.

Additional Readings

CR Aboul-Nasr R, et al: Comparison of touch imprints with aspirate smears for evaluating bone marrow specimens, *Am J Clin Pathol* (6)III:753-758, 1999.

Burke JM: *Dx/Rx: leukemia,* Boston, 2006, Jones and Bartlett.

CR Bain BJ: Bone marrow trephine biopsy, *J Clin Pathol* 54: 737-742, 2001.

CR DeVita VT, et al: *Cancer principles and practice,* ed 3, Philadelphia, 2001, Lippincott Williams & Wilkins.

CR Huyn BH, Stevenson AJ, Hanua CA: Fundamentals of bone marrow examination, *Hematol Oncol Clin North Am* 8:651-663, 1994.

CR Lawson S, et al: Trained nurses can obtain satisfactory bone marrow aspirates and trephine biopsies, *J Clin Pathol* 52:154-156, 1999.

CR Lin EM: *Advanced practice in oncology nursing: case studies and review,* Philadelphia, 2001, Saunders.

CR Litwack K: *Core curriculum for perianesthesia nursing,* ed 4, Philadelphia, 1999, Saunders.

CR Quinn DMD, Schick L: *Perianesthesia nursing core curriculum: preoperative, phase I and phase II PACU nursing,* Philadelphia, 2004, Saunders.

CR Ryan DH, Cohen HJ: *Bone marrow aspiration and morphology, hematology basic principles and practice,* ed 3, New York, 2000, Churchill Livingstone.

CR Trewhitt KG: Bone marrow aspirate and biopsy collection and interpretation, *Oncol Nurs Forum* 28:1409-1415, 2001.

Watson M, et al: *Oncology,* ed 2, New York, 2006, Oxford Press.

Donor Site Care

P U R P O S E :   Care of the donor site is performed to promote wound healing and maintain function. Pain control is a priority during donor site care.

Elizabeth A. Mann

Across the United States, diversity is found among burn units concerning policy, practice, and procedure in the care of thermal injuries. This in no way intimates that diversity in practice corresponds with diversity in quality. The burn care community, consisting of 127 burn units, regularly benchmarks among themselves, both formally and informally, to compare outcomes and update practices to ensure that patients receive optimum quality of care. As with any specialty, the effects of research and the trial of new techniques and products are always part of the search for best practice.

PREREQUISITE NURSING KNOWLEDGE

- A partial-thickness wound is surgically created when a donor site (Fig. 119-1) is harvested to obtain skin for a full-thickness defect. The more dermis moved with the skin graft, the less the graft shrinks with healing; therefore, deeper donor sites may be created to obtain skin for cosmetically significant areas such as the face or hands.[9] Depending on the percentage of dermis moved with the graft, donor sites created may be superficial or deep partial-thickness wounds that heal in 10 to 20 days (typically, 10 to 14 days; Fig. 119-2).[6]
- Factors that can disrupt or prolong healing include infection, desiccation, edema, adherent dressing changes, poor nutrition, hemodynamic instability, and a variety of preexisting medical conditions.[2]
- The longer a partial-thickness wound takes to heal, the more significant the scarring; therefore, donor sites can produce minimal or hypertrophic scars.[2] Donor sites

retain deep epidermal appendages, so they are generally capable of sweating and bearing hair after they heal. The donor site may be reharvested once healing is complete, but skin from the first harvest of a donor site is always of higher quality than that of repeat harvesting.
- Because the dermis is richly supplied with capillaries and nerve endings, donor sites are at risk for bleeding in the first 24 hours and are exquisitely tender to touch. They produce large volumes of serous exudate.
- Donor site treatment goals include minimizing bleeding, supporting reepithelialization, managing exudate, preventing infection, controlling pain, and minimizing scarring.[9] Epinephrine-soaked dressings, thrombin spray, or compression dressings may be applied in the operating room to attain stasis.[9] A compression dressing is usually used for the first 12 to 24 hours to ensure stasis.[8] After this initial period, compression may be applied for comfort.

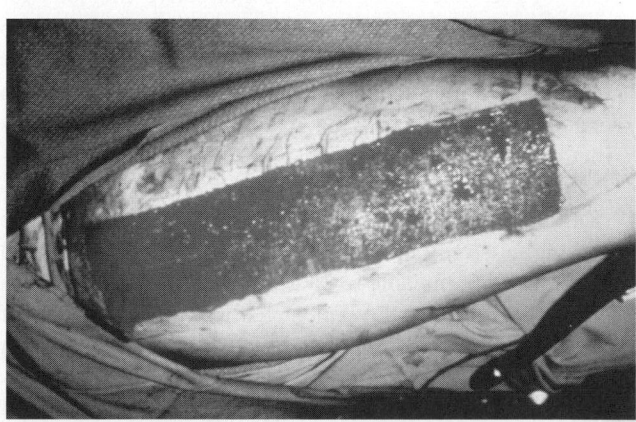

FIGURE 119-1   Fresh donor site.

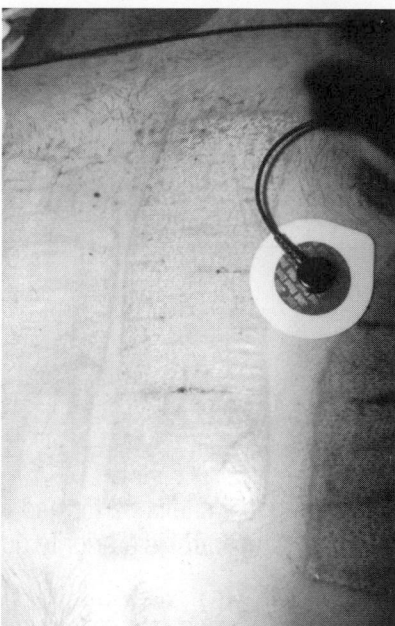

FIGURE 119-2   Donor sites.

- Wounds epithelialize most rapidly in a moist environment. If donor sites are small enough, use of a thin-film polyurethane or hydrocolloid dressing has been shown to promote rapid healing while providing comfort through dressing flexibility and occlusive coverage of nerve endings.[6] Occlusive dressings (sealed on all sides) can be difficult to maintain on larger donor sites because of the substantial volume of exudate.[6] A small drain (attached to a vacutainer and collection tube Becton, Dickinson and Co., Franklin Lakes, NJ) tube can be used to remove excess drainage from under a thin-film dressing. Calcium alginates have also been used successfully under occlusive dressings to mange exudate.[6]
- Multilayer occlusive dressings may also be used, with a nonstick dressing (e.g., greasy gauze, meshed silicone) applied next to the donor site and a bulky absorbent outer layer to maintain a moist environment and wick away excess drainage. The outer dressing may be changed periodically, leaving the inner dressing intact until the wound heals beneath it.
- One of the oldest and most cost-effective methods for treatment of donor sites is to apply mesh gauze, wrap with an outer wrap for 12 to 24 hours, and then remove the outer wrap and allow the inner dressing to remain exposed and dry until the wound heals beneath. This method has been done with fine mesh gauze and xeroform (McKesson Brand, San Francisco, CA)/xeroflo (Kendall Healthcare, Coviden, Mansfield, MA). The technique is only effective if the dressing dries well and becomes impermeable to bacteria, essentially acting as a scab.[11] Positioning the patient for maximal exposure of the donor sites, preventing prolonged donor site contact with sheets and clothing, and increasing airflow across the wound are important for this technique to work.[5] If the donor site is large, this procedure creates a rather stiff and uncomfortable protective layer.

- Biobrane (UDL Laboratories, Rockford, IL), a biosynthetic product, produces a more flexible donor site dressing. When exposed to air at 24 hours after harvesting, it dries to form a fibrous bond with the collagen in the wound. This dressing provides improved pain control, exudate management, and rate of healing when compared with a fine-mesh gauze dressing.[12]
- Antimicrobial creams or ointments have also been used on donor sites, essentially treating the wounds in the same way as partial-thickness burns are treated. The disadvantage to this approach is that it requires daily washing of the wound and reapplication of cream and dressings.[11]
- Slow-release silver dressings are gaining popularity for donor site use. These dressings are moistened twice daily with sterile water to release the silver. In highly exudating wounds, the wound moisture may be adequate to promote silver release without exogenously applied moisture. These dressings release silver for 3 or more days; ideally, they are placed on the donor site in the operating room, and the wound is allowed to heal beneath with infrequent or no dressing changes.[6,11]
- Donor sites need to be assessed daily for signs of infection, including periwound warmth and erythema, increased pain, and purulent drainage. Bacteria can delay healing and increase scarring or convert a partial-thickness donor site to a full-thickness wound.[2] Erythema should be outlined to monitor progression, with consideration of either removing the donor site dressing or applying a topical antimicrobial to penetrate the donor site dressing. Reopening or "melting" of epithelium in previously healed donor sites is often the result of colonization with gram-positive organisms and may require antibacterial intervention.[4] Heavy hair-bearing donor sites such as the scalp provide special challenges. Heavy hair growth can lead to matting of hair in the exudate, which can lead to accumulation of protein, proliferation of bacteria, and ingrowth of hair, a condition referred to as chronic folliculitis.[8] This problem can lead to chronic, nonhealing, inflamed wounds or conversion of partial-thickness donor sites to full-thickness wounds. Dressings that prevent drying and wick away the exudate work well.
- Donor sites are often very painful, with the amount of pain variable depending on the dressing technique used. Patients with donor sites usually need scheduled round-the-clock pain medication.[3,7]
- The donor site should not be exposed to the sun for a year after the burn. Apply full-spectrum sunblock to donor sites any time exposure to the sun is anticipated.[10]
- Protect fresh donor sites from dependent edema by wrapping with elastic bandages before sitting or ambulating.

EQUIPMENT

- Personal protective equipment (gown, mask, goggles as needed)
- Nonsterile gloves
- Scissors
- Replacement dressing as needed
- Pain and sedation medication (as prescribed)

PATIENT AND FAMILY EDUCATION

- Teach the patient and family that donor sites generally heal in 10 to 12 days with variable scarring. ➤➤*Rationale:* Realistic expectations about healing and scarring are provided.
- Provide donor site care instructions, and review them with the patient and family. Demonstrate how to assess and manage the donor site dressing, and have the patient and family return the demonstration. Encourage the patient and family to ask questions. Provide positive feedback. Arrange for home care or clinic visits to follow up on dressings and wound care. ➤➤*Rationale:* The patient's and family's understanding and ability to perform wound care are validated.
- Patients should be encouraged to avoid smoking. ➤➤*Rationale:* Smoking causes vasoconstriction, inhibits epithelialization, and decreases tissue oxygenation, all of which delay healing.[2]
- Explain to the patient about the pain and itching sensations associated with donor site healing.[1,7] ➤➤*Rationale:* Patients need to know that donor site pain and itching, although unpleasant, are normal and do not cause concern.
- Teach the patient and family about appropriate use of medications and nonpharmacologic interventions to manage pain and itching.[1] Encourage application of a topical moisturizer after healing.[7] ➤➤*Rationale:* Comfort is enhanced.
- Teach the patient and family about signs and symptoms of infection and the importance of reporting these in a timely manner.[4] ➤➤*Rationale:* The patient and family can recognize problems early so that appropriate measures can be instituted by the healthcare providers.
- Provide the patient and family with follow-up appointments and a contact to call with any problems. ➤➤*Rationale:* This information is necessary for further care and follow up.
- Assess the family's ability to provide care at home at each follow-up visit. ➤➤*Rationale:* Continued care of the wound is necessary after discharge.
- Stress the importance of wearing pressure garments if they are indicated. ➤➤*Rationale:* Pressure garments reduce scarring.[10]
- Inform the patient and family that the donor site should not be exposed to the sun for a year after the burn. Patients should wear clothing that covers wounds or a sunscreen with SPF higher than 15.[10] ➤➤*Rationale:* The patient and family are prepared for changes that occur after healing.

PATIENT ASSESSMENT AND PREPARATION

Patient Assessment

- Evaluate for signs of healing, as follows:
  - ❖ Decreased pain
  - ❖ Decreased edema
  - ❖ Dressing separation at wound edges with reepithelialization beneath it
  - ❖ Compare degree of healing with expected rate of healing based on number of days since skin harvested. ➤➤*Rationale:* Healing should occur within 10 to 12 days unless complications occur.
- Evaluate for signs and symptoms of infection, as follows:
  - ❖ Foul odor
  - ❖ Purulent drainage
  - ❖ Discoloration
  - ❖ Increased pain
  - ❖ Increasing edema
  - ❖ Cellulitis
  - ❖ Delayed healing
  - ❖ Fever or increasing white blood cell (WBC) count[4]
  - ➤➤*Rationale:* Donor site infection may necessitate antimicrobial intervention.[2]
- Evaluate the adequacy of the pain control by asking the patient to rate the pain on a scale of 0 to 10, both before and during wound care. ➤➤*Rationale:* An individualized plan for pain control should be in place for background and procedural pain.[3,7]
- Evaluate the patient's range of motion (ROM) in the vicinity of the donor site. Physical and occupational therapists may be consulted to assist the patient with maintaining ROM and with scar management. ➤➤*Rationale:* Wounds contract during healing; pain and tightness can decrease ROM. The patient should be encouraged to continue normal movement and ROM exercises.

Patient Preparation

- Ensure that the patient understands preprocedural teaching. Answer questions, and reinforce information as needed. ➤➤*Rationale:* Understanding of previously taught information is evaluated and reinforced.
- **VP** Premedicate the patient for pain and anxiety, as prescribed. Wait to perform the procedure until the medication has had time to work. ➤➤*Rationale:* Waiting allows time for the medication to take effect and promotes optimal comfort for the patient. Medication reduces pain and anxiety and encourages patient trust and compliance with procedure.

Procedure   for Care of Donor Sites

Steps	Rationale	Special Considerations
1. Prepare all necessary equipment and supplies. Treatment area should be warmed. Administer analgesic in advance of performing procedure.	Preparation facilitates efficient wound care and prevents needless delays. Warming the room decreases risk for hypothermia. Pain medications are effective for procedure.	
2. 🅷🅷		
3. 🅿🅴		
4. Remove gauze roll and any padding covering inner dressing.	Inner dressing is left in place until the wound heals unless a problem with infection occurs.	Gauze roll or outer dressing is usually removed after 24 hours if goal is for inner dressing layer to be exposed to air and dry.
5. Assess the donor site for signs of healing and complications; assess whether the inner dressing needs to be changed. **Proceed to Step 9** if inner donor dressing needs to be changed.	Validates the healing process and identifies complications. Avoid changing inner dressing to facilitate healing.	If inner dressing was stapled in place, staples need to be removed when inner dressing is fully adherent (generally between postoperative days 4 and 7).
6. Remove and discard gloves; apply a pair of clean gloves.	Handling the burn dressing contaminates examination gloves, and clean gloves are needed for wound care.	
7. Gently wash exudate from wound edges with warm tap water and pat dry.	Clears exudate that can harbor microorganisms from area of donor site. Keep covered donor site dry to improve healing.	
8. Use scissors to trim loose edges of donor site dressing. If inner dressing does not need to be changed, **proceed to Step 14** to complete donor site care.	Because dry inner dressing is not covered, loose edges of dressing can snag and displace inner dressing.	Assess need for outer dressing and apply as needed.

Inner Dressing Change

Steps	Rationale	Special Considerations
9. Remove inner dressing and discard it.		If dressing is adherent, soak with warm tap water to loosen.
10. Remove and discard gloves; apply a pair of clean gloves.	Handling the burn dressing contaminates examination gloves, and clean gloves are needed for wound care.	
11. Gently wash wound with mild pH-neutral soap, rinse with warm tap water, and pat dry.	Cleanses donor site.	Cleanse beyond donor site to reduce microbial count on surrounding tissue. Patients may do better if allowed to cleanse their own wounds.
12. Assess the donor site for progression of healing and complications; outline any inflammation with a marking pen.	Validates the healing process and identifies complications.	Notify healthcare providers from other disciplines who need to observe the wound ahead of time so that they can be present while the wound is uncovered.
13. Remove and discard gloves. Apply a pair of sterile or clean gloves.	Clean gloves are applied after washing a wound.	Sterile gloves may be used when applying dressings to large burn wounds.
14. Cut dressing to the size of donor site with sterile scissors, apply, and secure in place.	Ensures correct fit and adherence.	Dressing may be secured with tubular netting or cloth tape applied to the dressing margins.
15. Remove and discard gloves.	Reduces transmission of microorganisms.	
16. 🅷🅷		

Procedure   for Care of Donor Sites—*Continued*

Steps	Rationale	Special Considerations
17. Reapply bulky outer dressing if indicated.	Donor sites may be covered with bulky dressing to maintain moisture barrier, maintain a moist wound surface, or apply a topical antimicrobial soak.	Gauze roll or outer supportive dressing may be ordered over inner dressing until wound has healed.

Expected Outcomes

- Donor site heals within 2 weeks without complications
- Patient maintains a self-identified, acceptable level of pain relief
- Patient maintains comfort from measures taken for anxiety and itching
- Patient and family verbalize knowledge of patient condition and plan of care
- An optimal level of function is maintained or attained
- Patient and family response and interactions demonstrate adaptation to injury
- Patient and family collaborate in management of care
- At the time of discharge, patient and family verbalize and demonstrate an understanding of posthospital care

Unexpected Outcomes

- Bleeding
- Infection
- Conversion of donor site to deep partial-thickness or full-thickness wound

Patient Monitoring and Care

Steps	Rationale	Reportable Conditions
		These conditions should be reported if they persist despite nursing interventions.
1. Follow institutional standard for assessing pain. Administer analgesia as prescribed. Have the patient rate pain on a validated pain scale; check pain medication orders; and review patient's previous response to pain medication and assess the need to increase the dose. Incorporate non-pharmacologic pain relief techniques (e.g., relaxation techniques, massage therapy, music, visual imaging).	Identifies need for pain interventions. The donor site pain is minimized by an intact dressing that does not require a dressing change; the patient will have increased pain medication requirements if the dressing needs to be changed. Attention to the patient's pain fosters the patient's trust in healthcare provider.	- Continued pain despite pain interventions - Nonverbal indications of pain (e.g., restlessness, grimacing, teeth clenching) - Inability to cooperate with wound care - Increased respiratory rate - Verbalization of pain - Increased heart rate
2. Obtain baseline vital signs before procedure, monitor them throughout procedure, and check them for 30 minutes after procedure is complete.	Changes in vital signs can be a sign that the patient is experiencing pain or anxiety. Decreasing blood pressure, heart rate, and respiratory rate can be complications of pain medication (especially after dressing change is complete and stimulation has stopped).	- Increased or decreased blood pressure - Increased or decreased heart rate - Increased or decreased blood pressure - Increased or decreased respiratory rate - High peak pressures on ventilator
3. Assess the donor site for appearance (e.g., dressing wet or dry, dressing adherent, presence of drainage or bleeding, redness at edges) and progression toward healing (e.g., reepithelialization at wound edges).	Observe for usual progression of wound healing versus complications of infection, progression of donor site to deeper wound, and bleeding.	- Foul odor - Purulent or increased amounts of drainage - Cellulitis or edema - Healing tissue developing eschar - Discoloration of wound - Bleeding

Procedure continues on following page

Patient Monitoring and Care —*Continued*

Steps	Rationale	Reportable Conditions
4. Encourage exercise and activities of daily living; place patient in position of optimal function and assess need for pain medication to facilitate movement. Physical therapy may be necessary to maintain range of motion.[3,10] **(Level D*)**	Donor site wounds contract during the healing phase. Pain also inhibits movement.	

Documentation

Documentation should include the following:

- Patient and family education
- Date and time of wound care
- Appearance (e.g., dressing wet or dry, dressing adherence, presence of drainage or bleeding, redness at edges)
- Progression toward healing (e.g., reepithelialization at wound edges)
- Application of topical agents
- Type of dressing applied

- Pain assessment, interventions, and effectiveness
- Medications given for pain and sedation
- Other comfort measures used
- Patient's tolerance of the procedure
- Unexpected outcomes
- Nursing interventions

*Level D: Peer-reviewed professional organizational standards with clinical studies to support recommendations

References

1. Brooks JP, et al: Scratching the surface: managing the itch associated with burns: a review of current knowledge, *Burns* 34:751-760, 2008.
2. Broughton G, et al: Wound healing: an overview, *Plast Reconstr Surg* 117:1e-S-32e-S, 2006.
3. Faucher L, et al: Practice guidelines for the management of pain, *J Burn Care Res* 27:659-668, 2006.
4. Gallagher JJ, et al: Treatment of infections in burns. In Herndon D, editor: *Total burn care*, ed 3, London, 2007, Saunders Elsevier 136-176.
5. Hedman TL, et al: Two simple leg net devices designed to protect lower-extremity skin grafts and donor sites and prevent decubitus ulcer, *J Burn Care Res* 28:115-119, 2007.
CR 6. Honari S: Topical therapies and antimicrobials in the management of burn wounds, *Crit Care Nurs Clin North Am* 16:1-11, 2004.
7. Meyer WJ, et al: Management of pain and other discomforts in burned patients. In Herndon D, editor: *Total burn care*, ed 3, London, 2007, Saunders Elsevier, 797-818.
8. Mimoun M, et al: The scalp is an advantageous donor site for thin-skin grafts: a report on 945 harvested samples, *Plast Reconstr Surg* 118:369-373, 2006.

9. Muller M, et al: Operative wound management. In Herndon D, editor: *Total burn care*, ed 3, London, 2007, Saunders Elsevier,177-195.
10. Serghiou MA, et al: Comprehensive rehabilitation of the burn patient. In Herndon D, editor: *Total burn care*, ed 3, London, 2007, Saunders Elsevier, 620-651.
11. Stout LR: Burns. In Carlson KK, editor: *AACN advanced critical care nursing*, London, 2009, Saunders Elsevier, 1212-1260.
12. Whitaker IS, et al: A critical evaluation of the use of Biobrane as a biologic skin substitute: a versatile tool for the plastic and reconstructive surgeon, *Ann Plastic Surg* 60:333-337, 2008.

Additional Readings

CR Flynn MB, editor: Burn and wound care, *Crit Care Nurs Clin North Am* 16: 1-185, 2004.
Makic MBF, Mann E: Burn Injuries. In McQuillan K, Makic MBF, Whalen E, editors: *Trauma nursing: resuscitation through rehabilitation*, Philadelphia, 2009, Elsevier, 865-888.

Burn Wound Care

P U R P O S E :   Burn wound care is performed to promote healing, maintain function, and prevent infection and burn wound sepsis. A major focus must be on pain control.

Elizabeth A. Mann

PREREQUISITE NURSING KNOWLEDGE

- Burns destroy the structural integrity of the skin, disrupting its normal functions of regulating temperature, maintaining fluid status, protecting against infection, covering nerve endings, and establishing identity.[2] The skin is composed of two layers, the epidermis and the dermis, and is supported by a subcutaneous layer that is rich in blood vessels (Fig. 120-1).

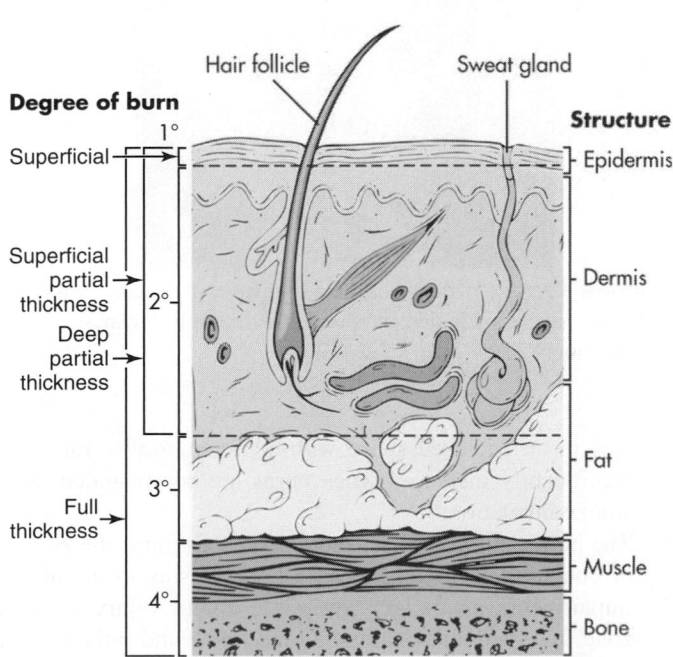

FIGURE 120-1   Cross section of skin with areas affected by partial-thickness and full-thickness burns. *(From Lewis SM, Cox IC: Medical-surgical nursing: assessment and management of clinical problems, ed 2, New York, 1987, McGraw-Hill.)*

- The *epidermis* is the outermost layer. It is capable of rapid regeneration through division of cells closest to the dermis; older epidermal cells are pushed outward as the epidermis is regenerated. The epidermis provides a barrier to the environment, containing melanocytes (protection from the sun) and Langerhans cells (protection against foreign organisms).
- The *dermis* contains blood vessels, sensory fibers (for pain, touch, pressure, and temperature), collagen, sebaceous glands, and sweat glands. Epidermal cells line deep dermal structures (hair follicles and sweat glands); these epidermal elements provide the ability for the skin to regenerate (the more epidermal cells remaining in the wound bed, the faster the healing).
- The depth of burns has historically been classified as first-degree (into epidermis), second-degree (into dermis), or third-degree (through skin into subcutaneous tissue; Table 120-1).[1,2]
  - *First-degree*, or superficial, *burns* extend only partially through the epidermis, thereby maintaining the barrier function of the skin. These burns are not included when estimating the percentage of total body surface area burned (%TBSA) because they do not result in an open wound.
  - *Second-degree burns* extend into the dermis and can be superficial (loss of the epidermis and part of the dermis) or deep (destruction of most of the dermis). They are also referred to as *partial-thickness burns* because they extend partially through the skin (Fig. 120-2). These wounds heal by epithelialization from epidermal cells remaining in the dermis. Shallow wounds are associated with rapid healing and less scarring. Deep wounds may result in slow-healing (more than 21 days) and fragile wounds prone to hypertrophic scarring. For that reason, surgical excision

TABLE 120-1	**Depth Characteristics of Burn Wounds**	
Type	Physical Characteristics	Healing
Superficial burn (first-degree): Destruction of epidermis, usually caused by overexposure to sun or brief exposure to hot liquid. This type of injury is not included in calculation of burn size.	Red; hypersensitive; no blisters.	Injured layers peel away from totally healed skin at 5 to 7 days without residual scarring.
Superficial partial-thickness burn (superficial second-degree): Destruction of epidermis and upper dermis. Usually results from scalding or brief contact with hot objects.	Blistered; very moist; red or pink in color; exquisitely painful; capillary refill intact.	Reepithelializes from epidermal appendages in 7 to 14 days. Usually has minimal scarring but variable repigmentation.
Deep partial-thickness burn (deep second-degree): Destruction of epidermis through to lower dermis. May result from grease or longer contact with hot objects.	Mottled pink to white; drier than superficial burns; less sensitive to pinprick; does not blanch to pressure; hair follicles and sweat glands intact.	Slower regeneration from epidermal elements: 14 to 21+ days in absence of grafting. Prone to hypertrophic scars and contracture formation. May require grafting to reduce healing time and complications.
Full-thickness burn (third-degree): Destruction of epidermis and all of dermis. Results from exposure to flames, chemicals that are not immediately washed, electrical injury, or prolonged contact with heat source.	Dry; leathery and firm to touch; pearly white, brown, or charred in appearance; no blanching to pressure; no pain, may see thrombosed vessels.	Incapable of self-regeneration. Preferred treatment is early excision and autografting.

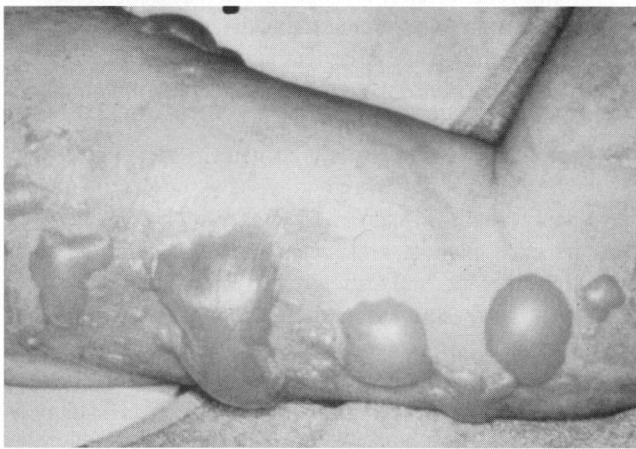

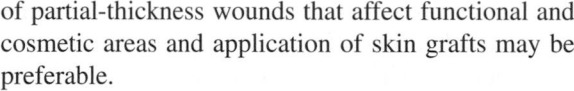

FIGURE 120-2 Blisters of a partial-thickness burn wound on the arm.

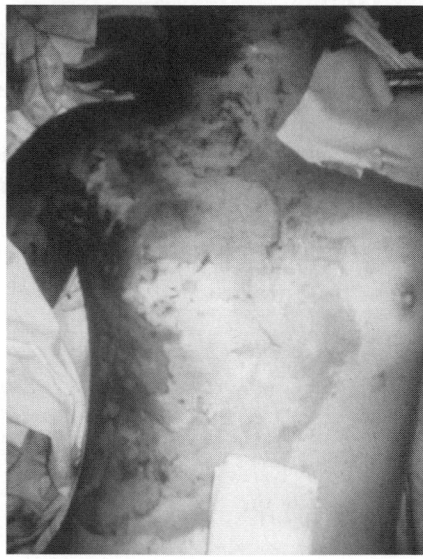

FIGURE 120-3 A fresh burn that is a partial-thickness burn toward the patient's left side and progresses to a full-thickness burn on the patient's right side.

of partial-thickness wounds that affect functional and cosmetic areas and application of skin grafts may be preferable.

❖ A *third-degree*, or *full-thickness*, *burn* involves complete destruction of the dermis. Because the skin is unable to regenerate, the dead tissue is removed and the wound is grafted with skin from another part of the patient's own body (autograft).[2] The grafted wound loses epidermal appendages and is unable to sweat, maintain lubrication, or protect from sun exposure after healing (Fig. 120-3).

• The depth of a burn wound is directly related to the temperature intensity and the duration of contact with the burning agent. The burning agent can be thermal (i.e., flame, contact, or scald), chemical, or electrical. An inhalation injury should always be suspected if the patient

was in an enclosed space with a fire; mortality rate is significantly increased when burns are compounded by smoke inhalation.[4]

• The burn injury produces three zones of injury: the zone of coagulation (cellular death), zone of stasis (vascular impairment, potentially reversible tissue injury), and zone of hyperemia (increased blood flow and inflammatory response). Decreased perfusion of the burn wound can cause the zone of stasis to deteriorate, deepening the initial wound. This progressive destruction can be minimized by providing adequate oxygenation and fluid resuscitation, alleviating pressure on the injured tissue, maintaining local and systemic warmth, and decreasing edema by elevating the burned area.[1]

- Assess for areas where full-thickness eschar is circumferential. Because of the inelastic nature of eschar, it may act like a tourniquet as edema develops, requiring surgical release (escharotomy) to prevent circulatory or respiratory compromise (Fig. 120-4).
- Monitor pulses, capillary refill, and sensation distal to circumferential eschar. Signs and symptoms that indicate a need for escharotomy include cyanosis of distal unburned skin, unrelenting deep tissue pain, progressive paresthesias, and progressive decrease or absence of pulse.[1]
- Adequacy of respiratory excursion must be assessed because circumferential eschar of the trunk can lead to decreased tidal volume and agitation (Fig. 120-5).[1]
- Escharotomy is performed at the bedside by a physician, with a scalpel or electrocautery used to cut the eschar longitudinally. Bleeding should be minimal because only dead tissue is cut; any bleeding can be controlled with sutures, silver nitrate sticks, collagen packing, or electrocautery. Pain is usually managed with small intravenous doses of opiates and benzodiazepines.

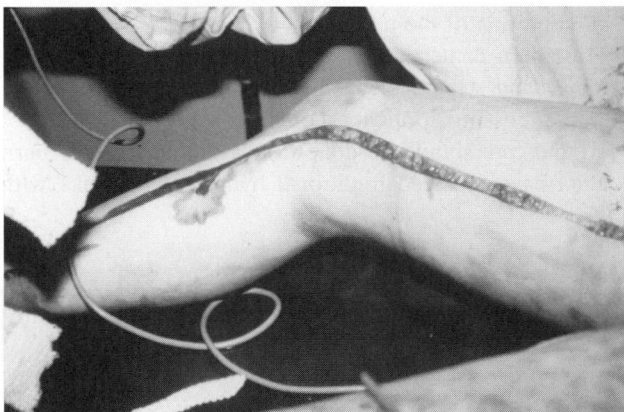

FIGURE 120-4   Escharotomy of the leg to improve circulation.

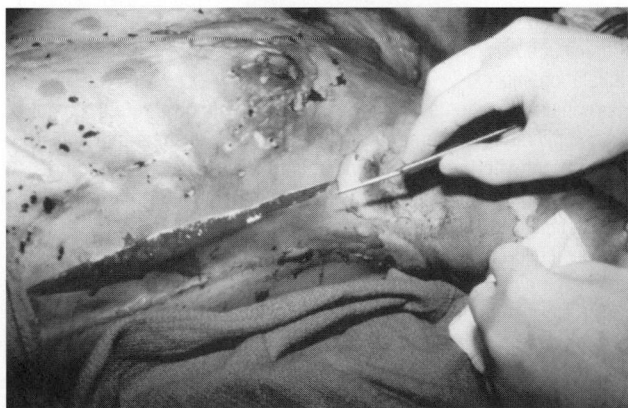

FIGURE 120-5   Full-thickness burn with chest escharotomy to improve chest expansion.

- Burn size may be determined with several methods.[20]
  - ❖ The *rule of nines* may be used to quickly calculate burn size. In an adult, the head and neck and each upper extremity represent 9% of the patient's body surface area. The anterior trunk, posterior trunk, and each leg represent 18% of the patient's body surface area. This rule only applies to adults; infants and young children have much larger heads in proportion to body size.
  - ❖ The *Lund and Browder chart* (Fig. 120-6) breaks the body into smaller areas and takes into consideration the proportional differences of persons of different ages.[12]
  - ❖ The *rule of the palm* notes that the patient's hand may be used as a template to represent roughly 1% of the TBSA.

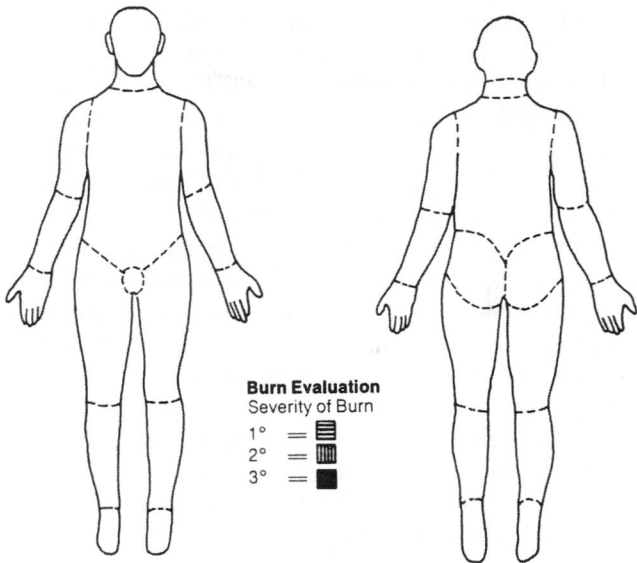

Burn Evaluation
Severity of Burn

1° = (hatched icon)
2° = (hatched icon)
3° = (solid icon)

Lund and Browder chart								
AREA	**AGE—YEARS**					**%** **2°**	**%** **3°**	**%** **TOTAL**
	0–1	**1–4**	**5–9**	**10–15**	**ADULT**			
Head	19	17	13	10	7			
Neck	2	2	2	2	2			
Ant. Trunk	13	17	13	13	13			
Post. Trunk	13	13	13	13	13			
R. Buttock	2½	2½	2½	2½	2½			
L. Buttock	2½	2½	2½	2½	2½			
Genitalia	1	1	1	1	1			
R.U. Arm	4	4	4	4	4			
L. U. Arm	4	4	4	4	4			
R.L. Arm	3	3	3	3	3			
L.L. Arm	3	3	3	3	3			
R. Hand	2½	2½	2½	2½	2½			
L. Hand	2½	2½	2½	2½	2½			
R. Thigh	5½	6½	8½	8½	9½			
L. Thigh	5½	6½	8½	8½	9½			
R. Leg	5	5	5½	6	7			
L. Leg	5	5	5 ½	6	7			
R. Foot	3½	3½	3½	3½	3½			
L. Foot	3½	3½	3½	3½	3½			
					Total			

FIGURE 120-6   The Lund and Browder chart is used to assess and graphically document size and depth of the burn wound.

- The inflammatory response causes a massive fluid shift to the interstitial space during the first 24 hours, with mobilization of fluid starting after 72 hours. Fluid resuscitation with a balanced salt solution is based on the patient's weight and burn size (partial-thickness and full-thickness wounds).[17] Large wounds are prone to huge evaporative water losses that require close monitoring of volume status.

- Effective resuscitation results in adequate urinary output (30 to 50 mL/hr or 0.5 to 1.0 mL/kg/hr) and mean arterial blood pressure of at least 60 mm Hg as surrogate markers of end-organ perfusion and hemodynamic stability.[17]

- Burns of specific anatomic areas need special consideration. Assess eyes for injury and treat chemical exposure with copious normal saline solution irrigation; treat burned ears with a topical antimicrobial cream and protect from pressure by eliminating use of pillows or dressings about the head; elevate burned extremities; consider the need for an indwelling urinary catheter in the patient with perineal burns; and shave hair growing through the burn wounds. Two burned surfaces that contact each other need dressings between them to prevent fusing as they heal (e.g., between toes, skin folds).

- Emergency treatment of thermal injuries includes initially cooling the burned skin with tepid water (never with ice) while recognizing the importance of preventing hypothermia.[1] In preparation for transfer, the airway should be assessed and 100% oxygen administered; large-bore intravenous (IV) access should be established and fluid resuscitation started; patients should be on nothing by mouth (NPO) status; wounds should be wrapped with a clean, dry sheet and possibly blanket; pain medication should be given in small IV doses, with recognition that coexisting injuries or medical conditions exacerbate the effects of opiates; tetanus prophylaxis should be administered; and all initial treatment should be documented.[1]

- Initial treatment of chemical burns includes removing saturated clothing, brushing off any powdered chemical, and continuously irrigating involved skin with copious amounts of water for 20 to 30 minutes. Neutralizing chemical burns with another chemical is contraindicated because the procedure generates heat. Burned eyes must be irrigated with large volumes of normal saline solution followed by an eye examination.[1] Some chemicals are absorbed systemically through burn wounds; contact the local poison control center to determine whether further treatment is indicated.[2] Ensure all providers wear appropriate personal protective equipment to prevent unintentional chemical exposure.

- Tar can be removed with mineral oil, a petrolatum-based ointment, or solvent.[16]

- Electrical injuries (Fig. 120-7) result when the body becomes part of the pathway for the electrical current. Deep burns may occur from tissue resistance where the patient contacted the electrical source and where the patient was grounded. Initially of greater concern than the burns is the high incidence of cardiac dysrhythmias, myoglobinuria

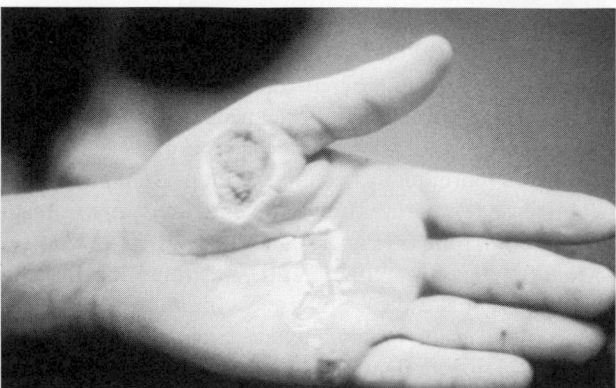

FIGURE 120-7   Entry site of an electrical burn.

resulting in acute tubular necrosis, and neurologic sequelae. Monitoring electrocardiographic (ECG) results, increasing urine output to 100 mL/hr in the presence of dark port-colored urine, assessing for associated trauma, and establishing baseline neurologic status are vital in the treatment of the electrical injury patient.[1,20]

- Criteria for transferring patients to a specialized burn care facility have been adopted by the American Burn Association and the American College of Surgeons. These criteria are listed in Table 120-2.

- Care of the burn wound and associated healing are determined by the extent and depth of the injury and the overall condition of the patient.

- Most burn centers use clean technique for dressing removal and wound cleansing, with sterile technique for sterile dressing application only.[2]

- Wound care should be done in a warm area. Many burn units have replaced traditional hydrotherapy tanks with

TABLE 120-2	**Criteria for Patient Transfer to a Specialized Burn Care Facility**

Partial-thickness burns on more than 10% TBSA

Burns that involve the face, hands, feet, genitalia, perineum, or major joints

Third-degree burns in any age group

Electrical burns, including lightning injury

Chemical burns

Inhalation injury

Burn injury in patients with preexisting medical disorders that could complicate management, prolong recovery, or affect mortality

Any patient with burns and concomitant trauma (such as fractures) in which the burn injury poses the greatest risk for morbidity or mortality

Burned children in hospitals without qualified personnel or equipment to care for children

Burn injury in patients who will need special social, emotional, or long-term rehabilitative intervention

(Adopted From Committee on Trauma, American College of Surgeons: Guidelines for the operation of burn centers resources for optimal care of the injured patient, Chicago, 2006, American College of Surgeons, 79-86).

shower tables for large wound care procedures to allow water run-off, thus decreasing leaching of electrolytes and minimizing wound exposure to perineal-contaminated water. Emergency equipment must always be immediately available during hydrotherapy procedures. As wounds decrease in size and patients approach discharge, bathtubs and showers offer reasonable options for wound cleansing.

- Initial wound cleansing requires thorough débridement of all devitalized tissue. Blisters are generally unroofed.[18] Use of dry gauze is effective to gently remove burned tissue, with use of a slow and deliberate wiping motion. Wash the wounds with gentle pH neutral liquid soap solution or wound cleanser and pat dry with clean towels.

- Topical antimicrobial agents limit bacterial proliferation and fungal colonization in burn wounds. The three most commonly used agents are 1% silver sulfadiazine (Silvadene, Monarch Pharmaceuticals, Inc., Bristol, TN), 10% mafenide acetate (Sulfamylon, UDL Laboratories, Inc., Rockford, IL), and 0.5% silver nitrate solution

(Table 120-3).[7] Systemic antibiotics are not routinely administered to burn patients because of the high risk for development of antibiotic resistance.[15]

- Eschar is a leathery layer of devitalized tissue that covers full-thickness burns. Bacterial action causes eschar to separate from the wound bed. However, the use of topical antimicrobial agents and early excision has minimized the nurse's involvement in eschar removal.

- Survival rates for burn patients are markedly improved with early excision and grafting.[6] The most important predictors of mortality are the patient age and the extent of the burn, with the presence of inhalation injury and comorbidity crucial factors. Although the burn wound has the most obvious potential for infection, the lower respiratory tract is the most common site of infection and carries the highest incidence of sepsis and death.[4]

- An autograft (skin graft taken from the patient) is the only treatment that can heal a full-thickness burn wound.[11] Wounds with higher than 105 organisms per gram of tissue impede graft adherence, so expedient grafting is desirable.[15]

TABLE 120-3	Topical Antimicrobial Agents		
Agent	**Activity**	**Advantages**	**Disadvantages**
Silver sulfadiazine 1% cream (Silvadine*)	Bactericidal effect on cell membrane and wall; excellent against *P. aeruginosa, S. aureus,* other burn flora, and yeast	Broad-spectrum antimicrobial coverage; low toxicity; no discomfort on application; easy to remove; rare hypersensitivity to sulfa component; may increase neovascularization	Poor eschar penetration; infrequent hypersensitivity; macerates surrounding tissues; contraindicated in pregnant women and newborns (risk for kernicterus); early transient neutropenia when applied to large burns
Mafenide acetate 10% cream (Sulfamylon‡)	Broad-spectrum against gram-positive and gram-negative organisms; not effective against yeast; diffuses through devascularized areas; is absorbed, metabolized, and excreted by kidneys	Highly soluble and penetrates eschar well; persistent activity against *Pseudomonas*	Pain on application of cream; systemically absorbed; may cause metabolic acidosis (through carbonic anhydrase inhibition); cutaneous hypersensitivity reactions occur; may see yeast overgrowth
Mafenide acetate (Sulfamylon) 5% solution	Broad-spectrum against gram-positive and gram-negative organisms; not effective against yeast	Moist dressings may be used over wounds, such as a new graft, when a liquid soak antibiotic is desired	Expensive; wet dressings often uncomfortable and may result in hypothermia
Silver nitrate, 0.5% in water (if dressing allowed to dry, concentration of silver nitrate increases and becomes caustic at 2%)	Bacteriostatic against many organisms; does not penetrate drainage or debris	Painless application; few organisms resistant to silver	Must be kept wet; poor penetration of eschar; stains unburned tissue and environment brown-black; hypotonicity of dressing may lead to hyponatremia and hypochloremia; requires thick dressings and resoaking every 4 hours to prevent drying
Silver nylon (a nonadherent nanocrystalline silver-coated dressing with sustained silver release for several days)	Lower minimal inhibitory concentration; a lower minimal bactericidal concentration; faster bacterial killing than other topicals	Decreases dressing changes by being left in place 3 days	Decreases ability to visualize wound

*Silvadene, Monarch Pharmaceuticals, Inc., Bristol, TN
‡Sulfamylon, UDL Laboratories, Inc., Rockford, IL

- Burn wound management accomplishes three primary goals: protect the wound, reduce metabolic demand, and provide comfort.
- A débrided full-thickness wound may be protected from infection and drying through the use of biologic dressings when donor sites are not available for autografting. Allograft, or homograft, refers to the use of "nonself" human skin grafts; such a graft becomes vascularized by the patient and risks rejection if it stays in place too long. Xenograft, or heterograft, is nonhuman skin obtained from commercial pigskin (porcine) processing companies; it forms a collagen bond with the wound and protects it for a period of time until donor sites are available for autografting. Porcine xenograft may be placed over clean partial-thickness wounds to protect the wound while it heals beneath the xenograft.[11]
- Integra (Integra Lifesciences Corporation, Plainsboro, NJ) is an acellular matrix composite graft that may be placed on débrided full-thickness burns. Capillaries and collagen grow into this matrix in about 3 weeks, forming a neodermis, which is then grafted with the patient's own epidermal cells. The matrix is slowly biodegradable and cannot be detected with wound biopsy after complete healing.[11] This allows for improved wound coverage and use of thinner donor sites but requires two surgeries. Thinner autografts allow more rapid healing of donor sites and produce less hypertrophic donor site scarring.
- Biosynthetic dressings such as Biobrane (UDL Laboratories, Inc., Rockford, IL) have been used to cover clean partial-thickness wounds to facilitate healing.[11,22] Biobrane is a two-layer, semisynthetic dressing composed of knitted-elastic nylon fabric that is mechanically bonded to a thin, Silastic, semipermeable membrane and coated with collagen polypeptides.[22] As the wound heals beneath, the dressing can be peeled away.[22]
- Topical antimicrobial agents are used to reduce wound colonization. Commonly used creams include silver sulfadiazine (Silvadene) and 10% mafenide acetate (Sulfamylon), antibacterial ointments such as bacitracin, and liquid soaks such as mafenide acetate 5% solution and 0.5% silver nitrate.[7] Creams and ointments are applied every 12 hours or as needed to cover the wound. Dry protective dressings prevent premature removal of the topical. Damp gauze dressings saturated with antimicrobial solution are changed every 24 hours, but dressings require moistening ("wet-down") every 4 to 6 hours to ensure activity of agent.
- Negative-pressure wound therapy may be used to maintain fresh graft placement, improve wound bed vascularization, and reduce microbial activity.[20]
- The burn patient's condition is hypermetabolic until burn wounds are closed and healing is complete. Increased caloric and protein requirements for wound healing are usually met through nasogastric or nasojejunal tube feeding to maintain mucosal integrity in large burns. Zinc and vitamin C have also been shown to be important in wound healing. Current research is evaluating the role of arginine and fish oil in decreasing infections,[13] glutamine's role in maintaining mucosal integrity and reducing infection,[13] and insulin's ability to preserve muscle mass.[21] Additional treatments include use of β-blockade[9] to reduce metabolic demand and oxandrolone[10] to increase anabolism.
- Burn patients should be encouraged to consume a high-protein diet. Supplementation with high-calorie nutritional drinks facilitates meeting energy needs. Large quantities of free water should be discouraged because risk for hyponatremia is high after a large burn.
- During wound care because heat lost through the wound, along with shivering, increases the metabolic rate.
- An individualized plan for pain control should be in place for both background pain (pain that is continuously present), breakthrough pain (associated with activity of daily living), and procedural pain (intermittent pain related to procedures).[5,14] Unrelieved pain can lead to stress-related immunosuppression, an increased potential for infection, delayed wound healing, and depression. Subcutaneous and intramuscular injections should be avoided because absorption is poor and unreliable as a result of edema. Intravenous administration of medication is preferred in critically ill patients; oral medication is preferred in noncritical patients with a functioning gastrointestinal system.[5,14] As the wound heals, the patient has more discomfort from itchiness and less discomfort from pain.[14] A moisturizing lotion prevents drying and reduces pruritus. Nonpharmacologic techniques can be learned to assist with the management of pain and itch.[3,5,14]
- Burn wounds contract during the healing phase. Self-care and range-of-motion exercises are encouraged. Stretching exercises and proper positioning are vital to prevent contractures and loss of function.[8] Static splinting is sometimes added to maintain sustained stretch.[8] Hypertrophic scar formation is countered through the use of topical silicone gel sheeting and pressure garments worn 24 hours a day until the scars mature and soften (6 to 18 months).[19] Keloids, if they form, may require surgery, steroid injections, and pressure treatment.[19]
- Grafts and donor sites on the lower extremities require support during healing when the patient is out of bed. Application of elastic bandages to extremities may prevent pooling of venous blood, permanent discoloration, or skin breakdown.
- The burn wound should not be exposed to the sun for a year because new scars sunburn easily.
- Patients should be instructed to select clothing that blocks sun and to use sunscreen on exposed grafts, generally for life.

EQUIPMENT

- Personal protective equipment as needed (e.g., gown, mask, goggles)
- Nonsterile gloves
- Sterile gloves
- Warm water
- Mild pH-neutral liquid soap, as ordered

- Normal saline (NS) solution
- Washcloths
- Towels
- Scissors and forceps (clean and sterile)
- Topical agents, as ordered
- Tongue depressors
- Sterile dressings as needed (e.g. gauze, Exu-dry [Smith & Nephew, St. Petersburgh, FL])
- Rolled dressing, gentle tape, or netting to secure dressings
- Pillows to elevate extremities
- Pain and sedation medication (as prescribed)

PATIENT AND FAMILY EDUCATION

- Provide detailed wound care instructions in writing or on videotape or DVD. Demonstrate wound care, and have patient and family return the demonstration before the planned discharge. Continue to involve patient and family in wound care for the remainder of the admission, and encourage them to ask questions. Provide positive feedback. Arrange for home care or clinic visits to follow up on wound care. ➵*Rationale:* Education validates patient and family understanding and ability to perform wound care and allows time for them to develop a level of comfort. The opportunity to reinforce important points is provided.
- Explore resources the patient will have for wound care at home (e.g., availability of running water, tub versus shower). ➵*Rationale:* This measure ensures that the patient is knowledgeable about care based on what adjustments need to be made at home.
- Simplify wound care and assess the family's ability to provide care at home. ➵*Rationale:* Continued care of the wound may be necessary after discharge.
- Teach patient and family about signs and symptoms of infection and the importance of reporting these in a timely manner. ➵*Rationale:* The patient and family can recognize problems early so that appropriate measures can be instituted by the healthcare provider.
- Teach patient and family about pain control; assess the patient's personal acceptable level of pain. ➵*Rationale:* Education and assessment decrease concerns about pain, facilitate individualized pain relief plan, and foster cooperation with care.
- Teach patient and family about pain management, including types of medications prescribed, timing of medications in relation to wound care, and nonpharmacologic pain strategies.[5] ➵*Rationale:* Comfort at home is supported.
- Provide instruction to the patient and family about the normal changes seen in the wound, including epithelial islands, healing margins, dryness on epithelialization, epidermal fragility on shearing, hypervascularization of the healed wound, and venous congestion in the dependent wound. ➵*Rationale:* Anxiety about appearance is reduced.
- Teach patient and family about care of healed burns, including medications to reduce itching,[3,14] use of nonperfumed moisturizers, protection from shear, and protection

from sun exposure for a minimum of a year. ➵*Rationale:* Education reduces complications and promotes patient satisfaction.
- Explain the rationale to the patient and family about the wearing and care of pressure garments. ➵*Rationale:* Pressure garments need to fit properly to reduce scar formation, and they can be difficult to apply.[19]
- Discuss the importance of mobility and proper positioning (e.g., splinting) on function. Self-care (activities of daily living) and range-of-motion exercises should be encouraged during the healing phase. ➵*Rationale:* Contractures associated with healing skin, improper positioning, and immobility are prevented.
- Identify caloric needs for healing and suggest appropriate nutritional supplements. ➵*Rationale:* Metabolic needs are increased for months after discharge, and a balanced diet facilitates gain of muscle mass versus adipose tissue.
- Inform patient and family that nightmares, alterations in body image, and psychologic disturbances are experienced by many burned patients.[20] Provide resources, including someone to follow up with, if desired. ➵*Rationale:* Information increases awareness of these problems and reassures patient and family that these experiences, although unpleasant, are not abnormal.
- Provide patient and family with follow-up appointments and someone to call with any problems. ➵*Rationale:* Necessary information for further care and follow-up is provided.

PATIENT ASSESSMENT AND PREPARATION
Patient Assessment

- Assess vital signs, including temperature. ➵*Rationale:* Baseline vital signs allow for comparison during and after the procedure to evaluate patient tolerance, normothermia, and adequacy of pain medication.
- Evaluate for signs of healing, including the following:
  - ❖ Decreased pain
  - ❖ Reepithelialization from epithelial islands within wound
  - ❖ Decreasing wound size
  - ❖ Decreased edema
  - ❖ Compare patient's level of healing with expected level of healing for number of days after burn.

  ➵*Rationale:* Healing should occur within a predictable time frame determined by the depth of burns, unless complications occur.
- Evaluate for the following signs and symptoms of infection[20]:
  - ❖ Foul odor
  - ❖ Purulent drainage
  - ❖ Increased pain
  - ❖ Increasing edema
  - ❖ Cellulitis
  - ❖ Fever
  - ❖ Development of eschar or early eschar separation
  - ❖ Wound discoloration
  - ❖ Increase in burn size or depth
  - ❖ Blurring of wound edges

➤➤*Rationale:* Infection can result in delayed wound healing, prolonged hospitalization, and death.

- Monitor for distal circulation (pulses, pain, color, sensation, movement, and capillary refill) to areas with circumferential burns and increased edema. ➤➤*Rationale:* Edema and circumferential burns impede distal circulation and cause worsening tissue perfusion and cell death.
- Determine patient's understanding of pain management strategies. Assess patient's pain level on a standardized pain scale (such as the 0 to 10 scale) before, during, and after the procedure. Explore discrepancies between the patient's level of pain and desired level of pain. ➤➤*Rationale:* An individualized plan for pain control should be in place for background, breakthrough, and procedural pain.[5,14] In addition to the traditional use of pain and anxiety medications, alternative therapies should be included (e.g., relaxation techniques, distraction, massage therapy, music therapy). The patient's needs change based on changes in the wound (e.g., healing, débridement, conversion to deeper wound).
- Evaluate patient's general level of function, particularly in burned areas. ➤➤*Rationale:* An individualized plan for range-of-motion exercises, positioning, and splinting should be made to optimize the patient's level of function. Burns contract during the healing phase, and immobility enhances loss of function.

Patient Preparation

- Ensure the patient understands procedural teaching. Answer questions as they arise and reinforce information as needed. ➤➤*Rationale:* Understanding of previously taught information is evaluated and reinforced.
- Notify other appropriate healthcare providers who need to assess the burn wound (e.g., physician) or perform a task (e.g., quantitative wound biopsies, range-of-motion exercises by physical therapist) of time of dressing change. ➤➤*Rationale:* Organization of care allows important assessment and intervention to take place without causing extra pain and stress to the patient.
- After checking previous requirements for patient comfort during the dressing change, premedicate the patient with pain medication and any sedative as prescribed, allowing an appropriate amount of time before starting wound care. ➤➤*Rationale:* Premedication allows time for medication to take effect and promotes optimal comfort for the patient.
- Consider synergistic effects of opioids, sedatives, and drugs that affect the central nervous system (CNS). Closely monitor patient 30 to 60 minutes after wound care procedure is completed. ➤➤*Rationale:* Stimulatory effects that counteract CNS depression are reduced after wounds are covered; decreased noxious stimuli and respiratory depression may occur.

Procedure   for Care of Burn Wounds

Steps	Rationale	Special Considerations
1. Prepare all necessary equipment and supplies. The treatment area should be warmed.	Preparation facilitates efficient wound care and prevents needless delays. Warming the room decreases risk for hypothermia.	
2. **HH**		
3. **PE**		
4. Remove old dressings and discard them in infectious waste container. Place towel or pad under exposed extremity.	Old dressings can contain large amounts of body secretions and blood. A clean field under the extremity allows the patient a place to rest the extremity during care.	Remove dressings only from areas that can be redressed within 20 to 30 minutes at one time. Finish wound care to these areas before moving to new areas (decreases heat loss and pain related to nerve endings being exposed to air).
5. Remove and discard gloves; apply a pair of clean gloves.	Used gloves are contaminated by handling of the burn dressing. Aseptic technique is necessary for wound care.	
6. Wash wound with mild pH-balanced soap solution or wound cleanser, rinse with warm tap water, and pat dry.	Cleanses wound of debris with mechanical débridement and reduces microorganisms.	Cleanse beyond wound to reduce microbial count on surrounding tissue. Patient tolerance may improve if allowed to cleanse one's own wounds.
7. Use scissors and forceps to remove loose necrotic tissue and any broken blister tissue. (**Level C***)	Bacteria proliferate in necrotic tissue.[18]	Typically, physicians perform this function in hospitals that do not specialize in burn wound care.

*Level C: Qualitative studies, descriptive or correlational studies, integrative reviews, systematic reviews, or randomized controlled trials with inconsistent results

Procedure | for Care of Burn Wounds—*Continued*

Steps	Rationale	Special Considerations
8. Assess the burn wound for color, size, odor, depth, drainage, bleeding, edema, cellulitis, epithelial budding, eschar separation, sensation, movement, peripheral pulses, and any signs of pressure areas from splints. For wet dressings, **proceed to Step 11.**	Validates the healing process and identifies complications.	Other healthcare providers who need to observe the wound should be notified ahead of time so that they can be present while the wound is uncovered.
9. Remove and discard gloves. Apply sterile gloves.	Gloves are contaminated from burn wound care. Sterile gloves should be used for application of the sterile dressing.	
10. *Creams:* Use sterile tongue depressor to remove required amount of topical agent from container. Place on sterile surface before applying $\frac{1}{16}$-inch layer directly to burn wound and covering with burn dressing, or apply $\frac{1}{16}$-inch layer on burn dressing and cover wound. *Ointments:* Apply thin layer to wound, apply dressing as needed.	Use of sterile tongue depressor and removal of only what is needed from container prevent contamination of topical agent. Dry dressings protect topical agent from premature removal.	If the area to be covered has folds and crevices, or if the wound consists of scattered areas, topical agents should be placed directly on the wound, rather than on the burn dressing (ensures good coverage without applying unnecessary amounts of an absorbable topical agent to uninjured areas).
11. *Soaks:* Pour prescribed solution into sterile bowl, and drop in sterile gauze pads. Squeeze out excess fluid and apply to wound. Apply protective veil to fresh graft as ordered.	Ideal moisture in dressing is similar to a damp sponge. Excess fluid may macerate tissue. Veil protects graft from adhering to dressing.	Wet dressings must be moistened every 4 to 6 hours. If dressing is adherent to epithelial buds or granulation tissue, wet the dressing with warm saline solution or sterile water to loosen.
12. Loosely wrap extremities with gauze rolls. Secure dressings with elastic net.	Holds dressings in place.	Wrap extremities from distal to proximal. Check pulses and capillary refill after wrapping to ensure circulation is not compromised.
13. Assess need for additional pain medication before continuing.	Patients have a right to good pain control. The success or failure of pain control for the current dressing change affects the way the patient responds to future dressing changes.	
14. **Repeat steps, starting at Step 4,** until all burn wounds have been cared for.	Isolating areas for dressing changes prevents unnecessary temperature loss, pain from increased nerve ending exposure to air movement, and cross contamination of wounds.	The size of the team doing the dressing and the amount of débridement time required determine how much of the wound should reasonably be exposed at any given time.
15. Apply splints as needed and elevate burned extremities with pillows or elastic net sling or both; elevate head of bed. **(Level C*)**	Maintains position of function, prevents contractures and pressure ulcers, and reduces edema. Elevation of donor sites and exposure to air facilitates healing.[8,19]	Do not bend knees if popliteal space is burned. Do not put pillow under head if neck or ears are burned. Do not inhibit movement with splints if patient is awake and able to use involved extremity.
16. Remove and discard gloves.		
17. **HH**		

*Level C: Qualitative studies, descriptive or correlational studies, integrative reviews, systematic reviews, or randomized controlled trials with inconsistent results

Procedure continues on following page

Expected Outcomes

- Wounds heal as expected without infectious complications
- Patient maintains a self-identified acceptable level of pain relief
- Patient attains comfort from measures taken for anxiety and itching
- Patient and family verbalize knowledge of patient condition and plan of care
- An optimal level of function is maintained or attained
- Patient and family response and interactions demonstrate adaptation to injury
- Patient and family collaborate in management of care
- At the time of discharge, patient and family verbalize and demonstrate an understanding of posthospital care

Unexpected Outcomes

- Wound converts to deeper injury
- Loss of allograft
- Wound infection or systemic sepsis occurs
- Wound heals with unnecessary loss of function

Patient Monitoring and Care

Steps	Rationale	Reportable Conditions
		These conditions should be reported if they persist despite nursing interventions.
1. Follow institutional standard for assessing pain. Administer analgesia as prescribed. Evaluate and treat the patient for pain. Ask the patient to rate pain on a scale of 0 to 10; check the orders for pain and sedation for dressing changes; check patient's medication requirements with previous dressing changes and have that amount of medication available in the room before starting the procedure; assess the need for more medication throughout the dressing change. Incorporate alternative pain relief techniques (e.g., relaxation techniques, massage therapy, distraction, music, visual imaging).	Identifies need for pain interventions. The burn patient has baseline pain that requires analgesia and increased pain medication requirements and possibly sedation requirements for the pain involved in dressing changes. Attention to the patient's pain fosters the patient's trust in healthcare personnel to control pain and promotes cooperation with future burn wound care. Goal of pain management is an alert patient who is able to cooperate and follow commands and respond to verbal stimuli.	• Continued pain despite pain interventions • Nonverbal indications of pain (restlessness, grimacing, teeth clenching) • Increased respiratory rate • Verbalization of pain • Inability to cooperate with dressing change • Increased heart rate • Increased or decreased blood pressure • Oversedation, depression of respiratory rate, unarousable
2. Obtain baseline vital signs before procedure, monitor throughout procedure, and check for 30 minutes after procedure is complete.	Changes in vital signs can be an indication that the patient is experiencing pain or anxiety. Decreasing blood pressure, heart rate, and respiratory rate can be complications of pain medication (especially after dressing change is complete and stimulation has stopped).	• Increased or decreased heart rate • Increased or decreased blood pressure • Increased or decreased respiratory rate; increased need for higher oxygen supplementation • High peak pressures on ventilator
3. Check patient's temperature before dressing change. Ensure patient's environment is warm; cover the portions of patient's body that are not involved in dressing change. Check temperature at end of dressing change.	Heat is lost through burn wounds. Hypermetabolism and shivering increase caloric demand.	• Hypothermia • Shivering

Patient Monitoring and Care —*Continued*

Steps	Rationale	Reportable Conditions
4. Monitor peripheral pulses and circulation in burned extremity during the dressing change, within 1 hour after applying dressing, and every 2 hours thereafter. Keep extremities elevated and assess for increased edema.	Circumferential burns can decrease or prevent blood flow to involved extremity. The dressing can be too tight, especially if edema increases.	• Increased peripheral edema • Pain or numbness in extremity • Prolonged or absent capillary refill in extremity • Decreased or absent pulses • Conversion to deeper burn wound
5. Assess the burn wound for color, size, odor, depth, drainage, bleeding, pain, early eschar separation, healing, and cellulitis in the surrounding tissue. Obtain wound biopsy as needed for suspected infection.	Observes for usual progression of wound healing versus complications of infection, progression of burn to deeper wound, and bleeding. Wound colonization is common. Histologic determination of level of organism invasion in presence of systemic symptoms is diagnostic for burn wound infection.	• Foul odor • Purulent or increased amounts of drainage • Elevated body temperatures • Cellulitis • Healthy granulation tissue developing eschar • Increasing necrosis, loss of graft • Blurring of burn wound edges • Discoloration of wound or presence of fungal elements • Early eschar separation • Bleeding
6. Encourage exercise and activities of daily living; perform range-of-motion exercises during dressing changes; place patient in position of optimal function, with splints used as needed, to maintain maximal function.[8,19] Use pain medication as needed to facilitate mobility.[14] **(Level C*)**	Burns and grafts contract during the healing phase if not correctly splinted and exercised; loss of function is a complication of immobility. Pain inhibits patients from moving.	• Contractures • Loss of function
7. Monitor patient's tolerance of tube feedings or patient's ingestion of a high-calorie and high-protein diet with supplements; encourage nutritious diet and discourage empty calories.[13,21] Limit free water intake. **(Level C)**	Nutrition is necessary for wound healing; burn patients are hypermetabolic. Protein-rich fluids promote healing; free water decreases intake of nutritional supplements and can lead to hyponatremia.	• Refusal to eat or inability to ingest adequate amount of nutrition • Poor wound healing

Documentation

Documentation should include the following:
• Patient and family education
• Date, time, and duration of wound care
• Areas of burn, other wounds, and pressure ulcers; weekly diagrams (or digital photographs) of unhealed wounds to monitor healing and wound changes
• Appearance of the wound (color, size, odor, depth, drainage, bleeding)
• Assessment of wound areas for level of pain (appropriate for depth and level of healing)
• Progression toward healing (e.g., presence of epithelial budding)
• Evidence of cellulitis around the wound (red, warm, tender)
• Assessment of peripheral pulses; color, movement, sensation, and capillary refill distal to a circumferential wound or an extremity wrapped in dressings
• Pain assessment, interventions, and effectiveness
• Medications given for pain, anxiety, and sedation
• Other comfort measures used
• Dressings and topical agents applied
• Patient's tolerance of the procedure
• Unexpected outcomes
• Nursing interventions

*Level C: Qualitative studies, descriptive or correlational studies, integrative reviews, systematic reviews, or randomized controlled trials with inconsistent results

References

CR 1. American Burn Association: *Advanced burn life support provider course*, Chicago, 2005, American Burn Association.

2. Bessey TQ: Wound care. In Herndon DN, editor: *Total burn care*, ed 3, London, 2007, Saunders Elsevier, 127-135.

3. Brooks JP, et al: Scratching the surface: managing the itch associated with burns: a review of current knowledge, *Burns* 34:751-760, 2008.

4. Demling RH: Smoke inhalation lung injury: an update, *Eplasty* 16:254-282, 2008.

5. Faucher L, et al: Practice guidelines for the management of pain, *J Burn Care Res* 27:659-668, 2006.

6. Guo F, et al: Management of burns over 80% of total body surface area: a comparative study, *Burns* doi:10.1016/j.burns.2008.05.021, 2008.

CR 7. Honari S: Topical therapies and antimicrobials in the management of burn wounds, *Crit Care Nurs Clin North Am* 16:1-11, 2004.

8. Huang T: Management of contractural deformities involving the axilla (shoulder), elbow, hip, knee, and ankle joints in burn patients. In Herndon DN, editor: *Total burn care*, ed 3, London, 2007, Saunders Elsevier, 727-740.

9. Ipaktchi K, Arbabi S: Advances in burn critical care, *Crit Care Med* 34:S239-S244, 2006.

10. Jeschke MG, et al: The effect of oxandrolone on the endocrinologic, inflammatory, and hypermetabolic responses during the acute phase postburn, *Ann Surg* 246:351-362, 2007.

11. Lineen E, et al: Biologic dressings in burns, *J Craniofac Surg* 19:923-928, 2008.

CR 12. Lund CC, Browder NC: The estimate of areas of burns, *Surg Gynecol Obstet* 79:352-358, 1944.

13. Masters B, Wood F: Nutrition support in burns: is there consistency in practice? *J Burn Care Res* 29:561-571, 2008.

14. Meyer WJ, et al: Management of pain and other discomforts in burned patients. In Herndon D, editor: *Total burn care*, ed 3, London, 2007, Saunders Elsevier, 797-818.

15. Polavarapu N, et al: Microbiology of burn wound infections, *J Craniofac Surg* 19:899-902, 2008.

16. Pham TN, et al: Evaluation of the burn wound: management decisions. In Herndon D, editor: *Total burn care*, ed 3, London, 2007, Saunders Elsevier, 119-126.

17. Pham TN: American Burn Association practice guidelines burn shock resuscitation, *J Burn Care Res* 29:257-266, 2008.

18. Sargent RL: Management of blisters in the partial-thickness burn: an integrative research review, *J Burn Care Res* 27:66-81, 2006.

19. Serghiou MA, et al: Comprehensive rehabilitation of the burn patient. In Herndon D, editor: *Total burn care*, ed 3, London, 2007, Saunders Elsevier, 620-651.

20. Stout LR: Burns. In Carlson KK, editor: *AACN advanced critical care nursing*, London, 2009, Saunders Elsevier, 1212-1260.

21. Wanek S, Wolf SE: Metabolic response to injury and role of anabolic hormones, *Curr Opin Clin Nutr Metab Care* 10:272-277, 2007.

22. Whitaker IS, et al: A critical evaluation of the use of Biobrane as a biologic skin substitute: a versatile tool for the plastic and reconstructive surgeon, *Ann Plastic Surg* 60:333-337, 2008.

Additional Readings

Broughton G, et al: Wound healing: an overview, *Plast Reconstr Surg* 117:1eS-32eS, 2006.

CR Flynn MB, editor: Burn and wound care, *Crit Care Nurs Clin North Am* 16: 1-185, 2004.

Makic MBF, Mann E: Burn injuries. In McQuillan K, Makic MBF, Whalen E, editors: *Trauma nursing: resuscitation through rehabilitation*, Philadelphia, 2009, Elsevier, 865-888.

Skin Graft Care

PURPOSE: Skin-graft care is performed to promote perfusion to the graft and to prevent infection. Successful graft transplant and care result in maximal function.

Dawn Lequatte Sculco

PREREQUISITE NURSING KNOWLEDGE

- Skin grafts, also called autografts, are sections of skin used to replace missing skin on a patient's body. An autograft is created by taking a donor graft from one area of a patient's body and transplanting it to a different area of the same patient's body. It involves the surgical removal of a section of the epidermis and a portion of the dermis.[1,8] This removal results in a new exposed wound area from which the donor graft was taken, called the donor site. The graft, a split-thickness skin graft (STSG), is applied over a clean, surgically excised wound that has been débrided of all nonviable tissue.

- An autograft is the only permanent treatment that can heal a large, full-thickness wound. Autografts may also be used to heal partial-thickness wounds with faster closure of the wound. The original wounds may be from a variety of causes (burns, infections, traumatic injury, etc).

- The autograft is harvested from an appropriate donor site on the patient's body with a dermatome, a surgical instrument that shaves layers of skin at different depths to be grafted over the wound bed.

- The STSG is commonly meshed (Fig. 121-1) so that it can be stretched to cover approximately 1.5 to 9 times more surface area than the original donor site. The ability to stretch the donor graft is important when there is a limited availability of suitable donor sites or when the wound area that requires grafting is extensive. Meshing the donor skin creates spaces, or interstices, that allow for fluid to escape, which can assist with graft adherence.

- Negative-pressure wound therapy (NPWT) is a mechanical wound care treatment that uses controlled negative pressure (via a machine, tubing, and sealed dressing) to accelerate wound healing. NPWT can also be used to enhance incorporation of a STSG mesh graft. The NPWT dressing is placed over the graft during surgery. A nonadherent dressing is used as a barrier for the graft to protect the graft from trauma and decrease overgrowth of granulation tissue formation.[1]

- Nonmeshed grafts, or sheet grafts, are used on the face, hands, and some joints because of cosmetic and functional concerns related to appearance and increased shrinkage.

- A sheet graft covers the same amount of surface area as the donor site. Pockets of serous fluid or blood tend to accumulate under these grafts (the interstices of meshed grafts allow the fluid to escape) and separate the graft from the wound bed, which is vital for blood supply, resulting in failure of the graft to adhere or "take" to the wound bed. Evacuation of this fluid is imperative. Sheet

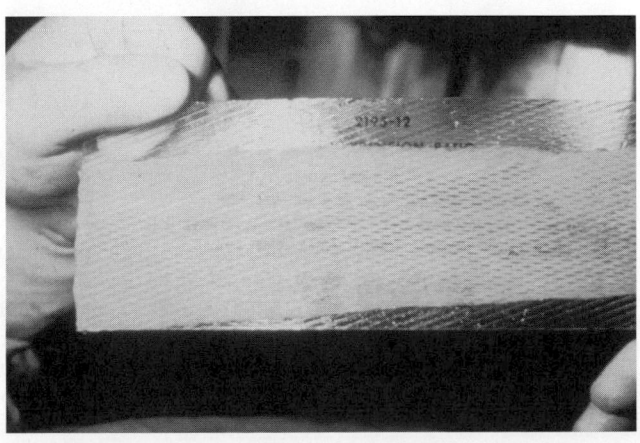

FIGURE 121-1   Meshed split-thickness skin graft.

grafts on the face, neck, and hands are generally inspected within the first 12 to 24 hours to look for fluid collections or graft dislodgement. If the sheet graft has been in place for less than 48 hours and the fluid is near the edge of sheet graft, the fluid can be rolled to the edge and out (Fig. 121-2).[2]

- Caution should be used when evacuating fluid after vascularization of the graft begins to avoid disruption of the graft attachment endangering graft take. A more safe practice for removing fluid involves making a small nick in the sheet graft directly over the area of fluid accumulation and gently expressing the fluid through the hole. In either case, the fluid should be gently dabbed away with gauze dampened with sterile normal saline solution or sterile water.[6] Seromas and hematomas tend to redevelop in the same areas, so careful charting should reflect location of any fluid pockets (blebs). Close monitoring of these areas should occur at least every 8 hours until bleb formation is no longer noted.
- In the operating room, all nonviable tissue is surgically excised to create a wound bed able to support a skin graft (Fig. 121-3); therefore, the grafted area should be observed for bleeding for the first 24 hours.

- The goals after a graft placement are to protect the wound bed from infection and desiccation and to ensure that no movement (shearing) of the graft occurs while it is becoming vascularized. Neovascularization begins within the first 24 hours of surgery as capillaries grow up into the graft, securing the graft permanently to its new site. Either a barrier dressing (e.g., Biobrane allograft [UDL Laboratories, Rockford, IL]) protects the wound (with or without a bulky dressing added), or a minimal nonadherent dressing (e.g., Xeroform [McKesson Brand, San Francisco]) is used with a bulky dressing over the grafted tissue to act as the barrier to infection, prevent drying and shearing. The newly grafted tissue must be well protected from shearing forces for 5 to 7 days to allow for graft adherence to the wound bed. With meshed skin grafts, the interstices of the autograft fill with granulation tissue and the epidermis of the autograft migrates over the granulation tissues. Successful grafting is often expressed as a percentage of graft "take," or adherence and vascularization of the graft to the new site.[1,5]
- Cultured epidermal autografts, most frequently used with burn injuries, are commercially available and are an option when the patient does not have enough unburned

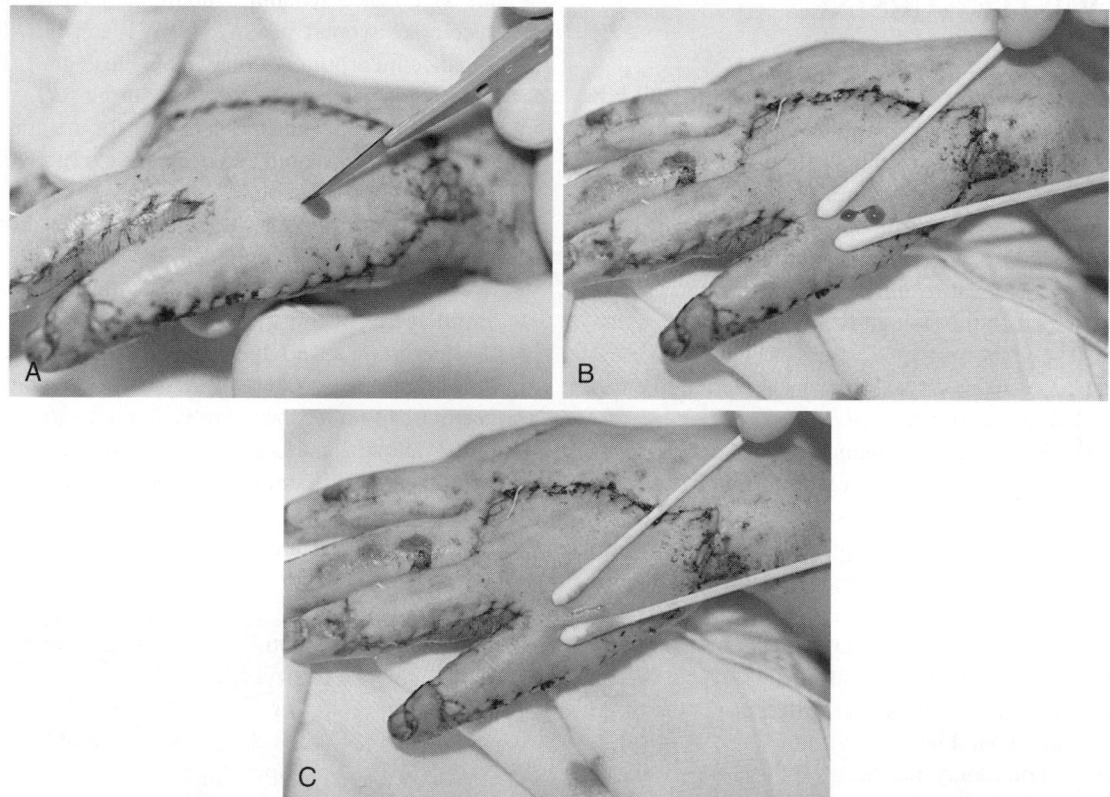

FIGURE 121-2   **A,** A no. 11 surgical blade and cotton-tipped applicator are used to blade a new sheet graft. Note that the blade is held so that the tip of the cutting surface comes into contact with only the graft. **B,** Cotton-tipped applicators are rolled gently over the graft toward the slit to express fluid that has collected between the graft and the wound bed surface. When deblebbing thick grafts, adequate-sized slits are important to avoid recurring buildup of fluid, which may jeopardize graft survivability and result in scarring. **C,** Blebs tend to recur in the same place. Vigilance about deblebbing at least once every 8 hours until bleb formation ceases is advisable. Documentation of bleb formation and location ensures that the next caregiver is aware of graft sites in need of close monitoring. *(From Carrougher GJ: Burn care and therapy, St Louis, 1998, Mosby.)*

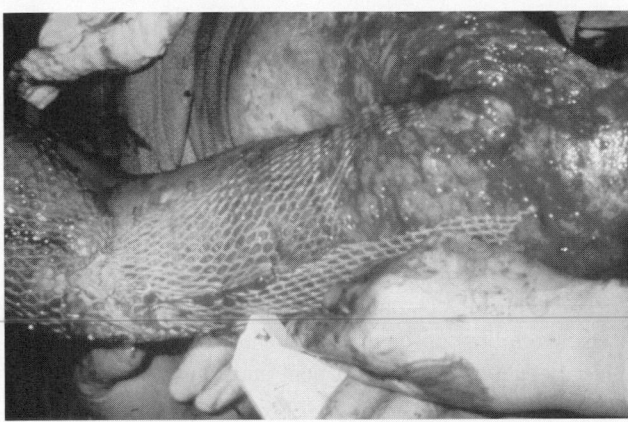

FIGURE 121-3 Meshed split-thickness skin graft covering the arm, with the remainder of the wound bed ready to be grafted.

tissue for donor sites to cover the burn in a reasonable period of time.[1,7] Cultured epidermal autografts are grown from a sample of the patient's own epidermal cells in a laboratory. However, the cost is prohibitive, the grafts are extremely fragile, and successful take of the graft is much more likely if the burn team has experience with this treatment.[3]

- The use of artificial skin and other options for wound coverage has expanded in recent years. Currently, the use of these wound coverings is limited to providing temporary wound coverage or allowing for dermal regeneration while waiting for suitable donor sites for definitive wound closure with autografting.

- Allografts, also called homografts, are fresh or cyropreserved grafts from human donors. Allografts are the gold standard for temporary coverage of wounds. Allograft benefits include prevention of wound desiccation, promotion of granulation tissue, and decreased water and heat loss.[1]

- The use of Integra® Dermal Regeneration Template (Ethicon Endo-Surgery, Inc, Cincinnati, Ohio) has been shown to decrease length of stay (LOS) in severely injured burned adults.[7] Integra® is a commercial bilayer dermal regeneration template system that is frequently used in burn centers to treat severe burns. Integra is composed of two layers. The first layer is made from cross-linked bovine collagen and chondroitin 6-sulfate (glycosaminoglycan) from shark collagen, which is a permanent dermal template that provides a scaffolding for the patient's own dermis to grow into. The second layer, the outer layer, is a temporary synthetic polysiloxane polymer (silicone)covering that acts as an artificial epidermis until the patient is ready for autografting, usually 2 to 3 weeks after the Integra is placed. Because of enhanced dermal regeneration, the graft bed requires only a very thin meshed donor graft from the patient to heal the wound. This allows quicker healing of donor sites and the ability to reharvest from the same donor site multiple times, if necessary, in a short time period. Clinical trials have shown that the epidermal autograft over Integra usually heals without the formation of the meshed appearance

typical of meshed autografts, thereby resulting in a better cosmetic outcome for the patient.[5]

- The graft is usually stapled or sutured in place, covered with a nonadherent dressing, and padded with a bulky bolster dressing to prevent mechanical dislodgement of the graft. Recent studies have shown that the use of fibrin sealants, a surgical hemostatic agent derived from human plasma, may be more effective than staples for adherence of sheet grafts.[4]

- After surgery, the graft is delicate, and care is taken to decrease trauma to the graft. If the graft is over a joint, the extremity may be immobilized to enhance graft take. The first dressing change is usually done after 3 to 5 days. Most centers use clean technique for dressing removal and donor-site cleansing and use sterile technique for dressing application only.[6]

- If a patient is allowed to mobilize after surgery, leg grafts must be supported with Ace wraps or other compressive dressings when the patient's legs are dependent for the first 3 to 5 days after surgery to prevent capillary engorgement and hematoma formation beneath the graft. Grafted extremities should be elevated when the patient is supine.

- Initial healing of the grafted area should occur in 7 to 10 days. The graft area is immobilized for 4 to 5 days to prevent dislocation and shearing. Splints and immobilizers are used during this time to prevent disruption of grafts and to provide therapeutic positioning of extremities.

- Signs of successful graft take include vascularization of the graft, reepithelialization of the interstices, decreased pain, and adherence of the graft. Signs of complications include graft necrosis, graft loss, cellulitis, purulent drainage, and fever.

- Skin grafts contract during the healing and remodeling phases. Continuing mobility and proper positioning are vital to prevent contractures and loss of function. Self-care and range-of-motion exercises should be encouraged as soon as the graft is adherent. Once the wounds heal, pressure garments may be ordered to be worn at all times, except during bathing, to reduce hypertrophic scar formation.[6]

- Pain related to care of wounds is complicated by several components: background pain (pain that is continuously present), procedural pain (intermittent pain related to procedures and routine care), and anxiety. Unrelieved pain can lead to stress-related immunosuppression, increased potential for infection, delayed wound healing, and depression. The management of pain should be a multidimensional approach, including pharmacologic and nonpharmacologic methods, tailored to individual patient needs.[8,9]

- Burns greater than 20% total body surface area (TBSA) cause a hypermetabolic response that results from a loss of glycogen stores, increased gluconeogenesis, and increased lipid metabolism. In addition, dressing changes, loss of normal thermoregulatory mechanisms, surgical débridement, pain, and infection exacerbate the hypermetabolic response to injury. Therefore, estimating and meeting a patient's nutritional needs is paramount to maximize wound healing.[3]

- Exposure of the healed skin graft to the sun should be avoided. The newly healed area is extremely sensitive to sunlight, and permanent discoloration can occur. To prevent discoloration, the patient should protect grafted areas with clothing or sunscreen. During the first year, as the patient's graft matures, the risk for skin discoloration slowly decreases.

EQUIPMENT

- Personal protective equipment (i.e., gowns, mask, goggles)
- Nonsterile gloves
- Sterile gloves
- Scissors and forceps
- Warm tap water (sometimes sterile water or sterile normal saline [NS] solution is used for first dressing change)
- Clean washcloths
- Staple remover
- Nonadherent dressing/gauze (e.g., Adaptic [Johnson and Johnson, New Brunswick, NJ], Xeroform)
- Secondary dressings, as needed
- Pain and antianxiolytic medication (as prescribed)
  Additional equipment, as needed, includes the following:
- Splints (to be secured with gauze roll, hook and loop closure [e.g., Velcro], elastic bandage such as ace wraps, or self-adherent wrap (e.g., Coban, 3M, St. Paul, MN)
- Towels or waterproof pads

PATIENT AND FAMILY EDUCATION

- Explain the procedure for skin graft care to patient and family. ➤*Rationale:* Explanation diminishes fear of the unknown and ensures that patient and family are knowledgeable about graft care.
- Inform patient and family that the grafted area needs to be protected for 5 to 7 days to encourage graft take and reduce the risk for mechanical trauma to graft site. ➤*Rationale:* Patient's and family's assistance in protecting the graft site is increased.
- Inform patient and family that the skin graft should not be exposed to the sun for approximately 1 year. Sunscreen and protective clothing should be used thereafter; some scarring and discoloration will occur but will improve over the first year. Explain that grafted area will not grow hair or be able to sweat because of permanent loss of these dermal appendages. ➤*Rationale:* The patient and family are prepared for changes that will be present after hospital discharge, and anxieties about body image are addressed.
- Discuss the importance of proper positioning. Explain the need for continuing mobility through self-care and range-of-motion exercises as soon as the graft is adherent and throughout the healing phase. ➤*Rationale:* Education prevents contractures and loss of function associated with healing skin grafts.

- Assess family's ability to provide care at home. ➤*Rationale:* Continued care of the wound is necessary after discharge.
- As appropriate, provide detailed wound care instructions in writing and review with patient and family. Demonstrate exactly what to do, and have patient and family return demonstrations before the planned discharge. Continue to involve patient and family in the wound care for the remainder of the admission, and encourage them to ask questions. Provide positive feedback. Arrange for home care or clinic visits to follow-up on dressings and wound care. ➤*Rationale:* Education validates patient and family understanding and ability to perform wound care independently and allows time for them to develop a level of comfort. The opportunity to reinforce important points is provided.
- Teach patient and family about pain and pruritus medications as prescribed. Provide the name of a water-based lotion to apply to healed areas. ➤*Rationale:* Comfort at home is supported.
- Teach patient and family about signs and symptoms of infection and the importance of reporting these in a timely manner. ➤*Rationale:* The patient and family can recognize problems early so that appropriate measures can be instituted by the healthcare team.
- Emphasize the importance of wearing pressure garments and splints. ➤*Rationale:* Scar formation and contractures are reduced.
- Schedule follow-up appointments and provide the name of someone to call with any problems. ➤*Rationale:* This information is necessary for further care and follow-up.
- Work with vocational rehabilitation counselor to formulate plan for patient's return to work. ➤*Rationale:* Depending on the severity of the patient's injuries, the patient may be physically unable to return to former employment or may need assistance with job modifications and accommodations. Developing a back-to-work plan based on any new limitations increases the patient's chance of successfully returning to work.

PATIENT ASSESSMENT AND PREPARATION

Patient Assessment

- Assess vital signs, including temperature. ➤*Rationale:* Baseline vital signs allow for comparison during and after the procedure to evaluate patient tolerance and need for pain medication.
- Evaluate for success of graft take: vascularization of the graft; reepithelialization of the interstices; decreased pain; adherence of the graft ➤*Rationale:* Graft success or adherence to wound is assessed with each episode of care to evaluate healing.
- Monitor for signs of complications: fever; elevated white blood cell count; cellulitis; increased purulent drainage or saturation of the secondary dressing. ➤*Rationale:* Baseline and ongoing assessment for signs of graft failure to include possible infection are important for early identification of complications to minimize graft loss.

- Compare patient's rate of healing with expected rate of wound of healing for number of days after skin graft. ➤➤*Rationale:* Initial healing of grafted area should occur in 7 to 10 days.
- Determine adequacy of the pain control regimen by asking the patient to rate the pain on a scale of 0 to 10 (or other scale as appropriate), both before wound care (background pain) and during the dressing change. ➤➤*Rationale:* An individualized plan for pain control should be in place for background and procedural pain. In addition to the traditional use of pain and anxiety medications, alternative therapies should be included (e.g., relaxation techniques, distraction, massage therapy, music therapy). The patient's medication requirements should decrease as the grafted area heals.
- Assess patient's level of function in the grafted area.[6] ➤➤*Rationale:* Skin grafts contract during the healing phase, and immobility enhances loss of function. The patient should be encouraged to continue normal movement and range-of-motion exercises after graft take has been established.[6]

Patient Preparation

- Ensure that patient understands preprocedural teachings. Answer questions as they arise, and reinforce information as needed. ➤➤*Rationale:* Understanding of previously taught information is evaluated and reinforced.
- Notify other appropriate healthcare providers who need to assess the graft (e.g., physician) or perform a task (e.g., range-of-motion exercises by physical therapist) of the time of dressing change. ➤➤*Rationale:* Organization of care allows important assessment and intervention to take place without causing extra pain and stress to the patient.
- Premedicate the patient with pain medication and any sedation and anxiolytic medications as prescribed. Allow an appropriate amount of time for medications to begin to take effect before starting wound care. ➤➤*Rationale:* Premedication reduces pain and anxiety and allows time for medication to take effect and promote optimal comfort for the patient. Patient trust and compliance with procedure are encouraged.

Procedure for Care of Skin Grafts

Steps	Rationale	Special Considerations
1. Prepare all necessary equipment and supplies.	Preparation facilitates efficient wound care and prevents needless delays.	Notify other disciplines that need to observe the wound ahead of time so that they can be present while the wound is uncovered.
2. **VP**		
3. **HH**		
4. **PE**		For larger graft dressing changes, all healthcare providers participating in the wound care should apply cap, mask, and gown. Smaller graft changes may require less personal protective equipment. If family is doing dressing change at home, mask, cap, and gown are not used.
5. Remove bulky, outer dressings and discard. Place towel or pad under exposed extremity.	Old dressings can contain large amounts of body secretions and blood. Towel allows a place for patient to rest extremity during care.	Initial dressing is commonly left in place for 3 to 5 days; bulky, outer dressings are changed while nonadherent gauze is left in place (check orders).
6. Remove and discard gloves; apply clean gloves.	Examination gloves are contaminated by handling the burn dressing; clean gloves are needed for wound care.	
7. If ordered, gently lift nonadherent gauze from grafted site, anchoring graft in place as needed. *Note:* Surgeon may staple on dressing that is to remain in place until skin graft heals (e.g., Biobrane).	Grafts are not firmly attached to the wound bed and can be pulled loose for up to 5 days after grafting.	Normal saline solution or warm tap water may be used to loosen dressings stuck to graft area.

Procedure continues on following page

Procedure for Care of Skin Grafts—*Continued*

Steps	Rationale	Special Considerations
8. Gently rinse graft site and surrounding tissue with normal saline solution or warm tap water with gauze or washcloths.	Cleanses wound of exudate and reduces microorganisms. Use pH-neutral cleansing agents.	Special care is necessary during cleansing process to not displace skin graft.
9. Use scissors and forceps to remove loose necrotic tissue. If the graft is a sheet graft, assess for and remove any pockets of fluid under the graft.	Clears debris that can harbor microorganisms. Pockets of fluid separate the graft from the wound bed, which is vital for blood supply, causing graft loss in that area.	Remove pockets of fluid. If the sheet graft has been in place for less than 48 hours and the fluid is near the edge of sheet graft, roll the fluid to the edge and out; otherwise, make a small nick in the sheet graft directly over the area of fluid accumulation and gently express the fluid through the hole. Gently remove exudate with gauze dampened with sterile normal saline solution or sterile water.
10. Remove staples that are no longer needed to hold graft or dressing in place.	Prevents embedding of staples, local irritation, infection, and scarring.	Staples can be removed starting 5 to 7 days after grafting. Removing a large number of staples may be very painful and may necessitate an anesthesia-assisted procedure.
11. Assess graft for progression of healing and for complications.	Validates the healing process and identifies complications.	
12. Apply nonadherent dressing (if interstices are open), cover with secondary dressings, and secure; or apply moisturizer to healed adherent graft areas where interstices are closed and cover with thin secondary dressings to promote mobility.	Protects graft while healing.	A water-based lotion is used to prevent drying and reduce itching when interstices are closed.
13. Remove and discard gloves; apply clean gloves.	Reduces transmission of microorganisms.	
14. Apply splints to appropriate limb and elevate the involved extremity. Hands and arms may be elevated with pillows or elastic net sling. Elevate head of bed.	Maintains position of function, prevents contractures, and reduces edema and pain.	If possible, prevent patient from lying on grafted areas. Consider use of pressure-reduction mattress for grafts or donor sites on posterior surfaces. After the initial period of immobilization, splints are used only when the patient is unable to participate in range-of-motion exercises or self-care.
15. Remove and discard personal protective equipment.		
16. **HH**		
17. Continue to monitor patient's vital signs.	Patient may be hypothermic or may experience respiratory complications after wound care.	Removal of painful stimuli may result in oversedation after wound care.

Expected Outcomes

- Graft take of greater than 90% is attained
- Patient maintains a self-identified acceptable level of pain relief
- Patient attains comfort from measures provided for anxiety and itching
- Patient and family verbalize knowledge of patient condition and plan of care
- An optimal level of function is maintained
- Patient and family response and interactions demonstrate adaptation to injury
- Patient and family collaborate in management of care
- At the time of discharge, patient and family verbalize and demonstrate an understanding of posthospital care

Unexpected Outcomes

- Bleeding
- Infection
- Graft failure

Patient Monitoring and Care

Steps	Rationale	Reportable Conditions
		These conditions should be reported if they persist despite nursing interventions.
1. Follow institution standard for assessing pain. Administer analgesia as prescribed. Ask the patient to rate pain on a scale of 0 to 10 (or other appropriate scale); check the orders for analgesic, sedative, and anxiolytic agents before dressing changes; evaluate the patient's medication requirements with previous dressing changes; and assess the need for more medication throughout the dressing change. Incorporate alternative pain relief techniques (e.g., relaxation techniques, distraction, massage therapy, music therapy, visual imaging).[9] **(Level D*)**	Identifies need for pain interventions. The patient with new skin grafts will have some baseline pain that requires pain medication; pain medication requirements may be increased and sedation or anxiolytic agents may also be necessary for the procedural pain involved in graft care.[9] Attention to the patient's pain fosters the patient's trust in healthcare personnel to control pain and promotes cooperation with future graft care.	• Continued pain despite pain interventions • Increased heart rate • Increased or decreased blood pressure • Increased respiratory rate • Verbalization of pain • Nonverbal indications of pain (restlessness, grimacing, teeth clenching) • Inability to cooperate with dressing change
2. Note baseline vital signs (including pulse oximetry, if narcotics were used). Monitor vital signs throughout the procedure, and continue to assess for 30 minutes after procedure is complete.	Changes in vital signs can be an indication that the patient is experiencing pain or anxiety. Decreasing blood pressure, heart rate, and respiratory rate can be complications of pain medication (especially after dressing change is complete and stimulation has stopped).	• Inability to verbally arouse patient • Increased or decreased heart rate • Increased or decreased blood pressure • Increased or decreased respiratory rate and depth of respirations • High peak pressures on ventilator

*Level D: Peer-reviewed, professional organizational standards with clinical studies to support recommendations

Procedure continues on following page

Patient Monitoring and Care —*Continued*

Steps	Rationale	Reportable Conditions
3. Assess graft site for appearance (e.g., color, drainage, bleeding, graft necrosis, graft loss, cellulitis) and progression toward healing (e.g., vascularization of the graft, reepithelialization of the interstices, decreased pain, adherence of the graft).	Observe for usual progression of wound healing versus complications.	• Foul odor • Purulent or increased amounts of drainage • Increased pain • Cellulitis • Hematoma or fluid collection under sheet grafts • Graft necrosis • Sloughing • Bleeding
4. Place patient in position of optimal function during initial period of immobilization of newly grafted areas, with splints used to maintain position. After the first 5 days, encourage exercise, activities of daily living, and range-of-motion exercises during dressing changes. Use pain medication as needed to facilitate mobility.[2] **(Level E*)**	Grafted skin contracts during the healing phase if not correctly splinted and exercised. Loss of function is a complication of immobility. Pain inhibits patients from moving.	• Contractures • Loss of function
5. Monitor patient's tolerance of tube feedings or ingestion of a high-calorie, high-protein diet with supplements[3]; encourage nutritious diet and discourage empty calories. Limit free water. **(Level D*)**	Nutrition is necessary for wound healing.[3] Burn patients are hypermetabolic.	• Poor wound healing • Graft failure
6. Continue to follow institution standard for assessing pain. Administer analgesia as prescribed.	Identifies need for pain interventions.	• Continued pain despite pain interventions

Documentation

Documentation should include the following:
- Patient and family education
- Date and time of graft care
- Appearance of graft site (e.g., color, drainage, bleeding, graft necrosis, sloughing, cellulitis)
- Progression toward healing (e.g., adherence and vascularization of the graft, reepithelialization of the interstices, decreased pain)
- Dressings and topicals applied
- Pain assessment, interventions, and effectiveness
- Medications given for pain and sedation
- Other comfort measures used
- Patient's tolerance of the procedure
- Unexpected outcomes
- Nursing interventions

*Level D: Peer-reviewed, professional organizational standards with clinical studies to support recommendations
*Level E: Multiple case reports, theory-based evidence from expert opinions, or peer-reviewed professional organizational standards without clinical studies to support recommendations

References

1. Bryant R, Nix D: *Acute & chronic wounds,* ed 3, St Louis, 2006, Mosby, 361-390.
CR 2. Carrougher GJ: *Burn care and therapy,* ed 1, St Louis, 1998, Mosby.
CR 3. Flynn MB: Nutritional support for the burn-injured patient, *Crit Care Nurs Clin North Am* 16(1): 139-144, 2004.
4. Gibran N, Luterman A, Herndon D, et al: Comparison of fibrin sealant and staples for attaching split-thickness autologous sheet grafts in patients with deep partial- or full-thickness burn wounds: a phase 1/2 clinical study, *J Burn Care Res* 28(3):401, 2007.
CR 5. Heimbach D, et al: Artificial dermis for major burns: a multicenter randomized clinical trial, *Ann Surg* 208:313-320, 1988.
CR 6. Honari S: Topical therapies and antimicrobials in the management of burn wounds, *Crit Care Nurs Clin North Am* 16(1): 1-11, 2004.
7. Jeng JC, Fidler PE, Sokolich JC, et al: Seven years' experience with Integra as a reconstructive tool, *J Burn Care Res* 28(1):120-126, 2007.

8. Makic MBF, Mann E: Burn injuries. In McQuillan K, Makic MBF, Whalen E, editors: *Trauma nursing: from resuscitation through rehabilitation*, ed 4, St Louis, 2009, Elsevier, 865-888.

CR 9. Montgomery RK: Pain management in burn injury, *Crit Care Nurs Clin North Am* 16(1):39-49, 2004.

Additional Readings

CR Barret JP, Herndon DN: Effects of burn wound excision on bacterial colonization and invasion, *Plast Reconstruct Surg* 111:744-750, 2003.

CR Branski LK, Herndon DN, Pereira C, et al, editors: Burn and wound care, *Crit Care Nurs Clin North Am* 16 (1): 2004.

Foster K, Richey K: Wound wise: the story on partial-thickness skin grafts, *Nurs Made Incredibly Easy* 6(2):19-21, 2008.

CR Heimbach DM, et al: Multicenter postapproval clinical trial of Integra Dermal Regeneration Template for burn treatment, *J Burn Care Rehab* 24:42-48, 2003.

Herndon DN, editor: *Total burn care,* ed 3, London, 2007, Saunders.

Integra Dermal Regeneration Template, retrieved January 14, 2010 from www.integra-ls.com/products.

Nowlin A: The delicate business of burn care, *RN* 69(1):52-58, 2006.

CR Osborn K: Critical care: nursing burn injuries, *Nurs Manage* 34(5):49-50, 52-56, 2003.

Pham C, Greenwood J, Cleland H, et al: Bioengineered skin substitutes for the management of burns: a systematic review, *Burns* 33(8):946-957, 2007.

Saffle JR: Covering massive burn injuries: integra-ting and interpreting the data, *Crit Care Med* 35(11):2661-2662, 2007.

Zhang X, Jeschke MG: Longitudinal assessment of integra in primary burn management: a randomised pediatric clinical trials, *Crit Care Med* 35(11):2615-2623, 2007.

PROCEDURE **122**

AP Intracompartmental Pressure Monitoring

PURPOSE: Compartment syndrome can occur within any confined anatomic region when elevations in tissue pressure are sufficient to cause neurovascular compromise of the tissues in that region or compartment. Typically, diagnosis of this syndrome is made with serial clinical examinations of the involved extremity. However, in patients with inconclusive physical findings or with an altered level of consciousness, direct measurement of the intracompartmental pressure is a useful diagnostic adjunct.

Christine A. Cottingham

PREREQUISITE NURSING KNOWLEDGE

- Nurses performing intracompartmental pressure monitoring (IPM) must have detailed knowledge of the anatomy of the involved limb compartments (Fig. 122-1), including external landmarks associated with each compartment. Compartment syndrome may also develop in the abdomen (abdominal compartment syndrome [ACS]). For directions on measurement of bladder pressure, refer to Procedure 106.
- All clinicians involved with performing and assisting with the procedure should have knowledge of aseptic technique.
- Nurses should be credentialed in performing IPM. This should include supervised training in the techniques used for IPM and opportunities to maintain clinical competence.
- Clinicians should have a high index of suspicion that the patient is at risk for developing compartment syndrome. Etiologies can be divided into internal and external sources. Examples of internal causes include fractures, contusions, and edema formation associated with crush injuries or reperfusion injuries. External sources are generally related to compression of the limb and include

such things as eschar from burn injuries, splints, casts, dressings, and immobility.[1] Definitive treatment may be as simple as releasing a splint, cast, or dressing. More advanced treatment may require release of the compartment with an escharotomy or fasciotomy.

- The pathophysiology of compartment syndrome is related to compromised perfusion. Blood flow to any tissue or organ requires a sufficient perfusion pressure, which is generally calculated as the mean arterial pressure minus the intracompartmental pressure and should be 70 to 80 mm Hg.[2] Therefore, as the mean arterial pressure decreases or the intracompartmental pressure increases, the perfusion to the tissue is reduced. Insufficient perfusion pressure may lead to ischemia and eventual necrosis of the tissues within the affected area.
- Normal compartment pressure within an unaffected compartment is considered less than 10 mm Hg.[3,4] Clinically significant pressure changes are generally defined in one of two ways:
  - ❖ An absolute value of more than 30 mm Hg in the presence of other signs and symptoms of compartment syndrome. However, injury of the area may lead to elevations of the intracompartmental pressure in the absence of actual compartment syndrome.[5] Positioning of the extremity may also cause elevations in intracompartmental pressure particularly when assessing dependent compartments.

Compartments of the Calf

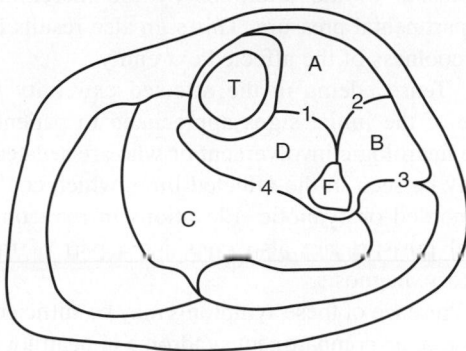

A   Anterior compartment
B   Lateral (peroneal) compartment
C   Superficial posterior compartment
D   Deep posterior compartment
T   Tibia
F   Fibula
1   Interosseous membrane
2   Anterior intermuscular septum
3   Posterior intermuscular septum
4   Intermuscular septum

Compartments of the Forearm

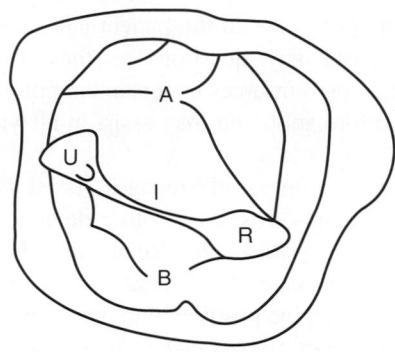

A   Volar (anterior) compartment
B   Dorsal (posterior) compartment
I   Interosseous membrane
R   Radius
U   Ulna

Compartments of the Thigh

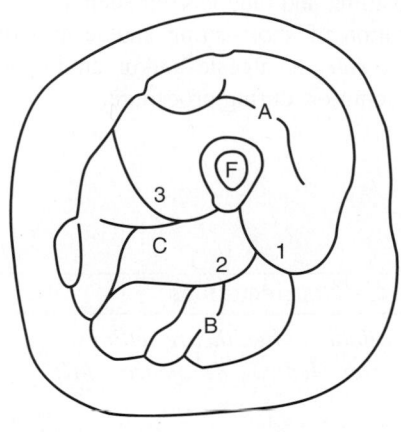

A   Anterior compartment
B   Posterior compartment
C   Medial compartment
F   Femur
1   Lateral intermuscular septum
2   Posterior intermuscular septum
3   Medial intermuscular septum

FIGURE 122-1 Muscle compartments of the calf, forearm, and thigh. *(Tiwari A, Haq AI, Myint F, Hamilton G: Acute compartment syndromes, Br J Surg 8:397-412, 2002.)*

❖ A delta compartment pressure (Δp) of less than 30 mm Hg: the diastolic blood pressure minus the intracompartmental pressure. This measurement may be a more reliable indicator of the risk for development of compartment syndrome because it takes into account blood pressure.[6,7]

- Acute compartment syndrome is a true orthopedic emergency. Signs and symptoms can develop in as little as 2 hours after injury. Ischemic damage to muscles and nerves can start in 4 to 6 hours, with permanent damage occurring in 12 to 24 hours.[3]

EQUIPMENT

- Electronic pressure monitoring device (bedside pressure monitor or a handheld monitoring device).
- Prefilled sterile saline solution syringe
- Dedicated disposable tubing with needle
- Chlorhexidine gluconate 1%
- 1% Lidocaine without epinephrine
- Sterile gloves
- Sterile dressing
- One roll of hypoallergenic tape

PATIENT AND FAMILY EDUCATION

- Explain the indications and rationale for performing this procedure to the patient and family. ➤➤*Rationale:* Explanation of the procedure may decrease patient and family anxiety and assist in patient cooperation.
- On the basis of institutional standard, obtain a formal consent, if the procedure is not emergent. ➤➤*Rationale:* Informed consent documents that the patient or family understands the explanation and need for the procedure.

PATIENT ASSESSMENT AND PREPARATION

Patient Assessment

- Review the patient's history for conditions associated with the development of compartment syndrome. ➤➤*Rationale:* This review raises the index of suspicion for diagnosis of compartment syndrome.
- Clinical presentation of the compartment syndrome is traditionally listed with a series of "P's"[1,8]:
  - ❖ *Pain:* Pain is the most commonly reported and earliest symptom of compartment syndrome but is often difficult to differentiate from that caused by the primary injury. Assessment of pain in patients with an altered level of consciousness is also difficult. Traditionally, pain is described as out of proportion to the injury or minimally responsive to analgesic interventions (e.g., intravenous narcotics). It is also exacerbated by active or passive stretching of the affected extremity.
  - ❖ *Parasthesia:* This sign precedes loss of motor function and occurs as pressure increases on the affected nerve. Early signs include loss of two point discrimination.
  - ❖ *Paresis* or *paralysis:* This sign is a late finding that occurs as result of pressure on the nerve or necrosis of the affected muscles.

- ❖ *Pulselessness:* Pulselessness is another late finding, from occlusion of the arterioles by the increasing intracompartmental pressure. This sign also results in pallor or coolness of the affected extremity.
- ❖ *Pressure:* Tense edema in the affected extremity is often one of the initial signs appreciated in patients who have neurologic involvement or who are sedated. Pallor may be seen in the affected limb, which could also be mottled or cyanotic. Elevations in intracompartmental pressure are also considered part of the confirmatory diagnosis.
- ➤➤*Rationale:* Presence of these symptoms may be sufficient to diagnose acute compartment syndrome in neurologically intact patients. In patients with an impaired level of consciousness (LOC), these symptoms signal the need for IPM.

Patient Preparation

- Explain steps of the procedure to the patient and family (if applicable). Answer any questions as they arise. ➤➤*Rationale:* Explanation reinforces understanding of previously presented information and may assist in allaying anxiety.
- Remove constricting dressings and bandages. Assist with the modification of splints, casts, and other devices on the affected extremity. ➤➤*Rationale:* Removal reduces external pressure on the tissue of the affected extremity.
- Place the patient in the supine position with the extremity at the level of the heart. ➤➤*Rationale:* Access to the affected compartment is provided. Positioning the extremity above the heart may impede circulation, placing it in a dependent position, and may worsen edema.
- Consider administration of short-acting analgesic and/or anxiolytic. ➤➤*Rationale:* Analgesic and/or anxiolytic decreases patient discomfort during procedure.

Procedure	for Intracompartmental Pressure Monitoring	
Steps	Rationale	Special Considerations

Many one-time and continuous intracompartmental pressure monitoring devices are available in healthcare settings. This procedure assumes the use of the Stryker Intracompartmental Pressure Sensor (Stryker Medical, Kalamazoo, MI; Fig. 122-2).

Steps	Rationale	Special Considerations
1. **HH**		
2. **PE**		

3. Before the intracompartmental measurement begins, comply with Universal Protocol requirements:
  A. Ensure all relevant documents and studies are available.
  B. Perform a pre-procedure verification and time out, if non-emergent.
	Ensures patient safety	

4. Clean insertion site with antiseptic solution (e.g. 1% chlorhexidine gluconate [CHG]).	Reduces bacterial flora on skin.	CHG must be dry for maximal effectiveness.

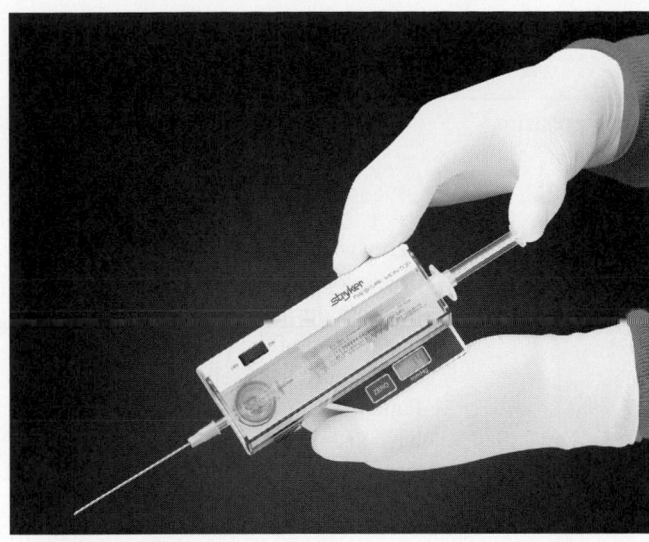

FIGURE 122-2 Stryker intracompartmental pressure monitor. *(Courtesy Stryker Instruments.)*

Procedure for Intracompartmental Pressure Monitoring—*Continued*

Steps	Rationale	Special Considerations
5. Remove gloves and assemble the dedicated disposable needle, prefilled sterile saline solution syringe, and pressure transducer.	Prepares the monitoring system.[7] **(Level M*)**	
6. Place the assembled disposable system into the pressure monitoring device. A. Ensure that the system is securely inserted and that the wings of the syringe are flat against the device. B. Close the cover until an audible click is heard.	Prepares the monitoring system.[7] **(Level M)**	
7. Tilt the device so that the needle is at least 45 degrees upward and purge the system with the saline solution.	Removes air bubbles and ensures an accurate reading.[7] **(Level M)**	
8. 🔲		
9. Apply clean gloves.		
10. Inject local anesthetic agent at site per institutional protocols.	Increases patient comfort.	Consider concomitant use of intravenous (IV) analgesics or anxiolytics if appropriate for patient's condition.
11. Determine landmarks for insertion.		Differences in insertion location can affect the measured value.
12. Estimate angle of insertion with the pressure monitoring device. Turn device on and press "zero" button. Wait until display shows that device is zeroed.	Eliminate atmospheric pressure, ensuring accurate reading.[7] **(Level M)**	
13. Remove needle cover and insert 1 to 3 cm depending on which compartment is being measured.		

*Level M: Manufacturer's recommendations only

Procedure continues on following page

Procedure | for Intracompartmental Pressure Monitoring—*Continued*

Steps	Rationale	Special Considerations
14. Inject 0.1 to 0.3 mL of saline solution into compartment.	Equilibrates device to tissue pressure.[7] **(Level M*)**	
15. Observe pressure reading displayed on the device.		
16. Verify placement by manually pressing on the tissue near the insertion site or by flexing and extending the extremity distal to the insertion site (e.g., ankle, wrist or knee).	Fluctuations in pressure readings verify correct placement of the needle.	Patients with normal compartment physiology have a rapid rise in pressure during palpation or contraction of the muscle with a rapid return to baseline pressure. Patients with compartment syndrome have a slow return to baseline pressure after relaxation of the muscle.
17. Remove and discard needle and syringe in appropriate receptacle. Apply an occlusive sterile dressing to the puncture site.	Reduces the risk of contamination.	
18. Discard used supplies.		
19. 🄷🄷		

Expected Outcomes

- Procedure completed without complications in a timely manner
- Minimal patient discomfort
- Pressure readings consistent with clinical presentation of the patient's extremity
- If compartment syndrome is present, a rapid fasciotomy of the involved compartment is required; obtain immediate surgical consult as necessary

Unexpected Outcomes

- Failure to recognize compartment syndrome, resulting in long-term morbidity for the patient
- Inaccurate pressure readings obtained
- Excessive bleeding from the catheter insertion site
- Signs and symptoms of procedure-related infection

Patient Monitoring and Care

Steps	Rationale	Reportable Conditions
		These conditions should be reported if they persist despite nursing interventions.
1. Complete a neurovascular assessment of the affected extremity hourly and as necessary.	Documentation and review of serial trends in assessment detect onset and development of compartment syndrome.	- Onset of pain or worsening of pain despite administration of analgesic agents - Paresthesia or hypothesia of the affected extremity - Changes in extremity skin color (mottling, cyanosis, pallor) and skin temperature - Decrease or loss of peripheral pulses - Paralysis of the affected extremity - Increase in circumference and tenseness of the extremity

*Level M: Manufacturer's recommendations only

Patient Monitoring and Care —*Continued*

Steps	Rationale	Reportable Conditions
2. Assess the insertion site for signs and symptoms of infection.	The needle insertion site may be a source of infection.	• Erythema, swelling, or drainage around the insertion site • Increase in skin warmth surrounding the insertion site • Increased pain and tenderness at the insertion site • Increase in white blood cell (WBC) count on complete blood count • Fever
3. Follow institution standard for assessing pain. Administer analgesia as prescribed.	Identifies need for pain interventions.	• Continued pain despite pain interventions

Documentation

Documentation should include the following:

• Consent information for the procedure, including potential complications
• Clinical findings before and after compartment pressure measurement
• Description of the compartments that were assessed
• Medications administered during procedure
• Results of the compartment pressure measurement

• The condition of the puncture site and dressing after the needle is removed
• Description of how the patient tolerated the procedure
• Development of unexpected outcomes
• Additional interventions
• Appropriate codes for billing

References

1. Heppenstall R, Scott R, Spaega A: A comparative study of the tolerance of skeletal muscle to ischaemia, *J Bone Joint Surg* 68-A:820-828, 1986.
2. Joint Commission: *Universal protocol for preventing wrong site, wrong procedure, wrong person surgery,* 2003, retrieved January 8, 2009, from http://www.jointcommission.org/PatientSafety/UniversalProtocol.
3. Kakar S, Firoozabodi R, McKean J, et al: Diastolic blood pressure in patients with tibia fractures under analgesia: implications for the diagnosis of compartment syndrome, *J Orthop Trauma* 21:99-103, 2007.
4. Ozkayin N, Aktuglu K: Absolute compartment pressure versus differential pressure for the diagnosis of compartment syndrome in tibial fractures, *Int Orthop* 29:396-401, 2005.
5. Prayson MJ, Chen JL, Hampers D, et al: Baseline compartment pressure measurements in isolated lower extremity fractures without clinical compartment syndrome, *J Trauma* 60:1037-1040, 2006.
6. Seiler JG, Womack S, De L'Aune WR, et al: Intracompartmental pressure measurements in the normal forearm, *J Orthop Trauma* 7:414-416, 1993.
7. Stryker Medical: *Intracomparmental pressure sensor,* from package insert.
8. Ulmer T: The clinical diagnosis of compartment syndrome of the lower leg: are clinical findings predictive of the disorder? *J Orthop Trauma* 16:572-577, 2002.

Additional Readings

Walsh CR: Musculoskeletal injuries. In McQuillan KA, Makic MBF, Whalen E, editors: *Trauma nursing: from resuscitation through rehabilitation,* ed 4, St Louis, 2009, Elsevier, 735.
Whiteside TE, Haney TC, Morimoto M, et al: Tissue pressure measurements as a determinant for the need of fasciotomy, *Clin Orthop Rel Res* 113:43-51, 1975.

Pressure Redistribution Surfaces: Continual Lateral Rotation Therapy and RotoRest™ Lateral Rotation Surface

P U R P O S E : The purpose of pressure redistribution surface (i.e., support surface) is to assist in the reduction of pressure over areas of the body and reduce the development of pressure ulcers and other skin breakdown.[9] Continual lateral rotation therapy provides dynamic rotation of a support surface to enhance mobilization and removal of pulmonary secretions for pulmonary benefit and to assist in preventing and treating physiologic complications of immobility. The RotoRest™ Lateral Rotation Surface is a unique kinetic therapy surface that can be perceived to be technically challenging to use. This surface is ideal for patients with traumatic injury, unstable spine, and traction and for patients who need aggressive rotation therapy.

Shannon Johnson

PREREQUISITE NURSING KNOWLEDGE

- Principles of prevention of pressure-induced injury should be understood, including high-risk areas for tissue injury in the critically ill patient.[12,13] High-risk areas of pressure injury include the occiput, coccyx, and heels.[11] Prolonged external pressure over bony prominences, shear and friction forces, and excessive moisture increase the risk of pressure ulcers.
- With use of a validated pressure ulcer risk assessment tool such as the Braden Scale, a patient's risk for a pressure ulcer should be assessed on admission to the intensive care unit (ICU), and at least every 12 to 24 hours thereafter, or with changes in patient condition. Interventions to prevent pressure ulcer development should target characteristics that put the patient at risk.[1,2]
- Redistribution of pressure includes frequent repositioning and use of support surfaces.[4,6]

- A pressure redistribution support surface is defined as a device designed for management of tissue loads, microclimate, or other therapeutic functions.[9]
  - ❖ Pressure redistribution support surfaces may be powered or nonpowered.
  - ❖ Newer acute care mattresses incorporate pressure reduction technology.
  - ❖ Preventive interventions, such as turning, monitoring nutrition, containing excessive moisture, and preventing shear and friction, are indicated with the use of a specialty surface.
  - ❖ Layers of linen placed on the surface should be limited to allow maximal benefit of the surface with the patient's skin.
- The many types of pressure redistribution surfaces range from the standard acute care foam mattress to air-filled or fluid-filled surfaces. Generally, the more specialized surfaces are indicated for certain wounds or patient conditions that result in excessive moisture, posterior grafts or wounds,

flaps, etc. Because the technology in pressure redistribution surfaces changes rapidly, practitioners should investigate the specific properties of available specialty mattresses to choose the correct surface for a patient.

- Bariatric pressure reduction surfaces provide similar properties to all special bed surfaces; however, they are wider, and the frame and surface are designed to accommodate heavier patients.
  - For maximal effects from pressure reduction therapy (low air loss, etc.), the weight of the patient must be tolerated by the surface.
  - Most ICU bed frames and specialty surfaces can support a patient up to 300 lbs. If the weight is greater than 300 lbs, the patient may need to move to a bariatric pressure reduction surface (refer to manufacturer's guidelines for maximum weight limit of ICU bed frame and support surface).
- Principles of wound healing should be understood and include evaluation of the patient's:
  - Overall risk as assessed with a valid risk assessment tool (i.e., Braden score)[2]
  - Nutritional status, including endpoint goals
  - Overall fluid management
  - Acid-base balance status
  - The presence of incontinence-associated moisture and effective management of diarrhea and urine
- Understanding of the pathophysiology of tissue ischemia is an important assessment parameter of the integumentary system in the complex critically ill patient. Tissue ischemia may be caused by direct pressure applied to tissues and by disease processes and medications (i.e., vasoactive medications).
- The terms *continual lateral rotation therapy* (CLRT) and *kinetic therapy* are often loosely used in a similar context.[5] *CLRT* is defined as the continuous turning of a patient from side to side with a less than 40-degree rotation; *kinetic therapy* is a 40-degree or greater rotation.[5]
- Support surfaces used to provide CLRT should have dynamic features to assist in pressure reduction over bony prominences. Special features may include:
  - Low air loss to assist in management of excessive moisture
  - Alternating pressure that provides pressure redistribution in a cyclic fashion to offload tissues
  - Multizoned surface in which different segments of the surface can have different pressure redistribution capabilities
- RotoRest™ (KCI Licensing, Inc, San Antonio, TX) lateral rotation surface is a kinetic therapy surface that does not incorporate low air loss into its technology, but if the patient is in continuous motion (rotation), pressure over bony prominences may be relieved during the continuous turning therapy. However, because of the aggressive degree of the turn, possible shear and friction injuries of the skin can occur during rotation.
- Knowledge is needed concerning the physiologic effects of immobility on body systems, including factors that contribute to impaired circulation. Potential complications in the critically ill patient include:
  - Venous stasis and thrombosis
  - Pulmonary and urinary stasis
  - Pressure ulcer formation with potential associated friction, moisture, and shear injury[4,8,13]
- Principles for successful use of CLRT therapy include clinician appreciation of the goals of therapy. For maximal benefit, the support surface should be in rotation more than 18 hours per day and at optimal rotation.[5,6]
  - The support surface should provide continuous rotation at varying degrees.
    - CLRT surfaces rotate up to 40 degrees.[5]
    - Kinetic therapy surfaces rotate up to 62 degrees.[7]
  - Surface provides continuous, slow, side-to-side turning of the patient with rotation of the therapeutic surface. The degree of rotation, and the time interval for rotation, is set by the clinician. The degree of rotation is set on each side, intermittently or constantly providing unilateral or bilateral rotation.
  - Serial skin assessments per institutional protocols are still required when patients are on rotational therapy surfaces.
  - The clinician should evaluate the patient's tolerance of CLRT/kinetic therapy and consider sedation and analgesics as appropriate.
- Indications for CLRT include critically ill patients who are at a higher risk of pulmonary complications such as:
  - Patients with increasing ventilatory support requirements
  - Patients at risk for ventilator-associated pneumonia (VAP)[14]
  - Patients who have clinical indications for acute lung injury or adult respiratory distress syndrome (ARDS)[3]:
    - Worsening Pao_2:Fio_2 (P:F) ratio
    - Presence of fluffy infiltrates via chest radiograph concomitant with pulmonary edema
    - Refractory hypoxemia
- Trauma diagnosis and spinal cord injury should be understood. Low air-loss surfaces are contraindicated for patients with unstable spine or pelvic injuries until the injury is stabilized. The RotoRest™ surface may be used with spinal injuries; additional care is necessary to place unstable spinal cord injuries or patients with pelvic instability on a RotoRest™ surface that has a firm, flat surface. Cervical traction and skeletal traction may be used with a RotoRest™ therapy surface.
- Patients should be placed on a pressure reduction surface as soon as possible to reduce the risk of pressure-associated tissue injury. Patients should be placed on a lateral rotation support surface as soon as possible to prevent negative effects of immobility and possible pulmonary complications.[4,8,13]
- When ordering a CLRT or kinetic therapy, the clinician should assess properties of the pressure redistribution surface and evaluate patient skin/tissue redistribution needs (i.e., moisture control, pressure redistribution).

- Regarding the CLRT support surface:
  - ❖ Several support surfaces are available for CLRT. Refer to hospital policy for types of support surfaces that may be used.
  - ❖ Evaluate the specific needs of the patient to include pulmonary indications for CLRT, including contraindications such as traction, unstable spine, and pelvic injuries.
  - ❖ Manufacturer-specific guidelines for implementing CLRT should be reviewed before the patient is placed on the support surface/bed frame.
- The RotoRest™ Delta Kinetic™ Therapy bed is shown in Figure 123-1.
- Noted principles in caring for a patient receiving kinetic therapy on a RotoRest™ Delta Kinetic™ Therapy bed include technical and clinical competence in the following:
  - ❖ The surface below the patient and the positioning packs consist of pressure-redistributing foam and a pad of nonliquid polymer gel with a low-friction, low-shear GORE medical fabric (KCI Licensing, Inc, San Antonio, Texas) cover that does not absorb body fluids.
  - ❖ The gel pads prevent the patient from bottoming out and transfer body heat evenly; they are radiographically transparent.
  - ❖ The bed provides continuous, slow, side-to-side turning of the patient by rotating the bed frame. Keeping the patient in maximal rotation assists with prevention of skin breakdown and provides the most effective therapy for pulmonary indications. The bed can turn up to 62 degrees on each side, either intermittently or constantly, providing unilateral or bilateral rotation.
  - ❖ The amount of time the patient is held at the rotation limit before rotating in the opposite direction can be adjusted from 7 seconds to 30 minutes.

- ❖ Head and shoulder packs provide cervical stability but should not be used as the primary means of stabilizing cervical spine fractures. Cervical traction, halo, and vest or internal fixation may be required. Lateral arm and leg hatches facilitate range of motion.
- ❖ Hatches underneath the bed (located in the cervical, thoracic, and rectal areas) provide access for skin care, catheter maintenance, and bladder and bowel management. Do not open thoracic and sacral hatches at the same time.
- ❖ The bed has a built-in scale with a maximal patient weight of 300 lbs.[7]
- ❖ An optional vibrator pack is available to provide chest physiotherapy to further mobilize pulmonary secretions.

EQUIPMENT

- Suggested personal protective equipment: Gloves
- Sheet or slide board to assist with moving patient onto the surface
- Transparent or foam protective dressings for areas prone to friction or shear
- Appropriate pressure redistribution surface, CLRT surface, or RotoRest™ lateral rotation surface

PATIENT AND FAMILY EDUCATION

- Explain to patient and family the adverse effects of pulmonary complications, tissue pressure, excessive moisture of the skin, and complications of immobility. ➥*Rationale:* Explanation encourages understanding when a different bed surface is needed based on the

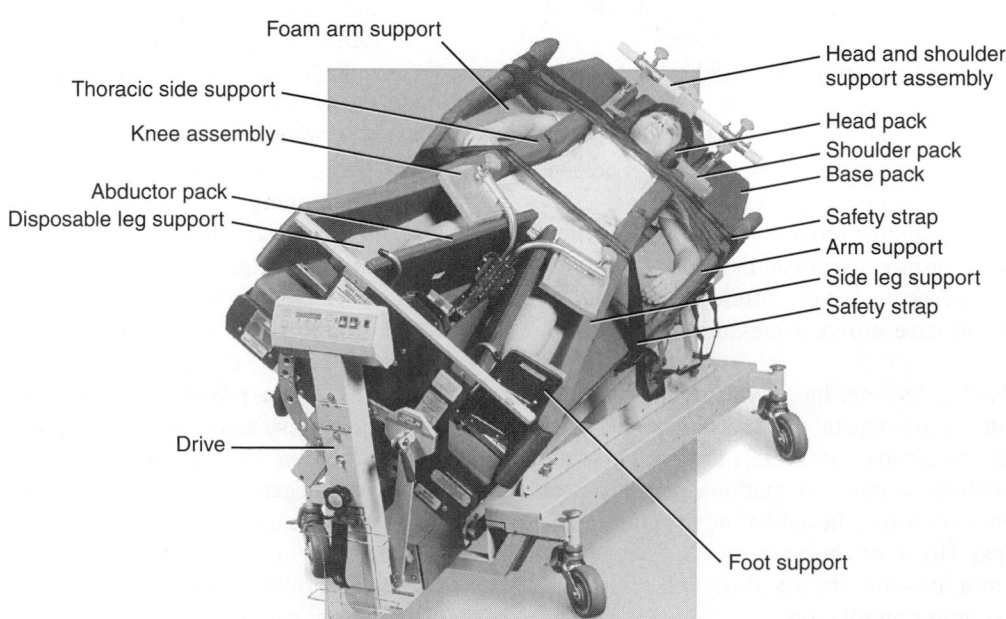

Figure 123-1   KCI RotoRest™ Delta Kinetic™ Therapy bed. *(Courtesy KCI Licensing, Inc, San Antonio, TX, 2008.)*

risk assessment of patient. The patient and family are able to ask questions.

- Explain how CLRT and properties of the support surface achieve pressure reduction. ➤➤*Rationale:* Understanding and cooperation are increased.
- Discuss the patient's need for long-term pressure redistribution strategies to include redistribution of weight while in a chair or bed and management of acute or chronic health problems, chronic pressure ulcers, or both. ➤➤*Rationale:* The family and patient are engaged in the plan of care, and the nurse can anticipate the need for patient discharge with pressure redistribution surface.
- When a support surface is used for the purpose of lateral rotation, explain how lateral rotation therapy is used to reduce the incidence of VAP and atelectasis. An added benefit is reduction of pressure on the skin. ➤➤*Rationale:* Understanding and cooperation are increased.
- Explain to patient and family the pulmonary benefit of CLRT in promoting dynamic movement of pulmonary secretions. ➤➤*Rationale:* Understanding of the role of pulmonary secretion mobility in the critically ill is encouraged.

PATIENT ASSESSMENT AND PREPARATION

Patient Assessment

- Assess the patient's risk for a pressure ulcer with an evidence-based practice assessment tool (i.e., Braden score).[1,2] ➤➤*Rationale:* Valid assessment tools assist in identification of patient risk for alterations in skin.
- Assess the patient's skin for evidence of pressure ulcer formation or alterations in skin on admission and throughout care based on institutional policy. ➤➤*Rationale:* Baseline and ongoing skin status data are provided.
- Assess the patient's wounds: location, size, stage of pressure ulcer, description of tissue in wound bed, type and amount of drainage, surrounding skin for maceration and inflammation, and pain on palpation of surrounding skin. ➤➤*Rationale:* Objective and thorough assessment of wounds on admission and throughout course of illness is necessary for measuring effectiveness of therapy and interventions.
- Assess the patient's vascular system: ensure hemodynamic stability is present, and assess for presence of edema in lower extremities and deep vein thrombosis (DVT) potential.[14] ➤➤*Rationale:* Baseline data are provided to measure and treat the ill effects of immobility.

- Assess the patient's pulmonary status to include the quality and presence of adventitious breath sounds, the rate and depth of respirations, cough, cyanosis, dyspnea, nasal flaring, arterial blood gas results, chest radiograph, mental status, and restlessness. ➤➤*Rationale:* Initial and ongoing evaluation of effectiveness of CLRT therapy on body systems is provided. Lateral movement provides postural drainage, mobilizes secretions, and enhances air exchange.[5]
- Assess the patient's bladder for complications associated with urinary stasis from immobility to include the presence of bladder distention, incomplete bladder emptying, or urinary infrequency. ➤➤*Rationale:* Baseline data are provided before implementation of lateral movement that decreases urinary stasis and associated complications.[14]
- Discuss goals for pressure redistribution and CLRT therapy with prescribing provider. ➤➤*Rationale:* The properties of the CLRT support surface are evaluated to match patient factors related to type of injury, moisture, and need for redistribution of pressure on skin and wounds.

Patient Preparation

- Ensure that the patient and family understand preprocedural teachings. Answer questions as they arise, and reinforce information as needed. ➤➤*Rationale:* Understanding of previously taught clinical information and rationale is evaluated and reinforced.
- Evaluate the properties of support surface to meet pulmonary needs, skin factors related to type of injury, moisture, and need for redistribution of pressure on skin and wounds. Order and inspect the bed functions before the patient is placed on the surface ➤➤*Rationale:* Support surface selection should match clinical indication for patient therapy. Relief of external pressure may decrease risk of pressure ulcer formation and facilitates wound healing.
- Verify correct patient with two identifiers. ➤➤*Rationale:* Prior to performing a procedure, the nurse should ensure the correct identification of the patient for the intended intervention.
- Organize moving the patient to the special surface, ensuring adequate personnel are available. Assist the patient to a supine position with the head of the bed elevated to 30 degrees (if not medically contraindicated) in preparation for move to specialty bed. ➤➤*Rationale:* Transfer of the patient from one bed to another is potentiated. Head of bed at 30 degrees minimizes shearing forces and protects airway.

Procedure | for Lateral Rotation Therapy

Steps	Rationale	Special Considerations
For framed CLRT surfaces, follow manufacturer guidelines for settings to include patient height, weight, and rotation settings; The RotoRest™ kinetic therapy surface is considered more challenging to use and thus is the only surface described in this section.		
Procedure for Kinetic Therapy with the RotoRest™ Surface		
	Rental beds may require a physician's order.	U.S. Food and Drug Administration (FDA) regulated. Ensures the properties of the specialty surface meet the patient's specific needs.
1. 🄷🄷		
2. 🄿🄴		
3. Ensure that bed is locked in horizontal position and that the drive is disengaged.	Ensures patient safety.	
4. Check all hatches to be certain they are properly latched; be sure castors are locked.	Prevents unplanned movement of bed.	
5. With use of a draw sheet, move the patient gently to the center of the surface while maintaining body alignment.[7] **(Level M*)**	Bouncing of patient can result in skin abrasions.	Pillar bars can be covered with a towel or folded paper sheet to avoid possibility of abrasion.
Positioning a Patient on a Kinetic Therapy Surface		
1. Center the patient on the bed by aligning the nose, umbilicus, and pubis with the center posts.[7] **(Level M)**	Facilitates proper balance. Rotating to one side indicates that the patient is not centered.	To initiate CPR, return the bed to the horizontal position and lock in place.
2. Place thoracic side supports in appropriate holes provided in the frame and ensure that they are tightened securely.	These are the main supporting apparatus.	The holes in the frame in which the side supports fit are near the surface of the base packs. Packs and supports are labeled for patient's right and left sides. Maintain 1-inch clearance between the end of the pack and the axilla.
3. Adjust the knee assembly to a position slightly above the patient's knee.	Provides support.	
4. Place the disposable leg support in a position under the thigh and calf so that it fits under the ankle and knee but not beneath the heel.	Decreases external pressure on the heels.	Leg supports should be changed with excessive moisture or when soiled.
5. Place the foot supports in the foot bracket assembly. The assembly should be positioned so that the footrest is in anatomic position. Tighten the foot assembly.[7] **(Level M)**	Maintains each foot in proper anatomic position.	The foot supports should not be left in place for longer than 2 hours at a time. A schedule of 2 hours on and 2 hours off should be maintained continuously. Side-to-side motion does not relieve pressure on the soles of the feet.
6. Install the abductor packs into the preset metal brackets.	Provides support.	
7. Place the side leg supports snugly against the patient's hips; tighten securely.	Provides support.	

*Level M: Manufacturer's recommendations only

Procedure | for Lateral Rotation Therapy—*Continued*

Steps	Rationale	Special Considerations
8. Install the knee pads in a position so that your hand just fits between the knee and the pack.[7] **(Level M*)**	Prevents pressure on the knee.	Knee packs can be adjusted to allow for variation in abduction and flexion of the patient's legs. They maintain proper posture of the lower limbs in the patient with spasticity, discouraging contracture formation.
9. Adjust the head and shoulder support assembly.	Provides further support.	
10. Place a hand on the patient's shoulder and adjust the shoulder pack to lightly touch your hand.[7] **(Level M)**	Prevents pressure ulcers.	A 1-inch (2.54-cm) clearance should always exist between the patient's shoulders and the shoulder packs. If cervical traction causes the patient to slide up on the bed during rotation, place the patient in the reverse Trendelenburg's position.
11. Adjust the head pack so that it does not touch the patient's ears or come into contact with the tongs of cervical traction. Tighten head and shoulder assemblies securely.	Provides support.	To remove the head and shoulder packs, loosen the handle of the shoulder pack and slide to the side or lift the entire assembly.
12. Tighten the clamps on the safety straps.	Provides support.	
13. Install the disposable foam arm supports.[7] **(Level M)**	Ensures that the patient's hands are in a position of function and that the ulnar nerve and elbows are protected.	
14. Secure the arm supports in the holes provided on the frame.	Provides support.	
15. Safety straps must be in place at all times. One safety strap is used to hold down the shoulder assembly. Place the other strap across the hip region.	Prevents falls and patient injury.	
16. Initiate therapy.		
17. Monitor patient hemodynamics with rotation therapy	Ensures that patient tolerates therapy	Changes in hemodynamics are expected; monitor patient's tolerance and hemodynamic goals (e.g. urine output, mentation, mean arterial pressure [MAP], intracranial pressure [ICP], etc). The patient may need time to acclimate to kinetic therapy. Interpret vital signs with knowledge of fixed transducer variation caused by degree of rotation (i.e., level may change, providing false data).[10]
18. Remove personal protective equipment, and perform hand hygiene.	Reduces transmission of microorganisms; Standard Precautions.	

*Level M: Manufacturer's recommendations only

Procedure continues on following page

Expected Outcomes

- Intact skin integrity
- Wound healing
- Absence of friction and shearing
- Absence of excessive skin moisture or dryness
- Improved peripheral circulation
- Improved urinary elimination
- Maximal pulmonary function achieved

Unexpected Outcomes

- Friction, shearing, motion sickness, agitation, disorientation, and falls from lateral movement of table if patient is not strapped in properly
- Pressure ulcer formation or further deterioration of existing pressure ulcers
- Desaturation or hemodynamic instability with rotation
- Dislodged invasive lines or tubes
- Development of urinary tract infection
- Development of worsening pulmonary status

Patient Monitoring and Care

Steps	Rationale	Reportable Conditions
		These conditions should be reported if they persist despite nursing interventions.
1. To initiate CPR, return the bed to the horizontal position by disengaging the clutch and lock in place with locking pin.	A flat, firm surface is necessary for CPR.	
2. Evaluate the patient's existing pressure areas and ulcers, wounds, flaps, and grafts for evidence of healing according to institutional guidelines.	Relief of external pressure facilitates healing.	• Deterioration or wounds fail to heal
3. Assess the skin for evidence of pressure (especially on the occiput, sacrum, and heels), friction, shearing, or moisture per hospital policy. Consider applying protective dressing to areas prone to friction or shear (i.e., transparent semiocculsive, hydrocolloid or foam dressings).	These factors contribute to pressure ulcer formation; kinetic therapy and other CLRT surfaces alone do not protect from pressure ulcer formation. Ensure that adequate skin assessment continues throughout therapy.	• Development of pressure ulcers or skin breakdown
4. Evaluate the patient's peripheral vascular circulation.	Lateral movement discourages venous stasis.	• Edema, decreased or absent pulses, discoloration, pain
5. Evaluate the patient's pulmonary function.	Lateral movement provides continuous postural drainage and mobilization of secretions.	• Adventitious breath sounds • Decreased respiratory rate and depth • Cough • Cyanosis • Dyspnea • Nasal flaring • Decreased oxygen saturation • Abnormal blood gases • Decreased mental acuity • Restlessness • Abnormal chest radiograph results
6. Evaluate the patient for urinary retention.	Lateral movement decreases urinary stasis.	• Decreased urine output • Bladder distention

Patient Monitoring and Care —*Continued*

Steps	Rationale	Reportable Conditions
7. Evaluate the patient's acceptance of and adaptation to the device (motion sickness, agitation, disorientation).	Increases cooperation and decreases anxiety.	• Intolerance to device
8. Monitor patient's tolerance and hemodynamic goals (e.g., urine output, mentation, MAP, ICP, etc.). The patient may need time to acclimate to kinetic therapy.	Lateral movement may alter hemodynamics because of the degree of rotation (turn) and changes in transducer positioning.	• Vital signs consistently below desired goal/parameters
9. Follow institutional standard for assessing pain. Administer analgesia as prescribed.	Identifies need for pain interventions.	• Continued pain despite pain interventions
10. Maintain bed in motion for 18 hours of every 24-hour period.[5,6] Target rotation on a kinetic therapy surface is 62 degrees.	Provides proper rotation and adequate mobility.	• Inability to rotate as per schedule
10. Maintain safety straps at all times.	Prevents falls and patient injury.	• Falls or injury
11. Maintain schedule for foot supports: 2 hours on and 2 hours off continuously.	Side-to-side movement does not relieve pressure on soles of feet.	• Breakdown on soles of feet
12. Determine when therapy should be discontinued. Reassess need every 24-hour period.	Lateral rotation therapy is no longer required.	

Documentation

Documentation should include the following:

- Patient and family education
- Date and time therapy is instituted
- Rationale for use of lateral rotation therapy surface
- Number of hours patient is in rotation mode per 24-hour period and degree of rotation achieved
- Safety straps in place, bed alarms engaged
- Complete a full skin assessment per institutional standards and as necessary
- Complete serial skin, pressure area, and wound assessments per institutional standards and as necessary

- Status of wound healing, if applicable
- Patient's response to therapy
- Any unexpected outcomes and interventions taken
- Phone number and name of company representative
- Pain assessment and management according to institutional guidelines

References

1. Ayello EA, Lyder CH: Protecting patients from harm: preventing pressure ulcers in hospital patients, *Nursing* 37(10):36-40, 2007.
CR 2. Braden BJ, Bergstrom N: Clinical utility of the Braden scale for predicting pressure sore risk, *Decubitus* 2(3):44-46,50-41, 1989.
CR 3. Bernard GR: Acute Respiratory distress syndrome: a historical perspective, *Am J Respir Crit Care Med* 172:798-802, 2005.
CR 4. Brienza DM, Geyer J: Using support surfaces to manage tissue integrity, *Adv Skin Wound Care* 18(3):151-157, 2005.

5. Goldhill DR, Imhoff M, McLean B, et al: Rotational bed therapy to prevent and treat respiratory complications: a review and meta-analysis, *Am J Crit Care* 16(1):50-62, 2007.
CR 6. Higgens Martin A: Should continuous lateral rotation therapy replace manual turning? *Nurs Manage* 32(8):41-45, 2001.
CR 7. Kinetic Concepts, Inc: *Roto-Rest Delta: operations and maintenance manual,* San Antonio, 1995, Kinetic Concepts.
CR 8. Maklebust J: Choosing the right support surface, *Adv Skin Wound Care* 18(3):158-160, 2005.
9. National Pressure Ulcer Advisory Panel: *Support surface standards initiative: terms and definitions related to support surfaces,* 2007, retrieved August 28, 2009, from www.npuap.org/npuap_S31_TD.

10. Rauen CA, Makic MB, Bridges E: Evidence-based practice habits: transforming research into bedside practice, *Crit Care Nurse* 29(2):46-59, 2009.

CR 11. Russell T, Logsdon A: Pressure ulcers and lateral rotation beds: a case study, *J Wound Ostomy Continence Nurs* 30(3):143-145, 2003.

12. Thompson P, Anderson J, Langeo D, et al: Support surfaces: definitions and utilization for patient care, *Adv Skin Wound Care* 21(6):264-266, 2008.

13. Turpin P, Pemberton V: Prevention of pressure ulcers in patients being managed on CLRT: is supplemental repositioning needed? *J Wound Ostomy Continence Nurs* 33(4):381-388, 2006.

CR 14. Washington GT, Macness CL: Evaluation of outcomes: the effects of continuous lateral rotation therapy, *J Nurse Care Qual* 20(3):273-282, 2005.

Additional Readings

Anderson J, Hanson D, Langeo D, et al: The evolution of support surfaces, *Adv Skin Wound Care* 19(3):130-132, 2006.

CR Agency for Health Care Policy and Research (AHCPR): *Pressure ulcers in adults: prediction and prevention,* AHCPR Publication 92-0047, Rockville, MD, 1992, US Department of Health and Human Services.

CR Agency for Health Care Policy and Research (AHCPR): *Treatment of pressure ulcers*, AHCPR Publication 95-0652, Rockville, MD, 1994, US Department of Health and Human Services.

National Pressure Ulcer Advisory Panel: www.npuap.org. Accessed September 2, 2009.

AP Wound Closure

P U R P O S E :   Wound closure is the process of holding body tissues together to promote wound healing. It is used to achieve hemostasis, approximate tissues separated by surgery or trauma, expedite healing with minimal scarring and without infection, provide strength until the natural tensile strength of the healing wound is sufficient to maintain closure, and maintain appropriate positioning of tubes or drains.

Tracey Anderson*

PREREQUISITE NURSING KNOWLEDGE

* The skin is the largest organ of the body and has two major tissue layers. The outermost layer, the epidermis, is made of stratified, squamous cells with keratin and melanin. This layer protects against environmental exposure, restricts water loss, and gives color. The inner layer, the dermis, is made of fibroelastic connective tissue with capillaries, lymphatics, and nerve endings and provides nourishment and strength. The layer beneath the dermis is the subcutaneous tissue, composed of areolar and fatty connective tissue to provide insulation, shock absorption, and calorie reserve.
* The natural components of wound healing include three overlapping phases of healing: inflammation, proliferation, and maturation.
  * *Inflammation:* Wound extends through the epidermis, disrupts blood vessels, and exposes collagen, activating the clotting cascade and inflammatory response. Vascular and cellular responses are designed to protect the body against foreign substances and limit blood loss via vasoconstriction and development of a clot providing hemostasis. The inflammatory response activates macrophages and clears the wound of cellular debris. Hemostasis with fibrin formation creates a protective wound scab. Kinins and prostaglandins produce local vasodilation and increase permeability of the vasculature, thereby promoting development of inflammatory exudate. Inflammation brings chemical stimuli for wound repair. Wounds left open for 3 hours show a dramatic increase in vascular permeability, which results in thick inflammatory exudate and may limit the therapeutic value of antibiotics.[5,21]
  * *Proliferation and epithelialization:* This phase of wound healing is characterized by generation of new tissue, angiogenesis, and collagen formation. After an incision, the divided parts of the epithelium are closed by cellular migration and mitosis, forming an epithelial bridge that protects the wound against bacteria. When the skin edges are slightly everted with suturing, epithelial bridging occurs within 18 to 24 hours. Wounds that have approximated skin edges may take 36 hours to epithelialize. If the edges are inverted, it may take up to 72 hours to completely epithelialize.[5]
  * Maturation is the remodeling phase of wound tissues during which collagen is reorganized to increase strength of the new tissue.
* Wound healing occurs via primary or secondary intention.
* Primary intention is used with limited tissue loss; the wound is clean, and the wound edges can be approximated and closed, frequently with sutures or staples.

AP   This procedure should be performed only by physicians, advanced practice nurses, and other healthcare professionals (including critical care nurses) with additional knowledge, skills, and demonstrated competence per professional licensure or institutional standard.

*Tracey Anderson would like to acknowledge the significant work done by the original chapter author, Peggy Kirkwood.

- Secondary intention is used when either a large amount of tissue has been lost or the wound is contaminated.[21] Wound dressing techniques are used to clean the wound and encourage development of granulation tissue and reepithelialization for wound closure.
- The goals of primary wound closure are to stop bleeding, prevent infection, preserve function, and restore appearance.
- Principles of proper wound closure include the following:
  - ❖ Elimination of dead space where serum and blood can accumulate, thus decreasing the risk for infection
  - ❖ Accurate approximation of deep tissue layers to each other with minimal tension on the surrounding tissues
  - ❖ Avoidance of tissue ischemia and strangulation from tying sutures too tightly
  - ❖ Decreased risk for infection by closing clean wounds within 3 to 8 hours of injury and using aseptic technique in all aspects of wound management
- Risk factors for surgical site infections include intrinsic factors (such as age, active skin condition, smoking status, body mass index, and comorbidities) and extrinsic factors (e.g., preoperative, perioperative, and postoperative patient care practices, such as preoperative skin preparation and postoperative dressings).[14] Risk factors for infection in a traumatic laceration include extremes of age, history of diabetes mellitus, chronic renal failure, jagged wound edges, stellate shape, visible contamination, injury deeper than the subcutaneous tissue, and presence of a foreign body.[10,15,18]
- Hair removal around suture site is not necessary before suturing unless the hair interferes with the procedure. Removal of hair has been associated with higher risk of infection. If hair must be removed, an electric clipper is preferred. A razor can cause abrasions and microscopic skin nicks that may increase the risk of infection.[6,14,16,19]
- Depending on the clinical setting, referral to an appropriate specialist (e.g., vascular, orthopedic, plastic, or general surgeon) may be warranted for wounds with damage to the blood supply, nerves, or joint; wounds on the face; or wounds with extensive tissue damage or infection.
- Wounds contaminated or infected with saliva, feces, or purulent exudate or that have been open longer than 8 hours may benefit from delayed closure on or after the fourth day to decrease the risk for infection.
- Wounds may be closed with several techniques: sutures, staples, adhesive skin strips (i.e., Steri-Strips, or skin adhesives.
  - ❖ Staples provide the strongest closure, skin adhesives and sutures are next strongest, and adhesive skin strips are the weakest.[1]
  - ❖ Stapling is faster, less expensive, and more cosmetically acceptable than suturing in the repair of many types of traumatic lacerations. Staples are useful for lacerations to the scalp, trunk, and extremities. They are slightly more painful to remove.
  - ❖ Adhesive skin strips (i.e., Steri-Strips) and skin adhesives are found to be equal in cosmetic outcomes and acceptability.[12,15] They are best used on wounds that are not under tension.

- Skin adhesives such as 2-octyl cyanoacrylate (Dermabond, Ethicon, Inc.) have been shown to be equivalent to sutures in repair of simple, clean wounds on children. Adhesives should not be used over joints; on hands, feet, lips, or mucosa; on infected, puncture, or stellate wounds; or in patients with poor circulation or a propensity to form keloids.[6] They are best suited for short (less than 6 to 8 cm), low-tension, clean-edged, straight to curvilinear wounds that do not cross joints or creases.[2,7,8]
- When considering suturing:
  - ❖ Curved needles are either tapered or cutting. Needles used for skin closure have an angle of 135 degrees.
  - ❖ Tapered needles are used in soft tissues (intestine, blood vessels, muscle, and fascia) and produce minimal tissue damage.
  - ❖ Cutting needles are used to approximate tougher tissue, such as skin. Reverse cutting needles have a cutting edge on the outside of the curve and provide a wall of tissue, rather than an incision, for the suture to rest against. This method resists suture cut-through and is therefore preferred.
  - ❖ Most needles are swaged, or molded, around the suture, providing convenience, safety, and speed in suture placement.
  - ❖ Needles should be handled only with needle holders to prevent needle damage to surrounding tissue and injury to the user.
  - ❖ Suture material is characterized by tissue reactivity, flexibility, knot-holding ability, wick action, and tensile strength. Suture size is indicated by "0." The higher the number that precedes "0," the smaller the suture (e.g., 4-0 is smaller than 3-0).
  - ❖ Sutures are absorbable or nonabsorbable, braided, or monofilament.
    - ○ Absorbable suture (i.e., natural gut, synthetic polymers) is used for layered closures. Gut suture is broken down via phagocytosis and induces a moderate inflammatory reaction. Chromic gut suture has increased strength and lasts longer in tissue, but it is not used on the skin because it can cause a severe tissue reaction. Synthetic absorbable sutures are favored over gut because of decreased infection rates and increased strength and longevity.[3]
    - ○ Nonabsorbable sutures are either natural fibers (i.e., silk, cotton, linen) or synthetic (i.e., nylon, Dacron, polyethylene) and are best for superficial lacerations because they are supple and easily handled and facilitate knot construction.
    - ○ Braided sutures are stronger, but the small spaces between the braids may harbor infection.
    - ○ Monofilament is best suited for skin closure because it produces less inflammatory response; however, the knots are less dependable.
    - ○ Nonabsorbable synthetic monofilament sutures (i.e., 4-0 or 5-0 nylon) are preferred for skin closure. Synthetic braided absorbable sutures provide the best closure for interrupted dermal sutures and ligation of bleeding vessels.

- ❖ Preferred knotting technique involves a square knot or double loop followed by a square knot tie.
- ❖ Injured tissue becomes edematous, and the suture tightens automatically within 12 to 24 hours; therefore, the practitioner must avoid tying the suture too tightly, which could produce tissue necrosis.
- ❖ The number of sutures required is the minimum needed to hold the wound edges exactly opposed without crimping. Tension should be minimized but not eliminated on the wound edges. The more tension on a wound, the closer the sutures should be placed.
- ❖ Lacerations are approximated with a variety of suturing techniques[5]:
  - ○ Simple interrupted dermal suture (Fig. 124-1) is used when the skin margins are level or slightly everted. The needle should enter and exit the skin surface at a right angle. The stitch should be as wide as the suture is deep and no closer than 2 mm apart. The knot should be tied with an instrument tie and repeated four or five times. The first suture is placed in the midportion of the wound. Additional sutures are placed in bisected portions of the wound until it is appropriately closed.
- • Subcutaneous suture with inverted knot or buried stitch (Fig. 124-2) is used for deeper wounds or wounds under tension. Absorbable sutures are used with the knot inverted below the skin margin. Begin at the bottom of the wound, come up and go straight across the incision to the base again, and tie. Deep, buried subcutaneous sutures are used to reduce the tension on skin sutures, close dead space beneath a wound, and allow for early suture removal.[9,13]
- • Vertical mattress suture (Fig. 124-3) promotes eversion of the skin, which promotes less prominent scarring.[13]

Mattress sutures are used when skin tension is present or where the skin is very thick (palms and soles of feet). This suture is identical to a simple suture, but an additional suture is taken very close to the edge of each side of the wound.

- • Three-point or half-buried mattress suture (Fig. 124-4) is used to close an acute corner of a laceration without impairing blood flow to the tip. The needle is inserted into the skin on the nonflap portion of the wound, passed transversely through the tip, and returned on the opposite side of the wound, paralleling the point of entrance. The suture is then tied, drawing the tip snugly in place.[9,13]
- • Subcuticular running suture (Fig. 124-5) is used for linear wounds under little or no tension and allows for edema formation. Wound approximation may not be as meticulous as with an interrupted dermal suture. An anchor suture is placed at one end of the wound, then continuous sutures are placed at right angles to the wound less than 3 mm apart. The wound is pulled together and the other end secured with either another square knot or tape under slight tension.
- ❖ Sutures must be completely removed in a timely fashion to avoid further tissue inflammation and possible infection. Sutures on extremities and the trunk should be removed in 8 to 14 days; those on the face should be removed in 3 to 5 days; and those on the palms, soles, back, and skin over mobile joints should be removed in 10 to 14 days.[5,17]

EQUIPMENT

- • Local anesthetic (with or without epinephrine)
- • Chlorhexidine solution[3] and sterile normal saline (NS) solution

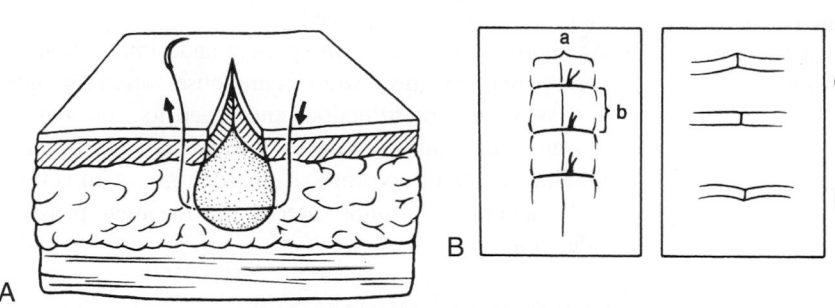

FIGURE 124-1 Interrupted dermal suture. **A,** Proper depth. **B,** Proper spacing (a=b). **C,** Proper final appearance. **D,** Improper final appearance. *(From Pfenninger JL, Fowler GC, editors: Pfenninger and Fowler's procedures for primary care, ed 2, St Louis, 2006, Mosby.)*

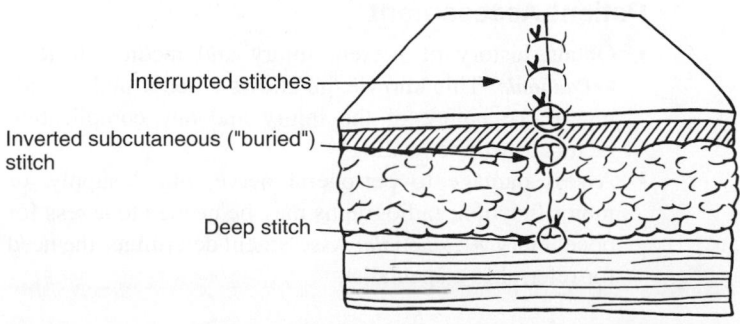

Interrupted stitches

Inverted subcutaneous ("buried") stitch

Deep stitch

FIGURE 124-2. Inverted subcutaneous suture. Also shown is layered closure. *(From Pfenninger JL, Fowler GC, editors: Pfenninger and Fowler's procedures for primary care, ed 2, St Louis, 2006, Mosby.)*

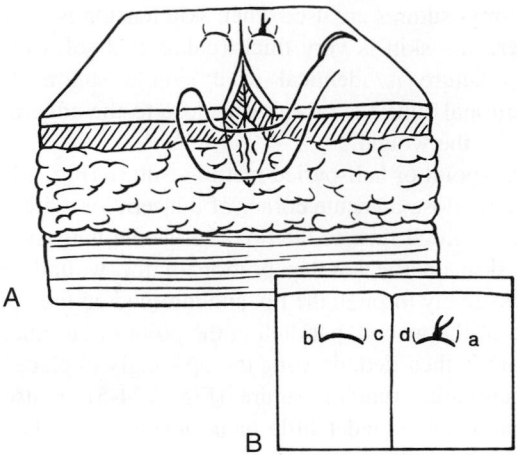

FIGURE 124-3 Vertical mattress suture. **A,** Cross section. **B,** Overhead view. Begin at *a,* and go under skin to *b.* Come out, go in at *c,* and exit at *d. (From Pfenninger JL, Fowler GC, editors: Pfenninger and Fowler's procedures for primary care, ed 2, St Louis, 2006, Mosby.)*

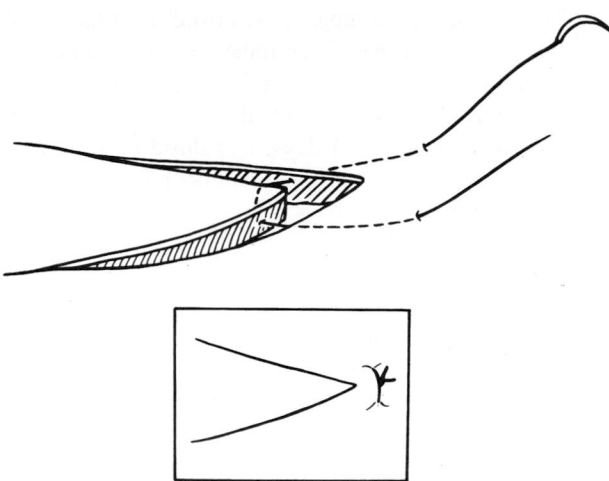

FIGURE 124-4 Three-point or half-buried mattress. *(From Pfenninger JL, Fowler GC, editors: Pfenninger and Fowler's procedures for primary care, ed 2, St Louis, 2006, Mosby.)*

- 8 to 10 4 × 4 gauze sponges
- Sterile metal prep basin
- 30- or 60-mL syringe and 18-gauge needle
- Sterile drape
- Fenestrated drape
- Sterile gloves, mask, eye protection
- Electric clippers (only if hair removal necessary)
- For suturing:
  - ❖ 6-inch needle holder
  - ❖ Suture material and needle
  - ❖ Curved dissecting scissors
  - ❖ Two mosquito hemostats: one curved, one straight
  - ❖ Suture scissors
  - ❖ Tissue forceps
  - ❖ Scalpel handle and no. 15 knife blade
  - ❖ Skin hooks (for atraumatic tissue handling)

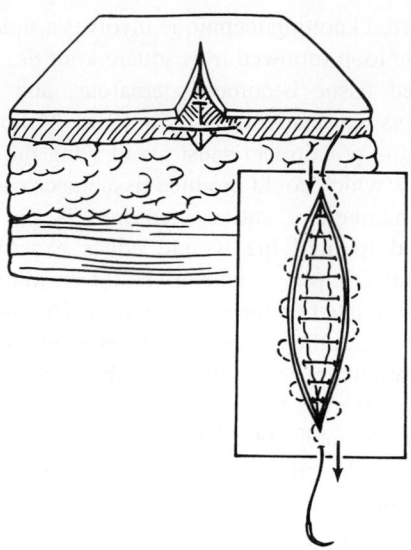

FIGURE 124-5 Subcuticular running suture. *(From Pfenninger JL, Fowler GC, editors: Pfenninger and Fowler's procedures for primary care, ed 2, St Louis, 2006, Mosby.)*

- For other wound closures:
  - ❖ Staple gun
  - ❖ Steri-Strips
  - ❖ Skin adhesive
- *Note:* Some hospitals use prepackaged suture kits; thus, it may be unnecessary to assemble all of the items listed here if such a kit is available.

PATIENT AND FAMILY EDUCATION

- Explain the procedure and risks and reassure the patient and family. ➡️*Rationale:* Explanation decreases patient anxiety and encourages patient and family cooperation and understanding of procedure.
- As appropriate, instruct the patient and family on aftercare: pain medication, wound care, observation for signs and symptoms of infection, and when to have wound closure material removed. ➡️*Rationale:* Instruction facilitates patient comfort, decreases risk for infection, and encourages prompt intervention to treat possible infection.

PATIENT ASSESSMENT AND PREPARATION
Patient Assessment

- Obtain history of present injury and medical history. ➡️*Rationale:* This knowledge allows a better understanding of the nature of the injury and any complicating factors to wound healing.
- Assess damage to peripheral nerve, blood supply, or motor function; radiographs may be needed to assess for bone injury. ➡️*Rationale:* Assessment determines the need for referral to a specialist.

Patient Preparation

- Ensure that patient understands preprocedural teachings and obtain consent. Answer questions as they arise, and reinforce information as needed. ➤➤*Rationale:* Suturing is an invasive procedure, so consent should be obtained before the procedure is started. Understanding of previously taught information is evaluated and reinforced.

- Administer pain medication as necessary. Consider moderate procedural sedation for laceration repair in children.[15] Consider use of LET (lidocaine, 4%; epinephrine, 0.1%; and tetracaine, 0.5%) topically for children. ➤➤*Rationale:* Pain medication reduces activity significantly during suturing to provide a stable field.
- Administer tetanus prophylaxis, if necessary (Table 124-1). ➤➤*Rationale:* Possibility of tetanus from unclean wound is prevented.

TABLE 124-1	**Guide to Tetanus Prophylaxis in Wound Management**			
History of Adsorbed Tetanus Toxoid (doses)	Clean Minor Wounds Tdap or Td[†]	Clean Minor Wounds TIG[‡]	All Other Wounds* Tdap or Td[†]	All Other Wounds* TIG[‡]
Less than 3 or unknown	Yes	No	Yes	Yes
3 or more doses[§]	No[¶]	No	No[**]	No

*Such as (but not limited to) wounds contaminated with dirt, feces, soil, and saliva; puncture wounds; avulsions; and wounds resulting from missiles, crushing, burns, and frostbite.

†For children younger than 7 years of age, DTaP is recommended; if pertussis vaccine is contraindicated, DT is given. For persons 7 to 9 years of age or 65 years or older, Td is recommended. For persons 10 to 64 years, Tdap is preferred to Td if the patient has never received Tdap and has no contraindication to pertussis vaccine. For persons 7 years of age or older, if Tdap is not available or not indicated because of age, Td is preferred to TT.

‡*TIG,* Human tetanus immune globulin. Equine tetanus antitoxin should be used when TIG is not available.

§If only three doses of fluid toxoid have been received, a fourth dose of toxoid, preferably an adsorbed toxoid, should be given. Although licensed, fluid tetanus toxoid is rarely used.

¶Yes, if it has been 10 years or longer since the last dose.

**Yes, if it has been 5 years or longer since the last dose. More frequent boosters are not needed and can accentuate side effects.

The appropriate use of tetanus toxoid and TIG in wound management is also important for the prevention of tetanus.

(Manual for the surveillance of vaccine-preventable diseases, ed 4, 2008, available at www.cdc.gov/vaccines/pubs/surv-manual/chpt16-tetanus.htm#9.)

Procedure	**for Wound Closure**	
Steps	**Rationale**	**Special Considerations**
1. **VP**		
2. Obtain consent.	Suturing is an invasive procedure; informed consent should be obtained before wound closure procedures.	
3. **HH**		
4. **PE**		
5. Anesthetize the wound. May proceed with infiltration with LET applied topically. Use local anesthetic with or without epinephrine and a 27- to 30-gauge needle to infiltrate the area.[1,18,20] **(Level C*)**	Provides for maximal patient comfort and cooperation during suturing.	Immobilization of site also aids in decreasing pain.
6. Examine wound thoroughly for foreign bodies, deep tissue layer damage, joint involvement, and injury to nerve, vessel, or tendon.	Prevents further damage. Assess need for referral.	Use aseptic technique to decrease contamination of wound. Radiographic imaging may be necessary to rule out retained foreign body before wound closure.

*Level C: Qualitative studies, descriptive or correlational studies, integrative reviews, systematic reviews, or randomized controlled trials with inconsistent results

Procedure continues on following page

Procedure for Wound Closure—*Continued*

Steps	Rationale	Special Considerations
7. Clean the wound.	Removes foreign substances and bacteria and reduces risk for infection.	
A. Mechanical: Wiping, brushing, and irrigating with copious amounts of high-pressure saline solution with a 30- or 60-mL syringe with 18-gauge needle.		Mechanical cleaning is important for prevention of infection. Wound must be properly cleaned and irrigated with high pressure. Care must be taken to avoid damage to the tissues.
B. Chemical: Antiseptic solution. Apply in concentric circles, moving toward the periphery.[14] **(Level A*)**	Chlorhexidine reduces bacterial colony counts.[3,14]	Use a cleansing solution that is nontoxic to tissues.
C. Only if necessary, remove any hair in the area with an electric clipper.[14,16] **(Level A)**	Do not remove hair at or around the suture site unless it interferes with the procedure.[4,6] Electric clippers (rather than razors) have been associated with significantly fewer infections.[4,6]	Consider use of hair apposition technique with longer hair to avoid shaving and promote wound closure without suturing.[11]
8. Remove nonsterile gloves, wash hands, and apply sterile gloves.		
9. Apply sterile drapes over and under the area as necessary.	Creates a sterile field. Reduces risk for infection.	
10. Examine the wound again for devitalized tissue that needs removal or débridement (see Procedure 127). Use a scalpel or sharp tissue scissors, if necessary.	Débridement may convert a jagged, contaminated wound into a clean surgical one and allow better approximation of tissues.	Débridement should be conservative and limited to removal of devitalized tissue that could act as a medium promoting bacterial growth.
11. If needed, loosen the wound from the subcutaneous tissue beneath the dermis with scissors or scalpel. *Note:* For wound closure methods other than suturing, **skip to Step 23.**	Allows the skin to glide together easily and aids approximation of skin edges.	
12. Select the appropriate needle and suture material according to type of wound.	Provides maximal support with the least amount of further tissue trauma.	
13. Arm the needle between the jaws of the needle holder (Fig. 124-6).	Prevents needle bending and provides for guided insertion.	The needle holder should be perpendicular to the needle and should grasp the needle 3 mm beyond the swaghole. The handle of the needle holder should be closed to first or second ratchet.
14. Grasp the needle holder (Fig. 124-7).	Correct grasp ensures smooth entry of needle and proper stitch placement with minimal manipulation.	
15. Position the free end of the suture away from operator.	Allows optimal visualization of the free end of the suture and ensures that it does not become entangled during knot construction.	
16. Pass the needle through the tissue until the needle point is visualized.		Hand should start prone; supination of the wrist passes needle in a direction toward person suturing and in the direction of the curvature of the needle.

*Level A: Meta-analysis of quantitative studies or metasynthesis of qualitative studies with results that consistently support a specific action, intervention, or treatment

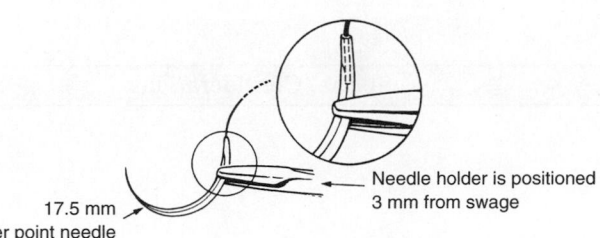

17.5 mm
Taper point needle

Needle holder is positioned
3 mm from swage

FIGURE 124-6 Because the laser-drilled hole is 15 mm long, this needle can be grasped by the needle holder 3 mm from the swage *(insert)*. Needle holder grasps the needle 3 mm from its swage. *(Copyright © 1996, 2010, Covidien. All rights reserved. Used with permission of Covidien.)*

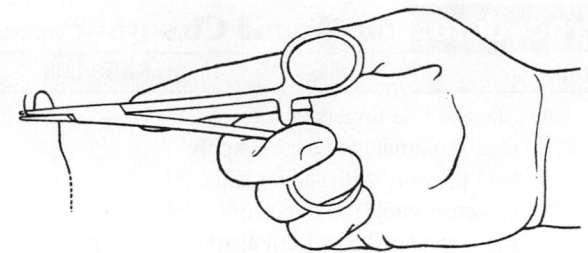

FIGURE 124-7 Thumb-ring finger grip of needle holder. *(Copyright © 1996, 2010, Covidien. All rights reserved. Used with permission of Covidien.)*

Procedure for Wound Closure—*Continued*

Steps	Rationale	Special Considerations
17. With use of tissue forceps to grasp the needle point, unclamp the needle holder jaws.	Stabilizes the needle to maintain its position in the tissue.	
18. Regrasp the needle between the needle holder jaws and pull the desired length of suture through the wound.	Prepares for tying knot.	Keep wrist in prone position.
19. Tie the suture knot. Edges should be slightly everted.		Secure the precise approximation of the wound edges without strangulating the tissue. The suture should be tied snugly, but gently.
A. Form suture loop: Wrap fixed suture end over and around needle holder twice.	Double wrap provides increased strength.	Keep length of free suture end less than 2 cm.
B. Pass free end of suture through the loop to create a throw.		Has a figure-8 shape.
C. Advance the throw to the wound surface by applying tension perpendicular to the wound.		
D. Repeat four or five times.		With each throw, your hands must reverse positions and apply equal and opposing tension to the suture ends in the same plane.
20. Cut suture by holding scissors blades perpendicular to the suture and keeping knot in view between the blades, allowing 3-mm tails to remain.	All knots slip to some degree. The ears of the knot must compensate for enlarged suture loop and prevent the knot from untying.	
21. Reposition knot away from wound edges.	Facilitates suture line care.	
22. **Repeat Steps 12 to 20** until wound is appropriately closed. Dress wound appropriately. **Go to Step 25.**		
23. Other wound closure techniques: Select wound closure technique to be used.		

Procedure continues on following page

Procedure for Wound Closure—*Continued*

Steps	Rationale	Special Considerations
A. Staples: Use fingers or forceps to approximate the edges. Apply firm pressure with stapler and dispense staples as directed. Place staples 0.5 to 1 cm apart. An assistant can help evert the wound edges while the primary operator uses the stapler.		
B. Adhesive skin strips (i.e., Steri-Strips): Ensure that skin is not oily or hairy and wound has minimal drainage. The strips should overlap the wound about 2 to 3 cm on each side of the wound. Start at the midpoint of the wound to approximate the sides and work out to the ends of the wound. Strips should be placed about 2 to 3 cm apart. Additional strips can be placed over the cross tapes to prevent the ends from coming loose.[1]	Skin that is not oily or hairy enhances proper adherence of Steri-Strips to skin.	Should not be used for large wounds or on patients who may remove them (confused, uncooperative, very young patients). Skin adherent (i.e., tincture of benzoin or Mastisol liquid adhesive) may be applied to the area to increase adhesion of skin strips.
C. Skin adhesive: Apply to dry, well-opposed wound edges. Use fingers or forceps to approximate wound edges. Open the product, saturate the porous applicator tip, and paint the edges of the wound with short brush strokes in a multilayering process. Allow 15 seconds between layers. Usually four layers are applied. Hold edges together for 30 to 60 seconds.		Obtaining an even, controlled flow of adhesive is critical to minimize drips and prevent complications. Do not place adhesive in the wound. It is ineffective and impairs healing and increases potential for foreign-body reaction.
24. Staples and adhesive skin strips (Steri-Strips): Cover wound with nonadherent dressing for the first 24 to 48 hours. Depending on institutional protocol, topical triple antibiotic ointment may be added before dressing application. Staples are removed with sterile technique and appropriate device.[5] **(Level C*)** Skin adhesive: Dressing is unnecessary, but a dry gauze pad may be used. Do not use ointments, creams, or tape strips. Do not soak, scrub, or expose to prolonged wetness. Patient may shower or gently bathe.[1] **(Level A*)**	Protects the wound from further injury; prevents microorganisms from colonizing[2]; minimizes bleeding, edema, and potential dead space; provides physiologic environment that is conducive to epithelial migration and scab formation; takes tension off the wound edges; cushions the wound from extraneous trauma; restricts motion, which decreases lymphatic flow and minimizes the spread of wound microflora.[5]	For continued oozing, apply a pressure dressing.
25. Dispose of equipment in appropriate receptacle.	Standard Precautions.	
26. **HH**		

*Level A: Meta-analysis of quantitative studies or metasynthesis of qualitative studies with results that consistently support a specific action, intervention, or treatment
*Level C: Qualitative studies, descriptive or correlational studies, integrative reviews, systematic reviews, or randomized controlled trials with inconsistent results

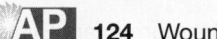

Expected Outcomes

- Bleeding is stopped
- Wound remains infection free
- Function is preserved
- Appearance is restored

Unexpected Outcomes

- Continued bleeding from the wound site or hematoma
- Wound infection and possible sepsis
- Skin necrosis
- Loss of function
- Abnormal appearance
- Wound dehiscence

Patient Monitoring and Care

Steps	Rationale	Reportable Conditions
		These conditions should be reported if they persist despite nursing interventions.
1. Monitor for evidence of infection.	Allows for early treatment and prevents systemic infection.	• Wound that is red, swollen, tender, or warm • Wound that drains or festers • Red streaks around the wound • Tender lumps in the groin or under the arm • Chills or fever

2. Administer prophylactic antibiotics if:
  A. Contamination of trauma site is suspected.
  B. Animal or human bite wounds exist.
  C. Preexisting medical conditions subject the patient to increased risk for infection (e.g., valvular heart disease, diabetes).
	Prevents wound infection.	

3. Follow institution standard for assessing pain. Administer analgesia as prescribed (agent and dose is determined by the extent of the trauma, the pain threshold of the patient, and the concerns of the patient and family).	Identifies need for pain interventions.	• Continued pain despite pain interventions
4. Splint wounds under considerable tension, as needed.	Decreases lymphatic flow, thereby decreasing the spread of wound bacteria. Provides support and limitation of movement to allow for proper wound healing and patient comfort.	
5. Keep wound and dressing clean and dry. If dressing gets wet, use sterile technique to remove it, blot dry with gauze pad, and reapply a clean, dry dressing.[14]	Decreases opportunity for infection from wicking action of a wet dressing.	
6. Keep dressed for 24 to 48 hours. If needed, clean with nontoxic cleaning solution, blot dry, apply triple antibiotic ointment, and reapply a sterile, nonadherent dressing.[5] **(Level B*)**	Decreases risk for wound contamination and infection. Beyond 48 hours, whether an incision must be covered by a dressing or whether showering or bathing is detrimental to healing is unclear.[14]	

*Level B: Well-designed controlled studies with results that consistently support a specific action, intervention, or treatment

Procedure continues on following page

Patient Monitoring and Care —*Continued*

Steps	Rationale	Reportable Conditions

7. Remove sutures or staples[5,17] (see Procedure 125)
  A. Facial wounds: 3 to 5 days
  B. Scalp and extremity wounds: 7 to 14 days
  C. Palms, soles, back, and skin over mobile joints: 10 to 14 days
	Prevents infection, enhances proper healing, and facilitates desirable cosmetic effects.	

8. Provide detailed patient and family education, including wound care, medications, signs and symptoms of infection, and follow-up appointments.	Facilitates patient and family cooperation.	

Documentation

Documentation should include the following:
- Patient and family education
- Location and appearance of wound
- Time since injury
- Procedure used to clean wound
- Procedure and technique used to close wound
- How patient tolerated the procedure

- Care of wound after closure
- Instructions given to patient and family
- Pain assessment and medication given
- Antibiotics given
- Tetanus status, if given
- Unexpected outcomes
- Nursing interventions

References

CR 1. Autio L, Olson KK: The four S's of wound management: staples, sutures, Steri-Strips, and sticky stuff, *Holist Nurs Pract* 16:80-88, 2002.

2. Beam JW: Tissue adhesives for simple traumatic lacerations, *J Athletic Training* 43(2):222-224, 2008.

CR 3. Chaiyakunapruk N, et al: Chlorhexidine compared with povidone-iodine solution for vascular catheter-site care: a meta-analysis, *Ann Intern Med* 136:792-801, 2002.

4. Cole E: Wound closure using adhesive strips, *Nurs Stand* 22:9:48-49, 2007.

CR 5. Edlich RF, Woods JA, Drake DB: *Scientific basis of wound closure techniques*, Norwalk, CT, 1996, Auto Suture Company.

CR 6. Edlich RF, et al: A scientific basis for choosing the technique of hair removal used prior to wound closure, *J Emerg Nurs* 26:134-139, 2000.

CR 7. Farion KJ, et al: Tissue adhesives for traumatic lacerations: a systematic review of randomized controlled trials, *Acad Emerg Med* 10:110-118, 2003.

CR 8. Farion KJ, Russell KF, Osmond MH, et al: Tissue adhesives for traumatic lacerations in children and adults, *Cochrane Database Syst Rev* 4:CD003326, DOI: 10.1002/14651858, CD003326, 2004.

CR 9. Hanasono MM, Hotchkiss RN: Locking horizontal mattress suture, *Dermatol Surg* 31:572-573, 2005.

10. Henry FP, Purcell EM, Eadie PA: The human bite injury: a clinical audit and discussion regarding the management of this alcohol fuelled phenomenon, *Emerg Med J* 23;455-458, 2007.

CR 11. Hock MO, et al: A randomized controlled trial comparing the hair apposition technique with tissue glue to standard suturing in scalp lacerations (HAT study), *Ann Emerg Med* 40:19-26, 2002.

CR 12. Khachemoune A, et al: Dehisced clean wound: resuture it or steri-strip it? *Dermatol Surg* 30:431-432, 2004.

CR 13. Krunic AL Weitzul S, Taylor RS: Running combined simple and vertical mattress suture: a rapid skin-everting stitch, *Dermatol Surg* 31:1325-1329, 2005.

CR 14. Mangram AJ, et al: Guideline for prevention of surgical site infection, 1999, *Infect Control Hosp Epidemiol* 20:247-278, 1999.

15. Moreira ME, Markovchick VJ: Wound management, *Emerg Med Clin North Am* 25:873-899, 2007.

CR 16. Moureau NL: Is your skin prep technique up-to-date? *Nursing* 33(11):17, 2003.

CR 17. Reilly J: Evidence-based surgical wound care on surgical wound infection, *Br J Nurs* 11(16 Suppl):S4,S6,S8,S10,S12, 2002.

18. Singer AJ, Dagum AB: Current management of acute cutaneous wounds, *N Engl J Med* 359:1037-1046, 2008.

19. Tanner J, Woodings D, Moncaster K: Preoperative hair removal to reduce surgical site infection, *Cochrane Database Syst Rev* 3:CD004122, DOI: 10.1002/1465185858, CD004122.pub3, 2006.

20. Waterbrook AL, Germann CA, Southall JC: Is epinephrine harmful when used with anesthetics for digital nerve blocks? *Ann Emerg Med* 50:472-475, 2007.
21. Zehtabchi S: The role of antibiotic prophylaxis for prevention of infection in patients with simple hand lacerations, *Ann Emerg Med* 49(5):682-689, 2007.

Additional Readings

Broughton G, Janis JE, Attinger CE: Wound healing: an overview, *Plast Reconstruct Surg* 117;7S:1eS-32eS, 2006.
Snell G: Laceration repair. In Pfenninger JL, Fowler GC, editors: *Pfenninger and Fowler's procedures for primary care*, ed 2, St Louis, 2006, Mosby, 12-19.

Suture and Staple Removal

P U R P O S E :   Sutures and staples are placed to approximate tissues that have been separated. When wound healing is sufficient to maintain closure, sutures and staples are removed.

Tracey Anderson

PREREQUISITE NURSING KNOWLEDGE

- Wound healing is a nonspecific response to injury. It involves the biologic processes of inflammation, collagen metabolism, and contraction in an overlapping, integrated continuum. Wound healing is divided into three phases: inflammatory, fibroblastic, and remodeling. The condition of the tissues and the mechanism of wound closure determine the relative duration of these phases and the end result of the healing process.
- Sutures and staples must be completely removed to avoid further tissue inflammation and possible infection.
- Timing of suture and staple removal depends on the following (Table 125-1):
  - ❖ Shape, size, and location of the incision
  - ❖ Absence of inflammation, drainage, and infection
  - ❖ Patient's general condition
- Timing of suture removal may be prolonged in patients with the following risk factors:
  - ❖ Steroid use
  - ❖ Irradiation treatment
  - ❖ Cytotoxic agent use
  - ❖ Diabetes
  - ❖ Rheumatoid arthritis
  - ❖ Trace element imbalance
  - ❖ Advanced age

EQUIPMENT

- Sterile gloves and mask
- Sterile towel or drape
- Sterile swab with antiseptic cleaning solution according to facility's policy (typically chlorhexidine)
- 4 × 4 gauze pads
- Suture removal kit with scissors and forceps (if no kit available, obtain sterile scissor and forceps)

  or
- Staple remover
- Skin tape or adhesive skin strips (Steri-Strips) of appropriate width
- Skin adherent (recommended as it helps with adherence and protects periwound area)

PATIENT AND FAMILY EDUCATION

- Explain the procedure and risks to the patient and family. Reassure the patient that he or she may feel a tickling or pulling sensation as the sutures or staples are removed. Assure the patient that the wound is healing properly and that removal of the sutures or staples does weaken the incision. ➤➤*Rationale:* Explanation decreases patient anxiety and encourages patient and family cooperation and understanding of procedure.
- Instruct the patient and family on aftercare: pain medication, wound care, activity restrictions, and observation for signs and symptoms of infection. ➤➤*Rationale:* Education facilitates patient comfort, decreases risk for infection, and encourages prompt follow-up for treatment of possible infection.

TABLE 125-1	Timing of Suture Removal
Location of Sutures	**Days Before Removal**
Extremities, scalp, and trunk	7-14
Face	3-5
Palms, soles, back, and skin over mobile joints	10-14

PATIENT ASSESSMENT AND PREPARATION

Patient Assessment

- Obtain history of present injury and medical history. ➤*Rationale:* This knowledge allows a better understanding of the nature of the injury and any complicating factors to suture or staple removal.
- Assess patient allergies, especially to adhesive tape and povidone-iodine or other topical solutions or medications. ➤*Rationale:* Further tissue damage can be prevented.
- After determining when sutures or staples were placed, observe wound for signs of gaping, drainage, inflammation, signs of infection, or embedded sutures. ➤*Rationale:* Findings may delay suture or staple removal.

Patient Preparation

- Ensure that patient understands preprocedural teachings. Answer questions as they arise, and reinforce information as needed. ➤*Rationale:* Understanding of previously taught information is evaluated and reinforced.
- Administer pain medication as prescribed. ➤*Rationale:* Pain medication reduces activity during suture or staple removal to provide a stable field.
- Provide privacy and position the patient for comfort without undue tension on the suture line or staples. ➤*Rationale:* Provides patient comfort and promotes cooperation during procedure.
- Adjust the light to shine directly on the suture line or staples. ➤*Rationale:* Light is used to provide ease of removal and patient comfort.
- Prepare sterile field. ➤*Rationale:* Sterile field is used to prevent contamination.

Procedure | for Suture Removal

Steps	Rationale	Special Considerations
1. Check order to confirm exact timing and other relevant information.	Ensures appropriate treatment.	Physician or physician extender may want to leave some sutures in place for an additional day or two to support the suture line.
2. **HH**		
3. **PE**		
4. Apply sterile drapes or towels over or under the area as needed.		
5. Gently tug on the sutures to test the wound line before removal to be sure the wound does not separate. If any doubt exists to the integrity of the suture line, apply a skin adherent and adhesive skin strips between sutures before removing them.	Ensures that wound is healed sufficiently before removal of sutures.	If patient has both retention and regular sutures in place, retention sutures may remain in place for 14 to 21 days.
6. Clean the suture line with antiseptic skin cleanser. The wound is considered clean, so when cleaning it, wipe from clean to dirty, moving from the inner aspect to outer margins of the wound.	Decreases the number of microorganisms and reduces the risk for infection.	Be particularly careful to clean the suture line before removing mattress sutures, especially if the visible, contaminated part of the stitch is too small to cut twice for sterile removal. Carefully remove encrusted drainage to allow visualization of all sutures to be removed.
7. Use sterile technique to remove running suture (Fig. 125-1)[1]: A. Use sterile forceps to grasp the knot and gently raise off the skin. B. Use rounded tip of sterile suture scissors to cut suture at the skin edge on one side of the visible part.	Visible part of suture is exposed to skin bacteria and is considered contaminated.	For running sutures, each individual section needs to be cut to prevent contaminated suture material from being pulled through the subcutaneous tissue.

Procedure continues on following page

Procedure | for Suture Removal—*Continued*

Steps	Rationale	Special Considerations
C. Remove the suture by lifting the visible end off the skin to avoid drawing contaminated portion through subcutaneous tissue.	Prevents pulling it through and contaminating subcutaneous tissue.[2]	
8. To remove mattress sutures (Fig. 125-2)[2]:		
A. Remove the small visible portion of the suture opposite the knot by cutting it at each visible end and lifting the small piece away from the skin.		
B. Remove the rest of the suture by pulling it out in the direction of the knot.		
C. If the visible portion is too small to cut twice, cut once and pull the entire suture out in the opposite direction.		
9. If the wound dehisces, apply butterfly adhesive strips or paper tape to support and approximate the edges and call the physician or physician extender.		Wound dehiscence is the premature opening of a wound along a suture line.[2] Adhesive strips may be used to reapproximate the wound edges until complete wound closure occurs.
10. Wipe incision line gently with gauze sponges soaked in antiseptic skin cleanser or prepackaged swab.[1] (**Level E***)	Removes serous or bloody drainage from the suture line.	
11. Apply adhesive skin strips or paper tape and a light, sterile gauze dressing, if desired. Leave strips in place for 3 to 5 days or as ordered.	Holds incision edges together, decreases transmission of microorganisms, and decreases irritation from clothing.	
12. Dispose of gloves and equipment in appropriate receptacle.		
13. 🄷🄷		

*Level E: Multiple case reports, theory-based evidence from expert opinions, or peer-reviewed professional organizational standards without clinical studies to support recommendations

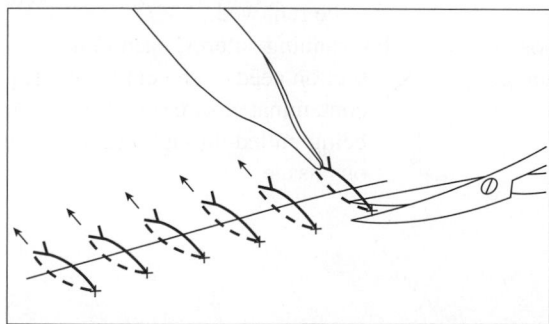

FIGURE 125-1 Removal of plain interrupted sutures with sterile forceps and scissors.

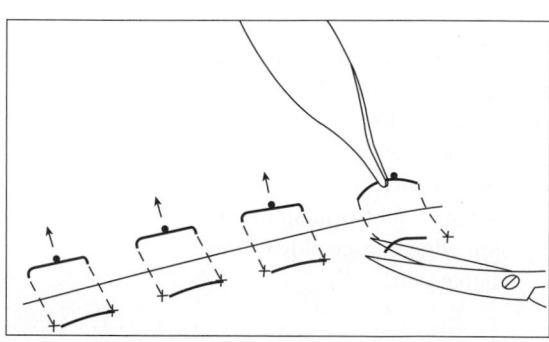

FIGURE 125-2 Removal of interrupted mattress sutures with sterile forceps and scissors.

Procedure | for Staple Removal

Steps	Rationale	Special Considerations
1. Check physician's order to confirm exact timing and other relevant information.	Ensures appropriate treatment.	Physician may want to leave some staples in place for an additional day or two to support the staple line.
2. **HH**		
3. **PE**		
4. Apply sterile drapes or towels over or under the area as needed.		
5. Gently test the wound line before removal of the staple to be sure the wound does not separate. If any doubt exists, apply a skin adherent and adhesive skin strips between staples before removing them.	Ensures that wound is healed sufficiently before removal of staples.	
6. Clean the staple line with antiseptic skin cleanser. The wound is considered clean, so when cleaning it, wipe from clean to dirty, moving from the inner aspect to outer margins of the wound.	Decreases the number of microorganisms and reduces the risk for infection.	Carefully remove encrusted drainage to allow visualization of all staples to be removed.

7. Use sterile technique to remove staples (Fig. 125-3).
  A. Gently place tip of staple remover under the staple at its center.
  B. Compress staple remover until staple bends in center and edges lift out of skin.
  C. Discard staple and proceed to next staple.		

8. If the wound dehisces, apply butterfly adhesive strips or paper tape to support and approximate the edges and call the physician.		
9. Wipe incision line gently with gauze sponges soaked in antiseptic skin cleanser or prepackaged swab.	Removes serous or bloody drainage from the staple line.	
10. Apply adhesive skin strips or paper tape and a light, sterile gauze dressing, if desired. Leave strips in place for 3 to 5 days or as ordered.	Holds incision edges together, decreases transmission of microorganisms, and decreases irritation from clothing.	
11. Dispose of gloves and equipment in appropriate receptacle.		
12. **HH**		

Procedure continues on following page

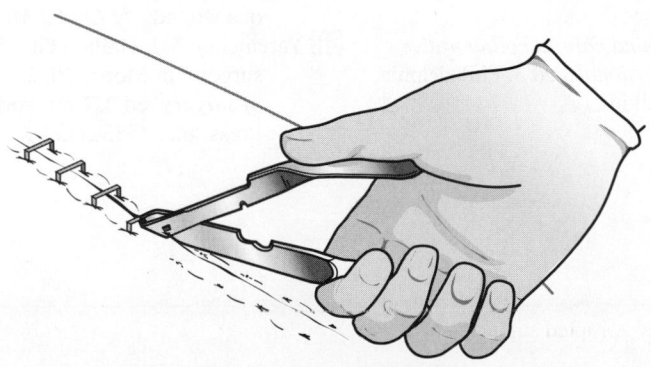

FIGURE 125-3 Staple removal.

Expected Outcomes

- Wound remains infection free
- Function is preserved
- Appearance is restored

Unexpected Outcomes

- Wound infection and possible sepsis
- Loss of function
- Abnormal appearance
- Wound dehiscence

Patient Monitoring and Care

Steps	Rationale	Reportable Conditions
		These conditions should be reported if they persist despite nursing interventions.
1. Retest range of motion and sensory perception after suture removal.	Ensures no further damage was imposed.	
2. Observe for wound discharge or other abnormal changes.	Allows for early treatment and prevents systemic infection.	• Wound that is red, swollen, tender, or warm • Wound that begins to drain or fester • Red streaks around the wound • Tender lumps in the groin or under the arm • Chills or fever • Redness that surrounds the incision and does not gradually disappear or show only a thin line after a few weeks[1]
3. Provide detailed patient and family education, including wound care, medications, signs and symptoms of infection, when the patient can get the incision wet, and follow-up instructions.	Facilitates patient and family cooperation.	
4. Follow institution standard for assessing pain. Administer analgesia as prescribed.	Identifies need for pain interventions.	• Continued pain despite pain interventions

Documentation

Documentation should include the following:
- Patient and family education and aftercare instructions
- Time since suturing
- Care of the wound after suture removal
- Location and appearance of wound
- Range of motion and sensory perception
- Pain assessment, interventions, and effectiveness

References

CR 1. Hrouda BS: How to remove surgical sutures and staples, *Nursing* 30:54-55, 2000.
2. Sussman C, Bates-Jensen B: *Wound care: a collaborative practice manual for health professionals*, ed 3, Philadelphia, 2006, Lippincott Williams & Wilkins.

Additional Readings

Singer AJ, Dagum AB: Current management of acute cutaneous wounds, *N Engl J Med* 359:1037-1046, 2008.
CR Yaremchuk MJ, Gallico GG: Principles and practice of plastic surgery. In Morris PJ, Wood WC, editors: *Oxford textbook of surgery*, ed 2, New York, 2000, Oxford University Press, Inc. 3533-3537.

Cleaning, Irrigating, Culturing, and Dressing an Open Wound

P U R P O S E :   Cleaning, irrigating, culturing, and dressing open wounds are performed to optimize healing. Wound culturing may be necessary to isolate and allow for treatment of organisms.

Marylou V. Robinson

PREREQUISITE NURSING KNOWLEDGE

- Goals of wound care must be clearly outlined so that proper wound care products are used.
- Wound care products should be matched to the patient and wound conditions. Although no specific dressing is considered superior to others,[9,13] properties of dressing products are different and should be assessed relative to wound treatment goals.[2,9]
  - ❖ Dressings may be categorized as semiocclusive or occlusive. Semiocclusive dressings are semipermeable to gases (O_2, CO_2, moisture) and are impermeable to liquids; they provide the moist wound healing environment that optimizes wound healing. Occlusive dressings lack permeability to gases and liquids.
  - ❖ Coarse gauze, used in a wet-to-dry dressing, nonselectively débrides the wound bed mechanically and absorbs wound fluid.
  - ❖ Dressings such as calcium alginates, foams, and hydrofibers enhance wound exudate absorption; hydrogels, hydrocolloids, and transparent films provide moisture to nondraining wounds with minimal absorption.
  - ❖ Wounds with excessive wound drainage also require protection of periwound skin (i.e., skin barrier wipes).
- Wounds heal by primary, secondary, or tertiary intention (Fig. 126-1).
  - ❖ Normal wound healing is often described as a progressive process that involves three overlapping phases: inflammation, proliferation, and maturation. The inflammatory phase is marked for hemostasis, increased vasodilation, and migration of neutrophils and macrophages to the area. The proliferation phase begins 2 to 4 days after injury and is the healing phase of the wound process in which epithelialization, angiogenesis, and collagen synthesis predominate.[8,9] The maturation phase involves the body remodeling collagen fiber and increasing tissue tensile strength.[8,9]
  - ❖ Most clean wounds heal by primary intention. Suturing each layer of tissue approximates the wound edges. These wounds typically heal quickly and require minimal wound care.
  - ❖ Open wounds heal by secondary intention by granulating from the base of the wound to the skin surfaces and contracting and epithelializing from the wound edges; care must be taken to allow for uniform granulation and prevention of open pockets or tunneling.
  - ❖ Tertiary intention involves a period of secondary healing to achieve edema reduction and decreased exudate production, followed by surgical closure for primary healing.
- Clean, moist wound beds allow for effective wound healing under the support of a dressing.
  - ❖ Openly granulating wounds heal more slowly, may result in drying of granulating tissue and tissue death, and may be more painful for the patient.
  - ❖ The presence of exudate is not synonymous with infection but is the natural result of the inflammatory response to maintain moisture and allow movement and replication of epithelial cells necessary for healing. A change in volume, color, or consistency of exudate may indicate impending infection.[2,4,12]

FIRST INTENTION (Primary union)   SECOND INTENTION (Granulation)   THIRD INTENTION (Secondary suture)

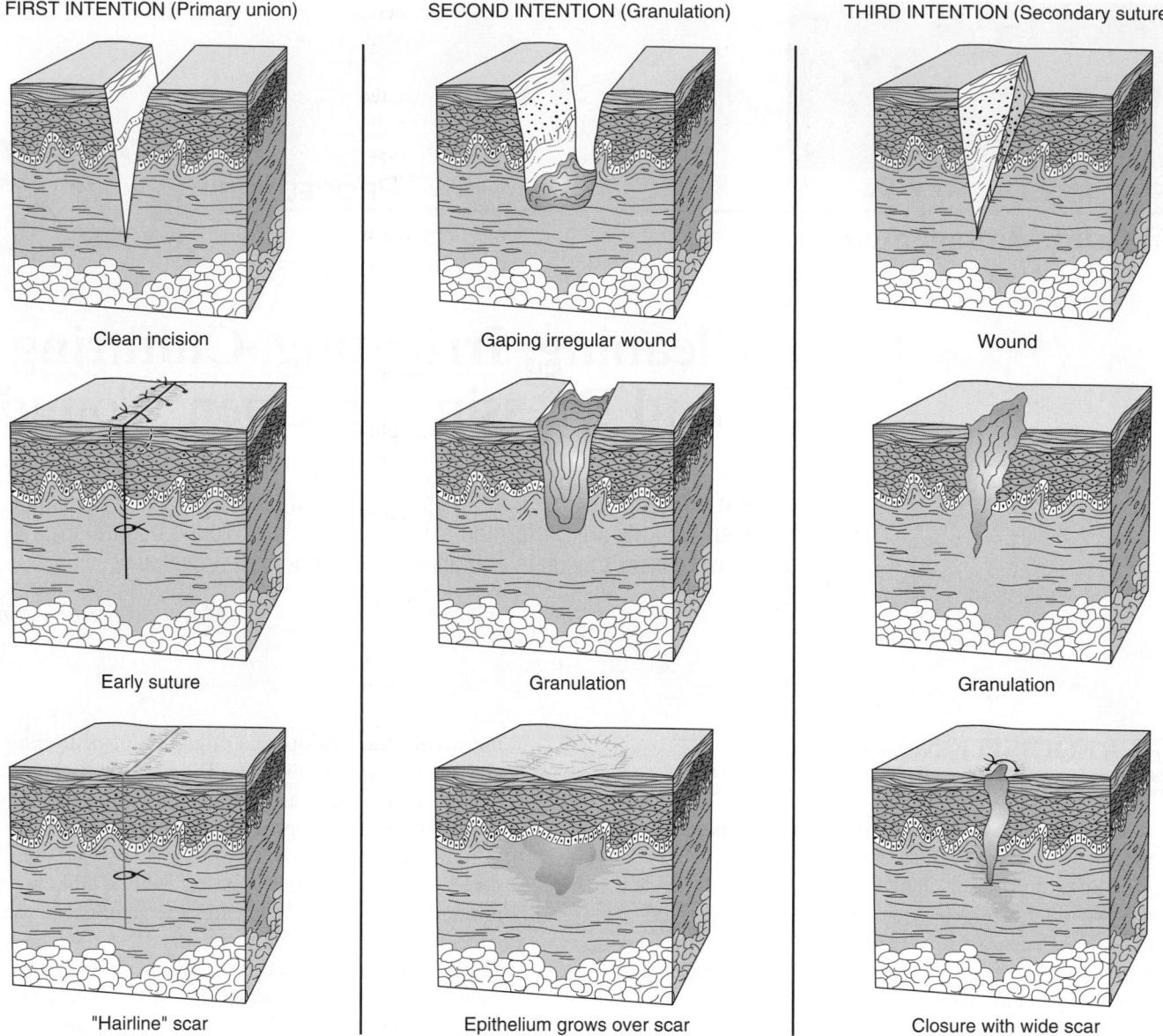

Clean incision	Gaping irregular wound	Wound
Early suture	Granulation	Granulation
"Hairline" scar	Epithelium grows over scar	Closure with wide scar

FIGURE 126-1   Wound healing by primary, secondary, and tertiary intention.

- Wound cleansing should be accomplished with minimal chemical or mechanical trauma.
  - Cytotoxic cleaning agents (i.e., chlorhexidine, iodine, hydrogen peroxide) should be limited because they can delay healing.[1,4,9,12]
  - Wound cleaning solutions should be pH neutral.
  - Normal saline (NS) solution is the cleaning agent of choice; however, tap water is safe and effective for cleaning of most acute and chronic wounds.[1,5,14]
  - The cleaning solution must be delivered with enough force to physically loosen foreign materials and bacteria without injuring the tissue. Effective wound cleaning is best achieved when solution is delivered at 8 to 13 psi (Fig. 126-2). A 35-mL syringe attached to an 18-gauge angiocatheter tip only delivers fluid at 8 psi. A 12-mL syringe with a 22-gauge angiocatheter tip provides 13 psi. (Increasing syringe size decreases the pressure of the stream, and increasing the bore of the

catheter tip increases the pressure.) Pressures greater than 15 psi may actually force bacteria and debris deeper into the wound bed.[2,8,9,12]
- Wound infections delay wound healing. Wound cultures (obtained before antibiotic therapy) may isolate organisms and differentiate between colonization and active infection.
  - Wound contamination is the presence of bacteria on the wound surface that are not actively multiplying. Signs and symptoms of infection are not present, and healing is not impaired.[4,12]
  - Colonization is the presence of bacteria in the wound that are actively multiplying or forming colonies. Colonization can delay healing but may not elicit signs of infection.
  - Wound infection is present if organisms are present at 105 colony-forming units per milliliter (103 for virulent organisms like β-hemolytic strep[4]) in conjunction

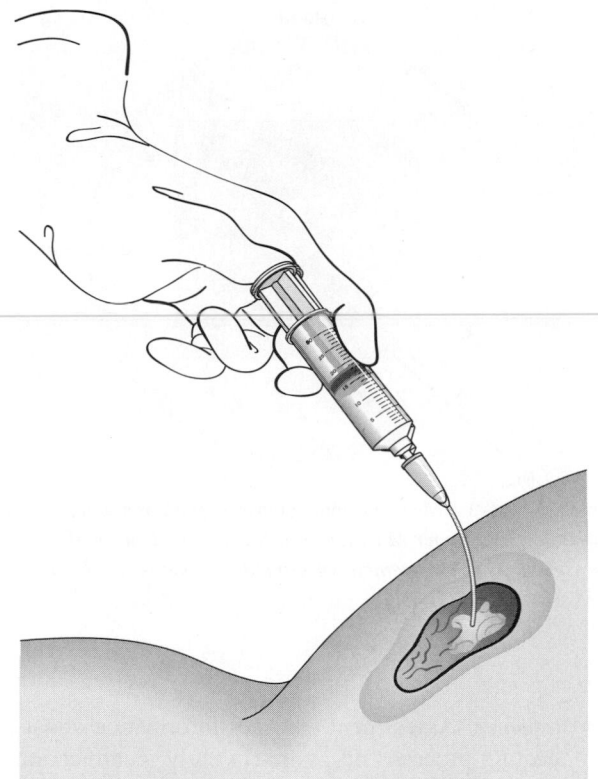

FIGURE 126-2   Irrigation of a wound.

with clinical findings such as erythema, edema, pain, purulence, fever, and leukocytosis.

❖ With the proliferation of organisms like methicillin-resistant *Staphylococcus aureus* (MRSA) and aggressive bacteria that cause necrotizing soft tissue infections (e.g., group A *Streptococci* and *Streptococcus pyogenes)*, the standard of empirically implementing antibiotic treatment without wound culture is being questioned. Knowledge of whether resistant strains of bacteria are present at the onset of treatment is critical to provide the optimal situation for healing and rapid intervention.[4,11]

❖ Bacterial invasion of wounds is managed with cleansing, débridement (see Procedure 127), and antibiotic therapy (local or systemic). Soaking can macerate wound and periwound tissues and may not improve bacterial counts.[14]

CRITICAL CARE DIMENSION

Critically ill patients commonly encounter factors that impair adequate wound healing, compounding the risks for poor patient outcomes. Nursing care should focus on early recognition and correction of underlying systemic disorders and patient-specific comorbidities that can impede wound healing goals.[2,8,9,12,13]

- Frequent comorbidities that can compromise optimal healing trajectories are diabetes mellitus, cardiovascular disease, chronic obstructive pulmonary disease, peripheral vascular disease, cancer, endocrine imbalances,

renal failure, cerebral vascular accident, nicotine addiction, alcohol abuse, neurovascular deficit, obesity, and ascites.

- Trauma-associated wound considerations include penetrating injuries that create anaerobic pockets and deep tissue injury; reperfusion of previously ischemic injuries that can trigger paradoxic injury extension; and possible contamination with organic and inorganic bodies that can inhibit effective wound healing, including feces, saliva, soils, and environmental vectors such as metal, rock, and glass.

- Sometimes medications and treatment interventions may jeopardize wound healing goals. Medications that impair tissue perfusion (i.e., vasoconstrictors) or the immune response (i.e., steroids, immunomodulators, antirejection drugs, antineoplastics) and treatments that impair tissue hydration (diuretics and fluid restrictions) may adversely affect wound healing.

- Poor nutritional status includes low serum protein, vitamin C, zinc, copper, and magnesium.

- Altered blood chemistries, especially hypokalemia and hyperglycemia (>200 mg/dL) and acid-base disturbances, should be assessed.

- Other factors that compound effective wound healing include hypothermia or hyperthermia, extended surgical procedures, intraoperative hypotension, immobility, hypoxemia, anemia, poor tissue oxygenation, sepsis, extremes of age, inadequate sleep or rest, uncontrolled pain, clotting abnormalities, mechanical friction on the wound, and the development of adhesions or hypertrophic or keloid scars.

EQUIPMENT

- Nonsterile and sterile gloves (two pairs); sterile field (depending on type and age of wound)
- Personal protective equipment (as needed)
- Two or three sterile cotton-tipped applicators for use in measurement
- (NS) solution or ordered irrigation solution
- Sterile basins
- Waterproof barriers
- Sterile 35-mL slip-tip syringe and 18-gauge angiocatheter sheath for irrigation (if necessary)
- Sterile gauze (4 × 4); possibly, ABD dressings (if the wound has excessive drainage, an absorptive dressing may be necessary; if the wound has minimal drainage, a moisture-enhancing dressing may be needed)
- Liquid skin barrier or wafer; apply around the wound edge to protect periwound tissue
- Hypoallergenic tape; tubular mesh bandage or one set of Montgomery straps

Additional equipment to have available, if needed, includes the following:

- Swab culture: two sterile serum-tipped swabs and culturettes
- Tissue biopsy: scalpel, forceps, gauze for hemostasis, and container **AP**

- Needle aspiration: 10-mL syringe, 22-gauge needle, and syringe cap **AP**

PATIENT AND FAMILY EDUCATION

- Explain the procedure and rationale that supports wound cleaning and dressing management. ➡️***Rationale:*** Patient anxiety and discomfort are decreased.
- Discuss patient's role in the procedure. ➡️***Rationale:*** Patient cooperation is elicited; patient is prepared for wound management on discharge (as appropriate).
- Explain the reason for obtaining a wound culture. ➡️***Rationale:*** Patient anxiety is decreased.
- Discuss signs and symptoms of local and systemic wound infection (erythema, pain, increased wound drainage, odor, fever) and inform when patient should consult a healthcare provider. ➡️***Rationale:*** The patient is prepared for wound management on discharge.

PATIENT ASSESSMENT AND PREPARATION

Patient Assessment

- Assess the following:
  - ❖ Wound drainage (amount, consistency, color, and possible odor)
  - ❖ Size, shape, length, width, and depth of wound bed, including pockets (Fig. 126-3)
  - ❖ Appearance of wound bed (color, presence of debris; i.e., necrotic or darkened areas on tissue bed are black; slough is green or cream yellow; and healthy tissue is red)
  - ❖ Condition of wound margins and periwound skin (intact versus maceration or xerosis; abnormal textures/undermining)
  - ❖ Pain or tenderness
  - ❖ Presence of erythema (blanches with pressure) or ecchymosis (does not blanch with pressure)
  - ❖ Elevated temperature or localized warmth at wound site
  - ❖ White blood cell count; may be elevated or show a change from baseline
  - ❖ With advance age, subtle changes in activity and cognition may be the only indications of infection[2,6]
  - ❖ Nutrition assessment

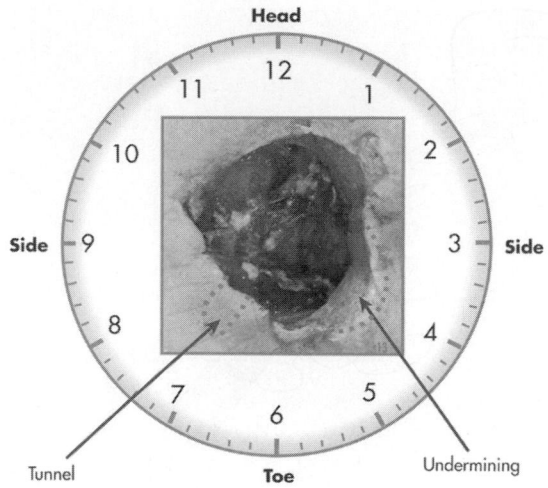

FIGURE 126-3 Measurement and assessment of a wound. *(From Lewis SL, Heitkemper MM, Dirksen SR: Medical-surgical nursing: assessment and management of clinical problems, ed 7, St Louis, 2007, Mosby, 204.)*

➡️***Rationale:*** Assessment provides information about the healing process and assists in early identification of wound infection. True wound bed assessment cannot be completed until after the wound bed has been cleansed.

Patient Preparation

- Ensure that patient understands preprocedural teachings. Answer questions as they arise, and reinforce information as needed. ➡️***Rationale:*** Understanding of previously taught information is evaluated and reinforced.
- Place patient in position of optimal comfort and visualization for wound care procedures. ➡️***Rationale:*** Proper positioning provides for effective wound visualization and enhances patient tolerance of procedure.
- Optimize lighting in room and provide privacy for patient. ➡️***Rationale:*** Lighting allows for optimal wound assessment, and privacy provides patient comfort.
- Administer premedication with prescribed analgesic, if indicated. ➡️***Rationale:*** Medication decreases patient anxiety and increases comfort. Pain and stress are recognized deterrents for healing.[3,13]

Procedure   for Cleaning, Irrigating, Culturing, and Dressing an Open Wound

Steps	Rationale	Special Considerations
Cleaning and Irrigating Wounds		
1. Wash hands; position patient to facilitate drainage and cleaning of wound.	Decreases contamination; uses gravity to direct flow of solution away from wound bed.	
2. Position waterproof barrier to collect drainage.	Controls flow of cleansing solution and minimizes solution contact with intact skin.	

Procedure for Cleaning, Irrigating, Culturing, and Dressing an Open Wound—*Continued*

Steps	Rationale	Special Considerations
3. Position wound-cleaning materials and soiled contamination container within reach of practitioner; conform to the principles of aseptic technique.	Decreases cross contamination during wound-cleaning process; enhances body mechanics for practitioner.	
4. **HH**		
5. **PE**		Face and eye barriers are strongly suggested with irrigation of wounds to protect healthcare provider against splash contaminate.[10]
6. Remove soiled dressing, noting any change in drainage and frequency of needed change. Discard in appropriate container.	Increasing drainage and frequency of change may indicate impending infection.[2,9,12,13]	
7. Assess condition of periwound skin and wound bed for shape and size, odor, and amount and consistency of drainage. Gently probe with cotton swab to note depth of tunnels and undermining. Remove soiled gloves.	Assesses for indications of healing or deterioration (see Fig. 126-3).	True wound bed assessment cannot be completed until after the wound bed has been cleansed. Measurements or photographs should be taken intermittently to document progression.
8. Establish sterile field; open sterile drape gauze; place sterile water or NS cleaning solution in sterile container. **(Level B*)**	Decreases cross contamination during the wound-cleaning process. Cleansing solution should not be cytotoxic.[1,2,4,5,8,9,12]	No evidence is found to support use of sterile technique when changing dressings on chronic wounds.[2,7]

9. If irrigation (see Fig. 126-2) is necessary, attach 18-gauge angiocatheter sleeve to syringe for irrigation.
  A. Apply sterile gloves.
  B. Draw up solution into syringe.
  C. Maintain 1- to 3-cm distance from wound surface.
  D. Direct solution onto wound bed from area of least contamination to greatest.
  E. Continue with irrigation until return solution is clear.
  (Level B)
	Irrigation reduces the bacterial population and removes excess debris to enhance healing. A 35-mL syringe with a 18-gauge needle provides approximately 8 psi, which is sufficient force to remove debris without creating wound bed damage. The smaller the syringe, the greater the psi.[1,14] Too great a force during irrigation can create tissue damage, drive bacteria deeper into the tissues, reinitiate the inflammatory process, and delay wound healing.[2,8,9,12]	Research does not support scrubbing or swabbing wounds.[14]
		Bulb syringes do not create enough psi to be effective.[9,14] Not all open wound beds need irrigation.

10. Cleaning a closed wound:
  A. With moistened gauze, cleanse from top of wound to base (or center of wound to edges).
  B. Discard gauze.
  C. Clean from area of least contamination to greatest (Fig. 126-4).
	Prevents wound contamination during the cleaning process.	If cleaning around a drain, clean from drain site outward in a circular motion; discard gauze with each circle.

11. Dry intact skin surrounding wound with gauze.	Limits maceration of healthy skin surrounding the wound.	

*Level B: Well-designed, controlled studies with results that consistently support a specific action, intervention, or treatment

Procedure continues on following page

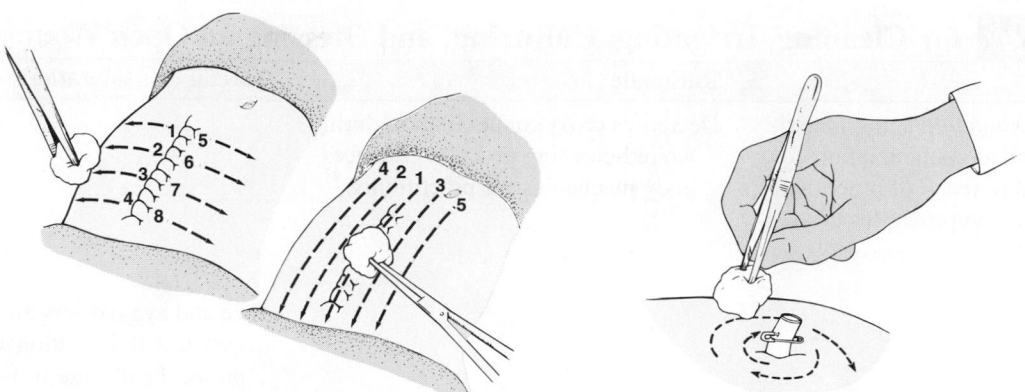

FIGURE 126-4   Cleaning of a wound. *(From Potter PA, Perry A: Basic nursing: essentials for practice, ed 5, St Louis, 2003, Mosby.)*

Procedure	for Cleaning, Irrigating, Culturing, and Dressing an Open Wound—*Continued*	
Steps	**Rationale**	**Special Considerations**

Culturing Wounds

Swab Culture

1. **VP**
2. Apply new sterile gloves and remove swab from culturette tube; maintain sterile technique. **(Level B*)** | Must clean wound before obtaining culture to ensure that debris contamination is not cultured.[12] | Wound culturing is a sterile procedure.
3. Swab firmly across the central surface of the wound in a zigzag manner, simultaneously rotating the swab between finger and thumb with gentle pressure to extract any tissue fluid. **(Level D*)** | Tissue fluid, not superficial exudate, is desired for proper results. Swabbing center of wound and not wound edges ensures collection of an adequate specimen.[12] | Culturing of wound edges may result in contamination from skin flora and wound debris.[2,12]
4. Carefully place saturated swab into culturette tube without touching swab or inside of container. | Enables adequate sample collection and prevents contamination. |
5. Crush ampule of medium in culturette and close securely; observe that culture medium surrounds swab. | Keeps specimen from drying and provides growth-supporting medium for culture. | With collection of an anaerobic culture, ensure tube is maintained upright to prevent carbon dioxide from escaping.
6. Label specimen with patient name, date, wound site; transport to laboratory as soon as possible. | Delays in culture transport increase risk of invalid testing from exposure to temperature changes. | Bacterial overgrowth occurs with delays in plating and analysis.[2,12]

Tissue Biopsy

1. **VP**
2. Apply sterile gloves; with sterile scalpel and forceps or punch biopsy, obtain a tissue sample approximately 1 to 2 mm in size (width and depth); apply pressure with sterile gauze to tissue sampling site. **(Level D)** | Ensures site markings have been made where appropriate. Ensures good tissue sample size free of necrotic tissue; provides for homeostasis of tissue bed. | Caution must be exercised in obtaining a tissue biopsy; consider local anesthetic to site before procedure; assess for excessive bleeding and damage to underlying and surrounding structures. Advanced training is recommended for nurses who perform this skill.

---

*Level B: Well-designed, controlled studies with results that consistently support a specific action, intervention, or treatment
*Level D: Peer-reviewed professional organizational standards with clinical studies to support recommendations

Procedure for Cleaning, Irrigating, Culturing, and Dressing an Open Wound—*Continued*

Steps	Rationale	Special Considerations
3. Place tissue sample in sterile container and close tightly; sample may be placed on agar plate, if indicated.	Prevents contamination of sample.	
4. Label specimen with patient name, date, wound site; transport to laboratory as soon as possible. **Proceed to Dressing Open Wounds.**		
Needle Aspiration		
1. **VP**		
2. Cleanse the skin, then apply sterile gloves; insert sterile needle on 10-mL syringe filled with 0.5 mL air into intact periwound tissue; aspirate fluid from several vectors with a fan technique approach and pull plunger rapidly to draw tissue fluid into the syringe.[2]	Ensures good specimen collection if two to four angles of aspiration are used.[2,12]	Goal is to obtain tissue fluid, not wound exudate. Caution required not to reinject fluid back into tissues.[2]
3. Express excess air out of syringe.		
4. With sterile technique, remove needle and replace with a blunt end cap.	Maintains Standard Precautions; prevents contamination.	
5. Label specimen with patient name, date, wound site; transport to laboratory as soon as possible.		
Dressing Open Wounds	Apply dressing appropriate to wound type and patient condition. Moisture-retentive dressings facilitate wound healing.	
1. Open sterile gauze 4 × 4 pads and saturate with NS solution; apply sterile gloves; wring out excessive moisture; apply 4 × 4s loosely over wound bed; gently pack gauze to wound edge but do not exceed wound edge. **(Level B*)**	Open moist gauze protects wound bed and allows for placement of dressing without creating open areas or pockets; dressing must be moist but not wet to allow for absorption.[1,9]	Moist dressing must stay within parameters of wound bed to prevent surrounding skin maceration. Dressings packed too firmly into wound compromise perfusion and wound healing. Wound care dressing products that absorb drainage or provide moisture may also be used. Gauze dressing may not control excessive wound exudate; alternative dressings to control exudate should be considered.
2. Place dry gauze 4 × 4s and ABDs over moist dressing.	Provides protection and absorption.	
3. Secure dressing.		

*Level B: Well-designed, controlled studies with results that consistently support a specific action, intervention, or treatment

Procedure continues on following page

Procedure for Cleaning, Irrigating, Culturing, and Dressing an Open Wound—*Continued*

Steps	Rationale	Special Considerations
A. Tubular mesh dressings: Sized to secure loose dressings underneath.	Conforming mesh dressings reduce the skin friction associated with tape removal and adhesive irritation. They allow airflow and increase security of coverage without added bulk.	Colorful binders may alleviate the visual distraction of wounds and facilitate a sense of normalcy, especially in pediatric populations.
B. Tape: Apply tape across the wound dressing, extending approximately 2 inches beyond dressing onto skin.	Hypoallergenic tape is less traumatic to noninjured skin; secures dressing in place.	
C. Montgomery straps (see Fig. 126-5):	Alternative if nonlatex mesh unavailable for sensitive clients.	The straps, tapes, or twill used must be replaced if they become soiled or moist because they become a reservoir for contamination.
(1) Apply a liquid or hydrocolloid barrier to surround skin where straps will be applied.	(1) Assists with providing a protective skin barrier and more effective anchoring of Montgomery straps.	
(2) Peel paper backing off straps and apply to skin surface with gentle, even pressure.	(2) Secures Montgomery straps to skin.	
(3) Lace the disposable ties (twill/trach tape; large rubber bands) through the holes in the straps in a crisscross fashion.	(3) Secures dressing in place beneath Montgomery strap.	

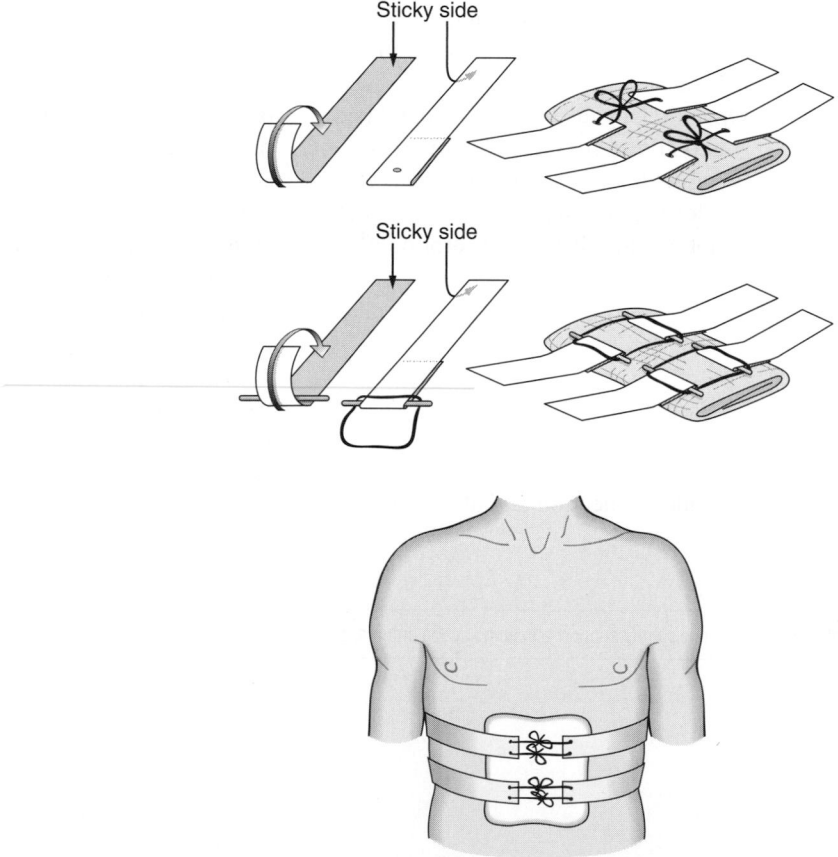

Figure 126-5   Montgomery straps.

Expected Outcomes

- Healed wound
- Wound bed is free of devitalized tissue
- Wound culture specimen obtained confirms and identifies causative organism of infection
- Wound heals uniformly without tunneling, abscess formation, or tracking
- Surrounding skin is free of maceration and erosion
- Wound is free of signs of infection or compromised perfusion

Unexpected Outcomes

- Cross contamination of wound
- Damage to wound bed (hemorrhage, dehiscence) from excessive force during irrigation
- Maceration or inflammation of surrounding skin
- Hemorrhage from tissue biopsy culture technique
- Signs of infection; changes in amount and character of wound drainage
- Wound healing (granulation and contraction) not noticeably progressing on a weekly basis
- Development of wound tunneling, abscess, or tracking

Patient Monitoring and Care

Steps	Rationale	Reportable Conditions
		These conditions should be reported if they persist despite nursing interventions.
1. Follow institution standard for assessing pain. Administer analgesia as prescribed.	Identifies need for pain interventions.	• Continued pain despite pain interventions
2. Assess patient, wound bed, and skin surrounding wound. **(Level B*)**	Continued assessment is essential; wounds must be free of infection to heal. Healthy granulation tissue is pink or red. Discoloration may indicate infection, necrotic tissue, or poor perfusion or hypoxemia at the wound bed site.	• Foul drainage or odor • Darkened or pale areas on tissue bed; red, green, or yellow tissue bed • Erythema; new ecchymosis • Pain • Change in wound drainage (amount, color, odor) • Elevated temperature • Elevated white blood cell count • Hyperglycemia in a patient with diabetes
3. Monitor wound dressing site for bleeding.	Capillary bed of a healing wound is fragile. Excessive stimulation during cleansing, culturing, or biopsy may disrupt the capillary integrity, creating excessive bleeding.	• Bleeding that does not stop with mild pressure to wound bed • Excessive bleeding
4. Assess wound bed and edges for undermining, pockets, or tunnels.	Healing by secondary intention increases risk for pockets or tunnels.	• Presence and depth of undermining, pocket, or tunnel

Documentation

Documentation should include the following:
- Patient and family education
- Pain assessment, premedication given, patient tolerance of procedure, and response to pain medication
- Wound cleaning and irrigation procedure completed; date; time
- Description of wound bed before and after cleaning or irritation; drainage and odors if appropriate; presence of necrotic and granulation tissue
- Description of surrounding skin (color, moisture, integrity)
- Weekly measurements of wound size (measure or trace wound area and depth when appropriate)

- Progression of difficult-to-heal or complex wounds (consider use of digital photography to document)
- Wound culture completed, date, time; type of culture obtained (swab, aerobic, anaerobic, needle aspiration, tissue biopsy)
- Description of approximate site where wound culture was obtained
- Description of wound drains, surrounding skin, and characteristics of wound drainage
- Type of dressing applied after wound care
- Unexpected outcomes
- Nursing interventions

*Level B: Well-de.signed, controlled studies with results that consistently support a specific action, intervention, or treatment

References

CR 1. Agency for Health Care Policy and Research: *Clinical practice guideline: treatment of pressure ulcers,* Rockville, MD, 1994, US Department of Health and Human Services.

2. Bates-Jensen BM, Ovington LG: Management of exudate and infection. In Sussman C, Bates-Jensen BM, editors: *Wound care: a collaborative practice manual,* ed 3, Philadelphia, 2007, Wolters Kluwer, 215-233.

CR 3. Broadbent E, Petrie K, Alley PG, et al: Psychological stress impairs early wound repair following surgery, *Psychosom Med* 65(5):865-869, 2003.

CR 4. Edwards R, Harding KG: Bacteria and wound healing, *Curr Opin Infect Dis* 17(2):91-96, 2004.

5. Fernandez R, Griffiths R: Water for wound cleansing, *Cochrane Database Syst Rev* 23(1):CD003861, 2008.

6. Johnson CB, Harper GM, Landsfeld CS: Geriatric medicine. In McPhee SJ, Papadakis MA, Tierney LM Jr, editors: *Current medical diagnosis and treatment,* ed 47, New York, 2008, Lange Medical Books/McGraw-Hill, 51-66.

CR 7. Lawson C, Juliano L, Ratilff CR: Does sterile or nonsterile technique make a difference in wounds healing by secondary intention? *Ostomy Wound Manage* 49(4): 56-60, 2003.

8. Makic MB, McQuillan KA: Wound healing and soft tissue injuries. In McQuillan KA, Makic MB, Whalen E, editors: *Trauma nursing: from resuscitation through rehabilitation,* ed 4, St Louis, 2009, Saunders Elsevier, 306-329.

9. Rolstad BS, Ovington LG: Principles of wound management. In Byrant RA, Nix CP, editors: *Acute and chronic wounds,* ed 3, Philadelphia, 2007, Mosby Elsevier, 391-426.

10. Siegel JD, Rhinehart E, Jackson M, et al: *Healthcare Infection Control Practices Advisory Committee, guideline for isolation precautions: preventing transmission of infectious agents in healthcare settings; transmission-based precautions,* Atlanta, 2007, Centers for Disease Control and Prevention.

11. Storr A: Inappropriate therapy for methicillin-resistant *Staphylococcus aureus:* resource utilization and cost implications, *Crit Care Med* 36(8):2335-2340, 2008.

12. Stotts N: Wound infection: diagnosis and management. In Byrant RA, Nix CP, editors: *Acute and chronic wounds,* ed 3, Philadelphia: 2007, Mosby Elsevier, 161-175.

13. Sussman C, Bates-Jensen B: Wound healing physiology: acute and chronic. In Sussman C, Bates-Jensen B, editors: *Wound care: a collaborative practice manual for health professionals,* ed 3, Philadelphia, 2007, Wolters Kluwer, 21-51.

14. The Joanna Briggs Institute: Solutions, techniques and pressure for wound cleansing, *Best Pract* 10(2):1-4, 2006, retrieved September 10, 2008, from www.joannabriggs.edu.au.

Additional Readings

Baranoski S: Choosing a wound dressing: part I, *Nursing* 38(1):60-616, 2008.

Baranoski S: Choosing a wound dressing: part II, *Nursing* 38(2):14-15, 2008.

Bates-Jensen BM, MacLean: Quality indicators for the care of pressure ulcers in vulnerable elders, *J Am Geriatr Soc* 55(Suppl 2):S409-S416, 2007.

Moore Z, Cowan S: A systematic review of wound cleansing for pressure ulcers, *J Clin Nurs* 17(15):1963-1972, 2008.

CR Wound Ostomy and Continence Nurses (WOCN) Society: *Guideline for prevention and management of pressure ulcers (series),* Glenview, IL, 2003, WOCN.

AP Débridement: Pressure Ulcers, Burns, and Wounds

P U R P O S E :   Wound débridement is the removal of necrotic nonviable tissue to promote wound healing.

Julie Lynn Henderson

PREREQUISITE NURSING KNOWLEDGE

- Before wound débridement, the patient and wound should be assessed for underlying causes, patient's physical condition, nutritional status, and current healthcare treatment plan, including medications.[3]
- Normal wound healing progresses through an orderly sequence of three overlapping phases: inflammation, proliferation, and reepithelialization and remodeling.
- The presence of necrotic tissue or debris interrupts the normal sequence of wound healing, retards healing processes, and provides a medium that promotes bacterial growth.[4]
- Acute wounds may be classified as either partial-thickness or full-thickness wounds. Partial-thickness wounds penetrate the epidermis and part of the dermis; partial-thickness wounds can be further described as superficial or deep partial-thickness wounds. Full-thickness wounds extend to all skin layers, the epidermis and dermis, and may penetrate subcutaneous tissues.[3]
- Pressure ulcers are defined as localized injury to the skin or underlying tissue usually over a bony prominence as a result of pressure.[7] The National Pressure Ulcer Advisory Panel (NPUAP) staging system is used to describe pressure ulcers.[1,7]
  - ❖ Stage I: Intact skin with nonblanchable redness of a localized area usually over a bony prominence. Darkly pigmented skin may not have visible blanching, but the area may differ in color from surrounding tissues.[7]

- ❖ Stage II: Presents as partial-thickness loss of dermis as a shallow open ulcer with a red-pink wound bed, without slough. May also present as an intact or open/ruptured serum-filled blister.[7]
- ❖ Stage III: Is described as full-thickness tissue loss. Subcutaneous fat may be visible; however, bone, tendon, and muscle are not exposed. Undermining and tunneling may also be present, as well as slough.[7]
- ❖ Stage IV: Presents as a full-thickness tissue injury to include exposed bone, tendon, or muscle. Slough or eschar may be present on some parts of the wound bed.
- ❖ Unstageable: Tissue injury that cannot be adequately assessed because of the slough or eschar covering the wound base. Wound débridement should occur before staging the tissue injury.[1,7]
- ❖ Suspected deep tissue injury: A purple or maroon localized area of discolored intact skin or blood-filled blister from damage of underlying soft tissue from pressure or shear. The area may be painful, boggy, warmer, or cooler as compared with adjacent tissue.[7]
- Necrotic tissue is nonviable tissue and may range in color from whitish gray, tan, yellow, and finally progressing to black. Necrotic tissue nourishes bacteria and slows healing by retarding the inflammatory phase.[4] It may lead to deeper penetration of bacteria into tissues, resulting in cellulites, osteomyelitis, and possible limb loss.[5]
- Débridement provides a mechanism of removal of necrotic tissue and reestablishes normal phases of wound healing.
- Vascular evaluation is essential before wound débridement. Inadequate perfusion may result in the wound extending into a deeper dermal or full-thickness wound after débridement.[9] Pressure ulcers, burns, and chronic wounds may develop necrotic tissue that requires débridement for wound healing to progress.

AP   This procedure should be performed only by physicians, advanced practice nurses, and other healthcare professionals (including critical care nurses) with additional knowledge, skills, and demonstrated competence per professional licensure or institutional standard.

- Débridement may be achieved with several methods[2]:
  - ❖ Surgical débridement: Fast and effective means of removal of devitalized tissue. Requires local anesthesia, use of sterile instruments, and conditions and availability of a qualified clinician.[2,9] Large amounts of necrotic tissue may be removed. This may be considered in burn patients with large amounts of eschar or with necrotizing soft tissue infections (i.e., necrotizing fasciitis).[5]
  - ❖ Sharp débridement: Similar to surgical debridement, but local anesthesia may or may not be administered. Sharp débridement procedures should be performed only by qualified physicians, advanced practice nurses, and other healthcare providers (including critical care nurses) with additional knowledge, skills, and demonstrated competence per professional licensure or institutional standard.[2,9] This kind of débridement may be done at the bedside, in a clinic, or at an office. Sharp débridement is best for adherent dry eschar with or without infection present. The bacterial count is rapidly reduced.[4] Sharp débridement may be difficult on hard, dry wounds. Consider enzymatic débridement as first option.[9] Sharp débridement should be discontinued in presence of pain, bleeding, or exposure of underlying structures.
  - ❖ Chemical (enzymatic) débridement: Highly selective method of removal of necrotic tissue. Relies on naturally occurring enzymes that are exogenously applied to the wound surface to degrade tissue. This is a slower process that requires a moist wound bed with adequate secondary dressing to absorb wound exudate. Enzymatic débriding agents may be selective or nonselective to viable tissues. Nonselective agents may be best for thick, leathery, adherent eschar. Selective agents may be best when excess protein buildup is present.[6] Examples of wounds that may benefit from chemical débridement are a partial-thickness burn wound or unstageable pressure ulcer.
  - ❖ Mechanical débridement: Method of physical removal of debris from the wound. Methods range from wet-to-dry gauze dressings, irrigation, pulsatile lavage, and whirlpool therapy. Débridement is nonselective, and healthy tissue and necrotic tissue and debris may be removed in the process, causing bleeding and pain.
  - ❖ Autolytic débridement: Uses the properties of moisture-interactive dressings to facilitate digestion of devitalized tissue by the body's own enzymes. Typically, if tissue autolysis does not begin to appear in the wound in 24 to 72 hours, another method of débridement should be considered.[2]
  - ❖ Physicians, advanced practice nurses, or physician extenders who have demonstrated knowledge and competency should perform surgical débridement.
- Sharp débridement should be performed by physicians, advanced practice nurses, registered nurses, and physical therapists with documented educational course completion and validation of knowledge and skill. One should check with state regulatory agencies before performing sharp wound débridement.[10]
- A key to successful safe sharp débridement is assessment and knowledge of anatomy.[5] All wound care procedures should adhere to principles of aseptic technique.
- Clinical judgment should be used in determining whether clean or sterile technique is indicated in the wound dressing procedure. Generally speaking, acute wounds may be cared for with sterile technique and chronic wounds may be cared for with clean technique.[1] The clinician must assess the patient, type or stage of wound, and type of procedure in deciding which technique should be used in wound care.

EQUIPMENT

- Sharp débridement:
  - ❖ Personal protective equipment (gown, goggles, mask)
  - ❖ Sterile gloves and field
  - ❖ Normal saline solution
  - ❖ Gauze 4 × 4 pads
  - ❖ Sterile instrument set (scissors, forceps, no. 10 scalpel)
  - ❖ Wound dressing
  - ❖ Tape
- Chemical débridement:
  - ❖ Normal saline solution or water to clean wound
  - ❖ Clean gloves or sterile gloves (depending on type and age of wound)
  - ❖ Enzymatic preparation or solution (prescribed)
  - ❖ Tongue blade
  - ❖ Filler dressing if needed; secondary absorptive dressing
  - ❖ No. 10 scalpel for crosshatching (optional)
  - ❖ Tape
- Mechanical débridement (wet-to-dry gauze dressing):
  - ❖ Clean or sterile gloves (depending on type and age of wound)
  - ❖ Normal saline solution
  - ❖ Gauze (rolled or 4 × 4 pads)
  - ❖ Secondary absorptive dressing
  - ❖ Tape
- Autolytic débridement:
  - ❖ Clean gloves
  - ❖ Normal saline solution or water to clean wound
  - ❖ Moisture-retentive dressing (transparent film, hydrocolloid dressing, hydrogels)
  - ❖ Secondary absorptive dressing as indicated
  - ❖ Tape

PATIENT AND FAMILY EDUCATION

- Explain procedure and reason for wound débridement; educate regarding potential complications such as bleeding if sharp débridement is the prescribed procedure. **➺Rationale:** Explanation decreases patient anxiety and comfort and informs patient.

PATIENT ASSESSMENT AND PREPARATION

Patient Assessment

- Vascular assessment should be completed before débridement. ➥*Rationale:* Poor perfusion may result in the extension of the wound after débridement.
- Assess tissues or underlying structures before sharp débridement. ➥*Rationale:* Sharp débridement is contraindicated if underlying structures such as muscle, bone, tendon, and blood vessels may be exposed.
- Assess for signs and symptoms of local and systemic infection. ➥*Rationale:* Débridement may seed bacteria into systemic circulation; appropriate antibiotics should be considered before débridement in at-risk patient populations.[8] Surgical débridement, the most aggressive type of débridement, is the method of choice when signs of severe cellulitis or sepsis are present.[1]
- Ensure that coagulation parameters are within normal limits. ➥*Rationale:* Coagulation abnormalities may result in unwanted bleeding complications from the débridement process.
- Assess the patient for pain and consider premedication. ➥*Rationale:* Medication decreases patient discomfort.

Patient Preparation

- Ensure that patient understands preprocedural teachings. Answer questions as they arise, and reinforce information as needed. ➥*Rationale:* Understanding of previously taught information is evaluated and reinforced.

- Verify correct patient with two identifiers. Obtain informed consent for surgical and sharp débridement.[2,11] ➥*Rationale:* Prior to performing a procedure, ensure the correct identification of the patient for the intended intervention. Informed consent ensures patient knowledge of procedure.
- Before the procedure, comply with Universal Protocol requirements.[11] Ensure all relevant studies and documents, including informed consent, are available. Ensure site markings have been made where appropriate. Prior to surgical or sharp débridement, perform a pre-procedure verification and time out, if non-emergent. ➥*Rationale:* Ensures patient safety.
- Premedicate patient with prescribed analgesic, if needed. Assess patient's response to analgesic before start of procedure. Reassess patient's need for additional analgesic agents throughout débridement procedure. Consider topical lidocaine solution. ➥*Rationale:* Patient anxiety and discomfort are decreased. Pain results in vasoconstriction of the cutaneous tissues from the increase in adrenergic activity. Adequate pain control improves tissue perfusion and results in improved healing.[3]
- Place patient in position of optimal comfort and visualization for dressing the wound. Keep the patient warm while the wound is exposed. ➥*Rationale:* Positioning provides for effective wound visualization and enhances patient tolerance of procedure. Keeping the patient warm prevents vasoconstriction that impairs wound healing.
- Optimize lighting in room and provide privacy for patient. ➥*Rationale:* Optimal wound assessment and patient comfort are provided.

Procedure for Débridement: Pressure Ulcers, Burns, and Wounds

Steps	Rationale	Special Considerations
Sharp Débridement	Fast and effective means of selective removal of devitalized tissue; should be performed by a qualified healthcare provider.	
1. **VP**		
2. Premedicate patient for pain.	Systemic analgesic may be administered before procedure and throughout procedure as needed for patient tolerance and compliance.	Assess patient response to analgesic.
3. Perform hand hygiene, then apply personal protective equipment (gown, goggles, and gloves) and clean wound.	Reduces transmission of microorganisms; Standard Precautions.	
4. Discard dirty gloves, perform hand hygiene, and apply clean gloves.	Reduces transmission of microorganisms; Standard Precautions.	
5. Prepare sterile drape and field of instruments, normal saline (NS) solution, gauze, and secondary dressing.	Maintains aseptic technique.	Gauze may be needed to provide hemostasis during procedure.
6. Discard clean gloves and apply sterile gloves.		

Procedure continues on following page

Procedure for Débridement: Pressure Ulcers, Burns, and Wounds—*Continued*

Steps	Rationale	Special Considerations
7. With forceps, lift eschar and gently cut with sterile scalpel or scissors. Débride tissue to line of demarcation of healthy tissue.	Goal of sharp débridement is removal of devitalized tissue without damage to healthy wound bed.	Pain and bleeding are signs of healthy tissue. Stop procedure if pain or bleeding is excessive or if there is impending bone, tendon, or proximity to fascial plane.[5]
8. Clean wound bed with NS solution.	Allows for removal of loose devitalized tissue and debris.	Reassess wound bed after procedure.
9. Apply moist wound dressing of choice.	Promotes wound healing of newly exposed tissues.	Assess for hemostasis before application of dressing.
10. Discard used supplies in appropriate receptacle and perform hand hygiene.		
Chemical Débridement	Selective débridement technique.	Requires prescription for desired enzyme preparation.
1. Perform hand hygiene, apply clean gloves, and clean wound.	Maintains aseptic technique.	
2. Discard dirty gloves and apply clean gloves.	Maintains clean technique.	
3. If wound eschar is hard and dry, no. 10 scalpel may be used to cross-hatch necrotic tissue. **(Level C*)**	Cross-hatching technique may allow better penetration of enzymatic agent and enhance enzyme activity.[5]	
4. Discard dirty gloves, perform hand hygiene, and apply clean gloves.	Maintains aseptic technique.	
5. Establish sterile field: enzymatic agent, NS solution, and secondary moist healing dressing.	Maintains aseptic technique.	
6. Apply enzymatic agent with tongue blade to eschar in the wound bed.	Assists with even application of enzymatic agent over necrotic wound tissue.	Concentrate enzymatic agent over nonviable tissue.
7. Place moisture-retentive dressing (typically, gauze moistened with NS solution) over wound.	Most enzymatic agents require a moist dressing to be applied over agent for effective action.	Other dressings that promote moist wound healing may be used.
8. Secure secondary dressing in place.	Secondary dressing is needed to absorb wound exudates.[9]	Assess periwound for irritation and breakdown from moisture. Consider application of liquid skin barrier to periwound edge.
9. Discard used supplies in appropriate receptacle and perform hand hygiene.		
Mechanical Débridement: Wet-to-Dry Gauze Dressing	Nonselective débridement technique.	Nonviable and viable tissue may be lost with this method of débridement.
1. Perform hand hygiene and apply clean gloves.	Maintains clean technique.	
2. Establish sterile field: gauze dressing moistened with NS solution.	Maintains aseptic technique.	
3. Clean wound.	Wound cleansing is a means of mechanical débridement; also removes nonadherent bacteria.	Remove any gauze particles left in the wound bed with gentle irrigation.
4. Apply new gloves.	Maintains aseptic technique.	

*Level C: Qualitative studies, descriptive or correlational studies, integrative reviews, systematic reviews, or randomized controlled trials with inconsistent results

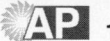

Procedure for Débridement: Pressure Ulcers, Burns, and Wounds—*Continued*

Steps	Rationale	Special Considerations
5. Place moistened gauze loosely into wound bed.	Excessive packing of gauze into wound bed may compromise perfusion.[7]	If more than one gauze dressing is used, place ends of two dressings close to each other for easy removal or consider use of a rolled gauze.
6. Cover wound with secondary absorptive dressing and secure.	Protects wound from external contamination and absorbs exudates.	Consider changing dressing if 75% or greater area of secondary dressing is saturated with wound drainage. Assess periwound area for maceration; consider use of liquid skin barrier or hydrocolloid to protect periwound skin.
7. Discard gloves and perform hand hygiene.		
8. After prescribed time interval, apply clean gloves and remove dressing to create mechanical débridement action.	Drying action of gauze adheres it to necrotic tissue, which is detached with dressing removal.	If dressing is dry and adherent to viable tissue, lightly moisten gauze to prevent excessive débridement of viable tissue and minimize pain.[2]
9. Discard used supplies in appropriate receptacle and perform hand hygiene.		
Autolytic Débridement	Selective débridement technique that uses the body's natural enzymes to break down necrotic tissue.	May not be effective for large wound surfaces.
1. Perform hand hygiene and apply clean gloves.		
2. Clean wound bed with NS solution or water.		
3. Apply moisture-retentive dressing.	Provides moist wound healing environment that enhances autolytic débridement process.	Assess dressing for absorptive properties. Consider changing dressing if 75% or greater area of the secondary dressing is saturated with wound drainage.
4. Apply secondary dressing as indicated.	Autolyic débridement results in production of wound exudates. Apply a secondary dressing to absorb exudate away from wound bed.	
5. Discard used supplies in appropriate receptacle and perform hand hygiene.		

Expected Outcomes

- Wound bed is free of necrotic tissue and debris
- Inflammatory progressing to proliferation stage of wound healing is reestablished, and wound healing progresses along normal trajectory
- Wound is free of infection or signs of compromised perfusion
- Wound hemostasis is established after sharp débridement

Unexpected Outcomes

- Depth of wound extends, and necrotic tissue recurs
- Normal wound healing process is not reestablished by removal of devitalized tissue and wound healing fails to progress[1-3]
- Bacterial infection is present; signs of local or systemic infection are present
- Excessive bleeding from lack of wound hemostasis

Procedure continues on following page

Patient Monitoring and Care

Steps	Rationale	Reportable Conditions
		These conditions should be reported if they persist despite nursing interventions.
1. Assess patient, wound bed, and surrounding skin for signs of infection. **(Level B*)**	Wound débridement may not effectively remove all bacteria; continued assessment for wound infection is essential for healing.[7,10]	• Erythema and warmth at wound site • Pain and tenderness • Edema • Change in wound drainage amount, color, odor • Fever • Elevated white blood cell count
2. Monitor dressing for signs of bleeding.	Wound débridement may disturb newly formed, fragile blood vessels and established blood vessels and cause bleeding.	• Bleeding that does not stop with mild pressure to wound bed • Excessive bleeding
3. Assess wound for signs of healing after débridement. **(Level B)**	Goal of necrotic tissue débridement is to establish wound healing in the form of granulation tissue and wound contracture.[2]	• Discoloration of wound bed noted (i.e., ecchymosis, ischemia) • Development of necrotic tissue in wound bed • Changed, diminished, or absent pulses distal to wound bed
4. Follow institution standard for assessing pain. Administer analgesia as prescribed.	Identifies need for pain interventions.	• Continued pain despite pain interventions

Documentation

Documentation should include the following:
- Patient and family education
- Description of wound bed before and after débridement
- Description of periwound skin assessment (color, maceration, integrity, evidence of infection, etc.)
- Size of wound after wound débridement procedure
- Description of dressing applied to wound bed (primary and secondary dressings as appropriate)
- Pain assessment, interventions, and effectiveness
- Premedication given, patient tolerance of procedure, and response to pain medication
- Description of wound débridement process and any unexpected complications
- Vascular assessment
- Description of established wound hemostasis obtained at completion of procedure
- Digital photography is recommended to document progression of wound healing[1]
- Obtain patient consent per institutional standards

*Level B: Well-designed controlled studies with results that consistently support a specific action, intervention, or treatment

References

CR 1. Agency for Health Care Policy and Research: *Treatment of pressure ulcers*, AHCPR Publication No. 95-0652, Rockville, MD, 1994, US Department of Health and Human Services.
2. Anderson I: Debridement methods in wound care, *Nurs Stand* 20(24):65-66,68,70,72, 2006.
3. Broughton G, et al: Wound healing: an overview, *Plast Reconstruct Surg* 117(7S):1e-s-32e-s, 2006.
4. Calianno C, et al: Wound bed preparation: laying the foundation for treating chronic wounds, part 1, *Wound Skin Care* 36(2):70, 2006.
5. Kirshen C, et al: Debridement: a vital component of wound bed preparation, *Adv Skin Wound Care* 19(9):506-517, 2006.
6. Kravitz S, et al: Management of skin ulcers: understanding the mechanism and selection of enzymatic debriding agents, *Adv Skin Wound Care* 21(2):72-74, 2008.
7. NPUAP: *Pressure ulcer stages revised*, retrieved September 24, 2008, from www.npuap.org.
CR 8. Ovington LG: Hanging wet-to-dry dressings out to dry, *Adv Skin Wound Care* 15:79-89, 2002.
CR 9. Rodeheaver GT: Pressure ulcer debridement and cleansing: a review of current literature, *Ostomy Wound Manage* 45:80-86, 1999.

CR 10. Thomaselli N: WOCN position statement: conservative sharp wound debridement for registered nurses, *J Wound Ostomy Continence Nurses* 22:32A, 1995.

CR 11. The Joint Commission: *Universal protocol for preventing wrong site, wrong procedure, wrong person surgery*, 2003, retrieved January 8, 2009, from www.jointcommission.org/PatientSafety/UniversalProtocol.

Additional Readings

Dryburgh N, Smith F, Donaldson J, et al: Debridement for surgical wounds, *Cochrane Database Syst Rev* 3:CD006214, DOI: 10.1002/14651858.CD006214.pub2, 2008.

Byrant RA, Nix CP, editors: *Acute and chronic wounds*, ed 3, Philadelphia, 2007, Mosby Elsevier.

Siegel JD, Rhinehart E, Jackson M, et al: *Healthcare Infection Control Practices Advisory Committee: 2007 guideline for isolation precautions: preventing transmission of infectious agents in healthcare settings: transmission-based precautions*, Atlanta, 2007, Centers for Disease Control and Prevention.

CR Sussman C, Fowler E, Wethe J: *Sharp debridement of wounds [video series]*, Torrance, CA, 1995, Sussman Physical Therapy, Inc.

Wound Management with Excessive Drainage

P U R P O S E : Management of wound exudate is an essential step in wound healing. Pouching may be used to contain excessive drainage. Drains may be placed in the wound for management of drainage.

Mary Beth Flynn Makic

PREREQUISITE NURSING KNOWLEDGE

- Wound exudate is produced in response to the inflammatory phase of the healing process. As wounds heal, the amount of exudate should diminish. Chronic, nonhealing wounds may produce exudate for prolonged periods of time, necessitating effective management of the fluid.[1,2,7,9-11]
- Goals of wound care must be clearly identified so that proper wound care products are used.[10] Wound healing is best achieved through adequate cleansing, débridement, and dressing of the wound bed on the basis of wound characteristics.
- Excessive wound fluid may create pressure in the wound bed and compromise perfusion. Excessive moisture may cause periwound tissue damage and extend the wound or skin injury.[5,6]
- Assessment of wound exudate should include the quantity, color, consistency, and odor of drainage. When changes in wound exudate occur, the cause should be explored. These changes along with other clinical signs and symptoms may indicate possible increase in bacterial burden or infection.
- Drains are placed in wounds to facilitate healing by providing an exit for excessive fluid accumulating in or near the wound bed. Most wound drains are surgically placed; drains may or may not be secured with sutures.
- Excessive wound fluid may provide a source for proliferation of microorganisms. Wound drains may be ports of microorganism entry; aseptic techniques must be strictly observed.

- Pouching is an effective means of collecting wound and fistula drainage.[3,8] Suction may be used with pouching systems to pull fluid away from the wound bed.[5]
- Excessive wound drainage is removed to allow for wound healing to occur without tissue congestion, microorganism proliferation, and skin maceration.
- Excessive wound drainage may need to be calculated into the assessment of a patient's daily intake and output.
- Negative-pressure wound therapy (see Procedure 131) stimulates tissue growth and promotes wound healing. The closed system also provides active withdrawal of excessive wound fluid to assist in the management of exudating wounds.[4]
- Assess the patient's nutritional needs, specifically for protein, with exudating wounds.
- Excessive wound exudate production may result in the loss of up to 100 g of protein daily in wound exudate.[2,9] Nutritional supplementation of protein is necessary for wound healing.

EQUIPMENT

- Nonsterile and sterile gloves; sterile field
- Personal protective equipment: gowns and face protection
- Sterile gauze (4 × 4 pads); abdominal pad (e.g., ABD) or other absorptive dressings may be needed
- Sterile water or normal saline (NS) solution for cleansing
- Liquid skin barrier, skin barrier wafers, paste, powder and sealant, or hydrocolloid to protect periwound surface
- Drainage bag or pouch: ostomy-type appliance
- Clean scissors; forceps, if appropriate
- Hypoallergenic tape

PATIENT AND FAMILY EDUCATION

- Explain the procedure and the reason for changing wound dressing; educate regarding potential odor during the procedure. ➤➤*Rationale:* Patient anxiety and discomfort are decreased.
- Discuss patient's role in dressing change procedure and maintenance of wound drains or pouches. ➤➤*Rationale:* Patient cooperation is elicited; patient is prepared for wound management on discharge.

PATIENT ASSESSMENT AND PREPARATION

Patient Assessment

- Monitor for signs and symptoms of wound infection, including the following:
  - ❖ Erythema
  - ❖ Edema
  - ❖ Increased pain
  - ❖ Elevated temperature and white blood cell count
  - ❖ Changes in wound drainage: amount, color, odor
  - ❖ Increased pressure or tenderness at wound site
  - ➤➤*Rationale:* Early detection of infection facilitates prompt and appropriate interventions.
- Assess patency of wound drainage system. ➤➤*Rationale:* Drains are frequently soft and pliable and thus can easily become kinked or blocked if wound drainage is fibrous in composition. Pouches with drainage systems may also become blocked with fibrous wound drainage; patency of the system is needed to ensure the wound drainage system moves exudate away from the wound.

Patient Preparation

- Verify correct patient with two identifiers. ➤➤*Rationale:* Prior to performing a procedure, the nurse should ensure the correct identification of the patient for the intended intervention.
- Ensure that patient understands preprocedural teachings. Answer questions as they arise, and reinforce information as needed. ➤➤*Rationale:* Understanding of previously taught information is evaluated and reinforced.
- Follow institutional standard for assessing pain. Administer analgesia as prescribed. ➤➤*Rationale:* Identifies need for pain interventions.
- Place patient in position of optimal comfort and visualization for dressing the wound. ➤➤*Rationale:* Positioning provides for effective wound visualization and enhances patient tolerance of procedure.
- Optimize lighting in room and provide privacy for patient. ➤➤*Rationale:* These measures allow for optimal wound assessment and patient comfort.

Procedure for Management of Wound Exudate with Drains and Pouches

Steps	Rationale	Special Considerations
Dressing Wounds with Drains		
1. **HH**		
2. **PE**		
3. Remove old dressing.	Maintains clean technique; Standard Precautions.	Use caution with dressing removal to ensure that drains are not dislodged.
4. Remove gloves. **HH**		
5. Establish sterile field.	Maintains sterile area for dressing supplies. Procedure for acute wounds should be completed with aseptic technique.	No evidence exists to support use of sterile technique when changing dressings on chronic wounds.
6. Clean and irrigate wound (see Procedure 126) as indicated.	Removes contaminated drainage and débris from wound.	Irrigation of wound drains should be performed only if indicated and only by physician or advanced practice nurse.[2,10]
7. Change gloves; open 4 × 4 gauze pads and apply on top of wound and around drains (Fig. 128-1). Avoid wrapping gauze around drain site.	Gauze absorbs drainage to keep underlying skin dry; wrapping gauze around drain may result in inadvertent drain removal with future dressing changes.	Drains are placed to remove excessive wound fluid. Apply a wound dressing capable of absorbing wound drainage and preventing moisture accumulation on surrounding healthy skin.[2,5]

Procedure continues on following page

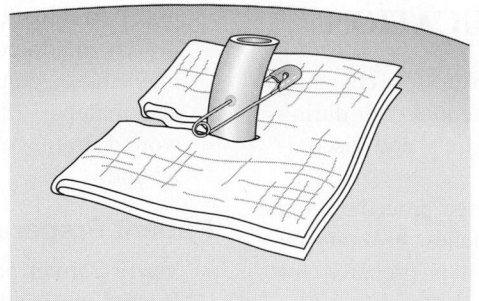

FIGURE 128-1   Dressing a wound with a drain.

Procedure for Management of Wound Exudate with Drains and Pouches—*Continued*

Steps	Rationale	Special Considerations
8. If necessary, apply secondary absorbent dressing (ABD; 4 × 4 gauze pads, foam dressings, etc.).	Secondary dressing absorbs drainage and protects clothing from drainage.	Wound exudate that leaks from edges or outer layer of dressing (strikethrough) creates a portal for bacteria to enter the wound. Dressings should be changed when they are 75% saturated or when strikethrough is present.[2,9]
9. Apply liquid skin barrier to periwound area and allow to dry. Apply hypoallergenic tape across the wound dressing extending approximately 2 inches beyond dressing onto skin. (**Level E***)	When tape is used to secure dressings, frequent dressing changes may result in skin irritation or disruption from the adhesive tape. Liquid skin barrier protects periwound tissue from the mechanical irritation of tape.[2,5] Hypoallergenic tape is less traumatic to noninjured skin; extend tape beyond dressing edges to anchor and secure dressing well.	Assess periwound edge for chemical and moisture irritation or skin breakdown from wound exudate.

Pouching a Wound with Exudate

Steps	Rationale	Special Considerations
1. **HH**		
2. **PE**		
3. If current drainage pouch has external opening, drain and measure content volume and discard.	Reduces transmission of microorganisms during dressing change; provides documentation of wound or fistula drainage.	Ensure that you have all needed supplies before removing old pouching system.
4. Gently remove old drainage pouch; support underlying skin with fingertips while drainage pouch is being removed; dispose of pouch.	Prevents tissue trauma to underlying skin.	A moist cloth may be applied to loosen edges of drainage pouch and assist with the removal process.
5. With wet gauze 4 × 4 pads, gently clean wound site from area of least contamination to greatest (see Procedure 126); clean and dry surrounding intact skin.	Maintains clean wound environment; surrounding skin should be free of moisture.	Inspect periwound skin for signs of maceration.
6. If ordered, irrigate wound or fistula (see Procedure 126) as ordered.	Cleans wound bed; decreases microorganism count.	

*Level E: Multiple case reports, theory-based evidence from expert opinions, or peer-reviewed professional organizational standards without clinical studies to support recommendations

Procedure for Management of Wound Exudate with Drains and Pouches—*Continued*

Steps	Rationale	Special Considerations
7. With wrapper from wound drainage pouch or wafer, create a template by drawing or measuring wound or fistula edge onto wrapper; cut out the center of the pattern on the wound skin barrier and drainage pouch (cut the pattern slightly larger than the tracing).	Irregular shapes and sizes of draining wounds are difficult to estimate; tracing wound onto wrapper allows for a better fit, with less potential for leaking on intact surrounding skin.	
8. Apply skin barrier (wafer, liquid, paste, sealant). **(Level E*)**	Assists in providing a good seal for the drainage pouch.[2,5]	A good seal is important to prevent moisture or wound exudate undermining the dressing and creating skin maceration.
9. Remove adhesive paper from drainage pouch; apply drainage pouch over wound, and with gentle, even pressure, secure pouch edges to skin barrier (Fig. 128-2).	Gentle, even pressure helps ensure a better seal from the drainage pouch to skin barrier; care must be taken to avoid development of wrinkles during pouch application; wrinkles in pouch barrier create a leak, and fluid is not contained within drainage pouch.[2,5]	If wrinkles are present, sealant paste may be added to drainage pouch edges to fill spaces created by wrinkles. Position pouch to maximize movement of exudate away from the wound. Carefully monitor wound management system for leaks. If leak develops, initiate wound management change. Trapped effluent can cause denudation within a short period of time.[12]

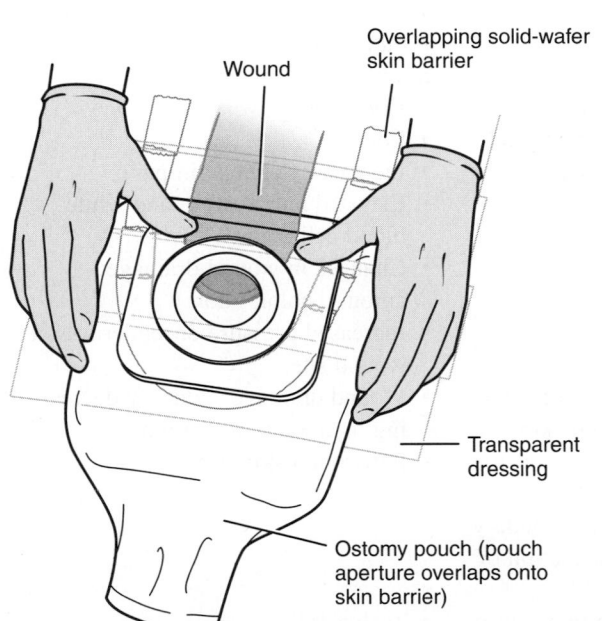

Wound

Overlapping solid-wafer skin barrier

Transparent dressing

Ostomy pouch (pouch aperture overlaps onto skin barrier)

FIGURE 128-2   Pouching a wound.

*Level E: Multiple case reports, theory-based evidence from expert opinions, or peer-reviewed professional organizational standards without clinical studies to support recommendations

Procedure continues on following page

Procedure for **Management of Wound Exudate with Drains and Pouches**—*Continued*

Steps	Rationale	Special Considerations
10. Close drainage pouch; wound exudate may be allowed to collect in pouch, or suction may be attached to end of pouch to pull fluid away from wound into a more distant collection container. **(Level D*)**	The type and amount of drainage coming from a wound determine whether or not suction is added to the drainage pouch.[1,2,5,9]	If suction is not used, empty the appliance regularly. Excessive exudate may create tension within the pouch, causing it to loosen the appliance.

Expected Outcomes

- Excessive exudate is removed from the wound bed
- Drains remain intact and patent
- Pouching system effectively collects and directs exudate away from wound bed
- Surrounding skin is dry and free of excessive wound drainage moisture (maceration)
- Wound drainage exit sites are clean and dry, without signs of infection or irritation
- Wound healing is enhanced because of effective wound drainage removal
- Wound drainage decreases in volume (over time) and is absent of foul odor or undesirable color

Unexpected Outcomes

- Wound drain becomes dislodged, blocked, or kinked
- Skin erosion or maceration occurs around wound edges
- Wound drain (if present) is dislodged during dressing or pouching procedure
- Wound is not healing efficiently because management of wound drainage is not effective
- Wound infection is suspected because of inadequate removal of wound drainage that allowed for bacterial growth

Patient Monitoring and Care

Steps	Rationale	Reportable Conditions
		These conditions should be reported if they persist despite nursing interventions.
1. Observe for signs of wound infection.	Drains assist with removal of excessive fluid but also provide a portal of entry of microorganisms.[5,9]	- Erythema - Edema - Increase or change in pain - Elevated temperature and white blood cell count - Changes in wound drainage: amount, color, odor - Increased pressure or tenderness at wound site
2. Assess for patency of wound drainage system and effective seal of pouching system.	Drains are frequently soft and pliable and thus can easily become kinked or blocked if wound drainage is fibrous in composition. Leakage from the pouch or secondary dressing may lead to maceration of the periwound skin.	- Wound drainage suddenly decreasing in amount or stopping - Periwound skin breakdown
3. Monitor amount of wound drainage relative to patient intake and output.	Excessive wound drainage may cause a fluid imbalance, necessitating intravenous or oral fluid replacements.	- Tachycardia - Hypotension - Oliguria - Increasing amounts of drainage

*Level D: Peer-reviewed professional organizational standards with clinical studies to support recommendations

Patient Monitoring and Care —*Continued*

Steps	Rationale	Reportable Conditions
4. Monitor caloric and protein intake in the presence of heavily draining wounds. Initiate a nutritional consult as needed.	Excessive wound drainage may result in the loss of 100 g of protein a day. Adequate protein needs to be replaced for wound healing.[2,9] Nutritional consult to replace protein loss from wound exudates may be indicated.	• Laboratory analysis suggestive of hypoalbuminemia
5. Follow institutional standard for assessing pain. Administer analgesia as prescribed.	Identifies need for pain interventions.	• Continued pain despite pain interventions

Documentation

Documentation should include the following:
• Patient and family education
• Premedication given, patient tolerance of procedure, and response to pain medication
• Wound cleansing, irrigation (if performed), and dressing change completed, with date and time

• Description of wound bed, drains, pouch, (suction if applied), surrounding skin, and characteristics of wound exudate (color, amount, odor)
• Dressing applied
• Unexpected outcomes
• Nursing interventions

References

1. Ayello EA: The TIME principles of wound bed preparation, *Adv Skin Wound Care* 22(Suppl 1):2-5, 2009.
2. Bates-Jensen BM, Ovington L: Management of exudate and infection. In Sussman C, Bates-Jensen BM, editors: *Wound care: a collaborative practice manual*, ed 3, Philadelphia, 2007, Lippincott Williams & Wilkins, 215-233.
3. Bates-Jensen BM, Seaman S: Management of malignant cutaneous wounds and fistulas. In Sussman C, Bates-Jensen BM, editors: *Wound care: a collaborative practice manual*, ed 3, Philadelphia, 2007, Lippincott Williams & Wilkins, 476-494.
4. Bovill E, et al: Topical negative pressure wound therapy: a review of its role and guidelines for its use in the management of acute wounds, *Int Wound J* 65(3): 722-731, 2008.
5. Bryant RA, Rolstad BS: Management of drain sites and fistulas. In Bryant RA, Nix DP, editors: *Acute & chronic wounds: current management concepts*, ed 3, Philadelphia, 2007, Mosby, 490-516.
6. Gray M, Weir D: Prevention and treatment of moisture-associated skin damage (maceration) in the periwound skin, *J Wound Ostomy Continence Nurs* 34(2):153-157, 2007.
CR 7. Hanson D, et al: Understanding wound fluid and the phases of healing, *Adv Skin Wound Care* 18(1):360-362, 2005.

8. Naude L: Exudate management: putting the patient first, *Pro Nurs Today* 12(5):29-32, 2008.
9. Nix DP: Patient assessment and evaluation of healing. In Bryant RA, Nix DP, editors: *Acute & chronic wounds: current management concepts*, ed 3, Philadelphia, 2007, Mosby.
CR 10. Ovington LG: Dealing with drainage: the what, why, and how of wound exudates, *Home Healthcare Nurse* 20:368-374, 2002.
11. Rolstad BS, Ovington LG: Principles of wound management. In Bryant RA, Nix DP, editors: *Acute & chronic wounds: current management concepts*, ed 3, Philadelphia, 2007, Mosby, 391-426.
12. Brindle CT, Blankenship J: Management of complex abdominal wounds with small bowel fistulae; isolation techniques and exudate control to improve outcomes, *J Wound Ostomy Continence Nurs* 36(4):396-404, 2009.

Additional Readings

Hocevar BJ, et al: Management of fistula in the abdominal region, *J Wound Ostomy Continence Nursing* 35(4): 417-423, 2008.
Skovgaard R, Keiding H: A cost-effectiveness analysis of fistula treatment in the abdominal region using a new integrated fistula and wound management system, *J Wound Ostomy Continence Nursing* 35(6):592-595, 2008.
Trevillion N: Cleaning wounds with saline or tap water, *Emerg Nurse* 16(2):24-26, 2008.

Drain Removal

P U R P O S E : Drain removal is performed when the drain is no longer needed for wound management.

Mary Beth Flynn Makic

PREREQUISITE NURSING KNOWLEDGE

- Goals of wound care should be clearly outlined so that proper wound care products are used after drain removal. The wound care products selected are based on the size, location, and care of the wound bed needs and include continued moisture management.
- Continue to monitor the wound bed after drain removal; mark dressing for presence of leakage after drain removal and continue to monitor.
- Apply appropriate dressing after drain removal. Coarse gauze absorbs wound fluid but may adhere to wound bed; calcium alginates, foams, and hydrofiber dressings enhance wound absorption; hydrogels provide moisture to nondraining wounds; hydrocolloids provide wound moisture with minimal absorption; and film dressings are for nonexudating wounds.[3-7]
- Drains are placed in wounds to facilitate healing by providing an exit for excessive fluid accumulation in or near the wound bed. Drains may be removed when drainage is considered to be minimal.[1,7]
- Type of drain, location, and how the drain is secured should be known before drain removal. Competence should be demonstrated by the clinician performing drain removal because significant tissue injury may result from an improperly removed drain.[1] With drain removal, never force removal of the drain. If resistance is felt, stop and notify healthcare provider.
- Common surgically placed wound drains include Hemovac (Zimmer Inc., Warsaw, IN), bulb suction drain (e.g. Jackson-Pratt or JP drain), and Penrose. Negative-pressure wound therapy devices may also be placed to assist with wound drainage.[2]

EQUIPMENT

- Nonsterile gloves
- Personal protective equipment (e.g., gowns and face protection)
- Sterile gauze 4 × 4 pads
- Dressing for exit site based on characteristics of wound
- Suture removal kit or sterile scissors
- Hypoallergenic tape

PATIENT AND FAMILY EDUCATION

- Explain the procedure and reason for drain removal. ➼*Rationale:* Patient anxiety and discomfort are decreased.
- Discuss patient's role in drain removal. ➼*Rationale:* Patient cooperation is elicited; patient is prepared for wound management on discharge.
- Provide patient education regarding monitoring wound for drainage. ➼*Rationale:* Patient is engaged in care of the wound site in preparation of discharge.

PATIENT ASSESSMENT AND PREPARATION

Patient Assessment

- Signs of wound infection at drain site include:
  - ❖ Change in the amount, odor, or characteristics of wound drainage
  - ❖ Erythema
  - ❖ Pain
  - ❖ Elevated temperature
  - ❖ Elevated white blood count
  - ❖ Foul drainage from exit site
  - ❖ Pressure or tenderness at drain exit site

➥*Rationale:* Drains are placed to remove excessive wound fluid and decrease the risk for infection. Changes in wound drainage may indicate presence of infection; early detection of infection facilitates prompt and appropriate interventions.

Patient Preparation

• Ensure that patient understands preprocedural teachings. Answer questions as they arise, and reinforce information as needed. ➥*Rationale:* Understanding of previously taught information is evaluated and rein forced.

• Premedicate patient with prescribed analgesic, if needed. ➥*Rationale:* Patients may not need premedication for drain removal; however, the patient's pain and need for analgesia should be assessed before the procedure and treated appropriately.

• Optimize lighting in room and provide privacy for patient. ➥*Rationale:* These measures allow for optimal assessment and patient comfort.

Procedure for Drain Removal

Steps	Rationale	Special Considerations
1. **HH**		
2. **PE**		
2. Open sterile scissors; cut any sutures, if present.	Releases drain from tissue suture anchors.	
3. Open gauze 4 × 4; place gauze close to drain skin exit site; instruct patient to take a deep, easy breath; withdraw drain swiftly and evenly. **(Level D*)**	Gauze is used to capture body fluids as the drain is removed. Deep breathing may decrease the pain the patient feels with drain removal.[6,7]	Do not force removal of drain. If resistance is felt, stop and notify healthcare provider.
4. Place sterile dressing over drain exit site and secure with tape.	Provides protection of open wound site; prevents entrance of microorganisms.	Monitor dressing for wound drainage.
5. Discard materials, drain, and personal protective equipment in appropriate receptacle.	Maintains infection control practices and decreases contamination; Standard Precautions.	
6. Perform hand hygiene.	Maintains infection control practices and decreases contamination; Standard Precautions.	

Expected Outcomes

• Intact drain is removed without resistance
• Wound drainage is minimal from exit site
• Drain exit site is free of signs of fluid accumulation, inflammation, or infection
• Wound healing continues to progress without presence of excessive wound fluid

Unexpected Outcomes

• Resistance is felt on drain removal, creating tissue trauma beneath skin surface
• Wound fluid accumulates beneath skin and drain exit site[1]
• Infection or inflammation occurs at drain exit site
• Poor approximation of skin edges occurs at drain exit site, requiring wound healing by secondary intention
• A portion of the drain remains in the wound tract

Patient Monitoring and Care

Steps	Rationale	Reportable Conditions
		These conditions should be reported if they persist despite nursing interventions.
1. Assess for presence of drainage from drain exit site.	Drainage should be minimal and cease within 24 hours. Continued drainage from drain exit site may indicate accumulation of wound fluid beneath the skin that needs to be evacuated.	• Continued drainage • Edema or pain at drain exit site

*Level D: Peer-reviewed, professional organizational standards with clinical studies to support recommendations

Procedure continues on following page

Procedure for Drain Removal—*Continued*

Steps	Rationale	Special Considerations
2. Monitor for signs of infection.	Drains are placed to remove excessive wound fluid and to decrease risk for infection.	• Erythema • Pain • Elevated temperature and white blood cell count • Change in wound drainage amount, color, odor • Pressure or tenderness at drain exit site
3. Follow institutional standard for assessing pain. Administer analgesia as prescribed.	Identifies need for pain interventions.	• Continued pain despite pain interventions

Documentation

Documentation should include the following:

- Patient and family education
- Type of drain removed, placement, date, time, and condition of the drain (i.e., intact drain)
- Amount of wound drainage documented in the last 24 hours before drain removal
- Premedication given, patient tolerance of procedure, and response to pain medication
- Type of dressing applied after drain removal
- Appearance of exit site
- Unexpected outcomes (i.e., resistance, nonintact drain on removal)
- Pain assessment, interventions, and effectiveness
- Nursing interventions

References

1. Bates-Jensen B, Woolfolk N: Acute surgical wound management. In Sussman C, Bates-Jensen B, editors: *Wound care: a collaborative practice manual for health professionals,* ed 3, Philadelphia, 2007, Lippincott Williams & Wilkins, 323-335.
2. Bovill E, Banwell PE, Teot L, et al: Topical negative pressure wound therapy: a review of its role and guidelines for its use in the management of acute wounds, *Int Wound J* 10:1-19, 2008.
3. Fleck CA: Wound assessment parameters and dressing selection, *Adv Skin Wound Care* 19:364-370, 2006.
4. Gray M, Wier D: Prevention and treatment of moisture-associated skin damage (maceration) in the periwound skin, *JWOCN* 43:153-157, 2007.
5. Sussman G: Management of the wound environment with dressings and topical agents. In Sussman C, Bates-Jensen B, editors: *Wound care: a collaborative practice manual for health professionals*, ed 3, Philadelphia, 2007, Lippincott Williams & Wilkins, 250-267.
6. Vuolo JC: Assessment and management of surgical wounds in clinical practice, *Nurs Stand* 20:46-56, 2006.
7. Walker J: Patient preparation for safe removal of surgical drains, *Nurs Stand* 21:39-41, 2007.

Additional Readings

Fleck CA: Managing wound pain, *Adv Skin Wound Care* 20:138-144, 2007.
CR Ovington LG: Dealing with drainage, *Home Healthcare Nurse* 20:368-375, 2002.
Trevillion N: Cleaning wounds with saline or tap water, *Emerg Nurse* 16:24-26, 2008.

Fecal Containment Devices and Bowel Management System

P U R P O S E : Fecal containment devices and bowel management systems may be used to divert liquid fecal matter associated with acute diarrhea. Containment of feces may assist with the prevention or treatment of incontinence-associated dermatitis, prevention of pressure ulcers, and contamination of perineal wounds.

Mary Beth Flynn Makic

PREREQUISITE NURSING KNOWLEDGE

- Critically ill patients have multiple risk factors that increase the chance of pressure ulcer development. A valid and reliable pressure ulcer risk assessment tool should be used to assess a patient's risk on admission and consistently throughout the hospitalization.[1]
- Patients with fecal incontinence and immobility are considered to be at increased risk of pressure ulcers.[13,17,20]
- Acutely ill patients are at high risk of fecal incontinence related to administration of a variety of mediations (i.e., antimicrobial, cardiovascular, central nervous system [CNS], and gastrointestinal agents),[19] enteral feeding,[2,22] disease processes (e.g., gastrointestinal, hepatic disease, spinal cord trauma, etc.), and enterotoxins (e.g., *Clostridium difficile*).[2]
- Personal protective equipment should be used when the source of the diarrhea is not identified, to avoid the possible spread of highly infectious organisms.
- Urinary and fecal incontinence results in skin breakdown.[5,6,8,22] Excessive moisture changes the skin's protective pH and increases the permeability of the skin, decreasing its protective function. Fecal content is more irritating than urine because digestive enzymes in feces contribute to erosion of skin.[13]
- Perineal skin damage may progress rapidly and ranges in severity, presenting with erythema, edema, weeping,

denuded skin, and pain.[8,9,13,16,23] Other negative outcomes may include skin ulceration and secondary infection, including bacterial *(Staphylococcus)* and yeast *(Candida albicans)* infections that increase discomfort and treatment costs.[8,13,15,16]
- Incontinence-associated dermatitis (IAD) is inflammation of the skin that occurs when urine or stool comes into contact with perineal or perigenital skin.[9] IAD is the clinical term used to describe incontinence-associated skin damage. IAD often occurs in conjunction with pressure and shear and friction forces that precipitate pressure ulcers.[9]
- It is well established that excessive moisture and incontinence, especially fecal incontinence, significantly increases the patient's risk of IAD and pressure ulcers; the research to guide fecal containment practice is limited.[1-3,6,9,14,17,22]
- Management of fecal incontinence should include the following elements:
  - ❖ Identification and treatment of the diarrhea. If the source of fecal incontinence cannot be eliminated, drug therapy may be used; however, the efficacy of these drugs is not known because randomized studies have focused on the management of chronic diarrhea in outpatients rather than acute diarrhea in hospitalized patients.[22]
  - ❖ Meticulous perineal skin care. Maintain clean, healthy skin by cleansing the skin with a pH-balanced no-rinse

skin cleansing solution after each episode of diarrhea. Avoid soap and water. Most soaps are alkaline, and the skin's pH is acidic (5.0 to 6.5); use of soap and water to cleanse the skin can further disrupt the skin's protective properties.[7]

❖ Apply a moisturizer with skin protectant. Moisturizers help hydrate intact skin, replace oils in the skin, and soothe skin irritation. Moisturizers that contain petrolatum, lanolin, dimethicone, or zinc can provide a protective barrier to protect and sooth denuded area.[8,10]

❖ Use absorbent underpads that wick effluent away from the skin and allow for circulation of air between the patient's skin and support surface. Avoid use of adult briefs and diapers that trap the moisture against the skin. Change underpads frequently.[16]

❖ Consider application of a fecal containment device or bowel management system.

• An external fecal containment device adheres directly to the perianal skin, moving feces away from the skin and into a drainage container. The device can remain in place for 1 to 2 days without leaking.[18] If the device is well adhered and not leaking, it may remain in place longer if clinically indicated. Care must be taken during removal of the device to prevent skin trauma or tears.

• The general agreement in the literature is that the perianal incontinence pouch offers many advantages over diapers and balloon rectal catheters and is the least invasive method of fecal containment.[11]

• Some authors have recommended short-term management of fecal incontinence with devices intended for other purposes.[14,16,22] Grogan and Kramer[11] studied the use of a nasopharyngeal trumpet inserted into the rectum and then connected to a drainage bag as an effective means to contain fecal material.

• Little research has been conducted to explore or recommend the use of a mushroom catheter with a soft flared tip or balloon-tipped catheter to divert stool.[21,22] Correct application of these products is important to prevent trauma to the rectum and internal structures. Adaptation of a device for an unapproved use may be associated with patient injury and concerns of increased liability if a problem arises.[22] The clinician should use US Food and Drug Administration (FDA)–approved fecal containment systems rather than adapting devices for management of liquid feces.

• Bowel management systems (BMS) are FDA-approved devices that may be inserted into the rectal vault for up to 29 days for the diversion of stool into a collection pouch (Figs. 130-1 and 130-2). Early research suggests the device does not harm the rectal mucosa but successfully diverts feces, allowing for perineal skin protection and healing.[3,6,14]

❖ Manufacturer-specific contraindications for BMS include allergies to product components; children; adults with strictured anal canals; and patients with impactions or recent rectal surgery (less than 6 weeks), severe hemorrhoids, localized inflammatory

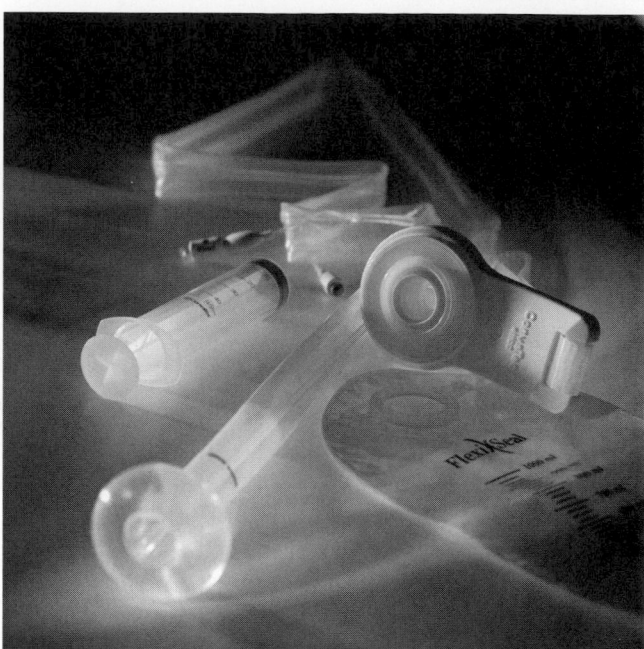

FIGURE 130-1   Flexi-Seal FMS, ConvaTec, Skillman, NJ. *(Copyright © 1996, 2010 Covidien. All rights reserved. Used with the permission of Covidien.)*

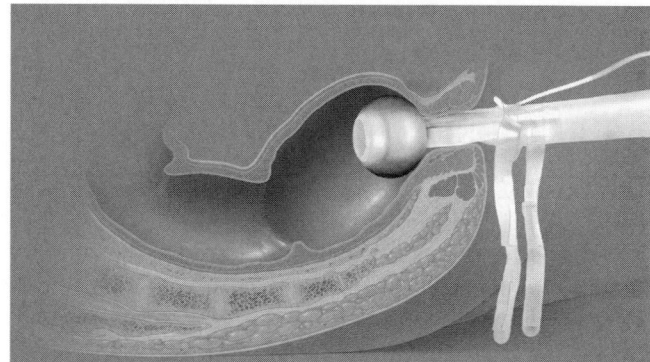

FIGURE 130-2   ActiFlow Indwelling Bowel Catheter. *(Courtesy of Hollister, Inc., Libertyville, IL.)*

process or disease, or an incompetent rectal sphincter.[4,12]

❖ The BMS may be inserted to manage existing diarrhea or provide fecal diversion away from existing wounds; however, the stool should be liquid or semiliquid.

❖ Use with caution in patients on anticoagulation therapy or with rectal varices, inflammatory bowel disease, low platelet count, or high international normalized ratio (INR).

• If blood is present in the rectum, ensure there is no evidence of pressure necrosis from the device. Discontinuation of use of the device is recommended if evident. Notify physician for any signs of bleeding.

- Avoid use of ointments or lubricants with petroleum base because they may compromise the integrity of the BMS device.[4,12]
- Transient fecal incontinence and diarrhea are common among hospitalized patients. Goals of a bowel management program should be clearly discussed among all healthcare providers, patient, and family. Goals should include treatment of the cause of the fecal incontinence if possible and prevention of perineal tissue injury and may not require a containment device.

EQUIPMENT

- Nonsterile gloves
- Personal protective equipment (e.g., gowns and face protection)
- Sterile water (or normal saline solution)
- Water-soluble lubricant
- Bowel management system
- Underpads
- Skin cleansing solution

PATIENT AND FAMILY EDUCATION

- Explain the procedure and rationale for insertion of a BMS. ➻*Rationale:* Patient anxiety and discomfort are decreased.
- Discuss goals of bowel management program and expected benefits of the intervention. ➻*Rationale:* The patient is prepared for placement of the BMS, possible odors, and perineal skin and wound care interventions.

PATIENT ASSESSMENT AND PREPARATION

Patient Assessment

- Review medical record and discuss medical history with patient for possible contraindications before placement of BMS. ➻*Rationale:* Possible complications associated with placement of device are avoided.
- Evaluate consistency of fecal contents; contents should be liquid to semiliquid to flow through the BMS. ➻*Rationale:* Liquid fecal consistency is important to prevent occlusion of the device.[3]
- Assess perineal skin for presence of open areas and pressure ulcers and apply moisture barrier creams. ➻*Rationale:* BMS may be used to prevent and treat IAD, and additional skin care products may be indicated to assist in perineal skin healing.[22]
- Evaluate the patient need for analgesia or sedation. ➻*Rationale:* Patient may tolerate procedure more comfortably.

Patient Preparation

- Ensure that patient understands preprocedural teachings. Answer questions as they arise, and reinforce information as needed. ➻*Rationale:* Understanding of previously taught information is evaluated and reinforced.
- Optimize lighting in room and provide privacy for patient. ➻*Rationale:* These measures allow for optimal assessment and patient comfort.
- Place patient in a left lateral position or position of optimal comfort and visualization for anus and rectum. ➻*Rationale:* Positioning provides for effective visualization and enhances patient tolerance of procedure.[3]

Procedure	**for Fecal Containment Device and Bowel Management System (BMS)**	
Steps	Rationale	Special Considerations
Fecal containment devices are commercially available. General principles for placement of the device are consistent between systems; however, the healthcare provider should read and follow manufacturer-specific guidelines for placement of device. Procedure may be most effectively performed with two healthcare providers.		
Fecal Containment Device		
1. [HH]		
2. [PE]		
3. Position patient in left lateral position with upper knee slightly flexed. **(Level D*)**	Assists with visualization and comfort of the patient for placement.[3]	
4. Cleans perineal area with no-rinse cleansing solution. Allow skin to dry thoroughly. **(Level D)**	Evaluate skin for presence of breakdown. Fecal containment device adheres better to dry skin.[2,6]	Do not apply device if perineal skin is not intact.[22]

*Level D: Peer-reviewed professional organizational standards with clinical studies to support recommendations

Procedure continues on following page

Procedure **for Fecal Containment Device and Bowel Management System (BMS)**—*Continued*

Steps	Rationale	Special Considerations
5. Working together, one healthcare provider should separate buttocks and the other healthcare provider should apply a no-sting/nonirritating skin protectant barrier solution; allow it to dry. **(Level D*)**	Application of containment device usually requires a pair of experienced healthcare providers to correctly position the patient and apply the device correctly.[18,22]	Avoid use of adhesive products that can cause discomfort or irritation to delicate perineal tissue.
6. Remove protective wrap and firmly apply fecal containment device around the anus; hold contact in place for approximately 1 minute.	Firm pressure and body heat allows the adhesive backing of the fecal containment device to adhere more effectively to the skin.	Opening of fecal containment device may need to be adjusted by healthcare provider to fit comfortably yet snuggly around the anal opening.
7. Attach collection bag to distal opening of the fecal containment device and place in a dependent position.	Collection device moves fecal material away from the skin.	
8. Monitor the volume, consistency, and color of fecal material. Fecal output needs to be evaluated as part of the patient's overall output assessment.	If diarrhea is excessive, fluids and electrolytes may be lost in the feces, resulting in dehydration and electrolyte imbalances.	
9. Change fecal containment device if leaking is noted or if stool is too thick to pass through device; if diarrhea has resolved, discontinue use.	Adequate seal is necessary for effective performance of the fecal containment device and protection of perineal skin.	Gently remove fecal containment device to avoid tearing skin. Use a nonirritating, no-sting adhesive remover to assist with removal of device.
10. Discard used supplies, remove gloves, and perform hand hygiene.	Maintains infection control practices and decreases contamination.	

Several systems are commercially available. General principles for placement of the device are consistent between systems; however, the healthcare provider should read and follow manufacturer-specific guidelines for placement of device.

Bowel Management System (BMS)
1. **HH**
2. **PE**

3. Administer prescribed analgesia or sedation agents if ordered.	May assist patient tolerance of procedure.	
4. Position patient in left lateral position with upper knee slightly flexed. **(Level D*)**	Assists with visualization and comfort of the patient for placement.[3]	
5. Apply water-soluble lubricant to a gloved finger and perform a manual digital rectal examination. **(Level D)**	Evaluates rectal vault for impacted stool.[3,14]	Perform digital disimpaction before continuing with placement of BMS.
6. Clean perineal area with no-rinse cleansing solution.	Evaluates skin for presence of breakdown and allows for better visualization.	
7. Open BMS kit and connect pieces according to manufacturer's instructions **(Level M*)**.	Functionality of the device should be assessed before placement.[4,12]	

*Level D: Peer-reviewed professional organizational standards with clinical studies to support recommendations
*Level M: Manufacturer's recommendations only

Procedure for Fecal Containment Device and Bowel Management System (BMS)—*Continued*

Steps	Rationale	Special Considerations
8. Apply water-soluble lubricant to the distal end of the BMS. With slow gentle pressure, advance the balloon through the anal sphincter.	Lubricant assists with insertion of the device gently through the anus and into the rectal vault.	Do not advance BMS if resistance is felt.
9. Inflate BMS balloon with water or normal saline solution per instruction guidelines.	Water or normal saline solution may be used to inflate the balloon and hold device in place.	Manufacturer may include prepackaged syringes. Do not exceed the manufacturer's recommended volume amount for balloon inflation. Additional fluid volume in the balloon can increase the amount of pressure on intestinal mucosa.
10. Gently pull the BMS back to ensure the balloon is in the rectum and positioned against the rectal floor (Fig. 130-3).	Device should rest on the rectal floor to collect fecal material and provide seal.	Some BMS manufacturers have a position indicator noted on the drainage tubing that should be visible after insertion.
11. Position the drainage bag in a dependent position.	Allows for effective flow of fecal material.	
12. Evaluate consistency of fecal material. Stool should be liquid to semiliquid. The BMS may be irrigated with water as necessary to ensure patency.[4,12] **(Level M*)**	Allows for effective flow of fecal material.	Slight leakage or smear of feces is often unavoidable. Do not exceed manufacturer's recommendations for fluid volume in the balloon.
13. Discard used supplies, remove protective equipment and gloves, and perform hand hygiene.	Maintains infection control practices.	

Expected Outcomes

- Containment of liquid feces
- Perineal skin remains intact or, if compromised before placement of BMS, healing of skin is evident
- Input and output balance are maintained

Unexpected Outcomes

- Injury to anal sphincter or rectal vault
- Fluid and electrolyte imbalances
- Infection
- Pressure necrosis
- Loss of sphincter tone

Patient Monitoring and Care

Steps	Rationale	Reportable Conditions
		These conditions should be reported if they persist despite nursing interventions.
1. Assess patient, perineal skin, and fecal drainage. **(Level C*)**	Continued assessment of patient IAD and possible development of pressure ulcers is essential because they may prolong the patient's hospitalization.[2,5,15,17]	• Foul drainage or odor • Worsening erythema and edema • Pain • Elevated temperature • Elevated white blood cell count

*Level C: Qualitative studies, descriptive or correlational studies, integrative reviews, systematic reviews, or randomized controlled trials with inconsistent results
*Level M: Manufacturer's recommendations only

Procedure continues on following page

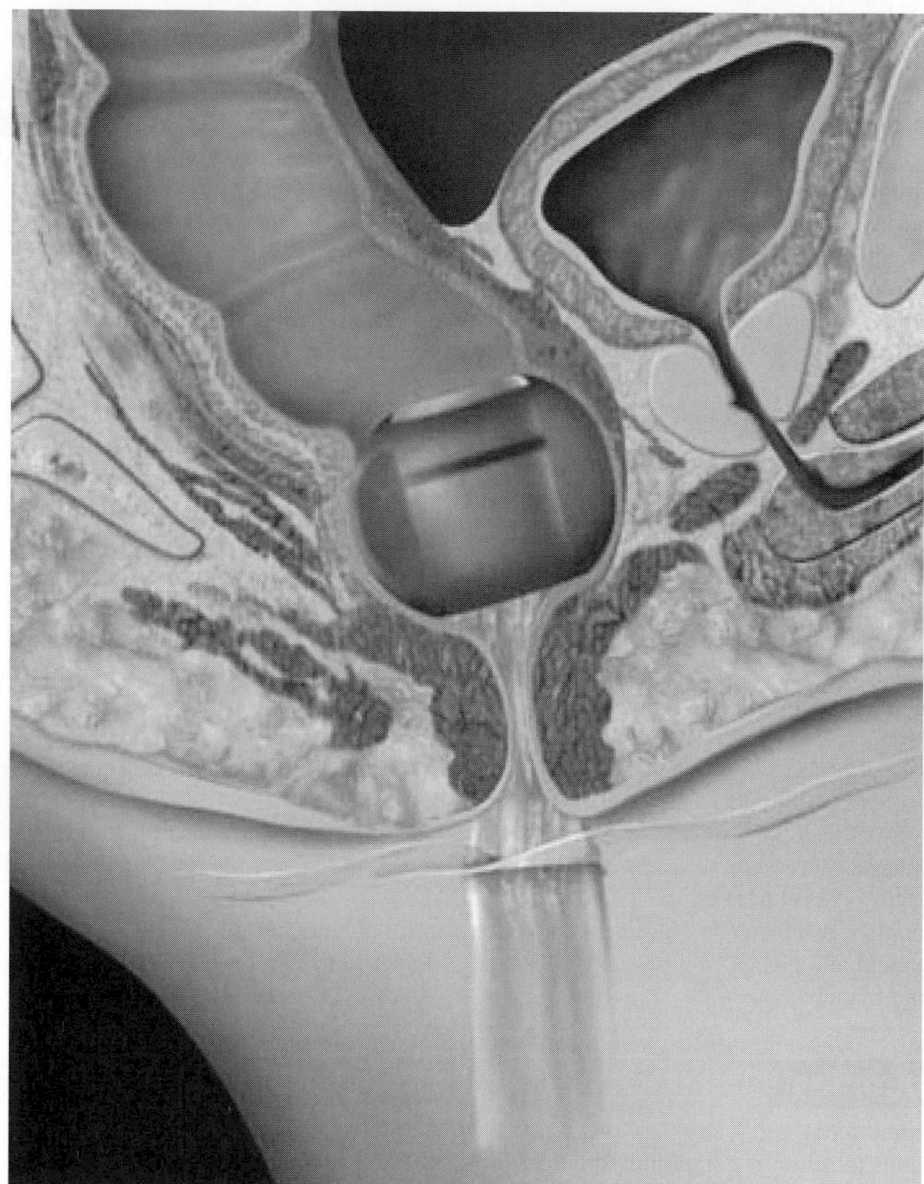

FIGURE 130-3   Correct placement of a bowel management system in the rectum. *(Courtesy of Hollister, Inc., Libertyville, IL.)*

Patient Monitoring and Care —*Continued*

Steps	Rationale	Reportable Conditions
2. Monitor fluid and electrolyte balances.	If diarrhea is excessive, fluids and electrolytes may be lost in the feces, resulting in dehydration and electrolyte imbalances.	• Output greater than input • Abnormal electrolyte laboratory analysis • Signs and symptoms of electrolyte imbalances (i.e., cardiac ectopy, neuromuscular symptoms, etc), tachycardia, decreased urine output, thirst, signs and symptoms of dehydration
3. Evaluate amount and consistency of fecal drainage.	Migration of catheter or change in fecal consistency may indicate obstruction or occlusion of BMS.	• Sudden change in amount of fecal drainage or consistency

Patient Monitoring and Care —*Continued*

Steps	Rationale	Reportable Conditions
4. Follow institution standard for assessing pain. Administer analgesia as prescribed.	Identifies need for pain interventions.	• Continued pain despite pain interventions

Documentation

Documentation should include the following:

- Patient and family education
- Description of perineal skin condition
- Patency of BMS
- Description and volume of feces
- Patient tolerance of procedure
- Progression of perineal wound healing
- Unexpected outcomes
- Pain assessment, interventions, and effectiveness

References

1. Ayello EA, Lyder CH: Protecting patients from harm: preventing pressure ulcers in hospital patients, *Nursing* 37:36-40, 2007.
2. Beitz JM: Fecal incontinence in acutely and critically ill patients: options in management, *Ostomy Wound Manage* 52:56-66, 2006.
3. Benoit RA, Watts C: The effect of a pressure ulcer prevention program and the bowel management system in reducing pressure ulcer prevalence in an ICU setting, *JWOCN* 34:163-175, 2007.
4. ConvaTec: *Flexi-Seal™ fecal management system,* retrieved December 12, 2008, from www.convaTec.com.
5. Doughty DB: Prevention and early detection of pressure ulcers in hospitalized patients, *JWOCN* 35:76-78, 2008.
6. Echols J, Friedman BC, Mullins RF, et al: Clinical utility and economic impact of introducing a bowel management system, *JWOCN* 34:664-670, 2007.
CR 7. Faria DT, Shwayder T, Krull EA: Perineal skin injury: extrinsic environmental risk factors, *Ostomy Wound Manage* 42:28-37, 1996.
8. Gray M: Incontinence-related skin damage: essential knowledge, *Ostomy Wound Manage* 53:28-31, 2007.
9. Gray M, Bliss DZ, Doughty DB, et al: Incontinence-associated dermatitis: a consensus, *JWOCN* 34:45-54, 2007.
10. Gray M, Bohacek L, Weir D, et al: Moisture vs pressure: making sense out of perineal wounds, *JWOCN* 43:134-142, 2007.
CR 11. Grogan T, Kramer D: The rectal trumpet: use of a nasopharyngeal airway to contain fecal incontinence in critically ill patients, *JWOCN* 29(1):193-201, 2002.
12. Hollister Incorporated: *Zassi™ bowel management system,* retrieved December 12, 2008, from www.holister.com.
13. Junkin J, Selekof JL: Prevalence of incontinence and associated skin injury in the acute care inpatient, *JWOCN* 34:260-269, 2007.
14. Keshava A, Renwick A, Stewart P, et al: A nonsurgical means of fecal diversion: the Zassi Bowel Management System, *Dis Colon Rectum* 50:1017-1022, 2007.

15. Newman DK: Double taboos: urinary and fecal incontinence: the state of the science, *Ostomy Wound Manage* 53:6-7, 2007.
16. Nix D: Prevedntion and treatment of perineal skin breakdown due to incontinence, *Ostomy Wound Manage* 52:26-28, 2006.
17. Padula CA, Osborne E, Williams J: Prevention and early detection of pressure ulcers in hospitalized patients, *JWOCN* 35:65-75, 2008.
CR 18. Palmieri B, Benuzzi, Bellini N: The anal bag: a modern approach to fecal incontinence management, *Ostomy Wound Manage* 51:44-52, 2005.
19. Roach M, Christie JA: Fecal incontinence in the elderly, *Geriatrics* 63:13-22, 2008.
20. Vollman KM: Ventilator-associated pneumonia and pressure ulcer prevention as targets for quality improvement in the ICU, *Crit Care Nurs Clin North Am* 18:453-467, 2006.
CR 21. Watterworth B, Ryzeuski J: Managing fecal incontinence, *JWOCN* 32:217-218, 2005.
22. Wishin J, Gallagher TJ, McCann E: Emerging options for the management of fecal incontinence in hospitalized patients, *JWOCN* 35:104-110, 2008.
23. Zulkowski K: Perineal dermatitis versus pressure ulcer: distinguishing characteristics, *Adv Skin Wound Care* 21:382-388, 2008.

Additional Readings

CR Bliss DZ, Stuart J, Savik K, et al: Fecal incontinence in hospitalized patients who are acutely ill, *Nurs Res* 49:101-108, 2000.
CR Gray M, Ratliff C, Donovan A: Perineal skin care for the incontinent patient, *Adv Skin Wound Care* 15:170-177, 2002.
Leandefel CS, Bowers BJ, Feld AD, et al: National Institutes of Health State-of-Science Conference Statement: prevention of fecal and urinary incontinence in adults, *Ann Intern Med* 148:449-460, 2008.

Negative-Pressure Wound Therapy

P U R P O S E :   The purpose of negative-pressure wound therapy is to apply controlled subatmospheric (negative) pressure to the wound bed for stimulation of granulation tissue and edema reduction, and thus, enhancement of wound healing.

Paula Gipp

PREREQUISITE NURSING KNOWLEDGE

- Negative-pressure wound therapy (NPWT) is an advanced wound care therapy that uses an occlusive wound dressing, tubing, and powered vacuum unit with a collection canister. Other terms found in the literature for NPWT include topical negative therapy (TPN) and subatmospheric pressure therapy.
- Many different U.S. Food and Drug Administration (FDA)–approved vacuum units are on the market for NPWT.[10] The Agency for Healthcare Research and Quality (AHRQ) provides a review of current NPWT manufacturers.[11] The most common devices seen in the acute care practice setting are ActiV.A.C.® and InfoV.A.C. Therapy Systems (KCI Licensing, Inc., San Antonio, TX; Fig. 131-1) and RENASYS EZ® (Smith & Nephew, St. Petersburg, FL[8]; Fig. 131-2). ActiV.A.C.® and Info V.A.C.®[12] use a patented open-cell foam wound contact dressing, and RENASYS EZ®[6] (and other newly developing units on the market) uses either an open-cell foam or the vacuum-pack method with an antimicrobial gauze packing dressing. The use of moistened gauze wound interface has also been reported in the literature as an effective dressing for NPWT.[7]
- Most randomized controlled studies and case studies on NPWT have been conducted with the V.A.C. therapy. No randomized controlled trials are found that compare the effectiveness of various NPWT techniques or systems.[11] Further clinical research to evaluate wound closure outcomes with the different NPWT units is needed.[5,8,10,11]

- NPWT assists with wound closure by applying a controlled subatmospheric (negative) pressure evenly over a wound bed. This mechanical stress creates a noncompressive force on the wound bed that dilates the arterioles, increasing the effectiveness of local circulation and enhancing the proliferation of granulation tissue.[1,4,5] NPWT enhances lymphatic flow and removal of excessive fluid, decreasing wound edema and bacterial load at the wound site, further aiding wound healing (Fig. 131-3).[1,2,4,5,9,10]
- Wound healing is best achieved through adequate cleansing, débridement, and dressing of the wound bed on the basis of patient and wound characteristics.

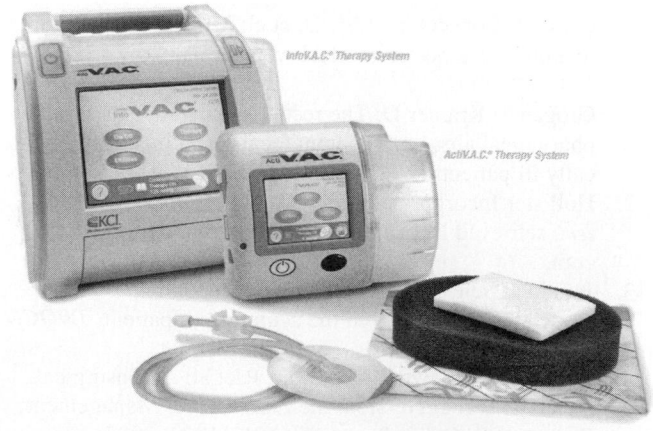

*Compared to V.A.C. ATS® Therapy System

FIGURE 131-1   Components of the Vacuum-Assisted Closure System: ActiV.A.C.® and InfoV.A.C.® Therapy Systems. *(Courtesy of KCI Licensing, Inc. 2009.)*

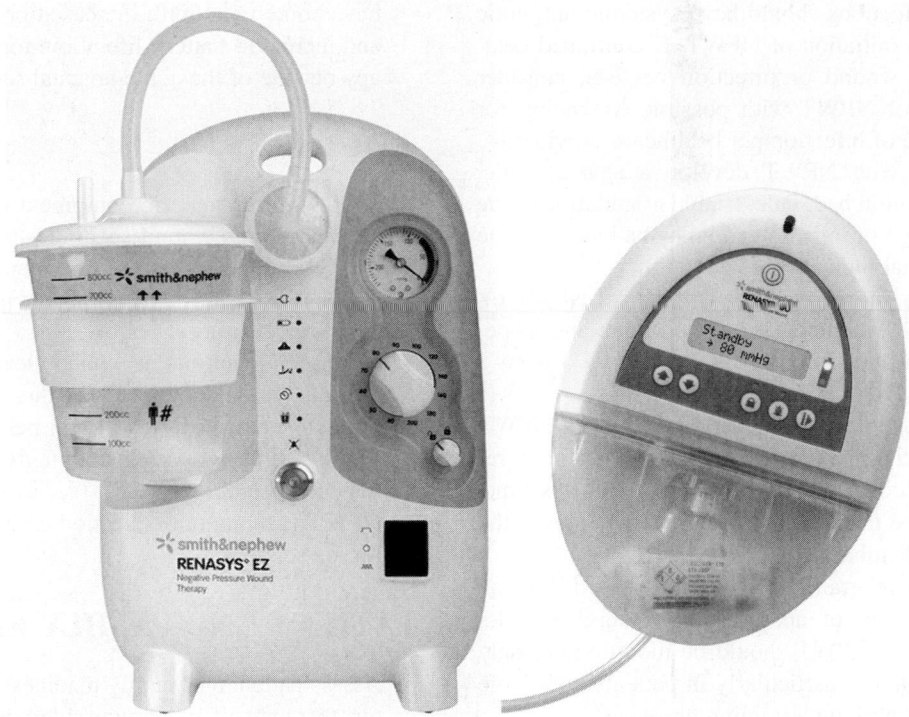

FIGURE 131-2   Components of RENASYS EZ® NPWT therapy. *(Courtesy of Smith & Nephew, Inc.)*

- Wounds heal by either primary or secondary intention (see Fig. 126-1). Most clean surgical wounds heal by primary intention. Suturing each layer of tissue approximates the wound edges. These wounds typically heal quickly and require minimal wound care. Contaminated surgical or traumatic wounds (open wounds) heal by secondary intention. Wounds that heal by secondary intention granulate from the base of the wound to the skin surfaces; care must be taken to allow for uniform granulation and prevention of open pockets or tunneling.
- Openly granulating wounds heal more slowly and must remain moist to enhance tissue granulation.

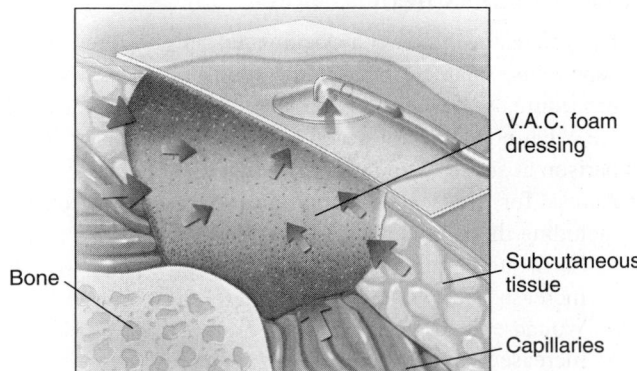

FIGURE 131-3   ActiV.A.C.® and InfoV.A.C.® Therapy Systems. Fluid, exudate, and debris removed from wound bed. *(Courtesy of KCI Lincensing, Inc. 2009)*

Wound care for these wounds focuses on maintaining a moist environment free of necrotic tissue, and decreasing pain.

- Open wounds may have excessive wound drainage that necessitates application of absorptive dressings, protection of periwound skin, and more frequent dressing changes to facilitate healing. NPWT provides wound drainage management and decreased frequency of dressing changes (most NPWT dressing changes are three times per week) with improved pain management.
- NPWT has been approved by the U.S. FDA for the following wounds:
  - ❖ Acute wounds (orthopedic trauma wounds, partial-thickness burns, abdominal wounds, surgical dehisced wounds, flaps, and grafts)
  - ❖ Chronic wounds (diabetic wounds, pressure ulcers, leg ulcers)
- Goals of NPWT in the management of wounds may include wound bed preparation for skin grafts, full wound closure, decrease in wound size, removal of wound edema for delayed primary closure, and increased perfusion to marginally viable flaps.
- The effectiveness of NPWT should be evaluated with each dressing change to include a comprehensive wound assessment and weekly wound measurements. If wound measurements have not improved at least 15% after 2 weeks of therapy, reevaluate the continuation of NPWT with reassessment of wound healing variables.[13]

- Wounds with infections should have systemic antibiotic treatment before initiation of NPWT. If continued deterioration of the wound or infection persists, consider discontinuation of NPWT with possible evaluation for surgical drainage of infection per healthcare provider.
- Wounds treated with NPWT develop a characteristic, beefy red granulation bed. Pale, friable granulation tissue is a secondary sign of infection and may be more reliable than the traditional indicators of infection.[3]
- Dehisced infected sternal wounds with use of NPWT require effective débridement of infected bone and a specific nonadherent wound contact layer before a NPWT dressing is placed.
- Successful management of enteric fistulae with NPWT with use of special application techniques has been reported in case studies but no clinical trials at this time. See NPWT device manuals for specific techniques in the management of fistulae.
- Rapid formation of granulation tissue with NPWT can lead to development of abscesses. The surgically dehisced wound with NPWT should be monitored closely for abscess formation, particularly in patients with large irregular wounds with undermining present.
- Transcutaneous oxygen pressure (Tcpo$_2$) evaluation should be considered before initiation of NPWT to lower extremity or toe wounds because of vascular flow requirements that are needed for optimal wound healing with NPWT.
- Contraindications to use of NPWT include malignancy disease in the wound, untreated osteomyelitis, nonenteric and unexplored fistulae, and necrotic tissue with eschar present.[10] See manufacturer NPWT manual for special precautions required with exposed blood vessels, organs, tendons, and nerves. Precautions should be used for wounds with active bleeding, for difficult wound hemostasis, and for patients undergoing anticoagulation therapy.
- For optimal NPWT with the V.A.C. device, at least 22 of 24 hours of daily uninterrupted therapy should be delivered. The newer vacuum units do not have research evidence at this time for required time duration of uninterrupted therapy for optimal wound healing. NPWT dressings are usually changed every 48 hours.[5,7-10] However, infected wound beds may require more frequent dressing changes (every 12 hours), and dressings over grafts may be changed less frequently (every 3 to 5 days).[5,8] The wound bed should be free of necrotic tissue and debris before application of the NPWT dressing.
- In highly exudative wounds, drainage from the wound bed may be significant in the first 24 to 48 hours of therapy. Studies have not suggested direct fluid replacements as necessary for ensuring homeostasis in highly exudative wounds.[1,3,4] Excessive bleeding should be noted for discontinuation of therapy.
- Nutritional requirements for wound healing are great. These needs must be assessed, met, and monitored frequently because poor nutrition can impede successful NPWT wound healing.
- The NPWT units discussed previously (ActiV.A.C.® and InfoV.A.C.® Therapy Systems and RENASYS EZ®)

have home units with increased portability. Smaller size and increased battery life allow for continuation of therapy outside of the acute hospital setting.

EQUIPMENT

The following is generic equipment used for most NPWT units. Device- and wound-specific variations may need to be considered by the healthcare provider.
- Standard Precautions equipment: gloves, gown, as indicated per institution policy
- Normal Precautions or wound cleanser with appropriate psi delivery device (see Procedure 126)
- Protective barrier film/wipe for periwound protection
- NPWT dressing with tubing/transparent drape kit (device-specific)
- NPWT vacuum unit/collection chamber (device-specific)
- Sterile scissors

PATIENT AND FAMILY EDUCATION

- Assess patient and family readiness to learn and any factors that may affect learning. Identification of the patient's preferred learning strategies (auditory, visualization, return demonstration) is also important. ➡*Rationale:* The nurse can develop the most appropriate teaching strategy for each patient.
- Provide information about NPWT, the procedure, and the equipment. ➡*Rationale:* Information may decrease or alleviate anxiety by assisting patient and family to understand the procedure, why it is needed, and the preferred outcomes.
- Explain the procedure and the reason for changing wound dressing. ➡*Rationale:* Patient anxiety and discomfort are decreased.
- Discuss patient's role during the dressing change procedure and in maintaining the NPWT system. ➡*Rationale:* Patient cooperation is elicited; patient is prepared for wound management on discharge.

PATIENT ASSESSMENT AND PREPARATION
Patient Assessment

- Fully assess wound with documentation of wound measurements, characteristics, and appropriateness for the procedure. ➡*Rationale:* Assessment ensures that use of NPWT is not contraindicated. Data are provided for comparison at successive dressing changes.
- Assess for signs and symptoms of wound infection, including the following:
  - Periwound erythema
  - Increased periwound warmth
  - Wound edema
  - Increased pain associated with wound
  - Increased odor and amount of wound exudate
  - Elevated temperature and white blood cell count

  ➡*Rationale:* Although NPWT assists with removal of excessive fluid, thus reducing the potential of bacteria in

the wound bed, assessment for signs and symptoms of wound infection is necessary, especially in patients with compromised conditions.

- Determine baseline pain assessment. ➻*Rationale:* Data are provided for comparison with past procedure assessment data. The nurse can plan for preprocedure and intraprocedure analgesia.
- Determine baseline nutritional and fluid volume status. ➻*Rationale:* Adequate fluids and protein are necessary for optimal wound healing with NPWT.
- Assess medical history, especially related to bleeding problems, fistula formation, or malignant disease. ➻*Rationale:* NPWT may be contraindicated in these conditions.
- Assess current medications specifically related to anticoagulant use. ➻*Rationale:* Possible areas of caution that should be monitored with NPWT use are identified.
- Assess current laboratory values, especially coagulation studies. ➻*Rationale:* Abnormalities possibly associated with risks related to NPWT use are identified.

Patient Preparation

- Verify correct patient with two identifiers. ➻*Rationale:* Prior to performing a procedure, the nurse should ensure the correct identification of the patient for the intended intervention.
- Ensure patient and family understanding of procedure. Reinforce teaching points as needed. ➻*Rationale:* Understanding of previously taught information is evaluated, and a conduit for questions is provided.
- Validate presence of patent intravenous access. ➻*Rationale:* Access may be needed for administration of intravenous analgesic medications.
- Position the patient in a manner that will ensure patient comfort and privacy and facilitate dressing application. ➻*Rationale:* Patient is prepared to undergo procedure.
- Administer prescribed analgesics if needed. ➻*Rationale:* Analgesics improve comfort level and tolerance of the procedure and decrease patient anxiety and discomfort.

Procedure | for Negative-Pressure Wound Therapy

Steps	Rationale	Special Considerations

General principles of NPWT are consistent across devices; however, wound-specific and device-specific guidelines need to be reviewed before NPWT. **Steps 1 to 8** *are generic to all NPWT applications.*
Procedure for KCI V.A.C. Therapy for Wounds; V.A.C. Application

Steps	Rationale	Special Considerations
1. 🅗🅗		
2. 🅟🅔		
3. Position the patient to facilitate wound cleansing with dressing application.	Provides for patient's comfort and allows for visualization and access to the wound.	

4. Assess, measure wound, and assemble supplies as indicated (Table 131-1).[4,5] **(Level D*)**	Select NPWT dressing type with appropriate size approximating wound size. Multiple types of V.A.C.-specialty size dressings are available (refer to manufacturer's manual):
	V.A.C.-specific Dressings:
	  a. Black polyurethane foam (Granu-Foam) has larger pores and is considered to be more effective in stimulating granulation tissue formation and wound contraction. It is the most frequently used.
	  b. White polyvinyl chloride foam (VersaFoam) is more dense, is premoistened, and has increased tensile strength. Because of its higher density, it requires higher pressure to obtain the same granulation rate as black foam.
	  c. Black polyurethane foam, Granu-Foam Silver, has antimicrobial silver and may reduce infections in wounds.[12]
		The black V.A.C. dressing does not hold moisture but allows exudates to pass through the dressing and be removed. Its design results in rapid growth of new granulation.
		The white V.A.C. dressing holds moisture but also allows exudate to be removed through it. It is nonadherent and can be used in tunnels and shallow undermining because of its higher tensile strength.

---

*Level D: Peer-reviewed professional organizational standards with clinical studies to support recommendations

Procedure continues on following page

TABLE 131-1	**Recommended Therapy Setting for KCI V.A.C. Therapy**	
Wound Characteristics	**Continuous Therapy**	**Intermittent Therapy**
Difficult dressing application	x	
Flap	x	
Highly exuding	x	
Grafts	x	
Painful wounds	x	
Tunnels or undermining	x	
Unstable structures	x	
Minimally exuding	x	x
Large wounds	x	x
Small wounds	x	x
Stalled wound healing progress	x	x
V.A.C. white foam dressing	x	x

Responsible physician or advanced practice nurse should be consulted for individual patient conditions. Consult device user manual and manufacturer's recommended guidelines before use.

(Adapted from Smith APS: V.A.C.® therapy clinical guidelines: a reference source for clinicians, San Antonio, TX, 2006, KCI Licensing, Inc.)

Procedure   for Negative-Pressure Wound Therapy—*Continued*

Steps	Rationale	Special Considerations
5. Cleanse the wound according to orders (see Procedure 126) or institutional protocol. **(Level B*)**	Wound bed cleansing and irrigation prepare the wound bed for application of dressing.[3,4]	
6. Physician or advanced practice nurse may débride (see Procedure 127) necrotic tissue or eschar if applicable.	NPWT assists with autolytic and mechanical débridement of surface slough; it should not be used as a primary means of débridement. Sharp débridement of necrotic tissue should be performed before initiation of therapy for optimal healing with NPWT.[5,6,13]	If extensive débridement is needed, surgical débridement in the operative suite may be necessary.
7. Prepare the periwound by cleansing with warm solution. Clip the hair around the wound. Dry skin and prepare the periwound tissue with a barrier protective film.[4] **(Level D*)**	Moisture from perspiration, oil, or body fluids may interfere with the drape's adherence. Barrier films act as a protectant against periwound maceration.	Potential for folliculitis with multiple removals of transparent drape may irritate hair follicles.
8. Remove gloves.		
9. **HH**		
10. Apply clean gloves		

*Level B: Well-designed, controlled studies with results that consistently support a specific action, intervention, or treatment
*Level D: Peer-reviewed professional organizational standards with clinical studies to support recommendations

Procedure for Negative-Pressure Wound Therapy—*Continued*

Steps	Rationale	Special Considerations
11. Open intact package and cut the V.A.C. foam with sterile scissors; do not cut foam directly over the wound.[10] **(Level E*)**	Prevents small particles of dressing from falling into the wound. The dressing should be cut to fit the size and shape of the wound, including tunnels and undermined areas. Tunneling can result in a cyst or abscess when vacuum pressure or granulation closes the entrance to the tunnel. Bacterial invasion and impaired healing result from unfilled dead space.[3]	Any exposed tendons, nerves, or blood vessels should be protected with placement of a layer of nonadherent dressing over them.
12. Gently place foam into wound, ensuring contact with all wound surfaces. Do not force foam dressing into any area of the wound. Always note total number of foam pieces used with notation on transparent drape and in patient's chart. **(Level E)**	Capillaries can be compressed if dressings are packed too tightly, and pressure on newly formed granulation tissue may prevent or delay healing.[10]	More than one dressing may be used to fill the wound bed. Foam pieces should be in contact but not overlapping each other to allow equalization of negative pressure applied to the wound bed by the suction device.[1,4]
13. Trim and place the V.A.C. transparent drape to cover the foam dressing and an additional 3 to 5 cm of intact periwound skin. Avoid stretching the drape over the wound.[12] **(Level M*)**	Avoids tension and shearing forces on surrounding tissue.	Bridging of wounds can be done for more than one wound of similar pathology in close proximity with one vacuum pump. See manufacturer-specific instructions.
14. Cut a 2-cm hole in the transparent drape, for fluid to pass through. Cut a hole rather than a slit because a slit may self-seal during therapy. Apply the T.R.A.C.® pad with tubing directly over the hole in the transparent drape. Apply gentle pressure around the pad to ensure complete adhesion.[12] **(Level M)**	The vacuum does not function without an occlusive seal. The drape may also help maintain a moist wound environment. The drape is vapor-permeable and allows for gas exchange. It also protects the wound from external contamination.	The foam contracts into wound bed if seal is obtained. If foam does not contract, reassess outer dressing for possible leaks in the system or dressing seal.[1,4]
15. Ensure the position of the T.R.A.C. tubing is not over bony prominences.[12] **(Level M)**	Minimizes the risk of pressure related to tubing placement.	Extra foams with drape can be used under the tubing to reduce pressure and stabilize the tubing.
16. Remove V.A.C. canister from packaging and insert into the vacuum unit. Connect T.R.A.C. pad tubing to canister tubing and ensure clamps are open.	Closed clamps prevent activation of the negative therapy.	
17. Turn on power to vacuum unit and select prescribed therapy setting. Assess dressing to ensure seal integrity. The dressing should collapse with a wrinkled appearance and no hissing sounds.[5] **(Level E)**	Setting options include continuous or intermittent negative-pressure therapy. The settings are determined by type of wound, exudate, and goals as ordered by the physician (see Table 131-1).	If dressing does not collapse, check tubing and transparent drape for leaks. Use additional drape to seal leaks as necessary.
18. Follow institutional standard for assessing pain.	Identifies need for management of discomfort associated with wound or NPWT system.	Report inability to manage patient's pain.

*Level E: Multiple case reports, theory-based evidence from expert opinions, or peer-reviewed professional organizational standards without clinical studies to support recommendations
*Level M: Manufacturer's recommendations only

Procedure continues on following page

Procedure for Negative-Pressure Wound Therapy—*Continued*

Steps	Rationale	Special Considerations
19. Discard used supplies; remove gloves.		
20. **HH**		
V.A.C. Dressing Removal Procedure		
1. **HH**		
2. **PE**		
3. To remove the dressing, raise the tubing connector above the level of the vacuum unit and tighten clamps on the dressing tubing. Disconnect the two tubings at the connection point.	Removes any remaining fluid from the tubing for purposes of infection control, preventing leakage.	
4. Allow the vacuum unit to pull the exudate through the canister tubing into the canister, then tighten clamp on the canister tube. Turn off vacuum unit. Remove canister from vacuum unit and discard.	Allows exudate to be contained; canister should be discarded per institutional policy.	
5. Allow foam to decompress. Gently stretch transparent drape horizontally to release adhesive from the skin. Do not peel vertically. Gently remove foam dressing from wound.[12] **(Level M*)**	Decreases patient discomfort and potential for skin and wound trauma.	
6. Discard used supplies; remove gloves.		
7. **HH**		

Expected Outcomes

- Wound healing or granulation enhanced by consistent negative-pressure therapy; early signs of contraction of wound margins
- Decreased volume of wound exudate (over time) and absence of foul odor or color
- Enhanced wound healing because of effective wound fluid or edema removal
- Decrease in size of wound with ability for surgical closure with flap/graft or skin graft; complete healing of wound
- Decreased time to satisfactory healing (may decrease hospital length of stay and cost)

Unexpected Outcomes

- Infection
- Bleeding
- Fistula formation
- Disruption of underlying tissue or structures
- Pain
- Misplacement over exposed vessel, ligaments, other structures
- Lack of improvement in wound after 1 to 2 weeks of therapy
- Tissue loss
- Ischemia and necrosis
- Periwound maceration

*Level M: Manufacturer's recommendations only

Patient Monitoring and Care

Steps	Rationale	Reportable Conditions
		These conditions should be reported if they persist despite nursing interventions. • Tissue breakdown
1. Assess location of V.A.C. T.R.A.C. tubing to avoid excessive pressure on surrounding tissue or structures.	Excessive pressure may result in tissue breakdown from tubing over bony prominences.	
2. Assess patency of V.A.C. system; drape has an occlusive seal, tubing is patent, and foam is compressed.	The V.A.C. dressing should be collapsed when seal is maintained and negative pressure is being delivered in a consistent manner. Alarms on the device indicate loss of seal; raised foam dressing indicates loss of negative-pressure therapy.	• Loss of seal • Raised foam dressing • Wound drainage suddenly decreasing in amount or stopping
3. Assess the amount and type the drainage.	Color of drainage can suggest bleeding, and rate of canister filling can alert the caregiver to wound problems.	• Bright red blood or rapid filling of the canister
4. Monitor condition of wound bed and periwound skin with dressing changes; observe for signs of wound infection.	Identifies any evidence of wound healing or any changes or abnormalities indicative of complications.	• Periwound erythema • Heat, edema, pain • Elevated temperature and white blood cell count • Cloudy or foul-smelling wound drainage • Increased wound drainage • Excess bleeding • Changes in tissue color within wound bed • Macerated periwound skin • New tunneling or undermining • Stool in the wound bed
5. Change the dressing every 48 hours. If infection is present, increase the frequency of dressing change to every 12 to 24 hours.[5] **(Level D*)**	Removes infectious material from the wound bed. If dressing adheres to the wound base, consider interfacing a single layer of nonadherent porous material (e.g., wide-meshed petrolatum-impregnated gauze) between the dressing and the wound when reapplying the dressing. If previous dressings were difficult to remove and painful, consider instillation into the tubing or dressing of a topical anesthetic agent such as 1% lidocaine without epinephrine ordered by physician or advanced practice nurse.	• Signs or symptoms of infection
6. Monitor the mode (continuous or intermittent) and level of suction. **(Level E*)**	Removal of edema and debris alleviates compressive forces, thus improving perfusion. Suctioning fluid from within the wound may remove wound fluid factors that inhibit healing.[3,4]	• Patient discomfort • Excess granulation tissue overgrowth into the dressing with removal • Continued edema within wound bed

*Level D: Peer-reviewed professional organizational standards with clinical studies to support recommendations

*Level E: Multiple case reports, theory-based evidence from expert opinions, or peer-reviewed professional organizational standards without clinical studies to support recommendations

Procedure continues on following page

Patient Monitoring and Care —*Continued*

Steps	Rationale	Reportable Conditions
	Application and release of negative pressure on the wound bed stimulate cell proliferation and protein synthesis. Mechanical stretch on the tissue by the negative pressure draws the wound toward the center, closing the defect.[12]	
7. Maintain an airtight seal.[12] **(Level M*)**	Loss of an airtight seal can result in a decreased amount of drainage removal and in desiccation of the wound.	
8. Label dressing with date and time of application and amount of foam pieces placed in wound.	V.A.C. foam dressings are not bioabsorbable. Ensure all pieces of foam are removed from the wound with each dressing change. Foam left in wound for greater than recommended time period may foster ingrowth of tissue into the foam.	• Foam left in wound for greater than recommended time period may foster ingrowth of tissue into the foam and create difficulty in removal of foam pieces from wound or lead to infection[12]
9. Change canister when full or at least weekly. Keep canister position level.	Controls odor.	
10. Monitor amount of wound drainage.[5] **(Level D*)**	If a wound produces excessive fluid, the patient may experience a fluid imbalance, requiring intravenous replacement. Excess drainage may also result in increased protein loss. A nutritional consult to replace protein loss from wound exudates may be indicated.	• Wound drainage that is foul-smelling and cloudy
11. Follow institution standard for assessing pain. Administer analgesia as prescribed. Pain can be associated with application of dressing, initiation of initial therapy, intermittent cycling, or removal of the dressing.	Identifies need for pain interventions. Use of analgesics at dressing changes can reduce the pain. Also, lowering the initial amount of negative pressure or maintaining the pressure at continual versus intermittent levels can assist in pain control.[3,4,7]	• Continued pain despite pain interventions

Documentation

Documentation should include the following:
- Patient and family education
- Patient tolerance of the procedure
- Condition of the wound bed and periwound skin description
- Characteristics of wound drainage
- Mode (continuous or intermittent) and degree (mmHg) of suction
- Nursing interventions
- Premedication given and patient's response to the pain medication

- Wound débridement procedure (if applicable); wound cleansing procedure completed, dated, and timed
- Size of the wound measured by length, width, and depth (consider obtaining a photograph of the wound, depending on institutional policy)
- Size and type of foam dressing applied and total number placed in the wound
- Unexpected outcomes, reportable conditions

*Level D: Peer-reviewed professional organizational standards with clinical studies to support recommendations
*Level M: Manufacturer's recommendations only

References

CR 1. Argenta LC, Morykwas MJ: Vacuum-assisted closure: a new method for wound control and treatment: clinical experience, *Ann Plastic Surg* 38:563-576, 1997.

CR 2. Armstrong D, et al: Proceedings from the 2003 National V.A.C. ® Education Conference, *Ostomy Wound Manage* 50(4A Suppl); 3S-27S; 2004.

CR 3. Bergstrom N, et al: *Treatment of pressure ulcers: clinical practice guideline, no. 15*, AHCPR publication no. 95-0652, Rockville, MD, 1994, US Department of Health and Human Services, Public Health Service, Agency for Healthcare Policy and Research.

4. Broughton G, et al: Wound healing: an overview, *Plast Reconstruct Surg* 117(7S Suppl):1e-s-32e-s, 2006.

5. Bovill E, et al: Topical negative pressure wound therapy: a review of its role and guidelines for its use in the management of acute wounds, *Int Wound J* 65(3):722-731, 2008.

6. Campbell P, Smith J, Smith G, editors: *Negative pressure wound therapy (NPWT) clinical case reports*, St Petersburg, FL, 2007, Smith & Nephew.

7. Chariker ME, Gerstle TL, Morrison CS: An algorithmic approach to the use of gauze-based negative-pressure wound therapy as a bridge to closure in pediatric extremity trauma, *Plast Reconstruct Surg* 123(5):1510-1520, 2009.

8. Gupta S: Differentiating negative pressure wound therapy devices: an illustrative case series, *Wounds J* 19(1 Suppl): 26S-28S;2007.

9. Koehler C, et al: Wound therapy using the vacuum-assisted closure device: clinical experience with novel indications, *J Trauma* 65(3):722-732, 2008.

10. Long MA, Blevins A: Options in negative pressure wound therapy: five case studies, *J Wound Ostomy Continence Nurs* 36(2):202-211, 2009.

11. Sullivan N, Snyder DL, Tipton K, et al: *Negative pressure wound therapy devices: technology assessment report, project ID: WNDT1108*, Rockville, MD. 2009, US Department of Health and Human Services, Agency for Healthcare Research Quality, available at www.ahrq.gov/clinic/ta/negpresswtd.

12. Smith APS: *V.A.C. ® therapy clinical guidelines: a reference source for clinicians*, San Antonio, TX, 2006, KCI Licensing, Inc.

13. World Union of Wound Healing Societies (WUWHS): *Principles of best practice: vacuum assisted closure: recommendation for use: a consensus document*, London, 2008, MEP Ltd.

Small-Bore Feeding Tube Insertion Using an Electromagnetic Guidance System (CORTRAK®)

P U R P O S E : The CORTRAK® system uses electromagnetic technology to enhance the safety of bedside placement of small-bore nasoenteric feeding tubes. The guidance system directs feeding tube placement by tracking the relative location of the tube as it proceeds down the alimentary tract. This visual guidance aids in avoiding intubation of the pulmonary system and facilitates postpyloric placement of feeding tubes.[1,5,8,12,15]

Karen A. Gilbert, Patricia H. Worthington

PREREQUISITE NURSING KNOWLEDGE

- Knowledge of upper respiratory and gastrointestinal anatomy and physiology is necessary.
- Proficiency is needed in physical assessment skills for lungs and abdomen.
- Clinical and technical competence is necessary in placement of small-bore feeding tubes and in use of the CORTRAK® (Corpak MedSystems, Wheeling, IL) device, based on institutional policies.
- Recognition is needed of risk factors associated with placement errors during insertion of small-bore feeding tubes: endotracheal intubation, advanced age, altered level of consciousness, and diminished reflexes for airway protection.[14]
- The benefits of enteral nutrition for the critically ill, including indications for postpyloric placement, should be understood.[6]

EQUIPMENT

- CORTRAK® feeding tube placement device (Fig 132-1)
- CORTRAK® feeding tube with transmitting stylet
- Irrigation tray

- 50-mL or larger catheter-tipped or Luer-Lok/slip syringe
- Water (tap water or sterile water based on institutional policy)
- Clean examination gloves
- Additional personal protective equipment, including gown and goggles
- Water-soluble lubricant
- Viscous lidocaine (optional)
- Water-absorbent barrier to protect patient's clothing
- Stethoscope
- Tape or other securing device

PATIENT AND FAMILY EDUCATION

- Explain the essential role adequate nutritional status plays in promoting wound healing and recovery from illness. ➤*Rationale:* Explanation may elicit cooperation and allay patient anxiety.
- Explain why a feeding tube is needed to ensure adequate nutritional intake. ➤*Rationale:* Explanation may elicit cooperation and facilitate tube insertion.
- Outline the steps in the procedure and the patient's role during feeding tube insertion (e.g., position, swallowing

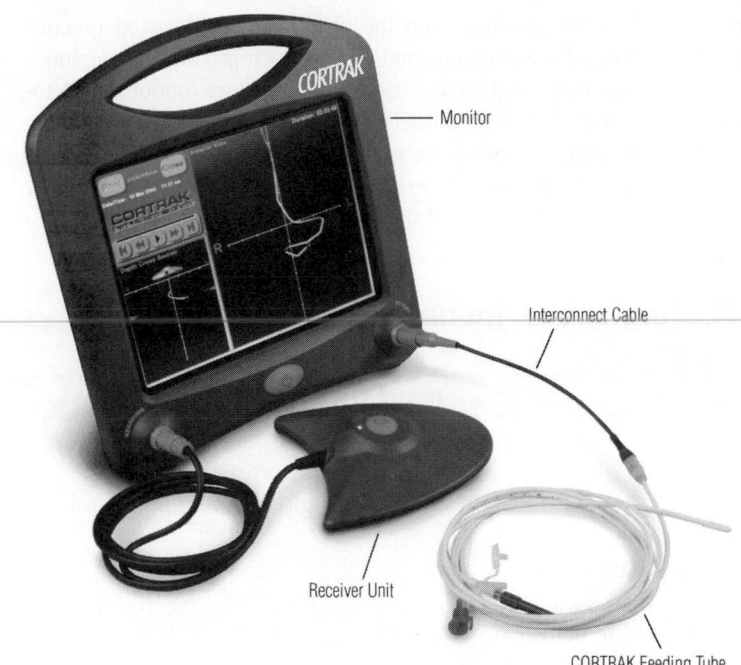

Monitor

Interconnect Cable

Receiver Unit

CORTRAK Feeding Tube

FIGURE 132-1 Electromagnetic Guidance System (COR-TRAK®). *(Courtesy of Corpak MedSystems, 2009.)*

as instructed). ➥*Rationale:* Patient cooperation may facilitate insertion.

- Describe the typical sensations experienced during feeding tube insertion. ➥*Rationale:* Explanation may alleviate anxiety and promote patient cooperation.
- Inform patient and family of the need for postinsertion radiograph. ➥*Rationale:* Information may provide reassurance regarding expected course of events.
- Reinforce the importance of using care when changing position or getting out of bed once the tube is placed. ➥*Rationale:* Emphasis may aid in preventing inadvertent dislodgment of the tube.

PATIENT ASSESSMENT AND PREPARATION

Patient Assessment

- Verify that the patient has no implanted medical devices that may be affected by electromagnetic fields. ➥*Rationale:* The CORTRAK® system is generally contraindicated for patients with implanted medical devices because of the potential for electromagnetic interference to impact the function of the implanted device or the CORTRAK®. However, *no* contraindication exists for defibrillators and pacemakers because extensive testing has shown that CORTRAK® does not affect the operation of these devices.[4]
- Assess the patient for the presence of absolute contraindications for nasal placement of small-bore feeding tubes, including basilar skull fracture; history of transsphenoidal surgery; facial, nasal, or sinus trauma; or severe clotting abnormalities. ➥*Rationale:* These conditions carry a high risk for complications from passage of the tube through the nasopharyngeal area. Intracranial placement of small-bore feeding tubes has occurred with

the nasal approach in patients with basilar skull fracture. The orogastric route is a safer alternative in this situation.[11]

- Evaluate the patient for relative contraindications for placement of either nasally or orally inserted small-bore feeding tubes, including esophageal varices with recent bleeding or ligation within 72 hours; esophageal stricture, tumor, recent esophageal surgery; history of gastrointestinal surgery with altered anatomic pathways; gastroesophageal reflux; and gastroparesis. ➥*Rationale:* These conditions may impede efforts to achieve optimal tip position for enteral nutrition.[6]
- Additional relative contraindications for nasal placement also include history of nasal polyps, septal abnormalities, sinusitis, and minor to moderate clotting abnormalities. ➥*Rationale:* These conditions carry a relative risk for complications from passage of the tube through the nasopharyngeal route. Placement of the tube may still be undertaken if the assessment of benefit outweighs risk.
- Assess gastrointestinal function. ➥*Rationale:* A functional gastrointestinal tract is essential for safe and effective tube feeding. The integrity and function of the gastrointestinal tract also guide decisions regarding the optimal location for delivery of nutrients (gastric versus postpyloric tip position).

Patient Preparation

- Reinforce the information previously covered during patient and family education. Respond to any additional questions or concerns the patient may have. ➥*Rationale:* Emphasis may enhance patient cooperation by reducing anxiety.
- Assess the need to remove any existing large-bore feeding tube. ➥*Rationale:* In some cases, the large-bore

tube may be kept in place to allow gastric decompression while delivery of enteral formula takes place in the small intestine. When the large-bore tube is to be replaced by a small-bore tube, the larger tube should be removed before the new tube is passed to avoid dislodging the small-bore tube during removal of the large-bore tube.

- Obtain an order from the physician or advanced practice nurse for the administration of metoclopramide 10 mg intravenously 10 minutes before the procedure (optional). Metoclopramide is used with caution because prolonged administration at higher doses is associated with the development of tardive dyskinesia. ➤➤*Rationale:* Enhanced gastric motility facilitates passage of the tube distal to the pylorus.[3]

Procedure	for Insertion of Small-Bore Feeding Tube with an Electromagnetic Guidance System (CORTRAK®)	
Steps	**Rationale**	**Special Considerations**
1. **HH**		
2. **PE**		Feeding tube insertion is a clean procedure; gloves should be worn.
3. Protect the patient's clothing.		
4. Place patient in a supine position with head of bed elevated to at least 30 degrees unless contraindicated.[10] **(Level B*)**	The patient should be as straight as possible for accurate tracking of the feeding tube. This position helps to facilitate the initial advancement of the tube into the esophagus.	
5. Press the orange power button to activate the CORTRAK® device (Fig. 132-2).		Hold button for approximately 2 seconds to turn on power.
6. Login by typing Username and Password.		
7. Press "New Placement."		
8. Enter the patient name and medical record number (optional).	The device can store a record of the insertion for future reference (Accounts Mode).	Placements can be performed without recording the procedure (Anonymous Mode).
9. Place the leading foot of the Receiver Unit over the patient's xiphoid process. The Receiver Unit cord heads toward the patient's feet (Fig. 132-3).	The Receiver Unit must be level with the spine and centered along midline to ensure reliable tracking of the tube during placement. If the Receiver Unit is placed too far below the xiphoid, the feeding tube appears to cross the horizontal axis too early, suggesting possible lung placement. If the Receiver Unit is placed too high over the sternum, lung placement may be missed.	A weighted band is available to place over the receiver unit for added stability. Do not reposition the Receiver Unit once it has been correctly placed on the xiphoid process. Movement of the Receiver Unit alters the alignment and the relationship of the track displayed on the Monitor Unit.
10. Determine the length of feeding tube to be inserted into stomach by measuring the length of the tube from the tip of the nose to the tip of an earlobe and to the bottom of the xiphoid process.[7] **(Level C*)**	The length of tube needed to reach the stomach ranges between 55 and 70 cm; the distal small bowel (ligament of Treitz) usually is located at 90 to 110 cm.[13]	
11. Move the stylet a few centimeters in and out the tube. Ensure that the stylet is firmly seated in the feeding tube.	Flushing the feeding tube before stylet removal to activate the lubricant inside the tube ensures that the stylet moves freely out of the tube once the desired position is achieved.	If the stylet is moving within the tube during the insertion, the tracing on the monitor is inaccurate.

*Level B: Well-designed, controlled studies with results that consistently support a specific action, intervention, or treatment
*Level C: Qualitative studies, descriptive or correlational studies, integrative reviews, systematic reviews, or randomized controlled trials with inconsistent results

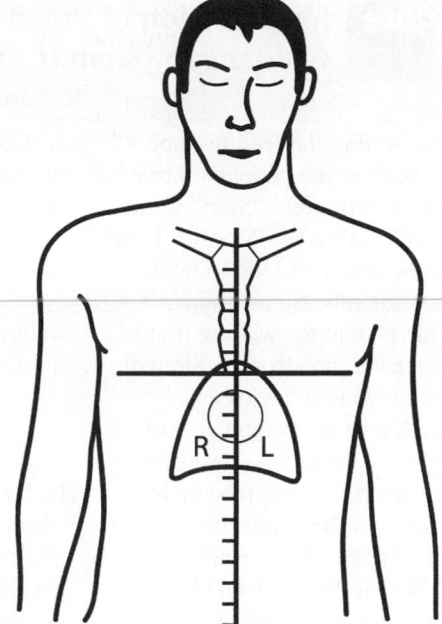

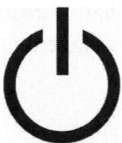

FIGURE 132-2   CORTRAK® power button. *(Courtesy of Corpak MedSystems, 2009.)*

FIGURE 132-3   CORTRAK® placement. *(Courtesy of Corpak MedSystems, 2009.)*

Procedure	**for Insertion of Small-Bore Feeding Tube with an Electromagnetic Guidance System (CORTRAK®)**—*Continued*	
Steps	**Rationale**	**Special Considerations**
12. Flush the feeding tube with water and dip the tip of the tube in water. Cap the medication port.	Observe for patency or leaks in the tube during flushing. Water activates a lubricant that has been applied to the internal and external surface of the tube. This ensures that the stylet moves freely out of the tube once the desired position is achieved.	
13. Connect the distal (orange) end of the feeding tube Transmitter Stylet to the Stylet Interconnect Cable on the lower right corner of the CORTRAK® Monitor Unit.	The CORTRAK® feeding tube uses a special stylet that transmits a signal during tube insertion.	Arrows that appear on both the stylet and the cable connectors act as a guide to prevent damage to the equipment during connection.
14. Lubricate the distal end of the tube with water-soluble jelly.[8,13] **(Level E*)** (Viscous lidocaine may be used if ordered by the physician or advanced practice nurse.)	Minimizes mucosal injury, facilitates insertion, and promotes patient comfort.	Oil-soluble lubricants should not be used because they are not absorbed by the pulmonary mucosa and may cause complications.
15. Insert the feeding tube into the nares and advance the tube gently along the base of the nostril.[8,13] **(Level E)**		

*Level E: Multiple case reports, theory-based evidence from expert opinions, or peer-reviewed professional organizational standards without clinical studies to support recommendations

Procedure continues on following page

Procedure	**for Insertion of Small-Bore Feeding Tube with an Electromagnetic Guidance System (CORTRAK®)**—*Continued*	

Steps	Rationale	Special Considerations
16. After inserting the feeding tube to the back of the patient's throat (10 to 15 cm), press "Start" either on the CORTRAK® Monitor Unit or on the Receiver Unit to begin to view the tube tip position.	An "Out of Range" message appears on the screen if the unit is started prematurely.	If the "Out of Range" message still appears at 30 to 35 cm, the tube is likely coiled in the mouth or throat.
17. Ask the patient to swallow if able. Advance the tube to coincide with the swallowing maneuver. If allowed, give the patient sips of water or ice chips.[8,13] **(Level E*)**	Swallowing assists passage of the tube into the esophagus.	
18. Follow the path of the tube tip by the tracing of the illuminated dot on the CORTRAK® Anterior View Screen (Fig. 132-4). Monitor the depth tracing on the Depth Cross-Section Screen simultaneously (Fig. 132-4).[5] **(Level M*)**	The Depth Cross-Section Screen shows the distance of tube tip from the sternum. The relatively posterior anatomic location of the esophagus and the duodenum is reflected by greater depth of these structures in relation to the stomach.	A deviation from the expected path may indicate placement error.
19. If the tracing veers sharply into the upper right or left quadrant at approximately 35 to 40 cm, slowly retract the feeding tube to 15 cm to erase the track and continue the placement procedure following the new track.[5] **(Level M)**	This finding may indicate a tube in the bronchus. Slowly pulling back the feeding tube clears the tracing of the placement attempt. A new track is visible as the placement resumes. If resistance is met, you should also withdraw the feeding tube at this point then continue to advance the feeding tube down the esophagus and into the stomach.	Restarting the device is not necessary. The feeding tube should slide down the esophagus quite easily. If resistance is met within the first 25 to 35 cm, the feeding tube may have passed into the bronchus.
20. In the stomach, if the feeding tube tip is not moving forward as the tube is inserted, slowly retract the feeding tube until the colored dot begins to move and then proceed with placement.[5] **(Level M)**	May indicate that the tube is coiling in the stomach rather than advancing. Coiled loops behind the transmitter are not visible on the monitor. The pathway through the stomach should resemble a backward "C" shape.	Instilling a bolus of air into the tube when the tip is nearing the pylorus may facilitate relaxation of the pylorus and aid in passage into the small bowel.
21. Assess configuration of the display pattern (pathway and depth) to determine whether appropriate position in the postpyloric region is likely (see Fig. 132-4).[5] **(Level M)**	The pathway through the duodenum often resembles a smaller, forward "C" shape.	A duodenum that is more posterior may show an upward curve in the Anterior View before it passes farther into the duodenum. The Depth Cross-Section indicates the depth of the feeding tube relative to the Receiver Unit/sternum. When the depth indicator is several notches below the horizontal axis, duodenal tube tip location is likely.
22. Maintain the stylet in place until the position of the tube is confirmed with abdominal radiograph.[5] **(Level M)**	The stylet aids in radiographic visualization. If the tube position is not optimal, the transmitter will be in place to allow further CORTRAK®-assisted repositioning.	The U.S. Food and Drug Administration has recently approved reinsertion of the Transmitting Stylet for periodic confirmation of tip location; however, clinical experience with this technique is limited.

*Level E: Multiple case reports, theory-based evidence from expert opinions, or peer-reviewed professional organizational standards without clinical studies to support recommendations

*Level M: Manufacturer's recommendations only

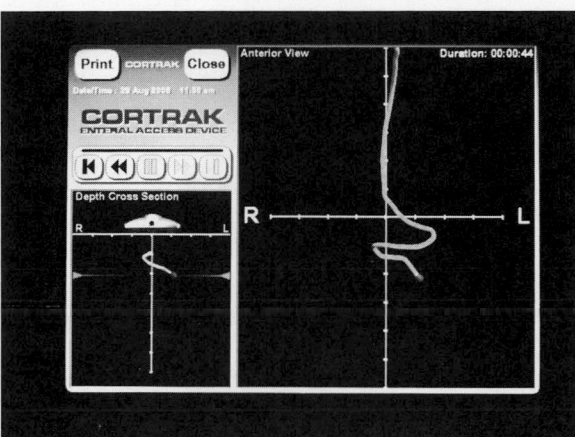

FIGURE 132-3 CORTRAK® screen. *(Courtesy of Corpak MedSystems, 2009.)*

Procedure for Insertion of Small-Bore Feeding Tube with an Electromagnetic Guidance System (CORTRAK®)—*Continued*

Steps	Rationale	Special Considerations
23. Press "End" on the monitor display or the orange button on the receiver.	Stops the recording/timing of the insertion procedure.	
24. Secure the feeding tube with tape or other commercial fixation device.	Decreases risk of inadvertent removal or change in position of the tube.	Avoid undue pressure on the naris from the tube because this can cause skin breakdown. Some practitioners advocate the use of a nasal bridle system to secure the tube against accidental removal with use of a loop of material through one naris, around the nasal septum, and back out of the other naris. A feeding tube is secured to this bridle.
25. Press "Print" to obtain a tracing of the placement (Fig. 132-5).	Printed tracing may be used as part of the documentation in the medical record.	
26. Disconnect the stylet from the interconnect cable.		Place or tape the long stylet beyond the patient's reach.
27. Press "Close" on the monitor unit; press "Shutdown."		
28. Obtain supine abdominal radiograph (Fig. 132-5).[2,10,11] **(Level A*)**	Radiographic confirmation is the most accurate method of determination of exact tube position after insertion.[2] The tip of the tube usually is not visible on chest radiograph.[2,10,11]	Gastric auscultation of an air bolus through the tube, aspiration of fluid from the tube, and placement of the proximal end of the feeding tube under water while observing for bubbles are all unreliable methods to confirm placement in the gastrointestinal (GI) tract. Numerous reports in the literature have documented false-positive results resulting in serious pulmonary complications.[10]

*Level A: Meta-analysis of quantitative studies or metasynthesis of qualitative studies with results that consistently support a specific action, intervention, or treatment

Procedure continues on following page

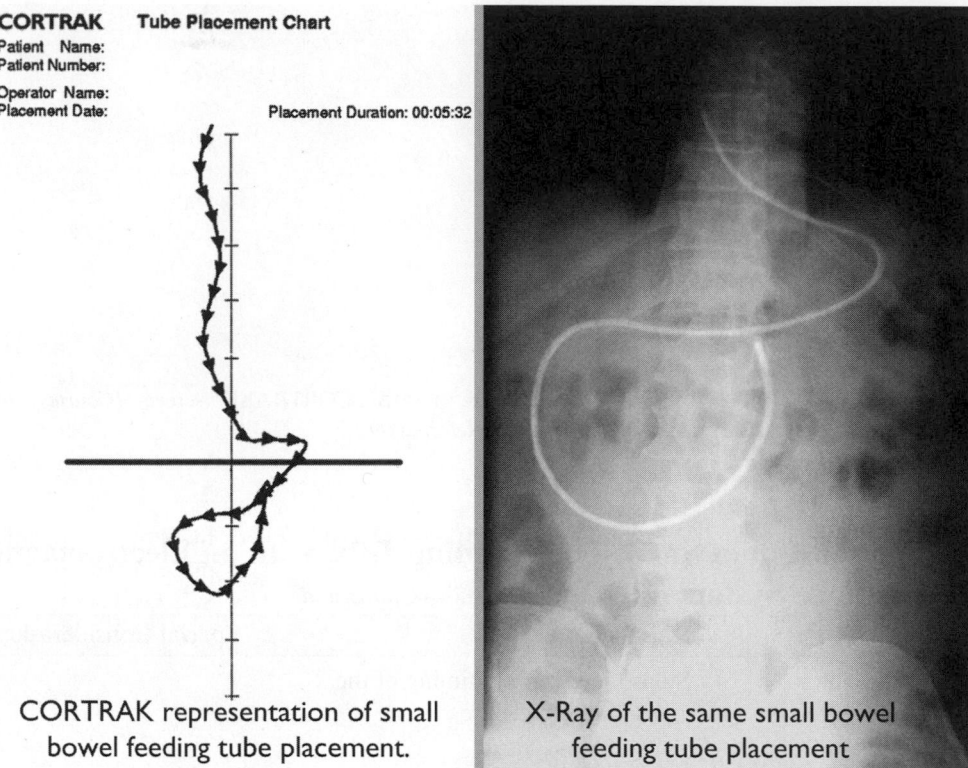

CORTRAK representation of small bowel feeding tube placement.

X-Ray of the same small bowel feeding tube placement

FIGURE 132-5   Printed tracing and radiograph. *(Courtesy of Corpak MedSystems, 2009.)*

Procedure	for Insertion of Small-Bore Feeding Tube with an Electromagnetic Guidance System (CORTRAK®)—*Continued*	
Steps	**Rationale**	**Special Considerations**
29. When proper location of the feeding tube is confirmed, flush with 5 to 10 mL of water.[5] **(Level M*)**	Activates internal lubrication to allow easier removal of stylet.	Failure to flush the feeding tube for stylet removal may damage the feeding tube.
30. Remove the stylet before administering feedings.[5] **(Level M)**		
31. Disinfect the CORTRAK® system components with a germicidal disposable cloth.		
32. *Important:* Label the tube with the date and time of confirmed placement. Note the centimeter marking on the tube at the tip of the patient's nose to identify the depth of tube placement. Record the tube depth in the patient's record.[10] **(Level B*)**	Once the initial tube placement has been confirmed radiographically, a simple bedside assessment for displacement is monitoring the tube for a change in the external length.[10]	This information lets other healthcare providers know whether the tube has been inadvertently pulled out of position.

*Level B: Well-designed, controlled studies with results that consistently support a specific action, intervention, or treatment
*Level M: Manufacturer's recommendations only

Expected Outcomes

- Distal tip of the feeding tube rests in the stomach or small intestine
- The CORTRAK® image generally correlates well with the radiograph
- The patient tolerates enteral feeding at rates that meet established goals
- The patient is able to swallow oral foods and fluids while the small-bore tube is in place, if appropriate
- The small-bore tube accepts enteral feedings, medications, and fluid

Unexpected Outcomes

- Coughing, dyspnea, oxygen desaturation, and restlessness indicate potential pulmonary placement
- Pneumothorax from inadvertent pleural placement
- Pulmonary aspiration of gastric contents
- Epistaxis or esophageal injury during passage of the tube
- Inadvertent tube dislodgment
- Skin irritation/necrosis at the nose
- Occluded feeding tube
- Sinusitis/otitis media

Patient Monitoring and Care

Steps	Rationale	Reportable Conditions
1. Monitor the length of the tube in the patient and tolerance to tube placement.[9]	Placement may be difficult in agitated patients. Change in tube length can indicate that the tip of tube may be in an unintended location. Coughing, vomiting, or respiratory symptoms may indicate tube dislodgment or aspiration.[8]	• Inability to cooperate with the tube placement • Self extubation (partial or complete) • Coughing, vomiting, dyspnea, or decrease in oxygen saturation
2. Assess the oral cavity and perform oral care per institutional policy.	Mouth breathing dries secretions, encouraging bacterial growth and mucosal breakdown.	
3. Assess the insertion site for drainage, bleeding, redness, swelling, or ulceration.	Pressure from the tube can compromise blood flow to the tissue and cause skin damage and infection.	• Drainage, bleeding, redness, swelling, or ulceration at the site

Documentation

Documentation should include the following:

- The type and size of tube inserted
- The length of tube inserted
- Patient response to the insertion
- Unexpected outcomes
- Radiographic confirmation of the tube position
- Nursing interventions
- Medications administered
- Patient and family education

References

1. Ackerman M, Mick DJ: Technologic approaches to determining proper placement of enteral feeding tubes, *AACN Adv Crit Care* 17:246-249, 2006.
2. Aguilar-Nescimento JE, Kudsk KA: Use of small bore feeding tubes: success and failures, *Curr Opin Clin Nutr Metab Care* 10:291-226, 2007.
3. Bankhead RR, Fang JC: Enteral access devices. In Gottschlich MM, editor: *The A.S.P.E.N. Nutrition Support Core Curriculum,* Silver Spring, MD, American Society for Parenteral and Enteral Nutrition, 2007, 233-245.
4. CORPAK MedSystems: *CORTRAK® contraindication statement,* Wheeling, IL, 2008, CORPACK MedSystems.
5. CORPAK Medsystems: *CORTRAK® enteral access system operator's guide,* Wheeling, IL, 2008, CORPAK Medsystems.
6. Cresci G, et al: Trauma, surgery, burns. In Gottschlich MM, editor: *The A.S.P.E.N. Nutrition Support Core Curriculum,* Silver Spring, MD, American Society for Parenteral and Enteral Nutrition, 2007, 455-476.
7. **CR** Ellett ML, et al: Predicting the insertion distance for placing gastric tubes, *Clin Nurs Res* 14:11-27, 2005.
8. Gray R, et al: Bedside electromagnetic-guided feeding tube placement: an improvement over traditional placement technique? *Nutr Clin Pract* 22:436-444, 2007.
9. **CR** Metheny NA, et al: Indicators of tube site during feedings, *J Neurosci Nurs* 37(6):320-325, 2005.
10. Metheny NA: Preventing respiratory complications of tube feedings: evidence based practice, *Am J Crit Care* 15(4):360-369, 2006.
11. Metheny NA, Meert KL, Clouse RE: Complications related to feeding tube placement, *Curr Opin Gastroenterol* 23:178-182, 2007.

12. Phang J, Marsh W, Prager R: Feeding tube placement with the aid of a new electromagnetic transmitter [abstract SO82], *JPEN J Parenter Enteral Nutr* 30:S48, 2006.

13. Roberts S, Echeverria P, Gabriel SA: Devices and techniques for bedside enteral feeding tube placement, *Nutr Clin Pract* 22:412-420, 2007.

14. Sorokin R, Gottlieb JE: Enhancing patient safety during feeding-tube insertion: a review of more than 2000 insertions, *JPEN J Parenter Enteral Nutr* 30:440-445, 2006.

15. Stockdale W, et al: Nasoenteric feeding tube insertion utilizing an electromagnetic tube placement system [abstract NP24], *Nutr Clin Pract* 22:118, 2007.

Additional Readings

Baskin WN: Acute complications associated with bedside placement of feeding tubes, *Nutr Clin Pract* 21:40-55,105, 2006.

Metheny NA, et al: Tracheal aspiration of gastric contents in critically ill tube-fed patients: frequency outcomes, and risk factors, *Crit Care Med* 34,1007-1015, 2006.

Percutaneous Endoscopic Gastrostomy (PEG), Gastrostomy, and Jejunostomy Tube Care

P U R P O S E :   Gastrostomy, percutaneous endoscopic gastrostomy, and jejunostomy tubes provide long-term access to the gastrointestinal tract for nutrition.

Margaret M. Ecklund

PREREQUISITE NURSING KNOWLEDGE

- Knowledge of the anatomy and physiology of the upper and lower gastrointestinal (GI) system is necessary.
- Patients who cannot have enteral tubes passed orally or nasally because of anatomy or surgery and those who need supplemental enteral nutrition support for longer than 4 weeks should be considered as candidates for long-term enteral access.
- The most commonly used long-term enteral access is the percutaneous endoscopic gastrostomy (PEG) tube. The PEG tube is inserted without general anesthesia. The use of a local anesthetic (i.e., 1% lidocaine injection) is used at the abdominal puncture site. A guidewire is threaded via endoscope through the oropharynx, esophagus, and stomach and brought out through the abdominal wall. The tube is then threaded over the guidewire and passed into the stomach. The tapered end of the tube is brought through a stab wound in the abdominal wall until the mushroomed end of the tube is set against the stomach wall. An adapter for infusion is attached to the end of the tube, and a disk on the tube is moved up to the abdominal wall to stabilize the tube in place.
- PEG tubes are large-bore catheters that range from 18 to 22 Fr and have a mushroom-shaped curved end in the stomach and a two-port distal end to instill enteral nutrition, medications, and fluid. Commercial PEG tubes have

disks, perpendicular to the tube, to hold the device close to the skin and lessen shift of tube in and out of the skin (Fig. 133-1).
- Relative contraindications for PEG placement include the following:
  - ❖ Previous gastric resection
  - ❖ Tumors that block the passage of the endoscope
  - ❖ Ascites

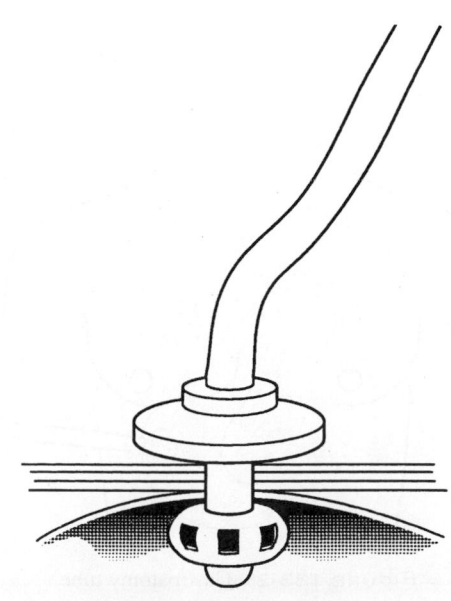

FIGURE 133-1   Percutaneous endoscopic gastrostomy.

* ❖ Morbid obesity
* ❖ Esophageal or gastric varices
* ❖ Esophageal stricture or narrowing
* Replacement gastrostomy tubes usually have a balloon in the intestinal lumen that is inflated with sterile water. This balloon prevents inadvertent dislocation. The distal end of the tube has an infusion port and a port for the balloon instillation (Fig. 133-2).
* A jejunostomy tube, which does not have a balloon, is indicated in those patients at risk for aspiration or who are unable to tolerate enteral feedings into the stomach. These tubes are routinely sutured in place for stability (Fig. 133-3). They are usually smaller bore, less than 14 Fr, and therefore are more prone to occlusion.
* If the tubes are inadvertently removed, reinsertion of the tubes is a routine procedure after the tunnel and stoma are healed (approximately 2 to 6 weeks after insertion).
* Because these tubes all enter through the abdominal wall, skin care at the site of insertion is important for skin integrity and prevention of infection.
* Consult with the multidisciplinary team to individualize nutrition goals. The nutrition plan is developed on the basis of the collaborative assessment of the nurse, dietitian, and physician or advance practice nurse.

EQUIPMENT

* Nonsterile gloves
* 4 × 4 gauze pads
* Cotton-tipped swabs
* 4 × 4 gauze pads, drain cut
* Protective skin barrier (e.g., vitamin A and D ointment)
* Silk tape (or paper tape if patient has a sensitivity to silk tape)
  Additional equipment to have available, as needed includes the following:
* Hydrogen peroxide
* Abdominal binder

PATIENT AND FAMILY EDUCATION

* Explain the purpose for the tube. ➤➤*Rationale:* Knowledge may decrease anxiety and fear of the unknown.
* Explain reason for skin care assessment and maintenance. ➤➤*Rationale:* Knowledge may decrease anxiety and fear of the unknown.
* Stress the importance of not pulling at the tube. ➤➤*Rationale:* Unnecessary pain and skin irritation may be avoided.
* Oral nutrition is possible with the long-term enteral access catheter. ➤➤*Rationale:* Knowledge may decrease anxiety and fear of the unknown.
* Long-term enteral access catheters can be removed when oral intake meets the needs of the individual. ➤➤*Rationale:* Knowledge may decrease anxiety and fear of the unknown. This also may be a goal for the patient to consume more via the oral route.
* Aspiration is a continued risk when the patient is positioned flat. ➤➤*Rationale:* Gastric residual volume can reflux and create a risk for pulmonary aspiration.

PATIENT ASSESSMENT AND PREPARATION
Patient Assessment

* Perform gastrointestinal assessment. ➤➤*Rationale:* A patient needs a functional gut to receive enteral nutrition.
* Assess skin condition at the feeding tube stoma; signs and symptoms of infection include the following:
  * ❖ Site redness or edema

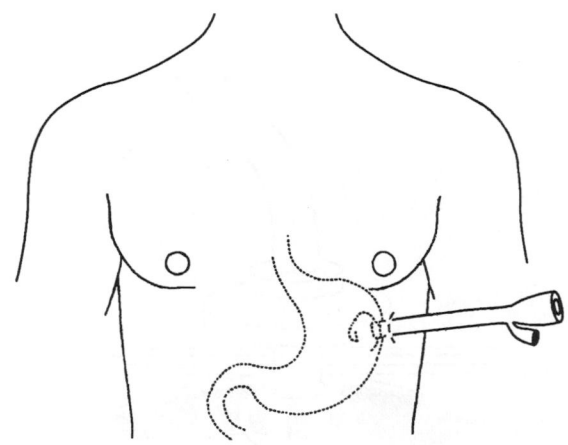

FIGURE 133-2   Gastrostomy tube.

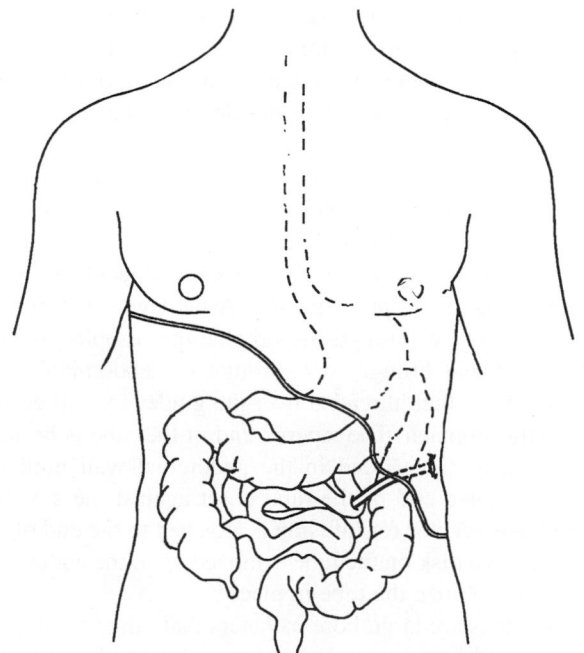

FIGURE 133-3   Jejunostomy tube placement.

❖ Warmth
❖ Purulent drainage
❖ Pain or tenderness
❖ Fever
➻*Rationale:* Intact skin integrity is a defense against infection. Early assessment of signs of infection promotes early, appropriate intervention.

Patient Preparation

• Ensure that patient understands preprocedural teachings. Answer questions as they arise, and reinforce information as needed. ➻*Rationale:* Understanding of previously taught information is evaluated and reinforced.
• Assist patient to position of comfort. ➻*Rationale:* Stoma of tube is easily accessible.

Procedure	for Percutaneous Endoscopic Gastrostomy (PEG), Gastrostomy, or Jejunostomy Tube Care	
Steps	**Rationale**	**Special Considerations**
1. ▣		
2. Apply nonsterile gloves.		
3. Use soap and warm water to moisten gauze pads and two cotton-tipped applicators. **(Level D*)**	Soap and water clean the skin surface at the stoma.[1-3]	Hydrogen peroxide, diluted to half strength with water, should be reserved for use for situations in which wound cleansing is a goal. Hydrogen peroxide dries skin at the stoma.[1-3]
4. Wipe the area closest to the tube (stoma) with the cotton-tipped applicators and proximal skin with the moistened gauze. Rinse with water. Displace the bumper to ensure cleaning and drying next to the skin at the stoma. Verify the bumper is not too tight against the skin. **(Level D)** One finger's breadth should fit between the bumper and the skin.	Moisture under the bumper can erode skin at tract.[3]	
5. Dry skin and stoma thoroughly with a dry gauze pad.	Prevents chafing and skin maceration.	
6. If significant moisture is found on the skin around the stoma, use cotton-tipped applicators to apply protective skin barrier (e.g., vitamin A and D ointment or other commercial topical moisture barrier products) in a circular motion around stoma. **(Level E*)**	Protective barrier ointment provides a moisture barrier for skin and assists wound healing. If purulent drainage is persistent, collaborate with healthcare practitioner to obtain and apply an antimicrobial ointment after skin cleansing.[1-3]	Increased moisture can cause a fungal infection that can be treated topically.[1,3]
7. Apply a 4 × 4 split gauze sponge around tube and secure with tape along edges. Change gauze every 12 hours or when soiled or moist. **(Level E)**	Gauze absorbs moisture from the stoma. If no drainage is present, gauze may be left off.[1-3]	
8. Anchor tube to skin at adjacent spot on abdomen. Site should be rotated to avoid skin damage from repeated taping. **(Level E)**	Reduces tension on the tube and avoids stoma erosion.[1-3]	

*Level D: Peer-reviewed, professional organizational standards with clinical studies to support recommendations
*Level E: Multiple case reports, theory-based evidence from expert opinions, or peer-reviewed professional organizational standards without clinical studies to support recommendations

Procedure continues on following page

Procedure for Percutaneous Endoscopic Gastrostomy (PEG), Gastrostomy, or Jejunostomy Tube Care—*Continued*

Steps	Rationale	Special Considerations
9. Adjust head of the bed to be at least 30 degrees when feedings are infusing. (**Level C***)	Minimizes the risk of aspiration.[4,5]	
10. Discard gloves and used supplies.		
11. 🅷🅷		

Expected Outcomes

- Intact skin at stoma of long-term enteral access device
- Long-term enteral access for enteral feeding and fluid administration remains patent

Unexpected Outcomes

- Infection at stoma
- Tube removal by patient or accidental dislodgment with patient movement
- Migration of tube into intestinal lumen
- Peritonitis
- Aspiration

Patient Monitoring and Care

Steps	Rationale	Reportable Conditions
		These conditions should be reported if they persist despite nursing interventions.
1. Assess skin integrity and quality of drainage from stoma.	Intact skin is the first line of prevention against infection.	• Erosion of stoma • Change in drainage • Increased volume of foul-smelling, purulent drainage from around stoma • Redness or pain at stoma
2. Ensure that the PEG tube has disk aligned next to the skin without pressure into the skin.	The disk helps prevent excess movement of the tube in and out of the skin. If the disk pushes with excess pressure, tissue injury may occur.[1-3]	• Pressure injury adjacent to stoma • Removal of tube by the patient • Clogging of the device • Buried bumper
3. Ensure that the patient does not remove long-term enteral access device. A loosely applied abdominal binder is helpful to deter a confused patient from pulling at the tube.	A tube removed before the tract is established is a potential surgical emergency and may necessitate immediate return to the operating room or endoscopy suite for repair and replacement. The immediate response is to place a replacement commercial tube or Foley catheter in the tract and notify the responsible healthcare provider. Consult the practitioner to determine the urgency of replacement. Tubes with established tracts can be replaced by the nurse at the bedside with a tube of comparable size and length.[1-3]	

*Level C: Qualitative studies, descriptive or correlational studies, integrative reviews, systematic reviews, or randomized controlled trials with inconsistent results

Patient Monitoring and Care —*Continued*

Steps	Rationale	Reportable Conditions
4. Note the distance of the tube from the infusion adapter to the entrance into the skin. Label the tube with the insertion date and the measurement at the entrance to the skin.	Facilitates future assessment for tube migration either inward or outward. Emesis or nausea may indicate pyloric obstruction from a tube migrating inward.[1-3]	• Length that has deviated significantly • Emesis or nausea
5. Evaluate wearing of the tube with ongoing use.	No routine change is indicated. Change of the tube is indicated with device failure.[3]	• Tube wearing

Documentation

Documentation should include the following:
- Patient and family education
- Condition of the stoma
- Any treatment rendered related to site complications
- Tube patency

- Type of tube and distance of the tube from the adapter to the entrance into the skin
- Unexpected outcomes
- Nursing interventions

References

1. Baskin WN: Acute complications associated with bedside placement of feeding tubes, *Nutr Clin Pract* 21:40-55, 2006.
CR 2. Loser C, Aschl G, Hebuterne, et al: ESPEN guidelines on artificial enteral nutrition-percutaneous endoscopic gastrostomy (PEG), *Clin Nutr* 24:845-861, 2005.
CR 3. McClave SA, Neff RL: Care and long term maintenance of percutaneous endoscopic gastrostomy tubes, *JPEN* 30:S27-S38, 2006.
CR 4. Metheny NA, Schallom ME, Edwards SJ: Effect of gastrointestinal motility and feeding tube site on aspiration risk in critically ill patients: a review, *Heart Lung* 33:131-145, 2004.

5. Metheny NA: Preventing respiratory complications of tube feedings: evidence-based practice, *Am J Crit Care* 15:360-369, 2006.

Additional Readings
CR Guenter P, Silkroski M: Tube feeding: practical guidelines and nursing protocols, Silver Spring, MD, 2001, Aspen Publishing.
CR Heiser M, Malaty H: Balloon type versus nonballoon type replacement percutaneous endoscopic gastrostomy: which is better? *Gastroenterol Nurs* 24:58-63, 2001.
CR Lord LM: Enteral access devices, *Nurs Clin North Am* 32: 685-702, 1997.

Small-Bore Feeding Tube Insertion and Care

P U R P O S E :   A small-bore feeding tube is inserted to provide access to the gastrointestinal tract for the patient who is unable to orally consume adequate calories. The tube can be used for administration of nutrients, fluid, and medications.

Margaret M. Ecklund

PREREQUISITE NURSING KNOWLEDGE

- Knowledge of the anatomy and physiology of the upper and lower gastrointestinal (GI) tract is needed.
- The GI tract should be functioning for gastric feedings to be digested and absorbed. Bowel sounds may not be audible, yet the GI tract is functional and enteral nutrition can be instituted safely and effectively and be well tolerated. Gastrointestinal findings that may affect the normal functioning of the tract and preclude gastric feeding are bowel obstruction, paralytic ileus, and some fistulas.
- Small-bore feeding tubes are preferable over larger-bore nasogastric tubes during the course of critical illness because the risk for tissue necrosis at the nares and sinusitis is lower. When small-bore feeding tubes are placed postpylorically, there is a reduced risk of aspiration.
- The small diameter of the tube allows simultaneous oral intake if the patient is able to consume orally without aspiration.
- Both weighted (tubes with an enlarged tip, filled with tungsten) and unweighted (bolus tip) small-bore nasogastric tubes are available. They typically are packaged with guidewires already in the lumen to assist passage of the tube. After successful placement, the guidewire is removed and discarded. The size of tubes range from 7 to 12 Fr.
- Unweighted-tip tubes migrate postpylorically into the duodenum more often than tubes with weighted tips. Weighted-tip tubes are harder for the patient with a compromised condition to swallow; ultimately, the

unweighted tube may be a more comfortable choice for the patient.
- Absolute contraindications for insertion of a nasogastric feeding tube are basilar skull fracture, transsphenoidal surgical approaches, and esophageal varices. Oral insertions are usually appropriate in these situations. Esophageal varices are a contraindication for any tube that transgresses the esophagus.
- Small-bore feeding tubes are not designed for drainage of gastric contents. If gastric decompression is desired, the small-bore nasogastric feeding tube should be replaced with a larger-bore nasogastric sump tube.
- It is important to review institutional standards regarding insertion of small-bore feeding tubes and complete competency for tube insertion.
- Some institutions restrict insertion to physicians and advanced practice nurses.

EQUIPMENT

- Small-bore feeding tube
- Small glass of water (bottle or tap, depending on institutional practice)
- 60-mL Luer-Lok tip, or catheter-tip syringe, appropriate for feeding tube (be sure size does not exceed recommended pressure limit for particular tube)
- Skin preparation agent
- Plastic adhesive or clear tape, or commercial fixation device
- Nonsterile gloves
- Water-soluble lubricant (if tube is not prelubricated)

PATIENT AND FAMILY EDUCATION

- Explain reason for insertion of tube and need for support of enteral nutrition. ➺*Rationale:* Knowledge may decrease anxiety and fear of the unknown.
- Explain how patient can assist with passage of the tube by positioning (e.g., sitting upright, head tipped forward and swallowing) when cued. ➺*Rationale:* Tube may pass more easily with patient cooperation.
- Explain the risk for gag reflex stimulation during insertion. ➺*Rationale:* Knowledge may decrease anxiety and fear of the unknown.
- Explain the reason for the radiograph after insertion. ➺*Rationale:* Knowledge may decrease anxiety and fear of the unknown.
- Discuss reasons for not pulling at the tube once it has been placed and secured. ➺*Rationale:* Leaving the tube in place avoids the need for reinsertion and another radiograph for verification. Reinsertion increases risk for trauma to nasopharyngeal passages. Dislodgment of the tube can increase the risk of aspiration.

PATIENT ASSESSMENT AND PREPARATION

Patient Assessment

- Assess for medical history of head and neck cancer and surgery, basilar skull fracture, esophageal cancer, decreased pharyngeal reflexes, or transsphenoidal pituitary

resection. ➺*Rationale:* These conditions prohibit safe passage of a tube nasally through the pharynx. Inadvertent intracranial placement of the small-bore feeding tube is possible with a basilar skull fracture.
- Assess patency of the nares for potential obstructions to feeding tube passage. ➺*Rationale:* A tube cannot pass through occlusion.
- Assess GI function. ➺*Rationale:* A functional gut is needed for administration of enteral feedings.

Patient Preparation

- Ensure that the patient understands preprocedural teachings. Answer questions as they arise, and reinforce information as needed. ➺*Rationale:* Understanding of previously taught information is evaluated and reinforced.
- If the patient has a large-bore nasogastric tube, it needs to be removed before placement of the small-bore nasogastric tube. ➺*Rationale:* Passing a small-bore tube is extremely difficult with an oral or nasal tube already in place. Removal of the large-bore tube after placement of the small-bore tube will likely cause displacement of the newly placed small tube.
- Perform oral care to moisten mucosa. Suction oropharyngeal area of excess secretions.[1] ➺*Rationale:* A moist, cleared oropharyngeal area facilitates patient comfort and passage of the tube.

Procedure for Small-Bore Feeding Tube Insertion and Care

Steps	Rationale	Special Considerations
1. **HH**		
2. **PE**		
3. Sit the patient upright and tip the head forward. **(Level E*)**	Facilitates passage of the tube into the esophagus. If the patient cannot tolerate upright positioning, position laterally to the right side to insert the tube.[3,6]	
4. Estimate the depth of tube insertion by measuring the tube from the tip of nose to the ear, then inferior to the stomach. **(Level E)**	Approximates the length of the tube to insert. If postpyloric placement is desired, add 10 to 15 cm to the length of tube measured.[3,6]	
5. Lubricate the tip of the tube with water. **(Level M*)**	Water activates a lubricant on the surface of the tube to facilitate passage through nares.	If the tube does not have self lubrication, a water-soluble lubricant can be applied to the tube.
6. Insert the tip of the tube into either naris; advance to the posterior pharynx until resistance is met. **(Level E)**	Once the tube is advanced through the nares, the oropharynx is reached and the tube meets resistance.[3,6]	
7. At this point, ask the patient to swallow. If the patient is able to cooperate, give small sips of water to attempt to trigger the swallow reflex and ease tube passage. **(Level E)**	Swallowing immediately assists passage of the tube into the esophagus. If the patient is unable to cooperate with swallowing, neck positioning may facilitate passage.[3,6]	If coughing begins immediately with advancement of the tube, immediately pull back to the nares and allow the patient to recover.

*Level E: Multiple case reports, theory-based evidence from expert opinions, or peer-reviewed professional organizational standards without clinical studies to support recommendations
*Level M: Manufacturer's recommendations only

Procedure continues on following page

Procedure   for Small-Bore Feeding Tube Insertion and Care—*Continued*

Steps	Rationale	Special Considerations
8. As the patient swallows, advance the tube to the desired marking. Remove the guidewire with one hand while holding the tube securely at the nares. **(Level M*)**	The initial swallow gets the tube into the esophagus, and the nurse can advance it to desired position without repeated swallowing. Removing the guidewire without holding the tube can cause the tube to pull out with the guidewire.	If the patient is unconscious or unable to cooperate, do not attempt to use water orally to pass tube. The guidewire may be left in and removed after radiographic verification. Caution is used because the tube may be displaced with stylet removal. The stylet should not be reinserted while tube is in the patient.
9. Apply skin preparation to the nose and securing surface of the face; allow to dry. **(Level D*)**	Prepares the surface of skin to help with the tape adhering.[4]	
10. Tape the tube securely to nose, with use of one half of a 3-cm strip. The lower portion of the tape is then split up to the tip of the nose and wrapped around the tube. **(Level D)**	The tape needs to hold the tube to prevent slipping it out. Pink plastic tape has shown an ability to stay secure for a greater length of time compared with other methods.[4]	Tape the tube so that it does not press against the skin. Excess pressure can cause breakdown. A commercial tube fixation device may be used, with the same securing principles.
11. Remove gloves.		
12. 🄷🄷		
13. Obtain a chest radiograph (lower chest view) to verify placement. **(Level D)**	Chest radiographic verification is the safest way to ensure correct placement. A lower chest view ensures the tip is in stomach or intestine.[2,3,6]	
14. If postpyloric placement is desired, tape additional length with coil in stomach. **(Level E*)**	The extra length can allow the migration of the tube past the pyloric valve.[2,3,5-7]	
15. Position the patient onto right side.	Assists with peristalsis. If the tube is in the stomach, peristalsis should move it beyond the sphincter.	Air insufflation techniques (with and without metoclopramide) have also been used to facilitate postpyloric placement of feeding tubes. This technique causes the stomach to distend with air injected by the practitioner and facilitates feeding tube passage through the pyloric sphincter.
16. Obtain abdominal radiograph. **(Level D)**	Abdominal radiographic verification is the standard of care to ensure correct placement.[2]	Postpyloric placement is verified with abdominal film to ensure tip is visualized.
17. If the tube has not migrated postpylorically, continue to position the patient onto the right side and recheck the radiograph. **(Level D)**	Right-side positioning potentially helps pass the tube postpyloric with the aid of peristalsis. The best location is at the beginning of the jejunum, or the fourth portion of the duodenum.[3,5,6]	
18. If the tube remains in the stomach, consult with the physician or advanced pratice nurse to prescribe metoclopramide intravenously and repeat radiograph after this drug is administered. **(Level D)**	Promotility agents have shown benefit in moving feeding tubes through the pyloric valve.[3,5-7]	Metoclopramide should be used with caution because prolonged administration at higher doses is associated with the development of tardive dyskinesia.

*Level D: Peer-reviewed, professional organizational standards with clinical studies to support recommendations
*Level E: Multiple case reports, theory-based evidence from expert opinions, or peer-reviewed professional organizational standards without clinical studies to support recommendations
*Level M: Manufacturer's recommendations only

Expected Outcomes

- The distal tip of tube is placed in either the stomach or the small bowel
- A patent tube that accepts enteral feedings, medications, and fluid
- The patient is able to swallow oral foods and fluids while the small-bore feeding tube is in place, if allowed

Unexpected Outcomes

- Coughing or dyspnea, indicating potential bronchial placement
- Pneumothorax from inadvertent pleural placement
- Tube coiled in esophagus or posterior pharynx
- Esophageal tear from trauma of tube passing
- Tube dislodging during therapy, necessitating removal and new tube placement
- Aspiration of stomach contents despite appropriate placement
- Clogging of enteral tube with medication fragments or enteral formula
- Skin irritation or breakdown at nose

Patient Monitoring and Care

Steps	Rationale	Reportable Conditions
		These conditions should be reported if they persist despite nursing interventions.
1. Monitor tolerance to tube placement.	Agitation may inhibit successful placement.	• Self-extubation • Agitation and inability to cooperate with tube placement • Recurrent vomiting • Continued coughing and dyspnea
2. Assess oral cavity and perform oral care every 2 to 4 hours and as needed.	Patients with orogastric or nasogastric tubes in place tend to mouth breathe, thus drying the mouth and increasing the risk for mucosal breakdown and ulceration. Tube presence also may predispose a patient to sinusitis or oral infections.	• Ulceration, drainage, foul odor
3. Monitor the insertion site of the tube for redness, swelling, drainage, bleeding, or skin breakdown. Use only water-soluble lubricants at site.	Many critically ill patients have fragile skin and have associated conditions that predispose them to skin breakdown. Frequent monitoring and subsequent repositioning of the tube can prevent serious damage.	• Redness • Swelling • Drainage • Bleeding • Skin breakdown at insertion site
4. Reposition and retape the tube every 24 hours or when the tape is soiled.	Decreases risk for tissue damage to mouth or nares.	

Documentation

Documentation should include the following:
- Patient and family education
- Size and type of tube placed
- Patient response to insertion
- Length of the tube external to the patient, from nose to the end of the tube
- Radiographic interpretation
- Unexpected outcomes
- Nursing interventions
- Medications administered

References

1. AACN Practice Alert: *Oral care in the critically ill,* 2007, from www.aacn.org accessed 01/03/10.
2. AACN Practice Alert: *Verification of feeding tube placement,* 2006, from www.aacn.org accessed 01/03/10.
3. Baskin WN: Acute complications associated with bedside placement of feeding tubes, *Nutr Clin Pract* 21:40-55, 2006.
CR 4. Burns SM, et al: Comparison of nasogastric tube securing methods and tube types in medical intensive care patients, *AJCC* 4:198-203, 1995.
CR 5. Metheny NA, Schallom ME, Edwards SJ: Effect of gastrointestinal motility and feeding tube site on aspiration risk in critically ill patients: a review, *Heart Lung* 33:131-145, 2004.
6. Metheny NA: Preventing respiratory complications of tube feedings: evidence-based practice, *Am J Crit Care* 15:360-369, 2006.
7. Sorokin R, Gottleib JE: Enhancing patient safety during feeding tube insertion: a review of more than 2000 insertions, *JPEN* 30:440-445, 2006.

Additional Readings

CR Guenter P, Silkroski M: *Tube feeding: practical guidelines and nursing protocols,* Silver Spring, MD, 2001, Aspen Publishers.
CR Lord LM, et al: Comparison of weighted vs unweighted enteral feeding tubes for efficacy of transpyloric intubation, *JPEN* 17:271-273, 1993.
CR Metheny N: Assessing placement of feeding tubes, *AJN* 101:36-45, 2002.

AP Determination of Death in Adult Patients

P U R P O S E : This procedure describes how death is determined. Institution policies and legislation governing declaration of death may vary across practice settings and states. However, standardized evidence-based criteria provide guidelines for practice involving the determination of cardiopulmonary and brain death.

Margaret L. Campbell

PREREQUISITE NURSING KNOWLEDGE

- Death is determined with either irreversible cessation of circulatory and respiratory functions or irreversible cessation of all functions of the entire brain, including the brain stem.
- Historically, death had been described as the cessation of circulation and respiration (cardiopulmonary death). The advent of mechanical ventilation and cardiovascular support, however, presented new challenges for determination of death in patients with catastrophic cerebral insults whose cardiopulmonary function could be preserved with complex technology.[3,5]
- Initial efforts to define death in an age of technologic advancement included the development of the Harvard criteria, which described determination of a condition known as irreversible coma, cerebral death, or brain death.[1]
- Since the initial introduction of the Harvard criteria, the Uniform Determination of Death Act (UDDA) was published in 1980 and was recommended by the President's Commission for the Study of Ethical Problems in Medicine and Biomedical and Biobehavioral Research as a model statute for state legislation defining death.[3]

AP This procedure should be performed only by physicians, advanced practice nurses, and other healthcare professionals (including critical care nurses) with additional knowledge, skills, and demonstrated competence per professional licensure or institutional standard.

- UDDA asserts that "an individual who has sustained either (1) irreversible cessation of circulatory and respiratory functions, or (2) irreversible cessation of all functions of the entire brain, including the brainstem, is dead. A determination of death must be made in accordance with accepted medical standards."[3]
- In cases of either cardiopulmonary or brain death, diagnosis of death requires both cessation of function and irreversibility.
- In cardiopulmonary death, cessation of function is determined with clinical examination.
- In cardiopulmonary death, irreversibility is confirmed with persistent cessation of functions during a period of observation.
- In brain death, cessation of function is determined when clinical evaluation discloses absence of both cerebral and brain stem function.
- In brain death, irreversibility is determined when the etiology of the coma is sufficient to account for the loss of brain function is established, the possibility of recovery of brain function is excluded, and the cessation of all brain function persists for a period of observation or therapy.[3,5]
- The concept of brain death continues to be a topic of international debate among clinicians, anthropologists, philosophers, and ethicists. This ongoing dialogue concerning the determination of death is a process of developing multidisciplinary consensus that is responsive to continually changing technology.[6,7]
- Although conceptualization of death continues to evolve, experts have generated clinical practice parameters for

brain death diagnosis that are grounded in empirical knowledge, supported by sufficiently rigorous research, and substantiated by high degrees of clinical certainty.[6,7]

- Cardinal findings in brain death include coma or unresponsiveness, apnea, absence of cerebral motor responses to pain in all extremities, and absence of brain stem reflexes, including pupillary signs, ocular movements, facial sensory and motor responses, and pharyngeal and tracheal reflexes.
- Legal responsibility for assessment and declaration of death varies by state. Some states permit registered nurses and advanced practice nurses to determine death.

EQUIPMENT

- For cardiopulmonary death determination:
  - ❖ Stethoscope
  - ❖ Electrocardiogram (ECG) monitor
  - ❖ ECG leads
  - ❖ ECG electrodes
  - ❖ Nonsterile gloves
- For brain death determination:
  - ❖ Flashlight
  - ❖ Laboratory testing supplies
  - ❖ Iced saline or water solution
  - ❖ 60-mL Luer-Lok syringe and 18- or 20-gauge angiocatheter with needle removed (or 60-mL Toomey syringe)
  - ❖ Small basin
  - ❖ Towels and protective bedding
  - ❖ Nonsterile gloves
  - ❖ Oxygen delivery via an endotracheal airway with a nasal cannula or straight tubing for oxygen delivery
  - ❖ Arterial blood gas kit supplies
  - ❖ Pulse oximeter
  - ❖ Blood pressure monitoring system

PATIENT AND FAMILY EDUCATION

- Assess family understanding of the death determination procedure and its purpose. ➤*Rationale:* Clarification and repeat explanation may assist in allaying some stress and anxiety for grief-stricken family members.
- Explain potential outcomes of the death determination procedure. ➤*Rationale:* Awareness of the duration and expectations of death determination procedures may allay some stress and anxiety in grief-stricken family members.
- Assess family understanding of the concept of "brain-dead" if testing for brain death. Give clear definition of brain death and death as synonymous and reinforce repeatedly with the family. ➤*Rationale:* The concept of brain death may be confusing to family members because the term "brain dead" may imply that only the brain is dead and the rest of the body is alive. Brain death must be described as death.

PATIENT ASSESSMENT AND PREPARATION
Patient Assessment

- Assess the patient's baseline cardiopulmonary and neurologic status in preparation for determination of death. ➤*Rationale:* In cardiopulmonary death, clinical examination discloses absence of responsiveness, heartbeat, and respiratory effort. In brain death, clinical examination reveals an absence of both cerebral and brain stem function.
- For brain death determination, the following prerequisites must also be met:
  - ❖ Acquire evidence of an acute catastrophic cerebral event consistent with the clinical diagnosis of brain death.
  - ❖ Exclude conditions that may confound the clinical assessment of brain death, such as acute metabolic or endocrine derangements or neuromuscular blockade.
  - ❖ Confirm the absence of drug intoxication or poisoning.
  - ❖ Maintain the patient's core body temperature greater than or equal to 32°C.
  - ➤*Rationale:* The brain death determination procedure must confirm both cessation and irreversibility of all brain function. The previous four criteria are required for the confirmation of irreversible cessation of brain function.

Patient Preparation

- Verify correct patient with two identifiers. ➤*Rationale:* Prior to performing a procedure, the nurse should ensure the correct identification of the patient for the intended intervention.
- Ensure that the family understands preprocedural teaching. Answer questions as they arise, and reinforce information as needed. ➤*Rationale:* This communication evaluates and reinforces understanding of previously taught information.
- Facilitate the discussion of organ donation by notifying the organ procurement organization (OPO). ➤*Rationale:* Centers for Medicare and Medicaid Services (CMS) require that all deaths be reported to the local OPO regardless of age or circumstances. Many OPOs have instituted the use of clinical triggers to initiate the referral. The triggers are based on OPO and hospital agreed-on physical examination findings. Patients who are brain dead are potential candidates for organ donation. Request for organ donation is the responsibility of representatives from the OPO or a specially trained designated hospital requester after consultation with the OPO (see Procedure 136).[2]
- Place the patient in a supine position. ➤*Rationale:* Positioning facilitates patient assessment, oculovestibular testing, and arterial puncture.

Procedure for Determination of Death

Steps	Rationale	Special Considerations
Determination of Cardiopulmonary Death		
1. **HH**		
2. **PE**		
3. Conduct a clinical examination: A. Assess level of consciousness. B. Assess airway. C. Assess breathing. D. Assess circulation.	The clinical examination in cardiopulmonary death reveals absence of responsiveness, heartbeat, and respiratory effort.	
4. Perform an ECG if available (see Procedures 57 and 60).	A confirmatory test such as ECG monitoring or 12-lead ECG may be performed to rule out reversible nonperfusing dysrhythmias.	
5. Confirm the irreversibility of the cessation of cardiopulmonary function.	Irreversibility is confirmed with persistent cessation of functions, including pulselessness, apnea, and loss of consciousness.	In clinical situations in which death is expected and the course has been gradual, the period of observation after cessation may be limited to the time needed to complete the examination. If ventricular fibrillation and cardiac standstill develop in a monitored patient and resuscitation is not undertaken or is unsuccessful, the required period of observation may be limited to the time needed to complete the examination. When a possible death is unobserved, unexpected, or sudden, the duration of the examination should be commensurate with continued resuscitative efforts. Declaration of death in patients who are first observed with rigor mortis may require only the period of observation necessary to establish that condition. In cases of donation after cardiac death, the duration of observation of cessation may be defined in policy or protocol (see Procedure 137).
6. Discard used supplies in an appropriate receptacle.	Removes and safely discards used supplies.	
7. **HH**		
Determination of Brain Death		
1. **HH**		
2. **PE**		
3. Ensure that the patient's core body temperature is at least 32°C at the time of the clinical examination for brain death determination.	Hypothermia may artificially alter the results of the neurologic examination, leading to confounding results regarding irreversible cessation of brain function.[6,7]	
4. Perform the necessary endocrine screenings as required for the individual patient to rule out reversible conditions, such as diabetic ketoacidosis.	Endocrine screening may exclude conditions that could confound the clinical assessment of brain death.[6,7]	

Procedure continues on following page

Procedure for Determination of Death—*Continued*

Steps	Rationale	Special Considerations
5. Perform the necessary toxicology screenings as required for the individual patient.	In cases in which the possibility of excessive sedation is present, toxicology screening for all likely drugs should be considered.[6,7]	If exogenous intoxication of drugs is determined to exist, death should not be declared until the intoxicant is metabolized or until confirmatory testing for cessation of intracranial circulation is considered.
6. In the presence of neuromuscular blockade use, assessment with a peripheral nerve stimulator is required before testing for cerebrally modulated motor responses (see Procedure 38).	Clinical brain death determination procedures cannot be undertaken in the presence of neuromuscular blockade. Neuromuscular blockade may confound motor testing in brain death because of pharmacologically induced motor weakness.	In cases in which neuromuscular blocking agents may have been previously used, testing with a peripheral nerve stimulator may determine whether adequate neuromuscular function is present for valid clinical brain death determination.
7. Establish evidence of coma or unresponsiveness.	In brain death, intense stimulation evokes no verbal or voluntary motor responses.	Spontaneous voluntary motor activity, shivering, posturing, and seizure activity are absent in brain death.
8. Assess the patient's cerebral motor responses to pain with central noxious stimulation such as a sternal rub or pinching the trapezius (Fig. 135-1).	Absence of cerebral motor responses to pain is a cardinal finding consistent with brain death.[6,7] Peripheral stimuli such as nail bed pressure may evoke a reflex arc as opposed to a true brain stem response.	Motor responses may occur spontaneously during apnea testing with the occurrence of hypoxia or hypotension and are considered to be of spinal reflex origin. Respiratory acidosis and brisk neck flexion also may generate spinal cord reflexes. Spinal reflex responses occur more frequently in young adults and include rapid spontaneous flexion and muscle stretch reflexes in the arms and legs, with resulting grasp-like walking movements. Spinal reflex movements are not cerebrally modulated. Spinal reflex movements may occur in the presence of brain death. Involuntary posturing movements are absent in brain death.

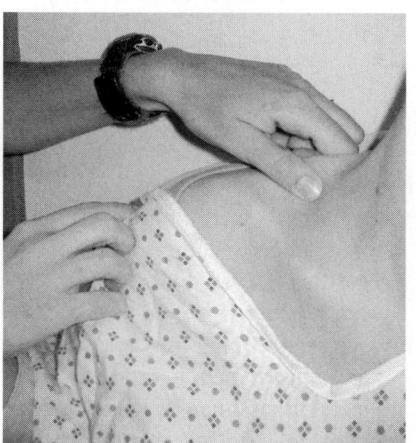

FIGURE 135-1   The trapezius pinch.

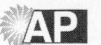

Procedure for Determination of Death—*Continued*

Steps	Rationale	Special Considerations
9. Assess the patient's pupillary size and bilateral response to light.	Round, oval, or irregularly shaped pupils are compatible with brain death. Pupillary light reflex must be absent in brain death. Absence of pupillary light reflexes, as a component of brain stem reflexes, is a cardinal finding consistent with brain death.[6,7] Most pupils are midposition size (4 to 6 mm) in brain death.	Dilated pupils may occur even in the presence of brain death because sympathetic cervical pathways connected to the pupillary dilator muscle may still be intact. Standard doses of atropine administered intravenously do not markedly affect pupillary response. Neuromuscular blocking agents do not significantly influence pupil size. Topical administration of medications and ocular trauma may influence pupillary size and reactivity. Preexisting ocular anatomic abnormalities may also confound pupillary assessment in brain death.
10. Assess the patient's corneal and jaw reflexes. A. Corneal reflexes should be tested with a cotton-tipped swab. B. Jaw reflexes are described as grimacing to pain and may be tested with application of deep pressure on the nail beds, the supraorbital ridge, or the temporomandibular joint.	Absence of facial and motor responses, as a component of brain stem reflexes, is a cardinal finding consistent with brain death. Corneal and jaw reflexes are absent in brain death.[6,7]	Severe facial trauma may inhibit interpretation of facial brain stem reflexes.
11. Assess the patient's gag and cough reflexes. A. The gag reflex may be elicited by stimulating the posterior pharynx with a tongue blade. B. The cough reflex may be tested with bronchial suctioning.	The absence of pharyngeal and tracheal reflexes, as a component of brain stem reflexes, is a cardinal finding consistent with brain death. Gag and cough reflexes are absent in brain death.[6,7]	Gag reflex may be difficult to evaluate in orally intubated patients.
12. Assess the patient's oculocephalic (doll's eye) reflexes (Fig. 135-2). A. Oculocephalic reflexes are elicited by rapidly and vigorously turning the head 90 degrees laterally on both sides. B. If the oculocephalic reflexes are intact, the patient's eyes deviate from the direction in which the patient's nose points. C. In brain death, oculocephalic reflexes are absent, with no eye movements occurring in response to head movements.	Absence of oculocephalic reflexes, as a component of brain stem reflexes, is a cardinal finding consistent with brain death.[6,7]	Contraindications to performance of oculocephalic reflex testing include suspicion of cervical spine fracture or instability.

Procedure continues on following page

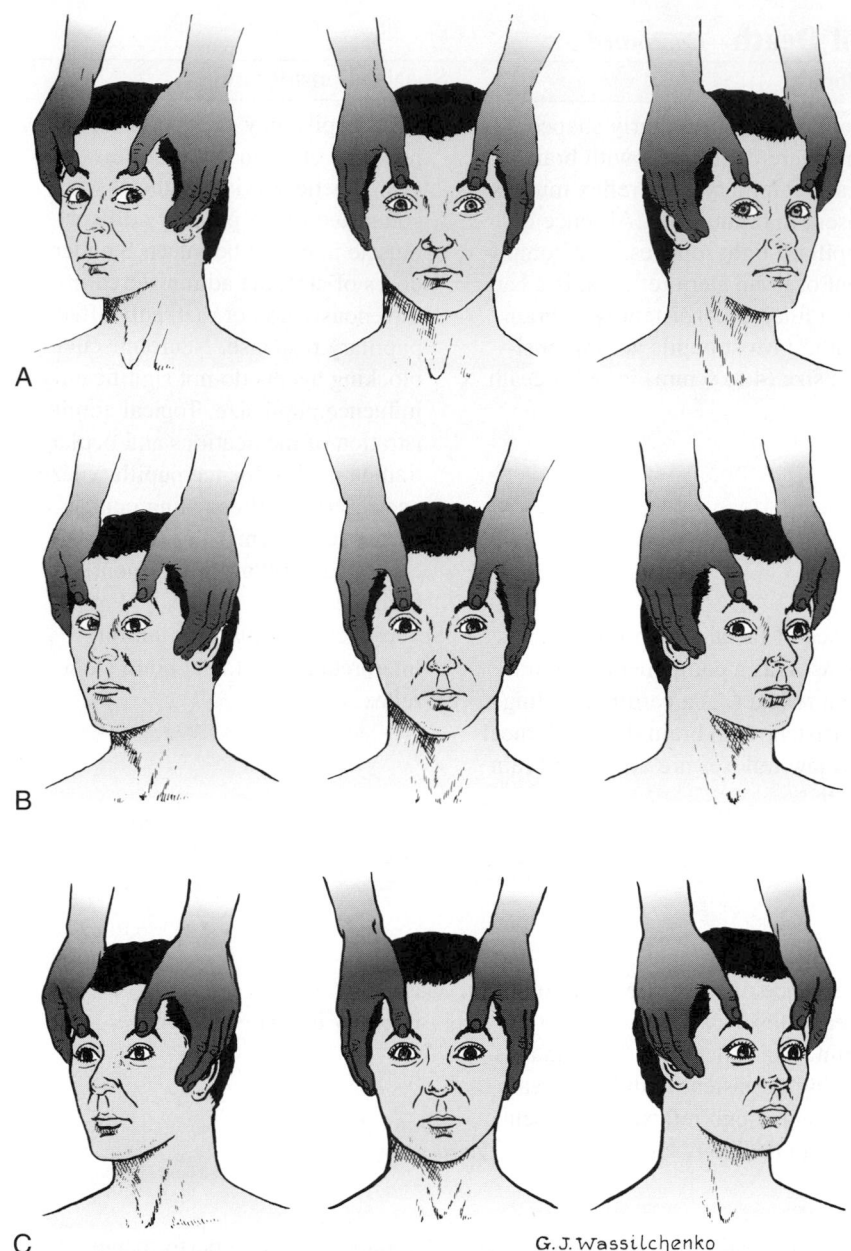

A

B

C

G. J. Wassilchenko

FIGURE 135-2 Oculocephalic reflex (doll's eyes). **A,** Normal. **B,** Abnormal. **C,** Absent. *(From Urden LD, Stacy KM, Lough ME, editors: Critical care nursing, ed 6, St Louis, 2010, Elsevier.)*

Procedure | for Determination of Death—*Continued*

Steps	Rationale	Special Considerations
13. Assess the patient's oculovestibular (caloric) reflexes (Fig. 135-3). A. Elevate the head of the bed to 30 degrees. B. Inspect the ear canals for patency. C. Instill 50 mL of iced water or saline solution into the ear over 30 seconds to 3 minutes. D. Observe the patient's eyes for 1 minute. E. After 5 minutes, perform the same procedure to the patient's other ear.	Absence of oculovestibular reflexes, as a component of brain stem reflexes, is a cardinal finding consistent with brain death.[6,7]	Contraindications to testing of oculovestibular reflexes include impaired integrity of the tympanic membranes. Several medications may diminish oculovestibular reflexes, such as sedatives, aminoglycosides, tricyclic antidepressants, anticholinergics, antiseizure agents, and neuromuscular blocking agents. Preexisting vestibular disease, preexisting cranial nerve disorders, and facial trauma involving the auditory canal and petrous bone also may inhibit oculovestibular reflex responses.

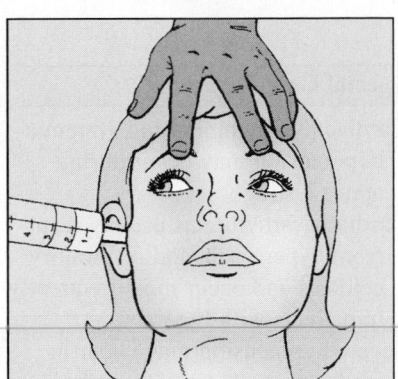

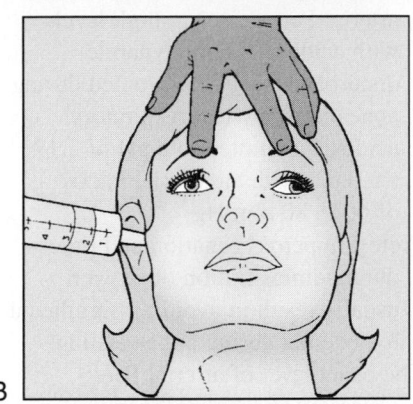

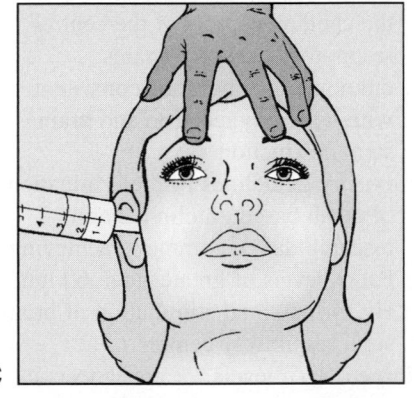

FIGURE 135-3 Oculovestibular reflex (cold caloric test). **A,** Normal. **B,** Abnormal. **C,** Absent. *(From Urden LD, Stacy KM, Lough ME, editors: Critical care nursing, ed 6, St Louis, 2010, Elsevier.)*

Procedure for Determination of Death—*Continued*

Steps	Rationale	Special Considerations
F. Observe the patient's eyes for 1 minute.		
G. In brain death, the oculovestibular reflexes are absent, with no deviation of the eyes in response to ear irrigation.		
14. Prepare for the performance of an apnea test.	A cardinal finding and essential component in the clinical determination of brain death is the demonstration of apnea. Loss of brain stem function definitively results in loss of centrally controlled breathing function, with resultant apnea.	

Procedure continues on following page

Procedure for Determination of Death—*Continued*

Steps	Rationale	Special Considerations

15. Achieve conditions necessary for apnea test precautions.[6,7]
  A. Maintain core body temperature greater than or equal to 32.0°C.
  B. Maintain systolic blood pressure greater than or equal to 90 mm Hg.
  C. Additional considerations include:
    1. Achieve euvolemia.
    2. Achieve eucapnea (arterial $Paco_2$ of greater than or equal to 40 mm Hg).
    3. Maintain/achieve hyperoxia (arterial Pao_2 of greater than or equal to 200 mm Hg). **(Level C*)**
	Apnea test precautions minimize cardiac dysrhythmias and systemic hypotension, which may occur during the apnea test.	Cardiac dysrhythmias and systemic hypotension may occur during apnea testing.[7]
		Cardiac dysrhythmias usually result from hypercarbia and respiratory acidosis and occur most frequently in patients with hypoxia.
		Severe hypotension may occur in well-oxygenated patients whose arterial $Paco_2$ rises to high levels with acidosis. Hemodynamic disturbances may be avoided during apnea testing when respiratory acidosis is limited to a pH of 7.17 ($\pm$ 0.02) with an arterial $Paco_2$ of 60 to 80 mm Hg.
		Pretest hyperoxygenation and procedural administration of oxygen usually result in avoiding significant hypoxemia during apnea testing.

16. Perform an apnea test:
  A. Obtain a baseline arterial blood gas (ABG) value.
  B. Disconnect the ventilator.
  C. Deliver 100% oxygen, 6 L/min. May place an oxygen cannula at the level of the carina.
  D. Observe closely for any respiratory movements, oxygenation changes (pulse oximetry), and hemodynamic instability.
  E. Obtain an ABG after approximately 8 minutes.
  F. If the $Paco_2$ is less than 60 mm Hg and the patient's condition is hemodynamically stable, wait an additional 2 minutes and redraw an ABG before reconnecting the ventilator.
  G. Reconnect the ventilator at a low respiratory rate and 1.0 fraction of inspired oxygen (Fio_2) while waiting for the ABG results.
	Determines the patient's respiratory status.
	If the apnea test must be repeated or the time of observation is extended, reconnect the ventilator at a low respiratory rate and 1.0 Fio_2 to maintain a high level of $Paco_2$ and hyperoxygenation.
		The exact level of arterial $Paco_2$ necessary to maximally stimulate the chemoreceptors of the central respiratory centers remains unknown in conditions consistent with hyperoxygenation and brain stem destruction.
		Advisory guidelines for determination of death based on clinical and research data recommend achieving $Paco_2$ levels of greater than 60 mm Hg for maximal stimulation of brain stem respiratory centers.[6]
		Target $Paco_2$ levels for apnea tests in brain death determination may be higher in patients with chronic hypercapnia.
		Hypocarbia may also occur in patients with acute catastrophic cerebral insults and may result from therapeutic hyperventilation or hypothermia.
		Although correction of hypocarbia should precede apnea testing, use of carbon dioxide admixtures should probably be avoided because of the associated consequences, including severe hypercarbia and respiratory acidosis.

*Level C: Qualitative studies, descriptive or correlational studies, integrative reviews, systematic reviews, or randomized controlled trials with inconsistent results

Procedure for Determination of Death—*Continued*

Steps	Rationale	Special Considerations
17. Abort the apnea test if hemodynamic instability occurs.	Cardiac arrest may result.	Cardiac arrest diminishes the possibility of successful organ retrieval or transplantation if the patient is a donor and results in aggressive resuscitative measures if the patient does not have a Do Not Resuscitate order.
18. Interpret the apnea test results (Table 135-1). A. Positive B. Negative C. Occurrence of cardiovascular or pulmonary instability D. Inconclusive	Aids in determination of brain death.[6,7]	
19. Facilitate compliance with institution recommendations regarding persistent observation in brain death determination.	Persistent observation further confirms irreversibility in the clinical determination of brain death. A repeat clinical evaluation of cardinal findings in brain death is recommended.	Most experts recommend an arbitrary interval of 6 hours between initial and repeat observations for the clinical determination of brain death in adults; however, a firm recommendation based on scientific literature cannot be given. All clinical tests of cardinal findings are equally essential in the declaration of brain death. The period of observation can be shortened if there is evidence of brain stem herniation or a catastrophic event can be supported with cerebral angiography or other tests of intracranial blood circulation.

Procedure continues on following page

TABLE 135-1	**Apnea Test Results**
Positive apnea test results	Respiratory movements are absent. Posttest arterial $Paco_2$ is $\geq$ 60 mm Hg. Supports clinical determination of brain death.
Negative apnea test results	Respiratory movements are observed regardless of arterial $Paco_2$ level. Does not support clinical determination of brain death; apnea test may be repeated after a change in clinical status is observed.
Apnea test results of cardiovascular or pulmonary instability	Systolic blood pressure falls below 90 mm Hg. Arterial oxygen desaturation below therapeutic levels occurs. Cardiac dysrhythmias occur. Immediately draw an arterial blood gas sample and reconnect the ventilator. Confirmatory test to finalize clinical determination of brain death may be performed.
Inconclusive apnea test results	No respiratory movements are observed. Posttest arterial $Paco_2$ is < 60 mm Hg without significant cardiovascular instability. Apnea test may be repeated with 10 minutes of apnea.

Procedure   for Determination of Death—*Continued*

Steps	Rationale	Special Considerations
20. Assist in obtaining confirmatory tests for brain death determination as indicated (Table 135-2). **(Level B*)**	Confirmatory testing may aid the diagnosis.[4,8] Although confirmatory tests are not mandatory in most situations, diagnostic testing may be necessary for the declaration of brain death with patients in whom specific components of clinical testing cannot be reliably evaluated. Clinical experience with confirmatory tests involves use of conventional angiography, electroencephalogram (EEG), transcranial Doppler ultrasound scan (TCD), and cerebral blood flow studies. The most reliable confirmatory test is cerebral angiography.[8]	
21. Discard used supplies in appropriate receptacles.	Removes and safely discards used supplies.	
22. 🅷🅷		

Expected Outcomes

- Clinical or diagnostic determination of death
- Declaration of death and notification of the family

Unexpected Outcomes

- Indecisive results regarding determination of death

Patient Monitoring and Care

Steps	Rationale	Reportable Conditions
		These conditions should be reported if they persist despite nursing interventions.
1. Assess family understanding of and response to the death determination procedure.	Family understanding of and response to the death determination situations may vary based on religious beliefs and cultural practices. Adequate assessment of the family provides the necessary foundation for the provision of support.	• Family confusion about brain death is common; the physician may need to be called back to answer questions and reiterate the findings

*Level B: Well-designed, controlled studies with results that consistently support a specific action, intervention, or treatment

TABLE 135-2	**Confirmatory Brain Death Test Results**
Cerebral angiography	No intracerebral filling at the level of the carotid bifurcation or circle of Willis External carotid circulation patent
Electroencephalogram (EEG)	No electrical activity during a period of at least 30 minutes of recording
Transcranial Doppler ultrasound scan	Absent diastolic or reverberating flow Flow only through systole or retrograde diastolic flow Small systolic peaks in early systole
Technetium 99m brain scan (cerebral blood flow scan)	No uptake of isotope in brain parenchyma ("hollow skull phenomenon")

Patient Monitoring and Care —*Continued*

Steps	Rationale	Reportable Conditions
2. Solicit family support (e.g., spiritual counselors, grief counselors, etc.).	Support may assist the family in the grieving process.	
3. Provide adequate private time for family members to visit with and grieve for the loss of their loved one.	Private visiting time provides family members with the opportunity for grieving and closure.	
4. Facilitate the discussion of organ donation options in cases of brain death.	The OPO screens the patient with brain death or devastating neurologic insults for possible organ donation and offers donation if the patient is medically suitable.	
5. Use grief resources available at hospital.	Families may benefit from having handprints or footprints made and retrieving a lock of hair. Family may wish to participate in a bereavement program.	
6. In cases in which brain death has not been confirmed but in which a grave prognosis is determined, be prepared to facilitate and provide support during discussions regarding possible withholding and withdrawing life-sustaining therapies (see Procedure 138).	Indecisive results regarding brain death determination may lead to consideration of other options, including withholding and withdrawing life-sustaining therapies. The healthcare team, in collaboration with the patient's family, may make decisions regarding continuation or initiation of resuscitation measures, provision of supportive care, and withholding and withdrawing life-sustaining therapies in cases of devastating neurologic insults without the occurrence of brain death. Organ donation after cardiac death may also be an option (see Procedure 137).	

Documentation

Documentation should include the following:
- Family education and support
- Description of the specific procedures performed for death determination, results of such procedures, and the patient's tolerance of procedures
- Clinical examination components consistent with the determination of death and the exact time of the death determination
- Time of brain death (documented as the time of the clinical diagnostic confirmation of complete and irreversible cessation of all brain function; not documented as the time of removal of mechanical ventilation or the time of organ donation)
- Time of cardiopulmonary death (documented as the time of clinical or diagnostic confirmation of complete and irreversible cessation of circulatory and respiratory function); ECG strips, if obtained, should be interpreted and included in the patient's permanent medical record
- The call to the OPO and the outcome of the referral on all deaths

References

CR 1. A definition of irreversible coma: report of the Ad Hoc Committee of the Harvard Medical School to Examine the Definition of Brain Death, *JAMA* 205(6): 337-340, 1968.

2. Center for Medicare and Medicaid Services: *Hospital conditions of participation about organ/tissue donation,* retrieved November 6, 2008, from www.cms.gov/manuals/downloads/som107ap_a_hospitals.pdf.

CR 3. Guidelines for the determination of death: report of the medical consultants on the diagnosis of death to the President's Commission for the Study of Ethical Problems in Medicine and Biomedical and Behavioral Research, *JAMA* 246(19):2184-2186, 1981.

4. Heran MK, Heran NS, Shemie SD: A review of ancillary tests in evaluating brain death, *Can J Neurol Sci* 35(4): 409-419, 2008.

CR 5. Practice parameters for determining brain death in adults (summary statement): the Quality Standards Subcommittee of the American Academy of Neurology, *Neurology* 45(5):1012-1014, 1995.

CR 6. Wijdicks EF: Determining brain death in adults, *Neurology* 45(5):1003-1011, 1995.

7. Wijdicks EF, Rabinstein AA, Manno EM, et al: Pronouncing brain death: contemporary practice and safety of the apnea test, *Neurology* 71(16):1240-1244, 2008.

8. Young GB, Shemie SD, Doig CJ, et al: Brief review: the role of ancillary tests in the neurological determination of death, *Can J Anaesth* 53(6):620-627, 2006.

Additional Reading

Medina J, Puntillo K: *AACN protocols for practice: palliative care and end-of-life issues in critical care,* Sudbury, MA, 2006, Jones and Bartlett Publishers.

Organ Donation: Identification of Potential Organ Donors, Request for Organ Donation, and Care of the Organ Donor

P U R P O S E : The purpose of this procedure is to outline the process of solid organ donation, with recognition for the care of donors and their families, the role of healthcare providers, the role of the regional organ procurement organization, and the importance of early referral.

D. Nathan Preuss

PREREQUISITE NURSING KNOWLEDGE

- Organ transplantation continues to improve every year. This success has led to the situation in which the demand for organs is greater than the supply.[4] From January 2009-January 2010, patients received 2,198 transplants. As of April 2010, there were 107,173 people on the waiting list.
- In 1968, the Uniform Anatomical Gift Act was created by the National Conference of Commissioners on Uniform State Laws. This document established a uniform Donor Card as a legal document for anyone 18 years or older to legally donate organs upon death.
- In 1980, the Uniform Determination of Death Act was passed into law; this act states that death may be declared with the cessation of circulatory and respiratory functions or with irreversible cessation of all functions of the entire brain, including the brain stem.
- In 1984, the National Organ Transplant Act established a nationwide computer registry operated by the United Network for Organ Sharing and authorized the funding of regional organ procurement organizations.
- As of 1998, every death or imminent death in a U.S. hospital must be reported to an organ procurement agency to meet the federal rules of the U.S. Department of Health and Human Services.[8]
- In 2005, the Organ Donation and Recovery Improvement Act provided additional funding for individuals making living donations, funded research to increase public awareness of the donation process, and funded programs to increase hospital donation activities.
- The two types of donors are heart-beating and non–heart-beating donors.
- Heart-beating donation occurs when an individual has sustained a devastating intracranial catastrophe that results in the death of all neurologic functioning, including the brain stem. After two independent neurologic examinations are passed, an individual is declared legally dead and can be considered for potential organ donation. These patients are the single largest source of transplantable organs.[10]
- Donation after cardiac death or non–heart-beating donation can be considered after a number of devastating illnesses or injuries that can be classified on the basis of the Maastricht classification.[1,2] Donation after cardiac death is a decision that can be made for a patient having life-sustaining therapy withdrawn. The patient is assessed to determine if he or she is a potential organ donor, and the family is approached for consent by an independent

team of healthcare providers (not the recovery team of healthcare providers). After the family has consented and said their final goodbyes, the withdrawal of life-sustaining therapy process occurs. After a predefined period of asystole, usually 2 to 5 minutes, the patient is pronounced dead by an independent physician and the organ recovery process is initiated (see Procedures 135 and 137).

• The Joint Commission has a set of standards specific to organ procurement and hospital policies and procedures and their relationship to the regional Organ Procurement Organization (OPO).[5,6]

• Various legal documents (i.e., advance directives, wills, and driver licenses) direct all those involved as to the wishes of the individual to donate. Most OPOs recognize the obligation to maximize the recovery of organs for the benefit of those recipients awaiting life-saving transplantation; however, the implementation of this process should be accomplished in a respectful manner that honors the donor's wishes. This process must include an approach that provides continuing support and care for the family while guiding them toward an understanding of their loved one's wishes.[7]

• The patient remains in the critical care unit while the organs to be donated are evaluated and suitable candidates are determined through regional and national registries.

• If the potential donor has a do not resuscitate (DNR) order in place and the family has given consent to donate organs, the DNR is revoked with the knowledge and consent of the family. Thus, if a cardiac arrest occurs, advanced cardiac life support (ACLS) is initiated. If resuscitation attempts fail and recovery teams are available, the recovery process takes place as soon as possible.

• Costs incurred are the responsibility of the regional OPO.

• Early referral to the local OPO is of prime importance. Two common recognition points are a Glasgow Coma Scale score of 5 or less and the absence of two or more brain stem reflexes, which are indicative of a poor outcome in at least 70% of the patients.[3]

• "First mention" and "decoupling" are two important concepts related to early referral and early intervention.

• *First mention* involves the healthcare provider providing an awareness of the possibility of donation. Early awareness of the possibility of organ donation correlates with family consent to donate organs, whereas families surprised by the possibility of organ donation are more likely to react negatively.[7] Thus, families may be more likely to donate if they are prepared that a request will be made.[3]

• *Decoupling* refers to the timing of the pronouncement of patient death (or the anticipation of death) and the request to consider donation of organs. The two events should not occur at the same time.

EQUIPMENT

• Thermometer
• Ventilator
• Central venous access (e.g., pulmonary artery or triple-lumen catheter)
• Blood pressure monitoring system (invasive or noninvasive)
• Intravenous (IV) infusion pumps
• Prescribed IV fluids
• Cardiac monitoring system
• Pulse oximetry
• Arterial blood gas kits
• Blood sampling tubes
• Consent forms
• Death certificates
• Request for anatomic gift certificates

Additional equipment, to have available as needed, includes the following:

• Medications as prescribed
• Pen light
• Tongue blade
• Cotton-tipped applicator
• Ice lavage
• 60-mL Toomey syringe

PATIENT AND FAMILY EDUCATION

• Inform the family of the patient's current condition. ➤*Rationale:* The family is kept informed and is prepared for realistic expectations of the patient's outcome.

• After the OPO has formally requested family consent for organ donation, collaborate with the OPO in answering important family questions. Family members may want information regarding which organ(s) can be donated, possible disfigurement, hospital costs, funeral arrangements, etc. ➤*Rationale:* This provides family members with important information and may decrease family anxiety regarding the donation process.

PATIENT ASSESSMENT AND PREPARATION

Patient Assessment

• Assess the patient's vital signs, hemodynamic parameters, and fluid status. ➤*Rationale:* Assessment provides baseline data and important data regarding the organ survivability to transplant.

• Assess the patient's current laboratory results (e.g., electrolyte, blood urea nitrogen, creatinine). ➤*Rationale:* Assessment provides baseline data and important data regarding the organ survivability to transplant.

• Assess oxygenation. ➤*Rationale:* Assessment provides baseline data and important data regarding the organ survivability to transplant.

• Obtain a thorough medical and social history from the family about the patient, including age, injuries, chronic diseases, and family, social, medical, and surgical history. Of particular interest is any history of renal, cardiac, liver, pulmonary, or pancreatic disease; malignant disease; hepatitis; diabetes; or human immunodeficiency virus (HIV) status. In the case of young female patients, pregnancy status should be determined before donation. In the case of young male patients, families should be aware of the possibility for sperm donation. ➤*Rationale:* This information assists the OPO transplant coordinator in assessment of the medical suitability of the patient for organ donation and possible patient-specific considerations.

- Assess the family members' understandings of the patient's current condition, prognosis, and plan of care. ➤*Rationale:* Assessment aids in determining family understanding. Organ donation should not be discussed until family members acknowledge their loved one's terminal status.[7]

Patient Preparation

- Verify correct patient with two identifiers. ➤*Rationale:* Prior to performing a procedure, the nurse should ensure the correct identification of the patient for the intended intervention.
- Ensure that the family understands preprocedural teaching. Answer questions as they arise, and reinforce information as needed. ➤*Rationale:* Understanding of previously taught information is evaluated and reinforced.
- When neurologic testing to determine clinical brain death begins, ensure that the patient is normothermic and that no sedating or paralyzing medications have been given. ➤*Rationale:* Hypothermia and sedating or paralyzing medications interfere with brain death testing.

- Facilitate the discussion of organ donation by notification of the OPO. ➤*Rationale:* The Centers for Medicare and Medicaid Services (CMS) require that all deaths be reported to the OPO regardless of age or circumstances. Many OPOs have instituted the use of clinical triggers to initiate the referral. The triggers are based on OPO and hospital agreed-upon physical examination findings.
- Patients who are brain dead are potential candidates for organ donation. Follow hospital policy regarding first mention. ➤*Rationale:* Request for organ donation is the responsibility of representatives from the OPO or a specially trained designated hospital requester after consultation with the OPO.[7]
- If a decision is made to donate organs, follow the plan of care determined by the OPO. ➤*Rationale:* The plan of care provides important care to promote organ survivability to transplant.
- An arterial catheter may be inserted, if not already in place. ➤*Rationale:* Assessment of blood pressure and ease of blood sampling are facilitated.
- Involve additional hospital resources (e.g., clergy, grief counselors, palliative care specialists). ➤*Rationale:* Additional family support is provided throughout the end-of-life process. Pastoral care may offer additional insights into faith, hope, and encouragement to those who may be experiencing despondency, remorse, guilt, or anger at this time.

Procedure	for Organ Donation: Identification of Potential Organ Donors, Request for Organ Donation, and Care of the Organ Donor	
Steps	**Rationale**	**Special Considerations**
Identification of Potential Donors		
1. Discuss as a healthcare team the patient's condition, prognosis, and plan of care.	Once a determination has been made as to the devastating nature of the patient's condition, all members of the team can speak with uniformity as a team and with the family members.	
2. Contact the OPO coordinator if the patient has a life-threatening illness or injury.	Early referral provides information about the potential for organ donation.	
3. **HH**		
4. **PE**		
5. Obtain laboratory samples as prescribed (e.g., complete blood cell [CBC] count, liver and renal function tests, electrolyte levels, hepatitis and HIV testing, etc.).	Provides data to assess organ function.	
6. Monitor vital signs.	Determines the presence of hemodynamic stability or instability. Decreased perfusion to the organs may alter organ donor potential.	
7. Monitor fluid status.	Determines kidney perfusion or hypoperfusion. Decreased urine output may alter organ donor potential.	

Procedure continues on following page

Procedure	**for Organ Donation: Identification of Potential Organ Donors, Request for Organ Donation, and Care of the Organ Donor**—*Continued*	
Steps	**Rationale**	**Special Considerations**
8. Assist with determination of brain death (see Procedure 135).	Facilitates the process and assesses whether the patient may be a possible organ donor.	
9. Assist the physician when the family is informed of the results of the determination of brain death.	Facilitates the process and offers support.	
10. Contact the OPO if the patient is declared brain dead.	The OPO coordinator will discuss possible organ donation with the family.	
11. Collaborate with the OPO coordinator to determine whether he or she wants the healthcare team to discuss the possibility of organ donation.	Families may be more likely to donate if they are prepared that a request will be made.[3,7]	
12. Discard used supplies in the appropriate receptacles.	Removes and safely discards used supplies.	
13. 🄷🄷		
Request for Organ Donation		
1. 🄷🄷		
2. Assist with determination of brain death (see Procedure 135).	Determines brain death.	
3. Consult the OPO coordinator when brain death testing begins.	Early assessment by the OPO coordinator determines whether the family is offered the option of donation.	
4. Ensure that the patient's family is told that the patient is brain dead.	Provides important information to the patient's family.	
5. Coordinate a meeting between the family, designated requestor, and OPO coordinator.	Facilitates the process.	The meeting is best done in a quiet, private setting.
6. If the patient's family decides to donate, the designated requestor or the OPO coordinator explains the process of recovery.	Informs the patient's family of the process that will occur.	
7. If the patient's family decides not to donate, the healthcare team can discuss with the family when life-sustaining therapy will be withdrawn.	Coordinates end-of-life care.	
8. Provide family support.	Supports the grieving family.	
9. 🄷🄷		
Care of the Organ Donor		
1. Ensure that brain death criteria have been met and proper documentation is in the chart (see Procedure 135).	A necessary criterion for organ donation.	
2. Ensure that the consent form for organ donation has been completed.	A necessary criterion for organ donation.	
3. 🄷🄷		

Procedure for Organ Donation: Identification of Potential Organ Donors, Request for Organ Donation, and Care of the Organ Donor—*Continued*

Steps	Rationale	Special Considerations
4. **PE**		
5. Obtain blood samples for laboratory analysis as prescribed by the OPO coordinator.	Determines organ function.	Common tests include CBC count; liver and kidney function; HIV and hepatitis screening; electrolyte levels; blood typing and screening; tissue typing; blood, urine, and sputum cultures; urinalysis.
6. Administer IV fluids and vasoactive medications if needed and as prescribed.	Provides necessary treatment.	
7. Administer medications such as triiodothyronine (T$_3$) and high-dose methylprednisolone as prescribed.	These medications may reduce inotropic requirements and the inflammatory response after brain stem death.	
8. Support the patient's family through the end-of-life process.	Assists the family with grieving.	
9. Assist with transfer of the patient to the operating room as directed by the OPO coordinator.	Prepares the patient for the donation process.	
10. Provide family support.	Facilitates family coping.	
11. Provide a mechanism for the family to obtain information about the organ recovery process.	Provides important family information.	
12. Discard used supplies in the appropriate receptacles.	Removes and safely discards used supplies.	
13. **HH**		

Expected Outcomes

- Determination of brain death
- OPO is notified of a patient determined to be brain dead
- The healthcare team works with the OPO coordinator to determine when and how the family should be approached regarding the option of organ donation
- The family understands the patient's status and prognosis
- The patient's wishes regarding organ donation are honored

Unexpected Outcomes

- The OPO is not notified of a patient determined to be brain dead
- The family does not understand that brain death has occurred
- The potential donor is not medically suitable for organ donation
- The patient's wishes regarding organ donation are not honored
- The recovered organs are not viable organs for transplantation

Patient Monitoring and Care

Steps	Rationale	Reportable Conditions
1. Assess the patient's vital signs every hour or more frequently as needed.	Determines cardiovascular stability.	• Abnormal vital signs
2. Continuously monitor cardiac rhythm.	Determines whether dysrhythmias are present.	• Dysrhythmias

Procedure continues on following page

Patient Monitoring and Care —*Continued*

Steps	Rationale	Reportable Conditions

3. Assess the patient's hemodynamic status if a pulmonary artery catheter is in place. Follow the goals of care as prescribed or recommended by the OPO coordinator,[4] such as:
  A. Goal for mean arterial pressure (MAP) between 60 and 80 mm Hg
  B. Goal for central venous pressure (CVP) between 4 and 10 mm Hg
  C. Goal for pulmonary artery occlusion pressure (PAOP) between 10 and 15 mm Hg
  D. Goal for cardiac index (CI) of greater than 2.1 L/min
	Determines hemodynamic stability. Assesses for a hyperdynamic phase characterized by sympathetic overactivity that causes a transient catecholamine surge, which increases heart rate, blood pressure, cardiac output, and systemic vascular resistance. Assesses for a cardiovascular collapse phase that is characterized by hypotension that results from loss of sympathetic tone, profound vasodilation, and myocardial depression.	• Abnormal blood pressure
		• Abnormal hemodynamic parameters

4. Continuously monitor pulse oximetry and obtain arterial blood gases as prescribed.	Determines oxygenation status.	• Abnormal pulse oximetry values • Abnormal arterial blood gas results
5. Monitor urine output every hour.	Determines perfusion to the kidneys.	• Urinary output less than 0.5 mL/kg/hr
6. Obtain laboratory samples as prescribed.	Determines organ function.	• Abnormal laboratory results
7. Assess the patient's body temperature every hour or as prescribed.	Determines whether interventions are needed to maintain normothermia.	• Elevated or decreased temperature
8. Consult with the grief counselor and pastoral care.	Provides family support.	

Documentation

Documentation should include the following:
- Family education
- Patient history and physical findings
- Vital signs, assessments, treatment, medication administration, and clinical status of the donor

- Intake and output
- Communication with the OPO coordinator
- Completed forms for consent to organ donation
- Unexpected outcomes
- Additional interventions

References

CR 1. Brook NR, Nicholson ML: Kidney transplant from non heart-beating donors, *Surg J Royal Coll Surg Edinb Ireland* 1:311-322, 2003.

CR 2. Doig CJ, Rocker G: Retrieving organs from non-heart-beating organ donors: a review of medical and ethical issues, *Can J Anesth* 50:1069-1076, 2003.

3. Ehrle R: Timely referral of potential organ donors, *Crit Care Nurse* 26:88-93, 2006.

CR 4. Intensive Care Society: *Guidelines for adult organ and tissue donation,* 2004, retrieved November 3, 2008, from www.ics.ac.uk.

5. Joint Commission: *JCAHO standards related to organ donation,* 2008, retrieved November 3, 2008, from www.jointcommission.org.

6. Joint Commission: Revisions to standard LD.3.110, *Joint Commission Perspect* 26:7, 2006.

CR 7. Metzger RA, et al: Research to practice: a national consent conference, *Prog Transplant* 15:1-6, 2005.

8. New York Organ Donor Network: *History of organ transplantation,* 2008, retrieved October 21, 2008, from www.donatelifeny.org.

9. OrganDonor.Gov: *Access to U.S. government information on organ & tissue donation and transplantation,* 2010, retrieved May 4, 2010 from www.organdonor.gov.

CR 10. Siminoff LA, et al: Factors influencing families' consent for donation of solid organs for transplantation, *JAMA* 286:71-77, 2001.

Additional Reading

Bernat JL, et al: Report of a national conference on donation after cardiac death, *Am J Transplant* 6:281-291, 2006.

Donation After Cardiac Death

P U R P O S E : The purpose of this procedure is to outline the process of donation of select organs after withdrawal of life-sustaining therapy and cardiopulmonary death.

Margaret L. Campbell

PREREQUISITE NURSING KNOWLEDGE

- Knowledge is needed of federal rules, state laws, organ procurement organization (OPO) policies, and hospital policies regarding donation after cardiac death. In 2007, The Joint Commission required hospitals, in coordination with the OPO, to create either donation after cardiac death (DCD) policies or justifications for opting out.[2,3]
- DCD occurs after irreversible cessation of cardiopulmonary function (see Procedure135).
- Donor criteria include:
  - ❖ A patient is ventilator-dependent, and not brain dead, and decisions have been made to withdraw mechanical ventilation.
  - ❖ Patient meets OPO designation for suitability for donation.
  - ❖ Cardiopulmonary death is likely to occur soon after withdrawal of mechanical ventilation (e.g., less than 90 minutes). The prescribed time interval may vary according to the transplant surgical team and organ.
  - ❖ Patient or surrogate has consented to donation.
- Families of patients considered for donation after cardiac death are dealing only secondarily with the request for organ donation. First, these families are dealing with the severe injury or illness of the patient that may have occurred suddenly.
- The decision to cease prolonged measures, including mechanical ventilation, must occur before the discussion about donation after cardiac death.
- The healthcare team that has cared for the potential donor must continue to care for the patient until cardiopulmonary death is pronounced.

- Palliative care is the treatment goal of the potential donor until death is pronounced. A palliative care consultant, if available, may participate in the predeath processes.[4]
- Palliative care continues if the donation is aborted for any reason after ventilation is withdrawn (e.g., the patient's death does not follow rapidly after ventilator withdrawal).

EQUIPMENT

- Consent forms
- Prepared operating room

PATIENT AND FAMILY EDUCATION

- Inform the family of the patient's current condition. ➡️***Rationale:*** The family is kept informed and is prepared for realistic expectations about the patient's expected outcome.
- Explain the medical and nursing care provided to the patient. ➡️***Rationale:*** The family understands therapies provided to treat and support the patient.
- Introduce the OPO designated requester when it is time to request organ donation. ➡️***Rationale:*** Request for organ donation is the responsibility of representatives from the OPO or a specially trained designated hospital requester.[3]

PATIENT ASSESSMENT AND PREPARATION
Patient Assessment

- With the critical care team, ascertain who is the patient's surrogate decision maker if the patient lacks capacity to make his or her own decisions. ➡️***Rationale:*** Hospital policy guides identification of the surrogate based on statute.

- Review with the family the medical and social history of the patient, including current age, injuries, chronic diseases, surgical history, familial history, and social habits. Of particular interest is a history of renal disease, hypertension, diabetes mellitus, malignant disease, hepatitis, and human immunodeficiency virus (HIV). ➤*Rationale:* This information is important so that the OPO transplant coordinator can assess the medical suitability of the patient for organ donation.
- Perform a physical assessment, with emphasis on old surgical scars, needle track marks, tattoos, body piercing, congenital anomalies, and injuries. ➤*Rationale:* These are indicators of physical conditions or social behaviors that may influence organ suitability for transplantation. Patients with recent tattoos and body piercings or fresh needle tracks are considered high risk and may not be accepted as a donor by the transplant team.
- Monitor pertinent patient data, including urine output, liver function studies, renal function studies, electrolytes, serum osmolality, coagulation panel, and urine studies, including specific gravity and culture results. ➤*Rationale:* Data are provided that may influence organ suitability for transplantation.
- Determine an accurate measurement of the patient's height and weight. ➤*Rationale:* This information is important for matching organs to a recipient of a corresponding body size.

Patient Preparation

- Verify correct patient with two identifiers. ➤*Rationale:* Prior to performing a procedure, the nurse should ensure the correct identification of the patient for the intended intervention.
- Ensure that the family understands preprocedural teaching. Answer questions as they arise, and reinforce information as needed. Families need special emotional consideration during all counseling and teaching. ➤*Rationale:* Understanding of previously taught information is evaluated and reinforced.
- Refer patients with a potentially life-threatening illness or injury to the OPO as early as possible for evaluation as a potential organ donor. Specific criteria do not exist for referral, unlike the case with the brain-dead organ donor. ➤*Rationale:* The OPO coordinator can evaluate the patient, and the critical care nurse is provided with information about the patient's potential as an organ donor.
- Involve additional hospital resources (e.g., clergy, grief counselors, palliative care specialists). ➤*Rationale:* Additional family support is provided throughout the end of the life process. Pastoral care may offer additional insights into faith, hope, and encouragement to those who may be experiencing despondency, remorse, guilt, or anger at this time.

Procedure	Donation After Cardiac Death	
Steps	**Rationale**	**Special Considerations**
1. Discuss the patient's prognosis with the healthcare team and confirm that the patient has a grave prognosis.	Early implementation of the process ensures that all involved can take the time needed for adequate decision making.	
2. Collaborate with the physician when he or she discusses the patient's prognosis with the family.	Prepares the family for the expected patient outcome and provides an opportunity to offer family support.	The purpose of this discussion is poor prognosis and withdrawal of life-sustaining treatments; no mention of organ donation should be made in this meeting. A designated requester from the OPO must make the offer of organ donation.[3]
3. Refer the patient to the OPO.	The OPO does an independent evaluation to determine eligibility for donation.	The process ceases here if the OPO indicates medical unsuitability.
4. Document the OPO referral and the OPO's recommendations.	The Centers for Medicare and Medicaid Services (CMS) and the OPO monitor hospital compliance with conditions of participation.	
5. Coordinate a meeting between the family, OPO coordinator, and clinical team if the patient is a candidate for donation.	Families are more likely to consent to organ donation when the OPO coordinator and the hospital staff collaborate in the consent process.	

Procedure	Donation After Cardiac Death—*Continued*	
Steps	**Rationale**	**Special Considerations**
6. Ensure that a request for donation is not made if there is evidence from the patient or surrogate that the patient would not want to be a donor.	The patient is his or her own decision maker, even when the patient is no longer able to communicate. Patient autonomy is respected when a patient's wishes (as appropriately communicated through an advance directive, informed surrogate, or driver's license) are honored.	
7. Ensure that the OPO coordinator is the person who discusses the option of organ donation with the patient's family.	Determines patient desires and family willingness to consider organ donation.	A member of the intensive care unit (ICU) team may also be present.
8. If the family consents to organ donation, the OPO coordinator will coordinate the process with the healthcare team.	OPO involvement increases the likelihood of successful procurement and transplantation. In addition, the OPO can provide guidance and support during the process.	Consent should be obtained from the medical examiner or the coroner before tissue or organ recovery if the patient's death is referred to the medical examiner or coroner. The OPO representative coordinates this consent process.
9. Allow the patient and family time to complete family affairs, communicate with each other, spend time together, and say goodbyes.	Facilitates family functioning and the grief process.	
10. Prepare families for what to expect during the withdrawal of life-sustaining therapy process, the dying process, and the cardiac donation process.	Helps family and friends to know what to expect.	
11. Determine the approximate time that the patient will be taken to the operating room or other designated area for ventilator withdrawal.	Allows for coordination and triage.	
12. Ensure that the ICU and operating room (OR) teams are prepared to have withdrawal of ventilation occur in or near the OR.	Circumstances around the donation may change rapidly and require accommodations that are unusual for the practice setting.	
13. Determine the roles of various personnel when the patient is taken to the designated area: A. OPO coordinator B. Anesthesiologist C. Critical care nurse D. OR nurse E. Physician F. Respiratory therapist G. Family support (e.g., clergy, grief counselor)	Determines who will be in the designated setting and defines healthcare provider responsibilities.	
14. Determine in advance who will withdraw life-sustaining therapy.	Facilitates the withdrawal of life-sustaining therapy process.	Someone from the critical care team or a palliative care consultant may conduct this process. No one from the transplant team or the OPO is involved in patient care until after cardiopulmonary death.

Procedure continues on following page

Procedure	**Donation After Cardiac Death**—*Continued*	
Steps	**Rationale**	**Special Considerations**
15. Determine family preference for physical presence or absence during the process of withdrawal of life-sustaining therapy.	Care of the dying patient and the family is of primary importance. Family members should be given the option to be present if they would like during the process of withdrawal of life-sustaining therapy.	Patients who will be donors after cardiac death are often taken to the OR or some other designated area for withdrawal of life-sustaining therapy. Accommodations for family presence must be made.
16. Initiate analgesia as prescribed (e.g., low dose of pain medication; less than 5 mg/hr of morphine) or continue prior symptom management medications. (**Level D***)	Promotes comfort.[1,5]	
17. Initiate anxiolytics as prescribed (e.g., low dose of medication; less than 5 mg/hr of midazolam). (**Level E***)	Decreases anxiety.[5]	
18. Transport the patient to the OR or designated area. Inform the appropriate hospital department (e.g., the admitting department) to hold the patient bed in the event the donation is aborted.	Prepares for the organ donation process. The patient will be transferred back to the ICU for continued palliative care if the donation is aborted.	Before the patient is transported, the process and timeline should be explained to the OR and the family should again be given the opportunity to be present before and at the time of withdrawal.
19. Prepping and draping may or may not occur before ventilator withdrawal. Hospital policy guides this process.	Prepares the patient for immediate surgery for organ retrieval after cardiopulmonary death.	
20. In some settings, femoral cannulation is done before ventilation is withdrawn to permit rapid chilling of the donor after death. Follow institutional standard.	Rapid chilling of the abdominal organs increases the probability of successful transplantation.	Femoral cannulation is an invasive procedure that does not benefit the patient and may be uncomfortable if the patient is conscious.
21. Withdraw mechanical ventilation and any other life-sustaining interventions (e.g., vasoactive medication).	Allows cardiopulmonary death to occur.	See Procedure 138.
22. Allow the family to spend as much time as they desire with the patient during ventilator withdrawal and until the time of cardiopulmonary death.	This is an important opportunity in the family's process of saying goodbye and beginning the grieving process.	
23. Administer interventions as needed to promote patient comfort (e.g., for symptoms of pain, dyspnea).	Promotes patient comfort.	
25. An interval of 2 or more minutes, as identified in institution policy, must occur before cardiopulmonary death is pronounced. Follow institutional guidelines.	Cardiopulmonary death is pronounced when there are no vital signs and irreversibility is identified.	See Procedure 135.
24. Transfer the patient back to the ICU if the donation is aborted.	Palliative care continues after an aborted donation.	Ensure that the family is aware of possible outcomes and bereavement resources.
25. Provide family support.	Supports the grieving family.	

*Level D: Peer-reviewed professional organizational standards with clinical studies to support recommendations
*Level E: Multiple case reports, theory-based evidence from expert opinions, or peer-reviewed professional organizational standards without clinical studies to support recommendations

Expected Outcomes

- The patient's wishes regarding donation are respected
- The patient's family is supported
- The patient dies within 90 minutes of ventilator withdrawal

Unexpected Outcomes

- The family does not agree with patient preferences
- The donation is aborted
- Distressing signs or symptoms

Patient Monitoring and Care

Steps	Rationale	Reportable Conditions
		These conditions should be reported if they persist despite nursing interventions.
1. Monitor the patient's temperature and intervene as necessary to achieve normothermia.	Minimizes coagulopathies.	• Temperature less than 96°F • Temperature greater than 101°F
2. Monitor the patient's cardiac and hemodynamic status continuously.	Determines hemodynamic stability.	• Systolic blood pressure (BP) less than 90 mm Hg • Changes in heart rate or other parameters set by the OPO coordinator
3. Monitor the patient's oxygenation status via continuous pulse oximetry and arterial blood gas results.	Determines the presence of hypoxemia.	• Pao_2 less than 100 mm Hg • Sao_2 less than or equal to 96% or other parameters as set by the OPO coordinator
4. Monitor the patient's urine output.	Determines renal function.	• Urine output less than 0.5 mL/kg/hr
5. Monitor laboratory studies as requested by the OPO coordinator (e.g., electrolyte levels, renal and liver function tests).	Determines organ function.	• Abnormal laboratory results
6. Follow institutional standard for assessing pain. Administer analgesia as prescribed.	Identifies need for pain interventions.	• Continued pain despite pain interventions
7. Provide family support. Incorporate the grief counselor and pastoral care.	Offers family resources during grieving.	• Ineffective family coping

Documentation

Documentation should include the following:

- Surrogate identification
- Family education
- Prognosis and family discussions
- Referral to OPO
- Knowledge of patient preferences, if any
- Completed consent form for organ donation and recovery
- Completed donor record, including vital signs, assessments, treatment, and the clinical status of the donor
- Plan for withdrawal of life-sustaining therapy
- Time of withdrawal of life-sustaining therapy
- Plan and implementation of symptom (e.g., pain, dyspnea) management
- Communication with the family, including summary of information provided and response of the family
- Time of transportation to the OR
- Pain assessment, interventions, and effectiveness
- Death pronouncement[1]
- Unexpected outcomes
- Family coping
- Additional interventions

References

CR 1. Campbell ML, Bizek KS, Thill MC: Patient responses during rapid terminal weaning from mechanical ventilation: a prospective study, *Crit Care Med* 27:73-77, 1999.

2. Center for Medicare and Medicaid Services: *Hospital conditions of participation about organ/tissue donation,* retrieved November 6, 2008, from www.cms.gov/manuals/downloads/som107ap_a_hospitals.pdf.

3. Fidler SA: Implementing donation after cardiac death protocols, *J Health Life Sci Law* 2(1):123,125-149, 2008.

4. Kelso CM, Lyckholm LJ, Coyne PJ, et al: Palliative care consultation in the process of organ donation after cardiac death, *J Palliat Med* 10(1):118-126, 2007.

5. Medina J, Puntillo K: *AACN protocols for practice: palliative care and end-of-life issues in critical care,* Sudbury, MA, 2006, Jones and Bartlett Publishers.

Additional Readings

American College of Critical Care Medicine, Society of Critical Care Medicine: Recommendations for non-heart-beating organ donation: a position paper by the ethics committee, *Crit Care Med* 29:1826-1831, 2001.

CR Arnold RM, Youngner SJ: Time is of the essence: the pressing need for comprehensive non-heart-beating cadaveric donation policies, *Transplant Proc,* 27:2913-2921, 1995.

CR D'Alessandro AM, Hoffman RM, Belzer FO: Non-heart-beating donors: one response to the organ shortage, *Transplantation Rev,* 9:168-176, 1995.

CR Edwards JM, Hasz RD, Robertson AM: Non-heart-beating organ donation: process and review, *AACN Clin Issues Crit Care,* 10:293-300, 1999.

CR Frader, J: Non-heart-beating organ donation: personal and institutional conflicts of interest, *Kennedy Inst Ethics J,* 3:189-198, 1993.

CR Institute of Medicine, Potts J, principal investigator: *Non-heart-beating organ transplantation: medical and ethics issues in procurement,* Washington, DC, 1997, National Academy Press.

CR Institute of Medicine: *Non-heart-beating organ transplantation: practice and protocols.* Washington, DC, 2000, National Academy Press.

CR Younger SJ, Arnold RM: Ethical, psychosocial, and public policy implications of procuring organs from non-heart-beating cadaver donors, *JAMA,* 269:2769-2774, 1993.

CR Van Norman GA: Another matter of life and death: what every anesthesiologist should know about the ethical, legal, and policy implications of the non-heart-beating cadaver organ donor, *Anesthesiology,* 98:763-773, 2003.

Withholding and Withdrawing Life-Sustaining Therapy

PURPOSE: This procedure is performed to assist patients and family members with the process of withholding or withdrawing life-sustaining therapy. Life-sustaining therapy may include nutrition, hydration, antibiotics, dialysis, ventilatory therapy, vasoactive therapy, implantable cardioverter-defibrillator therapy, intraaortic balloon pump therapy, ventricular assist device, and additional therapies.

Debra Lynn-McHale Wiegand, Margaret M. Mahon

PREREQUISITE NURSING KNOWLEDGE

- Withholding life-sustaining therapy (LST) is defined as "the considered decision not to institute a medically appropriate and potentially beneficial therapy, with the understanding that the patients will probably die without the therapy in question."[10]
- Withdrawal of LST is defined as "the cessation and removal of an ongoing medical therapy with the explicit intent not to substitute an equivalent alternative treatment; it is fully anticipated that the patient will die following the change in therapy."[10]
- Knowledge of state regulations, and hospital policies or procedures, regarding end-of-life decision making is essential.
- Hospitals should have policies that direct the process to withhold and withdraw LST.
- As much information as possible should be obtained from the patient regarding preferences about LST.
- If the patient is unable to communicate or chooses not to communicate, information should be obtained from the patient's designated surrogate, family, or healthcare providers regarding the patient's desired wishes about LST. This information may be ascertained from an advance directive or from verbal conversations with the surrogate, family, friends, or healthcare providers.
- Advance directives may exist in the form of a living will or a healthcare proxy.

- A living will is a document that identifies treatments a patient would or would not want under specific end-of-life situations. Most are specific to terminal illness, permanent state of unconsciousness, or persistent vegetative state.
- A healthcare proxy or a durable power of attorney for healthcare is a document that identifies a predetermined person who has been given the authority to represent the patient's preferences in healthcare decision making if the patient is unable to make decisions (e.g., comatose state) or chooses not to participate.
- Some patients have letters or other informal documents in which they convey their preferences for factors that should affect decision making and identify someone who can represent their wishes in decision making.
- Patients have a moral and legal right and responsibility to make decisions about their healthcare and the use of LST.
- Decision-making capacity is determined by an individual's ability to[2]:
  - Understand relevant information
  - Make a judgment about the information in light of his or her values
  - Intend a certain outcome
  - Communicate his or her decision to healthcare providers
- If a patient no longer has decision-making capacity, the patient's preferences should be represented by the patient's healthcare proxy. The ideal proxy, even if not specified within a legal framework, is the person who can

represent the patient's wishes, not the surrogate's. That is, decisions made by the healthcare proxy or surrogate should be based on the patient's previously stated wishes or, if there were no specific statements on presumed preferences, based on lifestyle and prior choices.

- Usually the patient's family is involved in the process of withholding and withdrawing LST. On occasion, the patient prefers that the family not be involved. If the patient does not want the family to be involved, the healthcare team should work with the patient to identify another person who can serve as the healthcare proxy or surrogate in the event that the patient loses decision-making capacity.
- Dialogue regarding end-of-life care should be comprehensive. Discussions should include the healthcare team, the patient, and the patient's family. Discussions should include what treatments are going to be withheld or withdrawn and should focus on patient wishes and medically appropriate goals of care. If the goal of care is a peaceful death, then all therapies that do not contribute toward this goal should be considered for discontinuation, including cessation of vasoactive agents, ventilatory therapy, assist devices, implantable cardioverter-defibrillator therapy, intravenous fluids, nutrition, laboratory studies, radiographs, extubation, etc.
- Therapies that support the goal of a peaceful death should be continued, such as administration of analgesia to promote comfort and anxiolytics to decrease anxiety.
- Patient comfort should also be promoted by ensuring a comfortable position, frequent skin and mouth care, and interventions to relieve signs and symptoms of distress.
- Families need to be supported throughout the end-of-life decision-making process.
- Families should be encouraged to say final goodbyes and to be present should they desire during the dying process.
- Patients, families, and healthcare providers often have different values.
- Healthcare providers are responsible for knowing how their personal beliefs affect their interactions with patients, families, and other healthcare providers.
- Patients and their families should be actively involved in all healthcare decisions, including end-of-life decisions (unless the patient requests that family members not be involved; see previous discussion).
- Family members involved in end-of-life decision making should be guided by their knowledge of what the patient wants or would want.
- If a critical care nurse cannot support the patient and family in the process of withholding or withdrawing LST, the critical care nurse should proceed through the appropriate channels to transfer care to another critical care nurse.
- It is recommended that paralyzing agents are discontinued and cleared from the patient's body before withdrawal of LST.[13]
- Maintenance of patient dignity and comfort is essential at all times, and especially at the end of life.
- Opioid administration to treat pain rarely causes respiratory depression when carefully titrated to a patient's distress.[3,7]

- Nurses should use effective doses of medications prescribed for symptom control; nurses have a moral obligation to advocate on behalf of the patient when prescribed medications are not sufficient to manage distressing symptoms.[1]
- Uncontrolled pain should be considered an emergency, with the entire healthcare team taking responsibility to provide relief.[6]
- Family meetings can be helpful in aiding patients, families, and healthcare providers in planning end-of-life care.
- Palliative care is interdisciplinary care that aims to relieve suffering and improve quality of life for patients with serious illness and their families.[9] Palliative care should be integrated into the care of acutely ill or injured patients in the intensive care unit (ICU).[15]
- Hospital ethics committees can be helpful in aiding patients, families, and healthcare providers when conflicts arise with decision making or during withholding or withdrawing LST discussions.

PATIENT AND FAMILY EDUCATION

- In collaboration with the physician and the critical care team, inform the patient and family of the patient's current condition and prognosis. ➤➤*Rationale:* The patient and family are informed of and prepared for anticipated outcomes.
- Explain resources available to aid with end-of-life decision making (e.g., nurses, physicians, social workers, pastoral care, grief counselors, palliative care team, ethics consultation, ethics committee). ➤➤*Rationale:* Additional resources and support are offered to assist the patient or family with end-of-life decisions.
- Describe how the patient is likely to respond to withholding or withdrawing of therapies, including expected outcomes and unexpected outcomes. ➤➤*Rationale:* The patient and family are prepared for the process. If death is anticipated, the dying process may progress quickly or slowly (e.g., occurring within minutes or lasting days). Although rare, death may not ensue after LST is withheld or withdrawn.
- Explain that analgesia and anxiolytics will be administered before withholding or withdrawing LST to prevent discomfort and after withholding or withdrawing LST to relieve any signs or symptoms of discomfort. ➤➤*Rationale:* Patient and family anxiety is decreased with the knowledge that patient comfort will be promoted.

PATIENT ASSESSMENT AND PREPARATION
Patient Assessment

- Assist the physician or advanced practice nurse in assessment of the patient's decision-making capacity. ➤➤*Rationale:* Patients with decision-making capacity should make their own therapy decisions.

- If patients do not have decision-making capacity, determine whether the patient has a designated healthcare proxy or surrogate. ⇒*Rationale:* The patient's healthcare proxy should make decisions for the patient if he or she no longer has decision-making capacity.
- If patients do not have decision-making capacity or a healthcare proxy, identify key individuals who can best represent patient preferences and who will be active participants in therapy decisions. ⇒*Rationale:* Family members must be able to communicate patient wishes for end-of-life care or be able to determine to the best of their knowledge what therapies the patient would or would not want. The patient may also have communicated therapy wishes to primary care providers and friends.

Patient Preparation

- Verify correct patient with two identifiers. ⇒*Rationale:* Prior to performing a procedure, the nurse should ensure the correct identification of the patient for the intended intervention.
- Ensure that the patient and family understand preprocedural teaching. Answer questions as they arise, and reinforce information as needed. ⇒*Rationale:* Understanding of previously taught information is evaluated and reinforced.
- Collaborate with the patient and family to plan the day and time that LST will be withheld or withdrawn.

⇒*Rationale:* Family and friends have time to spend with the patient and to arrive from out of town. The healthcare team has time to plan availability to be present during therapy changes.
- Identify family or friends whom the patient and family would like present during the withholding or withdrawal process. ⇒*Rationale:* The patient and family are involved in planning of the withholding or withdrawal of therapy, and patient preferences are respected.
- In addition to nursing, medicine, and possibly respiratory therapy, identify additional members of the healthcare team who the patient or family would like present during the withholding or withdrawal process (e.g., clergy, social worker, palliative care specialist, grief counselor). ⇒*Rationale:* The patient and family are provided control as they determine essential members of the healthcare team who should be involved with the withholding or withdrawing of therapy process.
- Encourage the patient and family to personalize the environment by bringing in music or other items that will make the room as the patient would want it to be. ⇒*Rationale:* An individualized, peaceful, caring environment is promoted.
- Establish or maintain a patent intravenous access. ⇒*Rationale:* Intravenous access is necessary for administration of analgesia and anxiolytics.

Procedure | for Withholding and Withdrawing Life-Sustaining Therapy

Steps	Rationale	Special Considerations
1. With the patient, family, and healthcare team, coordinate a comprehensive plan for the process of withholding or withdrawing LST.	Ensures that key individuals are aware of the end-of-life care plan. Addresses what aspects of therapy will be withheld and what aspects of therapy will be withdrawn.	The patient, family, and healthcare providers need to work together to facilitate the process. Thorough preplanning facilitates the process of end-of-life care.
2. Ensure that the patient, healthcare proxy, and family understand and agree to the process of withholding or withdrawing LST.	Ensures the understanding of what will be withheld or withdrawn, when it will be withheld or withdrawn, and in what order (or all at once).	Consult the ethics committee if conflicts arise.
3. Ensure that the patient, healthcare proxy, and family understand the probable outcome of withholding or withdrawing LST.	Ensures that no misperceptions exist regarding what will happen after therapy is withheld or withdrawn.	
4. Allow the patient and family time to complete family affairs, communicate with each other, spend time together, and say goodbyes.	Facilitates family functioning and the grief process.	
5. Prepare families for what to expect during the dying process: A. Variability of the dying process B. Changes in breathing pattern C. Noisy breathing D. Changes in color and temperature of skin	Family and friends know what to expect.	

Procedure continues on following page

Procedure for Withholding and Withdrawing Life-Sustaining Therapy—*Continued*

Steps	Rationale	Special Considerations
6. Ensure that key members of the healthcare team are actively involved in the process of withholding or withdrawing LST.	Presents a team approach to support the patient, family, and each other.	Predetermine who will withdraw therapy (e.g., ventilator, endotracheal tube, ventricular assist device, etc).
7. In collaboration with the physician, determine the type, route of administration, dosage, and time that analgesia and other medications (e.g., anxiolytics, anticholinergics, etc) will be initiated.	Allows time to ensure intravenous access and to obtain and prepare the medication.	Continuous intravenous infusion of the analgesia (e.g., morphine sulfate) and anxiolytic (e.g., midazolam) facilitates constant administration and ease of dosage adjustment.
8. In collaboration with the physician, determine how medications for pain and other symptoms will be titrated to signs of patient discomfort.	Provides a plan to promote patient comfort.	Pain medication should be titrated to increasing dosages only if signs or symptoms of patient discomfort are present. Signs and symptoms of discomfort include verbalization of pain, moaning, grimacing, increase in heart rate, increase in blood pressure, restlessness, diaphoresis, and labored breathing.
9. In collaboration with the physician, consider other medications and interventions that may promote comfort during the dying process.	Prevents distress.	For example, elevating the patient's head of the bed, oropharyngeal suctioning, reducing intravenous fluids, and administration of anticholinergic medications may decrease pulmonary sections; bronchodilators and benzodiazepines also may relieve dyspnea.[5,8,15]
10. Assist the patient to his or her preferred position of comfort.	Promotes comfort.	Place the patient in a comfortable position if he or she is unable to communicate. The supine position with the head of bed elevated may facilitate comfort and ease respirations.
11. Lower the side rails if family and friends are present.	Allows the family access to be close to the patient, hold his or her hand, or sit on the bed.	Side rails may need to be raised if the patient is moving, experiencing a seizure, etc.
12. Turn off all monitors.	Eliminates focus on the monitor.	Pulse can be checked via palpation. Blood pressure can be checked manually, if necessary, to assess whether additional pain medication is necessary. Some family members may prefer to observe heart rate and pulse oximetry. Follow institutional standard.
13. Ensure that the family is present.	Ensures that significant family members are there to support the patient and each other.	Some family members may choose to be close by but not in the room when LST is withheld or withdrawn.
14. Ensure that the environment is as the patient wants it or would want it.	Promotes patient and family involvement.	Consideration should be given to special cultural and religious preferences.
15. Ensure that key members of the healthcare team are present (e.g., critical care nurse, attending physician, respiratory therapist, pastor, palliative care specialist).	Presents a team approach to support the patient, family, and each other.	There may be healthcare providers who the patient or family specifically wish to be present.

Procedure	for Withholding and Withdrawing Life-Sustaining Therapy—*Continued*	
Steps	**Rationale**	**Special Considerations**
16. Initiate analgesia as prescribed (e.g., low dose of pain medication; less than 5 mg/hr of morphine) or continue prior symptom management medications. **(Level D*)**	Promotes comfort.[4,8]	If the patient is already receiving analgesia at a constant infusion, the same rate of infusion continues.
17. Initiate anxiolytics as prescribed (e.g., low dose of medication; less than 5 mg/hr of midazolam). **(Level E*)**	Decreases anxiety.[8]	If the patient is already receiving anxiolytics at a constant infusion, the same rate of infusion continues.
18. Withhold or withdraw therapy.	Discontinues unwanted therapy.	
19. Closely monitor the patient for signs or symptoms of distress. Signs and symptoms of patient discomfort during the dying process are distressing not only for the patient but also for the patient's family.[11,14] **(Level C*)**	Facilitates the process for the patient and family.	
20. Rapidly titrate intravenous analgesia and anxiolytics to signs and symptoms of patient distress.	Minimizes distress and promotes comfort.	Opioids have no ceiling for effectiveness; thus, titration is guided by patient symptoms of distress.[8]
21. Each time the infusion rate is titrated, a bolus dose should also be administered.[12] **(Level E)**	Achieves a rapid response.	
22. Provide basic comfort care to the patient, such as: A. Provide frequent mouth care B. Moisten the patient's mouth C. Apply a cool moist washcloth to the patient's forehead D. Wash and massage the patient with lotion E. Apply lip balm to the patient's lips F. Administer an antipyretic as prescribed to reduce a patient's fever G. Assist with turning to one's side supported by pillows	Promotes comfort.	
23. Support the patient and the family.	Provides essential care to the patient and family during the dying process.	Ensure that the environment is supportive for the family (e.g., comfortable chairs, tissues, etc).
24. Provide time for the patient and the family to be alone, if so desired.	Provides family time together during the dying process.	Check on the patient and family frequently.
25. Support the grieving family.	Aids family coping.	
26. If at all possible, do not transfer the patient from the ICU.[8,16] **(Level D)**	Transfers away from familiar staff interrupt the continuity of care and can increase family members' sense of abandonment.	

*Level C: Qualitative studies, descriptive or correlational studies, integrative reviews, systematic reviews, or randomized controlled trials with inconsistent results
*Level D: Peer-reviewed, professional organizational standards with clinical studies to support recommendations
*Level E: Multiple case reports, theory-based evidence from expert opinions, or peer-reviewed professional organizational standards without clinical studies to support recommendations

Procedure continues on following page

Expected Outcomes

- Patient wishes regarding end-of-life care are honored
- Therapies that are not wanted by the patient or family are withheld or withdrawn
- Patient dignity and comfort are achieved
- Family is actively involved in end-of-life care
- Patient and family receive needed support
- Patient death occurs (time frame may vary from minutes to hours to days)

Unexpected Outcomes

- The patient receives unwanted therapies
- The patient has discomfort
- Family members are not involved in end-of-life care
- Family conflicts arise regarding end-of-life therapy decisions
- Patient survives withholding or withdrawing of life support, necessitating consideration of a new plan of care and the possibility of long-term care

Patient Monitoring and Care

Steps	Rationale	Reportable Conditions
		These conditions should be reported if they persist despite nursing interventions.
1. Assess the patient for discomfort: A. Verbalization of pain B. Moaning C. Grimacing D. Tachycardia E. Hypertension F. Restlessness G. Diaphoresis H. Labored breathing I. Tachypnea J. Gasping K. Use of accessory muscles L. Delirium	Signs of discomfort indicate ineffective management of symptoms.	• Distressing symptoms that are not controlled with prescribed medications
2. Titrate analgesia or anxiolytics to comfort.	Promotes patient dignity and comfort.	• Distressing symptoms (e.g., dyspnea, anxiety) that are not controlled with prescribed medications
3. Assess vital signs before withholding or withdrawing LST, and then only as necessary to ensure that the patient is not experiencing discomfort.	Promotes patient dignity and comfort.	• Decreasing values of vital signs are normal and expected as LST is being withheld or withdrawn; thus, these should be reported only as needed to keep the health team informed • Increasing values of vital signs may indicate that analgesia and anxiolytic medications are insufficient
4. Support the patient and the family through the entire process.	Provides additional emotional support, promotes family functioning, and aids in the grief process.	• Ineffective family functioning or need for additional support services

Documentation

Documentation should include the following:
- Patient and family education
- Patient wishes regarding end-of-life care
- Coordination of the end-of-life process
- Patient, healthcare proxy, or family understanding of the withholding or withdrawing process and the anticipated outcome
- Involved family and healthcare team members
- When and how LST was withheld or withdrawn

- Patient level of comfort
- How comfort was promoted
- Medication administered
- Time of patient death
- Unexpected outcomes
- Additional interventions

References

CR 1. American Nurses Association: *American Nurses Association position statement on pain management and control of distressing symptoms in dying patients,* Washington, DC, 2003, ANA.

CR 2. Beauchamp TL, Childress JF: *Principles of biomedical ethics,* ed 5, New York, 2001, Oxford University Press.

3. Campbell ML: Treating distress at the end of life: the principle of double effect, *AACN Adv Crit Care* 19(3): 340-344, 2008.

CR 4. Campbell ML, Bizek KS, Thill MC: Patient responses during rapid terminal weaning from mechanical ventilation: a prospective study, *Crit Care Med* 27:73-77, 1999.

5. Clark K, Butler M: Noisy respiratory secretions at the end of life, *Curr Opin Support Palliat Care* 3(2):120-124, 2009.

6. Hospice and Palliative Nurses Association: *HPNA position statement: pain management,* Pittsburgh, 2008, HPNA.

7. Hospice and Palliative Nurses Association: *HPNA position statement: the ethics of opiate use within palliative care,* Pittsburgh, 2008, HPNA.

8. Medina J, Puntillo K: *AACN protocols for practice: palliative care and end-of-life issues in critical care,* Sudbury, MA, 2006, Jones and Bartlett Publishers.

9. National Consensus Project for Quality Palliative Care: Clinical practice guidelines for quality palliative care, ed 2, Pittsburgh, 2009.

CR 10. Prendergast TJ, Claessens MT, Luce JM: A national survey of end-of-life care for critically ill patients, *Am J Resp Crit Care Med* 158:1163-1167, 1998.

CR 11. Tolle SW, et al: Families reports of barriers to optimal care of the dying, *Nurs Res* 49(6):310-317, 2000.

12. Truog RD, Campbell ML, Curtis JR, et al: Recommendations for end-of-life care in the intensive care unit: a consensus statement by the American College of Critical Care Medicine, 36(3):953-963, *Crit Care Med,* 2008.

CR 13. Truog RD, Burns JP, Mitchell C, et al: Pharmacologic paralysis and withdrawal of mechanical ventilation at the end of life, *N Engl J Med* 342(7):508-511, 2000.

14. Wiegand DL, Petri L: Is a good death possible after withdrawal of life-sustaining therapy? *Crit Care Clin North Am.* In press.

15. Wiegand DL, Williams LD: End-of-life care. In Carlson K, editor: *AACN advanced critical care nursing,* Philadelphia, 2009, Elsevier, 1507-1525.

16. Wiegand DL: Withdrawal of life-sustaining therapy after sudden, unexpected life-threatening illness or injury: interactions between patients' families, healthcare providers, and the healthcare system, *Am J Crit Care* 15(2):178-187, 2006.

Additional Readings

CR Ballentine JM: Pacemaker and defibrillator deactivation in competent hospice patients: an ethical consideration, *Am J Hosp Palliat Med* 22:14-19, 2005.

CR Braun TC, Hagen NA, Hatfield RE, et al: Cardiac defibrillators in terminal care, *J Pain Symptom Manage* 18:126-131, 1999.

CR Campbell ML: Terminal dyspnea and respiratory distress, *Crit Care Clin North Am* 20:403-417, 2004.

CR Campbell ML: *Forgoing life-sustaining therapy,* Laguna Niguel, CA, 1998, AACN.

CR Daly BJ, Thomas D, Dyer MA: Procedures used in withdrawal of mechanical ventilation, *Am J Crit Care* 5(5)331-338, 1996.

Dudzinski DM: Ethics guidelines for destination therapy, *Ann Thorac Surg* 81:1185-1188, 2006.

CR Goldstein NE, Lampert R, Bradley E, et al: Management of implantable cardioverter defibrillators in end-of-life care, *Ann Intern Med* 141:835, 2004.

CR Grassman D: EOL considerations in defibrillator deactivation, *Am J Hospice Palliat Med* 22: 179-180, 2005.

CR The Hastings Center: *Guidelines on the termination of life sustaining treatment and the care of the dying,* Bloomington, IN, 1987, University Press.

Hospice and Palliative Nurses Association: *HPNA position statement: withholding and/or withdrawing life sustaining therapies,* Pittsburgh, 2008, HPNA.

Lampert R, et al: HRS expert consensus statement on the management of Cardiovascular Implantable Electronic Devices (CIEDs) in patients nearing end of life or requesting withdrawal of therapy. (In Press). *Heart Rhythm.*

Lewis WR, Luebke DL, Johnson NJ, et al: Withdrawing implantable defibrillator shock therapy in terminally ill patients, *Am J Med* 119:892, 2006.

CR Mayer SA, Kossoff SB: Withdrawal of life support in the neurological intensive care unit, *Neurology* 52(8):1602-1609, 1999.

CR Nambisan V, Chao D: Dying and defibrillation: a shocking experience, *Palliat Med* 18:482-483, 2004.

CR President's Commission for the Study of Ethical Problems in Medicine and Biomedical and Behavioral Research: *Deciding to forego life-sustaining treatment: a report on the ethical medical, and legal issues in treatment decisions,* Washington DC, 1983, US Government Printing Office.

MacIver J, Ross HJ: Withdrawal of ventricular assist device support, *J Palliat Care* 21:151-156, 2006.

CR Morreim EH: Surgically implanted devices: ethical challenges in a very different kind of research, *Thorac Surg Clin* 15:555-563, 2005.

CR Pellegrino ED: Decisions to withdraw life-sustaining treatment: a moral algorithm, *JAMA* 283:1065-1067, 2000.

CR Tilden VP, Tolle SW, Nelson CA, et al: Family decision making in foregoing life-extending treatments, *J Family Nurs* 5:426-442, 1999.

CR Tilden VP, Tolle SW, Garland MJ, et al: Decisions about life sustaining treatment: impact of physicians' behavior on the family, *Arch Intern Med* 155(6):633-638, 1995.

Wiegand DL: In their own time: the family experience during the process of withdrawal of life-sustaining therapy, *J Palliat Med* 11(8):1115-1121, 2008.

Wiegand DL, Deatrick JA, Knafl K: Family management styles related to withdrawal of life-sustaining therapy from adults who are acutely ill or injured, *J Family Nurs* 14(1):16-32, 2008.

Wiegand DL, Kalowes PG: Withdrawal of cardiac medications and devices, *AACN Adv Crit Care* 18(4):415-425, 2007.

Wiegand DL: Families and withdrawal of life-sustaining therapy: state of the science, *J Family Nurs* 12(2):165-184, 2006.

Calculating Doses and Flow Rates and Administering Continuous Intravenous Infusions

P U R P O S E : Calculation of doses and flow rates and administration of continuous intravenous infusions are performed to ensure accurate delivery of medications administered via the intravenous route. Many of the medications delivered via continuous intravenous infusion have potent effects and narrow margins of safety; therefore, accuracy in calculation and administration of these agents is imperative.

Shelley Burcat, Maribeth Kelly

PREREQUISITE NURSING KNOWLEDGE

- Knowledge of aseptic technique is necessary.
- Nurses must be aware of the indications, actions, side effects, dosages, administration/storage, assessment, and evaluation for medications administered.
- Many different types of medications are delivered as continuous intravenous (IV) infusions in acute and critical care settings. These medications include, but are not limited to, vasoactive, inotropic, antidysrhythmic, sedative, and analgesic agents. Hemodynamic assessment and electrocardiographic (ECG) monitoring are frequently necessary to evaluate the patient's response to the infusion. The nurse must be familiar with monitoring equipment such as cardiac monitors, arterial lines, pulmonary artery catheters, and noninvasive blood pressure cuffs.
- Titration is adjustment of the dose, either increasing or decreasing, to attain the desired patient response. Weaning is a gradual decrease of the dose when the medication is being discontinued.
- Alterations or interruptions of the flow rate can significantly affect the dose of medication being delivered and adversely affect the patient. For accurate delivery of IV

medications, volume-controlled infusion devices are required

- "Smart technologies" are electronic devices, such as computers, bedside monitors, and infusion pumps, that perform calculations of doses and flow rates after information is entered and programmed by the user. Although these devices are not universally available, their use may help to reduce medication errors.[4]
- Smart pumps are infusion pumps with comprehensive libraries of drugs and dose calculation software that can perform a "test of reasonableness" to check that programming is within preestablished institutional limits before the infusion can begin, which can reduce medication errors, improve workflow, and provide a source of data for continuous quality improvement.[10]
- Use of smart infusion pumps with activated dosage error reduction software alerts the practitioner when safe doses and infusion rates have been exceeded.[7] The clinician must use the technology consistently to avoid serious medication infusion errors.[6]
- Be aware that double key bounce and double keying errors may occur when pressing a number key once on an infusion pump, resulting in the unintended consequence of a repeat of that same number. This can result in infusing medications at a higher rate than expected.[5]

- Three factors are involved in the calculations for continuous IV infusions:
  - ◆ The concentration is the amount of medication diluted in a given volume of IV solution (e.g., 400 mg dopamine diluted in 250 mL normal saline [NS] solution, resulting in a concentration of 1.6 mg/mL; or 2 g lidocaine diluted in 500 mL 5% dextrose in water [D_5W], yielding a concentration of 4 mg/mL). The concentration is also expressed as amount of medication per milliliter of fluid.
  - ◆ The dose of the medication is the amount of medication to be administered over a certain length of time (e.g., dopamine 5 mcg/kg/min, lidocaine 2 mg/min, or diltiazem 5 mg/hr). The units of measure for the dose differ for various medications. The length of time is 1 minute or 1 hour. If the medication is weight-based, the dose of the medication is per kilogram of patient weight.
  - ◆ The flow rate is the rate of delivery of the IV fluid solution expressed as volume of IV fluid delivered per unit of time (e.g., 20 mL/hr). The unit of measure of the flow rate is milliliter per hour.
- All units of measure in the formula must be the same. It frequently is necessary to perform some conversions on the concentration before entering it into the formula. The units of measure of the concentration must be converted to the same units of measure of the dose (e.g., the concentration of dopamine is measured in milligrams, but the dose of dopamine is measured in micrograms).
- The mathematic formula for continuous IV infusion contains the three factors involved in continuous infusion (Table 139-1). When two factors are known, the third can be calculated with the basic formula. Therefore, when the concentration of the solution and the prescribed dose are known, the flow rate can be determined. When the concentration of the solution and the flow rate are known, the dose can be determined. Variations on the basic formula are used to allow for medications delivered per hour or per minute and for medications that are weight-based (Tables 139-2 and 139-3).
- Calculations for weight-based medications include the patient's weight in the formula. The choice of which weight to use can be challenging. Much disagreement and inconsistency are found in the literature as to which weight to use, ideal body weight, actual body weight, or dry body weight.[2,7] Distribution of specific medications across fat and fluid body compartments varies, thus affecting the therapeutic level. Because most medications are titrated to patient response and a desired clinical end point, a consistent approach is to use the patient's admission weight for initial dose calculations. The clinical pharmacist then should be consulted for obese patients and for medications that have potentially dangerous toxicities.
- Central IV access should be used for vasoconstrictive medications and medications that can cause tissue damage when extravasated.[3] Mechanisms and agents that may cause tissue damage include osmotic damage from hyperosmolar solutions, ischemic necrosis caused by vasoconstrictors and certain cation solutions, direct cellular toxicity caused by antineoplastic agents, direct tissue damage from pH strong acids and bases, and direct irritation.[9]
- The Joint Commission goal for medication safety includes standardization and limiting the number of drug concentrations available in organizations.[11] Standardized dosing methods for the same medications reduce IV infusion errors.[7]
- The Institute of Healthcare Improvement (IHI) recommendations for IV medication safety include conducting independent double checks, dose calculation aids on IV solution bag labels, use of IV smart infusion pumps with safety features, and use of premade dose and flow-rate charts.[1]
- Another recommendation identified the positive impact of regular drug administration updates and formal arithmetic testing on the frequency and cause of medication errors that are the result of lack of ability to calculate drug dosage correctly.[8]

TABLE 139-1 Basic Formula*

1. To determine an unknown flow rate:
$$\frac{\text{Dose (mg/hr or mcg/hr)}}{\text{Concentration (mg/mL or mcg/mL)}} = \text{Flow rate (mL/hr)}$$

2. To determine an unknown dose:
$$\text{Flow rate (mL/hr)} \times \text{Concentration (mg/mL or mcg/mL)} = \text{Dose (mg/hr or mcg/hr)}$$

3. To determine the concentration of drug in 1 mL of fluid:
$$\frac{\text{Total amount of drug (mg or mcg)}}{\text{Total volume of fluid (mL)}} = \text{Concentration}\frac{\text{(mg or mcg)}}{\text{(mL)}}$$

Example: When flow rate is unknown, diltiazem 125 mg/125 mL D_5W to be administered at 10 mg/hr.

A. Calculate concentration of drug in 1 mL of fluid:
$$\frac{125\ mg}{125\ mL} = \frac{1\ mg}{mL}$$

B. Enter known factors into the formula and solve:
$$\text{Flow rate (mL/hr)} \times \text{Concentration (mg or mcg/mL:)} = \text{Dose (mg or mcg/mL)}$$
$$\frac{10\ mL/hr}{1\ mg/mL} = 10\ mL/hr$$

Example: When dose is unknown, diltiazem 125 mg/125 mL D_5W is infusing at 15 mL/hr.

A. Calculate concentration of drug in 1 mL of fluid:
$$\frac{125\ mg}{125\ mL} = \frac{1\ mg}{mL}$$

B. Enter known factors into the formula and solve:
$$15\ mL/hr \times 1\ mg/mL = 15\ mg/hr$$

---

*Because there are units on the top of the equation and units on the bottom of the equation, to ensure that the final units are correct, the units on the bottom of the equation must be inverted and multiplied by the units of the top of the equation.

Example: $\dfrac{1800\ mcg/hr}{200\ mcg/mL} = \dfrac{9 \times mL}{hr} = 9\ mL/hr$

TABLE 139-2	**Variation for Medication Doses Measured per Minute (mg/min or mcg/min)***

1. To determine unknown flow rate:

$$\frac{\text{Dose (mg/min or mcg/min)} \times 60 \text{ min/hr}}{\text{Concentration (mg/mL or mcg/mL)}} = \text{Flow rate (mL/hr)}$$

2. To determine unknown dose:

$$\frac{\text{Flow rate (mL/hr)} \times \text{Concentration (mg/mL or mcg/mL)}}{60 \text{ min/hr}}$$
$$= \text{Dose (mg/min or mcg/min)}$$

Example: When flow rate is unknown, nitroglycerin 50 mg/250 mL D$_5$W to be administered at 30 mcg/min.

A. Convert the concentration to like units of measure:

$$\frac{50 \text{ mg}}{250 \text{ mL}} \times \frac{1000 \text{ mcg}}{1 \text{ mg}} = \frac{50,000 \text{ mcg}}{250 \text{ mL}}$$

B. Calculate concentration of drug in 1 mL of fluid:

$$\frac{50,000 \text{ mcg}}{250 \text{ mL}} = \frac{200 \text{ mcg}}{1 \text{ mL}}$$

C. Enter known factors into the formula and solve:

$$\frac{30 \text{ mcg/min} \times 60 \text{ min/hr}}{200 \text{ mcg/mL}} = 9 \text{ mL/hr}$$

Example: When dose is unknown, lidocaine 2 g/500 mL D5W is infusing at 30 mL/h.

A. Convert the concentration to like units of measure:

$$\frac{2 \text{ g}}{500 \text{ mL}} \times \frac{1000 \text{ mg}}{1 \text{ g}} = \frac{2000 \text{ mg}}{500 \text{ mL}}$$

B. Calculate concentration of drug in 1 mL of fluid:

$$\frac{2000 \text{ mg}}{500 \text{ mL}} = \frac{4 \text{ mg}}{\text{mL}}$$

C. Enter known factors into formula and solve:

$$\frac{30 \text{ mL/hr} \times 4 \text{ mg/mL}}{60 \text{ min/hr}} = 2 \text{ mg/min}$$

*The time factor of 60 min/hr must be added to the basic formula.

TABLE 139-3	**Variation for Weight-Based Medication Doses Measured per Minute (mcg/kg/min)***

1. To determine unknown flow rate:

$$\frac{\text{Dose (mcg/kg/min)} \times 60 \text{ min/hr} \times \text{Patient weight (kg)}}{\text{Concentration (mcg/mL)}} = \text{Flow rate (mL/hr)}$$

2. To determine unknown dose:

$$\frac{\text{Flow rate (mL/hr)} \times \text{Concentration (mcg/mL)}}{60 \text{ min/hr} \times \text{Patient weight (kg)}} = \text{Dose (mcg/kg/min)}$$

Example: When flow rate is unknown, dopamine 400 mg/250 mL D$_5$W to infuse at 5 mcg/kg/min. Patient weighs 100 kg.

A. Convert the concentration to like units of measure:

$$\frac{400 \text{ mg}}{250 \text{ mL}} \times \frac{1000 \text{ mcg}}{1 \text{ mg}} = \frac{400,000 \text{ mcg}}{250 \text{ mL}}$$

B. Calculate concentration of drug in 1 mL of fluid:

$$\frac{400,000 \text{ mcg}}{250 \text{ mL}} = \frac{1600 \text{ mcg}}{1 \text{ mL}}$$

C. Enter known factors into the formula and solve:

$$\frac{5 \text{ mcg/kg/min} \times 60 \text{ min/hr} \times 100 \text{ kg}}{1600 \text{ mcg/mL}} = 18.75 \text{ mL/hr}$$

Example: When dose is unknown, dobutamine 500 mg/250 mL D$_5$W is infusing at 15 mL/hr. Patient weighs 70 kg.

A. Convert the concentration to like units of measure:

$$\frac{500 \text{ mg}}{250 \text{ mL}} \times \frac{1000 \text{ mcg}}{\text{mg}} = \frac{50,000 \text{ mcg}}{250 \text{ mL}}$$

B. Calculate concentration of drug in 1 mL of fluid:

$$\frac{50,000 \text{ mcg}}{250 \text{ mL}} = \frac{2000 \text{ mcg}}{\text{mL}}$$

C. Enter known factors into the formula and solve:

$$\frac{15 \text{ mL/hr} \times 2000 \text{ mcg/mL}}{60 \text{ min/hr} \times 70 \text{ kg}} = 7.14 \text{ mcg/kg/min}$$

*The patient's weight in kilograms and the time factor of 60 min/hr must be added to the basic formula.

EQUIPMENT

- Prepared IV solution with medication to be administered
- IV tubing
- IV infusion device
- Nonsterile gloves
- Alcohol pads
- Calculator (optional)

PATIENT AND FAMILY EDUCATION

- Explain the indications and expected response to the pharmacologic therapy. ➨*Rationale:* Patients and families need explanations of the plan of care and interventions.
- Instruct the patient to report adverse symptoms, as indicated. Reportable symptoms include, but are not limited to, pain, burning, itching, or swelling at the IV site; dizziness; shortness of breath; palpitations; and chest pain.

➨*Rationale:* Reporting assists the nurse to evaluate the response to the pharmacologic therapy and to identify adverse reactions.

PATIENT ASSESSMENT AND PREPARATION

Patient Assessment

- Assess medication allergies. ➨*Rationale:* Assessment provides identification and prevention of allergic reactions.
- Obtain vital signs and hemodynamic parameters. ➨*Rationale:* The need for vasoactive agents is established, and baseline data are provided to evaluate the response to therapy.
- Assess the ECG results. ➨*Rationale:* Assessment establishes the need for antidysrhythmic therapy and provides baseline data.
- Obtain other assessments relevant to the medication being administered (e.g., sedation scale for continuous IV

sedatives). ➼*Rationale:* Patients are assessed for specific parameters that are affected by various medications in order to note the efficacy of the medications and to ensure their safe delivery.[2]

Patient Preparation

- Ensure that the patient and family understand preprocedural teachings. Answer questions as they arise, and reinforce information as needed. ➼*Rationale:* Understanding of previously taught information is evaluated and reinforced.

- Weigh the patient, if the medication is weight-based. ➼*Rationale:* Calculation of the correct dose based on patient weight is permitted. If the patient's weight has changed during hospitalization because of edema or other causes, use of the baseline admission weight is preferable.
- Verify patency or obtain patent, appropriate IV access. ➼*Rationale:* Delivery of the medication into the IV space is ensured. Some continuous infusion medications require central line access to prevent irritation or damage to smaller peripheral veins and to reduce the risk for extravasation.

Procedure	for Calculating Doses and Flow Rates and Administering Continuous Intravenous Infusions	
Steps	**Rationale**	**Special Considerations**
1. Verify the medication ordered by the prescribing practitioner.	Ensures accuracy of medication administration.	A medication order should include the medication, route, dose, and parameters for titration of the medication. The concentration of the solution and the diluent should be indicated in the order or determined by institutional policy.
2. **HH**		
3. **PE**		
4. Verify the five rights of medication administration: right patient, right drug, right dose, right time, and right route. Verify the correct patient with two identifiers.[1,2,3,11] **(Level E*)**	May reduce the potential for medication administration error.	
5. Connect and flush the IV solution (with prescribed medication) through the tubing system.	Prepares the infusion system.	
6. Place the IV infusion in the infusion device. There are two methods to perform the next step; **choose either Step 7 or Step 8 or both** as a double-check.		May refer to the infusion device user's manual for specific instructions on use of specific devices.
7. Determine the correct flow rate with manual mathematic calculation method.	The infusion device controls the consistent and accurate delivery of the flow rate.	Infusion devices are electrical equipment and may malfunction. Monitor the infusion for accuracy in flow rate.
A. Convert the concentration of the solution to the same units of measure as the dose.	All units of measure must be the same to perform the mathematic functions.	
B. Calculate the concentration of the medication per milliliter of fluid.	Necessary for the medication calculation.	
C. Enter the concentration and the dose into the formula and solve for the flow rate.	Necessary for the medication calculation. Entering information into the device is required for the device to infuse at the prescribed rate.	Use alternate formulas if medication dose is a per-minute or weight-based dose (see Tables 139-1, 139-2, and 139-3).

*Level E: Multiple case reports, theory-based evidence from expert opinions, or peer-reviewed professional organizational standards without clinical studies to support recommendations

Procedure for Calculating Doses and Flow Rates and Administering Continuous Intravenous Infusions—*Continued*

Steps	Rationale	Special Considerations
8. Determine the correct flow rate with electronic devices.	Prevents errors in medication administration.	Refer to the manufacturer's user guide for accurate programming of smart pump calculations. With the use of infusion devices with smart capabilities (i.e., Guard-rails, Alaris Medical Systems, San Diego, CA), refer to institutional policies for a review of medications that must be infused with the smart pump. May consider institutional competencies for nurses administering medications via a smart pump.
A. Enter the necessary information into the device, including, but not limited to, patient weight, drug name, concentration of solution, dose ordered. B. Program the device to electronically calculate the flow rate.	Ensures patient safety. Prevents mathematic errors or data entry and programming errors.	
9. Double-check the flow rate calculations or programming with another qualified individual.	Independent double-checks may reduce errors made when calculating dosages or programming pumps.	
10. Set the flow rate on the infusion pump.		
11. Connect the infusion system to the intended IV line or catheter. Initiate the infusion.	Initiates the therapy.	Alcohol should always be used to cleanse the IV port (hub) before the infusion is connected.
12. Discard used supplies.		
13. **HH**		

Expected Outcomes

- The desired patient response is achieved
- The correct dose of medication is administered
- The dose is titrated to achieve/maintain the desired patient response

Unexpected Outcomes

- Adverse reactions to the medication occur
- The incorrect dose of medication is administered
- The desired patient response is not achieved or maintained
- Infiltration or extravasation of medication occurs

Patient Monitoring and Care

Steps	Rationale	Reportable Conditions
		These conditions should be reported if they persist despite nursing interventions.
1. Evaluate the patient response by monitoring the indicated parameters for the medication being infused.	Medications given as continuous infusions often have potent effects and potentially serious adverse effects. Most medications given as continuous infusions have a quick onset of action. Frequent monitoring of parameters is necessary during initiation of the infusion.	• Adverse reactions • Hemodynamic instability • Cardiac dysrhythmias • Excessive sedation • Respiratory depression

Patient Monitoring and Care —*Continued*

Steps	Rationale	Reportable Conditions
2. If the patient response is inadequate, titrate the infusion as ordered until the prescribed parameters are met.	The patient's response to many continuous infusions is dose-dependent. To achieve the desired response, titration of the dose is necessary.	• Desired response not achieved within an acceptable dosage range
3. Assess the IV access for catheter placement, catheter patency, and signs of infiltration or extravasation every 1 to 4 hours and as needed.	Ensures delivery of the medication into the venous system. Prevents interruptions in delivery of the medication. Provides early recognition of complications.	• Extravasation of any medication • Intravenous line infiltration

Documentation

Documentation should include the following:
- Name of the medication and the type of solution in which the medication is diluted; concentration of the solution; dose; flow rate; and administration times
- Patient and family education

- Assessment of the IV access and site
- Parameters monitored and patient response
- Adverse reactions and interventions to treat the reaction
- Titration

References

1. Crimlisk J, Johnstone D, Sanchez G: Evidence-based practice, clinical simulations workshop, and intravenous medications: moving toward safer practice, *Med Surg Nurs* 18(3): 153-160, 2009.
2. Deglin JH, Vallerand AH: *Davis's drug guide for nurses*, ed 11, Philadelphia, 2009, F.A. Davis Co.
3. Ekle, E., & Sibley, A. editors: *Nurses handbook of IV drugs*, ed 3, Sudbury, MA, 2009, Jones & Bartlett Publishers.
CR 4. Institute for Safe Medication Practices (ISMP): *Medication safety alert: smart infusion pumps join CPOE and bar coding as important ways to prevent medications errors*, Huntington Valley, PA, 2002, Institute for Safe Medication Practices.
5. Institute for Safe Medication Practices (ISMP): *Medication safety alert nurse advise: ERR: double key bounce and double keying errors*, Huntington Valley, PA, 2006, Institute for Safe Medication Practices.
6. Institute for Safe Medication Practices (ISMP): Smart pumps are not smart on their own, *ISMP Medication Safety Alert* 12(8):1-2, 2007.
7. Institute for Safe Medication Practices (ISMP): *Medication safety alert nurse advise: ERR: lack of standard dosing methods contributes to IV infusion errors*, Huntington Valley, PA, 2008, Institute for Safe Medication Practices

8. Pentin J, Smith J: Drug calculations: are they safer with or without a calculator? *Br J Nurs* 15(14):778-781, 2006.
9. Polovich M, Whitford JM, Olsen M, editors: *Chemotherapy and biotherapy guidelines and recommendations for practice*, ed 3, Pittsburgh, 2009, ONS Publishing.
CR 10. Reves JG: *"Smart pump" technology reduces errors, 2003*, retrieved July 28, 2009, from http://www.apsf.org/resource_center/newsletter/2003/spring/smartpump.htm.
11. Spratto G, Woods A, editors: *2008 PDR nurse's drug handbook: patient safety goals [appendix 12]*, Clifton Park, NY, 2008, Thompson Healthcare Inc and Delmar Learning.

Additional Readings

CR Guiliano K, et al: A new strategy for calculating medication infusion rates, *Crit Care Nurs* 13:77-82, 1993.
CR Hadaway LC: How to safeguard delivery of high-alert IV drugs, *Nursing* 31:36-42, 2001.
CR Keohane C, Hayes J, Saniuk C, et al: Intravenous medication safety and smart infusion systems, *J Infusion Nurs* 28(5):321-328, 2005.
CR McMillen P: Calculating medication dosages, *Crit Care Nurs* 20:17-19, 2000.
CR Shilling-McCann, JA, executive publisher: *Springhouse's dosage calculations made incredibly easy*, ed 2, Springhouse, PA, 2000, Springhouse.

Index

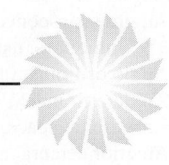

Page numbers followed by *f, t,* and *b* indicate figures, tables, and boxes, respectively.